THE COGNITIVE NEUROSCIENCES

THE COGNITIVE NEUROSCIENCES

Third Edition

Michael S. Gazzaniga, *Editor-in-Chief*

Section Editors: Emilio Bizzi

Ira B. Black

Alfonso Caramazza

Michael S. Gazzaniga

Scott T. Grafton

Todd F. Heatherton

Christof Koch

Joseph E. LeDoux

Nikos K. Logothetis

J. Anthony Movshon

Elizabeth A. Phelps

Pasko Rakic

Daniel L. Schacter

Anne Treisman

Brian Wandell

A BRADFORD BOOK
THE MIT PRESS
CAMBRIDGE, MASSACHUSETTS
LONDON, ENGLAND

MIT Press books may be purchased at special quantity discounts for business or sales promotional use. For information, please email special_sales@mitpress.mit.edu or write to Special Sales Department, The MIT Press, 5 Cambridge Center, Cambridge, MA 02142.

This book was set in Baskerville by SNP Best-set Typesetter Ltd., Hong Kong

Printed and bound in the United States of America.

Library of Congress Cataloging-in-Publication Data

The cognitive neurosciences / Michael S. Gazzaniga, editor-in-chief.—3rd ed.
       p. ; cm.
    "A Bradford book."
    Rev. ed. of: The new cognitive neurosciences. 2nd ed. c2000.
    Includes bibliographical references and index.
    ISBN 0-262-07254-8
    1. Cognitive neuroscience.   I. Gazzaniga, Michael S.
    II. New cognitive neurosciences.
    [DNLM: 1. Brain—physiology.   2. Mental Processes—physiology.   3. Neurosciences. WL 300 C6766 2004]
    QP360.5.N4986   2004
    612.8'2—dc22
                                    2004052587

CONTENTS

IX EMOTION AND SOCIAL NEUROSCIENCE   971

X CONSCIOUSNESS   1105

XI PERSPECTIVES AND NEW DIRECTIONS   1211

PREFACE

This book represents the combined efforts of more than a hundred brain scientists, each carefully chosen to illuminate one of dozens of problem areas within the field of cognitive neuroscience. Our initial meeting in 1993 launched this series of books, and with its success we met again in 1998. Each volume has served as a benchmark for where the field of cognitive neuroscience stands at each of these points in time. At the end of the 2003 meeting, the meeting that produced this new book, the field once again looked vibrant, energetic, and disciplined. Cognitive neuroscience will be around for a long time.

In late June of 2003, the Summer Institute in Cognitive Neuroscience convened at Lake Tahoe, in Squaw Valley, California, in preparation for the third edition of *The Cognitive Neurosciences*. Twenty-five fellows settled into their accommodations, and we began a grueling schedule of attending five to six talks every day for three weeks. Among our group of advanced graduate students, postdoctoral fellows, and early faculty, there was some initial apprehension concerning whether we could sustain vigilant concentration for the duration. Those fears were allayed within the first days. We were held in rapt attention as successive sections unfolded. All of the talks were structured to include cutting-edge research in support of a broader thesis. Yet, when placed in the context of an entire section, each talk's individual significance expanded as common themes and discrepancies emerged. Discussions sparked debates and collaborations that spilled out of the conference room into long lunches in the California sun, evening barbecues by the resort pool, and late-night poker games. In this rich environment, largely removed from the daily rigors and pressures of advancing laboratory progress, many of us rediscovered what initially drew us to the field of cognitive neuroscience. We spontaneously began to link seemingly unrelated questions and subdisciplines, excitedly discussing how a new generation of questions relating the brain and behavior could be addressed. Each of us left with a greater appreciation of how our individual research fit into a larger picture. Despite the institute's fast pace, we all left energized and excited, challenged and stimulated by the content of the chapters that follow. It is our hope that this book captures that energy, so that all may appreciate this comprehensive and current view of a field that is moving forward at lightning speed.

As usual, there are many to thank with deep gratitude. Each section editor did a magnificent job. A tremendous amount of work goes into both the selection of the contributors and reviewing each manuscript in this volume. Some of the section editors have been part of this project from the beginning. Others have joined along the way, and all have performed with distinction.

The conference itself is a complex event. The details of running a three-week conference fell to Donna Rocke of Dartmouth Medical School. Her unfailing good humor and caring nature kept both the faculty and fellows smiling at all times. Marin Gazzaniga, my magnificent daughter, served as managing editor of this enormous effort. She is a playwright, an actress, an author, an editor, and most of all a savvy, delightful, humorous, and patient soul who keeps all the troops pointed in the same direction. The book simply would not be possible without her.

The tragic death of Patricia Goldman-Rakic touched all of us in a profound way. Dr. Goldman-Rakic spoke at Lake Tahoe and gave a spectacular lecture. Some of the fellows had been her students, and all of us knew her very well. Indeed, her husband, Pasko Rakic, had launched the conference in the first days. To learn of her death days after the event left us all with a deep sense of loss. In the present volume her efforts were captured not only by her own hand but posthumously by her young colleagues. They were able to update her effort from the previous volume and include all of the new work she had achieved.

The depth of the intellectual questions that make up the field of cognitive neuroscience helps it attract the best and the brightest. I hope we have achieved our goal, which is to bring this sense of the excitement and content of the Lake Tahoe meeting to all students of the brain and mind. I think we have.

Michael S. Gazzaniga
Center for Cognitive Neuroscience
Dartmouth College
Hanover, New Hampshire

I EVOLUTION AND DEVELOPMENT

Introduction

PASKO RAKIC

THERE IS NO disagreement among neuroscientists that human cognitive abilities depend principally on the size and neuronal organization of the cerebral cortex. In the last 5 years, the field of developmental neurobiology has continued to make rapid progress toward understanding the genetic and molecular mechanisms underlying the development and evolution of this formidable organ. The chapters in this section summarize work elucidating the differences between human cortex and that of our nearest evolutionary relatives, as well as work illustrating the tight control over cortical patterning and the establishment of cortical connections. Although many have speculated whether the reductionist approaches of developmental neurobiology could ever be harmonized with the largely integrative approaches of cognitive neuroscience, it now appears as though that time is coming. In the last chapter, the known stages of human brain development are compared to the stages of human psychological development to argue that the biological changes associated with each stage can be mapped directly to cognitive changes. Thus, in this third edition of *The Cognitive Neurosciences*, it appears as though the gap between developmental neurobiology and developmental psychology has sufficiently narrowed that there is little doubt that it will eventually be bridged.

The chapters written from the developmental neurobiology perspective center on four major themes. The first chapter, by Preuss, addresses the question of what makes the human brain unique. Comparative studies have revealed that the human brain is distinguished by increased surface area, increased gestation time, and, some have argued, increased numbers of cortical areas, particularly in prefrontal cortex. Interestingly, the human brain does not differ from the brains of other primates in the number of genes regulating its development. However, recent work discussed by Preuss illustrates that certain genes appear to be up-regulated in the human brain, particularly those genes that increase the neuronal activity of pyramidal neurons. These increases in neuronal activity may be associated with increased cell signaling and bioenergetics. Thus, the human brain can be distinguished by changes in cortical structure as well as by increased genetic expression, resulting in changes in neuron dynamics.

The human brain can also be distinguished by its cortical neurogenesis, the second major theme of this section. Kornack points out that cell division during primate development is slower than in rodents (mice), but that the duration of neurogenesis is longer in primates. This subtle change in the temporal dynamics of neurogenesis could account for the expansion of the number of neurons in the upper cortical layers. Finally, it appears as though the human brain may also be distinguished by its inability to sustain neurogenesis throughout the life span. Although it has been argued that rodents and primates exhibit adult neurogenesis in the dentate gyrus and rostral migratory stream, the level of neuronal production is substantially smaller in the monkey than in the mouse, despite enlargement in overall size of the brain. Furthermore, recent studies in several laboratories have refuted findings from earlier and widely reported studies claiming that the primate cerebral cortex was also capable of generating new functional neurons into adulthood.

The third major theme has to do with human cortical patterning. Rakic and colleagues review recent work on the development of the cerebral cortex, specifically how neurons acquire their position by active migration from multiple sites of origin to their final, increasingly distant destinations. They have identified several families of genes and signaling molecules that control radial and tangential migration of neurons in the cerebral cortex. This work illustrates how understanding corticogenesis in the embryo provides hints of how spontaneous mutations that regulate the early developmental stages may have determined the species-specific size, parcellation of the map, and basic organization of the cerebral cortex. The next two chapters discuss the spatial control of neuronal migration, demonstrating that attractive and repulsive molecular cues can be found in gradients oriented along particular axes and functioning to shuttle neurons into their appropriate positions. Liu and Rao also discuss the temporal control of neuronal migration, demonstrating that the effect of these guidance molecules

changes across time, so that the neurons are more or less sensitive to their effects throughout cell migration. Finally, Garel and Rubenstein show that the establishment of these molecular gradients is tightly genetically controlled, reiterating Rakic's point that cortical development leaves no room for errors.

The final theme relates to the guidance of axonal projections from neurons that have found their appropriate cortical address. This process is similar to, but no less complex than, neuronal migration during cortical development. On a related topic, Chalupa and Huberman demonstrate that the segregation of left- and right-eye inputs to the dorsal lateral geniculate does not require normal retinal activity. These findings challenge the prevalent view that neuronal activity plays an instructive role in the formation of segregated ocular domains. Thus, the complexity of neuronal migration in cortical development is mirrored by the complexity of the cues required for the establishment of specific axonal projections.

The final chapter in this section attempts to show parallels between brain development and cognitive development. Kagan and Baird argue that the cognitive changes marking each major stage of psychological development can be associated with underlying neural changes. For example, at 2–3 months of age, infants lose particular brainstem-mediated reflex responses, presumably because axons from motor cortex begin to inhibit those from the brainstem. Similarly, the growth of interneurons and pyramidal cells in the prefrontal cortex, as well as the myelination of connections between the amygdala and frontal lobe, coincides with the appearance of fears of strangers and of separation, presumably because representations can be retrieved and compared with the present environment. Such parallels can be drawn throughout child development, thus illustrating that considerably more work needs to be directed toward showing causal connections between brain and cognitive development.

In summary, the work included in this section emphasizes the complexity and tight control of cortical development from neurogenesis to neuronal migration to axon guidance. At each stage there are spatial and temporal characteristics unique to humans, and these differences are in many cases regulated by unique levels of gene expression. Combined, these subtle yet dramatic differences in brain development result in a distinctly human brain that subserves distinctly human behavior.

1   What Is It Like to Be a Human?

TODD M. PREUSS

ABSTRACT Brain size increased remarkably following the divergence of the human and African ape lineages, but there is more to human brain evolution than enlargement: the comparative evidence indicates that humans underwent modifications of brain structure at many levels of organization. Higher-order cortex expanded disproportionately to primary areas, yet there is presently no clear evidence that humans evolved new cortical areas. The lack of detailed and reliable maps of human and ape cortex makes it difficult to compare the subdivisions of higher-order cortex across species, however. Humans clearly did modify the internal organization of certain cortical areas, evolving distinctive patterns of compartmentation and distinctive neuronal phenotypes. In addition, humans appear to exhibit greater degrees of hemispheric asymmetry than other primates. The development of new approaches to comparing humans and nonhuman primates, including comparative neuroimaging and genomics, promises to greatly enhance our understanding of the unique characteristics of the human brain.

People are strange

In a well-known essay, the philosopher Thomas Nagel invites us to consider what it is like to be a bat (Nagel, 1974). He uses this device to illustrate something about the nature of consciousness: bats are so strange, with their sonar and flying ability, that we cannot fully appreciate what it's like to be inside the skin of a bat; our comprehension of conscious experience is anchored in and limited by our own point of view. The merit of this example lies in Nagel's appreciation of the diversity of life, even of mental life. But whereas from our point of view bats may seem to be strange creatures, from an evolutionary standpoint all creatures are strange. Evolution is a branching tree; the processes of evolution result in descendant lineages becoming different, each in their distinctive ways, from the common ancestral population from which they sprang (figure 1.1). The mechanisms of evolutionary transformation ensure that every branch of the evolutionary tree is, in some respects, uniquely different from other lineages. Thus, the lesson of evolution is that people, too, are strange.

Our physical form and life history provide ample testimony to the strangeness of humans. Humans have a kind of locomotion—striding bipedalism—that is unique among

TODD M. PREUSS Center for Behavioral Neuroscience and Division of Neuroscience, Yerkes Primate Research Center, Emory University, Atlanta, Ga.

known animals, and our pelvis and lower limb have been radically remodeled in relation to this, to the point that we have lost one of the hallmarks of the primate order, a grasping big toe (Cartmill, 1992). Humans, even in hunter-gatherer societies, have unusually extensive fat deposits, and the form and distribution of hair in humans are bizarre. So peculiar are human fat and hair that some have explained them by proposing that human ancestors became aquatic for a time, and so converged on dolphins (Morgan, 1982). Alone among anthropoid primates, which subsist mainly on fruit and leaves, humans have included in their diets a substantial component of meat. Human females can survive for decades after menopause; in other primate species, the cessation of ovulatory cycling essentially coincides with senescence and death (O'Connell, Hawkes, and Blurton Jones, 1999). Humans, too, have the capacity to live much longer than other primates: under the best of circumstances, few chimpanzees or gorillas make it to age 50, whereas in hunter-gatherer societies, a woman who survives her childbearing years has a decent chance to live to age 65 (Blurton Jones, Hawkes, and O'Connell, 2002). In addition, the human disease profile differs in important respects from that of other primates (Olson and Varki, 2003). Even ignoring our intellectual abilities and cultural accretions, people are most peculiar beasts.

Although the strangeness of humans may be commonplace to anthropologists, it is not an idea that neuroscientists typically find easy to wrap their minds around. The neurosciences, along with many other branches of the biomedical sciences, have been extremely dependent on information derived from the study of nonhuman species for their understanding of human biology. The way these sciences conceive the relationship between humans and other species is reflected in the fact that they refer to nonhuman species as "models." In the model-animal paradigm, the study of nonhuman species is seen as the search for general facts or principles that are applicable to humans (Preuss, 2000a, 2001). I don't question that there are biological facts of considerable generality, nor do I question their great importance or the indispensable role of animal research in elucidating these facts. Nevertheless, the model-animal approach to human nature has important limitations. It fosters the view that humans, as well as the animals we use as proxies for understanding humans, are somehow typical, and thus it dignifies only the study of the ways in which animals resemble one

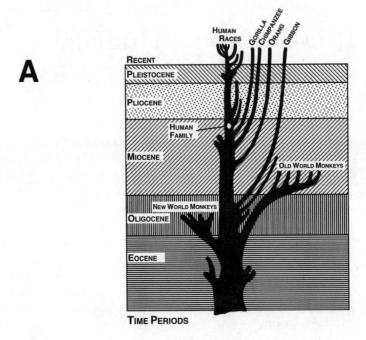

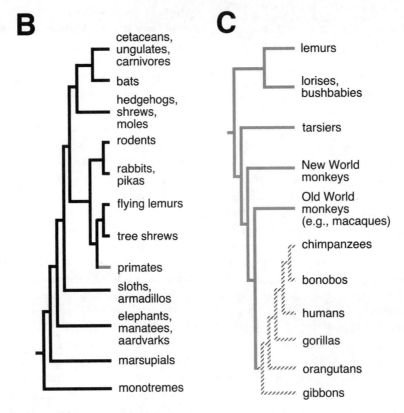

FIGURE 1.1 Contrasting classical Darwinian (*A*) and modern cladistic (*B*, *C*) conceptualizations of human evolution. Early treatments of human evolution, such as those of Elliot Smith (1924), a pioneering neuroanatomist and primatologist, depicted humans as the natural centerpiece of evolution (*A*). The path to humans is straight upward, while other species are set off on side branches. The Old World and New World monkeys are drawn as though they stopped evolving millions of years ago! In this view, humans are very much "at home in the universe," to borrow the phrase of Kauffman (1995). By contrast, modern views of mammalian (*B*) and primate (*C*) evolution treat humans as but one of many diverse outcomes of the evolutionary process. In this conception, evolution has no natural center; humans are, as it were, "home alone in the universe." This view of evolution encourages us to consider all species, including *Homo sapiens*, as distinctive in certain respects, rather than seeing the human species as merely an improved version of simpler ancestral forms. The tree in *B* is derived from recent comparative molecular studies of mammals (e.g., Murphy et al., 2001). *C* shows an expansion of the primate branch of evolution (Fleagle, 1999) derived from comparative molecular and morphological data. The hatched lines denote the hominoid group, which consists of humans, the "great apes" (chimpanzees, bonobos, gorillas, and orangutans), and the "lesser apes" (gibbons). Old World monkeys (including the familiar macaque monkeys) are the sister group of the hominoids.

another. (Surely it is what is *shared* among animals—what has been preserved in the crucible of evolutionary history—that is essential?) In the agenda of modern neuroscience, the evolutionary specializations of the human brain scarcely seem to rate a footnote. But if we dismiss human brain specializations as mere variations, we trivialize the very features of the brain that make us humans, rather than monkeys or mice or fruit flies. Evolutionary specializations are not trivia; they are the essence of human nature.

To be sure, nearly everyone acknowledges at least one specialization of the human brain: its enormous size. Perhaps (viewed from the neck up, at least) humans are really just brainier, more intelligent versions of other animals. Yet it is by no means clear that we can account for our cognitive and behavioral capacities as a simple consequence of brain expansion. We have no well-developed theory to explain how the tripling of brain volume in the human lineage in the 5–8 million years since humans last shared a common ancestor with the African apes relates mechanistically to our capacity for language, which is uniquely human (Wallman, 1992), nor to our more general capacity for symbolic representation (Deacon, 1997), nor to our ability to represent certain kinds of mental states (Povinelli and Preuss, 1995), nor to our propensity to represent the interactions of physical objects in terms of unobservable constructs like mass and force (Povinelli, 2000). Yes, our brains are larger than those of other primates, and in some sense they must be better, too. But humans don't merely think better than other animals, we think differently.

One bulwark of the "bigger, better" view of human brain evolution has been the widespread belief that there is little variation among mammals in the internal organization of the brain. The claim that there is a "basic uniformity" of cortical design—all mammalian cortex being a collection of "minicolumns" of essentially homogeneous cell composition, or, similarly, the claim that mammalian cortex possesses a common intrinsic circuitry across areas and across species, are expressions of this belief (e.g., Creutzfeldt, 1977; Rockel, Hiorns, and Powell, 1980). Again, I don't question the possibility, or even the likelihood, that certain features of cortical organization are shared widely among mammalian species. Logically, however, the presence of numerous characteristics that are widely shared among taxa does not imply the absence of important differences. In fact, evidence for cross-species variations in cortical structure at many levels of organization is accumulating rapidly (for general reviews, see Preuss, 2000a, 2001, in press; Kaas and Preuss, 2003). A few examples suffice to illustrate the remarkable diversity of mammalian cerebral cortex: Whereas thalamocortical projections in most mammals are largely uncrossed, at least one species has major crossed projections (Regidor and Divac, 1992). In primates, the densest cortical projections of the brainstem dopaminergic nuclei target the motor and pre-

motor cortex; in rodents, motors areas are nearly devoid of dopaminergic input (Berger and Gaspar, 1995; Williams and Goldman-Rakic, 1998). There are major differences in the laminar and regional distribution of other transmitter-containing fibers and receptor types (Gebhard et al., 1995; Sanchez et al., 1999; Young, Toloczko, and Inscl, 1999). The morphological and biochemical phenotypes of cortical neurons show some dramatic differences across species (Hof et al., 2000, 2001; Sherwood, Lee, et al., 2003). There are even major differences among mammalian groups in the developmental origins of interneurons (Letinic, Zoncu, and Rakic, 2002). There is, then, ample reason to suspect that there is more to human brain evolution than just enlargement.

Studying human brain specializations

What would we like to know about the human brain? Among other things, we would like to know how the ontogenetic program of the brain was modified to make it as big as it is; this must have involved changes early in embryogenesis that affect neuronal proliferation. We would also like to know what happened to the internal organization of the brain as it underwent expansion: Did the proportions of different subdivisions change? Do humans possess new cortical areas or subcortical nuclei? Were the patterns of interconnections among areas modified? Did humans undergo changes in the internal organization of structures that we share with other animals, such as changes in local circuitry or in the cell populations that make up particular areas? Were the morphologies and biochemical phenotypes of cells modified, and if so, were those changes local or global? Did humans evolve species-specific patterns of hemispheric asymmetry? And finally, how are evolutionary changes in the organization of the human brain related to changes in cognition and behavior?

This is a tall order, and before proceeding to review the available evidence bearing on these questions, it is useful to consider what kinds of information we would need to answer them. To understand humans we must study humans, and in this we face certain methodological handicaps: many of the physiological and anatomical techniques most widely used by neuroscientists require invasive procedures in living animals; with rare exceptions, these cannot be used in humans. Nor can genetic manipulations or breeding experiments be carried out in humans.

There is another obstacle to understanding human brain organization that might not be so obvious. To understand humans *as humans* requires comparing humans to other animals. The most informative comparisons with regard to human nature involve our closest relatives, the African great apes (chimpanzees, bonobos, and gorillas); what distinguishes us as a species are precisely those characteristics that distinguish humans from apes. (Comparing humans to macaque monkeys without considering other primate groups is not enough; macaque are too distantly related to humans, and human-macaque comparisons cannot distinguish human specializations from hominoid [ape plus human] specializations.) It is difficult enough to obtain high-quality human brain tissue, but that is largely a problem of the institutional barriers that separate pathologists and neuroscientists: there is no shortage of human brains. In obtaining ape brains, however, we face the additional problem that the resource is very scarce, and will only become more so as both wild and captive ape populations become ever smaller. When the apes are gone, we will forever lose a fundamental source of information about human nature. Moreover, certain key questions about human brain specializations— for example, how neurogenesis was enhanced in humans— will be difficult to answer without comparing fetal material from apes and humans, and it is unlikely that we will be able to obtain suitable tissue in the near future.

The situation is far from hopeless, however. There exist a variety of techniques that can be used very successfully in adult apes and humans, both in vivo and with postmortem tissue samples. These techniques include structural imaging, magnetic resonance spectroscopy, ligand-binding techniques (e.g., in situ hybridization and immunocytochemistry), and classical histochemical techniques. (In my experience, the use of ligand-binding and histochemical techniques with autopsied human tissue commonly produces very high-quality results, often rivaling the quality of results obtained with experimental animal material.) The recent development of genomics techniques make it possible to assess evolutionary changes in the structure and expression of genes, which in turn can guide the exploration of differences in brain structure and function. Also, the adaptation of functional imaging techniques for use in nonhuman primates facilitates the direct comparison of humans and other species. Most of the work done to date involves macaque monkeys, but the techniques are applicable to apes as well (Rilling et al., 2000). It remains the case that current techniques for studying connectivity in humans are less good than those used with nonhuman species, although methods continue to improve (Dai et al., 1998; Conturo et al., 1999; Sparks et al., 2000).

Candidate human brain specializations

ENLARGED ASSOCIATION CORTEX Most of the difference in brain size between humans and great apes is accounted for by the expansion of the cerebral cortex (Stephan, Frahm, and Baron, 1981). It has usually been supposed that this increase was not global but rather involved certain regions more than others, specifically the classical "association" areas of the parietal, temporal, and frontal cortex (e.g.,

Brodmann, 1909, 1912; Elliot Smith, 1924; Le Gros Clark, 1959; Blinkov and Glezer, 1968). Given its role in higher-level cognitive functions, much attention has been paid to the possibility that the frontal cortex, and in particular the prefrontal subregion, was differentially enlarged during human evolution (for reviews, see Falk, 1992; Semendeferi et al., 1997). Notably, Brodmann (1912) offered quantitative evidence of this, indicating that the prefrontal cortex (his *Regio frontalis*) occupies a larger proportion of the frontal lobe in humans than in other primates. The results of later quantitative architectonic studies by Blinkov and Glezer (1968) make the same point.

The special place of frontal cortex in human evolution has recently been challenged, however. Semendeferi and colleagues have carried out a series of structural magnetic resonance imaging (MRI) studies of humans, apes, and monkeys (Semendeferi and Damasio, 2000; Semendeferi et al., 1997, 2002) and have concluded that the frontal lobe, as a fraction of total cortical volume (about 35%), is at most marginally larger in humans than in the great apes. Thus, Semendeferi and colleagues conclude that the view that humans have an unusually or disportionately large frontal lobe is mistaken, and have suggested that the expansion of frontal cortex is not a hallmark of human evolution.

I do not wish to take issue with the morphometric results of Semendeferi and colleagues, but rather point out that their results can support a conclusion largely compatible with classical views. It comes down to being clear about the distinction between absolute and relative sizes and the distinction between frontal and prefrontal cortex. First, one would not expect *any* primate to have a brain the size of a human's: humans are way off the chart. The range of body size of the great apes (orangutans, gorillas, chimpanzees, and bonobos) overlaps human body size, but whereas these apes have brains on the order of 350–500 g, human brains average about 1300 g. We have far more brain than we should have, statistically speaking.

So there is no question that there was expansion of the brain in human evolution, and that this expansion involved the cortex especially. The question is, was this expansion global, affecting all areas equally or nearly so, or was there differential expansion of particular regions? To answer this question, we need data on the absolute sizes of individual cortical areas for the great apes and humans. Two areas that can be readily identified in all primate species and measured with some confidence are the primary visual area (V1; also called striate cortex and Brodmann's area 17) and the primary motor area (M1; Brodmann's area 4). It is instructive that the absolute sizes of both V1 (Frahm, Stephan, and Baron, 1984) and M1 (Blinkov and Glezer, 1968) are very similar in great apes and humans. Thus, the primary cortical areas of humans have the absolute size one would expect for a ape of our body size; it is all the other areas—mainly the higher-order or associational areas—that underwent expansion (Figure 1.2A, B).

The enlargement of higher-order areas is also apparent in recent mapping studies of visual cortex in humans and in Old World and New World monkeys. These studies strongly suggest that certain extrastriate (higher-order) visual areas in humans are relatively large in humans compared to area V1 (Sereno, 1998; Van Essen et al., 2001). With the enlargement of higher-order visual cortex on the lateral surface of the hemisphere, the primary visual area has been morphologically displaced in humans, so that is now largely confined to the medial portion of the occipital lobe. With respect to frontal cortex, it is noteworthy that the classical cytoarchitectonic studies of Brodmann (1912) and Bailey, Bonin, and McCulloch (1950) suggest that the primary motor cortex and premotor cortex occupy a much greater proportion of the frontal lobe in chimpanzees than in humans, which is to be expected if prefrontal cortex expanded in human evolution. In chimpanzees, the region of giant pyramidal cells (i.e., primary motor cortex) extends forward of the central sulcus, spanning the precentral gyrus and extending into the precentral sulcus, whereas in humans, the region of giant pyramidal cells is limited to the anterior bank of the central sulcus (see also Preuss et al., 1996, on humans, and Preuss et al., 1997, on chimpanzees).

The conclusion that higher-order areas expanded in human evolution, while primary areas retained more apelike proportions, is further buttressed by Armstrong's studies of neuron numbers in the various thalamic nuclei that project to the cerebral cortex (reviewed in Armstrong, 1982). Here, results indicate that the principal thalamic nuclei that project to primary visual, auditory, and somatosensory cortex (the lateral geniculate, medial geniculate, and ventrobasal nuclei, respectively) contain about the same numbers of neurons in humans and in the great apes. By contrast, the pulvinar, which projects to large portions of higher-order parietal, temporal, and prefrontal cortex, contains about twice as many neurons in humans as in apes, and the mediodorsal nucleus, which projects mainly to prefrontal cortex, has about three times as many neurons in humans as in apes (figure 1.2C).

So, it seems very likely that brain enlargement during human evolution involved primarily the disproportionate expansion of higher-order cortical areas, including the prefrontal cortex, which in humans comprises by far the largest portion of the frontal lobe. How can we reconcile this with the conclusions of Semendeferi and colleagues that the proportions of cerebral lobes have not changed markedly in human evolution? We can do so if we suppose that expansion was not limited to the prefrontal portion of the frontal lobe but also involved higher-order parietal, temporal, and occipital cortex: if these regions enlarged in rough proportion to the prefrontal region, the proportions of tissue devoted to the frontal, parietal, temporal, and occipital lobes in humans would have remained similar to those of apes.

New versus Modified Cortical Areas Was the evolutionary enlargement of the human brain accompanied by the appearance of new cortical areas? On the face of it, this seems a very likely prospect. The number of areas in the cortex varies across mammalian groups, and as a general rule, it seems that relatively encephalized groups have more cortical subdivisions than smaller-brained forms (Brodmann, 1909; Kaas, 1987; Allman, 1990; Kaas and Preuss, 2003). Thus, we should expect that humans, the most encephalized primates, have more cortical areas than other primates. Furthermore, neuroscientists tend to think of areas as processing modules with narrowly specified functional properties. If areas really do have narrow functional commitments, it makes sense that evolution would instantiate new functions by adding new areas to the cortex rather than by disrupting preexisting functions. Brodmann (1909), for example, considered the classical language areas of Broca and Wernicke to have no homologues in monkeys.

As sensible as this seems, there is at present no good evidence that humans do, in fact, possess uniquely human cortical areas. Brodmann's maps suggest that there are, but modern studies of human cortical areas generally emphasize the similarities between humans and nonhuman primates, and particularly macaque monkeys. For example, recent studies of frontal lobe areas, including the motor region, dorsolateral prefrontal region, and orbital and medial cortex, suggest something very close to an area-for-area match between humans and nonhuman primates (e.g., Petrides and Pandya, 1994; Rajkowska and Goldman-Rakic, 1995; Vogt et al., 1995; Baleydier, Achache, and Froment, 1997) (figure 1.3). Studies of visual cortex also emphasize the existence of a shared set of areas (Zilles and Clarke, 1997; Sereno, 1998; Van Essen et al., 2001).

In addition to the lack of direct evidence for new, human-specific cortical areas, there is a growing sense that some human-specific functions are represented in areas that have homologues in other primates (figure 1.4). It has long been argued that Broca's area, or at least a portion of it, has a homologue in nonhuman primates. Broca's area, which occupies the posterior part of the inferior frontal gyrus, corresponds to areas 44 and 45 of Brodmann (1909). Although Brodmann did not recognize areas 44 and 45 in nonhuman primates, many others have done so, including Walker (1940), whose map of macaque frontal cortex still provides the template for modern macaque research. Early arguments for a nonhuman homologue of Broca's area (reviewed by Preuss, 2000b) emphasized similarities in the location of the presumed homologue (in the ventral premotor region, immediately anterior to the orofacial representation of primary motor cortex), in cytoarchitecture (dysgranular; i.e.,

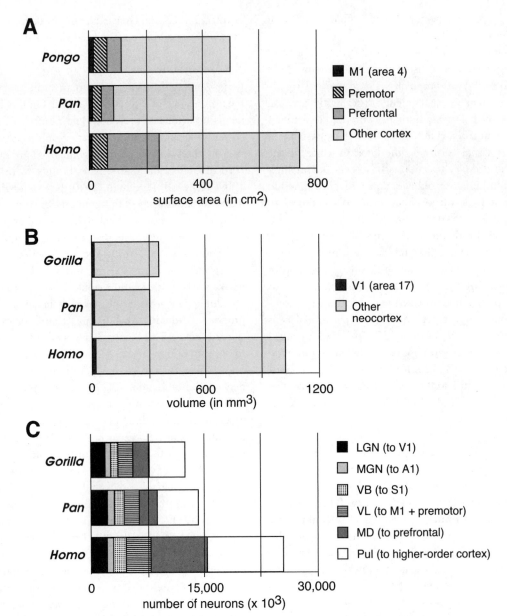

FIGURE 1.2 Absolute and relative dimensions of cortical and thalamic divisions in humans and great apes. (*A*) The cortical surface area devoted to the primary motor area (Brodmann's area 4) compared to the premotor cortex, prefrontal cortex, and other cortex in humans (*Homo*), chimpanzees (*Pan*), and orangutans (*Pongo*). Data are from Tables 194 and 196 of Blinkov and Glezer (1968). (*B*) The volume of the primary visual area and other neocortex in humans, chimpanzees, and gorillas, based on the data of Frahm et al. (1984). In both *A* and *B*, the dimensions of the primary areas are seen to be very similar in humans and apes, although the total dimensions of neocortex are much larger in humans. This suggests that the expansion of cortex in human evolution involved the nonprimary or associational regions particularly, while the primary areas changed relatively little. (*C*) Consideration of the number of neurons in the different thalamic nuclei of humans, chimpanzees, and gorillas yields a similar conclusion: evolutionary expansion involved higher-order structures, while primary structures remained similar in size (data from Armstrong, 1982). The lateral geniculate nucleus (LGN), medial geniculate nucleus (MGN), and ventrobasal nucleus (VB) project to the primary visual (V1), auditory (A1), and somatosensory (S1) cortical areas, respectively. These nuclei contain similar numbers of neurons in humans and apes. By contrast, the mediodorsal nucleus (MD), which projects mainly to the prefrontal association region, and the pulvinar nucleus (Pul), which projects to virtually all the nonprimary areas of primate cortex (including large regions of prefrontal, parietal, and temporal association cortex), are much larger in humans than in apes. (Human MD contains three times as many neurons as chimpanzee or gorilla MD.) The ventrolateral nucleus (VL), which projects to both the primary motor area (M1) and to higher-order, premotor cortex, is also enlarged in humans, but to a lesser extent than Pul and MD.

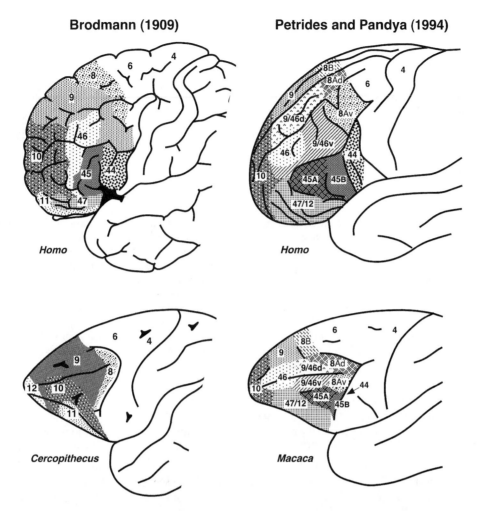

Brodmann (1909)

Homo

Cercopithecus

Petrides and Pandya (1994)

Homo

Macaca

FIGURE 1.3 The frontal lobe areas of humans (*Homo*) and Old World monkeys (*Cercopithecus* and *Macaca*) according to the cytoarchitectonic studies of Brodmann (1909) and Petrides and Pandya (1994). Brodmann concluded that the number of areas in the cerebral cortex increased during human evolution, whereas Petrides and Pandya depict humans and macaques as having the same complement of frontal lobe areas. Although Brodmann's map of the human brain remains the standard for localizing regions of functional activity in imaging studies, it is by no means clear that it corresponds closely to neurobiological reality. (Reproduced from Preuss, 2000b.)

intermediate between the agranular motor cortex and granular prefrontal cortex), and in nonlinguistic function (stimulation of the relevant region produces movements of the mouth and larynx). More recently, it has become clear that Broca's area in humans represents nonlinguistic movements of the hands as well as the mouth, and that the same is true of the presumed Broca's area homologue in macaques. Finally, the ventral premotor cortex of macaques contains so-called mirror neurons, neurons that respond when an animal either performs a particular movement or views the performance of the same movement, and Broca's area in humans has been shown to be activated under similar task conditions (Gallese et al., 1996).

The case has also been made that nonhuman primates possess homologues of posterior language areas, specifically Wernicke's area and the supramarginal and angular gyri. Although the argument is somewhat less well developed than

that for Broca's area, the form of the argument is the same: homologies between humans and nonhuman areas based on similarities in location within the cortical mantle (relative to better established areas), similarities in architectonic appearance, and similarities in nonlinguistic functions (for review, see Preuss, 2000b).

Human cognitive specializations are not limited to language. Behavioral and neuropsychological evidence suggests that humans have specialized ways of representing the behavioral interactions of physical objects, such as the manner of action of tools on other objects in the environment (Povinelli, 2000), and specialized representations of the manual actions involved in tool use (Johnson-Frey, 2003a). These functions probably involve portions of superior temporal cortex, in the case of object interactions, and subdivisions of posterior parietal cortex and ventral premotor cortex, in the case of tool manipulation (Johnson-Frey,

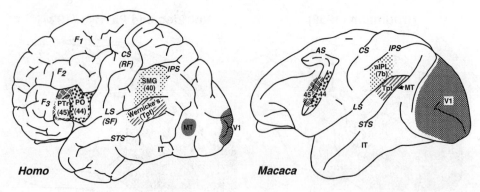

Homo

Macaca

FIGURE 1.4 Human cortical areas and their suggested homologues in macaques, based on architectonic and functional similarities. Broca's area in humans is located in the posterior part of the third frontal gyrus (F3) and includes two smaller gyri, pars opercularis (PO) and pars triangularis (PTr). These small gyri are occupied by areas 44 and 45 of Brodmann, respectively. In macaques, the ventral limb of the arcuate sulcus (AS) contains cortex that resembles humans areas 44 and 45 architectonically. Wernicke's area has been identified with architectonic area Tpt in humans, and there is a similar area in macaques. The cortex of the human supramarginal gyrus (SMG; Brodmann's area 40), which may be involved in language processing, resembles area 7b of macaques.

Note also the greater separation of area Tpt from the middle temporal (MT) and inferotemporal (IT) visual regions in humans compared to macaques. In macaques, area MT is situated in the posterior bank of the superior temporal sulcus (STS), whereas in humans it is located well inferior and posterior to the STS. It appears that expansion of the temporal association cortex has displaced the visual cortex inferiorly and posteriorly in the temporal and occipital lobes of humans compared to macaques. In humans, most of the primary visual area (V1) is located on the medial wall of the hemisphere. Additional abbreviations: CS, central sulcus; LS, lateral sulcus; SF, Sylvian fissure; RF, Rolandic fissure.

2003b). There is, however, no evidence that the emergence of these new functions entailed the emergence of new cortical areas; in fact, two of the areas that are crucially involved in manipulation, the ventral intraparietal area (VIP) and the posterior ventral premotor area (F4), are well known in macaques (Johnson-Frey, 2003b). In this instance, as in the case of language, there is some indication that the emergence of functional specialization was accompanied by hemispheric specialization rather than the evolution of new areas: tool manipulation activates cortex of the left hemisphere whether the manipulations are made with the right hand or the left hand (Johnson-Frey, 2003a).

Given the evidence summarized above, it is clear that we need to take seriously the possibility that evolution has modified the functions of the human brain at least in part by modifying the organization of existing areas rather than (or in addition to) adding new cortical areas. This should not be surprising: much of the work of evolution involves modifying existing organs to serve novel functions. Consider, for example, the many uses vertebrates have made of their forelimbs, including walking, swimming, flying, capturing prey, manipulating tools, and communicating.

Despite this, there are good reasons to be cautious about concluding that there really are no human-specific cortical areas. To make definitive conclusions about the evolution of cortical areas in human phylogeny, we would need (at a minimum) accurate and comprehensive cortical maps, obtained using comparable techniques, for humans, apes, and Old World monkeys. If we had these maps, we could in principle identify areas that are shared among these pri-

mates; any additional areas in humans would be human-specific. Furthermore, if we suspected that humans possessed functional specializations that involved particular areas, we could examine the relevant regions in greater detail in humans and nonhuman primates to determine whether humans possess a specialized bit of tissue that escaped the attention of mappers and that warrants designation as a new area. It would be very useful to examine the language regions of human cortex in this manner. If there were no evidence of a new area, we could then consider how evolution modified the size, internal organization, and connectivity of the area in question to support new or modified functions present in humans.

Alas, we don't have the maps to do this sort of analysis. Although cortical cartography is reasonably advanced in macaque monkeys, and although substantial portions of human cortex, especially frontal cortex and visual cortex, have been examined in considerable detail, large portions of human cortex remain to be explored. The fact that Brodmann's 1909 map of human cortex remains in widespread use, while his maps of other species have been extensively amended or discarded, is indicative of the sorry state of human cortical mapping. Moreover, information about apes (especially about chimpanzees, our closest relatives) is absolutely indispensable for identifying human cortical specialization, but there are no modern, comprehensive maps of ape cortex.

CEREBRAL ASYMMETRIES *Homo sapiens* has been referred to, with justice, as "the lopsided ape" (Corballis, 1991). One of

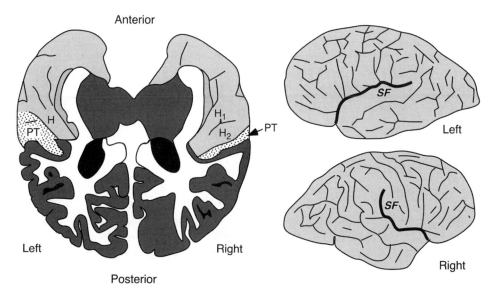

FIGURE 1.5 The left and right temporal lobes of humans are remarkably asymmetrical. The drawing on the left shows a brain sectioned in the horizontal plane to reveal the superior aspect of the temporal lobes; anterior is toward the top. (The cut surface of the cortex is represented by the dark gray fill.) The planum temporale (PT) is larger in the left hemisphere than the right in most people; in this individual, the right PT is scarcely evident. H_1 and H_2 are components of Heschl's gyrus, which corresponds to the primary auditory area. The drawings on the right illustrate the asymmetry in the course of the Sylvian fissure. In most individuals, the Sylvian fissure is shorter and flatter in the left hemisphere than in the right. Figures are based on photographs in Galaburda (1984).

the strangest things about humans is that for most activities that involve the use of a hand, a large majority of the members of our species will spontaneously use the right hand, which is mainly under the control of the left hemisphere. By contrast, while individual apes and monkeys may show a preference for one hand or the other in a particular activity, the preference is typically modest, and the individual may prefer to use a different hand in a different activity (McGrew and Marchant, 1997). Other aspects of human function are also strongly lateralized. In a large majority of humans, the left hemisphere carries out most of the neural functions involved in language. The right hemisphere is uniquely involved in aspects of visuospatial attention in humans (Corbetta and Shulman, 2002), and as a consequence, lesions of the right hemisphere are far more likely to result in hemispatial neglect than are lesions on the left. In macaque monkeys, by contrast, lesions of either hemisphere are about equally effective in producing neglect (Gaffan and Hornak, 1997). The strong population bias for left hemisphere control over the hand and language in humans suggests that our lopsidedness is the result of natural selection for genes that influence the functional commitments of each hemisphere (Annett, 1979; D. H. Geschwind et al., 2002).

Given the extent to which humans are functionally lateralized, one would expect humans to show corresponding structural asymmetries, and certainly a number of human brain asymmetries are now well documented (figure 1.5). Most notable, perhaps, is the asymmetry of the cortex located along the Sylvian fissure (lateral sulcus), which includes language-related cortex. In most humans the Sylvian fissure is longer on the left than on the right, and its posterior end typically has a distinct upward bend on the right (Galaburda, 1984). The cortex buried within the posterior part of the Sylvian fissure, extending from the posterior limit of the primary auditory region to the end of the fissure, is the so-called planum temporale (PT), which is usually considered to constitute a major portion of Wernicke's area. N. Geschwind and Levitsky (1968) reported that the left PT was larger than the right in 65% of individuals, and cytoarchitectonic area Tpt, which is located along the PT, is reported to be larger on the left than on the right (Galaburda and Sanides, 1980). With respect to Broca's area, it has been reported that the sulci of this region are longer and deeper on the left than on the right (Falzi, Perrone, and Vignolo, 1982; Albanese et al., 1989; Foundas, Leonard, and Heilman, 1995; Foundas et al., 1996), suggesting there is more cortex on the left, and Galaburda (1980) indicates that cytoarchitectonic area 44, which occupies the posterior part of Broca's area, is larger on the left than on the right.

Humans exhibit asymmetries at finer levels of organization as well. There are reports of left-right asymmetries in pyramidal cell size and dendritic morphology in Broca's and Wernicke's areas (Scheibel et al., 1985; Hayes and Lewis, 1993, 1995; Hutsler and Gazzaniga, 1996). Buxhoeveden and colleagues (2001) have recently reported that cell columns in human PT (i.e., Wernicke's area) are wider and more widely spaced on the left than on the right.

If there were a simple relationship between functional laterality and anatomical asymmetry, we would expect apes—which lack language and strong hand preferences—to lack the human pattern of cerebral asymmetries. Nevertheless, apes appear to be humanlike in several respects. Asymmetries of Sylvian fissure length (with the left longer than the right) are present in Old World monkeys and apes as well as in humans (see the review of Bradshaw and Rogers, 1993). Furthermore, in apes but not monkeys, the tip of the Sylvian fissure is usually higher on the right than on the left, as is the case in humans (LeMay and Geschwind, 1975; Yeni-Komshian and Benson, 1976). Recently it has been reported that chimpanzees possess PT asymmetries similar to those of humans (Gannon et al., 1998; Hopkins et al., 1998) and that, as in humans, the region of Broca's area is larger on the left than on the right in apes (Cantalupo and Hopkins, 2001). It is not clear, however, whether the magnitude of morphological asymmetry is as large in apes as in humans, and there is some evidence that it is not (Yeni-Komshian and Benson, 1976). Furthermore, the sulcal morphology of inferior frontal cortex is different in apes and humans, and, according to Sherwood and colleagues, there is very little relationship between the location of sulci and borders of Broca's area as determined histologically in apes, which renders inferences about the asymmetry of Broca's area problematic (Sherwood, Broadfield, et al., 2003). Finally, it is significant that Buxhoeveden and colleagues found that chimpanzees and macaque monkeys lack the left-right asymmetry of cell column size present in human PT (Buxhoeveden et al., 2001).

MODIFIED NEURONAL MORPHOLOGIES AND BIOCHEMISTRY
Great apes and humans possess two distinctive classes of pyramidal cells in layer 5 of anterior cingulate cortex. The first type are found deep in layer 5 and have a characteristic spindle-like shape. These spindle cells are much larger in humans than in apes, and are especially prone to degenerate in Alzheimer's disease (Nimchinsky et al., 1999). The second cell class is found in the upper part of layer 5 (Hof et al., 2001). These pyramidal cells are unusual in that they express calretinin, a calcium-binding protein that is typically expressed by GABAergic interneurons in the superficial layers of primate cortex, rather than in pyramidal cells. These cells are much more numerous in humans than in great apes (Hof et al., 2001). There are additional quantitative morphological differences between the pyramidal cells of humans and nonhuman primates. The giant pyramidal cells of primary motor cortex, the Betz cells, scale to brain size and body size, and humans have the largest Betz cells among primates (Sherwood, Lee, et al., 2003). Not all classes of pyramidal cells follow the same scaling principles, however. The distinction of having the largest Meynert cells, a group of deep pyramidal cells in primary visual cortex,

falls to several terrestrial species of Old World monkeys, specifically patas monkeys and baboons (Sherwood, Lee, et al., 2003); human Meynert cells are not outstandingly large. Meynert cells project to the superior colliculus, and Sherwood and colleagues (Sherwood, Lee, et al., 2003) suggest that their very large size in terrestrial monkeys, which are acutely responsive behaviorally to the proximity of predators, may be an adaptation to enhance motion detection. Humans and apes are also unusual among primates in that their layer 3 pyramidal cell population stains much more prominently for nonphosphorylated neurofilament protein than does the homologous cell group in Old World and New World monkeys; this difference can be seen throughout the cortical mantle (Preuss, Qi, and Kaas, 1999). It is likely that there are additional, region-specific specializations of pyramidal cell morphology in hominoids and in humans. For example, Elston, Benavides-Piccione, and DeFelipe (2001) report that the peak branching complexity of layer 3 pyramidal cell basal dendrites is markedly higher in the prefrontal cortex of humans than in macaques and marmosets, whereas the branching complexity in temporal and occipital cortex is similar in these species.

DeFelipe and colleagues have documented differences between macaques and humans in the biology of interneurons. The deep layers of human temporal cortex possess chandelier cells that co-express two calcium-binding proteins, parvalbumin and calbindin (del Río and DeFelipe, 1997). In macaques, by contrast, chandelier cells express only parvalbumin, and as a rule, mammalian interneurons typically express either parvalbumin or calbindin, but not both. In addition, the distinctive, candlestick-like terminals of chandelier cells that express parvalbumin are found throughout layers 2–6 in human temporal cortex and are especially numerous in the deep layers, whereas in macaques, these terminals are concentrated in superficial layers (DeFelipe et al., 2001). Unfortunately, we have no information about ape interneurons, so we cannot be certain whether these are human specializations or hominoid (ape-human) specializations.

Evolutionary changes in neuronal biology of the sort described above presumably reflect changes in the functional organization of the human brain, although for most brain regions we know too little about the functional contributions of different cell classes to understand how evolutionary changes in particular cell groups could be related to evolutionary changes in cognition and behavior. There is one neural domain, however, for which we have enough information to begin to frame some hypotheses about human functional specialization, and that is the visual system.

MODIFICATIONS OF THE VISUAL SYSTEM In visual neuroscience, the proposition that there are no important differences between macaques and humans is something close to an article of faith. Therefore, the visual system is perhaps the last place in the brain one might expect to have undergone significant modifications in human evolution. Nevertheless, there is abundant evidence of differences in visual system organization between humans, apes, macaques, and other nonhuman primates (reviewed by Preuss, 2003).

These differences are found across many levels of organization, starting with the retina. In the monkey species that have been examined, the ratio of long-wavelength (L) to medium-wavelength (M) cones is about 1:1 (Jacobs and Deegan, 1997), and the ratio in chimpanzees is about 1:3:1 (Jacobs, Deegan, and Moran, 1996). In humans, the L:M ratio averages approximately 2:1, although some individuals have much higher ratios (Jacobs and Deegan, 1997; Dobkins, Thiele, and Albright, 2000). In addition, the centralmost part of the human retina is virtually free of short-wavelength (S) cones, which is not the case in Old World and New World monkeys (Bumsted and Hendrickson, 1999). (The status of apes is unknown.) The large, parasol class of retinal ganglion cells (which project to the magnocellular, or M, layers of the lateral geniculate) have much larger dendritic fields in humans than in macaques, although the dendritic fields of midget cells (which project to the parvocellular, or P, layers of the geniculate) have similar dimensions in macaques and humans (Dacey and Petersen, 1992). These anatomical differences suggest that humans should be more sensitive in the long-wavelength part of the spectrum than macaques, and that humans and macaques should have different sensitivies to stimuli that activate the M pathway, such as flickering gratings. The psychophysical data are consistent with these expectations (Harwerth and Smith, 1985).

Recent studies have also identified evolutionary modifications of the primary visual area (V1), which are concentrated in layer 4A (figure 1.6). In macaques, layer 4A is a site of interaction between the magnocellular and parvocellular visual pathways. It receives direct inputs from the P layers of the LGN; these afferent fibers form a thin sheet in layer 4A, the location of which is marked by dense staining for cytochrome oxidase (CO). The sheet is interrupted by clusters of apical dendrites arising from pyramidal cell bodies located immediately below the sheet, which gives the sheet the appearance of a flattened honeycomb. The organization in other Old World and New World monkey species appears to be similar to that in macaques, with the exception of owl monkeys. Owl monkeys lack the direct P-geniculate projection to layer 4A present in other monkeys, along with the corresponding band of dense CO staining. (For a detailed review of the organization of layer 4A in monkeys, see Preuss and Coleman, 2002, and Preuss, 2003b.)

Studies in our laboratory indicate that the organization of layer 4A is very different in great apes and humans (Preuss, Qi, and Kaas, 1999; Preuss and Coleman, 2002).

Both great apes and humans lack a dense band of CO staining in layer 4A, which suggests that the direct P-geniculate projections are diminished in number or are more dispersed than in humans, so that they do not form a discrete, thin sheet. Layer 4A underwent additional modifications in the human lineage. Rather than having a system of apical dendrite bundles extending upward from layer 4B, human layer 4A is criss-crossed by a three-dimensional meshwork of tissue composed of small cell bodies embedded within bands of dendrites. These cell bodies (which are probably modified pyramidal cells) and dendrites stain densely with an antibody for nonphosphorylated neurofilament protein (NPNF). The same kind of meshlike pattern can be demonstrated by staining with the monoclonal antibody Cat-301, although Cat-301 labels primarily a different set of cell bodies and dendrites (multipolar interneurons and their processes) than those that stain for NPNF. Furthermore, the tissue bands that stain densely for NPNF and Cat-301 surround irregularly shaped territories densely packed with very small cells that stain for calbindin; these are probably inhibitory interneurons, although this has not yet been demonstrated.

By contrast to humans, Cat-301 and NPNF immunostaining is virtually absent from layer 4A of chimpanzees, Old World monkeys, and New World monkeys. Old World and New World monkeys also lack significant calbindin staining in layer 4A; chimpanzees have some calbindin-immunoreactive neurons in layer 4A, but these form an unbroken band; there is no evidence for the dual compartmentation seen in humans. This emphasizes the fact that humans do not simply differ from other primates in the biochemistry of layer 4A neurons, they also differ in the architecture of neurons and neurites that make up layer 4A.

It is difficult to interpret the functional significance of the structural specializations of layer 4A in apes and in humans, given the current state of our knowledge about the contributions of particular cell classes and compartments in V1 to visual function. However, Cat-301 staining is typically associated with elements of the M pathway, which suggests that the meshwork of tissue bands in human layer 4A could represent a modification of processing architecture related to the M pathway. Whatever the functional significance of human layer 4A modifications should ultimately prove to be, however, it is clear that area V1 underwent important changes in recent human evolution.

There is evidence for evolutionary change in extrastriate cortex as well, changes that also involve the M pathway and the dorsal (or parietal) processing stream, which receives strong inputs from the M pathway and which is involved in processing information about motion. The development of functional imaging techniques has made it possible for visual neuroscientists to examine the organization and functions of extrastriate cortex in humans and to compare human

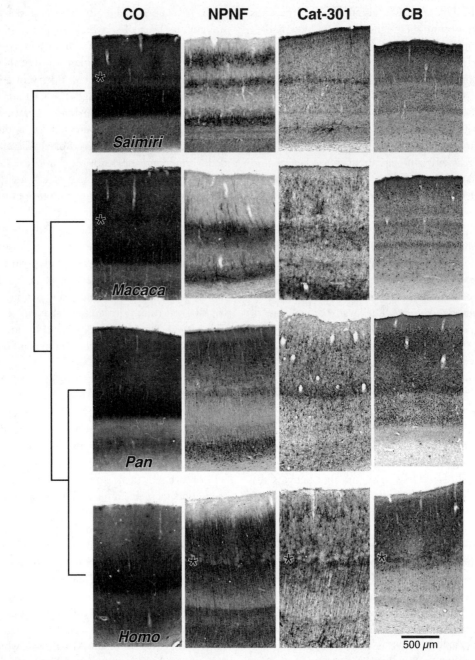

FIGURE 1.6 Evolutionary modifications of the primary visual area in ape and human evolution. New World and Old World monkeys, including squirrel monkeys (*Saimiri*) and macaque monkeys (*Macaca*), have a distinct band of cytochrome oxidase (CO) staining in layer 4A (asterisk) that is absent in chimpanzees (*Pan*) and humans (*Homo*). Humans have evolved a distinctive pattern of neu-ronal compartmentation in layer 4A (asterisks), marked by patchy staining for nonphosphorylated neurofilament protein (NPNF), the monoclonal antibody Cat-301, and calbindin (CB). The branching diagram on the left denotes the evolutionary relationships between these species.

organization with that of Old World and New World monkeys, which have been extensively studied using micro-electrode recording techniques. These imaging studies, in conjunction with histological studies, have demonstrated many similarities between humans and other primates, and the existence of a number of human extrastriate areas homologous to areas originally described in nonhuman primates is now well established. These include areas V2, V3, V3A, and the middle temporal area, MT (Sereno, 1998; Van Essen et al., 2001; Zilles and Clarke, 1997). Just as the human striate area (V1) differs in certain respects from its homologues in nonhuman primates, however, there are human-nonhuman differences in the characteristics of extrastriate areas. In macaques, microelectrode recording studies indicate that area V3 is highly responsive to motion, whereas area V3A (located immediately anterior to the dorsal part of area V3) is not. In humans, functional imaging studies report just the opposite result: V3A is more responsive to motion than area V3 (Tootell et al., 1997). That this is a real phyletic difference and not an artifact of technical differences was recently confirmed by a functional imaging study of macaques, which validated the microelectrode recording results: macaque V3 is more responsive to motion than V3A (Vanduffel et al., 2001).

Vanduffel and colleagues recently extended their comparative functional imaging investigations of motion processing, examining patterns of activation when human and macaque subjects view "structure-from-motion" stimuli (Vanduffel et al., 2002). These are two-dimensional dot arrays, moving in patterns that human observers interpret as a three-dimensional object rotating around an internal axis; comparison tasks involved patterns that are interpreted as simple two-dimensional movement. Vanduffel and colleagues reported that viewing structure-from-motion stimuli activated a number of extrastriate areas common to macaques and humans. However, humans also had several foci of activation in posterior parietal cortex that were not found in macaques under the same viewing conditions. These results could be interpreted in several ways. Humans might possess additional visual areas in parietal cortex that are absent in macaques. Alternatively, macaques and humans might possess the same complement of parietal areas, but humans have undergone evolutionary modifications of the functional properties of their parietal areas. If the latter is true, we might expect that macaques do not extract information about the three-dimension characteristics of objects in quite the same way that humans do (Preuss, 2003). This would not be surprising, given the evidence that humans represent object properties and interactions in ways that differ from nonhuman primates (Povinelli, 2000; Johnson-Frey, 2003b). Whatever the correct interpretation of these differences, the results of Vanduffel and colleagues (2002) provide additional evidence that the functional organization of the dorsal visual stream was modified in hominoid and/or human evolution.

New results from studies of gene sequences and gene expression

The differences in brain structure and function that distinguish humans from other animals presumably have correlates at the genetic level, involving some combination of changes in gene sequences, which alter the biochemical properties of the relevant gene products, and changes in gene expression, which involve the developmental timing and spatial patterning of gene expression as well as changes in the level of gene expression (i.e., changes in the number of mRNA transcripts produced from specific genes).

There are two general approaches one can take to the business of identifying the relationships between genes, on the one hand, and anatomy, physiology, and behavior, on the other. One can begin by identifying human specializations of brain organization and function and then try to isolate the genetic differences between humans and nonhumans that are responsible for the phenotypic differences. This is a daunting task, not least of all because of the impossibility of making interspecific crosses, although individual humans are occasionally identified with mutations that affect characteristics we regard as specifically human—for example, mutations that affect linguistic abilities—and pedigree analysis can then lead us to loci related to the human specializations.

The other approach begins at the molecular level, identifying species differences in gene sequences and differences in gene expression, and using that information to guide the exploration of phenotypic differences. This approach is founded upon our knowledge of the human genome sequence and the exploratory genomic techniques that exploit this sequence information. Some of these techniques are *in silico*, involving comparisons of sequence databases for multiple species to identify gene sequence differences, gene duplications, and insertion-deletion mutations. Other techniques involve comparing levels of expression of gene products from tissue samples obtained from different species. Once differentially expressed genes are identified, one can use molecular techniques to determine whether changes in gene expression are matched by changes in protein levels (they often are, although not always), as well as histological methods such as *in situ* hybridization and immunocyto-chemistry to determine where in the brain the products of differentially expressed genes are localized. Thus, information about genetic differences can provide a way to identify species differences in brain anatomy and physiology. This genomic approach has certain distinct advantages over classical genetic analysis. For one thing, it is possible to screen the entire genome for species differences quickly, and this in turn makes it possible to discover phenotypic differences between humans and nonhumans that were not previously known to exist. This can be particularly valuable when dealing with the brain and cognition, where our knowledge of human specializations is very rudimentary.

Given how often we are reminded that the gene sequences of humans and chimpanzees are about 99% identical, one might think that there is little to be learned about human specializations from the study of sequence differences. One must bear in mind, however, that there are somewhere on the order of 25,000 genes in humans and other anthropoid primates, with an average of roughly 1250 nucleotides per gene, so a difference of 1% adds up to more than 300,000 nucleotide differences in expressed gene sequences across the genome. A single nucleotide change can have a profound effect on the function of the resulting protein, for example, by creating a new phosphorylation site. Moreover, small changes in the noncoding, regulatory regions of the genome, such as transcription-factor binding sites, can also produce dramatic changes in gene expression.

SEQUENCE EVOLUTION OF FOXP2 Hurst and colleagues identified a family in Britain with an inherited developmental disorder that involves impairment of speech and language, especially aspects of syntax and phonology (Hurst et al., 1990). The disorder is not entirely language specific, as affected individuals also show intellectual deficits and impairment of orofacial praxis that are unrelated to language (Vargha-Khadem et al., 1995), although the linguistic impairment is severe. MRI studies suggest the existence of structural abnormalities in language-related brain structures (Watkins et al., 2002). Pedigree analysis of the KE family indicates that affected members share a point mutation of a transcription factor gene, FOXP2 (Lai et al., 2001).

The connection between FOXP2 and language prompted Enard and colleagues (Enard, Przeworski, et al., 2002) to compare the DNA and protein sequences of FOXP2 in humans, apes, rhesus macaques, and mice. They found FOXP2 to be a very conservative gene: the amino acid sequences of rhesus macaques, gorillas, and chimpanzees are identical. Humans, however, have mutations that result in two amino acid substitutions. These substitutions involve the replacement of a threonine residue with asparagine at one site, and an asparagine-to-serine replacement at the other. (These are not the sites affected in family KE, incidentally.) Since threonine and serine residues are targets for phosphorylation, these substitutions might well provide the FOXP2 transcription factor with different binding properties in humans. The fact that FOXP2 is otherwise so highly conserved evolutionarily suggests that the accumulation of two amino acid substitutions is not the result of random processes (drift to fixation) but rather is due to the action of natural selection (Enard, Przeworski, et al., 2002).

CHANGES IN GENE EXPRESSION The advent of gene microarrays makes it possible to rapidly screen the genome for human-specific changes in gene expression within the brain. Typical oligonucleotide microarrays contain sets of short sequences (25-mers) representing about 10,000 expressed human genes. To identify evolutionary differences in gene expression, one compares levels of hybridization obtained with RNA samples from the brains of humans and nonhuman primates. In practice, the technique is limited by the fact that the arrays are made with *human* sequences, and the RNA of nonhuman species will bind less well, owing to species differences in nucleotide sequences. This shortcoming can be compensated for to some extent by the parallel use of independent techniques, including cDNA arrays (which have longer sequence probes and thus are presumably less sensitive to small numbers of nucleotide differences) and the polymerase chain reaction (PCR) technique, which allows one to compare the expression levels of particular genes in different species to the levels of selected "housekeeping" genes, which are assumed to be expressed at similar levels across species. PCR is usually considered the most accurate and reliable technique for assessing differences in gene expression but is also more labor- and time-intensive than oligonucleotide or cDNA arrays.

Enard and colleagues (Enard, Khaitovich, et al., 2002) reported the first study of gene expression differences in the brains of humans compared to chimpanzees, orang, and macaque monkeys. They concluded that there was an acceleration of gene expression changes in human evolution, such that the human brain had accumulated more gene expression differences than did the chimpanzee brain in the period since humans and chimpanzees last shared a common ancestor. They also concluded that there was less change in the liver and blood, and that humans and chimpanzees exhibit about the same amount of change in these tissues.

A second study of gene expression differences in human brain evolution (Cáceres, Lachuer, et al., 2003) presents an account that differs in several important respects from that of Enard and colleagues (Enard, Khaitovich, et al., 2002). This study identified approximately 90 genes that are differentially expressed in the human cortex compared to chimpanzees and macaques, of which the large majority (about 90%) are up-regulated in humans. By comparison, the proportion of genes that are up-regulated and down-regulated in the liver and heart is close to 50:50. Furthermore, there are *fewer* gene expression changes in the brain than in other tissues. In summary, what is distinctive about the human cortex is the predominance of up-regulation: the great majority of genes that exhibit expression changes in humans are marked by increased levels of expression.

This study also specified the particular genes that underwent expression changes in human cortical evolution. These genes span a wide variety of functional groups. Among them are several genes required for the normal development and function of the nervous system, as indicated by the fact that deletions result in mental retardation. One example is the gene for general transcription factor II-i (*GTF2I*), which is among the genes deleted in Williams syndrome and which may be responsible for the deficits in visuospatial perception found in this form of mental retardation (Bellugi et al., 1999; Alberto and Jurado, 2003). The fact that *GTF2I* is up-regulated in human evolution is particularly interesting given the evidence (reviewed above) suggesting that the visuospatial processing systems related to the M pathway and the dorsal stream were modified in recent human evolution. The increased expression of *GTF2I* may therefore constitute part of the genetic foundation of human specializations of the visual system.

Other changes in human cortical evolution include the up-regulation of numerous genes related to neuronal signaling and neuronal activity. These include, for example, the gene for calcium/calmodulin-dependent protein kinase II alpha (*CAMK2A*), which mediates plasticity at glutamatergic synapses and is thought to be involved in long-term potentiation (Frankland et al., 2001), and which undergoes increased expression in experimental studies of the effects of increased neuronal activity (Ehlers, 2003). Also up-regulated is the gene for *CA2* (carbonic anhydrase II), an enzyme localized in astrocytes that is thought to play an important role in mediating the transport of lactate from glia to pyramidal cells, which use glia-derived lactate as a supplementary energy source during periods of increased activity (Deitmer, 2001). The fact that most of the gene expression changes in human cortical evolution involve the increased expression of neurons involved in neuronal activity suggests that a given volume of human cortex has a higher level of activity than a comparable volume of macaque cortex. Consistent with this, metabolic imaging in awake humans and macaques suggests that cortical glucose utilization rates are higher in humans than in macaques (compare, for example, Bentourkia et al., 2000, and Noda et al., 2002). This is otherwise a surprising result, as metabolic rates (per unit of tissue) typically decline with increasing brain size (Siesjö, 1978).

One might think it a good thing for humans to have evolved the ability to sustain unusually rates of cortical activity, but it must have come at a cost: higher rates of activity would result in higher rates of cellular and molecular damage, and thus accelerated aging. Yet humans are the longest-lived primates: it is common for human neurons to function adequately through eight decades of life. This is a neat trick, and it seems inescapable that human brain cells possess evolutionary modifications of the cellular and molecular repair mechanisms that retard aging. It is interesting, then, that among the genes exhibiting modified expression

in the human brain are several that have cytoprotective functions.

Conclusions

Humans are unusual in many aspects of their biology, yet neuroscientists have fostered the view that our brains are basically bigger, better versions of a generalized primate or mammalian brain. It is becoming increasingly clear that this is not that case, and that the brain underwent changes at many levels of organization during the recent evolutionary history of the human lineage. Neuroscientists have an expanding array of tools with which to explore human brain structure in detail, a project that, if carried out in an appropriate comparative framework, could shed new light on the nature of the human mind. Understanding what is distinctive about the human brain and mind is among the most fundamental of intellectual endeavors.

REFERENCES

ALBANESE, E., A. MERLO, A. ALBANESE, and E. GOMEZ, 1989. Anterior speech region: Asymmetry and weight-surface correlation. *Arch. Neurol.* 46:307–310.

ALBERTO, L., and P. JURADO, 2003. Williams-Beuren syndrome: A model of recurrent genomic mutation. *Horm. Res.* 59(Suppl. 1):106–113.

ALLMAN, J., 1990. Evolution of neocortex. In *Cerebral Cortex*, vol. B, *Comparative Structure and Evolution of Cerebral Cortex, Part II*, E. G. Jones and A. Peters, eds. New York: Plenum Press, pp. 269–283.

ANNETT, M., 1979. Family handedness in three generations predicted by the right shift theory. *Ann. Hum. Genet.* 42:479–491.

ARMSTRONG, E., 1982. Mosaic evolution in the primate brain: Differences and similarities in the hominoid thalamus. In *Primate Brain Evolution*, E. Armstrong and D. Falk, eds. New York: Plenum Press, pp. 131–161.

BAILEY, P., G. V. BONIN, and W. S. MCCULLOCH, 1950. *The Isocortex of the Chimpanzee*. Urbana: University of Illinois Press.

BALEYDIER, C., P. ACHACHE, and J. C. FROMENT, 1997. Neurofilament architecture of superior and mesial premotor cortex in the human brain. *Neuroreport* 8:1691–1696.

BELLUGI, U., L. LICHTENBERGER, D. MILLS, A. GALABURDA, and J. R. KORENBERG, 1999. Bridging cognition, the brain and molecular genetics: Evidence from Williams syndrome. *Trends Neurosci.* 22:197–207.

BENTOURKIA, M., A. BOL, IVANOIU, D. LABAR, M. SIBOMANA, A. COPPENS, C. MICHEL, G. COSNARD, and A. G. DE VOLDER, 2000. Comparison of regional cerebral blood flow and glucose metabolism in the normal brain: Effect of aging. *J. Neurol. Sci.* 181:19–28.

BERGER, B., and P. GASPAR, 1995. Comparative anatomy of the catecholaminergic innervation of rat and primate prefrontal cortex. In *Phylogeny and Ontogeny of Catecholamine Systems in the CNS of Vertebrates*, W. J. A. J. Smeets and A. Reiner, eds. Cambridge, England: Cambridge University Press, pp. 293–324.

BLINKOV, S., and I. GLEZER, 1968. *The Human Brain in Figures and Tables*. New York: Basic Books.

BLURTON JONES, N. G., K. HAWKES, and J. F. O'CONNELL, 2002. Antiquity of postreproductive life: Are there modern impacts on hunter-gatherer postreproductive life spans? *Am. J. Hum. Biol.* 14:184–205.

BRADSHAW, J. L., and L. J. ROGERS, 1993. *The Evolution of Lateral Asymmetries, Language, Tool Use, and Intellect.* San Diego, Calif.: Academic Press.

BRODMANN, K., 1909. *Vergleichende Lokalisationslehre der Grosshirnrinde.* Leipzig: Barth. Reprinted as *Brodmann's 'Localisation in the Cerebral Cortex,'* L. J. Garey, trans. ed. London: Smith-Gordon, 1994.

BRODMANN, K., 1912. Neue Ergibnisse über die vergleichende histologische Lokalisation der Grosshirnrinde mit besonderer Berücksichtigung des Stirnhirns. *Anat. Anz.* (Suppl.)41:157–216.

BUMSTED, K., and A. HENDRICKSON, 1999. Distribution and development of short-wavelength cones differ between *Macaca* monkey and human fovea. *J. Comp. Neurol.* 403:502–516.

BUXHOEVEDEN, D. P., A. E. SWITALA, M. LITAKER, E. ROY, and M. F. CASANOVA, 2001. Lateralization of minicolumns in human planum temporale is absent in nonhuman primate cortex. *Brain Behav. Evol.* 57:349–358.

CÁCERES, M., J. LACHUER, M. A. ZAPALA, J. C. REDMOND, L. KUDO, D. H. GESCHWIND, D. J. LOCKHART, T. M. PREUSS, and C. BARLOW, 2003. Elevated gene expression levels distinguish human from non-human primate brains. *Proc. Natl. Acad. Sci. U.S.A.* 100:13030–13035.

CANTALUPO, C., and W. D. HOPKINS, 2001. Asymmetric Broca's area in great apes. *Nature* 414:505.

CARTMILL, M., 1992. New views on primate origins. *Evol. Anthropol.* 1:105–111.

CONTURO, T. E., N. F. LORI, T. S. CULL, E. AKBUDAK, A. Z. SNYDER, J. S. SHIMONY, R. C. MCKINSTRY, H. BURTON, and M. E. RAICHLE, 1999. Tracking neuronal fiber pathways in the living human brain. *Proc. Natl. Acad. Sci. U.S.A.* 96:10422–10427.

CORBALLIS, M. C., 1991. *The Lopsided Ape.* New York: Oxford University Press.

CORBETTA, M., and G. L. SHULMAN, 2002. Control of goal-directed and stimulus-driven attention in the brain. *Nat. Rev. Neurosci.* 3:201–215.

CREUTZFELDT, O. D., 1977. Generality of functional structure of the neocortex. *Naturwissenschaften* 64:507–517.

DACEY, D. M., and M. R. PETERSEN, 1992. Dendritic field size and morphology of midget and parasol ganglion cells of the human retina. *Proc. Natl. Acad. Sci. U.S.A.* 89:9666–9670.

DAI, J., J. VAN DER VLIET, D. F. SWAAB, and R. M. BUIJS, 1998. Human retinohypothalamic tract as revealed by in vitro postmortem tracing. *J. Comp. Neurol.* 397:357–370.

DEACON, T. W., 1997. *The Symbolic Species.* New York: W. W. Norton.

DEFELIPE, J., J. I. ARELLANO, A. GOMEZ, E. C. AZMITIA, and A. MUNOZ, 2001. Pyramidal cell axons show a local specialization for GABA and 5-HT inputs in monkey and human cerebral cortex. *J. Comp. Neurol.* 433:148–155.

DEITMER, J. W., 2001. Strategies for metabolic exchange between glial cells and neurons. *Respir. Physiol.* 129:71–81.

DEL RÍO, M. R., and J. DEFELIPE, 1997. Colocalization of parvalbumin and calbindin D-28k in neurons including chandelier cells of the human temporal neocortex. *J. Chem. Neuroanat.* 12:165–173.

DOBKINS, K. R., A. THIELE, and T. D. ALBRIGHT, 2000. Comparison of red-green equiluminance points in humans and macaques: Evidence for different L:M cone ratios between species. *J. Opt. Soc. Am. A Opt. Image Sci. Vis.* 17:545–556.

EHLERS, M. D., 2003. Activity level controls postsynaptic composition and signaling via the ubiquitin-proteasome system. *Nat. Neurosci.* 6:231–242.

ELLIOT SMITH, G., 1924. *The Evolution of Man: Essays.* London: Oxford University Press.

ELSTON, G. N., R. BENAVIDES-PICCIONE, and J. DEFELIPE, 2001. The pyramidal cell in cognition: A comparative study in human and monkey. *J. Neurosci.* 21:RC163.

ENARD, W., P. KHAITOVICH, J. KLOSE, S. ZOLLNER, F. HEISSIG, P. GIAVALISCO, K. NIESELT-STRUWE, E. MUCHMORE, A. VARKI, R. RAVID, et al., 2002. Intra- and interspecific variation in primate gene expression patterns. *Science* 296:340–343.

ENARD, W., M. PRZEWORSKI, S. E. FISHER, C. S. LAI, V. WIEBE, T. KITANO, A. P. MONACO, and S. PAABO, 2002. Molecular evolution of FOXP2, a gene involved in speech and language. *Nature* 418:869–872.

FALK, D., 1992. *Evolution of the brain and cognition in hominids. Sixty-Second James Arthur Lecture on the Evolution of the Human Brain.* New York: American Museum of Natural History.

FALZI, G., P. PERRONE, and L. A. VIGNOLO, 1982. Right-left asymmetry in the anterior speech region. *Arch. Neurol.* 39:239–240.

FLEAGLE, J. G., 1999. *Primate Adaptation and Evolution,* 2nd ed. San Diego, Calif.: Academic Press.

FOUNDAS, A. L., C. M. LEONARD, R. GILMORE, E. FENNELL, and K. M. HEILMAN, 1996. The pars triangularis and speech and language lateralization. *Proc. Natl. Acad. Sci. U.S.A.* 93:719–722.

FOUNDAS, A. L., C. M. LEONARD, and K. M. HEILMAN, 1995. Morphologic cerebral asymmetries and handedness: The pars triangularis and planum temporale. *Arch. Neurol.* 52:501–508.

FRAHM, H. D., H. STEPHAN, and G. BARON, 1984. Comparison of brain structure volumes in Insectivora and Primates: V. Area striata (AS). *J. Hirnforsch.* 25:537–557.

FRANKLAND, P. W., C. O'BRIEN, M. OHNO, A. KIRKWOOD, and A. J. SILVA, 2001. Alpha-CaMKII-dependent plasticity in the cortex is required for permanent memory. *Nature* 411:309–313.

GAFFAN, D., and J. HORNAK, 1997. Visual neglect in the monkey: Representation and disconnection. *Brain* 120(Pt. 9):1647–1657.

GALABURDA, A. M., 1980. La région de Broca: Observations anatomiques faites un siècle aprés la mort de son découvreur. *Rev. Neurol. (Paris)* 136:609–616.

GALABURDA, A. M., 1984. Anatomical asymmetries. In *Cerebral Dominance,* N. Geschwind and A. M. Galaburda, eds. Cambridge, Mass.: Harvard University Press, pp. 11–25.

GALABURDA, A. M., and F. SANIDES, 1980. Cytoarchitectonic organization of the human auditory cortex. *J. Comp. Neurol.* 190:597–610.

GALLESE, V., L. FADIGA, L. FOGASSI, and G. RIZZOLATTI, 1996. Action recognition in the premotor cortex. *Brain* 119:593–609.

GANNON, P. J., R. L. HOLLOWAY, D. C. BROADFIELD, and A. R. BRAUN, 1998. Asymmetry of chimpanzee planum temporale: Humanlike pattern of Wernicke's brain language area homolog. *Science* 279:220–222.

GEBHARD, R., K. ZILLES, A. SCHLEICHER, B. J. EVERITT, T. W. ROBBINS, and I. DIVAC, 1995. Parcellation of the frontal cortex of the New World monkey *Callithrix jacchus* by eight neurotransmitter-binding sites. *Anat. Embryol.* 191:509–517.

GESCHWIND, D. H., B. L. MILLER, C. DECARLI, and D. CARMELLI, 2002. Heritability of lobar brain volumes in twins supports genetic models of cerebral laterality and handedness. *Proc. Natl. Acad. Sci. U.S.A.* 99:3176–3181.

GESCHWIND, N., and W. LEVITSKY, 1968. Left-right asymmetry in temporal speech region. *Science* 161:186–187.

HARWERTH, R. S., and E. L. SMITH, 1985. Rhesus monkey as a model for normal vision of humans. *Am. J. Optom. Physiol. Opt.* 62:633–641.

HAYES, T. L., and D. A. LEWIS, 1993. Hemispheric differences in layer III pyramidal neurons of the anterior language area. *Arch. Neurol.* 50:501–505.

HAYES, T. L., and D. A. LEWIS, 1995. Anatomical specialization of the anterior motor speech area: Hemispheric differences in magnopyramidal neurons. *Brain Lang.* 49:289–308.

HOF, P. R., I. I., GLEZER, E. A. NIMCHINSKY, and J. M. ERWIN, 2000. Neurochemical and cellular specializations in the mammalian neocortex reflect phylogenetic relationships: Evidence from primates, cetaceans, and artiodactyls. *Brain Behav. Evol.* 55:300–310.

HOF, P. R., E. A. NIMCHINSKY, D. P. PERL, and J. M. ERWIN, 2001. An unusual population of pyramidal neurons in the anterior cingulate cortex of hominids contains the calcium-binding protein calretinin. *Neurosci. Lett.* 307:139–142.

HOPKINS, W. D., L. MARINO, J. K. RILLING, and L. A. MACGREGOR, 1998. Planum temporale asymmetries in great apes as revealed by magnetic resonance imaging (MRI). *Neuroreport* 9:2913–2918.

HURST, J. A., M. BARAITSER, E. AUGER, F. GRAHAM, and S. NORELL, 1990. An extended family with a dominantly inherited speech disorder. *Dev. Med. Child Neurol.* 32:352–355.

HUTSLER, J. J., and M. S. GAZZANIGA, 1996. Acetylcholinesterase staining in human auditory and language cortices: Regional variation of structural features. *Cereb. Cortex* 6:260–270.

JACOBS, G. H., and J. F. DEEGAN, 2nd, 1997. Spectral sensitivity of macaque monkeys measured with ERG flicker photometry. *Vis. Neurosci.* 14:921–928.

JACOBS, G. H., J. F. DEEGAN, 2nd, and J. L. MORAN, 1996. ERG measurements of the spectral sensitivity of common chimpanzee (*Pan troglodytes*). *Vision Res.* 36:2587–2594.

JOHNSON-FREY, S. H., 2003a. Cortical mechanisms of tool use. In *Taking Action: Cognitive Neuroscience Perspectives on the Problem of Intentional Movements*, S. H. Johnson-Frey, ed. Cambridge, Mass.: MIT Press, pp. 185–217.

JOHNSON-FREY, S. H., 2003b. What's so special about human tool use? *Neuron* 39:201–204.

KAAS, J. H., 1987. The organization and evolution of neocortex. In *Higher Brain Function: Recent Explorations of the Brain's Emergent Properties*, S. P. Wise, ed. New York: John Wiley, pp. 347–378.

KAAS, J. H., and T. M. PREUSS, 2003. Human brain evolution. In *Fundamental Neuroscience*, 2nd ed., F. E. B. L. R. Squire, S. K. McConnell, J. L. Roberts, N. C. Spitzer, and M. J. Zigmond, eds. San Diego, Calif.: Academic Press, pp. 1147–1166.

KAUFFMAN, S., 1995. *At Home in the Universe*. New York: Oxford University Press.

LAI, C. S., S. E. FISHER, J. A. HURST, F. VARGHA-KHADEM, and A. P. MONACO, 2001. A forkhead-domain gene is mutated in a severe speech and language disorder. *Nature* 413:519–523.

LE GROS CLARK, W. E., 1959. *The Antecedents of Man*. Edinburgh: Edinburgh University Press.

LEMAY, M., and N. GESCHWIND, 1975. Hemispheric difference in the brains of great apes. *Brain Behav. Evol.* 11:48–52.

LETINIC, K., R. ZONCU, and P. RAKIC, 2002. Origin of GABAergic neurons in the human neocortex. *Nature* 417:645–649.

MCGREW, W. C., and L. F. MARCHANT, 1997. On the other hand: Current issues in and meta-analysis of the behavioral laterality of hand function in nonhuman primates. *Yearb. Phys. Anthropol.* 40:201–232.

MORGAN, E., 1982. *The Aquatic Ape: A Theory of Human Evolution*. New York, Stein and Day.

MURPHY, W. J., E. EIZIRIK, S. J. O'BRIEN, O. MADSEN, M. SCALLY, C. J. DOUADY, E. TEELING, O. A. RYDER, M. J. STANHOPE, W. W. DE JONG, and M. S. SPRINGER, 2001. Resolution of the early placental mammal radiation using Bayesian phylogenetics. *Science* 294:2348–2351.

NAGEL, T., 1974. What is it like to be a bat? *Philos. Rev.* 83:435–450.

NIMCHINSKY, E. A., E. GILISSEN, J. M. ALLMAN, D. P. PERL, J. M. ERWIN, and P. R. HOF, 1999. A neuronal morphologic type unique to humans and great apes. *Proc. Natl. Acad. Sci. U.S.A.* 96:5268–5273.

NODA, A., H. OHBA, T. KAKIUCHI, M. FUTATSUBASHI, H. TSUKADA, and S. NISHIMURA, 2002. Age-related changes in cerebral blood flow and glucose metabolism in conscious rhesus monkeys. *Brain Res.* 936:76–81.

O'CONNELL, J. F., K. HAWKES, and N. G. BLURTON JONES, 1999. Grandmothering and the evolution of homo erectus. *J. Hum. Evol.* 36:461–485.

OLSON, M. V., and A. VARKI, 2003. Sequencing the chimpanzee genome: Insights into human evolution and disease. *Nat. Rev. Genet.* 4:20–28.

PETRIDES, M., and D. N. PANDYA, 1994. Comparative architectonic analysis of the human and the macaque frontal cortex. In *Handbook of Neuropsychology*, F. Booler and J. Grafman, eds. Amsterdam: Elsevier, pp. 17–58.

POVINELLI, D. J., 2000. *Folk Physics for Apes: The Chimpanzee's Theory of How the World Works*. Oxford, England: Oxford University Press.

POVINELLI, D. J., and T. M. PREUSS, 1995. Theory of mind: Evolutionary history of a cognitive specialization. *Trends Neurosci.* 18:418–424.

PREUSS, T. M., 2000a. Taking the measure of diversity: Comparative alternatives to the model-animal paradigm in cortical neuroscience. *Brain Behav. Evol.* 55:287–299.

PREUSS, T. M., 2000b. What's human about the human brain? In *The New Cognitive Neurosciences*, 2nd ed. Cambridge, Mass.: MIT Press, pp. 1219–1234.

PREUSS, T. M., 2001. The discovery of cerebral diversity: An unwelcome scientific revolution. In *Evolutionary Anatomy of the Primate Cerebral Cortex*, D. Falk and K. Gibson, eds. Cambridge, England: Cambridge University Press, pp. 138–164.

PREUSS, T. M., 2003. Specializations of the human visual system: The monkey model meets human reality. In *The Primate Visual System*, J. H. Kaas and C. E. Collins, eds. Boca Raton, Fla.: CRC Press, pp. 231–259.

PREUSS, T. M., in press. Evolutionary specializations of primate brain systems. In *Primate Origins and Adaptations*, M. J. Ravoso and M. Dagosto, eds. New York: Kluwer Academic/Plenum Press.

PREUSS, T. M., and G. Q. COLEMAN, 2002. Human-specific organization of primary visual cortex: Alternating compartments of dense Cat-301 and calbindin immunoreactivity in layer 4A. *Cereb. Cortex* 12:671–691.

PREUSS, T. M., H. QI, and J. H. KAAS, 1999. Distinctive compartmental organization of human primary visual cortex. *Proc. Natl. Acad. Sci. U.S.A.* 96:11601–11606.

PREUSS, T. M., H.-X. QI, P. GASPAR, and J. H. KAAS, 1997. Histochemical evidence for multiple subdivisions of primary motor cortex in chimpanzees. *Soc. Neurosci. Abstr.* 23:1273.

PREUSS, T. M., I. STEPNIEWSKA, and J. H. KAAS, 1996. Movement representation in the dorsal and ventral premotor areas of owl monkeys: A microstimulation study. *J. Comp. Neurol.* 371:649–676.

RAJKOWSKA, G., and P. S. GOLDMAN-RAKIC, 1995. Cytoarchitectonic definition of prefrontal areas in the normal human cortex: I. Remapping of areas 9 and 46 using quantitative criteria. *Cereb. Cortex* 5:307–322.

REGIDOR, J., and I. DIVAC, 1992. Bilateral thalamocortical projection in hedgehogs: Evolutionary implications. *Brain. Behav. Evol.* 39:265–269.

RILLING, J., C. KILTS, S. WILLIAMS, M. BERAN, M. GIROUX, J. M. HOFFMAN, S. RAPOPORT, S. SAVAGE-RUMBAUGH, and D. RUMBAUGH, 2000. A comparative PET study of linguistic processing in humans and language-competent chimpanzees. *Am. J. Phys. Authropol.* (Suppl. 30):263–263.

ROCKEL, A. J., R. W. HIORNS, and T. P. S. POWELL, 1980. The basic uniformity of structure of the neocortex. *Brain* 103:221–224.

SANCHEZ, M. M., L. J. YOUNG, P. M. PLOTSKY, and T. R. INSEL, 1999. Autoradiographic and in situ hybridization localization of corticotropin-releasing factor 1 and 2 receptors in nonhuman primate brain. *J. Comp. Neurol.* 408:365–377.

SCHEIBEL, A. B., L. A. PAUL, I. FRIED, A. B. FORSYTHE, U. TOMIYASU, A. WECHSLER, A. KAO, and J. SLOTNICK, 1985. Dendritic organization of the anterior speech area. *Exp. Neurol.* 87:109–117.

SEMENDEFERI, K., and H. DAMASIO, 2000. The brain and its main anatomical subdivisions in living hominoids using magnetic resonance imaging. *J. Hum. Evol.* 38:317–332.

SEMENDEFERI, K., H. DAMASIO, R. FRANK, and G. W. VAN HOESEN, 1997. The evolution of the frontal lobes: A volumetric analysis based on three-dimensional reconstructions of magnetic resonance image scans of human and ape brains. *J. Hum. Evol.* 32:375–388.

SEMENDEFERI, K., A. LU, N. SCHENKER, and H. DAMASIO, 2002. Humans and great apes share a large frontal cortex. *Nat. Neurosci.* 5:272–276.

SERENO, M. I., 1998. Brain mapping in animals and humans. *Curr. Opin. Neurobiol.* 8:188–194.

SHERWOOD, C. C., D. C. BROADFIELD, R. L. HOLLOWAY, P. J. GANNON, and P. R. HOF, 2003. Variability of Broca's area homologue in African great apes: Implications for language evolution. *Anat. Rec.* 271A:276–285.

SHERWOOD, C. C., P. W. LEE, C. B. RIVARA, R. L. HOLLOWAY, E. P. GILISSEN, R. M. SIMMONS, A. HAKEEM, J. M. ALLMAN, J. M. ERWIN, and P. R. HOF, 2003. Evolution of specialized pyramidal neurons in primate visual and motor cortex. *Brain Behav. Evol.* 61:28–44.

SIESJÖ, B., 1978. *Brain Energy Metabolism.* Chichester, N.Y.: Wiley.

SPARKS, D. L., L. F. LUE, T. A. MARTIN, and J. ROGERS, 2000. Neural tract tracing using Di-I: A review and a new method to make fast Di-I faster in human brain. *J. Neurosci. Methods.* 103:3–10.

STEPHAN, H., J. FRAHM, and G. BARON, 1981. New and revised data on volumes of brain structures in insectivores and primates. *Folia Primatol.* 35:1–29.

TOOTELL, R. B., J. D. MENDOLA, N. K. HADJIKHANI, P. J. LEDDEN, A. K. LIU, J. B. REPPAS, M. I. SERENO, and A. M. DALE, 1997. Functional analysis of V3A and related areas in human visual cortex. *J. Neurosci.* 17:7060–7078.

VAN ESSEN, D. C., J. W. LEWIS, H. A. DRURY, N. HADJIKHANI, R. B. TOOTELL, M. BAKIRCIOGLU, and M. I. MILLER, 2001. Mapping visual cortex in monkeys and humans using surface-based atlases. *Vision Res.* 41:1359–1378.

VANDUFFEL, W., D. FIZE, J. B. MANDEVILLE, K. NELISSEN, P. VAN HECKE, B. R. ROSEN, R. B. TOOTELL, and G. A. ORBAN, 2001. Visual motion processing investigated using contrast agent-enhanced fMRI in awake behaving monkeys. *Neuron* 32:565–577.

VANDUFFEL, W., D. FIZE, H. PEUSKENS, K. DENYS, S. SUNAERT, J. T. TODD, and G. A. ORBAN, 2002. Extracting 3D from motion: Differences in human and monkey intraparietal cortex. *Science* 298:413–415.

VARGHA-KHADEM, F., K. WATKINS, K. ALCOCK, P. FLETCHER, and R. PASSINGHAM, 1995. Praxic and nonverbal cognitive deficits in a large family with a genetically transmitted speech and language disorder. *Proc. Natl. Acad. Sci. U.S.A.* 92:930–933.

VOGT, B. A., E. A. NIMCHINSKY, L. J. VOGT, and P. R. HOF, 1995. Human cingulate cortex: Surface features, flat maps, and cytoarchitecture. *J. Comp. Neurol.* 359:490–506.

WALKER, A. E., 1940. A cytoarchitectural study of the prefrontal area of the macaque monkey. *J. Comp. Neurol.* 73:59–86.

WALLMAN, J., 1992. *Aping Language.* Cambridge, England: Cambridge University Press.

WATKINS, K. E., F. VARGHA-KHADEM, J. ASHBURNER, R. E. PASSINGHAM, A. CONNELLY, K. J. FRISTON, R. S. FRACKOWIAK, M. MISHKIN, and D. G. GADIAN, 2002. MRI analysis of an inherited speech and language disorder: Structural brain abnormalities. *Brain* 125:465–478.

WILLIAMS, S. M., and P. S. GOLDMAN-RAKIC, 1998. Widespread origin of the primate mesofrontal dopamine system. *Cereb. Cortex* 8:321–345.

YENI-KOMSHIAN, G. H., and D. A. BENSON, 1976. Anatomical study of cerebral symmetry in the temporal lobe of humans, chimpanzees and rhesus monkeys. *Science* 192:387–389.

YOUNG, L. J., D. TOLOCZKO, and T. R. INSEL, 1999. Localization of vasopressin (V1a) receptor binding and mRNA in the rhesus monkey brain. *J. Neuroendocrinol.* 11:291–297.

ZILLES, K., and S. CLARKE, 1997. Architecture, connectivity, and transmitter receptors of human extrastriate cortex. *Cereb. Cortex* 12:673–742.

2 Adult Neurogenesis in the Primate Forebrain

DAVID R. KORNACK

ABSTRACT Most neurons of the mammalian brain are generated only during restricted periods of early development and are not normally replaced if lost to neurodegenerative disease or injury. Two exceptions—discovered in rodents nearly four decades ago— are granule neurons of the hippocampal dentate gyrus and interneurons of the olfactory bulb. These neurons are continually generated from dividing neural stem cells well into adulthood, and their proliferation, differentiation, and survival are influenced by a diverse array of environmental and epigenetic factors. Only recently has "adult neurogenesis" been documented in homologous brain regions in human and nonhuman primates, thus extending this interesting phenomenon into the realm of primate neurobiology and clinical neuroscience. These investigations have revealed similarities as well as differences between rodents and primates in neural stem cell biology and adult neurogenesis. These differences may reflect adaptations of stem cells to the environment of comparatively larger, longer-lived primate brains, and may have consequences for understanding mechanisms of neural plasticity in adulthood, as well as for developing neuronal replacement therapies.

The mammalian brain has traditionally been considered a nonrenewable organ. Unlike cells in most tissues, which undergo generation and replacement throughout life, the neurons in most brain regions are generated early on, during restricted periods of development, and are not replaced if lost. However, two exceptions to this general rule were discovered almost four decades ago in restricted regions of the rodent forebrain: the dentate gyrus of the hippocampal formation, and the subventricular zone, which generates interneurons of the olfactory bulb. Neurons in these regions continue to be generated throughout the lifetime of the animal.

Since the initial discovery of adult neurogenesis in rodents, the field has undergone a renaissance over the past 10 years and has generated widespread interest and enthusiasm, for at least two main reasons. First, beginning in the 1990s, with studies conducted mainly in rodents, neurogenesis in the adult dentate gyrus and subventricular zone has been found to be remarkably plastic, responding to a profound variety of environmental and epigenetic factors.

Second, more recently, work from several laboratories has demonstrated that adult neurogenesis is not a unique property of the rodent brain but also occurs in the brains of human and nonhuman primates. These findings raise the possibility that neurogenesis in humans may also be responsive to environmental factors and thus may represent a form of neuroplasticity in adulthood that has heretofore been unrecognized. Moreover, from a clinical standpoint, neural stem cells that generate neurons in the adult human brain may represent a resource that can be therapeutically harnessed in the service of brain repair. Recruiting a patient's own reserve of neural stem cells to replace neurons lost to injury or neurodegenerative disorders would bypass the need for invasive, allogeneic cell transplants from more controversial sources.

This chapter presents findings from recent studies that examined the possibility of neurogenesis in adult primate brains. These initial studies have been mostly descriptive, focusing on whether adult neurogenesis occurs in areas homologous to those neurogenic forebrain regions previously described in rodents. These investigations have revealed similarities as well as differences between the neurogenic systems of primates and rodents.

A brief historical view

Initially it was assumed that the generation of neurons was restricted to developmental periods in all mammals. Early investigations into the possible persistence of neurogenesis in the adult mammalian brain began in the 1960s by applying the method of [³H]thymidine autoradiography in rodents. When injected systemically, [³H]thymidine is incorporated into replicating DNA of dividing cells; thus labeled, these cells or their recent progeny can be detected in sections of brain tissue by using autoradiographic procedures. Studies performed using this method revealed that neurogenesis continues in adulthood in the hippocampal dentate gyrus and the subventricular zone and its rostral extension into the olfactory bulb (Altman and Das, 1965; Altman, 1969; Kaplan and Hinds, 1977; Kaplan and Bell, 1983).

These findings challenged the notion of stability in mature mammalian neuronal populations. Because of the potential functional implications of neurogenesis in both

DAVID R. KORNACK Center for Aging and Developmental Biology, Department of Neurobiology and Anatomy, University of Rochester School of Medicine and Dentistry, Rochester, N.Y.

normal and brain-injured individuals, it was imperative to determine whether new neurons are normally generated in adult primate brains as well. Accordingly, Rakic and colleagues carried out a series of studies in the 1980s on juvenile and adult rhesus monkeys (*Macaca mulatta*), using the same approach of [³H]thymidine autoradiography and morphological criteria to identify newly generated cells (Rakic and Nowakowski, 1981; Rakic, 1985; Eckenhoff and Rakic, 1988). Although continued gliogenesis and other nonneuronal cell division were detected in examined structures, which included the spinal cord, thalamus, neocortex, and hippocampus, no convincing evidence for newly generated neurons was found in adult monkeys.

These initial studies were limited by the sensitivity of the methods available at the time, allowing the possibility that low levels of neurogenesis might persist in adult monkeys that went undetected. Since then, improved methods have been introduced to detect and identify newly generated cells and to examine their possible origin and migratory pathways. Cell labeling with 5-bromodeoxyuridine (BrdU) is perhaps the most widely used method and has the advantages over [³H]thymidine autoradiography of being less expensive, nonradioactive, and faster to process (Miller and Nowakowski, 1988). The accessibility of this method has undoubtedly contributed to the resurrection of interest in adult neurogenesis among investigators. When systemically injected or added to drinking water, BrdU, a thymidine analogue, labels replicating DNA and can be detected in newly generated cells by using immunohistochemistry. Most important, this method can be combined with cell-type-specific immunohistochemical markers and confocal microscopic imaging, allowing high-resolution analysis and rigorous identification of newly generated cells. This method has been applied extensively to rodent models to examine factors that influence adult neurogenesis, and to probe the possible functional roles of new neurons in the mature brain. Most recently, these improved methods have prompted a reexamination of the possibility of neurogenesis in the adult brains of humans and nonhuman primates, since even a small capacity for adult neurogenesis could have profound implications for brain self-repair after injury or disease, or for circuit remodeling in response to experience.

Hippocampal neurogenesis

Neurogenesis in the adult hippocampal dentate gyrus has been most extensively characterized in rodents. In these animals, new granule neurons are generated from astrocyte-like progenitor cells that reside in the subgranular zone, which borders the hilus and granule cell layer (GCL) within the dentate gyrus (Seri and Alvarez-Buylla, 2002). Within 1 week after their generation, new neurons migrate a short distance into the GCL and express early neuronal markers such

as neuron-specific tubulin (TuJ1) and doublecortin (Kempermann et al., 2003). After about 1 week, most new neurons that survive have extended axons, receive synaptic input, and express markers that are characteristic of mature granule neurons, such as NeuN and calbindin (Stanfield and Trice, 1988; Hastings and Gould, 1999; Markakis and Gage, 1999). Although many newly generated cells do not survive much beyond their first week, some become functionally integrated with preexisting neurons (Van Praag et al., 2002) and survive as long as 11 months (Kempermann et al., 2003).

The previous [³H]thymidine autoradiographic studies in macaque monkeys suggested that neurogenesis in the dentate gyrus continued postnatally for several months, but appeared to cease well before sexual maturity (at 3–4 years), after which only newly generated astrocytes could be positively identified (Rakic and Nowakowski, 1981; Eckenhoff and Rakic, 1988). It was noted, however, that some small [³H]thymidine-labeled cells in the dentate gyrus of adult monkeys were difficult to positively classify, leaving open the possibility that a low level of neurogenesis might persist into adulthood. The more recent application of BrdU immunohistochemistry and cell-type immunomarkers has confirmed this possibility, indicating that adult neurogenesis occurs in the dentate gyrus of New World monkeys (Platyrrhini) (Gould et al., 1998) and Old World primates (Catarrhini), including humans (Eriksson et al., 1998; Gould, Reeves, Fallah, et al., 1999; Kornack and Rakic, 1999).

Similar to adult-generated neurons in rodents (Kaplan and Hinds, 1977), those in adult macaque monkeys appear to originate from progenitor cells in the subgranular zone, then migrate into the GCL, where they differentiate (Gould, Reeves, Fallah, et al., 1999; Kornack and Rakic, 1999). The immature, bipolar shape of BrdU/TuJ1 double-labeled cells in the adult monkey GCL resembles that of migrating young neurons during hippocampal development in this species (Nowakowski and Rakic, 1979; Eckenhoff and Rakic, 1984). The migration of these new neurons is most likely guided and supported in the adult—as it is during development—by radial glial fibers that penetrate through the GCL (Nowakowski and Rakic, 1979; Eckenhoff and Rakic, 1984). These astrocytic glia may also function as the neural progenitor cells in the adult dentate gyrus, generating the new neurons in primates as they do in rodents (Seri and Alvarez-Buylla, 2002). Within the monkey GCL, BrdU-labeled cells express mature neuronal markers, such as NeuN. Although the BrdU-labeled neurons described in adult human dentate gyrus had a mature morphology and the presence of immature neurons was not noted (Eriksson et al., 1998), the findings in macaque monkeys suggest that these cells in humans may also undergo a similar series of developmental stages and do not originate de novo from preexisting, mature neurons. Thus, adult-generated granule neurons in both rodents and primates undergo a similar sequence of generation, migration, and maturation. It remains to be determined whether in primates these new neurons make appropriate connections and become functionally incorporated into hippocampal circuitry. Moreover, the survival time of newly generated neurons in the primate dentate gyrus is also largely unknown. Some newly generated cells survive in the dentate gyrus at least 3 months in macaque monkeys (Kornack and Rakic, 1999; Gould et al., 2001) and as long as 2 years in humans (Eriksson et al., 1998); however, it was not established in these studies whether these labeled cells had a neuronal phenotype.

In addition to these similarities in adult dentate neurogenesis among species, there also appear to be significant differences. For example, estimated levels of neurogenesis are substantially lower in both humans and macaque monkeys than in rodents (Eriksson et al., 1998; Kornack and Rakic, 1999). Initially, it was not known whether the low levels in humans reflected a species difference or were due to the advanced age of the subjects used in the study, for even in rodents, levels of hippocampal neurogenesis decline with increasing age (Kuhn, Dickinson-Anson, and Gage, 1996). However, relatively low levels of neurogenesis have now been documented even in young adult macaque monkeys (Kornack and Rakic, 1999). Specifically, it has been estimated that approximately 0.004% of the neuronal population in the monkey dentate gyrus consists of new neurons generated per day, that is, one new neuron per 24,000 existing granule neurons per day. This fraction is an order of magnitude smaller than the estimate in mice of one new neuron in 2000 existing granule neurons generated per day (Kempermann, Kuhn, and Gage, 1997a). Thus, it is clear that levels of adult neurogenesis differ markedly among mammals. This is perhaps not surprising, given that rates of neural progenitor cell division are slower in primates than in rodents during cortical development (Kornack and Rakic, 1998; Kornack, 2000) and that levels of hippocampal neurogenesis differ even among genetically different strains of laboratory mice (Kempermann, Kuhn, and Gage, 1997a; Kempermann and Gage, 2002). It remains to be determined whether the reduced neurogenesis in these Old World primates reflects lower rates of neuronal production, survival, or both.

There may also be species differences regarding whether adult neurogenesis results in a continuous net accumulation of new neurons or instead reflects a turnover of neurons within the dentate gyrus. In rodents, new neurons are added to the neuronal population, resulting in a gradual increase in granule cell number during adulthood (Bayer, Yackel, and Puri, 1982; Crespo, Stanfield, and Cowan, 1986; Kempermann et al., 2003). Moreover, environmental enrichment and learning tasks can cause a further increase in the number of neurons in the GCL, suggesting a functional role for new neurons in adult brain plasticity (Kempermann,

Kuhn, and Gage, 1997b; Gould, Beylin, et al., 1999; Nilsson et al., 1999). In contrast, such neuronal accumulation may not occur in adult primates. Cell-counting studies indicate that the number of neurons in the normal human GCL remains relatively stable throughout most of postnatal life, despite a lifetime of enriched experiences (Seress, 1992; Simic et al., 1997; Harding, Halliday, and Kril, 1998). In macaques, too, the number of granule neurons and other neuronal elements in the dentate gyrus (e.g., the total number of synapses) remains stable from 4 to 35 years of age (Tiggs, Herndon, and Rosene, 1995; Keuker, Luiten, and Fuchs, 2003), suggesting that there is no increase in neuron number. This apparent lack of net accumulation of neurons in the primate dentate gyrus implies that the rate of neuronal production in adulthood is balanced by an equal rate of apoptosis and cell removal. Thus, in addition to differences in levels of neurogenesis, there may also be phyletic differences in the ultimate fate of new neurons and their functional role in the adult.

Although adult hippocampal neurogenesis has been known for nearly four decades in rodents, its functional significance in any mammal has remained elusive. Although initial investigations into possible functional roles showed correlations between increases in neurogenesis and improved performance on learning tasks (Kempermann, Kuhn, and Gage, 1997b; Gould, Beylin, et al., 1999), a direct causal link has been difficult to prove. Moreover, evidence from recent studies using other paradigms appears to argue against the existence of such a straightforward relationship (Feng et al., 2001; Lavenex, Lavenex, and Clayton, 2001; Bartolomucci et al., 2002; Bizon and Gallagher, 2003). It is thus becoming apparent that the role adult neurogenesis might play in hippocampal-dependent cognition is likely to be complex.

The reduction of adult neurogenesis in adult macaque monkeys and humans is in harmony with a general decline of adult neurogenesis during vertebrate evolution, which could be an adaptive strategy to maintain stable neuronal populations throughout life (Rakic and Nowakowski, 1981; Rakic and Kornack, 1993). This hypothesis is consistent with the restriction of adult neurogenesis in the mammalian brain to phylogenetically older structures—that is, the olfactory bulbs and hippocampal formation—and its absence in the more recently evolved neocortex. The reduced neurogenesis in the dentate gyrus of adult Old World primates may also be related to their prolonged period of adolescence and longer life span (Kornack and Rakic, 1999). Just as variations in forebrain anatomy across species have functional consequences, diversity in adult neurogenesis might also have consequences for species-typical behaviors and life history strategies that remain to be explored.

The demonstration of adult neurogenesis in humans and monkeys raises further questions regarding its role in long-lived primates with elaborate cognitive and social capacities. For example, the understanding and treatment of human brain disorders that implicate hippocampal dysfunction (e.g., temporal lobe epilepsy: Houser, 1992; Mathern et al., 1994; schizophrenia: Weinberger et al., 1992; Heckers et al., 1998) may require consideration of the status and potential involvement of ongoing neurogenesis in the dentate gyrus of affected patients. Indeed, a potential link between adult hippocampal neurogenesis and various psychiatric disorders, such as depression, is under active investigation (Eisch and Nestler, 2002; Santarelli et al., 2003).

Subventricular zone neurogenesis

Early experiments in rodents revealed the persistence of a second neurogenic region in the adult brain: the subventricular zone (SVZ) (Altman, 1969). The SVZ harbors the largest pool of dividing neural stem cells in the adult rodent brain (Alvarez-Buylla and García-Verdugo, 2002). These stem cells generate immature neurons that aggregate to form an extensive network of neuroblast chains along the lateral wall of the lateral cerebral ventricle (Doetsch and Alvarez-Buylla, 1996; Lois, García-Verdugo, and Alvarez-Buylla, 1996). These chains of neuroblasts coalesce anteriorly to form a highly restricted migratory route, called the *rostral migratory stream* (RMS), which extends from the anterior SVZ into the olfactory bulb. Unlike the radial glial-guided migration used by young neurons during early brain development (Rakic, 1990), neuroblasts undergoing "chain migration" in the adult SVZ/RMS migrate along one another via neurophilic interactions (Lois, García-Verdugo, and Alvarez-Buylla, 1996; Wichterle, García-Verdugo, and Alvarez-Buylla, 1997). These chains are ensheathed by tubes of flanking astrocytes, which delineate the RMS. Neuroblasts migrate rostrally within the RMS to enter the olfactory bulb, whereupon they differentiate into local interneurons (Corotto, Heneger, and Maruniak, 1993; Luskin, 1993; Lois and Alvarez-Buylla, 1994; Doetsch and Alvarez-Buylla, 1996). At least some of these cells become functionally integrated into preexisting circuitry (Carlén et al., 2002; Carleton et al., 2003).

Until recently, the question remained open of whether this SVZ/RMS neurogenic migratory system is peculiar to macrosmatic rodents, or also exists in microsmatic non-rodent species, particularly anthropoid primates (monkeys, apes, and humans). In rodents, which have relatively large olfactory bulbs and are predominantly nocturnal, this system is thought to play a role in odor discrimination (Gheusi et al., 2000; Petreanu and Alvarez-Buylla, 2002; Rochefort et al., 2002; Shingo et al., 2003). Compared to rodents, anthropoids have relatively small olfactory bulbs with elongated olfactory peduncles and are largely diurnal (Crosby and Humphrey, 1939). Moreover, both adult macaque monkeys

and humans appear to generate fewer new neurons in the hippocampal dentate gyrus than do adult mice (Eriksson et al., 1998; Kornack and Rakic, 1999), which perhaps might reflect an overall decline in adult neurogenesis in the Old World primate brain that would include the SVZ.

Initial hints about the possible existence of a neurogenic SVZ in adult primates came from studies—including those using BrdU or [³H]thymidine to label dividing cells—showing evidence for proliferative activity in the adult SVZ of the lateral ventricle in species ranging from New World monkeys (McDermott and Lantos, 1990) to Old World monkeys (Lewis, 1968; M. S. Kaplan, 1982; Rakic and Kornack, 1993) to humans (Eriksson et al., 1998; Kukekov et al., 1999). However, it was not determined whether these cells generate olfactory neuroblasts. The first indication that SVZ cells in adult primates could be neurogenic came from in vitro evidence that temporal lobe SVZ tissue from adult epileptic humans could generate cells with neuronal characteristics under tissue culture conditions (Kirschenbaum et al., 1994; Pincus et al., 1998; Kukekov et al., 1999). In support of these findings, other studies showed that some cells in the adult human anterior SVZ are immunopositive for markers associated with a neuroblast phenotype, including PSA-NCAM and TuJ1 (Bernier et al., 2000; Weickert et al., 2000). However, these immunohistochemical studies of postmortem tissue were unable to verify whether these cells were, in fact, newly generated, nor could the studies determine the cells' fate. Most recently, experiments using immunohistochemistry for BrdU and cell-type markers have indeed confirmed that dividing cells in the adult macaque monkey SVZ normally generate new neurons that migrate in chains to the olfactory bulb and differentiate into granule neurons, homologous to the SVZ/RMS in adult rodents (Kornack and Rakic, 2001a). Moreover, these SVZ-derived neurons appear to be restricted in their migration routes and do not populate the adult neocortex (Kornack and Rakic, 2001b). The existence of a neurogenic SVZ/RMS in the primate forebrain has subsequently been confirmed in neonatal and adult macaque monkeys (Pencea, Bingaman, Freedman, et al., 2001) and in adult squirrel monkeys (Bédard, Lévesque, et al., 2002). Together, these findings in both Old World and New World monkeys raise the possibility that an active SVZ/RMS system is also present in humans.

Similar to rodents, chains of neuroblasts in the SVZ and RMS of adult monkeys express the polysialic acid form of neural cell adhesion molecule (PSA-NCAM) (Bonfanti and Theodosis, 1994; Doetsch and Alvarez-Buylla, 1996; Doetsch, García-Verdugo, and Alvarez-Buylla, 1997; Kornack and Rakic, 2001a; Pencea, Bingaman, Freedman, et al., 2001; Bédard, Lévesque, et al., 2002), which has been shown, in mice, to mediate neuroblast migration to the olfactory bulb (Goldman and Luskin, 1998; Chazal et al., 2000).

This species similarity suggests that the very molecular cues that promote chain migration in the rodent olfactory stream also operate in the adult primate forebrain. It is also apparent that, as in rodents (Luskin, 1993; Lois, García-Verdugo, and Alvarez-Buylla, 1996; Doetsch, García-Verdugo, and Alvarez-Buylla, 1997), migrating neuroblasts in adult macaque monkeys are confined to the SVZ and RMS and do not penetrate into the surrounding striatal or septal parenchyma or overlying cortical white matter, suggesting the presence of guidance cues that spatially restrict migration. Specific molecules that may play such a restrictive role in directing neuroblast migration from the SVZ to the olfactory bulb have been identified in rodents (Hu and Rutishauser, 1996; Wu et al., 1999; Conover et al., 2000; Mason, Ito, and Corfas, 2001; Liu and Rao, 2003). By analogy to mechanisms that govern axonal pathfinding (Tessier-Lavigne and Goodman, 1996), it is likely that a combination of permissive and repulsive cues direct neuroblast migration in the adult mammalian brain and prevent widespread dispersion, even over the extended migratory distance of the primate RMS.

Despite the shared similarities, substantial differences exist between rodents and primate with regard to SVZ progenitor cell behavior and cytological organization (Kornack and Rakic, 2001a; Pencea, Bingaman, Freedman, et al., 2001). For example, in adult mice, new olfactory interneurons require a total of at least 15 days to be generated, migrate 3–5mm from the SVZ to the olfactory bulb, and develop a mature morphology (Lois and Alvarez-Buylla, 1994; Petreanu and Alvarez-Buylla, 2002). These cells migrate in the RMS at an average rate of 30 µm/hr. In adult macaque monkeys, the new granule neurons appear to require a much longer period for their generation, migration, and differentiation—between 75 and 97 days (Kornack and Rakic, 2001a). In the larger brains of these monkeys, the migratory route is considerably extended; the elongated olfactory peduncle alone is approximately 20mm long, which is longer than an entire mouse brain. Thus, even if rates of chain migration are comparable in mice and monkeys, one would not expect to see mature SVZ-derived neurons in the olfactory bulb of monkeys until at least 30 days after being labeled with BrdU in the SVZ. The fact that new granule neurons were not detected until after 75 postinjection days may reflect slower rates of neuronal generation, migration, or differentiation in the primate. Such protracted development is consistent with the longer neuronal generation times in macaque monkeys versus mice during fetal development (Kornack and Rakic, 1998) and with the observation that BrdU-labeled neuroblasts were still present in the adult monkey SVZ for as long as 97 days after injection (Kornack and Rakic, 2001a). It is also possible that new granule neurons that potentially arrived and differentiated earlier than 75 days after injection went undetected. Moreover,

because proliferating cells were observed in the olfactory bulb itself, it was proposed that at least some of these new granule neurons might be generated in situ, and differentiate over a protracted time period (Kornack and Rakic, 2001a). The presence of such local neural stem cells has recently been reported in the rodent olfactory bulb (Gritti et al., 2002).

In rodents, adult-generated olfactory neurons appear to be involved in olfactory information processing, including odor discrimination learning (Gheusi et al., 2000; Petreanu and Alvarez-Buylla, 2002; Rochefort et al., 2002; Shingo et al., 2003). Although primates have relatively smaller olfactory bulbs compared with overall brain size than do rodents, olfaction does play an important role in social communication for many primate species (Kaplan et al., 1977; Epple and Moulton, 1978; Zeller, 1987). In humans, the ability to discriminate odors declines with age, and impaired olfaction is among the first clinical signs of some neurodegenerative diseases, including Alzheimer's disease and idiopathic Parkinson's disease (Doty, 2001; Ramsden et al., 2001). However, whether adult neurogenesis actually participates in these olfactory functions and dysfunctions in human and nonhuman primates remains to be tested.

The existence of a large pool of dividing neural stem cells in the primate SVZ raises the possibility of harnessing these cells for therapeutic purposes. This possibility is strongly supported by experimental work in rodents, indicating that endogenous neural stem cells can be augmented in the adult brain to generated additional neurons (Rossi and Cattaneo, 2002). Moreover, although the destination of SVZ-derived neuroblasts is apparently normally restricted to the olfactory bulb, it may be possible to manipulate and redirect migrating neuroblasts to non-neurogenic brain regions suffering neuronal loss from trauma or neurodegenerative disease and to reestablish functional circuitry (Fallon et al., 2000). Indeed, experimental evidence suggests that endogenous SVZ-derived neuroblasts in adult mice can actually be induced in situ to repopulate injured neocortical areas, which are not normally neurogenic, and to establish axonal connections with appropriate thalamic targets (Arlotta, Magavi, and Macklis, 2003). Conceivably, this effect could be potentiated by, for example, expanding the SZ progenitor pool through the introduction of neurotrophic factors (Kuhn et al., 1997). For example, studies using rats indicate that experimentally increased levels of brain-derived neurotrophic factor (BDNF) can augment SVZ neuronal production and migration into both normal targets (RMS and olfactory bulb) and novel targets (e.g., striatum) (Zigova et al., 1998; Benraiss et al., 2001; Pencea, Bingaman, Wiegand, et al., 2001). Interestingly, the new neurons that stray into the striatum adopt a phenotype characteristic of medium spiny neurons, the cells that degenerate in Huntington's disease (Benraiss et al., 2001).

It remains unknown whether or to what extent neural stem cells in the intact adult primate forebrain are responsive to exogenous neurotrophic factors and whether similar mobilization to novel brain targets could be obtained over the longer migratory distances to be traversed by cells in the larger primate brain. Successfully coercing the adult brain's own neural progenitor cells to compensate for neuronal loss in humans would circumvent the ethical and immunological problems posed by therapeutic strategies that rely on transplants of cells from human fetuses or nonhuman species. For therapeutic applications in humans, it will be essential to assess the capacity of the adult primate SZ/RMS system for compensatory plasticity in response to neuronal loss in distant brain regions.

Other regions of adult neurogenesis?

The discovery of neurogenic regions in the adult primate brain homologous to those in rodents has spurred an interest in examining other brain regions for evidence of ongoing neurogenesis. Using BrdU and immunohistochemical cell labeling, a recent study reported that substantial numbers of new neurons are continually added to neocortical association areas in adult macaque monkeys (Gould, Reeves, Graziano, et al., 1999; Gould et al., 2001). Further, these neurons were proposed to be generated in the SVZ and then to migrate in streams through the subcortical white matter to the prefrontal, posterior parietal, and inferior temporal cortex. This report was exciting because it suggested a potential mechanism for cognitive function and cortical repair after injury that had previously not been recognized. However, it was also surprising because many previous studies using [³H]thymidine autoradiography indicated that neocortical neurons are generated before or shortly after birth in all species examined, including macaque monkeys (e.g., Angevine and Sidman, 1961; Berry and Rogers, 1965; Hicks and D'Amato, 1968; Caviness and Sidman, 1973; Rakic, 1974; Luskin and Shatz, 1985; Jackson, Peduzzi, and Hickey, 1989). The considerable conceptual and biomedical implications of adult cortical neurogenesis prompted other laboratories to investigate the robustness and reproducibility of this phenomenon in macaque monkeys, but these attempts could not confirm the original findings (Kornack and Rakic, 2001b; Koketsu et al., 2003). Although evidence for abundant non-neuronal cell proliferation in the monkey neocortex was obtained, convincing evidence for newly generated neurons was limited to the dentate gyrus and olfactory bulb. Nor could the presence of a migratory stream of neuroblasts through the subcortical white matter be verified. The reason for the discrepancy in the reports is unclear; the methods used in all studies were similar and the presence of new neurons in the hippocampus and olfactory bulb argued against the inability to detect new cortical neurons, if they were actually present in the numbers initially reported. However, it was noted in the subsequent studies that some cells on first inspection appeared to be BrdU-labeled neurons in the neocortex; these cells were ultimately resolved to consist of BrdU-positive satellite glia in close apposition to mature cortical neurons by using three-dimensional confocal microscopic analysis. Such cells have been identified in the rodent cortex and striatum as well (Kuhn et al., 1997), that had previously been interpreted as BrdU-labeled neurons (Craig et al., 1996). Consistent with these more recent findings in monkeys, studies with immunofluorescent double labeling of cortical cells with BrdU and NeuN in adult mice have also failed to detect neurogenesis under normal conditions (Arlotta, Magavi, and Macklis, 2003; Ehninger and Kempermann, 2003). The presence of newly generated neurons in other regions of the adult monkey brain has been reported (Bédard, Cossette, et al., 2002; Bernier et al., 2002), but these observations remain unconfirmed. A more detailed review of the caveats of the methods used, as well as a critique of the specific issues of these studies, is provided elsewhere (Nowakowski and Hayes, 2000; Grassi Zucconi and Giuditta, 2002; Rakic, 2002).

These most recent findings led to the conclusion that neocortical neurons are not normally renewed during the life span of macaque monkeys, which can last three decades; similar limits may exist in the human forebrain (Seress et al., 2001). Although preservation of neurons over a life span is considered important for memory and the storage of life-long experiences, the restricted capacity for neurogenesis in adulthood may be an impediment when the need arises to replace neurons lost to trauma or neurodegenerative disease (Rakic, 1998). Indeed, one could argue that the enormous present-day biomedical effort devoted to developing cell replacement therapies for neurological disorders is a testament to the remarkable resistance of the adult mammalian nervous system to renew itself (Snyder and Park, 2002). The challenge in the coming years will be to determine how to replace lost neurons in brain regions where they are not normally renewed and how to incorporate them into an adult brain environment to restore lost function (Björklund and Lindvall, 2000; Horner and Gage, 2000; Arlotta, Magavi, and Macklis, 2003).

REFERENCES

ALTMAN, J., 1969. Autoradiographic and histological studies of postnatal neurogenesis. IV. Cell proliferation and migration in the anterior forebrain, with special reference to persisting neurogenesis in the olfactory bulb. *J. Comp. Neurol.* 137:433–457.

ALTMAN, J., and G. D. DAS, 1965. Autoradiographic and histological evidence of postnatal hippocampal neurogenesis in rats. *J. Comp. Neurol.* 124:319–336.

ALVAREZ-BUYLLA, A., and J. M. GARCÍA-VERDUGO, 2002. Neurogenesis in adult subventricular zone. *J. Neurosci.* 22:629–634.

ANGEVINE, J. B., and R. L. SIDMAN, 1961. Autoradiographic study of cell migration during histogenesis of cerebral cortex in the mouse. *Nature* 192:766–768.

ARLOTTA, P., S. S. MAGAVI, and J. D. MACKLIS, 2003. Molecular manipulation of neural precursors in situ: Induction of adult cortical neurogenesis. *Exp. Gerontol.* 38:173–182.

BARTOLOMUCCI, A., G. DE BIURRUN, B. CZEH, M. VAN KAMPEN, and E. FUCHS, 2002. Selective enhancement of spatial learning under chronic psychosocial stress. *Eur. J. Neurosci.* 15:1863–1866.

BAYER, S. A., J. W. YACKEL, and P. S. PURI, 1982. Neurons in the rat dentate gyrus granular layer substantially increase during juvenile and adult life. *Science* 216:890–892.

BÉDARD, A., M. COSSETTE, M. LÉVESQUE, and A. PARENT, 2002. Proliferating cells can differentiate into neurons in the striatum of normal adult monkey. *Neurosci. Lett.* 328:213–216.

BÉDARD, A., M. LÉVESQUE, P. J. BERNIER, and A. PARENT, 2002. The rostral migratory stream in adult squirrel monkeys: Contribution of new neurons to the olfactory tubercle and involvement of the antiapoptotic protein Bcl-2. *Eur. J. Neurosci.* 16:1917–1924.

BENRAISS, A., E. CHMIELNICKI, K. LERNER, R. DONGYON, and S. A. GOLDMAN, 2001. Adenoviral brain-derived neurotrophic factor induces both neostriatal and olfactory neuronal recruitment from endogenous progenitor cells in the adult forebrain. *J. Neurosci.* 21:6718–6731.

BERNIER, P. J., A. BÉDARD, J. VINET, M. LÉVESQUE, and A. PARENT, 2002. Newly generated neurons in the amygdala and adjoining cortex of adult primates. *Proc. Natl. Acad. Sci. U.S.A.* 99: 11464–11469.

BERNIER, P. J., J. VINET, M. COSSETTE, and A. PARENT, 2000. Characterization of the subventricular zone of the adult human brain: Evidence for the involvement of Bcl-2. *Neurosci. Res.* 37:67–78.

BERRY, M., and A. W. ROGERS, 1965. The migration of neuroblasts in the developing cortex. *J. Anat.* 99:691–709.

BIZON, J. L., and M. GALLAGHER, 2003. Production of new cells in the rat dentate gyrus of the lifespan: Relation to cognitive decline. *Eur. J. Neurosci.* 18:215–219.

BJÖRKLUND, A., and O. LINDVALL, 2000. Cell replacement therapies for central nervous system disorders. *Nat. Neurosci.* 3:537–544.

BONFANTI, L., and D. T. THEODOSIS, 1994. Expression of polysialylated neural cell adhesion molecule by proliferating cells in the subependymal layer of the adult rat, in its rostral extension and the olfactory bulb. *Neuroscience* 62:291–305.

CARLÉN, M., R. M. CASSIDY, H. BRISMAR, G. A. SMITH, L. W. ENQUIST, and J. FRISÉN, 2002. Functional integration of adult-born neurons. *Curr. Biol.* 12:606–608.

CARLETON, A., L. T. PETREANU, R. LANSFORD, A. ALVAREZ-BUYLLA, and P.-M. LLEDO, 2003. Becoming a new neuron in the adult olfactory bulb. *Nat. Neurosci.* 6:507–518.

CAVINESS, V. S. J., and R. L. SIDMAN, 1973. Time of origin of corresponding cell classes in the cerebral cortex of normal and reeler mutant mice: An autoradiographic analysis. *J. Comp. Neurol.* 148:141–152.

CHAZAL, G., P. DURBEC, A. JANKOVSKI, G. ROUGON, and H. CREMER, 2000. Consequences of neural cell adhesion molecule deficiency on cell migration in the rostral migratory stream of the mouse. *J. Neurosci.* 20:1446–1457.

CONOVER, J. C., F. DOETSCH, J. M. GARCÍA-VERDUGO, N. W. GALE, G. D. YANCOPOULOS, and A. ALVAREZ-BUYLLA, 2000. Disruption of Eph/ephrin signaling affects migration and proliferation in the adult subventricular zone. *Nat. Neurosci.* 3:1091–1097.

COROTTO, F. S., J. A. HENEGER, and J. A. MARUNIAK, 1993. Neurogenesis persists in the subependymal layer of the adult mouse brain. *Neurosci. Lett.* 149:111–114.

CRAIG, C. G., V. TROPEPE, C. M. MORSHEAD, B. A. REYNOLDS, S. WEISS, and D. VAN DER KOOY, 1996. In vivo growth factor expansion of endogenous subependymal neural precursor cell populations in the adult mouse brain. *J. Neurosci.* 16:2649–2658.

CRESPO, D., B. B. STANFIELD, and W. M. COWAN, 1986. Evidence that late-generated granule cells do not simply replace earlier formed neurons in the rat dentate gyrus. *Exp. Brain Res.* 62: 541–548.

CROSBY, E. C., and T. HUMPHREY, 1939. Studies of the vertebrate telencephalon: The nuclear configuration of the olfactory and accessory olfactory formations and of the nucleus olfactorius anterior of certain reptiles, birds, and mammals. *J. Comp. Neurol.* 71:121–213.

DOETSCH, F., and A. ALVAREZ-BUYLLA, 1996. Network of tangential pathways for neuronal migration in adult mammalian brain. *Proc. Natl. Acad. Sci. U.S.A.* 93:14895–14900.

DOETSCH, F., J. M. GARCÍA-VERDUGO, and A. ALVAREZ-BUYLLA, 1997. Cellular composition and three-dimensional organization of the subventricular germinal zone in the adult mammalian brain. *J. Neurosci.* 17:5046–5061.

DOTY, R. L., 2001. Olfaction. *Annu. Rev. Psychol.* 52:423–452.

ECKENHOFF, M. F., and P. RAKIC, 1984. Radial organization of the hippocampal dentate gyrus: A Golgi, ultrastructural, and immunocytochemical analysis in the developing rhesus monkey. *J. Comp. Neurol.* 223:1–21.

ECKENHOFF, M. F., and P. RAKIC, 1988. Nature and fate of proliferative cells in the hippocampal dentate gyrus during the life span of the rhesus monkey. *J. Neurosci.* 8:2729–2747.

EHNINGER, D., and G. KEMPERMANN, 2003. Regional effects of wheel running and environmental enrichment on cell genesis and microglia proliferation in the adult murine neocortex. *Cereb. Cortex* 13:845–851.

EISCH, A. J., and E. J. NESTLER, 2002. To be or not to be: Adult neurogenesis and psychiatry. *Clin. Neurosci. Res.* 2:93–108.

EPPLE, G., and D. MOULTON, 1978. Structural organization and communicative functions of olfaction in nonhuman primates. In *Sensory Systems of Primates*, C. R. Noback, ed. New York: Plenum Press, pp. 1–22.

ERIKSSON, P. S., E. PERFILIEVA, T. BJÖRK-ERIKSSON, A. ALBORN, C. NORDBORG, D. A. PETERSON, and F. H. GAGE, 1998. Neurogenesis in the adult human hippocampus. *Nat. Med.* 4:1313–1317.

FALLON, J., S. REID, R. KINYAMU, I. OPOLE, R. OPOLE, J. BARATTA, M. KORC, T. L. ENDO, A. DUONG, G. NGUYEN, M. KARKEHABADHI, D. TWARDZIK, and S. LOUGHLIN, 2000. *In vivo* induction of massive proliferation, directed migration, and differentiation of neural cells in the adult mammalian brain. *Proc. Natl. Acad. Sci. U.S.A.* 97:14686–14691.

FENG, R., C. RAMPON, Y. P. TANG, D. SHROM, J. JIN, M. KYIN, B. SOPHER, G. M. MARTIN, S. H. KIM, R. B. LANGDON, S. S. SISODIA, and J. Z. TSIEN, 2001. Deficient neurogenesis in forebrain-specific *presenilin-1* knockout mice is associated with reduced clearance of hippocampal memory traces. *Neuron* 32:911–926.

GHEUSI, G., H. CREMER, H. MCLEAN, G. CHAZAL, J. D. VINCENT, and P. M. LLEDO, 2000. Importance of newly generated neurons in the adult olfactory bulb for odor discrimination. *Proc. Natl. Acad. Sci. U.S.A.* 97:1823–1828.

GOLDMAN, S. A., and M. B. LUSKIN, 1998. Strategies utilized by migrating neurons of the postnatal vertebrate forebrain. *Trends Neurosci.* 21:107–114.

GOULD, E., A. BEYLIN, P. TANAPAT, A. REEVES, and T. J. SHORS, 1999. Learning enhances adult neurogenesis in the hippocampal formation. *Nat. Neurosci.* 2:260–265.

GOULD, E., A. J. REEVES, M. FALLAH, P. TANAPAT, C. G. GROSS, and E. FUCHS, 1999. Hippocampal neurogenesis in adult Old World primates. *Proc. Natl. Acad. Sci. U.S.A.* 96:5263–5267.

GOULD, E., A. J. REEVES, M. S. A. GRAZIANO, and C. G. GROSS, 1999. Neurogenesis in the neocortex of adult primates. *Science* 286:548–552.

GOULD, E., P. TANAPAT, B. S. MCEWEN, G. FLUGGE, and E. FUCHS, 1998. Proliferation of granule cell precursors in the dentate gyrus of adult monkeys is diminished by stress. *Proc. Natl. Acad. Sci. U.S.A.* 95:3168–3171.

GOULD, E., N. VAIL, M. WAGERS, and C. G. GROSS, 2001. Adult-generated hippocampal and neocortical neurons in macaques have a transient existence. *Proc. Natl. Acad. Sci. U.S.A.* 98: 10910–10917.

GRASSI ZUCCONI, G., and A. GIUDITTA, 2002. Is it only neurogenesis? *Rev. Neurosci.* 13:375–383.

GRITTI, A., L. BONFANTI, F. DOETSCH, I. CAILLE, A. ALVAREZ-BUYLLA, D. A. LIM, R. GALLI, J. M. GARCIA-VERDUGO, D. G. HERRERA, and A. L. VESCOVI, 2002. Multipotent neural stem cells reside into the rostral extension and olfactory bulb of adult rodents. *J. Neurosci.* 22:437–455.

HARDING, A. J., G. M. HALLIDAY, and J. J. KRIL, 1998. Variation in hippocampal neuron number with age and brain volume. *Cereb. Cortex* 8:710–718.

HASTINGS, N. B., and E. GOULD, 1999. Rapid extension of axons into the CA3 region by adult-generated granule cells. *J. Comp. Neurol.* 413:146–154.

HECKERS, S., S. L. RAUCH, D. GOFF, C. R. SAVAGE, D. L. SCHACTER, A. J. FISCHMAN, and N. M. ALPERT, 1998. Impaired recruitment of the hippocampus during conscious recollection in schizophrenia. *Nat. Neurosci.* 1:318–323.

HICKS, S. P., and C. J. D'AMATO, 1968. Cell migrations to the isocortex in the rat. *Anat. Rec.* 160:619–709.

HORNER, P. J., and F. H. GAGE, 2000. Regenerating the damaged adult central nervous system. *Nature* 407:963–970.

HOUSER, C. R., 1992. Morphological changes in the dentate gyrus in human temporal lobe epilepsy. In *The Dentate Gyrus and Its Role in Seizures*, C. E. Ribak, C. M. Gall, and I. Mody, eds. *Epilepsy Res. Supppl.* 7:223–234.

HU, H., and U. RUTISHAUSER, 1996. A septum-derived chemorepulsive factor for migrating olfactory interneuron precursors. *Neuron* 16:933–940.

JACKSON, C. A., J. D. PEDUZZI, and T. L. HICKEY, 1989. Visual cortex development in the ferret. 1. Genesis and migration of visual cortical neurons. *J. Neurosci.* 9:1242–1253.

KAPLAN, J. N., D. CUBICCIOTTI, and W. K. REDICAN, 1977. Olfactory discrimination of squirrel monkey mothers by their infants. *Dev. Psychobiol.* 10:447–453.

KAPLAN, M. S., 1982. Proliferation of subependymal cells in the adult primate CNS: Differential uptake of DNA labelled precursors. *J. Hirnforsch.* 23:23–33.

KAPLAN, M. S., and D. H. BELL, 1983. Neuronal proliferation in the 9-month-old rodent: Radioautographic study of granule cells in the hippocampus. *Exp. Brain Res.* 52:1–5.

KAPLAN, M. S., and J. W. HINDS, 1977. Neurogenesis in the adult rat: Electron microscopic analysis of light radioautographs. *Science* 197:1092–1094.

KEMPERMANN, G., and F. H. GAGE, 2002. Genetic influence on phenotypic differentiation in adult hippocampal neurogenesis. *Dev. Brain. Res.* 134:1–12.

KEMPERMANN, G., D. GAST, G. KRONENBERG, M. YAMAGUCHI, and F. H. GAGE, 2003. Early determination and long-term persistence of adult-generated new neurons in the hippocampus of mice. *Development* 130:391–399.

KEMPERMANN, G., H. G. KUHN, and F. H. GAGE, 1997a. Genetic influence on neurogenesis in the dentate gyrus of adult mice. *Proc. Natl. Acad. Sci. U.S.A.* 94:10409–10414.

KEMPERMANN, G., H. G. KUHN, and F. H. GAGE, 1997b. More hippocampal neurons in adult mice living in an enriched environment. *Nature* 386:493–495.

KEUKER, J. I. H., P. G. M. LUITEN, and E. FUCHS, 2003. Preservation of hippocampal neuron numbers in aged rhesus monkeys. *Neurobiol. Aging* 24:157–165.

KIRSCHENBAUM, B., M. NEDERGAARD, A. PREUSS, K. BARAMI, R. A. R. FRASER, and S. A. GOLDMAN, 1994. In vitro neuronal production and differentiation by precursor cells derived from the adult human forebrain. *Cereb. Cortex* 6:576–589.

KOKETSU, D., A. MIKAMI, Y. MIYAMOTO, and T. HISATSUNE, 2003. Nonrenewal of neurons in the cerebral neocortex of adult macaque monkeys. *J. Neurosci.* 23:937–942.

KORNACK, D. R., 2000. Neurogenesis and the evolution of cortical diversity: Mode, tempo, and partitioning during development and persistence in adulthood. *Brain Behav. Evol.* 55:336–344.

KORNACK, D. R., and P. RAKIC, 1998. Changes in cell-cycle kinetics during the development and evolution of primate neocortex. *Proc. Natl. Acad. Sci. U.S.A.* 95:1242–1246.

KORNACK, D. R., and P. RAKIC, 1999. Continuation of neurogenesis in the hippocampus of the adult macaque monkey. *Proc. Natl. Acad. Sci. U.S.A.* 96:5768–5773.

KORNACK, D. R., and P. RAKIC, 2001a. The generation, migration, and differentiation of olfactory neurons in the adult primate brain. *Proc. Natl. Acad. Sci. U.S.A.* 98:4752–4757.

KORNACK, D. R., and P. RAKIC, 2001b. Cell proliferation without neurogenesis in adult primate neocortex. *Science* 294:2127–2130.

KUHN, H. G., H. DICKINSON-ANSON, and F. H. GAGE, 1996. Neurogenesis in the dentate gyrus of the adult rat: Age-related decrease of neuronal progenitor proliferation. *J. Neurosci.* 16: 2027–2033.

KUHN, H. G., J. WINKLER, G. KEMPERMANN, L. J. THAL, and F. H. GAGE, 1997. Epidermal growth factor and fibroblast growth factor-2 have different effects on neural progenitors in the adult rat brain. *J. Neurosci.* 17:5820–5829.

KUKEKOV, V. G., E. D. LAYWELL, O. SUSLOV, K. DAVIES, B. SCHEFFLER, L. B. THOMAS, T. F. O'BRIEN, M. KUSAKABE, and D. A. STEINDLER, 1999. Multipotent stem/progenitor cells with similar properties arise from two neurogenic regions of adult human brain. *Exp. Neurol.* 156:333–344.

LAVENEX, P. B., P. LAVENEX, and N. S. CLAYTON, 2001. Comparative studies of postnatal neurogenesis and learning: A critical review. *Avian Poulty Biol. Rev.* 12:103–125.

LEWIS, P. D., 1968. Mitotic activity in the primate subependymal layer and the genesis of gliomas. *Nature* 217:974–975.

LIU, G., and Y. RAO, 2003. Neuronal migration from the forebrain to the olfactory bulb requires a new attractant persistent in the olfactory bulb. *J. Neurosci.* 23:6651–6659.

LOIS, C., and A. ALVAREZ-BUYLLA, 1994. Long-distance neuronal migration in the adult mammalian brain. *Science* 264:1145–1148.

LOIS, C., J. M. GARCÍA-VERDUGO, and A. ALVAREZ-BUYLLA, 1996. Chain migration of neuronal precursors. *Science* 271: 978–981.

LUSKIN, M. B., 1993. Restricted proliferation and migration of postnatally generated neurons derived from the forebrain subventricular zone. *Neuron* 11:173–189.

LUSKIN, M. B., and C. J. SHATZ, 1985. Neurogenesis of the cat's primary visual cortex. *J. Comp. Neurol.* 242:611–631.

MARKAKIS, E. A., and F. H. GAGE, 1999. Adult-generated neurons in the dentate gyrus send axonal projections to field CA3 and are surrounded by synaptic vesicles. *J. Comp. Neurol.* 406:449–460.

MASON, H. A., S. ITO, and G. CORFAS, 2001. Extracellular signals that regulate the tangential migration of olfactory bulb neuronal precursors: Inducers, inhibitors, and repellents. *J. Neurosci* 21:7654–7663.

MATHERN, G. W., J. P. LEITE, J. K. PRETORIUS, B. QUINN, W. J. PEACOCK, and T. L. BABB, 1994. Children with severe epilepsy: Evidence of hippocampal neuron losses and aberrant mossy fiber sprouting during postnatal granule cell migration and differentiation. *Dev. Brain Res.* 78:70–80.

MCDERMOTT, K. W. G., and P. L. LANTOS, 1990. Cell proliferation in the subependymal layer of the postnatal marmoset, *Callithrix jacchus*. *Dev. Brain Res.* 57:269–277.

MILLER, M. W., and R. S. NOWAKOWSKI, 1988. Use of bromodeoxyuridine-immunohistochemistry to examine the proliferation, migration and time of origin of cells in the central nervous system. *Brain Res.* 457:44–52.

NILSSON, M., E. PERFLILIEVA, U. JOHANSSON, O. ORWAR, and P. ERIKSSON, 1999. Enriched environment increases neurogenesis in the adult rat dentate gyrus and improves spatial memory. *J. Neurobiol.* 39:569–578.

NOWAKOWSKI, R., and N. L. HAYES, 2000. New neurons: Extraordinary evidence or extraordinary conclusion? *Science* 288:771a.

NOWAKOWSKI, R. S., and P. RAKIC, 1979. The mode of migration of neurons to the hippocampus: A Golgi and electron microscopic analysis in foetal rhesus monkey. *J. Neurocytol.* 8:697–718.

PENCEA, V., K. D. BINGAMAN, L. J. FREEDMAN, and M. B. LUSKIN, 2001. Neurogenesis in the subventricular zone and rostral migratory stream of the neonatal and adult primate forebrain. *Exp. Neurol.* 172:1–16.

PENCEA, V., K. D. BINGAMAN, S. J. WIEGAND, and M. B. LUSKIN, 2001. Infusion of brain-derived neurotrophic factor into the lateral ventricle of the adult rat leads to new neurons in the parenchyma of the striatum, septum, thalamus, and hypothalmus. *J. Neurosci.* 21:6706–6717.

PETREANU, L., and A. ALVAREZ-BUYLLA, 2002. Maturation and death of adult-born olfactory bulb granule neurons: Role of olfaction. *J. Neurosci.* 22:6106–6113.

PINCUS, D. W., H. M. KEYOUNG, C. HARRISON-RESTELLI, R. R. GOODMAN, R. A. R. FRASER, M. EDGAR, S. SAKAKIBARA, H. OKANO, M. NEDERGAARD, and S. A. GOLDMAN, 1998. Fibroblast growth factor-2/brain-derived neurotrophic factor-associated maturation of new neurons generated from adult human subependymal cells. *Ann. Neurol.* 43:576–585.

RAKIC, P., 1974. Neurons in rhesus monkey visual cortex: Systematic relation between time of origin and eventual disposition. *Science* 183:425–427.

RAKIC, P., 1985. Limits of neurogenesis in primates. *Science* 227:1054–1056.

RAKIC, P., 1990. Principles of neural cell migration. *Experientia* 46:882–891.

RAKIC, P., 1998. Young neurons for old brains? *Nat. Neurosci.* 1:3–5.

RAKIC, P., 2002. Neurogenesis in adult primate neocortex: An evaluation of the evidence. *Nat. Rev. Neurosci.* 3:65–71.

RAKIC, P., and D. R. KORNACK, 1993. Constraints on neurogenesis in adult primate brain: An evolutionary advantage? In *Restorative Neurology*, vol. 6, *Neuronal Cell Death and Repair*, A. C. Cuello, ed. Amsterdam: Elsevier, pp. 257–266.

RAKIC, P., and R. S. NOWAKOWSKI, 1981. The time of origin of neurons in the hippocampal region of the rhesus monkey. *J. Comp. Neurol.* 196:99–128.

RAMSDEN, D. B., R. B. PARSONS, S. L. HO, and R. H. WARING, 2001. The aetiology of idiopathic Parkinson's disease. *J. Clin. Pathol. Mol. Pathol.* 54:369–380.

ROCHEFORT, C., G. GHEUSI, J. VINCENT, and P. LLEDO, 2002. Enriched odor exposure increases the number of newborn neurons in the adult olfactory bulb and improves odor memory. *J. Neurosci.* 22:2679–2689.

ROSSI, F., and E. CATTANEO, 2002. Neural stem cell therapy for neurological diseases: Dreams and reality. *Nat. Rev. Neurosci.* 3:401–409.

SANTARELLI, L., M. SAXE, C. GROSS, A. SURGET, F. BATTAGLIA, S. DULAWA, N. WEISSTAUB, C. BELZUNG, and R. HEN, 2003. Requirement of hippocampal neurogenesis for the behavioral effects of antidepressants. *Science* 301:805–809.

SERESS, L., 1992. Morphological variability and developmental aspects of monkey and human granule cells: Differences between the rodent and primate dentate gyrus. *Epilepsy Res. Suppl.* 7:3–28.

SERESS, L., H. ÁBRAHÁM, T. TORNÓCZKY, and G. KOSZTOLÁNYI, 2001. Cell formation in the human hippocampal formation from mid-gestation to the late postnatal period. *Neuroscience* 105:831–843.

SERI, B., and A. ALVAREZ-BUYLLA, 2002. Neural stem cells and the regulation of neurogenesis in the adult hippocampus. *Clin. Neurosci. Res.* 2:11–16.

SHINGO, T., C. GREGG, E. ENWERE, H. FUJIKAWA, R. HASSAM, C. GEARY, J. C. CROSS, and S. WEISS, 2003. Pregnancy-stimulated neurogenesis in the adult female forebrain mediated by prolactin. *Science* 299:117–120.

SIMIC, G., I. KOSTOVIC, B. WINBLAD, and N. BOGDANOVIC, 1997. Volume and number of neurons of the human hippocampal formation in normal aging and Alzheimer's disease. *J. Comp. Neurol.* 379:482–494.

SNYDER, E. Y., and K. I. PARK, 2002. Limitations in brain repair. *Nat. Med.* 8:928–930.

STANFIELD, B. B., and J. E. TRICE, 1988. Evidence that granule cells generated in the dentate gyrus of adult rodents extend axonal projections. *Exp. Brain Res.* 72:399–406.

TESSIER-LAVIGNE, M., and C. S. GOODMAN, 1996. The molecular biology of axon guidance. *Science* 274:1123–1131.

TIGGS, J., J. G. HERNDON, and D. L. ROSENE, 1995. Mild age-related changes in the dentate gyrus of adult rhesus monkeys. *Acta Anat.* 153:39–48.

VAN PRAAG, H., A. F. SCHINDER, B. R. CRISTIE, N. TONI, T. D. PALMER, and F. H. GAGE, 2002. Functional neurogenesis in the adult hippocampus. *Nature* 415:1030–1034.

WEICKERT, C. S., M. J. WEBSTER, S. M. COLVIN, M. M. HERMAN, T. M. HYDE, D. R. WEINBERGER, and J. E. KLEINMAN, 2000. Localization of epidermal growth factor receptors and putative neuroblasts in human subependymal zone. *J. Comp. Neurol.* 423:359–372.

WEINBERGER, D. R., K. F. BERMAN, R. SUDDATH, and E. F. TORREY, 1992. Evidence of a dysfunction of a prefrontal-limbic network in schizophrenia: A magnetic resonance imaging and regional cerebral blood flow study of discordant monozygotic twins. *Am. J. Psychiatry* 149:890–897.

WICHTERLE, H., J. M. García-Verdugo, and A. Alvarez-Buylla, 1997. Direct evidence for homotypic, glia-independent neuronal migration. *Neuron* 18:779–791.

Wu, W., K. Wong, J. Chen, Z. Jiang, S. Dupuis, J. Y. Wu, and Y. Rao, 1999. Directional guidance of neuronal migration in the olfactory system by the protein Slit. *Nature* 400:331–336.

Zeller, A. C., 1987. Communication by sight and smell. In *Primate Societies*, B. B. Smuts, D. L. Cheney, R. M. Seyfarth, R. W. Wrangham, and T. T. Struhsaker, eds. Chicago: University of Chicago Press, pp. 433–439.

Zigova, T., V. Pencea, S. J. Wiegad, and M. B. Luskin, 1998. Intraventricular administration of BDNF increases the number of newly generated neurons in the adult olfactory bulb. *Mol. Cell. Neurosci.* 11:234–245.

3 Setting the Stage for Cognition: Genesis of the Primate Cerebral Cortex

PASKO RAKIC, EUGENIUS S. B. C. ANG, AND JOSHUA BREUNIG

ABSTRACT Cerebral cortex provides biological substrate for human cognitive capacity and is arguably the part of the brain that sets us apart from any other species. Therefore, understanding the evolution and development of this complex structure is central to understanding human intelligence and creativity. Modern developmental neurobiology provides insight into how cerebral cortex may have evolved, how it develops in each individual, and how this finely tuned process may go astray, causing devastating disorders of highest brain functions. The initial developmental events, which are the subject of this review, invoke the genetic regulation involved in the production of proper number of neurons and their appropriate allocation and migration to final positions within the developing cortical plate. The genes and morphoregulatory molecules that control these early cellular events are being identified and their functions tested both in vitro and in vivo in transgenic animals. The data suggest that the early stages of corticogenesis set the stage for the subsequent formation of the neuronal connections and the pattern of synaptic architecture.

The human cerebral cortex is considered the crowning achievement of biological evolution. This imposing structure makes up about two-thirds of the neuronal mass of the brain and contains almost three-quarters of all our synapses. It is also the region of the brain that most distinctively sets us apart from other species. Therefore, the principles governing the development of the cerebral cortex may hold the key to explaining our cognitive capacity and the evolution of human intelligence and creativity. One of the most prominent features of the cerebral cortex in all species that is particularly prominent in primates is its parcellation into distinct laminar, radial, and areal domains (Eccles, 1984; Goldman-Rakic, 1987; Szentagothai, 1987; Rakic and Singer, 1988; Mountcastle, 1997). However, although the surface of the neocortex has expanded enormously during phylogeny (e.g., the surface of the human neocortex is 10 times larger than that of a macaque monkey and 1000 times larger than that of a rat), its thickness and its basic pattern of cytoarchitec-tonic organization have changed relatively little (Rakic, 1995b).

The development of the cerebral cortex and its expansion in size and complexity cannot be fully understand without answering some fundamental biological questions: When and where are cortical neurons generated? How is their number regulated in each species and in each individual? What accounts for the expansion of the cortical surface without a concomitant increase in thickness? How do postmitotic cells attain their proper laminar and areal position within the cortex? When and how are different cell phenotypes generated and the regional differences in the cerebral cortex established? Elucidation of these issues is an essential prerequisite for understanding the subsequent formation of the neuronal connections and synaptic architecture that underlie normal and abnormal cognitive capacity.

This chaper is based mainly on studies of neocortical development in the mouse, macaque, and human brain carried out in my laboratory over the past three decades. Although the principles of cortical development are similar in all three species, we believe that even small differences may provide clues as to how this structure has evolved. Since the functions of neurotransmitters, receptors, and ion channels do not change substantially over phylogenetic scale, the secret to the success of *Homo sapiens* is probably due mainly to an increased number of neurons, more elaborate connections, and functional specialization of cortical areas. This review will be limited to the early developmental events that lead to the formation of cellular constituents of the cortical plate. The subsequent formation of neuronal connections and synaptic junctions is described in other chapters in this volume.

Basic principles

The basic cellular events and main principles of cortical development are similar to those underlying the formation of other parts of the central nervous system (Sidman and Rakic, 1982; Rakic, 2000) and are diagrammatically

PASKO RAKIC, EUGENIUS S. B. C. ANG, and JOSHUA BREUNIG Department of Neurobiology, Yale University School of Medicine, New Haven, Conn.

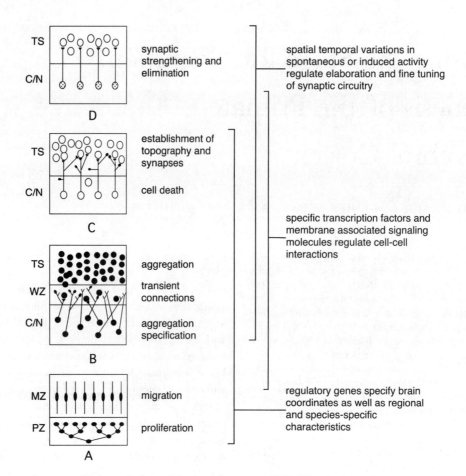

FIGURE 3.1 The complex organization of the adult central nervous system is the end product of sequential, interdependent cellular events that occur during embryonic development. Starting from the bottom (*A*) to the top of the diagram (*D*), individual neurons are generated in specific proliferative zones (VZ), and, after last cell division, migrate across the migratory zone (MZ) to attain their final locations, where they form cortical sheets or aggregate into nuclei (C/N). Some cells form transient connections in the waiting zones (WZ) before they enter their appropriate target structures (TS). The final set of neuronal connections, which are initially more numerous and diffuse, is established by elimination of cells and excess synapses, as shown at the top of the diagram. These basic cellular events can be observed in most regions of the developing brain. As indicated on the right side of the diagram, a major goal of modern developmental neurobiology is to uncover specific genes and molecules that regulate these cellular events in specific structures as well as to understand the mechanisms that enable the environment to influence the formation of neural connections.

illustrated in figure 3.1. Initial cellular events, such as the proliferation, migration, aggregation, and death of cells that form the brain, as well as the subsequent outgrowth of axons and the establishment of neuronal connections, proceed in an orderly fashion in each individual according to a species-specific timetable and are regulated by differential gene expression (figure 3.1*A*, *B*). In contrast, the later phases of development, which include the selective elimination of neurons, axons, and synapses and the shaping of the final circuits within topographical maps, are influenced by activity-dependent mechanisms that, after birth, involve individual experience (figure 3.1*C*, *D*). As indicated on the right side of the diagram, analysis of these events can be carried out at the genetic, molecular, and cellular levels. The present review will focus on only the selected aspects of the early events that are represented at the bottom of figure 3.1*A* and *B*.

Time and place of neuronal origin

Classical studies of neurogenesis based on light microscopic observations revealed lack of dividing and migrating neurons in the cerebral wall of the newborn child, suggesting that cortical neurons in human are likely to be generated before birth (e.g., Poliakov, 1959, 1965; reviewed in Sidman and Rakic, 1973, 1982; Rakic, 2002). However, the precise data on the onset and termination of corticogenesis could not be established with histological techniques (e.g., Conel, 1939). The use of sensitive and reliable methods in non-human primates to label dividing cells revealed that the neocortical neurons in the macaque monkey are produced mainly during the middle of gestation (Rakic, 1974, 1988a, 2002). This finding stands in contrast to what occurs in the cerebellum, olfactory bulb, and hippocampus, where neuronal addition continues after birth in this species (Rakic,

1973; Rakic and Nowakowski, 1981; Kornack and Rakic, 1999, 2001a). However, despite a comprehensive search in the adult monkey neocortex, no additional neurons have been found to be added during the animal's 30-year life span (Rakic, 1985; Kornack and Rakic, 2001b; Koketsu et al., 2003; reviewed in Rakic, 2002; see also Kornack, this volume). Comparative cytological analysis, as well as supravital labeling of dividing neurons in human embryos, indicates that neurons destined for the neocortex in our species are also generated during midgestation (Rakic and Sidman, 1968; Sidman and Rakic, 1973, 1982).

The observation of large numbers of mitotic figures situated near the lumen of the cerebral cavity of the embryonic human cerebrum and their paucity or absence in the cortical plate itself led to the suggestion that cortical neurons are produced in the germinal matrix situated at the ventricular surface (His, 1904). This hypothesis was substantiated by the application of modern methods for labeling dividing cells in mice (Angevine and Sidman, 1961), monkeys (Rakic, 1974), and humans (Rakic and Sidman, 1968; Letinic, Zoncu, and Rakic, 2002). Thus, while cortical projection neurons arise from these traditional germinal zones, recent studies in rodents have identified the presence of a population of bipolar, tangentially migrating neurons derived from the ganglionic eminence that negotiate the intermediate and marginal zone to eventually generate cortical interneurons (Lavdas et al., 1999; Marin and Rubenstein, 2001). Conversely, in what appears to be a significant species-specific difference, the majority of human cortical interneurons seem to originate in the ventricular and subventricular zones of the dorsal telecephalon, with only about one-third of them originating in the ganglionic eminence (Letinic, Zoncu, and Rakic, 2002). Proliferative cells in the ventricular zone are organized as a pseudostratified epithelium in which precursor cells divide asynchronously; their nuclei move away from the ventricular surface to replicate their DNA and then move back to the surface to undergo another mitotic cycle (reviewed in Sidman and Rakic, 1973; Rakic, 1988a). Electron microscopic and immunocytochemical analyses revealed the coexistence of neuronal and glial cell lines from the onset of corticogenesis (Rakic, 1972; Levitt, Cooper, and Rakic, 1981). Nevertheless, though it had been recognized that the primary or conversional radial glia phenotype could revert to the neuroepithelial form and generate neurons (Cameron and Rakic, 1991), increasing in vivo and in vitro evidence demonstrates that radial glia can also generate neuronal progenitors as well as neurons (Malatesta et al., 2000, 2003; Hartfuss et al., 2001; Noctor et al., 2001, 2002; Tamamaki et al., 2001; Fishell and Kriegstein, 2003; Tramontin et al., 2003). Recent studies in the rodent cerebrum suggest that the dividing radial glia can generate neuronal clones that migrate along the parental process into the cortical plate (Noctor et al., 2001), and the same has been found in primates (e.g., Rakic, 2003). However, subsequent observations have indicated the existence of a "transit-amplifying cell," a dedicated neuronal progenitor derived from the parent radial glial cell that does not inherit the pial fiber, similar to the situation observed in the developing primate germinal zone (Rakic, 2003; Haydar and Rakic, unpublished observations; A. Kriegstein, personal communication). In primates, early divergence of basic cell types that include radial glia and neuronal progenitors based on immunocytochemical analysis (Levitt, Cooper, and Rakic, 1981) has been confirmed using the retroviral gene transfer method, which enables the study of cell lineages in the developing mammalian telencephalon (Luskin, Pearlman, and Sanes, 1988; Cameron and Rakic, 1991; Kornack and Rakic, 1995). It appears that in the primate, the radial glial mother cell gives rise to a daughter cell that either directly or as a dedicated neuronal progenitor goes through several rounds of division to produce bipolar migrating neurons that will migrate up the radial process of the mother cell (see Rakic, 2003). However, it should be underscored that the large subventricular zone that in monkeys and humans generates the majority of interneurons (e.g., Letinic, Zoncu, and Rakic, 2002) is either very small or nonexistent in rodents.

Transient embryonic zones

Formation of the complex adult brain from the simple proliferative epithelium on the dorsal side of the embryo is an end product of a series of morphogenetic changes. Thus, during embryonic and fetal stages, the telencephalic wall consists of several cellular layers, or zones, that do not exist in the mature brain. Moving outward from the ventricle to the pial surface, these are, in order: ventricular, subventricular, intermediate, and subplate zones, the cortical plate, and the marginal zone (figure 3.2). Although most of these zones were described and characterized in the literature at the turn of the twentieth century (e.g., His, 1904), the subplate zone has been recognized as a separate entity only relatively recently (Kostovic and Molliver, 1974; reviewed in Kostovic and Rakic, 1990). This zone consists of early-generated subplate neurons scattered among numerous axons, dendrites, glial fibers, and migrating neurons. Most of these subplate neurons eventually degenerate, but some persist in the adult cerebrum as a set of interstitial cells (Kostovic and Rakic, 1980; Luskin and Shatz, 1985). Although it has been suggested that the subplate zone provides an opportunity for interactions between incoming afferent fibers and early-generated neurons, the significance of these transient contacts is not fully understood.

One possibility is that the subplate zone serves as a cellular substrate for competition among the initial contingent of

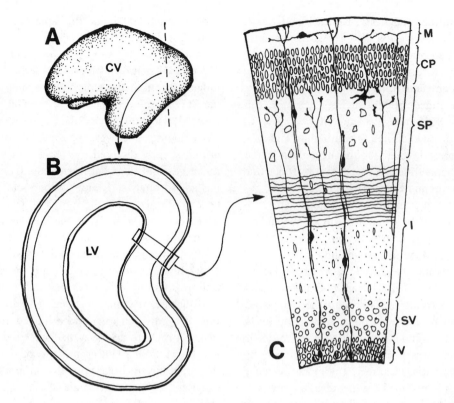

FIGURE 3.2   Cytological organization of the primate cerebral wall during the first half of gestation. (*A*) The cerebral vesicle of 60–65-day-old monkey fetuses is still smooth and lacks the characteristic convolutions that will emerge in the second half of gestation. (*B*) Coronal section across the occipital lobe at the level indicated by a vertical dashed line in A. The lateral cerebral ventricle at this age is still relatively large, and only the incipient calcarine fissure (CF) marks the position of the prospective visual cortex. (*C*) A block of tissue dissected from the upper bank of the calcarine fissure. At this early stage one can recognize six transient embryonic zones from the ventricular surface (bottom) to the pial surface (top): ventricular zone (V), subventricular zone (SV), intermediate zone (I), subplate zone (SP), cortical plate (CP), and marginal zone (M). Note the presence of spindle-shaped migrating neurons moving along the elongated radial glial fibers, which span the full thickness of the cerebral wall. The early afferents originating from the brainstem, thalamus, and other cortical areas invade the cerebral wall and accumulate initially in the subplate zone, where they make transient synapses before entering the overlying cortical plate. (Reprinted from Rakic, 1995b, by permission.)

cortical afferents and that this competition serves to regulate their distribution to appropriate regions of the overlying cortical plate (Rakic, 1976a, 1977; Kostovic and Rakic, 1984; McConnell, Ghosh, and Shatz, 1994). Subsequent autoradiographic, electron microscopic, and histochemical studies revealed that the axons observed in the subplate zone originate sequentially from the brainstem, basal forebrain, thalamus, and the ipsi- and contralateral cerebral hemispheres (Kostovic and Rakic, 1990). More recently, the subplate has been shown to be important for formation of functional architecture in the cortex, such as ocular dominance columns in the visual cortex, and also for ensuring the proper formation and strengthening of synapses in this area (Kanold et al., 2003). After a variable and partially overlapping period, these diverse fiber systems enter the cortical plate, and the subplate zone disappears, leaving only a vestige of cells scattered throughout the subcortical white matter that are known as interstitial neurons (Kostovic and Rakic, 1980; Chun and Shatz, 1989). A comparison among various species indicates that the size and role of this tran-

sient zone increase during mammalian evolution, culminating in the development of association areas of the human fetal cortex concomitant with enlargement of the cortico-cortical fiber systems (Kostovic and Goldman-Rakic, 1983; Kostovic and Rakic, 1990). The regional differences in the size, pattern, and resolution of the subplate zone also correlate with the pattern and elaboration of cerebral convolutions (Goldman-Rakic and Rakic, 1984).

Control of cortical size

The size of the cerebral cortex varies greatly among mammals and reaches a peak surface area in primates. Understanding the principles and mechanisms controlling the production of cells destined for the cerebral cortex may hold the key to understanding the evolution of human intelligence. Based on data on the time of cell origin and cell proliferation kinetics, we proposed that the number of cortical cells depends on the mode of mitotic division (symmetrical vs. asymmetrical), the duration of the cell cycle, and the degree of programmed cell death (PCD) in the proliferative zones (Rakic, 1988a, 1995b; Haydar, Ang, and Rakic, 2003). In the past few years technological advances have allowed us to study the regulation of these cellular events in transgenic mice as well as in nonhuman primates using the retroviral gene transfer method (e.g., Kornack and Rakic, 1995; Kuida et al., 1996, 1998; Zhong et al., 1996; Haydar et al., 1999). Because most genes and their products involved in cell production and fate determination seem to be preserved during evolution, one might expect that the control of neuronal number and differentiation would be basically similar in all species (Williams and Herrup, 1988). For example, one mechanism that regulates the number of cells produced in the ventricular zone is PCD, or apoptosis. Although PCD has been considered a major factor contributing to the formation of the vertebrate brain (Glucksmann, 1951), contemporary research has focused mainly on the histogenetic cell death involved in the elimination of inappropriate axonal connections at later stages of development (e.g., Rakic and Riley, 1983a,b; Oppenheim, 1991). However, the discovery of several classes of genes involved in PCD, which were initially identified in invertebrates, created the opportunity to study this phenomenon in the mammalian cerebrum. For example, a family of enzymes called caspases has been shown to play an important role in PCD in a variety of organs and tissues (Ellis and Horvitz, 1991). We have recently demonstrated that in mouse embryos deficient in caspase 9 and 3, fewer cells are eliminated than in their littermates (Kuida et al., 1996, 1998). A reduction of apoptosis in the knockout mice results in the formation of supernumerary founder cells in the cerebral ventricular zone. As a consequence, these mice form ectopic cells in the intermediate zone, as well as a larger cortical plate with more radial units. Correspondingly, diminishment of the clearance rate of apoptotic cells in transgenic mice lacking a receptor crucial for the recognition of dying cells results in enlarged proliferative zones that lead to the formation of ectopias, as well as an expanded cortical plate that begins to form convolutions (Li et al., 2003). Interestingly, mice expressing higher levels of β-catenin, which inhances the number of founder cells, experience the same type of cortical malformation (Chenn and Walsh, 2002, 2003). These studies provide examples of how convolutions in the cerebral cortex may have evolved, because mice engineered to lack caspases as well as to express β-catenin in neural precursors display a bigger cortical sheet and convolutions that form, seemingly passively, without any observable increase in thickness of the cortical plate (Haydar et al., 1999; Chenn and Walsh, 2002). These new approaches provide an example of how the mutation of a few genes that control the roduction of cells could result in the expansion of the cortex during evolution (Rakic, 1995b).

Neuronal cell migration

Since all cortical neurons originate near the ventricular surface of the cerebral vesicle, they must all move to their final positions in the cortex, which develops in the outer regions of the cerebral wall, just below the pia. Initially, while the cerebral wall is still thin, cells move only a short distance. Time-lapse imaging studies in the mouse forebrain have shown this short movement of the cell body, termed translocation, during the the early stages of cortical development (Nadarajah et al., 2003). The same has been seen in the human cerebral vesicle at the early stages (Sidman and Rakic, 1973). However, during the subsequent course of corticogenesis, the length of their pathway increases with enlargement of the cerebral hemispheres, particularly in the large primate cerebrum, in which, during midgestation, a massive migration of neurons occurs concomitantly with the rapid growth of the cerebral wall (reviewed in Sidman and Rakic, 1982; Rakic, 1988a). This magnitude of cell movement is perhaps the reason that neuronal cell migration was first observed in human embryos (His, 1874). In the early 1970s, advances in methods enabled the discovery that postmitotic neurons find their way to the cortex by following the elongated shafts of radial glial cells (figure 3.3; Rakic, 1972). Radial glial cells are particularly prominent in primates, including humans, where, in the late stages of corticogenesis, their fibers span the entire width of the large and convoluted cerebral hemispheres (Rakic, 1978; deAzevedo et al., 2003). For example, in the macaque monkey, radial glial cells transiently stop dividing during the peak of neuronal migration (Schmechel and Rakic, 1979). While moving along the glial surface, migrating neurons remain preferentially attached to curvilinear glial fibers, which suggested a "gliophilic" mode of migration (Rakic, 1985, 1990) that may be mediated by heterotypic adhesion molecules (Rakic, Cameron, and Komuro, 1994). As many as 30 migrating GFAP-negative neurons have been observed migrating along a single GFAP-positive radial glial fascicle in the human forebrain during midgestation (Rakic, 2003).

However, some postmitotic cells do not obey glial constraints and move along tangentially oriented axonal fascicles (e.g., the black, horizontally oriented cell aligned with TR in figure 3.3). We suggested the term *neurophilic* to characterize the mode of migration of this cell class (Rakic, 1985, 1990). Although lateral dispersion of postmitotic neurons was initially observed in Golgi-stained preparations (e.g., figure 3.1 of the report of the Boulder Committee, 1970), it has attracted renewed attention after the discovery that a specific, presumably neurophilic, cell class moves from the telencephalon to the olfactory bulb (Menezes and Luskin, 1994; Lois and Alvarez-Buylla, 1994) and from the ganglionic eminence to the dorsal neocortex

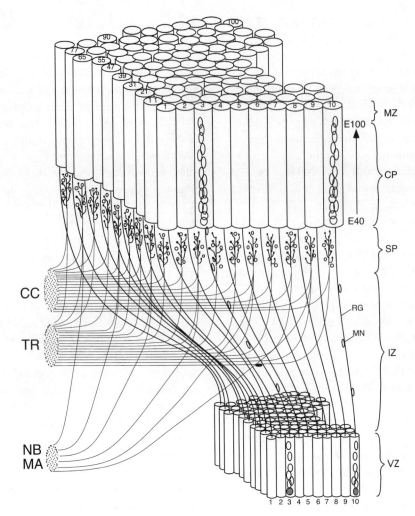

FIGURE 3.3 A three-dimensional illustration of the basic developmental events and types of cell-cell interactions occurring during the early stages of corticogenesis, before formation of the final pattern of cortical connections. This cartoon emphasizes radial migration, a predominant mode of neuronal movement which, in primates, underlies the elaborate columnar organization of the neocortex. After their last division, cohorts of migrating neurons (MN) first traverse the intermediate zone (IZ) and then the subplate zone (SP), where they have an opportunity to interact with "waiting" afferents arriving sequentially from the nucleus basalis and monoamine subcortical centers (NB, MA), from the thalamic radiation (TR), and from several ipsilateral and contralateral corticocortical bundles (CC). After the newly generated neurons bypass the earlier generated ones, which are situated in the deep cortical layers, they settle at the interface between the developing cortical plate (CP) and the marginal zone (MZ) and, eventually, form a radial stack of cells that share a common site of origin but are generated at different times. For example, neurons produced between E40 and E100 in radial unit 3 follow the same radial glial fascicle and form ontogenetic column 3. Although some cells, presumably neurophilic in their surface affinities, may detach from the cohort and move laterally, guided by an axonal bundle (e.g., the horizontally oriented, black cell leaving radial unit 3 and horizontally oriented fibers), most postmitotic cells are gliophilic—that is, they have an affinity for the glial surface and strictly obey constraints imposed by transient radial glial scaffolding (RG). This cellular arrangement preserves the relationships between the proliferative mosaic of the ventricular zone (VZ) and the corresponding protomap within the SP and CP, even though the cortical surface in primates shifts considerably during the massive cerebral growth encountered in midgestation (for details see Rakic, 1988).

(de Carlos, López-Mascaraque, and Valverde, 1996; Tamamaki et al., 1997). Studies in rodents also suggested a more widespread dispersion of clonally related cortical cells (reviewed in Rakic, 1995a; Reid, Liang, and Walsh, 1995; Tan et al., 1998). The majority of these cells migrating tangentially into the dorsal neocortex are inhibitory interneurons (reviewed in Marin and Rubenstein, 2001), as well as a minority that are oligodendrocytes (He et al., 2001). In humans, ganglionic eminence also contributes neurons to the dorsal thalamus (Letinic and Rakic, 2001).

It should be underscored, however, that clonal analysis in the convoluted primate cortex revealed that the majority of migrating cells obey the radial constraints imposed by the radial glial scaffolding (Kornack and Rakic, 1995; see also discussion under Radial Unit Hypothesis). Also, lineage analysis of transcription factors specific for either dorsal or ventral neocortex progenitor cells revealed that the majority of interneurons in the human are derived from the dorsal neocortex (Letinic, Zoncu, and Rakic, 2002). This strongly suggested that the primate cortex may confer species-specific differences in basic developmental events compared to other mammalian species.

Considerable progress has been made in understanding the molecular mechanisms behind neuronal migration and the physical displacement of cell perikarya during translocation of the cell nucleus and soma across the densely packed tissue. Initially, based on an in situ observation, it was proposed that a single pair of binding, complementary molecules with gliophilic properties can account for the recognition of glial guides (Rakic, 1981). In the last decade, however, several candidates for recognition and adhesion molecules have been discovered and are being tested (e.g., Hatten and Mason, 1990; Cameron and Rakic, 1994; Anton, Cameron, and Rakic, 1996; reviewed in Hatten, 2002). Recently, it was also shown that voltage- and ligand-gated ion channels on the leading process and cell soma of migrating neurons regulate the influx of calcium ions into migrating neurons (Komuro and Rakic, 1992, 1993, 1996; Rakic and Komuro, 1995). Calcium fluctuations in turn may trigger polymerization of cytoskeletal and contractile proteins essential for cell motility and translocation of the nucleus and surrounding cytoplasm (Rakic, Knyihar-Csillik, and Csillik, 1996). These studies indicate that neuronal migration is a multifaceted developmental event involving cell-cell recognition, differential adhesion, transmembrane signaling, and intracytoplasmic structural changes (Rakic, Cameron, and Komuro, 1994).

Molecules involved in the cytoskeletal rearrangement during migration have also been identified. Doublecortin and Lis1 have been shown to be involved in cytoskeletal dynamics during migration (Gleeson et al., 1999; reviewed in Feng and Walsh, 2001), and their mutation in humans has been implicated in certain brain abnormalities, such as double cortex (des Portes et al., 1998; Gleeson et al., 1998) and lissencephaly type I (Hattori et al., 1994).

A simple model of molecular components involved in cell migration is shown in figure 3.4. The discovery of the glial-guided radial migration led to the proposal of the radial unit hypothesis (Rakic, 1988a), which has served as a useful working model for research on the cellular and molecular mechanisms involved in normal and abnormal cortical development.

Radial unit hypothesis

The cellular mechanisms underlying expansion of cerebral cortex during individual development and evolution can be explained in the context of the radial unit hypothesis (Rakic, 1988a, 1995b). The neocortex in all species consists of an array of iterative neuronal groups (called, interchangeably, radial columns or modules) that share a common intrinsic and extrinsic connectivity and subserve the same function (Bugbee and Goldman-Rakic, 1983; Goldman-Rakic, 1987; Szentagothai, 1987; Mountcastle, 1997). The larger the cortex in a given species, the larger the number of participating columnar units (Rakic, 1978, 1995b). The radial unit hypothesis of cortical development postulates that the embryonic cortical plate forms from vertically oriented cohorts of neurons generated at the same site in the proliferative ventricular zone of the cerebral vesicle (Rakic, 1978). Each radial unit consists of several clones (polyclones) that migrate to the cortex following glial fascicles spanning the cerebral wall (Rakic, 1988a). In the cortical plate, later-generated cells bypass earlier-generated ones and settle in an inside-out gradient of neurogenesis (Rakic, 1974). Thus, the two-dimensional positional information of the proliferative units in the ventricular zone is transformed into a three-dimensional cortical architecture: the x- and y-axes of the cells are provided by their site of origin, whereas the z-axis is provided by their time of origin (see figure 3.3).

The radial unit hypothesis provides an explanation for the large expansion in cortical surface that occurred without a concomitant significant increase in thickness during phylogenetic and ontogenetic development (Rakic, 1988a). It also shows how the genes controlling the number of founder cells at the ventricular surface set a limit on the size of the cortical surface during individual development, as well as during the evolution of mammalian species (Rakic, 1995b). Thus, a relatively small change in the timing of developmental cellular events could have large functional consequences. For example, a minor increase in the length of the cell cycle or the magnitude of cell death in the ventricular zone could result in a large increase in the number of founder cells that form proliferative units (Rakic, 1988a). Since proliferation in the ventricular zone initially proceeds exponentially owing to the prevalence of symmetrical divisions, an additional

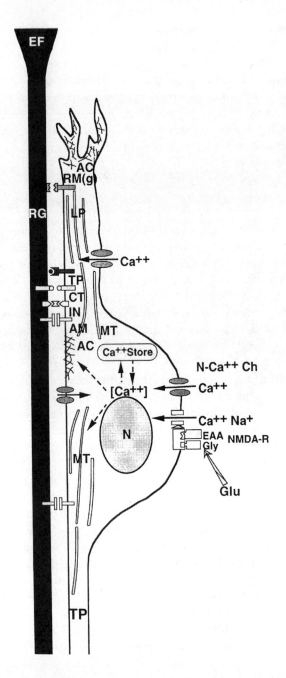

FIGURE 3.4 Model of a proposed cascade of cellular and molecular events that take place during the migration of postmitotic cells in the developing cerebral wall. After their last mitotic division in the ventricular zone, migrating cells extend a leading process (LP) that follows the contours of the radial glial fiber (RG) as it spans the expanding cerebral wall. The cytoskeleton within the LP and trailing process (TP) contain microtubules (MT) and actin-like contractile proteins (AC) that are involved in translocation of the cell nucleus (N) and the surrounding cytoplasm within the leading process until the cell enters the cortical plate. This system, maintained in vitro in slice preparations or imprint culture, provides an opportunity to examine the role of the various molecules that are engaged in recognition, adhesion, transmembrane signaling, and motility that underlie directed neuronal migration. The voltage-gated (N-type) and ligand-gated (NMDA-type) receptors/channels are thought to control calcium influx, which serves as messengers for execution of this movement. Abbreviations: AM, homotypic adhesion molecule; EAA, excitatory amino acid; EF, end foot of the radial glial fiber; Gly, glycine; LP, leading process; MT, microtubule; N, cell nucleus; TP, trailing process; RG, radial glial fiber; RM(g) gliophilic recognition molecule; TP, tyrosine phosphorylation. (Modified from Rakic, 1997.)

round of mitotic cycles during this phase doubles the number of founder cells and, consequently, the number of radial columns (figure 3.5; Rakic, 1995b). According to this model, fewer than four extra rounds of symmetric cell division in the ventricular zone before the onset of corticogenesis can account for a 10-fold difference in the size of the cortical surface. Because the mode of cell division changes to predominantly asymmetrical after the onset of corticogenesis, an extension of cell production in humans by about 2 weeks longer than in macaques should enlarge the cortical thickness by only 10%–15%, which is actually observed (Rakic, 1995b). Thus, as illustrated in figure 3.5, even a small delay in the onset of the second phase of corticogenesis

results in an order of magnitude larger cortical surface, due to the increasing number of founder cells at the ventricular zone.

The proposal that neurons composing a given radial column may be clonally related could be tested experimentally after the introduction of the retroviral gene transfer method for in vivo analysis of cell lineages in the mammalian brain (Sanes, 1989). Use of this approach suggested that most progenitors originating in the same site of the ventricular zone remain radially deployed in the cortex (Luskin, Pearlman, and Sanes, 1988; Kornack and Rakic, 1995; Tan et al., 1998; see, however, Reid, Liang, and Walsh, 1995). Furthermore, a number of studies in chimeric and transgenic mice have provided evidence that a majority of postmitotic, clonally related neurons move and remain radially distributed in the cortex (e.g., Nakatsuji, Kadokawa, and Suemori, 1991; Soriano et al., 1995; reviewed in Rakic, 1995a). Use of the retroviral gene transfer method in the embryonic primate brain has shown that even in the large and highly convoluted cerebrum, radial deployment of many clones is remarkably well preserved (Kornack and Rakic, 1995).

Protomap hypothesis

A major challenge to students of the cerebral cortex is how individual and species-specific cytoarchitectonic areas have emerged from the initially seemingly uniform ventricular zone and cortical plate. Both intrinsic and extrinsic factors have been suggested. One attractive hypothesis is that all cortical neurons are equipotential and that laminar and areal differences are induced by extrinsic influences exerted

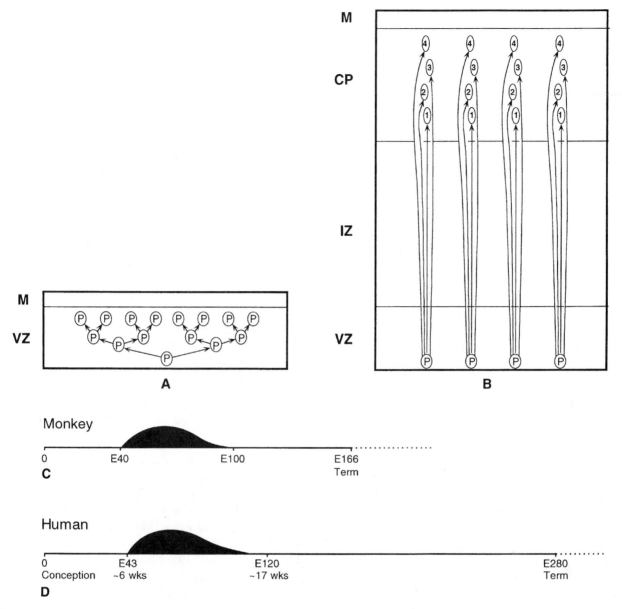

FIGURE 3.5 (A) Schematic model of symmetric cell divisions, which predominate before the E40. At this early embryonic age, the cerebral wall consists of only the ventricular zone (VZ), where all the cells are proliferating, and the marginal zone (M), into which some cells extend radial processes. Symmetric division produces two progenitors (P) during each cycle and causes rapid horizontal lateral spread. (B) Model of asymmetric or stem division, which becomes predominant in the monkey embryo after E40. During each asymmetric division, a progenitor (P) produces one postmitotic neuron that leaves the ventricular zone and another progenitor that remains within the proliferative zone and continues to divide. Postmitotic neurons migrate rapidly across the intermediate zone (IZ) and become arranged vertically in the cortical plate (CP) in reverse order of their arrival (1, 2, 3, 4). (C) Diagrammatic representation of the time of neuron origin in the macaque monkey. The data were obtained from ³H-thymidine autoradiographic analyses (Rakic, 1974). (D) Estimate of the time of neuron origin in the human neocortex based on the number of mitotic figures within the ventricular zone, supravital DNA synthesis in slice preparations of fetal tissue, and the presence of migrating neurons in the intermediate zone of the human fetal cerebrum. More recent study of brain slices from 20- to 25-day-old human fetal tissue indicates that the subventricular zone continues to produce interneurons during midgestational period (Letinic et al., 2003). (Reprinted from Rakic, 1995, by permission.)

via thalamic afferents (Creutzfeldt, 1977). However, there is also considerable evidence that the cells generated within the embryonic cerebral wall contain some intrinsic information about their prospective species-specific cortical organization. To reconcile existing experimental and descriptive data, we formulated a protomap hypothesis (Rakic, 1988a). This hypothesis suggests that the basic pattern of cytoarchitectonic areas emerges through synergistic, interdependent interactions between developmental programs intrinsic to cortical neurons and extrinsic signals supplied by specific inputs from subcortical structures. According to this hypothesis, neurons in the embryonic cortical plate—indeed, even in the proliferative ventricular zone where they originate—set up a primordial map that preferentially attracts appropriate afferents and has a capacity to respond to this input in a specific manner. The prefix proto- was introduced to emphasize the primordial, provisionary, and essentially malleable character of the protomap, which is subject to considerable modification by the extrinsic influences exerted at later stages (Rakic, 1988a).

The initial indication that developmental events in the proliferative ventricular zone foreshadow prospective regional differences in the overlying cerebral mantle comes from the observation that the neurogenesis of the primary visual cortex, which contains more neurons per radial unit than the adjacent areas, lasts longer (Rakic, 1976b). Furthermore, it has also been demonstrated that the mitotic index in the ventricular region subjacent to this area is higher than in adjacent regions (Dehay et al., 1993). Furthermore, initial establishment of cytoarchitectural and functional features specific to the visual cortex, such as ocular dominance columns, occurs independently of thalamic inputs to this area (Crowley and Katz, 2000). Therefore, certain region-specific differences in production of the ventricular zone can be detected even before neurons arrive at the cortex (Kennedy and Dehay, 1993; Algan and Rakic, 1997). Several lines of evidence indicate that, during the final cell division, one or both daughter cells start to express a variety of neuron class–specific signaling molecules (LoTurco et al., 1995; Lidow and Rakic, 1994). Postmitotic cells not only become committed to a neuronal fate but also become restricted in their repertoire of possible fates (McConnell, 1988). Numerous studies in which the cytology of postmitotic cells has been examined (e.g., Schwartz, Rakic, and Goldman-Rakic, 1991; LoTurco et al., 1995) and/or manipulated by variety of methods, such as spontaneous mutations (e.g., Caviness and Rakic, 1978; Rakic, 1995b), ionizing radiation (Algan and Rakic, 1997), retroviral gene transfer labeling (Parnavelas at al., 1991), transgenic mice (Kuida et al., 1996), and heterochromic transplantations (McConnell, 1988; McConnell and Kasanowski, 1991), all indicate that certain cell class–specific attributes are expressed before migrating neurons arrive at the corti-

cal plate and become synaptically connected. Remarkably, neurotransmitter secretion is unnecessary for proper brain formation (Verhage et al., 2000). In addition, retroviral tracing experiments and some clonal analyses suggest that the ventricular zone is comprised of a heterogeneous population of cells, and that cell lineage contributes substantially to the cell fate determination of neurons (Parnavelas et al., 1991; Aklin and van der Kooy, 1993; Kornack and Rakic, 1995; Williams and Price, 1995; Kuan et al., 1997; Laywell et al., 2000).

These findings raise the question of whether laminar and areal identities of cortical plate cells provide cues or chemotactic attractants for incoming afferent axons. Data from axonal tracing indicate that afferent connections from subcortical structures and other cortical regions find their way to the specific regions of the cortical plate either directly or via the subplate zone (Kostovic and Rakic, 1984, 1990; de Carlos and O'Leary, 1992; McConnell, Ghosh, and Shatz, 1994; Agmon et al., 1995; Catalano, Robertson, and Killackey, 1996; Richards et al., 1997), suggesting the existence of region-specific attractants for pathfinding and target recognition. In support of this idea, the development of correct topological connections in anophthalmic mice and in early enucleated animals indicates that basic connections and chemoarchitectonic characteristics can form in the absence of information from the periphery (e.g., Kaiserman-Abramoff, Graybiel, and Nauta, 1980; Olivaria and Van Sluyters, 1984; Rakic, 1988a; Kuljis and Rakic, 1990; Kennedy and Dehay, 1993; Rakic and Lidow, 1995; Miyashita-Lin et al., 1999). The gradients and/or region-specific distibution of various morphoregulatory molecules in the embryonic cerebral wall (e.g., Proteus et al., 1991; Arimatsu et al., 1992; Ferri and Levitt, 1993; Buffone et al., 1993; Cohen-Tannoudji, Babinet, and Wassef, 1994; Emerling and Lander, 1994; Levitt, Barbe, and Eagleson, 1997; Donoghue and Rakic, 1999; Bishop et al., 2000; Sestan, Rakic, and Donoghue, 2001) or layer-specific expression of POU-homeodomain genes (e.g., Frantz et al., 1994; Meissirel et al., 1997) may also contribute to the formation of specified axonal pathways. For example, recent methods such as electroporation of FGF8 applied before the beginning of the formation of thalamic connections have shown that morphoregulatory molecules can shift the anterior-posterior areal boundaries in the developing neocortex (Fukuchi-Shimogori and Grove, 2001). Thus, tangentially and radially distinct landmarks in the postmitotic cells facilitate axonal pathfinding and target recognition, which eventually lead to parcellation of the cerebral cortex.

It should be emphasized that although the embryonic cerebral wall exhibits gradients of several morphoregulatory molecules, as well as other area-specific molecular differences, the protomap within the embryonic cerebrum provides only a set of species-specific genetic instructions and biological constraints. The precise position of interareal borders, the overall size of each cytoarchitectonic area, and the details of their cellular and synaptic characteristics in the adult cerebral cortex are achieved through a cascade of reciprocal interactions between cortical neurons and the cues they receive from afferents arriving from a variety of extracortical sources (Rakic, 1988a). Such afferents may serve to coordinate and adjust the ratio of various cell classes with the subcortical structures, as has been shown in the primary visual system (Rakic, Suner, and Williams, 1991; Kennedy and Dehay, 1993; Rakic and Lidow, 1995; Meissirel et al., 1997). In summary, the concept of the cortical protomap includes the role of both intrinsic and extrinsic determinants in shaping the final pattern and relative sizes of the cytoarchitectonic areas.

Timing of cortical genesis in human

Since our ultimate goal is understanding the development of the neocortex in humans, a comparison of selected cellular features of the human cortex in different prenatal stages with those of the macaque monkey may help to determine the corresponding time and sequence of developmental events in these species. This is essential if we are to apply the findings obtained from experimental animals to the understanding of human cortical development (e.g., Chalupa and Wefers, 2000). To this end, Poliakov's comprehensive histological studies of cortical development in human fetuses, published originally in Russian (e.g., Poliakov, 1959, 1965), have been reviewed in more detail elsewhere (Sidman and Rakic, 1982). Here these data are summarized in figure 3.6 and compared with the timing of corresponding events in the macaque monkey.

Stage I. Initial formation of the cortical plate (from approximately the 6th to the 10th fetal weeks). During the 7th fetal week, postmitotic cells begin to migrate from the ventricular zone outward to form a new accumulation of cells at the junction of the intermediate and marginal zones. By the middle of this period, synapses of unknown origin are present above and below the cortical plate (Molliver, Kostovic, and Van der Loos, 1973; Zecevic, 1988). This stage corresponds approximately to the level of cortical development found in the monkey fetus between E40 and E54, depending on the region.

Stage II. Primary condensation of the cortical plate (through approximately the 10th and 11th fetal weeks). At this stage the cortical plate increases in thickness, becomes more compact, and is clearly demarcated from the fiber-rich part of the intermediate zone, which seems to have fewer cells per unit volume, indicating that the first major wave of migration is almost spent (figure 3.6). The end of this stage corresponds approximately to the E55–E59 period in the monkey, when the majority of efferent neurons of layers 5

and 6 are generated in most regions of the cortex (Sidman and Rakic, 1982; Marin-Padilla, 1988).

Stage III. Bilaminate cortical plate (most pronounced during the 11th to the 13th fetal week). The uniform and compact cortical plate of the second stage becomes subdivided into an inner zone, occupied mainly by cells with relatively large, somewhat widely spaced oval nuclei, and an outer zone of cells with densely packed, darker, bipolar nuclei (figure 3.6). This heterogeneity results from the more advanced maturation of the deep-lying neurons that had arrived at the cortical plate during earlier developmental stages, plus the addition of a new wave of somas of immature neurons that take up more superficial positions. This period is also characterized by the appearance of the cell-sparse, fiber-rich subplate zone situated below the cortical plate. This transient embryonic zone in the human fetus is particularly wide in the regions subjacent to the association areas (Kostovic and Rakic, 1990). The third stage corresponds roughly to the level of development achieved in the monkey between E59 and E64.

Stage IV. Secondary condensation (from the 13th to the 15th fetal week). During this period of gestation, the ventricular zone becomes progressively thinner while the subventricular zone remains relatively wide (figure 3.6). The cortical plate again becomes homogeneous in appearance and resembles, in a sense, a thickened version of stage II. The reason for this change may be that, in stage IV, most of the young neurons in the cortex become considerably larger as they differentiate, while relatively few new immature neurons enter the cortical plate. The result is a more uniform appearance. At the end of this stage, an accumulation of large cells appears below the cortical plate, and the subplate zone enlarges further (Kostovic and Rakic, 1990). Depending on the cortical region, this stage appears in the monkey between E64 and E75.

Stage V. Prolonged stage of cortical maturation (from the 16th fetal week and continuing well into the postnatal period). Morphological data are inadequate to determine for how long, or how many, neurons continue to migrate to the human neocortex after 16 weeks, and hence the line at the right side of the curve in figure 3.6 is dotted. By the fifth month, relatively few neuronal precursors seem to be proliferating in the reduced ventricular zone of the human cerebral hemispheres. However, interneurons, which continue to be generated in the subventricular zone and ganglionic eminence, are still being added to the cortex between the 20th and 25th week of gestation (Letinic, Zoncu, and Rakic, 2002), followed by a massive wave of gliogenesis (Badsberg Samuelsen et al., 2003). A comparison of the autoradiographic results in the monkey (Rakic, 1974, 1977) with comparable stages in the human (Rakic and Sidman, 1968; Marin-Padilla, 1988; Kostovic and Rakic, 1990) indicates that most neurons of the human neocortex are generated

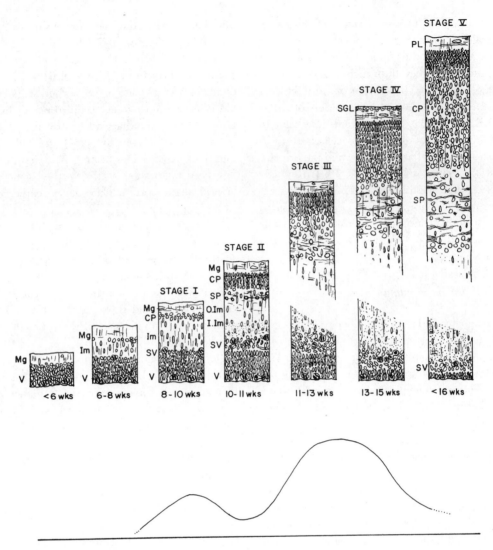

FIGURE 3.6 Semidiagrammatic drawings of the human cerebral wall at various gestational ages listed in fetal weeks below each column. The stages refer specifically to an arbitrarily chosen cortical area situated midway along the lateral surface of the hemisphere (detailed in Sidman and Rakic, 1982). In addition, the subplate zone, situated below the cortical plate, appears in the last three stages (Kostovic and Rakic, 1990). Because there is a gradient of maturation, as many as three of five stages of cortical development may be observed in different regions of the neocortex in the same fetal brain. In the three columns on the right, the inter-mediate zone is not drawn in full because the thickness of the cerebral wall has increased markedly compared with earlier stages and cannot fit into the drawing. The curve below the drawing schematically indicates waves of cell migration to the neocortex, assessed by the density of migrating neurons in the intermediate zone. Abbreviations: CP, cortical plate; Im, intermediate zone; I.Im and 0.Im, inner and outer intermediate zones, respectively; MG, marginal zone; PL, plexiform layer; SGL, subpial granular layer; SP, subplate zone; SV, subventricular zone; V, ventricular zone; wks, age in fetal weeks. (Reprinted from Rakic, 1988b, by permission.)

before the beginning of the third trimester of gestation. Toward term, the ventricular zone disappears, the subplate zone dissolves, and, as the intermediate zone transforms into the white matter, only a vestige of the subplate cells remains as interstitial neurons (Kostovic and Rakic, 1980). It should be emphasized that during as well after completion of neurogenesis, glial cells are generated and migrate across the cerebral wall (Badsberg Samuelsen et al., 2003). The stage of gliogenesis is particularly pronounced in the human forebrain, where glial cells, including oligos, outnumber neurons by severalfold. After all cortical neurons have been gener-ated and have attained their final positions, their differentiation, including the formation of synapses, proceeds for a long time, reaching a peak only during the second postnatal year. The subject of synaptogenesis in the cerebral cortex of both macaque monkey and human was reviewed in the second edition of this volume (Bourgeois, Goldman-Rakic, and Rakic, 2000), and not much new reseach has been done in this area since.

ACKNOWLEDGMENTS This work was supported by U.S. Public Health Service.

REFERENCES

AGMON, A. A., L. T. YANG, E. G. JONES, and D. K. DOWD, 1995. Topological precision in the thalamic projection to the neonatal mouse. *J. Neurosci.* 13:5365–5382.

AKLIN, S. E., and D. VAN DER KOOY, 1993. Clonal heterogeneity in the germinal zone of the developing telencephalon. *Development* 118:175–192.

ALGAN, O., and P. RAKIC, 1997. Radiation-induced area- and lamina-specific deletion of neurons in the primate visual cortex. *J. Comp. Neurol.* 381:335–352.

ANG, E. S. B. C., Jr., T. F. HAYDAR, V. GLUNCIC, and P. RAKIC, 2003. Areal- and laminar-specific distribution of GABAergic interneurons: Time-lapse multiphoton analysis in the embryonic mouse cortex. *J. Neurosci.* 23:5805–5815.

ANGEVINE, L. B., and R. L. SIDMAN, 1961. Autoradiographic study of cell migration during histogenesis of cerebral cortex in the mouse. *Nature* 192:766–768.

ANTON, S. A., R. S. CAMERON, and P. RAKIC, 1996. Role of neuron-glial junctional proteins in the maintenance and termination of neuronal migration across the embryonic cerebral wall. *J. Neurosci.* 16:2283–2293.

ARIMATSU, Y., M. MIYAMOTO, I. NIHONMATSU, K. HIRATA, Y. URATAINI, Y. HATANKA, and K. TAKIGUCHI-HOYASH, 1992. Early regional specification for a molecular neuronal phenotype in the rat neocortex. *Proc. Natl. Acad. Sci. U.S.A.* 89:8879–8883.

BADSBERG SAMUELSEN, G., K. BONDE LARSEN, N. BOGDANOVIC, H. LAURSEN, N. GREAM, J. F. LARSEN, and B. PAKKENBERG, 2003. The changing number of cells in the human fetal forebrain and its subdivisions: A stereological analysis. *Cereb. Cortex* 13:115–122.

BISHOP, K. M., G. GOUDREAU, and D. D. O'LEARY, 2000. Regulation of area identity in the mammalian neocortex by Emx2 and Pax6. *Science* 288:344–349.

BOULDER COMMITTEE, 1970. Embryonic vertebrate central nervous system: Revised terminology. *Anat. Rec.* 166:257–261.

BOURGEOIS, J. P., P. S. GOLDMAN-RAKIC, and P. RAKIC, 2000. Formation, elimination and stabilization of synapses in the primate cerebral cortex. In *Cognitive Neuroscience: A Handbook for the Field*, 2nd ed., M. S. Gazzaniga, ed. Cambridge, Mass.: MIT Press, pp. 23–32.

BUFFONE, A., H. J. KIM, L. PUELLES, M. H. PROTEUS, M. A. FROHMAN, G. R. MARTIN, and J. L. R. RUBINSTEIN, 1993. The mouse DLX-2 (Tes-1) Gbx-2 and Wnt-3 in the embryonic day 12.5 mouse forebrain defines potential transverse and longitudinal segmental boundaries. *Mech. Dev.* 40:129–140.

BUGBEE, N. M., and P. S. GOLDMAN-RAKIC, 1983. Columnar organization of cortico-cortical projections in squirrel and rhesus monkeys: Similarity of column width in species differing in cortical volume. *J. Comp. Neurol.* 220:355–364.

CAMERON, R. S., and P. RAKIC, 1991. Glial cell lineage in the cerebral cortex: Review and synthesis. *Glia* 4:124–137.

CAMERON, R. S., and P. RAKIC, 1994. Polypeptides that comprise the plasmalemmal microdomain between migrating neuronal and glial cells. *J. Neurosci.* 14:3139–3155.

CATALANO, S. M., R. T. ROBERTSON, and H. P. KILLACKEY, 1996. Individual axon morphology and thalamocortical topography in developing rat somatosensory cortex. *J. Comp. Neurol.* 366:36–53.

CAVINESS, V. S., Jr., and P. RAKIC, 1978. Mechanisms of cortical development: A view from mutations in mice. *Annu. Rev. Neurosci.* 1:297–326.

CHALUPA, L. M., and C. J. WEFERS, 2000. A comparative perspective on the formation of retinal connections in the mammalian brain. In *Cognitive Neuroscience: A Handbook for the Field*, 2nd ed., M. S. Gazzaniga, ed. Cambridge, Mass.: MIT Press, pp. 33–43.

CHENN, A., and C. A. WALSH, 2002. Regulation of cerebral cortical size by control of cell cycle exit in neural precursors. *Science* 297:365–369.

CHENN, A., and C. A. WALSH, 2003. Increased neuronal production, enlarged forebrains, and cytoarchitectural distortions in beta catenin overexpressing transgenic mice. *Cereb. Cortex* 13:599–606.

CHUN, J. M., and C. J. SHATZ, 1989. Interstitial cells of the adult neocortical white matter are the remnant of the early-generated subplate neuron population. *J. Comp. Neurol.* 282:555–569.

COHEN-TANNOUDJI, M., C. BABINET, and M. WASSEF, 1994. Early intrinsic regional specification of the mouse somatosensory cortex. *Nature* 368:460–463.

CONEL, J. L., 1939. *The Postnatal Development of the Human Cerebral Cortex: I. The Cortex of the Newborn.* Cambridge, Mass.: Harvard University Press.

CREUTZFELDT, O. D., 1977. Generality of the functional structure of the neocortex. *Naturwissenschaften* 64:507–517.

CROWLEY, J. C., and L. C. KATZ, 2000. Early development of ocular dominance columns. *Science* 290:1321–1324.

DE CARLOS, J. A., L. LÓPEZ-MASCARAQUE, and F. VALVERDE, 1996. Dynamics of cell migration from the lateral ganglionic eminence in the rat. *J. Neurosci.* 16:6146–6156.

DE CARLOS, J. A., and D. D. M. O'LEARY, 1992. Growth and targeting of subplate axons and establishment of major cortical pathways. *J. Neurosci.* 12:1194–1211.

DES PORTES, V., J. M. PINARD, P. BILLUART, M. C. VINET, A. KOULAKOFF, A. CARRIE, A. GELOT, E. DUPUIS, J. MOTTE, Y. BERWALD-NETTER, M. CATALA, A. KAHN, C. BELDJORD, and J. CHELLY, 1998. A novel CNS gene required for neuronal migration and involved in X-linked subcortical laminar heterotopia and lissencephaly syndrome. *Cell* 92:51–61.

DEAZEVEDO, L. C., C. FALLET, V. MOURA-NETO, C. DAUMAS-DUPORT, C. HEDIN-PEREIRA, and R. LENT, 2003. Cortical radial glial cells in human fetuses: Depth-correlated transformation into astrocytes. *J. Neurobiol.* 55:288–298.

DEHAY, C., P. GIROUD, M. BERLAND, I. SMART, and H. KENNEDY, 1993. Modulation of the cell cycle contributes to the parcellation of the primate visual cortex. *Nature* 366:464–466.

DONOGHUE, M. J., and P. RAKIC, 1999. Molecular evidence for the early specification of presumptive functional domains in the embryonic primate cerebral cortex. *J. Neurosci.* 19:5967–5979.

ECCLES, J. C., 1984. The cerebral neocortex: A theory of its operation. In *Cerebral Cortex* (vol. 2), E. G. Jones and A. Peters, eds. New York: Plenum Press, pp. 1–36.

ELLIS, R. E., and H. R. HORVITZ, 1991. Two *C. elegans* genes control the programmed deaths of specific cells in the pharynx. *Development* 112:591–603.

EMERLING, D. E., and A. D. LANDER, 1994. Laminar specific attachment and neurite outgrowth of thalamic neurons on cultured slices of developing cerebral cortex. *Development* 120:2811–2822.

FENG, Y., and C. A. WALSH, 2001. Protein-protein interactions, cytoskeletal regulation and neuronal migration. *Nat. Rev. Neurosci.* 2:408–416.

FERRI, R. T., and P. LEVITT, 1993. Cerebral cortical progenitors are fated to produce region-specific neuronal populations. *Cereb. Cortex* 3(3):187–198.

FISHELL, G., and A. R. KRIEGSTEIN, 2003. Neurons from radial glia: The consequences of asymmetric inheritance. *Curr. Opin. Neurobiol.* 13:34–41.

FRANTZ, G. D., A. P. BOHNER, R. M. AKERS, and S. K. MCCONNELL, 1994. Regulation of the POU domain gene SCIP during cerebral cortical development. *J. Neurosci.* 14:472–485.

FUKUCHI-SHIMOGORI, T., and E. A. GROVE, 2001. Neocortex patterning by the secreted signaling molecule FGF8. *Science* 294:1071–1074.

GLEESON, J. G., K. M. ALLEN, J. W. FOX, E. D. LAMPERTI, S. BERKOVIC, I. SCHEFFER, E. C. COOPER, W. B. DOBYNS, S. R. MINNERATH, M. E. ROSS, and C. A. WALSH, 1998. Doublecortin, a brain-specific gene mutated in human X-linked lissencephaly and double cortex syndrome, encodes a putative signaling protein. *Cell* 92:63–72.

GLEESON, J. G., P. T. LIN, L. A. FLANAGAN, and C. A. WALSH, 1999. Doublecortin is a microtubule-associated protein and is expressed widely by migrating neurons. *Neuron* 23:257–271.

GLUCKSMANN, A., 1951. Cell deaths in normal vertebrate ontogeny. *Biol. Rev.* 26:59–86.

GOLDMAN-RAKIC, P. S., 1987. Circuitry of primate prefrontal cortex and regulation of behavior by representational memory. In *Handbook of Physiology*, F. Plum and V. Mountcastle, eds. Bethesda, Md.: American Physiology Society, pp. 373–417.

GOLDMAN-RAKIC, P. S., and P. RAKIC, 1984. Experimental modification of gyral patterns. In *Cerebral Dominance: The Biological Foundation*, N. Geschwind and A. M. Galaburda, eds. Cambridge, Mass.: Harvard University Press, pp. 179–192.

HARTFUSS, E., R. GALLI, N. HEINS, and M. GOTZ, 2001. Characterization of CNS precursor subtypes and radial glia. *Dev. Biol.* 229:15–30.

HATTEN, M. E., 2002. Neuroscience: New directions in neuronal migration. *Science* 297:1660–1663.

HATTEN, M. E., and C. A. MASON, 1990. Mechanism of glial-guided neuronal migration *in vitro* and *in vivo*. *Experientia* 46:907–916.

HATTORI, M., H. ADACHI, M. TSUJIMOTO, H. ARAI, and K. INOUE, 1994. Miller-Dieker lissencephaly gene encodes a subunit of brain platelet-activating factor acetylhydrolase. *Nature* 370(6486):216–218.

HAYDAR, T. F., C.-Y. KUAN, R. A. FLAVELL, and P. RAKIC, 1999. The role of cell death in regulating the size and shape of the mammalian forebrain. *Cereb. Cortex* 9:621–626.

HAYDAR, T. F., E. S. B. C. ANG, JR., and P. RAKIC, 2003. Mitotic spindle rotation and mode of cell division in the developing telencephalon. *Proc. Natl. Acad. Sci. U.S.A.* 100:2890–2895.

HE, W., C. INGRAHAM, L. RISING, S. GODERIE, and S. TEMPLE, 2001. Multipotent stem cells from the mouse basal forebrain contribute GABAergic neurons and oligodendrocytes to the cerebral cortex during embryogenesis. *J. Neurosci.* 21:8854–8862.

HEBB, D. O., 1949. *The Organization of Behavior.* New York: Wiley.

HIS, W., 1874. *Unserer Körperform und das Physiologische Problem ihrer Enstehung.* Leipzig: Engelman.

HIS, W., 1904. *Die Entwicklung des Menschlichen Gehirns während der ersten Monate.* Leipzig: Hirzel.

KAISERMAN-ABRAMOFF, I. R., A. M. GRAYBIEL, and W. J. H. NAUTA, 1980. The thalamic projection to cortical area 17 in a congenitally anophthalmic mouse strain. *Neuroscience* 5:41–52.

KANOLD, P. O., P. KARA, R. C. REID, and C. J. SHATZ, 2003. Role of subplate neurons in functional maturation of visual cortical columns. *Science* 301:521–525.

KENNEDY, H., and C. DEHAY, 1993. Cortical specification of mice and men. *Cereb. Cortex* 3:171–186.

KOKETSU, D., A. MIKAMI, Y. MIYAMOTO, and T. HISATSUNE, 2003. Non-renewal of neurons in the cerebral neocortex of adult macaque monkeys. *J. Neurosci.* 23:937–942.

KOMURO, H., and P. RAKIC, 1992. Specific role of N-type calcium channels in neuronal migration. *Science* 257:806–809.

KOMURO, H., and P. RAKIC, 1993. Modulation of neuronal migration by NMDA receptors. *Science* 260:95–97.

KOMURO, H., and P. RAKIC, 1996. Calcium oscillations provide signals for the saltatory movement of CNS neurons. *Neuron* 17:257–285.

KORNACK, D. R., and P. RAKIC, 1995. Radial and horizontal deployment of clonally related cells in the primate neocortex: Relationship to distinct mitotic lineages. *Neuron* 15:311–321.

KORNACK, R. D., and P. RAKIC, 1999. Continuation of neurogenesis in the hippocampus of the adult macaque monkey. *Proc. Natl. Acad. Sci. U.S.A.* 96:5768–5773.

KORNACK, R. D., and P. RAKIC, 2001a. The generation, migration and differentiation of olfactory neurons in adult primate brain. *Proc. Natl. Acad. Sci. U.S.A.* 98:4752–4757.

KORNACK, R. D., and P. RAKIC, 2001b. Cell proliferation without neurogenesis in the adult primate neocortex. *Science* 294:2127–2130.

KOSTOVIC, I., and P. S. GOLDMAN-RAKIC, 1983. Transient cholinesterase staining in the mediodorsal nucleus of the thalamus and its connections in the developing human and monkey brain. *J. Comp. Neurol.* 219:431–447.

KOSTOVIC, I., and M. E. MOLLIVER, 1974. A new interpretation of the laminar development of cerebral cortex: Synaptogenesis in different layers of neopalium in the human fetus. *Anat. Rec.* 178:395.

KOSTOVIC, I., and P. RAKIC, 1980. Cytology and time of origin of interstitial neurons in the white matter in infant and adult human and monkey telencephalon. *J. Neurocytol.* 9:219–242.

KOSTOVIC, I., and P. RAKIC, 1984. Development of prestriate visual projections in the monkey and human fetal cerebrum revealed by transient acetylcholinesterase staining. *J. Neurosci.* 4:25–42.

KOSTOVIC, I., and P. RAKIC, 1990. Developmental history of transient subplate zone in the visual and somatosensory cortex of the macaque monkey and human brain. *J. Comp. Neurol.* 297:441–470.

KUAN, C., E. ELLIOT, R. FLAVELL, and P. RAKIC, 1997. Restrictive clonal allocation in the chimeric mouse brain. *Proc. Natl. Acad. Sci. U.S.A.* 94:3374–3379.

KUIDA, K., T. F. HAYDAR, C. KUAN, G. YONG, C. TAYA, H. KARASUYAMA, M. S.-S. SU, P. RAKIC, and R. A. FLAVELL, 1998. Reduced apoptosis and cytochrome c-mediated caspase activation in mice lacking Caspase-9. *Cell* 94:325–337.

KUIDA, K., T. S. ZHENG, S. NA, C. KUANG, D. YAN, H. KARASUYAMA, P. RAKIC, and R. A. FLAVELL, 1996. Decreased apoptosis in the brain and premature lethality in CPP32-deficient mice. *Nature* 384:368–372.

KULJIS, R. O., and P. RAKIC, 1990. Hypercolumns in the monkey visual cortex can develop in the absence of cues from photoreceptors. *Proc. Natl. Acad. Sci. U.S.A.* 87:5303–5306.

LAVDAS, A. A., M. GRIGORIOU, V. PACHNIS, and J. G. PARNAVELAS, 1999. The medial ganglionic eminence gives rise to a population of early neurons in the developing cerebral cortex. *J. Neurosci.* 19:7881–7888.

LAYWELL, E. D., P. RAKIC, V. G. KUKEKOV, E. HOLLAND, and D. STEINDLER, 2000. An identification of a multipotent astrocytic stem cell in the immature and adult mouse brain. *Proc. Natl. Acad. Sci. U.S.A.* 97:13883–13888.

LETINIC, K., and P. RAKIC, 2001. Telencephalic origin of human thalamic GABAergic neurons. *Nat. Neurosci.* 4:931–936.

LETINIC, K., R. ZONCU, and P. RAKIC, 2002. Origin of GABAergic neurons in the human neocortex. *Nature* 417:645–649.

LEVITT, P., 2000. Molecular determinants of the forebrain and cerebral cortex. In *Cognitive Neuroscience: A Handbook for the Field*, 2nd ed., M. S. Gazzaniga, ed. Cambridge, Mass.: MIT Press, pp. 23–32.

LEVITT, P., M. F. BARBE, and K. L. EAGLESON, 1997. Patterning and specification of the cerebral cortex. *Anno. Rev. Neurobiol.* 20:1–24.

LEVITT, P., M. L. COOPER, and P. RAKIC, 1981. Coexistence of neuronal and glial precursor cells in the cerebral ventricular zone of the fetal monkey: An ultrastructural immunoperoxidase analysis. *J. Neurosci.* 1:27–39.

LI, M., M. R. SARKISIAN, W. Z. MEHAL, P. RAKIC, and R. A. FLAVELL, 2003. Phosphatidylserine receptor is required for clearance of apoptotic cells. *Science* 302:1560–1563.

LIDOW, M. S., and P. RAKIC, 1992. Postnatal development of monoaminergic neurotransmitter receptors with primate neocortex. *Cereb. Cortex* 2:401–415.

LIDOW, M. S., and P. RAKIC, 1994. Unique profiles of $\alpha 1$-, $\alpha 2$-, and β-adrenergic receptors in the developing cortical plate and transient embryonic zones of the rhesus monkey. *J. Neurosci.* 14:4064–4078.

LOIS, C., and A. ALVAREZ-BUYLLA, 1994. Long-distance neuronal migration in the adult mammalian brain. *Science* 264:1145–1148.

LOTURCO, J. J., D. F. OWENS, M. J. S. HEATH, M. B. E. DAVIS, and A. R. KRIEGSTEIN, 1995. GABA and glutamate depolarize cortical progenitor cells and inhibit DNA synthesis. *Neuron* 15:1287–1298.

LU, S., L. D. BOGORAD, M. T. MURTHA, and F. RUDDLE, 1992. Expression pattern of a marine homeobox gene, Dbx, displays extreme spatial restriction in embryonic forebrain and spinal cord. *Proc. Natl. Acad. Sci. U.S.A.* 89:8053–8057.

LUSKIN, M. B., A. L. PEARLMAN, and J. R. SANES, 1988. Cell lineage in the cerebral cortex of the mouse studied in vivo and in vitro with a recombinant retrovirus. *Neuron* 1:635–647.

LUSKIN, M. B., and C. J. SHATZ, 1985. Studies of the earliest generated cells of the cat's visual cortex: Cogeneration of subplate and marginal zones. *J. Neurosci.* 5:1062–1075.

MALATESTA, P., M. A. HACK, E. HARTFUSS, H. KETTENMANN, W. KLINKERT, F. KIRCHOFF, and M. GOTZ, 2003. Neuronal or glial progeny: Regional differences in radial glia fate. *Neuron* 37:751–764.

MALATESTA, P., E. HARTFUSS, and M. GOTZ, 2000. Isolation of radial glial cells by fluorescent-activated cell sorting reveals a neuronal lineage. *Development* 127:5253–5263.

MARIN, O., and J. L. RUBENSTEIN, 2001. A long, remarkable journey: Tangential migration in the telencephalon. *Nat. Rev. Neurosci.* 2:780–790.

MARIN-PADILLA, M., 1988. Early ontogenesis of the human cerebral cortex. In *Cerebral Cortex: Development and Maturation of Cerebral Cortex*, A. Peters and E. G. Jones, eds. New York: Plenum Press, pp. 1–34.

McCONNELL, S. K., 1988. Development and decision-making in the mammalian cerebral cortex. *Brain Res. Dev.* 13:1–23.

McCONNELL, S. K., A. GHOSH, and C. J. SHATZ, 1994. Subplate pioneers and the formation of descending connections from cerebral cortex. *J. Neurosci.* 14:1892–1907.

McCONNELL, S. K., and C. E. KASANOWSKI, 1991. Cell cycle dependence of laminar determination in developing cerebral cortex. *Science* 254:282–285.

MEISSIREL, C., K. C. WIKLER, L. M. CHALUPA, and P. RAKIC, 1997. Early divergence of M and P visual subsystems in the embryonic primate brain. *Proc. Natl. Acad. Sci. U.S.A.* 94:5900–5905.

MENEZES, J. R. L., and M. B. LUSKIN, 1994. Expression of neuron-specific tubulin defines a novel population in the proliferative layers of the developing telencephalon. *J. Neurosci.* 14:5399–5416.

MIYASHITA-LIN, E. M., R. HEVNER, K. MONTZKA WASSARMAN, S. MARTINEZ, and J. L. R. RUBENSTEIN, 1999. Early neocortical regionalization in the absence of thalamic innervation. *Science* 285:906–909.

MOLLIVER, M. E., I. KOSTOVIC, and H. VAN DER LOOS, 1973. The development of synapses in cerebral cortex of the human fetus. *Brain Res.* 50:403–407.

MOUNTCASTLE, V., 1995. The evolution of ideas concerning the function of the neocortex. *Cereb. Cortex* 5:289–295.

MOUNTCASTLE, V. B., 1997. The columnar organization of the neocortex. *Brain* 120:701–722.

NADARAJAH, B., P. ALIFRAGIS, R. O. L. WANG, and J. G. PARNAVELAS, 2003. Neuronal migration in the developing cerebral cortex: Observations based on real-time imaging. *Cereb. Cortex* 13:607–611.

NAKATSUJI, M., Y. KADOKAWA, and H. SUEMORI, 1991. Radial columnar patches in the chimeric cerebral cortex visualized by use of mouse embryonic stem cells expressing β-galactosidase. *Dev. Growth Differ.* 33:571–578.

NOCTOR, S. C., A. C. FLINT, T. A. WEISMANN, R. S. DAMMERMAN, and A. R. KRIEGSTEIN, 2001. Neurons derived from radial glial cells establish radial units in neocortex. *Nature* 409:714–720.

NOCTOR, S. C., A. C. FLINT, T. A. WEISMANN, W. S. WONG, B. K. CLINTON, and A. R. KRIEGSTEIN, 2002. Dividing precursor cells of the embryonic ventricular zone have morphological and molecular characteristics of radial glia. *J. Neurosci.* 22:3161–3173.

OLIVARIA, J., and R. C. VAN SLUYTERS, 1984. Callosal connections of the posterior neocortex in normal-eyed, congenitally anophthalmic and neonatally enucleated mice. *J. Comp. Neurol.* 230:249–268.

OPPENHEIM, R. W., 1991. Cell death during development of the nervous system. *Annu. Rev. Neurosci.* 14:453–501.

PARNAVELAS, J. G., J. A. BARFIELD, E. FRANKE, and M. B. LUSKIN, 1991. Separate progenitor cells give rise to pyramidal and nonpyramidal neurons in the rat telencephalon. *Cereb. Cortex* 1:463–491.

POLIAKOV, G. I., 1959. Progressive neuron differentiation of the human cerebral cortex in ontogenesis. In *Development of the Central Nervous System*, S. A. Sarkisov and S. N. Preobrazenskaya, eds. Moscow: Medgiz, pp. 11–26 (in Russian).

POLIAKOV, G. I., 1965. Development of the cerebral neocortex during the first half of intrauterine life. In *Development of the Child's Brain*, S. A. Sarkisov, ed. Leningrad: Medicinam, pp. 22–52 (in Russian).

PROTEUS, M. H., E. J. BRICE, A. BUFFONE, T. B. USDIN, R. D. CIARANELLO, and J. R. RUBINSTEIN, 1991. Isolation and characterization of a library of cDNA clones that are preferentially expressed in the embryonic telencephalon. *Neuron* 7:221.

RAKIC, P., 1972. Mode of cell migration to the superficial layers of fetal monkey neocortex. *J. Comp. Neurol.* 145:61–84.

RAKIC, P., 1973. Kinetics of proliferation and latency between final cell division and onset of differentiation of cerebellar stellate and basket neurons. *J. Comp. Neurol.* 147:523–546.

RAKIC, P., 1974. Neurons in the monkey visual cortex: Systematic relation between time of origin and eventual disposition. *Science* 183:425–427.

RAKIC, P., 1976a. Prenatal genesis of connections subserving ocular dominance in the rhesus monkey. *Nature* 261:467–471.

RAKIC, P., 1976b. Differences in the time of origin and in eventual distribution of neurons in areas 17 and 18 of the visual cortex in the rhesus monkey. *Exp. Brain Res. Suppl.* 1:244–248.

RAKIC, P., 1977. Prenatal development of the visual system in the rhesus monkey. *Philos. Trans. R. Soc. London [Biol]* 278:245–260.

RAKIC, P., 1978. Neuronal migration and contact interaction in primate telencephalon. *J. Postgrad. Med.* 54:25–40.

RAKIC, P., 1981. Neuron-glial interaction during brain development. *Trends Neurosci.* 4:184–187.

RAKIC, P., 1985. Limits of neurogenesis in primates. *Science* 227:154–156.

RAKIC, P., 1988a. Specification of cerebral cortical areas. *Science* 241:170–176.

RAKIC, P., 1988b. Defects of neuronal migration and pathogenesis of cortical malformations. *Prog. Brain Res.* 73:15–37.

RAKIC, P., 1990. Principles of neuronal cell migration. *Experientia* 46:882–891.

RAKIC, P., 1995a. Radial versus tangential migration of neuronal clones in the developing cerebral cortex *Proc. Natl. Acad. Sci. U.S.A.* 92:11323–11327.

RAKIC, P., 1995b. A small step for the cell—a giant leap for mankind: A hypothesis of neocortical expansion during evolution. *Trends Neurosci.* 18:383–388.

RAKIC, P., 1997. Intra- and extracellular control of neuronal migration: Relevance to cortical malformations. In *Normal and Abnormal Development of the Cortex*, M. Galaburda and Y. Christen, eds. *Research and Perspectives in Neurosciences.* New York: Springer-Verlag, pp. 81–89.

RAKIC, P., 2000. Advantages of the mouse model: From spontaneous to induced mutations. In *The Mouse Brain Development*, A. Goffinet and P. Rakic, eds. New York: Springer-Verlag, pp. 1–19.

RAKIC, P., 2002. Neurogenesis in adult primate neocortex: An evaluation of the evidence. *Nat. Rev. Neurosci.* 3:65–71.

RAKIC, P., 2003. Elusive radial glial cells: Historical and evolutionary perspective. *Glia* 43:19–32.

RAKIC, P., R. S. CAMERON, and H. KOMURO, 1994. Recognition, adhesion, transmembrane signaling, and cell motility in guided neuronal migration. *Curr. Opin. Neurobiol.* 4:63–69.

RAKIC, P., E. KNYIHAR-CSILLIK, and B. CSILLIK, 1996. Polarity of microtubule assembly during neuronal migration. *Proc. Natl. Acad. Sci. U.S.A.* 93:9218–9222.

RAKIC, P., and H. KOMURO, 1995. The role of receptor-channel activity during neuronal cell migration. *J. Neurobiol.* 26:299–315.

RAKIC, P., and M. LIDOW, 1995. Distribution and density of neurotransmitter receptors in the absence of retinal input from early embryonic stages. *J. Neurosci.* 15:2561–2574.

RAKIC, P., and R. S. NOWAKOWSKI, 1981. Time of origin of neurons in the hippocampal region of the rhesus monkey. *J. Comp. Neurol.* 196:99–124.

RAKIC, P., and K. P. RILEY, 1983a. Overproduction and elimination of retinal axons in the fetal rhesus monkey. *Science* 209:1441–1444.

RAKIC, P., and K. P. RILEY, 1983b. Regulation of axon numbers in the primate optic nerve by prenatal binocular competition. *Nature* 305:135–137.

RAKIC, P., and R. L. SIDMAN, 1968. Supravital DNA synthesis in the developing human and mouse brain. *J. Neuropathol. Exp. Neurol.* 27:246–276.

RAKIC, P., and W. SINGER, 1988. *Neurobiology of the Neocortex.* New York: John Wiley & Sons.

RAKIC, P., L. J. STENSAAS, and E. P. SAYRE, 1974. Computer-aided three-dimensional reconstruction and quantitative analysis of cells from serial electronmicroscopic montages of fetal monkey brain. *Nature* 250:31–34.

RAKIC, P., I. SUNER, and R. W. WILLIAMS, 1991. Novel cytoarchitectonic areas induced experimentally within primate striate cortex. *Proc. Natl. Acad. Sci. U.S.A.* 88:2083–2987.

REID, C., I. LIANG, and C. WALSH, 1995. Systematic widespread clonal organization in cerebral cortex. *Neuron* 15:299–310.

RICHARDS, L. J., D. E. KOESTER, R. TUTTLE, and D. D. M. O'LEARY, 1997. Directed growth of early cortical axons is influenced by a chemoattractant released from an intermediate target. *J. Neurosci.* 17:2445–2458.

RUBENSTEIN, J. L. R., and P. RAKIC, 1999. Genetic control of cortical development. *Cereb. Cortex* 9:521–523.

SANES, J. R., 1989. Analyzing cell lineages with a recombinant retrovirus. *Trends Neurosci.* 12:21–28.

SCHMECHEL, D. E., and P. RAKIC, 1979. Arrested proliferation of radial glial cells during midgestation in rhesus monkey. *Nature* 227:303–305.

SCHWARTZ, M. L., P. RAKIC, and P. S. GOLDMAN-RAKIC, 1991. Early phenotype of cortical neurons: Evidence that a subclass of migrating neurons have callosal axons. *Proc. Natl. Acad. Sci. U.S.A.* 88:1354–1358.

SESTAN, N., P. RAKIC, and M. J. DONOGHUE, 2001. Independent parcellation of the embryonic visual cortex and thalamus revealed by combinatorial *Eph/ephrine* gene expression. *Curr. Biol.* 11:39–43.

SIDMAN, R. L., and P. RAKIC, 1973. Neuronal migration with special reference to developing human brain: A review. *Brain Res.* 62:1–35.

SIDMAN, R. L., and P. RAKIC, 1982. Development of the human central nervous system. In *Histology and Histopathology of the Nervous System*, W. Haymaker and R. D. Adams, eds. Springfield, Ill.: Charles C Thomas, pp. 3–145.

SORIANO, E., N. DUMESNIL, C. AULADELL, M. COHEN-TANNOUDJI, and C. SOTELO, 1995. Molecular heterogeneity of progenitors and radial migration in the developing cerebral cortex revealed by transgenic expression. *Proc. Natl. Acad. Sci. U.S.A.* 92:11676–11680.

SZENTAGOTHAI, J., 1987. The neuronal network of the cerebral cortex: A functional interpretation. *Prog. Brain Res.* 201:219–248.

TAMAMAKI, N., K. NAKAMURA, K. OKAMOTO, and T. KANEKO, 2001. Radial glia is a progenitor of neocortical neurons in the developing cerebral cortex. *Neurosci. Res.* 41:51–60.

TAN, S.-S., M. KALLONIATIS, K. STURM, P. P. L. TAM, B. E. REESE, and B. FAULKNER-JONES, 1998. Separate progenitors for radial and tangential cell dispersion during development of the cerebral neocortex. *Neuron* 21:295–304.

TRAMONTIN, A. D., J. M. GARCIA-VERDUGO, D. A. LIM, and A. ALVAREZ-BUYLLA, 2003. Postnatal development of radial glia and the ventricular zone (VZ): A continuum of the neural stem cell compartment. *Cereb. Cortex* 13:580–587.

VERHAGE, M., A. S. MAIA, J. J. PLOMP, A. B. BRUSSAARD, J. H. HEEROMA, H. VERMEER, R. F. TOONEN, R. E. HAMMER, T. K. VAN DEN BERG, M. MISSLER, H. J. GEUZE, and T. C. SUDHOF, 2000.

Synaptic assembly of the brain in the absence of neurotransmitter secretion. *Science* 287:864–869.

WILLIAMS, B. P., and J. PRICE, 1995. Evidence for multiple precursor cell types in the embryonic rat cerebral cortex. *Neuron* 14:1181–1188.

WILLIAMS, R. W., and K. HERRUP, 1988. Control of neuron number. *Annu. Rev. Neurosci.* 278:344–352.

ZECEVIC, N., 1998. Synaptogenesis in layer I of the human cerebral cortex in the first half of gestation. *Cereb. Cortex* 8:245–252.

ZECEVIC, N., and P. RAKIC, 2001. Development of layer I neurons in the primate cerebral cortex *J. Neurosci.* 21:5607–5619.

ZHONG, W., J. N. FEDER, M.-M. JIANG, L. Y. JAN, and Y. N. JAN, 1996. Asymmetric localization of a mammalian Numb homolog during mouse cortical neurogenesis. *Neuron* 17:43–53.

4 Neuronal Migration in the Brain

GUOFA LIU AND YI RAO

ABSTRACT Neuronal migration occurs in both developing and adult animals and is important in the formation, maintenance, and plasticity of the nervous system. Genetic defects in neuronal migration cause human diseases. Molecular studies have uncovered diffusible attractive and repulsive cues guiding the direction of radial and tangential migration. Intracellular pathways transduce extracellular signals through small GTPases to the cytoskeleton. Mechanisms for spatial control of neuronal migration are conserved with those for other somatic cells. Temporal control of neuronal migration is linked to spatial control through strategic positioning of spatial cues and changes in responsiveness to the cues. Neuronal migration and newly generated neurons may also play roles in sensory processing and behavioral plasticity.

Neuronal precursors in the brain have to migrate from their birthplace to sites of final residence and functioning. Proper neuronal migration is essential for the formation and normal functioning of the nervous system. The idea of neuronal migration was proposed after histological examinations of the neocortex by early embryologists, including Kolliker, His, Vignal, and Ramon y Cajal (reviewed in Hardesty, 1904; Cajal, 1911; Rakic, 1971, 1972; Bentivoglio and Mazzarello, 1999). However, there was a longstanding debate as to whether neurons actively migrated, because it was possible that neurons formed earlier were simply displaced by later-forming neurons (e.g., Tilney, 1933). In the spinal cord of chick embryos, Levi-Montalcini has shown that a subpopulation of neurons change their positions in a direction opposite to that expected from passive displacement, indicating that at least some neurons have to migrate actively (Levi-Montalcini, 1950). A convincing demonstration of active neuronal migration was obtained by Angevine and Sidman (1961) when they and others used autoradiographic tracing in the cerebrum of rodent embryos to reveal that newly formed neurons in the cortex are positioned in more superficial layers, thus leading to an inside-out sequence of neuronal positioning. This pattern is consistent with active neuronal migration and rules out passive displacement (Angevine and Sidman, 1961; Berry and Rogers, 1965; Hicks and D'Amato, 1968; Hinds, 1968; Rakic, 1971, 1972).

Reconstruction of electron microscopic examination of cerebellar and cerebral sections over different developmental stages led to the proposal of neuronal migration along the radially aligned glia cells (Rakic, 1971, 1972). Direct observations of neuronal migration in in vitro cultures of primary neurons and glia proved that neuronal cell bodies could actively migrate along glial fibers (Trenkner and Sidman, 1977; Hatten and Liem, 1981; Hatten, Liem, and Mason, 1984; Mason, Edmondson, and Hatten, 1988). A large amount of work based on histology, autoradiography, retroviral tracing, dye labeling, and modern imaging has established that most, if not all, neuronal precursor cells migrate in the developing CNS (Rakic, 1971, 1972; Nowakowski and Rakic, 1979; Levitt and Rakic, 1980; Gray, Leber, and Sanes, 1990; Hatten and Mason, 1990; Walsh and Cepko, 1990; Hatten and Heintz, 1998).

Modes of neuronal migration in the brain

Neuronal migration can be categorized by its relative direction as radial when cells migrate perpendicularly to the surface of the brain or tangential when cells migrate in a direction parallel to the surface of the brain (figure 4.1A).

Radial migration is the major mode for projection neurons in the developing telencephalon and the cerebellum (Hatten and Mason, 1990; Rakic, 1990; Parnavelas, 2000). In the embryonic cerebellum, Purkinje cells, the principal output neurons, migrate outward to form the Purkinje cell layer (PCL) beneath the external germinal layer (EGL). In the postnatal cerebellum of rodents, neuronal precursor cells in the EGL migrate internally across the PCL into the internal granule layer (IGL). The behavior of radially migrating neurons can be divided into locomotion and translocation (Book and Morest, 1990). Translocation is a common mode in early stages of neocortical development, whereas locomotion becomes more common in later stages (Nadarajah et al., 2001) (figure 4.1B, C).

During locomotion, the entire cell, including the soma and the leading and trailing processes, moves synchronously (Edmondson and Hatten, 1987; Noctor et al., 2001) (figure 4.1C). Cells that undergo locomotion display a saltatory pattern of migration: periods of rapid forward movements are interspersed with long stationary phases (Nadarajah et al., 2001).

Translocation can be further divided into somal translocation and nuclear translocation (nucleokinesis). Cells undergoing somal translocation extend a long leading process that terminates at the pial surface and a short (or no) trailing

GUOFA LIU and YI RAO Department of Anatomy and Neurobiology, Washington University School of Medicine, St. Louis, Mo.

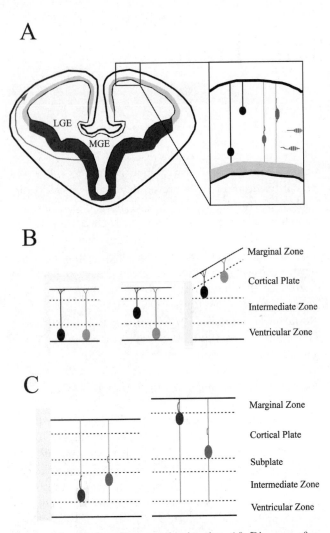

Tangential migration of neurons was observed in the 1960s (Altman and Das, 1966; Rakic and Sidman, 1969). Studies in the late 1980s and the 1990s rekindled interest in tangential migration (Kishi, 1987; Van Eden et al., 1989; Gray, Leber, and Sanes, 1990; Walsh and Cepko, 1990; O'Rourke et al., 1992, 1995; Fishell, Mason, and Hatten, 1993; Luskin, 1993; Tan and Breen, 1993; Lois and Alvarez-Buylla, 1994; DeDiego, Smith-Fernandez, and Fairen, 1994; Hu et al., 1996; Lois, García-Verdugo, and Alvarez-Buylla, 1996; Anderson et al., 1997; reviewed in Alvarez-Buylla and Kirn, 1997; Luskin, 1998). Major sources of neurons that undergo tangential migration are the upper rhombic lip (URL) in the cerebellar primordium (Wingate and Hatten, 1999) and the ventral telencephalon (reviewed in Parnavelas, 2000; Corbin, Nery, and Fishell, 2001; Marin et al., 2001). Migration of precursor cells from the URL along the surface of the embryonic cerebellar primordium contributes to the formation of the EGL in rodents (Adler, Cho, and Hatten, 1996; Wingate and Hatten, 1999).

There are three ganglionic eminences (GEs) in the ventral telencephalon: the lateral GE (LGE), the medial GE (MGE), and the caudal GE (CGE) (Corbin, Nery, and Fishell, 2001; Marin et al., 2001). Neuronal precursor cells from the LGE in the embryo migrate to the striatum, the nucleus accumbens, and the olfactory bulb (Wichterle et al., 2001); cells from the MGE migrate to the neocortex (Van Eden et al., 1989; DeDiego, Smith-Fernandez, and Fairen, 1994; De Carlos, Lopez-Mascaraque, and Valverde, 1996; Anderson et al., 1997; Tamamaki, Fujimori, and Takauji, 1997; Lavdas et al., 1999; Wichterle et al., 2001); and cells from the CGE migrate to the posterior dorsal telencephalon (Nery, Fishell, and Corbin, 2002).

Tangential migration has also been observed in the hypothalamus, the pons, and the spinal cord.

Unlike radial migration, tangential migration does not rely on glial fibers. Although astrocytes have been implicated in forming tubular structures through which chains of neurons migrate in the adult rostral migratory stream (RMS) (Lois, García-Verduga, and Alvarez-Buylla, 1996), these chains do not exist in the neonatal RMS (Menezes et al., 1995). It is not clear whether there is distinction between translocation and locomotion as distinct modes for tangentially migrating neurons (e.g., figure 4.2C).

Some cells can undergo both tangential and radial migration. For example, cells in the EGL of the cerebellum migrate tangentially before they change the migration mode to radial migration (Komuro et al., 2001). After EGL cells radially migrate into the IGL, these new granule cells can detach from the radial glial cells (Bergmann glia) and migrate further in a radial direction, but in a manner independent of the Bergmann glial fibers (Komuro and Rakic,

FIGURE 4.1 Modes of neuronal migration. (*A*) Diagram of a coronal section of the embryonic forebrain. Arrow shows the direction of neuronal migration from the MGE to the neocortex. The right panel shows radial migration and tangential migration in the neocortex. (*B*) Somal translocation in the cortex. These three panels show different stages of the same two neurons. The earlier neuron (in black) ends up inside, whereas the later neuron (in gray) ends up outside. The leading processes of both neurons shorten over time. (*C*) Locomotion in the cortex. The two panels show different stages of the same two neurons. The earlier neuron (in black) ends up inside, whereas the later neuron (in gray) ends up outside. Both the leading processes and the cell bodies move from the ventricular zone to the cortical plate.

process (Brittis et al., 1995; Nadarajah et al., 2001). The leading process of somal translocating cells shortens as the soma moves toward the pia. The speed of migration is steady and continuous, which is markedly different from that of locomotion (Nadarajah et al., 2001). Cells undergoing locomotion can switch over to somal translocation when the leading process contacts the pia (Nadarajah et al., 2001). In nuclear translocation, the nucleus moves within the cell from one end to the other. Cells undergoing nucleus translocation end up with a shorter leading process and a longer

1998). It is unclear what determines the migratory mode that a neuronal precursor cell takes and how the transition between different modes is regulated.

Spatial control of neuronal migration

We will use tangential migration in the RMS as a model to discuss the spatial control of neuronal migration. The major interneurons in the olfactory bulb (OB), the periglomerular and granule cells, are derived from neuronal precursor cells migrating from the embryonic LGE and postnatal subventricular zone (SVZa) in the lateral ventricles of the anterior forebrain (Hinds, 1968; Altman, 1969; Bayer, 1983; Corotto, Henegar, and Maruniak, 1993; Luskin, 1993; Lois and Alvarez-Buylla, 1994; Lois, García-Verdugo, and Alvarez-Buylla, 1996; Wichterle et al., 2001) (figure 4.2A). The generation of SVZa neurons and their migration to the OB through the RMS are continuous in adult mammals, including rodents (Altman and Das, 1966; Hinds, 1968; Altman, 1969; Bayer, 1983; Lois and Alvarez-Buylla, 1994; Lois,

García-Verdugo, and Alvarez-Buylla, 1996) and primates, including New World monkeys (McDermott and Lantos, 1990), Old World monkeys (Lewis, 1968; Kaplan, 1983; Gould et al., 1999; Kornack and Rakic, 2001; Pencea et al., 2001), and humans (Pincus et al., 1998; Kukekov et al., 1999; Weickert et al., 2000). In primates, SVZa neurons have to migrate several centimeters to reach the OB (Kornack and Rakic, 2001; Pencea et al., 2001). Persistent neuronal migration has also been demonstrated in other regions of the brain (see, e.g., Eriksson et al., 1998); the RMS therefore provides a useful model to understand a process of general importance in the brain.

Our studies of neuronal migration led to the suggestion that there are attractive and repulsive guidance cues that control SVZa migration to the OB. These cues are diffusible proteins that are secreted by cells at specific locations and act on the SVZa cells. Neither the glial nor the neuronal fibers along which neuronal precursor cells migrate provide sufficient directional information. Instead, secreted molecular cues have been shown to play important roles in guiding

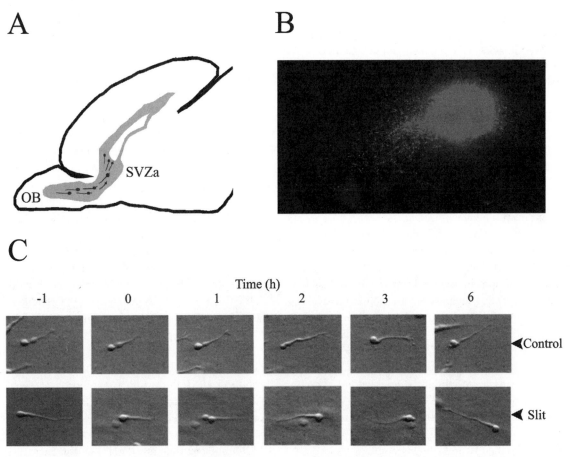

FIGURE 4.2 Neuronal migration in the RMS and guidance by Slit. (*A*) Diagram of a sagittal section of the neonatal forebrain. The anterior subventricular zone (SVZa) is the origin of the precursor cells that migrate through the rostral migratory stream (RMS) into the olfactory bulb (OB). (*B*) DiI labeling of cells in the RMS that migrate toward the OB. DiI was injected into the RMS of a slice of the neonatal rat brain and the image was made 24 hours after in vitro culture. (*C*) A repulsive role for Slit on migrating SVZa cells in vitro. Explants were cultured alone for 24 hours before being cocultured with either Slit or control aggregates. Time-lapse microscopy was used to track neuronal migration. The Slit/control aggregates were placed on the right.

neuronal migration. The first cue found to guide neuronal migration in the mammalian brain was the protein Slit (Wu et al., 1999). The Slit gene was firstly identified in *Drosophila* (Nusslein-Volhard, Wieschaus, and Kluding, 1984). The *Drosophila* Slit protein contains an N-terminal signal peptide, four leucine-rich repeats (LRRs), seven EGF repeats, a laminin G domain, and a C-terminal cysteine-rich motif (or cysteine knot) (Rothberg et al., 1988, 1990). Vertebrate Slit proteins are similar to the *Drosophila* orthologue except that they contain nine EGF repeats. In 1999, Slit was shown to be a repellent for axons projecting from different regions of the nervous system (Brose et al., 1999; Kidd, Bland, and Goodman, 1999; Li et al., 1999).

The ability of Slit to repel migrating neurons was first found in the RMS (Wu et al., 1999). The initial experiment involved cocultures of SVZa explants and cell lines secreting Slit and observation of the distribution of SVZa cells around the circumferences of the explants (Wu et al., 1999). It could not distinguish between repulsion and inhibition. A different group suggested that Slit played an inhibitory but not a repulsive role in neuronal migration (Mason, Ito, and Corfas, 2001). A series of experiments that included time-lapse microscopy have now provided definitive evidence that Slit functions primarily as a repellent for SVZa neurons (Ward et al., 2003). Slit repulsion of SVZa cells requires the presence of a gradient of the Slit protein (Wu et al., 1999; Chen et al., 2001; Ward et al., 2003).

A diffusible activity has been discovered recently in the OB that can attract SVZa cells (Liu and Rao, 2003). Removal of the region secreting this activity significantly reduces, but does not eliminate, the migration of SVZa cells toward the OB (Liu and Rao, 2003). The molecular nature of the OB attractant is unknown at present, but it appears to be different from the known attractants.

Ephrins, which function through the Eph tyrosine kinase receptors (Flanagan and Vanderhaeghen, 1998; O'Leary and Wilkinson, 1999; Palmer and Klein, 2003), may also control RMS migration. Because ephrins are not diffusible, they may act by creating regions that are nonpermissive to migrating neurons. EphB1–3 and EphA4 and their transmembrane ligands, ephrins-B2/3, have been implicated in SVZa migration (Conover et al., 2000). When the extracellular parts of either EphB2 or ephrin-B2 were introduced into the lateral ventricles to inhibit the interaction between endogenous ephrin and Eph, the migration of SVZa cells was disrupted (Conover et al., 2000).

It is unclear how many guidance cues are required for SVZa migration to the OB and whether and how they coordinate neuronal migration along the entire RMS.

Other regions of the brain also use guidance cues to control neuronal migration. In the cerebellum, the secreted protein netrin is an attractant for neurons migrating toward the basilar pons (Yee et al., 1999; Alcantara et al., 2000). Pre-cursor cells from the MGE can migrate into either the striatum or the neocortex to become GABAergic interneurons. Guidance by Slit may be important in initiating their migration (Zhu et al., 1999), whereas the repulsive semaphorins are important for directing some interneurons into the neocortex and others into the striatum (Marin et al., 2001).

Signal transduction pathways involved in neuronal migration

The signal transduction mechanisms for guidance cues are thought to be similar between axon guidance and neuronal migration (Kolodkin and Ginty, 1997; Flanagan and Vanderhaeghen, 1998; O'Leary and Wilkinson, 1999; Kennedy, 2000; Merz and Culotti, 2000; Raper, 2000; Wong et al., 2002; Palmer and Klein, 2003). We will discuss the Slit-Robo pathway, since it has been directly studied in context in neuronal migration. The receptor of Slit is the transmembrane protein Roundabout (Robo) (Kidd et al., 1998; Zallen, Yi, and Bargmann, 1998; Brose et al., 1999; Kidd, Bland, and Goodman, 1999; Li et al., 1999). Robo was discovered for axon guidance in *Drosophila* and *C. elegans* (Seeger et al., 1993; Kidd et al., 1998; Zallen, Yi, and Bargmann, 1998). Studies in *Drosophila* indicate that *slit* and *robo* mutations interact genetically (Kidd, Bland, and Goodman, 1999). Biochemical studies of mammalian Slit and Robo proteins provide direct evidences that Slit binds to Robo (Brose et al., 1999; Li et al., 1999), and functional studies indicate that the extracellular part of Robo blocks the repulsive effect of Slit on migrating neurons (Wu et al., 1999; Zhu et al., 1999).

Robo is a single-pass transmembrane protein with five immunoglobulin (Ig) domains and three fibronectin type III (FNIII) repeats in its extracellular part. Biochemical experiments showed that the Ig domains in Robo are sufficient to interact with the LRR in Slit (Battye et al., 2001; Chen et al., 2001; Nguyen Ba-Charvet et al., 2001). The large intracellular region of *Drosophila* Robo and the three mammalian Robos contains four identifiable conserved motifs: CC0, CC1, CC2, and CC3 (Taguchi et al., 1996; Kidd et al., 1998; Zallen, Yi, and Bargmann, 1998; Brose et al., 1999; Yuan et al., 1999). The cytoplasmic domain of Robo determines the repulsive response (Bashaw and Goodman, 1999). Deletion of each of the CC motifs leads to a partial *robo* phenotype (Bashaw et al., 2000), whereas expression of each of these deletion mutants failed to rescue the *robo* phenotype, suggesting an additive effect of these motifs (Bashaw et al., 2000). The CC2 motif is a consensus binding site for Ena-VASP-homology domain (EVH1) of Enabled (Ena), and in vitro binding experiments showed Ena interaction with Robo through CC2 and CC1 (Bashaw et al., 2000). The Abelson kinase (Abl) can phosphorylate a tyrosine residue in CC1 in vitro and seems either to antagonize (Bashaw et al., 2000) or to synergize with the activity of Robo in *Drosophila*

(Wills et al., 2002). It is unknown whether Slit can regulate the activities of Abl and Ena. Work in *Drosophila* has suggested the involvement of protein tyrosine phosphatases (PTPases) in the Slit-Robo pathway (Sun et al., 2000). Mutations in two receptor PTPase genes, *PTP10D* and *PTP69D*, interact genetically with *slit* and *robo*. Phenotypic analyses suggest that PTPases increase the sensitivity to Slit.

The CC3 motif of Robo1 interacts with a novel subfamily of GTPase-activating proteins (GAPs), the srGAPs (Wong et al., 2001). srGAPs 1 and 2 are expressed in regions responsive to Slit and in a pattern similar to that of Robo1 (Wong et al., 2001). Extracellular interaction between Slit and Robo increases the intracellular interaction between the CC3 motif of Robo and the SH3 motif of the srGAPs. Slit treatment of either a mammalian cell line or the primary SVZa cells reduces the amount of the active form of the Rho GTPase Cdc42 (Wong et al., 2001). The functional role of Cdc42 in neuronal migration has been demonstrated because the repulsive effect of Slit on migrating SVZa cells was blocked by a constitutively active mutant of Cdc42 (Wong et al., 2001).

Because the active form of Cdc42 activates the intracellular protein N-WASP, which promotes actin branching by activation of the Arp2/3 complex, a working hypothesis for Slit-mediated repulsion of migrating neurons has been proposed (Wong et al., 2001). This pathway begins with the extracellular interaction of Slit with Robo, resulting in increased intracellular interaction of Robo with srGAPs and the inactivation of Cdc42. The relatively lower level of Cdc42 activity on the side of the cell proximal to a higher concentration of Slit leads to relatively lower activities of N-WASP and the Arp2/3 complex on the proximal side. Actin polymerization will therefore be polarized, with less polymerization on the proximal side and more on the distal side of the cell (Wong et al., 2001). This is a working model, and the relationship of Abl, Ena, PTPases, and possibly other components to the model remains to be examined.

Temporal control of neuronal migration

A major model for neuronal migration in the brain is the migration of cells from EGL into the IGL in the cerebellum (Rakic, 1971, 1990; Hatten and Heintz, 1998; Pearlman et al., 1998) (figure 4.3*A*, *B*). In the embryo, EGL cells are derived from cells in the URL (Adler, Cho, and Hatten, 1996; Wingate and Hatten, 1999). Cells in the URL migrate tangentially to form the EGL (Wingate and Hatten, 1999) (figure 4.3*A*). Once in the EGL, the URL-derived cells do not migrate toward the IGL in the embryo. Postnatally, EGL cells are induced to proliferate by the sonic hedgehog (SHH) protein secreted from the Purkinje cells underlying the EGL cells (Wechsler-Reya and Scott, 1999). Postnatal EGL cells migrate radially from the more superficial layer through the

Purkinje cell layer to IGL, giving rise to the granule cells (Rakic, 1971) (figure 4.3*B*). The migration of EGL cells toward the IGL in vivo is thought to depend on radially aligned glial fibers (Rakic, 1971). In vitro, EGL cells can bind to and migrate along the glial fibers (Hatten and Liem, 1981; Edmondson and Hatten, 1987; Mason, Edmondson, and Hatten, 1988; Hatten and Mason, 1990). The binding of EGL cells to the glial fiber requires the cell adhesion molecule astrotactin (Edmondson et al., 1988; Zheng, Heintz, and Hatten, 1996). Because the same neuron can migrate in both directions along the same glial fiber (Hatten and Liem, 1981; Edmondson and Hatten, 1987; Mason, Edmondson, and Hatten, 1988), the glial fibers do not provide information to guide the direction of neuronal migration.

During our investigation of the mechanisms underlying temporal and spatial control of EGL migration, which we sought to understand by studying the migration of embryonic and postnatal EGL cells in rodents, we found that temporal control of cell migration is accomplished by regulation of spatial control (Zhu et al., 2002). Our results make it possible to propose a mechanistic model for the temporal and spatial control of neuronal migration in the cerebellum (figure 4.3*C*, *D*). Cerebellar migration is controlled by strategic positioning of multiple attractive and repulsive cues and developmental changes in cellular responses to these cues. In the embryo, the meninges contain both attractants and repellents, and the embryonic EGL cells respond predominantly to the meningeal attractant. There is also a diffusible repellent from the neuroepithelium. The combination of the meningeal attractant and the neuroepithelial repellent prevents the EGL cells from migrating into the internal layers in the embryo (figure 4.3*C*). Postnatally, the inner layers in the cerebellum are not repulsive. However, both the attractant and the repellent are still present in the postnatal meninges. Postnatal EGL cells respond to the repellent in the meninges but not to the attractive activity in the meninges (figure 4.3*D*).

The meningeal attractant is the chemokine SDF-1, which was previously known as a chemotactic factor for leukocytes. In vitro cocultures of embryonic EGL explants with either purified SDF-1 protein or a mammalian cell line that secretes SDF-1 protein indicate SDF-1 attracts embryonic but not postnatal EGL cells (figure 4.3*E*, *F*) (Klein et al., 2001; Lu et al., 2001; Zhu et al., 2002). SDF-1 is present in embryonic and postnatal meninges, whereas its receptor CXCR4 is present in the EGL. Our analysis of explants from mice lacking the SDF-1 gene indicates that SDF-1 is the predominant, if not the sole, attractant in the meninges (Zhu et al., 2002). When either SDF-1 or the *CXCR4* gene was knocked out, cerebellar granule cells were found in the internal layers prematurely in the embryo (Ma et al., 1998; Tachibana et al., 1998; Zou et al., 1998). The molecular identities of the repellents in the meninges and the neuro-epithelium are not known.

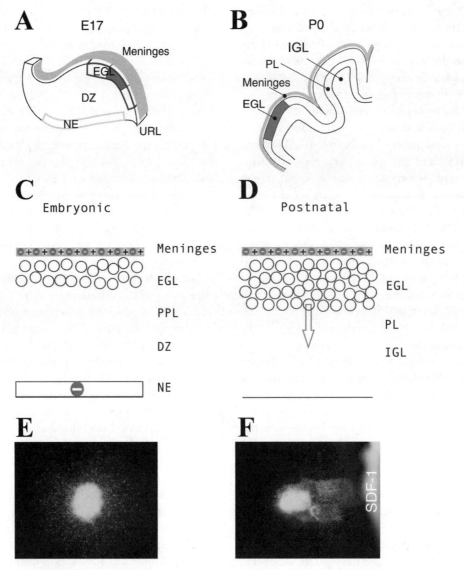

FIGURE 4.3 Spatial and temporal control of neuronal migration in the cerebellum. (*A*) Diagram of E17 rat cerebellar primordium showing the relative positions of the EGL, the differentiation zone (DZ), and the neuroepithelium (NE). (*B*) Diagram of part of the neonatal cerebellum, showing the EGL, the Purkinje cell layer (PL), and the internal granule layer (IGL). (*C*) The left panel is a diagram of the embryonic cerebellum. Diffusible attractant (+) and repellent (−) are present in the embryonic meninges. The embryonic EGL cells respond to the attractive cue in the meninges. There is a diffusible repulsive activity in the neuroepithelium (NE). The combination of the meningeal attractant and the neuroepithelial repellent prevents the EGL cells from migrating into the internal layers in the embryo. PPL, prospective Purkinje layer. (*D*) The right panel is a diagram of the postnatal cerebellum. Both the attractive and repulsive cues are still present in the postnatal meninges. However, the postnatal EGL cells respond predominantly to the repulsive cue in the meninges. The neuroepithelium is not present in the postnatal cerebellum, and there is no repulsive activity in the Purkinje layer (PL) and the IGL. EGL cells will thus migrate toward the IGL. (*E*) In vitro culture of a control embryonic EGL explant whose nuclei were revealed by staining with the Hoechst 33258 dye. Note cells migrating out of the explant are distributed symmetrically around the circumference of the explant. (*F*) Coculture of an embryonic EGL explant with HEK cells expressing SDF-1. The number of cells migrating out of the explant toward the source of SDF-1 is much higher than the number migrating from the source of SDF-1.

The model in figure 4.3C and D has several interesting features. It indicates that an active anchoring mechanism is required to prevent the embryonic EGL cells from premature migration into the IGL, that there is a signaling role for the meninges in neural development, and that a chemokine and its receptor functioning through the heterotrimeric G proteins are essential in neuronal migration. A crucial temporal change is that EGL cells change their responsiveness to the meningeal attractant SDF-1 (Zhu et al., 2002). The molecular mechanism underlying this developmental change comes from studies of reverse signaling by Eph tyrosine kinase receptors and their transmembrane ligands the ephrins (Lu et al., 2001). It was found that the intracellular domain of an ephrin B ligand could bind to a regulator of G proteins (RGS), which inhibits SDF-1 activation of CXCR4 (Lu et al., 2001). Because the expression of both Eph and ephrin are up-regulated postnatally (Lu et al., 2001), Eph-ephrin signaling may thus underlie the developmental change in EGL responsiveness.

Genes affecting cortical lamination in mice

Genetic studies combined with molecular cloning in mice have revealed new molecules that are involved in cortical lamination. *Reeler* mutant mice have abnormal lamination of cerebral and cerebellar cortexes. Histological studies of *reeler* mice show that an approximate inversion of the normal inside-out pattern of cortical migration, with all major morphological cell classes present in the *reeler* cortex (Falconer, 1951; Caviness and Sidman, 1973a, 1973b). Although the preplate develops normally in *reeler* mutant mice, the cohorts of migrating neurons fail to invade the preplate and split it into the marginal zone and the subplate during the formation of the cortical plate (Goffinet, 1979; Pinto and Caviness, 1979; Caviness, 1982; Ogawa et al., 1995; Sheppard and Pearlman, 1997). The *reeler* mice are defective in positioning of neurons within specific layers, especially during cortical plate formation. In the cerebellum, *reeler* mice show abnormal lamination of the Purkinje cells (Mariani et al., 1977).

A major advance in our understanding of *reeler* gene function is the identification of its product Reelin, a large secreted protein (D'Arcangelo et al., 1995). It is expressed primarily in the Cajal-Retzius (CR) cells in the marginal zone of the neocortex and in the nuclear transitory zone (NTZ) and the EGL of the cerebellum (D'Arcangelo et al., 1995; Miyata et al., 1996; Schiffmann, Bernier, and Goffinet, 1997). Multimerization of Reelin may be required to initiate Reelin signaling (Utsunomiya-Tate et al., 2000). Genetic and biochemical studies have demonstrated that two members of the low-density lipoprotein (LDL) family of lipoproteins, the very-low-density lipoprotein receptor (VLDLR) and the low-density lipoprotein receptor-related

protein 8 (LRP8, also known as the apolipoprotein E receptor-2 or ApoER2), are the receptors for Reelin (Trommsdorff et al., 1999; D'Arcangelo et al., 1999). Mice lacking VLDLR show *reeler* phenotype in the cerebellum, whereas ApoER2 single knockout mice match the *reeler* phenotype in the cortex. Mice lacking both genes exhibit anatomical defects almost identical to *reeler* (Trommsdorff et al., 1999). The significance of additional hypothetical Reelin receptors such as the cadherin-related neuronal receptors and integrin α3β1 is unclear (Senzaki, Ogawa, and Yagi, 1999; Dulabon et al., 2000).

Other spontaneously occurring mutant mice such as *scrambler* (Sweet et al., 1996) and *yotari* (Yoneshima et al., 1997) have been described, and their phenotype is remarkably similar to that of *reeler*. Both of them were caused by mutations in the mouse homologue of *Drosophila disabled* (*Dab-1*) (Howell, Gertler, and Cooper, 1997; Sheldon et al., 1997; Ware et al., 1997). Similar to VLDLR and ApoER2, *Dab-1* is expressed in the Reelin-responsive cortical plate neurons and the Purkinje cells. Dab-1 protein is a cytoplasmic protein and can bind to the intracellular part of VLDLR and ApoER2 (Trommsdorff et al., 1999). Tyrosine phosphorylation of Dab-1 is increased by Reelin stimulation, and the level of Dab-1 tyrosine phosphorylation is reduced in *reeler* mice (Howell, Herrick, and Cooper, 1999). Mutations in the phosphorylation sites of Dab-1 cause ataxia due to abnormalities in cell positioning in the cerebral and cerebellar corteces (Howell et al., 2000). These biochemical and genetic evidences suggest Reelin signal through the transmembrane receptors VLDLR and ApoER2 to Dab-1 phosphorylation in controlling neuronal position.

Several hypotheses have been proposed to explain Reelin function in laminar positioning. A popular one is that Reelin might act as a stop signal for radially migrating neurons (Frotscher, 1997; Sheppard and Pearlman, 1997; Dulabon et al., 2000). Reelin may promote detachment of migrating neurons from the processes of radial glial cells (Dulabon et al., 2000). Reelin has also been proposed to directly regulate the function of radial glia scaffold, which is important for cortical lamination (Super et al., 2000).

There are other mouse mutants defective in cortical lamination. Mice lacking the cyclin-dependent kinase 5 (cdk5) show defective migration in the cerebral and cerebellar cortexes (Ohshima et al., 1996). These defects are not identical to those in *reeler*. The migrating cells could split the preplate into the marginal zone and the subplate in *cdk5* mutants, but late-born neurons do not show the inside-out pattern in that they accumulate under the subplate (Dhavan, Tsai, and Tsai, 2001). Cdk5 is a ubiquitously expressed serine-threonine kinase that requires p35 and p39 proteins for activation. Mice lacking both p35 and p39 show a cortical phenotype similar to that in *cdk5* mutant mice (Ko et al., 2001). In vitro studies suggest that Cdk5 regulates cytoskeleton dynamics through the phosphorylation of the Pak kinase and micro-tubule-associated proteins (Nikolic et al., 1998; Sobue et al., 2000). The expression of p35 and p39 in migrating cortical neurons is regulated cell-autonomously by the POU domain transcription factors Brn1 and Brn2, whose mutation also leads to cortical inversion (McEvilly et al., 2002).

Members of the neurotrophin family, brain-derived neurotrophic factor (BDNF) and neurotrophin-4 (NT-4), have been shown to promote the migration of cortical neurons by interacting with the TrkB receptor (Behar et al., 1997). Infusion of NT-4 or BDNF into the lateral ventricle or application of these proteins to slices of the developing cortex results in neuronal heterotopias that appear to be the result of increased neuronal migration (Brunstrom et al., 1997; Ringstedt et al., 1998). BDNF is highly expressed in the developing cerebellum, with the strongest expression in the IGL. BDNF is motogenic and attractive for neurons migrating from the EGL (Borghesani et al., 2002). The migration of cerebellar granule cells out of the EGL is impaired in BDNF mutant mice. BDNF−/− granule cells are defective in initiation of migration along glial fibers in vitro; this situation can be rescued by exogenous BDNF.

The epidermal growth factor receptor (EGFR) and its ligands, including heparin-binding EGF (HB-EGF) and TGF, are highly expressed in the developing cortex (Kornblum et al., 1997; Nakagawa et al., 1998). Neuronal precursors are accumulated in telencephalic proliferative zones in mice lacking EGFR (Threadgill et al., 1995). Overexpression of EGFR in the embryonic cortex enhances radial migration (Burrows et al., 1997; Caric et al., 2001).

Disorders of neuronal migration in humans

Multiple human diseases are caused by defects in neuronal migration (Barth, 1987; Volpe, 1987; Reiner et al., 1993; Hattori et al., 1994b; Pinard et al., 1994; Norman et al., 1995; Eksioglu et al., 1996; Gordon, 1996; Gunay and Aysun, 1996; Flint and Kriegstein, 1997; des Portes et al., 1998; Pearlman et al., 1998). These include lissencephaly (Jellinger and Rett, 1976), periventricular heterotopia (Huttenlocher, Taravath, and Mojtahedi, 1994), subcortical band heterotopia (SBH) (Barkovich, Jackson, and Boyer, 1989), Zellweger cerebrohepatorenal syndrome (Volpe and Adams, 1972), and some forms of congenital muscular dystrophy (Fenichel, 1988).

Patients with classic or type I lissencephaly and double cortex (DC) display mild to severe mental retardation and epilepsy. Although patients are usually asymptomatic at birth, developmental delay and seizures are obvious in later stages. The degree of mental impairment varies widely, but most patients display moderate mental retardation, with IQs in the 50–90 range (Barkovich, Jackson, and Boyer, 1989;

Gleeson et al., 2000). Seizure types include mixed artial, tonic clonic, or atypical absence (Ricci et al., 1992; Soucek et al., 1992).

The pathological and radiographic defects in classic lissencephaly are the absence of gyria and sulci with abnormally thick gray matter in the cortex (Kuchelmeister, Bergmann, and Gullotta, 1993). There are additional abnormalities in cerebellum and brainstem. Although the outer cortex appears normal in DC, overaccumulation of neurons in the subcortical white matter suggests a defect in ongoing neuronal migration (Barkovich, Jackson, and Boyer, 1989; Harding, 1996).

Mutations in either the lissencephaly-1 (*LIS1*) or the doublecortin (*DCX*) genes can cause lissencephaly. Most of the identifiable mutations in *LIS1* are de novo deletion of one copy of *LIS1* (Reiner et al., 1993). Most of the identifiable mutations in the *DCX* gene are single base mutations (Gleeson et al., 1998, 1999). *LIS1* mutations are haploinsufficient in that a 50% decrease in LIS1 protein levels is sufficient to produce the lissencephaly phenotype. DC is on the X-chromosome, and the phenotype is more severe in affected males than females. DC is generally regarded as a cell-autonomous mosaic phenotype in females, owing to random inactivation of the X-chromosome. The Lis-1 protein is the regulatory subunit of brain platelet-activating factor acetylhydrolase (PAF-AH) (Hattori et al., 1994b), which deacetylates and inactivates PAF, a potent proinflammatory phospholipid (Hanahan, 1986). PAF-AH is expressed in CR cells and the ventricular zone of the developing neocortex (Clark et al., 1997). PAF causes neurite retraction (Clark et al., 1995; McNeil et al., 1999) and regulates the migration of cerebellar granule cells (Bix and Clark, 1998). It is not known whether Lis-1 function is related to PAF, though. More suggestively, Lis-1 is similar to Nudf protein, which is crucial for nuclear translocation in the filamentous fungi *Aspergillus* (Xiang et al., 1995; Morris, Efimov, and Xiang, 1998). Lis-1 can stabilize microtubules (Sapir, Elbaum, and Reiner, 1997). Biochemically, Lis-1 can bind to cytoplasmic dynein and mammalian homologues of *Aspergillus* Nudc and Nudf (Feng et al., 2000; Niethammer et al., 2000; Sasaki et al., 2000; Smith et al., 2000). Subcellularly, Lis-1 is associated with the centrosome, and the precise mechanism of how Lis-1 is involved in neuronal migration is unclear (Feng et al., 2000; Niethammer et al., 2000; Sasaki et al., 2000; Smith et al., 2000).

The *DCX* gene has been cloned (Gleeson et al., 1998; des Portes et al., 1998), and its product is a microtubule-associated protein (Francis et al., 1999; Gleeson et al., 1999), which can promote the microtubule assembly (Gleeson et al., 1999).

A second form of lissencephaly is cobblestone lissencephaly (also known as type II lissencephaly), which includes three distinct human disorders, muscle-eye-brain

(MEB) disease, Fukuyama-type muscular dystrophy (FCMD), and Walker-Warburg syndrome (WWS). In addition to mental retardation and epilepsy, patients with cobblestone lissencephaly are often defective in eye and muscle development (Fukuyama, Osawa, and Suzuki, 1981; Santavuori et al., 1989; Lichtig et al., 1993). Pathologically, the cortex in cobblestone lissencephaly is similar to that of classic lissencephaly in lacking gyria and sulci, but the cortical surface has a roughened, "cobbleslone" appearance that is thought to result from neuronal migration out of the developing brain through breaches in the superficial basement membrane (Squier, 1993; Gelot et al., 1995). The gene for FCMD has been identified and named *fukutin*. It encodes a glycoprotein or glycolipid-modifying enzyme (Kobayashi et al., 1998; Aravind and Koonin, 1999). Recent evidence suggests that fukutin may function as a stop signal for migrating neurons (Saito et al., 2000). MEB has recently been shown to be caused by mutations in POMGnT1, the gene encoding O-mannosyl-β-1,2-N-acetylglucosaminyltransferanse (Yoshida et al., 2001), which may be required for α-dystroglycan binding to laminin, an extracellular matrix protein (Chiba et al., 1997).

Another form of lissencephaly is known as lissencephaly with cerebellar hypoplasia (LCH). Most patients have acquired microcephaly and severe cognitive developmental delay, with little or no language and inability to sit or stand unsupported. Seizures are frequent. Additional clinical features vary. There are six subtypes of LCH. Although the cortex in patients with LCH is similar in appearance to the cortex in classic lissencephaly, the cerebellum is severely diminished. Hong and colleagues (2000) identified a mutation in the *reelin* gene in two families, indicating that mutations in *reelin* are responsible for one subtype of LCH (LCHb). It is not surprising that the defect in LCH is similar to the defects observed in the *reeler* mouse.

The pathological and radiographic defect in periventricular heterotopia (PH) is a striking collection of neurons that line the lateral ventricles, suggesting a migration disorder in which many neurons destined for the cortical plate fail to migrate and instead accumulate close to the progenitor zones of the cerebral cortex (Eksioglu et al., 1996). In addition to the heterotopic collection of neurons, there is a normal-appearing outer cortex, suggesting that some neurons migrate normally. The symptoms of patients with PH are quite different. Some have mild or no symptoms, whereas others may have mild mental retardation, epilepsy, psychiatric symptoms, or other systemic features.

PH shows X-linked dominant inheritance, with affected females displaying PH and affected males unable to survive gestation (Huttenlocher, Taravath, and Mojtahedi, 1994). The gene responsible for PH is located on the X-chromosome and encodes filamin 1 (FLN1), an actin-binding/cross-linking protein (Fox et al., 1998).

Other childhood neurological disorders, such as Zellweger syndrome and tuberous sclerosis, have been associated with defects in neuronal migration. Zellweger syndrome manifests with a cortical dysplasia resembling polymicrogyria of cerebral and cerebellar cortex, sometimes with pachygyria around the sylvian fissure, and focal subcortical and subependymal heterotopia (Takashima et al., 1992). In Zellweger syndrome, there is a generalized defect in neuronal migration (Volpe and Adams, 1972), and the mutated genes are involved in peroxisome formation (Shimozawa et al., 1992; Baes et al., 1997; Faust and Hatten, 1997). The connection between peroxisome formation and neuronal migration is unclear. Tuberous sclerosis affects multiple organs. A defect in neuronal migration is typically present in focal sites of cortical dysplasia (Palmini et al., 1991; Raymond et al., 1995; Frater et al., 2000), with atypical or underdifferentiated neurons (Ferrer et al., 1984; Chou and Chou, 1989). It is caused by mutations in the tuberous sclerosis complex (TSC) genes 1 and 2, which encode hamartin and tuberin (van Slegtenhorst et al., 1997). Interestingly, both hamartin and tuberin can interact with the ezrin-radixin-moesin family of actin-binding proteins and activate the Rho GTPase (Lamb et al., 2000; Astrinidis et al., 2002). Hamartin and tuberin can also interact with each other and inhibit the mammalian target of rapamycin (mTOR) (Inoki et al., 2002).

Roles of neuronal migration and newly generated neurons in behavior and neural plasticity

Neuronal migration is essential for postnatal behavior changes in birds (Nottebohm, 1981; Goldman and Nottebohm, 1983; reviewed in Alvarez-Buylla and Kirn, 1997; Goldman and Luskin, 1998; Nottebohm, 2002). Findings of neurogenesis and adult neural stem cells suggest that neuronal migration is important in the brains of adult mammals, including humans (Reynolds and Weiss, 1992; Richards, Kilpatrick, and Bartlett, 1992; Suhonen et al., 1996; Brustle et al., 1997; Olsson et al., 1997; Eriksson et al., 1998; Gage, 1998). Because neuronal stem cells give rise to neurons during neural plasticity (Greenough, West, and DeVoogd, 1978; Kempermann, Kuhn, and Gage, 1997; Van Praag et al., 1999, 2002; Shors et al., 2001; Gage, 2002; Kempermann, 2002), neuronal migration is likely to be essential for neural plasticity. However, it is not known whether migration plays a regulatory role in plasticity.

In the OB, newly generated neurons and their migration are important for odor discrimination (Gheusi et al., 2000) and can potentially play a role in plasticity (Gheusi et al., 2000; Cecchi et al., 2001). In the hippocampus, newly generated neurons and their migration have been proposed to be important in associative learning (Shors et al., 2001). More studies are needed before we know the precise roles of neuronal migration in the functioning of the brain and in neural plasticity.

It should also be noted that a role for neuronal migration in brain evolution has been proposed by Rakic and colleagues. Humans have the largest pulvinar nucleus in the dorsal thalamus among the primates. Rakic and Sidman (1969) found two phases of pulvinar development in the human brain. The early phase of pulvinar growth results from cell proliferation in the diencephalon, whereas the late phase results from migration of neuronal precursor cells from the ganglionic eminence (GE) in the telencephalon to the pulvinar nucleus (Rakic and Sidman, 1969). In monkeys, by contrast, there is only the early phase of pulvinar development, and the telencephalon did not seem to have contributed any neurons to the pulvinar nucleus (Ogren and Rakic, 1981). Neurons migrated from the GE to the dorsal thalamus in human brain but not in monkey or mouse brains (Letinic and Rakic, 2001). These comparative studies of neuronal migration led to the suggestion that establishment of new routes of neuronal migration might have contributed to the evolution of the human brain (Ogren and Rakic, 1981; Letinic and Rakic, 2001; reviewed in Rao and Wu, 2001). Regions connected to each other anatomically and functionally are thought to co-evolve during the evolution of the mammalian brain (Barton and Harvey, 2000). The telencephalon is connected to the thalamus, and establishment of the migratory pathway from the telencephalon GE to the dorsal thalamus may contribute to the co-evolution of the frontal cortex and the thalamic nuclei (Letinic and Rakic, 2001).

REFERENCES

ALCANTARA, S., M. RUIZ, F. DE CASTRO, E. SORIANO, and C. SOTELO, 2000. Netrin 1 acts as an attractive or as a repulsive cue for distinct migrating neurons during the development of the cerebellar system. *Development* 127:1359–1372.

ALDER, J., N. K. CHO, and M. E. HATTEN, 1996. Embryonic precursor cells from the rhombic lip are specified to a cerebellar granule neuron identity. *Neuron* 17:389–399.

ALTMAN, J., 1969. Autoradiographic and histological studies of postnatal neurogenesis. IV. Cell proliferation and migration in the anterior forebrain, with special reference to persisting neurogenesis in the olfactory bulb. *J. Comp. Neurol.* 137:433–458.

ALTMAN, J., and G. D. DAS, 1966. Autoradiographic and histological studies of postnatal neurogenesis. I. A longitudinal investigation of the kinetics, migration and transformation of cells incorporating tritiated thymidine in neonate rats, with special reference to postnatal neurogenesis in some brain regions. *J. Comp. Neurol.* 127:337–390.

ALVAREZ-BUYLLA, A., and J. R. KIRN, 1997. Birth, migration, incorporation, and death of vocal control neurons in adult songbirds. *J. Neurobiol.* 33:585–601.

ANDERSON, S. A., D. D. EISENSTAT, L. SHI, J. L. R. RUBENSTEIN, 1997. Interneuron migration from the basal forebrain to the neocortex: Dependence on Dlx genes. *Science* 278:474–476.

ANGEVINE, J. B., JR., and R. L. SIDMAN, 1961. Autoradiographic study of cell migration during histogenesis of cerebral cortex in the mouse. *Nature* 192:766–768.

ARAVIND, L., and E. V. KOONIN, 1999. The fukutin protein family–predicted enzymes modifying cell-surface molecules. *Curr. Biol.* 9:R836–R837.

ASTRINIDIS, A., T. P. CASH, D. S. HUNTER, C. L. WALKER, J. CHERNOFF, and E. P. HENSKE, 2002. Tuberin, the tuberous sclerosis complex 2 tumor suppressor gene product, regulates Rho activation, cell adhesion and migration. *Oncogene* 21:8470–8476.

BAES, M., P. GRESSENS, E. BAUMGART, P. CARMELIET, M. CASTEELS, M. FRANSEN, P. EVRARD, D. FAHIMI, P. E. DECLERCQ, P. P. VAN VELDHOVEN, and G. P. MANNAERTS, 1997. A mouse model for Zellweger syndrome. *Nat. Genet.* 17:49–57.

BARKOVICH, A. J., D. E. JACKSON, JR., and R. S. BOYER, 1989. Band heterotopias: A newly recognized neuronal migration anomaly. *Radiology* 171:455–458.

BARTH, P. G., 1987. Disorders of neuronal migration. *J. Neurol. Sci.* 14:1–16.

BARTON, A. R., and P. H. HARVEY, 2000. Mosaic evolution of brain structure in mammals. *Nature* 405:1055–1058.

BASHAW, G. J., and C. S. GOODMAN, 1999. Chimeric axon guidance receptors: The cytoplasmic domains of slit and netrin receptors specify attraction versus repulsion. *Cell* 97:917–926.

BASHAW, G. J., T. KIDD, D. MURRAY, T. PAWSON, and C. S. GOODMAN, 2000. Repulsive axon guidance: Abelson and Enabled play opposing roles downstream of the roundabout receptor. *Cell* 101:703–715.

BATTYE, R., A. STEVENS, R. L. PERRY, and J. R. JACOBS, 2001. Repellent signaling by Slit requires the leucine-rich repeats. *J. Neurosci.* 21:4290–4298.

BAYER, S. A., 1983. ^{3}H-thymidine-radiographic studies of neurogenesis in the rat olfactory bulb. *Exp. Brain Res.* 50:329–340.

BEHAR, T. N., M. M. DUGICH-DJORDJEVIC, Y. X. LI, W. MA, R. SOMOGYI, X. WEN, E. BROWN, C. SCOTT, R. D. MCKAY, and J. L. BARKER, 1997. Neurotrophins stimulate chemotaxis of embryonic cortical neurons. *Eur. J. Neurosci.* 9:2561–2570.

BENTIVOGLIO, M., and P. MAZZARELLO, 1999. The history of radial glia. *Brain Res. Bull.* 49:305–315.

BERRY, M., and A. W. ROGERS, 1965. The migration of neuroblasts in the developing cerebral cortex. *J. Anat.* 99:691–709.

BIX, G. J., and G. D. CLARK, 1998. Platelet-activating factor receptor stimulation disrupts neuronal migration in vitro. *J. Neurosci.* 18:307–318.

BOOK, K. J., and D. K. MOREST, 1990. Migration of neuroblasts by perikaryal translocation: Role of cellular elongation and axonal outgrowth in the acoustic nuclei of the chick embryo medulla. *J. Comp. Neurol.* 297:55–76.

BORGHESANI, P. R., J. M. PEYRIN, R. KLEIN, J. RUBIN, A. R. CARTER, P. M. SCHWARTZ, A. LUSTER, G. CORFAS, and R. A. SEGAL, 2002. BDNF stimulates migration of cerebellar granule cells. *Development* 129:1435–1442.

BRITTIS, P. A., K. MEIRI, E. DENT, and J. SILVER, 1995. The earliest patterns of neuronal differentiation and migration in the mammalian central nervous system. *Exp. Neurol.* 134:1–12.

BROSE, K., K. S. BLAND, K. H. WANG, D. ARNOTT, W. HENZEL, C. S. GOODMAN, M. TESSIER-LAVIGNE, and T. KIDD, 1999. Evolutionary conservation of the repulsive axon guidance function of Slit proteins and of their interactions with Robo receptors. *Cell* 96:795–806.

BRUNSTROM, J. E., M. R. GRAY-SWAIN, P. A. OSBORNE, and A. L. PEARLMAN, 1997. Neuronal heterotopias in the developing cerebral cortex produced by neurotrophin-4. *Neuron* 18: 505–517.

BRUSTLE, O., A. C. SPIRO, K. KARRAM, K. CHOUDHARY, S. OKABE, and R. D. McKAY, 1997. In vitro-generated neural precursors participate in mammalian brain development. *Proc. Natl. Acad. Sci. U.S.A.* 94:14809–14814.

BURROWS, R. C., D. WANCIO, P. LEVITT, and L. LILLIEN, 1997. Response diversity and the timing of progenitor cell maturation are regulated by developmental changes in EGFR expression in the cortex. *Neuron* 19:251–267.

CAJAL, S., and Y. RAMON, 1911, 1995. *Histology of the Nervous System*, N. Swanson and L. W. Swanson, *trans.* New York: Oxford University Press.

CARIC, D., H. RAPHAEL, J. VITI, A. FEATHERS, D. WANCIO, and L. LILLIEN, 2001. EGFRs mediate chemotactic migration in the developing telencephalon. *Development* 128:4203–4016.

CAVINESS, V. S., JR., 1982. Neocortical histogenesis in normal and reeler mice: A developmental study based upon [3H]thymidine autoradiography. *Brain Res.* 256:293–302.

CAVINESS, V. S., JR., and R. L. SIDMAN, 1973a. Retrohippocampal, hippocampal and related structures of the forebrain in the reeler mutant mouse. *J. Comp. Neurol.* 147:235–254.

CAVINESS, V. S., JR., and R. L. SIDMAN, 1973b. Time of origin or corresponding cell classes in the cerebral cortex of normal and reeler mutant mice: An autoradiographic analysis. *J. Comp. Neurol.* 148:141–151.

CECCHI, G. A., L. T. PETREANU, A. ALVAREZ-BUYLLA, and M. O. MAGNASCO, 2001. Unsupervised learning and adaptation in a model of adult neurogenesis. *J. Comput. Neurosci.* 11:175–182.

CHEN, J. H., L. WEN, S. DUPUIS, J. Y. WU, and Y. RAO, 2001. The N-terminal leucine-rich regions in Slit are sufficient to repel olfactory bulb axons and subventricular zone neurons. *J. Neurosci.* 21:1548–1556.

CHIBA, A., K. MATSUMURA, H. YAMADA, T. INAZU, T. SHIMIZU, S. KUSUNOKI, I. KANAZAWA, A. KOBATA, and T. ENDO, 1997. Structures of sialylated O-linked oligosaccharides of bovine peripheral nerve alpha-dystroglycan: The role of a novel O-mannosyl-type oligosaccharide in the binding of alpha-dystroglycan with laminin. *J. Biol. Chem.* 272:2156–2162.

CHOU, T. M., and S. M. CHOU, 1989. Tuberous sclerosis in the premature infant: A report of a case with immunohistochemistry on the CNS. *Clin. Neuropathol.* 8:45–52.

CLARK, G. D., R. S. McNEIL, G. J. BIX, and J. W. SWANN, 1995. Platelet-activating factor produces neuronal growth cone collapse. *Neuroreport* 6:2569–2575.

CLARK, G. D., M. MIZUGUCHI, B. ANTALFFY, J. BARNES, and D. ARMSTRONG, 1997. Predominant localization of the LIS family of gene products to Cajal-Retzius cells and ventricular neuroepithelium in the developing human cortex. *J. Neuropathol. Exp. Neurol.* 56:1044–1052.

CONOVER, J. C., F. DOETSCH, J. M. GARCIA-VERDUGO, N. W. GALE, G. D. YANCOPOULOS, and A. ALVAREZ-BUYLLA, 2000. Disruption of Eph/ephrin signaling affects migration and proliferation in the adult subventricular zone. *Nat. Neurosci.* 3:1091–1097.

CORBIN, J. G., S. NERY, and G. FISHELL, 2001. Telencephalic cells take a tangent: Non-radial migration in the mammalian forebrain. *Nat. Neurosci.* 4 Suppl:1177–1182.

COROTTO, F. S., J. A. HENEGAR, and J. A. MARUNIAK, 1993. Neurogenesis persists in the subependymal layer of the adult mouse brain. *Neurosci. Lett.* 149:111–114.

D'ARCANGELO, G., R. HOMAYOUNI, L. KESHVARA, D. S. RICE, M. SHELDON, and T. CURRAN, 1999. Reelin is a ligand for lipoprotein receptors. *Neuron* 24:471–479.

D'ARCANGELO, G., G. G. MIAO, S.-C. CHEN, H. D. SOARES, J. I. MORGAN, and T. CURRAN, 1995. A protein related to extracellular matrix proteins deleted in the mouse mutant reeler. *Nature* 374:719–723.

DE CARLOS, J. A., L. LOPEZ-MASCARAQUE, and F. VALVERDE, 1996. Dynamics of cell migration from the lateral ganglionic eminence in the rat. *J. Neurosci.* 16:6146–6156.

DE DIEGO, I., K. KYRIAKOPOULOU, D. KARAGOGEOS, and M. WASSEF, 2002. Multiple influences on the migration of precerebellar neurons in the caudal medulla. *Development* 129:297–306.

DE DIEGO, I., N. SMITH-FERNANDEZ, and A. FAIREN, 1994. Cortical cells that migrate beyond area boundaries: Characterization of an early neuronal population in the lower intermediate zone of prenatal rats. *Eur. J. Neurosci.* 6:983–997.

DES PORTES, V., F. FRANCIS, J. M. PINARD, I. DESGUERRE, M. L. MOUTARD, I. SNOECK, L. C. MEINERS, F. CAPRON, R. CUSMAI, S. RICCI, J. MOTTE, B. ECHENNE, G. PONSOT, O. DULAC, J. CHELLY, and C. BELDJORD, 1998. Doublecortin is the major gene causing X-linked subcortical laminar heterotopia (SCLH). *Hum. Mol. Genet.* 7:1063–1070.

DHAVAN, R., L. H. TSAI, and L. H. TSAI, 2001. A decade of cdk5. *Nat. Rev. Mol. Cell Biol.* 2:749–759.

DULABON, L., E. C. OLSON, M. G. TAGLIENTI, S. EISENHUTH, B. McGRATH, C. A. WALSH, J. A. KREIDBERG, and E. S. ANTON, 2000. Reelin binds alpha3beta1 integrin and inhibits neuronal migration. *Neuron* 27:33–44.

EDMONDSON, J. C., and M. E. HATTEN, 1987. Glial-guided granule neuron migration in vitro: A high-resolution time-lapse video microscopic study. *J. Neurosci.* 7:1928–1934.

EDMONDSON, J. C., R. K. LIEM, J. E. KUSTER, and M. E. HATTEN, 1988. Astrotactin: A novel neuronal cell surface antigen that mediates neuron-astroglial interactions in cerebellar microcultures. *J. Cell Biol.* 106:505–517.

EKSIOGLU, Y. Z., I. E. SCHEFFER, P. CARDENAS, J. KNOLL, F. DIMARIO, G. RAMSBY, M. BERG, K. KAMURO, S. F. BERKOVIC, G. M. DUYK, J. PARISI, P. R. HUTTENLOCHER, and C. A. WALSH, 1996. Periventricular heterotopia: An X-linked dominant epilepsy locus causing aberrant cerebral cortical development. *Neuron* 16:77–87.

ERIKSSON, P. S., E. PERFILIEVA, T. BJÖRK-ERIKSSON, A. ALBORN, C. NORDBORG, D. A. PETERSON, and F. H. GAGE, 1998. Neurogenesis in the adult human hippocampus. *Nat. Med.* 4:1313–1317.

FALCONER, D. S., 1951. Two new mutants, "trembler" and "reeler," with neurological actions in the house mouse. *J. Genet.* 50: 192–201.

FAUST, P. L., and M. E. HATTEN, 1997. Targeted deletion of the pex2 peroxisome assembly gene in mice provides a model for Zellweger syndrome, a human neuronal migration disorder. *J. Cell Biol.* 139:1293–1306.

FENICHEL, G. M., 1988. Congenital muscular dystrophies. *Neurol. Clin.* 6:519–528.

FENG, G., E. C. OLSON, P. T. STUKENBUERG, L. A. FLANAGAN, M. W. KIRSCHNER, and C. A. WALSH, 2000. LIS1 regulates CNS lamination by interacting with mNudE, a central component of the centrosome. *Neuron* 28:665–679.

FERRER, I., I. FABREGUES, J. COLL, T. RIBALTA, and A. RIVES, 1984. Tuberous sclerosis: A Golgi study of cortical tuber. *Clin. Neuropathol.* 3:47–51.

FISHELL, G., C. A. MASON, and M. E. HATTEN, 1993. Dispersion of neural progenitors within the germinal zones of the forebrain. *Nature* 362:636–638.

FLANAGAN, J. G., and P. VANDERHAEGHEN, 1998. The ephrins and Eph receptors in neural development. *Annu. Rev. Neurosci.* 21: 309–345.

FLINT, A. C., and A. R. KRIEGSTEIN, 1997. Mechanisms underlying neuronal migration disorders and epilepsy. *Curr. Opin. Neurobiol.* 10:92–97.

FOX, J. W., E. D. LAMPERTI, Y. Z. EKLU, S. E. HONG, Y. FENG, D. A. GRAHAM, I. E. SCHEFFER, W. B. DOBYNS, B. A. HIRSCH, R. A. RADTKE, S. F. BERKOVIC, P. R. HUTTENLOCHER, and C. A. WALSH, 1998. Mutations in filamin 1 prevent migration of cerebral cortical neurons in human periventricular heterotopia. *Neuron* 21:1315–1325.

FRANCIS, F., A. KOULAKOFF, D. BOUCHER, P. CHAFEY, B. SCHAAR, M. C. VINET, G. FRIOCOURT, N. McDONNELL, O. REINER, A. KAHN, S. K. McCONNELL, Y. BERWALD-NETTER, P. DENOULET, and J. CHELLY, 1999. Doublecortin is a developmentally regulated, microtubule-associated protein expressed in migrating and differentiating neurons. *Neuron* 23:247–256.

FRATER, J. L., R. A. PRAYSON, H. H. MORRIS III, and W. E. BINGAMAN, 2000. Surgical pathologic findings of extratemporal-based intractable epilepsy: A study of 133 consecutive resections. *Arch. Pathol. Lab. Med.* 124:545–549.

FROTSCHER, M., 1997. Dual role of Cajal-Retzius cells and reelin in cortical development. *Cell Tissue Res.* 290:315–322.

FUKUYAMA, Y., M. OSAWA, and H. SUZUKI, 1981. Congenital progressive muscular dystrophy of the Fukuyama type: Clinical, genetic and pathological considerations. *Brain Dev.* 3:1–29.

GAGE, F. H., 1998. Stem cells of the central nervous system. *Curr. Opin. Neurobiol.* 8:671–676.

GAGE, F. H., 2002. Neurogenesis in the adult brain. *J. Neurosci.* 22:612–613.

GELOT, A., T. BILLETTE DE VILLEMEUR, C. BORDARIER, M. M. RUCHOUX, C. MORAINE, and G. PONSOT, 1995. Developmental aspects of type II lissencephaly: Comparative study of dysplastic lesions in fetal and post-natal brains. *Acta Neuropathol. (Berl.)* 89:72–84.

GHEUSI, G., H. CREMER, H. McLEAN, G. CHAZAL, J. D. VINCENT, and P. M. LLEDO, 2000. Importance of newly generated neurons in the adult olfactory bulb for odor discrimination. *Proc. Natl. Acad. Sci. U.S.A.* 97:1823–1828.

GLEESON, J. G., K. M. ALLEN, J. W. FOX, E. D. LAMPERTI, S. BERKOVIC, I. SCHEFFER, E. C. COOPER, W. B. DOBYNS, S. R. MINNEROTH, M. E. ROSS, C. A. WALSH, 1998. Double cortin, a brain-specific gene mutated in human X-linked lissencephaly and double cortex syndrome, encodes a putative signaling protein. *Cell* 92:63–72.

GLEESON, J. G., P. T. LIN, L. A. FLANAGAN, and C. A. WALSH, 1999. Doublecortin is a microtubule-associated protein and is expressed widely by migrating neurons. *Neuron* 23:257–271.

GLEESON, J. G., S. MINNERATH, R. I. KUZNIECKY, W. B. DOBYNS, I. D. YOUNG, M. E. ROSS, and C. A. WALSH, 2000. Somatic and germline mosaic mutations in the doublecortin gene are associated with variable phenotypes. *Am. J. Hum. Genet.* 67: 574–581.

GOFFINET, A. M., 1979. An early development defect in the cerebral cortex of the reeler mouse: A morphological study leading to a hypothesis concerning the action of the mutant gene. *Anat. Embryol. (Berl.)* 157:205–216.

GOLDMAN, S. A., and M. B. LUSKIN, 1998. Strategies utilized by migrating neurons of the postnatal vertebrate forebrain. *Trends Neurosci.* 21:107–114.

GOLDMAN, S. A., and F. NOTTEBOHM, 1983. Neuronal production, migration and differentiation in a vocal control nucleus of the adult female canary brain. *Proc. Natl. Acad. Sci. U.S.A.* 80:2390–2394.

GORDON, N., 1996. Epilepsy and disorders of neuronal migration. II. Epilepsy as a symptom of neuronal migration defects. *Dev. Med. Child Neurol.* 38:1131–1134.

GOULD, E., A. J. REEVES, M. S. A. GRAZIANO, and C. G. GROSS, 1999. Neurogenesis in the neocortex of adult primates. *Science* 286:548–552.

GRAY, G. E., S. M. LEBER, and J. R. SANES, 1990. Migratory patterns of clonally related cells in the developing central nervous system. *Experientia* 46:929–940.

GREENOUGH, W. T., R. W. WEST, and T. J. DEVOOGD, 1978. Postsynaptic plate perforations: Changes with age and experience in the rat. *Science* 202:1096–1098.

GUNAY, M., and S. AYSUN, 1996. Neuronal migration disorders presenting with mild clinical symptoms. *Pediatr. Neurol.* 14:153–154.

HAGER, G., H. U. DODT, W. ZIEGLGANSBERGER, and P. LIESI, 1995. Novel forms of neuronal migration in the rat cerebellum. *J. Neurosci. Res.* 40:207–219.

HANAHAN, D. J., 1986. Platelet activating factor: A biologically active phosphoglyceride. *Annu. Rev. Biochem.* 55:483–509.

HARDESTY, I., 1904. On the development and nature of the neuroglia. *Am. J. Anat.* 3:229–268.

HARDING, B., 1996. Grey matter heterotopia. In *Dysplasias of Cerebral Cortex and Epilepsy*, R. Gerrini, F. Andermann, R. Canapicchi, J. Roger, B. G. Zifkin, and P. Pfanner, eds. Philadelphia: Lippincott-Raven, pp. 81–88.

HATTEN, M. E., and N. HEINTZ, 1998. Neurogenesis and migration. In *Fundamentals of Neuroscience*, M. Zigmond, ed. New York: Academic Press.

HATTEN, M. E., R. H. K. LIEM, and C. A. MASON, 1984. Two forms of glial cells interact differently with neurons in vitro. *J. Cell Biol.* 98:193–204.

HATTEN, M. E., and R. H. K. LIEM, 1981. Astroglia provide a template for the positioning of developing cerebellar neurons in vitro. *J. Cell Biol.* 90:622–630.

HATTEN, M. E., and C. A. MASON, 1990. Mechanisms of glial-guided neuronal migration in vitro and in vivo. *Experientia* 46: 907–916.

HATTORI, M., H. ADACHI, M. TSUJIMOTO, H. ARAI, and K. INOUE, 1994a. The catalytic subunit of bovine brain platelet-activating factor acetylhydrolase is a novel type of serine esterase. *J. Biol. Chem.* 269:23150–29155.

HATTORI, M., H. ADACHI, M. TSUJIMOTO, H. ARAI, and K. INOUE, 1994b. Miller-Dieker lissencephaly gene encodes a subunit of brain platelet-activating factor acetylhydrolase. *Nature* 370: 216–218.

HICKS, S. P., and C. J. D'AMATO, 1968. Cell migrations to the isocortex in the rat. *Anat. Rec.* 160:619–634.

HINDS, J. W., 1968. Autoradiographic study of histogenesis in the mouse olfactory bulb. II. Cell proliferation and migration. *J. Comp. Neurol.* 134:305–322.

HONG, S. E., Y. Y. SHUGART, D. T. HUANG, S. A. SHAHWAN, P. E. GRANT, J. O. HOURIHANE, N. D. MARTIN, and C. A. WALSH, 2000. Autosomal recessive lissencephaly with cerebellar hypoplasia is associated with human RELN mutations. *Nat. Genet.* 26:93–96.

HOWELL, B. W., F. B. GERTLER, and J. A. COOPER, 1997. Mouse disabled (mDab1): A src binding protein implicated in neuronal development. *EMBO J.* 16:121–132.

HOWELL, B. W., R. HAWKES, P. SORIANO, and J. A. COOPER, 1997. Neuronal position in the developing brain is regulated by mouse disabled-1. *Nature* 389:733–736.

HOWELL, B. W., T. M. HERRICK, and J. A. COOPER, 1999. Reelin-induced tryosine phosphorylation of disabled 1 during neuronal positioning. *Genes Dev.* 13:643–648.

HOWELL, B. W., T. M. HERRICK, J. D. HILDEBRAND, Y. ZHANG, and J. A. COOPER, 2000. Dab1 tyrosine phosphorylation sites relay positional signals during mouse brain development. *Curr. Biol.* 10:877–885.

HU, H., H. TOMASIEWICS, T. MAGNUSON, and U. RUTISHAUSER, 1996. The role of polysialic acid in migration of olfactory bulb interneuron precursors in the subventricular zone. *Neuron* 16:735–743.

HUTTENLOCHER, P. R., S. TARAVATH, and S. MOJTAHEDI, 1994. Periventricular heterotopia and epilepsy. *Neurology* 44:51–55.

INOKI, K., Y. LI, T. ZHU, J. WU, and K. L. GUAN, 2002. TSC2 is phosphorylated and inhibited by Akt and suppresses mTOR signaling. *Nat. Cell. Biol.* 4:648–657.

JELLINGER, K., and A. RETT, 1976. Agyria-pachygyria (lissencephaly syndrome). *Neuropadiatrie* 7:66–91.

KAPLAN, M. S., 1983. Proliferation of subependymal cells in the adult primate CNS: Differential uptake of DNA labeled precursors. *J. Hirnforsch.* 24:23–33.

KEMPERMANN, G., 2002. Why new neurons? Possible functions for adult hippocampal neurogenesis. *J. Neurosci.* 22:635–638.

KEMPERMANN, G., H. G. KUHN, and F. H. GAGE, 1997. More hippocampal neurons in adult mice living in an enriched environment. *Nature* 386:493–495.

KENNEDY, T. E., 2000. Cellular mechanisms of netrin function: Long-range and short-range actions. *Biochem. Cell Biol.* 78:569–575.

KIDD, T., K. S. BLAND, and C. S. GOODMAN, 1999. Slit is the midline repellent for the Robo receptor in *Drosophila*. *Cell* 96:785–794.

KIDD, T., K. BROSE, K. J. MITCHELL, R. D. FETTER, M. TESSIER-LAVIGNE, C. S. GOODMAN, and G. TEAR, 1998. Roundabout controls axon crossing of the CNS midline and defines a novel subfamily of evolutionarily conserved guidance receptors. *Cell* 92:205–215.

KISHI, K., 1987. Golgi studies on the development of granule cells of the rat olfactory bulb with reference to migration in the subependymal layer. *J. Comp. Neurol.* 258:112–124.

KLEIN, R. S., J. B. RUBIN, H. D. GIBSON, E. N. DEHAAN, X. ALVAREZ-HERNANDEZ, R. A. SEGAL, and A. D. LUSTER, 2001. SDF-1α induces chemotaxis and enhances Sonic hedgehog-induced proliferation of cerebellar granule cells. *Development* 128:1971–1981.

KO, J., S. HUMBERT, R. T. BRONSON, S. TAKAHASHI, A. B. KULKARNI, E. LI, and L. H. TSAI, 2001. p35 and p39 are essential for cyclin-dependent kinase 5 function during neurodevelopment. *J. Neurosci.* 21:6758–6771.

KOBAYASHI, K., Y. NAKAHORI, M. MIYAKE, K. MATSUMURA, E. KONDO-IIDA, Y. NOMURA, M. SEGAWA, M. YOSHIOKA, K. SAITO, M. OSAWA, K. HAMANO, Y. SAKAKIHARA, I. NONAKA, Y. NAKAGOME, I. KANAZAWA, Y. NAKAMURA, K. TOKUNAGA, and T. TODA, 1998. An ancient retrotransposal insertion causes Fukuyama-type congenital muscular dystrophy. *Nature* 394:388–392.

KOLODKIN, A. L., and D. D. GINTY, 1997. Steering clear of semaphorins: Neuropilins sound the retreat. *Neuron* 19:1159–1162.

KOMURO, H., and P. RAKIC, 1993. Modulation of neuronal migration by NMDA receptors. *Science* 260:95–97.

KOMURO, H., and P. RAKIC, 1998. Distinct modes of neuronal migration in different domains of developing cerebellar cortex. *J. Neurosci.* 18:1478–1490.

KOMURO, H., E. YACUBOVA, E. YACUBOVA, and P. RAKIC, 2001. Mode and tempo of tangential cell migration in the cerebellar external granular layer. *J. Neurosci.* 21:527–540.

KORNACK, D. R., and P. RAKIC, 1995. Radial and horizontal deployment of clonally related cell in the primate neocortex: Relationship to distinct mitotic lineages. *Neuron* 15:311–321.

KORNACK, D. R., and P. RAKIC, 2001. The generation, migration, and differentiation of olfactory neurons in the adult primate brain. *Proc. Natl. Acad. Sci. U.S.A.* 98:4752–4757.

KORNBLUM, H. I., R. J. HUSSAIN, J. M. BRONSTEIN, C. M. GALL, D. C. LEE, and K. B. SEROOGY, 1997. Prenatal ontogeny of the epidermal growth factor receptor and its ligand, transforming growth factor alpha, in the rat brain. *J. Comp. Neurol.* 380:243–261.

KUCHELMEISTER, K., M. BERGMANN, and F. GULLOTTA, 1993. Neuropathology of lissencephalies. *Childs Nerv. Syst.* 9:394–399.

KUKEKOV, V. G., E. D. LAYWELL, O. SUSLOV, K. DAVIES, B. SCHEFFLER, L. B. THOMAS, T. F. O'BRIEN, M. KUSAKABE, and D. A. STEINDLER, 1999. Multipotent stem/progenitor cells with similar properties arise from two neurogenic regions of adult human brain. *Exp. Neurol.* 156:333–344.

LAMB, R. F., C. ROY, T. DIEFENBACH, H. VINTERS, M. JOHNSON, D. G. JAY, and A. HALL, 2000. The TSC1 tumour suppressor hamartin regulates cell adhesion through ERM proteins and the GTPase Rho. *Nat. Cell Biol.* 2:281–287.

LAVDAS, A. A., M. GRIGORIOU, V. PACHNIS, and J. G. PARNAVELAS, 1999. The medial ganglionic eminence gives rise to a population of early neurons in the developing cerebral cortex. *J. Neurosci.* 19:7881–7888.

LETINIC, K., and P. RAKIC, 2001. Telencephalic origin of human thalamic GABAergic neurons. *Nat. Neurosci.* 4:931–936.

LEVI-MONTALCINI, R., 1950. The origin and development of the visceral system in the spinal cord of the chick embryo. *J. Morphol.* 86:253–278.

LEVITT, P., and P. RAKIC, 1980. Immunoperoxidase localization of glial fibrillary acidic protein in radial glial cells and astrocytes of the developing rhesus monkey brain. *J. Comp. Neurol.* 193:815–840.

LEWIS, P. D., 1968. Mitotic activity in the primate subependymal layer and the genesis of gliomas. *Nature* 217:974–975.

LI, H. S., J. H. CHEN, W. WU, T. FAGALY, W. L. YUAN, L. ZHOU, S. DUPUIS, Z. JIANG, W. NASH, C. GICK, D. ORNITZ, J. Y. WU, and Y. RAO, 1999. Vertebrate Slit, a secreted ligand for the transmembrane protein roundabout, is a repellent for olfactory bulb axons. *Cell* 96:807–818.

LICHTIG, C., R. M. LUDATSCHER, H. MANDEL, and R. GERSHONI-BARUCH, 1993. Muscle involvement in Walker-Warburg syndrome: Clinicopathologic features of four cases. *Am. J. Clin. Pathol.* 100:493–496.

LIU, G., and Y. RAO, 2003. Neuronal migration from the forebrain to the olfactory bulb requires a new attractant persistent in the olfactory bulb. *J. Neurosci.* 23:6651–6659.

LOIS, C., and A. ALVAREZ-BUYLLA, 1994. Long-distance neuronal migration in the adult mammalian brain. *Science* 264:1145–1148.

LOIS, C., J.-M. GARCÍA-VERDUGO, and A. ALVAREZ-BUYLLA, 1996. Chain migration of neuronal precursors. *Science* 271:978–981.

LU, Q, E. SUN, R. S. KLEIN, and J. G. FLANAGAN, 2001. Ephrin-B reverse signaling is mediated by a novel PDZ-RGS protein and selectively inhibits G protein-coupled chemoattraction. *Cell* 105:69–79.

LUSKIN, M. B., 1993. Restricted proliferation and migration of postnatally generated neurons derived from the forebrain subventricular zone. *Neuron* 11:173–189.

Luskin, M. B., 1998. Neuroblasts of the postnatal mammalian forebrain: Their phenotype and fate. *J. Neurobiol.* 36:221–233.

Ma, Q., D. Jones, P. R. Borghesani, R. A. Segal, T. Nagasawa, T. Kishimoto, R. T. Bronson, and T. A. Springer, 1998. Impaired B-lymphopoiesis, myelopoiesis, and derailed cerebellar neuron migration in CXCR4- and SDF-1-deficient mice. *Proc. Natl. Acad. Sci. U.S.A.* 95:9448–9453.

Mariani, J., F. Crepel, K. Mikoshiba, J. P. Changeux, and C. Sotelo, 1977. Anatomical, physiological and biochemical studies of the cerebellum from Reeler mutant mouse. *Philos. Trans. R. Soc. Lond. B. Biol. Sci.* 281:1–28.

Marin, O., A. Yaron, A. Bagri, M. Tessier-Lavigne, and J. L. Rubenstein, 2001. Sorting of striatal and cortical interneurons regulated by semaphorin-neuropilin interactions. *Science* 293:872–875.

Mason, C. A., J. C. Edmondson, and M. E. Hatten, 1988. The extending astroglial process: Development of glial cell shape, the growing tip, and interactions with neurons. *J. Neurosci.* 8: 3124–3134.

Mason, H. A., S. Ito, and G. Corfas, 2001. Extracellular signals that regulate the tangential migration of olfactory bulb neuronal precursors: Inducers, inhibitors, and repellents. *J. Neurosci.* 21: 7654–7663.

McDermott, K. W. G., and P. L. Lantos, 1990. Cell-proliferation in the subependymal layer of the postnatal marmoset, Callithrix-Jacchus. *Dev. Brain Res.* 57:269–277.

McEvilly, R. J., M. O. de Diaz, M. D. Schonemann, F. Hooshmand, and M. G. Rosenfeld, 2002. Transcriptional regulation of cortical neuron migration by POU domain factors. *Science* 295:1528–1532.

McNeil, R. S., J. W. Swann, B. R. Brinkley, and G. D. Clark, 1999. Neuronal cytoskeletal alterations evoked by a platelet-activating factor (PAF) analogue. *Cell. Motil. Cytoskel.* 43:99–113.

Menezes, J. R., C. M. Smith, K. C. Nelson, and M. B. Luskin, 1995. The division of neuronal progenitor cells during migration in the neonatal mammalian forebrain. *Mol. Cell. Neurosci.* 6:496–508.

Merz, D. C., and J. G. Culotti, 2000. Genetic analysis of growth cone migrations in *Caenorhabditis elegans*. *J. Neurobiol.* 44:281–288.

Miyata, T., K. Nakajima, J. Aruga, S. Takahashi, K. Ikenaka, K. Mikoshiba, and M. Ogawa, 1996. Distribution of a reeler gene–related antigen in the developing cerebellum: An immuno-histochemical study with an allogeneic antibody CR-50 on normal and reeler mice. *J. Comp. Neurol.* 372:215–228.

Morris, N. R., V. P. Efimov, and X. Xiang, 1998. Nuclear migration, nucleokinesis and lissencephaly. *Trends Cell Biol.* 8:467–470.

Nadarajah, B., J. E. Brunstrom, J. Grutzendler, R. O. Wong, and A. L. Pearlman, 2001. Two modes of radial migration in early development of the cerebral cortex. *Nat. Neurosci.* 4: 143–150.

Nakagawa, T., M. Sasahara, Y. Hayase, M. Haneda, H. Yasuda, R. Kikkawa, S. Higashiyama, and F. Hazama, 1998. Neuronal and glial expression of heparin-binding EGF-like growth factor in central nervous system of prenatal and early-postnatal rat. *Brain Res. Dev. Brain Res.* 108:263–272.

Nery, S., G. Fishell, and J. G. Corbin, 2002. The caudal ganglionic eminence is a source of distinct cortical and subcortical cell populations. *Nat. Neurosci.* 5:1279–1287.

Nguyen, Ba-Charvet, K. T., K. Brose, L. Ma, K. H. Wang, V. Marillat, C. Sotelo, M. Tessier-Lavigne, and A. Chedotal, 2001. Diversity and specificity of actions of Slit2 proteolytic fragments in axon guidance. *J. Neurosci.* 21:4281–4289.

Niethammer, M., D. S. Smith, R. Ayala, J. Peng, J. Ko, M. S. Lee, M. Morabito, and L. H. Tsai, 2000. NUDEL is a novel Cdk5 substrate that associates with LIS1 and cytoplasmic dynein. *Neuron* 28:697–711.

Nikolic, M., M. M. Chou, W. Lu, B. J. Mayer, and L. H. Tsai, 1998. The p35/Cdk5 kinase is a neuron-specific Rac effector that inhibits Pak1 activity. *Nature* 395:194–198.

Noctor, S. C., A. C. Flint, T. A. Weissman, R. S. Dammerman, and A. R. Kriegstein, 2001. Neurons derived from radial glial cells establish radial units in neocortex. *Nature* 409:714–720.

Norman, M. G., B. C. McGillivray, D. K. Kalousek, A. Hill, and K. J. Poskitt, 1995. Neuronal migration disorders and cortical dysplasias. Part I. Migration disorders. In *Congenital Malformations of the Brain: Pathologic, Embryological, Clinical, Radiological and Genetic Aspects*, M. G. Norman, ed. New York: Oxford University Press, pp. 223–277.

Nottebohm, F., 1981. A brain for all seasons: cyclical anatomical changes in song control nuclei of the canary brain. *Science* 214:1368–1370.

Nottebohm, F., 2002. Why are some neurons replaced in adult brain? *J. Neurosci.* 22:24–28.

Nowakowski, R. S., and P. Rakic, 1979. The mode of migration of neurons to the hippocampus: A Golgi and electron microscopic analysis in foetal rhesus monkey. *J. Neurocytol.* 8:697–718.

Nusslein-Volhard, C., E. Wieschaus, and H. Kluding, 1984. Mutations affecting the pattern of the larval cuticle in *Drosophila melanogaster*. I. Zygotic loci on the second chromosome. *Rouxs Arch. Dev. Biol.* 193:67–282.

Ogawa, M., T. Miyata, K. Nakajima, K. Yagyu, M. Seike, K. Ikenaka, H. Yamamoto, and K. Mikoshiba, 1995. The reeler gene–associated antigen on Cajal-Retzius neurons is a crucial molecule for laminar organization of cortical neurons. *Neuron* 14:899–912.

Ogren, M. P., and P. Rakic, 1981. The prenatal development of the pulvinar in the monkey: ^{3}H-thymidine autoradiographic and morphometric analyses. *Anat. Embryol.* 162:1–20.

Ohshima, T., J. M. Ward, C. G. Huh, G. Longenecker, Veeranna, H. C. Pant, R. O. Brady, L. J. Martin, and A. B. Kulkarni, 1996. Targeted disruption of the cyclin-dependent kinase 5 gene results in abnormal corticogenesis, neuronal pathology and perinatal death. *Proc. Natl. Acad. Sci. U.S.A.* 93:1173–11178.

O'Leary, D. D., and D. G. Wilkinson, 1999. Eph receptors and ephrins in neural development. *Curr. Opin. Neurobiol.* 9:65–73.

Olsson, M., C. Bentlage, K. Wictorin, K. Campbell, and A. Bjorklund, 1997. Extensive migration and target innervation by striatal precursors after grafting into the neonatal striatum. *Neuroscience* 79:57–78.

O'Rourke, N. A., M. E. Dailey, S. J. Smith, and S. K. McConnell, 1992. Diverse migratory pathways in the developing cerebral cortex. *Science* 258:99–302.

O'Rourke, N. A., D. P. Sullivan, C. E. Kaznowski, A. A. Jacobs, and S. K. McConnell, 1995. Tangential migration of neurons in the developing cerebral cortex. *Development* 121:2165–2176.

Palmer, A., and R. Klein, 2003. Multiple roles of ephrins in morphogenesis, neuronal networking, and brain function. *Genes Dev.* 17:1429–1450.

Palmini, A., F. Andermann, A. Olivier, D. Tampieri, Y. Robitaille, E. Andermann, and G. Wright, 1991. Focal neuronal migration disorders and intractable partial epilepsy: A study of 30 patients. *Ann. Neurol.* 30:741–749.

Parnavelas, J. G., 2000. The origin and migration of cortical neurones: New vistas. *Trends Neurosci.* 23:126–131.

PEARLMAN, A. L., P. L. FAUST, M. E. HATTEN, and J. E. BRUNSTROM, 1998. New directions for neuronal migration. *Curr. Opin. Neurobiol.* 8:5–54.

PENCEA, V., K. D. BINGAMAN, L. J. FREEDMAN, and M. B. LUSKIN, 2001. Neurogenesis in the subventricular zone and rostral migratory stream of the neonatal and adult primate forebrain. *Exp. Neurol.* 172:1–16.

PINARD, J. M., J. MOTTE, C. CHIRON, R. BRIAN, E. ANDERMANN, and O. DULAC, 1994. Subcortical laminar heterotopia and lissencephaly in two families: A single X linked dominant gene. *J. Neurol. Neurosurg. Psychiatry* 57:14–20.

PINCUS, D. W., H. M. KEYOUNG, C. HARRISON-RESTELLI, R. R. GOODMAN, R. A. R. FRASER, M. EDGAR, S. SAKAKIBARA, H. OKANO, M. NEDERGAARD, and S. A. GOLDMAN, 1998. Fibroblast growth factor-2/brain-derived neurotrophic factor-associated maturation of new neurons generated from adult human subependymal cells. *Ann. Neurol.* 43:576–585.

PINTO, LORD, M. C., and V. S. CAVINESS, JR., 1979. Determinants of cell shape and orientation: A comparative Golgi analysis of cell-axon interrelationships in the developing neocortex of normal and reeler mice. *J. Comp. Neurol.* 187:49–69.

RAKIC, P., 1971. Neuron-glia relationship during granule cell migration in developing cerebellar cortex. *J. Comp. Neurol.* 141:383–312.

RAKIC, P., 1972. Mode of cell migration to the superficial layers of fetal monkey neocortex. *J. Comp. Neurol.* 145:81–84.

RAKIC, P., 1990. Principles of neural cell migration. *Experientia* 46:882–891.

RAKIC, P., and R. L. SIDMAN, 1969. Telencephalic origin of pulvinar neurons in the fetal human brain. *Z. Anat. Entwicklungsgesch.* 129:3–82.

RAKIC, P., and V. S. CAVINESS, 1995. Cortical development: View from neurological mutants two decades later. *Neuron* 14:1101–1104.

RAO, Y., and J. Y. WU, 2001. Neuronal migration and the evolution of the human brain. *Nat. Neurosci.* 4:860–862.

RAPER, J. A., 2000. Semaphorins and their receptors in vertebrates and invertebrates. *Curr. Opin. Neurobiol.* 10:88–94.

RAYMOND, A. A., D. R. FISH, S. M. SISODIYA, N. ALSANJARI, J. M. STEVENS, and S. D. SHORVON, 1995. Abnormalities of gyration, heterotopias, tuberous sclerosis, focal cortical dysplasia, microdysgenesis, dysembryoplastic neuroepithelial tumour and dysgenesis of the archicortex in epilepsy: Clinical, EEG and neuroimaging features in 100 adult patients. *Brain* 118:629–660.

REINER, O., R. CARROZZO, Y. SHEN, M. WEHNERT, F. FAUSTINELLA, W. B. DOBYNS, C. T. CASKEY, and D. H. LEDBETTER, 1993. Isolation of a Miller-Dieker lissencephaly gene containing G protein beta-subunit-like repeats. *Nature* 364:717–721.

REYNOLDS, B. A., and S. WEISS, 1992. Generation of neurons and astrocytes from isolated cells of the adult mammalian central nervous system. *Science* 255:1707.

RICCI, S., R. CUSMAI, G. FARIELLO, L. FUSCO, and F. VIGEVANO, 1992. Double cortex: A neuronal migration anomaly as a possible cause of Lennox-Gastaut syndrome. *Arch. Neurol.* 49:61–64.

RICHARDS, L. J., T. J. KILPATRICK, and P. F. BARTLETT, 1992. De novo generation of neuronal cells from the adult mouse brain. *Proc. Natl. Acad. Sci. U.S.A.* 89:8591–8595.

RINGSTEDT, T., S. LINNARSSON, J. WAGNER, U. LENDAHL, Z. KOKAIA, E. ARENAS, P. ERNFORS, and C. F. IBANEZ, 1998. BDNF regulates reelin expression and Cajal-Retzius cell development in the cerebral cortex. *Neuron* 21:305–315.

ROTHBERG, J. M., D. A. HARTLEY, Z. WALTHER, and S. ARTAVANIS-TSAKONAS, 1988. Slit: An EGF-homologous locus of *D.*

melanogaster involved in the development of the embryonic central nervous system. *Cell* 55:1047–1059.

ROTHBERG, J. M., J. R. JACOB, C. S. GOODMAN, and S. ARTAVANIS-TSAKONAS, 1990. Slit: An extracellular protein necessary for the development of midline glia and commissural axon pathways contains both EGF and LRR domains. *Genes Dev.* 4:2169–2187.

SAITO, Y., M. MIZUGUCHI, A. OKA, and S. TAKASHIMA, 2000. Fukutin protein is expressed in neurons of the normal developing human brain but is reduced in Fukuyama-type congenital muscular dystrophy brain. *Ann. Neurol.* 47:756–764.

SANTAVUORI, P., H. SOMER, K. SAINIO, J. RAPOLA, S. KRUUS, T. NIKITIN, L. KETONEN, and J. LEISTI, 1989. Muscle-eye-brain disease (MEB). *Brain Dev.* 11:147–153.

SAPIR, T., A. CAHANA, R. SEGER, S. NEKHAI, and O. REINER, 1999. LIS1 is a microtubule-associated phosphoprottin. *Eur. J. Biochem.* 265(1):181–188.

SAPIR, T., M. ELBAUM, and O. REINER, 1997. Reduction of microtubule catastrophe events by LIS1, platelet-activating factor acetylhydrolase subunit. *EMBO J.* 16:6977–6984.

SASAKI, S., A. SHIONOYA, M. ISHIDA, M. J. GAMBELLO, J. YINGLING, A. WYNSHAW-BORIS, and S. HIROTSUNE, 2000. A LIS1/NUDEL/cytoplasmic dynein heavy chain complex in the developing and adult nervous system. *Neuron* 28:681–696.

SCHIFFMANN, S. N., B. BERNIER, and A. M. GOFFINET, 1997. Reelin mRNA expression during mouse brain development. *Eur. J. Neurosci.* 9:1055–1071.

SEEGER, M., G. TEAR, D. FERRES-MARCO, and C. S. GOODMAN, 1993. Mutations affecting growth cone guidance in *Drosophila*: Genes necessary for guidance toward or away from the midline. *Neuron* 10:19–26.

SENZAKI, K., M. OGAWA, and T. YAGI, 1999. Proteins of the CNR family are multiple receptors for Reelin. *Cell* 99:635–647.

SHELDON, M., D. S. RICE, G. D'ARCANGELO, H. YONESHIMA, K. NAKAJIMA, K. MIKOSHIBA, B. W. HOWELL, J. A. COOPER, D. GOLDOWITZ, and T. CURRAN, 1997. Scrambler and yotari disrupt the disabled gene and produce a reeler-like phenotype in mice. *Nature* 389:730–733.

SHEPPARD, A. M., and A. L. PEARLMAN, 1997. Abnormal reorganization of preplate neurons and their associated extracellular matrix: An early manifestation of altered neocortical development in the reeler mutant mouse. *J. Comp. Neurol.* 378:173–179.

SHIMOZAWA, N., T. TSUKAMOTO, Y. SUZUKI, T. ORII, Y. SHIRAYOSHI, T. MORI, and Y. FUJIKI, 1992. A human gene responsible for Zellweger syndrome that affects peroxisome assembly. *Science* 255:1132–1134.

SHORS, T. J., G. MIESEGAES, A. BEYLIN, M. ZHAO, T. RYDEL, and E. GOULD, 2001. Neurogenesis in the adult is involved in the formation of trace memories. *Nature* 410:372–376.

SMITH, D. S., M. NIETHAMMER, Y. ZHOU, M. J. GAMBELLO, A. WYNSHAW-BORIS, and L.-H. TSAI, 2000. Regulation of cytoplasmic dynein behavior and microtubule organization by mammalian Lis1. *Nat. Cell Biol.* 2:767–775.

SNOW, R. L., and J. A. ROBSON, 1995. Migration and differentiation of neurons in the retina and optic tectum of the chick. *Exp. Neurol.* 134:13–24.

SOBUE, K., A. AGARWAL-MAWAL, W. LI, W. SUN, Y. MIURA, and H. K. PAUDEL, 2000. Interaction of neuronal Cdc2-like protein kinase with microtubule-associated protein tau. *J. Biol. Chem.* 275:16673–16680.

SOUCEK, D., G. BIRBAMER, G. LUEF, S. FELBER, E. KRISTMANN, and G. BAUER, 1992. Laminar heterotopic grey matter (double cortex) in a patient with late onset Lennox-Gastaut syndrome. *Wien. Klin. Wochenschr.* 104:607–608.

SQUIER, M. V., 1993. Fetal type II lissencephaly: A case report. *Childs Nerv. Syst.* 9:400–402.

SUHONEN, J. O., D. A. PETERSON, J. RAY, and F. H. GAGE, 1996. Differentiation of adult hippocampus-derived progenitors into olfactory neurons in vivo. *Nature* 383:624–627.

SUN, Q., S. BAHRI, A. SCHMID, W. CHIA, and K. ZINN, 2000. Receptor tyrosine phosphatases regulate axon guidance across the midline of the *Drosophila* embryo. *Development* 127:801–812.

SUPER, H., J. A. DEL RIO, A. MARTINEZ, P. PEREZ-SUST, and E. SORIANO, 2000. Disruption of neuronal migration and radial glia in the developing cerebral cortex following ablation of Cajal-Retzius cells. *Cereb. Cortex* 10:602–613.

SWEET, H. O., R. T. BRONSON, K. R. JOHNSON, S. A. COOK, and M. T. DAVISSON, 1996. Scrambler, a new neurological mutation of the mouse with abnormalities of neuronal migration. *Mamm. Genome* 71:798–802.

TACHIBANA, K., S. HIROTA, H. IIZASA, H. YOSHIDA, K. KAWABATA, Y. KATAOKA, Y. KITAMURA, K. MATSUSHIMA, N. YOSHIDA, S. NISHIKAWA, T. KISHIMOTO, and T. NAGASAWA, 1998. The chemokine receptor CXCR4 is essential for vascularization of the gastrointestinal tract. *Nature* 393:591–594.

TAGUCHI, A., A. WANAKA, T. MORI, K. MATSUMOTO, Y. IMAI, T. TAGAKI, and M. TOHYAMA, 1996. Molecular cloning of novel leucine-rich repeat proteins and their expression in the developing mouse nervous system. *Brain Res. Mol. Brain Res.* 35:31–40.

TAKASHIMA, S., S. HOUDOU, J. KAMEI, M. HASEGAWA, T. MITO, Y. SAZUKI, and K. MAEDA, 1992. Neuropathology of peroxisomal disorder; Zellweger syndrome and neonatal adrenoleukodystrophy. *No To Hattatsu* 24:186–193.

TAMAMAKI, N., K. E. FUJIMORI, and R. TAKAUJI, 1997. Origin and route of tangentially migrating neurons in the developing neocortical intermediate zone. *J. Neurosci.* 17:8313–8323.

TAN, S. S., and S. BREEN, 1993. Radial mosaicism and tangential cell dispersion both contribute to mouse neocortical development. *Nature* 362:638–640.

THREADGILL, D. W., A. A. DLUGOSZ, L. A. HANSEN, T. TENNENBAUM, U. LICHTI, D. YEE, C. LAMANTIA, T. MOURTON, K. HERRUP, R. C. HARRIS, et al., 1995. Targeted disruption of mouse EGF receptor: Effect of genetic background on mutant phenotype. *Science* 269:230–234.

TILNEY, F., 1933. Behavior in its relation to the development of the brain. Part II. Correlation between the development of the brain and behavior in the albino rat from embryonic states to maturity. *Bull. Neurol. Inst. N.Y.* 3:252–358.

TRENKNER, E., and R. SIDMAN, 1977. Histogenesis of mouse cerebellum in microwell cultures: Cell reaggregation and migration, fiber and synapse formation. *J. Cell Biol.* 75:915–940.

TROMMSDORFF, M., M. GOTTHARDT, T. HIESBERGER, J. SHELTON, W. STOCKINGER, J. NIMPF, R. E. HAMMER, J. A. RICHARDSON, and J. HERZ, 1999. Reeler/Disabled-like disruption of neuronal migration in knockout mice lacking the VLDL receptor and ApoE receptor 2. *Cell* 97:689–701.

UTSUNOMIYA-TATE, N., K. KUBO, S. TATE, M. KAINOSHO, E. KATAYAMA, K. NAKAJIMA, and K. MIKOSHIBA, 2000. Reelin molecules assemble together to form a large protein complex, which is inhibited by the function-blocking CR-50 antibody. *Proc. Natl. Acad. Sci. U.S.A.* 97:9729–9734.

VAN EDEN, C. G., L. MRZLJAK, P. VOORN, and H. B. M. UYLINGS, 1989. Prenatal development of GABA-ergic neurons in the neocortex of the rat. *J. Comp. Neurol.* 289:213–227.

VAN PRAAG, H., B. R. CHRISTIE, T. J. SEJNOWSKI, and F. H. GAGE, 1999. Running enhances neurogenesis, learning and long-term potentiation in mice. *Proc. Natl Acad. Sci. U.S.A.* 96:13427–13431.

VAN PRAAG, H., A. F. SCHINDER, B. R. CHRISTIE, N. TONI, T. D. PALMER, and F. H. GAGE, 2002. Functional neurogenesis in the adult hippocampus. *Nature* 415:1030–1034.

VAN SLEGTENHORST, M., R. DE HOOGT, C. HERMANS, M. NELLIST, B. JANSSEN, S. VERHOEF, D. LINDHOUT, A. VAN DEN OUWELAND, D. HALLEY, J. YOUNG, et al., 1997. Identification of the tuberous sclerosis gene TSC1 on chromosome 9q34. *Science* 277:805–808.

VOLPE, J., 1987. *Neurology of the Newborn*, 2nd ed. Philadelphia: Saunders.

VOLPE, J. J., and R. D. ADAMS, 1972. Cerebro-hepato-renal syndrome of Zellweger: An inherited disorder of neuronal migration. *Acta Neuropathol (Berl.)* 20:175–198.

WALSH, C. A., 1999. Genetic malformations of the human cerebral cortex. *Neuron* 23:19–29.

WALSH, C., and C. CEPKO, 1990. Cell lineage and cell migration in the developing cerebral cortex. *Experientia* 46:940–947.

WARD, M., C. MCCANN, M. DEWULF, J. Y. WU, and Y. RAO, 2003. Distinguishing between directional guidance and motility regulation in neuronal migration. *J. Neurosci.* 23:5170–5177.

WARE, M. L., J. W. FOX, J. L. GONZALEZ, N. M. DAVIS, C. L. DE ROUVROIT, C. J. RUSSO, S. C. CHUA, A. M. GOFFINET, and C. A. WALSH, 1997. Aberrant splicing of a mouse disabled homolog, mdab1, in the scrambler mouse. *Neuron* 19:239–249.

WECHSLER-REYA, R. J., and M. P. SCOTT, 1999. Control of neuronal precursor proliferation in the cerebellum by Sonic Hedgehog. *Neuron* 22:103–114.

WEICKERT, C. S., M. J. WEBSTER, S. M. COLIN, M. M. HERMAN, T. M. HYDE, D. R. WEINBERGER, and J. E. KLEINMAN, 2000. Localization of epidermal growth factor receptors and putative neuroblasts in human subependymal zone. *J. Comp. Neurol.* 423:359–372.

WICHTERLE, H., D. H. TURNBULL, S. NERY, G. FISHELL, and A. ALVAREZ-BUYLLA, 2001. In utero fate mapping reveals distinct migratory pathways and fates of neurons born in the mammalian basal forebrain. *Development* 128:3759–3771.

WILLS, Z., M. EMERSON, J. RUSCH, J. BIKOFF, B. BAUM, N. PERRIMON, and D. VAN VACTOR, 2002. A Drosophila homolog of cyclase-associated proteins collaborates with the Abl tyrosine kinase to control midline axon pathfinding. *Neuron* 36:611–622.

WINGATE, R. J. T., and M. E. HATTEN, 1999. The role of the rhombic lip in avian cerebellum development. *Development* 126:4395–4404.

WONG, K., X. R. REN, Y. Z. HUANG, Y. XIE, G. LIU, H. SAITO, H. TANG, L. WEN, S. M. BRADY-KALNAY, L. MEI, J. Y. WU, W. C. XIONG, and Y. RAO, 2001. Signal transduction in neuronal migration: Roles of GTPase activating proteins and the small GTPase Cdc42 in the Slit-Robo pathway. *Cell* 107:209–221.

WONG, K., H. T. PARK, J. Y. WU, and Y. RAO, 2002. Slit proteins: guidance cues for cells ranging from neurons to leukocytes. *Curr. Opin. Genet. Dev.* 12:583–591.

WU, W., K. WONG, J. H. CHEN, Z. H. JIANG, S. DUPUIS, J. Y. WU, and Y. RAO, 1999. Directional guidance of neuronal migration in the olfactory system by the secreted protein Slit. *Nature* 400:331–336.

XIANG, X., A. H. OSMANI, S. A. OSMANI, M. XIN, and N. R. MORRIS, 1995. NudF, a nuclear migration gene in Aspergillus-nidulans, is similar to the human LIS-1 gene required for neuronal migration. *Mol. Biol. Cell* 6:297–310.

YEE, K. T., H. H. SIMON, M. TESSIER-LAVIGNE, and D. O. M. O'LEARY, 1999. Extension of long leading processes and neuronal migration in the mammalian brain directed by the chemoattractant Netrin-1. *Neuron* 24:607–622.

YONESHIMA, H., E. NAGATA, M. MATSUMOTO, M. YAMADA, K. NAKAJIMA, T. MIYATA, M. OGAWA, and K. MIKOSHIBA, 1997. A novel neurological mutation of mouse, yotari, which exhibits a reeler-like phenotype but expresses reelin. *Neurosci. Res.* 29: 217–223.

YOSHIDA, A., K. KOBAYASHI, H. MANYA, K. TANIGUCHI, H. KANO, M. MIZUNO, T. INAZU, H. MITSUHASHI, S. TAKAHASHI, M. TAKEUCHI, R. HERRMANN, V. STRAUB, B. TALIM, T. VOIT, H. TOPALOGLU, T. TODA, and T. ENDO, 2001. Muscular dystrophy and neuronal migration disorder caused by mutations in a glycosyltransferase, POMGnT1. *Dev. Cell* 1:717–724.

YUAN, W., L. ZHOU, J. CHEN, J. Y. WU, Y. RAO, and D. ORNITZ, 1999. The mouse Slit family: Secreted ligands for Robo expressed in patterns that suggest a role in morphogenesis and axon guidance. *Dev. Biol.* 212:290–306.

ZALLEN, J. A., B. A. YI, and C. I. BARGMANN, 1998. The conserved immunoglobulin superfamily member SAX-3/Robo directs multiple aspects of axon guidance in *C. elegans*. *Cell* 92: 217–227.

ZHENG, C., N. HEINTZ, and M. E. HATTEN, 1996. CNS gene encoding astrotactin, which supports neuronal migration along glial fibers. *Science* 272:417–419.

ZHU, Y., H. S. LI, L. ZHOU, J. Y. WU, and Y. RAO, 1999. Cellular and molecular guidance of GABAergic neuronal migration from the striatum to the neocortex. *Neuron* 23:473–485.

ZHU, Y., T. YU, X. C. ZHANG, T. NAGASAWA, J. Y. WU, and Y. RAO, 2002. Role of the chemokine SDF-1 as the meningeal attractant for embryonic cerebellar neurons. *Nat. Neurosci.* 5:719–720.

ZHU, Y., T. YU, X.-C. ZHANG, T. NAGASAWA, J. Y. WU, and Y. RAO, 2002. Role of the chemokine SDF-1 as the meningeal attractant for embryonic cerebellar neurons. *Nat. Neurosci.* 5:719–720.

ZOU, Y. R., A. H. KOTTMANN, M. KURODA, I. TANIUCHI, and D. R. LITTMAN, 1998. Function of the chemokine receptor CXCR4 in haematopoiesis and in cerebellar development. *Nature* 393: 595–599.

5 Patterning of the Cerebral Cortex

SONIA GAREL AND JOHN L. R. RUBENSTEIN

ABSTRACT The cerebral cortex is characterized by a modular functional organization: distinct cortical areas with specific patterns of input and output projections are devoted to different functions. Whereas this precise areal organization is shaped and modified by experience, its elaboration begins during embryogenesis. For several decades, the role of nature versus nurture in cortical development has been debated. Recent experiments have shown that cortical regionalization occurs early in embryogenesis, independently of extrinsic input. These observations contribute the elaboration of a new model of cortical development where early intrinsic patterning of the cerebral cortex plays a key role in the emergence of cortical areas.

The functioning of the mammalian cerebral cortex, which regulates most aspects of perception, cognition, and behavior, relies on a precise organization that forms during embryonic and postnatal development (O'Leary, Schlaggar, and Tuttle, 1994; Monuki, Porter, and Walsh, 2001; Pallas, 2001; Ragsdale and Grove, 2001; Ruiz i Altaba, Gitton, and Dahmane, 2001; Sur and Leamey, 2001; O'Leary and Nakagawa, 2002; Lopez-Bendito and Molnar, 2003). Different regions of the cortex are dedicated to distinct functions (Brodmann, 1909). For instance, rostral regions regulate motor and executive functions, caudal regions process somatosensory, auditory, and visual inputs, and ventral regions process olfaction. These different cortical areas are defined by a specific histology, molecular identity, and connectivity pattern, particularly with the dorsal thalamus, which provides the main input to the cerebral cortex.

Over several decades, two models of cortical regionalization have been debated. The protocortex model proposes that cortical areas are defined by the input they receive from the dorsal thalamus ("extrinsic" patterning; O'Leary, 1989). An extension of this model proposes that the nature of the input, for instance visual, is the key parameter. Support for this view comes from axonal rerouting experiments showing that the auditory cortex can process a visual input (Pallas, 2001; Sur and Leamey, 2001). On the other hand, the protomap model proposes that molecular determinants intrinsic to the cortical primordium generate cortical subdivisions with histologically and functionally distinct properties (Rakic, 1988). This model is supported by numerous recent studies, described herein, that demonstrate the role of patterning signals and transcription factors in defining the map of the developing cortex. The weight of the data suggests that both a protomap and the pattern of cortical inputs contribute to the emergence of cortical areas. In this chapter, we present evidence for this unified model, focusing on recent findings that have identified embryonic events controlling regionalization of the neocortex in mice.

Embryonic development of the cerebral cortex: A brief overview

ONTOGENIC ORIGIN OF THE CEREBRAL CORTEX To understand regionalization of the cerebral cortex, we must consider the processes that control early development of the telencephalon. The telencephalon is induced in the rostrolateral neural plate (Cobos et al., 2001). Its molecular regionalization is coupled with a series of major morphological changes, including neurulation (neural tube closure) and evagination of the telencephalic vesicles. The cerebral cortex develops from the "dorsal" part of the telencephalic vesicles, or pallium (figure 5.1). The pallium is further subdivided into medial (MP), dorsal (DP), lateral (LP), and ventral pallium (VP), which will give rise respectively to the hippocampal formation (limbic lobe), the neocortex, the olfactory/piriform cortex, and the claustrum (figure 5.1) (Puelles et al., 2000; Marin and Rubenstein, 2002; Rubenstein and Puelles, 2003). Each of these large domains is subdivided into subdomains, such as the areas of the neocortex (figure 5.1) or the hippocampal fields.

In parallel with these morphogenetic processes, cortical progenitors located in the proliferative neuroepithelium initiate the production of postmitotic neurons that radially migrate toward the pial surface (Marin and Rubenstein, 2002; Rubenstein and Puelles, 2003). In mice, these neurons differentiate into glutamatergic projection neurons, whereas GABAergic interneurons mainly derive from the subpallium proliferative epithelium (Marin and Rubenstein, 2001, 2003). In humans, the cortical proliferative zone generates some GABAergic neurons as well (Letinic, Zoncu, and Rakic, 2002). In the cortex, early-born neurons give rise to subplate neurons, layer I neurons (Cajal-Retzius cells), and deep layer neurons (layers V and VI in the neocortex) (Marin

SONIA GAREL INSERM U368, Département de Biologie, Ecole Normale Supérieure, Paris, France.

JOHN L. R. RUBENSTEIN Nina Ireland Laboratory of Developmental Neurobiology, University of California, San Francisco, Calif.

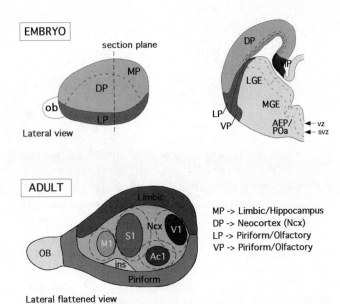

EMBRYO

section plane

MP

DP

ob

LP

Lateral view

DP

LGE

MGE

LP

VP

AEP/
POa

vz

svz

ADULT

Limbic

Ncx

S1

V1

M1

OB

ins

Ac1

Piriform

Lateral flattened view

MP -> Limbic/Hippocampus
DP -> Neocortex (Ncx)
LP -> Piriform/Olfactory
VP -> Piriform/Olfactory

FIGURE 5.1 The development of cortical subdivisions. Schema at top left represents a lateral view of an E14 embryonic telencephalic vesicle showing the lateral (LP; intermediate gray) and dorsal pallium (DP; light gray). The medial pallium (MP) is located on the other side of the vesicle (dotted line). Top right schema represents a cross-section of the same telencephalic vesicle at the level indicated on the left. The ventral and lateral pallium (light gray), dorsal pallium (intermediate gray) and medial pallium (dark gray) subdivide the "dorsal" part of the vesicle, while the lateral and medial ganglionic eminence (LGE, MGE), the anterior entopeduncular region (AEP), and the preoptic area (POa) subdivide the "ventral" part. Schema at bottom represents a flattened lateral view of an adult telencephalic vesicle (i.e., a projection of the lateral view, which includes the normally hidden limbic or medial wall). The correspondence between embryonic and adult structures is indicated in the list. Furthermore, the relative positions of neocortical areas are represented by ovals surrounded by solid lines for primary areas or dotted lines for nonprimary areas. Nonlabeled neocortex is multimodal.

Abbreviations: Ac1, primary auditory cortex; AEP, anterior entopeduncular area; DP, dorsal pallium; ins, insular cortex; LGE, lateral ganglionic eminence; LP, lateral; M1, primary motor cortex; MGE, medial ganglionic eminence; MP, medial pallium; Ncx, neocortex; OB, olfactory bulb; POa, preoptic area; S1, primary somatosensory area; SVZ, subventricular zone; V1, primary visual area; VP, ventral pallium; VZ, ventricular zone. (Figure compiled from Marin and Rubenstein, 2002; Rubenstein and Puelles, 2003.)

and Rubenstein, 2002). Later-born neurons migrate past layers 5 and 6 to form more superficial layers of the cortical plate (layers II to IV in the neocortex).

FORMATION OF THALAMOCORTICAL INTERCONNECTIONS Distinct cortical areas have unique patterns of connectivity. In particular, they exhibit specific connections with nuclei of the dorsal thalamus, which relays information from the periphery (O'Leary, Schlaggar, and Tuttle, 1994; Monuki, Porter, and Walsh, 2001; Pallas, 2001; Ragsdale and Grove, 2001; Ruiz i Altaba, Gitton, and Dahmane, 2001;

Sur and Leamey, 2001; O'Leary and Nakagawa, 2002; Lopez-Bendito and Molnar, 2003).

Dorsal thalamus neurons begin to send axonal projections during embryogenesis. These axons travel through the ventral thalamus and the basal ganglia before reaching the intermediate zone of the cortex (figure 5.2) (Catalano, Robertson, and Killackey, 1991; Miller, Chou, and Finlay, 1993; Molnar, Adams, and Blakemore, 1998; Auladell et al., 2000). Conversely, corticofugal axons from the subplate, layer V and VI, leave the cortex, enter the basal ganglia, and then split into two tracts as they approach the telencephalic-diencephalic boundary: corticothalamic axons (layer VI neurons) run through the ventral thalamus into the dorsal thalamus, and corticospinal axons (layer V neurons) join the cerebral peduncule and innervate subcortical targets such as the superior colliculus, the pons, and the spinal cord (figure 5.2) (Jones, 1984; De Carlos and O'Leary, 1992; Miller, Chou, and Finlay, 1993; Auladell et al., 2000). Corticofugal and thalamocortical axons running through the basal ganglia together form the fiber tracts of the internal capsule.

Once thalamocortical axons from a given thalamic nucleus reach the appropriate cortical region, they transiently synapse on subplate cells (Herrmann, Antonini, and Shatz, 1994). Then, after a short waiting period, thalamic axons grow branches into the cortical plate (Catalano, Robertson, and Killackey, 1991; Miller, Chou, and Finlay, 1993; Molnar, Adams, and Blakemore, 1998; Auladell et al., 2000). On reaching layer IV, they elaborate terminal arbors and synapse upon cortical neurons (Senft and Woolsey, 1991; Agmon et al., 1993; Kageyama and Robertson, 1993; Catalano, Robertson, and Killackey, 1996; Rebsam, Seif, and Gaspar, 2002).

Different thalamic nuclei project to a specific cortical areas in a domain-specific manner (figure 5.2) (Kageyama and Robertson, 1993; O'Leary, Schlaggar, and Tuttle, 1994; Schlaggar and O'Leary, 1994; Agmon et al., 1995; Sur and Leamey, 2001; Lopez-Bendito and Molnar, 2003). This feature is clearly illustrated by the sensory thalamic nuclei: the dorsal lateral geniculate nucleus (dLGN), the ventrobasal nucleus (VB), and the medial geniculate nucleus (MG). These nuclei receive peripheral input from the retina, from skin sensory receptors, and from the cochlea; thalamic nuclei, in turn, project to visual, somatosensory, and auditory cortical areas, respectively. Thus, ascending sensory projections of different modalities (e.g., vision, audition, somatosensory perception) are relayed through specific nuclei of the dorsal thalamus and ultimately to precise cortical areas. Conversely, cortical neurons reciprocally project to the same thalamic nuclei that innervate the area they are located in.

Within each area, a second level of topographic organization is observed: thalamocortical projections form a physical map representing the entire sensory field or space

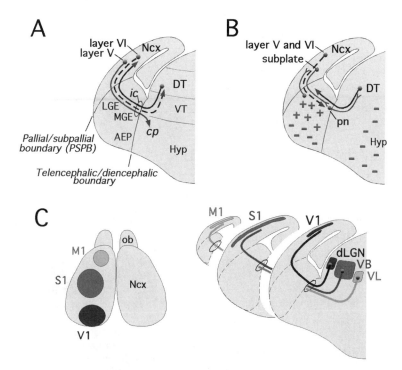

FIGURE 5.2 The formation of thalamocortical interconnections. (*A*) Schematic representation of the embryonic axon tracts formed by thalamocortical (solid dark gray), corticothalamic (dotted dark gray) and corticospinal (solid light gray). In the lateral and medial ganglionic eminences (LGE, MGE), these axons form the internal capsule (ic), and at the telencephalic/diencephalic boundary, corticothalamic and corticospinal tracts diverge; corticospinal axons join the cerebral peduncule (cp). (*B*) Schematic representation of some cues involved in the pathfinding of thalamic and cortical axons; these include attractive (+) and repulsive (−) axon guidance cues as well as transient axonal projections from the basal ganglia (including the perireticular nucleus, pn) and the cortical subplate (thin gray line). (*C*) Cortical primary areas (on the left) receive specific thalamic input (series of rostrocaudal coronal sections on the right). The primary motor cortex (M1) receives projections from the ventrolateral (VL) thalamic nucleus (light gray), the primary somatosensory cortex (S1) receives projections from the ventrobasal (VB) complex (intermediate gray), and the primary visual cortex (V1) receives projections from the dorsolateral geniculate nucleus (dLGN) (dark gray).

Abbreviations: AEP, anterior entopeduncular region; cp, cerebral peduncule; dLGN, dorsolateral geniculate nucleus; DT, dorsal thalamus; Hyp, hypothalamus; ic, internal capsule; LGE, lateral ganglionic eminence; M1, primary motor cortex; MGE, medial ganglionic eminence; Ncx, neocortex; ob, olfactory bulb; pn, perireticular nucleus; S1, primary somatosensory cortex; V1, primary visual cortex; VB, ventrobasal complex; VL, ventrolateral nucleus; VT, ventral thalamus. (Compiled from Metin and Godement, 1996; Molnar, Adams, and Blakemore, 1998; Braisted, Tuttle, and O'Leary, 1999; Bagri et al., 2002; Marin et al., 2002; Lopez-Bendito and Molnar, 2003.)

(O'Leary, Schlaggar, and Tuttle, 1994; Monuki and Walsh, 2001; Ragsdale and Grove, 2001; Sur and Leamey, 2001; O'Leary and Nakagawa, 2002; Lopez-Bendito and Molnar, 2003). For instance, sensory input from individual mouse facial whiskers are processed in specific positions within the barrel field of the somatosensory cortex (Schlaggar and O'Leary, 1993; Killackey, Rhoades, and Bennett-Clarke, 1995; Erzurumlu and Kind, 2001). Topographic sensory maps form postnatally, and their organization is plastic, that is, it is modified in response to activity (Erzurumlu and Kind, 2001). On the contrary, domain-specific thalamocortical and corticothalamic projections are initiated early during embryonic development and appear to form independently of peripheral input (Godement, Saillour, and Imbert, 1979; Kaiserman-Abramof, Graybiel, and Nauta, 1980) and of evoked neuronal activity (Molnar et al., 2002).

Early "intrinsic" regionalization of the cerebral cortex

MOLECULAR PARCELLATION OF THE EMBRYONIC NEOCORTEX The initial evidence supporting the protomap model came from experimental manipulations in primate embryos (Rakic, 1988). Subsequently, the expression patterns of different genes revealed the existence of molecular boundaries within the developing cortex. These genes include the somatosensory cortex H-2Z1 transgene (Cohen-Tannoudji, Babinet, and Wassef, 1994; Gitton, Cohen-Tannoudji, and Wassef, 1999b), cell surface proteins (LAMP: Zacco et al., 1990; latexin: Hatanaka et al., 1994; cadherins: Suzuki et al., 1997; Nakagawa, Johnson, and O'Leary, 1999; Eph/ Ephrin: Gao et al., 1998; Donoghue and Rakic, 1999; Mackarehtschian et al., 1999; Miyashita-Lin et al., 1999; Sestan, Rakic, and Donoghue, 2001; Takemoto et al., 2002;

Yun et al., 2003; and transcription factors [Tbr1, Id2, RZR-beta]: Bulfone et al., 1995; Nothias, Fishell, and Ruiz i Altaba, 1998; Rubenstein et al., 1999).

Notably a number of these molecules showed restricted expression patterns before the arrival of thalamic axons, supporting the existence of a "prethalamic" molecular parcellation of the neocortex (Mackarehtschian et al., 1999; Nakagawa, Johnson, and O'Leary, 1999; Rubenstein and Rakic, 1999). Analyses of *Gbx-2* and *Mash1* knockout mice, which lack thalamocortical input, have demonstrated that early steps in cortical molecular regionalization are independent of thalamic innervation (Miyashita-Lin et al., 1999; Nakagawa, Johnson, and O'Leary, 1999; Yun et al., 2003). Consistently, the expression of the H-2Z1 transgene is induced in cortical explants that do not receive thalamic inputs (Gitton, Cohen-Tannoudji, and Wassef, 1999b), and the expression of latexin is induced in isolated cortical cells (Arimatsu et al., 1999). Finally, heterotopic transplantation experiments showed that the expression patterns of H-2Z1 and LAMP are specified early in development (Barbe and Levitt, 1991; Cohen-Tannoudji, Babinet, and Wassef, 1994). Together these experiments have established that the cerebral cortex is intrinsically regionalized from very early stages of embryogenesis.

EARLY PATTERNING OF THE CORTEX BY SIGNALING CENTERS

Discrete signaling centers producing secreted molecules are implicated in early cortical regionalization. These centers are localized along and flanking the midline of the telencephalic vesicles (figure 5.3) (Rubenstein and Rakic, 1999; Wilson and Rubenstein, 2000; Monuki and Walsh, 2001; Ragsdale and Grove, 2001; Ruiz i Altaba, Gitton, and Dahmane, 2001; O'Leary and Nakagawa, 2002). Dorsally, molecules of the bone morphogenetic protein (BMP) and WNT families control patterning of the medial and dorsal pallium, such as the hippocampus, choroid plexus, and neocortex. Indeed, inactivation of *Wnt3a*, or of the Wnt signaling factor *Lef-1*, severely disrupts the formation of the hippocampus (Galceran et al., 2000; Lee et al., 2000). Ectopic expression and conditional inactivation of the BMP signaling pathway alter respectively the patterning of the dorsal pallium and the development of dorsal midline structures development of the dorsal midline structures (Hebert, Mishina, and McConnell, 2002), as well as a broader patterning of the dorsal pallium (Furuta, Piston, and Hogan, 1997; Golden et al., 1999; Panchision et al., 2001; Ohkubo, Chiang, and Rubenstein, 2002). At the rostral margin of the telencephalon, a source of FGF8 positively regulates telencephalic outgrowth and rostrocaudal regionalization within the cortex (Crossley and Martin, 1995; Shimamura and Rubenstein, 1997; Meyers, Lewandoski, and Martin, 1998; Reifers et al., 1998; Crossley et al., 2001; Fukuchi-Shimogori and Grove, 2001; Garel, Huffman, and Rubenstein, 2003; Storm, Rubenstein, and Martin, 2003). Finally, sources of

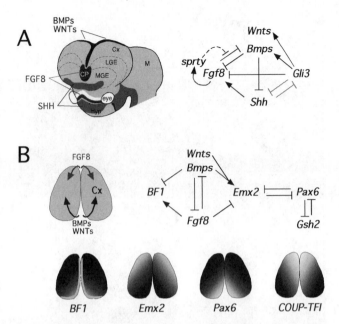

FIGURE 5.3 Signaling centers pattern the telencephalic vesicles. (*A*) A schematic frontal view of an E10.5 brain shows the expression domains of selected *Wnts* (e.g., Wnt3a) and *Bmps* (e.g., BMP4) (dark gray), *Fgfs* (e.g., *Fgf8*) (intermediate gray) and *Shh* (light gray). On the right is a summary of some of the epistatic relations between the different signaling molecules. Dotted lines indicate a hypothetical relationship and light gray lines between *Shh* and *Gli3* indicate a mutual repression of their signaling pathways. (*B*) Role of FGF8 and BMPs/WNTs in controlling the expression of transcription factors in the cerebral cortex. On the left is a schematic diagram of an E11.5 telencephalon and the relative action of secreted midline molecules on the patterning of the cerebral cortex. On the right are some of the known epistatic relationships between secreted molecules and transcription factors. The lower panel shows the resulting rostrocaudal and mediolateral gradients of expression of *BF-1* (*Foxg1*), *Emx2*, *Pax6*, and *COUP-TFI* in the dorsal telencephalon.

Abbreviations: CP, commissural plate; Cx, cerebral cortex; Hyp, hypothalamus; LGE, lateral ganglionic eminence; M, midbrain; MGE, medial ganglionic eminence. (Compiled from Chiang et al., 1996; Gulisano et al., 1996; Furuta, Piston, and Hogan, 1997; Shimamura and Rubenstein, 1997; Theil et al., 1999; Bishop, Goudreau, and O'Leary, 2000; Tole, Ragsdale, and Grove, 2000; Toresson, Potter, and Campbell, 2000; Crossley et al., 2001; Yun, Potter, and Rubenstein, 2001; Anderson et al., 2002; Aoto et al., 2002; Kobayashi et al., 2002; Marin and Rubenstein, 2002; Ohkubo, Chiang, and Rubenstein, 2002; Rallu, Machold, et al., 2002; Theil et al., 2002; Storm, Rubenstein, and Martin, 2003.)

sonic hedgehog (Shh) in the ventral forebrain are essential to the regionalization of the "ventral" telencephalon and might play a role in the patterning of the pallium as well (Chiang et al., 1996; Kohtz et al., 1998; Ohkubo, Chiang, and Rubenstein, 2002; Rallu, Corbin, and Fishell, 2002; Rallu, Machold, et al., 2002). Thus, an array of at least three midline patterning centers is involved in the establishment of regional differences in the telencephalon. The potential for other signaling centers that could be mediated by retinoids (LaMantia et al., 2000; Schneider et al.,

2001; Smith et al., 2001; Halilagic, Zile, and Studer, 2003), the WNT pathway (Kim, Lowenstein, and Pleasure, 2001), or the FGF/EGF pathway (Gimeno et al., 2002; Assimacopoulos, Grove, and Ragsdale, 2003) remains.

The activities of these patterning molecules are regulated by inhibitors and/or repressors of their transduction pathways. For instance, secreted inhibitors of BMPs and WNTs, such as Noggin, Chordin, and sFRPs, are present in the medial and dorsal pallium, and their patterns of expression are consistent with a role in restricting the extent of BMPs and WNTs signaling inside pallium subregions (Shimamura et al., 1995; McMahon et al., 1998; Klingensmith et al., 1999; Kim, Lowenstein, and Pleasure, 2001; Anderson et al., 2002). Similarly, *sprouty* genes, which encode negative regulators of the FGF pathway (Hacohen et al., 1998; Furthauer et al., 2001; Hanafusa et al., 2002), have an expression pattern that overlaps the *Fgf8* domain (Chambers and Mason, 2000; Furthauer et al., 2002; Storm, Rubenstein, and Martin, 2003). Finally, *Gli3*, a repressor of the Shh pathway, is expressed in the pallium, and its inactivation in mouse leads to ventralization of the cortex (Franz, 1994; Grove et al., 1998; Theil et al., 1999; Tole, Ragsdale, and Grove, 2000; Rallu, Corbin, and Fishell, 2002; Rallu, Machold, et al., 2002).

Another level of complexity is added by the fact that these different signaling centers regulate each other's activity (figure 5.3). For instance, ectopic BMP application (Golden et al., 1999; Ohkubo, Chiang, and Rubenstein, 2002) or a reduction in the level of BMP antagonists Chordin and Noggin (Anderson et al., 2002) both negatively regulate *Fgf8* and *Shh* expression in the telencephalon. Furthermore, a reduction in FGF8 activity leads to an increase in *Bmp4* expression and a reduction in *Shh* expression (Schneider et al., 2001; Storm, Rubenstein, and Martin, 2003). Loss of *Shh* expression leads to loss of *Fgf8* expression and an apparent expansion of BMP signaling (Ohkubo, Chiang, and Rubenstein, 2002). In addition, in *Gli3* mutant mice, *Bmps* and *Wnts* expression levels are drastically down-regulated, whereas *Fgf8* expression is up-regulated (Grove et al., 1998; Theil et al., 1999, 2002; Aoto et al., 2002). Thus, multiple levels of cross-regulation and negative feedback loops are likely to create a specific dosage of active secreted molecules and provide precise positional information during development. As such, a subtle imbalance in the *active* levels of these important signaling molecules could affect cortical regionalization.

Signaling Centers Regulate Proliferation, Cell Death, and the Expression of Transcription Factors   Members of the WNT, BMP, and FGF families or their antagonists have been shown to modulate telencephalic morphogenesis, in part by regulating cell proliferation and cell death. For instance, *Wnt3a* inactivation drastically reduces proliferation in the medial pallium, leading to a failure in hippocampus development (Lee et al., 2000). Conversely, the BMP pathway is implicated in dorsal midline cell death (Hebert, Mishina, and McConnell, 2002). Finally, *Fgf8* loss-of-function experiments have shown that this factor is a positive regulator of telencephalic outgrowth via modulation of cell death and proliferation (Meyers, Lewandoski, and Martin, 1998; Reifers et al., 1998; Shanmugalingam et al., 2000; Garel, Huffman, and Rubenstein, 2003; Storm, Rubenstein, and Martin, 2003). These effects appear to function in part through transcription factors. For instance, *BF-1* (*Foxg1*), a member of the winged helix family, has been shown to regulate telencephalic outgrowth (Xuan et al., 1995; Dou, Li, and Lai, 1999), and its expression is regulated positively by FGF8 (Shimamura and Rubenstein, 1997; Kobayashi et al., 2002; Storm, Rubenstein, and Martin, 2003) and negatively by BMP4 (Furuta, Piston, and Hogan, 1997; Ohkubo, Chiang, and Rubenstein, 2002). Similarly, *Msx* genes, which act as positive regulators of apoptosis, are induced in response to BMP4 (Furuta, Piston, and Hogan, 1997).

More generally, it has been proposed that a balanced input of these patterning signals regulates by synergy or competition the graded or localized expression of transcription factors in the cortical neuroepithelium, which in turn controls pallium development and regionalization (figure 5.3). Such a mechanism would account for the observation that a relatively normal sensory map is formed on a surgically reduced cortical sheet in marsupials (Huffman et al., 1999). In particular, two genes encoding homeodomain transcription factors, *Emx2* and *Pax6*, have been shown to play key roles in cortical regionalization and will be presented in detail in the following section. These genes are expressed in gradients along the mediolateral (dorsoventral) and rostrocaudal axes of the cerebral cortex (Simeone, Acampora, et al., 1992; Simeone, Gulisano, et al., 1992; Stoykova and Gruss, 1994; Gulisano et al., 1996; Stoykova et al., 2000; Toresson, Potter, and Campbell, 2000; Yun, Potter, and Rubenstein, 2001; Muzio et al., 2002b), and their expression is likely regulated by patterning centers. In particular, promoter analysis has shown that *Emx2* is a direct target of BMP and WNT signaling pathways in the cortical primordium (Theil et al., 2002). Furthermore, both ectopic FGF8 and a reduction in *Fgf8* levels have shown that FGF8 negatively regulates *Emx2* expression (Crossley et al., 2001; Garel, Huffman, and Rubenstein, 2003; Storm, Rubenstein, and Martin, 2003). Finally, when *Fgf8* levels are severely reduced, *Pax6* expression is down-regulated (Garel et al., 2003; E. Storm, S. Garel, and J. Rubenstein, unpublished observations). Thus, there is accumulating evidence that signaling centers regulate cell proliferation, cell death, and the expression of key transcription factors in the cortical primordium. However, the epistatic relationship between these three downstream events remains largely unexplored.

Role of Transcription Factors in Defining Positional Information Within the Cerebral Cortex Primordium

Localized expression of transcription factors specify cortical domains
Several transcription factors with restricted or graded expression within the pallial neuroepithelium have been shown to control the specification of cortical domains. For instance, cortical progenitors in mutants of the LIM transcription factor Lhx2 acquire the molecular fate of the dorsalmost region of the telencephalic vesicle (Bulchand et al., 2001; Monuki, Porter, and Walsh, 2001). Furthermore, the opposing activities of the *Pax6* and *Gsh2* homeobox genes regulate the formation of the ventral pallium (VP) and its boundaries (Corbin et al., 2000; Toresson, Potter, and Camphell, 2000; Yun, Potter, and Rubenstein, 2001). The domains of strong expression of these two genes meet at the boundary between the VP and the adjacent dorsal lateral ganglionic eminence (dLGE). In *Gsh2−/−* embryos, the dLGE is respecified into a VP-like territory, whereas in *Pax6* mutant embryos, the VP is transformed into a dLGE-like structure.

In addition to these genes, some factors are implicated in controlling the size of cortical domains. For instance, inactivation of *Emx2* severely impairs medial pallium growth, leading to an absence or severe reduction of the hippocampus at birth (Pellegrini et al., 1996; Yoshida et al., 1997; Tole, Goudreau, et al., 2000). Overall, these analyses suggest that cortical patterning is generated via combinations of transcription factors that establish the identity, boundaries, and sizes of cortical domains.

Gradients of transcription factors regulate neocortical regionalization
Emx2 and *Pax6* are expressed in gradients along the medio-lateral and rostrocaudal axis of the cerebral cortex. *Emx2* is expressed in a high mediocaudal to low laterorostral gradient, whereas *Pax6* is expressed in an opposite gradient within the proliferating cortical neuroepithelium (Simeone, Acampora, et al., 1992; Simeone, Gulisano, et al., 1992; Stoykova and Gruss, 1994; Gulisano et al., 1996; Stoykova et al., 2000; Toresson, Potter, and Campbell, 2000; Yun, Potter, and Rubenstein, 2001; Muzio et al., 2002b). In *Emx2−/−* mice, molecularly defined caudal cortical areas are severely reduced and more rostral areas expand caudally (figure 5.4) (Bishop, Goudreau, and O'Leary, 2000; Mallamaci et al., 2000; Bishop et al., 2002). In particular, the occipital cortex (presumptive visual cortex) in *Emx2−/−* mutant newborns adopts a molecular fate characteristic of the parietal neocortex (figure 5.4) (presumptive somatosensory cortex). This molecular shift correlates with a corresponding shift in thalamic projections (figure 5.5), suggesting that the relative size of functional cortical areas is modified in these mutants. Contrary to the phenotype observed in *Emx2−/−* mice, rostral cortical areas acquire a molecular

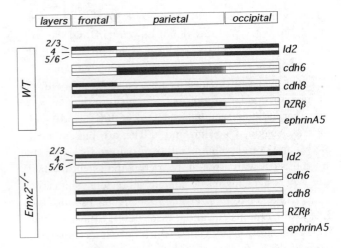

FIGURE 5.4   Regional and layer-specific expression of molecular markers define cortical molecular subdomains at birth. Expression of *Id2*, cadherin 6 (*cdh6*), *cdh8*, *RZRβ*, and *ephrinA5* in different cortical layers and frontal, parietal, or occipital cortical domains is presented in wild type and *Emx2−/−* newborns. A coherent caudal shift in the boundaries of their expression is detected in *Emx2−/−* mutant newborns. (Compiled from Mackarehtschian et al., 1999; Nakagawa, Johnson, and O'Leary, 1999; Rubenstein et al., 1999; Bishop, Goudreau, and O'Leary, 2000; Mallamaci et al., 2000; Bishop et al., 2002.)

identity characteristic of more caudal ones in *Pax6* mutant mice (Bishop, Goudreau, and O'Leary, 2000; Bishop, Rubenstein, and O'Leary, 2002). However, since thalamic axons do not reach the cortex in *Pax6* mutant embryos, the pattern of connectivity of these molecularly modified cortical areas cannot be determined (Kawano et al., 1999; Pratt et al., 2000, 2002; Hevner, Miyashita-Lin, and Rubenstein, 2002; Jones et al., 2002). Finally, another gene encoding an orphan nuclear receptor, *COUP-TFI*, is expressed in a strong to weak, laterocaudal to mediorostral gradient (Wang et al., 1991; Jonk et al., 1994; Qiu et al., 1994; Liu, Dwyer, and O'Leary, 2000). In *COUP-TFI−/−* mice, molecular aspects of cortical regionalization are modified (Zhou, Tsai, and Tsai, 2001). In particular, caudal neocortical areas acquire the molecular identity of more rostral ones, and this molecular shift correlates with a change in the organization of thalamic projections.

Do these factors interact? *Emx2* expression expands in *Pax6* mutants, and vice versa (Muzio et al., 2002b), suggesting that EMX2 and PAX6 repress each other's activity. Furthermore, EMX2 and PAX6 have been implicated in early patterning of the cortex (Muzio and Mallamaci, 2003), as well as in cortical proliferation and outgrowth (Heins et al., 2001; Estivill-Torrus et al., 2002; Muzio et al., 2002a; Shinozaki et al., 2002; Bishop et al., 2003; Muzio and Mallamaci, 2003). Thus, it is possible that counteracting gradients of *Emx2* and *Pax6* regulate the relative size and/or specification of caudomedial and rostrolateral cortical domains, respectively.

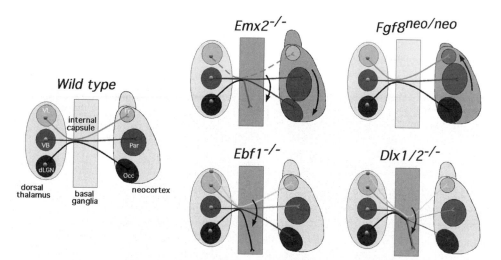

FIGURE 5.5 Cortical regionalization and thalamocortical target-ing in *Emx2−/−*, *Fgf8neo/neo*, *Ebf1−/−* and *Dlx1/2−/−* mutant embryos. The initial targeting of VL, VB, and dLGN axons to the frontal, parietal, and occipital cortex is schematically represented by solid lines of light, intermediate, and dark gray, respectively. The connected thalamic nuclei and cortical subdomains are indicated by the same color code. Changes in the molecular properties of a structure are indicated by gray shading. In *Emx2−/−* mutant embryos, defects in cortical regionalization (black arrow) and axonal pathfinding in the basal ganglia lead to a caudal shift in thalamocortical projections (black arrow over the axons). In *Fgf8neo/neo* mutant embryos, a rostral shift of molecular properties

(black arrow) is observed, whereas thalamocortical projections appear normal. On the contrary, basal ganglia defects in *Ebf1−/−* and *Dlx1/2−/−* mutant embryos affect thalamic axons pathfinding in this region and induce a caudal shift in the organization of thalamocortical projections (black arrows).

Abbreviations: dLGN, dorsolateral geniculate nucleus; Fr, frontal cortex; Occ, occipital cortex; Par, parietal cortex; VB, ventrobasal complex; VL, ventrolateral nucleus. (Compiled from Bishop, Goudreau, and O'Leary, 2000; Mallamaci et al., 2000; Bishop, Rubenstein, and O'Leary, 2002; Garel et al., 2002; Lopez-Bendito et al., 2002; Garel, Huffman, and Rubenstein, 2003.)

Initial targeting of thalamocortical projections: Role of intermediate structures

THALAMOCORTICAL PROJECTIONS: REACHING THEIR TARGET STRUCTURE   Cortical areas are in part defined by their pattern of connection with the dorsal thalamus. Thalamo-cortical and reciprocal corticothalamic projections begin to form during embryogenesis (see earlier discussion under "Ontogenetic Origin of the Cerebral Cortex"), raising the question of what mechanisms control the specificity of this early innervation.

Before reaching their final target, thalamic and corticofu-gal axons grow through intermediate structures, where they undergo abrupt changes of trajectory and growth cone morphology (Miller, Chou, and Finlay, 1993; Metin and Godement, 1996; Molnar, Adams, and Blakemore, 1998; Braisted, Tuttle, and O'Leary, 1999; Auladell et al., 2000; Skaliora, Adams, and Blakemore, 2000). In vitro explant experiments and analyses of mutant mice have shown that guidance molecules and transient cell populations or axons located along axon pathways play a key role in regulating axon outgrowth and pathfinding (see figure 5.2). For instance, attractive guidance cues, including the secreted molecule netrin-1, regulate the turning of thalamic axons into basal ganglia at the diencephalic-telelecephalic bound-ary (Metin et al., 1997; Richards et al., 1997; Braisted,

Tuttle, and O'Leary, 1999; Braisted et al., 2000). Conversely, the secreted factors slit-1 and slit-2 repel axons from the hypothalamus and prevent them from growing toward the midline and ventral territories of the basal ganglia (Bagri et al., 2002). Furthermore, the inactivation of *sema6A*, a transmembrane molecule of the semaphorin family, per-turbs the navigation of thalamic axons at the diencephalic-telencephalic boundary (Leighton et al., 2001). Finally, patterning defects of the preoptic area due to inactivation of the transcription factor gene *Nkx2.1* affect pathfinding of corticofugal axons at the telencephalic-diencephalic boundary, whereas corticothalamic axons behave normally (Marin et al., 2002). These observations point to a key role of the embryonic basal ganglia in organizing afferent and efferent cortical projections.

Independently, transient cell populations located in the basal ganglia mantle, which extend projections into the thal-amus or the neocortex, have been proposed to guide thala-mocortical and corticofugal axons into the basal ganglia (see figure 5.2) (Mitrofanis and Baker, 1993; Mitrofanis and Guillery, 1993; Metin and Godement, 1996). Supporting this hypothesis, *Mash1* or *Pax6* mutant mice, which lack some of these transient cell populations, exhibit abnormal thalamocortical axonal pathfinding (Tuttle et al., 1999; Jones et al., 2002). Cortical subplate neurons also represent a transient cell population that regulates early aspects of corticothalamic connectivity. Subplate axons are the first cortical projections to grow toward the thalamus, and they interact closely with thalamic axons (McConnell, Ghosh, and Shatz, 1989; Ghosh et al., 1990; Shatz et al., 1990; Ghosh and Shatz, 1992; Molnar, Adams, and Blakemore, 1998). Ablation of subplate cells in a cortical subregion induces pathfinding mistakes in the corresponding cortical projection and prevents thalamic innervation of the lesioned region (Ghosh et al., 1990; Ghosh and Shatz, 1993; McConnell, Ghosh, and Shatz, 1994). These observations provided a basis for the "handshake hypothesis" which proposes that converging cortical and thalamic axons meet in the basal ganglia and use each other to reach their target (Molnar and Blakemore, 1991, 1995; Molnar, Adams, and Blakemore, 1998). Consistently, thalamic and cortical axons grow in close contact within the internal capsule (Molnar, Adams, and Blakemore, 1998) and thalamic axons project to a displaced "subplate" in *reeler* mutant mice (Molnar, Adams, Goffinet, et al., 1998). Analyses of mutants with major subplate axonal defects, such as *Tbr1−/−*, *COUP−TFI−/−*, or *Emx1−/−*; *Emx2−/−* mice (Zhou et al., 1999; Hevner et al., 2001; Hevner, Miyashita-Lin, and Rubenstein, 2002; Bishop et al., 2003), or with an impaired thalamic projection, such as *Gbx2−/−* mice (Miyashita-Lin et al., 1999; Hevner, Miyashita-Lin, and Rubenstein, 2002), have shown that defects in one projection have a corresponding effect on the reciprocal thalamic or cortical projection. Similarly, in *p75−/−* mice, in which subplate axons of the occipital cortex show an abnormal outgrowth, the thalamic innervation of the occipital cortex is specifically reduced (McQuillen et al., 2002). Thus, although some experiments have suggested that thalamic and cortical axons do not fasciculate in vitro (Bagnard et al., 2001), there is accumulating evidence that these axons grow in close vicinity in vivo and require each other to reach their respective targets. These interactions could play a key role in the regulating reciprocity of thalamocortical projections in vivo.

Thus, long-distance attractive and repulsive cues, as well as contact-mediated interactions with cell populations and perhaps their axons, guide thalamic and cortical axons to their target structures. However, so far these activities cannot fully account for the domain-specific organization of thalamocortical projections.

THE FORMATION OF DOMAIN-SPECIFIC PROJECTIONS A prevailing model for the formation of topographically organized projections stipulates that these projections are generated through the restricted or graded expression of complementary cues within the projecting and targeted structure. Evidence for this model, known as the chemo-affinity model, comes from the mapping of retinotectal system (Sperry, 1963; Drescher, Bonhoeffer, and Muller, 1997; Goodhill and Richards, 1999; Feldheim et al., 2000).

Support for this mechanism in the formation of thalamocortical maps comes from the cortical expression of Eph/Ephrins (Gao et al., 1998; Donoghue and Rakic, 1999; Mackarehtschian et al., 1999; Vanderhaeghen et al., 2000; Sestan, Rakic, and Donoghue, 2001; Takemoto et al., 2002; Uziel et al., 2002; Yun et al., 2003) and from the phenotypes of *Emx2−/−* and *COUP-TFI−/−* mice, where early changes in cortical molecular regionalization correlate with a shift in thalamic projections (figure 5.5) (Bishop, Goudreau, and O'Leary, 2000; Mallamaci et al., 2000; Zhou, Tsai, and Tsai, 2001). These results suggested that *Emx2* and *COUP-TFI* regulate the restricted neocortical expression of guidance molecules that would control the targeting of thalamic axons.

However, localized attractive or repulsive cortical cues, which could account for the formation of domain-specific thalamocortical projections, have not been identified in vitro yet. Indeed, while localized factors have been shown to regulate the differential innervation of the limbic cortex versus neocortex (Barbe and Levitt, 1991, 1992; Levitt, Barbe, and Eagleson, 1997; Mann et al., 1998), thalamic axons can grow in vitro into any neocortical region without showing a preference (Molnar and Blakemore, 1991). Furthermore, the study of *Fgf8* hypomorphic mice suggests that early cortical regionalization might not strictly control the initial targeting of thalamic axons (figure 5.5), that is, the positioning of thalamic axons within the cortical intermediate zone (Garel, Huffman, and Rubenstein, 2003). Indeed, in these mutants, early gradients of *Emx2* and *COUP-TFI* expression are shifted rostrally and, rostral cortical domains adopt the molecular identity of more caudal cortical regions. However, the initial targeting of thalamic axons in *Fgf8* hypomorphic mutants was indistinguishable from the one observed in wild-type newborns.

Furthermore, the analysis of *Ebf1−/−* and *Dlx1/2−/−* embryos has revealed that the initial domain-specific organization of thalamocortical projections can be shifted along the rostrocaudal axis in the absence of cortical or thalamic regionalization defects (figure 5.5) (Garel et al., 2002). *Ebf1* and *Dlx1/2* inactivation impair different aspects of basal ganglia mantle formation. In both mutants, the shift in thalamocortical targeting was preceded by a shift in the rostrocaudal trajectory of thalamic axons within the basal ganglia. Indeed, in both *Ebf1* and *Dlx1/2* mutants, the trajectory of thalamic axons is shifted as soon as they cross the diencephalic-telencephalic boundary and enter the basal ganglia. Thus, these observations indicate that the trajectory of thalamic axons within the basal ganglia participates in the initial targeting of thalamic axons to different rotrocaudal cortical domains. This idea is supported by the observations that in *Emx2* and *COUP-TFI* mutant mice, the first defects in thalamic axonal navigation are also observed at the telencephalic-diencephalic boundary and within the basal ganglia (figure 5.5) (Zhou et al., 1999; Zhou, Tsai, and Tsai, 2001; Lopez-Bendito et al., 2002). Overall, these results indicate a role for intermediate targets in the guidance and initial targeting of thalamocortical projections. However, these experiments do not investigate the mechanisms regulating the later steps of thalamocortical outgrowth, such as the invasion of the cortical plate, the targeting of axons to layer IV, or the survival of these projections.

Arealization of the cerebral cortex

INTRINSIC DETERMINANTS AND THE GUIDANCE OF THALAMO-CORTICAL AXONS WITHIN THE NEOCORTEX   Although the initial domain-specific targeting of thalamic axons might not be strictly controlled by the cortex, there is a large body of evidence that cortical cues control the guidance and behavior of thalamic axons once they reach the cerebral cortex. For instance, coculture experiments have shown that thalamic axons recognize the layer IV of the neocortex by stopping and branching (Yamamoto, Kurotani, and Toyama, 1989; Molnar and Blakemore, 1991; Bolz, Novak, and Staiger, 1992; Yamamoto et al., 1992; Yamamoto, Higashi, and Toyama, 1997; Yamamoto, Inui et al., 2000; Yamamoto, Matsuyama, et al., 2000; Yamamoto, 2002). Furthermore, extracellular matrix and adhesion molecules are implicated in regulating the outgrowth of thalamic axons into the intermediate zone and cortical plate (Bicknese et al., 1994; Emerling and Lander, 1994, 1996; Miller et al., 1995; Mann et al., 1998).

Recently, members of the ephrin/Eph family, which show a localized expression in the cerebral cortex and dorsal thalamus, have been implicated in regulating the patterns of thalamic innervation (Flanagan and Vanderhaeghen, 1998; Gao et al., 1998; Donoghue and Rakic, 1999; Mackarehtschian et al., 1999; Vanderhaeghen et al., 2000; Sestan, Rakic, and Donoghue, 2001; Takemoto et al., 2002; Uziel et al., 2002; Yun et al., 2003). In vitro experiments have suggested that the expression of *ephrinB3* in the amygdala and limbic cortex (Takemoto et al., 2002) and of *ephrinA5* in the limbic cortex (Gao et al., 1998) might prevent neurite outgrowth of nonlimbic axons into these areas. Analysis of *ephrinA5* mutant mice has confirmed the role of this factor in preventing the outgrowth of thalamic somatosensory axons into the limbic cortex (Uziel et al., 2002). Furthermore, *ephrinA5* mutants have a distorted somatosensory map, suggesting a role for this factor in cortical map formation (Vanderhaeghen et al., 2000). Finally, in vitro coculture experiments also support that these molecules are important in the targeting of thalamic axons to layer IV (Mann et al., 2002). Thus, the restricted expression and layer-specific expression of Eph and ephrins in the neocortex may, as in the retinotectal system, regulate the formation of collaterals and the final innervation of the cortical plate by thalamic axons.

Additional factors, such as cadherins and neurotrophins, are implicated in the formation and refinement of thalamocortical projections. For instance, N-cadherin-blocking antibodies inhibit the ability of thalamic axons to stop in the layer IV of cortical explants (Poskanzer et al., 2003). Furthermore, genetic ablation of neurotrophin-3 in the cerebral cortex results in a decrease of thalamic innervation of the retrosplenial and visual cortex, which are two sites of neurotrophin-3 expression (Ma et al., 2002). Since neurotrophin-3 regulates axonal survival and sprouting, these results support a role for local neurotrophin activity in the establishment of thalamic innervation.

In addition to these local activities that apparently control thalamic outgrowth, branching, and potentially survival, there is evidence that a guidance activity can regulate the directionality of thalamic axons within the neocortex. Heterotopic transplantation experiments in the cortex of newborn rats have shown that, in some cases, the grafted tissue receives thalamic inputs characteristic of their cortical region of origin (Levitt, Barbe, and Eagleson, 1997; Frappe, Roger, and Gaillard, 1999; Gaillard and Roger, 2000). The factors responsible for this activity remain to be determined.

Thus, restricted cortical cues regulate the establishment of an initial thalamocortical innervation pattern, which is further refined in response to activity.

A MAJOR ROLE OF CORTICAL "INTRINSIC" REGIONALIZATION IN AREA MATURATION   While the approximate locations of presumptive cortical areas can be identified at birth, functional cortical areas can only be defined postnatally. Key experiments have demonstrated the role of thalamic input in the maturation and plasticity of the cortical areal map (Rakic, Suner, and Williams, 1991; Catalano and Shatz, 1998). These experiments have recently been reviewed and will not be presented here (Pallas, 2001; Ptito et al., 2001; Sur and Leamey, 2001). However, recent experiments have shown that early patterning molecules are also essential to the functional organization of a neocortical area (Fukuchi-Shimogori and Grove, 2001).

In utero electroporation has been used to alter the levels and spatial distribution of FGF8 signaling while not seriously affecting the postnatal viability of the mice (Fukuchi-Shimogori and Grove, 2001). In these experiments, rostral electroporations of *Fgf8* or of a dominant-negative *Fgf8* receptor at early stages of embryonic development modify the rostrocaudal position of the somatosensory cortex, similar to what is observed in *Fgf8* mutant mice (Garel, Huffman, and Rubenstein, 2003). Unlike the *Fgf8* mutants, the electroporated mice survive and show a rostral displacement of the somatosensory barrel cortex, whose development depends both on intrinsic properties of the cortex and

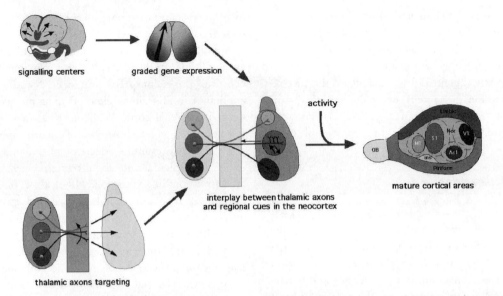

signalling centers

graded gene expression

activity

thalamic axons targeting

interplay between thalamic axons
and regional cues in the neocortex

mature cortical areas

FIGURE 5.6 A model for the formation of cortical areas. Sequential steps in convergent pathways involved in the development of cortical areas are shown. The top pathway controls the regionalization of the cortical neuroepithelium via the effects of secreted molecules from patterning centers that control the graded expression of transcription factors. The bottom pathway controls thalamic development and the subsequent growth of thalamic axons through the diencephalon and basal ganglia to distinct regions of the cerebral cortex. The pathways converge when thalamic axons encounter regional cues within the cortex that direct their growth and branching into appropriate cortical areas. Finally, activity drives the further maturation of cortical areas.

on thalamic activity. Strikingly, an ectopic caudal source of FGF8 induced a partial mirror-image duplication of the barrel field (Fukuchi-Shimogori and Grove, 2001). This remarkable duplication reproduces the phenomenon by which new cortical areas have emerged during evolution: duplication of central representation and reverse symmetry (mirror image). Together these experiments point out a key role of localized secreted factors in the emergence of functional cortical areas. The mechanisms involved, however, remain to be fully elucidated.

THE PATTERN OF THALAMIC INNERVATION IN EARLY CORTICAL AREALIZATION   While activity and input can modify cortical areas properties (Pallas, 2001; Ptito et al., 2001; Sur and Leamey, 2001), some observations conversely suggest that thalamic input may regulate or refine some early aspects of cortical molecular regionalization (O'Leary, Schlaggar, and Tuttle, 1994; Paysan et al., 1997; Gitton, Cohen-Tannoudji, and Wassef, 1999a; Dehay et al., 2001; Gurevich, Robertson, and Joyce, 2001; Polleux et al., 2001). For instance, whereas the activation of the H-2Z1 transgene in the somatosensory cortex is independent of thalamic input, it is not independently expressed once thalamic axons have reached the neocortex (Gitton, Cohen-Tannoudji, and Wassef, 1999a,b). Similarly, in the cortex of *Mash1* mutants, which lack thalamic input, *ephrinA5* expression is modified, although this could be due to the expression of *Mash1* in cortical progenitors (Yun et al., 2003).

A model of cortical arealization

The data reviewed herein suggest an integrated model of cortical arealization (figure 5.6). During embryogenesis, the cerebral cortex primordium is regionalized by discrete sources of secreted molecules that regulate the localized or graded expression of transcription factors. Interactions between these secreted molecules or transcription factors control the relative growth of cortical domains and delimit the boundaries between cortical territories. In a subsequent step, the positional information in the cortical progenitors is imprinted in radially migrating postmitotic neurons. In parallel, thalamic axons grow through the diencephalon and then basal ganglia, where their relative positioning is regulated; from there they enter distinct parts of the cortex. Once in the cortex, thalamic axons sense local cues that control their outgrowth and branching into appropriate regions. Determining the respective roles of intrinsic and extrinsic factors in the emergence of mature cortical areas remains an essential step in our understanding of cortical patterning and development.

ACKNOWLEDGMENTS   We dedicate this work to the memory of Patricia Goldman-Rakic, a pioneer in the studies of cortical anatomy and its functions. Work was supported by the Human Frontiers Science Program (S.G.) and by Nina Ireland, the Sandler Foundation, and the NIH (NINDS grant no. NS34661-01A1 and NIMH grant no. K02 MH01046-01) (J.R.).

REFERENCES

AGMON, A., L. T. YANG, E. G. JONES, and D. K. O'DOWD, 1995. Topological precision in the thalamic projection to neonatal mouse barrel cortex. *J. Neurosci.* 15:549–561.

AGMON, A., L. T. YANG, D. K. O'DOWD, and E. G. JONES, 1993. Organized growth of thalamocortical axons from the deep tier of terminations into layer IV of developing mouse barrel cortex. *J. Neurosci.* 13:5365–5382.

ANDERSON, R. M., A. R. LAWRENCE, R. W. STOTTMANN, D. BACHILLER, and J. KLINGENSMITH, 2002. Chordin and noggin promote organizing centers of forebrain development in the mouse. *Development* 129:4975–4987.

AOTO, K., T. NISHIMURA, K. ETO, and J. MOTOYAMA, 2002. Mouse GLI3 regulates *Fgf8* expression and apoptosis in the developing neural tube, face, and limb bud. *Dev. Biol.* 251:320–332.

ARIMATSU, Y., M. ISHIDA, K. TAKIGUCHI-HAYASHI, and Y. URATANI, 1999. Cerebral cortical specification by early potential restriction of progenitor cells and later phenotype control of postmitotic neurons. *Development* 126:629–638.

ASSIMACOPOULOS, S., E. A. GROVE, and C. W. RAGSDALE, 2003. Identification of a Pax6-dependent epidermal growth factor family signaling source at the lateral edge of the embryonic cerebral cortex. *J. Neurosci.* 23:6399–6403.

AULADELL, C., P. PEREZ-SUST, H. SUPER, and E. SORIANO, 2000. The early development of thalamocortical and corticothalamic projections in the mouse. *Anat. Embryol. (Berl.)* 201:169–179.

BAGNARD, D., N. CHOUNLAMOUNTRI, A. W. PUSCHEL, and J. BOLZ, 2001. Axonal surface molecules act in combination with semaphorin 3a during the establishment of corticothalamic projections. *Cereb. Cortex* 11:278–285.

BAGRI, A., O. MARIN, A. S. PLUMP, J. MAK, S. J. PLEASURE, J. L. RUBENSTEIN, and M. TESSIER-LAVIGNE, 2002. Slit proteins prevent midline crossing and determine the dorsoventral position of major axonal pathways in the mammalian forebrain. *Neuron* 33:233–248.

BARBE, M. F., and P. LEVITT, 1991. The early commitment of fetal neurons to the limbic cortex. *J. Neurosci.* 11:519–533.

BARBE, M. F., and P. LEVITT, 1992. Attraction of specific thalamic input by cerebral grafts depends on the molecular identity of the implant. *Proc. Natl. Acad. Sci. U.S.A.* 89:3706–3710.

BICKNESE, A. R., A. M. SHEPPARD, D. D. O'LEARY, and A. L. PEARLMAN, 1994. Thalamocortical axons extend along a chondroitin sulfate proteoglycan-enriched pathway coincident with the neocortical subplate and distinct from the efferent path. *J. Neurosci.* 14:3500–3510.

BISHOP, K. M., S. GAREL, Y. NAKAGAWA, J. L. RUBENSTEIN, and D. D. O'LEARY, 2003. Emx1 and Emx2 cooperate to regulate cortical size, lamination, neuronal differentiation, development of cortical efferents, and thalamocortical pathfinding. *J. Comp. Neurol.* 457:345–360.

BISHOP, K. M., G. GOUDREAU, and D. D. O'LEARY, 2000. Regulation of area identity in the mammalian neocortex by Emx2 and Pax6. *Science* 288:344–349.

BISHOP, K. M., J. L. RUBENSTEIN, and D. D. O'LEARY, 2002. Distinct actions of Emx1, Emx2, and Pax6 in regulating the specification of areas in the developing neocortex. *J. Neurosci.* 22:7627–7638.

BOLZ, J., N. NOVAK, and V. STAIGER, 1992. Formation of specific afferent connections in organotypic slice cultures from rat visual cortex cocultured with lateral geniculate nucleus. *J. Neurosci.* 12:3054–3070.

BRAISTED, J. E., S. M. CATALANO, R. STIMAC, T. E. KENNEDY, M. TESSIER-LAVIGNE, C. J. SHATZ, and D. D. O'LEARY, 2000. Netrin-1 promotes thalamic axon growth and is required for proper development of the thalamocortical projection. *J. Neurosci.* 20:5792–5801.

BRAISTED, J. E., R. TUTTLE, and D. D. O'LEARY, 1999. Thalamocortical axons are influenced by chemorepellent and chemoattractant activities localized to decision points along their path. *Dev. Biol.* 208:430–440.

BRODMANN, K., 1909. *Vergleichende Lokalisationslehre der Grosshirnrinde in ihren Prinzipien dargestellt auf Grund des Zellenbaues* (Localization in the cerebral cortex). Leipzig, Germany: Barth.

BULCHAND, S., E. A. GROVE, F. D. PORTER, and S. TOLE, 2001. LIM-homeodomain gene *Lhx2* regulates the formation of the cortical hem. *Mech. Dev.* 100:165–175.

BULFONE, A., S. M. SMIGA, K. SHIMAMURA, A. PETERSON, L. PUELLES, and J. L. RUBENSTEIN, 1995. T-brain-1: A homolog of Brachyury whose expression defines molecularly distinct domains within the cerebral cortex. *Neuron* 15:63–78.

CATALANO, S. M., R. T. ROBERTSON, and H. P. KILLACKEY, 1991. Early ingrowth of thalamocortical afferents to the neocortex of the prenatal rat. *Proc. Natl. Acad. Sci. U.S.A.* 88:2999–3003.

CATALANO, S. M., R. T. ROBERTSON, and H. P. KILLACKEY, 1996. Individual axon morphology and thalamocortical topography in developing rat somatosensory cortex. *J. Comp. Neurol.* 367:36–53.

CATALANO, S. M., and C. J. SHATZ, 1998. Activity-dependent cortical target selection by thalamic axons. *Science* 281:559–562.

CHAMBERS, D., and I. MASON, 2000. Expression of *sprouty2* during early development of the chick embryo is coincident with known sites of FGF signalling. *Mech. Dev.* 91:361–364.

CHIANG, C., Y. LITINGTUNG, E. LEE, K. E. YOUNG, J. L. CORDEN, H. WESTPHAL, and P. A. BEACHY, 1996. Cyclopia and defective axial patterning in mice lacking Sonic hedgehog gene function. *Nature* 383:407–413.

COBOS, I., K. SHIMAMURA, J. L. RUBENSTEIN, S. MARTINEZ, and L. PUELLES, 2001. Fate map of the avian anterior forebrain at the four-somite stage, based on the analysis of quail-chick chimeras. *Dev. Biol.* 239:46–67.

COHEN-TANNOUDJI, M., C. BABINET, and M. WASSEF, 1994. Early determination of a mouse somatosensory cortex marker. *Nature* 368:460–463.

CORBIN, J. G., N. GAIANO, R. P. MACHOLD, A. LANGSTON, and G. FISHELL, 2000. The Gsh2 homeodomain gene controls multiple aspects of telencephalic development. *Development* 127:5007–5020.

CROSSLEY, P. H., and G. R. MARTIN, 1995. The mouse Fgf8 gene encodes a family of polypeptides and is expressed in regions that direct outgrowth and patterning in the developing embryo. *Development* 121:439–451.

CROSSLEY, P. H., S. MARTINEZ, Y. OHKUBO, and J. L. RUBENSTEIN, 2001. Coordinate expression of Fgf8, Otx2, Bmp4, and Shh in the rostral prosencephalon during development of the telencephalic and optic vesicles. *Neuroscience* 108:183–206.

DE CARLOS, J. A., and D. D. O'LEARY, 1992. Growth and targeting of subplate axons and establishment of major cortical pathways. *J. Neurosci.* 12:1194–1211.

DEHAY, C., P. SAVATIER, V. CORTAY, and H. KENNEDY, 2001. Cell-cycle kinetics of neocortical precursors are influenced by embryonic thalamic axons. *J. Neurosci.* 21:201–214.

DONOGHUE, M. J., and P. RAKIC, 1999. Molecular evidence for the early specification of presumptive functional domains in the embryonic primate cerebral cortex. *J. Neurosci.* 19:5967–5979.

DOU, C. L., S. LI, and E. LAI, 1999. Dual role of brain factor-1 in regulating growth and patterning of the cerebral hemispheres. *Cereb. Cortex* 9:543–550.

DRESCHER, U., F. BONHOEFFER, and B. K. MULLER, 1997. The Eph family in retinal axon guidance. *Curr. Opin. Neurobiol.* 7:75–80.

EMERLING, D. E., and A. D. LANDER, 1994. Laminar specific attachment and neurite outgrowth of thalamic neurons on cultured slices of developing cerebral neocortex. *Development* 120:2811–2822.

EMERLING, D. E., and A. D. LANDER, 1996. Inhibitors and promoters of thalamic neuron adhesion and outgrowth in embryonic neocortex: Functional association with chondroitin sulfate. *Neuron* 17:1089–1100.

ERZURUMLU, R. S., and P. C. KIND, 2001. Neural activity: Sculptor of "barrels" in the neocortex. *Trends Neurosci.* 24:589–595.

ESTIVILL-TORRUS, G., H. PEARSON, V. VAN HEYNINGEN, D. J. PRICE, and P. RASHBASS, 2002. Pax6 is required to regulate the cell cycle and the rate of progression from symmetrical to asymmetrical division in mammalian cortical progenitors. *Development* 129:455–466.

FELDHEIM, D. A., Y. I. KIM, A. D. BERGEMANN, J. FRISEN, M. BARBACID, and J. G. FLANAGAN, 2000. Genetic analysis of ephrin-A2 and ephrin-A5 shows their requirement in multiple aspects of retinocollicular mapping. *Neuron* 25:563–574.

FLANAGAN, J. G., and P. VANDERHAEGHEN, 1998. The ephrins and Eph receptors in neural development. *Annu. Rev. Neurosci.* 21:309–345.

FRANZ, T., 1994. Extra-toes (Xt) homozygous mutant mice demonstrate a role for the Gli-3 gene in the development of the forebrain. *Acta Anat. (Basel)* 150:38–44.

FRAPPE, I., M. ROGER, and A. GAILLARD, 1999. Transplants of fetal frontal cortex grafted into the occipital cortex of newborn rats receive a substantial thalamic input from nuclei normally projecting to the frontal cortex. *Neuroscience* 89:409–421.

FUKUCHI-SHIMOGORI, T., and E. A. GROVE, 2001. Neocortex patterning by the secreted signaling molecule FGF8. *Science* 294:1071–1074.

FURTHAUER, M., W. LIN, S. L. ANG, B. THISSE, and C. THISSE, 2002. Sef is a feedback-induced antagonist of Ras/MAPK-mediated FGF signalling. *Nat. Cell Biol.* 4:170–174.

FURTHAUER, M., F. REIFERS, M. BRAND, B. THISSE, and C. THISSE, 2001. Sprouty4 acts in vivo as a feedback-induced antagonist of FGF signaling in zebrafish. *Development* 128:2175–2186.

FURUTA, Y., D. W. PISTON, and B. L. HOGAN, 1997. Bone morphogenetic proteins (BMPs) as regulators of dorsal forebrain development. *Development* 124:2203–2212.

GAILLARD, A., and M. ROGER, 2000. Early commitment of embryonic neocortical cells to develop area-specific thalamic connections. *Cereb. Cortex* 10:443–453.

GALCERAN, J., E. M. MIYASHITA-LIN, E. DEVANEY, J. L. RUBENSTEIN, and R. GROSSCHEDL, 2000. Hippocampus development and generation of dentate gyrus granule cells is regulated by LEF1. *Development* 127:469–482.

GAO, P. P., Y. YUE, J. H. ZHANG, D. P. CERRETTI, P. LEVITT, and R. ZHOU, 1998. Regulation of thalamic neurite outgrowth by the Eph ligand ephrin-A5: Implications in the development of thalamocortical projections. *Proc. Natl. Acad. Sci. U.S.A.* 95:5329–5334.

GAREL, S., K. J. HUFFMAN, and J. L. RUBENSTEIN, 2003. Molecular regionalization of the neocortex is disrupted in Fgf8 hypomorphic mutants. *Development* 130:1903–1914.

GAREL, S., K. YUN, R. GROSSCHEDL, and J. L. RUBENSTEIN, 2002. The early topography of thalamocortical projections is shifted in Ebf1 and Dlx1/2 mutant mice. *Development* 129:5621–5634.

GHOSH, A., A. ANTONINI, S. K. MCCONNELL, and C. J. SHATZ, 1990. Requirement for subplate neurons in the formation of thalamocortical connections. *Nature* 347:179–181.

GHOSH, A., and C. J. SHATZ, 1992. Pathfinding and target selection by developing geniculocortical axons. *J. Neurosci.* 12:39–55.

GHOSH, A., and C. J. SHATZ, 1993. A role for subplate neurons in the patterning of connections from thalamus to neocortex. *Development* 117:1031–1047.

GIMENO, L., R. HASHEMI, P. BRULET, and S. MARTINEZ, 2002. Analysis of Fgf15 expression pattern in the mouse neural tube. *Brain. Res. Bull.* 57:297–299.

GITTON, Y., M. COHEN-TANNOUDJI, and M. WASSEF, 1999a. Role of thalamic axons in the expression of H-2Z1, a mouse somatosensory cortex-specific marker. *Cereb. Cortex* 9:611–620.

GITTON, Y., M. COHEN-TANNOUDJI, and M. WASSEF, 1999b. Specification of somatosensory area identity in cortical explants. *J. Neurosci.* 19:4889–4898.

GODEMENT, P., P. SAILLOUR, and M. IMBERT, 1979. Thalamic afferents to the visual cortex in congenitally anophthalmic mice. *Neurosci. Lett.* 13:271–278.

GOLDEN, J. A., A. BRACILOVIC, K. A. MCFADDEN, J. S. BEESLEY, J. L. RUBENSTEIN, and J. B. GRINSPAN, 1999. Ectopic bone morphogenetic proteins 5 and 4 in the chicken forebrain lead to cyclopia and holoprosencephaly. *Proc. Natl. Acad. Sci. U.S.A.* 96: 2439–2444.

GOODHILL, G. J., and L. J. RICHARDS, 1999. Retinotectal maps: Molecules, models and misplaced data. *Trends Neurosci.* 22: 529–534.

GROVE, E. A., S. TOLE, J. LIMON, L. YIP, and C. W. RAGSDALE, 1998. The hem of the embryonic cerebral cortex is defined by the expression of multiple Wnt genes and is compromised in Gli3-deficient mice. *Development* 125:2315–2325.

GULISANO, M., V. BROCCOLI, C. PARDINI, and E. BONCINELLI, 1996. *Emx1* and *Emx2* show different patterns of expression during proliferation and differentiation of the developing cerebral cortex in the mouse. *Eur. J. Neurosci.* 8:1037–1050.

GUREVICH, E. V., R. T. ROBERTSON, and J. N. JOYCE, 2001. Thalamo-cortical afferents control transient expression of the dopamine D(3) receptor in the rat somatosensory cortex. *Cereb. Cortex* 11:691–701.

HACOHEN, N., S. KRAMER, D. SUTHERLAND, Y. HIROMI, and M. A. KRASNOW, 1998. Sprouty encodes a novel antagonist of FGF signaling that patterns apical branching of the *Drosophila* airways. *Cell* 92:253–263.

HALILAGIC, A., M. H. ZILE, and M. STUDER, 2003. A novel role for retinoids in patterning the avian forebrain during presomite stages. *Development* 130:2039–2050.

HANAFUSA, H., S. TORII, T. YASUNAGA, and E. NISHIDA, 2002. Sprouty1 and Sprouty2 provide a control mechanism for the Ras/MAPK signalling pathway. *Nat. Cell Biol.* 4:850–858.

HATANAKA, Y., Y. URATANI, K. TAKIGUCHI-HAYASHI, A. OMORI, K. SATO, M. MIYAMOTO, and Y. ARIMATSU, 1994. Intracortical regionality represented by specific transcription for a novel protein, latexin. *Eur. J. Neurosci.* 6:973–982.

HEBERT, J. M., Y. MISHINA, and S. K. MCCONNELL, 2002. BMP signaling is required locally to pattern the dorsal telencephalic midline. *Neuron* 35:1029–1041.

HEINS, N., F. CREMISI, P. MALATESTA, R. M. GANGEMI, G. CORTE, J. PRICE, G. GOUDREAU, P. GRUSS, and M. GOTZ, 2001. Emx2 promotes symmetric cell divisions and a multipotential fate in precursors from the cerebral cortex. *Mol. Cell Neurosci.* 18:485–502.

HERRMANN, K., A. ANTONINI, and C. J. SHATZ, 1994. Ultrastructural evidence for synaptic interactions between thalamocortical axons and subplate neurons. *Eur. J. Neurosci.* 6:1729–1742.

HEVNER, R. F., E. MIYASHITA-LIN, and J. L. RUBENSTEIN, 2002. Cortical and thalamic axon pathfinding defects in Tbr1, Gbx2, and Pax6 mutant mice: Evidence that cortical and thalamic axons interact and guide each other. *J. Comp. Neurol.* 447:8–17.

HEVNER, R. F., L. SHI, N. JUSTICE, Y. HSUEH, M. SHENG, S. SMIGA, A. BULFONE, A. M. GOFFINET, A. T. CAMPAGNONI, and J. L. RUBENSTEIN, 2001. Tbr1 regulates differentiation of the preplate and layer 6. *Neuron* 29:353–366.

HUFFMAN, K. J., Z. MOLNAR, A. VAN DELLEN, D. M. KAHN, C. BLAKEMORE, and L. KRUBITZER, 1999. Formation of cortical fields on a reduced cortical sheet. *J. Neurosci.* 19:9939–9952.

JONES, L., 1984. Laminar distribution of cortical efferent cells. In *Cerebral Cortex*, vol. I, *Cellular Components of the Cerebral Cortex*, A. Peters and E. G. Jones, eds. New York: Plenum Press, pp. 521–553.

JONES, L., G. LOPEZ-BENDITO, P. GRUSS, A. STOYKOVA, and Z. MOLNAR, 2002. Pax6 is required for the normal development of the forebrain axonal connections. *Development* 129:5041–5052.

JONK, L. J., M. E. DE JONGE, C. E. PALS, S. WISSINK, J. M. VERVAART, J. SCHOORLEMMER, and W. KRUIJER, 1994. Cloning and expression during development of three murine members of the COUP family of nuclear orphan receptors. *Mech. Dev.* 47:81–97.

KAGEYAMA, G. H., and R. T. ROBERTSON, 1993. Development of geniculocortical projections to visual cortex in rat: Evidence of early ingrowth and synaptogenesis. *J. Comp Neurol.* 335:123–148.

KAISERMAN-ABRAMOF, I. R., A. M. GRAYBIEL, and W. J. NAUTA, 1980. The thalamic projection to cortical area 17 in a congenitally anophthalmic mouse strain. *Neuroscience* 5:41–52.

KAWANO, H., T. FUKUDA, K. KUBO, M. HORIE, K. UYEMURA, K. TAKEUCHI, N. OSUMI, K. ETO, and K. KAWAMURA, 1999. Pax-6 is required for thalamocortical pathway formation in fetal rats. *J. Comp. Neurol.* 408:147–160.

KILLACKEY, H. P., R. W. RHOADES, and C. A. BENNETT-CLARKE, 1995. The formation of a cortical somatotopic map. *Trends Neurosci.* 18:402–407.

KIM, A. S., D. H. LOWENSTEIN, and S. J. PLEASURE, 2001. Wnt receptors and Wnt inhibitors are expressed in gradients in the developing telencephalon. *Mech. Dev.* 103:167–172.

KLINGENSMITH, J., S. L. ANG, D. BACHILLER, and J. ROSSANT, 1999. Neural induction and patterning in the mouse in the absence of the node and its derivatives. *Dev. Biol.* 216:535–549.

KOBAYASHI, D., M. KOBAYASHI, K. MATSUMOTO, T. OGURA, M. NAKAFUKU, and K. SHIMAMURA, 2002. Early subdivisions in the neural plate define distinct competence for inductive signals. *Development* 129:83–93.

KOHTZ, J. D., D. P. BAKER, G. CORTE, and G. FISHELL, 1998. Regionalization within the mammalian telencephalon is mediated by changes in responsiveness to Sonic Hedgehog. *Development* 125:5079–5089.

LAMANTIA, A. S., N. BHASIN, K. RHODES, and J. HEEMSKERK, 2000. Mesenchymal/epithelial induction mediates olfactory pathway formation. *Neuron* 28:411–425.

LEE, S. M., S. TOLE, E. GROVE, and A. P. MCMAHON, 2000. A local Wnt-3a signal is required for development of the mammalian hippocampus. *Development* 127:457–467.

LEIGHTON, P. A., K. J. MITCHELL, L. V. GOODRICH, X. LU, K. PINSON, P. SCHERZ, W. C. SKARNES, and M. TESSIER-LAVIGNE, 2001. Defining brain wiring patterns and mechanisms through gene trapping in mice. *Nature* 410:174–179.

LETINIC, K., R. ZONCU, and P. RAKIC, 2002. Origin of GABAergic neurons in the human neocortex. *Nature* 417:645–649.

LEVITT, P., M. F. BARBE, and K. L. EAGLESON, 1997. Patterning and specification of the cerebral cortex. *Annu. Rev. Neurosci.* 20:1–24.

LIU, Q., N. D. DWYER, and D. D. O'LEARY, 2000. Differential expression of COUP-TFI, CHL1, and two novel genes in developing neocortex identified by differential display PCR. *J. Neurosci.* 20:7682–7690.

LOPEZ-BENDITO, G., C. H. CHAN, A. MALLAMACI, J. PARNAVELAS, and Z. MOLNAR, 2002. Role of Emx2 in the development of the reciprocal connectivity between cortex and thalamus. *J. Comp. Neurol.* 451:153–169.

LOPEZ-BENDITO, G., and Z. MOLNAR, 2003. Thalamocortical development: How are we going to get there? *Nat. Rev. Neurosci.* 4:276–289.

MA, L., T. HARADA, C. HARADA, M. ROMERO, J. M. HEBERT, S. K. MCCONNELL, and L. F. PARADA, 2002. Neurotrophin-3 is required for appropriate establishment of thalamocortical connections. *Neuron* 36:623–634.

MACKAREHTSCHIAN, K., C. K. LAU, I. CARAS, and S. K. MCCONNELL, 1999. Regional differences in the developing cerebral cortex revealed by ephrin-A5 expression. *Cereb. Cortex* 9:601–610.

MALLAMACI, A., L. MUZIO, C. H. CHAN, J. PARNAVELAS, and E. BONCINELLI, 2000. Area identity shifts in the early cerebral cortex of *Emx2*−/− mutant mice. *Nat. Neurosci.* 3:679–686.

MANN, F., C. PEUCKERT, F. DEHNER, R. ZHOU, and J. BOLZ, 2002. Ephrins regulate the formation of terminal axonal arbors during the development of thalamocortical projections. *Development* 129:3945–3955.

MANN, F., V. ZHUKAREVA, A. PIMENTA, P. LEVITT, and J. BOLZ, 1998. Membrane-associated molecules guide limbic and nonlimbic thalamocortical projections. *J. Neurosci.* 18:9409–9419.

MARIN, O., J. BAKER, L. PUELLES, and J. L. RUBENSTEIN, 2002. Patterning of the basal telencephalon and hypothalamus is essential for guidance of cortical projections. *Development* 129:761–773.

MARIN, O., and J. L. RUBENSTEIN, 2001. A long, remarkable journey: Tangential migration in the telencephalon. *Nat. Rev. Neurosci.* 2:780–790.

MARIN, O., and J. L. RUBENSTEIN, 2002. Patterning, regionalization and cell differentiation in the forebrain. In *Mouse Development*, J. Rossant and P. Tam, eds. New York: Academic Press, pp. 75–106.

MARIN, O., and J. L. RUBENSTEIN, 2003. Cell migration in the forebrain. *Annu. Rev. Neurosci.* 26:441–483.

MCCONNELL, S. K., A. GHOSH, and C. J. SHATZ, 1989. Subplate neurons pioneer the first axon pathway from the cerebral cortex. *Science* 245:978–982.

MCCONNELL, S. K., A. GHOSH, and C. J. SHATZ, 1994. Subplate pioneers and the formation of descending connections from cerebral cortex. *J. Neurosci.* 14:1892–1907.

MCMAHON, J. A., S. TAKADA, L. B. ZIMMERMAN, C. M. FAN, R. M. HARLAND, and A. P. MCMAHON, 1998. Noggin-mediated antagonism of BMP signaling is required for growth and patterning of the neural tube and somite. *Genes Dev.* 12:1438–1452.

MCQUILLEN, P. S., M. F. DEFREITAS, G. ZADA, and C. J. SHATZ, 2002. A novel role for p75NTR in subplate growth cone complexity and visual thalamocortical innervation. *J. Neurosci.* 22:3580–3593.

METIN, C., D. DELEGLISE, T. SERAFINI, T. E. KENNEDY, and M. TESSIER-LAVIGNE, 1997. A role for netrin-1 in the guidance of cortical efferents. *Development* 124:5063–5074.

METIN, C., and P. GODEMENT, 1996. The ganglionic eminence may be an intermediate target for corticofugal and thalamocortical axons. *J. Neurosci.* 16:3219–3235.

MEYERS, E. N., M. LEWANDOSKI, and G. R. MARTIN, 1998. An *Fgf8* mutant allelic series generated by Cre- and Flp-mediated recombination. *Nat. Genet.* 18:136–141.

MILLER, B., L. CHOU, and B. L. FINLAY, 1993. The early development of thalamocortical and corticothalamic projections. *J. Comp. Neurol.* 335:16–41.

MILLER, B., A. M. SHEPPARD, A. R. BICKNESE, and A. L. PEARLMAN, 1995. Chondroitin sulfate proteoglycans in the developing cerebral cortex: The distribution of neurocan distinguishes forming afferent and efferent axonal pathways. *J. Comp. Neurol.* 355:615–628.

MITROFANIS, J., and G. E. BAKER, 1993. Development of the thalamic reticular and perireticular nuclei in rats and their relationship to the course of growing corticofugal and corticopetal axons. *J. Comp. Neurol.* 338:575–587.

MITROFANIS, J., and R. W. GUILLERY, 1993. New views of the thalamic reticular nucleus in the adult and the developing brain. *Trends Neurosci.* 16:240–245.

MIYASHITA-LIN, E. M., R. HEVNER, K. M. WASSARMAN, S. MARTINEZ, and J. L. RUBENSTEIN, 1999. Early neocortical regionalization in the absence of thalamic innervation. *Science* 285:906–909.

MOLNAR, Z., R. ADAMS, and C. BLAKEMORE, 1998. Mechanisms underlying the early establishment of thalamocortical connections in the rat. *J. Neurosci.* 18:5723–5745.

MOLNAR, Z., R. ADAMS, A. M. GOFFINET, and C. BLAKEMORE, 1998. The role of the first postmitotic cortical cells in the development of thalamocortical innervation in the reeler mouse. *J. Neurosci.* 18:5746–5765.

MOLNAR, Z., and C. BLAKEMORE, 1991. Lack of regional specificity for connections formed between thalamus and cortex in coculture. *Nature* 351:475–477.

MOLNAR, Z., and C. BLAKEMORE, 1995. How do thalamic axons find their way to the cortex? *Trends Neurosci.* 18:389–397.

MOLNAR, Z., G. LOPEZ-BENDITO, J. SMALL, L. D. PARTRIDGE, C. BLAKEMORE, and M. C. WILSON, 2002. Normal development of embryonic thalamocortical connectivity in the absence of evoked synaptic activity. *J. Neurosci.* 22:10313–10323.

MONUKI, E. S., F. D. PORTER, and C. A. WALSH, 2001. Patterning of the dorsal telencephalon and cerebral cortex by a roof plate-Lhx2 pathway. *Neuron* 32:591–604.

MONUKI, E. S., and C. A. WALSH, 2001. Mechanisms of cerebral cortical patterning in mice and humans. *Nat. Neurosci.* 4 Suppl.: 1199–1206.

MUZIO, L., B. DIBENEDETTO, A. STOYKOVA, E. BONCINELLI, P. GRUSS, and A. MALLAMACI, 2002a. Conversion of cerebral cortex into basal ganglia in *Emx2(−/−) Pax6(Sey/Sey)* double-mutant mice. *Nat. Neurosci.* 5:737–745.

MUZIO, L., B. DIBENEDETTO, A. STOYKOVA, E. BONCINELLI, P. GRUSS, and A. MALLAMACI, 2002b. Emx2 and Pax6 control regionalization of the pre-neuronogenic cortical primordium. *Cereb. Cortex* 12:129–139.

MUZIO, L., and A. MALLAMACI, 2003. Emx1, emx2 and pax6 in specification, regionalization and arealization of the cerebral cortex. *Cereb. Cortex* 13:641–647.

NAKAGAWA, Y., J. E. JOHNSON, and D. D. O'LEARY, 1999. Graded and areal expression patterns of regulatory genes and cadherins in embryonic neocortex independent of thalamocortical input. *J. Neurosci.* 19:10877–10885.

NOTHIAS, F., G. FISHELL, and A. RUIZ I ALTABA, 1998. Cooperation of intrinsic and extrinsic signals in the elaboration of regional identity in the posterior cerebral cortex. *Curr. Biol.* 8:459–462.

O'LEARY, D. D., 1989. Do cortical areas emerge from a protocortex? *Trends Neurosci.* 12:400–406.

O'LEARY, D. D., and Y. NAKAGAWA, 2002. Patterning centers, regulatory genes and extrinsic mechanisms controlling arealization of the neocortex. *Curr. Opin. Neurobiol.* 12:14–25.

O'LEARY, D. D., B. L. SCHLAGGAR, and R. TUTTLE, 1994. Specification of neocortical areas and thalamocortical connections. *Annu. Rev. Neurosci.* 17:419–439.

OHKUBO, Y., C. CHIANG, and J. L. RUBENSTEIN, 2002. Coordinate regulation and synergistic actions of BMP4, SHH and FGF8 in the rostral prosencephalon regulate morphogenesis of the telencephalic and optic vesicles. *Neuroscience* 111:1–17.

PALLAS, S. L., 2001. Intrinsic and extrinsic factors that shape neocortical specification. *Trends Neurosci.* 24:417–423.

PANCHISION, D. M., J. M. PICKEL, L. STUDER, S. H. LEE, P. A. TURNER, T. G. HAZEL, and R. D. MCKAY, 2001. Sequential actions of BMP receptors control neural precursor cell production and fate. *Genes Dev.* 15:2094–2110.

PAYSAN, J., A. KOSSEL, J. BOLZ, and J. M. FRITSCHY, 1997. Area-specific regulation of gamma-aminobutyric acid type A receptor subtypes by thalamic afferents in developing rat neocortex. *Proc. Natl. Acad. Sci. U.S.A.* 94:6995–7000.

PELLEGRINI, M., A. MANSOURI, A. SIMEONE, E. BONCINELLI, and P. GRUSS, 1996. Dentate gyrus formation requires Emx2. *Development* 122:3893–3898.

POLLEUX, F., C. DEHAY, A. GOFFINET, and H. KENNEDY, 2001. Pre- and post-mitotic events contribute to the progressive acquisition of area-specific connectional fate in the neocortex. *Cereb. Cortex* 11:1027–1039.

POSKANZER, K., L. A. NEEDLEMAN, O. BOZDAGI, and G. W. HUNTLEY, 2003. N-cadherin regulates ingrowth and laminar targeting of thalamocortical axons. *J. Neurosci.* 23:2294–2305.

PRATT, T., J. C. QUINN, T. I. SIMPSON, J. D. WEST, J. O. MASON, and D. J. PRICE, 2002. Disruption of early events in thalamocortical tract formation in mice lacking the transcription factors Pax6 or Foxg1. *J. Neurosci.* 22:8523–8531.

PRATT, T., T. VITALIS, N. WARREN, J. M. EDGAR, J. O. MASON, and D. J. PRICE, 2000. A role for Pax6 in the normal development of dorsal thalamus and its cortical connections. *Development* 127: 5167–5178.

PTITO, M., J. F. GIGUERE, D. BOIRE, D. O. FROST, and C. CASANOVA, 2001. When the auditory cortex turns visual. *Prog. Brain Res.* 134:447–458.

PUELLES, L., E. KUWANA, E. PUELLES, A. BULFONE, K. SHIMAMURA, J. KELEHER, S. SMIGA, and J. L. RUBENSTEIN, 2000. Pallial and subpallial derivatives in the embryonic chick and mouse telencephalon, traced by the expression of the genes Dlx-2, Emx-1, Nkx-2.1, Pax-6, and Tbr-1. *J. Comp. Neurol.* 424:409–438.

QIU, Y., A. J. COONEY, S. KURATANI, F. J. DEMAYO, S. Y. TSAI, and M. J. TSAI, 1994. Spatiotemporal expression patterns of chicken ovalbumin upstream promoter-transcription factors in the developing mouse central nervous system: Evidence for a role in segmental patterning of the diencephalon. *Proc. Natl. Acad. Sci. U.S.A.* 91:4451–4455.

RAGSDALE, C. W., and E. A. GROVE, 2001. Patterning the mammalian cerebral cortex. *Curr. Opin. Neurobiol.* 11:50–58.

RAKIC, P., 1988. Specification of cerebral cortical areas. *Science* 241:170–176.

RAKIC, P., I. SUNER, and R. W. WILLIAMS, 1991. A novel cytoarchitectonic area induced experimentally within the primate visual cortex. *Proc. Natl. Acad. Sci. U.S.A.* 88:2083–2087.

RALLU, M., J. G. CORBIN, and G. FISHELL, 2002. Parsing the prosencephalon. *Nat. Rev. Neurosci.* 3:943–951.

RALLU, M., R. MACHOLD, N. GAIANO, J. G. CORBIN, A. P. MCMAHON, and G. FISHELL, 2002. Dorsoventral patterning is established in the telencephalon of mutants lacking both Gli3 and Hedgehog signaling. *Development* 129:4963–4974.

REBSAM, A., I. SEIF, and P. GASPAR, 2002. Refinement of thalamocortical arbors and emergence of barrel domains in the primary somatosensory cortex: A study of normal and monoamine oxidase A knock-out mice. *J. Neurosci.* 22:8541–8552.

REIFERS, F., H. BOHLI, E. C. WALSH, P. H. CROSSLEY, D. Y. STAINIER, and M. BRAND, 1998. Fgf8 is mutated in zebrafish acerebellar (ace) mutants and is required for maintenance of midbrain-hindbrain boundary development and somitogenesis. *Development* 125:2381–2395.

RICHARDS, L. J., S. E. KOESTER, R. TUTTLE, and D. D. O'LEARY, 1997. Directed growth of early cortical axons is influenced by a chemoattractant released from an intermediate target. *J. Neurosci.* 17:2445–2458.

RUBENSTEIN, J. L., S. ANDERSON, L. SHI, E. MIYASHITA-LIN, A. BULFONE, and R. HEVNER, 1999. Genetic control of cortical regionalization and connectivity. *Cereb. Cortex* 9:524–532.

RUBENSTEIN, J. L., and L. PUELLES, 2003. Development of the Nervous System. In *Molecular Basis Of Inborn Errors of Development*, C. J. Epstein, R. P. Erikson, and A. Wynshaw-Boris, eds. New York: Oxford University Press, chapter 7.

RUBENSTEIN, J. L., and P. RAKIC, 1999. Genetic control of cortical development. *Cereb. Cortex* 9:521–523.

RUIZ I ALTABA, A., Y. GITTON, and N. DAHMANE, 2001. Embryonic regionalization of the neocortex. *Mech. Dev.* 107:3–11.

SCHLAGGAR, B. L., and D. D. O'LEARY, 1993. Patterning of the barrel field in somatosensory cortex with implications for the specification of neocortical areas. *Perspect. Dev. Neurobiol.* 1:81–91.

SCHLAGGAR, B. L., and D. D. O'LEARY, 1994. Early development of the somatotopic map and barrel patterning in rat somatosensory cortex. *J. Comp. Neurol.* 346:80–96.

SCHNEIDER, R. A., D. HU, J. L. RUBENSTEIN, M. MADEN, and J. A. HELMS, 2001. Local retinoid signaling coordinates forebrain and facial morphogenesis by maintaining FGF8 and SHH. *Development* 128:2755–2767.

SENFT, S. L., and T. A. WOOLSEY, 1991. Growth of thalamic afferents into mouse barrel cortex. *Cereb. Cortex* 1:308–335.

SESTAN, N., P. RAKIC, and M. J. DONOGHUE, 2001. Independent parcellation of the embryonic visual cortex and thalamus revealed by combinatorial Eph/ephrin gene expression. *Curr. Biol.* 11:39–43.

SHANMUGALINGAM, S., C. HOUART, A. PICKER, F. REIFERS, R. MACDONALD, A. BARTH, K. GRIFFIN, M. BRAND, and S. W. WILSON, 2000. Ace/Fgf8 is required for forebrain commissure formation and patterning of the telencephalon. *Development* 127:2549–2561.

SHATZ, C. J., A. GHOSH, S. K. MCCONNELL, K. L. ALLENDOERFER, E. FRIAUF, and A. ANTONINI, 1990. Pioneer neurons and target selection in cerebral cortical development. *Cold Spring Harb. Symp. Quant. Biol.* 55:469–480.

SHIMAMURA, K., D. J. HARTIGAN, S. MARTINEZ, L. PUELLES, and J. L. RUBENSTEIN, 1995. Longitudinal organization of the anterior neural plate and neural tube. *Development* 121:3923–3933.

SHIMAMURA, K., and J. L. RUBENSTEIN, 1997. Inductive interactions direct early regionalization of the mouse forebrain. *Development* 124:2709–2718.

SHINOZAKI, K., T. MIYAGI, M. YOSHIDA, T. MIYATA, M. OGAWA, S. AIZAWA, and Y. SUDA, 2002. Absence of Cajal-Retzius cells and subplate neurons associated with defects of tangential cell migra-

tion from ganglionic eminence in Emx1/2 double mutant cerebral cortex. *Development* 129:3479–3492.

SIMEONE, A., D. ACAMPORA, M. GULISANO, A. STORNAIUOLO, and E. BONCINELLI, 1992. Nested expression domains of four homeobox genes in developing rostral brain. *Nature* 358:687–690.

SIMEONE, A., M. GULISANO, D. ACAMPORA, A. STORNAIUOLO, M. RAMBALDI, and E. BONCINELLI, 1992. Two vertebrate homeobox genes related to the *Drosophila* empty spiracles gene are expressed in the embryonic cerebral cortex. *Embo. J.* 11:2541–2550.

SKALIORA, I., R. ADAMS, and C. BLAKEMORE, 2000. Morphology and growth patterns of developing thalamocortical axons. *J. Neurosci.* 20:3650–3662.

SMITH, D., E. WAGNER, O. KOUL, P. MCCAFFERY, and U. C. DRAGER, 2001. Retinoic acid synthesis for the developing telencephalon. *Cereb. Cortex* 11:894–905.

SPERRY, R. W., 1963. Chemoaffinity in the orderly growth of nerve fiber patterns and connections. *Proc. Natl. Acad. Sci. U.S.A.* 50:703–710.

STORM, E. E., J. L. RUBENSTEIN, and G. R. MARTIN, 2003. Dosage of Fgf8 determines whether cell survival is positively or negatively regulated in the developing forebrain. *Proc. Natl. Acad. Sci. U.S.A.* 100:1757–1762.

STOYKOVA, A., and P. GRUSS, 1994. Roles of Pax-genes in developing and adult brain as suggested by expression patterns. *J. Neurosci.* 14:1395–1412.

STOYKOVA, A., D. TREICHEL, M. HALLONET, and P. GRUSS, 2000. Pax6 modulates the dorsoventral patterning of the mammalian telencephalon. *J. Neurosci.* 20:8042–8050.

SUR, M., and C. A. LEAMEY, 2001. Development and plasticity of cortical areas and networks. *Nat. Rev. Neurosci.* 2:251–262.

SUZUKI, S. C., T. INOUE, Y. KIMURA, T. TANAKA, and M. TAKEICHI, 1997. Neuronal circuits are subdivided by differential expression of type-II classic cadherins in postnatal mouse brains. *Mol. Cell. Neurosci.* 9:433–447.

TAKEMOTO, M., T. FUKUDA, R. SONODA, F. MURAKAMI, H. TANAKA, and N. YAMAMOTO, 2002. Ephrin-B3-EphA4 interactions regulate the growth of specific thalamocortical axon populations in vitro. *Eur. J. Neurosci.* 16:1168–1172.

THEIL, T., G. ALVAREZ-BOLADO, A. WALTER, and U. RUTHER, 1999. Gli3 is required for *Emx* gene expression during dorsal telencephalon development. *Development* 126:3561–3571.

THEIL, T., S. AYDIN, S. KOCH, L. GROTEWOLD, and U. RUTHER, 2002. Wnt and Bmp signalling cooperatively regulate graded *Emx2* expression in the dorsal telencephalon. *Development* 129:3045–3054.

TOLE, S., G. GOUDREAU, S. ASSIMACOPOULOS, and E. A. GROVE, 2000. *Emx2* is required for growth of the hippocampus but not for hippocampal field specification. *J. Neurosci.* 20:2618–2625.

TOLE, S., C. W. RAGSDALE, and E. A. GROVE, 2000. Dorsoventral patterning of the telencephalon is disrupted in the mouse mutant extra-toes(J). *Dev. Biol.* 217:254–265.

TORESSON, H., S. S. POTTER, and K. CAMPBELL, 2000. Genetic control of dorsal-ventral identity in the telencephalon: Opposing roles for Pax6 and Gsh2. *Development* 127:4361–4371.

TUTTLE, R., Y. NAKAGAWA, J. E. JOHNSON, and D. D. O'LEARY, 1999. Defects in thalamocortical axon pathfinding correlate with altered cell domains in Mash-1-deficient mice. *Development* 126:1903–1916.

UZIEL, D., S. MUHLFRIEDEL, K. ZARBALIS, W. WURST, P. LEVITT, and J. BOLZ, 2002. Miswiring of limbic thalamocortical projections in the absence of ephrin-A5. *J. Neurosci.* 22:9352–9357.

VANDERHAEGHEN, P., Q. LU, N. PRAKASH, J. FRISEN, C. A. WALSH, R. D. FROSTIG, and J. G. FLANAGAN, 2000. A mapping label required for normal scale of body representation in the cortex. *Nat. Neurosci.* 3:358–365.

WANG, L. H., N. H. ING, S. Y. TSAI, B. W. O'MALLEY, and M. J. TSAI, 1991. The *COUP*-TFs compose a family of functionally related transcription factors. *Gene Expr* 1:207–216.

WILSON, S. W., and J. L. RUBENSTEIN, 2000. Induction and dorsoventral patterning of the telencephalon. *Neuron* 28: 641–651.

XUAN, S., C. A. BAPTISTA, G. BALAS, W. TAO, V. C. SOARES, and E. LAI, 1995. Winged helix transcription factor BF-1 is essential for the development of the cerebral hemispheres. *Neuron* 14: 1141–1152.

YAMAMOTO, N., 2002. Cellular and molecular basis for the formation of lamina-specific thalamocortical projections. *Neurosci. Res.* 42:167–173.

YAMAMOTO, N., S. HIGASHI, and K. TOYAMA, 1997. Stop and branch behaviors of geniculocortical axons: A time-lapse study in organotypic cocultures. *J. Neurosci.* 17:3653–3663.

YAMAMOTO, N., K. INUI, Y. MATSUYAMA, A. HARADA, K. HANAMURA, F. MURAKAMI, E. S. RUTHAZER, U. RUTISHAUSER, and T. SEKI, 2000. Inhibitory mechanism by polysialic acid for lamina-specific branch formation of thalamocortical axons. *J. Neurosci.* 20:9145–9151.

YAMAMOTO, N., T. KUROTANI, and K. TOYAMA, 1989. Neural connections between the lateral geniculate nucleus and visual cortex in vitro. *Science* 245:192–194.

YAMAMOTO, N., Y. MATSUYAMA, A. HARADA, K. INUI, F. MURAKAMI, and K. HANAMURA, 2000. Characterization of factors regulating lamina-specific growth of thalamocortical axons. *J. Neurobiol.* 42:56–68.

YAMAMOTO, N., K. YAMADA, T. KUROTANI, and K. TOYAMA, 1992. Laminar specificity of extrinsic cortical connections studied in coculture preparations. *Neuron* 9:217–228.

YOSHIDA, M., Y. SUDA, I. MATSUO, N. MIYAMOTO, N. TAKEDA, S. KURATANI, and S. AIZAWA, 1997. *Emx1* and *Emx2* functions in development of dorsal telencephalon. *Development* 124:101–111.

YUN, K., S. POTTER, and J. L. RUBENSTEIN, 2001. *Gsh2* and *Pax6* play complementary roles in dorsoventral patterning of the mammalian telencephalon. *Development* 128:193–205.

YUN, M. E., R. R. JOHNSON, A. ANTIC, and M. J. DONOGHUE, 2003. EphA family gene expression in the developing mouse neocortex: Regional patterns reveal intrinsic programs and extrinsic influence. *J. Comp. Neurol.* 456:203–216.

ZACCO, A., V. COOPER, P. D. CHANTLER, S. FISHER-HYLAND, H. L. HORTON, and P. LEVITT, 1990. Isolation, biochemical characterization and ultrastructural analysis of the limbic system-associated membrane protein (LAMP), a protein expressed by neurons comprising functional neural circuits. *J. Neurosci.* 10:73–90.

ZHOU, C., Y. QIU, F. A. PEREIRA, M. C. CRAIR, S. Y. TSAI, and M. J. TSAI, 1999. The nuclear orphan receptor COUP-TFI is required for differentiation of subplate neurons and guidance of thalamocortical axons. *Neuron* 24:847–859.

ZHOU, C., S. Y. TSAI, and M. J. TSAI, 2001. COUP-TFI: An intrinsic factor for early regionalization of the neocortex. *Genes Dev.* 15:2054–2059.

6 A New Perspective on the Role of Activity in the Development of Eye-Specific Retinogeniculate Projections

LEO M. CHALUPA AND ANDREW D. HUBERMAN

ABSTRACT Eye-specific projections to the visual thalamus (eye-specific layers of the dorsal lateral geniculate nucleus) and striate cortex (ocular dominance columns) represent prominent model systems for studying neural circuit development. It has been widely assumed that during development correlated activity of adjacent retinal ganglion cells plays a vital role in the segregation of initially overlapped left and right eye projections via a Hebbian-type mechanism. Here we discuss new evidence that challenges this view. The results of recent studies indicate that neural activity may simply permit rather than instruct the formation of eye-specific projections. These findings suggest that yet to be identified axon guidance cues drive the patterning of eye-specific projections.

In all mammalian species, the inputs of the two eyes to the dorsal lateral geniculate nucleus (dLGN) are segregated into separate eye-specific domains or "layers" at maturity (Jones, 1985). In turn, axons from neurons in eye-specific dLGN layers project to primary visual cortex (V1) in alternating, nonoverlapping domains called ocular dominance columns. For almost four decades, these eye-specific patterns of connections have served as a model system for studies dealing with the development and plasticity of sensory circuits in the mammalian brain.

Early in development, binocular inputs to the dorsal lateral geniculate nucleus (dLGN) (Rakic, 1976; Linden, Guillery, and Cucchiaro, 1981; Shatz, 1983; Godement, Salaun, and Imbert, 1984) and visual cortex (Rakic, 1976; Hubel, Wiesel, and LeVay, 1977; LeVay, Stryker, and Shatz, 1978; Levay, Wiesel, and Hubel, 1980) are intermingled extensively, before gradually segregating into their respective eye-specific territories. This process is thought to require neuronal activity. It is important to note that the pattern of activity, as opposed to the mere presence of spontaneous discharges, has been hypothesized to "instruct" the segregation process (Crair, 1999; Feller, 1999; Stellwagen and Shatz, 2002).

LEO M. CHALUPA and ANDREW D. HUBERMAN Department of Ophthalmology, School of Medicine; Section of Neurobiology, Physiology and Behavior, Division of Biological Sciences; and Center for Neuroscience; University of California, Davis, Calif.

In this chapter we first provide a brief historical account of the experimental evidence that gave rise to the idea that patterned neural activity plays an instructive role in the formation of segregated visual projections. Next, we describe the results of experiments that challenge traditional theories of how separated left- and right-eye domains form. Finally, we will review the results of recent studies that tested directly whether patterns of neural activity could provide the instructive cues required for the segregation of eye-specific retinogeniculate projections to the dLGN.

Development of ocular dominance columns

The idea that neuronal activity has a profound influence on the development of visual system connections stems from the pioneering studies of Wiesel and Hubel. Their work showed that closure of one eye during a critical period in postnatal life rendered that eye permanently incapable of driving cortical cells (Wiesel and Hubel, 1965a,b). Subsequently it was shown that this physiological effect was accompanied by a marked reduction in the amount of cortical territory innervated by geniculocortical axons representing the deprived eye and a dramatic expansion of the geniculocortical axons representing the nondeprived eye (Hubel, Wiesel, and LeVay, 1977; Shatz and Stryker, 1978). These deprivation studies demonstrated that activity-mediated competition between axons representing the two eyes can determine the allocation of postsynaptic space in V1. Not surprisingly, there is an ongoing effort to understand the molecular basis of critical period plasticity (for a recent review, see Berardi et al., 2003).

It is important to stress that these visual deprivation studies did not directly address the issue of how ocular dominance columns (ODCs) are formed. The development of visual circuits and the plasticity of those circuits later in life are often treated as synonymous events in which activity-based competition is involved (Berardi et al., 2003). This assumption derives in large part from studies that relied on transneuronal tracing of retinal-dLGN-V1 connections to assess the presence or absence of ODCs during early development. Monocular injections of transneuronal tracers indicated that early in development, axons representing the two eyes are extensively overlapped in layer 4 of V1 (Hubel, Wiesel, and LeVay, 1977; LeVay, Stryker, and Shatz, 1978; LeVay, Wiesel, and Hubel, 1980; Rakic, 1976) before gradually segregating into left- and right-eye ODCs. A role for retinal activity in ODC segregation was supported by the finding that abolishing action potentials in both eyes with intraocular injections of tetrodotoxin (TTX) prevented the emergence of ODCs in the visual cortex (Stryker and Harris, 1986). Thus, near the turn of the century, the generally accepted model was that early in development, the projections of the two eyes overlapped in the visual cortex, and the formation of separate left- and right-eye ODCs reflected activity-mediated competition between the two eyes.

The notion that activity-mediated events drive the initial formation of ODCs was first challenged by Crowley and Katz (1999). These investigators removed both eyes of postnatal ferrets weeks before geniculocortical axons invade V1, and then, after the animals reached adulthood, injected anterograde tracers into one or the other eye-specific layer in the dLGN. Surprisingly, they found normal ODCs in these animals. Obviously, the formation of ODCs could not be due to retinal activity. Moreover, this early eye removal is known to result in severely altered patterns of spontaneous activity in the remaining geniculocortical pathway (Weliky and Katz, 1999). The authors therefore concluded that the formation of ODCs "relies primarily on activity-independent cues, rather than on specific patterns of correlated activity" (Crowley and Katz, 1999).

In a subsequent study, these investigators used the same tracing method to demonstrate that ODCs are present in the ferret cortex very shortly after geniculocortical axons innervate layer IV and are refractory to imbalances in retinal activity during this time (Crowley and Katz, 2000). The results of these studies impied that the "overlap" of eye-specific dLGN inputs to V1 seen in the earlier transneuronal experiments was spurious, reflecting leakage of transneuronal tracer into opposite-eye layers in the dLGN. The results of Crowley and Katz therefore raised serious doubt that activity instructs the initial formation of ODCs.

Development of eye-specific inputs to the dLGN

Rakic (1976) pioneered the exploration of the prenatal visual system and was the first to show that in the embryonic macaque monkey, the projections of the two eyes are initially overlapped in the dLGN before segregating into eye-specific layers. Subsequently, this was found to be the case in other species when tested using a variety of tracing methods (mouse: Godement, Salaun, and Imbert, 1984; ferret:

Linden, Guillery, and Cucchiaro, 1981; Hahm, Cramer, and Sur, 1999; Huberman, Stellwagen, and Chapman, 2002; Huberman et al., 2003; cat: Shatz, 1983). Rakic (1981) also showed that fetal monocular enucleation results in the maintenance of a widespread projection from the remaining eye to the dLGN and the visual cortex, thus demonstrating the importance of prenatal binocular interactions in this process. Similar results have been obtained following monocular enucleation in the fetal cat (Chalupa and Williams, 1984; Shook and Chalupa, 1985).

The cellular and molecular mechanisms underlying binocular competitive interactions were not directly addressed in these studies, but, generalizing from the literature dealing with the plasticity of cortical ODCs, it was reasonable to assume that prenatal binocular competition is also activity mediated. To test this idea, Shatz and Stryker (1988) infused TTX into the brain of fetal cats before retinal segregation occurred. This caused the projections of the two eyes to remain widespread and overlapping. An obvious implication of this study was that retinal ganglion cells are capable of discharging action potentials even before these cells can be activated by light.

This was soon demonstrated by Galli and Maffei (1988), who recorded in vivo from retinal ganglion cells of the embryonic rat. These experiments also showed that neighboring ganglion cells exhibit correlated discharges (Maffei and Galli-Resta, 1990). Subsequent in vitro patch-clamp recordings documented the ontogeny of excitable membrane properties in retinal ganglion cells from the fetal cat (Skaliora, Scobey, and Chalupa, 1993; Skaliora et al., 1995) and rat (Wang et al., 1997). The introduction of in vitro multi-electrode-array recordings (Meister et al., 1991) and optical recording of intracellular calcium allowed the simultaneous recording of hundreds of retinal cells (Feller et al., 1996; Wong, Meister, and Shatz, 1993). These studies revealed that the spontaneous bursts of correlated ganglion cell activity propagate across the developing retina in a wavelike manner. Such retinal waves have been now reported in many species, including chick, turtle, mouse, rabbit, rat, ferret, and cat (reviewed in Wong, 1999), suggesting that they are a common feature of retinal development. Based on their specific spatial-temporal properties, retinal waves have been hypothesized to play an essential role in the segregation of left- and right-eye inputs to the dLGN (Feller, 1999; Cohen-Corey, 2002; Sengpiel and Kind, 2002), the establishment of retinotopic order in the superior colliculus (Butts and Rokshar, 2001), and the segregation of ON and OFF ganglion cell projections to the dLGN (Wong and Oakley, 1996).

How could retinal waves drive eye-specific segregation? Eye-specific segregation is thought to occur because the correlated discharges of spatially adjacent ganglion cells in one eye are better capable of depolarizing neurons in the dLGN than are uncorrelated inputs stemming from the two eyes. In accordance with the Hebbian postulate (Hebb, 1949), co-active inputs are preferentially stabilized relative to temporally uncorrelated inputs (Bi and Poo, 2001; Zhang and Poo, 2001).

Three lines of evidence have been invoked in support of this "fire-together, wire-together" idea. First, the occurrence of waves coincides with the segregation of retinal projections (mouse: Muir-Robinson, Hwang, and Feller, 2002; ferret: Penn et al., 1998; Huberman, Stellwagen, and Chapman, 2002; Huberman et al., 2003). Second, abolishing all retinal activity prevents the formation of eye-specific projection patterns (Penn et al., 1998; Huberman, Stellwagen, and Chapman, 2002; Muir-Robinson, Hwang, and Feller, 2002; Huberman et al., 2003). Third, inducing an imbalance in the overall activity levels of the two eyes causes the more active eye to innervate more dLGN territory at the expense of the less active eye (Penn et al., 1998; Stellwagen and Shatz, 2002).

However, none of these lines of research has directly tested the idea that correlated retinal ganglion cell discharges are essential for the formation of eye-specific projections. To do so would require a means for perturbing the correlated activity of adjacent retinal ganglion cells without affecting the overall discharge levels of these neurons. The studies that blocked retinal waves did so by abolishing all ganglion cell discharges (Penn et al., 1998; Huberman, Stellwagen, and Chapman, 2002; Muir Robinson, Hwang, and Feller, 2002), and the studies that altered the balance of waves in the two eyes either significantly increased or decreased the frequency of ganglion cell action potentials (Penn et al., 1998; Stellwagen and Shatz, 2002). Thus, it has remained an open question whether the changes in eye-specific projections observed in these experiments were due to altering the pattern, as opposed to the level, of spontaneous retinal activity.

A direct test of the role of correlated activity

An opportunity to resolve this issue was provided by the manufacture of a novel immunotoxin designed to selectively target cholinergic neurons (Gunhan et al., 2002). Although the cellular basis of retinal waves remains unclear, it is known that during the developmental phase when eye-specific segregation is occurring, spontaneous discharges of retinal ganglion cells are caused by acetylcholine released by starburst amacrine cells (Feller et al., 1996; Zhou and Zhou, 2000). We reasoned that immunotoxin depletion of starburst amacrine cells would disrupt the correlated discharges of ganglion cells without completely blocking the activity of these neurons or significantly changing their overall levels of activity (Huberman et al., 2003).

This strategy was applied to newborn ferrets. In this species retinogeniculate projections are extensively overlapped at birth, segregating gradually to attain their adult-like state by postnatal day 10 (P10) (Linden, Guillery, and Cucchiaro, 1981; Penn et al., 1998; Huberman, Stellwagen, and Chapman, 2002; Huberman et al., 2003). Binocular injections of the immunotoxin were made on the day of birth (P0), and within 48 hours this resulted in the elimination of approximately 80% of the starburst amacrine cells (compare figure 6.1A and F).

To assess the effects of this manipulation on the firing patterns of these neurons, whole-cell patch-clamp recordings were made from P2–P10 retinal ganglion cells. These recordings showed that ganglion cells were in fact spontaneously active in the cholinergic cell–depleted retinas. However, their discharge properties were markedly aberrant; some cells fired spikes very infrequently compared to those in normal retinas, while others manifested a firing frequency that was much higher than normal. Of note, while the discharges of individual cells were abnormal, the overall firing rate of the sample of cells recorded was not statistically different from normal in the immunotoxin-treated retinas (see figure 3 in Huberman et al., 2003).

To test directly whether correlated discharges were perturbed by starburst amacrine cell depletion, dual patch-clamp recordings were made from neighboring ganglion cells (less than $25\,\mu m$ apart) (figure 6.1B and G). In the normal P2–P10 retinas, all ganglion cells showed highly correlated spiking and membrane potential activity, irrespective of cell class (figure 6.1C–E) (Huberman et al., 2003; Liets et al., 2003). By contrast, not a single ganglion cell pair in the immunotoxin-treated retinas showed any significant correlated activity (figure 6.1H–J), and this was the case for every age retina examined, from P2 to P10. These electrophysiological findings demonstrated that depletion of starburst amacrine cells rapidly eliminated the correlated discharges of neighboring retinal ganglion cells without significantly altering the overall activity levels of these neurons.

Now for the key issue: Did elimination of correlated ganglion cell activity disrupt the segregation of left- and right-eye retinogeniculate projections? To answer this question, we examined the pattern of retinogeniculate connections in normal developing ferrets at ages P2 and P10 and compared these with P10 animals that had received intraocular injections of the cholinergic immunotoxin on P0. As mentioned above, an injection of immunotoxin on P0 eliminated the correlated firing of neighboring ganglion cells by P2, an age when binocular retinogeniculate inputs are still intermingled extensively (figure 6.2A).

Remarkably, in the ferrets injected with immunotoxin, normal eye-specific segregation of retinogeniculate connections still formed (compare figure 6.2B and C). Indeed, quantitative comparison of the extent of overlap for left- and right-eye axons indicated that the degree and the pattern of segregation were the same for control and experimental P10 animals (figure 6.2E, F).

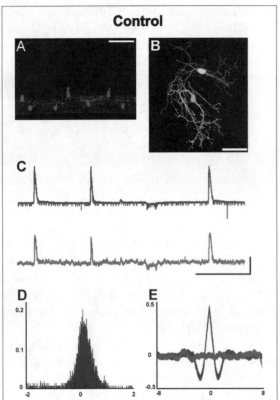

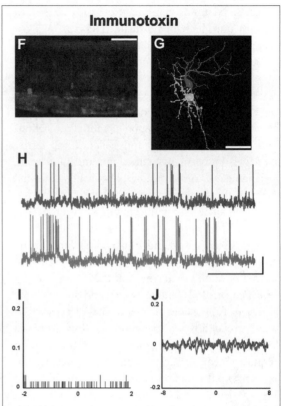

FIGURE 6.1 (*A*) Photomicrograph of a P10 ferret retina injected with saline on P0. Regularly spaced starburst amacrine cells are shown in red after labeling by anti-choline acetyletransferase (ChAT) immunohistochemistry. Ganglion cell layer is to the bottom and photoreceptor layer is to the top of the photomicrograph. Scale bar = 100 μm.

(*B*) Two neighboring ganglion cells in a control retina. One was filled with a green dye and the other with a red dye, during the paired patch-clamp recording session. Scale bar = 25 μm.

(*C*) An example of current-clamp recordings from two neighboring ganglion cells in a control retina. Green trace shows the activity of one ganglion cell and red trace shows that of the neighboring cell. Highly correlated, periodic bursts of activity are clearly present. Horizontal scale = 1 minute, vertical scale = 20 mV.

(*D*) Cross-correlation of spiking activity for two neighboring control ganglion cells (shown in blue). There is a prominent peak near zero time lag. Red indicates the cross-correlation resulting from a random shuffle of the same spike data. This and all other ganglion cell pairs recorded in control P2–P10 retinas showed statistically significant correlations (n = 15 pairs).

(*E*) Cross-correlation of the membrane potential activity for two neighboring control ganglion cells (shown in blue). There is a prominent peak near zero time lag. Red indicates the cross-correlation of a random shuffle of the same membrane potential data. This and all other ganglion cell pairs recorded in control P2–P10 retinas showed statistically significant correlations in their activity patterns (n = 15 pairs).

(*F*) Photomicrograph of a P10 ferret retina that was injected with immunotoxin on P0. Most starburst amacrine cells are ablated.

However, a single starburst cell can be seen in red. Ganglion cell layer is to the bottom and photoreceptor layer is to the top. Scale bar = 100 μm.

(*G*) Two neighboring ganglion cells in an immunotoxin retina. One was filled with a green dye and the other with a red dye during the paired patch-clamp recording session. Scale bar = 25 μm.

(*H*) An example of current-clamp recordings from two neighboring ganglion cells in an immunotoxin-treated retina. Green trace shows the activity of one ganglion cell and red trace shows the activity of the neighboring cell. The spiking activity of these two cells does not appear correlated. Horizontal scale = 1 minute, vertical scale = 20 mV.

(*I*) Cross-correlation of spiking activity for two neighboring ganglion cells in an immunotoxin-treated retina (shown in blue). There is no peak in the correlation at any time lag, and the correlation resembles that of a random shuffle of the same spike data (shown in red). Neither this nor any other ganglion cell pair recorded from immunotoxin-treated P2–P10 retinas showed statistically significant correlations (n = 15 pairs).

(*J*) Cross-correlation of the membrane potential activity for two neighboring ganglion cells in an immunotoxin-treated retina (shown in blue). There is no peak in the correlation at any time lag and the correlation resembles that of a random shuffle of the same membrane potential data (shown in red). Neither this nor any other ganglion cell pair recorded from immunotoxin-treated P2–P10 retinas showed statistically significant correlations (n = 15 pairs). (All panels adapted from Huberman et al., 2003.) (See color plate 1.)

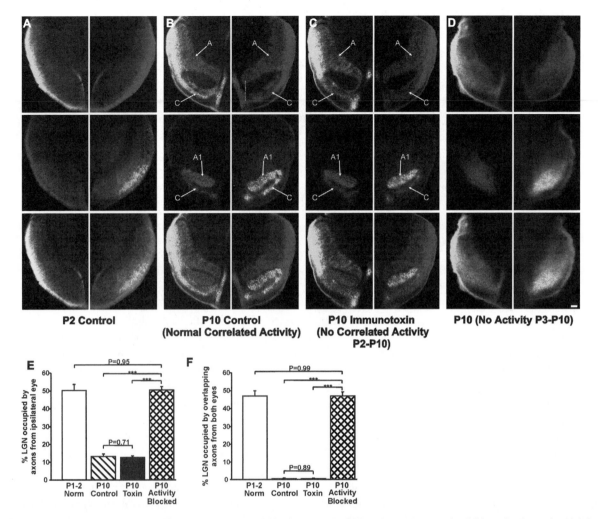

P2 Control

**P10 Control
(Normal Correlated Activity)**

**P10 Immunotoxin
(No Correlated Activity
P2-P10)**

P10 (No Activity P3-P10)

FIGURE 6.2 Development of eye-specific layers in the dLGN of (A) normal P2, (B) control P10, (C) P10 immunotoxin-treated, and (D) epibatidine-treated ferrets. (A–D) Axons from the right eye are shown in green and axons from the left eye are shown in red. Contralateral (top panels) and ipsilateral (middle panels) retinal inputs to the dLGN, and their merged representation (bottom panels) are shown. Tissue sections are in the horizontal plane: rostral is to the top and medial is to the center of each panel. Scale bar in A = 150 μm; scale bar in B–D = 100 μm. (All panels adapted from Huberman et al., 2003.)

(A) A normal P2 ferret. Inputs from the two eyes are still overlapped at this age; the contralateral eye projection is found throughout the nucleus, where it intermingles with axons from the ipsilateral eye.

(B) A control P10 ferret. Axons from the two eyes are completely segregated by this age. Arrows indicate the complementary "A" (contralateral eye) and A1 (ipsilateral eye) layers. C layers are also seen.

(C) A P10 ferret that received binocular intravitreal injections of immunotoxin on P0. Axons from the two eyes are segregated normally in these animals. Arrows indicate the complementary and "A" (contralateral eye) and A1 (ipsilateral eye) layers. Normal C layers are also evident.

(D) A P10 ferret that received binocular intravitreal injections of epibatidine (which blocks all retinal activity) every 48 hours from P3 to P10. Projections from the two eyes overlapped; there is no gap in the contralateral eye's projection, and the ipsilateral eye's projection is dramatically expanded.

(E and F) Quantification of the percent of dLGN area occupied by the ipsilateral eye projection (E) and overlapping axons from the two eyes (F) in the four treatment groups. Open bars: normal P1/2 ferrets (n = 8), hatched bars = control P10 ferrets (n = 12), black bars = P10 ferrets that received binocular injections of immunotoxin on P0 (n = 14), cross hatched bars = P10 ferrets that received binocular injections of epibatidine from P3 to P10 (n = 14). ***P < 0.0001; t-test; ±SEM. (See color plate 2.)

These results showed for the first time that correlated activity of neighboring ganglion cells is not required for the segregation of eye-specific retinogeniculate projections.

We also assessed the effects of blocking all ganglion cell discharges, beginning on P3, using cholinergic agents. When the state of retinogeniculate projections was examined in these animals at P10, left- and right-eye inputs appeared to be intermingled to the same extent as in newborn animals (figure 6.2D–F). Thus, as reported previously (Penn et al., 1998), pharmacological blockade of all ganglion cell activity prevented segregation of retinogeniculate projections.

A new perspective on the role of retinal activity

Collectively, our results indicate that the formation of eye-specific inputs to the dLGN is not dependent on correlated activity of retinal ganglion cells. Thus, the widely held belief that retinal waves instruct the formation of eye-specific domains appears to be incorrect.

Why, then, are retinal waves present during early development? Correlated activity of spatially adjacent ganglion cells may play a role in refining other key features of the developing visual system. As mentioned earlier, retinotopy and segregated ON/OFF dLGN sublaminae might be refined by retinal waves (Wong and Oakley, 1996; Butts and Rokshar, 2001). With respect to ON/OFF segregation, it is relevant to note that blockade of NMDA receptors in the developing ferret dLGN perturbs the formation of ON/OFF sublaminae (Hahm, Langdon, and Sur, 1991; Hahm, Cramer, and Sur, 1999). Since NMDA receptors are considered to provide the cellular mechanism by which correlated activity acts to stabilize developing synapses (Bi and Poo, 2001; Cohen-Cory, 2002), this is in accord with the notion that correlated ganglion cell discharges play a role in the formation of ON/OFF segregated inputs to the ferret dLGN. Interestingly, blocking NMDA receptors in the developing ferret dLGN does not prevent eye-specific segregation (Smetters, Hahm, and Sur, 1994), which is in line with our findings that correlated activity does not drive this process. It would be worthwhile to examine the retinotopic organization and ON/OFF sublamination in the dLGN of animals treated with the cholinergic immunotoxin. This would provide a direct test of the hypothesis that correlated ganglion cell activity is required for the normal development of these salient features of the mature visual system.

The fact that complete blockade of all ganglion cell discharges prevented the segregation of left- and right-eye projections indicates that such activity is necessary for these projections to form normally. The degree of intermingling of left- and right-eye projections in P10 animals that had all retinal activity blocked from P3 to P10 was found to be equivalent to that of P0–P2 ferrets (figure 6.2A and D, 6.2E and F). This does not mean, however, that when all ganglion cell discharges are blocked, retinogeniculate projections remain "frozen" in their immature state. In fact, the growth and innervation pattern of individual retinogeniculate fibers is markedly abnormal in activity-blocked retinas (Sretavan, Shatz, and Stryker, 1988). This suggests that activity blockade alters axon morphology through mechanisms that are unrelated to the disruption of competitive interactions between developing retinogeniculate axons. Collectively, our results point to a permissive rather than an instructive role for retinal activity in the formation of segregated eye-specific projection patterns.

What does account for the stereotyped pattern of eye-specific layers in the dLGN? The fact that early in development, the projections from the two eyes are intermingled in the dLGN does not rule out the expression of molecular cues that define eye-specific regions in this structure. The presence of eye-specific molecules in the dLGN would neatly account for the highly regular contralateral and ipsilateral eye pattern of layers seen in this nucleus (Jones, 1985). Such stereotypy is difficult to reconcile with an activity-based mechanism. Indeed, a purely activity-dependent sorting should result in randomly distributed patterns of right- and left-eye inputs to the dLGN (Huberman, Stellwagen, and Chapman, 2002). Thus, some bias for one or the other layer by the two eyes must exist (Sanes and Yamagata, 1999). Activity-dependent proponents have speculated that the stereotyped pattern of layering in the dLGN reflects the earlier arrival of contralateral-eye versus ipsilateral-eye axons. The use of sensitive anatomical tracers indicates, however, that axons from both eyes are present throughout the dLGN from very early times (figure 6.2A) (Penn et al., 1998; Huberman, Stellwagen, and Chapman, 2002; Huberman et al., 2003).

A new perspective is that soon after retinal axons have innervated the dLGN, a cadre of left- and right-eye molecular cues is expressed, resulting in the retraction of terminals situated in inappropriate territories and the elaboration of terminals located in the appropriate eye-specific zone. Such cues could be layer-specific, with a strong preference for nasal versus temporal ganglion cell axons, or they may be expressed in gradients that force the preferential removal of one eye's exuberant projections. A molecular scheme that focuses on differential recognition of nasal versus temporal ganglion cell axons is bolstered by the finding that in achiasmatic dogs, axons arising from nasal retina and temporal retina in the same eye segregate into distinct zones identical to eye-specific layers (Williams, 1994). Once eye-specific connections are formed, retinal activity appears to be required for their maintenance (Chapman, 2000), but the mechanism by which such a stabilizing action is mediated is as yet unknown.

Studies aimed at identifying eye-specific molecules in the dLGN and the genes that act downstream of activity to regulate axonal growth are currently under way in several laboratories. It remains to be established whether the results of such studies will validate our new perspective on the development of eye-specific retinogeniculate projections.

ACKNOWLEDGEMENT This work was supported by grants from the National Eye Institute of the National Institutes of Health, and a Research to Prevent Blindness Award.

REFERENCES

BERARDI, N., T. PIZZORUSSO, G. M. RATTO, and L. MAFFEI, 2003. Molecular basis of plasticity in the visual cortex. *Trends Neurosci.* 26:369–378.

BI, G., and M. POO, 2001. Synaptic modification by correlated activity: Hebb's postulate revisited. *Annu. Rev. Neurosci.* 24:139–166.

BUTTS, D. A., and D. S. ROKSHAR, 2001. The information content of spontaneous retinal waves. *J. Neurosci.* 21:961–973.

CHALUPA, L. M., and R. W. WILLIAMS, 1984. Organization of the cat's lateral geniculate nucleus following interruption of prenatal binocular competition. *Hum. Neurobiol.* 3:103–107.

CHAPMAN, B., 2000. Necessity for afferent activity to maintain eye-specific segregation in ferret lateral geniculate nucleus. *Science* 287:2479–2482.

COHEN-CORY, S., 2002. The developing synapse: Construction and modulation of synaptic structures and circuits. *Science* 298:770–776.

CRAIR, M. C., 1999. Neuronal activity during development: Permissive or instructive? *Curr. Opin. Neurobiol.* 9:88–93.

CROWLEY, J. C., and L. C. KATZ, 1999. Development of ocular dominance columns in the absence of retinal input. *Nat. Neurosci.* 2:1125–1130.

CROWLEY, J. C., and L. C. KATZ, 2000. Early development of ocular dominance columns. *Science* 290:1321–1324.

FELLER, M. B., 1999. Spontaneous correlated activity in developing neural circuits. *Neuron* 22:653–656.

FELLER, M. B., D. P. WELLIS, D. STELLWAGEN, F. WERBLIN, and C. J. SHATZ, 1996. Requirement for cholinergic synaptic transmission in the propagation of spontaneous retinal waves. *Science* 272:1182–1187.

GALLI, L., and L. MAFFEI, 1988. Spontaneous impulse activity of rat retinal ganglion cells in prenatal life. *Science* 242:90–91.

GODEMENT, P., J. SALAUN, and M. IMBERT, 1984. Prenatal and postnatal development of retinogeniculate and retinocollicular projections in the mouse. *J. Comp. Neurol.* 230:552–575.

GUNHAN, E., P. V. CHOUDARY, T. E. Landerholm, and L. M. CHALUPA, 2002. Depletion of cholinergic amacrine cells by a novel immunotoxin does not perturb the formation of segregated on and off cone bipolar cell projections. *J. Neurosci.* 22: 2265–2273.

HAHM, J. O., K. S. CRAMER, and M. SUR, 1999. Pattern formation by retinal afferents in the ferret lateral geniculate nucleus: Developmental segregation and the role of *N*-methyl-D aspartate receptors. *J. Comp. Neurol.* 411:327–345.

HAHM, J. O., R. B. LANGDON, and M. SUR, 1991. Disruption of retinogeniculate afferent segregation by antagonists to NMDA receptors. *Nature* 351:568–570.

HEBB, D. O., 1949. *Organization of Behavior: A Neuropsychological Theory.* New York: John Wiley and Sons.

HUBEL, D. H., T. N. WIESEL, and S. LEVAY, 1977. Plasticity of ocular dominance columns in monkey striate cortex. *Philos. Trans. R. Soc. Lond. B Biol. Sci.* 278:377–409.

HUBERMAN, A. D., D. STELLWAGEN, and B. CHAPMAN, 2002. Decoupling eye-specific segregation from lamination in the lateral geniculate nucleus. *J. Neurosci.* 22:9419–9429.

HUBERMAN, A. D., G. Y. WANG, L. C. LIETS, O. A. COLLINS, B. CHAPMAN, and L. M. CHALUPA, 2003. Eye-specific retinogeniculate segregation independent of normal neuronal activity. *Science* 300:994–998.

JONES, E. G., 1985. *The Thalamus.* New York: Plenum Press.

LIETS, L. C., B. A. OLSHAUSEN, G. Y. WANG, and L. M. CHALUPA, 2003. Spontaneous activity of morphologically identified ganglion cells in the developing ferret retina. *J. Neurosci.* 23: 7343–7350.

LEVAY, S. M., P. STRYKER, and C. J. SHATZ, 1978. Ocular dominance columns and their development in layer IV of the cat's visual cortex: A quantitative study. *J. Comp. Neurol.* 179:223–224.

LEVAY S. M., T. N. WIESEL, and D. H. HUBEL, 1980. The development of ocular dominance columns in normal and visually deprived monkeys. *J. Comp. Neurol.* 191:1–51.

LINDEN, D. C., R. W. GUILLERY, and J. CUCCHIARO, 1981. The dorsal lateral geniculate nucleus of the normal ferret and its postnatal development. *J. Comp. Neurol.* 203:189–211.

MAFFEI, L., and L. GALLI-RESTA, 1990. Correlation in the discharges of neighboring rat retinal ganglion cells during prenatal life. *Proc. Natl. Acad. Sci. U.S.A.* 87:2861–2864.

MEISTER, M., R. O. WONG, D. A. BAYLOR, and C. J. SHATZ, 1991. Synchronous bursts of action potentials in ganglion cells of the developing mammalian retina. *Science* 252:939–943.

MUIR-ROBINSON, G., B. J. HWANG, and M. B. FELLER, 2002. Retinogeniculate axons undergo eye-specific segregation in the absence of eye-specific layers. *J. Neurosci.* 22:5259–5264.

PENN, A. A., P. A. RIQUELME, M. B. FELLER, and C. J. SHATZ, 1998. Competition in retinogeniculate patterning driven by spontaneous activity. *Science* 279:2108–2112.

RAKIC, P., 1976. Prenatal genesis of connections subserving ocular dominance in the rhesus monkey. *Nature* 261:467–471.

RAKIC, P., 1981. Development of visual centres in the primate brain depends on binocular competition before birth. *Science* 214:928–931.

SANES, J. R., and M. YAMAGATA, 1999. Formation of lamina-specific synaptic connections. *Curr. Opin. Neurobiol.* 9:79–87.

SENGPIEL, F., and P. C. KIND, 2002. The role of activity in development of the visual system. *Curr. Biol.* 12:R818–R826.

SHATZ, C. J., 1983. The prenatal development of the cats retinogeniculate pathway. *J. Neurosci.* 3:482–499.

SHATZ, C. J., and M. P. STRYKER, 1978. Ocular dominance in layer IV of the cat's visual cortex and the effects of monocular deprivation. *J. Physiol.* 281:267–283.

SHATZ, C. J., and M. P. STRYKER, 1988. Prenatal tetrodotoxin infusion blocks segregation of retinogeniculate afferents. *Science* 242:87–89.

SHOOK, B. L., and L. M. CHALUPA, 1986. Organization of geniculocortical connections following prenatal interruption of binocular interactions. *Dev. Brain Res.* 393:47–62.

SKALIORA, I., P. R. SCOBEY, and L. M. CHALUPA, 1993. Prenatal development of excitability in cat retinal ganglion cells: Action potentials and sodium currents. *J. Neurosci.* 13:313–323.

SKALIORA, I., D. W. ROBINSON, R. P. SCOBEY, and L. M. CHALUPA, 1995. Properties of K^+ conductances in cat retinal ganglion cells during the period of activity-mediated refinements in retinofugal pathways. *Eur J. Neurosci.* 7:1558–1568.

Smetters, D. K., J. Hahm, and M. Sur, 1994. An *N*-methyl-D-aspartate receptor antagonist does not prevent eye-specific segregation in the ferret retinogeniculate pathway. *Brain Res.* 658:168–178.

Sretavan, D. W., C. J. Shatz, and M. P. Stryker, 1988. Modification of retinal ganglion cell axon morphology by prenatal infusion of tetrodotoxin. *Nature* 336:468–471.

Stellwagen, D., C. J. Shatz, 2002. An instructive role for retinal waves in the development of retinogeniculate connectivity. *Neuron* 33:357–367.

Stryker, M. P., and W. A. Harris, 1986. Binocular impulse blockade prevents the formation of ocular dominance columns in cat visual cortex. *J. Neurosci.* 6:2117–2133.

Wang, G. Y., G. Ratto, S. Bisti, and L. M. Chalupa, 1997. Functional development of intrinsic properties in ganglion cells of the mammalian retina. *J. Neurophysiol.* 78:2895–2903.

Weliky, M., and L. C. Katz, 1999. Correlational structure of spontaneous neuronal activity in the developing lateral geniculate nucleus in vivo. *Science* 285:599–604.

Wiesel, T. N., and D. H. Hubel, 1965a. Comparison of the effects of unilateral and bilateral eye closure on cortical unit responses in kittens. *J. Neurophysiol.* 28:1029–1040.

Wiesel, T. N., and D. H. Hubel, 1965b. Extent of recovery from the effects of visual deprivation in kittens. *J. Neurophysiol.* 28:1060–1072.

Williams, R. W., 1994. Target recognition and visual maps in the thalamus of achiasmatic dogs. *Nature* 367:637–639.

Wong, R. O., 1999. Retinal waves and visual system development. *Annu. Rev. Neurosci.* 22:29–47.

Wong, R. O., and D. M. Oakley, 1996. Changing patterns of spontaneous bursting activity of on and off retinal ganglion cells during development. *Neuron* 16:1087–1095.

Wong, R. O., M. Meister, and C. J. Shatz, 1993. Transient period of correlated bursting activity during development of the mammalian retina. *Neuron* 11:923–938.

Zhang, L. I., and M. M. Poo, 2001. Electrical activity and development of neural circuits. *Nat. Neurosci.* 4 Suppl:1207–1214.

Zhou, Z. J., and D. Zhou, 2000. Coordinated transitions in neurotransmitter systems for the initiation and propagation of spontaneous retinal waves. *J. Neurosci.* 20:6570–6577.

7 Brain and Behavioral Development During Childhood

JEROME KAGAN AND ABIGAIL BAIRD

ABSTRACT This chapter summarizes what has been learned about the correspondences between brain maturation and the ontogeny of human psychological competences from birth to puberty. Significant maturational transitions occur at 2–3 months, 7–12 months, 12–24 months, 4–8 years, and puberty.

This chapter summarizes some of the temporal correspondences between the emergence of select human psychological properties and changes in brain anatomy and function across the first dozen years of human development. Although we will suggest, albeit tentatively, some theoretical bases for the correspondences, we recognize that the meaning of every conclusion must be evaluated in light of the source of evidence. The information provided by an apparatus or procedure represents only a partial picture of the whole phenomenon that scientists wish to comprehend. On many occasions, a psychological and a biological measure of a construct lead to different conclusions. For example, a majority of a group of 10-year-olds shown pictures of children they had played with 3–6 years earlier, along with pictures of unfamiliar children, failed to recognize most of the faces of their former playmates when asked to say whether they had ever seen the child in the photograph. However, many of these children, not all, produced a galvanic skin response to pictures of the children they had known earlier, but not to photographs of strangers (Newcombe and Fox, 1994). Thus, the answer to the question, "Do 10-year-olds remember their playmates after a 6-year interval?" depends on the method. This restraining principle applies to statements describing the relation between brain and psychological properties.

The conceptualization of change has been a perennial node of debate because of uncertainty over whether to treat development as continuous or as a sequence of qualitatively different stages marked by transitions. Scientists attribute a stage to an era of growth when a correlated cluster of features, displayed across a class of relevant contexts, changes its pattern of organization. However, it is usually

the case that a period of time must pass before all the components assume their new organization and are displayed across a broad envelope of situations. That is why we prefer the word *phase* to *stage*, because the former term implies that the process of transformation was gradual.

The presence of temporal correlations between the maturational state of the brain and the psychological properties of children does not imply a strict determinacy, because experience is a participant in most behaviors. The brain changes that occur between 12 and 24 months are necessary for the emergence of speech, but children will not speak if they are not exposed to any language. The fundamental premise of this chapter is that brain maturation constrains the time of emergence of the psychological characteristics of our species and, although necessary, it is not sufficient for the actualization of the psychological phenomena.

Infancy

We consider first the correspondences between brain growth and psychological development during the first year, with an emphasis on the changes that occur during the transitions between 2 and 3 months and between 7 and 12 months of age. We assume that the maturational processes are occurring in infants who are exposed regularly to the objects, events, and people characteristic of all but the most depriving environments. We describe first the psychological changes, and then the brain events believed to contribute to the former.

TRANSITION AT 2–3 MONTHS The disappearance of a number of newborn reflexes, including the palmar grasp and the Babinski reflex, is a reliable sign of the first transition. Most scientists believe that this phenomenon is due to cortical inhibition of brainstem neurons (Brodal, 1981; Volpe, 1995). Projections from the supplementary motor cortex to the brainstem and spinal cord inhibit activity in the brainstem neurons (Bates and Goldman-Rakic, 1993; Galea and Darian-Smith, 1995). Although these axons reached the brainstem and spinal cord prenatally, actual synaptic contacts do not appear until 2–3 months (Kostovic, 1990; Fitzgerald, 1991). It is also relevant that GABAergic and glycinergic inhibitory interneurons in the spinal cord

JEROME KAGAN Department of Psychology, Harvard University, Cambridge, Mass.
ABIGAIL BAIRD Department of Psychology, Dartmouth College, Hanover, N.H.

undergo enhanced growth during the first 3 months (Akert, 1994; Ralston, 1994).

This first transition is also marked by an obvious reduction in crying and an increase in social smiling (deWeerth and Geert, 2002). The former could be the result of cortical inhibition of the brainstem nuclei that mediate crying (especially the reticular formation, central gray, nucleus solitarius, and parabrachial nucleus) (Fitzgerald, 1991; Zilles and Rehkamper, 1994).

A third characteristic of the transition is the ascendance of a psychological basis for recruiting and sustaining attention to a stimulus. Duration of attention to a visual event during the first 7–8 weeks is guided primarily by its physical features, especially size, contour density, and motion. After the transition, duration of attention is modulated to a greater degree by the relation between the event and the infant's acquired schema for that event (Kagan, 1970).

A schema is the first psychological form to emerge from the brain activity evoked by an event. The psychological definition of a schema is a pattern of the event's physical features. Thus, the vocabulary that describes a schema for a visual event contains words like "contour density," "color," "shape," and "motion" and differs from the vocabulary of terms that describe the neural activity that represents the foundation of the schema. One reason why recruitment of attention to a discrepant event is not automatic before 2 months is that infants must relate the event to an acquired schema, and this process is fragile during the first 2 months of life. Further, the function relating duration of attention to discrepancy is not linear but resembles an inverted U, where moderately discrepant events recruit longer bouts of attention than very familiar or very novel events (Kagan, Kearsley, and Zelazo, 1978). For example, 4-month-olds will look longer at the face of an unfamiliar person than at a familiar face or a totally novel event (e.g., an irregularly shaped piece of polyfoam). Although there can be no absolute answer to the question, How long does an infant's schema for an event last? it is possible to estimate the duration of preservation for a particular experimental procedure and for infants of a particular age. The evidence suggests an enhancement in the duration of a schema for a new event at 2–3 months (Boller et al., 1996; Rose, Feldman, and Jankowski, 2002).

It is likely that hippocampal maturation contributes to the improved ability of 2-month-olds to recognize an event following a delay because the greatest increase in the velocity of growth of the hippocampus occurs between 2 and 3 months (Kretschman et al., 1986). Specifically, the mossy cells of the hippocampal dentate gyrus undergo a spurt of differentiation (Seress and Mrzljak, 1992). The hippocampal growth might also make it possible for 3-month-olds to establish visual expectations (Haith, 1994). Infants, lying supine, looked up at two monitors. Each monitor displayed, alternately, a chromatic picture of a face or design for 700 ms, followed by an interval of 1100 ms when both monitors were dark, after which a different stimulus appeared on the second monitor. This alternation continued for about 1.5 minutes. About one-fifth of $3\frac{1}{2}$-month-olds, but no 2-month-olds, anticipated the appearance of a stimulus by moving their head to the monitor on which a picture was about to appear during the interval when both monitors were dark.

TRANSITION AT 7–12 MONTHS   The transition that occurs in most healthy infants between 7 and 12 months is accompanied by the ability to retrieve schemata from past events that are no longer in the perceptual field and to hold them along with the current perception in a working memory circuit while they try to assimilate the latter to the former. Four-month-olds can recognize that an event in their perceptual field was experienced in the past, but have difficulty retrieving a schema for a past event that is no longer present and performing cognitive operations on it.

Support for this generalization comes from a longitudinal study of infants who were assessed every 2 weeks from 6 to 14 months. In one procedure the examiner hid an attractive object under one of two identical cylinders, placed an opaque screen between the infant and the cylinder for delays of either 1, 3, or 7 sec, and then removed the screen to allow the infant to reach toward one of the cylinders. There was a linear increase with age in the probability of reaching to the hidden object as the delay increased. No 7-month-old reached to the correct location with a delay of 7 sec; however, most 12-month-olds solved that problem easily (Fox, Kagan, and Weiskopf, 1979). Comparable studies of infant monkeys affirm an improvement in the ability to retrieve a hidden object following increasingly long delays at 2–3 months of age, which corresponds to 7–10 months in the human infant (Diamond and Goldman-Rakic, 1989; Diamond, 1990). The transition at 7–12 months also marks the time when schematic concepts for the phonemes of the infant's language (Kuhl, 1991), temporal sequences of syllables (Marcus et al., 1999), and spontaneous imitation following a long delay appear (Bauer, 2002).

The enhancement of working memory is accompanied by a spurt of growth and differentiation in both pyramidal and inhibitory interneurons in the prefrontal cortex between 7 and 12 months. Specifically, double bouquet interneurons in layer III show a broader distribution of dendrites and their axons display numerous ascending and descending collaterals (Mrzljak et al., 1990). This growth is accompanied by increased glucose uptake (measured by PET) in the lateral and the dorsolateral prefrontal cortex (Huttenlocher, 1979, 1990; Chugani, 1994; Kostovic, Skavic, and Strinovic, 1998). Further, changes in oxygenated and deoxygenated hemoglobin in the blood supply to the frontal lobe, based on optical scanning, affirm the role of the prefrontal cortex in working memory (Baird et al., 2002). It is also relevant that hippocampal volume approaches adult size between 10 and 12 months (Kretschman et al., 1986), due in part to the number of spines and extra large excrescences on the proximal dendrites of pyramidal cells in the CA3 region of Ammon's horn (Seress and Mrzljak, 1992). These anatomical changes are accompanied by faster alpha frequencies (6–9 Hz) between 7 and 12 months (Bell, 1998).

The integrity of the hippocampal formation, but not the prefrontal cortex, is necessary for holding a representation in a short-term memory store for periods of less than 10 sec. However, the integrity of the prefrontal cortex is necessary for successful performance on the Piagetian A not B task, even with short delays (Diamond, Zola-Morgan, and Squire, 1989). As a result, some scientists distinguish between the concept of a short-term memory store and the concept of working memory; the latter implies that some cognitive activity was imposed on the information.

THE APPEARANCE OF FEAR TO DISCREPANCY   The improvement in working memory after 7 months permits infants to attempt assimilation of an event discrepant from their experience to a retrieved schema. If the discrepant event cannot be assimilated, and if the infant has no coping response, she may become fearful and cry (Bronson, 1968; Gunnar-Von Gnechten, 1978; Kagan, Kearsley, and Zelazo, 1978). The phenomenon of separation fear is illustrative. The unexpected departure of the mother, especially if the infant is in an unfamiliar place, is a discrepant event. The older infant retrieves a schema for her former presence and tries to relate it to the current perception of her absence. If the infant cannot assimilate the mother's absence to the schema for her former presence, he may become fearful and cry. The ability to hold the retrieved schema of the mother's prior presence with her current absence in a working memory circuit requires the brain maturation described earlier. Patterns of growth in the amygdala and prefrontal cortex are also likely to be relevant to both separation and stranger fear. The amygdala is activated by both unexpected and discrepant events, and projections from the amygdala to the cortex, through axons within the capsula interna, develop mature myelin between 7 and 10 months, the time when both fear of strangers and separation from a caretaker emerge (Chrousos and Gold, 1992).

The transition at 7–12 months is also accompanied by an enhanced ability to adjust sensory motor structures in the service of attaining a goal. For example, 5-month-olds use both hands to reach toward an object, whether small or large, while 8-month-olds reach with one hand toward small objects but with both hands toward large objects (Clifton et al., 1991; Rochat and Senders, 1991). The neuronal ensembles in motor cortex that mediate a class of motor action

are comparable to words in the child's vocabulary. One ensemble is activated when a monkey prepares to grasp a small object with thumb and forefinger; a different ensemble is activated when the whole hand must be used to grasp larger objects (Rizzolatti, Fogassi, and Gallese, 2000).

In sum, the central feature of the behavioral changes between 7 and 12 months is the ability to retrieve schemata and hold them and the current situation in a working memory circuit for 20–30 s while comparisons are being made or additional cognitive operations are performed. We suggest that the biological foundation for these advances rests in part on growth and differentiation of neurons in the prefrontal cortex and enhanced connectivity between the prefrontal cortex and the amygdala, hippocampus, and temporal lobe. The parallels between brain and biological growth in monkeys and human infants add credibility to this view.

The second year

The second year is distinguished by four psychological competences that might depend, in part, on a particular set of changes in the brain. The new properties include (1) the ability to comprehend and to express meaningful speech, (2) the capacity to infer selected mental and feeling states in others, (3) representations of the actions that are prohibited by adults, and (4) the first signs of conscious awareness of the self's feelings and intentions.

SPEECH   The brain bases for the new language competence are embedded in broad corticocortical networks that link the auditory pathway and temporal cortex to the parietal, frontal, and cerebellar regions involved in representations of temporal sequences. It may not be a coincidence that the first words emerge in most children between 12 and 15 months, the time that rapid dendritic growth occurs in the left orofacial section of Broca's area (Simonds and Scheibel, 1989). There is also an increase in the cerebellar volume, due in part to extensive lengthening of dendrites in the dentate nucleus of the cerebellum (Yamaguchi, Goto, and Yamamoto, 1989), and levels of glucose uptake attain 175% of adult values by the second birthday (Schmahmann and Pandy, 1997). Although Wernicke's area plays a greater role in the perceptual aspects of speech comprehension and Broca's area plays a greater role in the motor components of speech, both areas participate in these as well as other psychological functions (Devlin, Matthews, and Rushworth, 2003).

We suggest that the growth of neurons in cortical layer III, whose axons constitute the corpus callosum, contributes to the emergence of speech. This growth is accompanied by peak levels of glutamate binding, as well as a spurt in GABA activity in inhibitory interneurons of layer III, during the second year of life (Mrzljak et al., 1990; Slater et al., 1992; Huttenlocher and Dabholkar, 1997). Most scientists are friendly to the hypothesis that perceptual schemata representing objects and events are more fully represented in the right hemisphere, while lexical structures are more fully represented in the left (Lauder, 1983). If the layer III changes made callosal transfer more efficient, the perceptual schemata activated upon seeing a cup on a table would be integrated more rapidly with the lexical representation for the object, represented more fully in the left hemisphere, and the child might say "cup." It is of interest that a compromised ability in older adults to retrieve a name for a familiar person is accompanied by callosal thinning, suggesting the waning of a process in the elderly that is waxing in the second year (Sullivan et al., 2002).

INFERENCE The ability to infer selected thoughts and feelings of others, a second competence of the second year, might be aided by the same aspects of brain growth. A particularly clear demonstration of this talent is observed when an adult hides a toy under one of three covers behind a barrier so that the child cannot see where the toy is hidden. If, after removing the barrier, the adult directs her gaze toward the place where the toy is located, 2-year-olds, but not 1-year-olds, will look in the direction of the adult's orientation and reach toward that place, suggesting they inferred that the adult was looking at the correct location (Kagan, 1981). When infants 8–19 months of age saw an adult turn her head toward an interesting sight, only the 18- and 19-month-olds reliably used the direction of the adult gaze to guide the direction of their orientation toward a target (Moore and Corkum, 1998; Tomasello, 1999). The ability to infer what is in the minds of others is also revealed in behavioral signs of empathy upon perceiving distress in another person (Zahn-Waxler, Robinson, and Emde, 1992; Young, Fox, and Zahn-Waxler, 1999). The growth in layer III neurons would permit the rapid integration of the schematic representations of the somatic sensations experienced when in distress, which are stored primarily in the right hemisphere, with semantic representations of the state of the other, represented primarily in the left hemisphere. As a result, empathy would occur.

REPRESENTATIONS OF PROHIBITED ACTIONS Children first acquire schematic concepts for prohibited actions during the second year. Most 2-year-olds will hesitate if a parent asks them to perform an act that violates a family norm, such as pouring cranberry juice on a clean tablecloth, and will show behavioral signs of concern when they see an object whose integrity is flawed. (Kagan, 1981). Parents living on isolated atolls in the Fijian chain, who recognize this advance, believe that their children acquire *vakayala*, meaning good sense, soon after their second birthday (Kagan, 1981).

This phenomenon, too, could be facilitated by the more efficient coordination of information between the two hemispheres. Specifically, the visceral schemata that represent the feeling of uncertainty that follows parental criticism or punishment, more fully represented in the right hemisphere, will be integrated with the semantic representations for prohibited behaviors, mediated more fully in the left hemisphere.

SELF-AWARENESS Finally, initial signs of self-awareness appear in the second year. For example, infants now recognize their reflection in the mirror, direct adults to act in particular ways, show signs of distress when they cannot imitate the behavior of another but signs of pride if they can, and describe in speech what they are doing as they are doing it (Kagan, 1981). The enhanced connectivity between the two hemispheres could contribute to these phenomena as well. The representations of the child's feeling tone, which varies from moment to moment and is an important foundation of self-awareness, is represented primarily in the right hemisphere. When this information is integrated with the semantic categories for self's name, thoughts, and intentions, represented primarily in the left, a consciousness of self's feelings and intentions could emerge.

OTHER BRAIN EVENTS In addition to the enhanced integration of information from the two hemispheres, other maturational changes in the second year could contribute to the psychological competences of this era. For example, peak levels of glutamate binding, activity of glutamate decarboxylase, required for the synthesis of GABA, as well as a spurt in GABA activity in inhibitory interneurons of layer III occur between 1 and 2 years of age (Slater et al., 1992; Huttenlocher and Dabholkar, 1997). GABA mediates inhibitory functions, and all observers of children recognize the increased ability of 2-year-olds to regulate their behavior. In addition, the activity of choline acetyltransferase increases sharply during the second year, when pyramidal neurons begin to express acetylcholine in cell bodies and fibrillary networks (Decker and McGaugh, 1991; Court et al., 1993). Finally, there is a spurt in EEG coherence between the left parietal and left temporal areas in the middle of the second year, implying greater functional connectivity among noncontiguous cortical areas (Thatcher, 1994).

The behaviors and cognitive functions of 1-year-olds are similar to those of chimpanzees. Both species show enhanced working memory and fear to discrepant events that cannot be assimilated. However, by the end of the second year the differences between the two species become more distinct. No observer would confuse a 2-year-old child with a chimpanzee of any age because of the emergence of language, inference, awareness of prohibited acts, and self-consciousness.

The belief that a set of universal psychological properties emerges after the second birthday, accelerates between 5 and 8 years of age, and plateaus from age 8 to puberty is present in essays written centuries earlier (see White, 1996, for a review). Even nonliterate parents who are uncertain of their child's age begin to assign chores when their children reach 6 or 7 years. Parents now expect their children to be able to care for young infants, tend animals, work in the field, and conform to community mores because they have noticed that their children have become teachable, responsible, capable of understanding what others want, and able to understand rational explanations. The maturing abilities of this prolonged era include (1) active integration of past with present, (2) enhanced reliance on semantic networks, and (3) detection of shared relations between categories.

INTEGRATION OF PAST WITH PRESENT   One sign of this developmental phase, usually observed by the fourth birthday, is the automatic and more reliable activation of past representations in order to interpret the present moment (Loken, Leichtman, and Kagan, 2002). This ability is the phenomenon that Jean Piaget (1950) called conservation. In a classic demonstration of this competence, an examiner shows a child two identical balls of clay and asks whether the two balls have the same amount of clay, or whether one ball has more clay than the other. All children acknowledge that the two balls have equivalent amounts of clay. The examiner then rolls one of the two balls into a sausage shape and asks the child again, "Which one has more clay?" Four-year-olds treat the question as if it were independent of the first, and, since the sausage appears to have more substance, they say that the sausage has more clay. By contrast, 7-year-olds regard the sausage as part of a temporal sequence that began when the examiner showed the child the two identical balls and asked the first conservation question. The 7-year-olds understood that after the examiner transformed one ball into the sausage the examiner intended to ask, "Given the sequence you have seen over the last minute or two, which ball has more clay?" The older child treats the second question as part of a coherent temporal sequence.

This competence motivates children to wonder about causal connections between events. The implicit question, "Why did this event occur?" provokes children to retrieve structures that might represent possible antecedents of a current situation (Povinelli et al., 1999). Thus, 7-year-olds who harm a person or damage property relate that outcome to a prior intention, or to their clumsy behavior, and, as a result, are vulnerable to a feeling of remorse. For the same reason, 7-year-old children are usually reflective on a problem following a mistake because they recognize that their error was due to a failure to consider all the alternative solutions carefully.

SEMANTIC NETWORKS   A second significant feature of this era is an expanded reliance on semantic networks to categorize experience. One reason for the phenomenon called infantile amnesia is that young children do not regularly use semantic structures to code their experiences, and therefore cannot report a salient event experienced in the past (Simock and Hayne, 2002). The application of semantic categories to experience influences the way children organize and retrieve knowledge. If a list of 12 words containing two semantic categories (for example, animals and foods) is read to children 4 and 7 years old, only the older children cluster words that belong to the same semantic category in their recall. This phenomenon could only occur if older children had an automatic tendency to group words that were members of the same semantic category. The improvement in memory functioning over the years 2 through 8 is due, in part, to the use of language to structure experience (Nelson, 1996).

SHARED RELATIONS   Detection of shared relations between or among categories of events is a third competence that emerges after age 4 or 5 years. Children under 6 years can detect a physical feature, function, or name that is shared by two or more events. However, younger children do not detect a shared semantic relation between events that belong to different categories (for example, the loudest of six noises shares the semantic relation of magnitude with the sweetest of six tastes). The reason for the late appearance of this competence is that the shared relation is not given immediately in perception, as is true for shape or motion, but must be inferred with a semantic form.

Seven-year-old children understand that the semantic concepts "smaller" and "bigger" are not absolute properties of any object but refer to a relation between objects. Similarly, older, but not younger, children understand that right and left refer to relations between objects and are not fixed properties of any object (Kuenne, 1946). The ability to detect relations shared by different events allows children to assign an object to a category based on multiple dimensions. For example, 7-year-olds but not 4-year-olds will sort a pile of toys that vary in size and hue into four groups (Piaget, 1950).

The psychological competences described above require the participation of many brain sites acting coordinately. One relevant fact is that the human brain attains 90% of its adult weight between 4 and 8 years (Giedd et al., 1996), with the rate of increase in cortical surface greatest between 2 and 6 years. This growth is accompanied by increased glucose uptake in both cortical and subcortical structures (Chugani, 1994, 1998).

The balance between the number of synapses formed and the number eliminated shifts after 5 or 6 years to a ratio that favors the latter. The reduction in extra synapses is assumed to reflect consolidation of the active synaptic networks that represent new learning. Synaptic density reaches its peak earlier in layer IV than in layers II and III; the latter mediate associative activity. Maximum synaptic density in the prefrontal cortex is not attained until 3–4 years of age (Huttenlocher and Dabholkar, 1997).

Dopamine concentrations, as well as the density of dopamine D_1 receptors in the monkey prefrontal cortex, approach adult values between 2 and 3 years, corresponding to 6–9 years in children. Although dopamine does not show as clear a developmental change as norepinephrine, dopaminergic fibers attain maximal extension in layer III of the monkey's prefrontal cortex at about 3 years of age, comparable to about 9–10 years in humans (Rosenberg and Lewis, 1994). Although the synthesis of serotonin peaks at 3 years, serotonin receptors do not reach maximum density in the basal ganglia, hippocampus, and cerebellum until 5 or 6 years. Finally, acetylcholinesterase-positive pyramidal neurons, believed to be restricted to apes and humans, first appear in layer III in the frontal, motor, and association cortices and the hippocampus between 4 and 5 years (Kostovic, Skavic, and Strinovic, 1988; Mesulam and Geula, 1988).

The connectivity of the brain, which is the central feature of this developmental era, is also revealed in enhanced myelination and improved EEG coherence. The axons of the anterior corpus callosum show their most rapid growth of myelin between 3 and 6 years, and the longer tracts, which link noncontiguous sites within a hemisphere, display a spurt of myelination after the third birthday. This process continues at a slower rate into adulthood (Yakovlev and Lecour, 1967; Curnes et al., 1988). As a result, the ratio of white to gray matter in layers II and III, which favored the latter during the first 3 years, is now reversed and white matter exceeds gray matter for the first time.

There is also an increase between 3 and 4 years in the magnitude of coherence of EEG frequency bands between frontal sites, on the one hand, and temporal areas, on the other (Ornitz, 2002). Finally, blood flow, which was greater in the right than in the left parietal-temporal cortex in the first 4 years, becomes greater in the left hemisphere by the fifth birthday (Takahashi et al., 1999).

The salient feature of the psychological advances observed between ages 2 and 7 is the almost automatic evocation of representations that are relevant to an incentive or context. The most fundamental brain change during this time is a massive interconnectedness involving both hemispheres, anterior and posterior cortical sites, and cortical and subcortical structures. Two facts are of special importance. The first is a shift in blood flow from the right temporal and parietal areas to homologous areas in the left hemisphere.

The second is the fact that the number of synapses eliminated exceeds that of new synapses formed, first in sensory and later in frontal areas, reflecting the strengthening of circuits that have proven adaptive.

Adolescence

Although most cognitive processes are functional by 8–10 years of age, the capacity for abstract thought, logical reasoning, planning, and cognitive flexibility are enhanced after puberty and during the adolescent years (Piaget, 1950). One obvious hallmark of adolescence is the ability to detect logical contradiction or semantic inconsistency among beliefs, or between feelings and beliefs, that belong to a network. For example, recognition of disloyal thoughts about a friend ("I'm a good person, but I hope my friend fails the examination") can elicit a moment of dissonance or guilt, even if the friend is not hurt by those thoughts. The young child is less likely to recognize this inconsistency. The detection of inconsistencies in beliefs pertaining to a theme motivates youth to try to integrate their past knowledge with current experience in order to understand their present circumstances more completely. It is likely that behaviors that were issued without reflection in early childhood come under increasing control of conscious reflective processes during adolescence. For example, young children, who can distinguish among different facial expressions, often find it difficult to think about human emotions abstractly. Adolescents, by contrast, can make sophisticated inferences about a person's emotional state from that person's facial expression or posture. This may be one reason why medieval Europeans did not permit youth younger than 13 or 14 years old to take monastic vows.

The frontal cortex contributes in a major way to these cognitive capacities. Although medial temporal structures are functionally mature early in development, the frontal lobes do not reach full functional maturity until after puberty, and the anterior frontal regions mature later than posterior regions (Giedd et al., 1999; Sowell, Thompson, Holmes, Batth, et al., 1999; Sowell, Thompson, Holmes, Jernigan, et al., 1999). In addition, there is continued synaptic pruning through adolescence into the second decade (Casey et al., 2000). These advances are probably influenced by changes in neurophysiology as well (Baird et al., 1999).

The increased myelination of the anterior cingulate, which mediates emotional, attentional, and cognitive functions (Vogt, Finch, and Olson, 1992; Casey et al., 1997), should result in improved corticocortical and corticosubsortical connections. Projections from cortical and subcortical regions to the cingulate facilitate the coordination and regulation of psychological processes; unfortunately, we do not know the details of this developmental phenomenon. Research on rodent brains may shed light on this issue because projections from the rat amygdala to the cingulate appear at puberty (Amaral and Insausti, 1992). Cunningham, Battacharyya, and Benes (2002) using antero-grade tracers in the amygdala, discovered a sharp increase in the density of labeled fibers originating in the amygdala and synapsing on the cingulate and medial prefrontal regions at puberty.

Finally, it is of interest that the volumes of subcortical structures in female adolescents (especially the amygdala and hippocampus) are very similar to adult volumes. By contrast, these subcortical volumes are larger in adolescent boys than in adult men, suggesting the different effects of male and female hormones on the pruning of synapses in these areas (Giedd, Snell, et al., 1996; Paus, et al., 2001).

In sum, the psychological changes that occur during the adolescent years are correlated with the pruning of synapses in prefrontal cortex, myelination of axons connecting the prefrontal cortex to the rest of the brain, and the firmer inclusion of the cingulate cortex in circuits involving the amygdala and the prefrontal cortex.

Synthesis and controversy

The evidence indicates that the times of emergence of the universal psychological features of human development are constrained by maturation of the central nervous system, even though the brain changes do not guarantee the new psychological structures. Almost all 1-year-olds, regardless of their cultural setting, are able to retrieve past representations and maintain them and their perception of the current context in a working memory circuit for intervals as long as 30 sec, in some cases longer. The fact that pyramidal neurons in frontal sites display accelerated growth from 7 to 12 months supports the suggestion that the behavioral phenomena require the biological changes.

The hidden sequence during the first 12–13 years is from (1) establishing an initial connectivity among sensory, limbic, and medial temporal structures to (2) improved integration of the two hemispheres to (3) connecting the frontal lobe to the above sites and, finally, to (4) a massive connectivity among all brain sites as the child prepares for school or, in villages without schools, for assumption of family responsibilities.

However, despite these facts, we remain frustrated in our attempt to answer three significant questions: (1) How do psychological phenomena emerge from brain activity? (2) How does experience influence brain growth? (3) Which experiences accelerate and which retard the emergence of the milestones once the brain has attained the appropriate level of growth? A wrinkled guru who knows the answers to these questions might shake her head after reading this chapter and mutter that all we have done is to describe some roughly temporal correspondences between brain and behavior and assume, with insufficient caution, a causal connection.

THE IMPORTANCE OF SPECIFICITY The stark contrast between the specificity of brain function and the generality of many popular psychological constructs is a paradox. Almost every time a biologist posits a relation between two aspects of brain function, or between brain function and a psychological product, other scientists discover that the original claim was too general. The facts of nature force most neuroscientists to be splitters. By contrast, psychiatrists and psychologists tend to be lumpers, preferring more abstract to more constrained concepts. The profiles of change in dopamine concentration in three sites in the rat brain reveal the problem with an ambitious striving for generality. Dopamine concentrations produced by two different sweet-tasting substances were assessed in the prefrontal cortex, as well as in the shell and core of the nucleus accumbens (Bassareo, De Luca, and De Chiara, 2002). The taste of sucrose produced an increase in dopamine in the prefrontal cortex exclusively, but a combination of sucrose and choco-late, which is an unfamiliar stimulus for rats, produced a dopamine increase in all three sites. Even though both sub-stances were "sweet," each elicited a different brain state.

Developmental psychologists are just beginning to appreciate the significance of tiny details in a procedure. For example, preschool children tested in a small room (4 × 6 feet) without any windows failed to use a landmark (a single blue wall) to find an object they saw an adult hide in the corner of the room. However, the same children used the blue wall as a landmark if they were tested in a larger room (8 × 12 feet). Simply changing the size of the room led to a different inference about the child's ability to use a landmark (Learmonth, Nadel, and Newcombe, 2002). We suggest that scientists should parse the broad constructs that dominate current psychological theory, for example, reward, fear, intel-ligence, and memory, into a number of more restricted con-cepts that are in closer accord with what is known about the brain. This suggestion is not a defense of reductionism but a plea for consistency in the level of specificity in the descrip-tions of brain and mind.

LOCALIZATION The notion that a particular psychological process emerges from activity in a particular site remains attractive (Blanke et al., 2002). Although the ability to inhibit an inappropriate response and the ability to hold informa-tion in working memory require the integrity of the frontal lobe, neither function is localized in this site, for most psy-chological processes recruit structures from diverse sites. There is no single place in the brain where the memory of a past automobile accident or a feeling of vitality is recog-nized, even though some sites contribute more and others less to the psychological phenomenon. After a review of 275 studies that used PET or fMRI, Duncan and Miller (2002) concluded that mapping a defined cognitive process on a well-defined brain region may not be possible. The prefrontal cortex may be a general computational resource that is relied on to solve different cognitive problems.

The most significant maturational event occurring over the first dozen years is an increasing connectivity of the prefrontal cortex with the rest of the brain. The expansion of the human prefrontal cortex to one-third of the total cortical surface, compared with only one-tenth in the gorilla, appears to be a seminal reason for the display of the psychological properties that differentiate humans from all other primates. We suggest that eight distinctive human properties are (1) an expanded working memory; (2) the ability to maintain a representation of a goal, despite distractions, due to the inhibition of thoughts and responses irrelevant to the goal; (3) the ability to retrieve representations of events from the distant past, including the incentive and its temporal and spatial properties, a process called episodic memory; (4) the ability to generate representations of events that might occur in the distant future; (5) conscious awareness of self's feelings, thoughts, and properties; (6) creation of the concept of prohibited acts, understanding the semantic categories "good" and "bad," and capacities for anxiety or shame over violations of a standard; (7) the seeking of new experiences that can be understood or coped with effectively; and (8) the ability to invent relations of similarity and difference among varied classes of representations. These eight competences require participation of the prefrontal cortex and its connections to other brain sites, and therefore require coherence among brain regions.

Coda

We end by asking whether it is possible, in principle, to translate sentences describing the psychological phenomena discussed in this chapter into sentences containing only biological words. The answer is uncertain at the present time, but there are reasons to be skeptical of the possibility of a complete translation. Roald Hoffman (2001) reminds us that scientists cannot even translate a chemical description of the oxidation of iron into the vocabulary of physics without losing the central meaning of "oxidative state of a molecule."

We doubt, for example, whether scientists will be able to replace the psychological term *reward* with biological words describing only brain activity, because *preference* and *pleasure* are psychological properties of whole animals, not of neuronal circuits. One reason for the incommensurability between the languages of neuroscience and psychology is that the complete semantic network of a neurobiological term is different from the network of the same word when

used to name psychological phenomena. Even the French word *douce* and the English word *sweet* have different networks (Kuhn, 2000). Although a piece of cake is called *douce* by the French and *sweet* by Americans, only the French use the word *douce* to name a bland-tasting soup and only Americans use the word *sweet* to describe a young pretty girl. Thus, *douce* and *sweet* have related but not synonymous meanings.

The semantic network for the term *fear* among neuroscientists has salient nodes for "amygdala," "freezing," "startle," and "electric shock." The salient nodes of the network for this word when used by psychologists are "worry," "uncertain," "evaluative," "vigilant," and "symptom."

The complete semantic network for a concept is analogous to the physicist's notion of a phase space, because a collection of gas molecules in a vessel can assume a very large number of states, only one of which can be measured at a given time. For example, a picture of a snake can activate many different representations, depending on the context, and no member of that family is knowable until an investigator intervenes with a probe to measure it. Therefore, the pattern of brain activation in a person lying in an fMRI scanner and looking at pictures of snakes is not the only profile these stimuli could provoke. These pictures would probably create a different brain state if the person were looking at them on a television screen at home. Every conclusion regarding the neural profile that accompanies a psychological event is valid for the class of contexts in which the measurement was made. That is why Bohr believed that scientists can never know what nature is; they only know what their measurements permit them to infer.

A behavior, thought, or feeling is the final product of a series of cascades that began with an external stimulus, thought, or spontaneous biological event. The number of cascades varies with the psychological outcome of interest. However, the biological and psychological forms that make up each cascade must be described with a distinct vocabulary. Genes, chromosomes, neurons, organisms, and species have unique functions that are linked to distinct predicates. Genes mutate, chromosomes separate, neurons depolarize, organisms mate, and species evolve.

There is an increase in order and a loss of determinism as we move from the forms and functions of one cascade to those of the next—for example, from neuronal excitation in motor cortex to a child reaching toward a rattle—because there are fewer possible ways a child can reach for an object than possible states of the relevant neuronal ensembles. Hence, it is not possible to predict the exact direction and speed of a child's arm reaching for a rattle from complete knowledge of the immediately preceding neuronal profile. As the human brain matures, the links between one stage of psychological functioning and the next become a little less predictable because of the increasing importance of the child's past experiences. Neuronal change and human experience interact to create a reciprocally influential process that recapitulates across development. This growth eventually enables most adolescents to appreciate that, like the different perceptions of a Monet painting from 1 versus 20 feet away, there is more than one way to interpret an event.

ACKNOWLEDGMENTS   This work was supported by a grant from the Bial Foundation. Some ideas presented in this chapter are part of a book-length manuscript by Jerome Kagan and Norbert Hershkowitz of the University of Bern.

REFERENCES

AKERT, K., 1994. Limbisches system. In *Benninghoff Anatomie*, D. Drenckhahn and W. Zenker, eds. Munich: Urban and Schwarzenberg, pp. 493–526.

AMARAL, D. G., and R. INSAUSTI, 1992. Retrograde transport of B-³H aspartate injected into the monkey amygdaloid complex. *Exp. Brain Res.* 88:375–388.

BAIRD, A. A., S. A. GRUBER, D. A. FEIN, L. C. MASS, R. J. STEINGARD, P. F. RENSHAW, B. M. COHEN, and D. A. YURGELIN-TODD, 1999. Functional magnetic resonance imaging of facial affect recognition in children and adolescents. *J. Am. Acad. Child Adolesc. Psychiatry* 38:195–199.

BAIRD, A. A., J. KAGAN, T. GAUDETTE, K. A. WALZ, N. HERSHLAG, and D. A. BOAS, 2002. Frontal lobe activation during object permanence. *NeuroImage* 16:1120–1126.

BASSAREO, V., M. A. DE LUCA, and G. DE CHIARA, 2002. Differential expression of motivational stimulational properties by dopamine in nucleus accumbens vs. core and prefrontal cortex. *J. Neurosci.* 22:4709–4719.

BATES, J. F., and P. S. GOLDMAN-RAKIC, 1993. Prefrontal connections of medial motor areas in the rhesus monkey. *J. Comp. Neurol.* 336:211–228.

BAUER, P. J., 2002. Long term recall memory. *Curr. Direct. Psychol. Sci.* 11:137–141.

BELL, M. A., 1998. Search for valid infant EEG rhythms. *Psychophysiology* 35:S19.

BLANKE, O., S. ORTIGUE, T. LANDIS, and M. SEECK, 2002. Stimulating illusory own body perceptions. *Nature* 22:4709–4719.

BOLLER, K., C. ROVEE-COLLIER, M. GULYA, and K. PRETA, 1996. Infants' memory for context. *J. Exp. Child Psychol.* 63:583–602.

BRODAL, A., 1981. Grasp reflex. In *Neurological Anatomy in Relation to Clinical Medicine*. New York: Oxford University Press, p. 241.

BRONSON, G. W., 1968. The development of fear in man and other animals. *Child Dev.* 39:409–431.

CASEY B. J., K. M. THOMAS, R. B. BADGAIYAM, C. H. ECCARD, J. R. JENNINGS, and E. A. CRONE, 2000. Dissociation of response conflict and attentional selection and expectancy with functional magnetic resonance imaging. *Proc. Nat. Acad. Sci. U.S.A.* 97:8728–8733.

CASEY, B. J., R. TRAINOR, J. N. JIDD, Y. VAUSS, C. K. VAITUZIS, S. D. HAMBURGER, P. KOZUCH, and J. L. RAPPAPORT, 1997. The role of the interior cingulate and automatic and control processes. *Dev. Psychobiol.* 30:61–69.

CHROUSOS, G. P., and P. W. GOLD, 1992. The concepts of stress and stress system disorders. *JAMA* 267:1244–1252.

CHUGANI, H. T., 1994. Development of regional brain glucose metabolism. In *Human Behavior and the Developing Brain*, G. Dawson and K. Fischer, eds. New York: Guilford Press, pp. 153–175.

CHUGANI, H. T., 1998. A critical period of brain development. *Prevent. Med.* 27:184–188.

CLIFTON, R. K., P. ROCHAT, R. Y. LITOVSKY, and E. E. PERRIS, 1991. Object representation guides infants' reaching in the dark. *J. Exp. Psychol. Hum. Percept. Perform.* 17:323–329.

COURT, J. A., E. K. PERRY, M. JOHNSON, M. PIGGOT, J. A. KERWIN, R. H. PERRY, and P. G. INCE, 1993. Regional patterns of cholinergic and glutamate activity in the developing and aging human brain. *Brain Res. Dev. Brain Res.* 74:73–82.

CUNNINGHAM, M. E., S. BHATTACHARYYA, and F. M. BENES, 2002. Amygdalo-cortical sprouting continues into early adulthood. *Comp. Neurol.* 453:116–130.

CURNES, J. T., P. C. BURGER, W. T. DJANG, and O. B. BOYKO, 1988. MR imaging of compact white matter pathways. *Am. J. Neuroradiol.* 9:1061–1068.

DE WEERTH, C., and V. GEERT, 2002. Changing patterns of infant behavior in mother-infant interaction. *Infant Behav. Dev.* 24:347–371.

DECKER, M. W., and J. MCGAUGH, 1991. The role of interactions between the cholinergic system and other neuro-modulatory systems in learning and memory. *Synapse* 7:151–168.

DEVLIN, J. T., P. M. MATTHEWS, and M. F. S. RUSHWORTH, 2003. Semantic processing in the left inferior prefrontal cortex. *J. Cogn. Neurosci.* 15:71–84.

DIAMOND, A., 1990. Rate of maturation of the hippocampus and the developmental progression of children's performance on the delayed nonmatching to sample in visual paired comparison tasks. *Ann. N. Y. Acad. Sci.* 608:394–426.

DIAMOND, A., and P. S. GOLDMAN-RAKIC, 1989. Comparison of human infants and rhesus monkeys on Piaget's AB task. *Exp. Brain Res.* 74:24–40.

DIAMOND, A., S. ZOLA-MORGAN, and L. R. SQUIRE, 1989. Successful performance by monkey with lesions of the hippocampal formation on A not B and object retrieval, two tasks that mark developmental changes in human infants. *Behav. Neurosci.* 108:526–537.

DUNCAN, J., and E. K. MILLER, 2002. Cognitive focus through adaptive neural coding in the primate prefrontal cortex. In *Principles of Frontal Lobe Function*, D. T. Stuss and R. T. Knight, eds. New York: Oxford University Press, pp. 278–291.

FITZGERALD, M., 1991. The development of descending brain stem control of spinal cord sensory processing. In *Fetal and Neonatal Brain Stem*, M. A. Hanson, ed. Cambridge, England: Cambridge University Press, pp. 127–136.

FOX, N., J. KAGAN, and S. WEISKOPF, 1979. The growth of memory during infancy. *Genet. Psychol. Monogr.* 99:91–130.

GALEA, M. P., and I. DARIAN-SMITH, 1995. Post-natal maturation of a direct cortico-spinal projections in the macaque monkey. *Cereb. Cortex* 5:518–540.

GIEDD, J. N., J. BLUMENTHAL, N. O. JEFFRIES, F. X. CASTELLANOS, H. LIU, A. ZIJDENBOS, T. PAUS, A. C. EVANS, and J. L. RAPAPPORT, 1999. Brain development during childhood and adolescence: *Nat. Neurosci.* 2:861–863.

GIEDD, J. N., J. W. SNELL, N. LANGE, J. C. RAJAPAKSE, B. J. CASEY, P. L. KOZUCH, A. C. VAITUZIS, Y. C. VAUSS, S. D. HAMBURGER, D. KAYSEN, and J. L. RAPOPORT, 1996. Quantitative magnetic resonance imaging of human brain development: Ages 4 to 18. *Cereb. Cortex* 6:551–560.

Giedd, J. N., S. Vaituzis, S. Hamburger, N. Lange, J. C. Rajapakse, D. Kaysen, Y. Vauss, and J. L. Rapaport, 1996. Quantitative MRI of the temporal lobe, amygdala, and hippocampus in normal human development in ages 4 to 8. *J. Comp. Neurol.* 366:223–230.

Gunnar-Von Gnechten, M., 1978. Changing of frightening toy into a pleasant toy by allowing the infant to control its actions. *Dev. Psychol.* 14:157–162.

Haith, M. M., 1994. Visual expectations as the first step toward the development of future oriented processes. In *The Development of Future Oriented Processes*, M. M. Haith, J. B. Benson, R. J. Roberts, and B. F. Pennington, eds. Chicago: University of Chicago Press, 11–38.

Hoffmann, R., 2001. Hi O Silver. *Am. Sci.* 89:311–313.

Huttenlocher, P., 1979. Synaptic density in human frontal cortex. *Brain Res.* 163:195–205.

Huttenlocher, P. R., 1990. Morphometric study of human cerebral cortex development. *Neuropsychologia* 28:517–527.

Huttenlocher, P. R., and A. S. Dabholkar, 1997. Regional differences in synaptogenesis in human cerebral cortex. *J. Comp. Neurol.* 387:167–178.

Kagan, J., 1970. The determinants of attention in the infant. *Am. Sci.* 58:298–306.

Kagan, J., 1981. *The Second Year.* Cambridge, Mass.: Harvard University Press.

Kagan, J., R. B. Kearsley, and P. Zelazo, 1978. *Infancy.* Cambridge, Mass.: Harvard University Press.

Kostovic, I., 1990. Structural and histochemical reorganization of the human prefrontal cortex during perinatal and postnatal life. *Prog. Brain Res.* 85:223–240.

Kostovic, I., J. Skavic, and D. Strinovic, 1988. Acetylcholinesterase in the human frontal associative cortex during the period of cognitive development. *Neurosci. Lett.* 90:107–112.

Kretschmann, H. J., G. Kammradt, I. Krauthausen, B. Sauer, and F. Wingert, 1986. Growth of the hippocampal formation in man. *Bibl. Anat.* 28:27–52.

Kuenne, M., 1946. Experimental investigation of the relation of language to transposition behavior in young children. *J. Exp. Psychol.* 36:471–490.

Kuhl, P. K., 1991. Human adults and human infants show a perceptual magnet effect for the prototypes of speech categories, monkeys do not. *Percept. Psychophys.* 50:93–107.

Kuhn, T. S., 2000. *The Road Since Structure*, J. Conant and J. Haugeland, eds. Chicago: University of Chicago Press.

Lauder, J. M., 1983. Hormonal and humoral influences on brain development. *Psychoneuroendocrinology* 8:121–155.

Learmonth, A. E., L. Nadel, and N. S. Newcombe, 2002. Children's use of landmarks. *Psychol. Sci.* 13:337–341.

Loken, E., M. D. Leichtman, and J. Kagan, 2002. *Integration of Past and Present.* Unpublished manuscript.

Marcus, G. F., S. Vijayan, S. Bandi Rao, and P. M. Vishton, 1999. Rule learning by seven month old infants. *Science* 283:77–80.

Mesulam, M. M., and C. Geula, 1988. Acetylcholinesterase-rich pyramidal neurons in the human neocortex and hippocampus. *Ann. Neurol.* 24:765–773.

Moore, C., and V. Corkum, 1998. Infant gaze following based on eye direction. *Br. J. Dev. Psychol.* 16:495–503.

Mrzljak, L., H. B. Uylings, C. G. van Eden, and M. Judas, 1990. Neuronal development in human prefrontal cortex in prenatal and postnatal stages. *Prog. Brain Res.* 85:185–222.

Nelson, K., 1996. Memory development from 4 to 7 years. In *The Five to Seven Year Shift*, A. J. Sameroff and M. M. Haith, eds. Chicago: University of Chicago Press, pp. 141–160.

Newcombe, N., and N. A. Fox, 1994. Infantile amnesia. *Child Dev.* 65:31–40.

Ornitz, M. E., 2002. Developmental aspects of neurophysiology. In *Child and Adolescent Psychiatry*, M. Lewis, ed. Philadelphia: Lippincott, Williams, and Wilkins, pp. 60–74.

Paus, T., D. L. Collins, A. C. Evans, G. Leonard, B. Pike, and A. Zijdenbos, 2001. Maturation of white matter in the human brain. *Brain Res. Bull.* 54:255–266.

Piaget, J., 1950. *Psychology of Intelligence.* London: Rutledge and Kegan-Paul.

Povinelli, D. J., A. M. Landry, L. A. Theall, B. R. Clark, and C. M. Castille, 1999. Development of young children's understanding that the recent past is causally bound to the present. *Dev. Psychol.* 35:1426–1439.

Ralston, D. D., 1994. Cortico-rubral synaptic organization in *Macaca fasicularis. J. Comp. Neurol.* 350:657–673.

Rizzolatti, G., G. Fogassi, and V. Gallese, 2000. Cortical mechanisms subsuming object grasping and action recognition. In *The New Cognitive Neurosciences*, M. S. Gazzaniga, ed. Cambridge, Mass.: MIT Press, pp. 539–582.

Rochat, P., and S. J. Senders, 1991. Active touch in infancy. In *Newborn Attention*, M. J. S. Weiss and P. R. Zelazo, eds. Norwood, N.J.: Ablex, pp. 412–442.

Rose, S. A., J. F. Feldman, and J. J. Jankowski, 2002. Processing speed in the first year of life. *Dev. Psychol.* 38:895–902.

Rosenberg, D. R., and D. A. Lewis, 1994. Changes in the dopaminergic innervation of monkey prefrontal cortex during late post-natal development. *Biol. Psychiatry* 36:272–277.

Schmahmann, J. D., and D. M. Pandy, 1997. Anatomic substrates. In *The Cerebellum and Cognition*, J. D. Schmahmann, ed. San Diego, Calif.: Academic Press, pp. 31–55.

Seress, L., and L. Mrzljak, 1992. Postnatal development of mossy cells in the human dentate gyrus. *Hippocampus* 2:127–142.

Simcock, G., and H. Hayne, 2002. Breaking the barrier. *Psychol. Sci.* 13:225–231.

Simonds, R. J., and A. B. Scheibel, 1989. The postnatal development of the motor speech area. *Brain Lang.* 37:42–58.

Slater, P., S. McConnell, S. W. D'Souza, A. J. Barson, M. D. Simpson, and A. C. Gilchrist, 1992. Age related changes in binding to excitatory amino acid uptake site in temporal cortex of the human brain. *Brain Res. Dev. Brain Res.* 65:157–160.

Sowell, E. R., P. M. Thompson, C. J. Holmes, R. Batth, T. L. Jernigan, and A. W. Toga, 1999. Localizing age-related changes in brain structure between childhood and adolescents using statistical parametric mapping. *NeuroImage* 9:587–597.

Sowell, E. R., P. M., Thompson, C. J. Holmes, T. L. Jernigan, and A. W. Toga, 1999. In vivo evidence for post-adolescent brain maturation and striatal regions. *Nat. Neurosci.* 2:859–861.

Sullivan, E. V., A. Pfefferbaum, S. M. E. Adelstein, G. E. Swan, and D. Carmell, 2002. Differential rates of regional brain change in callosal and ventricular size. *Cereb. Cortex* 12:438–445.

Takahashi, T., R. Shirane, S. Sato, and T. Yoshimoto, 1999. Developmental changes in cerebral blood flow and oxygen metabolism in children. *Am. J. Neuroradio.* 20:917–922.

Thatcher, R. W., 1994. Cyclic cortical reorganization. In *Human Behavior and the Developing Brain*, G. Dawson and K. Fischer, eds. New York: Guilford Press, 232–266.

Tomasello, M., 1999. *The Cultural Origins of Human Cognition.* Cambridge, Mass.: Harvard University Press.

Vogt, B. A., D. M. Finch, and C. R. Olson, 1992. Functional heterogeneity in cingulate cortex. *Cereb. Cortex* 2:435–443.

Volpe, J. J., 1995. *Neurology of the Newborn*, 3rd ed. Philadelphia: Saunders.

White, S. H., 1996. The child's entry into the age of reason. In *The Five to Seven Year Shift*, A. G. Sameroff and M. M. Haith, eds. Chicago: University of Chicago Press, pp. 17–32.

Yakovlev, P. I., and A. R. Lecour, 1967. The myelogenetic cycles of regional maturation of the brain. In *Regional Development of the Brain in Early Life*, A. Minkowski, ed. Oxford, England: Blackwell Scientific, pp. 3–70.

Yamaguchi, K., N. Goto, and T. Y. Yamamoto, 1989. Development in the human cerebellar nuclei. *Acta Anat.* 136:61–68.

Young, S. K., N. A. Fox, and C. Zahn-Waxler, 1999. The relation between temperament and empathy in two year olds. *Dev. Psychol.* 35:1189–1197.

Zahn-Waxler, C., J. L. Robinson, and R. N. Emde, 1992. The development of empathy in twins. *Dev. Psychol.* 28:1038–1047.

Zilles, K., and G. Rehkamper, 1994. *Funktionelle Neuroanatomie*. Berlin: Springer Lehrbuch.

II PLASTICITY

Introduction

IRA B. BLACK

FIVE YEARS AGO, in the second edition of *The New Cognitive Neurosciences*, we could state with confidence that plasticity, the collective mechanisms underlying brain adaptability, emerges at multiple levels of the neuraxis. Molecular, synaptic, growth factor, and hormonal mechanisms, for example, were complemented by cortical map formation and mutability. In the ensuing half decade, however, a newly recognized source of plasticity has swept through neuroscience—the genesis of new neurons and glia throughout life. This discovery has fundamentally altered our view of brain and mind adaptability. The present section introduces this new level of plasticity in the context of traditional analysis.

To set the classic context, we initially focus on the synapse as the paradigmatic locus of plasticity. Modification of synaptic strength is thought to underlie alterations in cognitive function. Crozier and colleagues elaborate a theory of synaptic plasticity, indicating that only active synapses undergo modification. Synapses are bidirectionally modifiable, resulting in strengthening, long-term potentiation (LTP) or weakening, long-term depression (LTD). The specialized glutamate NMDA receptor acts as a trigger for synaptic strengthening and weakening. Activity that increases postsynaptic responses strengthens the synapse, whereas activity that fails to elicit responses results in depression. The participation of other glutamate receptors, and associated molecular mechanisms, are discussed in detail. Considerations of the central role of synaptic plasticity in cognition must now be viewed against the background of ongoing neurogenesis in the brain.

Van Praag and colleagues describe the remarkable fact of neurogenesis in the mammalian (including human) brain. Neurogenesis occurs in the dentate gyrus of the hippocampus and in the olfactory bulb. The process consists of mitosis, survival, migration, differentiation, and integration into host

107

systems. Neurogenesis arises from stem cells in the brain. These elements self-renew through cell division, and can differentiate into multiple specialized cell types. Notably, the component processes are highly regulated by experience, environmental conditions, genetics, aging, and disease. Consequently, environment and experience can access brain structure, and potentially function at this fundamental level. Indeed, the functions of the newly generated cells in brain plasticity are the subject of intense investigation.

Which neurogenetic mechanisms are potentially subject to plastic regulation? Nowakowski and Hayes describe the dynamics of proliferation in the brain. The productive potential of proliferating populations is proportional to the number of proliferating cells, inversely proportional to cell cycle length, and critically dependent on cell fate decisions, such as reentry into the cell cycle or exit to differentiate. Control of these processes and, consequently, the regulation of plasticity is presently the subject of intense investigation.

Neurogenesis within the brain is now complemented by the emerging concept of adult stem cell plasticity. It is apparent that stem cell populations are widely distributed in the adult, residing in many peripheral organs, including bone marrow, muscle, liver, and skin. Many of these cells are notably plastic, capable of differentiating across traditional lineage boundaries. For example, bone marrow stromal cells, mesodermal derivatives, have been differentiated into presumptive neurons (ectodermal) by means of a simple in vitro procedure, and can populate the brain, expressing neuronal traits. In sum, environmental signals elicit the expression of potentialities that extend well beyond the fate restrictions of cells originating in classic embryonic germ layers. Consequently, intrinsic genomic mechanisms of commitment and

cell fate are apparently mutable. How do systemic sources of neurons and glia affect brain function, if at all? Do neural elements derived from the periphery normally populate the brain? More generally, do peripheral adult stem cells participate in brain plasticity itself?

How does the environment, through systemic factors, integrate and regulate plasticity expressed by the foregoing synaptic and neurogenetic mechanisms? McEwen focuses on the hippocampus, which subserves certain forms of learning and memory. Stress and sex hormones, in conjunction with excitatory transmitters, regulate three types of structural plasticity in the adult hippocampus: synaptogenesis, dendritic reorganization, and neurogenesis in the dentate gyrus. For example, estrogens regulate synapse formation in adult hippocampus of ovariectomized females, but not in castrated males. Chronic stress suppresses neurogenesis and remodeling of dendrites. McEwen describes sex differences in the plastic responses of the brain to stress. This work is beginning to indicate how psychosocial factors alter brain and mind function through the mediation of hormones and transmitters.

As always, periods of discovery and transition are marked by more questions than answers, by controversy as well as unanimity. The chapters in this section attempt to relate the excitement as well as the areas of uncertainty and debate. Hopefully, the reader will appreciate the fertile foment of a dynamic field in transition. Our view of 5 years ago, that plasticity emerges at multiple levels of the neuraxis, has been more than vindicated. In fact, plasticity may be regarded as a systemic process involving environment as well as organism. The psychosocial milieu interacts with experience and behavior to regulate the genes, hormones, and transmitters that govern synaptic and neurogenetic mechanisms.

8 Long-Term Plasticity of Glutamatergic Synaptic Transmission in the Cerebral Cortex

ROBERT A. CROZIER, BENJAMIN D. PHILPOT,
NATHANIEL B. SAWTELL, AND MARK F. BEAR

ABSTRACT   Experience modifies synapses in the brain. It is widely hypothesized that these changes are critically involved in fine-tuning sensory and motor systems, as well as in cognitive processes such as learning and memory. A major goal in neurobiology is to understand the cellular and biochemical mechanisms underlying synaptic modifications and to relate these to systems-level functions of the brain. In this chapter we discuss some of the processes that establish long-term, activity-dependent synaptic modifications in the hippocampus in vitro. Longlasting modifications in synaptic transmission—that is, "plasticity"—can be produced experimentally by the appropriate amounts of presynaptic and postsynaptic activities at many glutamatergic synapses in the central nervous system. The best-characterized forms of activity-dependent synaptic plasticity in the cortex are long-term potentiation (LTP) and long-term depression (LTD). In this chapter we discuss the experimental methodology, induction parameters, and expression mechanisms that result in LTP and LTD in vitro. The chapter ends with a brief discussion of how LTP and LTD might relate to experience-dependent plasticity in vivo.

Background and methodology

The elementary properties of glutamatergic synaptic transmission and plasticity have been most extensively studied in the hippocampus, a structure critically involved in learning and memory (Squire, 1992). The hippocampus has a well-characterized laminar organization that is advantageous for electrophysiological, anatomical, and biochemical studies. Because of this organization, electrophysiologists can stimulate a fairly homogeneous population of axons and record their monosynaptic responses. The most often studied and best-characterized synapse is the Schaffer collateral axons projecting from the cornu ammonis 3 (CA3) cells that connect with the dendrites of CA1 cells (figure 8.1). Further, because the synaptic architecture of the hippocampus is well preserved in vitro, the hippocampal slice preparation (figure 8.1) is ideally suited for studies of synaptic transmission and plasticity. Although several forms of synaptic plasticity exist throughout the brain, available data suggest that the Schaffer collateral–CA1 synapse is a reasonable model for many other cortical synapses. Therefore, synaptic plasticity in CA1 will be our focus.

Fast excitatory synaptic transmission at the Schaffer collateral–CA1 synapse is primarily mediated by glutamate-gated ion channels, which are responsible for the excitatory postsynaptic potential (EPSP). Two subtypes of glutamate receptor considered here are: AMPA and NMDA receptors (figure 8.2). The receptors get their names from their selective pharmacological agonists: α-amino-3-hydroxy-5-methylisoxazole-propionic acid (AMPA), and N-methyl-D-aspartate (NMDA). In the hippocampus, AMPA receptors are responsible for the initial and largest component of the EPSP. The contribution of NMDA receptors to EPSPs is more variable, owing to a block of the channel by magnesium at hyperpolarized membrane potentials. These receptors are strongly activated only when there is coincident presynaptic release of glutamate coupled with a postsynaptic depolarization to remove the magnesium blockade (Mayer, Westbrook, and Guthrie, 1984; Nowak et al., 1984).

A brief note on the experimental methodology commonly used to study LTP may be a useful preface to our discussion. LTP/LTD in the hippocampus is studied both in the intact animal and in brain slice preparations (figure 8.1). Numerous electrophysiological recording techniques are used to measure the changes in synaptic potentials associated with LTP/LTD. The most common is the extracellular field potential, which primarily reflects the excitatory synaptic activity of a population of neurons. Experimentally, the Schaffer collaterals are stimulated and recordings are made in the stratum radiatum (apical dendrites) of CA1 pyramidal cells. The negative-going field potential reflects currents

ROBERT A. CROZIER and MARK F. BEAR   The Picower Center for Learning and Memory, Massachusetts Institute of Technology, Cambridge, Mass.
BENJAMIN D. PHILPOT   Department of Cell and Molecular Physiology, University of North Carolina, Chapel Hill, N.C.
NATHANIEL B. SAWTELL   Neurological Sciences Institute, Oregon Health and Science University, Beaverton, Ore.

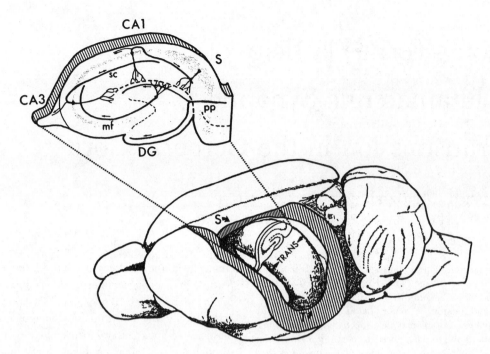

FIGURE 8.1   A drawing of the rodent brain, oriented so that anterior is to the left, demonstrating the location of the hippocampus. The long axis of the hippocampus extends from the septum (S) to the temporal cortex (T). A segment of the hippocampus taken in a transverse axis (TRANS) is shown in detail with a schematic of the trisynaptic loop. Abbreviations: DG, dentate gyrus; CA3, CA1, cornu ammonis fields of the hippocampus; S, subiculum; pp, per- forant path fibers from the entorhinal cortex; mf, mossy fibers from the granule cells; sc, Schaffer collaterals connecting CA3 to CA1. (Reprinted from *Neuroscience*, vol. 31, D. G. Amaral and M. P. Witter, The three-dimensional organization of the hippocampal forma- tion: A review of anatomical data, pp. 571–591, Copyright 1989, with permission from Elsevier.)

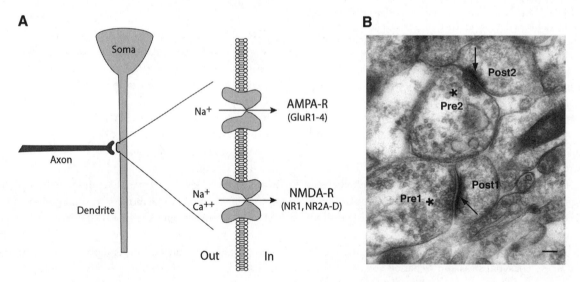

FIGURE 8.2   The glutamatergic synapse. (A) Schematic demon- strating AMPA and NMDA types of glutamate receptor. The AMPA receptor, composed of GluR1-4 subunits, conducts Na$^+$ and K$^+$ ions. The NMDA receptor, composed of the obligatory NR1 subunit and modulatory NR2A-D subunits, can conduct Ca^{++} ions along with Na$^+$ and K$^+$. In addition to glutamate binding, activa- tion of NMDA receptors requires removal of a magnesium ionophore block by depolarization and binding of the co-agonist glycine (not pictured). (B) Electron micrograph demonstrating presynaptic (Pre) terminals containing round vesicles and corre- sponding postsynaptic elements on dendritic spines. Asterisks denote synaptic vesicles and arrows indicate postsynaptic densities. (Electron micrograph courtesy of Dr. Michelle A. Adams.)

flowing from extracellular to intracellular compartments during synaptic activation. LTP/LTD can also be observed with intracellular recordings in which EPSPs are measured from a single postsynaptic neuron (e.g., a CA1 pyramidal cell). Whole-cell voltage-clamp recordings are now common and allow one to resolve excitatory postsynaptic currents (EPSCs) elicited by the release of neurotransmitter.

Using these electrophysiological methods, three major protocols have been developed for inducing LTP or LTD: (1) tetanic (repetitive) stimulation at various frequencies, (2) pairing presynaptic stimulation while holding postsynaptic voltage constant at different values, and (3) pairing presynaptic stimulation with electrically evoked postsynaptic spikes of varying delays. LTP and LTD induced by these methods are likely to use overlapping if not identical mechanisms, because all depend on activation of NMDA receptors for induction (Shouval, Bear, and Cooper, 2002).

In frequency-dependent plasticity (figure 8.3), changes in synaptic strength are induced by varying the rate of presynaptic stimulation of a population of axons (Dudek and Bear, 1992; Kirkwood et al., 1993). LTD, for example, is typically induced by low-frequency stimulation (LFS, e.g., 900 pulses at 1 Hz). In contrast, the induction of LTP is usually achieved with high-frequency stimulation (HFS). Theta-burst stimulation (10–15 trains delivered at 5 Hz, each train consisting of four pulses delivered at 100 Hz) is commonly used to induce LTP; this stimulation pattern mimics endogenous theta rhythms in the hippocampus that occur during some forms of learning and exploratory behavior (Larson, Wong, and Lynch, 1986). The intensity (which determines the number of axons recruited) and the temporal patterns of HFS can be crucial in activating NMDA receptors sufficiently to produce the calcium transients necessary for LTP and/or LTD.

The pairing protocol consists of providing presynaptic stimulation coincident with steady depolarization of the postsynaptic cell (Kelso, Ganong, and Brown, 1986). During baseline recording, test stimuli are delivered at a low frequency (e.g., 0.05 Hz) and the membrane potential of the postsynaptic cell is clamped near −70 mV—a potential that is predominantly AMPA receptor mediated. During pairing, the stimulation rate is increased to 1 Hz, and if the postsynaptic cell is depolarized to approximately 0 mV, then LTP is induced. Conversely, when the postsynaptic cell is held at approximately −40 mV, LTD is induced (Selig et al., 1995). Notably, pairing-induced plasticity demonstrates the importance of the magnitude of postsynaptic depolarization in directing the valence of plasticity.

More recently, spike timing–dependent plasticity (STDP) has been demonstrated by pairing evoked EPSPs with precisely timed postsynaptic, back-propagating action potentials (Magee and Johnston, 1997; Markram et al., 1997; Zhang et al., 1998; Feldman, 2000; Froemke and Dan, 2002; Nelson, Sjostrom, and Turrigiano, 2002). If the EPSP con-sistently precedes the spike within a 50-ms window, then LTP is induced, whereas LTD is induced if the EPSP closely follows the action potential. STDP has been observed in both the hippocampus (Magee and Johnston, 1997; Bi and Poo, 1998; Debanne, Gahwiler, and Thompson, 1998) and neocortex (Markram et al., 1997; Egger, Feldmeyer, and Sackmann, 1999; Feldman, 2000; Froemke and Dan, 2002). Of the methods for LTP/LTD induction, STDP might most closely mimic naturally occurring synaptic events. However, other methods of LTP/LTD induction are typically used for mechanistic studies because of their high reliability and reproducibility. The methods used to study LTP/LTD therefore depend on the questions being addressed.

Long-term potentiation in the CA1 region of hippocampus

LTP can be induced in many brain regions, including the hippocampus and neocortex, and the increase in synaptic strength can persist for hours and perhaps even for a lifetime (figure 8.3) (Abraham et al., 2002; for review, see Bliss and Collingridge, 1993). The mechanisms by which HFS produces a longlasting potentiation of synaptic transmission vary from one brain location to another. For the purposes of this chapter we will focus primarily on the LTP that requires activation of postsynaptic NMDA receptors, but the reader should be aware that non-NMDAR forms of LTP exist (Grover and Teyler, 1990).

Research has largely focused on three questions. First, how are LTP/LTD induced? Repeated synaptic activation sets in motion a series of biochemical reactions that ultimately trigger the expression of synaptic potentiation or depression. Second, how are LTP/LTD expressed? Enhancement or depression of synaptic transmission in principle can result from several types of modifications on both sides of the synapse. Third, how are LTP/LTD maintained? In vivo, LTP/LTD can last for many weeks and possibly a lifetime, and somehow this selective synaptic change is maintained in the face of molecular turnover. Our discussion is primarily concerned with the first two questions, as less is known about the long-term maintenance of synaptic plasticity.

LTP INDUCTION   One of the key properties of LTP is input specificity, which means that synaptic pathways that receive conditioning stimulation (e.g., HFS) show the plasticity, while there are no changes in the synaptic weights of other non-conditioned pathways synapsing onto the same postsynaptic neurons. Another key property is associativity, which means that a weak input that would normally be incapable of producing LTP can strengthen if conditioning stimulation is provided to the weak input concurrently with a stronger set of inputs. As such, the weak input is "associated" with the stronger inputs during conditioning stimulation.

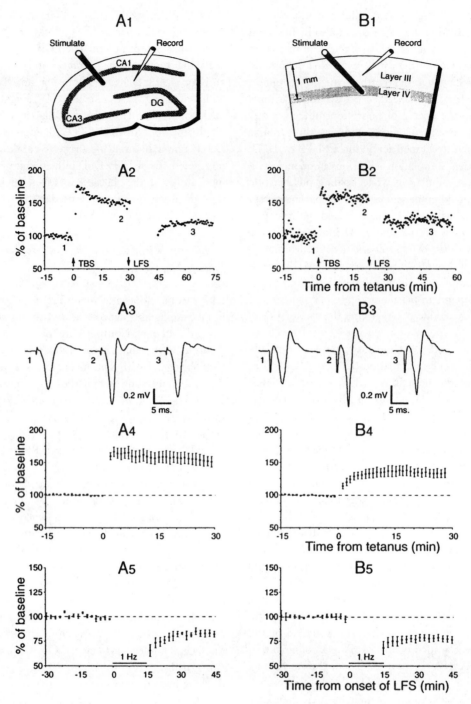

FIGURE 8.3 Bidirectional synaptic plasticity is a common feature throughout the brain. Shown here are in vitro models of plasticity in the rat hippocampus (A) and visual cortex (B). Row 1 schematizes the stimulation and recording configurations. Row 2 demonstrates a plot over time of the change in normalized field EPSP magnitude induced by theta-burst stimulation (TBS; three trains of 10 bursts delivered at 200-ms intervals, with each burst consisting of four pulses at 100 Hz) and by low-frequency stimulation (LFS) consisting of 900 pulses delivered at 1 Hz (A_2) or 3 Hz (B_2). Row 3 shows averages of four consecutive field potentials taken from the experiment shown in row 2. Row 4 demonstrates the average change in field EPSP magnitude after TBS, and row 5 depicts the average response magnitude after LFS. Abbreviations: DG, dentate gyrus; CA1, CA3, fields of the hippocampus. (Modified with permission from A. Kirkwood et al., Common forms of synaptic plasticity in the hippocampus and neocortex in vitro. *Science* 260:1518–1521. © 1993, American Association for the Advancement of Science.)

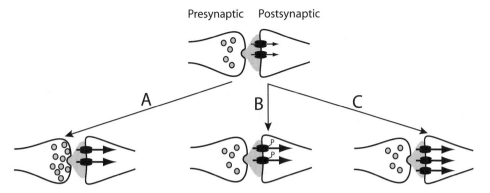

Presynaptic   Postsynaptic

FIGURE 8.4 Model of non-mutually exclusive mechanisms for LTP expression. Calcium entry through NMDA receptors triggers LTP that might be expressed presynaptically (A) and/or postsynaptically (B, C). (A) LTP expressed as an increase in the presynaptic release of neurotransmitter. One possibility is that a retrograde messenger increases the probability of neurotransmitter release by increasing the size of the readily releasable pool of neurotransmitter vesicles. Thus, enhanced transmitter release over time can be reflected as a larger postsynaptic depolarization (depicted as larger arrows; compare with top row). (B) The phosphorylation of AMPA receptors can increase synaptic strength by enhancing channel open probability and/or single channel conductance. (C) Synaptic efficacy can be enhanced by an increase in the number of functional postsynaptic AMPA receptors.

The initial steps in LTP induction are well characterized (for review, see Bear and Malenka, 1994) and depend on a transient but large increase in intracellular calcium through NMDA receptors. Sufficient activation of NMDA receptors occurs either by summation of EPSCs or by direct depolarization with an intracellular recording electrode. With the displacement of Mg^{2+} from the channel by depolarization, calcium entry is then permitted into the postsynaptic dendritic spine. The rise in the concentration of intracellular calcium is thought to be a necessary and perhaps sufficient trigger for LTP (Malenka, Kauer, Perkel, and Nicoll, 1989; Malenka, 1991; Yang, Tang, and Zucker, 1999). The evidence in support of these statements has been extensively reviewed (Madison, Malenko, and Nicoll, 1991; Siegelbaum and Kandell, 1991; Bliss and Collingridge, 1993; Malenka and Nicoll, 1999) and includes the following findings: first, specific NMDA receptor antagonists block the induction of LTP; second, LTP can be elicited by temporally pairing low-frequency afferent stimulation with postsynaptic depolarization; third, LTP is prevented by loading CA1 cells with calcium chelators, which presumably buffer any rise in intracellular calcium concentration; and finally, directly increasing calcium in CA1 cells causes a synaptic enhancement.

How does a large increase in intracellular calcium translate into an enhancement of synaptic strength? There is good evidence that this event activates certain protein kinases, including calcium/calmodulin-dependent protein kinase II (CaMKII) and protein kinase C (PKC) (for review, see Kelly, 1991; Muller et al., 1991; Lisman, 1994). These kinases phosphorylate specific substrate proteins, which ultimately manifests as enhanced synaptic efficacy, but precisely how and where synaptic effectiveness is increased remains controversial. These issues will be discussed next.

LTP EXPRESSION   Although a general consensus exists regarding the induction mechanisms of LTP (i.e., a large, transient elevation of postsynaptic calcium), multiple mechanisms of LTP expression have been observed. Generally, there are several ways in which a synapse could be made stronger (figure 8.4): (1) an increased probability of presynaptic glutamate release or an increased number of release sites; (2) enhanced postsynaptic responsiveness due to an increase in the functional properties; (3) a change in the number of postsynaptic glutamate receptors or a change in their localization; and (4) extrasynaptic changes, such as a decrease in glutamate clearance in the synaptic cleft. The pursuit of answers to the question of how LTP is expressed has led to a much deeper understanding of synaptic function in the brain. Instead of providing an exhaustive review of the literature on the topic, we will summarize evidence supporting a presynaptic change, followed by evidence supporting a postsynaptic change.

(a) *Presynaptic reliability hypothesis.* Since neurotransmitter release is probabilistic, a straightforward way to enhance synaptic efficacy is to increase the likelihood that neurotransmitter will be released. One method for assessing changes in presynaptic release probability is to measure paired-pulse facilitation (PPF) before and after inducing LTP. PPF occurs in CA1 because, on average, synapses have a low resting release probability (i.e., an action potential frequently fails to induce transmitter release) that increases when two pulses are given in rapid succession. As resting release probability is increased, PPF is decreased (Manabe and Nicoll, 1994). Thus, if LTP were manifest as an increase in release probability, then an accompanying decrease in PPF would be expected. It is important to add, however, that a change in PPF need not only reflect a change in release probability because postsynaptic variables also contribute to PPF (Wang and Kelly, 1997).

The data examining changes in PPF as a consequence of LTP are contradictory. Most groups find that LTP produces no change in PPF, but some do (Malinow, Schulman, and Tsien, 1989; Malinow and Tsien, 1990). There appears to be a relationship between the initial amount of PPF and the change after LTP. If PPF is very pronounced under baseline conditions (reflecting a low glutamate release probability), then it is likely that LTP will be associated with a decrease in PPF. However, if PPF is modest under baseline conditions, then there is generally no change in PPF despite induction of LTP (Schulz, Cook, and Johnston, 1994, 1995; Sokolov et al., 1998). Some of these data may be reconciled by evidence of insertion of a subsynaptic, latent pool of AMPA receptors into the synaptic membrane, which is discussed later in the chapter in the section on AMPA receptor trafficking.

Further evidence for an enhancement in presynaptic release comes from "minimal stimulation" experiments (Stevens and Wang, 1994). By adjusting stimulation intensity to a minimal level such that a stimulus often fails to evoke a postsynaptic current, two components of synaptic strength can be separately assessed: (1) reliability, or the fraction of stimuli that produce a postsynaptic response, and (2) potency, which is the average amplitude of a postsynaptic response when release does occur. Stevens and Wang (1994) report a decrease in the rate of failures (i.e., increased reliability) and no change in potency following induction of LTP in the hippocampus. Thus, these results support a presynaptic locus of LTP expression.

In contrast to these findings, other investigators do report changes in potency following LTP induction (Oliet, Malenka, and Nicoll, 1996). Oliet, Maleuka, and Nicoll (1996) found an increase in the amplitude and a small but significant increase in the frequency of quantal events following LTP induction. An increase in quantal amplitude likely reflects a postsynaptic modification, namely a change in the number or properties of AMPA receptors. Traditionally, affecting the frequency of quantal events is interpreted as a presynaptic modification resulting from an increase in the probability of neurotransmitter release or an increase in the number of release sites. However, as we will address in our discussion of AMPA receptor trafficking, failures of synaptic transmission and changes in the frequency of quantal events may also result from a postsynaptic change in the number of functional receptors.

(b) *The phosphorylation hypothesis.* Phosphorylation of postsynaptic proteins plays an essential role in the induction of LTP in the hippocampus (Browning, Huganir, and Greengard, 1985). In addition to CaMKII (Kelly, 1991; Lisman, 1994), several other major second messenger–dependent kinases have been implicated in LTP. They are the calcium/phospholipid-dependent protein kinase C (PKC) (Muller et al., 1991), cAMP-dependent protein kinase (PKA) (Schulman, 1995), the family of tyrosine kinases (O'Dell, Kandel, and Grant, 1991; Grant et al., 1992; Yu et al., 1997), and mitogen-activated protein (MAP) kinase (Kornhauser and Greenberg, 1997; Zhu et al., 2002). Many of these enzymes are spatially restricted within the synapse to an area just below the postsynaptic membrane known as the postsynaptic density (PSD). The PSD is a protein-rich region that contains enzymes, scaffolding molecules, and receptors. Thus, by containing enzyme localization it is possible to restrict the activity of these enzymes to specific substrates.

Influx of calcium through NMDA receptors can activate one or more of these kinases, which in turn phosphorylates target proteins. The most direct scheme for the induction and expression of plasticity is for these kinases to directly phosphorylate AMPA and/or NMDA receptors. These ligand-gated ion channels contain large, C-terminal intracellular tails with many consensus sites for phosphorylation. The effects of phosphorylation on these channels include regulation of receptor desensitization rate, channel open probability, channel conductance properties, regulation of subunit assembly, and regulation of receptor aggregation or insertion at the synapse. All of these levels of regulation could play important roles in modifying synaptic efficacy.

Several properties of CaMKII make it an especially attractive candidate as a molecular mechanism for LTP (for reviews, see Kelly, 1991; Schulman, 1993). (1) CaMKII is a prominent constituent of the PSD, comprising approximately 2.7% of total PSD protein (Kennedy, 1997). (2) Each CaMKII holoenzyme contains 10–12 catalytic subunits, each of which has 3–4 phosphorylation sites, thus providing the holoenzyme with multiple points of regulation. (3) CaMKII has an unusual property: in the presence of sufficient levels of calcium and calmodulin, CaMKII catalytic subunits may become autophosphorylated. Once autophosphorylated, the enzyme's affinity for calmodulin increases dramatically (a process known as calmodulin trapping). (4) CaMKII subunits activated by autophosphorylation exhibit some degree of constitutive, calcium-independent activity (Schulman, 1993). Thus, CaMKII activity can outlive the original signal inducing its activation. Together, these observations suggest that CaMKII is well situated to detect calcium influx through NMDA receptors, and to induce and maintain LTP.

There is a large body of evidence implicating CaMKII in LTP at hippocampal CA1 synapses. On a molecular level, the amount of phosphorylated CaMKII protein at the synapse increases after the induction of LTP (Fukunaga et al., 1993; Fukunaga, Muller, and Miyamoto, 1995; Ouyang et al., 1997), and in situ hybridization studies demonstrate an increase in CaMKII mRNA in cell bodies and dendrites of hippocampal neurons following LTP induction (Thomas et al., 1994; Roberts et al., 1996). Pharmacological inhibition of endogenous CaMKII prevents the induction of LTP (Malenka, Kauer, Perkel, Mauk, et al., 1989; Malinow, Schulman, and Tsien, 1989; Ito, Hidaka, and Sugiyama, 1991; Yasuda et al., 2003), and transgenic mice lacking the α isoform of CaMKII exhibit deficits in LTP and in spatial learning (Silva, Paylor, et al., 1992; Silva, Stevens, et al., 1992). Conversely, manipulations that enhance CaMKII activity cause synaptic strengthening. For example, introduction of constitutively active CaMKII into hippocampal neurons either acutely through the recording pipette (Lledo et al., 1995) or by transfection (Petit, Perlman, and Malinow, 1994) results in an increase in basal synaptic transmission that occludes tetanus-induced LTP, and drives GluR1 receptors into synapses (Hayashi et al., 2000; Shi et al., 2001; Poncer, Esteban, and Malinow, 2002; Esteban et al., 2003).

Recently, researchers identified a CaMKII phosphorylation site on the GluR1 subunit of AMPA receptors that is likely modified during LTP. Phosphorylation of serine residue 831 (Ser831) on GluR1 increases the single-channel conductance of AMPA receptors (Barria et al., 1997; Mammen et al., 1997; Derkach, Barria, and Soderling, 1999), which can also occur after LTP induction (Benke et al., 1998; Lee et al., 2000). Finally, recent data suggest that LTP is impaired in adult mice that were genetically modified to lack normal Ser831 phosphorylation (Lee et al., 2003). Therefore, CaMKII phosphorylation of Ser831 might provide a molecular mechanism for the enhanced AMPA receptor function associated with LTP (figure 8.5). Additionally but not mutually exclusively, CaMKII activity may regulate the trafficking of a latent pool of AMPA receptors into the synaptic membrane as a mechanism for LTP expression and maintenance (discussed below).

(c) *AMPA receptor trafficking.* Phosphorylation can affect the signaling properties of receptors already present in the synaptic membrane, but recent data demonstrate that dendrites also contain a latent population of subsynaptic receptors that are poised for membrane insertion. The regulation of AMPA receptor insertion (and removal) is controlled by a number of factors, including phosphorylation, activity levels, and endo- and exocytosis. AMPA receptor trafficking can have effects on both LTP and LTD.

Evidence that AMPA receptors may be actively inserted into the postsynaptic membrane originated from studies of so-called silent synapses (figure 8.6). The silent synapse hypothesis postulates that a subset of synapses contains NMDA receptors but few or no functional AMPA receptors. Such synapses are "silent" at resting membrane potential because NMDA receptors pass little current at rest. LTP induction causes the conversion of synapses from silent to functional. The most likely mechanism for this is "AMPAfication," which is the insertion of latent clusters of AMPA receptors into the postsynaptic membrane (Kullmann, 1994; Isaac, Nicoll, and Malenka, 1995; Liao, Hessler, and Malinow, 1995; Durand, Kovalchuk, and Konnerth, 1996).

The silent synapse hypothesis is elegant in its simplicity and has gained repute. Similar observations have been made in neocortex and culture, and evidence from developmental studies confirms the presence of NMDA receptor-only synapses in immature animals and subsequent AMPAfication of these synapses with maturation (Isaac et al., 1997; Gomperts et al., 1998; Rumpel, Hatt, and Gottmann, 1998; Liao et al., 1999; Petralia et al., 1999). As discussed in the next section, the unsilencing of synapses segues into the

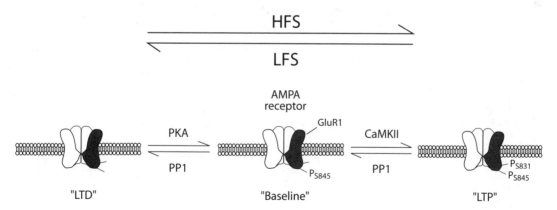

FIGURE 8.5   Model depicting changes in the phosphorylation state of the GluR1 AMPA receptor subunit during bidirectional, NMDA receptor–dependent plasticity. High-frequency stimulation (HFS) activates CaMKII to increase phosphorylation on Ser831 (CaMKII site; P$_{S831}$) from the basal state. Low-frequency stimulation (LFS) activates protein phosphates, such as PP1, which dephosphorylates Ser845 (PKA site; P$_{S845}$). "Dedepression" of a previously depressed synapse can activate PKA to phosphorylate Ser845.

"Depotentiation" of previously potentiated synapses can activate phosphatases such as PP1 to dephosphorylate Ser831. The phosphorylation state of the AMPA receptor can alter single-channel properties and/or AMPA receptor trafficking (see text). (Modified with permission from H. K. Lee et al., Regulation of distinct AMPA receptor phosphorylation sites during bidirectional synaptic plasticity. *Nature* 405:955–959. © 2000 *Nature* [*Nature* Publishing Group].)

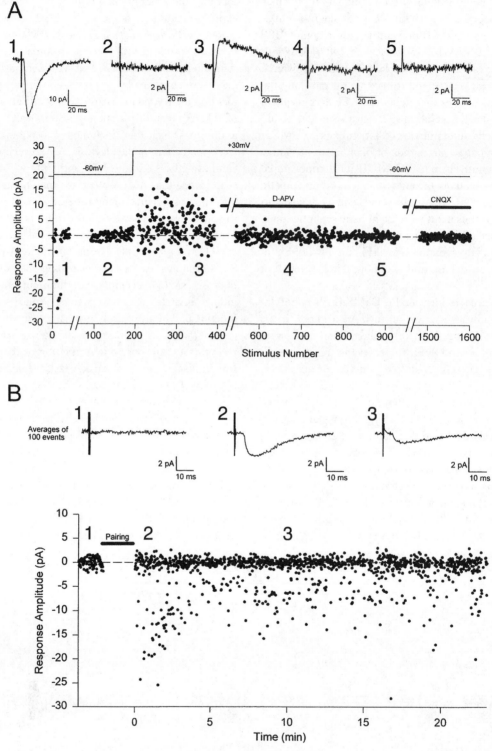

FIGURE 8.6 Silent synapses in the hippocampus. (A) Example experiment demonstrating that at high stimulation intensities AMPA receptor–mediated currents can be observed at a voltage-clamped holding potential of −60 mV (1), while minimal stimulation can be applied such that no AMPA currents are observed (2). NMDA receptor–mediated currents can be observed with the same minimal stimulation intensity if the cell is clamped at +30 mV to remove the magnesium block of the NMDA receptor (3; note that currents are outward at this holding potential). The NMDA receptor antagonist blocks NMDA currents observed at +30 mV (4). At −60 mV, no currents are observed (5), and the absence of AMPA-mediated currents was confirmed by the absence of an effect of the AMPA receptor antagonist CNQX. Waveforms represent averages taken at the indicated times. (B) Example experiment demonstrating that silent synapses can exhibit LTP. At −60 mV, no AMPA-mediated currents are observed with minimal stimulation. After a pairing protocol in which afferent stimulation is paired with depolarization of the cell to −10 mV, AMPA receptor EPSCs are now clearly observed. Waveforms represent averages taken at the indicated times. (Modified with permission from J. T. R. Isaac et al., Evidence for silent synapses: Implications for the expression of LTP and LTD. *Neuron* 15:427–434. © *Neuron*, 1995.)

broader theme of the subunit-specific regulation of AMPA receptor trafficking.

EXPRESSION AND MAINTENANCE OF LTP THROUGH AMPA RECEPTOR TRAFFICKING First proposed by Lynch and Baudry (1984), the trafficking of glutamate receptors provides an elegant means of producing stable, long-term biochemical changes in synaptic efficacy by including (or excluding) more receptors in the synaptic membrane.

AMPA receptors are heteromers comprised of subunits that can be broadly distinguished based on the length of their cytoplasmic C-tails. Long-tail subunits are GluR1, GluR4, and GluR2L (a splice variant of GluR2). Short-tail subunits are GluR2, GluR3, and GluR4c (a splice variant of GluR4). The emerging picture is that long-tail subunits impart the property of activity-dependent receptor delivery (for detailed review, see Malinow and Malenka, 2002; Song and Huganir, 2002). In contrast, AMPARs containing short-tail subunits are constituitively recycled (figure 8.7).

GluR1 receptors, like GluR4 receptors, are driven into synapses by activity; however, the mechanisms for insertion differ. Experiments performed on organotypic hippocampal slice cultures infected with GluR1-GFP were observed optically to contain diffuse GFP expression in dendrites, with little fluorescence in spines; however, following LTP induction, spines were subsequently filled with GFP (Shi et al., 1999). This·observation suggests that LTP delivers GluR1 to spines. Though intriguing, that report did not demonstrate that GluR1 was actually inserted into synapses. This issue was subsequently answered electrophysiologically. Overexpressed GluR1 homomeric AMPARs can be distinguished from native receptors by their unique biophysical property. Studies exploiting this property demonstrated that GluR1-containing AMPA receptors are incorporated into the synapse in response to LTP-inducing stimuli, and that this process requires NMDA receptor and CaMKII activation (Hayashi et al., 2000). Biochemical studies also confirm that native GluR1 is delivered to synapses after LTP induction in vivo (Heynen et al., 2000). Interestingly, while GluR1 delivery requires strong tetanization that leads to LTP, spontaneous activity is sufficient for GluR4 delivery (Zhu et al., 2000; Esteban et al., 2003). This delivery is still NMDA receptor dependent, but it depends on activation of PKA rather than CaMKII, and was proposed to predominate early in development, when circuits are first being established (Zhu and Malinow, 2002).

Long-term depression in the CA1 region of hippocampus

If synapses only had the ability to strengthen, neural networks would lose malleability because all synapses would eventually strengthen to a point of saturation. In order for network properties to remain dynamic and still efficiently store information, synapses must have the ability to be finely tuned in a bidirectional manner. Thus, it is satisfying that the functional inverse of LTP, known as LTD, appears to be a common feature throughout the brain (reviewed in Bear and Malenka, 1994; Malinow and Malenka, 2002; Song and Huganir, 2002). LTD, a lasting decrease in synaptic weight, can be induced by patterned electrical stimulation (Dudek and Bear, 1992; Mulkey and Malenka, 1992; Christie, Kerr, and Abraham, 1994; Linden and Connor, 1995; Bear and Abraham, 1996). Classically, LTD is divided into two types: homosynaptic and heterosynaptic. Homosynaptic LTD is input-specific; that is, only those afferents that receive conditioning stimulation concurrent with weak postsynaptic depolarization are depressed. Heterosynaptic LTD is not input-specific but rather describes a generalized decrease in the synaptic efficacy of a group of afferents possibly resulting from an overall attenuation in postsynaptic excitability. The typically observed forms of LTD require elevation of intracellular free calcium, although the source of calcium entry may vary; calcium usually enters via voltage-dependent calcium channels for heterosynaptic LTD and through NMDA receptors for homosynaptic LTD. Heterosynaptic LTD is prominent in the dentate gyrus of the hippocampus in vivo, though it may occur in other brain regions under certain experimental conditions (Levy and Steward, 1979; Abraham and Goddard, 1983; Abraham and Wickens, 1991). Homosynaptic LTD has been observed throughout the mammalian brain, both in vitro and in vivo (Bear and Malenka, 1994). Because homosynaptic LTD is most thoroughly characterized in the CA1 region of the hippocampus, CA1 LTD will be the focus of our discussion.

The standard method for inducing homosynaptic LTD in the CA1 region is to apply low-frequency stimulation (LFS) to the Schaffer collaterals (e.g., 900 pulses delivered at 1 Hz; see figure 8.3). The main properties of homosynaptic LTD are as follows (for review, see Bear and Abraham, 1996): (1) LTD is input-specific—only synapses undergoing the conditioning stimulation become depressed, while convergent but inactive afferents are unaffected. (2) LFS-induced LTD is frequency dependent. Stimulation in the range of 0.5–3 Hz is generally sufficient to induce LTD, whereas delivering the same number of pulses at a higher frequency may result in no change or in LTP. (3) Under most experimental conditions, LTD is blocked by NMDA receptor antagonists. (4) LTD may be developmentally regulated. In most areas of the brain, the magnitude of LTD diminishes with age. (5) LTD is saturable and reversible. Repeated episodes of LFS result in a depression that saturates. LTD can be reversed by high-frequency stimulation, showing that the depression is not the result of cell damage or death.

LTD INDUCTION Remarkably, the induction of LTD has many of the same requirements as the induction of LTP.

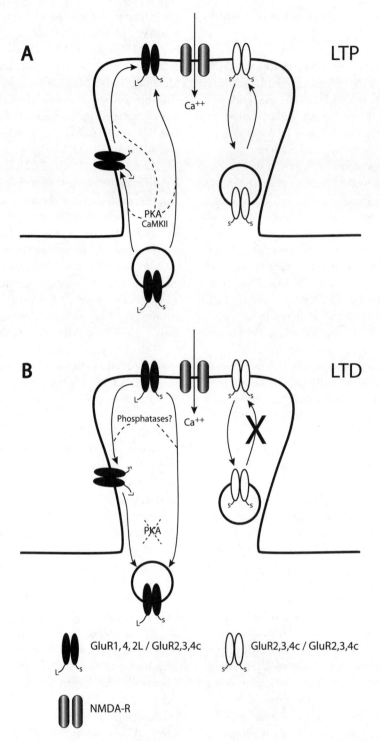

A   LTP

Ca++

PKA
CaMKII

L   S

B   LTD

Phosphatases?   Ca++

X

PKA

L   S

GluR1, 4, 2L / GluR2,3,4c   GluR2,3,4c / GluR2,3,4c

NMDA-R

FIGURE 8.7 Putative mechanisms of AMPA receptor trafficking. (A) During the induction of LTP, protein kinases such as PKA and CaMKII are likely involved in the molecular cascade that promotes the insertion and/or translocation of AMPA receptors toward synaptic sites. Notably, AMPA receptors containing a subunit with a long cytoplasmic tail (i.e., GluR1, GluR4, and GluR2L) are actively inserted into the synapses, whereas AMPA receptors comprised solely of subunits with short cytoplasmic domains (i.e., GluR2 and GluR3) are involved in constitutive replacement of receptors. (B) During the induction of LTD, protein phosphatases might trigger the active internalization and/or translocation of AMPA receptors away from synaptic sites. In addition, PKA activity may be disrupted (denoted by the dotted X), and consequently AMPA receptors may be internalized. LTD might also be expressed by preventing the constitutive replacement of AMPA receptors (denoted by large X). (Modified with permission from R. Malinow and R. C. Malenka, AMPA receptor trafficking and synaptic plasticity. *Annual Review of Neuroscience* 25:103–126. © 2002 by *Annual Reviews*, www.annualreviews.org.)

As with LTP, both in vitro (Dudek and Bear, 1992) and in vivo (Heynen, Abraham, and Bear, 1996) experiments demonstrate that NMDA receptor activation is required for the induction of most forms of LTD. Moreover, the influx of calcium through NMDA receptors is the critical component for the induction of LTD (Mulkey and Malenka, 1992). Postsynaptic injections of calcium chelators such as BAPTA block the induction of LTD, while the photolysis of caged calcium in the postsynaptic cell can induce LTD in the absence of presynaptic activity (Neveu and Zucker, 1996).

Although it may seem paradoxical that increases in intracellular free calcium can lead to both LTD and LTP, this observation can be reconciled by two primary observations. First, the time course and the magnitude of calcium elevations can differ dramatically during the induction of LTP and LTD. For example, the induction of LTD can occur with modest ($\sim 0.7 \mu M$) but enduring ($\sim 60 s$) calcium elevations, while LTP can occur with high ($\sim 10 \mu M$) but brief ($\sim 3 s$) elevations in intracellular calcium (Yang, Tang, and Zucker, 1999). Second, calcium-sensitive enzymes at the synapse vary greatly in their affinity for calcium. For example, the protein phosphatase calcineurin has a much greater calcium affinity than the protein kinase CaMKII (figure 8.8). Thus the kinetics and magnitude of the calcium signal can initiate markedly different biochemical cascades. John Lisman (1989) incorporated these two observations into a model suggesting that LTD is a consequence of protein phosphatases that are activated with low concentrations of calcium, while LTP is a consequence of a relative shift toward protein kinase activity that occurs at higher calcium levels. There is now cumulative experimental support for the basic tenets of the Lisman model. Data suggest that the moderate rise in intracellular calcium associated with LTD activates the calcium-dependent phosphatase calcineurin (also known as PP2B). Calcineurin, in turn, dephosphorylates inhibitor 1, thus activating protein phosphatase 1 (PP1). Considerable evidence demonstrates that this phosphatase cascade is required for the induction of LTD (Bear and Abraham, 1996; Morishita et al., 2001).

Although we focused our attention on NMDA receptor–dependent forms of LTD, it is important to acknowledge other forms of synaptic depression. For example, changing either the extracellular milieu or the pattern of conditioning stimulation has revealed a distinct form of LTD that relies on activation of metabotropic glutamate receptors (Kemp and Bashir, 1997, 1999; Oliet et al., 1997; Huber, Kayser, and Bear, 2000; Huber, Roder, and Bear, 2001).

LTD EXPRESSION AND MAINTENANCE   As for LTP, several non-mutually exclusive possibilities exist for the expression of LTD. LTD can occur through (1) a presynaptic reduction in neurotransmitter release, (2) a postsynaptic attenuation of receptor channel conductances, and/or (3) a postsynaptic loss in the number of synaptically expressed receptors. We will briefly discuss these possibilities.

Controversy exists as to whether there is a presynaptic locus of LTD. Some studies have used quantal analysis to demonstrate that LTD is a consequence of reduced presynaptic neurotransmitter release (Bolshakov and Siegelbaum, 1994; Stevens and Wang, 1994). These studies suggested that the induction of LTD results in decreased reliability of synaptic transmission without affecting potency. However, Oliet, Malenka, and Nicoll (1996) found that LTD is associated with a decrease in miniature EPSC amplitude, as would be expected from a postsynaptic locus for LTD. As mentioned earlier, the interpretation of quantal analysis is clouded by observations that synaptic reliability is subject to AMPA receptor number as well as changes in presynaptic release. Newer techniques, nevertheless, continue to support the possibility that LTD may be, at least in part, a consequence of reduced presynaptic release. For example, a chemically induced form of LTD suppresses evoked release of the presynaptic fluorescent indicator dye FM1-43, suggesting that LTD attenuates neurotransmitter release (Stanton, Heinemann, and Muller, 2001).

While a presynaptic locus for LTD remains a contentious point, there is now a general consensus that NMDA receptor–dependent LTD modifies postsynaptic AMPA receptor responses. NMDA receptor–dependent LTD induced chemically by the application of NMDA or synaptically by LFS causes a persistent dephosphorylation of GluR1 in CA1 of the hippocampus (see figure 8.5; Kameyama et al., 1998; Lee et al., 1998, 2000). The dephosphorylation is specific to Ser845, a site phosphorylated by PKA (Kameyama et al., 1998; Lee et al., 2000). These authors also demonstrated that inhibitors of postsynaptic PKA cause a synaptic depression that occludes LTD, and that chemically and synaptically induced LTD are inhibited by activators of PKA. Furthermore, peptides that disrupt PKA localization at the synapse cause a rundown in synaptic transmission that occludes LTD (Robert A. Crozier and Mark F. Bear, unpublished observations). Finally, mice with mutations of both the PKA and CaMKII phosphorylation sites on GluR1 fail to express NMDA receptor–dependent LTD (Lee et al., 2003). Together, there is strong evidence that postsynaptic dephosphorylation of the AMPA receptor may underlie the expression of NMDA receptor–dependent homosynaptic LTD.

What are the consequences of AMPA receptor dephosphorylation at the PKA site? One direct effect of dephosphorylation of Ser845 on GluR1 is a reduction in peak open probability of AMPA receptor channels, thus impairing AMPA currents (Banke et al., 2000). Additionally, recent data suggest that Ser845 dephosphorylation of GluR1 promotes AMPA receptor internalization, reducing the number

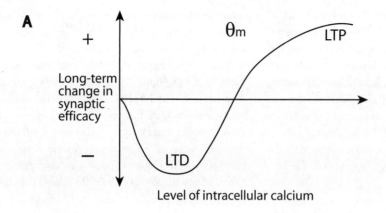

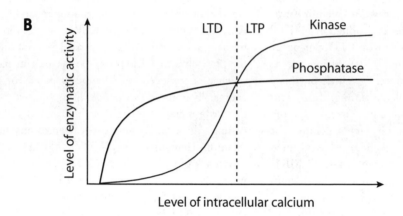

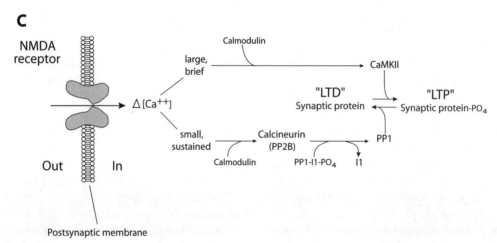

FIGURE 8.8 Model of the induction mechanisms involved in homosynaptic long-term potentiation (LTP) and long-term depression (LTD). (A) The BCM theory (Bienenstock et al., 1982) accounts for bidirectional plasticity. The theory states that the amount of postsynaptic depolarization and thus calcium influx via NMDA receptors determines the valence of the plasticity. Lower levels of calcium influx result in LTD, while LTP results from greater amounts of calcium influx. The crossover point, or modification threshold, between LTD and LTP is termed θ_m. (B) Phosphatases involved in LTD induction might have a relatively greater affinity for activation by calcium, whereas kinases are activated at higher concentrations of calcium. As such, LTD can be induced by phosphatase activity at low concentrations of calcium; the balance shifts

to relatively greater kinase activity, and thus LTP, at high concentrations of calcium. (Modified with permission from J. E. Lisman, A mechanism for the Hebb and the anti-Hebb processes underlying learning and memory. *Proc. Natl. Acad. Sci. U.S.A.* 86:9574–9578. © 1985 by John Lisman.) (C) A model demonstrating the cascade of events involved with synaptic plasticity induced by calcium entry through the NMDA receptor. High, transient increases of calcium bind to calmodulin to activate calcium/calmodulin-dependent kinase II (CaMKII) to induce LTP. Low, sustained increases in calcium activate the phosphatase calcineurin (a.k.a. PP2B), which in turn dephosphorylates inhibitor 1 (I1) to activate protein phosphatase 1 (PP1). The phosphatase activity of PP1 induces LTD.

of functional AMPA receptors at the synapse (see figure 8.7). The following evidence supports the possibility that Ser845 dephosphorylation leads to AMPA receptor internalization: (1) LTD induces AMPA receptor internalization both in vitro (Carroll et al., 1999; Beattie et al., 2000; Man et al., 2000) and in vivo (Heynen et al., 2000); (2) internalized receptors are dephosphorylated at Ser845 (Ehlers, 2000); and (3) AMPA receptor internalization is blocked in a mutant mouse deficient in normal Ser845 phosphorylation/dephosphorylation (Lee et al., 2003).

Although the mechanisms underlying the induction and expression of LTD are relatively well characterized, less is known about the requirements for long-term maintenance (i.e., many hours to days) of LTD. Notably, a form of LTD has been described in the cerebellum that requires protein synthesis for long-term maintenance (Linden, 1996). To date, there is no information on the biochemical requirements for LTD maintenance in the cerebral cortex. LTD in vivo appears to be very stable, however, and can last for days (Staubli and Scafidi, 1997; Manahan-Vaughan, 1998).

Functional significance of LTP and LTD

LTP and LTD are currently the leading candidate synaptic mechanisms for learning and memory as well as for experience-driven organization of neural networks. However, unequivocal proof of the significance of LTP/LTD has remained elusive (Stevens, 1998). We will briefly review some of the evidence linking LTP and LTD to experience-dependent plasticity in the hippocampus; for a more thorough discussion, see Bear (1998).

To directly prove that the mechanisms of LTP/LTD can account for some types of memory, several conditions must be met (Stevens, 1998): (1) the cellular mechanisms of LTP/LTD must be similar to those underlying learning and memory; (2) LTP/LTD must naturally occur with learning and be crucial for memory; and (3) blocking LTP/LTD must also block learning and memory. We will discuss several experimental strategies that have been devised to address these requirements. Although only briefly mentioned here, there are also numerous arguments against a role for LTP/LTD in learning and memory (Goda and Stevens, 1996; Nosten-Bertrand et al., 1996; Meiri et al., 1998; Okabe et al., 1998; reviewed by Shors and Matzel, 1997; Bear, 1998).

If learning and memory require the induction of LTP/LTD, then the formation of memories should be blocked by manipulations that disrupt LTP/LTD (Izquierdo and Medina, 1995). Because many forms of LTP/LTD require activation of NMDA receptors, one approach is to block NMDA receptors in the hippocampus and test for deficits in learning spatial tasks. NMDA receptors can be pharmacologically blocked by administering antagonists into the lateral ventricles or into the hippocampus itself. In general, such studies suggest that NMDA receptor activation is required for hippocampus-dependent tasks, such as spatial learning. For example, infusions of the NMDA receptor antagonist APV into the lateral ventricles prevented the induction of LTP in the dentate gyrus, and also impaired learning of a spatial water maze task (Morris et al., 1986). Moreover, the degree of LTP impairment may correlate with the degree of memory impairment (Davis, Butcher, and Morris, 1992). Injections of an NMDA receptor antagonist into the hippocampus itself can also impair memory. For example, posttraining infusions of an NMDA receptor antagonist into the hippocampus impair memory of an inhibitory avoidance task (Izquierdo et al., 1992). Collectively, these data support the hypothesis that NMDA receptor activation is required for at least some types of memory formation, possibly via the mechanisms of LTP/LTD. However, these interpretations are confounded by the possibility that APV causes motor and sensory deficits and alters the pattern of activity in CA1 (Abraham and Kairiss, 1988; Caramanos and Shapiro, 1994; Shors and Matzel, 1997). Moreover, some studies have reported an enhancement in learning following blockade of NMDA receptor–dependent LTP (Mondadori et al., 1989).

Use of genetic technology has allowed researchers to ablate or modify a candidate memory molecule and compare the consequences on LTP and LTD with naturally occurring learning and memory. Silva and colleagues (Silva, Paylor, et al., 1992; Silva, Stevens, Tonegawa, and Wang, 1992a) used this technique to delete an isoform of CaMKII. These mice have impaired hippocampal LTP and exhibit specific deficits in a spatial learning task (Silva, Paylor, et al., 1992). Conversely, genetic enhancement of NMDA receptor function can potentiate the expression of LTP and improve learning and memory (Tang et al., 1999). Because these studies had a gene that was perturbed in every cell, a limitation is the inability to rule out abnormal development as the cause of the observed deficits or the possibility that remaining function is due to compensatory developmental changes. Now more refined techniques are overcoming these limitations, and genetic manipulations can be restricted both developmentally and regionally. For example, reports from the Tonegawa laboratory describe a transgenic mouse with a deletion of the obligatory NR1 subunit of the NMDA receptor that occurs exclusively in CA1 pyramidal cells only after postnatal day 17 (Tsien et al., 1996). These mice have deficits in LTP/LTD in CA1 and impaired spatial memory. To date, these correlations represent some of the most convincing evidence that the mechanisms underlying NMDA receptor–dependent LTP and LTD are also involved in learning and memory.

If LTP is necessary for memory, then manipulations that saturate LTP should occlude further LTP and memory formation. Several studies suggest that this is indeed the case. A common procedure in these studies is to implant electrodes chronically into the perforant path/dentate gyrus and to give repeated tetani over many days. Using such an approach, LTP saturation can impair learning of spatial memory tasks that involve the hippocampus (McNaughton et al., 1986; Castro et al., 1989). Moreover, after LTP saturation, the ability to perform a spatial task recovers at a rate similar to the decay in synaptic enhancement (Castro et al., 1989). However, these studies have proved difficult to replicate, possibly because of incomplete saturation of inputs (for example, Robinson, 1992). To overcome this problem, multielectrode stimulating arrays were used and residual LTP from naive pathways was tested (Moser et al., 1998). In this study, spatial memory was impaired in animals with no residual LTP but remained in animals capable of appreciable LTP. The interpretation of these studies is clouded by the possibility that the repetitive electrical stimulation necessary to saturate LTP might disrupt normal cellular and synaptic function. Thus, the observed deficits in spatial memory may reflect nonspecific effects of electrical stimulation rather than a specific disruption of LTP.

Although the hippocampus has classically been the subject of intense research investigating the role of LTP/LTD in learning and memory, studies in the amygdala may provide the best link between LTP and memory and thus should be briefly mentioned (reviewed by Stevens, 1998). The amygdala is a site for associative fear learning. When a mild foot shock (unconditioned stimulus) is paired with a tone (conditioned stimulus), rats learn a fear-conditioned freezing response to the tone. The essential amygdala pathways can exhibit LTP (Clugnet and LeDoux, 1990; Maren and Fanselow, 1995; Rogan and LeDoux, 1995), and blockade of LTP impairs fear conditioning (Miserendino et al., 1990; Fanselow and Kim, 1994). Moreover, there is now convincing evidence that auditory fear conditioning results in a significant synaptic enhancement of the thalamoamygdaloid pathway involved in memory formation (McKernan and Shinnick-Gallagher, 1997; Rogan, Staubli, and LeDoux, 1997). The resemblance of the learning-induced enhancement to LTP is remarkable. However, to equate LTP with memory formation, an additional demonstration is required; LTP of the auditory inputs should be able to substitute for the conditioning tone to produce the fearful memory (Stevens, 1998).

Summary

Although our discussion has largely focused on the hippocampus, the frequency with which LTP/LTD is observed in other parts of the brain suggests that these are widespread cellular phenomena. Moreover, LTP and LTD are useful constructs, on both theoretical and experimental levels, to explain diverse experience-dependent modifications in the brain. LTP and LTD remain the most viable synaptic mechanisms for learning and memory. Despite the intense interest in LTP and LTD, there remains a great deal of debate about the mechanisms underlying these phenomenona as well as their physiological role.

ACKNOWLEDGMENTS Support was provided by the Howard Hughes Medical Institute, the Human Frontier Science Program, the National Science Foundation, and the National Institutes of Health (M. Bear), and by the Whitehall Foundation (B. Philpot). Dr. Mary Lynn Mercado provided a critical reading of an earlier version of the manuscript.

REFERENCES

ABRAHAM, W. C., and G. V. GODDARD, 1983. Asymmetric relationships between homosynaptic long-term potentiation and heterosynaptic long-term depression. *Nature* 305:717–719.

ABRAHAM, W. C., and E. W. KAIRISS, 1988. Effects of the NMDA antagonist 2AP5 on complex spike discharge by hippocampal pyramidal cells. *Neurosci. Lett.* 89:36–42.

ABRAHAM, W. C., B. LOGAN, J. M. GREENWOOD, and M. DRAGUNOW, 2002. Induction and experience-dependent consolidation of stable long-term potentiation lasting months in the hippocampus. *J. Neurosci.* 22:9626–9634.

ABRAHAM, W. C., and J. R. WICKENS, 1991. Heterosynaptic long-term depression is facilitated by blockade of inhibition in area CA1 of the hippocampus. *Brain Res.* 546:336–340.

AMARAL, D. G., and M. P. WITTER, 1989. The three-dimensional organization of the hippocampal formation: A review of anatomical data. *Neuroscience* 31:571–591.

BANKE, T. G., D. BOWIE, H. LEE, R. L. HUGANIR, A. SCHOUSBOE, and S. F. TRAYNELIS, 2000. Control of GluR1 AMPA receptor function by cAMP-dependent protein kinase. *J. Neurosci.* 20:89–102.

BARRIA, A., D. MULLER, V. DERKACH, L. C. GRIFFITH, and T. R. SODERLING, 1997. Regulatory phosphorylation of AMPA-type glutamate receptors by CaM-KII during long-term potentiation. *Science* 276:2042–2045.

BEAR, M. F., 1998. The role of LTD and LTP in development and learning. In *Mechanistic Relationships between Development and Learning*, T. J. Carew, R. Menzel, and C. J. Shatz, eds. New York: John Wiley and Sons.

BEAR, M. F., and W. C. ABRAHAM, 1996. Long-term depression in hippocampus. *Annu. Rev. Neurosci.* 19:437–462.

BEAR, M. F., and R. C. MALENKA, 1994. Synaptic plasticity: LTP and LTD. *Curr. Opin. Neurobiol.* 4:389–399.

BEATTIE, E. C., R. C. CARROLL, X. YU, W. MORISHITA, H. YASUDA, M. VON ZASTROW, and R. C. MALENKA, 2000. Regulation of AMPA receptor endocytosis by a signaling mechanism shared with LTD. *Nat. Neurosci.* 3:1291–1300.

BENKE, T. A., A. LUTHI, J. T. ISAAC, and G. L. COLLINGRDIGE, 1998. Modulation of AMPA receptor unitary conductance by synaptic activity. *Nature* 393:793–797.

BI, G. Q., and M. M. POO, 1998. Synaptic modifications in cultured hippocampal neurons: Dependence on spike timing, synaptic strength, and postsynaptic cell type. *J. Neurosci.* 18:10464–10472.

BIENENSTOCK, E. L., L. N. COOPER, and P. W. MUNRO, 1982. Theory for the development of neuronal selectivity: Orientation specificity and binocular interaction in visual cortex. *J. Neurosci.* 2:32–48.

BLISS, T. V. P., and G. L. COLLINGRIDGE, 1993. A synaptic model of memory: Long-term potentiation in the hippocampus. *Nature* 361:31–39.

BOLSHAKOV, V. Y., and S. A. SIEGELBAUM, 1994. Postsynaptic induction and presynaptic expression of hippocampal long-term depression. *Science* 264:1148–1152.

BROWNING, M. D., R. HUGANIR, and P. GREENGARD, 1985. Protein phosphorylation and neuronal function. *J. Neurochem.* 45:11–23.

CARAMANOS, Z., and M. L. SHAPIRO, 1994. Spatial memory and *N*-methyl-D-aspartate antagonists APV and MK-801: Memory inpairments depend on familiarity with the environment, drug dose, and training duration. *Behav. Neurosci.* 108:30–43.

CARROLL, R. C., D. V. LISSIN, M. VON ZASTROW, R. A. NICOLL, and R. C. MALENKA, 1999. Rapid redistribution of glutamate receptors contributes to long-term depression in hippocampal cultures. *Nat. Neurosci.* 2:454–460.

CASTRO, C. A., L. H. SILBERT, B. L. MCNAUGHTON, and C. A. BARNES, 1989. Recovery of spatial learning deficits after decay of electrically induced synaptic enhancement in the hippocampus. *Nature* 342:545–548.

CHRISTIE, B. R., D. S. KERR, and W. C. ABRAHAM, 1994. The flip side of synaptic plasticity: Long-term depression mechanisms in the hippocampus. *Hippocampus* 4:127–135.

CLUGNET, M. C., and J. E. LEDOUX, 1990. Synaptic plasticity in fear conditioning circuits: Induction of LTP in the lateral nucleus of the amygdala by stimulation of the medial geniculate body. *J. Neurosci.* 10:2818–2824.

DAVIS, S., S. P. BUTCHER, and R. G. MORRIS, 1992. The NMDA receptor antagonist D-2-amino-5-phosphonopentanoate (D-AP5) impairs spatial learning and LTP in vivo at intracerebral concentrations comparable to those that block LTP in vitro. *J. Neurosci.* 12:21–34.

DEBANNE, D., B. H. GAHWILER, and S. M. THOMPSON, 1998. Long-term synaptic plasticity between pairs of individual CA3 pyramidal cells in rat hippocampal slice cultures. *J. Physiol.* 507(Pt. 1):237–247.

DERKACH, V., A. BARRIA, and T. R. SODERLING, 1999. Ca^{2+}/calmodulin-kinase II enhances channel conductance of alpha-amino-3-hydroxy-5-methyl-4-isoxazolepropionate type glutamate receptors. *Proc. Natl. Acad. Sci. U.S.A.* 16:3269–3274.

DUDEK, S. M., and M. F. BEAR, 1992. Homosynaptic long-term depression in area CA1 of hippocampus and effects of *N*-methyl-D-aspartate receptor blockade. *Proc. Natl. Acad. Sci. U.S.A.* 89:4363–4367.

DURAND, G. M., Y. KOVALCHUK, and A. KONNERTH, 1996. Long-term potentiation and functional synapse induction in developing hippocampus. *Nature* 381:71–75.

EGGER, V., D. FELDMEYER, and B. SAKMANN, 1999. Coincidence detection and changes of synaptic efficacy in spiny stellate neurons in rat barrel cortex. *Nat. Neurosci.* 2:1098–1105.

EHLERS, M. D., 2000. Reinsertion or degradation of AMPA receptors determined by activity-dependent endocytic sorting. *Neuron* 28:511–525.

ESTEBAN, J. A., S. H. SHI, C. WILSON, M. NURIYA, R. L. HUGANIR, and R. MALINOW, 2003. PKA phosphorylation of AMPA receptor subunits controls synaptic trafficking underlying plasticity. *Nat. Neurosci.* 6:136–143.

FANSELOW, M. S., and J. J. KIM, 1994. Acquisition of contextual Pavlovian fear conditioning is blocked by application of an NMDA receptor antagonist D,L-2-amino-5-phosphonovaleric

acid to the basolateral amygdala. *Behav. Neurosci.* 108:210–212.

FELDMAN, D. E., 2000. Timing-based LTP and LTD at vertical inputs to layer II/III pyramidal cells in rat barrel cortex. *Neuron* 27:45–56.

FROEMKE, R. C., and Y. DAN, 2002. Spike-timing-dependent synaptic modification induced by natural spike trains. *Nature* 416:433–438.

FUKUNAGA, K., D. MULLER, and E. MIYAMOTO, 1995. Increased phosphorylation of Ca^{2+}/calmodulin-dependent protein kinase II and its endogenous substrates in the induction of long-term potentiation. *J. Biol. Chem.* 270:6119–6124.

FUKUNAGA, K., L. STOPPINI, E. MIYAMOTO, and D. MULLER, 1993. Long-term potentiation is associated with an increased activity of Ca^{2+}/calmodulin-dependent protein kinase II. *J. Biol. Chem.* 268:7863–7867.

GODA, Y., and C. F. STEVENS, 1996. Synaptic plasticity: The basis of particular types of learning. *Curr. Biol.* 6:375–378.

GOMPERTS, S. N., A. RAO, A. M. CRAIG, R. C. MALENKA, and R. A. NICOLL, 1998. Postsynaptically silent synapses in single neuron cultures. *Neuron* 21:1443–1451.

GRANT, S. G., T. J. O'DELL, K. A. KARL, P. L. STEIN, P. SORIANO, and E. R. KANDEL, 1992. Impaired long-term potentiation, spatial learning, and hippocampal development in fyn mutant mice. *Science* 258:1903–1910.

GROVER, L. M., and T. J. TEYLER, 1990. Two components of long-term potentiation induced by different patterns of afferent activation. *Nature* 347:477–479.

HAYASHI, Y., S. H. SHI, J. A. ESTEBAN, A. PICCINI, J. C. PONCER, and R. MALINOW, 2000. Driving AMPA receptors into synapses by LTP and CaMKII: Requirement for GluR1 and PDZ domain interaction. *Science* 287:2262–2267.

HEYNEN, A. J., W. C. ABRAHAM, and M. F. BEAR, 1996. Bidirectional modification of CA1 synapses in the adult hippocampus *in vivo*. *Nature* 381:163–166.

HEYNEN, A. J., E. M. QUINLAN, D. C. BAE, and M. F. BEAR, 2000. Bidirectional, activity-dependent regulation of glutamate receptors in the adult hippocampus in vivo. *Neuron* 28:527–536.

HUBER, K. M., M. S. KAYSER, and M. F. BEAR, 2000. Role for rapid dendritic protein synthesis in hippocampal mGluR-dependent long-term depression. *Science* 288:1254–1257.

HUBER, K. M., J. C. RODER, and M. F. BEAR, 2001. Chemical induction of mGluR5- and protein synthesis–dependent long-term depression in hippocampal area CA1. *J. Neurophysiol.* 86:321–325.

ISAAC, J. T., M. C. CRAIR, R. A. NICOLL, and R. C. MALENKA, 1997. Silent synapses during development of thalamocortical inputs. *Neuron* 18:269–280.

ISAAC, J. T. R., R. A. NICOLL, and R. C. MALENKA, 1995. Evidence for silent synapses: Implications for the expression of LTP and LTD. *Neuron* 15:427–434.

ITO, I., H. HIDAKA, and H. SUGIYAMA, 1991. Effects of KN-62, a specific inhibitor of calcium/calmodulin-dependent protein kinase II, on long-term potentiation in the rat hippocampus. *Neurosci. Lett.* 121:119–121.

IZQUIERDO, I., C. DA CUNHA, R. ROSAT, D. JERUSALINSKY, M. B. FERREIRA, and J. H. MEDINA, 1992. Neurotransmitter receptors involved in post-training memory processing by the amygdala, medial septum, and hippocampus of the rat. *Behav. Neural. Biol.* 58:16–26.

IZQUIERDO, I., and J. H. MEDINA, 1995. Correlation between the pharmacology of long-term potentiation and the pharmacology of memory. *Neurobiol. Learn. Mem.* 63:19–32.

KAMEYAMA, K., H. K. LEE, M. F. BEAR, and R. L. HUGANIR, 1998. Involvement of a postsynaptic protein kinase A substrate in the expression of homosynaptic long-term depression. *Neuron* 21:1163–1175.

KELLY, P. T., 1991. Calmodulin-dependent protein kinase II: Multifunctional roles in neuronal differentiation and synaptic plasticity. *Mol. Neurobiol.* 5:153–177.

KELSO, S. R., A. H. GANONG, and T. BROWN, 1986. Hebbian synapses in the hippocampus. *Proc. Natl. Acad. Sci. U.S.A.* 83:5326–5330.

KEMP, N., and Z. I. BASHIR, 1997. NMDA receptor-dependent and -independent long-term depression in the CA1 region of the adult rat hippocampus in vitro. *Neuropharmacology* 36:397–399.

KEMP, N., and Z. I. BASHIR, 1999. Induction of LTD in the adult hippocampus by the synaptic activation of AMPA/kainate and metabotropic glutamate receptors. *Neuropharmacology* 38:495–504.

KENNEDY, M. B., 1997. The postsynaptic density at glutamatergic synapses. *Trends Neurosci.* 20:264–268.

KIRKWOOD, A., S. M. DUDEK, J. T. GOLD, C. D. AIZENMAN, and M. F. BEAR, 1993. Common forms of synaptic plasticity in the hippocampus and neocortex in vitro. *Science* 260:1518–1521.

KORNHAUSER, J. M., and M. E. GREENBERG, 1997. A kinase to remember: Dual roles for MAP kinase in long-term memory. *Neuron* 18:839–842.

KULLMANN, D. M., 1994. Amplitude fluctuations of dual-component EPSCs in hippocampal pyramidal cells: Implications for long-term potentiation. *Neuron* 12:1111–1120.

LARSON, J., D. WONG, and G. LYNCH, 1986. Patterned stimulation at the theta frequency is optimal for the induction of hippocampal long-term potentiation. *Brain Res.* 368:347–350.

LEE, H. K., M. BARBAROSIE, K. KAMEYAMA, M. F. BEAR, and R. L. HUGANIR, 2000. Regulation of distinct AMPA receptor phosphorylation sites during bidirectional synaptic plasticity. *Nature* 405:955–959.

LEE, H. K., K. KAMEYAMA, R. L. HUGANIR, and M. F. BEAR, 1998. NMDA induces long-term synaptic depression and dephosphorylation of the GluR1 subunit of AMPA receptors in hippocampus. *Neuron* 21:1151–1162.

LEE, H. K., K. TAKAMIYA, J. S. HAN, H. MAN, C. H. KIM, G. RUMBAUGH, S. YU, L. DING, C. HE, R. S. PETRALIA, R. J. WENTHOLD, M. GALLAGHER, and R. L. HUGANIR, 2003. Phosphorylation of the AMPA receptor GluR1 subunit is required for synaptic plasticity and retention of spatial memory. *Cell* 112:631–643.

LEVY, W. B., and O. STEWARD, 1979. Synapses as associative memory elements in the hippocampal formation. *Brain Res.* 175:233–245.

LIAO, D., N. A. HESSLER, and R. MALINOW, 1995. Activation of postsynaptically silent synapses during pairing-induced LTP in CA1 region of hippocampal slice. *Nature* 375:400–404.

LIAO, D., X. ZHANG, R. O'BRIEN, M. D. EHLERS, and R. L. HUGANIR, 1999. Regulation of morphological postsynaptic silent synapses in developing hippocampal neurons. *Nat. Neurosci.* 2:37–43.

LINDEN, D. J., 1996. A protein synthesis-dependent late phase of cerebellar long-term depression. *Neuron* 17:483–490.

LINDEN, D. J., and J. A. CONNOR, 1995. Long-term synaptic depression. *Annu. Rev. Neurosci.* 18:319–357.

LISMAN, J. E., 1989. A mechanism for the Hebb and the anti-Hebb processes underlying learning and memory. *Proc. Natl. Acad. Sci. U.S.A.* 86:9574–9578.

LISMAN, J., 1994. The CaM kinase II hypothesis for the storage of synaptic memory. *Trends Neurosci.* 17:406–412.

LLEDO, P.-M., G. O. HJELMSTAD, S. MUKHERJI, T. R. SODERLING, R. C. MALENKA, and R. A. NICOLL, 1995. Calcium/calmodulin-dependent kinase II and long-term potentiation enhance synaptic transmission by the same mechanism. *Proc. Natl. Acad. Sci. U.S.A.* 92:11175–11179.

LYNCH, G. S., and M. BAUDRY, 1984. The biochemistry of memory: A new and specific hypothesis. *Science* 224:1057–1063.

MADISON, D. V., R. C. MALENKA, and R. A. NICOLL, 1991. Mechanisms underlying long-term potentiation of synaptic transmission. *Annu. Rev. Neurosci.* 14:379–397.

MAGEE, J. C., and D. JOHNSTON, 1997. A synaptically controlled, associative signal for Hebbian plasticity in hippocampal neurons. *Science* 275:209–213.

MALENKA, R. C., 1991. The role of postsynaptic calcium in the induction of long-term potentiation. *Mol. Neurobiol.* 5:289–295.

MALENKA, R., J. KAUER, D. PERKEL, M. MAUK, P. KELLY, R. NICOLL, and M. WAXHAM, 1989. An essential role for postsynaptic calmodulin and protein kinase activity in long-term potentiation. *Nature* 340:554–557.

MALENKA, R. C., J. A. KAUER, D. J. PERKEL, and R. A. NICOLL, 1989. The impact of postsynaptic calcium on synaptic transmission: Its role in long-term potentiation. *Trends Neurosci.* 12:444–450.

MALENKA, R. C., and R. A. NICOLL, 1999. Long-term potentiation: A decade of progress? *Science* 285:1870–1874.

MALINOW, R., and R. C. MALENKA, 2002. AMPA receptor trafficking and synaptic plasticity. *Annu. Rev. Neurosci.* 25:103–126.

MALINOW, R., H. SCHULMAN, and R. W. TSIEN, 1989. Inhibition of postsynaptic PKC or CaMKII blocks induction but not expression of LTP. *Nature* 245:862–865.

MALINOW, R., and R. W. TSIEN, 1990. Presynaptic enhancement shown by whole-cell recordings of long term potentiation in hippocampal slices. *Nature* 346:177–180.

MAMMEN, A. L., K. KAMEYAMA, K. W. ROCHE, and R. L. HUGANIR, 1997. Phosphorylation of the alpha-amino-3-hydroxy-5-methylisoxazole4-propionic acid receptor GluR1 subunit by calcium/calmodulin-dependent kinase II. *J. Biol. Chem.* 272:32528–32533.

MAN, H. Y., J. W. LIN, W. H. JU, G. AHMADIAN, L. LIU, L. E. BECKER, M. SHENG, and Y. T. WANG, 2000. Regulation of AMPA receptor-mediated synaptic transmission by clathrin-dependent receptor internalization. *Neuron* 25:649–662.

MANABE, T., and R. A. NICOLL, 1994. Long-term potentiation: Evidence against an increase in transmitter release probability in the CA1 region of the hippocampus. *Science* 265:1888–1892.

MANAHAN-VAUGHAN, D., 1998. Priming of group 2 metabotropic glutamate receptors facilitates induction of long-term depression in the dentate gyrus of freely moving rats. *Neuropharmacology* 37:1459–1464.

MAREN, S., and M. S. FANSELOW, 1995. Synaptic plasticity in the basolateral amygdala induced by hippocampal formation stimulation in vivo. *J. Neurosci.* 15:7548–7564.

MARKRAM, H., J. LUBKE, M. FROTSCHER, and B. SAKMANN, 1997. Regulation of synaptic efficacy by coincidence of postsynaptic APs and EPSPs. *Science* 275:213–215.

MAYER, M. C., G. L. WESTBROOK, and P. B. GUTHRIE, 1984. Voltage dependent block by magnesium of NMDA responses in spinal cord neurones. *Nature* 309:261–267.

MCKERNAN, M. G., and P. SHINNICK-GALLAGHER, 1997. Fear conditioning induces a lasting potentiation of synaptic currents in vitro. *Nature* 390:607–611.

McNaughton, B. L., C. A. Barnes, G. Rao, J. Baldwin, and M. Rasmussen, 1986. Long-term enhancement of hippocampal synaptic transmission and the acquisition of spatial information. *J. Neurosci.* 6:563–571.

Meiri, N., M. K. Sun, Z. Segal, and D. L. Alkon, 1998. Memory and long-term potentiation (LTP) dissociated: Normal spatial memory despite CA1 LTP elimination with Kv1.4 antisense. *Proc. Natl. Acad. Sci. U.S.A.* 95:15037–15042.

Miserendino, M. J., C. B. Sananes, K. R. Melia, and M. Davis, 1990. Blocking of acquisition but not expression of conditioned fear-potentiated startle by NMDA antagonists in the amygdala. *Nature* 345:716–718.

Mondadori, C., L. Weiskrantz, H. Buerki, F. Petschke, and G. E. Fagg, 1989. NMDA receptor antagonists can enhance or impair learning performance in animals. *Exp. Brain Res.* 75:449–456.

Morishita, W., J. H. Connor, H. Xia, E. M. Quinlan, S. Shenolikar, and R. C. Malenka, 2001. Regulation of synaptic strength by protein phosphatase 1. *Neuron* 32:1133–1148.

Morris, R. G. M., E. Anderson, G. S. Lynch, and M. Baudry, 1986. Selective impairment of learning and blockade of long-term potentiation by an *N*-methyl-D-aspartate receptor antagonist, APV. *Nature* 319:774–776.

Moser, E. I., K. A. Krobert, M. B. Moser, and R. G. Morris, 1998. Impaired spatial learning after saturation of long-term potentiation. *Science* 281:2038–2042.

Mulkey, R. M., and R. C. Malenka, 1992. Mechanisms underlying induction of homosynaptic long-term depression in area CA1 of the hippocampus. *Neuron* 9:967–975.

Muller, D., P. A. Buchs, L. Stoppini, and H. Boddeke, 1991. Long-term potentiation, protein kinase C, and glutamate receptors. *Mol. Neurobiol.* 5:277–288.

Nelson, S. B., P. J. Sjostrom, and G. G. Turrigiano, 2002. Rate and timing in cortical synaptic plasticity. *Philos. Trans. R. Soc. Lond. B Biol. Sci.* 357:1851–1857.

Neveu, D., and R. S. Zucker, 1996. Postsynaptic levels of $[Ca^{2+}]i$ needed to trigger LTD and LTP. *Neuron* 16:619–629.

Nosten-Bertrand, M., M. L. Errington, K. P. S. J. Murphy, Y. Tokugawa, E. Barboni, E. Kazlova, D. Michalovich, R. G. M. Morris, J. Silver, C. L. Stewart, T. V. P. Bliss, and R. J. Morris, 1996. Normal spatial learning despite regional inhibition of LTP in mice lacking Thy-1. *Nature* 379:826–829.

Nowak, L., P. Bregostovski, P. Ascher, A. Herbert, and A. Prochiantz, 1984. Magnesium gates glutamate-activated channels in mouse central neurones. *Nature* 307:462–465.

O'Dell, T. J., E. R. Kandel, and S. G. Grant, 1991. Long-term potentiation in the hippocampus is blocked by tyrosine kinase inhibitors. *Nature* 353:558–560.

Okabe, S., C. Collin, J. M. Auerbach, N. Meiri, J. Bengzon, M. B. Kennedy, M. Segal, and R. D. McKay, 1998. Hippocampal synaptic plasticity in mice overexpressing an embryonic subunit of the NMDA receptor. *J. Neurosci.* 18:4177–4188.

Oliet, S. H., R. C. Malenka, and R. A. Nicoll, 1996. Bidirectional control of quantal size by synaptic activity in the hippocampus. *Science* 271:1294–1297.

Oliet, S. H., R. C. Malenka, and R. A. Nicoll, 1997. Two distinct forms of long-term depression coexist in CA1 hippocampal pyramidal cells. *Neuron* 18:969–982.

Ouyang, Y., D. Kantor, K. M. Harris, E. M. Schuman, and M. B. Kennedy, 1997. Visualization of the distribution of autophosphorylated calcium/calmodulin-dependent protein kinase II after tetanic stimulation in the CA1 area of the hippocampus. *J. Neurosci.* 17:5416–5427.

Petit, D., S. Perlman, and R. Malinow, 1994. Potentiated transmission and prevention of further LTP by increased CaMKII activity in postsynaptic hippocampal slice neurons. *Science* 266:1881–1885.

Petralia, R. S., J. A. Esteban, Y. X. Wang, J. G. Partridge, H. M. Zhao, R. J. Wenthold, and R. Malinow, 1999. Selective acquisition of AMPA receptors over postnatal development suggests a molecular basis for silent synapses. *Nat. Neurosci.* 2:31–36.

Poncer, J. C., J. A. Esteban, and R. Malinow, 2002. Multiple mechanisms for the potentiation of AMPA receptor-mediated transmission by alpha-Ca^{2+}/calmodulin-dependent protein kinase II. *J. Neurosci.* 22:4406–4411.

Roberts, L. A., M. J. Higgins, C. T. O'Shaughnessy, T. W. Stone, and B. J. Morris, 1996. Changes in hippocampal gene expression associated with the induction of long-term potentiation. *Mol. Brain Res.* 42:123–127.

Robinson, G. B., 1992. Maintained saturation of hippocampal long-term potentiation does not disrupt acquisition of the eight-arm radial maze. *Hippocampus* 2:389–395.

Rogan, M. T., and J. E. LeDoux, 1995. LTP is accompanied by commensurate enhancement of auditory-evoked responses in a fear conditioning circuit. *Neuron* 15:127–136.

Rogan, M. T., U. V. Staubli, and J. E. LeDoux, 1997. Fear conditioning induces associative long-term potentiation in the amygdala. *Nature* 390:604–607.

Rumpel, S., H. Hatt, and K. Gottmann, 1998. Silent synapses in the developing rat visual cortex: Evidence for postsynaptic expression of synaptic plasticity. *J. Neurosci.* 18:8863–8874.

Schulman, H., 1993. The multifunctional Ca^{2+}/calmodulin-dependent protein kinases. *Curr. Opin. Cell. Biol.* 5:247–253.

Schulman, H., 1995. Protein phosphorylation in neuronal plasticity and gene expression. *Curr. Opin. Neurobiol.* 5:375–381.

Schulz, P. E., E. P. Cook, and D. Johnston, 1994. Changes in paired-pulse facilitation suggest presynaptic involvement in long-term potentiation. *J. Neurosci.* 14:5325–5337.

Schulz, P. E., E. P. Cook, and D. Johnston, 1995. Using paired-pulse facilitation to probe the mechanisms for long-term potentiation (LTP). *J. Physiol. (Paris)* 89:3–9.

Selig, D., G. Hjelmstad, C. Herron, R. Nicoll, and R. Malenka, 1995. Independent mechanisms for long-term depression of AMPA and NMDA responses. *Neuron* 15:417–426.

Shi, S., Y. Hayashi, J. A. Esteban, and R. Malinow, 2001. Subunit-specific rules governing AMPA receptor trafficking to synapses in hippocampal pyramidal neurons. *Cell* 105:331–343.

Shi, S. H., Y. Hayashi, R. S. Petralia, S. H. Zaman, R. J. Wenthold, K. Svoboda, and R. Malinow, 1999. Rapid spine delivery and redistribution of AMPA receptors after synaptic NMDA receptor activation. *Science* 284:1811–1816.

Shors, T. J., and T. J. Matzel, 1997. Long-term potentiation: What's learning got to do with it? *Behav. Brain Sci.* 20:597–614.

Shouval, H. Z., M. F. Bear, and L. N. Cooper, 2002. A unified model of NMDA receptor-dependent bidirectional synaptic plasticity. *Proc. Natl. Acad. Sci. U.S.A.* 99:10831–10836.

Siegelbaum, S. A., and E. R. Kandell, 1991. Learning-related synaptic plasticity: LTP and LTD. *Curr. Opin. Neurobiol.* 1:113–120.

Silva, A., R. Paylor, J. Wehner, and S. Tonegawa, 1992. Impaired spatial learning in α-calcium-calmodulin kinase II mutant mice. *Science* 257:206–211.

Silva, A. J., C. F. Stevens, S. Tonegawa, and Y. Wang, 1992a. Deficient hippocampal long-term potentiation in alpha-calcium-calmodulin kinase II mutant mice. *Science* 257:201–206.

SILVA, A., C. STEVENS, S. TONEGAWA, and Y. WANG, 1992b. Deficient hippocampal long-term potentiation in α-calcium-calmodulin kinase II mutant mice. *Science* 257:206–211.

SOKOLOV, M. V., A. V. ROSSOKHIN, T. BEHNISCH, K. G. REYMANN, and L. L. VORONIN, 1998. Interaction between paired-pulse facilitation and long-term potentiation of minimal excitatory postsynaptic potentials in rat hippocampal slices: A patch-clamp study. *Neuroscience* 85:1–13.

SONG, I., and R. L. HUGANIR, 2002. Regulation of AMPA receptors during synaptic plasticity. *Trends Neurosci.* 25:578–588.

SQUIRE, L. R., 1992. Memory and the hippocampus: A synthesis from findings with rats, monkeys and humans. *Psychol. Rev.* 99:195–231.

STANTON, P. K., U. HEINEMANN, and W. MULLER, 2001. FM1-43 imaging reveals cGMP-dependent long-term depression of presynaptic transmitter release. *J. Neurosci.* 21:RC167.

STAUBLI, U., and J. SCAFIDI, 1997. Studies on long-term depression in area CA1 of the anesthetized and freely moving rat. *J. Neurosci.* 17:4820–4828.

STEVENS, C. F., 1998. A million dollar question: Does LTP = memory? *Neuron* 20:1–2.

STEVENS, C. F., and Y. WANG, 1994. Changes in reliability of synaptic function as a mechanism for plasticity. *Nature* 371:704–707.

TANG, Y. P., E. SHIMIZU, G. R. DUBE, C. RAMPON, G. A. KERCHNER, M. ZHUO, G. LIU, and J. Z. TSIEN, 1999. Genetic enhancement of learning and memory in mice. *Nature* 401:63–69.

THOMAS, K. L., S. LAROCHE, M. L. ERRINGTON, T. V. BLISS, and S. P. HUNT, 1994. Spatial and temporal changes in signal transduction pathways during LTP. *Neuron* 13:737–745.

TSIEN, J. Z., D. F. CHEN, D. GERBER, C. TOM, E. H. MERCER, D. J. ANDERSON, M. MAYFORD, E. R. KANDEL, and S. TONEGAWA, 1996. Subregion- and cell-type-restricted gene knockout in mouse brain. *Cell* 87:1317–1326.

WANG, J. H., and P. T. KELLY, 1997. Attenuation of paired-pulse facilitation associated with synaptic potentiation mediated by postsynaptic mechanisms. *J. Neurophysiol.* 78:2707–2716.

YANG, S. N., Y. G. TANG, and R. S. ZUCKER, 1999. Selective induction of LTP and LTD by postsynaptic $[Ca^{2+}]i$ elevation. *J. Neurophysiol.* 81:781–787.

YASUDA, H., A. L. BARTH, D. STELLWAGEN, and R. C. MALENKA, 2003. A developmental switch in the signaling cascades for LTP induction. *Nat. Neurosci.* 6:15–16.

YU, X. M., R. ASKALAN, G. N. KEIL, and M. W. SALTER, 1997. NMDA channel regulation by channel-associated protein tyrosine kinase Src. *Science* 275:674–678.

ZHANG, L. I., H. W. TAO, C. E. HOLT, W. E. HARRIS, and M. POO, 1998. A critical window for cooperation and competition among developing retinotectal synapses. *Nature* 395:37–44.

ZHU, J. J., J. A. ESTEBAN, Y. HAYASHI, and R. MALINOW, 2000. Postnatal synaptic potentiation: Delivery of GluR4-containing AMPA receptors by spontaneous activity. *Nat. Neurosci.* 3:1098–1106.

ZHU, J. J., and R. MALINOW, 2002. Acute versus chronic NMDA receptor blockade and synaptic AMPA receptor delivery. *Nat. Neurosci.* 5:513–514.

ZHU, J. J., Y. QIN, M. ZHAO, L. VAN AELST, and R. MALINOW, 2002. Ras and Rap control AMPA receptor trafficking during synaptic plasticity. *Cell* 110:443–455.

9 Neurogenesis in the Adult Mammalian Brain

HENRIETTE VAN PRAAG, XINYU ZHAO, AND FRED H. GAGE

ABSTRACT Over the past decades, it has become well established that neurogenesis occurs in the adult mammalian brain. The new neurons arise from stem or progenitor cells that exist throughout the central nervous system. In culture, stem cells can give rise to neurons, glia and oligodendrocytes. In vivo local factors restrict the genesis of new neurons to the olfactory bulb and hippocampus. The production of new cells in these areas is regulated by a variety of environmental, pharmacological, hormonal, and genetic factors. Although factors that increase neurogenesis have been correlated with improved cognition and mood, the functional significance of the birth of new cells in the adult brain remains unknown at this time.

Historical perspective

Until quite recently it was assumed that neurogenesis, or the production of new neurons, occurred only during development, and never in the adult organism. The famous neuroanatomist Cajal stated that "Once development was ended, the fonts of growth and regeneration of the axons and dendrites dried up irrevocably. In adult centers, the nerve paths are something fixed and immutable: everything may die, nothing may be regenerated." This statement holds true for most regions of the adult brain. However, there are two adult brain areas in which neurogenesis is observed: the subventricular zone of the anterior lateral ventricles, which give rise to cells that become neurons in the olfactory bulb, and the subgranular zone in the dentate gyrus of the hippocampus, a brain region that is important for learning and memory, which generates new granule cell neurons.

The initial studies that suggested that the adult brain could generate new neurons were largely ignored. In the 1960s, Joseph Altman and co-workers published a series of papers reporting that some dividing cells in the adult brain survived and differentiated into cells with a morphology similar to that of neurons (Altman and Das, 1965). The technique they used to label the cells was tritiated thymidine autoradiography. Tritiated thymidine is incorporated into the DNA of dividing cells. The highest density of labeling was in the subventricular zone and in the dentate gyrus of the hippocampus. It was known that the dentate gyrus of the hippocampus is essentially devoid of glia. Therefore, the labeling in this region was attributed to the uptake of thymidine by dentate granule cells. However, it could not be proved that the adult-generated cells were neurons rather than glia, since no phenotypic markers were available that could be used in conjunction with thymidine autoradiography. The absence of specific markers for neurons and glia and continued skepticism surrounding the concept of adult neurogenesis limited further development of the research.

In the mid-1970s and the early 1980s, these initial observations were reexamined using the electron microscope, with substantial confidence growing that neurogenesis could occur in the adult brain. By combining electron microscopy and tritiated thymidine labeling, researchers were able to show that labeled cells in the rat dentate gyrus have ultrastructural characteristics of neurons, such as dendrites and synapses (Kaplan and Hinds, 1977). However, this finding was not considered to be evidence of significant neurogenesis in adult mammals by most researchers. It was still not possible to prove definitively that the new cells were neurons. In addition, the concept that there may be brainstem cells that could proliferate, migrate, and then differentiate into new neurons had not yet been introduced. It was therefore thought that mature neurons would have to replicate, an idea that most researchers found incredible. Furthermore, the possible relevance of the findings for humans was underestimated because there was no evidence of neurogenesis in adult primates.

In the mid-1980s this fledgling field was stimulated by astonishing findings in adult canaries. It was discovered that neurogenesis occurs in brain areas that mediate song learning (Goldman and Nottebohm, 1983). Using a combination of tritiated thymidine autoradiography and ultrastructural and electrophysiological techniques, researchers provided evidence that the new cells were neurons (Paton and Nottebohm, 1984). In addition, they showed that there is a peak in the production of new neurons at the time of year birds acquire songs (Barnea and Nottebohm, 1994). It was also shown that neurogenesis in the hippocampal complex of adult chickadees is correlated with seed-storing behavior. In

HENRIETTE VAN PRAAG and FRED H. GAGE The Salk Institute for Biological Studies, La Jolla, Calif.

XINYU ZHAO University of New Mexico School of Medicine, Albuquerque, N.M.

fact, the hippocampus is relatively larger in seed-storing than in non-storing birds and appears to play an important role in spatial learning. Chickadees store seeds in the fall and then retrieve them after days or weeks. In one of the studies the birds were captured at different times of the year, injected with tritiated thymidine, released, and recaptured 6 weeks later. It was found that there was significant seasonality in the number of hippocampal cells labeled with tritiated thymidine. Birds that had received the label in October had more labeled cells than chickadees that had received the label at other times of the year (Barnea and Nottebohm, 1994). Taken together, these results raised the possibility that new neurons play a functional role in the mature brain, and led to a revival of interest in possible neurogenesis in adult mammals.

Despite the observations of neurogenesis in the adult avian brain, confusion over the mechanism of origin of cell genesis in the adult brain persisted. However, in the early 1990s it was revealed that cells with stem cell properties could be isolated and expanded in culture (Reynolds and Weiss, 1992). In a variety of culture conditions with differ-ent factors, these isolated cells can be induced to proliferate and differentiate into glia or neurons (see later discussion under Neural Stem Cells in vitro). These in vitro observa-tions suggested a mechanism for neurogenesis in the adult brain in vivo. Mature committed neurons were not dividing, but rather a population of immature stem cell-like cells exists in the brain, and it is likely that it is the proliferation and dif-ferentiation of this population that results in neurogenesis. Interestingly, immature or stem cells that can divide and give rise to neurons in culture can be isolated from many areas of the adult brain and spinal cord, not only neurogenic regions such as the subventricular zone and hippocampus but also areas that are non-neurogenic, such as the septum, striatum, substantia nigra, spinal cord, cerebral cortex, corpus callosum, and optic nerve and eye (Palmer et al., 1999; Lie et al., 2002). In culture, these cells are multipotent and can give rise to neurons and glia. This suggests that the potential for neurogenesis exists throughout the adult mam-malian nervous system but that the signals necessary for neurogenesis have been lost, or inhibitory mechanisms may prevent its occurrence.

Following the discovery of the mechanism by which new neurons could arise in the adult brain in vivo, great con-ceptual and technical progress was made. The thymidine analogue 5-bromo-3′-deoxyuridine (BrdU), a traceable analogy of uridine that is incorporated into the genome of cells undergoing cell division, was used to label new cells in vivo. The advantage of BrdU over thymidine autoradiogra-phy is that the cells can be visualized using immunocyto-chemistry. This method allows for a more accurate estimate of the number of new cells using stereological techniques. In addition, BrdU immunocytochemistry can be used in combination with now available specific markers for neurons, such as NeuN and Calbindin, and for glia, such as S100β and glial fibrillary acidic protein (GFAP). Double labeling for BrdU and NeuN has been used extensively over the past decade to demonstrate whether a newborn cell has become a neuron (Kuhn, Dickinson-Anson, and Gage, 1996; Gage, 2002). By this method it has also been shown that there is a time course over which neurogenesis occurs. When BrdU-labeled cells were examined a few days after the last BrdU injection, the majority of the cells did not acquire colabel for any of the mature neuronal or glial markers, suggesting that these are immature, proliferating cells. Four weeks after the last BrdU injection about 60% of the BrdU-positive cells colabeled with the neuronal marker NeuN, suggesting it takes about a month for newly born cells to become a neuron (Kuhn, Dickinson-Anson, and Gage, 1996). These findings were recently confirmed and extended using retroviral labeling selective for dividing cells. Using this method, researchers demonstrated that although new neurons have acquired the functional and morphological characteristics of neurons at 1 month, they continue to increase in size and complexity for several months (van Praag et al., 2002).

Until recently, studies that provided evidence of neurogen-esis were considered irrelevant to the primate or human brain. It was assumed that neurogenesis became restricted throughout evolution as the brain became more intricate. Thus, lizards and other reptiles can regenerate and replace neurons following damage, whereas in the complex human brain, the addition of new neurons could conceivably disturb the intricate wiring of neuronal connections. However, it has now been reported that neurogenesis occurs in the hippocampus of nonhuman primates (Gould et al., 1999; Kornack and Rakic, 1999). At about the same time the possible occurrence of neurogenesis in humans was studied. Administering BrdU and then examining cell pro-liferation in tumor biopsies is occasionally used to monitor tumor progression in patients with cancer. Because BrdU is a small, soluble molecule, it is distributed throughout the body, including the brain, and thus can be a marker for cell division and neurogenesis in humans. It was reported that in five cancer patients who had received BrdU between 15 days and more than 2 years earlier, all showed neurogenesis as revealed by colabeling of BrdU with markers of mature neurons in the dentate gyrus. These studies clearly demon-strated that neurogenesis, at least in the dentate gyrus, is a process that persists throughout life in mammalian species, including humans (Eriksson et al., 1998; Kornack and Rakic, 1999; Gage, 2002).

Although neurogenesis in the dentate gyrus of the hip-pocampus of adult mammals is now a generally accepted phenomenon, the functional significance of the new neurons remains unclear. In fact, until very recently it was not known whether the newborn neurons are functionally integrated into the hippocampal circuitry. All the evidence in mammals described so far is based on morphological studies, since use of ³H-thymidine and BrdU requires extensive processing of the tissue to visualize the cells. Moreover, only the soma can be observed with these methods. In a recent study that used a retrovirus expressing green fluorescent protein (GFP) that only infects dividing cells, newly born cells were visualized directly in live hippocampal slices. It was demonstrated that new granule neurons in the hippocampus exhibit neuronal morphology (GFP is expressed in the cytoplasm) and have passive membrane potentials, action potentials, and synaptic inputs that are similar to those of mature dentate neurons (van Praag et al., 2002). A subsequent study using similar methodology showed how new olfactory bulb neurons become integrated and functional (Carleton et al., 2003).

Regulation of neurogenesis in vivo

It is now well established that neurogenesis occurs in the adult mammalian nervous system. However, the function of the new cells remains unclear. Interestingly, a variety of environmental, behavioral, genetic, neuroendocrine, and neurochemical factors can influence the proliferation and survival of newborn cells. Treatments and manipulations that enhance the production of new cells have been associated with enhanced cognition and mental health, whereas reductions in number of new cells correlate with impaired memory, stress, and depression. Several of these factors are discussed here and outlined in table 9.1.

GENETIC BACKGROUND Mice of different genetic backgrounds have different levels of neurogenesis. For example, mice of varying genetic backgrounds display different levels of cell proliferation and cell survival. When C57B/L6, BALB/c, CD1, and 129/SvJ strains of mice are compared, C57BL6 mice have the highest proliferation rate, whereas CD1 mice have the highest cell survival rate. 129/SvJ mice have the lowest proliferation rate and survival rate and also the lowest neuronal differentiation and the most gliogenesis of all these mice. (Kempermann, Kuhn, and Gage, 1997a). Interestingly these mice also do not perform as well on spatial learning tasks as C57Bl/6 mice (Kempermann, Brandon, and Gage, 1998). Furthermore, among A/J, C3H/HeJ, and DBA/2J mice, A/J mice have a significantly higher proliferation rate, whereas 3H/HeJ have the highest survival rate. DBA/2J mice also have significantly lower neurogenesis and higher astrocyte genesis than other strains (Kempermann and Gage, 2002). A second major difference demonstrated in different strains of mice is their response to environmental stimulation. When housed in an enriched environment, C57BL6 mice have increased cell survival without a change in cell proliferation, whereas 129Sv/J have

increases in both proliferation and survival. In both C57B1/6 and 129Sv/J mice, environmental enrichment is associated with improved learning (Kempermann, Kuhn, and Gage, 1997a; Kempermann, Brandon, and Gage, 1998).

GROWTH FACTORS AND TROPHIC FACTORS Several growth factors and trophic factors have been shown to affect adult neurogenesis, including basic fibroblast growth factor (FGF-2), epidermal growth factor (EGF), brain-derived neurotrophic factor (BDNF), and insulin-like growth factor I (IGF-I). Two of the major growth factors that influence neural progenitor cell (NPC) proliferation both in vivo and in vitro are FGF-2 and EGF. Intracerebroventricular (ICV) infusion of FGF-2 and EGF results in increased neurogenesis in the subventricular zone (SVZ) but not in dentate gyrus (DG) of the hippocampus (Craig et al., 1996; Kuhn et al., 1997; Wagner et al., 1999). ICV administration of BDNF increased the number of new neurons in adult olfactory bulb (Zigova et al., 1998), whereas ICV vascular endothelial growth factor (VEGF) enhanced cell proliferation in both SVZ and DG (Jin et al., 2002). In addition, peripheral infusion of IGF-I increases adult neurogenesis (Aberg et al., 2000) and reverses the aging-related reduction in new cells (Lichtenwalner et al., 2001). Physical exercise results in enhanced neurogenesis (van Praag, Christie et al., 1999; van Praag, Kempermann et al., 1999) and elevated expression of BDNF, FGF-2, and IGF-I (Russo-Neustadt et al., 2000) (Carro et al., 2000; Gomez-Pinilla, Dao, and So, 1997). The exercise-induced stimulation of hippocampal neurogenesis may be mediated in part by greater uptake of IGF-I and VEGF into brain from serum (Trejo, Carro, and Torres-Alemán, 2001; Fabel et al., 2003). Dietary restriction also results in enhanced cell proliferation and survival in DG and increased expression of BDNF and NT-3 (Lee, Seroogy, and Mattson, 2002). Increased neurogenesis in adult songbirds is also associated with elevated levels of BDNF, VEGF, and VEGF receptor (R2) (Louissaint et al., 2002).

NEUROTRANSMITTERS Neurotransmitters also play important roles in regulating adult neurogenesis. Glutamate receptor agonists have been shown to inhibit cell proliferation in DG, whereas the NMDA receptor antagonists enhance cell genesis (Cameron, McEwen, and Gould, 1995; Cameron, Tanapat, and Gould, 1998). However, a recent report indicates that an AMPA receptor potentiator increases hippocampal cell proliferation (Bai, Bergeron, and Nelson, 2003). Prolonged exposure to monoamines can enhance the level of cell proliferation in rats. In particular, serotonergic antidepressants have been shown to stimulate granule cell production (Malberg et al., 2000), whereas administration of the serotonin 5-HT (1A) receptor antagonists decreases cell proliferation in the DG (Radley and Jacobs, 2002). Moreover, it has been shown that serotonin 1A receptor–null mice

TABLE 9.1

Factors affecting in vivo cell proliferation and neurogenesis in adult hippocampus and SVZ/olfactory bulb

Factor	Proliferation	Glial Genesis	Neurogenesis	References
Genetic background	Yes	Yes	Yes	Kempermann and Gage (2002), Kempermann et al. (1997a)
FGF-2	—	—	—	Kuhn et al. (1997)
	↑*	↑*	↑*	Wagner et al. (1999)
EGF	—	↑	↓	Craig et al. (1996), Kuhn et al. (1997)
IGF	↑	—	↑	Aberg et al. (2000)
VEGF	↑	n.d.	↑	Jin et al. (2002)
BDNF	↑*	n.d.	↑*	Lee et al. (2002)
Serotonin	↑	n.d.	↑	Jacobs et al. (2000)
Norepinephrine	↑	—	—	Kulkarni et al. (2002)
Glutamate	↓	n.d.	n.d.	Cameron et al. (1995), Gould (1994)
(Antagonist: MK801)	↑	n.d.	↑	Cameron et al. (1998)
Serotonin	↑	n.d.	↑	Gould et al. (1999), Jacobs et al. (2000)
Stress	↓	n.d.	n.d.	Gould et al. (1997)
Glucocorticoids	↓	n.d.	n.d.	Cameron and Gould (1994)
Adrenalectomy	↑	n.d.	↑	Cameron and McKay (1999)
Estrogen	↑	—	—	Tanapat et al. (1999)
Prolactin	↑*	n.d.	↑*	Shingo et al. (2003)
CAMP/CREB	↑	n.d.	—	Nakagawa et al. (2002)
Methamphetamine	↓	n.d.	n.d.	Teuchert-Noodt et al. (2000)
Opiate/heroin/morphine	↓	n.d.	n.d.	Eisch et al. (2000)
Enriched environment	—	—	↑	Kempermann et al. (1997b)
Wheel running	↑	—	↑	van Praag et al. (1999)
Learning	—	n.d.	↑	Gould et al. (1999)
			—	van Praag et al. (1999)
Dietary restriction	↑	n.d.	n.d.	Lee et al. (2002)
Aging	↓	n.d.	↓	Kuhn et al. (1996)
Vitamin E deficiency	↑	n.d.	n.d.	Ciaroni et al. (1999)
Traumatic brain injury	↑	↑	↑	Kernie et al. (2001)
Epilepsy	↑	n.d.	↑	Parent et al. (1997)
Stroke/ischemia	↑	n.d.	↑	Liu et al. (1998), Nakatomi et al. (2002)
γ-Irradiation	↓	↑	↓	Monje et al. (2002)
Lesion (cortex)†	↑†	↑†	↑†	Magavi et al. (2000)

Abbreviation: n.d., not determined.

*In SVZ/olfactory bulb only.

†In cortex only.

were insensitive to the neurogenic and behavioral effects of the serotonin reuptake inhibitor fluoxetine (Santarelli et al., 2003). Thus, the antidepressant effect of serotonin may be mediated by its neurogenic properties (Jacobs, van Praag, and Gage, 2000). It is likely that the mechanism of serotonergic action could be mediated through the cAMP second messenger cascade (Mendez et al., 1999). Increased second messenger cAMP and phosphorylation of its downstream effector, CREB, have been shown to increase cell proliferation in the dentate gyrus (Nakagawa et al., 2002). Other monoamines may also play a role in neurogenesis. Deletion

of norepinephrine by neurotoxin DSP-4 results in a 63% reduction in DG cell proliferation with no influence on percentage of new cells that become neurons (Brezun and Daszuta, 1999; Kulkarni et al., 2002). Administration of the dopaminergic antagonist haloperidol, however, enhanced hippocampal neurogenesis in gerbils (Dawirs, Hildebrandt, and Teuchert-Noodt, 1998). The neuromodulator nitric oxide can promote cell proliferation and migration in both SVZ and DG (Zhang et al., 2001). Opiates, on the other hand, reduce hippocampal cell genesis (Eisch et al., 2000).

HORMONAL FACTORS   Stress and the concomitant increase in glucocorticoid levels can reduce the level of cell proliferation in adult rodents (Gould et al., 1992; McEwen, 1999) and primates (Fuchs and Flugge, 1998), whereas adrenalectomy enhances cell proliferation (Gould et al., 1992). Adult neurogenesis in SVZ (Tropepe et al., 1997) and DG (Seki and Arai, 1995; Kuhn, Dickinson-Anson, and Gage, 1996) decreases with age in rodents. This aging-associated decline can be restored by reducing corticosteroid levels by an adrenalectomy (Cameron and McKay, 1999). Testosterone has been shown to increase neurogenesis in birds (Louissaint et al., 2002). Estrogen, on the other hand, causes a transient increase in cell proliferation levels in rats (Tanapat et al., 1999; Ormerod, Lee, and Galea, 2003), possibly via the 5-HT pathway (Banasr et al., 2001). Increased prolactin levels during pregnancy have been associated with enhanced neurogenesis in SVZ of mice (Shingo et al., 2003). Thyroid hormone promotes in vitro differentiation of adult neural stem cells (Palmer, Ray, and Gage, 1995).

ENVIRONMENT AND EXERCISE   In an experimental setting, an enriched environment is "enriched" in relation to standard laboratory housing conditions when animals are kept in larger cages and in larger groups, with the opportunity for more complex social interactions. In addition, the environment includes tunnels, nesting material, toys, and the opportunity to perform voluntary physical activity on running wheels. Enrichment has behavioral, morphological, and molecular effects that have been studied extensively (van Praag, Kempermann, and Gage, 2000). In a fairly recent study it was discovered that housing animals in an enriched environment enhances the survival of newborn neurons in the adult mouse hippocampus (Kempermann, Kuhn, and Gage, 1997b). In a subsequent study several components of the enriched environment, such as exercise and learning, were isolated and their effects on neurogenesis were studied. It was found that similar to the effects of environmental enrichment, voluntary exercise in a running wheel enhanced the survival of newborn neurons in the dentate gyrus. Learning a hippocampus-dependent task (the Morris water maze) did not influence cell proliferation or neurogenesis (van Praag, Kempermann, and Gage, 1999). Both enrichment and exercise enhance learning and increase growth factors, neurotransmitters, and possibly synaptic plasticity in a similar manner (van Praag, Christie et al., 1999; van Praag, Kempermann, and Gage, 1999). However, it remains to be determined whether exercise is the critical component of enrichment or whether enriched living has additional unique features. Despite the similarities, the mechanisms underlying the changes in cell genesis may be different. Enrichment increases new cell survival in adult DG but does not affect cell proliferation level, whereas physical exercise increases both, with comparable effects on neurogenesis (Kempermann, Kuhn, and Gage, 1997a; van Praag, Christie et al., 1999). Moreover, the effects of enrichment and exercise are selective for the DG and do not affect SVZ neurogenesis (Brown et al., 2003).

DISEASES/INJURY CONDITIONS AND DRUG ABUSE   Neurogenesis levels change during the course of CNS diseases and following insults. Ischemia increases cell proliferation in both SVZ and DG, and such an increase is FGF-2 dependent (Liu et al., 1998; Yoshimura et al., 2001; Nakatomi et al., 2002). Seizures have been shown to increase neurogenesis in DG (Parent et al., 1997) and in area CA1 ((Nakatomi et al., 2002). In DG, epilepsy leads to the production of ectopic granule cells. The seizure-induced cells may lead to aberrant circuitry and further abnormal excitability of the hippocampus (Parent et al., 1997; Scharfman, 2000). Furthermore, CNS injuries can induce neurogenesis in normally non-neurogenic regions such as cortex (Magavi, Leavitt, and Macklis, 2000). Traumatic brain injury induces astrocytogenesis at the proximal site and increases neurogenesis at the distal site in DG (Kernie, Erwin, and Parada, 2001). Irradiation reduces NPC proliferation and neuronal differentiation in rat hippocampus (Monje et al., 2002). Drugs of abuse, such as methamphetamine, transiently decrease cell proliferation in the DG of adult gerbil (Teuchert-Noodt, Dawirs, and Hildebrandt, 2000). Chronic administration of morphine or heroin can reduce neurogenesis in adult hippocampus (Eisch et al., 2000), a finding that may explain why long-term drug abusers have poor memory function (Guerra et al., 1987).

FUNCTIONS OF DEVELOPMENTAL GENES IN ADULT NEUROGENESIS   Genes that are currently best known for their roles in development acquire new and important roles in adulthood, including the regulation of adult neural stem cell function. However, overexpression or ablation of such genes can cause developmental problems that prevent studying their role in adulthood. For example, Sonic hedgehog (Shh) was first discovered as a crucial regulator of nervous system and limb development (Jessell and Lumsden, 1997). However, the homozygous null-Shh mutation is embryonically lethal (Chiang et al., 1996), and transgenic mice overexpressing Shh are susceptible to tumor formation early in development (Oro et al., 1997). In a recent study, an adeno-associated viral vector was used to overexpress Shh in the adult rat hippocampus. It was found that the number of proliferating cells and newborn neurons was tripled. Furthermore, cyclopamine, a pharmacological inhibitor of Shh signaling (Berman et al., 2002), reduced the number of proliferating cells in the hippocampal subgranular zone by a factor of 2. This study indicates that Shh regulates adult neurogenesis, one of its few known roles beyond development (Lai et al., 2003).

Genes important during development can regulate not only progenitor cell proliferation but also their differentiation. Noggin is a polypeptide that binds to bone morphogenetic proteins (BMPs) and inhibits their function. It was originally identified for its regulation of *Xenopus* neurulation (Smith and Harland, 1992) and has subsequently been found to be important in the development of the neural tube and somite (McMahon et al., 1998). Alvarez-Bullya and colleagues found that BMPs cell-autonomously repress neuronal and promote glial differentiation of adult progenitors in the SVZ. Furthermore, the overexpression of noggin using an adenoviral vector promoted the neuronal differentiation of progenitors grafted into the striatum (Lim et al., 2000).

KNOWLEDGE OBTAINED FROM TRANSGENIC MICE STUDIES In addition to ectopic overexpression, genetic ablation approaches have also led to the identification of several novel regulators of neurogenesis (table 9.2). Transgenic mutant mice have been used to study the roles of several extracellular signaling molecules. The analysis of FGF-2 mutant knockout mice showed that FGF-2 may be necessary for cell genesis after ischemic insult. In the injured FGF-2 knockout mice, the neurogenic response is markedly reduced (Yoshimura et al., 2001). In addition, a study of heterozygous BDNF knockouts reported decreased cell proliferation and survival in the hippocampus (Lee, Seroogy, and Mattson, 2002). Furthermore, mCD24, a glycosylphosphatidylinositol-anchored protein widely expressed during development, but only in neurogenic regions of the adult CNS, is believed to be involved in cell migration and signaling. mCD24−/− mutant mice exhibited significantly higher rates of progenitor cell proliferation both in the DG and SVZ, indicating that this signaling molecule represses progenitor expansion by an unknown mechanism (Belvindrah, Rougon, and Chazal, 2002).

The presenilins, known for their involvement in the etiology of Alzheimer's disease, may also play a role in the regulation of neurogenesis. Homozygous mutant presenilin-1 (PS1) animals suffer from severe embryonic abnormalities and embryonic death (Shen et al., 1997). Therefore, Tsien and colleagues employed the *Cre-loxP* system, with *Cre* expression driven from the α-calcium/calmodulin-dependent kinase II (CaMKII) promoter, to delete PS1 in the postmitotic neurons in the forebrain. Under basal conditions, no changes in neurogenesis were observed in these animals; however, the neurogenic response to environmental enrichment was reduced (Feng et al., 2001). A subsequent study showed that transgenic mice overexpressing PS1 had decreased numbers of hippocampal progenitors (Wen et al., 2002).

In addition to extracellular signaling molecules, intracellular signal transducers and cell cycle regulators have been implicated in controlling adult neural stem cell proliferation. CREB is well recognized for its role in learning and memory and neuronal survival signal transduction (Silva et al., 1998). Nakagawa and colleagues placed the tetracycline-regulated transactivator under the control of the CamKII promoter in order to inducibly express a dominant negative CREB in the forebrain, which resulted in a 35% reduction in the number of proliferating cells in the DG (Nakagawa et al., 2002). Another transcription factor, E2F1, also appears to be responsible for implementing proliferative signals in progenitor cells. The E2F family of transcription factors acts downstream of mitogenic signals (Zhu et al., 2003) and controls the expression of key cell cycle regulators including cyclins and enzymes involved in nucleotide biosynthesis and DNA replication (Trimarchi and Lees, 2002). Homozygous null-E2F1 mutants have significantly reduced progenitor cell proliferation in both the DG and SVZ (Cooper-Kuhn et al., 2002). Furthermore, ablation of p27Kip1, an inhibitor of cyclin-dependent kinase 2, results in faster proliferation of transit-amplifying cells in the SVZ. This increased proliferation is accompanied by higher levels of apoptosis and also appears to occur at the expense of lineage progression to neuroblasts (Doetsch et al., 2002).

TABLE 9.2

Studies involving transgenic animals to study cell proliferation and neurogenesis in adult hippocampus and SVZ

Gene	Transgenic Type	Phenotype	Reference
FGF-2	Homozygous null	Reduced DG proliferation upon injury	Yoshimura et al. (2001)
mCD24	Homozygous null	Increased DG and SVZ proliferation	Belvindrah et al. (2002)
PS-1	Conditional null	Reduced DG proliferation in enriched environment	Feng et al. (2001)
PS-1	Overexpression	Reduced DG proliferation	Wen et al. (2002)
CREB	Conditional dom. neg.	Reduced DG proliferation	Nakagawa et al. (2002)
E2F1	Homozygous null	Reduced DG and SVZ proliferation	Cooper-Kuhn et al. (2002)
P27Kip1	Homozygous null	Increased SVZ proliferation	Doetsch et al. (2002)
CCg	Homozygous null	Reduced DG proliferation	Taupin et al. (2000)
TLX	Homozygous null	Reduced proliferation	Shi et al. (2004)
MBD1	Homozygous null	Decreased neurogenesis	Zhao et al. (2003)

Recently, the methyl-CpG binding protein (MBD) family has been shown to be involved in neurogenesis. Binding of MBDs and further recruitment of histone deacetylase (HDAC) repressor complexes result in histone deacetylation and inactivation of chromatin structures that are repressive for transcription (Bird, 2002). By studying mice lacking MBD1, a member of the MBD family, a link between DNA methylation, genomic stability, and hippocampal neurogenesis was made. MBD1−/− mice have reduced neurogenesis, impaired spatial learning, and a significant reduction in long-term potentiation in the DG of the hippocampus (Zhao et al., 2003).

Finally, a very important role for TLX, a gene initially identified as an orphan nuclear receptor, has been established. TLX is expressed in vertebrate forebrains during development and is highly expressed in the adult brain. The brains of TLX-null mice have been reported to have no obvious defects during embryogenesis; however, mature mice suffer from retinopathies, severe limbic defects, aggressiveness, reduced copulation, and progressively violent behavior. Interestingly, TLX mutant mice show a loss of cell proliferation and reduced labeling of nestin in neurogenic areas in the adult brain. Although stem cells can still be isolated from the brains of TLX-null mice, they fail to proliferate in culture. Reintroducing TLX into TLX-null cells rescues their ability to proliferate and to self-renew (Shi et al., 2004).

Neural stem cells in vitro

The identification and isolation of multipotent NPCs from the adult CNS have yielded an explanation of the cellular basis for adult neurogenesis. To date, NPCs can be isolated from many different brain regions (Weiss et al., 1996; Palmer, Takahashi, and Gage, 1999; Shihabuddin et al., 2000; Lie et al., 2002). Clonal analysis indicates that these cells are multipotent in in vitro culture systems (Shihabuddin et al., 2000). However, when grafted into the adult brain, these cells differentiate into neurons only in the DG and SVZ (Shihabuddin et al., 2000; Lie et al., 2002).

FGF-2 and EGF are two potent mitogens for NPCs. During early development, NPCs are responsive only to FGF-2, not EGF. At later stages of development, EGF-responsive NPCs appear (Represa et al., 2001; Temple, 2001); EGF-responsive NPCs can be isolated from SVZ (Morshead et al., 1994). FGF-2 is a potent mitogen for NPCs isolated from adult hippocampus and other brain regions (Palmer et al., 1999). EGF and FGF-2 have synergistic proliferation effects on NPCs isolated from adult mouse brain (J. Ray, unpublished observations).

Both conditioned media and FGF-2 are required for NPCs to survive when cultured at low density. A glycosylated form of Cystatin (CCg) has been shown to be an essential component of the conditioned media. CCg is expressed in the subgranular layer of the DG in adult hippocampus, and exogenous CCg can increase NPC cell proliferation both in vitro and in vivo (Taupin et al., 2000; Taupin and Gage, 2002). Other growth factors, such as NT-3 and BDNF, have been shown to mildly increase neuronal differentiation without changing the proliferation rate of cultured NPCs (Palmer, Takahashi, and Gage, 1995). NGF has been shown to affect NPC proliferation/differentiation in vitro (Cameron, Hazel, and McKay, 1998). IGF-1 can increase NPC cell proliferation in vitro and can also influence NPC cell fate in terms of what type of neurotransmitters the differentiated neurons secrete (Anderson et al., 2002). TGF-β family members and its subfamily, BMPs, have been shown to affect the NPC cell fate (Cameron, Hazel, and McKay, 1998).

Regional selectivity of neurogenesis in the adult brain

Apart from understanding how neurogenesis is regulated, it is of interest to study why neurogenesis exists only in restricted areas in the adult mammalian brain. At the molecular level, there are two possible explanations: (1) differences in the intrinsic properties of different NPCs residing in the neurogenic region versus the non-neurogenic region, and (2) different environmental cues elicited by the neurogenic environment versus the non-neurogenic environment dictate NPC fate.

Both mechanisms may play critical roles in the process. NPCs isolated from non-neurogenic regions of the brain had to be cultured in the presence of FGF-2 for several passages before they differentiated into neurons, whereas NPCs isolated from DG could differentiate into neurons immediately after being isolated from the brain (Palmer et al., 1999). However, in a recent study it was reported that cells from the non-neurogenic substantia nigra could differentiate into neurons directly (Lie et al., 2002). Furthermore, NPCs isolated from the hippocampus could differentiate into neurons, astrocytes, and oligodendrocytes when treated with RA and 0.5% FBS for 2 weeks, resulting in about 10% neurons and 10%–20% oligodendrocytes (Palmer, Takahashi, and Gage, 1997). NPCs isolated from spinal cord treated with the same condition, however, gave rise to over 50% oligodendrocytes, 10% neurons, and less than 10% astrocytes (Gage laboratory observation). These observations indicate that even though multipotent NPCs can be isolated from many different brain regions, there are some intrinsic differences in freshly isolated NPCs. Such differences can be diminished in cell culture in the presence of growth factors.

Environmental factors appear to be critical in determining NPC fate. First, when cultured multipotent NPCs isolated from spinal cord (SC) were grafted back into the brain, they differentiated into neurons only in DG and SVZ. In SC and other non-neurogenic brain regions, grafted NPCs only differentiated into glia, indicating that local environments play critical roles in determining NPC cell fate (Shihabuddin et al., 2000; Lie et al., 2002). Second, coculture of GFP-labeled NPCs with primary astrocytes showed that astrocytes isolated from the hippocampus and SC of newborns and adults have distinct effects on NPC neuronal differentiation in vitro. Astrocytes from the newborn hippocampus have the strongest neuronal lineage-promoting effect, whereas the astrocytes from adult SC have the strongest neurogenesis-inhibiting effects (Song, Stevens, and Gage, 2002).

Conclusions

We now know something about the remarkable process of neurogenesis in the adult brain. Neurogenesis is a process that includes cell proliferation, survival, migration, fate choices, differentiation, and integration. Neurogenesis occurs in the olfactory bulb and DG of the hippocampus in all mammals studied, from mouse to man. The cells that become neurons are generated from stem cells that exist throughout life in the adult brain. The local environment where the cells are born determines to a large extent the fate of the cells. We also know that the process of neurogenesis is highly regulated by experience and disease. We are only at the very beginning of understanding all the factors that affect neurogenesis, but certainly genetics and aging are key factors. We do know that the newly born cells are functional upon integration, but the time course of integration is longer than the parallel process in development.

There is much to learn about this remarkable process, including the nature and identity of the authentic stem cell that gives rise to the new neurons. We also need a detailed molecular understanding of the cellular and molecular controls of the process. However, the biggest task is to understand the systems function of neurogenesis. Why has neurogenesis been selected for evolutionarily, and why does it occur only in limited areas of the brain? Finally, are there lessons that we can learn about the process of neurogenesis in the limited regions where it does occur that could inform us about how to generate new neurons in other parts of the brain?

REFERENCES

ABERG, M. A., N. D. ABERG, H. HEDBACKER, J. OSCARSSON, and P. S. ERIKSSON 2000. Peripheral infusion of IGF-I selectively induces neurogenesis in the adult rat hippocampus. *J. Neurosci.* 20:2896–2903.

ALTMAN, J., and G. D. DAS, 1965. Autoradiographic and histological evidence of postnatal neurogenesis in rats. *J. Comp. Neurol.* 124:319–335.

ANDERSON, M. F., M. A. ABERG, M. NILSSON, and P. S. ERIKSSON, 2002. Insulin-like growth factor-I and neurogenesis in the adult mammalian brain. *Brain Res. Dev. Brain Res.* 134:115–122.

BAI, F., M. BERGERON, and D. L. NELSON, 2003. Chronic AMPA receptor potentiator (LY451646) treatment increases cell proliferation in adult rat hippocampus. *Neuropsychopharmacology* 44:1013–1021.

BANASR, M., M. HERY, J. M. BREZUN, and A. DASZUTA, 2001. Serotonin mediates oestrogen stimulation of cell proliferation in the adult dentate gyrus. *Eur. J. Neurosci.* 14:1417–1424.

BARNEA, A., and F. NOTTEBOHM, 1994. Seasonal recruitment of hippocampal neurons in adult free-ranging black-capped chickadees. *Proc. Natl. Acad. Sci. U.S.A.* 91:11217–11221.

BELVINDRAH, R., G. ROUGON, and G. CHAZAL, 2002. Increased neurogenesis in adult mCD24-deficient mice. *J. Neurosci.* 22:3594–3607.

BERMAN, D. M., S. S. KARHADKAR, A. R. HALLAHAN, J. I. Pritchard, C. G. Eberhart, D. N. Watkins, J. K. Chen, M. K. Cooper, J. Taipale, J. M. Olson, and P. A. Beachy, 2002. Medulloblastoma growth inhibition by hedgehog pathway blockade. *Science* 297:1559–1561.

BIRD, A., 2002. DNA methylation patterns and epigenetic memory. *Genes Dev.* 16:6–21.

BREZUN, J. M., and A. DASZUTA, 1999. Depletion in serotonin decreases neurogenesis in the dentate gyrus and the subventricular zone of adult rats. *Neuroscience* 89:999–1002.

BROWN, J., C. M. COOPER-KUHN, G. KEMPERMANN, H. VAN PRAAG, J. WINKLER, F. H. GAGE, and H. G. KUHN, 2003. Enriched environment and physical activity stimulate hippocampal but not olfactory bulb neurogenesis. *Eur. J. Neurosci.* 17(10):2042–2046.

CAMERON, H. A., and E. GOULD, 1994. Adult neurogenesis is regulated by adrenal steroids in the dentate gyrus. *Neuroscience* 61(2):203–209.

CAMERON, H. A., T. G. HAZEL, and R. D. McKAY, 1998. Regulation of neurogenesis by growth factors and neurotransmitters. *J. Neurobiol.* 36:287–306.

CAMERON, H. A., B. S. McEWEN, and E. GOULD, 1995. Regulation of adult neurogenesis by excitatory input and NMDA receptor activation in the dentate gyrus. *J. Neurosci.* 15:4687–4692.

CAMERON, H. A., and R. D. McKAY, 1999. Restoring production of hippocampal neurons in old age. *Nat. Neurosci.* 2:894–897.

CAMERON, H. A., P. TANAPAT, and E. GOULD, 1998. Adrenal steroids and N-methyl-D-aspartate receptor activation regulate neurogenesis in the dentate gyrus of adult rats through a common pathway. *Neuroscience* 82:349–354.

CARLETON, A., L. T. PETREANU, R. LANSFORD, A. ALVAREZ-BUYLLA and P. M. LLEDO, 2003. Becoming a new neuron in the adult olfactory bulb. *Nat. Neurosci.* 6(5):507–518.

CARRO, E., A. NUNEZ, S. BUSIGUINA, and I. TORRES-ALEMAN, 2000. Circulating insulin-like growth factor I mediates effects of exercise on the brain. *J. Neurosci.* 20:2926–2933.

CHIANG, C., Y. LITINGTUNG, E. Lee, K. E. YOUNG, J. L. CORDEN, H. WESTPHAL, and P. A. BEACHY, 1996. Cyclopia and defective axial patterning in mice lacking Sonic hedgehog gene function. *Nature* 383:407–413.

CIARONI, S., R. CUPPINI, T. CECCHINI, P. FERRI, P. AMBROGINI, C. CUPPINI, P. DEL GRANDE, 1999. Neurogenesis in the adult rat dentate gyrus is enhanced by vitamin E deficiency. *J. Comp. Neurol.* 411(3):495–502.

COOPER-KUHN, C. M., M. VROEMEN, J. BROWN, H. YE, M. A. THOMPSON, J. WINKLER, and H. G. KUHN, 2002. Impaired adult neurogenesis in mice lacking the transcription factor E2F1. *Mol. Cell Neurosci.* 21:312–323.

CRAIG, C. G., V. TROPEPE, C. M. MORSHEAD, B. A. REYNOLDS, S. WEISS, and D. VAN DER KOOY, 1996. In vivo growth factor expansion of endogenous subependymal neural precursor cell populations in the adult mouse brain. *J. Neurosci.* 16:2649–2658.

DAWIRS, R. R., K. HILDEBRANDT, G. TEUCHERT-NOODT, 1998. Adult treatment with haloperidol increases dentate granule cell proliferation in the gerbil hippocampus. *J. Neural Transm.* 105:317–312.

DOETSCH, F., J. M. VERDUGO, I. CAILLE, A. ALVAREZ-BUYLLA, M. V. CHAO, and P. CASACCIA-BONNEFIL, 2002. Lack of the cell-cycle inhibitor p27Kip1 results in selective increase of transit-amplifying cells for adult neurogenesis. *J. Neurosci.* 22:2255–2264.

EISCH, A. J., M. BARROT, C. A. SCHAD, D. W. SELF, and E. J. NESTLER, 2000. Opiates inhibit neurogenesis in the adult rat hippocampus. *Proc. Natl. Acad. Sci. U.S.A.* 97:7579–7584.

ERIKSSON, P. S., E. PERFILIEVA, T. BJORK-ERIKSSON, A. M. ALBORN, C. NORDBORG, D. A. PETERSON, and F. H. GAGE, 1998. Neurogenesis in the adult human hippocampus. *Nat. Med.* 4:1313–1317.

FABEL, K., K. FABEL, B. TAM, D. KAUFER, A. BAIKER, N. SIMMONS, C. J. KUO, T. D. PALMER, 2003. VEGF is necessary for exercise-induced adult hippocampal neurogenesis. *Eur. J. Neurosci.* 18:2803–2812.

FENG, R., C. RAMPON, Y. P. TANG, D. SHROM, J. JIN, M. KYIN, B. SOPHER, M. W. MILLER, C. B. WARE, G. M. MARTIN, et al., 2001. Deficient neurogenesis in forebrain-specific presenilin-1 knockout mice is associated with reduced clearance of hippocampal memory traces. *Neuron* 32:911–926.

FUCHS, E., and G. FLUGGE, 1998. Stress, glucocorticoids and structural plasticity of the hippocampus. *Neurosci. Biobehav. Rev.* 23:295–300.

GAGE, F. H., 2002. Neurogenesis in the adult brain. *J. Neurosci.* 22:612–613.

GOLDMAN, S. A., and F. NOTTEBOHM, 1983. Neuronal production, migration, and differentiation in a vocal control nucleus of the adult female canary brain. *Proc. Natl. Acad. Sci. U.S.A.* 80:2390–2394.

GOMEZ-PINILLA, F., L. DAO, and V. SO, 1997. Physical exercise induces FGF-2 and its mRNA in the hippocampus. *Brain Res.* 764:1–8.

GOULD, E., H. A. CAMERON, D. C. DANIELS, C. S. WOOLLEY, and B. S. MCEWEN, 1992. Adrenal hormones suppress cell division in the adult rat dentate gyrus. *J. Neurosci.* 12:3642–3650.

GOULD E., B. S. MCEWEN, P. TANAPAT, L. A. GALEA, and E. FUCHS, 1997. Neurogenesis in the dentate gyrus of the adult tree shrew is regulated by psychosocial stress and NMDA receptor activation. *J. Neurosci.* 17(7):2492–2498.

GOULD, E., A. J. REEVES, M. FALLAH, P. TANAPAT, C. G. GROSS, and E. FUCHS, 1999. Hippocampal neurogenesis in adult Old World primates. *Proc. Natl. Acad. Sci. U.S.A.* 96:5263–5267.

GUERRA, D., A. SOLE, J. CAMI, and A. TOBENA, 1987. Neuropsychological performance in opiate addicts after rapid detoxification. *Drug Alcohol Depend.* 20:261–270.

JACOBS, B. L., H. VAN PRAAG, and F. H. GAGE, 2000. Adult brain neurogenesis and psychiatry: A novel theory of depression. *Mol. Psychiatry* 5:262–269.

JESSELL, T. M., and A. LUMSDEN, 1997. Inductive signals and the assignment of cell fate in the spinal cord and hindbrain. In *Molecular and Cellular Approaches to Neural Development*, W. M. Cowan, T. M. Jessell, and S. L. Zipursky, eds. Oxford, England: Oxford University Press.

JIN, K., Y. ZHU, Y. SUN, X. O. MAO, L. XIE, and D. A. GREENBERG, 2002. Vascular endothelial growth factor (VEGF) stimulates neurogenesis in vitro and in vivo. *Proc. Natl. Acad. Sci. U.S.A.* 99:11946–11950.

KAPLAN, M. S., and J. W. HINDS, 1977. Neurogenesis in the adult rat: Electron microscopic analysis of light radioautographs. *Science* 197:1092–1094.

KEMPERMANN, G., E. P. BRANDON, and F. H. GAGE, 1998. Environmental stimulation of 129/SvJ mice causes increased cell proliferation and neurogenesis in the adult dentate gyrus. *Curr. Biol.* 8:939–942.

KEMPERMANN, G., and F. H. GAGE, 2002. Genetic influence on phenotypic differentiation in adult hippocampal neurogenesis. *Brain Res. Dev. Brain Res.* 134:1–12.

KEMPERMANN, G., H. G. KUHN, and F. H. GAGE, 1997a. Genetic influence on neurogenesis in the dentate gyrus of adult mice. *Proc. Natl. Acad. Sci. U.S.A.* 94:10409–10414.

KEMPERMANN, G., H. G. KUHN, and F. H. GAGE, 1997b. More hippocampal neurons in adult mice living in an enriched environment. *Nature* 386:493–495.

KERNIE, S. G., T. M. ERWIN, and L. F. PARADA, 2001. Brain remodeling due to neuronal and astrocytic proliferation after controlled cortical injury in mice. *J. Neurosci. Res.* 66:317–326.

KORNACK, D. R., and P. RAKIC, 1999. Continuation of neurogenesis in the hippocampus of the adult macaque monkey. *Proc. Natl. Acad. Sci. U.S.A.* 96:5768–5773.

KORNACK, D. R., and P. RAKIC, 2001. Cell proliferation without neurogenesis in adult primate neocortex. *Science* 294:2127–2130.

KUHN, H. G., H. DICKINSON-ANSON, and F. H. GAGE, 1996. Neurogenesis in the dentate gyrus of the adult rat: Age-related decrease of neuronal progenitor proliferation. *J. Neurosci.* 16:2027–2033.

KUHN, H. G., J. WINKLER, G. KEMPERMANN, L. J. THAL, and F. H. GAGE, 1997. Epidermal growth factor and fibroblast growth factor-2 have different effects on neural progenitors in the adult rat brain. *J. Neurosci.* 17:5820–5829.

KULKARNI, V. A., S. JHA, and V. A. VAIDYA, 2002. Depletion of norepinephrine decreases the proliferation, but does not influence the survival and differentiation, of granule cell progenitors in the adult rat hippocampus. *Eur. J. Neurosci.* 16:2008–2012.

LAI, K., B. K. KASPAR, F. H. GAGE, and D. V. SCHAFFER, 2003. Sonic hedgehog regulates adult neural progenitor proliferation in vitro and in vivo. *Nat. Neurosci.* 6:21–27.

LEE, J., K. B. SEROOGY, and M. P. MATTSON, 2002. Dietary restriction enhances neurotrophin expression and neurogenesis in the hippocampus of adult mice. *J. Neurochem.* 80:539–547.

LICHTENWALNER, R. J., M. E. FORBES, S. A. BENNETT, C. D. LYNCH, W. E. SONNTAG, and D. R. RIDDLE, 2001. Intracerebroventricular infusion of insulin-like growth factor-I ameliorates the age-related decline in hippocampal neurogenesis. *Neuroscience* 107:603–613.

LIE, D. C., G. DZIEWCZAPOLSKI, A. R. WILLHOITE, B. K. KASPAR, C. W. SHULTS, and F. H. GAGE, 2002. The adult substantia nigra contains progenitor cells with neurogenic potential. *J. Neurosci.* 22:6639–6649.

LIM, D. A., A. D. TRAMONTIN, J. M. TREVEJO, D. G. HERRERA, J. M. GARCIA-VERDUGO, and A. ALVAREZ-BUYLLA, 2000. Noggin antagonizes BMP signaling to create a niche for adult neurogenesis. *Neuron* 28:713–726.

LIU, J., K. SOLWAY, R. O. MESSING, and F. R. SHARP, 1998. Increased neurogenesis in the dentate gyrus after transient global ischemia in gerbils. *J. Neurosci.* 18:7768–7778.

LOUISSAINT, A., JR., S. RAO, C. LEVENTHAL, and S. A. GOLDMAN, 2002. Coordinated interaction of neurogenesis and angiogenesis in the adult songbird brain. *Neuron* 34:945–960.

MAGAVI, S. S., B. R. LEAVITT, and J. D. MACKLIS, 2000. Induction of neurogenesis in the neocortex of adult mice. *Nature* 405:951–955.

MALBERG, J. E., A. J. EISCH, E. J. NESTLER, and R. S. DUMAN, 2000. Chronic antidepressant treatment increases neurogenesis in adult rat hippocampus. *J. Neurosci.* 20:9104–9110.

McEWEN, B. S., 1999. Stress and the aging hippocampus. *Front. Neuroendocrinol.* 20:49–70.

McMAHON, J. A., S. TAKADA, L. B. ZIMMERMAN, C. M. FAN, R. M. HARLAND, and A. P. McMAHON, 1998. Noggin-mediated antagonism of BMP signaling is required for growth and patterning of the neural tube and somite. *Genes Dev.* 12:1438–1452.

MENDEZ, J., T. M. KADIA, R. K. SOMAYAZULA, K. I. EL-BADAWI, and D. S. COWEN, 1999. Differential coupling of serotonin 5-HT1A and 5-HT1B receptors to activation of ERK2 and inhibition of adenylyl cyclase in transfected CHO cells. *J. Neurochem.* 73:162–168.

MONJE, M. L., S. MIZUMATSU, J. R. FIKE, and T. D. PALMER, 2002. Irradiation induces neural precursor-cell dysfunction. *Nat. Med.* 8:955–962.

MORSHEAD, C. M., B. A. REYNOLDS, C. G. CRAIG, M. W. McBURNEY, W. A. STAINES, D. MORASSUTTI, S. WEISS, and D. VAN DER KOOY, 1994. Neural stem cells in the adult mammalian forebrain: A relatively quiescent subpopulation of subependymal cells. *Neuron* 13:1071–1082.

NAKAGAWA, S., J. E. KIM, R. LEE, J. E. MALBERG, J. CHEN, C. STEFFEN, Y. J. ZHANG, E. J. NESTLER, and R. S. DUMAN, 2002. Regulation of neurogenesis in adult mouse hippocampus by cAMP and the cAMP response element-binding protein. *J. Neurosci.* 22:3673–3682.

NAKATOMI, H., T. KURIU, S. OKABE, S. YAMAMOTO, O. HATANO, N. KAWAHARA, A. TAMURA, T. KIRINO, and M. NAKAFUKU, 2002. Regeneration of hippocampal pyramidal neurons after ischemic brain injury by recruitment of endogenous neural progenitors. *Cell* 110:429–441.

ORMEROD, B. K., T. T. LEE, and L. A. GALEA, 2003. Estradiol initially enhances but subsequently suppresses (via adrenal steroids) granule cell proliferation in the dentate gyrus of adult female rats. *J. Neurobiol.* 55:247–260.

ORO, A. E., K. M. HIGGINS, Z. HU, J. M. BONIFAS, E. H. EPSTEIN, JR., and M. P. SCOTT, 1997. Basal cell carcinomas in mice overexpressing sonic hedgehog. *Science* 276:817–821.

PALMER, T. D., E. A. MARKAKIS, A. R. WILLHOITE, F. SAFAR, and F. H. GAGE, 1999. Fibroblast growth factor-2 activates a latent neurogenic program in neural stem cells from diverse regions of the adult CNS. *J. Neurosci.* 19:8487–8497.

PALMER, T. D., J. RAY, and F. H. GAGE, 1995. FGF-2-responsive neuronal progenitors reside in proliferative and quiescent regions of the adult rodent brain. *Mol. Cell. Neurosci.* 6:474–486.

PALMER, T. D., J. TAKAHASHI, and F. H. GAGE, 1997. The adult rat hippocampus contains primordial neural stem cells. *Mol. Cell. Neurosci.* 8:389–404.

PARENT, J. M., T. W. YU, R. T. LEIBOWITZ, D. H. GESCHWIND, R. S. SLOVITER, and D. H. LOWENSTEIN, 1997. Dentate granule cell neurogenesis is increased by seizures and contributes to aberrant network reorganization in the adult rat hippocampus. *J. Neurosci.* 17:3727–3738.

PATON, J. A., and F. N. NOTTEBOHM, 1984. Neurons generated in the adult brain are recruited into functional circuits. *Science* 225:1046–1048.

RADLEY, J. J., and B. L. JACOBS, 2002. 5-HT1A receptor antagonist administration decreases cell proliferation in the dentate gyrus. *Brain Res.* 955:264–267.

REPRESA, A., T. SHIMAZAKI, M. SIMMONDS, and S. WEISS, 2001. EGF-responsive neural stem cells are a transient population in the developing mouse spinal cord. *Eur. J. Neurosci.* 14:452–462.

REYNOLDS, B. A., and S. WEISS, 1992. Generation of neurons and astrocytes from isolated cells of the adult mammalian central nervous system. *Science* 255:1646.

RUSSO-NEUSTADT, A. A., R. C. BEARD, Y. M. HUANG, and C. W. COTMAN, 2000. Physical activity and antidepressant treatment potentiate the expression of specific brain-derived neurotrophic factor transcripts in the rat hippocampus. *Neuroscience* 101:305–312.

SANTARELLI, L., M. SAXE, C. GROSS, A. SURGET, F. BATTAGLIA, S. DULAWA, N. WEISSTAUB, J. LEE, R. DUMAN, O. ARANCIO, C. BELZUNG, and R. HEN, 2003. Requirement of hippocampal neurogenesis for the behavioral effects of antidepressants. *Science* 301:805–809.

SCHARFMAN, H. E., J. H. GOODMAN, A. L. SOLLAS, 2000. Granule-like neurons at the hilar/CA3 border after status epilepticus and their synchrony with area CA3 pyramidal cells: Functional implications of seizure-induced neurogenesis. *J. Neurosci.* 20:6144–6158.

SEKI, T., and Y. ARAI, 1995. Age-related production of new granule cells in the adult dentate gyrus. *Neuroreport* 6:2479–2482.

SHEN, J., R. T. BRONSON, D. F. CHEN, W. XIA, D. J. SELKOE, and S. TONEGAWA, 1997. Skeletal and CNS defects in Presenilin-1-deficient mice. *Cell* 89:629–639.

SHI Y., D. CHICHUNG LIE, P. TAUPIN, K. NAKASHIMA, J. RAY, R. T. YU, F. H. GAGE, and R. M. EVANS, 2004. Expression and function of orphan nuclear receptor TLX in adult neural stem cells. *Nature* 427(6969):78–83.

SHIHABUDDIN, L. S., P. J. HORNER, J. RAY, F. H. GAGE, 2000. Adult spinal cord stem cells generate neurons after transplantation in the adult dentate gyrus. *J. Neurosci.* 20:8727–8735.

SHINGO, T., C. GREGG, E. ENWERE, H. FUJIKAWA, R. HASSAM, C. GEARY, J. C. CROSS, and S. WEISS, 2003. Pregnancy-stimulated neurogenesis in the adult female forebrain mediated by prolactin. *Science* 299:117–120.

SILVA, A. J., J. H. KOGAN, P. W. FRANKLAND, and S. KIDA, 1998. CREB and memory. *Annu. Rev. Neurosci.* 21:127–148.

SMITH, W. C., and R. M. HARLAND, 1992. Expression cloning of noggin, a new dorsalizing factor localized to the Spemann organizer in *Xenopus* embryos. *Cell* 70:829–840.

SONG, H., C. F. STEVENS, and F. H. GAGE, 2002. Astroglia induce neurogenesis from adult neural stem cells. *Nature* 417:39–44.

TANAPAT, P., N. B. HASTINGS, A. J. REEVES, and E. GOULD, 1999. Estrogen stimulates a transient increase in the number of new neurons in the dentate gyrus of the adult female rat. *J. Neurosci.* 19:5792–5801.

TAUPIN, P., and F. H. GAGE, 2002. Adult neurogenesis and neural stem cells of the central nervous system in mammals. *J. Neurosci. Res.* 69:745–749.

TAUPIN, P., J. RAY, W. H. FISCHER, S. T. SUHR, K. HAKANSSON, A. GRUBB, and F. H. GAGE, 2000. FGF-2-responsive neural stem cell proliferation requires CCg, a novel autocrine/paracrine cofactor. *Neuron* 28(2):385–397.

TEMPLE, S., 2001. The development of neural stem cells. *Nature* 414:112–117.

TEUCHERT-NOODT, G., R. R. DAWIRS, and K. HILDEBRANDT, 2000. Adult treatment with methamphetamine transiently decreases dentate granule cell proliferation in the gerbil hippocampus. *J. Neural Transm.* 107:133–143.

TREJO, J. L., E. CARRO, and I. TORRES-ALEMÁN, 2001. Circulating insulin-like growth factor I mediates exercise-induced increases in the number of new neurons in the adult hippocampus. *J. Neurosci.* 21:1628–1634.

TRIMARCHI, J. M., and J. A. LEES, 2002. Sibling rivalry in the E2F family. *Nat. Rev. Mol. Cell. Biol.* 3:11–20.

TROPEPE, V., C. G. CRAIG, C. M. MORSHEAD, and D. VAN DER KOOY, 1997. Transforming growth factor-alpha null and senescent mice show decreased neural progenitor cell proliferation in the forebrain subependyma. *J. Neurosci.* 17:7850–7859.

VAN PRAAG, H., B. R. CHRISTIE, T. J. SEJNOWSKI, and F. H. GAGE, 1999. Running enhances neurogenesis, learning, and long-term potentiation in mice. *Proc. Natl. Acad. Sci. U.S.A.* 96: 13427–13431.

VAN PRAAG, H., G. KEMPERMANN, and F. H. GAGE, 1999. Running increases cell proliferation and neurogenesis in the adult mouse dentate gyrus. *Nat. Neurosci.* 2:266–270.

VAN PRAAG, H., G. KEMPERMANN, and F. H. GAGE, 2000. Neural consequences of environmental enrichment, *Nat. Rev. Neurosci.* 1:191–198.

VAN PRAAG, H., A. F. SCHINDER, B. R. CHRISTIE, N. TONI, T. D. PALMER, and F. H. GAGE, 2002. Functional neurogenesis in the adult hippocampus. *Nature* 415:1030–1034.

WAGNER, J. P., I. B. BLACK, and E. DICICCO-BLOOM, 1999. Stimulation of neonatal and adult brain neurogenesis by subcutaneous injection of basic fibroblast growth factor. *J. Neurosci.* 19:6006–6016.

WEISS, S., C. DUNNE, J. HEWSON, C. WOHL, M. WHEATLEY, A. C. PETERSON, and B. A. REYNOLDS, 1996. Multipotent CNS stem cells are present in the adult mammalian spinal cord and ventricular neuroaxis. *J. Neurosci.* 16:7599–7609.

WEN, P. H., X. SHAO, Z. SHAO, P. R. HOF, T. WISNIEWSKI, K. KELLEY, V. L. FRIEDRICH, JR. L. HO, G. M. PASINETTI, J. SHIOI, et al., 2002. Overexpression of wild type but not an FAD mutant presenilin-1 promotes neurogenesis in the hippocampus of adult mice. *Neurobiol. Dis.* 10:8–19.

YOSHIMURA, S., Y. TAKAGI, J. HARADA, T. TERAMOTO, S. S. THOMAS, C. WAEBER, J. C. BAKOWSKA, X. O. BREAKEFIELD, and M. A. MOSKOWITZ, 2001. FGF-2 regulation of neurogenesis in adult hippocampus after brain injury. *Proc. Natl. Acad. Sci. U.S.A.* 98:5874–5879.

ZHANG, R., L. ZHANG, Z. ZHANG, Y. WANG, M. LU, M. LAPOINTE, and M. CHOPP, 2001. A nitric oxide donor induces neurogenesis and reduces functional deficits after stroke in rats. *Ann. Neurol.* 50:602–611.

ZHAO, X., T. UEBA, B. R. CHRISTIE, B. BARKHO, M. J. MCCONNELL, K. NAKASHIMA, E. S. LEIN, B. EADIE, J. CHUN, K. LEE, and F. H. GAGE, 2003. Methyl-CpG binding protein 1 is important for neurogenesis and genomic stability in adult neural stem cells. *Proc. Natl. Aca. Sci. U.S.A.* 100:6777–6782.

ZHU, Y., K. JIN, X. O. MAO, and D. A. GREENBERG, 2003. Vascular endothelial growth factor promotes proliferation of cortical neuron precursors by regulating E2F expression. *FASEB J.* 17:186–193.

ZIGOVA, T., V. PENCEA, S. J. WIEGAND, and M. B. LUSKIN, 1998. Intraventricular administration of BDNF increases the number of newly generated neurons in the adult olfactory bulb. *Mol. Cell. Neurosci.* 11:234–245.

10 Stress, Deprivation, and Adult Neurogenesis

ELIZABETH GOULD

ABSTRACT   Perhaps the most basic of all structural changes in the brain is the addition of new neurons, a phenomenon known as neurogenesis. Although this process was once believed to be restricted to the embryonic or early postnatal period, neurogenesis is now recognized as a substantial process in some regions of the adult brain. In fact, the dentate gyrus adds thousands of new neurons every day throughout adulthood, raising intriguing questions about the regulation and significance of this phenomenon. The incorporation of new neurons into preexisting circuitry results in a cascade of structural changes that further increase the structural plasticity of this region. For example, new neurons elaborate axons and dendrites and undergo synaptogenesis. These progressive events are typically followed by a series of regressive phenomena, such as cell death, and probably process retraction and synapse elimination.

Coincident with the growing acceptance of adult neurogenesis as a significant phenomenon in the mammalian brain, numerous studies have identified several conditions that regulate its occurrence. These findings suggest possible functions for adult-generated neurons. This chapter considers the phenomenon of adult neurogenesis in the mammalian brain, with an emphasis on the dentate gyrus. It then reviews the regulation of dentate gyrus neurogenesis by both hormones and experience, with an emphasis on the impact of negative experiences such as stress and deprivation. Finally, the potential role these new cells may play in aspects of hippocampal function, such as learning, anxiety regulation, and control of endocrine systems, is explored. Some recent evidence suggesting unique properties of immature neurons is considered in light of the hypothesis that a continual influx of these cells to hippocampal circuitry has important functional consequences.

Brief historical overview of adult neurogenesis in the mammalian brain

About 40 years ago, the first evidence that new neurons are produced in the adult mammalian brain was reported. In a series of papers, Altman provided evidence that cells labeled in adulthood with the marker of DNA synthesis, ^{3}H-thymidine, had the morphological characteristics of neurons. These new neurons were observed in the dentate gyrus (DG), the olfactory bulb, and the neocortex of adult rats and cats (reviewed in Gross, 2000; Gould and Gross, 2002). This work had very little impact on the field at the time, as did a series

of studies that replicated and extended the work about 15 years later. At that time, Kaplan and colleagues reported ^{3}H-thymidine-labeled cells with the ultrastructural characteristics of neurons, including synapses on cell bodies and dendrites in these same brain regions (the DG, the olfactory bulb, and the neocortex) of adult rats. Despite the rather large number of papers published on this subject by the mid-1980s, adult neurogenesis in the mammalian brain did not gain credence until the late 1990s, when it was rediscovered using newer techniques (reviewed in Gross, 2000). At this time, multiple papers from several groups were published providing new evidence for adult neurogenesis in the DG of rats, mice, tree shrews, marmosets, macaques, and humans (Eriksson et al., 1998; reviewed in Gross, 2000). At around the same time, adult neurogenesis in the olfactory bulb was also substantiated. The case for the neocortex and other regions remains controversial. Some studies have reported new cells with neuronal characteristics in the neocortex of adult rodents and primates (Kaplan, 1981; Gould, Reeves, et al., 1999; Gould et al., 2001; Bernier et al., 2002; Galvez et al., 2002; Dayer, Cleaver, et al., 2003), while others have not (Kornack and Rakic, 2001; Koketsu et al., 2003). Recent reports have presented evidence for adult neurogenesis in additional areas, including the striatum (Bedard, Cossette, et al., 2002), the olfactory tubercle (Bedard, Levesque, et al., 2002), and the substantia nigra (Zhao et al., 2003), suggesting that neuron addition may be a feature of many brain regions, but these observations await confirmation.

Methodological considerations related to adult neurogenesis

To show that a new neuron has been produced in the adult brain, cell division must first be demonstrated. The traditional method for identifying cells that were generated at certain times is ^{3}H-thymidine autoradiography. For in vivo studies, this technique requires injecting ^{3}H-thymidine into live animals and then examining their brains at different survival times after injection. ^{3}H-thymidine is incorporated into cells during DNA synthesis in preparation for mitosis, and at long enough survival times, various techniques can be used to determine the phenotype of the daughter cells. This is the technique that was used by Altman and Kaplan in their pioneering work on adult neurogenesis. Although this

ELIZABETH GOULD   Department of Psychology, Program in Neuroscience, Princeton University, Princeton, N.J.

139

method is very powerful, it has some drawbacks, including that when used in combination with thick tissue sections it is incompatible with stereological methods for cell counting and it is difficult to determine the phenotype of the new cells without an electron microscope. To circumvent some of these problems, the bromodeoxyuridine (BrdU) labeling method has been used for studies of adult neurogenesis. Like ³H-thymidine, BrdU is incorporated into cells in S phase and can be used to label proliferating cells and their progeny. Unlike ³H-thymidine, however, BrdU is visualized using immunohistochemical methods and is amenable to stereological estimates of the total number of new cells as well as the unequivocal demonstration that new cells are colabeled with cell-type-specific markers. BrdU labeling has significantly advanced our understanding of adult neurogenesis and has shown, at least for the DG and olfactory bulb, that adult neurogenesis is substantial. However, a recent study has made it clear that our understanding of this technique was based on erroneous assumptions derived from developmental studies, and thus this phenomenon continues to be underestimated and, perhaps, misinterpreted. Cameron and McKay (2001) showed that the modal dose of BrdU for studies of adult neurogenesis (50 mg/kg) labels less than 50% of the total cells in S phase. When used during development, this dose appears to label all cells in S phase. Although BrdU is a small molecule, differences in metabolism or blood-brain barrier permeability prevent the adult animal from incorporating it at the same rate as in the developing animal. Higher doses of BrdU (up to 600 mg/kg) label more proliferating cells, do not label nonspecifically, and are not toxic to the cells or animals (Cameron and McKay, 2001). Using higher doses of BrdU, these authors showed that approximately 9000 new cells are generated every day in the DG of the adult rat; most differentiate into neurons. They estimate that every month, enough new granule cells are produced to compose approximately 6% of the total granule cell population.

Once cell division has been demonstrated, the neuronal phenotype of the new cells must be established. Support for adult neurogenesis can be obtained by showing that the adult-generated cells receive synaptic input, extend axons, express biochemical markers of neurons, and exhibit electrophysiological characteristics of neurons. All of these lines of evidence have now been reported for adult neurogenesis in the DG and olfactory bulb of adult rodents. The case for other brain regions is less complete and remains debated. If adult neurogenesis does occur in the neocortex and other regions, such as the striatum and substantia nigra, why was it overlooked until recently and not universally observed by all groups searching for similar evidence? One possible explanation is methodological differences related to BrdU labeling and staining for cell-type-specific markers. Technical variations, including the use of frozen tissue and harsh

pretreatments associated with some BrdU labeling protocols, may diminish the ability to visualize new cells with neuronal staining characteristics, particularly in regions where the level of neurogenesis is lower than that observed in the DG and olfactory bulb. Clearly, resolution of the question of how widespread adult neurogenesis is throughout the brain will require continued work in the area and the application of additional methods to the problem.

Adult neurogenesis in the dentate gyrus

In the DG, new cells originate from progenitor cells located in the structure itself. The progenitor cells have some characteristics of astroglia (Seri et al., 2001) and are primarily concentrated in the subgranular zone, the region between the granule cell layer and the hilus. The subgranular zone is not a distinct layer but rather a sporadic collection of progenitor cell clusters lining the deep aspect of the granule cell layer. Cells in this region divide, presumably asymmetrically, to produce some daughter cells that retain the ability to divide and others that become either neurons or glia. The new cells migrate the short distance to the granule cell layer and differentiate into neurons. Adult neurogenesis has been observed in the DG of virtually every mammalian species examined, including mice, voles, rats, cats, rabbits, guinea pigs, tree shrews, marmosets, macaques, and humans (reviewed in Gould and Gross, 2002), but it has been studied most extensively in rats. In this species, new cells have been shown to receive synaptic input, extend axons into the CA3 region, and express several biochemical markers of granule neurons, including NeuN, NSE, calbindin, MAP-2, and Tuj1. Adult-generated cells in the mouse DG have been shown to generate action potentials and exhibit other electrophysiological characteristics associated with granule cells (van Praag et al., 2002). A recent study has shown that some newly generated cells in the DG of adult rats, unlike granule cells, have the functional properties of inhibitory neurons (Liu et al., 2003). Although these findings may suggest that two subpopulations of new neurons exist in this brain region (one with excitatory properties and the other with inhibitory properties), an alternative possibility is that new neurons temporarily exhibit characteristics of inhibitory neurons as part of a natural process of maturation.

Given the magnitude of new neuron addition to the DG, the fact that over many decades neuroanatomists did not report other evidence for structural change in this intensively studied brain region is puzzling. If approximately 9000 new cells are added to the DG every day and if most of these cells extend axons, elaborate dendrites, and undergo synaptogenesis, some evidence of massive structural change should have been noticed. There are probably several reasons for this major oversight. First, neuron number in the DG appears to be tightly regulated. In addition to massive cell production, neurite extension, and synaptogenesis, there is also massive cell death, and probably neurite retraction, and synapse elimination. Traditional histological methods may have failed to reveal these dynamic processes because they do not result in changes in the size or shape of the brain region or in the numbers of cells, dendritic elements, or synapses. Second, because the prevailing view has been that structural change is a developmental, and not adult, phenomenon, evidence for such change was usually interpreted otherwise. A good example of this can be seen with descriptions of mossy fiber terminals in the CA3 region. Detailed neuroanatomical descriptions of the specialized synapses of mossy fibers on CA3 pyramidal cells, called excrescences, have described numerous morphological types of these terminals. Previously, these different types of terminals were presented as evidence that mossy fiber synapses were unusually complex. Given our current understanding of neurogenesis in the region, it seems reasonable to consider the possibility that these different types of synapses reflect different maturational stages of connections formed by newly generated granule cells.

Turnover of adult-generated cells

Recent studies have shown that several thousand new neurons are generated every day in the adult rat (Cameron and McKay, 2001). The addition of such a large number of new neurons in adulthood raises the issue of whether the hippocampal formation (and other regions that appear to add new neurons) continues to grow throughout life. Recent data suggest that there is substantial death of adult-generated cells in control rodents and primates that may offset the continual addition of new cells. The presence of pyknotic or degenerating cells in the DG, olfactory bulb, and frontal cortex supports this view. Do the new cells replace cells that were born during development or those born in adulthood? Recent evidence suggests that both of these possibilities may be the case. In the DG, cells generated during the first postnatal week of life, as well as those generated in adulthood, decrease in number with time following mitosis (Dayer, Ford, et al., 2003). However, the majority of dying cells appear to be generated in adulthood. Pyknotic cells within the DG are located primarily in the subgranular zone or deep in the granule cell layer, regions that contain progenitor cells and immature neurons. In addition, BrdU and ³H-thymidine labeling studies in adults suggest that the originally labeled population expands due to mitosis and then drops off in number. Coincident with the decrease in labeled cell number is the appearance of BrdU-labeled pyknotic cells (Gould, Beylin, et al., 1999). However, as discussed subsequently, the longevity of adult-generated neurons may be affected by environmental conditions, raising the question of whether information on the turnover

of newly produced cells is confounded by the abnormal conditions under which laboratory control animals exist. Thus, the natural life span of adult-generated neurons in the mammalian brain remains unknown.

Neurogenesis following damage

Several lines of evidence suggests that the ongoing processes of cell death and cell proliferation in the adult brain are causally linked. First, endocrine manipulations that alter survival of granule cells also affect the production of new cells in a similar fashion. For example, removal of circulating adrenal steroids by adrenalectomy results in massive death of granule cells, as well as an enhanced proliferation of granule cell precursors (Cameron and Gould, 1994). Second, specific lesion of the granule cell layer, created by mechanical or excitotoxic means, results in a compensatory increase in the proliferation of granule cell precursors and, ultimately, the production of new neurons (Gould and Tanapat, 1997). Third, experimental conditions associated with granule cell death, such as ischemia and seizures, result in increased granule cell neurogenesis (reviewed in Kozorovitskiy and Gould, 2003). Similar increases in neurogenesis have been observed in other brain regions, including the neocortex and striatum, following damage. These findings suggest two, not mutually exclusive scenarios: (1) dying granule cells send signals to progenitors to divide at a faster rate, or (2) the death of mature neurons releases progenitor cells from inhibition by eliminating a neurogenesis inhibitory signal. Both of these mechanisms, as well as the molecules responsible for stimulating and inhibiting neurogenesis, have been identified in other systems (reviewed in Hastings and Gould, 2003), but the relevance of these results to the adult DG remains unknown.

Hormonal regulation of adult neurogenesis

The hippocampal formation is a brain region that is particularly sensitive to hormones. Many cell types in the hippocampal formation contain hormone receptors, and this area responds to experimental hormone manipulations in adulthood with dramatic biochemical, molecular, and structural changes (reviewed in McEwen, 2002). Several studies have shown that the production of new neurons in the DG is sensitive to levels of circulating steroid hormones. This regulation can be in a negative direction, with the net effect being a decrease in the number of immature granule neurons, or in a positive direction, with the net effect being an increase in the number of new neurons (figure 10.1).

NEGATIVE EFFECTS: GLUCOCORTICOIDS Several studies have indicated that glucocorticoids inhibit the production of new neurons by decreasing the proliferation of granule cell precursors (Gould et al., 1992). During development, treating

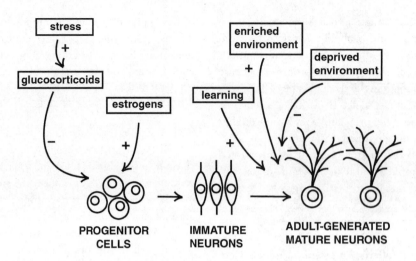

FIGURE 10.1 Some endocrine and experiential modulators of adult neurogenesis in the dentate gyrus. Estrogens, glucocorticoids, and stress affect proliferation of progenitor cells, whereas learning and environmental complexity may enhance the survival of neurons produced in adulthood.

rat pups with corticosterone decreases the production of new granule cells. In adulthood, removal of circulating adrenal steroids by adrenalectomy increases the proliferation of granule cell precursors and ultimately the production of new neurons. This phenomenon also occurs in aged animals in which granule cell production has diminished. Removal of adrenal steroids restores young adult levels of cell proliferation in the DG of old rats (Cameron and McKay, 1999).

The levels of circulating glucocorticoids change at different times of development, with experience, and across the diurnal rhythm, presenting the possibility that glucocorticoid inhibition of cell proliferation may reflect naturally occurring processes relevant to hippocampal function. A good example of this may be in observed in the DG of the meadow vole. Meadow voles are seasonal breeders, and the breeding season is associated with higher levels of circulating glucocorticoids in females; cell proliferation is suppressed at this time (Galea and McEwen, 1999).

POSITIVE EFFECTS: ESTROGEN   The ovarian steroid estrogen has a positive effect on the production of new cells in the DG of adult rats (Tanapat et al., 1999). Removal of estrogen by ovariectomy decreases the proliferation of new cells, while replacement of estrogen prevents this effect. Moreover, a natural fluctuation in the proliferation of granule cell precursors is evident across the estrous cycle; cell proliferation is highest during proestrus, the time of maximal estrogen levels. The stimulation of cell proliferation by estrogen results in a sex difference favoring females in the production of immature neurons. However, estrogen-related increases in the production of new cells are transient: by a few weeks after BrdU injection, no difference in the number of new cells can be detected. This raises the possibility that an understanding of the impact of estrogen-related differ-

ences in new neuron production is confounded by the manner in which laboratory animals are housed. Rodents living in the wild are unlikely to experience continual estrous cycles. The more likely hormonal profile for a wild rodent would be a single estrous cycle followed by pregnancy, parturition, and lactation. Thus, naturally occurring changes in the levels of ovarian steroids are more likely to be relevant under conditions such as pregnancy, puberty, or aging.

Regulation by experience

NEGATIVE REGULATION: STRESS   Many studies have shown that stressful experiences decrease the production of new granule cells during development and in adulthood (table 10.1). These studies have examined three different mammalian species, using species-relevant, naturalistic stressors. Exposure of postnatal and adult rats to the odors of natural predators decreases the rate of cell proliferation in the DG (Tanapat et al., 2001). This effect appears to be dependent on a stress-induced rise in adrenal hormones. Similar studies have been carried out in adult tree shrews and marmosets using stress paradigms of social subordination (Gould et al., 1997) and resident-intruder (Gould et al., 1998). In all cases, stress has been shown to decrease the proliferation of granule cell precursors and ultimately the production of immature neurons in the DG. Recent work suggests that certain types of stressors can persistently dampen neurogenesis even in adulthood. Malberg and Duman (2003) have shown that while both escapable and inescapable shock diminish cell proliferation in the DG, the inescapable version of this paradigm continues to inhibit new cell formation for more than a week after the stressor has subsided.

Table 10.1

Table 10.1

Studies examining effects of stress on cell proliferation in the dentate gyrus of late juvenile and adult animals

Stressor	Species	Effect on Cell Proliferation	References
Social stress (acute and chronic)	Tree shrews, marmosets	Diminished	Gould et al., 1997, 1998; Czéh et al., 2001
Predator odor	Rats	Diminished	Tanapat et al., 2001; Falconer and Galea, 2003
Electric shock	Rats	Diminished	Malberg and Duman, 2003
Restraint (chronic)	Rats	Diminished	Pham et al., 2003
Prenatal restraint	Rats	Diminished	Lemaire et al., 2000
Prenatal acoustic startle	Macaques	Diminished	Coe et al., 2003
Maternal separation	Rats	Diminished	Mirescu, Peters, and Gould, in press

Recent studies have demonstrated that developmental stress has a persistent impact on the later production of granule cells. In both rodents and monkeys, prenatal and early postnatal stress results in a persistent dampening of the proliferation of granule cell precursors in later life (Lemaire et al., 2000; Coe et al., 2003; Mirescu, Peter, and Gould, in press). Prenatal and postnatal stress are associated with persistent changes in the hypothalamic-pituitary-adrenal (HPA) axis, including the development of an inefficient shut-off mechanism for glucocorticoids. These findings present the possibility that new cell production is persistently inhibited in animals exposed to early life stressors because these animals experience higher than normal levels of glucocorticoids. The results also underscore the importance of knowing and controlling the developing environment of experimental animals. This may be particularly relevant to studies of nonhuman primates, which often involve animals without known developmental histories or even known birth dates. Unintended early life stress may result in persistently diminished neurogenesis and perhaps explain, in part, some of the quantitative as well as qualitative discrepancies in the literature on this subject.

Collectively, these findings support the view that the production of immature neurons in the DG varies depending on exposure to stressful experiences. Thus, the pool of immature neurons in the DG may be an important substrate by which stress has a longlasting effect on hippocampal function. However, to understand the potential impact of stress on hippocampal structure and function, it may be necessary to examine these issues in animals living in more natural environments. Animals living in laboratory control conditions appear to lose a larger proportion of adult-generated cells than those living in more complex environments (Kempermann, Kuhn, and Gage, 1997; Nilsson et al., 1999). Thus far, the effects of chronic stress on animals living in naturalistic, relatively complex environments have not been explored.

POSITIVE REGULATION: ENVIRONMENTAL COMPLEXITY AND LEARNING   The first evidence that environmental complex-

ity influences new hippocampal neurons in the adult was published by Barnea and Nottebohm (1994). This study showed that black-capped chickadees living in the wild maintained a higher number of new hippocampal neurons than those living in captivity. Similar findings were reported in the mouse and rat using the "enriched environment" paradigm; rodents living in enriched environments maintained more new granule cells than those living in standard laboratory cages (Kempermann, Kuhn, and Gage, 1997; Nilsson et al., 1999). There are many variables that differ between living in the wild and living in captivity, or between living in an enriched environment and living in a standard laboratory cage; among them are levels of stress, social interaction, physical activity, and learning. In addition to the report that birds living in complex environments have more new hippocampal neurons, a seasonal difference in new neuron number has been correlated with a seasonal difference in seed caching and retrieval. Since these behaviors are likely to involve spatial navigation learning, a function attributed to the hippocampal formation, a causative link between learning and new neurons has been proposed. Subsequently, it was shown that the number of new hippocampal neurons can be increased by engaging birds in learning tasks that involve this brain region (Patel, Clayton, and Krebs, 1997). Studies have shown a similar phenomenon in rodents: learning hippocampal-dependent tasks enhances the number of new granule cells, while other types of learning do not have such an effect (Gould, Beylin, et al., 1999). Specifically, the number of immature neurons in the DG is increased following spatial, but not visual, training in a Morris water maze. Similarly, trace eyeblink conditioning, but not delay eyeblink conditioning, increases the number of new granule cells in the DG (Gould, Beylin, et al., 1999; Leuner et al., in press). Although some evidence suggests that the effect of learning on the number of new neurons is the result of enhanced cell survival, the possibility that cell proliferation is additionally affected has not been ruled out (Lemaire et al., 2000). Because the hippocampus-dependent versions of the Morris water maze and eyeblink conditioning take more trials to acquire than the hippocampus-independent versions of these same tasks, it is possible that new cells respond especially to tasks that are more difficult. Although no study has yet matched task difficulty of hippocampus-dependent and independent learning paradigms and examined new cell number, it is potentially instructive to consider the fact that place learning in a Morris water maze (a hippocampus-dependent task) is considerably easier (in terms of number of trials required to reach criterion) than delay eyeblink conditioning (a hippocampus-independent task).

ENRICHMENT OR DEPRIVATION? Numerous studies have investigated structural changes in the brain associated with rearing or living in "enriched" environments. These studies have found several differences in brain regions of animals living in the more complex environment (see Jones et al., 1997). In these rodent studies, the enriched environment typically consists of a larger living space, more conspecifics, toys, tunnels, exercise equipment, and often a more varied diet than that available to controls. Living in this type of environment enhances performance on learning tasks and also increases the number of dendrites, the number of glial cells, and the number of new granule cells compared with controls. The most common interpretation of these findings is that brain structure and function are responsive to environmental complexity. A converse interpretation is that these are deprivation effects, that is, that the brain and behavior of control animals are abnormal due to the absence of normal stimulation. This puzzle could be solved by providing evidence for differences in animals living in super-complex versus complex environments. No evidence like this exists. These studies may indicate that standard control animals, be they birds living in aviaries or rodents living in laboratory cages, are living in a very deprived state. Given the social requirements of primates, it is likely that monkeys living in standard laboratory cages are having grossly abnormal and deprived experiences. To date, no studies have demonstrated the effects of environmental enrichment on adult neurogenesis in primate brains. Differences in the living conditions of nonhuman primates in various laboratories may result in differences in the numbers of new neurons produced in the brains of these animals. The extent to which such differences explain discrepancies in the literature regarding adult neurogenesis remains to be determined.

Features of adult-generated cells

Although a substantial number of new neurons are produced in the DG in adulthood, the majority of granule cells originate during development. Thus, the granule cell layer consists of neurons ranging in age from hours to years. Although many thousands of new neurons are added to this area every day, this is a relatively small proportion of cells when considered in relation to the large number of mature granule neurons produced during development (the total number of granule neurons is approximately 1–2 million in the adult rat). For these cells to have an impact on hippocampal function, they must have unique functional properties that empower them in a way that is unequal to the impact of mature granule cells. Some evidence suggests that this may be the case.

STRUCTURAL CHARACTERISTICS OF ADULT-GENERATED NEURONS Adult-generated neurons are likely to have structural characteristics that differ from those of developmentally generated neurons. These structural differences may enable a relatively small number of immature neurons to have a proportionately larger effect on hippocampal physiology than the same number of mature neurons. For example, adult-generated cells are capable of undergoing rapid structural change, as evidenced by the fact that they have axons in distal CA3 within 4–10 days after mitosis (Hastings and Gould, 1999). This suggests a great capacity to form new connections, presumably under the appropriate environmental conditions. Recent retrograde tracer studies have reported differences in the axon terminal fields of granule neurons produced at different developmental time points; granule cells produced during development have axons that diverge longitudinally within the CA3 region, whereas those produced in adulthood may have more concentrated projections (Hastings et al., 2002). Although existing evidence suggests structural differences between mature and immature granule cells, more research is needed to determine the extent to which cells produced at different time points form different types of circuits within the hippocampal formation.

FUNCTIONAL CHARACTERISTICS OF ADULT-GENERATED NEURONS Evidence suggests that immature neurons may have different electrophysiological characteristics than mature neurons. For example, long-term potentiation (LTP) in the developing hippocampal formation lasts considerably longer than that in the adult hippocampal formation. Moreover, developing neurons have been shown to exhibit giant depolarizing action potentials and respond to GABA with depolarization instead of hyperpolarization. These data from developing hippocampal slices have presented the possibility that adult-generated cells are transiently developmental in nature, at least for a short time after their generation. Indeed, recent evidence suggests this is the case. Immature granule cells in the DG of the adult rat may have longer lasting LTP than mature granule cells (Wang, Scott, and Wojtowicz, 2000). Moreover, this form of LTP is insensitive to inhibition by GABA, unlike that of mature granule cells (Snyder, Kee, and Wojtowicz, 2001; Schmidt-Hieber, Jonas, and Bischofberger, 2004). These findings support the view that a relatively small population of immature granule cells could exert a substantial functional influence over the hippocampal formation. However, this research remains in its infancy. Much work is needed to determine the functional characteristics of new neurons in the DG.

Possible functions of new neurons

The daily production of thousands of new granule cells and their incorporation into the existing circuitry is costly in terms of energy expenditure. It is likely that these new cells are not produced merely to replace older cells that die, because existing evidence suggests that a substantial amount of cell death occurring in this region involves the adult-generated population. Thus, the continual influx of new cells may provide an important mechanism for some aspect of hippocampal function that cannot be achieved with a structure consisting of mature neurons exclusively.

A ROLE IN LEARNING? The existence of a large pool of immature neurons in a brain region that is important for certain types of learning and memory raises the possibility that these new cells participate in such a function. Although most theories of learning do not involve new neurons, many ideas about hippocampal function are compatible with a role for new granule neurons. One idea is that the hippocampal formation acts to associate discontiguous events, that is, stimuli that are separated by space or time (Wallenstein, Eichenbaum, and Hasselmo, 1998). A persisting addition of new neurons, accompanied by rapid synapse formation, may play a role in connecting stimuli with discontiguous parameters. Several studies support the view that the hippocampal formation plays a temporary role in storing new memories. This idea is supported by data showing that recent, but not remote, memories for certain information are eliminated by lesions of the hippocampal formation (Squire and Zola-Morgan, 1991). A rapidly changing population of adult-generated neurons with unique functional properties may serve as a substrate for a temporary role of the hippocampal formation in information storage. Neurons produced in adulthood might play a role in information processing during a short time after their generation. The new cells might degenerate or undergo changes in connectivity, gene expression, or both, around the time that the hippocampal formation no longer plays a role in the storage of that particular memory. A temporary role for adult-generated granule neurons in learning has been suggested in canaries, in which seasonal changes in song correlate with the transient recruitment of more new neurons into the relevant circuitry (Nottebohm, 1985).

Thus, some theories of hippocampal learning are consistent with a role for new neurons but do any data exist to support this possibility? Several studies have presented interesting positive correlations between the number of new hip-

pocampal neurons and learning. For example, conditions that increase the number of new granule neurons also improve performance on hippocampal-dependent tasks (Gould, Beylin, et al., 1999). Among the factors that enhance the number of new neurons as well as hippocampal-dependent learning are estrogen treatment and living in an enriched environment. Conversely, situations that decrease the number of new hippocampal neurons have been shown to impair performance on these tasks. Among the factors that diminish the number of new neurons and learning are glucocorticoid treatment and stress.

However, some recent studies have found either no relationship between learning and the number of new neurons or, in fact, an inverse relationship. With regard to the first case, aging is associated with a decline in new cell production in the hippocampus, and yet this decrease does not appear to be associated with impaired performance on hippocampus-dependent tasks (Merrill et al., 2003). With regard to the second case, chronic stress has been shown to persistently inhibit neurogenesis in tree shrews, and yet this experience was associated with improved, not impaired, performance on a specific spatial navigation learning task (Bartolomucci et al., 2002). Do these negative findings indicate that new neurons are not involved in learning? Perhaps, but they may indicate that new neurons only affect hippocampal function under certain conditions. Since stress, aging, and environmental complexity all influence multiple brain measures, in addition to neurogenesis, it is possible that changes in new neuron number relate to learning only when imposed upon a particular neural background and under certain learning circumstances. For example, declining new neuron number may fail to correlate with learning impairments because of other age-associated changes, such as diminished numbers of synapses (Morrison and Hof, 2002).

When examining data related to the issue of adult neurogenesis and learning, it is important to note that new cells are likely to require some time for integration into existing circuitry. Thus, acute changes in cell proliferation are not likely to influence hippocampal function until a certain time period has passed. Similarly, chronic changes in cell proliferation are more likely to have functional consequences because their effects may be additive and thus larger. This particular point may be well-illustrated by considering the acute and chronic effects of stress. Acute and chronic stress have been shown to diminish the proliferation of granule cell precursors in the DG. However, acute stress has been shown (with certain paradigms) to enhance learning, whereas chronic stress typically impairs learning (Shors, Chua, and Falduto, 2001; McEwen, 2002; but see Bartolomucci et al., 2002).

A more direct link between new neurons and learning has recently been reported. Treatment with the antimitotic agent methylmethazoxymethanol acetate (MAM) for 2 weeks diminishes the pool of new neurons by about 80%. If we assume that approximately 9000 new cells are produced every day in the dentate gyrus (126,000 per 2 weeks), then an 80% reduction is likely to result in a decrease of approximately 100,800 new cells during this time (about 5%–10% of the total number of granule cells). This form of treatment impairs performance on trace eyeblink conditioning (Shors, Mieseagaes, et al., 2001). By contrast, delay eyeblink conditioning, the hippocampus-independent version of the same task, is not affected by MAM treatment. Replenishment of immature neurons after cessation of MAM treatment results in the recovery of hippocampal function in the form of normal trace eyeblink conditioning. Two recent studies support these findings by demonstrating that focal irradiation, a treatment that inhibits cell proliferation in the DG, impairs hippocampus-dependent learning (Madsen et al., 2003; Raber et al., 2004). These results are particularly surprising, given that studies searching for behavioral changes following gross lesion of the hippocampus rarely find a learning impairment unless a very large percentage of the total hippocampal formation is destroyed. However, if the adult-generated cells have unusual properties that increase their efficacy compared with that of their developmentally generated counterparts, then this relatively small group of neurons may have a significant impact.

A recent study has demonstrated that other forms of hippocampus-dependent learning tasks are insensitive to a decrease in the number of new neurons. For example, spatial learning in a Morris water maze is unaffected by MAM treatment, as is contextual fear conditioning (a learning paradigm that may require the hippocampal formation) (Shors et al., 2002). Because both spatial learning in a Morris water maze and context fear conditioning are more rapidly acquired than trace eyeblink conditioning, the possibility that new cells are important only for training on difficult tasks is raised. This suggests either that new DG cells participate only in certain types of hippocampus-dependent learning (e.g., those that involve associating stimuli separated in time) or that some other effect of the drug is impairing this specific task through another mechanism. Collectively, these findings suggest that new neurons may play a role in certain types of learning but not others. Definitive information awaits the development of better methods for knocking out new neurons in the absence of nonspecific potentially deleterious effects.

A ROLE IN ANXIETY AND ENDOCRINE REGULATION? In addition to its widely recognized role as a brain region involved in learning and memory, the hippocampal formation plays a less publicized role in the regulation of anxiety and endocrine function. Lesions of the hippocampus significantly alter performance on measures of anxiety in rats, suggesting that this brain region is involved in modulating reaction in potentially threatening situations (Bannerman et al., 2003). Lemaire and colleagues (1999) have noted an interesting negative correlation between the rate of cell proliferation in the hippocampus and reaction to novelty, a possible measure of anxiety. A recent study suggests that adult-generated neurons may be involved in regulating anxiety responses to antidepressant treatment (Santorelli et al., 2003). In this study, adult mice that had reduced neurogenesis in the hippocampus as a result of focal irradiation did not show the normal antidepressant-induced alleviation of anxiety symptoms. These findings present the possibility that new neurons may be involved in some of the therapeutic actions of antidepressants, an idea previously suggested by the work of Duman, Nakagawa, and Malberg (2001).

Lesions of the hippocampus have also revealed that this brain structure participates in the endocrine response to stress. That is, destruction of the hippocampal formation prevents the efficient return of glucocorticoid levels to their basal state after stress (Feldman and Conforti, 1980). Research into the effects of early stressors on the development of the HPA axis and adult neurogenesis has revealed potential links between adult-generated neurons and this hippocampal function. That is, prenatal and postnatal stress results in persistent changes in the HPA axis in the form of inefficient shut-off of the stress response in adulthood. Early stressors have additionally been shown not only to diminish cell proliferation in an acute manner but also to permanently dampen the production of new neurons, even in adulthood (Lemaire et al., 2000; Coe et al., 2003; Mirescu et al., in press). These findings raise the as yet untested possibility that adult-generated neurons play an important role in regulating the HPA axis. Studies designed to examine the effects of specific depletion of adult-generated neurons on the shut-off of the stress response could test this view.

Most research on the development of the HPA axis has been based on observations that individuals suffering from psychiatric conditions, such as depression and posttraumatic stress disorder, show signs of HPA axis dysregulation and diminished hippocampal volume on MRI studies (Bremner et al., 1995; Sheline et al., 1996; Newport, Stowe, and Nemeroff, 2002; Manji et al., 2003). Although the mechanisms that underlie diminished hippocampal volume in these conditions are unknown, it is possible that persistently decreased neurogenesis contributes to this clinical finding. Interestingly, these conditions are also associated with impaired learning, but the mechanisms that underlie these cognitive changes remain unknown.

Conclusions

Several decades after the first series of reports of adult neurogenesis in the mammalian brain, the phenomenon has been verified for the DG and olfactory bulb (the case for other brain regions remains open for further investigation). In the DG, the number of new granule cells produced in adulthood is substantial. The production and survival of these cells appear to be under the influence of various factors, including hormones, stress, environmental complexity, deprivation, and learning. These observations may provide clues to the potential function of adult neurogenesis. Although these studies are in their infancy and await the development of novel techniques, initial attempts to investigate the influence of a lack of new neurons on hippocampal function have suggested that these cells may play a role in certain types of learning, anxiety regulation, and possibly regulation of the stress response.

REFERENCES

BANNERMAN, D. M., M. GRUBB, R. M. DEACON, B. K. YEE, J. FELDON, and J. N. RAWLINS, 2003. Ventral hippocampal lesions affect anxiety but not spatial learning. *Behav. Brain Res.* 139: 197–213.

BARNEA, A., and F. NOTTEBOHM, 1994. Seasonal recruitment of hippocampal neurons in adult free-ranging black-capped chickadees. *Proc. Natl Acad. Sci. U.S.A.* 91:11217–11221.

BARTOLOMUCCI, A., G. DE BIURRUN, B. CZÉH, M. VAN KAMPEN, and E. FUCHS, 2002. Selective enhancement of spatial learning under chronic psychosocial stress. *Eur. J. Neurosci.* 15:1863–1866.

BEDARD, A., M. COSSETTE, M. LEVESQUE, and A. PARENT, 2002. Proliferating cells can differentiate into neurons in the striatum of normal adult monkey. *Neurosci. Lett.* 16328:213–216.

BEDARD, A., M. LEVESQUE, P. J. BERNIER, and A. PARENT, 2002. The rostral migratory stream in adult squirrel monkeys: Contribution of new neurons to the olfactory tubercle and involvement of the antiapoptotic protein Bcl-2. *Eur. Neurosci.* 16:1917–1924.

BERNIER, P. J., A. BEDARD, J. VINET, M. LEVESQUE, and A. PARENT, 2002. Newly generated neurons in the amygdala and adjoining cortex of adult primates. *Proc. Natl. Acad. Sci. U.S.A.* 99: 11464–11469.

BREMNER, J. D., P. RANDALL, T. M. SCOTT, R. A. BRONEN, J. P. SEIBYL, S. M. SOUTHWICK, R. C. DELANEY, G. MCCARTHY, D. S. CHARNEY, and R. B. INNIS, 1995. MRI-based measurement of hippocampal volume in patients with combat-related posttraumatic stress disorder. *Am. J. Psychiatry* 152:973–981.

CAMERON, H. A., and E. GOULD, 1994. Adult neurogenesis is regulated by adrenal steroids in the dentate gyrus. *Neuroscience* 61:203–209.

CAMERON, H. A., and R. D. MCKAY, 1999. Restoring production of hippocampal neurons in old age. *Nat. Neurosci.* 2:894–897.

CAMERON, H. A., and R. D. MCKAY, 2001. Adult neurogenesis produces a large pool of new granule cells in the dentate gyrus. *J. Comp. Neurol.* 435:406–417.

COE, C. L., M. KRAMER, B. CZÉH, E. GOULD, A. J. REEVES, C. KIRSCHBAUM, and E. FUCHS, 2003. Prenatal stress diminishes neurogenesis in the dentate gyrus of juvenile rhesus monkeys. *Biol. Psychiatry* 54:1025–1034.

CZÉH, B., T. MICHAELIS, T. WATANABE, J. FRAHM, G. DE BIURRUN, M. VAN KAMPEN, A. BARTOLOMUCCI, and E. FUCHS, 2001. Stress-induced changes in cerebral metabolites, hippocampal volume, and cell proliferation are prevented by antidepressant treatment with tianeptine. *Proc. Natl. Acad. Sci. U.S.A.* 98:12796–12801.

DAYER, A. G., K. M. CLEAVER, T. G. ABOUANTOUN, and H. A. CAMERON, 2003. Newborn neurons in the adult neocortex and striatum may be generated from different precursor populations. *SFN Abstracts* 671.1.

DAYER, A. G., A. A. FORD, K. M. CLEAVER, M. YASSAEE, and H. A. CAMERON, 2003. Short-term and long-term survival of new neurons in the rat dentate gyrus. *J. Comp. Neurol.* 9460:563–572.

DUMAN, R. S., S. NAKAGAWA, and J. MALBERG, 2001. Regulation of adult neurogenesis by antidepressant treatment. *Neuropsychopharmacology* 25:836–844.

ERIKSSON, P. S., E. PERFILIEVA, T. BJORK-ERIKSSON, A. M. ALBORN, C. NORDBORG, D. A. PETERSON, and F. H. GAGE, 1998. Neurogenesis in the adult human hippocampus. *Nat. Med.* 4:1313–1317.

FALCONER, E. M., and L. A. GALEA, 2003. Sex differences in cell proliferation, cell death and defensive behavior following acute predator odor stress in adult rats. *Brain Res.* 975:22–36.

FELDMAN, S., and N. CONFORTI, 1980. Participation of the dorsal hippocampus in the glucocorticoid feedback effect on adrenocortical activity. *Neuroendocrinology* 30:52–55.

GALEA, L. A., and B. S. MCEWEN, 1999. Sex and seasonal differences in the rate of cell proliferation in the dentate gyrus of adult wild meadow voles. *Neuroscience* 89:955–964.

GALVEZ, R., P. SOSKIN, J. CHO, A. GROSSMAN, and W. GREENOUGH, 2002. Voluntary exercise increases the number of new neurons in the adult rat motor cortex in a time dependent fashion. *SFN Abstr.* 442.1.

GOULD, E., A. BEYLIN, P. TANAPAT, A. REEVES, and T. J. SHORS, 1999. Learning enhances adult neurogenesis in the hippocampal formation. *Nat. Neurosci.* 2:260–265.

GOULD, E., H. A. CAMERON, D. C. DANIELS, C. S. WOOLLEY, and B. S. MCEWEN, 1992. Adrenal hormones suppress cell division in the adult rat dentate gyrus. *J. Neurosci.* 12:3642–3650.

GOULD, E., and C. G. GROSS, 2002. Neurogenesis in adult mammals: Some progress and problems. *J. Neurosci.* 22:619–623.

GOULD, E., B. S. MCEWEN, P. TANAPAT, L. A. GALEA, and E. FUCHS, 1997. Neurogenesis in the dentate gyrus of the adult tree shrew is regulated by psychosocial stress and NMDA receptor activation. *J. Neurosci.* 17:2492–2498.

GOULD, E., A. J. REEVES, M. S. GRAZIANO, and C. G. GROSS, 1999. Neurogenesis in the neocortex of adult primates. *Science* 286: 548–552.

GOULD, E., and P. TANAPAT, 1997. Lesion-induced proliferation of neuronal progenitors in the dentate gyrus of the adult rat. *Neuroscience* 80:427–436.

GOULD, E., P. TANAPAT, B. S. MCEWEN, G. FLUGGE, and E. FUCHS, 1998. Proliferation of granule cell precursors in the dentate gyrus of adult monkeys is diminished by stress. *Proc. Natl. Acad. Sci. U.S.A.* 95:3168–3171.

GOULD, E., N. VAIL, M. WAGERS, and C. G. GROSS, 2001. Adult-generated hippocampal and neocortical neurons in macaques have a transient existence. *Proc. Natl. Acad. Sci. U.S.A.* 98: 10910–10917.

GROSS, C. G., 2000. Neurogenesis in the adult brain: Death of a dogma. *Nat. Rev. Neurosci.* 1:67–73.

HASTINGS, N. B., and E. GOULD, 1999. Rapid extension of axons into the CA3 region by adult-generated granule cells. *J. Comp. Neurol.* 413:146–154.

HASTINGS, N. B., and E. GOULD, 2003. Neurons inhibit neurogenesis. *Nat. Med.* 9:264–266.

HASTINGS, N. B., M. I. SETH, P. TANAPAT, T. A. RYDEL, and E. GOULD, 2002. Granule neurons generated during development extend divergent axon collaterals to hippocampal area CA3. *J. Comp. Neurol.* 452:324–333.

Jones, T. A., A. Y. Klintsova, V. L. Kilman, A. M. Sirevaag, and W. T. Greenough, 1997. Induction of multiple synapses by experience in the visual cortex of adult rats. *Neurobiol. Learn. Mem.* 68:13–20.

Kaplan, M. S., 1981. Neurogenesis in the 3-month-old rat visual cortex. *J. Comp. Neurol.* 195:323–338.

Kempermann, G., H. G. Kuhn, and F. H. Gage, 1997. More hippocampal neurons in adult mice living in an enriched environment. *Nature* 386:493–495.

Koketsu, D., A. Mikami, Y. Miyamoto, and T. Hisatsune, 2003. Nonrenewal of neurons in the cerebral neocortex of adult macaque monkeys. *J. Neurosci.* 23:937–992.

Kornack, D. R., and P. Rakic, 2001. Cell proliferation without neurogenesis in adult primate neocortex. *Science* 294:2127–2130.

Kozorovitskiy, Y., and E. Gould, 2003. Adult neurogenesis: A mechanism for brain repair? *J. Clin. Exp. Neuropsychol.* 25:721–732.

Lemaire, V., C. Aurousseau, M. Le Moal, and D. N. Abrous, 1999. Behavioural trait of reactivity to novelty is related to hippocampal neurogenesis. *Eur. J. Neurosci.* 11:4006–4014.

Lemaire, V., M. Koehl, M. Le Moal, and D. N. Abrous, 2000. Prenatal stress produces learning deficits associated with an inhibition of neurogenesis in the hippocampus. *Proc. Natl. Acad. Sci. U.S.A.* 97:11032–11037.

Leuner, B., S. Mendola-Loffredo, Y. Kozorovitskiy, D. Samburg, E. Gould, and T. J. Shors, in press. Learning enhances the survival of new neurons beyond the time when the hippocampus is required for memory. *J. Neurosci.*

Liu, S., J. Wang, D. Zhu, Y. Fu, K. Lukowiak, and Y. Lu, 2003. Generation of functional inhibitory neurons in the adult rat hippocampus. *J. Neurosci.* 23:732–736.

Madsen, T. M., P. E. Kristjansen, T. G. Bolwig, and G. Wortwein, 2003. Arrested neuronal proliferation and impaired hippocampal function following fractionated brain irradiation in the adult rat. *Neuroscience* 119:635–642.

Malberg, J. E., and R. S. Duman, 2003. Cell proliferation in adult hippocampus is decreased by inescapable stress: Reversal by fluoxetine treatment. *Neuropsychopharmacology* 28:1562–1571.

Manji, H. K., J. A. Quiroz, J. Sporn, J. L. Payne, K. A. Denicoff, N. Gray, C. A. Zarate, Jr., and D. S. Charney, 2003. Enhancing neuronal plasticity and cellular resilience to develop novel, improved therapeutics for difficult-to-treat depression. *Biol. Psychiatry* 53:707–742.

McEwen, B. S., 2002. Sex, stress and the hippocampus: Allostasis, allostatic load and the aging process. *Neurobiol. Aging* 23:921–939.

Merrill, D. A., R. Karim, M. Darraq, A. A. Chiba, and M. H. Tuszynski, 2003. Hippocampal cell genesis does not correlate with spatial learning ability in aged rats. *J. Comp. Neurol.* 459:201–207.

Mirescu, C., J. D. Peters, and E. Gould, in press. Early life experience alters response of adult neurogenesis to stress. *Nat. Neurosci.*

Morrison, J. H., and P. R. Hof, 2002. Selective vulnerability of corticocortical and hippocampal circuits in aging and Alzheimer's disease. *Prog. Brain Res.* 136:467–486.

Newport, D. J., Z. N. Stowe, and C. B. Nemeroff, 2002. Parental depression: Animal models of an adverse life event. *Am. J. Psychiatry* 159:1265–1283.

Nilsson, M., E. Perfilieva, U. Johansson, O. Orwar, and P. S. Eriksson, 1999. Enriched environment increases neurogenesis in the adult rat dentate gyrus and improves spatial memory. *J. Neurobiol.* 39:569–578.

Nottebohm, F., 1985. Neuronal replacement in adulthood. *Ann. N.Y. Acad. Sci.* 457:143–161.

Patel, S. N., N. S. Clayton, and J. R. Krebs, 1997. Spatial learning induces neurogenesis in the avian brain. *Behav. Brain Res.* 89:115–128.

Pham, K., J. Nacher, P. R. Hof, and B. S. McEwen, 2003. Repeated restraint stress suppresses neurogenesis and induces biphasic PSA-NCAM expression in the adult rat dentate gyrus. *Eur. J. Neurosci.* 17:879–886.

Raber, J., R. Rola, A. LeFevour, D. Morhardt, J. Curley, S. Mizumatsu, S. R. VandenBerg, and J. R. Fike, 2004. Radiation-induced cognitive impairments are associated with changes in indicators of hippocampal neurogenesis. *Radiat. Res.* 162:39–47.

Santorelli, L., M. Saxe, C. Gross, A. Surget, F. Battaglia, S. Sulawa, N. Weisstaub, J. Lee, R. Duman, O. Arancio, C. Belzung, and R. Hen, 2003. Requirement of hippocampal neurogenesis for the behavioral effects of antidepressants. *Science* 301:805–809.

Schmidt-Hieber, C., P. Jonas, and J. Bischofberger, 2004. Enhanced synaptic plasticity in newly generated granule cells of the adult hippocampus. *Nature* 429:184–187.

Seri, B., J. M. Garcia-Verdugo, B. S. McEwen, and A. Alvarez-Buylla, 2001. Astrocytes give rise to new neurons in the adult mammalian hippocampus. *J. Neurosci.* 21:7153–7160.

Sheline, Y. I., P. W. Wang, M. H. Gado, J. G. Csernansky, and M. W. Vannier, 1996. Hippocampal atrophy in recurrent major depression. *Proc. Natl. Acad. Sci. U.S.A.* 93:3908–3913.

Shors, T. J., C. Chua, and J. Falduto, 2001. Sex differences and opposite effects of stress on dendritic spine density in the male versus female hippocampus. *J. Neurosci.* 21:6292–6297.

Shors, T. J., G. Miesegaes, A. Beylin, M. Zhao, T. Rydel, and E. Gould, 2001. Neurogenesis in the adult is involved in the formation of trace memories. *Nature* 410:372–376.

Shors, T. J., D. A. Townsend, M. Zhao, Y. Kozorovitskiy, and E. Gould, 2002. Neurogenesis may relate to some but not all types of hippocampal-dependent learning. *Hippocampus* 12:578–584.

Snyder, J. S., N. Kee, and J. M. Wojtowicz, 2001. Effects of adult neurogenesis on synaptic plasticity in the rat dentate gyrus. *J. Neurophysiol.* 85:2423–2431.

Squire, L. R., and S. Zola-Morgan, 1991. The medial temporal lobe memory system. *Science* 253:1380–1386.

Tanapat, P., N. B. Hastings, A. J. Reeves, and E. Gould, 1999. Estrogen stimulates a transient increase in the number of new neurons in the dentate gyrus of the adult female rat. *J. Neurosci.* 19:5792–5801.

Tanapat, P., N. B. Hastings, T. A. Rydel, L. A. Galea, and E. Gould, 2001. Exposure to fox odor inhibits cell proliferation in the hippocampus of adult rats via an adrenal hormone-dependent mechanism. *J. Comp. Neurol.* 437:496–504.

van Praag, H., A. F. Schinder, B. R. Christie, N. Toni, T. D. Palmer, and F. H. Gage, 2002. Functional neurogenesis in the adult hippocampus. *Nature* 415:1030–1034.

Wallenstein, G. V., H. Eichenbaum, and M. E. Hasselmo, 1998. The hippocampus as an associator of discontiguous events. *Trends Neurosci.* 21:317–323.

Wang, S., B. W. Scott, and J. M. Wojtowicz, 2000. Heterogenous properties of dentate granule neurons in the adult rat. *J. Neurobiol.* 42:248–257.

Zhao, M., S. Momma, K. Delfani, M. Carlen, R. M. Cassidy, C. B. Johansson, H. Brismar, O. Shupliakov, J. Frisen, and A. M. Janson, 2003. Evidence for neurogenesis in the adult mammalian substantia nigra. *Proc. Natl. Acad. Sci. U.S.A.* 100:7925–7930.

11 Quantitative Analysis of Fetal and Adult Neurogenesis: Regulation of Neuron Number

RICHARD S. NOWAKOWSKI AND NANCY L. HAYES

ABSTRACT The proliferative populations in fetal and adult brain differ in fundamental ways. In both, the productive potential is proportional to the number of proliferating cells, inversely proportional to the cell cycle length, and highly influenced by cell fate decisions, i.e., re-entry into the cell cycle (P) vs exit to differentiate (Q). In the developing neocortex, the proliferative population is large but transient. Neuron production lasts ~6 days or 11 cell cycles. During this time the cell cycle lengthens from ~8 to ~18 hours, Q increases from 0 to1, and P decreases from 1 to 0. The neurons produced migrate to the cortical plate where ~25% die during the early postnatal period. In contrast, in the adult dentate gyrus, the proliferative population is small, consisting of ~1800 cells in a C57BL/6J mouse at P60, and persists for most of the lifetime of the animal, which means that P = Q = ~0.5. The cell cycle is about 12–14 hours long, so there are ~1000 cell cycles during the lifetime of a mouse. For each cell cycle, on average, 1 postproliferative cell is produced for each proliferating cell. In the postproliferative population, cell death begins within hours and lasts for 5–6 weeks with a half-life of ~8 days, and only ~30% of the postproliferative cells survive for 5–6 weeks. We estimate that in C57BL/6J mouse about 35% of these new cells become neurons for a net production of ~150–300 neurons per day. In addition, there is considerable genetic variation in all of these processes in different inbred strains of mice.

The properties of the proliferative populations in fetal and adult central nervous system (CNS) differ in fundamental ways, and a thorough understanding of neurogenesis requires a quantitative characterization of the dynamic aspects of each of these stem/progenitor populations. Both during development and in the adult brain, neurogenesis is tightly regulated by events surrounding and associated with cell proliferation in stem/progenitor populations. This is because the neurons in the adult brain are nonproliferative and have made an irreversible exit from the cell cycle during development (figure 11.1). This is in contrast to some other cell types of the body that either are formed by continuous cell proliferation (e.g., blood cells by the bone marrow, the

epithelium of the gut) or that can be prodded to reenter the cell cycle and to proliferate in response to an injury or other insult (see figure 11.1).

The key to understanding neurogenesis is the recognition that the productive capacity of any proliferating population is proportional to the number of proliferating cells, inversely proportional to the cell cycle length, and highly influenced by cell fate decisions, that is, either reentry into the cell cycle (P) or exit from the cell cycle to differentiate (Q). The cells of a proliferating population move through the cell cycle, synthesizing DNA to replicate their genomes, and then divide at mitosis into two daughter cells (figure 11.2). After each cell division, some of the daughters leave the cell cycle to mature into neurons or glia, but some remain in the proliferative population to divide again. At the level of the single dividing cell, one, both, or neither of the daughter cells can reenter the cell cycle (see figure 11.2). Hence, there are three kinds of cell division. If both daughter cells have the same proliferative fate, the cell division is said to be symmetrical. There are two types of symmetrical cell divisions: either both daughter cells can reenter the cell cycle (symmetrical nonterminal) or both can exit the cell cycle (symmetrical terminal). When one daughter cell reenters the cell cycle and one exits the cell cycle, the cell division is said to be asymmetrical.

The detection of a proliferating population is most commonly achieved with exogenous S phase markers. The most frequently used S phase markers are tritiated thymidine (^{3}H-TdR) and bromodeoxyuridine (BrdU), although other halogenated uridines (e.g., iododeoxyuridine [IUdR]) can also be used. These molecules are all analogues of the nucleotide thymidine, and because they are therefore incorporated into newly synthesized DNA, they are markers for DNA synthesis and not for proliferation per se. Because DNA synthesis occurs during the S phase of the cell cycle, proliferating cells are labeled by these markers. However, DNA synthesis also occurs during DNA repair (Katchanov et al., 2001), preapoptotically (Yang, Geldmacher, and Herrup, 2001), and in association with gene amplification (Kirsanova and Anisimov, 2001). Any cell that is synthesizing DNA during

RICHARD S. NOWAKOWSKI and NANCY L. HAYES Department of Neuroscience and Cell Biology, UMDNJ-Robert Wood Johnson Medical School, Piscataway, N.J.

149

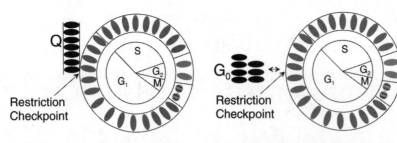

"Irreversible" exit from cell cycle (CNS, PNS, Cardiac Muscle)

Continuously Cycle (Bone Marrow, Gut, Skin) or Reversible Re-entry (Liver, Wound Healing)

FIGURE 11.1   During development the stem/progenitor cells in the CNS and a few other organs make an irreversible commitment to exit the cell cycle (left-hand side). In contrast, in many other tissues, cells retain the ability to proliferate either by remaining in the cell cycle (e.g., bone marrow, gut, skin) or by maintaining a G_0 state that allows them to reenter the cell cycle (right-hand side).

the time that the marker is available will take up that label and incorporate it into the new DNA. For cells in S phase of the proliferative cell cycle, only a short exposure to the marker is necessary to label the cells to a detectable level. For example, for either ^{3}H-TdR or BUdR, cells in S phase are detectably labeled within 10–15 minutes after a single exposure to the marker (Hayes and Nowakowski, 2000). The precursors themselves persist in the tissue longer than this period of time, and, depending on the method of detection, they can persist in concentrations large enough to label cells entering the S phase anywhere from about 30 minutes to several hours later (Nowakowski and Rakic, 1974; Takahashi, Nowakowski, and Caviness, 1992; Hayes and Nowakowski, 2000).

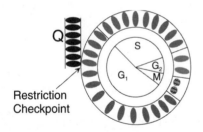

One, neither, or both daughter cells can re-enter the cell cycle

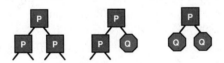

FIGURE 11.2   During the G_1 phase of the cell cycle, proliferating cells decide whether to reenter the S phase and divide again or to leave the cell cycle. The cells that exit the cell cycle are called Q cells (for "quiescent" or "quitting"); the cells that remain in the cell cycle are P cells (for "proliferating"). Because there are two daughter cells for each mitotic division, there are three possible combinations of fates with respect to the exit from the cell cycle: neither, one, or both daughter cells can exit the cell cycle. These types of cell division are called symmetrical nonterminal (S/NT), asymmetrical (A), and symmetrical terminal (S/T), respectively.

The method of detection of the exogenous S phase markers is an important consideration not just as an experimental detail but because different methods of detection can significantly affect the interpretation of the experiment. The main considerations here are (1) how sensitive the detection method is and (2) whether or not it is stoichiometric (figure 11.3). ^{3}H-TdR is detected autoradiographically. This method involves depositing a photographic emulsion on top of the tissue directly on the microscope slide (Rogers, 1973). The slide is then exposed for several days or even weeks, during which time the tritium decays and emits beta particles that activate the silver halide crystals in the emulsion; the silver halide crystals are then reduced to silver metal particles using standard photographic developers (Rogers, 1973). The number of silver grains over the nucleus is related to the number of tritium (^{3}H) atoms in the underlying DNA, the exposure time, the emulsion and developer used, and so on, but it is relatively linear over a wide range of conditions (Rogers, 1973). This means that the detection of ^{3}H-TdR is approximately stoichiometric; that is, the signal detected is approximately proportional to the amount of ^{3}H-TdR that is present. BUdR is detected immunohistochemically. This method involves several steps. In the first step a monoclonal antibody is used; this primary antibody recognizes the conformational changes that BUdR produces in single-stranded DNA that are not present when the native nucleotide thymidine is there (Gratzner, 1982). In the next steps, the bound primary antibody is detected, usually with a method that involves some amplification of the signal. For example, in one commonly used technique, a biotinylated secondary antibody and an avidin-biotin complex are used to multiply the number of reaction sites available to a final substrate (Hsu, Raine, and Fanger, 1981). By virtue of this molecular scaffold and the extraordinarily high affinity of avidin for biotin, the signal is amplified severalfold, but not stoichiometrically.

In the developing brain, there is extensive cell proliferation as the neurons and glial cells of the brain are produced. The proliferative populations are large but transient, and at

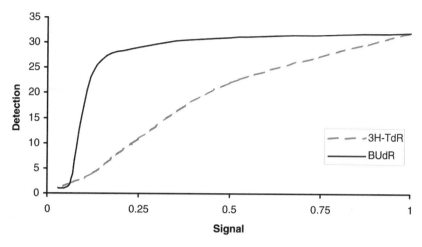

FIGURE 11.3   A schematic diagram of the difference between stoichiometric (for ³H-TdR) and nonstoichiometric (for BrdU) detection. For stoichiometric methods, the amount of substance detected (on the *y*-axis) is approximately proportional to the amount present in the tissue (*x*-axis). For nonstochiometric methods, the relationship is distinctly nonlinear, and there is no clear way to discern how much signal is actually present.

the end of the developmental period essentially all of the neurons of the adult brain have been produced (for review, see Nowakowski et al., 2002). In contrast, in the adult CNS there is only a small amount of continued cell proliferation, and it is generally accepted (for reviews, see Gage, 2002; Rakic, 2002; Taupin and Gage, 2002) that there are only two regions of the adult mammalian CNS in which both cell proliferation and neuron production continue. These regions are the subventricular zone (SVZ) surrounding the lateral ventricles and the subgranular zone of the hilus of the dentate gyrus (DG).

With respect to plasticity in the adult brain, it is essential to understand the behaviors of these proliferative populations and the contributions of their progeny to the structure and function of the brain. In the DG, we know that cells in the proliferating population divide and that some of the progeny become neurons and glia that persist and become incorporated into the granule cell layer. What is not known, however, is the magnitude of this phenomenon. How large is the proliferative population? What is the contribution of the progeny with respect to the extant neuronal population? We have begun to address these issues using some of the quantitative methods that we have developed to characterize proliferating populations and neuron production in the developing neocortex (Nowakowski et al., 2002). For our studies of cell proliferation in the adult brain, we have focused on the intrahilar region of the DG because its location is well-defined and well-circumscribed anatomically. These properties make it amenable to quantification.

Criteria for detecting cell proliferation

It is necessary to establish criteria for the detection of both cell proliferation and changes in cell proliferation. In most contemporary work, the detection of cell proliferation in the developing and adult brain is reported from labeling with BUdR. During normal development and in well-established normal adult situations (e.g., in the DG), this is probably adequate. However, caution must be used in equating changes observed in BUdR labeling in pathological or experimentally produced conditions. There are two reasons for this. First, BUdR labeling detects DNA synthesis, and although DNA synthesis is an integral part of proliferation, it also occurs in other situations, notably during DNA repair (Katchanov et al., 2001) and in a preapoptotic, abortive round of DNA replication (Yang, Geldmacher, and Herrup, 2001). It may also occur during gene amplification (Kirsanova and Anisimov, 2001), which may or may not exist in the brain. Second, pathological or other experimental conditions may modify the proliferative behavior of the cells being studied (e.g., may change the length of the cell cycle or some of its component phases). These two cautionary notes also apply to the use of antibodies directed against molecules involved in the cell cycle itself. Thus, it is clear that additional criteria are needed to establish that cell proliferation occurs. For BrdU studies, it is essential to show (1) that the labeled cells actually divide, and (2) that the number of cells that divide is commensurate with the number that are labeled. There are quite simple ways to do this. First, one could show that at an appropriate time after labeling with BrdU there are labeled mitotic figures, that is, cells exhibiting the chromosomal arrangements associated with metaphase. Indeed, within a few hours (i.e., the length of the $G_2 + M$ phases of the cell cycle), 100% of the mitotic figures should be labeled (Cai, Hayes, and Nowakowski, 1997b). The labeled mitotic figures should continue to be present for a time at least equal to the length of the S phase. An alternative is simply to show that after a survival time appropri-

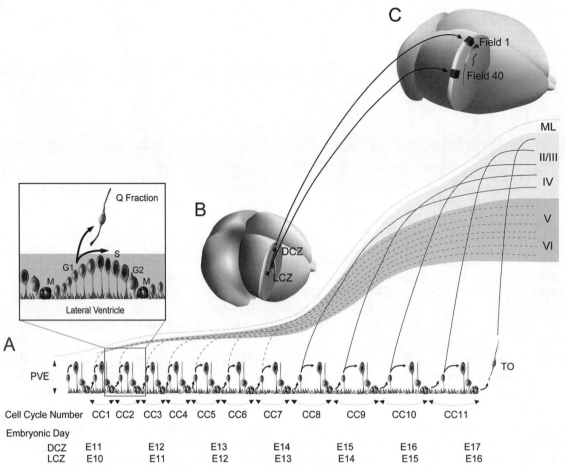

Cell Cycle Number

| | CC1 | CC2 | CC3 | CC4 | CC5 | CC6 | CC7 | CC8 | CC9 | CC10 | CC11 |

Embryonic Day

DCZ	E11		E12		E13		E14		E15	E16	E17
LCZ	E10		E11		E12		E13		E14	E15	E16

FIGURE 11.4 Summary of neocortical development. Histogenesis of the neocortex is initiated with cell proliferation in the pseudostratified ventricular epithelium (PVE) of the ventricular zone (VZ). During a preneuronogenetic phase (pre-NI), the founder population proliferates through a series of cycles during which no cells exit the cycle (Q = 0, P = 1.0). The onset of the neuronogenetic interval (NI) corresponds to CC1, the first cycle at which Q becomes greater than 0, and postmitotic cells exit the cycle as young neurons. The cells of the PVE then execute a series of 11 cell cycles in the mouse (CC1–CC11). As young neurons of the Q fraction exit the proliferative population at each cell cycle, they migrate across the embryonic cerebral wall where they are assembled into neocortex more or less in inside-to-outside order. Thus, the earliest-formed cells are destined for layer VI of the cortex while later-formed cells will take up positions in progressively more superficial layers V–II. Lines (for granular/supragranular layers) and dashed lines (for infragranular layers) schematically indicate the cell cycle of neuron origin in approximate relation to laminar destination. At the conclusion of migration, a substantial proportion of young neurons is eliminated by cell death, while surviving neurons grow, differentiate, and become integrated into cortical circuitry. (Modified from Takahashi, Nowakowski, and Caviness, 2001.)

ate to allow for the labeled cells to divide, there is an increase (approximately twofold) in the number of labeled cells.

Brief review of cell proliferation in the fetal brain

In the developing mouse neocortex (figure 11.4) the proliferative cells occupy a specific layer of the developing hemispheric wall that is known as the ventricular zone (VZ). The VZ is the main proliferative population, and there is a 6-day period during which virtually all of the neurons of the adult neocortex are produced by the proliferating cells of the VZ. During this period the cell cycle of the VZ cells lengthens (figure 11.5) from about 8 hours to about 18 hours (Caviness, Takahashi, and Nowakowski, 1991, 1995;

Nowakowski, Takahashi, and Caviness, 1993). It is known that the range of cell cycle lengths present in the population during this period is relatively narrow (±7%) (Cai, Hayes, and Nowakowski, 1997b), and thus, from the lengthening cell cycle, it can be calculated that a total of approximately 11 cell cycles occur during this 6-day period (Caviness, Takahashi, and Nowakowski, 1995). Moreover, with each passage through the cell cycle (see figure 11.5) a progressively greater proportion of the daughter cells leave the cell cycle (Q cells) as opposed to reentering S (P cells) (Takahashi, Nowakowski, and Caviness, 1994, 1996a).

The two daughter cells resulting from a mitotic division make the decision to exit (Q) or reenter (P) the cell cycle sometime during the G_1 phase of the cell cycle. An impor-

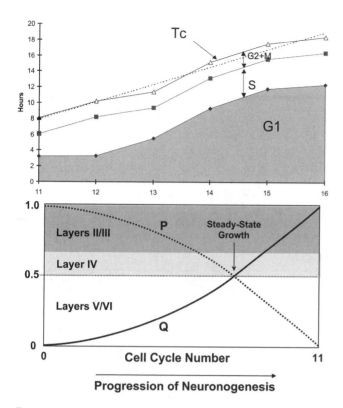

FIGURE 11.5 During the development of the neocortex, the cell cycle lengthens on each of the 6 days of neuron production (top diagram). At the same time (bottom diagram), the proportion of daughter cells that exit the cell cycle (Q) increases and the proportion that remain in the cell cycle (P) decreases. Note that at all times, P + Q = 1 (bottom diagram).

tant issue is whether they make this decision independently of each other or whether the fates of the two daughter cells are correlated (figure 11.6). Using a retroviral method that labels single proliferating cells at a known time during the proliferative period, we have shown that cells in a lineage remain clustered through several passes through the cell cycle, producing a mosaic of lineages of different sizes in the pseudostratified ventricular epithelium (PVE) (Cai, Hayes, and Nowakowski, 1997a). In figure 11.7 a comparison of the size distributions of these clusters of retrovirally labeled cells with models derived from the repeated application of binomial probabilities (i.e., a Markov chain model; see Cai et al., 2002) based on the P/Q measurements obtained from the S phase marker experiments (Takahashi, Nowakowski, and Caviness, 1996a; Miyama et al., 1997) is shown. These data showed that the two daughter cells make their P/Q decisions independently, and thus that the changing values of P and Q are directly related to the changing proportions of symmetrical and asymmetrical cell divisions that occur as development proceeds (Cai et al., 2002).

There is also a lateral to medial gradient in neocortical development (Miyama et al., 1997), and finally, after neuron production has ended (Gilmore et al., 2000), about 25% of the cells produced die (Verney et al., 2000). Using all of these data, from multiple experiments and viewpoints, a conceptual (and quantitative) framework has been assembled that accounts for a substantial portion of our factual knowledge about neocortical development in mice and other species (for reviews, see Caviness, Takahashi, and Nowakowski, 1995, 1999, 2000; Takahashi, Nowakowki, and Caviness, 1999; Nowakowski et al., 2002). This conceptual framework has been used to analyze the influence of cell cycle regulators on cortical development and P/Q pathways (Caviness et al., 2003).

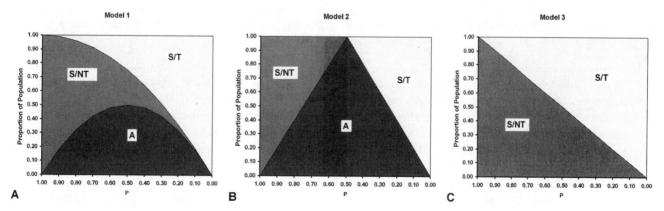

FIGURE 11.6 Schematic diagrams of changes in the proportions of symmetrical nonterminal (S/NT), symmetrical terminal (S/T), and asymmetrical (A) cell divisions as a function of changes in P (abscissa) during the neuronogenetic interval. At any given time the sum of the proportions of the three types of cell division adds up to 1.0 (ordinate). The frequency histograms shown in figure 11.7 show that if the proportion of three types of cell division is assumed to be independently determined for each of the two daughter cells (Model 1), then observed retroviral clone sizes are well accounted for (for details, see Cai et al., 2002).

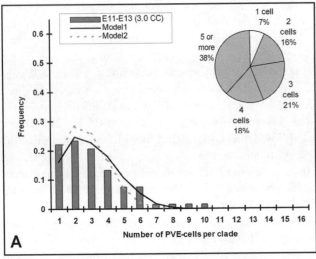

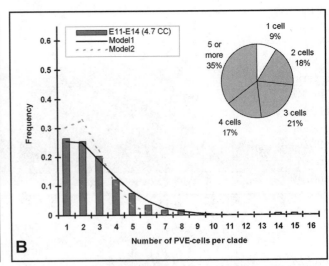

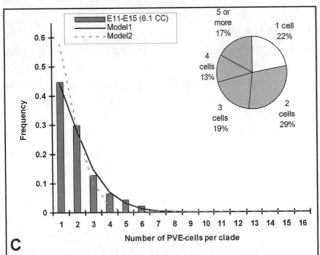

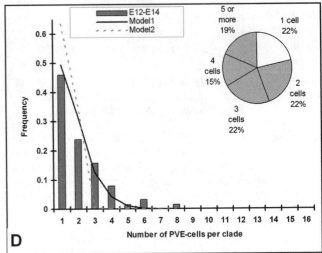

FIGURE 11.7   Frequency histogram of the PVE clades for the E11–E13 (*A*), E11–E14 group (*B*), E11–E15 group (*C*), and E12–E14 group (*D*). The mean size of the PVE clades (indicated by the arrows) decreases with a longer survival time and with more cell cycles (3.0 cell cycles for E11–E13, 4.7 cell cycles for E11–E14, 6.1 cell cycles for E11–E15, and 2.8 cell cycles for E12–E14). Each pie chart inset shows the proportion of AP-labeled cells that reside in each clade size. The two curves in each histogram are the predicted size distribution calculated from independent data using Model 1 (solid line) and Model 2 (dashed line). A χ^2 goodness-of-fit test shows that the distributions obtained with Model 1 do not differ from the experimental data, whereas those obtained with Model 2 are highly significantly different ($P < 10^{-8}$). Thus, Model 1 accounts for the observed data better, indicating that the cell fates are determined independently. (Modified from Cai et al., 2002.)

In the developing neocortex, essentially all of the cells in the VZ are proliferating; that is, the "growth fraction" is close to 1. Thus, by this measure, proliferative capacity is high at all stages. However, the changes in the length of the cell cycle (and the finite life span of the VZ) clearly indicate that a proliferative cell has a greater capacity to produce progeny at E11, when the cell cycle is short, than at E15, when the cell cycle is much longer. Changes in the cell cycle mean capacity is higher at E11 and lower at E16, but changes in P/Q mean that expansion is favored early and output is favored later. Thus, as a useful concept to compare proliferating cell populations, we define *proliferative capacity* as proportional to the number of proliferating cells and inversely proportional (but not linearly) to the length of the cell cycle. Similar considerations of changes in P/Q indicate that the output from these populations is changing. If P is high, there is expansion rather than output. If Q is high, there is output at the expense of the size of the population (i.e., the size of the population decreases, and with it, capacity). Importantly, when P = Q = 0.5, there is a balance between output and proliferation, and the proliferative population remains at a constant size (i.e., steady state) and produces a constant number of Q cells per cell cycle.

Brief history of adult neurogenesis

The presence of a proliferating population of stem and progenitor cells in the DG of mammals was first described in the mouse (Angevine, 1964, 1965) and rat (Kaplan and Hinds, 1977; Bayer, 1982; Bayer, Yackel, and Puri, 1982; Stanfield and Trice, 1988). Since that time the presence of this proliferative population in adults has been confirmed in a variety of other mammals, including monkeys (Kornack and Rakic, 1999) and humans (Eriksson et al., 1998). It has been shown that during the adult period, the number of DG granule cells increases (Bayer, 1982; Bayer, Yackel, and Puri, 1982), the newly produced granule cells displace earlier generated granule cells (Crespo, Stanfield, and Cowan, 1986), and they grow an axon into the molecular layer of CA3 (Stanfield and Trice, 1988). These axons make normal synapses (Markakis and Gage, 1999) that are functional (van Praag et al., 2002).

Proliferative capacity and cell cycle during adult neurogenesis in the dentate gyrus

The proliferative population in the DG of the adult mammal exhibits several differences from the VZ of the developing fetus. First, it is a permanent proliferative population that seems to persist for the life of the animal, whereas the VZ disappears at the end of the developmental period. The permanence of the proliferating population means that for its cells (on average, i.e., at the population level), P and Q must be approximately 0.5. If P were larger than 0.5, there would be an ever increasing proliferative population and, perhaps, tumors. If P were significantly smaller than 0.5, the proliferative population would disappear. Second, the cells produced are a mixture of neurons and glia, whereas the VZ produces mostly neurons. Third, most of the newly produced cells in the adult DG die within a few weeks after their production, whereas in the neocortex, most of the neurons produced during the developmental period persist for the life of the animal. Fourth, in the adult DG the postproliferative daughters and the proliferating cells are intermingled, whereas in the developing neocortex the migrating young neurons leave the VZ in less than one cell cycle (Takahashi, Nowakowski, and Caviness, 1996b).

It is the third difference that made it necessary to develop a new cell cycle measuring method for use in the adult DG. We needed a method that did not depend on the ability to discriminate between BUdR-labeled cells that were still proliferating and those that were no longer proliferating. To do this we developed the "saturate-and-survive" method (figure 11.8). In this method, the entire proliferative population is labeled by cumulative exposure to BUdR. Then the change of the number of labeled cells is monitored over several cell

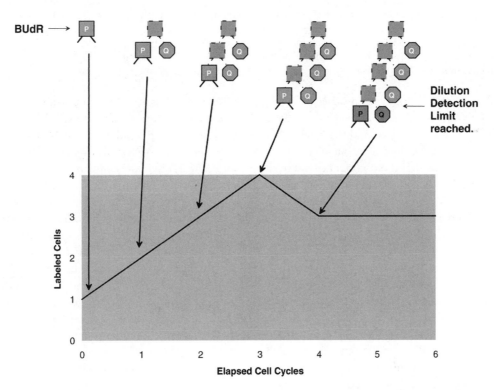

FIGURE 11.8   The principles of the "saturate-and-survive" method (SSM) in the absence of cell death. At the onset of the experimental period, BUdR is given for several hours (i.e., Tc-Ts hours) to label all of the proliferating cells (gray square with white P in the first column). At the end of this period these cells divide, producing on average one P cell and one Q cell; that is, there are now twice as many labeled cells as before. This process is repeated in each successive cell cycle, producing more Q cells but retaining only one P cell. Finally, after three to four cell cycles, the last remaining P cell divides and, because the label is reduced below detection, its two daughter cells no longer appear as labeled (shown as gray figures with black P or Q).

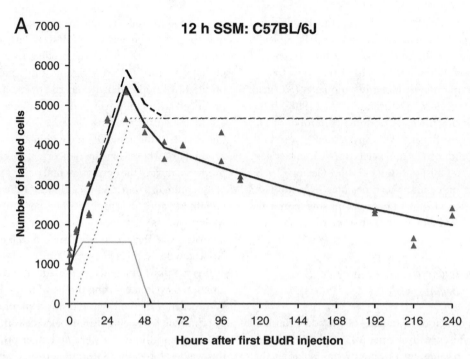

FIGURE 11.9 Interpretation of the SSM curve. A mathematical model of the behavior of the proliferating population in the adult dentate gyrus was based on the assumption of steady-state dynamics, a Ts value measured independently, and a least-squares fit to the data collected from a 12-hour saturation paradigm in C57BL/6J. Labeling of the proliferating population (P; gray line) is complete in less than 12 hours after the first BUdR injection; the number of labeled P cells remains constant until the dilution detection limit (DDL) is reached, after which it drops rapidly to 0. The number of labeled postmitotic cells (Q) produced (dotted line) rises linearly to a peak approximately coincident with the DDL, after which, in the absence of cell death, that number would remain constant. Thus, in the absence of any cell death, the expected number of labeled cells at any point (dashed line) is equal to the sum of P and Q. Any deviation of the curve fit to the data (heavy black line) from the expected number of labeled cells (dashed line) is most likely attributable to cell death in the newly produced cells. Values for the total number of proliferating cells, Tc, Ts, and the incidence of cell death per unit time can be calculated from the curve. (Modified from Hayes and Nowakowski, 2002.)

cycles. In the absence of cell death, the number of labeled cells will increase to a peak as both daughter cells—that is, the Q cell, which leaves the cell cycle, and the P cell, which continues to proliferate—are visibly labeled and counted by the experimenter. However, after three to four cell cycles, the P cell dilutes the BUdR label below the ability of the methods used to detect it, and it "disappears" (i.e., is no longer visibly labeled), leaving behind only labeled Q cells. This means that for each one labeled cell produced during the saturation period at the start of the experiment there will be produced three to four labeled progeny (one per cell cycle) before the proliferating cell finally dilutes its label below detectability. Thus, after the peak is reached, there is an abrupt fall as the P cells disappear from view, and then a plateau is reached (see figure 11.8). In actual experiments the presence of cell death among the newly produced cells markedly affects the shape of the SSM curve, particularly after the peak (figure 11.9). However, the rate of cell death can be modeled mathematically, and a half-life of the newly produced Q cells can be estimated. Using these methods, we have shown that for C57BL/6J mice the cell cycle in the adult DG is approximately 12–14 hours long, there are approximately 1800 proliferating cells per DG, and about 80% of the newly produced cells disappear (presumably die) with a half-life of about 8 days (Hayes and Nowakowski, 2002).

How do these numbers compare if other inbred strains are examined? A clear difference is seen when C57BL/6J and BALB/cByJ are compared (figure 11.10). There are clearly fewer S phase cells in BALB/cByJ and also fewer labeled cells at what should be the peak of the SSM curve. Is this an issue of a different cell cycle length? Or of fewer proliferating cells? When the SSM method is applied to BALB/cByJ, we find that there is no change in the cell cycle length, but there is a decrease by about 50% in the number of proliferating cells (Hayes and Nowakowski, 2002). There is also no change in the half-life of the newly produced Q cells, and when examined 5–6 weeks after saturation labeling, we find that a similar proportion of the newly produced cells have survived in both strains; this number remains stable for at least 5 months (Hayes and Nowakowski, unpublished data). Since inbred strains differ primarily in their genetic composition (Silver, 1995), this means that there are genetic controls on the number of proliferating cells in the DG. When integrated over the life span of the mouse, the potential significance of these differences is clearer. Estimating that about one-third of the cells produced become

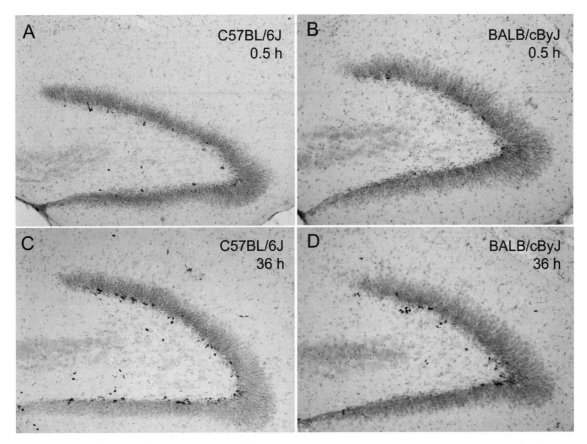

FIGURE 11.10 BrdU labeling in adult DG of C57BL/6J and BALB/cByJ male mice. Sacrifice 0.5 hours after a single injection of BrdU shows that the number of cells in S phase is greater in C57 (*A*) than in BALB/c mice (*B*), but in both strains most of the labeled cells are found in the subgranular zone. The maximal number of labeled cells following a 12-hour saturation paradigm occurs at approximately 36 hours in both strains and is greater in C57 (*C*) than in BALB/c (*D*). At 36 hours in both strains, the labeled cells in the subgranular zone are frequently arranged in clusters of about 5–8 cells. (Modified from Hayes and Nowakowski, 2002.)

neurons, and using a cell cycle of 12 hours, a $Q = 0.5$, and the surviving population 5–6 weeks after saturation labeling, we estimate that there are about 108 neurons that have survived per cell cycle in C57BL/6J, or about 216 neurons per day. In BALB/cByJ there would be only about 63 neurons per cell cycle, or about 126 per day. Extrapolating over an estimated 500-day life span, and assuming no decrease in the proliferating population, this would be approximately 108,000 neurons in C57BL/6J, versus only about 63,000 in BALB/cByJ. Interestingly, both of these numbers are far less than the 250,000–350,000 granule cells in a mouse DG (Wimer et al., 1978; Wimer and Wimer, 1989). These life span estimates would be even lower if the reported fall in the number of proliferating cells in the DG (Kempermann, Kuhn, and Gage, 1998; Kempermann, Gast, and Gage, 2002) is considered.

Summary and conclusions

The properties of the proliferative populations in fetal and adult CNS differ in fundamental ways, and a thorough understanding of neurogenesis requires a quantitative characterization of the dynamic aspects and behaviors of stem/progenitor populations. The key to understanding neurogenesis is recognition that the productive capacity of any proliferating population is proportional to the number of proliferating cells, inversely proportional to the cell cycle length, and highly influenced by cell fate decisions—that is, reentry into the cell cycle (P) or exit to differentiate (Q). Overall, it should be recognized that neurogenesis is a complex process with numerous control points involved in regulating the cell cycle, cell fate decisions (P/Q), cell death, and neuronal differentiation. Cell cycle length varies during development, and there are genetically based differences in the size of the proliferating populations of stem/progenitor cells in the adult DG. The net number of "new" neurons added per day is relatively small and insufficient to replace the DG even over the entire life span of a mouse. There is undoubtedly additional genetic variation, both in the number of proliferating cells and in their ability to survive, that is waiting to be discovered. Each of these control points could be influenced by environmentally produced signals.

At present the functional role of adult neurogenesis is unknown, but an understanding of its function needs to consider, at a minimum, both the size of the proliferative population and the size and survival of the output. The dynamic aspects of this process mean that at any given time, the entire spectrum of proliferating cells and "new" cells in various stages of maturation are present in the adult DG, and it is not hard to imagine that these different, representative portions of the neurogenetic process play different functional roles. Finally, we point out that the existence of genetic diversity in the proliferative population and in the survival of its output provides a significant new lever for addressing the possible roles of adult neurogenesis in behavior and cognition.

REFERENCES

ANGEVINE, J. B., JR., 1964. Autoradiographic study of histogenesis in the area dentata of the cerebral cortex in the mouse. *Anat. Rec.* 148:255.

ANGEVINE, J. B., JR., 1965. Time of neuron origin in the hippocampal region: An autoradiographic study in the mouse. *Exp. Neurol. Suppl.* 2:1–71.

BAYER, S. A., 1982. Changes in the total number of dentate granule cells in juvenile and adult rats: A correlated volumetric and ^{3}H-thymidine autoradiographic study. *Exp. Brain Res.* 46:315–323.

BAYER, S. A., J. W. YACKEL, and P. S. PURI, 1982. Neurons in the rat dentate gyrus granular layer substantially increase during juvenile and adult life. *Science* 216:890–892.

CAI, L., N. L. HAYES, and R. S. NOWAKOWSKI, 1997a. Synchrony of clonal cell proliferation and contiguity of clonally related cells: Production of mosaicism in the ventricular zone of developing mouse neocortex. *J. Neurosci.* 17:2088–2100.

CAI, L., N. L. HAYES, and R. S. NOWAKOWSKI, 1997b. Local homogeneity of cell cycle length in developing mouse cortex. *J. Neurosci.* 17:2079–2087.

CAI, L., N. L. HAYES, T. TAKAHASHI, V. S. CAVINESS, JR., and R. S. NOWAKOWSKI, 2002. Size distribution of retrovirally marked lineages matches prediction from population measurements of cell cycle behavior. *J. Neurosci. Res.* 69:731–744.

CAVINESS, V., T. TAKAHASHI, and R. NOWAKOWSKI, 1995. Numbers, time and neocortical neuronogenesis: A general developmental and evolutionary model. *Trends Neurosci.* 18:379–383.

CAVINESS, V. S., JR., T. GOTO, T. TARUI, T. TAKAHASHI, P. G. BHIDE, and R. S. NOWAKOWSKI, 2003. Cell output, cell cycle duration and neuronal specification: A model of integrated mechanisms of the neocortical proliferative process. *Cereb. Cortex* 13:592–598.

CAVINESS, V. S., JR., T. TAKAHASHI, and R. S. NOWAKOWSKI, 1991. Cytokinetic parameters of the ventricular zone in developing mouse neocortex. *Soc. Neurosci. Abstr.* 17:29.

CAVINESS, V. S., JR., T. TAKAHASHI, and R. S. NOWAKOWSKI, 1993. Regulated and non-regulated parameters of cell proliferation in the developing neocortex. *Soc. Neurosci. Abstr.* 17:29.

CAVINESS, V. S., JR., T. TAKAHASHI, and R. S. NOWAKOWSKI, 1999. The G1 restriction point as critical regulator of neocortical neuronogenesis. *Neurochem. Res.* 24:497–506.

CAVINESS, V. S., JR., T. TAKAHASHI, and R. S. NOWAKOWSKI, 2000. Neuronogenesis and the early events of neocortical histogenesis. *Results Probl. Cell Differ.* 30:107–143.

CRESPO, D., B. B. STANFIELD, and W. M. COWAN, 1986. Evidence that late-generated granule cells do not simply replace earlier formed neurons in the rat dentate gyrus. *Exp. Brain Res.* 62: 541–548.

ERIKSSON, P. S., E. PERFILIEVA, T. BJORK-ERIKSSON, A. M. ALBORN, C. NORDBORG, D. A. PETERSON, and F. H. GAGE, 1998. Neurogenesis in the adult human hippocampus [see comments]. *Nat. Med.* 4:1313–1317.

GAGE, F. H., 2002. Neurogenesis in the adult brain. *J. Neurosci.* 22:612–613.

GILMORE, E. C., R. S. NOWAKOWSKI, V. S. CAVINESS, JR., and K. HERRUP, 2000. Cell birth, cell death, cell diversity and DNA breaks: How do they all fit together? *Trends Neurosci.* 23:100–105.

GRATZNER, H. G., 1982. Monoclonal antibody to 5-bromo and 5-iododeoxyuridine: A new reagent for detection of DNA replication. *Science* 218:474–478.

HAYES, N. L., and R. S. NOWAKOWSKI, 2000. Exploiting the dynamics of S-phase tracers in developing brain: Interkinetic nuclear migration for cells entering versus leaving the S-phase. *Dev. Neurosci.* 22:44–55.

HAYES, N. L., and R. S. NOWAKOWSKI, 2002. Dynamics of cell proliferation in the adult dentate gyrus of two inbred strains of mice. *Brain Res. Dev. Brain Res.* 134:77–85.

HSU, S. M., L. RAINE, and H. FANGER, 1981. Use of avidin-biotin-peroxidase complex (ABC) in immunoperoxidase techniques: A comparison between ABC and unlabeled antibody (PAP) procedures. *J. Histochem. Cytochem.* 29:577–580.

KAPLAN, M. S., and J. W. HINDS, 1977. Neurogenesis in the adult rat: Electron microscopic analysis of light radioautographs. *Science* 197:1092–1094.

KATCHANOV, J., C. HARMS, K. GERTZ, L. HAUCK, C. WAEBER, L. HIRT, J. PRILLER, R. VON HARSDORF, W. BRUCK, H. HORTNAGL, U. DIRNAGL, P. G. BHIDE, and M. ENDRES, 2001. Mild cerebral ischemia induces loss of cyclin-dependent kinase inhibitors and activation of cell cycle machinery before delayed neuronal cell death. *J. Neurosci.* 21:5045–5053.

KEMPERMANN, G., D. GAST, and F. H. GAGE, 2002. Neuroplasticity in old age: Sustained fivefold induction of hippocampal neurogenesis by long-term environmental enrichment. *Ann. Neurol.* 52: 135–143.

KEMPERMANN, G., H. G. KUHN, and F. H. GAGE, 1998. Experience-induced neurogenesis in the senescent dentate gyrus. *J. Neurosci.* 18:3206–3212.

KIRSANOVA, I. A., and A. P. ANISIMOV, 2001. [Somatic polyploidy in neurons of the gastropod molluscs. II. Dynamics of DNA synthesis in the process of postnatal growth of CNS neurons in Succineid snail]. *Tsitologiia* 43:437–445.

KORNACK, D. R., and P. RAKIC, 1999. Continuation of neurogenesis in the hippocampus of the adult macaque monkey. *Proc. Natl. Acad. Sci. U.S.A.* 96:5768–5773.

MARKAKIS, E. A., and F. H. GAGE, 1999. Adult-generated neurons in the dentate gyrus send axonal projections to field CA3 and are surrounded by synaptic vesicles. *J. Comp. Neurol.* 406:449–460.

MIYAMA, S., T. TAKAHASHI, R. S. NOWAKOWSKI, and V. S. CAVINESS, JR., 1997. A gradient in the duration of the G1 phase in the murine neocortical proliferative epithelium. *Cereb. Cortex* 7:678–689.

NOWAKOWSKI, R. S., and P. RAKIC, 1974. Clearance rate of exogenous ^{3}H-thymidine from the plasma of pregnant rhesus monkeys. *Cell Tissue Kinetics* 7:189–194.

NOWAKOWSKI, R. S., T. TAKAHASHI, and V. S. CAVINESS, JR., 1993. Expansion and output of the neocortical PVE during the neuronogenetic period. *Soc. Neurosci. Abstr.* 19:29.

Nowakowski, R. S., V. S. Caviness, Jr., T. Takahashi, and N. L. Hayes, 2002. Population dynamics during cell proliferation and neuronogenesis in the developing murine neocortex. In *Cortical Development: From Specification to Differentiation (Results and Problems in Cell Differentiation*, vol. 39), C. Hohmann, ed. New York: Springer-Verlag, pp. 1–22.

Rakic, P., 2002. Neurogenesis in adult primate neocortex: An evaluation of the evidence. *Nat. Rev. Neurosci.* 3:65–71.

Rogers, A. W., 1973. *Techniques of Autoradiography*, 2nd ed. New York: Elsevier Scientific.

Silver, L., 1995. *Mouse Genetics: Concepts and Applications.* Oxford, England: Oxford University Press.

Stanfield, B. B., and J. E. Trice, 1988. Evidence that granule cells generated in the dentate gyrus of adult rats extend axonal projections. *Exp. Brain Res.* 72:399–406.

Takahashi, T., R. S. Nowakowski, and V. S. Caviness, Jr., 1992. BUdR as an S-phase marker for quantitative studies of cytokinetic behaviour in the murine cerebral ventricular zone. *J. Neurocytol.* 21:185–197.

Takahashi, T., R. S. Nowakowski, and V. S. Caviness, Jr., 1994. Mode of cell proliferation in the developing mouse neocortex. *Proc. Natl. Acad. Sci. U.S.A.* 91:375–379.

Takahashi, T., R. S. Nowakowski, and V. S. Caviness, Jr., 1996a. The leaving or Q fraction of the murine cerebral proliferative epithelium: A general model of neocortical neuronogenesis. *J. Neurosci.* 16:6183–6196.

Takahashi, T., R. S. Nowakowski, and V. S. Caviness, Jr., 1996b. Interkinetic and migratory behavior of a cohort of neocortical neurons arising in the early embryonic murine cerebral wall. *J. Neurosci.* 16:5762–5776.

Takahashi, T., R. S. Nowakowski, and V. S. Caviness, Jr., 1999. Cell cycle as operational unit of neocortical neuronogenesis. *Neuroscientist* 5:155–163.

Takahashi, T., R. S. Nowakowski, and V. S. Caviness, Jr., 2001. Neocortical neuronogenesis: Regulation, control points and a strategy of structural variation. In *Handbook of Cognitive Developmental Neuroscience*, C. A. Nelson and M. Luciana, eds. Cambridge, MA: MIT Press, pp. 3–22.

Taupin, P., and F. H. Gage, 2002. Adult neurogenesis and neural stem cells of the central nervous system in mammals. *J. Neurosci. Res.* 69:745–749.

van Praag, H., A. F. Schinder, B. R. Christie, N. Toni, T. D. Palmer, and F. H. Gage, 2002. Functional neurogenesis in the adult hippocampus. *Nature* 415:1030–1034.

Verney, C., T. Takahashi, P. G. Bhide, R. S. Nowakowski, and V. S. Caviness, Jr., 2000. Independent controls for neocortical neuron production and histogenetic cell death. *Dev. Neurosci.* 22:125–138.

Wimer, C. C., and R. E. Wimer, 1989. On the sources of strain and sex differences in granule cell number in the dentate area of house mice. *Brain Res. Dev. Brain Res.* 48:167–176.

Wimer, R. E., C. C. Wimer, J. E. Vaughn, R. P. Barber, B. A. Balvanz, and C. R. Chernow, 1978. The genetic organization of neuron number in the granule cell layer of the area dentata in house mouse. *Brain Res.* 157:105–122.

Yang, Y., D. S. Geldmacher, and K. Herrup, 2001. DNA replication precedes neuronal cell death in Alzheimer's disease. *J. Neurosci.* 21:2661–2668.

12 Stem Cell Plasticity: Overview and Perspective

DALE WOODBURY AND IRA B. BLACK

ABSTRACT Increasing evidence suggests that adult stem cells are far more plastic than expected, able to generate cells outside accepted lineages. Under appropriate conditions, even traditional germ layer constraints can be traversed. Neural stem cells can generate mesodermal blood cells, while peripheral stem cell populations give rise to neurons and glia. These unexpected discoveries have fueled extensive research into stem cell biology, focused predominantly on regenerative medicine. The consequences of stem cell plasticity at the organismal level have received less attention. In this chapter we examine adult stem cell plasticity, focusing on the ability of peripheral stem cells to differentiate into neural elements in vitro and in vivo. Evidence for the integration of cells derived from peripheral sources into the brain parenchyma is examined, as is the potential role in brain plasticity. Finally, controversies, prospects, and challenges of this nascent field are considered.

The ability to respond to the environment is a hallmark of the animal brain. Learning and memory are particularly important in mammals, allowing acclimatization to diverse environmental niches. Because widespread neurogenesis is generally restricted to periods of embryonic development, adaptation is primarily accomplished not through the generation of new cells but through the modification of existing neurons. New synaptic connections between neurons form rapidly during postnatal development. For example, the hippocampus of the neonatal rat contains less than 1% of the synaptic connections that will exist in adulthood (Marrone and Petit, 2002). Active connections are strengthened and enlarged, and inactive connections are eliminated (Cohen-Cory, 2002). Such plasticity allows organisms to adapt to changing conditions in the absence of ongoing neurogenesis. Does this mean that neurogenesis cannot play a role in plasticity?

Evidence for the role of adult neurogenesis in brain plasticity came initially from the study of songbirds. Singing in male canaries is controlled by a number of interconnected brain nuclei. The volume of these nuclei undergoes seasonal changes, being significantly greater during times of increased vocalization. Evidence suggests that newborn neurons are recruited to song nuclei, where they replace older neurons. The neural plasticity required to learn complex song patterns may rely in part on the integration of these replacement neurons (Nottebohm, 1981; Goldman and Nottebohm, 1983; Nottebohm, Nottebohm, and Crane, 1986).

Adult neurogenesis in mammals does not occur on the grand scale observed in songbirds. In fact, the existence of extensive neurogenesis in adult mammals remains highly controversial. Evidence that the mammalian brain contains a stem cell population (neural stem cell, or NSC) capable of generating neurons in vitro was not provided until 1992 (Reynolds, Tetzlaff, and Weiss, 1992).

Stem cell populations are present in many adult tissues, including intestine, liver, muscle, and bone marrow. In fact, adult bone marrow contains two distinct stem cell populations, hematopoietic stem cells (HSCs) and marrow stromal cells (MSCs), which generate disparate progeny. Stem cells can be thought of as remnants of development, retaining a relatively undifferentiated state. When adjacent differentiated cells require replacement, stem cells divide and generate a mature cell dedicated to a particular function. The best-studied stem cell population is the HSC. All components of the blood, from platelets to red blood cells, can be derived from a single HSC. The complex control mechanisms underlying fate determination have been extensively studied and elucidated.

Because of their relatively recent discovery, NSCs are less well characterized. NSCs, first isolated from embryonic striatal tissue, differentiate into neurons and glia in culture. Subsequent studies have revealed that the adult rodent brain also contains NSCs, suggesting that the mature brain has the ability to generate differentiated cells anew when necessary (Vescovi et al., 1993). Since these early studies, NSCs have been cultured from multiple brain regions, as well as from the spinal cord of adult rodents. More recently, NSCs have been derived from human brains. These cells can be maintained in an immature state for more than 2 years in culture and retain the capacity for neuronal and glial differentiation (Svendsen, Caldwell, and Ostenfeld, 1999; Vescovi et al., 1999). The presence of NSCs suggests that the human brain may respond to environmental challenges not only by

DALE WOODBURY and IRA B. BLACK Stem Cell Research Center, Department of Neuroscience & Cell Biology, University of Medicine & Dentistry of New Jersey, Robert Wood Johnson Medical School, Piscataway, N.J.

modifying interactions between existing cells, but also through cell proliferation.

The existence of stem cells in the adult brain was unexpected. The extent of their differentiative capacity was even more startling. Upon introduction into recipient mice, long-term cultured NSCs differentiated into hematopoietic cells (Bjornson et al., 1999). The differentiation of one cell into another not along an established lineage is referred to as *transdifferentiation*. Because neural tissues and hematopoietic tissues derive from different embryonic germ layers, this transdifferentiation event was termed *transgermal differentiation*. This finding implied that distinctions between embryonic germ layers were less rigid than previously thought, and sparked a wave of studies investigating stem cell potential.

In this chapter we examine evidence of stem cell plasticity, with a particular focus on the ability of peripheral stem cells to undergo neural differentiation. Evidence for and against transgermal differentiation will be considered.

Characteristics of neural stem cells

NSCs reside deep within the brain, in the region surrounding the ventricles, but the precise origin of NSCs remains controversial (Morshead and van der Kooy, 2001). Early reports suggested that NSCs were derived from the ependymal cells that line the ventricles. More recently, NSC activity has been attributed to astrocyte-like cells in the subependymal zone (Chiasson et al., 1999; Laywell et al., 2000).

NSCs can be grown in culture from the embryonic and adult brain in the presence of peptide growth factors. Under these conditions, clusters of cells called neurospheres emerge. Neurospheres are complex structures that contain cells at various stages of differentiation (Mokry, Subrtova, and Nemecek, 1996). When separated into individual cells, a small percentage can give rise to secondary spheres, indicating the maintenance of stem cells within the neurosphere. Spheres derived from rodents have been maintained in culture for more than 4 years, twice the lifetime of the donor animal. Despite extended culture, NSCs are capable of differentiation into neurons and glia (Zhou and Chiang, 1998; Zhou et al., 2000).

NEURAL STEM CELLS DIFFERENTIATE INTO HEMATOPOIETIC ELEMENTS: START OF A REVOLUTION? Stem cells fall into two broad classes, embryonic stem cells (ESCs) and adult stem cells (ASCs). Aside from their origins, one characteristic was known to distinguish the two types: ESCs were pluripotent, whereas ASCs were severely limited in differentiative potential. It was accepted that ESCs could differentiate into all cells making up an organism. It was also accepted that ASCs could give rise only to mature cells derived from the same tissue. For example, HSCs could differentiate into components of the blood, exclusively. Similarly, the progeny of NSCs was limited to neurons and glia. Or was it? Under appropriate conditions, long-term cultured adult NSCs exhibited far greater plasticity than imagined.

NSCs grown in culture maintained their neural differentiation competence in vitro. When growth factors were removed, the neurospheres produced neurons and glia, as expected. Concomitantly, other neurospheres from this culture (sister-spheres) were injected into the blood of host mice. The transplanted cells were later identified by the expression of unique genetic markers, and their fates were examined. Surprisingly, the bone marrow of recipient animals contained NSC-derived hematopoietic cells, suggesting that the NSCs had transdifferentiated into HSCs. Moreover, the spleens of the transplanted animals contained mature blood cells derived from the exogenous NSCs (Bjornson et al., 1999).

These results suggested that NSCs in particular, and perhaps ASCs in general, have far more potential than had been appreciated. More surprisingly, the ability of ectodermal NSCs to differentiate into mesodermal hematopoietic cells implied that distinctions between embryonic germ layers were potentially flexible. Evidence that NSCs can generate skeletal and smooth muscle in vitro adds support to this contention (Galli et al., 2000; Oishi et al., 2002). Were ASCs totipotent? Could they differentiate into any cell, irrespective of lineage? Could peripheral stem cells differentiate into neural elements? If so, might stem cells residing both inside and outside the central nervous system (CNS) contribute to brain plasticity and cognition?

HOW PLASTIC IS PLASTIC? ADULT STEM CELLS CONTRIBUTE TO TISSUES DERIVED FROM ALL EMBRYONIC GERM LAYERS Demonstration of the pluripotency of ESCs has relied primarily on their response to the permissive environment of the blastocyst. ESCs grown in culture can be transplanted into the early embryo, where they participate in normal development. The resultant pups can be examined at various prenatal and postnatal stages to determine the degree of ESC contribution. Animals derived in this fashion demonstrate varying degrees of chimerism. However, it is clear that ESCs can participate in the formation of every tissue extant in the embryonic and postnatal animal. Generation of fully chimeric animals is de facto evidence of the pluripotency of ESCs.

Recently, attempts to repeat these studies utilizing ASCs have been undertaken. Cultured NSCs were introduced into blastocysts and the resultant embryos were analyzed for chimerism. Exogenous NSCs contributed to multiple tissues, including brain, spinal cord, heart, liver, and intestine, derivatives of all three germ layers. The incorporated NSCs expressed proteins consistent with their tissue of residence, suggestive of appropriate integration. NSCs may therefore display plasticity similar to that possessed by ESCs when subjected to a permissive environment such as the blastocyst (Clarke et al., 2000).

Pluripotency is not limited to ASCs derived from the brain. Multipotent adult progenitor (MAP) cells can be cultured from the bone marrow and copurify with marrow stromal cells. The relationship of MAP cells to MSCs is presently unclear, but they share many similarities and express common antigenic markers. Single MAP cells introduced into blastocysts result in the generation of chimeric animals that survive to adulthood with no apparent abnormalities. Organs of ectodermal, endodermal, and mesodermal derivation contained MAP cells to varying degrees. Cells in the bone marrow, lung, liver, heart, muscle, and brain could be traced back to a single exogenous MAP cell. Aside from unresolved germ-line transmission, MAP cells display plasticity similar to that seen with ESCs (Jiang, Jahagirdar et al., 2002; Keene et al., 2003).

PERIPHERAL STEM CELLS DIFFERENTIATE INTO NEURAL ELEMENTS IN VITRO   The demonstration that NSCs can undergo transgermal differentiation prompted intense study of peripheral stem cells. If NSCs can become mesoderm, could easily accessible mesodermal stem cells become neuroectoderm? If so, the implications for the treatment of degenerative neurological diseases such as Parkinson's disease and Alzheimer's disease would be profound. Moreover, the prospect that peripheral stem cells might be capable of generating functional brain cells in adult animals required exploration.

The earliest efforts centered on the mesenchymal stem cell or marrow stromal cell (MSC), a stem cell population residing in the bone marrow. MSCs fulfill the basic criteria of stem cells. They are able to self-renew (give rise to another MSC) and differentiate into multiple mature cell types, including osteoblasts, chondrocytes, tenoblasts, and adipocytes (Dennis et al., 1999, 2002; Pittenger, Mosca, and McIntosh, 2000). The relative accessibility of MSCs, combined with their rapid growth in culture, made them promising candidates for studies of stem cell plasticity.

Two reports published almost simultaneously suggested that MSCs were capable of neural differentiation. Perhaps indicative of their inherent plasticity, MSCs in culture were shown to express nestin, a marker of neuroepithelial precursor cells (Sanchez-Ramos et al., 2000; Woodbury et al., 2000). Treatment of MSCs with retinoic acid and the neurotrophin brain-derived neurotrophic factor (BDNF) for 14 days affected neural gene expression in a small number of MSCs. Coculture of treated MSCs with primary brain cells significantly increased the percentage of MSCs expressing neural genes. Under optimal conditions, 5% of the MSCs expressed NeuN, a marker of postmitotic neurons, while 8% expressed the astrocytic marker GFAP. Consistent with dif-

ferentiation, the expression of nestin decreased in treated cells. Apparently, MSCs in culture can express neural proteins, suggestive of transgermal differentiation (Sanchez-Ramos et al., 2000). It appears that neural cells in vitro produce factors that enhance the differentiation of MSCs into neural elements. Interestingly, it has been demonstrated that neurons derived from NSCs also require glial factors to mature appropriately (Song, Stevens, and Gage, 2002). What if peripheral stem cells migrate to the brain in intact organisms? Exposed to similar factors, might they differentiate into neural cells and contribute to brain plasticity?

Alternative methods have been used to induce neural differentiation of MSCs. Rat MSCs exposed to a chemically defined neuronal induction media undergo rapid morphological transformations, assuming neural characters in less than 60 minutes (Woodbury, Schwartz, Prockop, and Black, 2000) (figure 12.1). In a typical response, the cell body retracts, yielding process-like peripheral extensions. Morphological differentiation continues at a rapid rate, ultimately generating a contracted and refractile cell body with emanating extensions. Diverse neuronal morphologies are obtained within a single culture and include bipolar, multipolar, and pyramidal cell types (figure 12.2). Subsets of responding cells express the neuronal markers neuron-specific enolase (NSE), neurofilament-M (NF-M), tau, and NeuN. Under appropriate conditions, close to 80% of treated MSCs display neural morphologies and express NSE or NF-M. Human MSCs respond to the differentiation pro-

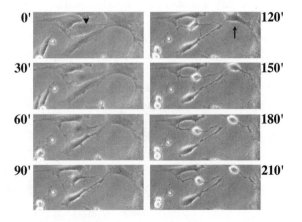

FIGURE 12.1 Differentiation to putative neurons is rapid and dramatic. Neuronal induction media is added to cultured MSCs displaying stromal morphologies (arrowhead in 0′). The cell body rapidly retracts, leaving peripheral process-like extensions (arrow in 120′). With time, the cell body becomes increasingly refractile and the putative processes become more evident, yielding a cell that is morphologically neuronal and not stromal. (Reprinted with permission from D. Woodbury et al., Adult rat and human bone marrow stromal cells differentiate into neurons. *J. Neurosci. Res.* 61:364–370. © 2000 by John Wiley and Sons, Inc.)

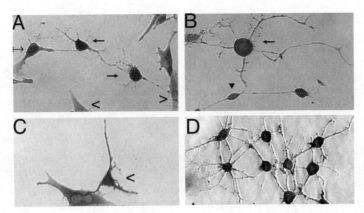

FIGURE 12.2   MSC-derived neurons display varying morphologies and form networks. (A) After a 5-hour exposure to neural induction media, some MSCs remain nonresponsive (<), some respond fully (thick arrows), displaying contracted cell bodies and process-like extensions, and others exhibit both stromal and neuronal characteristics (thin arrow). (B) MSC-derived neurons display multipolar (arrow) and simple bipolar (arrowhead) morphologies. (C) Rare cells are morphologically pyramidal in appearance (<). (D) MSC-derived neurons form networks with each other and with nonresponsive cells retaining stromal morphologies (lower left). (Reprinted with permission from D. Woodbury et al., Adult rat and human bone marrow stromal cells differentiate into neurons. *J. Neurosci. Res.* 61:364–370. © 2000 by John Wiley and Sons, Inc.)

tocol in a similar manner, consistent with findings described earlier.

Subsequent reports confirmed the ability of MSCs to adopt neuronal traits in vitro. Treatment of MSCs with chemical agents that raised intracellular cAMP levels, or overexpression of the neuralizing agent noggin, caused differentiation of MSCs into presumptive neurons (Deng et al., 2001; Kohyama et al., 2001). In addition to expressing neural proteins, induced MSCs responded to depolarizing stimuli in a manner consistent with neuronal differentiation.

A second peripheral stem cell, derived from the dermis of mammalian skin, also possesses the ability to undergo neural differentiation. These cells, termed skin-derived progenitors (SKPs), give rise to putative neurons (NF-M or β-III-tubulin positive) and glial cells in culture. Interestingly, this neuroectodermal stem cell population could also generate mesodermal adipocytes and smooth muscle cells through transgermal differentiation (Toma et al., 2001).

Thus, peripheral stem cell populations were shown to have the capacity to differentiate into presumptive neurons under artificial, in vitro conditions. However, relevance to the living organism remained to be established. Could transgermal differentiation of peripheral stem cells into neurons occur in vivo, contributing to brain plasticity?

MARROW CELLS MIGRATE INTO THE BRAIN AND DIFFERENTIATE   The influence of the brain on peripheral systems is particularly evident in complex behaviors such as locomotion. When the connection between the brain and peripheral systems is compromised, as in spinal cord injury, intact peripheral organs lose function. However, brain-body communication is not unidirectional. Peripheral inputs can influence events within the brain, although the consequences are less obvious. For example, physical exercise increases neurogenesis in the hippocampus of laboratory animals (van Praag et al., 1999). In contrast, high stress levels depress neurogenesis. Can the periphery influence neurogenesis, and perhaps cognition, through additional mechanisms?

Several studies have demonstrated that marrow-derived cells routinely migrate into the brain and begin expressing neural markers. To track the movement of exogenous bone marrow cells, cells from a divergent donor strain were transplanted into a neonatal host animal (Brazelton et al., 2000; Mezey and Chandross, 2000; Mezey et al., 2000). Donor cells populated the marrow and expressed appropriate blood-related antigens, as expected (Brazelton et al., 2000). Surprisingly, however, some donor cells migrated into the brain and became morphologically indistinguishable from surrounding host cells. Donor cells integrated into the brain parenchyma, expressed neuron-specific antigens (NeuN, β-III-tubulin, NF-H), and ceased expression of blood-related proteins. Thus, it appears that on exposure to the neural environment, peripherally derived cells can differentiate into neurons and glia, consistent with preceding in vitro studies.

Similarly, transplantation of bone marrow cells into lethally irradiated adult mice results in colonization of the marrow by donor cells. Analysis of recipient animals indicated the presence of donor cells in the parenchyma of the cerebellum, a late-developing brain structure. The number of donor cells in the cerebellum increased with time, suggesting that engraftment was ongoing. Donor cells displayed the unmistakable morphology of Purkinje cells, the output neurons of the cerebellar cortex, and expressed genes suggestive of functional integration (Priller et al., 2001).

In sum, rare bone marrow–derived cells take up residence in the brain parenchyma in vivo. Subsets respond to their new environment by decreasing expression of blood-specific proteins and initiating expression of neural proteins in a site-specific manner. Moreover, it appears that this infiltration is an ongoing event. The route of migration from the periphery into the brain is unknown, but a likely site of entry is through the vasculature. Interestingly, it has been established that neurogenesis is most prevalent around blood vessels, occurring in a "vascular niche" in the hippocampus (Palmer, Willhoite, and Gage, 2000). Is it possible that some of the participating stem cells are derived from the periphery?

Evidence also exists for the migration of circulating MSCs into the demyelinated spinal cord. In contrast to the preceding studies, a specific lesion was created prior to introduction of donor stem cells. Exogenous marrow-derived cells (MSCs and HSCs) delivered intravenously to host animals localized to the site of the spinal cord lesion. Significant remyelination occurred, demonstrating characteristics of both peripheral and CNS myelination. Conductance across the lesion was partially restored, indicative of partial repair. In contrast, intravenous administration of Schwann cells (peripheral myelin-producing cells) or olfactory ensheathing cells did not result in repair of the damaged spinal cord. In this model system, only marrow-derived stem cells were shown to exit the circulation, target sites of injury within the CNS, and participate in repair. Evidently, in a pathological condition, cues from the CNS can recruit cells from the periphery that then participate in repair (Akiyama, Radtke, and Kocsis, 2002). Might similar cues, expressed at lower levels, be responsible for the ongoing migration of marrow-derived cells into the uncompromised brain? Even more speculatively, could recruitment vary in response to stress or exercise, influencing acclimatization to external events?

DIRECT TRANSPLANTATION OF BONE MARROW CELLS INTO THE CNS In the absence of a lesion, only a miniscule fraction of systemically administered marrow cells reach the CNS, owing to a host of intervening variables. Consequently, analysis of neural differentiation is extremely difficult. To circumvent this impediment, bone marrow cells have been transplanted directly into the brain and spinal cord. For example, MSCs derived from adult animals have been transplanted into the ventricles of neonatal mice. Recipient animals were analyzed 12 or 45 days after transplantation to assess migration and differentiation of donor cells. Infused MSCs were found in multiple brain regions, including the hippocampus, striatum, and cerebellum. Introduced cells displayed neural morphologies and expressed markers consistent with differentiation to astrocytes (GFAP positive) and neurons (NF-H positive). Donor cells appeared in much higher numbers in the brain than seen with peripheral injection strategies, with no evidence of increased mortality or morbidity (Kopen, Prockop, and Phinney, 1999). Such studies suggest that access to the brain through normal

migration may serve to limit participation of peripheral stem cells in neural plasticity. Direct infusion circumvents this obstacle, allowing large numbers of introduced cells to assume neural characters. Such an approach is clearly more relevant to studies of neurodegenerative disease, but implies that access to the CNS, not the potential of peripheral stem cells, limits participation in brain plasticity.

Apparent transgermal differentiation in humans

Several studies have suggested that transgermal differentiation occurs in humans. For example, donor bone marrow cells integrated into the buccal epithelia of patients following therapeutic bone marrow transplants. The contribution of donor cells was significant, varying from 0.8% to greater than 12% of the cells examined. The rapid turnover of buccal cells may explain the high level of chimerism detected. Differentiation of mesodermal bone marrow cells (MSCs and/or HSCs) to ectodermal epithelial cells suggests that transgermal differentiation is a common event in humans (Tran et al., 2003).

Similarly, bone marrow cells can contribute to neuronal populations in the adult brain. Posthumous analysis of bone marrow recipients revealed donor cells residing in the brain. The majority of donor cells were non-neuronal, but subsets of NeuN-positive neurons were found in the cerebellum and hippocampus. Neurons often appeared in clusters, suggesting infiltration of a single cell, with subsequent mitosis and neural differentiation. In contrast to the robust colonization of the buccal epithelium, less than 7 out of every 10,000 analyzed neurons were donor-derived. Nevertheless, it is clear that in humans as well as in rodents, peripheral cells migrate into the brain and subsequently differentiate into neural cells (Mezey et al., 2003). Perhaps stem cells normally located outside the CNS can participate in brain plasticity, even in humans.

Potency of adult stem cells: Possible explanations

A plausible explanation for the apparent plasticity of ASCs has been proposed, based on the biology of MAP cells. As described earlier, MAP cells copurify with MSCs and have been isolated from both rodents and humans. This stem cell population is capable of differentiation into derivatives of all three embryonic germ layers, a plasticity evocative of ESCs (Jiang, Jahagirdar, Reinhardt, et al., 2002).

Cells with characteristics similar to those of MAP cells have now been isolated from brain and muscle, in addition to bone marrow. Cells from these dissimilar organs can be propagated in culture under identical conditions. When appropriately treated, MAP cells derived from each of these tissues differentiate into endothelial cells, hepatocytes, and neural cells—representatives from each germ layer.

Similarities between MAP cells derived from different organs goes beyond their differentiative capacity. Phenotypic analysis by fluorescence activated cell sorting (FACS) techniques revealed a similar pattern of gene expression: MAP cells from each tissue were CD13+, c-kit−, CD44−, CD45−, and MHC-I− and MHC-II−. Microarray analysis of the three MAP populations demonstrated highly homologous expression patterns for more than 99% of the genes analyzed (more than 12,000 in total). Potentially, a single population of MAP cells circulates and can integrate in these disparate tissues (Jiang, Vaessen, Lenuik, et al., 2002). Restricted in vivo differentiation potential may reflect limitations imposed on MAP cells by the resident tissue. Additional potential may be revealed when MAP cells are removed from this environment, as in culture. Similar potential might be unmasked if, for example, peripheral MAP cells migrate into the brain. Exposed to a new environment with novel cues, MAP cells may differentiate into neural cells, contributing to brain plasticity.

CULTURED MSCs ARE MULTIDIFFERENTIATED Further insight into possible mechanisms of transgermal differentiation has come from gene expression analysis of cultured MSCs. MSCs grown in vitro are highly proliferative and retain the capacity for neuronal and osteogenic differentiation. Expression profiles demonstrated that proliferating MSCs are not "blank slates," expressing limited numbers of genes. On the contrary, MSCs appear to be multidifferentiated, expressing genes representative of all three embryonic germ layers and of germinal tissues.

Not unexpectedly, MSCs in culture transcribe prototypical mesodermal genes such as myosin, leptin, and the smooth muscle–specific gene SM22α. In addition, MSCs express the endodermal gene ceruloplasmin and neuroectodermal genes such as NSE, syntaxin 13, amyloid precursor protein (APP), and brain-specific aldolase C. Most surprisingly, protamine2, a germ-line–specific protein, is highly expressed in proliferating MSCs. Differentiation to specific fates may be accomplished in part by modulating expression of active genes rather than by comprehensive up-regulation of lineage-specific transcripts (Woodbury, Reynolds, and Black, 2002). This mechanism would be consistent with the rapid acquisition of neural morphologies that has been reported. Multidifferentiated cells may be "primed" for differentiation to a number of lineages while still retaining proliferative capacity.

MSCs EXPRESS NEURONAL DETERMINATION FACTORS Neuronal differentiation is initiated and propagated by transcription factors of the basic helix-loop-helix (bHLH) family. Neurogenic bHLH genes are expressed in a defined temporal fashion, resulting in a cascade of expression that activates neuronal cell fate programs. NeuroD, an intermediary in the neurogenic cascade, is expressed at high levels in proliferating MSCs. Adoption of neural morphologies is accompanied by a decrease in expression of NeuroD, recapitulating the pattern seen in vivo. In concert, neuron-specific tau and NF-M gene expression is up-regulated (Woodbury, Reynolds, and Black, 2002).

It is not clear why MSCs that express NeuroD do not undergo neuronal differentiation in the absence of exogenous signals. Perhaps inhibitory molecules block the actions of NeuroD in undifferentiated MSCs. Inactivation of these inhibitory molecules may allow preexisting NeuroD to rapidly affect neuronal differentiation. Such an underlying mechanism may explain why diverse treatment paradigms have been successful in converting MSCs to putative neurons. Similarly, exposure to a new environment, such as the CNS, may allow NeuroD to initiate neuronal differentiation, thus contributing to plasticity.

Transgermal differentiation: Is it real?

The transgermal differentiation of adult stem cells is the subject of lively debate. There have been some difficulties replicating original studies that demonstrated plasticity. Moreover, additional evidence has suggested alternative explanations for the observed differentiative capacity.

A comprehensive study attempted to verify the observation that NSCs introduced into the blood can regenerate the damaged hematopoietic system. Neurospheres of varying passage numbers were injected into sublethally irradiated mice. Despite rigorous analysis, not a single event of transgermal differentiation to hematopoietic lineages could be documented. Moreover, analysis of high-passage NSCs provided evidence of changes in growth factor dependence and gene expression. The authors concluded that transgermal differentiation of NSCs to hematopoietic lineages is an extremely rare event, and may reflect genetic and epigenetic alterations acquired during culture (Morshead et al., 2002). In keeping with this contention, freshly isolated (noncultured) NSCs fail to transdifferentiate into hematopoietic lineages in vivo (Magrassi et al., 2003).

More disturbing than difficulties reproducing claims of transgermal differentiation is evidence that stem cells can acquire unexpected phenotypes through fusion to differentiated cells. Bone marrow cells grown in culture with ESCs acquired enhanced differentiative capacity, suggesting that coculture with ESCs unmasked latent stem cell potency in the bone marrow cells. However, karyotypic analysis revealed that the ES-like cells were polyploid, generated by direct fusion of a bone marrow cell with an ESC (Terada et al., 2002). While rare, such fusion events could explain in part some reports of transgermal differentiation.

Evidence suggests that fusion of donor and host cells also occurs in vivo. Several studies have demonstrated the transgermal differentiation of HSCs to hepatic oval cells. In one model, donor HSCs rescued mutant mice afflicted with fatal liver dysfunction. There is now clear evidence that the donor HSCs fused with host cells in the liver, correcting the fatal deficiency. Interestingly, the fused cells expressed hepatocyte-specific genes, while repressing expression of hematopoietic markers. Nevertheless, in this model, correction of the genetic defect is achieved through cell fusion, not through transgermal differentiation of donor stem cells (Wang et al., 2003).

At present it is unclear how the incidence of donor-to-host cell fusion affects previous reports of transgermal differentiation in vivo. The degree of cell fusion likely varies from organ to organ. Demonstration of cell fusion between host and donor cells appears to be most prominent in the liver. In contrast, studies centered on human buccal epithelial cells demonstrated that while up to 12.7% of examined cells were donor-derived, only 0.01% were multinucleated (Tran et al., 2003). In this case, cell fusion does not account for the observed transgermal differentiation. Together, the data suggest that bone marrow–derived cells can contribute to disparate tissues through transgermal differentiation and/or fusion. The principal mechanism will likely vary from tissue to tissue. In the brain, multinucleated Purkinje cells can be generated through donor-host fusion events. This mechanism may serve to rescue compromised neurons while maintaining established contacts (Weimann et al., 2003). In contrast, karyotypically normal, donor-derived Purkinje neurons may represent newborn cells not shackled by prior connections (Mezey et al., 2003).

Perspectives

Stem cell populations exist in many organs in the adult animal, including the brain. Historically it was accepted that adult stem cells were limited in their differentiative capacity, giving rise only to cells within their resident tissue. However, recent evidence indicates that ASCs retain remarkable plasticity and are capable of differentiating into unexpected cell types, including derivatives of other germ layers. Ectodermal NSCs give rise to mesodermal blood cells, while marrow-derived stem cells differentiate into putative neural cells. Such plasticity is not limited to isolated cells grown in a culture dish but occurs in living organisms, including humans. This newly appreciated plasticity of ASCs has profound biological implications, particularly for the brain. Once thought constrained with a circumscribed neuronal population, it is now accepted that regions of the adult brain support neurogenesis throughout life, fueled by resident stem cells. The evidence presented in this chapter raises the prospect that extraneural stem cells may also contribute to neurogenesis and play a role in brain plasticity. In fact, one may hypothesize that the preponderance of neurogenesis surrounding vascular structures reflects entry into the brain parenchyma of blood-borne peripheral stem cells.

As is true of any fledgling field, reports of ASC plasticity have been greeted with skepticism and have raised more questions than they have answered. What is the mechanism behind the reported plasticity? What cues mediate differentiation of exogenous cells? In the brain, can newly differentiated neurons integrate and contribute to established circuits? Answers to these and other pending questions will require extensive study. Nevertheless, it appears that ASCs should be considered more than niche players contributing solely to their resident tissues.

REFERENCES

AKIYAMA, Y., C. RADTKE, and J. D. KOCSIS, 2002. Remyelination of the rat spinal cord by transplantation of identified bone marrow stromal cells. *J. Neurosci.* 22:6623–6630.

BJORNSON, C. R., R. L. RIETZE, B. A. REYNOLDS, M. C. MAGLI, and A. L. VESCOVI, 1999. Turning brain into blood: A hematopoietic fate adopted by adult neural stem cells in vivo. *Science* 283:534–537.

BRAZELTON, T. R., F. M. ROSSI, G. I. KESHET, and H. M. BLAU, 2000. From marrow to brain: Expression of neuronal phenotypes in adult mice. *Science* 290:1775–1779.

CHIASSON, B. J., V. TROPEPE, C. M. MORSHEAD, and D. VAN DER KOOY, 1999. Adult mammalian forebrain ependymal and subependymal cells demonstrate proliferative potential, but only subependymal cells have neural stem cell characteristics. *J. Neurosci.* 19:4462–4471.

CLARKE, D. L., C. B. JOHANSSON, J. WILBERTZ, B. VERESS, E. NILSSON, H. KARLSTROM, U. LENDAHL, and J. FRISEN, 2000. Generalized potential of adult neural stem cells. *Science* 288:1660–1663.

COHEN-CORY, S., 2002. The developing synapse: Construction and modulation of synaptic structures and circuits. *Science* 298:770–776.

DENG, W., M. OBROCKA, I. FISCHER, and D. J. PROCKOP, 2001. In vitro differentiation of human marrow stromal cells into early progenitors of neural cells by conditions that increase intracellular cyclic AMP. *Biochem. Biophys. Res. Commun.* 282:148–152.

DENNIS, J. E., J. P. CARBILLET, A. I. CAPLAN, and P. CHARBORD, 2002. The STRO-1+ marrow cell population is multipotential. *Cells Tissues Organs* 170:73–82.

DENNIS, J. E., A. MERRIAM, A. AWADALLAH, J. U. YOO, B. JOHNSTONE, and A. I. CAPLAN, 1999. A quadripotential mesenchymal progenitor cell isolated from the marrow of an adult mouse. *J. Bone Miner. Res.* 14:700–709.

GALLI, R., U. BORELLO, A. GRITTI, M. G. MINASI, C. BJORNSON, M. COLETTA, M. MORA, M. G. DE ANGELIS, R. FIOCCO, G. COSSU, and A. L. VESCOVI, 2000. Skeletal myogenic potential of human and mouse neural stem cells. *Nat. Neurosci.* 3:986–991.

GOLDMAN, S. A., and F. NOTTEBOHM, 1983. Neuronal production, migration, and differentiation in a vocal control nucleus of the adult female canary brain. *Proc. Natl. Acad. Sci. U.S.A.* 80:2390–2394.

JIANG, Y., B. N. JAHAGIRDAR, R. L. REINHARDT, R. E. SCHWARTZ, C. D. KEENE, X. R. ORTIZ-GONZALEZ, M. REYES, T. LENVIK, T. LUND, M. BLACKSTAD, J. DU, S. ALDRICH, A. LISBERG, W. C. LOW, D. A. LARGAESPADA, and C. M. VERFAILLIE, 2002. Pluripotency of mesenchymal stem cells derived from adult marrow. *Nature* 418:41–49.

JIANG, Y., B. VAESSEN, T. LENVIK, M. BLACKSTAD, M. REYES, and C. M. VERFAILLIE, 2002. Multipotent progenitor cells can be isolated from postnatal murine bone marrow, muscle, and brain. *Exp. Hematol.* 30:896–904.

KEENE, C. D., X. R. ORTIZ-GONZALEZ, Y. JIANG, D. A. LARGAESPADA, C. M. VERFAILLIE, and W. C. LOW, 2003. Neural differentiation and incorporation of bone marrow–derived multipotent adult progenitor cells after single cell transplantation into blastocyst stage mouse embryos. *Cell Transplant.* 12:201–213.

KOHYAMA, J., H. ABE, T. SHIMAZAKI, A. KOIZUMI, K. NAKASHIMA, S. GOJO, T. TAGA, T. OKANO, J. HATA, and A. UMEZAWA, 2001. Brain from bone: Efficient "meta-differentiation" of marrow stroma–derived mature osteoblasts to neurons with Noggin or a demethylating agent. *Differentiation* 68:235–244.

KOPEN, G. C., D. J. PROCKOP, and D. G. PHINNEY, 1999. Marrow stromal cells migrate throughout forebrain and cerebellum, and they differentiate into astrocytes after injection into neonatal mouse brains. *Proc. Natl. Acad. Sci. U.S.A.* 96:10711–10716.

LAYWELL, E. D., P. RAKIC, V. G. KUKEKOV, E. C. HOLLAND, and D. A. STEINDLER, 2000. Identification of a multipotent astrocytic stem cell in the immature and adult mouse brain. *Proc. Natl. Acad. Sci. U.S.A.* 97:13883–13888.

MAGRASSI, L., S. CASTELLO, L. CIARDELLI, M. PODESTA, A. GASPARONI, L. CONTI, S. PEZZOTTA, F. FRASSONI, and E. CATTANEO, 2003. Freshly dissociated fetal neural stem/progenitor cells do not turn into blood. *Mol. Cell. Neurosci.* 22:179–187.

MARRONE, D. F., and T. L. PETIT, 2002. The role of synaptic morphology in neural plasticity: Structural interactions underlying synaptic power. *Brain Res. Brain Res. Rev.* 38:291–308.

MEZEY, E., and K. J. CHANDROSS, 2000. Bone marrow: a possible alternative source of cells in the adult nervous system. *Eur. J. Pharmacol.* 405:297–302.

MEZEY, E., K. J. CHANDROSS, G. HARTA, R. A. MAKI, and S. R. MCKERCHER, 2000. Turning blood into brain: Cells bearing neuronal antigens generated in vivo from bone marrow. *Science* 290:1779–1782.

MEZEY, E., S. KEY, G. VOGELSANG, I. SZALAYOVA, G. D. LANGE, and B. CRAIN, 2003. Transplanted bone marrow generates new neurons in human brains. *Proc. Natl. Acad. Sci. U.S.A.* 100:1364–1369.

MOKRY, J., D. SUBRTOVA, and S. NEMECEK, 1996. Differentiation of epidermal growth factor-responsive neural precursor cells within neurospheres. *Acta Med.* 39:7–20.

MORSHEAD, C. M., P. BENVENISTE, N. N. ISCOVE, and D. VAN DER KOOY, 2002. Hematopoietic competence is a rare property of neural stem cells that may depend on genetic and epigenetic alterations. *Nat. Med.* 8:268–273.

MORSHEAD, C. M., and D. VAN DER KOOY, 2001. A new "spin" on neural stem cells? *Curr. Opin. Neurobiol.* 11:59–65.

NOTTEBOHM, F., 1981. A brain for all seasons: Cyclical anatomical changes in song control nuclei of the canary brain. *Science* 214:1368–1370.

NOTTEBOHM, F., M. E. NOTTEBOHM, and L. CRANE, 1986. Developmental and seasonal changes in canary song and their rela-tion to changes in the anatomy of song-control nuclei. *Behav. Neural Biol.* 46:445–471.

OISHI, K., Y. OGAWA, S. GAMOH, and M. K. UCHIDA, 2002. Contractile responses of smooth muscle cells differentiated from rat neural stem cells. *J. Physiol.* 540:139–152.

PALMER, T. D., A. R. WILLHOITE, and F. H. GAGE, 2000. Vascular niche for adult hippocampal neurogenesis. *J. Comp. Neurol.* 425:479–494.

PITTENGER, M. F., J. D. MOSCA, and K. R. MCINTOSH, 2000. Human mesenchymal stem cells: Progenitor cells for cartilage, bone, fat and stroma. *Curr. Top. Microbiol. Immunol.* 251:3–11.

PRILLER, J., D. A. PERSONS, F. F. KLETT, G. KEMPERMANN, G. W. KREUTZBERG, and U. DIRNAGL, 2001. Neogenesis of cerebellar Purkinje neurons from gene-marked bone marrow cells in vivo. *J. Cell Biol.* 155:733–738.

REYNOLDS, B. A., W. TETZLAFF, and S. WEISS, 1992. A multipotent EGF-responsive striatal embryonic progenitor cell produces neurons and astrocytes. *J. Neurosci.* 12:4565–4574.

SANCHEZ-RAMOS, J., S. SONG, F. CARDOZO-PELAEZ, C. HAZZI, T. STEDEFORD, A. WILLING, T. B. FREEMAN, S. SAPORTA, W. JANSSEN, N. PATEL, D. R. COOPER, and P. R. SANBERG, 2000. Adult bone marrow stromal cells differentiate into neural cells in vitro. *Exp. Neurol.* 164:247–256.

SONG, J. H., C. F. STEVENS, and F. H. GAGE, 2002. Neural stem cells from adult hippocampus develop essential properties of functional CNS neurons. *Nat. Neurosci.* 15:15.

SVENDSEN, C. N., M. A. CALDWELL, and T. OSTENFELD, 1999. Human neural stem cells: Isolation, expansion and transplantation. *Brain Pathol.* 9:499–513.

TERADA, N., T. HAMAZAKI, M. OKA, M. HOKI, D. M. MASTALERZ, Y. NAKANO, E. M. MEYER, L. MOREL, B. E. PETERSEN, and E. W. SCOTT, 2002. Bone marrow cells adopt the phenotype of other cells by spontaneous cell fusion. *Nature* 416:542–545.

TOMA, J. G., M. AKHAVAN, K. J. FERNANDES, F. BARNABE-HEIDER, A. SADIKOT, D. R. KAPLAN, and F. D. MILLER, 2001. Isolation of multipotent adult stem cells from the dermis of mammalian skin. *Nat. Cell Biol.* 3:778–784.

TRAN, S. D., S. R. PILLEMER, A. DUTRA, A. J. BARRETT, M. J. BROWNSTEIN, S. KEY, E. PAK, R. A. LEAKAN, A. KINGMAN, K. M. YAMADA, B. J. BAUM, and E. MEZEY, 2003. Differentiation of human bone marrow-derived cells into buccal epithelial cells in vivo: A molecular analytical study. *Lancet* 361:1084–1088.

VAN PRAAG, H., B. R. CHRISTIE, T. J. SEJNOWSKI, and F. H. GAGE, 1999. Running enhances neurogenesis, learning, and long-term potentiation in mice. *Proc. Natl. Acad. Sci. U.S.A.* 96:13427–13431.

VAN PRAAG, H., G. KEMPERMANN, and F. H. GAGE, 1999. Running increases cell proliferation and neurogenesis in the adult mouse dentate gyrus. *Nat. Neurosci.* 2:266–270.

VESCOVI, A. L., E. A. PARATI, A. GRITTI, P. POULIN, M. FERRARIO, E. WANKE, P. FROLICHSTHAL-SCHOELLER, L. COVA, M. ARCELLANA-PANLILIO, A. COLOMBO, and R. GALLI, 1999. Isolation and cloning of multipotential stem cells from the embryonic human CNS and establishment of transplantable human neural stem cell lines by epigenetic stimulation. *Exp. Neurol.* 156:71–83.

VESCOVI, A. L., B. A. REYNOLDS, D. D. FRASER, and S. WEISS, 1993. bFGF regulates the proliferative fate of unipotent (neuronal) and bipotent (neuronal/astroglial) EGF-generated CNS progenitor cells. *Neuron* 11:951–966.

WANG, X., H. WILLENBRING, Y. AKKARI, Y. TORIMARU, M. FOSTER, M. AL-DHALIMY, E. LAGASSE, M. FINEGOLD, S. OLSON, and M.

GROMPE, 2003. Cell fusion is the principal source of bone-marrow-derived hepatocytes. *Nature* 422:897–901.

WEIMANN, J. M., C. A. CHARLTON, T. R. BRAZELTON, R. C. HACKMAN, and H. M. BLAU, 2003. Contribution of transplanted bone marrow cells to Purkinje neurons in human adult brains. *Proc. Natl. Acad. Sci. U.S.A.* 100:2088–2093.

WOODBURY, D., K. REYNOLDS, and I. B. BLACK, 2002. Adult bone marrow stromal stem cells express germline, ectodermal, endodermal, and mesodermal genes prior to neurogenesis. *J. Neurosci. Res.* 69:908–917.

WOODBURY, D., E. J. SCHWARZ, D. J. PROCKOP, and I. B. BLACK, 2000. Adult rat and human bone marrow stromal cells differentiate into neurons. *J. Neurosci. Res.* 61:364–370.

ZHOU, F. C., and Y. H. CHIANG, 1998. Long-term nonpassaged EGF-responsive neural precursor cells are stem cells. *Wound Repair Regen.* 6:337–348.

ZHOU, F. C., M. R. KELLEY, Y. H. CHIANG, and P. YOUNG, 2000. Three to four-year-old nonpassaged EGF-responsive neural progenitor cells: Proliferation, apoptosis, and DNA repair. *Exp. Neurol.* 164:200–208.

13 How Sex and Stress Hormones Regulate the Structural and Functional Plasticity of the Hippocampus

BRUCE S. McEWEN

ABSTRACT The hippocampal formation, which expresses high levels of adrenal steroid receptors and a smaller number of receptors for gonadal hormones, is a resilient brain structure that is important for certain types of learning and memory. It is also vulnerable to insults such as stroke, seizures, and head trauma. The hippocampus is also sensitive and vulnerable to the effects of stress and stress hormones, and it is responsive to the actions of sex hormones as well, both during development and during adult life. Stress and sex hormones regulate three types of structural plasticity in the adult hippocampus: synaptogenesis, reorganization of dendrites, and neurogenesis in the dentate gyrus; they do so acting in concert with excitatory amino acid neurotransmitters and other endogenous modulators. Estrogens regulate synapse formation in the adult hippocampus of ovariectomized females but not in adult-castrated males. Chronic, and even sometimes acute, psychosocial stress causes suppression of neurogenesis and remodeling of dendrites in the hippocampus and the amygdala, another brain region that is closely connected to fear and stress. Developmentally programmed sex differences are also seen that determine how these forms of plasticity are manifested.

The brain is sensitive to hormones secreted by the adrenal cortex, gonads, and thyroid in adult life, as well as in early development. The earliest evidence for the hormone responsiveness of the nervous system came from the direct implantation of steroid hormones into the brain (Lisk, 1962; Barfield, 1969). Those initial studies in the 1960s used sex hormones because reproductive behaviors were known to be regulated by gonadal steroids. With the introduction of tritiated steroid hormones in the 1960s, it became possible to map the location of steroid hormone receptors in brain tissue by autoradiography and in vitro binding assays (Morrell and Pfaff, 1978; McEwen et al., 1979). This mapping was based on a model of steroid hormone action introduced in the 1960s that centered on intracellular receptors that regulate genes by binding directly to DNA and are located in the cell nucleus (Jensen and Jacobson, 1962). The model of steroid action contributed greatly to understanding the regulation of gene transcription in eukaryotes (Yamamoto, 1985; Evans, 1988; Beato and Sanchez-Pacheco, 1996). This model not only provided a clear cellular target for localizing steroid receptors in brain cells but also indicated how a chemical messenger could produce longlasting effects on neuronal structure and function.

Yet the model has changed. First, many of these hormone effects do not occur alone but rather in the context of ongoing neuronal activity. In particular, excitatory amino acids and N-methyl-D-aspartate (NMDA) receptors play an important role in the functional and structural changes produced in the hippocampal formation by estrogens and glucocorticoid hormones. At the same time, excitatory amino acids and NMDA receptors are involved in the destructive actions of stress and trauma on the hippocampus, and one of the challenges for future research is to understand what triggers the transition from adaptive plasticity to permanent damage. Second, there is increasing evidence that steroid hormone receptors not only signal the genome directly but also have indirect effects on the genome and on cellular activity through second messenger systems. This chapter reviews the adaptive plasticity in the hippocampus produced by circulating adrenocortical and gonadal hormones acting in many cases in concert with excitatory amino acid neurotransmitters. It also considers the mechanistic basis of sex differences in these responses.

Salient features of hippocampal neuroanatomy

The hippocampus has two major regions, Ammon's horn and the dentate gyrus. The principal synaptic pathways include input to the granule cells of the dentate gyrus from the entorhinal cortex via the perforant pathway. These

BRUCE S. McEWEN Harold and Margaret Milliken Hatch Laboratory of Neuroendocrinology, Rockefeller University, New York, N.Y.

171

pathways in turn project via the mossy fibers to the CA3 pyramidal cells, which then project via the Schaffer collaterals to the CA1 pyramidal cells. Within the CA3 region are a number of features that have considerable significance for its functional activity and vulnerability to damage. These features include the collaterals to other CA3 neurons, as well as recurrent projections from CA3 neurons lying closest to the dentate gyrus back to the dentate gyrus (Li et al., 1994). Both of these collateral systems contribute to the bursting pattern of CA3 neuronal activity that is a contributing factor to seizure-induced destruction of CA3 pyramidal neurons (Sloviter, 1994).

Besides the principal neurons, the hippocampal formation contains a variety of nonprincipal cells, including the excitatory mossy cells of the dentate hilus and the inhibitory interneurons that express a variety of neurochemical features in addition to producing γ-aminobutyric acid (GABA). These neurons play an important role in regulating excitability within the hippocampus (Freund and Buzsaki, 1996).

Finally, the dentate gyrus is unique within the brain in having continued neurogenesis of granule neurons during adult life (Gould et al., 2000; Cameron and McKay, 2001). The dentate gyrus is formed later than Ammon's horn, and maturation of the dentate gyrus in the first 2 weeks of life in the newborn rat (Cameron and Gould, 1996) is related to the development of emotionality, as seen in the effects of neonatal handling (Meaney et al., 1988) and in the appearance of "behavioral inhibition" (Takahashi, 1995; Gould and Cameron, 1997). The dentate gyrus, as well as the CA1 region of the hippocampus, is anatomically and functionally connected to the amygdala (Petrovich, Canteras, and Swanson, 2001), and lesions of the basolateral amygdala impair the formation of long-term potentiation in the dentate gyrus (Ikegaya, Saito, and Abe, 1997; Petrovich, Canteras, and Swanson, 2001). We next turn our attention to the modulatory effects of circulating gonadal and adrenal hormones on the structure and function of the hippocampus.

Sex hormones and the hippocampus

EXCITATORY SYNAPSE FORMATION IN THE HIPPOCAMPUS: AN EXAMPLE OF GENOMIC AND NONGENOMIC EFFECTS Estrogen treatment increases dendritic spine density on CA1 pyramidal neurons (Woolley, 1999; McEwen et al., 2001). As observed by electron microscopy, treatment of ovariectomized adult rats with estrogen also induces new synapses on spines and not on dendritic shafts of CA1 neurons, without affecting dendrite length or branching. Progesterone treatment acutely enhanced spine formation but caused the down-regulation of estrogen-induced synapses over the next 24 hours (Woolley and McEwen, 1993).

Estrogens do not act alone, and in fact, ongoing excitatory neurotransmission is required for synapse induction (Woolley, 1999; McEwen et al., 2001). This was shown by means of NMDA receptor antagonists, which blocked estrogen-induced synaptogenesis on dendritic spines in ovariectomized female rats. Furthermore, estrogen treatment increased the density of NMDA receptors in the CA1 region of the hippocampus (Woolley et al., 1997). Thus, the activation of NMDA receptors by glutamate is an essential factor in causing new excitatory synapses to develop, and the NMDA receptor system is regulated by estrogen treatment.

Spines are occupied by asymmetrical, excitatory synapses. They are sites of Ca^{2+} ion accumulation and contain NMDA receptors (Horner, 1993). NMDA receptors are expressed in large amounts in CA1 pyramidal neurons and can be imaged by conventional immunocytochemistry techniques as well as by confocal imaging, in which individual dendrites and spines can be studied for colocalization with other markers (Gazzaley et al., 1996). Confocal microscopic imaging showed that estrogen treatment up-regulates immunoreactivity for the largest NMDA receptor subunit, NR1, on dendrites and cell bodies of CA1 pyramidal neurons, whereas NR1 mRNA levels did not change after estrogen treatment that induces new synapses (Gazzaley et al., 1996). This suggests the possibility that NR1 expression is regulated posttranscriptionally by estrogen. Recent evidence suggests that muscarinic cholinergic transmission plays a critical role in the up-regulation of NMDA receptor expression by estrogen (Daniel and Dohanich, 2001).

Other recent evidence indicates that in young female rats, estrogen induction of NR1 is proportional to the induction of new spines, so that NMDA receptor density per spine is not increased; however, in the aging female rat, there is NR1 induction without an increase in dendritic spines (Adams et al., 2001). This might make the aging hippocampus more vulnerable to excitotoxic damage, for example by stroke or seizures.

Where are the estrogen receptors that mediate these effects? Adult CA1 pyramidal cells of the dorsal hippocampus do not express detectable cell nuclear estrogen receptors when assessed by tritium autoradiography and light microscopic immunocytochemistry (Weiland, Orikasa et al., 1997), whereas they express low levels of ERα and ERβ mRNA by in situ hybridization (Shughrue and Merchenthaler, 2000; McEwen and Magarinos, 2001). Instead, immunocytochemistry for ERα showed cell nuclear estrogen receptors in sparsely distributed interneurons in the CA1 region, as well as in other regions of Ammon's horn and the dentate gyrus, with a greater density in the ventral than in the dorsal hippocampus (see McEwen and Alves, 1999, for references). Autoradiography with ^{125}I estrogen was used to label estrogen receptors with a higher specific radioactivity and showed binding sites not previously detected in hippocampus using

³H estradiol (Shughrue and Merchenthaler, 2000). This may indicate locations of estrogen actions in hippocampal pyramidal cells, particularly in the ventral hippocampus.

Besides cell nuclear estrogen receptors, there is increasing evidence for non-nuclear estrogen receptors that interact with second messenger pathways (Razandi et al., 1999; Kelly and Levin, 2001). Stimulated by this evidence, we used electron microscopy to examine ERα localization in rat hippocampal formation (Milner et al., 2001). We were able to see at the electron microscopic level the cell nuclear labeling seen on light microscopy in some GABA interneurons. In the stratum radiatum of CA1, we found half of the total ERα immunoreactivity in unmyelinated axons and axon terminals containing small synaptic vesicles, an observation consistent with evidence that estrogen can influence neurotransmitter release (Gibbs, Hashash, and Johnson, 1997). Around 25% of the ERα immunoreactivity was found in dendritic spines of principal cells, where it was often associated with spine apparatus and/or postsynaptic densities, suggesting that estrogen might act locally to regulate calcium availability, phosphorylation, or protein synthesis. Finally, the remaining 25% of ERα immunoreactivity was found in astrocytic profiles, often located near the spines of principal cells.

The close association between ERα immunoreactivity and dendritic spines supports a possible local, nongenomic role for this estrogen receptor in the regulation of dendritic spine density via second messenger systems. Initial in vivo and in vitro studies in the hippocampus of one second messenger pathway, the phosphorylation of CREB, have indicated that estrogen has rapid effects that are evident within as little as 15 minutes to increase phosphoCREB immunoreactiviy in cell nuclei of hippocampal pyramidal neurons (Lee et al., 2000). One pathway by which CREB phosphorylation may occur involves the phosphoinositol-3 (PI3) kinase, or Akt, system (Datta, Brunet, and Greenberg, 1999). Indeed, the Akt system is activated rapidly by estrogen in vitro and in vivo and participates in the rapid initiation of translation of PSD-95 mRNA in vitro (Akama and McEwen, 2003; Znamensky et al., 2003). Moreover, estrogen receptor–mediated activation of second messenger systems in dendritic spines and presynaptic endings might lead to retrograde signal transduction back to the cell nucleus, perhaps via Akt or CREB, providing another pathway through which estrogen could regulate gene expression.

How can the nuclear and non-nuclear actions of estrogen work together in the hippocampus? There is strong evidence both in vivo and in vitro supporting an indirect GABAergic mediation of estrogen's actions on synapse formation involving the ERα-containing inhibitory interneurons (Murphy et al., 1998; Rudick and Woolley, 2000). The in vitro evidence comes from in vitro studies of estrogen-induced synapse for-

mation, in which estrogen induces spines on dendrites of dissociated hippocampal neurons by a process that is blocked by an NMDA receptor antagonist and not by an AMPA/kainate receptor blocker (Murphy and Segal, 1996). Furthermore, estrogen treatment was found to increase expression of phosphorylated CREB, and a specific antisense to CREB prevented both the formation of dendritic spines and the elevation in phosphoCREB immunoreactivity (Murphy and Segal, 1997). The cellular location of ERα in the cultures, resembling the in vivo localization, was in putative inhibitory interneurons, that is, glutamic acid decarboxylase (GAD)-immunoreactive cells, which constituted around 20% of the total neuronal population. Estrogen treatment caused decreases in GAD content and the number of neurons expressing GAD, and mimicking this decrease with mercaptopropionic acid, an inhibitor of GABA synthesis, caused an up-regulation of dendritic spine density, paralleling the effects of estrogen (Murphy et al., 1998). Thus, estrogen-induced synapse formation may involve the suppression of GABA inhibitory input to the pyramidal neurons where the synapses are being generated.

ANDROGENS AND THE HIPPOCAMPUS The hippocampus expresses androgen receptors that are prominently localized in CA1 pyramidal neurons (Kerr et al., 1995). Androgens positively regulate androgen receptor mRNA levels in CA1 (Kerr et al., 1995). In turn, androgen treatment induces changes in NMDA receptor expression and alters neuronal activity mediated by NMDA receptors in CA1 pyramidal neurons. Electrophysiologically, chronic treatment of castrated rats with the potent androgen, dihydrotestosterone (DHT), increased the action potential duration of CA1 pyramidal neurons and decreased the amplitude of the fast hyperpolarization; moreover, DHT treatment promoted recovery of the membrane potential after depolarization with NMDA (Pouliot, Handa, and Beck, 1996). Binding of the antagonist MK801 to NMDA receptors in the CA1 region was elevated by castration, and this increase was prevented by DHT treatment, indicating that the antagonist-binding form of the NMDA receptor is affected by androgen treatment (Kus et al., 1995).

Castration increased levels of mRNA for the gonadotropin-releasing hormone (GnRH) receptor on CA1 pyramidal neurons, but also in the CA3 region and the dentate gyrus; curiously, however, castration decreased the second messenger response to GnRH in hippocampal slices (Jennes et al., 1995). Except for electrophysiological studies, there is nothing to suggest a function for GnRH receptors in the hippocampus.

Androgens also have an influence on the adrenocortical response system of the hippocampus. Androgen treatment suppressed expression of type II (glucocorticoid) receptor mRNA but had no effect on type I (mineralocorticoid) receptor mRNA levels (Kerr, Beck, and Handa, 1996a). In this connection, castration has been reported to increase reactivity of the hypothalamo-pituitary-adrenal (HPA) axis (Handa et al., 1993). One possible reason for this is that castration increases the reactivity of neural circuits involved in regulating HPA function. Consistent with this notion is the finding that castration increased, and androgen replacement suppressed, the immediate early gene responses to novelty in the CA1 region of the hippocampus, but not in CA3 or the dentate gyrus (Kerr, Beck, and Handa, 1996b). We next turn our attention to the effects of stress and adrenal steroids on the hippocampus.

Androgen treatment also induces spine synapses in CA1 pyramidal neurons of adult castrated male rats (Leranth, Petnehazy, and Maclusky, 2003). This effect is produced over several days by treatment with DHT, but not by treatment with estradiol. The lack of an estrogen effect agrees with a previous report that also showed that blocking aromatization of testosterone at birth in male rats renders the adult male rat brain responsive to estrogens in inducing spine synapses (Lewis, McEwen, and Frankfurt, 1995). Thus, estrogens at birth "defeminize" the capability of the hippocampus to respond to estrogens for synapse formation. It remains to be seen how sensitivity to androgens is regulated by the neonatal gonadal hormone milieu.

The androgen effect on spine synapse formation in male rats may underlie the recent finding that an acute restraint-shock stress increases spine synapses within 24 hours in the CA1 region of the hippocampus (Shors, Chua, and Falduto, 2001). The response to the stressor includes a surge in testosterone levels in blood, which could contribute to the synapse formation.

Adrenal steroids and the hippocampus

ROLES OF STRESS-RELATED HORMONES IN ADAPTATION The amygdala and hippocampus are both involved in contextual fear conditioning and in passive avoidance learning, and adrenal steroids have a biphasic influence on these processes. In fear conditioning, glucocorticoids enhance learned fear (Corodimas et al., 1994), and they play an important role in forming the memory of context in contextual fear conditioning, but not of the actual effect of foot shock in rats that are already familiar with the context where the shock is administered (Pugh, Fleshner, and Rudy, 1997; Pugh, Tremblay, et al., 1997). This finding suggests that the hippocampal role in contextual fear conditioning is enhanced by moderate levels of glucocorticoids, but the fear conditioning either is not so dependent on glucocorticoids or is so strong that glucocorticoid influences are hard to demonstrate. Yet there is evidence for an influence of glucocorticoids on the flow of information within the amygdala.

Glucocorticoids potentiate serotonin inhibition of the processing of excitatory input to the lateral amygdala from the thalamus, suggesting that there is a mechanism for containing, or limiting, the sensory input that is important for fear conditioning (Stutzmann, McEwen, and Ledoux, 1998). Thus, adrenal steroids may regulate the nature of the signals that reach the amygdala and allow for greater discrimination of the most salient cues for learning.

Moreover, in passive avoidance, both catecholamines and glucocorticoids play a role in facilitating the learning (Cahill et al., 1994; Roozendaal, 2000). Catecholamines work outside of the blood-brain barrier, and their effects can be blocked by β-adrenergic-blocking agents that do not cross the blood-brain barrier (Cahill et al., 1994). Glucocorticoids enter the brain, and local implants of exogenous corticosterone into hippocampus, amygdala, and nucleus tractus solitarii are all able to enhance passive avoidance learning (Roozendaal, 2000).

Adrenal steroids also play a supporting role in the learning of a spatial navigation task in mice (Oitzl et al., 2001). Adrenalectomy impairs the acquisition of the memory of a hidden platform location in the Morris water maze and glucocorticoid administration restores the normal learning curve; however, in mice in which the glucocorticoid receptor (GR) was deleted and replaced with a GR that did not dimerize, so it could not bind to DNA, glucocorticoids had no effect in improving task acquisition (Oitzl et al., 2001). This finding illustrates a role for GRs acting on the genome in a task that is known to depend on the hippocampus. Interestingly, other actions of glucocorticoids via GRs are known to involve the protein-protein interactions that are not prevented in mice carrying the GR defective in the DNA-binding domain (Reichardt and Schutz, 1998).

Other evidence for glucocorticoid actions supports an inverted U-shaped dose-response curve in which low to moderate levels of adrenal steroids enhance acquisition of tasks that involve the hippocampus, whereas high levels of glucocorticoids disrupt task acquisition (Diamond et al., 1992, 1999; Pugh, Tremblay et al., 1997; Conrad, Lupien, and McEwen, 1999). Adrenal steroids have biphasic effects on the excitability of hippocampal neurons, which may underlie their biphasic actions on memory and recall (Diamond et al., 1992; Pavlides et al., 1994, 1995; Pavlides and McEwen, 1999).

ADAPTIVE STRUCTURAL PLASTICITY One of the ways that stress hormones modulate function within the brain is by changing the structure of neurons. Within the hippocampus, the input from the entorhinal cortex to the dentate gyrus is ramified by the connections between the dentate gyrus and the CA3 pyramidal neurons. One granule neuron innervates, on average, 12 CA3 neurons; each CA3 neuron innervates, on average, 50 other CA3 neurons via axon collaterals, as well as 25 inhibitory cells via other axon collaterals (Feng et al., 2001). The net result is a 600-fold amplification of excitation, as well as a 300-fold amplification of inhibition, that provides some degree of control of the system. The dentate gyrus–CA3 system is believed to play a role in the memory of sequences of events, although long-term storage of memory occurs in other brain regions.

There is structural plasticity within the DG-CA3 system in that new neurons continue to be produced in the dentate gyrus throughout adult life (Gould et al., 2000) and CA3 pyramidal cells undergo remodeling of their dendrites (McEwen, 1999; McEwen et al., 2001). The subgranular layer of the dentate gyrus contains cells that have the properties of astrocytes (e.g., expression of glial fibrillary acidic protein) that give rise to granule neurons (Seri et al., 2001). After bromodeoxyuridine (BrdU) administration to label the DNA of dividing cells, these newly born cells appear as clusters in the inner part of the granule cell layer, where a substantial number of them will go on to differentiate into granule neurons within as little as 7 days. The new granule neurons appear to be quite excitable and capable of participating in long-term potentiation. In the adult rat, 9000 new neurons are born per day and survive with a half-life of 28 days (Altman and Das, 1965).

There are many hormonal and neurochemical modulators of neurogenesis and cell survival in the dentate gyrus (Aberg et al., 2000; Gould et al., 2000; Malberg et al., 2000; Czeh et al., 2001; Trejo, Carro, and Torres-Aleman, 2001). Neurogenesis in the adult dentate gyrus is enhanced by the hormone, IGF-1, and by serotonin and a number of antidepressant drugs. Estradiol accelerates cell proliferation in female rats. IGF-1 is the mediator of the ability of exercise to increase cell proliferation in the dentate gyrus. Lack of IGF-1 and insulin in diabetes has the opposite effect and decreases cell proliferation.

Neurogenesis and/or survival of newly born cells is increased by putting mice in a complex ("enriched") environment (Kempermann, Kuhn, and Gage, 1997). It is increased by a form of classical conditioning that activates the hippocampus ("trace conditioning") and prolongs the survival of newly born dentate gyrus neurons (Gould, Beylin, et al., 1999; Shors, Chua, and Falduto, 2001). Certain types of acute stress and many chronic stressors suppress neurogenesis or cell survival in the dentate gyrus, and the mediators of these inhibitor effects include excitatory amino acids acting via NMDA receptors and endogenous opioids (Cameron, Tanapat, and Gould, 1998; Gould and Tanapat, 1999; McEwen, 1999; Eisch et al., 2000).

Another form of structural plasticity is the remodeling of dendrites in the hippocampus (McEwen et al., 2001). This can be seen in rats undergoing adaptation to psychosocial stress in the visible burrow system (VBS). The VBS is an apparatus with an open chamber with a supply of food and

water and several tunnels and chambers (Blanchard, McKittrick, and Blanchard, 2001). Rats can be observed from above by a video camera in this apparatus. In the VBS, male rats housed with several females establish a dominance hierarchy within several days. Over the course of the next week, a few subordinate males may die, and others (bearing scars from bite marks) will show enlarged adrenals, low testosterone levels, and many changes in brain chemistry. The dominant male has the fewest scars and the highest level of testosterone, but also has somewhat larger adrenal glands than caged control rats.

Regarding changes in brain structure, we were surprised when we looked at the branching of dendrites within the CA3 region. It was the dominant rat that had a more extensive pattern of debranching of the apical dendrites of the CA3 pyramidal neurons in the hippocampus, whereas the subordinate rats had reduced branching compared to the caged controls (McKittrick et al., 2000). We will examine this phenomenon in more detail in the discussion of chronic stress, but what the VBS result emphasizes is that it is not adrenal size or presumed amount of physiological stress per se that determines dendritic remodeling but a complex set of other factors that modulate neuronal structure. We refer to the phenomenon as dendritic remodeling, and we generally find that it is a reversible process. In hibernating hamsters, it occurs in a matter of hours and reverses itself just as quickly when hibernating animals are aroused from torpor (A. M. Magarinos, B. S. McEwen, and P. Pevet, unpublished observations).

REPEATED STRESS AND STRUCTURAL CHANGES IN THE HIPPOCAMPUS AND AMYGDALA   In the VBS example, the subordinate rats showed remodeling of dendrites relative to caged controls (McKittrick et al., 1996; Blanchard et al., 1998). Since the adrenal glands are enlarged in dominant animals as well as subordinates in the VBS, stress is a factor in the dendritic remodeling that is found in this paradigm. We now turn to the application of several forms of repeated stress to ascertain what happens to neurons within the hippocampus. We will also introduce new findings on how neurons in the amygdala respond to repeated stress.

One type of stress involves repeated restraint stress. We have restrained rats for 6 hours per day during their rest period, from 10 A.M. to 4 P.M., during the normal resting period, and we have continued this treatment for up to 6 weeks. Although this form of stress appears to be a relatively innocuous and mild, rats react with a number of behavioral changes and structural alterations in the hippocampus and amygdala. A single restraint stress session has no effect on dentate gyrus cell proliferation, with BrdU used to label new cells, but 21 days of repeated restraint stress suppresses cell proliferation; however, we have found that continuing daily restraint out to 6 weeks results in decreased dentate gyrus neuron number and volume, and a reduction by half in the survival of cells born during the period of daily stress (K. Pham et al., unpublished observations).

Besides suppressing neurogenesis, 21 days of daily restraint stress reduces branching and total length of apical dendrites of CA3 neurons (Magarinos and McEwen, 1995a, 1995b). The basal dendritic tree is not altered by repeated restraint stress. Repeated stress has also been reported to decrease the length and branching of dentate gyrus granule neurons and CA1 pyramidal neurons (Sousa et al., 2000). Dendritic remodeling is also produced by daily exposure to elevated corticosterone levels (Magarinos, Deslandes, and McEwen, 1999; McEwen, 1999; Sousa et al., 2000). Both stress- and glucocorticoid-induced remodeling are reversible (Conrad, Magarinos et al., 1999; Magarinos, Deslandes, and McEwen, 1999).

Although glucocorticoids are able to mimic the effects of repeated stress on remodeling of dendrites, glucocorticoids do not act alone, and their effects can be blocked by agents that interfere with glutamate and serotonin actions, respectively (McEwen, 1999). Excitatory amino acids play a major role in structural plasticity, and they may be responsible for suppressing neurogenesis in the dentate gyrus, as well as participating in the remodeling of dendrites (Gould and Tanapat, 1999; McEwen, 1999). During restraint stress, extracellular levels of glutamate are elevated in the hippocampus, as shown by microdialysis (Lowy, Gault, and Yamamoto, 1993; Moghaddam et al., 1994). An amino acid, taurine, that is not synaptically localized was not increased extracellularly during restraint stress. The most important finding was that adrenalectomy prevented the increased levels of extracellular glutamate seen during restraint stress (Lowy, Gault, and Yamamoto, 1993). This implies that adrenal secretions modulate the extracellular levels of glutamate.

There are multiple and interacting mediators for dendritic remodeling in the CA3 region of the hippocampus. This has been shown by blocking the stress-induced remodeling with agents for different pathways (McEwen et al., 2001). Blocking glucocorticoid secretion, for example, each day during daily restraint stress prevents dendritic remodeling. Similarly, blocking NMDA receptors also blocks remodeling. Excitatory amino acids are implicated by another drug. Using the antiseizure medication phenytoin also prevented stress-induced remodeling, as well as remodeling caused by daily glucocorticoid treatment. Phenytoin produces its antiseizure effects by blocking sodium and t-type calcium channels (see Magarinos et al., 1996; McEwen, 1999).

Another way of preventing both stress- and glucocorticoid-induced remodeling is by daily administration of a tricyclic antidepressant, tianeptine, which enhances serotonin reuptake. Serotonin release is known to be increased by stress, and this may feed into the excitatory amino acid pathway by modulating NMDA receptor sensitivity (McEwen et al., 2001). Finally, enhancing inhibitory tone with a benzodiazepine prevents stress-induced dendritic remodeling (Magarinos, Deslandes, and McEwen, 1999).

Although other areas of the hippocampus are affected by repeated stress and glucocorticoids, the CA3 region seems to be among the most sensitive. This is because CA3 neurons excite each other when they are excited by mossy fiber input, as was discussed earlier. Moreover, they stimulate further excitatory input by sending collaterals back to mossy cells in the dentate gyrus. As a result of this feedforward excitability, the CA3 is vulnerable to kainic acid–induced seizures. Cell death ensues because the cells overexcite each other. Repeated stress may be activating the same mechanism, but in a more controlled manner. Here the outcome is retraction of dendrites, which may be a protective mechanism that reduces excitatory input and spares neurons from death.

Since there are many interacting pathways that appear to contribute to the remodeling of dendrites in CA3, there are also many points at which glucocorticoids interact to affect the various neurochemical systems that are involved (McEwen, 1999; McEwen et al., 2001). We have seen, for example, that adrenal secretions promote the stress-induced increase of extracellular glutamate levels. Glucocorticoids also increase expression of NMDA receptor subunits in the hippocampus and increase certain types of calcium currents (Weiland, Orchinik, and Tanapat, 1997). They also facilitate serotonin turnover and in some brains areas increase expression of 5-HT2A receptors, while down-regulating inhibitory 5-HT1A receptors (McKittrick et al., 1996). Finally, glucocorticoids modulate subunit composition of GABAa receptors in hippocampus and alter the efficacy of the GABAa receptors in different subfields of the hippocampus (Orchinik et al., 2001). Although the details of how these effects culminate to alter dendritic morphology are not clear, the nature of these effects is consistent with the hypothesis that glucocorticoids tip the balance toward excitation over inhibition within the hippocampus.

Repeated restraint stress has a number of effects on behavior after 21 days or longer. These effects include cognitive impairment on spatial recognition memory tests and increased anxiety in an open field, as well as increased fear conditioning (Luine et al., 1994; Conrad et al., 1996; Conrad, Magarinos, et al., 1999) and increased aggression toward animals in the same cage that is manifested progressively during the dark period following the daily restraint stress (G. E. Wood, L. T. Young, and B. S. McEwen, unpublished observations). The cognitive impairment is likely to be related to the structural changes in the hippocampus described earlier, whereas the anxiety, fear, and aggression may be due to changes in the amygdala. A neural correlate of the increased anxiety, fear, and aggression is the recently reported hypertrophy of neurons in the amygdala (Chattarji et al., 2000) and the recently reported actions of acute stress to induce plasticity in the mouse amygdala (Pawlak et al., 2003).

An animal model of chronic psychosocial stress has been very influential and informative in showing that the hippocampal structural plasticity after chronic restraint stress can be generalized to another species and to a stressful situation that has consequences that are reminiscent of depressive illness (Czeh et al., 2001). Tree shrews (*Tupia belangeri*) are solitary animals, and placing an intruder to live next to a known dominant animal results in considerable psychosocial stress to the intruder in terms of threats and scuffles. Housing the intruder next to the dominant animal for 28 days and allowing a 1-hour period each day when the cage door between them is open results in considerable physiological stress. Body weight declines and cortisol and catecholamine levels in the urine are increased, compared with observations in caged controls not exposed to a dominant.

Repeated psychosocial stress for 28 days causes remodeling of dendrites of CA3 neurons (Magarinos et al., 1996), very much like that found after repeated restraint stress and also like that seen in dominant and subordinate rats in the VBS studies described earlier. Unfortunately, we do not know what happens to dendritic remodeling in the dominant tree shrews! The remodeling of CA3 dendrites can be prevented by daily treatment of intruder tree shrews with phenytoin.

Chronic psychosocial stress also causes reduced neurogenesis in the dentate gyrus (Czeh et al., 2001; Gould, McEwen, et al., 1997). The effects of psychosocial stress to suppress neurogenesis can be prevented by daily treatment with the antidepressant tianeptine. Other antidepressants have been reported to increase neurogenesis in the dentate gyrus (Malberg et al., 2000), but so far the recent study on the tree shrew is the only one to use an antidepressant to counteract the effects of an ongoing stress (Czeh et al., 2001). Tree shrews show behavioral alterations—anhedonia and reduced exploratory activity—that are prevented by treatment with antidepressants (van Kampen et al., 2002). Therefore, these results have some relevance to what antidepressants may be doing in depressive illness. For a further discussion of these issues, the reader is referred to a number of recent reviews (Duman et al., 2000; Gould et al., 2000; McEwen, 2000; Sapolsky, 2000).

SEX DIFFERENCES The effects of stress in the hippocampus and amygdala occur in an environment influenced by sex hormones and developmentally programmed sex differences. Neurogenesis in the dentate gyrus of female rats is decreased by ovariectomy and increased by estrogen treatment (Tanapat et al., 1999). Stress-induced remodeling of apical dendrites of CA3 neurons occurs in male rats but not in females (Galea et al., 1997). Thus, the circulating levels of estrogens must be considered along with the developmental programming of morphology and function. Indeed, developmentally programmed sex differences have been seen in the hippocampus as well as in other extrahypothalamic brain structures.

Male and female rats differ in their responses to acute stress and its effects on classical conditioning of the eyeblink response to a puff of air. Males show enhancement of conditioning, whereas females show a suppression (Wood and Shors, 1998). In males, acute stress increases the growth of spines on CA1 pyramidal neurons, whereas it suppresses it in females (Shors et al., 2001). Treatment of newborn females with testosterone produced a male pattern of response to acute stress, whereas interfering with androgen action in utero in males had the opposite effect (Shors and Miesegaes, 2002). In female rats, estrogens reduce the acquistion of conditioned avoidance responses and fear conditioning (Diaz-Veliz et al., 1989, 1991; Gupta et al., 2001).

The hippocampal formation shows subtle sex differences in structure and function. One series of studies has pointed to sex differences in hippocampal morphology that are dependent on the rearing environment (Jursaka, 1991). Other sex differences are revealed by the effects of hormone treatment. In the CA1 region of males, estrogen treatment fails to induce as large a number of spine synapses as in females, but blockage at birth of the aromatizaton of testosterone to estradiol in male neonates increases the amount of spine synapses induced by estrogen treatment in adulthood (Lewis, McEwen, and Frankfurt, 1995). This suggests that the responsiveness of the hippocampus to estrogenic regulation of synapse formation is defeminized in males by the neonatal actions of testosterone. On the other hand, in the eyeblink conditioning described earlier, it appears to be the actions of androgens before birth that play a significant role in the masculinization of the response of the adult hippocampus to acute stress (Shors and Miesegaes, 2002).

How do these sex differences come about during development? Like the cerebral cortex, the rat hippocampus transiently expresses estrogen receptors during perinatal development (O'Keefe and Handa, 1990; O'Keefe et al., 1995). The story regarding androgen receptors is less clear. The presence of estrogen receptors in the hippocampus coincides with the transient expression of the aromatizing enzyme system that converts testosterone to estradiol (MacLusky et al., 1987); as a result, estrogen receptors in male rats would be exposed to locally generated estradiol, and this could lead to sexual differentiation of hippocampal structure and function. Consistent with this scenario are data showing that, while neonatal castration of male rats produced female-like learning curves in a Morris water maze, the administration of estradiol to newborn female rats produced a malelike learning curve (Williams and Meck, 1991).

These cognitive sex differences are not necessarily due solely to what goes on in the CA1, because sex differences in the hippocampus are not confined to the CA1 region. For example, there are sex differences in the density of apical dendritic excrescences and branching of dendrites of CA3 pyramidal neurons. Treatment with triiodothyronine (T3) during the first week of postnatal life enhanced these differences (Gould et al., 1990). Excrescences on the proximal region of apical dendrites receive input from mossy fiber synapses from granule neurons of the dentate gyrus. Therefore, the greater density of excrescences in males is consistent with a report that male rats have a greater number of mossy fiber synapses than females (Parducz and Garcia-Segura, 1993).

In contrast to the story for apical dendrites, female rats have more branch points than males on basal dendrites of CA3 pyramidal neurons, suggesting that they have more synaptic input (Galea et al., 1997). As noted earlier, however, females show atrophy of basal dendritic processes after 21 days of daily restraint stress, whereas males show atrophy of apical dendrites (Galea et al., 1997; Magarinos and McEwen, 1995b). Moreover, pyramidal neuron loss was evident in subordinate male vervet monkeys but not in females after prolonged psychosocial stress (Uno et al., 1989), and evidence of neuronal damage in rats undergoing cold swim stress was evident in males but not in females (Mizoguchi et al., 1992). However, after estrogens are absent, the female hippocampus may be vulnerable to functional impairment, judging from the report that women who showed an increase in overnight urinary cortisol over 2.5 years showed declines in cognitive performance on hippocampal-related memory tasks (Seeman et al., 1997).

Conclusions

The brain is a resilient organ that is capable of considerable structural remodeling in adult life. This chapter has provided a glimpse into one aspect of this plasticity involving the hippocampus and amygdala and the actions of adrenal steroids and gonadal hormones acting in concert with excitatory amino acid neurotransmitters and other modulators. In these types of plasticity, increasing evidence reveals that male and female brains differ in their responses to these agents, including different responses to both acute and chronic stressors. Some of these sex differences may be developmentally programmed, whereas others may reflect the interactions between gonadal hormones and ongoing stress. This is an exciting area of inquiry that is highly relevant to stress-related disorders, including major anxiety-related disorders and depressive illness (McEwen, 2003). It is also of fundamental interest for neuroscience because the ability of some nerve cells to undergo remodeling is clearly dependent on the hormonal milieu and on developmental processes in which hormones play a role.

REFERENCES

ABERG, M. A., N. D. ABERG, H. HEDBACKER, J. OSCARSSON, and P. S. ERIKSSON, 2000. Peripheral infusion of IGF-1 selectively induces neurogenesis in the adult rat hippocampus. *J. Neurosci.* 20:2896–2903.

ADAMS, M. M., R. A. SHAH, W. G. M. JANSSEN, and J. H. MORRISON, 2001. Different modes of hippocampal plasticity in response to estrogen in young and aged female rats. Proc. *Natl. Acad. Sci. U.S.A.* 98:8071–8076.

AKAMA, K. T., and B. S. MCEWEN, 2003. Estrogen stimulates post-synaptic density-95 rapid protein synthesis via the Akt/protein kinase B pathway. *J. Neurosci.* 23:2333–2339.

ALTMAN, J., and G. D. DAS, 1965. Autoradiographic and histological studies of postnatal neurogenesis. I. A longitudinal investigation of the kinetics, migration and transformation of cells incorporating tritiated thymidine in neonate rats, with special reference to postnatal neurogenesis in some brain regions. *J. Comp. Neurol.* 126:337–390.

BARFIELD, R., 1969. Activation of copulatory behavior by androgen implanted into the preoptic area of the male fowl. *Horm. Behav.* 1:37–52.

BEATO, M., and A. SANCHEZ-PACHECO, 1996. Interaction of steroid hormone receptors with the transcription initiation complex. *Endocr. Rev.* 17:587–609.

BLANCHARD, R. J., M. HEBERT, R. R. SAKAI, C. MCKITTRICK, A. HENRIE, E. YUDKO, B. S. MCEWEN, and D. C. BLANCHARD, 1998. Chronic social stress: Changes in behavioral and physiological indices of emotion. *Aggress. Behav.* 24:307–321.

BLANCHARD, R. J., C. R. MCKITTRICK, and D. C. BLANCHARD, 2001. Animal models of social stress: Effects on behavior and brain neurochemical systems. *Physiol. Behav.* 73:261–271.

CAHILL, L., B. PRINS, M. WEBER, and J. L. MCGAUGH, 1994. Beta-adrenergic activation and memory for emotional events. *Nature* 371:702–704.

CAMERON, H. A., and E. GOULD, 1996. The control of neuronal birth and survival. In *Receptor Dynamics in Neural Development*, C. A. Shaw, ed. New York: CRC Press, pp. 141–157.

CAMERON, H. A., and R. D. G. MCKAY, 2001. Adult neurogenesis produces a large pool of new granule cells in the dentate gyrus. *J. Comp. Neurol.* 435:406–417.

CAMERON, H. A., P. TANAPAT, and E. GOULD, 1998. Adrenal steroids and N-methyl-D-aspartate receptor activation regulate neurogenesis in the dentate gyrus of adult rats through a common pathway. *Neuroscience* 82:349–354.

CHATTARJI, S., A. VYAS, R. MITRA, and B. S. S. RAO, 2000. Effects of chronic unpredictable and immobilization stress on neuronal plasticity in the rat amygdala and hippocampus. *Soc. Neurosci. Abs.* 26:571.9, 1533.

CONRAD, C. D., L. A. M. GALEA, Y. KURODA, and B. S. MCEWEN, 1996. Chronic stress impairs rat spatial memory on the Y-maze and this effect is blocked by tianeptine pre-treatment. *Behav. Neurosci.* 110:1321–1334.

CONRAD, C. D., S. J. LUPIEN, and B. S. MCEWEN, 1999. Support for a bimodal role for type II adrenal steroid receptors in spatial memory. *Neurobiol. Learn. Mem.* 72:39–46.

CONRAD, C. D., A. M. MAGARINOS, J. E. LEDOUX, and B. S. MCEWEN, 1999. Repeated restraint stress facilitates fear conditioning independently of causing hippocampal CA3 dendritic atrophy. *Behav. Neurosci.* 113:902–913.

CORODIMAS, K. P., J. E. LEDOUX, P. W. GOLD, and J. SCHULKIN, 1994. Corticosterone potentiation of learned fear. *Ann. N. Y. Acad. Sci.* 746:392.

CZEH, B., T. MICHAELIS, T. WATANABE, J. FRAHM, G. DE BIURRUN, M. VAN KAMPEN, A. BARTOLOMUCCI, and E. FUCHS, 2001. Stress-induced changes in cerebral metabolites, hippocampal volume and cell proliferation are prevented by antidepressant treatment with tianeptine. *Proc. Natl. Acad. Sci. U.S.A.* 98: 12796–12801.

DANIEL, J. M., and G. P. DOHANICH, 2001. Acetylcholine mediates the estrogen-induced increase in NMDA receptor binding in CA1 of the hippocampus and the associated improvement in working memory. *J. Neurosci.* 21:6949–6956.

DATTA, S. R., A. BRUNET, and M. E. GREENBERG, 1999. Cellular survival: A play in three Akts. *Genes Dev.* 13:2905–2927.

DIAMOND, D. M., M. C. BENNETT, M. FLESHNER, and G. M. ROSE, 1992. Inverted-U relationship between the level of peripheral corticosterone and the magnitude of hippocampal primed burst potentiation. *Hippocampus* 2:421–430.

DIAMOND, D. M., C. R. PARK, K. L. HEMAN, and G. M. ROSE, 1999. Exposing rats to a predator impairs spatial working memory in the radial arm water maze. *Hippocampus* 9:542–552.

DIAZ-VELIZ, G., F. URRESTA, N. DUSSAUBAT, and S. MORA, 1991. Effects of estradiol replacement in ovariectomized rats on conditioned avoidance responses and other behaviors. *Physiol. Behav.* 50:61–65.

DIAZDIAZ-VELIZ, G., V. SOTO, N. DUSSAUBAT, and S. MORA, 1989. Influence of the estrous cycle, ovariectomy and estradiol replacement upon the acquisition of conditioned avoidance responses in rats. *Physiol. Behav.* 46:397–401.

DUMAN, R. S., J. MALBERG, S. NAKAGAWA, and C. D'SA, 2000. Neuronal plasticity and survival in mood disorders. *Biol. Psychiatry* 48:732–739.

EISCH, A. J., M. BARROT, C. A. SCHAD, D. W. SELF, and E. J. NESTLER, 2000. Opiates inhibit neurogenesis in the adult rat hippocampus. *Proc. Natl. Acad. Sci. U.S.A.* 97:7579–7584.

EVANS, R., 1988. The steroid and thyroid hormone receptor superfamily. *Science* 240:889–895.

FENG, R., C. RAMPON, Y.-P. TANG, D. SHROM, J. JIN, M. KYIN, B. SOPHER, G. M. MARTIN, S.-H. KIM, R. B. LANGDON, S. S. SISODIA, and J. Z. TSIEN, 2001. Deficient neurogenesis in forebrain-specific presenilin-1 knockout mice is associated with reduced clearance of hippocampal memory traces. *Neuron* 32:911–926.

FREUND, T. F., and G. BUZSAKI, 1996. Interneurons of the hippocampus. *Hippocampus* 6:345–470.

GALEA, L. A. M., B. S. MCEWEN, P. TANAPAT, T. DEAK, R. L. SPENCER, and F. S. DHABHAR, 1997. Sex differences in dendritic atrophy of CA3 pyramidal neurons in response to chronic restraint stress. *Neuroscience* 81:689–697.

GAZZALEY, A. H., N. G. WEILAND, B. S. MCEWEN, and J. H. MORRISON, 1996. Differential Regulation of NMDAR1 mRNA and protein by estradiol in the rat hippocampus. *J. Neurosci.* 16:6830–6838.

GIBBS, R. B., A. HASHASH, and D. A. JOHNSON, 1997. Effect of estrogen on potassium-stimulated acetylcholine release in the hippocampus and overlying cortex of adult rats. *Brain Res.* 749:143–146.

GOULD, E., A. BEYLIN, P. TANAPAT, A. REEVES, and T. J. SHORS, 1999. Learning enhances adult neurogenesis in the hippocampal formation. *Nat. Neurosci.* 2:260–265.

GOULD, E., and H. A. CAMERON, 1997. Early NMDA receptor blockade impairs defensive behavior and increases cell proliferation in the dentate gyrus of developing rats. *Behav. Neurosci.* 111:49–56.

GOULD, E., B. S. MCEWEN, P. TANAPAT, L. A. M. GALEA, and E. FUCHS, 1997. Neurogenesis in the dentate gyrus of the adult tree shrew is regulated by psychosocial stress and NMDA receptor activation. *J. Neurosci.* 17:2492–2498.

GOULD, E., and P. TANAPAT, 1999. Stress and hippocampal neurogenesis. *Biol. Psychiatry* 46:1472–1479.

GOULD, E., P. TANAPAT, T. RYDEL, and N. HASTINGS, 2000. Regulation of hippocampal neurogenesis in adulthood. *Biol. Psychiatry* 48:715–720.

GOULD, E., A. WESTLIND-DANIELSSON, M. FRANKFURT, and B. S. MCEWEN, 1990. Sex differences and thyroid hormone sensitivity of hippocampal pyramidal neurons. *J. Neurosci.* 10:996–1003.

GUPTA, R. R., S. SEN, L. L. DIEPENHORST, C. N. RUDICK, and S. MAREN, 2001. Estrogen modulates sexually dimorphic contextual fear conditioning and hippocampal long-term potentiation (LTP) in rats. *Brain Res.* 888:356–365.

HANDA, R. J., K. M. NUNLEY, S. A. LORENS, J. P. LOUIE, R. F. MCGIVERN, and M. R. BOLLNOW, 1993. Androgen regulation of adrenocorticotropin and corticosterone secretion in the male rat following novelty and foot shock stressors. *Physiol. Beh.* 55:117–124.

HORNER, C. H., 1993. Plasticity of the dendritic spine. *Prog. Neurobiol.* 41:281–321.

IKEGAYA, Y., H. SAITO, and K. ABE, 1997. The basomedial and basolateral amygdaloid nuclei contribute to the induction of long-term potentiation in the dentate gyrus *in vivo*. *Eur. J. Neurosci.* 8:1833–1839.

JENNES, L., B. BRAME, A. CENTERS, J. A. JANOVICK, and P. M. CONN, 1995. Regulation of hippocampal gonadotropin releasing hormone (GnRH) receptor mRNA and GnRH-stimulated inositol phosphate production by gonadal steroid hormones. *Mol. Brain Res.* 33:104–110.

JENSEN, E., and H. JACOBSON, 1962. Basic guides to the mechanism of estrogen action. *Rec. Prog. Horm. Res.* 18:387–408.

JURSAKA, J., 1991. Sex differences in "cognitive" regions of the rat brain. *Psychoneuroendocrinology* 16:105–119.

KELLY, M. J., and E. R. LEVIN, 2001. Rapid actions of plasma membrane estrogen receptors. *Trends Endocrinol. Metab.* 12:152–156.

KEMPERMANN, G., H. G. KUHN, and F. H. GAGE, 1997. More hippocampal neurons in adult mice living in an enriched environment. *Nature* 586:493–495.

KERR, J. E., R. J. ALLORE, S. G. BECK, and R. J. HANDA, 1995. Distribution and hormonal regulation of androgen receptor (AR) and AR messenger ribonucleic acid in the rat hippocampus. *Endocrinology* 136:3213–3221.

KERR, J. E., S. G. BECK, and R. J. HANDA, 1996a. Androgens modulate glucocorticoid receptor mRNA, but not mineralocorticoid receptor mRNA levels, in the rat hippocampus. *J. Neuroendocrinol.* 8:439–447.

KERR, J. E., S. G. BECK, and R. J. HANDA, 1996b. Androgens selectively modulate C-FOS messenger RNA induction in the rat hippocampus following novelty. *Neuroscience* 74:757–766.

KUS, L., R. J. HANDA, J. M. HAUTMAN, and A. J. BEITZ, 1995. Castration increases [^{125}I]MK801 binding in the hippocampus of male rats. *Brain Res.* 683:270–274.

LEE, S. J., J. C. DUNLOP, S. E. ALVES, W. G. BRAKE, and B. S. MCEWEN, 2000. PCREB immunoreactivity in the rat hippocampus following estrogen treatment: In vivo and in vitro studies. *Soc. Neurosci. Abstr.* 26:294.

Leranth, C., O. Petnehazy, and N. J. MacLusky, 2003. Gonadal hormones affect spine synaptic density in the CA1 hippocampal subfield of male rats. *J. Neurosci.* 23:1588–1592.

Lewis, C., B. S. McEwen, and M. Frankfurt, 1995. Estrogen-induction of dendritic spines in ventromedial hypothalamus and hippocampus: Effects of neonatal aromatase blockade and adult castration. *Dev. Brain Res.* 87:91–95.

Li, X. G., P. Somogyi, A. Ylinen, and G. Buzsaki, 1994. The hippocampal CA3 network: An in vivo intracellular labeling study. *J. Comp. Neurol.* 339:181–208.

Lisk, R., 1962. Diencephalic placement of estradiol and sexual receptivity in female rat. *Am. J. Physiol.* 203:493–496.

Lowy, M. T., L. Gault, and B. K. Yamamoto, 1993. Adrenalectomy attenuates stress-induced elevations in extracellular glutamate concentrations in the hippocampus. *J. Neurochem.* 61:1957–1960.

Luine, V., M. Villegas, C. Martinez, and B. S. McEwen, 1994. Repeated stress causes reversible impairments of spatial memory performance. *Brain Res.* 639:167–170.

MacLusky, N., A. S. Clark, F. Naftolin, and P. S. Goldman-Rakic, 1987. Oestrogen formation in the mammalian brain: Possible role of aromatase in sexual differentiation of the hippocampus and neocortex. *Steroids* 50:459–474.

Magarinos, A. M., A. Deslandes, and B. S. McEwen, 1999. Effects of antidepressants and benzodiazepine treatments on the dendritic structure of CA3 pyramidal neurons after chronic stress. *Eur. J. Pharm.* 371:113–122.

Magarinos, A. M., and B. S. McEwen, 1995a. Stress-induced atrophy of apical dendrites of hippocampal CA3c neurons: Comparison of stressors. *Neuroscience* 69:83–88.

Magarinos, A. M., and B. S. McEwen, 1995b. Stress-induced atrophy of apical dendrites of hippocampal CA3c neurons: Involvement of glucocorticoid secretion and excitatory amino acid receptors. *Neuroscience* 69:89–98.

Magarinos, A. M., B. S. McEwen, G. Flugge, and E. Fuchs, 1996. Chronic psychosocial stress causes apical dendritic atrophy of hippocampal CA3 pyramidal neurons in subordinate tree shrews. *J. Neurosci.* 16:3534–3540.

Malberg, J. E., A. J. Eisch, E. J. Nestler, and R. S. Duman, 2000. Chronic antidepressant treatment increases neurogenesis in adult rat hippocampus. *J. Neurosci.* 20:9104–9110.

McEwen, B. S., 1999. Stress and hippocampal plasticity. *Annu. Rev. Neurosci.* 22:105–122.

McEwen, B. S., 2000. The neurobiology of stress: From serendipity to clinical relevance. *Brain Res.* 886:172–189.

McEwen, B. S., 2003. Mood disorders and allostatic load. *Biol. Psychiatry* 54:200–207.

McEwen, B. S., K. Akama, S. Alves, W. G. Brake, K. Bulloch, S. Lee, C. Li, G. Yuen, and T. A. Milner, 2001. Tracking the estrogen receptor in neurons: Implications for estrogen-induced synapse formation. *Proc. Natl. Acad. Sci. U.S.A.* 98:7093–7100.

McEwen, B. S., and S. H. Alves, 1999. Estrogen actions in the central nervous system. *Endocr. Rev.* 20:279–307.

McEwen, B. S., P. G. Davis, B. Parsons, and D. W. Pfaff, 1979. The brain as a target for steroid hormone action. *Annu. Rev. Neurosci.* 2:65–112.

McEwen, B. S., and A. M. Magarinos, 2001. Stress and hippocampal plasticity: Implications for the pathophysiology of affective disorders. *Hum. Psychopharmacol.* 16:S7–S19.

McKittrick, C. R., A. M. Magarinos, D. C. Blanchard, R. J. Blanchard, B. S. McEwen, and R. R. Sakai, 1996. Chronic social stress decreases binding to 5HT transporter sites and reduces dendritic arbors in CA3 of hippocampus. *Soc. Neurosci Abstr.* 22:809.18, 2060.

McKittrick, C. R., A. M. Magarinos, D. C. Blanchard, R. J. Blanchard, B. S. McEwen, and R. R. Sakai, 2000. Chronic social stress reduces dendritic arbors in CA3 of hippocampus and decreases binding to serotonin transporter sites. *Synapse* 36:85–94.

McKittrick, C. R., and B. S. McEwen, 1996. Regulation of serotonergic function in the CNS by steroid hormones and stress. In *CNS Neurotransmitters and Neuromodulators Neuroactive Steroids*, T. W. Stone, ed. New York: CRC Press, pp. 37–76.

Meaney, M., D. Aitken, H. Berkel, S. Bhatnagar, and R. Sapolsky, 1988. Effect of neonatal handling of age-related impairments associated with the hippocampus. *Science* 239:766–768.

Milner, T. A., B. S. McEwen, S. Hayashi, C. J. Li, L. Reagen, and S. E. Alves, 2001. Ultrastructural evidence that hippocampal alpha estrogen receptors are located at extranuclear sites. *J. Comp. Neurol.* 429:355–371.

Mizoguchi, K., T. Kunishita, D. H. Chui, T. Tabira, 1992. Stress induces neuronal death in the hippocampus of castrated rats. *Neurosci. Lett.* 138:157–160.

Moghaddam, B., M. L. Boliano, B. Stein-Behrens, R. Sapolsky, 1994. Glucocorticoids mediate the stress-induced extracellular accumulation of glutamate. *Brain Res.* 655:251–254.

Morrell, J., and D. W. Pfaff, 1978. A neuroendocrine approach to brain function: Localization of sex steroid concentrating cells in vertebrate brains. *Am. Zool.* 18:447–460.

Murphy, D. D., N. B. Cole, V. Greenberger, M. Segal, 1998. Estradiol increases dendritic spine density by reducing GABA neurotransmission in hippocampal neurons. *J. Neurosci.* 18:2550–2559.

Murphy, D. D., M. Segal, 1996. Regulation of dendritic spine density in cultured rat hippocampal neurons by steroid hormones. *J. Neurosci.* 16:4059–4068.

Murphy, D. D., M. Segal, 1997. Morphological plasticity of dendritic spines in central neurons is mediated by activation of cAMP response element binding protein. *Proc. Natl. acad. Sci. U.S.A.* 94:1482–1487.

O'keefe, J. A., and R. J. Handa, 1990. Transient elevation of estrogen receptors in the neonatal rat hippocampus. *Dev. Brain Res.* 57:119–127.

O'keefe, J. A., Y. Li, L. H. Burgess, and R. J. Handa, 1995. Estrogen receptor mRNA alterations in the developing rat hippocampus. *Mol. Brain Res.* 30:115–124.

Oitzl, M. S., H. M. Reichardt, M. Joels, and E. R. De Kloet, 2001. Point mutation in the mouse glucocorticoid receptor preventing DNA binding impairs spatial memory. *Proc. Natl. Acad. Sci. U.S.A.* 98:12790–12795.

Orchinik, M., S. S. Carroll, Y.-H. Li, B. S. McEwen, and N. G. Weiland, 2001. Heterogeneity of hippocampal GABA$_A$ receptors: Regulation by corticosterone. *J. Neurosci.* 21:330–339.

Parducz, A., and L. M. Garcia-Segura, 1993. Sexual differences in the synaptic connectivity in the rat dentate gyrus. *Neurosci. Lett.* 161:53–56.

Pavlides, C., A. Kimura, A. M. Magarinos, and B. S. McEwen, 1994. Type I adrenal steroid receptors prolong hippocampal long-term potentiation. *Neuroreport* 5:2673–2677.

Pavlides, C., and B. S. McEwen, 1999. Effects of mineralocorticoid and glucocorticoid receptors on long-term potentiation in the CA3 hippocampal field. *Brain Res.* 851:204–214.

Pavlides, C., Y. Watanabe, A. M. Magarinos, and B. S. McEwen, 1995. Opposing role of adrenal steroid Type I and Type II receptors in hippocampal long-term potentiation. *Neuroscience* 68:387–394.

PAWLAK, R., A. M. MAGARINOS, J. MELCHOR, B. McEWEN, and S. STRICKLAND, 2003. Tissue plasminogen activator in the amygdala is critical for stress-induced anxiety-like behavior. *Nat. Neurosci.* 6:168–174.

PETROVICH, G. D., N. S. CANTERAS, and L. W. SWANSON, 2001. Combinatorial amygdalar inputs to hippocampal domains and hypothalamic behavior systems. *Brain Res. Rev.* 38:247–289.

POULIOT, W. A., R. J. HANDA, and S. G. BECK, 1996. Androgen modulates *N*-methyl-D-aspartate-mediated depolarization in CA1 hippocampal pyramidal cells. *Synapse* 23:10–19.

PUGH, C. R., M. FLESHNER, and J. W. RUDY, 1997. Type II glucocorticoid receptor antagonists impair contextual but not auditory-cue fear conditioning in juvenile rats. *Neurobiol. Learn. Mem.* 67:75–79.

PUGH, C. R., D. TREMBLAY, M. FLESHNER, and J. W. RUDY, 1997. A selective role for corticosterone in contextual-fear conditioning. *Behav. Neurosci.* 111:503–511.

RAZANDI, M., A. PEDRAM, G. L. GREENE, and E. R. LEVIN, 1999. Cell membrane and nuclear estrogen receptors (ERs) originate from a single transcript: Studies of ERα and ERβ expressed in Chinese hamster ovary cells. *Mol. Endocrinol.* 13:307–319.

REICHARDT, H. M., G. SCHUTZ, 1998. Glucocorticoid signalling: multiple variations of a common theme. *Mol. Cell. Endocrinol.* 146:1–6.

ROOZENDAAL, B., 2000. Glucocorticoids and the regulation of memory consolidation. *Psychoneuroendocrinology* 25:213–238.

RUDICK, C. N., and C. S. WOOLLEY, 2000. Estradiol induces a phasic Fos response in the hippocampal CA1 and CA3 regions of adult female rats. *Hippocampus* 10:274–283.

SAPOLSKY, R. M., 2000. The possibility of neurotoxicity in the hippocampus in major depression: A primer on neuron death. *Biol. Psychiatry* 48:755–765.

SEEMAN, T. E., B. S. McEWEN, B. H. SINGER, M. S. ALBERT, and J. W. ROWE, 1997. *Increase in urinary cortisol excretion and memory declines*: MacArthur studies of successful aging. *J. Clin. Endocrinol. Metab.* 82:2458–2465.

SERI, B., J. M. GARCIA-VERDUGO, B. S. McEWEN, and A. ALVAREZ-BUYLLA, 2001. Astrocytes give rise to new neurons in the adult mammalian hippocampus. *J. Neurosci.* 21:7153–7160.

SHORS, T. J., C. CHUA, and J. FALDUTO, 2001. Sex differences and opposite effects of stress on dendritic spine density in the male versus female hippocampus. *J. Neurosci.* 21:6292–6297.

SHORS, T. J., and G. MIESEGAES, 2002. Testosterone in utero and at birth dictates how stressful experience will affect learning in adulthood. *Proc. Natl. Acad. Sci. U.S.A.* 99:13955–13960.

SHORS, T. J., G. MIESEGAES, A. BEYLIN, M. ZHAO, T. RYDEL, and E. GOULD, 2001. Neurogenesis in the adult is involved in the formation of trace memories. *Nature* 410:372–376.

SHUGHRUE, P. J., and I. MERCHENTHALER, 2000. Evidence for novel estrogen binding sites in the rat hippocampus. *Neuroscience* 99:605–612.

SLOVITER, R. S., 1994. The functional organization of the hippocampal dentate gyrus and its relevance to the pathogenesis of temporal lobe epilepsy. *Ann. Neurol.* 35:640–654.

SOUSA, N., N. V. LUKOYANOV, M. D. MADEIRA, O. F. X. ALMEIDA, and M. M. PAULA-BARBOSA, 2000. Reorganization of the morphology of hippocampal neurites and synapses after stress-induced damage correlates with behavioral improvement. *Neuroscience* 97:253–266.

STUTZMANN, G. E., B. S. McEWEN, and J. E. LEDOUX, 1998. Serotonin modulation of sensory inputs to the lateral amygdala: Dependency on corticosterone. *J. Neurosci.* 18:9529–9538.

TAKAHASHI, L. K., 1995. Glucocorticoids, the hippocampus, and behavioral inhibition in the preweanling rat. *J. Neurosci.* 15:6023–6034.

TANAPAT, P., N. B. HASTINGS, A. J. REEVES, and E. GOULD, 1999. Estrogen stimulates a transient increase in the number of new neurons in the dentate gyrus of the adult female rat. *J. Neurosci.* 19:5792–5801.

TREJO, J. L., E. CARRO, and I. TORRES-ALEMAN, 2001. Circulating insulin-like growth factor I mediates exercise-induced increases in the number of new neurons in the adult hippocampus. *J. Neurosci.* 21:1628–1634.

UNO, H., T. ROSS, J. ELSE, M. SULEMAN, and R. SAPOLSKY, 1989. Hippocampal damage associated with prolonged and fatal stress in primates. *J. Neurosci.* 9:1705–1711.

VAN KAMPEN, M., M. KRAMER, C. HIEMKE, G. FLUGGE, and E. FUCHS, 2002. The chronic psychosocial stress paradigm in male tree shrews: Evaluation of a novel animal model for depressive disorders. *Stress* 5:37–46.

WEILAND, N. G., M. ORCHINIK, and P. TANAPAT, 1997. Chronic corticosterone treatment induces parallel changes in *N*-methyl-D-aspartate receptor subunit messenger RNA levels and antagonist binding sites in the hippocampus. *Neuroscience* 78:653–662.

WEILAND, N. G., C. ORIKASA, S. HAYASHI, and B. S. McEWEN, 1997. Distribution and hormone regulation of estrogen receptor immunoreactive cells in the hippocampus of male and female rats. *J. Comp. Neurol.* 388:603–612.

WILLIAMS, C. L., and W. H. MECK, 1991. The organizational effects of gonadal steroids on sexually dimorphic spatial ability. *Psychoneuroendocrinology* 16:155–176.

WOOD, G. E., and T. J. SHORS, 1998. Stress facilitates classical conditioning in males, but impairs classical conditioning in females through activational effects of ovarian hormones. *Proc. Natl. Acad. Sci. U.S.A.* 95:4066–4071.

WOOLLEY, C., and B. S. McEWEN, 1993. Roles of estradiol and progesterone in regulation of hippocampal dendritic spine density during the estrous cycle in the rat. *J. Comp. Neurol.* 336:293–306.

WOOLLEY, C. S., 1999. Effects of estrogen in the CNS. *Curr. Opin. Neurobiol.* 9:349–354.

WOOLLEY, C. S., N. G. WEILAND, B. S. McEWEN, and P. A. SCHWARTZKROIN, 1997. Estradiol increases the sensitivity of hippocampal CA1 pyramidal cells to NMDA receptor-mediated synaptic input: Correlation with dendritic spine density. *J. Neurosci.* 17:1848–1859.

YAMAMOTO, K., 1985. Steroid receptor regulated transcription of specific genes and gene networks. *Annu. Rev. Genet.* 19:209–252.

ZNAMENSKY, V., K. T. AKAMA, B. S. McEWEN, and T. A. MILNER, 2003. Estrogen levels regulate the subcellular distribution of phosphorylated Akt in hippocampal Ca1 dendrites. *J. Neurosci.* 23:2340–2347.

III SENSORY
SYSTEMS

Introduction

J. ANTHONY MOVSHON AND
BRIAN WANDELL

THE TASK OF SENSORY systems is to provide a faithful representation of biologically relevant events in the external environment. Over the years, we have learned that the physical signals transduced by receptors are very different from the biologically important information in the environment. The receptor signals are a list of numerical values, such as the number of pixels in an image or a list of the instantaneous pressure levels in a sound. This list defines much about the stimulus, but knowing only the list gives little understanding of the *information* it contains. The sensitivity and precision of sensory transduction are remarkable, but, as Helmholtz taught us, making accurate inferences from receptor signals is the true challenge of sensory systems.

These inferences are at the same time enormously richer and enormously simpler than the basic measurements of light intensity, force, and chemical composition made by sensory receptors. The inferences are richer because they contain representations of objects, states, and events that are abstracted from the primitive sensory signals; they are simpler because they represent the distillation of the vast quantities of raw measurement information offered to the central nervous system by each sensory surface. The fundamental questions of sensory neuroscience, then, are the following: What are the computations that extract meaning from incoming receptor data? What neural mechanisms perform these computations? In what ways do different sensory systems operate differently, and in what ways are they the same?

This section on sensory systems includes chapters with a variety of perspectives on the inferences and neural mechanisms of the senses of sight, hearing, smell, and touch. Different chapters explore levels of function, from early stages of encoding to high levels of perceptual inference.

The levels of analysis cover the gamut from cell biology to behavior.

A recurrent theme in recent sensory studies is that the need for efficient neural coding should have implications for the nature of neural computation. But apart from a general sense that less is more, the need for efficiency was not clearly articulated until Laughlin and others took the trouble to work through the energy demands of neural computation and discovered how extraordinarily expensive it is to carry out neural signaling. Laughlin's conclusions are broadly relevant to neuroscience beyond sensory systems, but they are particularly relevant to sensory systems because of their extraordinary data processing demands. Another chapter whose relevance spans the sensoria is that by Simoncelli and colleagues, who present an elegant method for analyzing neuronal responses. They show how applying these methods in the visual system can uncover previously unseen aspects of neural computation.

The basic wiring of a neural system is intimately related to its function. In his chapter Dacey reviews the exquisite architecture of multiple parallel visual networks that originate in the retina. These networks send their signals to distinct locations in the brain, so that we learn that the parallel nature of brain computation begins at the first sensory synapse. The theme of parallel organization continues in the chapters of Horton and Sincich, and Hackett and Kaas, who discuss, respectively, the cortical architecture of the visual and auditory pathways. The similarities between the organizational structures of cortical processing in these senses are striking and suggest that much cortical processing is organized according to a single basic plan.

The neural circuits that perform the basic computations of sensation are best understood using microelectrode measurements. Carandini, Doupe, Ferster, Maunsell, and Romo and their colleagues each describe insightful methods for learning about the neural computations in a variety of systems. Carandini and Boudreau examine the computational principles in visual cortex that refine the representation of the early visual signal. Maunsell studies how the signals in single units are influenced by attention. Doupe describes the neural circuits that participate in the generation of birdsong, a system remarkable for its intimate relationship to both sensory and motor systems. Romo describes a remarkable series of experiments in which he traces how single units code information about somatosensory discriminations and how these signals can explain behavioral performance.

Theorists seek to explain human perception using computational models based on electrophysiological recordings in animals. In recent years, neuroimaging has augmented such computational modeling by providing a glimpse of the neural responses in the human brain. In their chapters, McDermott and Adelson, Heeger and Ress, Recanzone, Yost, and Sobel and colleagues seek to identify the basic properties of human sensation through the use of computation and careful quantification of sensory signals. McDermott and Yost, describing work in vision and hearing, emphasize the broad rules of perception that are the targets of computational modeling. Heeger and Ress, Sobel, and Recanzone describe analyses that link neural measurements and behavior. The chapter by Heeger and Ress describes how neuroimaging measurements can be used to understand visual attention; Sobel's review of olfaction, an area that is developing at a rapid pace, spans neuroimaging, behavior, and computation; Recanzone examines the interactions between the senses through a set of intriguing experiments that include animal behavior and single-unit recording.

One might wonder how such a substantial representation of the senses finds its way into a volume on cognitive neuroscience. Each of the chapters in this section provides a different kind of answer to that question. Cognitive systems must act on data provided by the senses, and the nature of sensory function is a fundamental constraint on cognitive function. The key issues in these chapters have wide relevance to cognitive processes, and many of the chapters cross the traditional borders between sensation, perception, cognition, and action. Together this work is producing a new and integrated view of the relations between perceptual processes and the other processes that form the neural basis of cognition.

14 The Implications of Metabolic Energy Requirements for the Representation of Information in Neurons

SIMON B. LAUGHLIN

ABSTRACT Brains are metabolically demanding tissues, and the fact that neural signaling consumes much of this metabolic energy is exploited widely in functional imaging. Cortical energy budgets suggest that the rate at which cortical circuits consume energy increases with firing rate. Most of this energy is used to drive action potentials along axon collaterals and to generate postsynaptic potentials. Thus the high metabolic rate of cortical gray matter is a direct consequence of its ability to integrate information from many sources. Because these energy demands place a severe limitation on the rate at which a population of neurons can fire, the cortex uses energy-efficient circuits and codes. Efficiency is improved by combining analog signals (postsynaptic potentials) and digital signals (spikes) in hybrid circuits, by splitting signals into parallel channels, by eliminating inputs from redundant synapses, by using adaptation and opponency to remove redundancy, by adopting energy efficient distributions of firing rate, and by using sparse distributed codes to represent information. Thus energy efficiency is one of the many factors that guide us toward a better understanding of cortical function.

The batteries in our mobile phones and notebook computers constantly remind us that energy is used to transmit and process information. Indeed, profound physical relationships define the minimum quantities of energy required to acquire information and compute, and the development of this line of inquiry from Szilard's treatment of Maxwell's demon is nicely summarized in Leff and Rex (1990). The brain is no exception to the rule that practical computation requires energy, but does the brain's energy usage influence the way in which it operates? Work on neuro-energetics is primarily directed toward understanding and treating the damage caused when the energy supply is reduced in anoxia and stroke (Ames, 1997). In the last 20 years the field has been stimulated by the success of functional imaging, which infers changes in neural activity from changes in metabolic rate (e.g., positron emission tomography [PET]) and in the vas-

SIMON B. LAUGHLIN Department of Zoology, University of Cambridge, Cambridge, England.

cular supply of oxygen (e.g., blood oxygen level-dependent functional magnetic resonance imaging [BOLD fMRI]). However, when it comes to the question, does energy usage influence how the brain represents and processes information, the transition from speculation to analysis is a recent event (Levy and Baxter, 1996). Nonetheless, there is now clear evidence that the brain needs to be energy efficient and that this need can guide us to a better understanding of the neural circuits that represent events and action.

We start by briefly reviewing data on retinal and cerebral metabolism to show that sense organs and brains use significant quantities of metabolic energy for maintenance and signaling. We then examine how energy is used by signaling mechanisms, such as action potentials and synapses, and show that usage limits the number of action potentials in neocortex. Finally, we consider neural circuit designs and representations that improve energy efficiency. These energy-efficient strategies include the use of dendritic computation and spike transmission to implement hybrid "analog-digital" processing, split or parallel coding, redundancy reduction, and the formation of sparse distributed representations.

Brains and sense organs use significant quantities of energy to process information

Brain is metabolically expensive tissue whose energy demands have constrained its evolution and function, particularly in primates (Aiello, Bates, and Joffe, 2001). Both invertebrate and vertebrate brains typically have specific metabolic rates (metabolic rates per gram) that are 10–30 times the body's resting average, and the rates of mammalian retina and cortical gray matter equal the metabolic rate of heart muscle (Ames, 2000; Schreiber et al., 2002). Like a heart, a brain continuously uses energy, and consequently, neural consumption has a significant impact on an animal's energy budget. For example, the adult human brain is responsible for 20% of resting oxygen consumption, despite accounting for just 2% of body mass. In general, significant energy costs promote the evolution of economical mechanisms (Weibel, 2000). To examine the metabolic efficiency of nervous systems, we must relate energy consumption to neural function.

The human brain consumes energy at a high rate that is little changed by mental activity, and function rapidly fails without oxygen. Sokoloff and co-workers used radioactive [^{14}C]-deoxyglucose to measure local rates of glucose uptake from autoradiograms of mammalian brains, and discovered large regional differences in energy consumption. The lowest rates are in white matter and the highest are in auditory areas, such as inferior colliculus and auditory cortex. In rat and monkey cerebral cortex, the specific metabolic rate of gray matter varies by approximately one-third, according to cortical area. The average for gray matter is approximately 50% higher than the specific metabolic rate of the whole brain. Moreover, the specific metabolic rate increases locally with neural activity (Clarke and Sokoloff, 1999). When an animal views gratings moving in one direction, the accumulation of [^{14}C]-deoxyglucose picks out orientation columns in V1 (Hubel, Wiesel, and Stryker, 1978).

Measurements of the effects of anesthesia on metabolic rate also demonstrate that energy consumption depends on neural activity. The effects are large and robust, but it should be remembered that anesthetics can act at many sites and neurons can adapt quickly to changes in signal level by regulating signaling mechanisms. Deep anesthesia abolishes electrical activity and reduces the metabolic rate of the whole brain by 50%, suggesting that, on average, energy consumption is equally divided between neural signaling and maintenance. Blocking the Na/K pump suggests that signaling usage is dominated by the need to restore the ions that generate electrical responses in axons and at synapses (Siesjö, 1978; Astrup, Sorensen, and Sorensen, 1981).

Cortical gray matter apparently uses more energy for signaling than most other regions of the brain. The noninvasive in vivo technique of magnetic resonance spectroscopy (MRS) measures the passage of labeled atoms through identified intermediates in metabolic pathways in relatively small brain volumes. The data are entered into metabolic models to estimate the rate of glucose consumption and the turnover of the excitatory neurotransmitter glutamate. When electrical activity is progressively depressed by increasing the depth of anesthesia, the rates of glucose consumption and glutamate turnover in gray matter fall in step. Because approximately 90% of cortical synapses use glutamate, the correlation between glucose consumption and glutamate turnover associates changes in metabolic rate with changes in neural activity. The deepest anesthesia abolishes both electrical activity and the turnover of glutamate, and

depresses glucose consumption by 80%–90% (Rothman et al., 2003). This high signal-dependent fraction of energy usage can be reconciled with the lower value of 50% for the brain as a whole if the higher than average specific metabolic rate of gray matter is attributed to signaling (Attwell and Laughlin, 2001). This assumption produces a signaling fraction of approximately 75% in cortical gray matter that agrees well with theory and approaches the 80%–90% derived in vivo by MRS.

These studies underpin functional imaging by linking the changes in metabolic rate measured by PET to changes in neural activity and suggesting that the changes in blood flow and oxygenation that generate the BOLD response in fMRI cater to the changing demands of neural activity. Experiments support this conclusion. In primate visual cortex (Logothetis et al., 2001) and rat cortical barrels (Smith et al., 2002), the BOLD signal correlates approximately linearly both with the firing rate of neurons and with the amplitude of the local field potentials (these potentials indicate spike and synaptic activity in local connections). It is this strong dependence of energy usage on signaling, together with the sensitivity of the sophisticated instrumentation and data analysis techniques, that allows functional imagers to detect where and when neural representations change as the brain operates. How can we reconcile the vivid patterns of activation displayed in functional images with the longstanding finding that the conscious brain's total oxygen consumption does not change with the level of mental activity? Activation is localized to a small fraction of the cerebral volume, and, because BOLD is sensitive, vivid responses represent relatively small changes in local metabolic rate. When these small local increases are superimposed on a high background level of metabolic activity throughout the brain and are accompanied by reductions in other areas, they will have little effect on the total metabolic rate.

In conclusion, a variety of measurements have linked energy consumption to neural activity. To look more deeply at the neural basis of functional images and to understand energy efficiency, we must relate energy usage to signaling in neural circuits.

Assigning energy consumption to neural mechanisms

The quantities of energy consumed by the different activities of a nervous system have been measured directly in experiments and estimated theoretically in energy budgets.

Experiments It is difficult to measure the quantities of energy consumed by a given set of neurons under normal operating conditions, and it is especially difficult to attribute consumption to specific mechanisms operating at particular sites. Measuring the concentrations of metabolites is relatively straightforward, but measuring the fluxes that change these concentrations is not. One can track the passage of labeled atoms through a metabolic pathway (as in MRS) or measure the rates at which substrates and products are consumed or generated, but the spatiotemporal resolution of these techniques is limited. It is also difficult to assign energy consumption to particular signaling mechanisms, such as action potentials, synapses, and second messengers, because blocking one mechanism in a circuit usually alters the rate at which others operate. Finally, if one uses in vitro systems to improve access and resolve structures under the microscope, how can one drive the system with the appropriate natural signals? For these reasons there is a shortage of measurements of the energy used by identified neurons and neural mechanisms in CNS, under normal conditions (Ames, 2000).

The most comprehensive and reliable measurements of neural energy usage come from the mammalian retina (Ames and Li, 1992; Ames et al., 1992), where both neural circuits and their responses to optical stimuli are known. Ames exploited these advantages by developing a retinal perfusion system and was able to measure fluxes, introduce blockers, and control neural activity with light. In the dark, approximately 50% of retinal energy is used by the Na/K pump. Light reduces total consumption by 40%, by shutting off the large dark current in rod photoreceptors. In darkness, rat rods have a specific metabolic rate equal to that of rat cardiac muscle, $30\,\mu$mol ATP/g/min (Ames, 2000). Synaptic consumption is significant. Application of blockers suggests that glutamatergic synapses (e.g., tonically active photoreceptor synapses) account for approximately 15% of the retina's dark consumption, and in the light, stimulation with optical patterns increases consumption. The synthesis of macromolecules (proteins, DNA, RNA, and lipids) accounts for less than 3% of dark consumption. Approximately 40% of retinal consumption was unaccounted for, and labeling experiments suggested that this usage involves GTP rather than ATP (Ames et al., 1992).

Given that the analysis of a favorable system, retina, is incomplete and that CNS is more difficult to experiment on, theoretical methods have been developed. These "bottom-up" energy budgets are instructive but are no substitute for experiments. New preparations and experimental techniques are urgently required to monitor consumption in identified cells under well-controlled conditions.

THEORETICAL APPROACHES: "BOTTOM-UP" ENERGY BUDGETS FOR NEURAL SIGNALING To construct a "bottom-up" energy budget for a system, one calculates the energy used by each of its components. Three types of data are used: biophysical and biochemical, anatomical, and physiological. The biophysical and biochemical data specify the energy used to operate a particular signaling mechanism, such as the amount of ATP required to pump back the Na^+, K^+, and

Ca^{2+} ions that generated an excitatory postsynaptic potential (EPSP) at a synapse. Because these data are mainly molecular, energy consumption is derived as ATP molecules hydrolyzed to $ADP + P_i$. Anatomical data specify the number and size of the sites at which these mechanisms operate (e.g., the number of synapses, the area of membrane invaded by a spike) and, by describing circuits, define the pathways that couple signaling at different sites. Physiological data confirm the anatomical data on coupling between sites, quantify the strength of interactions, and convert energy usage per operation into a rate of consumption by defining the number of times that a mechanism normally operates. The method was initiated in fly retina (Laughlin, de Ruyter van Steveninck, and Anderson, 1998), expanded and improved by application to the gray matter of rodent cortex (Attwell and Laughlin, 2001), and extended to human cortex (Lennie, 2003).

Calculating the energy used to drive a neuron presents a problem. A neuron's firing rate does not specify the magnitudes of the synaptic currents that drive firing, because membrane potential depends on the ratio between excitatory and inhibitory conductances. Thus a weak synaptic input from an excitatory region of a neuron's receptive field will produce the same firing rate as the combination of a strong excitatory input with a strong input from an inhibitory region. The ideal solution to this problem is to use anatomical and physiological data to estimate the synaptic drive (Laughlin, de Ruyter van Steveninck, and Anderson, 1998), but this involves an exceptionally detailed knowledge of circuitry that is not yet available in cortex.

Cortical energy budgets circumvent this problem by considering the average cortical neuron firing at the average rate because it is being driven by the average number of synapses. This sweeping generalization works because, to a first approximation, the cerebral cortex is a closed system (the number of intrinsic connections greatly exceeds the number of inputs to the cortex; Braitenberg and Schüz, 1998). Consequently the average number of input synapses per neuron equals the average number of output synapses per neuron. Under this condition, the energy used for signaling by the average neuron is the energy used pre- and postsynaptically at its output synapses, plus the energy used to transmit an action potential through its axonal arbor to stimulate those synapses, plus a contribution from the resting potential (Attwell and Laughlin, 2001). The synaptic energy consumption is derived from data on presynaptic transmitter release and recycling and data on postsynaptic ion currents and second messenger responses. To circumvent the problem that current flow at a particular synapse is influenced by activity in its circuit (it depends on the postsynaptic membrane potential and hence on inputs from other synapses), one considers the average synapse. The average synaptic current is determined by two sets of measurements, the average conductances and open times of postsynaptic ion channels and the driving force for the relevant ions, given by their reversal potentials and the average membrane potential of a cortical neuron.

The resting consumption, 3.42×10^8 ATP/s/rat neuron, is estimated from measurements of the average membrane potential and input resistance of neurons when synaptic inputs are blocked. Similar calculations for the glial cells associated with each rat neuron give 1.02×10^8 ATP/s. The values for human cortical cells, obtained by multiplying the rat values by the ratios of the surface areas, are 6.6×10^8 ATP/s for a neuron and 3.1×10^8 ATP/s for associated glia.

The energy required to propagate the action potential through a pyramidal cell is calculated from anatomical measurements of the membrane areas of dendrites, the cell body, and the axonal arbor in gray matter (axon collaterals) (Attwell and Laughlin, 2001). Multiplying these areas (Braitenberg and Schüz, 1998) by the specific capacitance of membrane and the amplitude of the action potential (100 mV) gives the minimum charge, and hence sodium ion influx, required to depolarize the membrane to the peak of the action potential. This capacitive sodium influx is multiplied by 4 to account for K^+ ions leaving the cell through potassium channels as Na^+ ions enter. Corrections are made for the partial depolarization of dendrites by backpropagating action potentials, and account is taken of the involvement of Ca^{2+} ions in dendritic depolarization. Based on these calculations, it takes 3.84×10^8 ATP molecules to propagate an action potential through a rat pyramidal cell, and 9.2×10^8 ATP molecules through a human neuron. With 4 cm of axon collateral in a rat pyramidal cell (Braitenberg and Schüz, 1998) and 10 cm in a human neuron (Lennie, 2003), most of this ATP is used to transmit the action potential laterally through gray matter.

The ATP used when an action potential causes an output synapse to signal by releasing a vesicle is calculated from biophysical and biochemical data on synaptic transmission (Attwell and Laughlin, 2001). Presynaptically, 12,000 Ca^{2+} ions enter to stimulate vesicle release and 12,000 ATP molecules are used to remove them. The vesicle releases 4000 molecules of glutamate, and recycling this neurotransmitter via glia uses 2.66 ATP molecules per glutamate, giving a total consumption of 11,000 ATP molecules per vesicle. The numbers of molecules associated with vesicle fusion and recycling suggest a consumption of 1000 ATP molecules per vesicle. Thus 24,000 ATP molecules are used presynaptically when a vesicle is released.

The postsynaptic responses to the glutamate released by the vesicle consume 140,000 ATP molecules, and most of this ATP is used by the Na/K pump to restore the ions that generated the postsynaptic current. Only 3000 ATP molecules are required to support the metabotropic response to glutamate—a Ca^{2+} transient in the postsynaptic spine.

Metabotropic responses are generally very economical because they involve micromolar concentrations of second messenger in small compartments. The total amount of energy used when a synapse signals by releasing a vesicle is the sum of pre- and postsynaptic consumption, calculated earlier as 24,000 ATP molecules + 140,000 ATP molecules = 164,000 ATP molecules. The estimates of presynaptic usage (calcium entry, vesicle fusion and retrieval, and glutamate recycling) are reliable, but the postsynaptic consumption is uncertain because reports of the numbers of ion channels activated by a vesicle vary considerably (Attwell and Laughlin, 2001). In the absence of equivalent data on synaptic transmission in primate cortex, rat values have been applied to the synapses of human pyramidal cells (Lennie, 2003).

The energy used when a single pyramidal cell fires an action potential is obtained by multiplying the amount of energy used when a synapse releases a vesicle by the number of output synapses that released, and then adding the energy required to propagate the action potential. The average rat pyramidal cell makes 8000 output synapses. At the mean firing rate in rat cortex (4 Hz), the probability that an action potential releases a vesicle at a synapse is 0.25. Thus, 2000 synapses are activated per pyramidal cell per action potential, giving a synaptic consumption of 3.28×10^8 ATP molecules. Note that we need only consider the pyramidal cell's output synapses. In a closed system the current delivered by its input synapses is already accounted for as the output synapses of other neurons. Adding the energy used to propagate the action potential, 3.84×10^8 ATP molecules, gives a total signaling cost of 7.1×10^8 ATP molecules per pyramidal cell per action potential for the rat (Attwell and Laughlin, 2001). A human pyramidal cell makes 17,500 synapses, which are tentatively assigned a vesicle release probability of 0.5. With 8750 activated synapses, the consumption is 1.4×10^9 ATP molecules, and adding the cost of a spike gives a total of 2.4×10^9 ATP molecules per human pyramidal cell per action potential (Lennie, 2003). The cost per human neuron is higher than rat because it is larger and activates four times as many synapses. The human cell's higher probability of vesicle release increases the contribution of synapses relative to action potentials (figure 14.1). Note that the total cost of firing an action potential (including synapses) has a significant impact on local energy demands because it is equivalent to maintaining the resting potential of the neuron and associated glia for 1.6 s in the rat and 2.2 s in humans.

The metabolic impact of neural signaling is assessed by calculating the energy required to sustain signaling at a given rate. The mean firing rate of neurons in rat cortex appears to be around 4 Hz (Attwell and Laughlin, 2001). Multiplying the consumption per neuron per action potential by this mean rate, and adding the resting rate, gives a total rate of

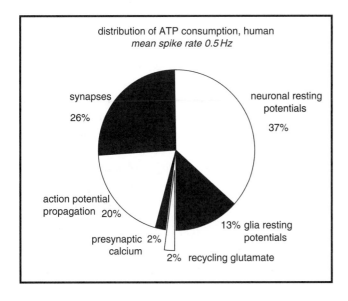

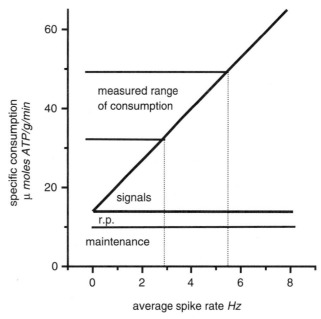

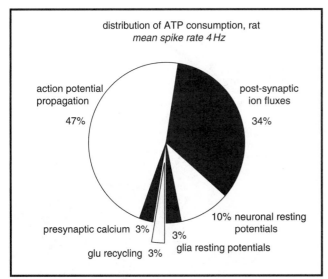

FIGURE 14.1 Estimated distributions of the energy used by signaling mechanisms in the gray matter of rat and human cortex. The figures are based on "bottom-up" energy budgets, assuming a mean spike rate in cortical neurons of 4 Hz in rat and 0.5 Hz in human. The rat spike rate was estimated from published data (Attwell and Laughlin, 2001). The human rate was estimated by dividing the energy used per spike into an estimate of the energy available for signaling (Lennie, 2003), and the value used here is in the middle of the predicted range (0.16–0.9 Hz). A higher firing rate decreases the percentage devoted to resting potentials and leaves the ratio of energy used in synapses and action potentials unchanged.

FIGURE 14.2 The specific consumption (rate of consumption of ATP/g) as a function of spike rate in rat cortical gray matter. The maintenance consumption is the metabolic rate for whole brain when electrical activity is abolished (see text for further details). The consumption by the resting potentials of neurons and glia (r.p.) and the spike-dependent signaling consumption are estimated by "bottom-up" budgeting (Attwell and Laughlin, 2001). The range of measured consumptions is taken from the work of Sokoloff and colleagues (Clarke and Sokoloff, 1999). The measured range of energy consumption constrains the mean spike rate to approximately 3.0–5.5 Hz.

consumption of 3.29×10^9 ATP molecules/s for a rat cortical neuron and its associated glia. Multiplying the rate per neuron by the average density of neurons in rat cortex, 9.2×10^7 neurons/cm³ (Braitenberg and Schüz, 1998), gives a consumption of 3.0×10^{17} ATP molecules/cm³/s, which, converting to the units used in experimental studies of metabolic rate, is 30 μmol ATP/g/min. This estimate lies just below the measurements of rates of total consumption in different cortical areas, 33–50 μmol ATP/g/min, and the shortfall can be assigned to maintenance costs. As discussed earlier, 50% of the brain's total energy consumption has been assigned to maintenance, but the proportion is thought to be lower in cortical gray matter. Given an average specific consumption of 21 μmol ATP/g/min for the whole brain, maintenance amounts to approximately 10 μmol ATP/g/min. Subtracting this maintenance rate from the rates measured in cortical gray matter gives a signaling consumption of 23–40 μmol ATP/g/min. The predictions of the budget fall squarely in the middle in this range (figure 14.2). Note that in multiplying the metabolic rate per pyramidal cell by the total density of neurons, one assumes that a pyramidal cell represents all types of cortical neuron. Because 80% of cortical neurons are pyramidal cells and 90% of cortical synapses use glutamate, other neurons (e.g., inhibitory neurons, local interneurons) will have to perform very differently from pyramidal cells to significantly change the energy budget.

As first suggested by Lennie, the number of spikes in cortex is severely limited by metabolic rate (Lennie, 1998). In rat, the mean spike rate of 4 Hz accounts for much of the high metabolic rate of cortical gray matter (Attwell and Laughlin, 2001). The mean rate cannot be increased by very much within the limits of energy supply, because energy demand increases in proportion to firing rate (figure 14.2). The severity of this energy limit on mean firing rate is directly related to the ability of the cortex to correlate and associate events. Some 47% of signaling energy goes to propagate action potentials in extensive collaterals and 40% goes to drive numerous synapses (see figure 14.1). This pattern of usage is reflected in the distribution of mitochondria (Wong-Riley, 1989; Attwell and Laughlin, 2001).

Lennie (2003) calculates that the metabolic constraint on spike rate is much more severe in human. The specific metabolic rate measured in human cortex is half the rat's, as expected from Kleiber's law, which states that specific metabolic rate declines with body mass (Kleiber, 1975). Lennie assumes that in human cortex the synaptic vesicle release probability is twice that in rat cortex ($P = 0.5$, cf. $P = 0.25$) because mean firing rate is metabolically limited to a lower value. The combination of a reduction in energy supply and an increase in demand lowers the metabolic limit on firing rate in human cortex to between 0.16 Hz and 0.9 Hz, depending on the variations in the parameters used to make this estimate (Lennie, 2003). The lower mean firing rate increases the relative contribution of resting potentials to total energy consumption (see figure 14.1).

In summary, the best available estimates of neural energy usage demonstrate a severe metabolic limit to the number of action potentials in cortex. This limit will influence how neurons represent information. Action potentials must be used sparingly (Lennie, 1998). Ongoing studies suggest that this metabolic constraint has influenced two intimately related aspects of neural function: the design of neurons and neural circuits, and the structure of neural codes and representations.

Energy-efficient neurons and circuits

Recent studies suggest three ways to improve energy efficiency: combining analog synapses with digital spikes in hybrid circuits, using split coding to divide information among pathways of low capacity, and eliminating redundant synapses.

COMBINING ANALOG AND DIGITAL IN HYBRID CIRCUITS Analog neural signals (graded changes in membrane potential produced by synapses) transmit information at higher rates over short distances than spike trains (de Ruyter van Steveninck and Laughlin, 1996). In addition, an analog device is usually more energy efficient at processing information (Sarpeshkar, 1998), because analog directly implements a powerful set of linear and nonlinear operations. In neurons these operations are performed rapidly using elec-

trical current flow, and more slowly, or more locally, with highly economical second messenger systems (Koch, 1999). The problem with analog is noise. Each analog component generates noise, which it feeds into the circuit, and the accumulated noise from many components kills signals in complicated circuits (Sarpeshkar, 1998). Noise accumulation is a particularly serious constraint in analog nervous systems because graded (analog) synapses constantly release synaptic vesicles. Although the effects of noise can be reduced by using more synapses and signaling molecules to transfer and process signals, this lowers metabolic efficiency by increasing energy consumption out of proportion to information rate (see below and figure 14.3). The more efficient solution is to eliminate noise by abandoning analog for "digital" with, for example, synapses that release one vesicle per incoming spike (Laughlin et al., 2000).

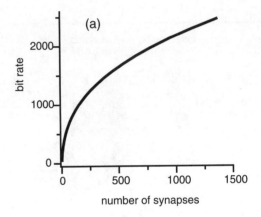

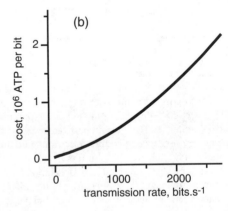

FIGURE 14.3 Information is coded more economically (i.e., at a lower energy cost) in neural systems of low capacity. (*a*) The bit rate of an array of synapses connecting two neurons increases sublinearly with the number of synapses. Each synapse transmits the same signal but injects independent noise (e.g., from vesicle release). (*b*) The unit cost of the information transmitted by the array increases with the transmission rate. Data in *a* and *b* are calculated using the signal-to-noise ratio, bit rate, and energy consumption of a photoreceptor output synapse in blowfly retina (Laughlin, de Ruyter van Steveninck, and Anderson, 1998).

Sarpeshkar (1998) analyzed the relationships between signal quality, component size, and power consumption in analogue and digital electronics and, using these relationships, invented practical circuits (e.g., a silicon cochlear) that are energy efficient because they judiciously combine the advantages of analog and digital. An operation is performed efficiently by a small group of analog components and then, to avoid noise accumulation, the result is digitized for noise-free transmission to the next stage, where digital is reconverted to analogue for further processing. Sarpeshkar considers neurons as hybrid devices, processing and integrating analogue synaptic signals and converting them to "digital" spike trains, and he suggests that their hybrid architecture contributes to the remarkable energy efficiency of the human brain (Sarpeshkar, 1998). Sarpeshkar also shows that it is more efficient to process information with a larger number of components of lower information capacity than with a smaller number of components of higher capacity. As discussed in the next section, the brain implements this efficient design by splitting information into low-capacity lines.

SPLITTING SIGNALS INTO PARALLEL LINES   Neural information is cheaper in components of lower capacity. The analog signals of blowfly photoreceptors and their postsynaptic interneurons code 1000 bits/s and 1600 bits/s, respectively, at a unit cost of over 1,500,000 ATP molecules/bit. By comparison, one of the 220 chemical synapses connecting a photoreceptor to an interneuron transmits 55 bits/s for just 40,000 ATP molecules/bit. The synapse is limited to 55 bits/s by synaptic noise. Using many such synapses in parallel improves the signal-to-noise ratio (SNR) roughly in proportion to the $\sqrt{}$(number of synapses), and the rate of information transfer rises nonlinearly with the number of synapses (figure 14.3a). However, the metabolic cost of synaptic transmission rises in proportion to the number of synapses, leading to a pronounced decline in metabolic efficiency with increasing bit rate (figure 14.3b). Consequently, a metabolically efficient nervous system will avoid using neurons of high capacity by dividing information among a number of neurons of low capacity (Laughlin, de Ruyter van Steveninck, and Anderson, 1998).

Brains apparently use many small neurons of low capacity, but are there more concrete examples of information being divided among neurons to improve efficiency? This strategy has been independently formulated as split coding to explain the division of the retinal data stream into ON and OFF pathways (von der Twer and MacLeod, 2001). If a neuron encodes its input with A action potentials subject to noise $\sqrt{A}$, it can transmit $\sqrt{A}$ discriminable output levels. When A = 100 action potentials are used by one neuron, 10 signal levels are coded. When the input is split between an ON neuron and an OFF neuron, 100 action

potentials specify $2 \times \sqrt{50} \approx 14$ levels, a 40% improvement in efficiency. Sensory information is commonly divided among parallel neural pathways, but the extent to which this improves metabolic efficiency is an open question. Ideally, signals should be split into statistically independent parts because correlation reduces efficiency by introducing redundancy, but making a clean division is not always as simple as separating ON and OFF. If an imperfect division into neurons with overlapping sensitivities is more efficient than no division at all, the widespread strategy of dividing sensory inputs into parallel streams contributes to metabolic efficiency.

MATCHING COMPONENTS AND ELIMINATING REDUNDANT SYNAPSES   Because energy is used to receive and transmit signals, the information capacity of the inputs and outputs should be matched to avoid wasteful bottlenecks and overcapacity (Levy and Baxter, 2002; Schreiber et al., 2002). Retinal photoreceptors and interneurons that carry less reliable signals make fewer synapses (Schreiber et al., 2002). A cortical pyramidal cell presents an extreme mismatch (Levy and Baxter, 2002). Several thousand input synapses produce spikes in a single output axon, and because most input synapses come from other pyramidal cells, each input synapse delivers as much information, on average, as the axon outputs. Consequently the number of effective input synapses can be reduced by lowering the probability of vesicle release without losing information, and this will reduce energy consumption. With so many synapses in cortex, regulating vesicle release has a large effect on energy usage. In rat cortex, increasing the probability of vesicle release from 0.25 to 1.0 almost doubles the energy used per spike (Attwell and Laughlin, 2001). Levy and Baxter (2002) calculated the release probabilities that optimize metabolic efficiency. Their treatment emphasizes the value of applying information theory, connects synaptic failures to metabolic efficiency, and shows that measured vesicle release probabilities are in the metabolically efficient "ballpark." However, there is no compelling reason why the input synapses all have to have the same release probability. Would an efficient system preferentially use those synapses that are most likely to contribute to function, such as those whose activation is most likely to coincide with other inputs?

It is worth reiterating that any means of reducing the number of effective synapses and the lengths of connection in cortex will improve energy efficiency (Attwell and Laughlin, 2001). We have seen how one form of synaptic plasticity, a change in vesicle release probability, is very effective at reducing cortical signaling costs. The layout of neurons in gray matter also plays a role. Topographic mapping and columnar organization reduce the length of connections by placing neurons with related responses closer together. It must be emphasized that metabolic efficiency need not be the only reason for adopting a good design. Plasticity is a hallmark of neural function, and maps make it easier to extract higher-order parameters such as shape and movement, and to interpolate (Knudsen, du Lac, and Esterly, 1987).

Energy-efficient neural codes and representation

A highly effective means of increasing efficiency is to reduce the number of action potentials used to represent events, because this reduces the energy used by both action potentials and synapses. "Economy of impulses" has many other advantages: concise messages lay out information more clearly and are easier to process (Barlow, 1972; Field, 1994). Economy is achieved by at least three related means: the energy-efficient distribution of firing rates, redundancy reduction, and the use of sparse and distributed codes.

ENERGY-EFFICIENT FIRING RATES   An energy-efficient code minimizes the number of spikes required to code a given amount of information or maximizes the information coded by a given number of spikes. The firing rates of some cortical neurons satisfy this requirement by following a Boltzmann distribution (Baddeley et al., 1997). In other cortical neurons and in salamander retinal ganglion cells, the distribution falls below the Boltzmann at low rates, and these cells are adhering to a distribution of firing rates that optimizes energy efficiency in the presence of intrinsic noise (Balasubramanian, Kimber, and Berry, 2001; Garcia de Polavieja, 2002). The low rates are being used less frequently because, with fewer spikes per interval, they are less reliable. The distribution measured in a salamander retinal ganglion cell is tailored to the noise recorded in that particular cell (Balasubramanian and Berry, 2002).

REDUNDANCY REDUCTION   Many retinal and cortical neurons adapt to steady stimuli and use antagonism within the receptive field to eliminate background signals. These properties save energy by reducing the amplitude and duration of signals. Furthermore, the savings can be made without loss of information when adaptation and antagonism reduce redundancy, that is, remove those signal components that can be predicted from preceding and neighboring inputs (Barlow, 1961a). Redundancy reduction is commonly implemented in sensory pathways by matching adaptation, filtering, and antagonism to the statistics of natural signals, so that only predictable components are eliminated (Olshausen and Field, 2000; Simoncelli and Olshausen, 2001). Because it removes the uninformative, redundancy reduction improves several measures of efficiency (Attneave, 1954; Barlow, 1961b). These include a measure that can go against the economy of impulses (Levy and Baxter, 1996), making the best use of a limited number of neurons by maximizing the quantity of information coded by each.

SPARSE DISTRIBUTED CODING   Contrary to the principles of eliminating redundancy discussed in the previous section, metabolic efficiency can be improved by increasing the number of neurons used for representation and reducing the probability that each neuron signals (Levy and Baxter, 1996). This strategy achieves a high representational capacity because there are many different ways in which a small amount of activity can be distributed over a large population of neurons. Levy and Baxter (1996) used information theory to determine the representational capacity of neurons as a function of the proportion of time that they are active. They then divided this capacity by the total cost of representation, which is the cost of maintaining neurons in readiness (the fixed cost) and the cost of activating them (the signaling cost). There is an optimum proportion of active cells that maximizes metabolic efficiency, and this optimum depends on the ratio between the signaling cost and the fixed cost (figure 14.4). The published estimates of costs predict that an energy-efficient system will activate between 1% and 16% of neurons at any one time, with the lowest percentage for human cortex, where the cost per action potential per neuron is higher (Levy and Baxter, 1996; Attwell and Laughlin, 2001; Lennie, 2003).

This metabolically efficient tactic, activating neurons infrequently, is called sparse coding. Sparse coding is implemented by neurons that respond strongly but highly selectively to localized features of sensory input or motor output (Field, 1994; Hahnloser, Kozhevnikov, and Fee, 2002). Because a single neuron rarely encounters its feature, it fires in short bursts, sparsely distributed in time. Activity is sparsely distributed in space (across the population of neurons) because at any given time, only a small fraction of neurons encounter their feature. There is strong evidence that natural images are sparsely represented in primary visual cortex, V1. Models that minimize the number of active neural channels required to code natural images generate sets of oriented spatial filters that resemble the receptive fields of V1 neurons (Olshausen and Field, 1996). Conversely, when linear models of V1 receptive fields are applied to natural images, they generate sparse representations (Willmore and Tolhurst, 2001). Most important, sparse activity is recorded from neurons in V1 in response to natural stimuli (Vinje and Gallant, 2000; Weliky et al., 2003).

Metabolic efficiency is just one of the advantages of sparse coding. Reducing the number of active neurons used to specify a particular event simplifies pattern recognition, pattern generation, classification, and coincidence detection (Field, 1994). However, sparseness and distribution also make it more difficult for neuroscientists to determine the form and function of neural representations.

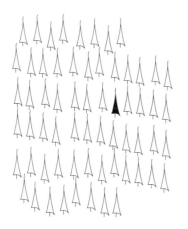 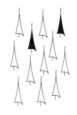 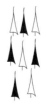

	1 active, 63 at rest capacity = 64			2 active, 10 at rest capacity = 66			4 active, 4 at rest capacity = 70		
cost ratio signalling:fixed	costs			costs			costs		
	signalling	fixed	total	signalling	fixed	total	signalling	fixed	total
100:1	100	64	*164	200	12	212	400	8	408
10:1	10	64	74	20	12	*32	40	8	48
5:1	5	64	69	10	12	*22	20	8	28
1:1	1	64	65	2	12	14	4	8	*12

FIGURE 14.4 The dependence of the metabolic efficiency of neural representation on the sparseness of neural activity. These three populations of neurons have almost identical representational capacities (at least 64 different states) and achieve their capacities by activating 1 neuron out of 64, 2 out of 10, and 4 out of 8 (active neurons are shown in gray). The signaling, fixed, and total costs of each of these representations is tabulated below, for four cost ratios, fixed:signaling. The population representing information at the lowest cost is marked for each ratio. As the fixed:signaling ratio rises, the sparseness of the most economical code declines. (Modified from Laughlin [2001] after Levy and Baxter [1996] and Attwell and Laughlin [2001].)

Conclusion and prospect

The energy required for signaling limits the number of action potentials available to the brain, and the brain counters this limitation with energy-efficient circuits, codes, and representations. Energy efficiency can help us discover how sensory information is represented by neurons. We face a serious technical problem. We can detect where and when information about an event is represented using a variety of electrophysiological (Makeig, 2002) and imaging techniques (e.g., single-unit recordings, evoked potentials, BOLD), but it is much more difficult to discover how information is represented and processed by neural circuits. Neurons have such prodigious abilities to interact that a large number of hypothetical networks are capable of processing information according to behavioral requirements. The number of hypotheses to be entertained and tested can be reduced by examining the factors that constrain neural representation. This approach, hypothesis reduction by constraint analysis, has been successfully applied to the uptake of visual information in the periphery by considering natural image statistics, noise, and dynamic range. A better understanding of energy efficiency will eliminate unreasonable hypotheses and suggest more likely alternatives.

REFERENCES

AIELLO, L. C., N. BATES, and T. H. JOFFE, 2001. In defence of the expensive tissue hypothesis. In *Evolutionary Anatomy of the Primate Cerebral Cortex*, D. Falk and K. R. Gibson, eds. Cambridge, England: Cambridge University Press, pp. 57–78.

AMES, A., 1997. Energy requirements of brain function: When is energy limiting? In *Mitochondria and Free Radicals in Neurodegenerative Disease*, M. F. Beal, N. Howell, and I. Bodis-Wollner, eds. New York: Wiley-Liss, pp. 17–27.

AMES, A., 2000. CNS energy metabolism as related to function. *Brain Res. Rev.* 34:42–68.

AMES, A., and Y. Y. LI, 1992. Energy-requirements of glutamatergic pathways in rabbit retina. *J. Neurosci.* 12:4234–4242.

AMES, A., Y. Y. LI, E. C. HEHER, and C. R. KIMBLE, 1992. Energy-metabolism of rabbit retina as related to function: High cost of Na^+ transport. *J. Neurosci.* 12:840–853.

ASTRUP, J., P. M. SORENSEN, and H. R. SORENSEN, 1981. Oxygen and glucose consumption related to Na^+-K^+ transport in canine brain. *Stroke* 12:726–730.

ATTNEAVE, F., 1954. Informational aspects of visual processing. *Psychol. Rev.* 61:183–193.

ATTWELL, D., and S. B. LAUGHLIN, 2001. An energy budget for signalling in the grey matter of the brain. *J. Cereb. Blood Flow Metab.* 21:1133–1145.

BADDELEY, R., L. F. ABBOTT, M. C. A. BOOTH, F. SENGPIEL, T. FREEMAN, E. A. WAKEMAN, and E. T. ROLLS, 1997. Responses of neurons in primary and inferior temporal visual cortices to natural scenes. *Proc. R. Soc. Lond. B.* 264:1775–1783.

BALASUBRAMANIAN, V., and M. J. BERRY, 2002. A test of metabolically efficient coding in the retina. *Network* 13:531–552.

BALASUBRAMANIAN, V., D. KIMBER, and M. J. BERRY, 2001. Metabolically efficient information processing. *Neural Comput.* 13:799–816.

BARLOW, H. B., 1961a. Possible principles underlying the transformation of sensory messages. In *Sensory Communication*, W. A. Rosenblith, ed. Cambridge, Mass.: MIT Press, pp. 217–234.

BARLOW, H. B., 1961b. The coding of sensory messages. In *Current Problems in Animal Behaviour*, W. H. Thorpe and O. L. Zangwill, eds. Cambridge, England: Cambridge University Press, pp. 331–360.

BARLOW, H. B., 1972. Single units and perception. *Perception* 1:371–394.

BRAITENBERG, V., and A. SCHÜZ, 1998. *Cortex: Statistics and Geometry of Neuronal Connectivity*, 2nd ed. Berlin: Springer.

CLARKE, D. D., and L. SOKOLOFF, 1999. Circulation and energy metabolism of the brain. In *Basic Neurochemistry: Molecular, Cellular and Medical Aspects*, 6th ed., G. J. Siegel, B. W. Agranoff, R. W. Albers, S. K. Fisher, and M. D. Uhler, eds. Philadelphia: Lippincott-Raven, pp. 637–669.

DE RUYTER VAN STEVENINCK, R. R., and S. B. LAUGHLIN, 1996. The rate of information-transfer at graded-potential synapses. *Nature* 379:642–645.

FIELD, D. J., 1994. What is the goal of sensory coding? *Neural Comput.* 6:559–601.

GARCIA DE POLAVIEJA, G., 2002. Errors drive the evolution of biological signalling to costly codes. *J. Theor. Biol.* 214:657–664.

HAHNLOSER, R., A. KOZHEVNIKOV, and M. FEE, 2002. An ultrasparse code underlies the generation of neural sequences in a songbird. *Nature* 419:65–70.

HUBEL, D. H., T. N. WIESEL, and M. P. STRYKER, 1978. Anatomical demonstration of orientation columns in macaque monkey. *J. Comp. Neurol.* 177:361–379.

KLEIBER, M., 1975. *The Fire of Life: An Introduction to Animal Energetics*, rev. ed. Huntington, N.Y.: Krieger.

KNUDSEN, E. I., S. DU LAC, and S. D. ESTERLY, 1987. Computational maps in the brain. *Ann. Rev. Neurosci.* 10:41–67.

KOCH, C., 1999. *Biophysics of Computation*. Oxford, England: Oxford University Press.

LAUGHLIN, S. B., J. C. ANDERSON, D. C. O'CARROLL, and R. R. DE RUYTER VAN STEVENINCK, 2000. Coding efficiency and the metabolic cost of sensory and neural information. In *Information Theory and the Brain*, R. Baddeley, P. Hancock, and P. Foldiak, eds. Cambridge, England: Cambridge University Press, pp. 41–61.

LAUGHLIN, S. B., R. R. DE RUYTER VAN STEVENINCK, and J. C. ANDERSON, 1998. The metabolic cost of neural information. *Nat. Neurosci.* 1:36–41.

LEFF, H. S., and A. F. REX, 1990. *Maxwell's Demon: Entropy, Information, Computing*. Bristol, England: Adam Hilger.

LENNIE, P., 1998. Single units and visual cortical organization. *Perception* 27:889–935.

LENNIE, P., 2003. The cost of cortical computation. *Curr. Biol.* 13:493–497.

LEVY, W. B., and R. A. BAXTER, 1996. Energy-efficient neural codes. *Neural Comput.* 8:531–543.

LEVY, W. B., and R. A. BAXTER, 2002. Energy-efficient neuronal computation via quantal synaptic failures. *J. Neurosci.* 22: 4746–4755.

LOGOTHETIS, N. K., J. PAULS, M. AUGATH, T. TRINATH, and A. OELTERMANN, 2001. Neurophysiological investigation of the basis of the fMRI signal. *Nature* 412:150–157.

MAKEIG, S., 2002. Response: Event-related brain dynamics: Unifying brain electrophysiology. *Trends Neurosci.* 25:390.

OLSHAUSEN, B. A., and D. J. FIELD, 1996. Emergence of simple-cell receptive-field properties by learning a sparse code for natural images. *Nature* 381:607–609.

OLSHAUSEN, B. A., and D. J. FIELD, 2000. Vision and the coding of natural images. *Am. Sci.* 88:238–245.

ROTHMAN, D. L., K. L. BEHAR, F. HYDER, and R. G. SHULMAN, 2003. In vivo NMR studies of the glutamate neurotransmitter flux and neuroenergetics. *Ann. Rev. Physiol.* 65:401–427.

SARPESHKAR, R., 1998. Analog versus digital: Extrapolating from electronics to neurobiology. *Neural Comput.* 10:1601–1638.

SCHREIBER, S., C. K. MACHENS, A. V. M. HERZ, and S. B. LAUGHLIN, 2002. Energy efficient coding with discrete stochastic events. *Neural Comput.* 14:1323–1346.

SIESJÖ, B., 1978. *Brain Energy Metabolism*. New York: Wiley.

SIMONCELLI, E. P., and B. A. OLSHAUSEN, 2001. Natural image statistics and neural representation. *Ann. Rev. Neurosci.* 24: 1193–1216.

SMITH, A. J., H. BLUMENFELD, K. L. BEHAR, D. L. ROTHMAN, and R. G. SHULMAN, 2002. Cerebral energetics and spiking frequency: The neurophysiological basis of fMRI. *Proc. Natl. Acad. Sci. U.S.A.* 99:10765–10770.

VINJE, W. E., and J. L. GALLANT, 2000. Sparse coding and decorrelation in primary visual cortex during natural vision. *Science* 287:1273–1276.

VON DER TWER, T., and D. I. MACLEOD, 2001. Optimal nonlinear codes for the perception of natural colours. *Network* 12:395–407.

WEIBEL, E. R., 2000. *Symmorphosis: On Form and Function in Shaping Life*. Cambridge, Mass.: Harvard University Press.

WELIKY, M., J. FISER, R. H. HUNT, and D. N. WAGNER, 2003. Coding of natural scenes in primary visual cortex. *Neuron* 37:703–718.

WILLMORE, B., and D. J. TOLHURST, 2001. Characterizing the sparseness of neural codes. *Network* 12:255–270.

WONG-RILEY, M. T. T., 1989. Cytochrome oxidase: An endogenous metabolic marker for neuronal activity. *Trends Neurosci.* 12: 94–101.

15 Somatosensory Discrimination: Neural Coding and Decision-Making Mechanisms

RANULFO ROMO, VICTOR DE LAFUENTE, AND
ADRIÁN HERNÁNDEZ

ABSTRACT This chapter addresses the question of which components of the evoked neuronal activity in somatosensory cortex represent vibrotactile stimuli. We review experiments that probe how these representations determine the limits of vibrotactile discrimination. We also discuss recent results that suggest how vibrotactile stimuli are represented in areas central to primary somatosensory cortex (S1) during working memory. Finally, we review data from areas central to S1 that show neural correlates of a decision-making process during vibrotactile discrimination.

From the most stereotyped behavior of invertebrates to the most elaborate behavior of primates, a central issue in neuroscience is the elucidation of how sensory information is used to generate behavioral actions. In principle, this process can be understood as a chain of three basic neural operations. The representation of the physical attributes of the environment (i.e., sensory coding) and the execution of motor commands can be regarded as the end points of this chain of operations. In the middle of the chain is a crucial processing step in which the sensory representations are analyzed and transformed in such a way that the nervous system is able to choose the adequate motor response from an enormous repertoire of possible behavioral responses.

To study the neural basis of perceptual decisions, Romo and colleagues (Romo et al., 1999, 2003; Romo and Salinas, 2001; Romo, Hernández, Zainos, Brody, et al., 2002) analyzed neuronal responses in several areas of somatosensory cortex in trained monkeys performing a sensory discrimination task (Mountcastle et al., 1990; Hernández et al., 1997). In this task, monkeys must compare the frequency of two vibratory stimuli applied consecutively to their fingertips, and then use their free hand to push one of two response buttons to indicate which stimulus was of higher or lower frequency (figure 15.1). The discrimination task, although apparently simple, is designed so that it can only be executed correctly when a minimum number of neuronal operations or cognitive steps is performed: encoding the two stimulus frequencies, holding the first stimulus frequency in working memory, comparing the second stimulus frequency with the memory trace of the first stimulus frequency, and, finally, executing a motor response to indicate discrimination. Thus, the discrimination task allows us to investigate a wide range of essential processes of perceptual decision making.

The results obtained to date show that the changes in the firing patterns of neurons from several cortical areas (figure 15.2) provide enough information to support the operations required to solve the discrimination task (Romo and Salinas, 2001, 2003; Romo, Hernández, Zainos, Brody, et al., 2002). One interesting and unexpected observation is that in each studied cortical area central to primary somatosensory cortex (S1), there are two complementary neuronal populations with opposite tuning properties (Romo et al., 1999; Salinas et al., 2000; Hernández, Zainos, and Romo, 2002; Romo, Hernández, Zainos, Lemus, et al., 2002). The responses of these two populations can be understood as the neural representation of two perceptual categories that, at all levels of the processing hierarchy (sensory, association, and motor areas), encode the stimulus frequencies and the behavioral decisions. The responses of these two complementary populations are not aftereffects of peripheral sensory encoding. In fact, populations of neurons with opposite responses are not observed in S1 (Salinas et al., 2000; Romo, Hernández, Zainos, Lemus, et al., 2002). Given that this coding scheme is found only in areas central to S1, it is likely that these opposite responses reflect the nature of the processing operations implemented by the brain to solve the discrimination task. This dual encoding mechanism is also of interest because a simple subtraction operation between this dual sensory representation may generate a decision signal that, in the vibrotactile discrimination task, would indicate whether the frequency of the second stimulus was higher or lower than that of the first (Romo et al., 2003). To review the evidence supporting these conjectures, we analyze the neuronal activity associated with the diverse components of the discrimination task.

RANULFO ROMO, VICTOR DE LAFUENTE, and ADRIÁN HERNÁNDEZ Instituto de Fisiología Celular, Universidad Nacional Autónoma de México, Mexico City, Mexico.

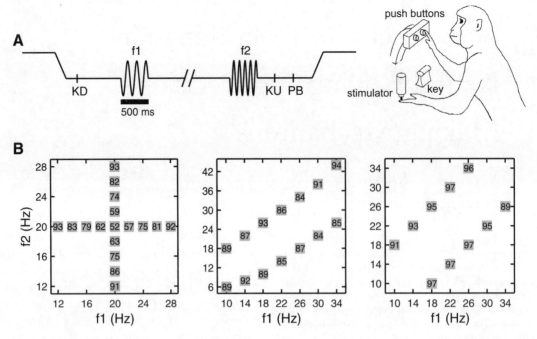

FIGURE 15.1 Flutter discrimination task. (*A*) Sequence of events during discrimination trials. The mechanical probe is lowered, indenting the fingertip of one digit of the restrained hand; the monkey places its free hand on an immovable key (KD); and the probe oscillates vertically at the base stimulus frequency (f_1). After a delay, a second mechanical vibration is delivered at the comparison frequency (f_2). The monkey releases the key (KU) and presses either a medial or a lateral push-button (PB) to indicate whether the comparison frequency was lower or higher than the base. (*B*) Stimulus sets used during recording sessions. Each box indicates a base/comparison frequency pair, with numbers inside the boxes showing overall percent of correct discriminations. The stimulus sets shown were used to determine discrimination thresholds (left) and to study working memory (middle) and comparison (right) processes during the task. The three sets were often used during any given recording session.

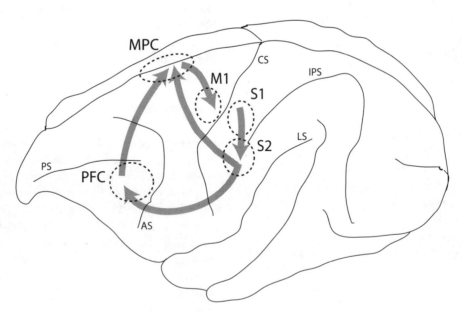

FIGURE 15.2 Monkey cortical areas activated during the somatosensory discrimination task. The schematic of the brain shows the approximate location of each cortical (broken lines). Gray arrows indicate a suggested but still uncertain sequential cortical processing scheme. The schematic of the brain also shows the region of approach to secondary somatosensory cortex (S2), which is hidden, in the lateral sulcus. AS, arcuate sulcus; CS, central sulcus; IPS, intraparietal sulcus; LS, lateral sulcus; M1, primary motor cortex; MPC, medial premotor cortex; PFC, prefrontal cortex; PS, principal sulcus; S1, primary somatosensory cortex.

Peripheral and central encoding of vibrotactile stimuli

The first step in the chain of neuronal operations involved in the vibrotactile discrimination task is the transduction of mechanical stimuli into electrical activity susceptible to be analyzed by the central nervous system (CNS). The way in which mechanical stimuli are encoded by the firing patterns of the primary afferents (ending in mechanoreceptor organs) is critical because the characteristics of the transduction process constrain all subsequent operations that the brain may perform to represent the stimulus properties (Talbot et al., 1968).

In a classic study, using an experimental approach that combined electrophysiology and psychophysics, Mountcastle and colleagues (1967) demonstrated that activity elicited by skin vibrations of low (5–50 Hz) and high frequencies (60–300 Hz) are transmitted to the CNS by two distinct groups of primary afferents (Talbot et al., 1968). On one hand, they quantified the responses of primary afferents to different frequencies to estimate sensory tuning curves. These curves showed the amplitude, as a function of frequency, to which the afferents responded "in phase" with the stimuli, that is, by emitting a spike, or a group of them, for each sinusoidal wave of the stimulus (with a probability of 0.9). On the other hand, these authors estimated in human subjects the amplitude detection thresholds as a function of frequency. By comparing neuronal and psychophysical tuning curves, Mountcastle and colleagues were able to establish that activity in the rapidly adapting fibers (RA), which end in the Meissner corpuscles of the glabrous skin, explained the human detection thresholds for frequencies in the 5–50 Hz range (the sensation of "flutter"). Using the same methods, they also established that activity in the afferent fibers terminating in the pacinian corpuscles (PC) explained the human detection thresholds for frequencies in the 60–300 Hz range (the sensation of "vibration"). This and other studies of the response properties of primary afferents (Johansson, Landstrom, and Lundstrom, 1982; Johansson and Vallbo, 1983; Vallbo and Johansson, 1984; Johnson, 2001), established that during our vibrotactile discrimination task (in the 5–50 Hz range), the first neuronal signals that encode the stimuli are transmitted to the CNS by the RA primary afferents.

Primary afferents relay in second-order neurons at the dorsal column nucleus of the spinal cord, which in turn project to the posterior ventrolateral nucleus of the thalamus (Mountcastle, 1984). The somatic thalamic neurons, then, project to S1 (Mountcastle, 1984). How are vibrotactile stimuli encoded in S1 neurons? In anesthetized monkeys, and later in awake monkeys performing the vibrotactile discrimination task, Mountcastle and colleagues found that responses of S1 neurons with RA properties, similar to RA afferents, were "phase-locked" with the mechanical stimuli; that is, they fired an action potential (or a group of them) for each sinusoidal wave (Mountcastle et al., 1969, 1990). In addition, they found that S1 neurons with slowly adapting properties (SA) also responded to low-frequency stimulation, producing trains of periodic spikes. Microstimulation studies, however, had previously revealed that electrical microstimulation of the SA afferents evoked a sustained pressure sensation (Ochoa and Torebjork, 1983). The fact that higher stimulation frequencies produced increasing pressure sensations indicates that firing rates of SA neurons signal not the frequency but the intensity of the pressure on the skin. These results suggested that only the activity of neurons with RA properties was responsible for the perception of low-frequency stimuli (5–50 Hz).

Mountcastle and colleagues then posed a fundamental question: What is the code these neurons use to transmit information about the stimulus frequency? In other words, which features of the spike trains can be used by neurons central to S1 to estimate the stimulus frequency? Mountcastle's studies indicated that firing rates of RA neurons did not seem to be significantly modulated by the frequency of the stimuli (though a sample of only 17 neurons was analyzed). Therefore, and because of the exquisite temporal precision with which RA neurons responded to each sinusoidal wave of the stimulus, Mountcastle and colleagues suggested that areas central to S1 could use the periodicity of the spike trains to estimate the frequency of the stimuli (Mountcastle, Steinmetz, and Romo, 1990).

Periodicity and firing rate as neural codes for the frequency of vibrotactile stimuli

The role of cortical somatosensory neurons in the discrimination task has recently been re-addressed. A specific objective of these studies was to provide evidence to support or refute the hypothesis of the periodicity of S1 neurons' responses as the coding signal of the frequency of vibrotactile stimuli. To achieve this, Hernández, Zainos, and Romo (2000) recorded the activity of single S1 neurons while monkeys performed the vibrotactile discrimination task. They found, as Mountcastle and colleagues (1990) had before, that the majority of S1 neurons emitted spike trains that reflected the regularity of sinusoidal stimuli (figure 15.3A). In addition, they also found S1 neurons that modulated their firing rates (figure 15.3D) as a function of the stimulus frequency (Salinas et al., 2000). They used signal detection theory to assess how much about stimulus frequency is present in the neuronal firing rate (Green and Swets, 1966). The appeal of this form at analysis, known as receiver operating curve (ROC) analysis, is that the neurometric curve calculated from the neuronal response distributions is analogous to, and can be directly compared with, the psychophysical performance. This analysis showed that

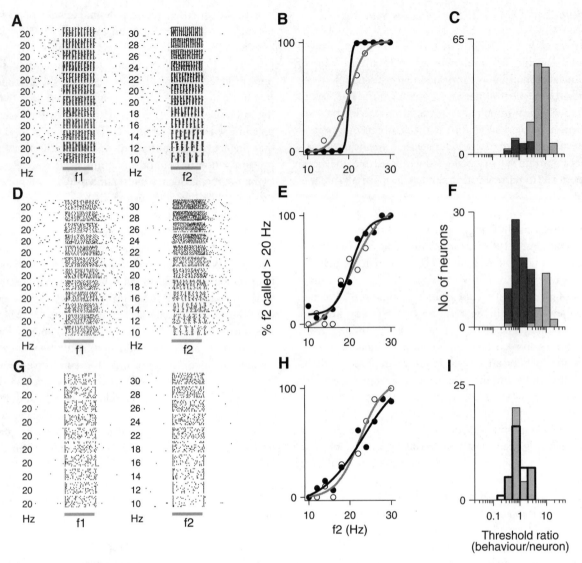

FIGURE 15.3 Comparison between S1 activity and psychophysical performance. *A*, *D*, and *G* show responses of three area 1 neurons recorded during discrimination. Each line represents a trial and each dot an action potential. Trials were delivered randomly. Gray horizontal bars at the bottom of each raster plot mark stimulation periods; first (f_1) and second (f_2) stimulus frequencies are indicated. (*A*) Responses showing little rate modulation but faithfully reflecting the periodicity of the stimuli. (*D*) Responses showing strong rate modulation but little regularity in spike timing relative to the periodic stimuli. (*G*) Responses to aperiodic stimuli. *B*, *E*, and *H* show psychometric and neurometric curves. On the *y*-axis is shown percentage of trials in which f_2 was called higher than f_1, where f_1 was 20 Hz. Open circles and gray curves correspond to the monkey's performance. Filled circles and black curves indicate the performance of an ideal observer that based his decisions on

the responses of a single neuron. Continuous lines are sigmoidal fits to the data; the discrimination threshold is inversely proportional to maximum steepness. (*B*) Performance of the ideal observer was based on the periodicity of the neuron in *A*. (*E* and *H*) Performance of the ideal observer was based on the firing rates of the neurons in *D* and *G*, respectively. *C*, *F*, and *I* indicate numbers of S1 neurons with the indicated threshold ratios. (*C* and *F*) Neurometric thresholds based on spike-train periodicity (light gray bars) were much smaller than those based on mean firing rate modulation (dark gray bars) and matched the behavioral thresholds. (*I*) Threshold ratios based on mean firing rates evoked by aperiodic stimuli (light gray bars) were similar to those obtained with periodic stimuli (open bars). (Modified from Hernández, Zainos, and Romo, 2000.)

neurometric discrimination curves calculated from firing rate modulations were indistinguishable from the psychometric curves (figure 15.3E, F) that resulted from the discrimination responses of the monkeys (Hernández, Zainos, and Romo, 2000). This evidence suggested that changes in the firing rate form a potential code of stimulus frequency.

What is the relationship between the periodicity of the neuron's responses and the animal's performance? Can periodicity of spike trains be used to estimate the stimulus frequency? Further studies demonstrated that the information contained in the power spectral density (PSD) of the spike trains could allow an ideal observer to attain performance levels far superior to those achieved by the animals (Hernández, Zainos, and Romo, 2000; Salinas et al., 2000). The fact that animals could have achieved higher levels of performance (and therefore more reward) if they had used periodicity information cast doubt on the capacity of neurons from areas central to S1 to extract frequency information from the periodicity (figure 15.3B, C). However, we must also consider that the information extracted by means of the PSD analysis constitutes an upper limit, and that the neuronal mechanisms that could implement an approximation of PSD analysis may not be able to attain the precision of numerical methods. So far, then, we can only suggest that information contained in the periodicity and in firing rate could be used to estimate the stimulus frequency.

The role of periodicity as a possible source of information for estimating stimulus frequency was further tested using an aperiodic version of the vibrotactile stimuli (Romo et al., 1998; Hernández, Zainos, and Romo, 2000; Salinas et al., 2000). In this configuration, the time between each sinusoidal wave varied randomly to reduce the periodic component of the stimuli. As might be expected if monkeys were using the number of pulses per unit of time to estimate the stimulus frequency, they did not need to be retrained to solve the aperiodic variant of the discrimination task. Although the interpulse intervals varied considerably, the monkeys were able to successfully extract and compare the average frequency of the two stimuli (Romo et al., 1998; Hernández, Zainos, and Romo, 2000; Salinas et al., 2000). As expected, the activity of S1 neurons reflected the aperiodic structure of the stimuli (figure 15.3G), and the neurometric thresholds calculated from the firing rates matched the psychophysical thresholds (figure 15.3H, I; Hernández, Zainos, and Romo, 2000). Salinas and colleagues (2000) then demonstrated that the stimulus frequency could not be estimated from the temporal structure of the responses of these neurons, but only from their firing rate modulations.

Additional evidence supporting a firing rate code for frequency discrimination was obtained by analyzing the responses of S1 neurons at psychophysical thresholds. In this condition, the behavioral responses to the same stimulus can be predicted from variations in the neuronal responses. Any proposed neural code should be capable of predicting behavior from neuronal activity. By comparing neuronal response variations of both firing rate and periodicity during correct and incorrect discriminations, Salinas and colleagues (2000) found that only variations in the number of spikes (firing rate), and not the temporal regularity of the spike trains, covaried with the monkey's behavioral responses on a trial-by-trial basis.

The evidence discussed so far points to firing rate as a strong candidate for the signal that neurons in the somatosensory areas may use to code the frequency of mechanical stimuli. However, it must be noted that humans, and probably monkeys, are able to distinguish two stimuli with equal average frequency but distinct temporal structures. This observation suggests that, when necessary, the somatosensory cortex can extract the temporal structure of the stimuli. Recordings of S1 neurons during the discrimination task revealed a continuous distribution of neurons that exquisitely represent the temporal structure of the stimuli and those that only increase their average firing rate as a function of the frequency. This distribution probably reflects a processing hierarchy among neurons in S1: Neurons with "phase-locked" responses are probably located closer to thalamic inputs than neurons that only modulate their firing rate and do not reflect the temporal structure of the stimuli. The firing rate–modulated neurons could be integrating the information of periodic-response neurons and transforming them into a firing rate code (Hernández, Zainos, and Romo, 2000).

Probing the neural coding efficiency by S1 microstimulation

Neurophysiological studies often reveal close associations between neuronal activity and sensory events, but does such activity have an impact on perception and subsequent behavior? We typically assume so, but this is hard to verify. To verify whether the evoked neuronal activity in the RA circuit of S1 is sufficient for vibrotactile discrimination, Romo and colleagues (1998, 2000) manipulated the S1 representation of the vibrotactile stimulus by injecting current bursts of electrical stimuli at the same mechanical frequencies.

A first approach was to manipulate the comparison stimulus frequency during the discrimination task (Romo et al., 1998). In half of the trials, microstimulation of area 3b substituted for the mechanical, comparison stimulus frequency. Artificial stimuli consisted of periodic or aperiodic current bursts delivered at the same comparison frequencies as the mechanical comparison stimuli. Microstimulation sites in area 3b were selected to have RA neurons with receptive fields on the fingertip at the location of the mechanical stimulating probe (Sur, Wall, and Kaas, 1984). Remarkably, the

FIGURE 15.4 Psychophysical performance in frequency discrimination with natural, mechanical stimuli delivered to the fingertips and with artificial, electrical stimuli delivered directly to S1 neurons. Monkeys were first trained to compare two mechanical stimuli presented sequentially on the fingertips (see figure 15.1). Then some of the mechanical stimuli were replaced by trains of electrical current bursts microinjected into clusters of RA neurons in area 3b. Each burst consisted of two biphasic current pulses. Current bursts were delivered at the same comparison frequencies as natural stimuli. In half of the trials the monkeys compared two mechanical vibrations delivered on the skin; in the other half one or both stimuli were replaced by microstimulation. The two trial types were interleaved, and frequencies always changed from trial to trial. The diagrams on the left show the four protocols used. The curves on the right show the animals' performance in the situations illustrated on the left. Filled and open circles indicate mechanical and electrical stimuli, respectively; continuous lines are fits to the data points. (A) All stimuli were periodic; the comparison stimulus could be either mechanical or electrical. (B) The base stimulus was periodic and the comparison aperiodic; the comparison could be mechanical or electrical. (C) All stimuli were periodic; the base stimulus could be mechanical or electrical. (D) All stimuli were periodic; on microstimulation trials both base and comparison stimuli were artificial. Vibrotactile stimuli were either sinusoids or trains of short mechanical pulses, each consisting of a single-cycle sinusoid lasting 20 ms. Monkeys' performance was practically the same with natural and artificial stimuli. (Modified from Romo et al., 1998, 2000.)

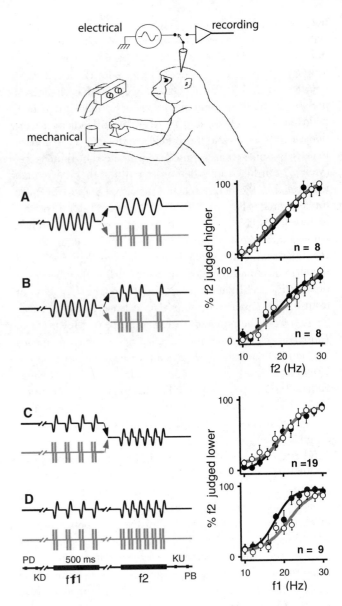

monkeys could discriminate between the mechanical (base) and the electrical (comparison) signals with performance profiles indistinguishable from those obtained with natural periodic or aperiodic stimuli (figure 15.4A, B).

Romo and colleagues (2000) then wondered whether, in addition to using artificial stimuli during the comparison period of the task, monkeys could store and use a quantitative trace of an electrical stimulus delivered to clusters of RA neurons in S1 cortex in place of the first mechanical stimulus. They also wondered whether monkeys could perform the entire task on the basis of purely artificial stimuli (Romo et al., 2000). This would demonstrate that activation of the RA circuit of S1 was sufficient to initiate the entire cognitive process involved in the task.

Again, the mixed mechanical/microstimulation protocol was used, in which microstimulation trials were randomly intermixed with standard, purely mechanical trials. The frequency pairs and event sequence were the same in both mechanical and microstimulation trials, except that in microstimulation trials the first or both mechanical stimuli were substituted by trains of current pulses injected in S1 and delivered at the frequency of the mechanical stimulus they were replacing. The stimulus set was designed to ensure exploration of the working memory component of the task and determination of discrimination thresholds.

Psychophysical performance with electrical microstimulation patterns in S1 cortex at the mechanical base stimulus

frequencies they were replacing was similar to that measured with the mechanical stimulus (figure 15.4C). These results show that monkeys were able to memorize the base artificial stimulus frequency and compare the second stimulus with the memory trace left by the artificial stimulus. As for substituting electrical patterns for the comparison stimulus, monkeys could not reach the usual level of performance when clusters of SA neurons were microstimulated (Romo et al., 2000). Nor they could discriminate when microstimulation patterns were made at the border between RA and SA clusters. These control experiments tell us about the specificity of the RA circuit in flutter discrimination (Romo et al., 2000). Finally, in most sessions in which the two mechanical stimuli were replaced by microstimulated patterns, monkeys were able to reach discrimination levels close to those measured with mechanical stimuli delivered to the fingertips (figure 15.4D). This indicates that microstimulation elicits quantitative memorizable and discriminable percepts, and shows that activation of the RA circuit of S1 is sufficient to initiate the entire subsequent neural process associated with vibrotactile discrimination.

Relevant to interpreting the S1 microstimulation results, previous studies have shown that activity in a single cutaneous afferent fiber could produce localized somatic sensations, and frequency microstimulation of RA afferents linked to Meissner's corpuscles produced the sensation of flutter (Vallbo, 1995). These observations strongly support the notion that the activity initiated in specific mechanoreceptors is read out by S1; this reading is then widely distributed to those anatomical structures that are linked to S1. The whole sequence of events associated with this sensory discrimination task must depend on this distributed neural signal. As discussed in the following section, a transformation of the coding scheme is observed as information flows from S1 to the secondary somatosensory cortex (S2).

Coding vibrotactile stimuli in areas central to S1

Coding Vibrotactile Stimuli in S2 Anatomical (Burton, Fabri, and Alloway, 1995) and electrophysiological (Pons et al., 1987) evidence suggests that S1 and S2 are connected serially in monkeys (Iwamura, 1998). Lesions in the hand representation of S1 selectively deactivate responses of the hand representation in S2 (Pons et al., 1987). During the frequency discrimination task, S2 neurons respond approximately 10 ms after S1 neurons, a finding that is also consistent with a serial flow of information from S1 to S2 (a difference of approximately 10 ms between each processing stage has also been observed in the visual system; Thorpe and Fabre-Thorpe, 2001). In addition, the majority of the responses of S2 neurons are not phase-locked with the temporal structure of the stimuli, and it has been shown that the temporal structure of spike trains of S2 neurons could not provide enough information to estimate the stimulus frequency (Salinas et al., 2000). As shown for S1, comparisons of activity during correct and error trials showed that only firing rate variations covaried with discrimination responses (Salinas et al., 2000).

How, then, is the stimulus frequency represented in the somatosensory cortex? The results reviewed suggest that the neural representation of the stimulus frequency is achieved by a two-step mechanism. First, information of the number of pulses, the time intervals between them, and the total duration of the stimulus is represented in the spike trains produced by S1 neurons, particularly in RA neurons of S1. This information is transmitted to S2, and it is transformed in such a way that the temporal structure of the stimulus is no longer represented in the response spike trains. Second, almost half of the S2 neurons are preferentially activated by low stimulus frequencies: they show negative monotonic

responses as a function of the increasing stimulus frequencies. Thus, in addition to the positive monotonic responses (like those observed in S1), in S2 there is a complementary population of neurons with opposite responses. This dual encoding has also been observed in S2 of monkeys trained in texture discrimination (Sinclair and Burton, 1991, 1993). As discussed later in this chapter, the frequency representation based on two sets of neurons with opposite tuning properties (slopes) seems to have a beneficial effect for the stimulus encoding and for discrimination performance (Romo et al., 2003). The cellular and network properties responsible for the transformation observed between S1 and S2 are not known, but the existence of two complementary types of responses at early stages may also be useful for interfacing with more central structures involved in motor processes like those studied by Gold and Shadlen (2001).

Coding Vibrotactile Stimuli in Frontal Cortex During the first stimulus presentation, in addition to the activity in S1 and S2, sensory responses have been observed in the prefrontal (PFC) and medial premotor (MPC) cortices (Romo et al., 1998; Hernández, Zainos, and Romo, 2002), with response latencies slightly higher than S2 and S1. As for S2, the PFC and MPC neurons encode the stimulus frequency by two classes of neurons with opposite slopes. In PFC and MPC, subtraction can also enhance information about the stimulus frequency.

What is the role of these sensory representations located in areas central to S2? Current viewpoints on the cortical hierarchy of information processing propose that neuronal activity proximal to the motor cortex can be related to the preparation and execution of motor commands. However, the role of sensory responses in PFC and PMC is difficult to explain in motor terms because monkeys cannot make predictions about the direction of the response movement based on the first stimulus information (Romo et al., 1998; Hernández, Zainos, and Romo, 2002). Crick and Koch (1995) have suggested that conscious perception of sensory stimuli requires activation of frontal cortices. Moreover, it has been proposed that higher sensory representations need to be fed back to lower-level sensory areas in order to be perceived (Pascual-Leone and Walsh, 2001). According to this hypothesis, neural activation of frontal cortices during the first stimulus presentation would be related to the conscious perception of the stimulus. However, this conjecture remains to be proved.

Coding vibrotactile stimuli during working memory

To adequately solve the vibrotactile discrimination task, the frequency of the first stimulus must be compared with the frequency of the second stimulus. The presence of this interstimulus delay requires the use of working memory mechanisms to hold in time the frequency of the first stimulus. Unlike other psychophysical tasks, in which certain features of a single stimulus must be evaluated according to a previously learned criterion (acquired during training and stored in long-term memory), on the discrimination task the reference value (first stimulus) changes on every trial, forcing the monkeys to use working memory mechanisms (Hernández et al., 1997). Where and how is the first stimulus frequency stored? The ability to retain behaviorally meaningful sensory information for a brief time interval has been associated with activation of PFC neurons (Funahashi, Bruce, and Goldman-Rakic, 1989; Fuster, 1989; Miller and Cohen, 2001).

To explore the role of the PFC in the discrimination task, Romo and colleagues (1999) studied the activity of neurons in the inferior convexity of the PFC. In addition to the sensory responses, neurons in this area manifested firing rate modulations during the delay period between the two stimuli. Did the delay activity of these neurons carry information about the first stimulus frequency? To answer this question, Romo and colleagues (1999) calculated the delay period during which firing rates can be adequately modeled by a linear function of the first stimulus frequency, that is, the period of time in which delay activity carries sensory information. The activation patterns proved to be anything but static. Based on activation dynamics, most of the neurons in the PFC can be sorted into three categories. "Early" neurons provide stimulus frequency information during the first third of the delay period. The dependence of firing rates to stimulus frequency is evident toward the end of the delay period in "late" neurons. Finally, neurons classified as "persistent" carry information about the stimulus frequency throughout the entire delay period (figure 15.5E, F). During this period, approximately half of the neurons increased their firing rate as a positive monotonic function (positive slope) of the increasing stimulus frequency, while the other half of the neurons decreased their firing rate (negative slope) as a function of the increasing stimulus frequency. Thus, analysis of the activation dynamics of PFC neurons revealed that during the delay period, stimulus frequency—an analogue scalar value—seems to be coded directly in the firing rate (also a scaled analogue value) of two complementary populations of neurons.

Is PFC the only cortical area involved in working memory during vibrotactile discrimination? Certainly not. But the PFC may play a crucial role. This became evident when we contrasted the neuronal activity of other cortical areas in the same task (figure 15.5). For example, S2 neurons retain information only during the early component of the delay period (figure 15.5C, D). The MPC, which includes the pre-SMA (presupplementary area) and the SMA proper, contain an important fraction of neurons that encode the first stimulus frequency during the delay period (figure 15.5G, H;

Hernández, Zainos, and Romo, 2002). As in the PFC, neural activity in MPC was not static and could be sorted into early, late, and persistent categories. In the MPC, however, approximately 60% of neurons code stimulus frequency during the final third of the delay period (late responses). Similar to S2 and PFC, approximately half of MPC neurons are preferentially activated by low stimulus frequencies and the other half by high stimulus frequencies. An interesting finding was that none of the S1 neurons studied during the vibrotactile discrimination task showed information about the first stimulus during the delay period (figure 15.5A, B).

The temporal dynamics of frequency-encoding delay activity in S2, PFC, and PMC are consistent with the cortical hierarchy of information processing (Brody et al., 2002; Romo and Salinas, 2003): neurons in S2 encode the stimulus frequency during the early component of the delay period. PFC neurons maintain this information during the entire delay period, allowing it to be fed back to lower-level sensory areas or to be forwarded to movement-related areas. Finally, toward the end of the delay period, as the stimuli comparison operation and movement execution become imminent, neurons in MPC activate strongly.

Is the delay activity of MPC and PFC neurons coding the first stimulus frequency or, instead, reflecting preparatory activity related to the forthcoming motor response? The stimuli sets used in the discrimination task were designed in such a way that the frequency of the first stimulus on its own did not allow prediction of the response movement beyond chance levels. Given that monkeys achieved 84%–94% correct responses, significantly above the 50% chance level, it is possible to state that the delay activity observed in MPC and PCF neurons is not exclusively related to a motor plan.

Comparison and decision-making processes

The second (comparison) stimulus is presented after the delay period. Monkeys then have to compare this stimulus with the memory trace of the first stimulus and decide whether it has a higher or lower frequency. Where and how is the neuronal operation of comparison and decision-making executed? Gold and Shadlen (2001) have shown that only a subtraction operation between the responses of two neurons tuned with opposite stimulus characteristics is necessary to generate a decision signal favoring a particular sensory hypothesis. Supporting this proposal, they have found decision-making neural activity that seems to arise from responses of direction-sensitive neurons in the parietal visual cortex of monkeys (Gold and Shadlen, 2000; Shadlen and Newsome, 2001).

Extending Gold and Shadlen's proposal to the vibrotactile discrimination task, the sign resulting from subtraction of the responses of neurons with opposite tuning curves may indicate whether the second stimulus was of a higher or

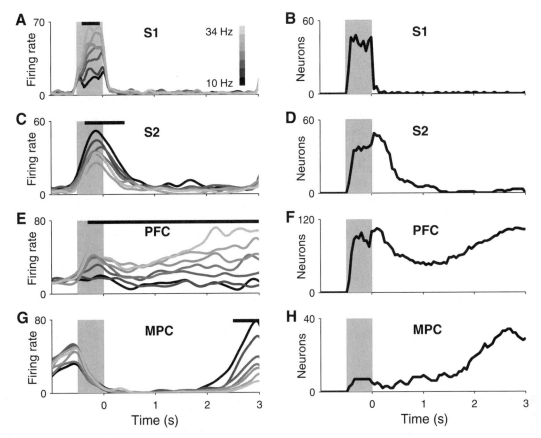

FIGURE 15.5 Neuronal responses observed during the delay period in four areas. *A, C, E,* and *G* show spike density functions from four single neurons. Dark bars above each plot indicate times during which the neuron's firing rate carried a significant ($P < 0.01$) monotonic signal about the base stimulus. Gray densities are used to sort responses according to base frequency, as indicated by the scale gradient. (*A* and *E*) These neurons fired most strongly with high stimulus frequencies. (*C* and *G*) These neurons fired most strongly with low frequencies. (*B, D, F,* and *H*) Numbers of recorded neurons carrying a significant signal about the base stimulus, as a function of time relative to the beginning of the delay period; only data collected from runs with a fixed delay of 3s are included. Abbreviations: S1, primary somatosensory cortex; S2, secondary somatosensory cortex; MPC, medial premotor cortex; PFC, prefrontal cortex. (Modified from Romo et al., 1999; Salinas et al., 2000; Hernández, Zainos, and Romo, 2002.)

lower frequency than the first. It is possible that the subtraction operation could be implemented between the sensory representation of the second stimulus and the mnemonic reference of the first stimulus frequency. Is there any evidence indicating that this operation is performed during the discrimination task? To answer this question, Romo and colleagues (Romo, Hernández, Zainos, Lemus et al., 2002) studied the responses of S2 and MPC neurons (Hernández, Zainos, and Romo, 2002) during the 500-ms period of the second stimulus presentation, that is, during the period in which the comparison operation takes place.

In addition to the massive afferents originating in S1 areas (3a, 3b, 1, and 2), S2 is reciprocally connected with the insular cortex, with areas 5 and 7b in the parietal cortex, and with areas 6, 4, PFC, and SMA proper in the frontal cortices (Cipolloni and Pandya, 1999). This connectivity, in principle, allows S2 to integrate both sensory information (bottom-up) and information fed back from more central areas (top-down). For this reason, S2 may be well-suited to

participate in the comparison and decision-making process. Consistent with this hypothesis, Romo and colleagues (Romo, Hernández, Zainos, Lemus et al., 2002) found that the responses of S2 neurons to the second stimulus were modulated not only by the frequency of the stimulus being presented, but also by the frequency of the first stimulus applied some seconds before. This fact is illustrated by the neural responses to the final 200-ms period of the second stimulus (f_2), where it can be observed that activity is not related to specific frequency values of f_2 or f_1. Instead, the neural responses indicate whether $f_2 > f_1$ or $f_2 < f_1$ (Romo, Hernández, Zainos, Brody, et al., 2000).

To study these observations quantitatively, Romo and colleagues (Romo, Hernández, Zainos, Brody, et al., 2002) analyzed the response of neurons by means of a multiple linear regression of the type: firing rate = $a_1 \cdot f_1 + a_2 \cdot f_2 +$ constant. The coefficients a_1 and a_2 measure the strength of the relationship between a neuron's firing rate and the frequency of the first (f_1) and second (f_2) stimuli, respectively. Fitting this equation to neuronal responses in successive time windows and plotting a_2 as a function of a_1 allows an appreciational the time dynamics of the neuron's response dependence on the frequency of f_1 and f_2 (figure 15.6). Three lines on this graph are of particular interest. Points falling on the $a_2 = 0$ line illustrate neural responses that are function of f_1 only. Points on $a_1 = 0$ indicate responses that are exclusively a function of f_2. Points along the diagonal $a_1 = -a_2$ illustrate neural responses that are the result of the difference between f_2 and f_1. Applying multiple linear regression analysis through a sliding time window throughout the second stimulus period revealed the temporal dynamics of the dependence of the neuron's firing rate on the first and second stimuli. It was found that the temporal dynamics of individual neurons were highly variable, but the population showed a clear tendency. Initially, firing rates were mainly a function of f_1 or f_2 frequency. However, toward the end of the 500-ms period of the second stimulus, firing rates were no longer a function of f_1 or f_2 but only of the sign resulting from the subtraction of $f_2 - f_1$. Thus, the activity of the S2 neurons during the second stimulus reflected the comparison process between f_1 and f_2. In principle, this operation could be generated by the subtraction of the mnemonic reference of f_1 (maintained by PFC or other higher areas) and the sensory representation of f_2 (originating in S1). The symmetrical point distribution in the first and fourth quadrants indicates the existence of two neuronal populations with opposite responses (figure 15.6B). Points in the first quadrant are from neurons that prefer (i.e., fire strongly during) the condition $f_2 > f_1$, while points in the fourth quadrant come from $f_2 < f_1$ selective neurons. In this manner, decision signals resulting from the comparison operation are coded by means of two neuronal populations with opposite responses, that is, by means of a dual representation.

An important issue concerning the selective responses observed toward the end of the second stimulus is whether they arise from a comparison operation or instead are exclusively related to the preparation of a motor response. To answer this question, 17 neurons of area S2 were studied while monkeys performed a control task on which they executed the same response movements, but instead of being guided by the result of the comparison process they were visually instructed to press the illuminated button for reward. In this control task, the correct response button was illuminated at the beginning of the trial, so that somatosensory information and the comparison process were unnecessary for reward. During this control experiment, most of the response's dependence on f_1 and f_2 was lost, suggesting that it is related to the comparison operation and not necessarily to the motor response.

The evidence discussed to this point suggests that S2 is involved in the comparison process. However, recent findings have shown that other structures may also be involved.

It is possible that the decision signals observed in S2 are only a copy of decision-making processes elaborated in other cortical areas. As we shall see below, decision-related signals are observed in MPC before they appear in S2. Moreover, preliminary results indicate that decision signals may be generated in the PFC (unpublished observations) even earlier than in MPC and S2.

It has consistently been found that MPC activity is related to movement preparation (Shima and Tanji, 2000). Given that the ultimate objective of the discrimination task is to generate a response movement (to obtain a reward), and because this can be correctly achieved only after comparing the first and second stimuli, is the MPC involved in the sensory-to-motor transformation achieved by the comparison operation? Romo and colleagues (Romo, Hernández, Zainos, Brody, et al., 2002) found that about half of the neurons recorded in MPC during the discrimination task showed activity during the second stimulus. Of these neurons, a vast majority showed selective responses that indicated whether $f_2 > f_1$ or $f_2 < f_1$ (figure 15.6D). An ROC analysis, which estimates the probability of an ideal observer, looking at single neuron responses, of correctly distinguishing the $f_2 > f_1$ or $f_2 < f_1$ conditions, was used to quantitatively study the strength of the selective responses. A 0.5 valued ROC index indicates that the response of the neuron is similar for both conditions and that is unable to indicate, beyond chance level, if $f_2 > f_1$ or $f_2 < f_1$ had occurred. In contrast, a 1.0 ROC index indicates that the neuron is able to indicate, on each trial, whether $f_2 > f_1$ or $f_2 < f_1$ had occurred. To study the temporal dynamics of this selective activity, ROC indices for each neuron were calculated in a 100-ms-wide sliding window, displaced in 20-ms steps, beginning 1 s before the second stimulus presentation and ending 1 s after the stimulus presentation (figure 15.7). During the comparison process, approximately half the neurons showed ROC indices that deviated above 0.5 (indicating selective activity for the $f_2 > f_1$ condition), while the other half deviated below 0.5 (indicating selective activity for the $f_2 < f_1$ condition). These results indicate that, just as in the neural representation of sensory stimuli, two complementary neuronal populations code decision signals indicating the result of the comparison process.

To quantitatively measure the neural response's dependence on the frequency of the first and second stimuli, just as in S2 neurons, a multiple linear regression analysis was carried. Romo and colleagues (Hernández, Zainos, and Romo, 2002) found that during the first 100 ms of the second stimulus, the activity of some neurons was mainly a function of f_1 frequency (figure 15.8A). This finding is consistent with a "memory recall" of the base stimulus frequency. However, what is typically observed in MPC is that, during the second stimulus, some neurons initially code f_1 or f_2 frequency, and later these and other neurons code whether $f_2 > f_1$ or $f_2 < f_1$

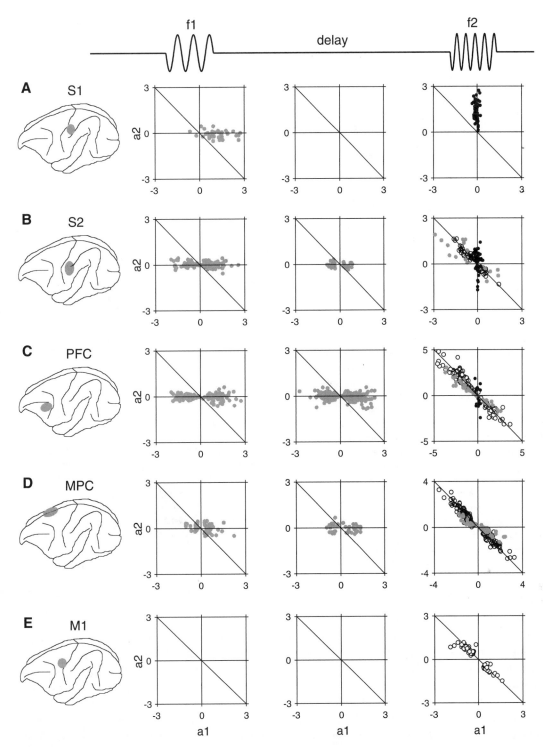

FIGURE 15.6 Population dynamics in different cortical areas during the flutter discrimination task. Each data point represents one neuron. For each, responses were fit to the equation: firing rate = $a_1 \times f_1 + a_2 \times f_2$ + constant. The coefficients a_1 and a_2 were computed from responses at different times during the task. Points that fall on the $a_1 = 0$ axis represent responses that depend on f_2 only (black circles); points that fall on the $a_2 = 0$ axis represent responses that depend on f_1 only (gray circles); points that fall on the $a_2 = -a_1$ line represent responses that are functions of $f_2 - f_1$ (open circles). The data shown are significantly different from (0, 0) in at least one of the epochs analyzed. (A) S1 responses during the first stimulation period (f_1; left), the interstimulus period (delay; middle), and the second stimulation period (f_2; right). These neurons were active only during stimulation; most of them increased their rates with increasing frequency (positive a_1 and a_2). (B) S2 neurons

respond to f_1 (left) and exhibit a modest but significant amount of delay activity (middle). Positive and negative coefficients indicate rates that increase and decrease as functions of frequency, respectively. During the initial part of f_2 (right), neurons may have significant a_1 coefficients (gray circles) or may respond exclusively to f_2 (black circles), as computed from the first 200 ms after stimulus onset. Later on, the coefficients cluster around the line $a_2 = -a_1$ (open circles), as computed from the last 300 ms before stimulus offset. Brain diagram shows region of approach to S2, which is hidden in the lateral sulcus. (C) Data from PFC. Coefficients are calculated as in B. (D) Data from MPC. Coefficients are calculated as in B. (E) Data from M1. Coefficients are calculated as in B. (Modified from Romo et al., 1999; Hernández, Zainos, and Romo, 2000; Salinas et al., 2000; R. Romo et al., unpublished observations.)

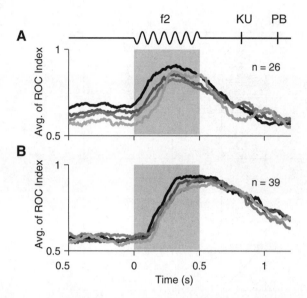

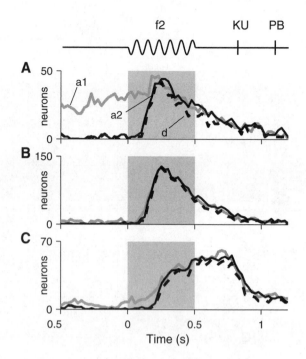

FIGURE 15.7 Discrimination capacity of MPC neurons. Vertical axes show the ROC index averaged across neurons. This measures the average strength of the differential response (i.e., one arm movement versus the other) regardless of whether it corresponds to $f_2 > f_1$ or $f_2 < f_1$. This quantity is shown as a function of time. Differences between f_1 and f_2 are indicated by dark to light gray levels, from 0 (light line) to 2, 4, and 8 Hz (dark line). Traces were computed from trials with different f_1 but fixed f_2 (see figure 15.1C, left). (A) ROC indices computed from neurons carrying a significant signal about f_1 during the delay. Note that differential activity increases during the comparison period (f_2), and that it rises earlier as the difference between f_1 and f_2 increases. (B) ROC indices for MPC neurons that did not carry a significant signal about f_1 during the delay period. These neurons do not show significant ROC indices during the delay. Differential activity develops during the comparison but later than in A, and with comparable magnitude for various frequency differences. (Modified from Hernández et al., 2002.)

FIGURE 15.8 Timing of differential activity in MPC. (A) Numbers of neurons with significant coefficients a_1 (gray line) and a_2 (black line), as functions of time; d (dashed line) indicates cases where a_1 and a_2 had similar magnitudes but opposite signs (points near the diagonal in figure 15.5D). (A) Data are from neurons that carried a significant amount of information about f_1 during the delay period. (B) As in A, but for neurons that had no significant delay activity and fired most strongly during the comparison period. The differential response (d) is slightly delayed with respect to A. (C) As in B, but for neurons that fired most strongly after the comparison, during the reaction-time period. The differential response (d) is delayed with respect to B. (Modified from Hernández, Zainos, and Romo, 2002.)

(figure 15.8A–C). These results show that during the second stimulus presentation, the dynamics of MPC neurons are very similar to those observed in S2 neurons and are consistent with a stimuli comparison operation.

As in S2, a crucial question is whether the differential responses observed in MPC are exclusively related to motor planning or instead arise from the stimuli comparison operation. Error trial analysis indicates that they code the decision motor output (figure 15.9). However, during the visual instruction task (discussed earlier), all neurons attenuated their responses (to ROC values close to 0.5), suggesting that the differential activity observed during the comparison period depended on the comparison operation and did not merely reflect the planning of a motor response (Hernández, Zainos, and Romo, 2002).

As we have seen, the decision-making process is widely distributed through the cortex—S2, MPC, and PFC (R. Romo et al., unpublished observations). To what extent the decision responses are generated de novo in each area or arise from shared inputs remains an open question that needs to be further explored.

Decision motor responses

We have seen that both S2 and MPC show neural dynamics consistent with a frequency comparison operation. What is the role of the primary motor cortex (M1)? It has been shown that M1 neurons code parameters such as the strength and direction of movements (Georgopoulos, Schwartz, and Kettner, 1986). This might lead us to think that M1 receives neural signals resulting from the comparison operation (binary signals that should trigger arm movements to either of the response buttons). However, recordings of M1 neurons in monkeys performing the frequency discrimination task showed that these neurons are activated during the second stimulus presentation about 600 ms before response movement initiation. In addition, multiple linear regression analysis (discussed earlier) showed that these responses are grouped very close to the diagonal

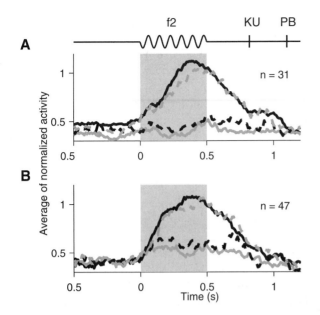

FIGURE 15.9 Analysis of error trials for MPC neurons. Curves show mean normalized responses as functions of time for neurons with (A) and without (B) significant delay activity. Separate traces are shown for correct trials in the preferred condition (continuous black line) and nonpreferred condition (continuous gray line). Broken lines correspond to error trials. The preferred condition is either $f_2 > f_1$ or $f_2 < f_1$, whichever produces a stronger response for a given neuron. Traces were calculated from trials with differences of 4 Hz between f_1 and f_2. Activities were normalized with respect to the highest firing rate during correct trials. (Modified from Hernández et al., 2002.)

$a_2 = -a_1$, indicating that this activity depends on the result of the comparison of the stimuli (figure 15.6E). The pattern of M1 activity is quite similar to the differential responses observed in S2 and MPC (figure 15.6B–E). This observation opens the possibility that the differential responses observed in these cortical area could be just a copy of the activity generated in M1. To test this hypothesis, Romo and colleagues (Romo, Hernández, Zainos, Brody et al., 2002) compared response latencies in these three areas. The results showed that differential responses in M1 are the last to appear (295 ± 20 ms), and that comparison and decision-making activity in S2 (236 ± 21 ms) and in MPC (201 ± 66 ms) preceded the activity of M1 neurons.

Just as in S2, PFC and MPC neurons with selective activity in M1 can be sorted into two populations. Those that activate more when $f_2 > f_1$ are plotted in the first quadrant (regression analysis) and those that activate maximally when $f_2 < f_1$ are plotted in the fourth quadrant of figure 15.6E. We should not forget that we have observed this dual coding in all the cortical areas studied central to S1, and in all the operations required to solve the discrimination task (figure 15.6).

What is the role of the differential activity observed in M1? Does it constitute only a mirror image of decision signals originated in other areas, or does it instead play an active role in information processing? To study the role of M1 in decision-making processes, Salinas and Romo (1998) studied responses of M1 neurons in monkeys trained to categorize the speed of movement of a mechanical probe moving along one of their fingertips. By pressing one of the two response buttons, monkeys had to indicate whether movement speed was high or low, based on arbitrary categories learned during training (Romo et al., 1993, 1996, 1997). Movement speed was systematically varied in order to produce psychophysical categorization curves. As expected, the majority of M1 neurons showed movement-related activity that did not indicate the stimulus speed of motion. However, one fifth of these neurons showed selective activity that was a function of both stimulus speed and the stimulus category (high or low). One important observation is that the differences in firing rates of these neurons (that indicated the selectivity for one category or the other) are not explained exclusively by the differences in the direction of response movement. This conclusion is supported by results obtained by Schwartz, Kettner, and Georgopoulos (1988), who implied that the 11° response button separation would only produce a 1 spike/s difference in the response of a movement direction-selective neuron. The selectivity of M1 neurons and their ability to code (through two complementary populations) the sensory component of the stimuli (velocity of movement) suggests the existence of subpopulations of M1 neurons that may be involved in the conversion of sensory information into response movements (Salinas and Romo, 1998).

Discussion

We have analyzed the neuronal activity from multiple cortical areas during the diverse components of the vibrotactile discrimination task. The responses of RA neurons in S1 show enough information to support frequency discrimination with performance levels similar to those obtained by monkeys. Moreover, artificial activation of these neurons probed their causal relation to the neural representation of the somestesic stimuli used in the discrimination task.

During the first stimulus (figure 15.6), sensory responses that are a function of stimulus frequency are also observed in S2, MPC, and PFC (R. Romo et al., unpublished observations). Sensory responses in these cortical areas, central to S1, may be related to the extraction of abstract qualities (frequency) and to the analysis of the behavioral meaning of the stimuli. The fact that delay activity of S2 and MPC neurons carry first stimulus frequency information led us to think that they may be involved in the working memory component of the comparison task (figure 15.6B, D). However, because only PFC activity is maintained throughout the delay period, this area may be key to retaining frequency information of the first stimulus in working memory (figure 15.5*E*, figure 15.6*C*). During the second stimulus presentation, when the stimuli comparison operation is performed, the dynamics of firing rates of S2, PFC, and MPC neurons are consistent with the implementation of a subtraction operation (figure 15.6). The temporal evolution of activity during the second stimulus results in a binary signal that predicts which of the two response buttons will be pressed by the monkeys.

Although there are differences in the number of neurons responding during each component of the discrimination task, the similarity of the temporal dynamics of S2, PFC, and MPC activation is surprising (figure 15.6). Before these results, we thought that each area would be specifically involved in a particular component of the discrimination task. The fact that multiple cortical areas at different levels of the processing hierarchy show similar activation dynamics constitutes an unexpected finding. However, the comparison between stored and ongoing sensory information takes place to varying degrees across those cortical areas central to S1.

Contrasting with other psychophysical tasks in which sensory stimuli are briefly presented (lasting < 100 ms), in the vibrotactile discrimination task the stimuli are presented for a long period (500 ms). In addition, monkeys are allowed to initiate their motor response in a large time window. We can state, therefore, that comparison and decision operations performed during the discrimination task are not limited to serial processing by the feedforward connections between cortical areas (Lamme and Roelfsema, 2000). It is probable that recurrent flow of information between multiple areas is key to the processes involved in performing the discrimination task. To what extent the activity of each area is necessary and sufficient for explaining the processes of stimulus coding, memorization, and decision making, however, remains an open question.

An interesting finding is the existence of neural populations with opposite responses, or, more precisely, of populations with tuning curves of opposite sign. One of the simplest ways in which neurons could encode the frequency of vibratory stimuli is by means of a tuning curve in which particular firing rate values encoded particular stimulus frequencies, determined by any arbitrary function. Then, if all neurons of a given area had similar responses, pooling of individual responses could provide an accurate estimate of the stimulus frequency (the fidelity of this estimate would be determined by the correlation values among neurons; Shadlen and Newsome, 1998). Instead of this simple coding scheme, the results showed that, in all areas central to S1, there is not a single, but a dual stimulus encoding. Given that the slopes are of opposite signs (antagonistic responses), pooling the activity of these two groups of neurons would not give any useful information about the stimulus frequency. Therefore, well-structured cortical circuits are necessary to

keep the information of each separated population. As we have seen, this dual encoding is preserved along the processing levels, from S2 and MPC to PFC. What is the role of this dual representation? We speculate about two possible complementary answers.

First, it has been shown that responses of individual S2 neurons provide less information about the stimulus frequency than do the individual responses of S1 neurons (Salinas et al., 2000). Unlike S1, where the information provided by individual neurons is enough to explain the monkeys' discrimination thresholds, neurometric curves obtained from individual responses of S2 neurons are well below the discrimination thresholds of monkeys. Is sensory information degraded as it flows from S1 to S2? At first sight, this may seem to be the case. However, combining the responses of neurons with opposite slopes could compensate for the loss of information. Romo and colleagues (2003) have shown that it is possible to recover the information apparently lost between S1 and S2 by means of a subtraction operation between pairs of neurons with opposite tuning curves. This operation, which can be thought of as a contrast enhancement mechanism, is particularly useful when neurons show positive correlation coefficients: subtracting the activity of two positively correlated neurons cancels correlated random modulations. Thus, the existence of neuronal populations with opposite signs constitutes a mechanism for representing sensory information along the successive processing stages of cortex, even though significant levels of positive correlation exist among the activity of the neurons.

A second indication of the possible role of dual representations can be obtained from findings of other sensory stimuli comparison tasks. Freedman and colleagues (2001) trained monkeys to compare two images, separated by an interstimulus period, and to indicate if the second image belonged, or not, to the same category as the first (arbitrary categories learned during training). Recordings from PFC neurons revealed distinct neuronal populations that responded selectively to the images belonging to a given category. Similar to what is found in the discrimination task, visual stimuli are encoded in the cortex by means of the activity of groups of oppositely tuned neurons. The responses of categorical neurons may be interpreted as the arbitrary classification of stimuli into behaviorally significant groups.

Also in the PFC, Nieder and colleagues (Nieder, Freedman, and Miller, 2002; Nieder and Miller, 2003) found groups of neurons whose firing rates were functions of the number of items contained in a visual image. In this experiment, monkeys had to indicate whether the number of items in a first image was equal to the number of items in a second image presented 1 s later. Given that each image could contain up to five items, the authors found five populations of neurons whose firing rates were tuned to the number of items in each image. It is important to note that this coding scheme (one group of neurons for each number) would be inefficient for counting large quantities of items. Insofar as humans can count infinitely large numbers of items, it is probable that the monkeys were not "counting" in the same sense as humans do. Instead, similar to what is observed during the discrimination task and during the categorization of visual stimuli, monkeys were apparently grouping the images into categories defined by their *numerosity* (the quantity of items that each image contained).

Are neurons with categorical responses located exclusively in the PFC? In the vibrotactile discrimination task, as we have shown, complementary populations of neurons can be observed in S2 and MPC, as well as in PFC. Studying the activity of S2 neurons during a tactile texture comparison task, Sinclair and Burton (1991) also found neuronal populations with opposite tuning curves. In addition, Carpenter, Georgopoulos, and Pellicer (1999) observed that categorical responses could also be found in M1. These investigators trained monkeys to recall the order of appearance of serially presented visual stimuli located at random positions around a central area. To solve this task, the animals had to remember the order in which as many as five stimuli were presented. The results showed that in M1, there are neuronal populations that are activated by a stimulus appearing in a given spatial and temporal position. These neuronal responses may be interpreted as signaling information of the type, "the lower right stimulus was the second to appear." In this way, they found groups of neurons differently activated by each spatial and temporal combination of stimuli. As these results show, rules defining the behavioral meaning of neuronal responses can be highly abstract; that is, they can show little if any relation to the physical qualities of the stimuli.

In the vibrotactile discrimination task, monkeys were not explicitly trained to classify the stimuli into two categories. However, in light of the findings just discussed, we think that the existence of two populations of neurons with opposite responses may indicate that the cortex of the discriminating monkeys could be evaluating whether each stimulus frequency belonged to a "high" or "low" category.

Classifying images according to the number of items they contain supposes a behavioral rule different from that of classifying images according to their degree of similarity to a standard image, which is also different from recalling the serial order in which a certain number of stimuli appear. The frequency discrimination task, in turn, demands different rules from those mentioned above. Surprisingly, in all mentioned tasks we observe neuronal populations whose activity can be associated with categories by means of which the brain codes the behavioral meaning of each sensory stimulus.

As discussed earlier, Gold and Shadlen (2001) have shown the theoretical value, and provided physiological evidence, of the role of opposite sensory responses in decision making. Romo and colleagues (2003), on the other hand, demonstrated the role of opposite representations as a mechanism that preserves information in successive processing stages and avoids the adverse effects of positively correlated responses. We therefore are tempted to suggest that neuronal populations with antagonistic responses showing abstract characteristics of the stimuli may indicate a general processing strategy in the service of two basic operations during perception: (1) to encode sensory stimuli with behavioral meaning, and (2) through a subtraction operation, to drive behavioral decisions.

Conclusion

Recordings from single neurons in the cortex of monkeys performing a vibrotactile discrimination task revealed the existence of two complementary neuronal responses during the diverse components of the task. This dual representation is found in physically distant areas, located at distinct levels of the processing hierarchy (S2, PFC, and PMC). This encoding scheme has also been found in the cortices of monkeys performing tasks that require behavioral decisions based on a comparison operation.

How responses emerge in each cortical area and to what extent the activity of each group of neurons is necessary and sufficient to explain perceptual processes are issues that need to be further explored. It is likely that perceptual process require large-scale, recurrent, dynamic interactions of distant neuronal populations distributed at different levels of the processing hierarchy. This emphasizes the importance of studying multiple cortical areas during the same behavioral task (Romo and Salinas, 2003).

ACKNOWLEDGMENTS   This work was supported by an International Research Scholars Award from the Howard Hughes Medical Institute and by grants from the Millennium Science Initiative-CONACYT and DGAPA-UNAM (R.R.).

REFERENCES

BRODY, C. D., A. HERNÁNDEZ, A. ZAINOS, L. LEMUS, and R. ROMO, 2002. Analysing neuronal correlates of the comparison of two sequentially presented stimuli. *Philos. Trans. R. Soc. Lond. B Biol. Sci.* 357:1843–1850.

BURTON, H., M. FABRI, and K. ALLOWAY, 1995. Cortical areas within the lateral sulcus connected to cutaneous representations in areas 3b and 1: A revised interpretation of the second somatosensory area in macaque monkeys. *J. Comp. Neurol.* 355:539–562.

CARPENTER, A. F., A. P. GEORGOPOULOS, and G. PELLICER, 1999. Motor cortical encoding of serial order in a context-recall task. *Science* 283:1752–1757.

CIPOLLONI, P. B., and D. N. PANDYA, 1999. Cortical connections of the frontoparietal opercular areas in the rhesus monkey. *J. Comp. Neurol.* 403:431–458.

CRICK, F., and C. KOCH, 1995. Are we aware of neural activity in primary visual cortex? *Nature* 375:121–123.

DECHARMS, R. C., and A. ZADOR, 2000. Neural representation and the cortical code. *Annu. Rev. Neurosci.* 23:613–647.

FREEDMAN, D. J., M. RIESENHUBER, T. POGGIO, and E. K. MILLER, 2001. Categorical representation of visual stimuli in the primate prefrontal cortex. *Science* 291:312–316.

FUNAHASHI, S., C. J. BRUCE, and P. S. GOLDMAN-RAKIC, 1989. Mnemonic coding of visual space in the monkey's dorsolateral prefrontal cortex. *J. Neurophysiol.* 61:331–349.

FUSTER, J. M., 1989. *The Prefrontal Cortex.* New York: Raven Press.

GEORGOPOULOS, A. P., A. B. SCHWARTZ, and R. R. KETTNER, 1986. Neuronal population coding of movement direction. *Science* 233:1416–1419.

GOLD J. I., and M. N. SHADLEN, 2000. Representation of a perceptual decision in developing oculomotor commands. *Nature* 404:390–394.

GOLD, J. I., and M. N. SHADLEN, 2001. Neural computations that underlie decisions about sensory stimuli. *Trends Cogn. Sci.* 5:10–16.

GREEN, D. M., and J. A. SWETS, 1966. *Signal Detection Theory and Psychophysics.* New York: Wiley.

HERNÁNDEZ, A., E. SALINAS, R. GARCIA, and R. ROMO, 1997. Discrimination in the sense of flutter: New psychophysical measurements in monkeys. *J. Neurosci.* 17:6391–6400.

HERNÁNDEZ, A., A. ZAINOS, and R. ROMO, 2000. Neuronal correlates of sensory discrimination in the somatosensory cortex. *Proc. Natl. Acad. Sci. U.S.A.* 97:6191–6196.

HERNÁNDEZ, A., A. ZAINOS, and R. ROMO, 2002. Temporal evolution of a decision-making process in medial premotor cortex. *Neuron* 33:959–972.

IWAMURA, Y., 1998. Hierarchical somatosensory processing. *Curr. Opin. Neurobiol.* 8:522–528.

JOHANSSON, R. S., U. LANDSTROM, and R. LUNDSTROM, 1982. Responses of mechanoreceptive afferent units in the glabrous skin of the human hand to sinusoidal skin displacements. *Brain Res.* 244:17–25.

JOHANSSON, R. S., and A. B. VALLBO, 1983. Tactile sensory coding in the glabrous skin of the human hand. *Trends Neurosci.* 6:27–32.

JOHNSON, K. O., 2001. The roles and functions of cutaneous mechanoreceptors. *Curr. Opin. Neurobiol.* 11:455–461.

LAMME, V. A., and P. R. ROELFSEMA, 2000. The distinct modes of vision offered by feedforward and recurrent processing. *Trends Neurosci.* 23:571–579.

MERCHANT, H., A. ZAINOS, A. HERNÁNDEZ, E. SALINAS, and R. ROMO, 1997. Functional properties of primate putamen neurons during the categorization of tactile stimuli. *J. Neurophysiol.* 77:1132–1154.

MILLER, E. K., and J. D. COHEN, 2001. An integrative theory of prefrontal cortex function. *Annu. Rev. Neurosci.* 24:167–202.

MOUNTCASTLE, V., 1984. Central nervous system mechanisms in mechanoreceptive sensibility. In *Handbook of Physiology*, Section 1, vol. III, Pt. 2, S. R. Geiger, I. Darian-Smith, J. M. Brookhart, and V. Mountcastle, eds. Baltimore: Waverly, pp. 789–878.

MOUNTCASTLE, V. B., R. H. LAMOTTE, and G. CARLI, 1972. Detection thresholds for stimuli in humans and monkeys: Comparison with threshold events in mechanoreceptive afferent nerve fibers innervating the monkey hand. *J. Neurophysiol.* 35:122–136.

MOUNTCASTLE, V. B., M. A. STEINMETZ, and R. ROMO, 1990. Frequency discrimination in the sense of flutter: Psychophysical measurements correlated with postcentral events in behaving monkeys. *J. Neurosci.* 10:3032–3044.

MOUNTCASTLE, V. B., W. H. TALBOT, I. DARIAN-SMITH, and H. H. KORNHUBER, 1967. Neural basis of the sense of flutter-vibration. *Science* 155:597–600.

MOUNTCASTLE, V. B., W. H. TALBOT, H. SAKATA, and J. HYVARINEN, 1969. Cortical neuronal mechanisms in flutter-vibration studied in unanesthetized monkeys: Neuronal periodicity and frequency discrimination. *J. Neurophysiol.* 32:452–484.

NIEDER, A., D. J. FREEDMAN, and E. K. MILLER, 2002. Representation of the quantity of visual items in the primate prefrontal cortex. *Science* 297:1708–1711.

NIEDER, A., and E. K. MILLER, 2003. Coding of cognitive magnitude: Compressed scaling of numerical information in the primate prefrontal cortex. *Neuron* 37:149–157.

OCHOA, J., and E. TOREBJORK, 1983. Sensations evoked by intraneural microstimulation of single mechanoreceptor units innervating the human hand. *J. Physiol.* 342:633–654.

PASCUAL-LEONE, A., and V. WALSH, 2001. Fast backprojections from the motion to the primary visual area necessary for visual awareness. *Science* 292:510–512.

PONS, T. P., P. E. GARRAGHTY, D. P. FRIEDMAN, M. MISHKIN, 1987. Physiological evidence for serial processing in somatosensory cortex. *Science* 237:417–420.

ROMO, R., C. D. BRODY, A. HERNÁNDEZ, and L. LEMUS, 1999. Neuronal correlates of parametric working memory in the prefrontal cortex. *Nature* 399:470–473.

ROMO, R., A. HERNÁNDEZ, A. ZAINOS, C. D. BRODY, and L. LEMUS, 2000. Sensing without touching: Psychophysical performance based on cortical microstimulation. *Neuron* 26:273–278.

ROMO, R., A. HERNÁNDEZ, A. ZAINOS, C. BRODY, and E. SALINAS, 2002. Exploring the cortical evidence of a sensory-discrimination process. *Philos. Trans. R. Soc. Lond. B Biol. Sci.* 357:1039–1051.

ROMO, R., A. HERNÁNDEZ, A. ZAINOS, L. LEMUS, and C. D. BRODY, 2002. Neuronal correlates of decision-making in secondary somatosensory cortex. *Nat. Neurosci.* 5:1217–1225.

ROMO, R., A. HERNÁNDEZ, A. ZAINOS, and E. SALINAS, 1998. Somatosensory discrimination based on cortical microstimulation. *Nature* 392:387–390.

ROMO, R., A. HERNÁNDEZ, A. ZAINOS, and E. SALINAS, 2003. Correlated neuronal discharges that increase coding efficiency during perceptual discrimination. *Neuron* 38 649–657.

ROMO, R., H. MERCHANT, A. ZAINOS, and A. HERNÁNDEZ, 1996. Categorization of somaesthetic stimuli: Sensorimotor performance and neuronal activity in primary somatic sensory cortex of awake monkeys. *Neuroreport* 7:1273–1279.

ROMO, R., H. MERCHANT, A. ZAINOS, and A. HERNÁNDEZ, 1997. Categorical perception of somesthetic stimuli: Psychophysical measurements correlated with neuronal events in primate medial premotor cortex. *Cereb. Cortex* 7:317–325.

ROMO, R., S. RUIZ, P. CRESPO, A. ZAINOS, and H. MERCHANT, 1993. Representation of somatosensory stimuli in primate supplementary motor area. *J. Neurophysiol.* 70:2690–2694.

ROMO, R., and E. SALINAS, 2001. Touch and go: Decision mechanisms in somatosensation. *Annu. Rev. Neurosci.* 24:107–137.

ROMO, R., and E. SALINAS, 2003. Flutter discrimination: Neural codes, perception, memory and decision making. *Nat. Rev. Neurosci.* 4:203–218.

ROMO, R., E. SCARNATI, and W. SCHULTZ, 1992. Role of primate basal ganglia and frontal cortex in the internal generation of movements. II. Movement-related activity in the anterior striatum. *Exp. Brain Res.* 91:385–395.

SALINAS, E., A. HERNÁNDEZ, A. ZAINOS, and R. ROMO, 2000. Periodicity and firing rate as candidate neural codes for the frequency of vibrotactile stimuli. *J. Neurosci.* 20:5503–5515.

SALINAS, E., and R. ROMO, 1998. Conversion of sensory signals into motor commands in primary motor cortex. *J. Neurosci.* 18:499–511.

SCHULTZ, W., and R. ROMO, 1992. Role of primate basal ganglia and frontal cortex in the internal generation of movements. I. Preparatory activity in the anterior striatum. *Exp. Brain Res.* 91:363–384.

SCHWARTZ, A. B., R. E. KETTNER, and A. P. GEORGOPOULOS, 1988. Primate motor cortex and free arm movements to visual targets in three-dimensional space. I. Relations between single cell discharge and direction of movement. *J. Neurosci.* 8:2913–3927.

SHADLEN, M. N., and W. T. NEWSOME, 2001. Neural basis of a perceptual decision in the parietal cortex (area LIP) of the rhesus monkey. *J. Neurophysiol.* 86:1916–1936.

SHIMA, K., and J. TANJI, 2000. Neuronal activity in the supplementary and presupplementary motor areas for temporal organization of multiple movements. *J. Neurophysiol.* 84:2148–2160.

SINCLAIR, R. J., and H. BURTON, 1991. Neuronal activity in the primary somatosensory cortex in monkeys (*Macaca mulatta*) during active touch of textured surface gratings: Responses to groove width, applied force, and velocity of motion. *J. Neurophysiol.* 66:153–169.

SINCLAIR, R. J., and H. BURTON, 1993. Neuronal activity in the second somatosensory cortex of monkeys (*Macaca mulatta*) during active touch of gratings. *J. Neurophysiol.* 70:331–350.

SUR, M., J. T. WALL, and J. H. KAAS, 1984. Modular distribution of neurons with slowly adapting and rapidly adapting responses in area 3b of somatosensory cortex in monkeys. *J. Neurophysiol.* 51:724–744.

TALBOT, W. H., I. DARIAN-SMITH, H. H. KORNHUBER, and V. B. MOUNTCASTLE, 1968. The sense of flutter-vibration: Comparison of the human capacity with response patterns of mechanoreceptive afferents from the monkey hand. *J. Neurophysiol.* 31:301–334.

THORPE, S. J., and M. FABRE-THORPE, 2001. Neuroscience: Seeking categories in the brain. *Science* 291:260–263.

VALLBO, A. B., 1995. Single-afferent neurons and somatic sensation in humans. In *The Cognitive Neuroscience*, M. S. Gazzaniga, ed. Cambridge, Mass.: MIT Press, pp. 237–252.

VALLBO, A. B., and R. S. JOHANSSON, 1984. Properties of cutaneous mechanoreceptors in the human hand related to touch sensation. *Hum. Neurobiol.* 3:3–14.

16   Auditory Cortex in Primates: Functional Subdivisions and Processing Streams

TROY A. HACKETT AND JON H. KAAS

ABSTRACT   The auditory cortex of primates includes those areas of the cerebral cortex that receive inputs from a collection of auditory nuclei in the thalamus, including the medial geniculate complex and posterior group. The auditory cortical areas comprise a network of three interconnected regions (core, belt, and parabelt) that process inputs in serial and parallel. The belt and parabelt regions project to auditory-related areas of the temporal, posterior parietal, and prefrontal cortex. These areas tend to be sites of multisensory convergence, where modality-specific information related to the spatial or nonspatial characteristics of the sensory environment is integrated and subsequently used to guide goal-directed behavior. Neural imaging and advanced electrophysiological techniques are beginning to reveal the functional properties of these information streams and define the roles of the various elements involved. The model of the primate auditory cortex described in this chapter incorporates observations from studies involving nonhuman primates and humans spanning several decades. Although many of its features await validation, the key components of the model form the foundation of a comprehensive description of the cortical auditory system.

One goal of auditory neuroscience is to describe how the auditory areas of the brain process information about sound so that other parts of the brain can make use of it. By the time that information reaches the level of cortex, the original acoustic signal will have been transformed by the middle ear, inner ear, and at least four major nuclei in the brainstem and thalamus. At each level of processing a given sound is represented by the activity of neurons in that region. The neural representation at each level is derived from the inputs that converge upon it. Ultimately, at some level or levels of processing, perhaps in cortex, a code is derived from the neural representation that influences behavior. Collectively, auditory researchers are moving toward a comprehensive theory of auditory processing in the brain, but the picture is far from complete in any species studied to date. Yet what has been learned is sufficient for the construction of rea-

sonable models that can be tested and modified over time. The model described in this chapter is primarily based on studies of auditory cortex in nonhuman primates conducted in many laboratories over several decades. An exhaustive description of the primate literature is beyond the scope of this chapter, and the interested reader is referred to a number of excellent reviews, from which a more comprehensive view can be gained (Woolsey and Walzl, 1982; Newman, 1988; Aitkin, 1990; Hackett, 2002; Hackett and Kaas, 2002; Hall et al., 2002; Scott and Johnsrude, 2003).

Early insights into the organization of auditory cortex in humans and nonhuman primates in the late 1800s and early 1900s were derived from lesion studies and the classic anatomical descriptions of the cerebral cortex. The detailed parcellations of the superior temporal region of von Economo, Brodmann, and Beck were tremendously influential and remain embedded in current models (see Hackett, 2002). The emergence of electrophysiological techniques in the mid-1900s made it possible to record electrical potentials and the activity of single neurons evoked by acoustic stimulation. From these techniques it has been possible to understand, in part, how sound is represented in the activity of neurons in cortical and subcortical structures. More recently, functional imaging techniques have made it possible to indirectly examine auditory activity in the brain of animals and humans. In addition to being noninvasive, these techniques allow us to index auditory-related activity throughout the entire brain as it develops over time. Although each technique contributes unique information to the data set, it is important to relate the results to a common frame of reference. For our purposes here, that reference is the areal map of the superior temporal cortex in macaque monkeys, which depicts the location and extent of the auditory cortical areas that have been identified or proposed (figure 16.1).

In recent years, we have been developing a working model of the primate auditory cortex based on the collective findings in New World and Old World primates (Hackett, Stepniewska, and Kaas, 1998a; Kaas and Hackett, 1998, 2000; Kaas, Hackett, and Tramo, 1999). This model shares

TROY A. HACKETT   Department of Hearing and Speech Sciences, Vanderbilt University School of Medicine, Nashville, Tenn.

JON H. KAAS   Department of Psychology, Vanderbilt University, Nashville, Tenn.

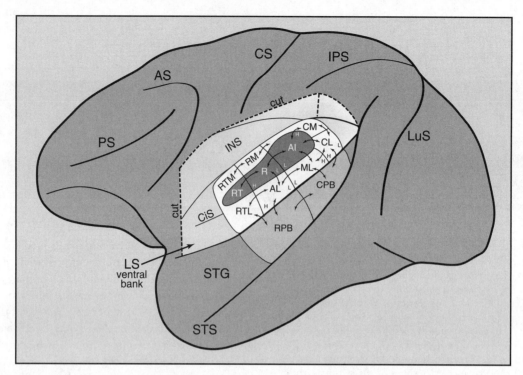

FIGURE 16.1 Schematic view of the macaque left hemisphere showing the location of auditory cortical areas and local connections. The dorsal bank of the lateral sulcus has been removed (line marked "cut") to expose the superior temporal plane (LS ventral bank). The floor and outer bank of the circular sulcus (CiS) have been flattened to show the medial auditory belt fields. The core region (dark shading) contains three subdivisions (AI, R, RT). In the belt region (no shading), seven subdivisions are proposed (CM, CL, ML, AL, RTL, RTM, RM). The subdivisions of the parabelt region (RPB, CPB; no shading) occupy the exposed surface of the superior temporal gyrus (STG). The core fields project to surrounding belt areas (arrows). Inputs to the parabelt arise from the lateral and medial belt subdivisions. Connections between the parabelt and medial belt fields are not illustrated, to improve clarity. Tonotopic gradients in the core and lateral belt fields are indicated by the letters H (high frequency) and L (low frequency). (Adapted from Hackett, Preuss, and Kaas, 2001.) (A1, primary auditory area 1 (core); AL, anterolateral area (belt); AS, arcuate sulcus; CiS, circular sulcus of the sylvian fissure; CL, caudolateral area (belt); CM, caudomedial area (belt); CPB, caudal parabelt area; CS, central sulcus; H, high frequency stimulus; INS, insula; IPS, intraparietal sulcus; L, low frequency stimulus; LS, lateral sulcus; LuS, lunate sulcus; PL, posterolateral area (belt); PS, principal sulcus; R, rostral primary auditory area (core); RL, rostrolateral area (belt); RM, rostromedial area (belt); RPB, rostral parabelt area; RT, rostrotemporal primary auditory area (core); RTL, lateral rostrotemporal area (belt); RTM, medial rostrotemporal area (belt); STG, superior temporal gyrus; STS, superior temporal sulcus; Tpt, temporoparietal area).

many features with extant models of the human auditory cortex (see Hackett, 2002). This is not surprising, given the close phylogenetic relationship of these mammals. However, because a comprehensive description of the primate auditory system is not at hand, and because most of what is known about auditory processing in mammals comes from studies in mammals other than primates, few extensions can safely be made to humans. Moreover, even if a reasonably complete description of the nonhuman primate auditory system were available, it would certainly be an incomplete representation of the human, given the expanded auditory abilities of humans in speech recognition and related processing. Therefore, comparisons between human and nonhuman primate cortex should not be overstated.

Our working model represents those anatomical and physiological features that have consistently been found across primate species and laboratories. The model does not address detailed physiological mechanisms. Rather, it should be viewed as a schematic diagram that represents the flow of information into and out of the auditory cortical system. At the very least, the model provides a structural framework for the formulation of hypotheses that will ultimately enable revision of its components. It also allows testable theories to be generated concerning the roles of a particular field, and provides a basis for comparison with models of sensory processing for other modalities and other taxa.

Auditory and auditory-related cortex

We define auditory cortex to include those cortical areas that are the preferential targets of neurons in either the ventral (MGv) or dorsal (MGd) divisions of the medial geniculate complex. By this definition, a large portion of the superior temporal cortex in primates is occupied by the auditory cortex (figure 16.1). The medial boundaries lie within the lateral sulcus at the junction with the insula (rostrally) and parietal operculum (caudally). The lateral boundary on the surface of the superior temporal gyrus (STG) is poorly defined, but appears to extend to edge of the superior temporal sulcus (STS) or slightly onto its dorsal bank. The caudal boundary is located near the junction of the lateral and superior temporal sulci at the border of the temporoparietal temporal area (Tpt). Rostrally, auditory cortex occupies most of the STG except for the rostral third of the temporal lobe. There are, of course, numerous cortical regions outside the boundaries of auditory cortex that also process auditory information. Since these fields receive inputs from some portion of auditory cortex, and generally do not receive significant inputs from the auditory thalamus (medial geniculate complex), they are referred to as *auditory-related cortex*. These regions include the temporal pole and portions of the STS, intraparietal sulcus, and prefrontal cortex.

Organization of auditory cortex

REGIONAL DIVISIONS OF AUDITORY CORTEX   One major feature of the model is that auditory cortex can be divided into three functional regions: core, belt, and parabelt (figure 16.1). Although these regions are distinguished on the basis of anatomical and physiological features, they are not structurally or functionally homogeneous. Rather, each region contains a variable number of subdivisions bound by a common set of features. Brief descriptions of the major features follow for each region of auditory cortex.

The *core region* in primates contains two or three subdivisions, including A1, which is commonly known as the primary auditory cortex. Although the number of auditory areas differs between species, an area called A1 has been identified in all studied mammals. In prosimian and simian primates, the position of the core varies systematically relative to the edge of the sylvian fissure. In New World monkeys the core occupies the dorsal gyrus of the temporal lobe and extends only a short distance (1–3 mm) into the lateral sulcus (Forbes and Moskowitz, 1974; Imig et al., 1977; Fitzpatrick and Imig, 1980; Aitkin, Kudo, and Irvine, 1988; Luethke, Krubitzer, and Kaas, 1989; Morel and Kaas, 1992). In Old World macaques, chimpanzees, and humans, the core is contained completely in the depths of the sulcus, covered by the overlying frontal and parietal opercula (see Hackett, Preuss, and Kaas, 2001). The region corresponding to the core in humans is much of area 41 of Brodmann (1909), located on the medial two-thirds of the first transverse gyrus of Heschl (see figure 16.4; for more detailed descriptions, see Galaburda and Sanides, 1980; Rademacher et al., 1993; Hackett, Preuss, and Kass, 2001; Hackett, 2002). The architecture of the core region is characterized by granulous (koniocellular) cytoarchitecture and dense myelination from layers III through VI. The chemoarchitecture features dense expression of several markers in a band spanning laminae IIIc and IV (i.e., cytochrome oxidase, acetylcholinesterase, parvalbumin). Marker expression in this band is higher in the core than in surrounding regions of auditory cortex (Jones et al., 1995; Kosaki et al., 1997; Hackett, Stepniewska, and Kaas, 1998a). The principal thalamic inputs to the core originate in the laminated ventral division of the MGv. The corticocortical connections of the core region are primarily limited to the surrounding belt region.

Surrounding the core is a narrow band of areas known as the *belt region*. For convenience, we refer to the areas bordering the medial and lateral borders of the core as the medial belt and lateral belt, respectively. In all primates the medial belt areas adjoin insular cortex rostrally and posterior parietal cortex caudally. The medial belt region corresponds most closely to area 52 of Brodmann (1908, 1909). In New World monkeys the lateral belt areas are located on the surface of the STG adjacent to the core. In Old World monkeys, including macaques, the lateral belt areas extend from the core on the superior temporal plane to the edge of the lateral sulcus, and often slightly onto the dorsal surface of the STG. In chimpanzees and humans, however, cortex that corresponds to the lateral belt lies posterolateral to Heschl's gyri within the sylvian fissure (Hackett, Preuss, and Kaas, 2001). Thus, the lateral belt region of monkeys corresponds most closely to area 42 of Brodmann (see figure 16.4), and includes some portion of the planum temporale (see Hackett, 2002). The architectonic features of the belt differ from the core in two general ways. First, compared to the core, there is a significant reduction in granularity and cell density in the outer layers, and an increase in the size of pyramidal cells in lower layer III. Second, fiber density is greatly diminished, such that horizontal bands of fibers in layers IV and Vb can be resolved (i.e., bistriate). With respect to chemoarchitecture, the expression of acetylcholinesterase, cytochrome oxidase, and parvalbumin is significantly reduced in both lateral and medial belt regions compared to the core, particularly in the layer IIIc/IV band. Connections of the belt region include the dorsal division of MGd, the core and parabelt regions of auditory cortex, and auditory-related cortex.

The *parabelt region* adjoins the lateral portion of the belt region ventrolaterally on the surface of the STG in macaque monkeys. The territory occupied by the parabelt has long been associated with homotypical cortex of the STG in humans and other primates, but the parabelt is likely to correspond to only part of the classically defined regions, such as TA or area 22, that cover the STG (see figures 16.1 and 16.4). This comparison should be considered tentative, however, because the expansion of this region in humans may represent the addition of areas not presently accounted for. The architecture of the parabelt region resembles that of the lateral belt, a fact that has likely contributed to ambiguity in the identification of the latter (see Hackett, 2002). A prominent feature of the cytoarchitecture is that neurons are arranged in distinct radial columns from layer VI to layer II. The pyramidal cells in layer III are more uniform in size, often appearing to be stacked atop one another in distinct columns. The term "organ pipe" formation, introduced by von Economo and Koskinas (1925) to describe this structural feature of area TA in humans, is commonly used in cytoarchitectonic descriptions of the parabelt region in monkeys (Pandya and Sanides, 1973; Galaburda and Pandya, 1983; Hackett, Stepniewska, and Kaas, 1998a.). Myelination is of the bistriate type but is slightly less dense overall than the belt. Acetylcholinesterase, cytochrome oxidase, and parvalbumin are expressed at low levels in the parabelt, compared to the moderate levels characteristic of the lateral belt. Thalamic inputs to the parabelt include the MGd, suprageniculate, limitans, and medial pulvinar, but not the MGv (Hackett, Stepniewska, and Kaas, 1998b). Cortical inputs originate in the medial and lateral belt regions, but not the core. The absence of significant connections with the core is a key difference in the functional organization of the belt and parabelt regions.

AREAL DIVISIONS OF AUDITORY CORTEX A second feature of the model is that within each of the three major auditory cortical regions, two or more *areas* or *subdivisions* have been proposed (see figure 16.1). The subdivisions of the core are A1, the rostral primary auditory area (R), and the rostrotemporal primary auditory area (RT). The subdivisions of the belt region are the caudomedial area (CM), rostromedial area (RM), medial rostrotemporal area (RTM), caudolateral area (CL), mediolateral area (ML), anterolateral area (AL), and lateral rostrotemporal area (RTL). The subdivisions of the parabelt are the rostral (RPB) and caudal (CPB) parabelt areas. Unfortunately, the nomenclature varies between laboratories and is no small source of confusion in the literature. The nomenclature adopted for use with our model retains conventions established in earlier studies (e.g., Merzenich and Brugge, 1973; Imig et al., 1977), with recent modifications. Whereas the core, belt, and parabelt regions can be reliably distinguished on the basis of prominent architectonic features and patterns of connections, the establishment of individual subdivisions within a given region depends on the identification of subsets of unique features. Accordingly, supportive data vary by area, and some areas included in the model are based on minimal information. Areas that are not adjacent, such as CM and AL, can be reliably distinguished on the basis of unique architectonic features or patterns of connections. However, because areas within a region tend to have similar architectonic features and connections, the identification of borders is frequently ambiguous. For these areas, borders tend to be defined by

neuron response properties rather than anatomical features. Within the core, for example, A1 and R have similar architecture and connections. At present, the only clear distinction between them is receptive field organization. The frequency organization of the cochlea is represented in both A1 and R, but the tonotopic gradients run in opposite directions from a common low-frequency border (see figure 16.1) (Merzenich and Brugge, 1973; Imig et al., 1977; Brugge, 1982; Aitkin et al., 1986; Luethke, Krubitzer, and Kaas, 1989; Morel and Kaas, 1992; Morel, Garraghty, and Kaas, 1993; Rauschecker, Tian, and Hauser, 1995; Kosaki et al., 1997; Rauschecker et al., 1997; Recanzone, Guard, and Phan, 2000; Cheung et al., 2001; Tian et al., 2001). Microelectrode recordings in the belt areas surrounding the core have also provided evidence of tonotopic organization that has been useful in supporting anatomically defined subdivisions. In these experiments pure tones and narrow-band noise stimuli were used to demonstrate that the tonotopic gradients in the lateral belt areas (AL, ML) parallel the adjacent core areas (see figure 16.1) (Rauschecker, Tian, and Hauser, 1995; Kosaki et al., 1997), whereas the tonotopic gradients in CM and CL mirror that of A1 (Recanzone, Guard, and Phan, 2000; Kajikawa et al., 2003; Selezneva et al., 2003). Thus, an independent representation of the cochlea, or absence thereof, is an important criterion in the establishment of auditory cortical areas where anatomical features are ambiguous.

SERIAL PROCESSING OF INFORMATION A third feature of the model is that the core, belt, and parabelt regions represent successive stages (figure 16.2) in the processing of auditory information in cortex (Kaas and Hackett, 1998; Kaas, Hackett, and Tramo, 1999). This hierarchy was introduced to account for the observation that the parabelt region receives corticocortical inputs from the belt but not the core (Hackett, Stepniewska, and Kaas, 1998a), and thalamocortical inputs from the MGd but not the MGv (Hackett, Stepniewska, and Kaas, 1998b). Thus, the flow of primary information out from the core terminates in the belt region, which projects widely to the parabelt and auditory-related cortex. This does not imply that processing in auditory cortex is strictly serial. Each area is connected with several other areas, and the inputs from the medical geniculate complex (MGC) distribute in parallel across areas and regions. Nevertheless, there is an underlying serial component in the flow of information. This is consistent with physiological recordings in monkeys that reveal increasing spectrotemporal integration in the lateral belt region (Rauschecker, Tian, and Hauser, 1995; Rauschecker, 1998).

PARALLEL PROCESSING OF INFORMATION A fourth feature of the model is that the subdivisions within a given region

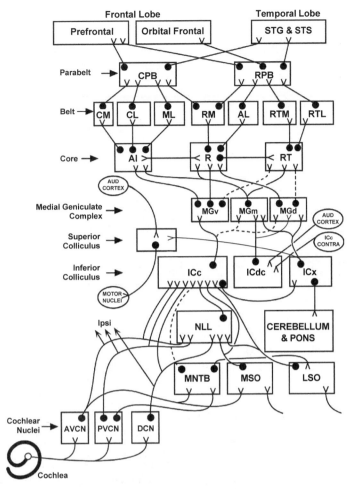

FIGURE 16.2 The primate auditory pathway. Schematic diagram shows major and some minor brainstem pathways from the contralateral cochlea to the subcortical nuclei and cortical auditory areas. Subdivisions of the nuclear complexes and their major con-

nections are also shown. See list of abbreviations for decoding of nomenclature. (MGd, dorsal division of the medial geniculate complex; MGm, magnocellular division of the medial geniculate complex; MGv, ventral division of the medial geniculate complex).

receive parallel inputs from lower and higher stages of processing (figure 16.2). Within the core, for example, each subdivision receives parallel inputs from the MGv, and has reciprocal connections with more than one belt area. In the belt region, all subdivisions receive inputs from the MGd and have reciprocal connections with one or more subdivisions within the core and parabelt. Thus, the flow of information from core to parabelt is not strictly serial, as several subdivisions at each stage appear to be processing common inputs in parallel. However, this parallel arrangement is not known to constrain activity in different areas to the simultaneous processing of identical information. Neurophysiological support for serial and parallel processing can be found in the study by Rauschecker and colleagues (1997). After ablation of the core area, A1, responses to pure-tone stimulation in the adjacent belt area, CM, were abolished, while responses to broadband stimuli were not. Responses in the adjacent core area, R, were not affected. This indicates that inputs to R from MGv were independent of the inputs to A1 (paral-

lel connection), whereas responses in CM required intact connections with A1 (serial connection).

CORRESPONDENCE OF AUDITORY CORTICAL FIELDS IN HUMANS AND NONHUMAN PRIMATES   Much is being discovered concerning the processing of auditory information in the cerebral cortex of both humans and nonhuman primates. A looming question is the extent to which findings in one species can be generalized to the other. What are the common features of auditory cortical organization? What are the differences? A basic understanding of the similarities and differences in auditory cortical organization would establish valuable links between the animal and human research literature, and contribute significantly to our understanding of auditory cortex. Unfortunately, comparative studies of the auditory cortex are rare. Experiments tend to be conducted in single species, and methodological differences limit direct comparisons. Yet some progress has been made, with the promise of additional advances in the future.

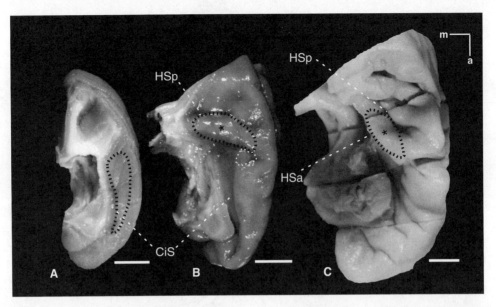

FIGURE 16.3   Orientation of the core region. Dorsolateral views of the left superior temporal plane showing position of the core region in macaque monkey (*A*), chimpanzee (*B*), and human (*C*). Black dashed ovoids in all panels indicate boundaries of the core. Dashed straight white lines designate sulcal landmarks. CiS, circu-lar sulcus; HSa, anterior Heschl's sulcus; HSp, posterior Heschl's sulcus; a, anterior, m, medial. Temporal lobe specimens are not to scale. Human specimen scaled down. Scale bars = 5 mm. (Adapted from Hackett, Preuss, and Kaas, 2001.)

In one recent study the architectonic criteria used to iden-tify the core region in macaque monkeys were used to iden-tify the location and extent of the core in chimpanzees and humans (Hackett, Preuss, and Kaas, 2001). Although the architectonic profiles were not identical across these taxo-nomic groups, coherence of the major features of the core allowed unambiguous identification of the region in each species (figure 16.3). Beyond the core, where direct anatom-ical comparisons are not yet available, the results of previ-ous studies form the sole basis for comparative analyses. One such attempt has been made to identify common features of auditory cortex in humans and nonhuman primates by ret-rospective analysis of the classic and modern accounts of the architecture and connections (Hackett, 2002). Excluding dif-ferences in nomenclature and in the identification of minor subdivisions, the analyses revealed that a core–belt–parabelt scheme is a reasonable approximation of the data for both humans and nonhuman primates (figure 16.4). With few exceptions (e.g., Brodmann, 1905, 1908; Mauss, 1908; Lashley and Clark, 1946), an elongated central core region (area 41) has been independently identified in all primate species. The core is flanked by belts of cortex, variably sub-divided, that separate the core from parietal and insular cortex medially and from the remaining superior temporal cortex laterally. As figure 16.4 indicates, the human medial belt region corresponds most closely to area 52 of Brod-mann, whereas the lateral belt region corresponds to area 42. In studies by different researchers, the corresponding regions are designated by other nomenclatures but are oth-erwise comparable (see Hackett, 2002). The remaining supe-

rior temporal cortex, especially the portion lateral and pos-terior to area 42, is a large heterogeneous region commonly known as area 22 of Brodmann. The boundaries of area 22 are currently not well defined, and it is likely that several dis-tinct areas constitute this territory, including parts of the planum temporale and STG (e.g., Rivier and Clarke, 1997; Wallace, Johnston, and Palmer, 2002). In relative position and basic cytoarchitecture, much of area 22 appears to cor-respond to the parabelt region identified in monkeys, yet it is important to emphasize that confidence in the correspon-dence between auditory fields identified in monkeys and humans diminishes with distance from the core. The expan-sion of the auditory areas in humans, particularly in the planum temporale and the remainder of area 22, makes a one-to-one correspondence unlikely.

One additional consideration with direct relevance to functional studies in humans concerns the orientation of the auditory cortical regions with respect to the anatomical axes of the brain (figure 16.3). In macaque monkeys, the core is elongated along the rostrocaudal (anteroposterior) axis. In chimpanzees the orientation of the core varies. In some chimpanzee specimens the core is elongated along a promi-nent transverse temporal gyrus (TTG) oriented from caudo-medial to rostrolateral, as in humans. In other specimens the core is elongated along the dorsolateral bank of the circular sulcus, as in macaques, and is less obvious as a "transverse" gyrus. In humans, one or more TTGs extend from postero-medial to anterolateral. In specimens with a single TTG, the core is elongated along the gyrus. In specimens with two or more TTGs, the core usually occupies portions of the two

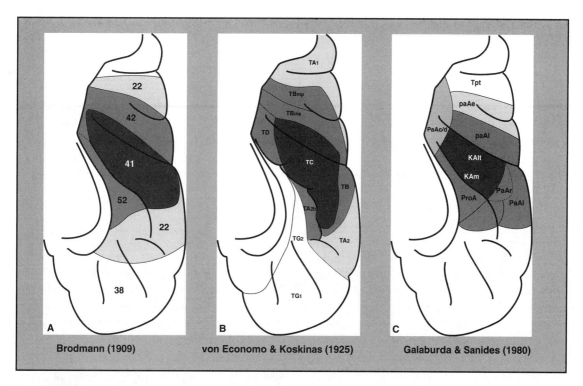

A	B	C
Brodmann (1909)	von Economo & Koskinas (1925)	Galaburda & Sanides (1980)

FIGURE 16.4 Regional parcellation of the human temporal cortex. In each panel, major divisions of auditory cortex, as defined in three different investigations, are fitted to a standardized drawing of the superior temporal plane. Only the superior tempo-ral plane and dorsal edge of the superior temporal gyrus are visible. Areas corresponding to the core region are darkly shaded. Belt areas are moderately shaded, and putative parabelt areas are lightly shaded. (Adapted from Hackett, 2002.)

most anterior gyri, but maintains the same orientation from posteromedial to anterolateral. The significance of these gross anatomical distinctions becomes crucial when comparisons are made between monkeys and humans. For example, the likely correlates of the caudal (posterior) auditory areas of the macaque monkey lie posteromedial in the sylvian fissure of humans. Accordingly, the rostral (anterior) auditory areas of monkeys would correspond to anterolateral territory in the superior temporal plane in humans.

FUNCTIONAL STUDIES IN HUMANS Several of the features that compose the core–belt–parabelt scheme are consistent with patterns of auditory-evoked activations seen on functional imaging studies of human auditory cortex. A variety of techniques have been employed, including neuroimaging—functional magnetic resonance imaging (fMRI) or position emission tomography (PET)—and electrophysiology—electroencephalography (EEG) and magnetoencephalography (MEG). The results clearly indicate that both simple and complex acoustic stimuli generate activity in the core and surrounding belt cortex, as well as more distant cortical areas. From these techniques researchers are learning much about the processing of sound in auditory and auditory-related cortex of humans (for reviews, see Johnsrude, Giraud, and Frackowiak, 2002; Hall, Hart, and Johnsrude, 2003; Scott and Johnsrude, 2003). Numerous

studies have focused on the identification of cortical areas involved in the processing of complex stimuli, such as speech or moving sounds. Others have emphasized basic features of functional organization, such as the representation of stimulus frequency or harmonic complexes. To some extent these findings are in line with the primate model.

Within the core, there is a broad range of evidence supporting the existence of tonotopic organization along Heschl's gyrus (electrophysiology: Verkindt et al., 1995; Howard et al., 1996; magnetoencephalography: Elberling et al., 1982; Pantev et al., 1988, 1995; Bertrand, Perrin, and Pernier, 1991; Yamamoto et al., 1992; Romani, Williamson, and Kaufman, 1982; Tiitinen et al., 1993; Huotilainen et al., 1995; Langner et al., 1997; Hoke, Ross, and Hoke, 1998; Lutkenhoner and Steinstrater, 1998; Rosburg et al., 1998; Fujioka et al., 2003; positron emission tomography: Lauter et al., 1985; de Rossi et al., 1996; Ottaviani et al., 1997; Lockwood et al., 1999; functional magnetic resonance imaging: Strainer et al., 1997; Wessinger et al., 1997; Bilecen et al., 1998; Talavage et al., 1997, 2000; Di Salle et al., 2001; Engelien et al., 2002; Schonwiesner, von Cramon, and Rubsamen, 2002; Formisano et al., 2003). The tonotopic gradient most often identified places the representation of high frequencies medially and low frequencies laterally. Although this field most likely corresponds to A1, additional tonotopic representations are sometimes identified in fields outside of

A1. In many of these studies, however, the demonstration of a tonotopic gradient was less than clear. One reason for these difficulties is the limited spatial resolution of the noninvasive techniques compared with the single-electrode techniques used in animal studies in which tonotopic maps are robust. A second confound concerns the relatively high stimulus presentation levels frequently used in studies in humans. In animal studies, the characteristic frequency of single neurons or neuronal clusters in a given recording site is defined by responses to tonal stimuli at or near threshold, often less than 20–30 dB sound pressure level. By contrast, stimulus levels used in most of the neuroimaging and MEG studies have been 60 dB or greater. In auditory cortex the receptive field (i.e., frequency range) of most neurons tends to widen with increasing intensity above threshold. Thus, as stimulus level is increased above threshold, the frequency-specific activation of a restricted cortical volume is likely to diminish, blurring the tonotopic gradients. Although these difficulties have clouded results so far, recent methodological advances suggest that tonotopic patterns of organization in human auditory cortex will become clearer (Formisano et al., 2003).

Both neuroimaging (Petersen et al., 1988; Wise et al., 1991; Price et al., 1992; Binder et al., 1996; Talavage et al., 2000; Di Salle et al., 2001) and electrophysiogical (Liegeois-Chauvel et al., 1995; Pantev et al., 1995; Lutkenhoner and Steinstrater, 1998; Engelien et al., 2000; Howard et al., 2000) studies in humans indicate that multiple auditory cortical fields make up the belt cortex posterolateral to the core in humans. To some extent the active loci identified match recent anatomical parcellations of the superior temporal region in humans (Galaburda and Sanides, 1980; Rivier and Clarke, 1997; Wallace, Johnston, and Palmer, 2002). Seifritz and colleagues (2002) reported that sustained components of the blood oxygen level-dependent (BOLD) signal activated sources in the core region, while transient components of the BOLD signal activated sources in the adjacent belt regions. Although the results are suggestive of functional distinctions between core and belt regions, it is not yet clear how sustained and transient BOLD responses relate to sustained and transient single-unit activity in these or other auditory cortical fields (Seifritz et al., 2003; Zatorre, 2003). Their results may relate to a number of neuroimaging studies in humans that provide support for a processing hierarchy in auditory cortex involving a centralized core and surrounding belt regions. Whereas the cortex of Heschl's gyrus is activated by a broad range of simple and complex sounds compared to silence, the cortical territory outside this core is typically more selective for sounds with spectral and temporal structure, including speech (Griffiths et al., 1998; Mummery et al., 1999; Binder et al., 2000; Giraud et al., 2000; Hall et al., 2000, 2002; Scott et al., 2000; Thivard et al., 2000; Goncalves et al., 2001; Wessinger et al., 2001; Patterson

et al., 2002; Scott and Johnsrude, 2003). The core may also be more sensitive than belt areas to stimulus intensity differences (Hart, Palmer, and Hall, 2002). These findings are consistent with increasing stimulus specificity at later stages of processing in areas outside the core, and in some respects are analogous to anatomical (Morel, Garraghty, and Kass, 1993) and physiological evidence of increasing spectrotemporal integration in the belt region of monkeys (Rauschecker, Tian, and Hauser, 1995; Recanzone, Guard, and Phan, 2000; Recauzone, Guard, Phan, et al., 2000).

Organization of auditory-related cortex

AUDITORY PROCESSING IN PREFRONTAL CORTEX The relationship between auditory cortical areas and auditory-related areas in prefrontal and posterior parietal cortex is becoming more clear, both from studies of connections and from studies of neuronal responsiveness. Early studies of macaque monkeys revealed that nonprimary auditory areas projected to prefrontal cortex (Mettler, 1935; Ward, Peden, and Sugar, 1946; Sugar, French, and Chusid, 1948; Hurst, 1959) and that the rostral and caudal auditory fields projected to functionally distinct prefrontal domains (Pandya, Hallett, and Mukherjee, 1969; Pandya and Kuypers, 1969). The connection patterns have since been elucidated in greater detail (Hackett, Stepniewska, and Kaas, 1999; Romanski, Bates, and Goldman-Rakic, 1999; Romanski, Tian, et al., 1999; Petrides and Pandya, 2002). The rostral belt and parabelt fields are most densely connected with orbitofrontal cortex, areas 10, 12, 45, and rostral 46 within the inferior convexity, and area 10 in frontopolar cortex (figure 16.5). Caudal belt and parabelt fields are primarily connected with the dorsolateral periprincipal region (e.g., caudal 46) and dorsal prearcuate cortex (e.g., area 8a), regions thought to be involved in directing eyes or attention toward objects or sounds in space. Thus, rostral auditory fields target prefrontal areas thought to be involved in non-spatial auditory processing, while the caudal auditory fields target prefrontal areas involved in multimodal spatial tasks. The segregation of pathways is not complete, however, as there are connections between rostral and caudal auditory areas, as well as overlapping projections to the dorsal STS and prefrontal area 46 (principal sulcus region). Thus, there are numerous opportunities for interaction between pathways (see Kaas and Hackett, 1999). The anatomical studies further revealed that the corticocortical connections linking auditory domains in temporal and prefrontal cortex are reciprocal. Although the laminar input/output patterns have not been quantified, it is likely that the activity of neurons in auditory cortex are modulated by the feedback projections of their prefrontal targets.

Microelectrode recordings have revealed unimodal and multimodal neurons responsive to auditory, visual, and

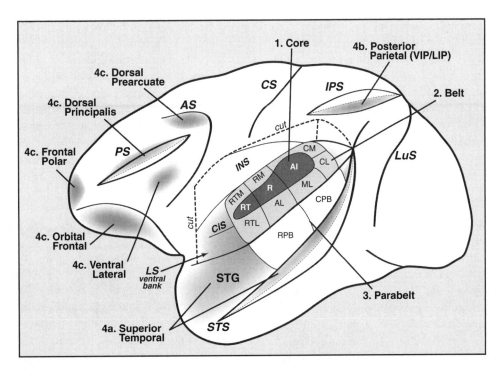

FIGURE 16.5 Auditory and auditory-related cortex in the macaque monkey. Shaded areas in temporal, posterior parietal, and prefrontal cortex indicate regions with auditory cortex connections. Major sulci have been opened to show extension of auditory-related cortex within each sulcus. Levels of auditory cortical pro-cessing are indicated by numbers for each region: level 1, core; level 2, belt; level 3, parabelt; level 4a, superior temporal; level 4b, posterior parietal; level 4c, prefrontal. (LIP, lateral intraparietal area; VIP, ventral intraparietal area).

somatic stimulation throughout the temporal lobe in monkeys, but few studies have been devoted to the significance of auditory activity in prefrontal cortex (see Hackett and Kaas, 2002). The influence of auditory stimuli has most often been studied in the context of visually related tasks, so little is actually known about auditory processing in conditions that relate more specifically to audition. Auditory stimuli clearly play a role in spatially related tasks mediated by neurons in the frontal eye fields and dorsal periarcuate region (Ito, 1982; Azuma and Suzuki, 1984; Suzuki, 1985; Vaadia et al., 1986; Vaadia, 1989; Russo and Bruce, 1994). Many periarcuate neurons, for example, respond to passive auditory stimulation, but auditory and visual responses are more likely in active spatial tasks. Further, during active localization, many units were tuned to one or more spatial locations (i.e., 0°, 30°, 60°, or 90° contralateral), whereas the same units exhibited little spatial tuning in the passive detection task. These findings suggest that location encoding mechanisms in this region are not necessarily based on location-specific units but on the coordinated activity of multiple neurons that have broad spatial tuning (Vaadia et al., 1986). Neurons in orbitofrontal cortex respond to auditory and visual stimuli during nonspatial tasks, such as cross-modal matching (Benevento et al., 1977; Thorpe, Rolls, and Maddison, 1983). Recording from neurons in ventrolateral areas 12/45, Romanski and Goldman-Rakic (2002) found

responses to macaque monkey vocalizations. This area overlapped partially with a region just anterior to the ventral arcuate sulcus in which neurons were responsive to visual stimuli.

While this brief survey of the physiological literature supports the functional segregation of auditory activity in prefrontal cortex, as inferred from the connectivity, this distinction has not been the aim of any study. Studies involving auditory stimuli in the periprincipal and precarcuate regions tend to involve spatial tasks, while studies of ventrolateral and orbitofrontal areas do not. Thus, impressions of functional specificity are not free of bias. Indeed, unimodal and bimodal units active in passive and nonspatial tasks have been found within periprincipal, prearcuate, postarcuate, and ventrolateral areas (Wollberg and Sela, 1980; Watanabe, 1982). Further, while the connectional patterns are indicative of functional heterogeneity in the pathways that target the prefrontal cortex, some caution is needed in interpreting the functional roles of the prefrontal pathways until studies include systematic comparisons of neurons in various prefrontal areas.

Functional imaging studies in humans have so far not led to the identification of functional modules in the frontal lobe, whereas studies involving auditory and speech-related tasks consistently reveal activations in circumscribed regions of frontal and prefrontal cortex. Areas activated in auditory perceptual tasks, especially those including speech, are rather task dependent but most often include the middle, superior, and inferior frontal gyri, in addition to large portions of the STG and STS (Demonet et al., 1992; Binder et al., 1996, 2000; Schlapeske et al., 1999; Belin et al., 2000; Hickock and Poeppel, 2000; Martinkauppi et al., 2000; Scott et al., 2000; Wise et al., 2001; Griffiths and Warren, 2002). Areas activated in speech production are also task dependent and most often include bilateral motor and premotor areas, STS, posterior inferior frontal gyrus, anterior insula, posterior inferior parietal, anterolateral and medial temporal, and the posterior supratemporal plane (Paulesu, Frith, and Frackowiak, 1993; Klein et al., 1995; Petrides, Alivisatos, and Evans, 1995; Fiez and Petersen, 1998; Wise et al., 1999, 2001; Braun et al., 2001; Blank et al., 2002). In these studies, coactivation within and beyond the classic language areas of Broca and Wernicke (e.g., superior and middle temporal, cingulate, and inferior parietal cortical regions) is a common finding, suggesting that a distributed network of areas is engaged. These findings are generally consistent with inferences that can be drawn, in part, from studies in monkeys (e.g., Romanski and Goldman-Rakic, 2002).

AUDITORY PROCESSING IN POSTERIOR PARIETAL CORTEX
The posterior parietal cortex contains several functionally distinct areas that contribute to a multimodal representation of space used by motor structures to guide movements (see Andersen et al., 1997). The ventral intraparietal area (VIP) has widespread connections with visuospatial, vestibular, motor, and somatosensory networks, particularly those that involve the upper body, whereas the connections of the lateral intraparietal area (LIP) favor visual cortical areas. A number of studies have described connections linking LIP and especially VIP with the caudal STG, including the caudal parabelt, CM, and Tpt (Pandya and Kuypers, 1969; Divac et al., 1977; Hyvarinen, 1982; Lewis and Van Essen, 2000). The connections suggest that auditory cortex contributes to multisensory integration in posterior parietal cortex, consistent with recent physiological studies of auditory responsiveness in this region (Mazzoni et al., 1996; Stricanne et al., 1996; Grunewald, Linden, and Andersen, 1999; Linden, Grunewald, and Andersen, 1999; Schlack, 2002; Cohen, Cohen, and Gifford, 2004). The most striking feature of the auditory projections to posterior parietal cortex is the absence of inputs from rostral areas of the belt or parabelt (figure 16.5). When considered along with the segregation of inputs to prefrontal cortex, the suggestion that the caudal auditory fields contribute to spatially related activity in the brain takes on added significance. Functional imaging studies in humans indicate that posterior parietal cortex, particularly in the right hemisphere, is active during tasks requiring active localization of sounds (Griffiths et al.,

1998; Bushara et al., 1999; Zatorre et al., 1999, 2002; Weeks et al., 2000; Alain et al., 2001; Bremmer et al., 2001; Maeder et al., 2001). The deep portion of the human intraparietal sulcus, which may correspond to the macaque VIP, is active in the multisensory processing of moving stimuli (Bremmer et al., 2001). In this study fMRI was used to measure activations associated with moving auditory, tactile, and visual stimuli. Activations common to all three modalities included the VIP region bilaterally, the right ventral premotor cortex, and a posterior inferior parietal area bilaterally on the upper bank of the sylvian fissure. Overall, the findings of these many studies are consistent with the view that auditory inputs to the posterior parietal cortex contribute to networks of sensory and premotor areas devoted to multisensory processing of spatially related information.

AUDITORY PROCESSING IN THE SUPERIOR TEMPORAL SULCUS
The cortex of the STS represents a significant portion of the lateral temporal lobe in both macaque monkeys and humans. The deep sulcus contains several architectonic regions that have reciprocal connections (figure 16.5) with nonprimary auditory, somatic, and visual sensory cortices (Seltzer and Pandya, 1978, 1991, 1994; Desimone and Ungerleider, 1986; Neal, Pearson, and Powell, 1990; Barnes and Pandya, 1992; Cusick et al., 1995; Seltzer et al., 1996; Saleem et al., 2000). Although the lower bank of the STS appears to be involved largely with visual processing, the areas that occupy the fundus and upper bank of the STS are multisensory (Benevento et al., 1977; Bruce, Desimone, and Gross, 1981; Baylis, Rolls, and Leonard, 1987; Hikosaka et al., 1988; Mistlin and Perrett, 1990). These areas comprise the superior temporal polysensory region (STP), which corresponds to the architectonic area TPO. With respect to audition, the lateral belt and parabelt regions have dense connections with the STP (Pandya, Hallett, and Mukherjee, 1969; Galaburda and Pandya, 1983; Cipolloni and Pandya, 1989; Hackett, Stepniewska, and Kass, 1998a). Unfortunately, little is known concerning the functional significance of these inputs, as neuronal activity in the STS associated with auditory stimulation has not been systematically studied in monkeys. On functional imaging and MEG studies the human STS is activated on a wide range of auditory tasks, especially those involving speech and language (Mummery et al., 1999; Binder et al., 2000; Belin et al., 2000, 2002; Scott et al., 2000; Jancke et al., 2002; Wong et al., 2002; Papanicolaou et al., 2003). In addition, there is some evidence of multisensory integration in the human STS, as found in monkeys (e.g., Calvert et al., 2000, 2001; Campbell et al., 2001). How the STS in humans corresponds to that of monkeys is not known. The anatomical and physiological evidence is supportive of some level of correspondence, yet the superior temporal cortex is greatly expanded in humans, including the addition of the middle temporal

gyrus and sulcus, which is also active during language-related tasks in humans (see Price, 2000).

MULTISENSORY INTEGRATION IN AUDITORY CORTEX
Although multisensory integration is a well-established feature of posterior parietal cortex and the STS, recent studies have started to reveal evidence of multisensory inputs to cortical regions long considered to be unimodal. With respect to auditory cortex, several studies can be pieced together to support the hypothesis that sensory processing in auditory cortex is directly influenced by visual and somatosensory inputs. Robinson and Burton (1980a,b) found neurons responsive to auditory and/or somatic sensory stimulation in two fields on the lower bank of the lateral sulcus, caudal to A1, in macaque monkeys. One of those fields, PA (Jones and Burton, 1976), corresponds closely to the caudomedial belt area (CM) in our model of auditory cortex. A second field, RI, lies caudal and medial to PA and may correspond partially to VS of Krubitzer et al. (1995). The connections of CM with auditory cortex are typical of the auditory belt areas, except for the recent observation that CM may be the only belt field that projects to the VIP area within the intraparietal sulcus. More recently, Schroeder et al. (2001) and Fu et al. (2003) sampled single- and multi-unit responses from sites in A1 and CM. Neurons in CM were found to be responsive to both auditory and somesthetic stimulation elicited by electrical stimulation of the median nerve in the hand or mechanical stimulation of the upper body. The source of somatosensory input to CM has not been determined, but preliminary data indicate that the somatosensory cortical areas RI, S2, and several multisensory nuclei of the thalamus project to CM (de la Mothe et al., 2002). In addition to CM, Werner-Reise and colleagues (2003) found that eye position modulated the responses of a subpopulation of A1 neurons to sound, echoing previous findings from the same laboratory from recordings in the inferior colliculus (Groh et al., 2001). Although the anatomical basis for these effects is not clear, recent anatomical studies indicate that infragranular neurons in the caudal areas of the core, belt, and parabelt auditory regions project to parts of area 17 devoted to peripheral and paracentral vision (Falchier et al., 2002), establishing previously unknown links between auditory and visual cortex. Overall, these surprising results indicate that multisensory interactions in cortex are not limited to known multisensory regions (e.g., intraparietal sulcus, STS) but are much more widespread, extending even to the primary sensory cortex.

PROCESSING STREAMS IN AUDITORY CORTEX?   A prominent theme in recent studies of auditory cortex in nonhuman primates and humans concerns the controversial proposal that auditory information is segregated into functional streams specialized for the processing of spatial (where) and non-spatial (what) information (see Romanski, Tian, et al., 1999; Kaas and Hackett, 2000; Rauschecker and Tian, 2000; Recanzone, 2001; Tian et al., 2001; Maeder et al., 2001; Middlebrooks, 2002; Zatorre et al., 2002). This is conceptually analogous to the dorsal and ventral streams of processing identified in the visual system (Ungerleider and Mishkin, 1982). Partial support for the dual streams hypothesis comes from anatomical studies showing that the caudal and rostral portions of auditory cortex target functionally distinct domains in auditory related cortex (figure 16.6) that mediate spatial and nonspatial processing (Rauschecker, 1998; Hackett, Stepniewska, and Kaas, 1999a; Romanski, Bates, and Goldman-Rakic, 1999; Romanski, Tian, et al., 1999; Lewis and Van Essen, 2000). In addition to projections to visual cortex, the caudal subdivisions of the belt and parabelt are preferentially connected with regions in the posterior parietal cortex and prefrontal cortex associated with the processing of spatially related (where) information. In contrast, the rostral subdivisions of the belt and parabelt have no known connections with visual or posterior parietal cortex but are strongly connected with the temporal pole and regions of the prefrontal cortex associated with the processing of nonspatial (what) information.

Whereas the anatomical data clearly reveal the presence of divergent rostral and caudal pathways in monkeys, the physiological significance of those projections remains controversial, especially concerning the processing of spatial and object-related information within areas of auditory cortex (see Recanzone, this volume). Support for the segregation of function by rostral and caudal divisions of auditory cortex can be found in a recent study of neurons in the lateral belt fields (Tian et al., 2001). Macaque monkeys were systematically presented with one of seven communication calls presented at one of seven different azimuth locations. Neurons in the rostral belt area, A1, were found to be more selective for a particular macaque monkey call than neurons in the caudal belt area, CL, which were more selective for the spatial location (azimuth) of the call. These results are consistent with those of Recanzone, Guard, Phan, and colleagues (2000), in which A1 neurons were found to be less sensitive to spatial location than neurons in the caudomedial belt field, CM. Findings in monkeys appear to conflict with the results of intensive neurophysiological studies of other species, which have not produced evidence of maps of auditory space or differences in spatially related processing among auditory cortical areas. Middlebrooks and colleagues contend that information about sound source location and identity is encoded in the firing patterns of individual neurons distributed across auditory cortical areas of cats with no areal specificity (see Middlebrooks, 2002). Because it is not known how spatial location or the identity of auditory objects is encoded by neurons in auditory cortex, the extent to which spatial and nonspatial processing is mediated by different

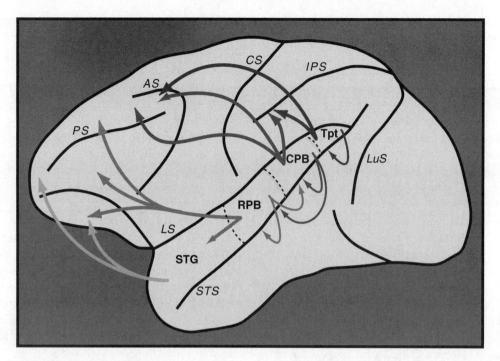

FIGURE 16.6   Topography of auditory-related projections. Projections to the prefrontal cortex from auditory cortex and auditory-related fields of the superior temporal gyrus. Subdivisions of belt and parabelt/STG fields (shaded arrows) project topographically to segregated regions of superior temporal, posterior parietal, and prefrontal cortex. Connectional patterns indicate a propensity for rostral and caudal auditory areas to target functionally distinct domains in prefrontal cortex. Connections with posterior parietal cortex arise only from caudal auditory cortex. Projections to superior temporal sulcus from rostral and caudal auditory fields are overlapping. (Modified from Kaas and Hackett, 2000.)

cortical areas or groups of areas remains unclear. Additional studies are needed to reveal the functional differences between these anatomically distinct areas.

In the functional imaging literature, support for what and where streams also varies. A number of functional imaging and lesion studies have provided support for the segregation of spatial and nonspatial auditory processing in the human brain (Alain et al., 2001; Maeder et al., 2001; Scott et al., 2000; Martinkauppi et al., 2000; Kikuchi-Yorioka and Sawaguchi, 2000; Clarke et al., 2002; Warren et al., 2002), while other results contradict or only partially support the hypothesis (e.g., Cohen and Wessinger, 1999; Belin and Zatorre, 2000; Zatorre et al., 2002). Bushara and colleagues (1999) found evidence of separate subsystems of spatial attention for the visual and auditory localization tasks in the superior parietal and middle frontal gyri bilaterally. Activation was overlapping in the lateral intraparietal, medial frontal, and inferior temporal cortex, suggesting multisensory or supramodal activity related to spatial and nonspatial processes. Maeder and colleagues (2001) showed a clear dissociation between cortical areas activated in sound localization and recognition tasks. The middle temporal and left inferior frontal gyri showed greater activation on the sound recognition task than on the localization task, which activated the lower inferior parietal lobe and posterior middle and inferior frontal gyri bilaterally. Several studies have linked activation of posterior auditory cortical areas to moving stimuli (Baumgart et al., 1999; Griffiths et al., 2000; Thivard et al., 2000; Bremmer et al., 2001; Warren et al., 2002; Hall and Moore, 2003). Zatorre and colleagues (2002) provide evidence consistent with the dual streams and distributed streams hypotheses. They found that posterior auditory areas in the planum temporale and temporoparietal operculum were specifically responsive to spatial location, but only when the auditory stimuli contained object-related features, indicating that neurons in these fields were sensitive to spectrotemporal features related to what and where.

Anatomical evidence of significant interactions between caudal and rostral auditory areas suggests that the processing of spatial and nonspatial auditory information is not mediated by completely segregated streams in cortex. Moreover, other processing streams are likely to arise from auditory cortex. The anatomical heterogeneity of the superior temporal region in humans and nonhuman primates suggests that multiple functions could be subserved by neurons within and between areas. The posterior portion of the STG known as Wernicke's area, although poorly defined, is anatomically heterogeneous, encompassing numerous auditory cortical areas of varied functional significance, including speech perception, production, and lexical access (Wise et al., 2001). Scott and Johnsrude (2003) point to numerous functional distinctions that can be made between auditory processing that occurs in systems of cortical fields that lie anterior and posterior to the core region in humans. In particular, they review evidence for an anterior system of auditory and auditory-related areas that may be involved in mapping phonetic cues onto lexical representations, and a posterior system of areas linked to motor-related representations of speech. The human planum temporale, which probably includes cortex corresponding to the lateral belt and parabelt regions of monkeys, has been linked to multiple processes, including activation by speech and nonspeech sounds, silent and spoken articulation, sound localization, and sound motion (Griffiths and Warren, 2002). Griffiths and Warren (2002) proposed that the planum temporale can be modeled as a computational hub that is engaged in the analysis of a variety of complex sounds for the purpose of matching spectrotemporal patterns of sounds with learned representations. In this way the planum temporale would direct subsequent processing in areas that mediate identification and perception. Thus, while the anterior and posterior auditory areas may contribute to different processing streams in cortex, multiple processing streams may be represented within each system of areas.

Summary

The organization of the primate auditory cortex is gradually becoming clearer as structural and functional studies in humans and nonhuman primates become available. Although many uncertainties remain, much progress has been made by integrating classic and modern studies. In this chapter, the functional organization of the primate auditory cortex was described in the form of a model based on the collective findings of the field. According to this model, the processing of auditory information in the cerebral cortex spans at least four levels of processing, involving a network of auditory and auditory-related areas. Auditory cortex is comprised of three regions (core, belt, parabelt), arranged in a processing hierarchy, that receive thalamocortical inputs from one or more divisions of the medial geniculate complex. Each region contains a variable number of subdivisions that process information in parallel. Thus, processing in auditory cortex incorporates both serial and parallel elements. Auditory-related fields in prefrontal, posterior parietal, occipital, and superior temporal cortex are the targets of neurons in the belt and parabelt regions of auditory cortex, but receive no inputs from the auditory thalamus. Inputs from auditory, somatic, and visual sensory modalities tend to adjoin or overlap in auditory-related cortex, consistent with multisensory integration in these regions. In addition, the rostral and caudal areas of auditory cortex target functionally distinct sectors of auditory-related cortex that mediate the processing of nonspatial and spatially related information. The divergence of rostral and caudal auditory pathways forms the basis of the dual streams hypothesis, in which the outputs of auditory cortex are segregated into functional streams specialized for the processing of nonspatial (what) and spatial (where) information.

REFERENCES

AITKIN, L. M., 1990. *The Auditory Cortex, Structural and Functional Bases of Auditory Perception*. London: Chapman and Hall.

AITKIN, L. M., M. KUDO, and D. R. R. IRVINE, 1988. Connections of the primary auditory cortex in the common marmoset (*Callithrix jacchus jacchus*). *J. Comp. Neurol.* 269:235–248.

AITKIN, L. M., M. M. MERZENICH, D. R. F. IRVINE, J. C. CLAREY, and J. E. NELSON, 1986. Frequency representation in auditory cortex of the common marmoset (*Callithrix jacchus jacchus*). *J. Comp. Neurol.* 252:175–185.

ALAIN, C., S. R. ARNOTT, S. HEVENOR, S. GRAHAM, and C. L. GRADY, 2001. "What" and "where" in the human auditory system. *Proc. Natl. Acad. Sci. U.S.A.* 98:12301–12306.

ANDERSON, R. A., L. H. SYNDER, D. C. BRADLEY, and J. XING, 1997. Multimodal representation of space in the posterior parietal cortex and its use in planning movements. *Anno. Rev. Neurosci.* 20:303–330.

AZUMA, M., and H. SUZUKI, 1984. Properties and distribution of auditory neurons in the dorsolateral prefrontal cortex of the alert monkey. *Brain Res.* 90:57–73.

BARNES, C. L., and D. N. PANDYA, 1992. Efferent cortical connections of multimodal cortex of the superior temporal sulcus in the rhesus monkey. *J. Comp. Neurol.* 318:222–244.

BAUMGART, F., B. GASCHLER-MARKEFSKI, M. G. WOLDORFF, H. J. HEINZE, and H. SCHEICH, 1999. A movement-sensitive area in auditory cortex. *Nature* 400:724–726.

BAYLIS, G. C., E. T. ROLLS, and C. M. LEONARD, 1987. Functional subdivisions of the temporal lobe neocortex. *J. Neurosci.* 7:330–342.

BENEVENTO, L. A., J. FALLON, B. J. DAVIS, and M. REZAK, 1977. Auditory-visual interaction in single cells in the cortex of the superior temporal sulcus and the orbital frontal cortex of the macaque monkey. *Exp. Neurol.* 57:849–872.

BELIN, P., and R. J. ZATORRE, 2000. "What," "where" and "how" in auditory cortex. *Nat. Neurosci.* 3:965–966.

BELIN, P., R. J. ZATORRE, and P. AHAD, 2002. Human temporal-lobe response to vocal sounds. *Brain Res. Cogn. Brain Res.* 13:17–26.

BELIN, P., R. J. ZATORRE, P. LAFAILLE, P. AHAD, and B. PIKE, 2000. Voice-selective areas in human auditory cortex. *Nature* 403:309–312.

BERTRAND, O., F. PERRIN, and J. PERNIER, 1991. Evidence for a tonotopic organization of the auditory cortex observed with electrical evoked potentials. *Acta Otolaryngol. Suppl.* 491:116–123.

BILECEN, D., K. SCHEFFLER, N. SCHMID, K. TSCHOPP, and J. SEELING, 1998. Tonotopic organization of the human auditory cortex as detected by BOLD-FMRI. *Hear. Res.* 126:19–27.

BINDER, J. R., J. A. FROST, T. A. HAMMEKE, S. M. RAO, and R. W. COX, 1996. Function of the left planum temporale in auditory and linguistic processing. *Brain* 119:1239–1347.

BINDER, J. R., J. A. FROST, T. A. HAMMER, P. S. F. BELLGOWAN, J. A. SPRINGER, J. N. KAUFMAN, and E. T. POSSING, 2000. Human temporal lobe activation by speech and nonspeech sounds. *Cereb. Cortex* 10:514–528.

BLANK, S. C., S. K. SCOTT, K. MURPHY, W. WARBURTON, and R. J. S. WISE, 2002. Speech production: Wernicke, Broca and beyond. *Brain* 125:1829–1838.

BRAUN, A. R., A. GUILLEMIN, L. HOSEY, and M. VARGA, 2001. The neural organization of discourse: An H$_2^{15}$O-PET study of narrative production in English and American sign language. *Brain* 124:2028–2044.

BREMMER, F., A. SCHLACK, N. J. SHAH, O. ZAFIRIS, M. KUBISCHIK, K.-P. HOFFMANN, K. ZILLES, and G. R. FINK, 2001. Polymodal motion processing in posterior parietal and premotor cortex: A human fMRI study strongly implies equivalencies between humans and monkeys. *Neuron* 29:287–296.

BRODMANN, K., 1905. Beitrage zur histologischen Lokalisation der Grosshirnrinde. Dritte Mitteilung. Die Rinderfelder der niederen Affen. *J. Psych. Neurol.* 4:177–226.

BRODMANN, K., 1908. Beitrage zur histologischen Localisation der Grosshirnrinde: Die cytoarchitektonische Cortexgliederung der Halbaffen (*Lemuriden*). *J. Psych. Neurol.* 10:287–334.

BRODMANN, K., 1909. *Vergleichende Lokalisationslehre der Grosshirnrinde.* Leipzig: Barth.

BRUCE, C., R. DESIMONE, and C. G. GROSS, 1981. Visual properties of neurons in a polysensory area in superior temporal sulcus of the macaque. *J. Neurophysiol.* 46:369–384.

BRUGGE, J. F., 1982. Auditory cortical areas in primates. In *Cortical Sensory Organization*, vol. 3, C. N. Woolsey, ed. Clifton, N. J.: Humana Press, pp. 59–70.

BUSHARA, K. O., R. A. WEEKS, K. ISHII, M. J. CATALAN, B. TIAN, J. P. RAUSCHECKER, and M. HALLETT, 1999. Modality-specific frontal and parietal areas for auditory and visual spatial localization in humans. *Nat. Neurosci.* 2:759–766.

CALVERT, G. A., R. CAMPBELL, and J. F. BRAMMER, 2000. Evidence from functional magnetic resonance imaging of crossmodal binding in the human heteromodal cortex. *Curr. Biol.* 10:649–657.

CALVERT, G. A., P. C. HANSEN, S. D. IVERSON, and M. J. BRAMMER, 2001. Detection of audio-visual integration sites in humans by application of electrophysiological criteria to the BOLD effect. *NeuroImage* 14:427–438.

CAMPBELL, R., M. MacSWEENEY, S. SURGULADZE, G. CALVERT, P. McGUIRE, J. SUCKLING, M. J. BRAMMER, and A. S. DAVIS, 2001. Cortical substrates for the perception of face actions: An fMRI study of the specificity of activation for seen speech and for meaningless lower-face acts (gurning). *Brain Res. Cogn. Brain Res.* 12:233–243.

CHEUNG, S. W., P. H. BEDENBAUGH, S. S. NAGARAJAN, and C. E. SCHREINER, 2001. Functional organization of squirrel monkey primary auditory cortex: Responses to pure tones. *J. Neurophysiol.* 85:1732–1749.

CIPOLLONI, P. B., and D. N. PANDYA, 1989. Connectional analysis of the ipsilateral and contralateral afferent neurons of the superior temporal region in the rhesus monkey. *J. Comp. Neurol.* 281:567–585.

CLARKE, S., A. BELLMANN-THIRAN, P. MAEDER, M. ADRIANI, O. VERNET, L. REGLI, O. CUISENAIRE, and J. P. THIRAN, 2002. What and where in human audition: Selective deficits following focal hemispheric lesions. *Exp. Brain Res.* 147:8–15.

COHEN, Y. E., I. S. COHEN, and G. W. GIFFORD III, 2004. Modulation of LIP activity by predictive auditory and visual cues. *Cereb. Cortex* [Epub ahead of print].

COHEN, Y. E., and C. N. WESSINGER, 1999. Who goes there? *Neuron* 24:769–771.

CUSICK, C. G., B. SELTZER, M. COLA, and E. GRIGGS, 1995. Chemoarchitectonics and corticortical terminations within the superior temporal sulcus of the rhesus monkey: Evidence for subdivisions of superior temporal polysensory cortex. *J. Comp. Neurol.* 360:513–535.

DE LA MOTHE, L. A., S. BLUMELL, Y. KAJIKAWA, and T. A. HACKETT. 2002. Connections of auditory medial belt cortex in marmoset monkeys. Program No. 261.6. 2002 Abstract Viewer/Itinerary Planner. Washington, DC: Society for Neuroscience. Online.

DE ROSSI, G., G. PALUDETTI, W. DI NARDO, M. L. CALCAGNI, D. DI GUIDA, G. ALMADORI, and J. GALLI, 1996. SPET monitoring of perfusion changes in auditory cortex following mono- and multi-frequency stimuli. *Nuklearmedizin* 35:112–115.

DEMONET, J.-F., F. CHOLLET, S. RAMSAY, D. CARDEBAT, J. L. NESPOULOUS, R. WISE, A. RASCOL, and R. FRACKOWIAK, 1992. The anatomy of phonological and semantic processing in normal subjects. *Brain* 115:1753–1768.

DESIMONE, R., and L. G. UNGERLEIDER, 1986. Multiple visual areas in the caudal superior temporal sulcus of the macaque. *J. Comp. Neurol.* 248:164–189.

DI SALLE, F., E. FORMISANO, E. SEIFRITZ, D. E. LINDEN, K. SCHEFFLER, C. SAULINO, G. TEDESCHI, F. E. ZANELLE, A. PEPINO, R. GOEBEL, and E. MARCIANO, 2001. Functional fields in human auditory cortex revealed by time-resolved fMRI without interference of EPI noise. *NeuroImage* 13:328–338.

DIVAC, I., J. H. LAVAIL, P. RAKIC, and K. R. WINTSON, 1977. Heterogeneous afferents to the inferior parietal lobule of the rhesus monkey revealed by the retrograde transport method. *Brain Res.* 123:197–207.

DUNCAN, J., and A. M. OWEN, 2000. Common regions of the human frontal lobe recruited by diverse cognitive demands. *Trends Neurosci.* 23:475–483.

ELBERLING, C., C. BAK, B. KOFOED, J. LEBECK, and K. SAERMARK, 1982. Auditory magnetic fields: Source location and "tonotopical organization" in the right hemisphere of the human brain. *Scand. Audiol.* 11:61–65.

ENGELIEN, A., M. SCHULZ, B. ROSS, V. AROLT, and C. PANTEV, 2000. A combined functional in vivo measure for primary and secondary auditory cortices. *Hear. Res.* 148:153–160.

FALCHEIR, A., S. CLAVAGNIER, P. BARONE, and H. KENNEDY, 2002. Anatomical evidence of multimodal integration in primate striate cortex. *J. Neurosci.* 22:5749–5759.

FIEZ, J. A., and S. E. PETERSEN, 1998. Neuroimaging studies of word reading. *Proc. Natl. Acad. Sci. U.S.A.* 95:914–921.

FITZPATRICK, K. A., and T. J. IMIG, 1980. Auditory cortico-cortical connections in the owl monkey. *J. Comp. Neurol.* 177:537–556.

FORBES, B. F., and N. MOSKOWITZ, 1974. Projections of auditory responsive cortex in the squirrel monkey. *Brain Res.* 67:239–254.

FORMISANO, E., D.-S. KIM, F. DISALLE, P.-F. VAN DE MOORTELE, K. UGURBIL, and R. GOEBEL, 2003. Mirror-symmetric tonotopic maps in human primary auditory cortex. *Neuron*, 40:859–869.

FU, K. M., T. A. JOHNSTON, A. S. SHAH, L. ARNOLD, J. SMILEY, T. A. HACKETT, P. E. GARRAGHTY, and C. E. SCHROEDER, 2003. Auditory cortical neurons respond to somatosensory stimulation. *J. Neurosci.* 23:7510–7515.

FUJIOKA, T., B. ROSS, H. OKAMOTO, Y. TAKESHIMA, R. KAKIGI, and C. PANTEV, 2003. Tonotopic representation of missing fundamental complex sounds in the human auditory cortex. *Eur. J. Neurosci.* 18:432–440.

GALABURDA, A. M., and D. N. PANDYA, 1983. The intrinsic architectonic and connectional organization of the superior temporal region of the rhesus monkey. *J. Comp. Neurol.* 221:169–184.

GALABURDA, A. M., and F. SANIDES, 1980. Cytoarchitectonic organization of the human auditory cortex. *J. Comp. Neurol.* 190:597–610.

GIRAUD, A.-L., C. LORENZI, J. ASHBURNER, J. WABLE, I. JOHNSRUDE, R. FRACKOWIAK, and A. KLEINSCHMIDT, 2000. Representation of the temporal envelope of sounds in the human brain. *J. Neurophysiol.* 84:1588–1598.

GONCALVES, M. S., D. A. HALL, I. S. JOHNSRUDE, and M. P. HAGGARD, 2001. Can meaningful effective connectivities be obtained between auditory cortical regions? *NeuroImage* 14:1353–1360.

GRIFFITHS, T. D., C. BUCHEL, R. S. J. FRACKOWIAK, and R. D. PATTERSON, 1998. Analysis of temporal structure in sound by the human brain. *Nat. Neurosci.* 1:422–427.

GRIFFITHS, T. D., G. G. GREEN, A. REES, and G. REES, 2000. Human brain areas involved in the analysis of auditory movement. *Hum. Brain Mapp.* 9:72–80.

GRIFFITHS, T. D., and J. D. WARREN, 2002. The planum temporale as a computational hub. *Trends Neurosci.* 25:348–353.

GROH, J. M., A. S. TRAUSE, A. M. UNDERHILL, K. R. CLARK, and S. INATI, 2001. Eye position influences auditory responses in primate inferior colliculus. *Neuron* 29:509–518.

GRUNEWALD, A., J. F. LINDEN, and R. A. ANDERSEN, 1999. Responses to auditory stimuli in macaque lateral intraparietal area. I. Effects of training. *J. Neurophysiol.* 82:330–342.

HACKETT, T. A., 2002. The comparative anatomy of the primate auditory cortex. In *Primate Audition: Behavior and Neurobiology*, A. Ghazanfar, ed. Boca Raton, Fla.: CRC Press, pp. 199–226.

HACKETT, T. A., and J. H. KAAS, 2002. Auditory processing in the primate brain. In *Handbook of Psychology*, Vol. 3, *Biological Psychology*, M. Gallagher and R. J. Nelson, eds. New York: John Wiley and Sons.

HACKETT, T. A., T. M. PREUSS, and J. H. KAAS, 2001. Architectonic identification of the core region in auditory cortex of macaques, chimpanzees, and humans. *J. Comp. Neurol.* 441:197–222.

HACKETT, T. A., I. STEPNIEWSKA, and J. H. KAAS, 1998a. Subdivisions of auditory cortex and ipsilateral cortical connections of the parabelt auditory cortex in macaque monkeys. *J. Comp. Neurol.* 394:475–495.

HACKETT, T. A., I. STEPNIEWSKA, and J. H. KAAS, 1998b. Thalamocortical connections of parabelt auditory cortex in macaque monkeys. *J. Comp. Neurol.* 400:271–286.

HACKETT, T. A., I. STEPNIEWSKA, and J. H. KAAS, 1999. Prefrontal connections of the auditory parabelt cortex in macaque monkeys. *Brain Res.* 817:45–58.

HALL, D. A., M. P. HAGGARD, M. A. AKEROYD, A. Q. SUMMERFIELD, A. R. PALMER, M. R. ELLIOTT, and R. W. BOWTELL, 2000. Modulation and task effects in auditory processing measured using fMRI. *Hum. Brain Mapp.* 10:107–119.

HALL, D. A., H. C. HART, and I. S. JOHNSRUDE, 2003. Relationships between human auditory cortical structure and function. *Audiol. Neurootol.* 8:1–18.

HALL, D. A., I. S. JOHNSRUDE, M. P. HAGGARD, A. R. PALMER, M. A. AKEROYED, and A. Q. SUMMERFIELD, 2002. Spectral and temporal processing in human auditory cortex. *Cereb. Cortex* 12:140–149.

HALL, D. A., and D. R. MOORE, 2003. Auditory neuroscience: The salience of looming sounds. *Curr. Biol.* 13:R91–R93.

HART, H. C., A. R. PALMER, and D. A. HALL, 2002. Heschl's gyrus is more sensitive to tone level than non-primary auditory cortex. *Hear. Res.* 171:177–190.

HICKOCK, G., and D. POEPPEL, 2000. Towards a functional neuroanatomy of speech perception. *Trends Cogn. Sci.* 4:131–138.

HIKOSAKA, K., E. IWAI, H. SAITO, and K. TANAKA, 1988. Polysensory properties of neurons in the anterior bank of the caudal superior temporal sulcus of the macaque monkey. *J. Neurophysiol.* 60:1615–1637.

HOKE, E. S., B. ROSS, and M. HOKE, 1998. Auditory afterimage: Tonotopic representation in the auditory cortex. *Neuroreport* 9:3065–3068.

HOWARD, M. A., I. O. VOLKOV, P. J. ABBAS, H. DAMASIO, M. C. OLLENDIECK, and M. A. GRANNER, 1996. A chronic microelectrode investigation of the tonotopic organization of human auditory cortex. *Brain Res.* 724:260–264.

HOWARD, M. A., I. O. VOLKOV, R. MIRSKY, P. C. GARELL, M. D. NOH, M. GRANNER, H. DAMASIO, M. STEINSCHNEIDER, R. A. REALE, J. E. HIND, and J. F. BRUGGE, 2000. Auditory cortex on the human posterior superior temporal gyrus. *J. Comp. Neurol.* 416:79–82.

HURST, E. M., 1959. Some cortical association systems related to auditory functions. *J. Comp. Neurol.* 112:103–119.

HYVARINEN, J., 1982. Posterior parietal lobe of the primate brain. *Physiol. Rev.* 62:1060–1129.

IMIG, T. J., M. A. RUGGERO, L. M. KITZES, E. JAVEL, and J. F. BRUGGE, 1977. Organization of auditory cortex in the owl monkey (*Aotus trivirgatus*). *J. Comp. Neurol.* 171:111–128.

ITO, S.-I., 1982. Prefrontal unit activity of macaque monkeys during auditory and visual reaction time tasks. *Brain Res.* 247:39–47.

JANCKE, L., T. WUSTENBERG, K. SCHULZE, and H. J. HEINZE, 2002. Asymmetric hemodynamic responses of the human auditory cortex to monaural and binaural stimulation. *Hear. Res.* 170: 166–178.

JOHNSRUDE, I. S., A. L. GIRAUD, and R. S. J. FRACKOWIAK, 2002. Functional imaging of the auditory system: The use of positron emission tomography. *Audiol. Neurootol.* 7:251–276.

JONES, E. G., and H. BURTON, 1976. Areal differences in the laminar distribution of thalamic afferents in cortical fields of the insular, parietal and temporal regions of primates. *J. Comp. Neurol.* 168:197–247.

JONES, E. G., M. E. DELL'ANNA, M. MOLINARI, E. RAUSELL, and T. HASHIKAWA, 1995. Subdivisions of macaque monkey auditory cortex revealed by calcium-binding protein immunoreactivity. *J. Comp. Neurol.* 362:153–170.

KAAS, J. H., and T. A. HACKETT, 1998. Subdivisions and levels of processing in primate auditory cortex. *Audiol. Neurootol.* 3:73–85.

KAAS, J. H., and T. A. HACKETT, 1999. "What" and "where" processing in auditory cortex. *Nat. Neurosci.* 2:1045–1047.

KAAS, J. H., and T. A. HACKETT, 2000. Subdivisions of auditory cortex and processing streams in primates. *Proc. Nat. Acad. Sci. U.S.A.* 97:11793–11799.

KAAS, J. H., T. A. HACKETT, and M. J. TRAMO, 1999. Auditory processing in primate cerebral cortex. *Curr. Opin. Neurobiol.* 9:164–170.

KAJIKAWA, Y., L. DE LA MOTHE, S. BLUMELL, and T. A. HACKETT, 2003. Response properties of neurons in core and medial belt auditory cortex of marmoset monkeys. *Assoc. Res. Otolaryngol. Abstr.* 972.

KLEIN, D., B. MILNER, R. J. ZATORRE, E. MEYER, and A. C. EVANS, 1995. The neural substrates underlying word-generation: A bilingual functional imaging study. *Proc. Natl. Acad. Sci. U.S.A.* 92:2899–2903.

KIKUCHI-YORIOKA, Y., and T. SAWAGUCHI, 2000. Parallel visuospatial and audiospatial working memory processes in the monkey dorsolateral prefrontal cortex. *Nat. Neurosci* 3:1075–1076.

Kosaki, H., T. Hashikawa, J. He, and E. G. Jones, 1997. Tonotopic organization of auditory cortical fields delineated by parvalbumin immunoreactivity in macaque monkeys. *J. Comp. Neurol.* 386:304–316.

Krubitzer, L., J., Clarey, R. Tweedale, G. Elston, and M. Calford, 1995. A redefinition of somatosensory areas in the lateral sulcus of macaque monkeys. *J. Neurosci.* 15:3821–3839.

Langner, G., M. Sames, P. Heil, and H. Schultze, 1997. Frequency and periodicity are represented in orthogonal maps in the human auditory cortex: Evidence from magnetoencephalography. *J. Comp. Physiol. A* 181:665–676.

Lashley, K. S., and G. Clark, 1946. The cytoarchitecture of the cerebral cortex of Ateles: A critical examination of architectonic studies. *J. Comp. Neurol.* 85:223–306.

Lauter, J. L., P. Herscovitch, C. Formby, M. E. Raichle, 1985. Tonotopic organization in human auditory cortex revealed by positron emission tomography. *Hear. Res.* 2:199–205.

Lewis, J. W., and D. C. Van Essen, 2000. Corticocortical connections of visual, sensorimotor, and multimodal processing areas in the parietal lobe of the macaque monkey. *J. Comp. Neurol.* 428:112–137.

Liegeois-Chauvel, C., Laguitton, V., J. M. Badier, D. Schwartz, and P. Chauvel, 1995. Cortical mechanisms of auditive perception in man: Contribution of cerebral potentials and evoked magnetic fields by auditive stimulations. *Rev. Neurol. (Paris)* 151:495–504.

Linden, J. F., A. Grunewald, A., and R. A. Andersen, 1999. Responses to auditory stimuli in macaque lateral intraparietal area II: Behavioral modulation. *J. Neurophysiol.* 82:343–358.

Lockwood, A. H., R. J. Salvi, M. L. Coad, S. A. Arnold, D. S. Wack, B. W. Murphy, and R. F. Burkard, 1999. The functional anatomy of the normal human auditory system: Responses to 0.5 and 4.0 kHz tones at varied intensities. *Cereb. Cortex* 9:65–76.

Luethke, L. E., L. A. Krubitzer, and J. H. Kaas, 1989. Connections of primary auditory cortex in the New World monkey, Saguinus. *J. Comp. Neurol.* 285:487–513.

Lutkenhoner, B., and O. Steinstrater, 1998. High-precision neuromagnetic study of the functional organization of the human auditory cortex. *Audiol. Neurootol.* 3:191–213.

Maeder, P. P., R. A. Meuli, M. Adriani, A. Bellmann, E. Fornari, J. P. Thiran, A. Pittet, and S. Clarke, 2001. Distinct pathways involved in sound recognition and localization: A human fMRI study. *NeuroImage* 14:802–816.

Martinkauppi, S., P. Rama, J. H. Aronen, A. Korvenoja, and S. Carlson, 2000. Working memory of auditory localization. *Cereb. Cortex* 10:889–898.

Mauss, T., 1908. Die faserarchitektonische Gliederung der Grosshirnrinde bei den niederen Affen. *J. Psych. Neurol.* 13:263–325.

Mazzoni, P., R. M. Bracewell, S. Barash, and R. A. Andersen, 1996. Spatially tuned auditory responses in area LIP of macaques performing delayed memory saccades to acoustic targets. *J. Neurophysiol.* 75:1233–1241.

Merzenich, M. M., and J. F. Brugge, 1973. Representation of the cochlear partition on the superior temporal plane of the macaque monkey. *Brain Res.* 50:275–296.

Mettler, F. A., 1935. Corticofugal fiber connections of the cortex of *Macaca mulatta*: The temporal region. *J. Comp. Neurol.* 61:25–47.

Middlebrooks, J. C., 2002. Auditory space processing: Here, there or everywhere? *Nat. Neurosci.* 5:824–826.

Mistlin, A. H., and D. L. Perrett, 1990. Visual and somatosensory processing in the macaque temporal cortex: The role of "expectation". *Exp. Brain Res.* 82:437–450.

Morel, A., P. E. Garraghty, and J. H. Kaas, 1993. Tonotopic organization, architectonic fields, and connections of auditory cortex in macaque monkeys. *J. Comp. Neurol.* 335:437–459.

Morel, A., and J. H. Kaas, 1992. Subdivisions and connections of auditory cortex in owl monkeys. *J. Comp. Neurol.* 318:27–63.

Mummery, C. J., J. Ashburner, S. K. Scott, and R. J. S. Wise, 1999. Functional neuroimaging of speech perception in six normal and two aphasic subjects. *J. Acoust. Soc. Am.* 106:449–547.

Neal, J. W., R. C. Pearson, and T. P. Powell, 1990. The connections of area PG, 7a, with cortex in the parietal, occipital, and temporal lobes of the monkey. *Brain Res.* 532:249–264.

Newman, J. D., 1988. Primate hearing mechanisms. In *Comparative Primate Biology*, H. D. Steklis and J. Erwin, eds. vol. 4, New York: Alan R. Liss, pp. 469–499.

Ottaviani, F., S. Di Girolamo, G. Briglia, G. de Rossi, D. Di Giuda, and W. Di Nardo, 1997. Tonotopic organization of human auditory cortex analyzed by SPET. *Audiology* 36:241–248.

Pandya, D. N., M. Hallett, and S. K. Mukherjee, 1969. Intra- and interhemispheric connections of the neocortical auditory system in the rhesus monkey. *Brain Res.* 14:49–65.

Pandya, D. N., and H. G. J. M. Kuypers, 1969. Cortico-cortical connections in the rhesus monkey. *Brain Res.* 13:13–36.

Pandya, D. N., and F. Sanides, 1973. Architectonic parcellation of the temporal operculum in rhesus monkey and its projection pattern. *Z. Anat. Entwickl. Gesch.* 139:127–161.

Pantev, C., O. Bertand, C. Eulitz, C. Verkindt, S. Hampson, G. Schuierer, and T. Elbert, 1995. Specific tonotopic organizations of different areas of the human auditory cortex revealed by simultaneous magnetic and electric recordings. *Electroencephalog. Clin. Neurophysiol.* 94:26–40.

Pantev, C., M. Hoke, K. Lehnertz, B. Lutkenhoner, G. Anogianakis, and W. Wittkowski, 1988. Tonotopic organization of the human auditory cortex revealed by transient auditory evoked magnetic fields. *Electroencephalog. Clin. Neurophysiol.* 69:160–170.

Papanicolaou, A. C., E. Catillo, J. I. Breier, R. N. Davis, P. G. Simos, and R. L. Diehl, 2003. Differential brain activation patterns during perception of voice and tone onset time series: A MEG study. *NeuroImage* 18:448–459.

Patterson R. D., S. Uppenkamp, I. S. Johnsrude, and T. D. Griffiths, 2002. The processing of temporal pitch and melody information in auditory cortex. *Neuron* 36:767–776.

Paulesu, E., C. D. Frith, and R. S. J. Frackowiak, 1993. The neural correlates of the verbal component of working memory. *Nature* 362:342–345.

Petersen, S. E., P. T. Fox, M. I. Posner, M. Mintun, and M. E. Raichle, 1988. Positron emission tomographic studies of the cortical anatomy of single-word processing. *Nature* 331:585–589.

Petrides, M., B. Alivisatos, and A. C. Evans, 1995. Functional activation of the human ventrolateral frontal cortex during mnemonic retrieval of verbal information. *Proc. Natl. Acad. Sci. U.S.A.* 92:5803–5807.

Petrides, M., and D. N. Pandya, 2002. Comparative cytoarchitectonic analysis of the human and the macaque ventrolateral prefrontal cortex and corticocortical connection patterns in the monkey. *Eur. J. Neurosci.* 16:291–310.

Price, C. J, 2000. The anatomy of language: Contributions from functional imaging. *J. Anat.* 197:335–359.

Price, C., R. Wise, S. Ramsay, K. Friston, D. Howard, K. Patterson, and R. Frackowiak, 1992. Regional response differences within the human auditory cortex when listening to words. *Neurosci. Lett.* 146:179–182.

RADEMACHER, J., V. CAVINESS, H. STEINMETZ, and A. GALABURDA, 1993. Topographical variation of the human primary cortices: Implications for neuroimaging, brain mapping and neurobiology. *Cereb. Cortex* 3:313–329.

RAUSCHECKER, J. P., and B. TIAN, 2000. Mechanisms and streams for processing of "what" and "where" in auditory cortex. *Proc. Natl. Acad. Sci. U.S.A.* 97:11800–11806.

RAUSCHECKER, J. P., 1998. Parallel processing in the auditory cortex of primates. *Audiol. Neurootol.* 3:86–103.

RAUSCHECKER, J. P., B. TIAN, and M. HAUSER, 1995. Processing of complex sounds in the macaque nonprimary auditory cortex. *Science* 268:111–114.

RAUSCHECKER, J. P., B. TIAN, T. PONS, and M. MISHKIN, 1997. Serial and parallel processing in rhesus monkey auditory cortex. *J. Comp. Neurol.* 382:89–103.

RECANZONE, G. H., 2000. Spatial processing in the auditory cortex of the macaque monkey. *Proc. Natl. Acad. Sci. U.S.A.* 97: 11829–11835.

RECANZONE, G. H., 2001. Spatial processing in the primate auditory cortex. *Audiol. Neurootol.* 6:178–181.

RECANZONE, G. H., D. C. GUARD, and M. L. PHAN, 2000. Frequency and intensity response properties of single neurons in the auditory cortex of the behaving macaque monkey. *J. Neurophysiol.* 83:2315–2331.

RECANZONE, G. H., D. C. GUARD, M. L. PHAN, and T. I. K. SU, 2000. Correlation between the activity of single auditory cortical neurons and sound-localization behavior in the macaque monkey. *J. Neurophysiol.* 83:2723–2739.

RIVIER, F., and S. CLARKE, 1997. Cytochrome oxidase, acetylcholinesterase, and NADPH-diaphorase staining in human supratemporal and insular cortex: Evidence for multiple auditory areas. *NeuroImage* 6:288–304.

ROBINSON, C. J., and H. BURTON, 1980a. Organization of somatosensory receptive fields in cortical areas 7b, retroinsula, postauditory and granular insula of *M. fascicularis. J. Comp. Neurol.* 192:69–92.

ROBINSON, C. J., and H. BURTON, 1980b. Somatic submodality distribution within the second somatsensory (SII), b, retroinsular, postauditory, and granular insular cortical areas of *M. fascicularis. J. Comp. Neurol.* 192:93–108.

ROMANI, G. L., S. J. WILLIAMSON, and L. KAUFMAN, 1982. Tonotopic organization of the human auditory cortex. *Science* 216:1339–1340.

ROMANSKI, L. M., J. F. BATES, and P. S. GOLDMAN-RAKIC, 1999. Auditory belt and parabelt projections to the prefrontal cortex in the rhesus monkey. *J. Comp. Neurol.* 403:141–157.

ROMANSKI, L. M., B. TIAN, J. FRITZ, M. MISHKIN, P. GOLDMAN-RAKIC, and J. P. RAUSCHECKER, 1999. Dual streams of auditory afferents target multiple domains in the primate prefrontal cortex. *Nat. Neurosci.* 2:1131–1136.

ROMANSKI, L. M., and P. S. GOLDMAN-RAKIC, 2002. An auditory domain in primate prefrontal cortex. *Nat. Neurosci.* 5:15–16.

ROSBURG, T., I. KREITSCHMANN-ANDERMAHR, E. EMMERICH, H. NOWAK, and H. SAUER, 1998. Hemispheric differences in frequency dependent dipole orientation of the human auditory evoked field component N100m. *Neurosci. Lett.* 258:105–108.

RUSSO, G. S., and C. J. BRUCE, 1989. Auditory receptive fields of neurons in frontal cortex of rhesus monkey shift with direction of gaze. *Soc. Neurosci. Abstr.* 15:1204.

SALEEM, K. S., W. SUZUKI, K. TANAKA, and T. HASHIKAWA, 2000. Connections between anterior inferotemporal cortex and superior temporal sulcus regions in the macaque monkey. *J. Neurosci.* 20:5083–5101.

SCHLACK, A., 2002. *Multimodal Encoding of Space and Motion in Primate Ventral Intraparietal Area.* Doctoral dissertation, Ruhr University, Bochum.

SCHLAPESKE, J., S. L. ROSSELL, P. W. R. WOODRUFF, and A. S. DAVID, 1999. The planum temporale: A systematic, quantitative review of its structural, functional and clinical significance. *Brain Res. Rev.* 29:26–49.

SCHONWIESNER, M., D. Y. VON CRAMON, and R. RUBSAMEN, 2002. Is it tonotopy after all? *NeuroImage* 17:1144–1161.

SCHROEDER, C. E., R. W. LENDSLEY, C. SPECHT, A. MARCOVICI, J. F. SMILEY, and D. C. JAVITT, 2001. Somatosensory input to auditory association cortex in the macaque monkey. *J. Neurophysiol.* 85:1322–1327.

SCOTT, S. K., C. C. BLANK, S. ROSEN, and R. J. S. WISE, 2000. Identification of a pathway for intelligible speech in the left temporal lobe. *Brain* 123:2400–2406.

SCOTT, S. K., and I. S. JOHNSRUDE, 2003. The neuroanatomical and functional organization of speech perception. *Trends Neurosci.* 26:100–107.

SEIFRITZ, E., F. ESPOSITO, F. HENNEL, H. MUSTOVID, J. G. NEUHOFF, D. BILECEN, G. TEDESCHI, K. SCHEFFLER, and F. DI SALLE, 2002. Spatio-temporal pattern of neural processing in the human auditory cortex. *Science* 297:1706–1708.

SEIFRITZ, E., F. ESPOSITO, J. G. NEUHOFF, and F. DI SALLE, 2003. Response: Sound analysis in auditory cortex—from temporal decomposition to perception. *Trends Neurosci.* 26:231–232.

SELEZNEVA, E., S. HENNING, E. BUDINGER, and M. BROSCH, 2003. Spatial organisation of response properties in the primary and the caudomedial field of monkey's auditory cortex. *Assoc. Res. Otolaryngol. Abstr.* 338.

SELTZER, B., and D. N. PANDYA, 1978. Afferent cortical connections and architectonics of the superior temporal sulcus and surrounding cortex in the rhesus monkey. *Brain Res.* 149: 1–24.

SELTZER, B., and D. N. PANDYA, 1991. Post-rolandic cortical projections of the superior temporal sulcus in the rhesus monkey. *J. Comp. Neurol.* 312:625–640.

SELTZER, B., and D. N. PANDYA, 1994. Parietal, temporal, and occipital projections to cortex of the superior temporal sulcus in the rhesus monkey: A retrograde tracer study. *J. Comp. Neurol.* 343:445–463.

SELTZER, B., M. G. COLA, C. GUTIERREZ, M. MASSEE, C. WELDON, and C. G. CUSICK, 1996. Overlapping and nonoverlapping cortical projections to cortex of the superior temporal sulcus in the rhesus monkey: Double anterograde tracer studies. *J. Comp. Neurol.* 370:173–190.

STRAINER, J. C., J. L. ULMER, F. Z. YETKIN, V. M. HAUGHTON, D. L. DANIELS, S. J. MILLEN, 1997. Functional MR of the primary auditory cortex: An analysis of pure tone activation and tone discrimination. *Am. J. Neuroradiol.* 18:601–610.

STRICANNE, B., and R. A. ANDERSON, 1996. Eye-centered, head-centered, and intermediate coding of remembered sound locations in area LIP. *J. Neurophysiol.* 76:2071–2076.

SUGAR, O., J. D. FRENCH, and J. G. CHUSID, 1948. Corticocortical connections of the superior surface of the temporal operculum in the monkey (*Macaca mulatta*). *J. Neurophysiol.* 11:175–184.

SUZUKI, H., 1985. Distribution and organization of visual and auditory neurons in the monkey prefrontal cortex. *Vis. Res.* 25:465–469.

TALAVAGE, T. M., P. J. LEDDEN, R. R. BENSON, B. R. ROSEN, and J. R. MELCHER, 2000. Frequency-dependent responses exhibited by multiple regions in human auditory cortex. *Hear. Res.* 150:225–244.

TALAVAGE, T. M., P. J. LEDDEN, M. I. SERENO, B. R. ROSEN, and A. M. DALE, 1997. Multiple phase-encoded tonotopic maps in human auditory cortex. *NeuroImage* 5:S8.

THIVARD, L., P. BELIN, M. ZILBOVICIOUS, J.-B. POLINE, and Y. SAMSON, 2000. A cortical region sensitive to auditory spectral motion. *Neuroreport* 11:2969–2972.

THORPE, S. J., E. T. ROLLS, and S. MADDISON, 1983. The orbitofrontal cortex: Neuronal activity in the behaving monkey. *Exp. Brain Res.* 49:93–115.

TIAN, B., D. RESER, A. DURHAM, A. KUSTOV, J. P. RAUSCHECKER, 2001. Functional specialization in rhesus monkey auditory cortex. *Science* 292:290–293.

TIITINEN, H., K. ALHO, R. HUOTILAINEN, R. J. ILMONIENI, J. SIMOLA, and R. NAATANEN, 1993. Tonotopic auditory cortex and the magnetoencephalographic (MEG) equivalent of the mismatch negativity. *Psychophysiology* 30:S537–S540.

UNGERLEIDER, L. G., and M. MISHKIN, 1982. Two cortical visual systems. In *Analysis of Visual Behavior*, D. J. Ingle, M. A. Goodale, and R. J. W. Mansfield, eds. Cambridge, Mass.: MIT Press, pp. 549–586.

VAADIA, E., 1989. Single-unit activity related to active localization of acoustic and visual stimuli in the frontal cortex of the rhesus monkey. *Brain Behav. Evol.* 33:127–131.

VAADIA, E., D. A. BENSON, R. D. HEINZ, and M. H. GOLDSTEIN JR., 1986. Unit study of monkey frontal cortex: Active localization of auditory and of visual stimuli. *J. Neurophysiol.* 56:934–952.

VERKINDT, C., O. BERTRAND, F. PERRIN, J. F. ECHALLIER, and J. PERNIER, 1995. Tonotopic organization of the human auditory cortex: N100 topography and multiple dipole model analysis. *Electroencaphalog. Clin. Neurophysiol.* 96:143–156.

VON ECONOMO, C., and G. N. KOSKINAS, 1925. *Die Cytoarchitectonik der Hirnrinde des erwachsenen Menschen.* Berlin: Julius Springer.

WALLACE, M. N., P. W. JOHNSTON, and A. R. PALMER, 2002. Histochemical identification of cortical areas in the auditory region of the human brain. *Exp. Brain Res.* 143:499–508.

WARD, A. A., JR., J. K. PEDEN, and O. SUGAR., 1946. Cortico-cortical connections in the monkey with special reference to area 6. *J. Neurophysiol.* 9:453–461.

WARREN, J. D., B. A. ZIELINSKI, G. G. GREEN, J. P. RAUSCHECKER, and T. D. GRIFFITHS, 2002. Perception of sound-source motion by the human brain. *Neuron.* 34:139–148.

WATANABE, M., 1992. Frontal units of the monkey coding the associative significance of visual and auditory stimuli. *Exp. Brain Res.* 89:233–247.

WEEKS, R. A., A. AZIZ-SULTAN, K. O. BUSHARA, B. TIAN, C. M. WESSINGER, N. DANG, J. P. RAUSCHECKER, and M. HALLETT, 1999. A PET study of human auditory spatial processing. *Neurosci. Lett.* 262:155–158.

WERNER-REISS, U., K. A. KELLY, A. S. TRAUSE, A. M. UNDERHILL, and J. M. GROH, 2003. Eye position affects activity in primary auditory cortex of primates. *Curr. Biol.* 13:554–562.

WESSINGER, C. M., M. H. BUONOCORE, C. L. KUSSMAUL, and G. R. MANGUN, 1997. Tonotopy in human auditory cortex examined with functional magenetic resonance imaging. *Hum. Brain Mapp.* 5:18–25.

WESSINGER, C. M., J. VANMETER, B. TIAN, J. VAN LARE, J. PEKAR, and J. P. RAUSCHECKER, 2001. Hierahical organization of the human auditory cortex revealed by functional magnetic resonance imaging. *J. Cogn. Neurosci.* 13:1–7.

WISE, R., F. CHOLLET, U. HADAR, K. FRISTON, E. HOFFNER, and R. FRACKOWIAK, 1991. Distribution of cortical neural networks involved in word comprehension and word retrieval. *Brain* 114:1803–1817.

WISE, R. J., J. GREENE, C. BUCHEL, and S. K. SCOTT, 1999. Brain regions involved in articulation. *Lancet* 353:1057–1061.

WISE, R. J., S. K. SCOTT, S. C. BLANK, C. J. MUMMERY, K. MURPHY, and E. A. WARBURTON, 2001. Separate neural subsystems within "Wernicke's area." *Brain* 124:83–95.

WOLLBERG, Z., and J. SELA, 1980. Frontal cortex of the awake squirrel monkey: Responses of single cells to visual and auditory stimuli. *Brain Res.* 198:216–220.

WOOLSEY, C. N., and E. M. WALZL, 1982. Cortical auditory area of *Macaca mulatta* and its relation to the second somatic sensory area (Sm II). In *Cortical Sensory Organization. Multiple Auditory Areas*, C. N. Woolsey, ed. New Jersey: Humana, pp. 231–256.

WONG, D., D. B. PISONI, J. LEARN, J. T. GANDOUR, R. T. MIYAMOTO, and G. D. HUTCHINS, 2002. PET imaging of differential cortical activation by monaural speech and nonspeech stimuli. *Hear. Res.* 166:9–23.

YAMAMOTO, T., T. UEMURA, R. LLINAS, 1992. Tonotopic organization of human auditory cortex revealed by multi-channel SQUID system. *Acta Otolaryngol.* 112:201–204.

ZATORRE, R. J., 2003. Sound analysis in auditory cortex. *Trends Neurosci.* 26:229–230.

ZATORRE, R. J., M. BOUFFARD, P. AHAD, and P. BELIN, 2002. Where is "where" in the human auditory cortex? *Nat. Neurosci.* 5:905–909.

ZATORRE, R. J., T. A. MONDOR, and A. C. EVANS, 1999. Auditory attention to space and frequency activates similar cerebral systems. *NeuroImage* 10:544–554.

17 A New Foundation for the Visual Cortical Hierarchy

JONATHAN C. HORTON AND LAWRENCE C. SINCICH

ABSTRACT The primate visual system is often schematized into dorsal (magno) and ventral (parvo, konio) streams. This dichotomy is based, in part, on the pattern of projections from V1 to V2 established nearly 20 years ago by tracer studies. These early studies showed just three V1 outputs, proposed to convey information about a single visual attribute (color, form, or motion) to a single V2 compartment (thin, pale, or thick stripe). New data reveal a more complex innervation pattern, with projections arising from multiple layers (2, 3, 4A, 4B, 5, 6) to each stripe compartment in V2. In the upper layers, these projections are divided by cytochrome oxidase: patches to thin stripes, interpatches to pale and thick stripes. These studies suggest extensive intermingling of parvo/magno signals in pale/thick stripes, and provide a new foundation for the segregation of visual information in the cortical hierarchy.

Our most enduring concepts about the brain are founded on the bedrock of anatomy. One can always debate the interpretation of a physiological response: How should a neuron's receptive field be mapped and defined? What does it mean when a cell fires? Anatomy does not trifle with ambiguity. It provides physical facts about the nervous system. These facts can seem tedious, even trivial, but they supply a tangible basis for understanding brain function.

A generation ago, visual neuroscience was in the throes of a debate about how information is disseminated from the primary visual cortex (V1) to higher visual areas in the primate brain. Traditionalists believed that the visual image is first digested in V1, and then passed essentially intact through a series of higher cortical areas for further processing to elaborate perceptions. Revisionists proposed that images are broken down by V1 into components of color, form, and motion. These components are then distributed via parallel projections to extrastriate areas specialized for their analysis. The matter was settled by a series of landmark studies conducted by Livingstone and Hubel (1984, 1987). First, they identified three compartments in V1 corresponding to color, form, and motion. Second, they demonstrated that each compartment sends a segregated projection to a distinct compartment in the next visual area (V2). Finally,

they showed that the compartments in V2 are also divided by color, form, and motion.

Livingstone and Hubel's work furnished powerful support for the idea that color, form, and motion can be assigned to distinct cortical compartments in V1 and V2. Their studies were particularly compelling because they were built on a foundation of anatomy. We have undertaken a reexamination of the projections from V1 to V2 and have discovered a pattern of connections that conflicts with Livingstone and Hubel's original description. The discrepancies highlighted by our new anatomical data cast doubt on their account of the projections from V1 to V2 and force a reconsideration of how color, form, and motion are segregated in the early visual cortex.

Color, form, and motion: The prevailing view

To a student consulting any standard neuroscience textbook, the basic organization of the central visual pathways appears to be clearly established. The pathway serving perception begins with a projection from the retina to a thalamic relay station called the lateral geniculate body. It supplies the primary visual cortex with input from two major cell classes, parvocellular and magnocellular. These cell classes have distinctive receptive field properties that reflect a fundamental dichotomy in the visual system (Shapley, 1995). The receptive fields of parvo cells are color-coded and have high spatial resolution. These units convey information about color and form along a ventral stream to an area in the prelunate gyrus called V4, and ultimately to the temporal lobe, where object recognition takes place. The receptive fields of magno cells are color-blind, but have excellent contrast sensitivity and temporal resolution. These cells transmit information about motion and depth along a dorsal stream to an area in the superior temporal sulcus called MT, and to other parietal lobe areas concerned with spatial localization and movement. Although the primate visual system is daunting in its complexity, in conceptual terms it has been distilled to "what" (ventral) versus "where" (dorsal) systems, generated predominately by parvo and magno cells, respectively (Ungerleider and Mishkin, 1982; Van Essen, 1985; Maunsell and Newsome, 1987; Livingstone and Hubel, 1988; Zeki and Shipp, 1988; Van Essen and Gallant, 1994).

JONATHAN C. HORTON and LAWRENCE C. SINCICH Beckman Vision Center, University of California, San Francisco, Calif.

This conventional picture has required slight modification following the discovery of a koniocellular class of cells in the lateral geniculate body. This third class is defined by immunostaining for the α subunit of type II calmodulin-dependent protein kinase (Hendry and Yoshioka, 1994). Why konio cells preferentially express this enzyme is unknown, but it serves as a handy label to identify a previously neglected population. It has become clear that konio cells are a remarkably diverse group of neurons in their receptive field properties. Some konio cells in ventral geniculate laminae, for example, have magno-like responses. Many in dorsal laminae have blue-ON/yellow-OFF receptive fields (Hendry and Reid, 2000), raising the possibility that the blue/yellow color axis is handled by konio cells, whereas the red/green axis is mediated by parvo cells. Textbooks either have ignored the existence of konio cells (Kandel, Schwartz, and Jessel, 2000; Purves et al., 2001) or have elected to lump them with parvo cells, because both classes contribute to color processing (Nicholls et al., 2001). According to updated schemes, the ventral stream is supplied by parvo/konio cells and the dorsal stream is fed by magno cells.

Functional compartments revealed by cytochrome oxidase

Convincing evidence for the model outlined above has come from studies that have traced the connections of magno, parvo, and konio channels through the early stages of the visual system. In this endeavor, the mitochrondrial enzyme cytochrome oxidase (CO) has proved a valuable tool (Wong-Riley, 1989). It has revealed in V1 a regular array of dark patches (also called blobs or puffs) in tangential sections (Horton and Hubel, 1981). These patches form interrupted pillars, visible in cortex from white matter to pial surface, except in layers 4C and 4A (Horton, 1984). Livingstone and Hubel (1984) reported, based on tangential electrode penetrations through the superficial layers, that patch cells have center-surround, color-opponent receptive fields. Subsequently it was observed that individual patches are dedicated to a single type of color opponency: red/green or blue/yellow (Ts'o and Gilbert, 1988). These physiological studies have provided persuasive evidence that patches constitute a specialization for color processing in the primate visual system. It also has been shown that all patches in the upper layers receive a direct projection from geniculate konio cells (Hendry and Yoshioka, 1994). This reinforces the notion that patches represent color, but raises a new question: Why is blue/yellow (konio) input not detectable in patches devoted to red/green? It also remains to be determined how red/green parvo color information reaches the patches in the upper layers. Parvocellular input to V1 terminates diffusely in layer 4Cβ. Presumably, red/green color signals are conveyed selectively to the patches in the upper layers via intracortical circuits (Callaway, 1998).

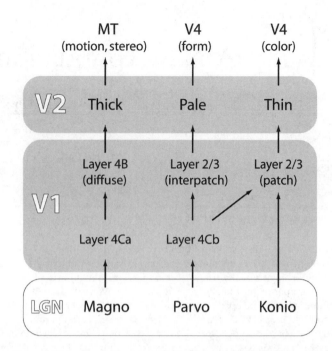

FIGURE 17.1   Prevailing view of the flow of visual signals through the early portions of the central visual pathway in primates, showing three channels in the lateral geniculate nucleus (LGN) that are propagated to extrastriate cortex. The crucial feature of this scheme is that each class of V2 stripe gets input from a single V1 source. Signals concerning motion/stereo, form, and color are segregated in V1, V2, and higher visual areas.

The cortex between patches, known colloquially as the interpatch or interblob compartment, has been assigned the role of processing information about form. Livingstone and Hubel (1984) reported that interpatch cells are selective for stimulus orientation, thereby qualifying them for the task of recognizing shapes. Interpatch cells were also characterized as not "explicitly color-coded," although "they probably receive their inputs from explicitly color-coded parvocellular geniculate cells" (Livingstone and Hubel, 1988). Thus, color and form were proposed to be encoded separately in patches and interpatches, respectively, leading to the idea of separate processing of these attributes (figure 17.1).

The magno input to V1 terminates in layer 4Cα. This layer projects strongly to layer 4B. Livingstone and Hubel described cells in layer 4B as oriented, direction selective, and lacking color selectivity (Livingstone and Hubel, 1984). This magno dominated layer was deemed to constitute the motion and stereo channel in V1.

Soon after patches were discovered in V1, the CO method was applied to V2. It yielded another surprising pattern: coarse parallel stripes stretching across V2 from the V1 border to the V3 border, organized in repeating cycles of pale-thick-pale-thin (Tootell et al., 1983; Horton, 1984). No prior anatomical or physiological studies had given a hint of this striking feature of the functional architecture in V2. Once V1 patches and V2 stripes were identified, it became paramount to probe their links. Livingstone and Hubel (1984) undertook this challenge by making injections of a retrograde tracer, wheat germ–conjugated horseradish peroxidase (WGA-HRP), into individual V2 stripes. They found retrogradely labeled cells only in layers 2/3 of V1, clustered with an impressive degree of specificity. Patches projected to thin stripes, interpatches to pale stripes, and both patches and interpatches to thick stripes. In a subsequent report, Livingstone and Hubel (1987) retracted the finding of an upper layer projection to thick stripes and reported instead that thick stripes are supplied exclusively by layer 4B. Their final version of the projections was: layers 2/3 patches → thin stripes; layers 2/3 interpatches → pale stripes; layer 4B patches and interpatches → thick stripes (figure 17.1).

These anatomical studies by Livingstone and Hubel, identifying three parallel V1 inputs to the three classes of V2 stripes, furnished the strongest evidence in favor of the idea that color, form, and motion/stereo are segregated in the cortex. Further corroboration was provided by subsequent analysis of the efferent projections from V2 to higher areas in the visual cortical hierarchy (DeYoe and Van Essen, 1985; Shipp and Zeki, 1985). Thin (color) stripes were found to connect to V4, an area associated previously with color perception (Zeki, 1980). Thick (stereo and motion) stripes were reported to project to MT, an area thought to be specialized for motion perception. Finally, pale (form) stripes were determined to connect to V4, within subregions distinct from those supplied by thin stripes (DeYoe et al., 1994). A consensus emerged that form, color, and motion are indeed processed by separate pathways that originate early in the visual system (figure 17.1). This view has prevailed for the past 20 years, with only a few murmurs of dissent (Martin, 1988; Merigan and Maunsell, 1993).

Exploring connections in flatmounts

We have undertaken a systematic reexamination of the pattern of connections from V1 to the three types of CO stripes in V2. At first glance, this project seems quite straightforward. Several technical obstacles, however, conspire to make it a difficult proposition. In macaques, only a narrow strip of V2 lies on the surface of the cortex. Consequently, sections cut tangentially to the exposed occipital surface (known as the operculum) capture only a small portion of the V2 stripe pattern, located near the V1 border. From this fragment it is often difficult to decide if a stripe should be classified as pale, thin, or thick. To mitigate this problem, we have adopted the approach of unfolding and flattening the cortex prior to histological processing (Olavarria and Van Sluyters, 1985; Tootell and Silverman, 1985). Figure 17.2 shows an example of a flatmount of the entire cerebral cortex from a macaque. The preparation of such flatmount specimens represents a valuable innovation in neuro-

anatomy, because it enables one to trace the connections from a given area throughout the entire cerebral cortex in only about 20 tangential sections. One can also correlate neuronal connections with the functional architecture of individual cortical areas, revealed by using a wide variety of staining techniques (Sincich, Adams, and Horton, 2003). For studies involving only V1 and V2, we generally flatmount only the operculum and lunate sulcus, to save time and to make sections smaller for handling. In such preparations, one can visualize the whole pattern of CO staining in dorsal V2, making it easier to identify stripes reliably.

As mentioned above, only a thin strip of V2 located near the V1 border is exposed on the cortical surface, where injections can be made under direct visualization. Therefore, tracer injections must be small to prevent spillover into V1. They must also be tightly confined, to avoid contamination of adjacent stripes, because individual stripes are quite narrow (~1 mm). In this setting, gold-conjugated cholera toxin B subunit (CTB) is ideal because it diffuses less than other commonly employed tracers, such as horseradish peroxidase conjugates or fluorescent compounds. It also has the advantage of leaving a tiny purple mark at the injection site. One can determine by inspection if this "witness mark" is situated in a thin, pale, or thick stripe after the section has been reacted for CO but before the silver intensification step.

It is important to make an irrevocable assignment of each tracer injection to a V2 stripe class before silver intensification, for two reasons. First, silver intensification obscures CO staining at the injection site, making stripe identification more difficult. Second, at this stage of the experiment the results are still unknown, so one is not swayed by knowledge of the outcome in making stripe assignments. In some macaques, one cannot distinguish readily between stripe classes. The poor differentiation of stripes in some macaques is a mystery; it may reflect a genuine, natural variation in their expression from animal to animal. At any rate, it means that reliable identification of V2 stripe type in macaques is sometimes impossible. Faced with an injection in a dark stripe of uncertain ilk, it is tempting to conclude that it must have been located in a thin stripe, because patches were filled in V1. To avoid the trap of employing such circular logic, one must assign each injection to a stripe type before examining the pattern of retrograde labeling in V1.

A final virtue of CTB is that the silver intensification step is compatible with CO histochemistry, eliminating the need to process alternate sections, one for CO and one for the retrograde tracer (Livingstone and Hubel, 1984). This eliminates the potential alignment problems associated with comparing patterns in adjacent sections. The yield of data is also doubled, because every section can be reacted for both CO and CTB. In the *same* section, CO staining is visible in light-field and CTB label is visible in dark-field with crossed polarizing filters.

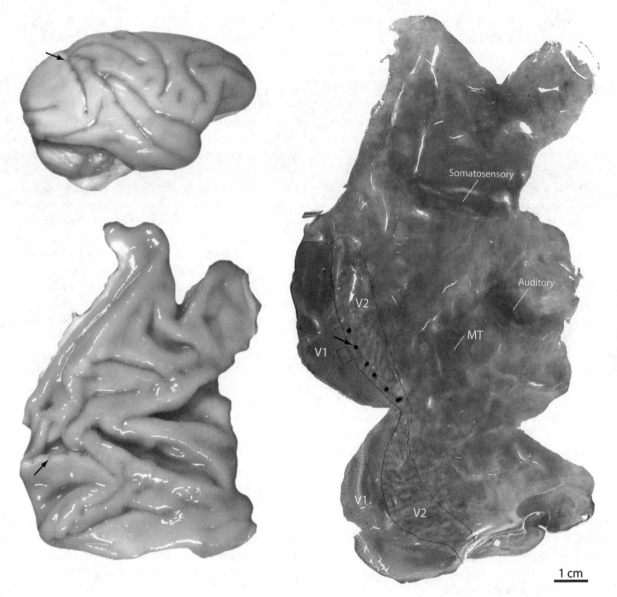

FIGURE 17.2 Unfolding the cortex aids in mapping connections between the multitude of different areas postulated in the macaque brain (Felleman and Van Essen, 1991). It also facilitates the correlation of projection patterns and columnar architecture. Here the intact right hemisphere of a macaque brain is flattened to yield tan-

gential sections of the entire cortex (Sincich, Adams, and Horton, 2003). A string of six CTB injections in V2 is visible in the CO-stained section. The arrow shows a single tracer injection in V2, with its retrograde labeling located in the boxed region in V1. This injection is featured at higher power in figure 17.3.

In 17 macaque monkeys we made 187 tracer injections, placed blindly into V2. As emphasized above, in every case the assignment of stripe type and the decision to include an injection in our data set were made before the transport results were known. Our strategy was to confine our analysis to injections that landed in a single stripe of unambiguous identity. This made it necessary to exclude the majority of injections. Of the 187 tracer injections, 110 were rejected because they were made in a stripe of uncertain identity, straddled two stripes, spread into V1, or were too small for transport. This left only 77 injections confined to a single stripe. However, from this subset a clear picture of the V1 to V2 projections emerged (Sincich and Horton, 2002a).

Reexamination of V1 to V2 projections

Figure 17.3 shows a pale stripe injection. This particular macaque is a prime example of an animal without clearly recognizable thin and thick stripes. In such cases only pale stripe injections could be used. This pale stripe injection yielded retrogradely filled cells in layers 2/3. They were concentrated in interpatches. In addition, we observed strong labeling in layer 4B. In this layer the label usually showed a strong tendency to cluster into interpatches, but there was variation from animal to animal. Here we show a case where the label was quite diffuse in layer 4B. In 31 of 33 cases, pale stripe injections yielded interpatch label in layers 2/3 and in

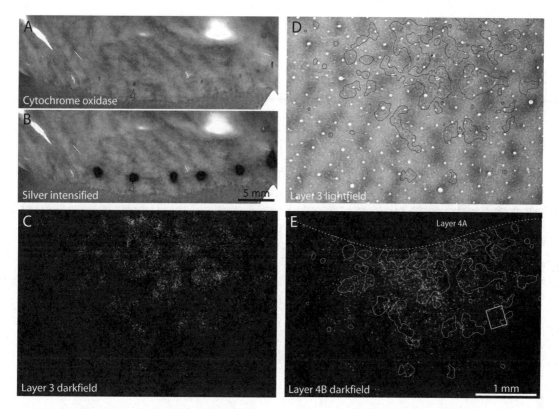

FIGURE 17.3   Pale stripe injection. (*A*) V2 stripes prior to silver intensification. The arrowhead shows an injection site in a pale stripe. In this animal, the dark stripes cannot be classified as "thin" or "thick." (*B*) Same section after silver intensification. (*C*) Retrogradely filled cells in V1, within the boxed region shown in figure 17.2. (*D*) Same section, showing the relationship between the CO patches and the clumps of labeled cells, represented by contour outlines. The cells are concentrated in the interpatches. (*E*) A deeper section, cut through layer 4B, showing more diffuse labeling. In most animals the layer 4B label was aggregated into interpatches, but this tendency is little evident in this case. Boxed region is shown in figure 17.6*A*.

layer 4B. In two cases, we observed patch label in layers 2/3. We assume that these two cases were misclassified thin stripes.

Figure 17.4 shows a case of a thin stripe injection from a different animal. There were patches of labeled cells in layers 2/3. These patches coincided perfectly with the CO patches. In addition, there was a sparse population of small cells labeled in layer 4B. These cells were located preferentially within CO patches. Thin stripe injections resulted in patch label in layers 2/3 in 17 of 17 cases and in layer 4B in 16 of 17 cases.

Figure 17.5 shows a thick stripe injection, from another animal. Labeled cells were abundant in the interpatches in layers 2/3. There were also labeled cells in layer 4B, but fewer. The layer 4B cells were large and tended to be localized to interpatches, but less strongly than the cells in layers 2/3. In all 27 cases, thick stripe injections produced interpatch label in layers 2/3 and layer 4B.

Labeled cells were also observed in layer 4A (Van Essen et al., 1986; Rockland, 1992; Levitt, Yoshioka, and Lund, 1994). After tracer injection into pale stripes and thick stripes, most labeled cells were located in areas that coincided with interpatches in other layers. After injection into thin stripes, labeled cells were most numerous in portions of layer 4A in register with patches.

Finally, large cells were labeled at the junction of layers 5/6 (Kennedy and Bullier, 1985; Van Essen et al., 1986; Rockland, 1992). These cells were distributed diffusely after tracer injection into all three classes of V2 stripes. We observed no tendency for clustering into patches or interpatches.

To summarize, we found that layers 2/3, 4A, 4B, and 5/6 projected from V1 to V2. Only layers 1 and 4C did not project to V2. In the superficial layers of V1, these projections were divided by CO: interpatches connected to pale and thick stripes, patches connected to thin stripes. To determine if segregated (but physically intermingled) interpatch populations supply either pale stripes or thick stripes, we made paired injections of different retrograde tracers into V2. In three cases we succeeded in placing injections into adjacent pale and thick stripes. Up to a third of the retrogradely filled cells in V1 were double-labeled, indicating that many interpatch cells project indiscriminately to both pale and thick stripes. In contrast, two cases of paired injections into thin and pale stripes produced only a handful of double-labeled cells out of potentially thousands.

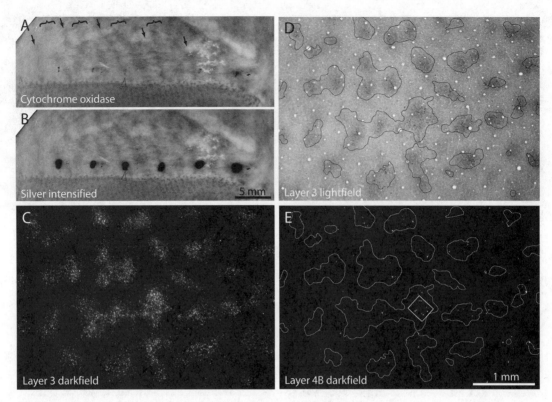

FIGURE 17.4 Thin stripe injection. (*A*) In this animal, the thin (arrows) and thick (brackets) stripes can be differentiated. The arrowhead marks the thin stripe injection featured in the subsequent panels. (*B*) Same section, after silver intensification. (*C*) Ret-rogradely filled cells in V1. (*D*) Same section, showing outlines of the retrogradely filled cells, which coincide with patches. (*E*) Cells in layer 4B are sparse, but located in patches. Boxed region is shown in figure 17.6*B*.

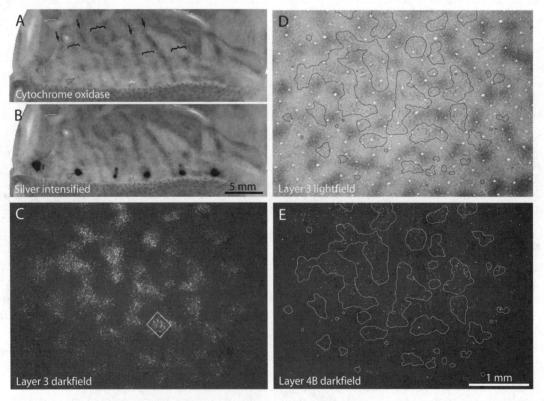

FIGURE 17.5 Thick stripe injection. (*A*) Injection site, marked by an arrowhead. Note that the second thin stripe from the left bifur-cates to form a λ. Such anomalies are common, underscoring the importance of examining the whole CO pattern in V2 before attempting to assign stripe identities. (*B*) After silver intensification. (*C*) Labeled cells in V1. Boxed region is shown in figure 17.6*C*. (*D*) Outlines, showing that labeled cells are located in interpatches. (*E*) In layer 4B, labeled cells are more numerous in interpatches.

Projections from layers 2/3 originated from separate compartments: patches and interpatches. This compartmentalization was revealed by restricting the data analysis to tracer injections that were sharply confined to single stripe types. Xiao and Felleman (2004) have reported that patches and interpatches project equally to thin stripes. Their conclusion was based on three injections thought to be in thin stripes. Their anomalous result can be explained by contamination of flanking pale stripes, which yields a mix of cell labeling in patches and interpatches. In cases where tracer injection is rigorously confined to thin stripes (e.g., figure 17.4), the labeling in V1 is overwhelmingly in patches. The dual tracer experiments mentioned above show that the segregation of patch and interpatch projections from layer 2/3 is nearly perfect (Horton and Sincich, 2004).

A new view of the V1 to V2 pathway

These studies have identified numerous projections from V1 to V2 that were previously unknown. They include outputs from layer 4B to pale stripes, layer 4B to thin stripes, and layers 2/3 to thick stripes (figure 17.6). Layers 4A and 5/6 also send projections to V2. This new account of the V1 to V2 pathway is difficult to reconcile with the prior model (figure 17.1) based on the idea that only three projections exist from V1 to V2. The old model proposed that each projection carried information about color, form, and motion to thin, pale, and thick stripes, respectively. Instead, we find that each V2 stripe type is richly supplied by all output layers of V1 (figure 17.7).

Previously, it was reported that layer 4B is a magno-dominated layer that projects exclusively to thick stripes. Although it is true that layer 4B receives strong input from magno-recipient layer 4Cα (Fitzpatrick, Lund, and Blasdell, 1985), it also receives major parvo input (Yabuta, Sawatari, and Callaway, 2001). Moreover, our data show that layer 4B projects to all stripe types in V2. In light of these facts, it is inaccurate to construe layer 4B as simply a magno channel for conveying motion information to extrastriate cortex.

Movshon and Newsome (1996) used antidromic stimulation to characterize the physiological properties of layer 4B neurons that project directly to area MT. The units were oriented and highly direction-selective. Thus, it appears that at least one subset of neurons in layer 4B does convey

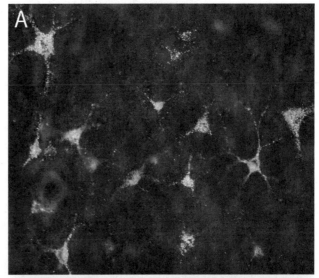
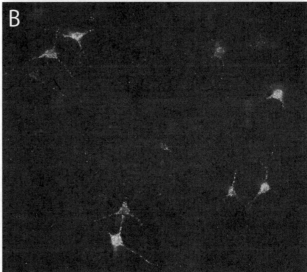
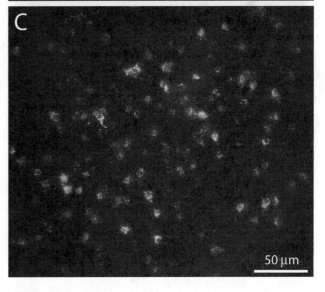

FIGURE 17.6 New projections from V1 to V2. (*A*) Layer 4B contains many large neurons that project to pale stripes. (*B*) Layer 4B also contains small neurons that project to thin stripes. Their diminutive size and location within patches suggest that they are a distinct population from layer 4B cells that project to pale or thick stripes. (*C*) Layer 2/3 interpatches send a dense projection to thick stripes. All panels to scale.

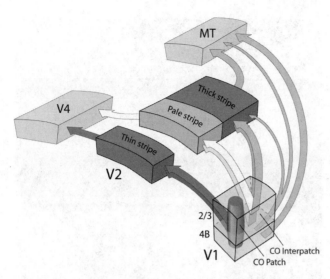

FIGURE 17.7 New model of projections from V1 to extrastriate cortex. These are divided by CO compartment: patches (layers 2, 3, 4A, 4B) → thin stripes; interpatches (layers 2, 3, 4A, 4B) → pale and thick stripes. In addition, large cells at the layer 5/6 junction project diffusely to all three stripe types (not shown). Two additional populations arise from layer 4B: one projects uniquely to area MT and the other sends a branching axon to V2 and MT.

information about motion direction to area MT. Do these same units project to area V2? To address this issue, we injected MT and V2 with different tracers and examined the retrogradely filled cells in layer 4B (Sincich and Horton, 2003). Only about 5% of cells were double-labeled. This result means that distinct populations of cells in layer 4B supply areas V2 and MT, underscoring the specificity of intercortical connections. The next step is to test the receptive field properties of 4B cells that project to V2. It is possible they are magno-dominated and direction-selective, as suggested by Livingstone and Hubel (1988). In that case, one is faced with the dilemma that layer 4B cells project to both pale and thick stripes, but only thick stripes project to area MT. Perhaps cells in layer 4B are more heterogeneous than previously conceived, with magno-dominated units going to thick stripes and parvo/konio-dominated units to pale stripes. Such an arrangement might rescue the concept that motion and form channels are strictly segregated in the V1 to V2 pathway, at least in layer 4B. It remains to be determined what signals are carried by the small population of layer 4B cells in patches that project to thin stripes.

In the upper layers of V1 it is more difficult to sustain the idea that motion and form signals are well segregated. Livingstone and Hubel (1988) proposed a form pathway comprised of parvo signals that flows from layer 4Cβ via layer 2/3 interpatches to V2 pale stripes. This model has been contradicted by subsequent studies showing that interpatches in the upper layers receive a mixed parvo/magno input (Lachica, Beck, and Casagrande, 1992; Yoshioka, Levitt, and Lund, 1994; Callaway and Wiser, 1996). We now

show that interpatch neurons project to both pale and thick stripes, rather than just to pale stripes. Of course, segregation of form and motion could still be preserved at the level of individual neurons. For example, parvo-dominated "form" neurons might project to pale stripes and magno-dominated "motion" neurons to thick stripes. This notion, however, is difficult to reconcile with our double-label experiment showing that the axons of individual interpatch cells often terminate in both pale stripes and thick stripes.

The most striking feature uncovered by our experiments is that V1 projections to V2 are defined by CO: patches → thin stripes, interpatches → pale stripes and thick stripes. This compartmentalization in V1 is strong for the upper layers, weak in layers 4A and 4B, and absent in layers 5/6. The crucial issue is to identify what properties are being segregated by CO. Livingstone and Hubel (1984, 1988) have proposed that the function of patches is color processing. Although cells within patches certainly contribute to color processing, there is substantial evidence to suggest that patches do not represent a specialization for color. First, patches are also present in the owl monkey, bush baby, and cat (Horton, 1984; Murphy, Jones, and Van Sluyters, 1995). These species have rudimentary color vision. Second, patches receive major input from layer 4Cα (Lachica, Beck, and Casagrande, 1992; Yoshioka, Levitt, and Lund, 1994; Yabuta and Callaway, 1998). If patches are for color, it is not easy to explain why they receive such strong magno input. Third, in the bush baby and owl monkey, there is no difference in the orientation tuning of cells in patches versus interpatches (DeBruyn et al., 1993; O'Keefe et al., 1998). This undermines the notion that patches contain exclusively nonoriented, color-coded units. Perhaps species variation, or the poor color vision of the bush baby and owl monkey, explains this contradictory result. But at least one study in macaque has found no relationship between CO staining, color tuning, and orientation selectivity (Leventhal et al., 1995). Fourth, color-coded cells in macaque V1 often demonstrate a high degree of orientation selectivity (Johnson, Hawken, and Shapley, 2001). Such units, according to Livingstone and Hubel (1984), should be located outside patches, because they are oriented.

Our findings help explain the controversy surrounding the correlation of receptive field properties with stripe type in V2. Perpetuating the purported divisions of V1, Hubel and Livingstone (1987) reported segregation of form, color, and stereopsis in V2. They found oriented, end-stopped cells in pale stripes, which they concluded are part of the parvocellular system. Unoriented, color-opponent cells were described in thin stripes. Oriented, disparity-tuned, direction-selective neurons were located in thick stripes, designated part of the magnocellular system. Stimuli were used selectively in the assessment of receptive fields in these studies. For example, color properties were not evaluated in oriented cells, contributing to the impression that "none showed overt color coding."

Subsequently, no fewer than six studies have reexamined the segregation of form, color, and stereopsis in V2 (Peterhans and von der Heydt, 1993; Levitt, Kiper, and Movshon, 1994; Roe and Ts'o, 1995; Gegenfurtner, Kiper, and Fenstemaker, 1996; Ts'o, Roe, and Gilbert, 2001; Shipp and Zeki, 2002). The verdict has been decidedly mixed, with varying reports of segregation by stripe type. A roadblock faced by all investigators has been the considerable difficulty of reconstructing electrode tracks in CO-stained sections to correlate recording sites with unambiguously identified pale, thin, and thick stripes. It is worth pointing out that the first systematic study of form, color, and disparity in V2 was carried out prior to the discovery of CO stripes (Burkhalter and Van Essen, 1986). No segregation of these receptive field modalities was noticed. This suggests that any compartmentalization of these parameters, if present, is not obvious on physiological grounds alone.

Optical imaging provides a powerful means for exploring columnar segregation in the cortex, because it provides data regarding the net response of large ensembles of neurons to a given stimulus. It has been used in V2 to garner evidence for specialization with stripe classes. Orientation domains shun thin stripes, but at the same time, they do not coincide exactly with pale and thick stripes (Malach, Tootell, and Malonek, 1994; Xu et al., 2002). Color stimuli appear to activate selectively V2 subregions, but the correlation with thin stripes is problematic (Xiao, Wang, and Felleman, 2003). Roe and Ts'o (1995) and Ts'o, Roe, and Gilbert (2001) have emphasized the difficulty of correlating compartments, defined by physiological criteria and optical imaging, with the CO stripe pattern in V2. Nonetheless, optical imaging is likely to provide further clues, especially when applied to primate species, such as squirrel monkeys, that lack a lunate sulcus. Such species are ideal for optical imaging because V2 is flat and located on the brain surface.

Conclusions

The pattern of projections that we report from V1 to V2 vitiates a sharp division of form, color, and motion/stereopsis by CO stripe class. Localization of form, color, and motion perception certainly occurs in extrastriate cortex, at least in some primates. Achromatopsia in humans, for example, provides compelling evidence that color is localized to the fusiform and lingual gyri. Our point is that form, color, and motion should not be equated with pale, thin, and thick V2 stripes, respectively. Moreover, it is misleading to associate parvo and konio with the "ventral" pathway and magno with the "dorsal" pathway. Because interpatches project to both pale stripes and thick stripes, it is likely that parvo and magno inputs are distributed to both V4 and MT. This explains why mixed parvo and magno inputs have been detected in V4 by selective blockade of individual geniculate laminae (Ferrera, Nealey, and Maunsell, 1992). It is puzzling, however, that relatively little effect has been seen in MT after parvocellular blockade (Maunsell, Nealey, and DePriest, 1990).

Our study of the V1 to V2 projection in macaques reconfigures the most widely accepted model for the partitioning of functional streams early in the primate visual system. This model, however, was based on an incomplete description of the pathways from the lateral geniculate body to V1 and on to V2. It would be satisfying at this point to propose an alternative scheme, but too many uncertainties persist. We do not know what purpose, if any, is served by patches in V1 or stripes in V2. It is conceivable that they have a trivial basis (Purves, Riddle, and LaMantia, 1992), like the ocular dominance columns in squirrel monkeys (Adams and Horton, 2003). The stripes in V2 might arise simply from the interdigitation of V1 and pulvinar inputs (Levitt, Yoshioka, and Lund, 1995; Sincich and Horton, 2002b), and therefore play no role in the purported segregation of form, color, and motion/stereo. It is disconcerting that in many macaques, dark stripes in V2 cannot be differentiated into thick and thin. Until better data are available, one hesitates to correlate columns and compartments of the visual cortex with specific visual functions. Rather than present another model, we provide a new foundation for future studies.

REFERENCES

Adams, D. L., and J. C. Horton, 2003. Capricious expression of cortical columns in the primate brain. *Nat. Neurosci.* 6:113–114.

Burkhalter, A., and D. C. Van Essen, 1986. Processing of color, form and disparity information in visual areas VP and V2 of ventral extrastriate cortex in the macaque monkey. *J. Neurosci.* 6:2327–2351.

Callaway, E. M., 1998. Local circuits in primary visual cortex of the macaque monkey. *Annu. Rev. Neurosci.* 21:47–74.

Callaway, E. M., and A. K. Wiser, 1996. Contributions of individual layer 2–5 spiny neurons to local circuits in macaque primary visual cortex. *Vis. Neurosci.* 13:907–922.

DeBruyn, E. J., V. A. Casagrande, P. D. Beck, and A. B. Bonds, 1993. Visual resolution and sensitivity of single cells in the primary visual cortex (V1) of a nocturnal primate (bush baby): Correlations with cortical layers and cytochrome oxidase patterns. *J. Neurophysiol.* 69:3–18.

DeYoe, E. A., D. J. Felleman, D. C. Van Essen, and E. McClendon, 1994. Multiple processing streams in occipitotemporal visual cortex. *Nature* 371:151–154.

DeYoe, E. A., and D. C. Van Essen, 1985. Segregation of efferent connections and receptive field properties in visual area V2 of the macaque. *Nature* 317:58–61.

Felleman, D. J., and D. C. Van Essen, 1991. Distributed hierarchical processing in the primate cerebral cortex. *Cereb. Cortex* 1:1–47.

Ferrera, V. P., T. A. Nealey, and J. H. R. Maunsell, 1992. Mixed parvocellular and magnocellular geniculate signals in visual area V4. *Nature* 358:756–758.

FITZPATRICK, D., J. S. LUND, and G. G. BLASDEL, 1985. Intrinsic connections of macaque striate cortex: Afferent and efferent connections of lamina 4C. *J. Neurosci.* 5:3329–3349.

GEGENFURTNER, K. R., D. C. KIPER, and S. B. FENSTEMAKER, 1996. Processing of color, form, and motion in macaque area V2. *Vis. Neurosci.* 13:161–172.

HENDRY, S. H., and R. C. REID, 2000. The koniocellular pathway in primate vision. *Annu. Rev. Neurosci.* 23:127–153.

HENDRY, S. H., and T. YOSHIOKA, 1994. A neurochemically distinct third channel in the macaque dorsal lateral geniculate nucleus. *Science* 264:575–577.

HORTON, J. C., 1984. Cytochrome oxidase patches: A new cytoarchitectonic feature of monkey visual cortex. *Philos. Trans. R. Soc. Lond. B. Biol. Sci.* 304:199–253.

HORTON, J. C., and D. H. HUBEL, 1981. Regular patchy distribution of cytochrome oxidase staining in primary visual cortex of macaque monkey. *Nature* 292:762–764.

HORTON, J. C., and L. C. SINCICH, 2004. How specific is V1 input to V2 thin stripes? *Soc. Neurosci. Abstr.* 34 (submitted).

HUBEL, D. H., and M. S. LIVINGSTONE, 1987. Segregation of form, color, and stereopsis in primate area 18. *J. Neurosci.* 7:3378–3415.

JOHNSON, E. N., M. J. HAWKEN, and R. SHAPLEY, 2001. The spatial transformation of color in the primary visual cortex of the macaque monkey. *Nat. Neurosci.* 4:409–416.

KANDEL, E. R., J. H. SCHWARTZ, and T. M. JESSEL, eds., 2000. *Principles of Neural Science*, 4th ed. New York: McGraw-Hill.

KENNEDY, H., and J. BULLIER, 1985. A double-labeling investigation of the afferent connectivity to cortical areas V1 and V2 of the macaque monkey. *J. Neurosci.* 5:2815–2830.

LACHICA, E. A., P. D. BECK, and V. A. CASAGRANDE, 1992. Parallel pathways in macaque monkey striate cortex: Anatomically defined columns in layer III. *Proc. Natl. Acad. Sci. U.S.A.* 89:3566–3570.

LEVENTHAL, A. G., K. G. THOMPSON, D. LIU, Y. ZHOU, and S. J. AULT, 1995. Concomitant sensitivity to orientation, direction, and color of cells in layers 2, 3, and 4 of monkey striate cortex. *J. Neurosci.* 15:1808–1818.

LEVITT, J. B., D. C. KIPER, and J. A. MOVSHON, 1994. Receptive fields and functional architecture of macaque V2. *J. Neurophysiol.* 71:2517–2542.

LEVITT, J. B., T. YOSHIOKA, and J. S. LUND, 1994. Intrinsic cortical connections in macaque visual area V2: Evidence for interaction between different functional streams. *J. Comp. Neurol.* 342:551–570.

LEVITT, J. B., T. YOSHIOKA, and J. S. LUND, 1995. Connections between the pulvinar complex and cytochrome oxidase-defined compartments in visual area V2 of macaque monkey. *Exp. Brain Res.* 104:419–430.

LIVINGSTONE, M. S., and D. H. HUBEL, 1984. Anatomy and physiology of a color system in the primate visual cortex. *J. Neurosci.* 4:309–356.

LIVINGSTONE, M. S., and D. H. HUBEL, 1987. Connections between layer 4B of area 17 and the thick cytochrome oxidase stripes of area 18 in the squirrel monkey. *J. Neurosci.* 7:3371–3377.

LIVINGSTONE, M. S., and D. H. HUBEL, 1988. Segregation of form, color, movement, and depth: Anatomy, physiology, and perception. *Science* 240:740–749.

MALACH, R, R. B. TOOTELL, and D. MALONEK, 1994. Relationship between orientation domains, cytochrome oxidase stripes, and intrinsic horizontal connections in squirrel monkey area V2. *Cereb. Cortex* 4:151–165.

MARTIN, K. A. C., 1988. From enzymes to perception: A bridge too far? *Trends Neurosci.* 11:380–387.

MAUNSELL, J. H., T. A. NEALEY, and D. D. DEPRIEST, 1990. Magnocellular and parvocellular contributions to responses in the middle temporal visual area (MT) of the macaque monkey. *J. Neurosci.* 10:3323–3334.

MAUNSELL, J. H., and W. T. NEWSOME, 1987. Visual processing in monkey extrastriate cortex. *Annu. Rev. Neurosci.* 10:363–401.

MERIGAN, W. H., and J. H. R. MAUNSELL, 1993. How parallel are the primate visual pathways? *Annu. Rev. Neurosci.* 16:369–402.

MOVSHON, J. A., and W. T. NEWSOME, 1996. Visual response properties of striate cortical neurons projecting to area MT in macaque monkeys. *J. Neurosci.* 16:7733–7741.

MURPHY, K. M., D. G. JONES, and R. C. VAN SLUYTERS, 1995. Cytochrome-oxidase blobs in cat primary visual cortex. *J. Neurosci.* 15:4196–4208.

NICHOLLS, J. G., A. R. MARTIN, B. G. WALLACE, and P. A. FUCHS, eds., 2001. *From Neuron to Brain*, 4th ed. Sunderland, Mass.: Sinauer Associates.

O'KEEFE, L. P., J. B. LEVITT, D. C. KIPER, R. M. SHAPLEY, and J. A. MOVSHON, 1998. Functional organization of owl monkey lateral geniculate nucleus and visual cortex. *J. Neurophysiol.* 80:594–609.

OLAVARRIA, J. F., and R. C. VAN SLUYTERS, 1985. Unfolding and flattening the cortex of gyrencephalic brains. *J. Neurosci. Methods* 15:191–202.

PETERHANS, E., and R. VON DER HEYDT, 1993. Functional organization of area V2 in the alert macaque. *Eur. J. Neurosci.* 5:509–524.

PURVES, D., G. J. AUGUSTINE, D. FITZPATRICK, L. C. KATZ, A. S. LAMANTIA, J. O. MCNAMARA, and S. M. WILLIAMS, 2001. *Neuroscience*, 2nd ed. Sunderland, Mass.: Sinauer Associates.

PURVES, D., D. R. RIDDLE, and A. S. LAMANTIA, 1992. Iterated patterns of brain circuitry (or how the cortex gets its spots). *Trends Neurosci.* 15:362–368.

ROCKLAND, K. S., 1992. Laminar distribution of neurons projecting from area V1 to V2 in macaque and squirrel monkeys. *Cereb. Cortex* 2:38–47.

ROE, A. W., and D. Y. TS'O, 1995. Visual topography in primate V2: Multiple representation across functional stripes. *J. Neurosci.* 15:3689–3715.

SHAPLEY, R., 1995. Parallel neural pathways and visual function. In *The Cognitive Neurosciences*, 1st ed. M. Gazzaniga, ed. Cambridge, Mass.: MIT Press, pp. 315–324.

SHIPP, S., and S. ZEKI, 1985. Segregation of pathways leading from area V2 to areas V4 and V5 of macaque monkey visual cortex. *Nature* 315:322–325.

SHIPP, S., and S. ZEKI, 2002. The functional organization of area V2. I. Specialization across stripes and layers. *Vis. Neurosci.* 19:187–210.

SINCICH, L. C., D. L. ADAMS, and J. C. HORTON, 2003. Complete flatmounting of the macaque cerebral cortex. *Vis. Neurosci.* 20:663–686.

SINCICH, L. C., and J. C. HORTON, 2002a. Divided by cytochrome oxidase: A map of the projections from V1 to V2 in macaques. *Science* 295:1734–1737.

SINCICH, L. C., and J. C. HORTON, 2002b. Pale cytochrome oxidase stripes in V2 receive the richest projection from macaque striate cortex. *J. Comp. Neurol.* 447:18–33.

SINCICH, L. C., and J. C. HORTON, 2003. Independent projection streams from macaque striate cortex to the second visual area and middle temporal area. *J. Neurosci.* 23:5684–5692.

TOOTELL, R. B., and M. S. SILVERMAN, 1985. Two methods for flatmounting cortical tissue. *J. Neurosci. Methods* 15:177–190.

TOOTELL, R. B. H., M. S. SILVERMAN, R. L. DE VALOIS, and G. H. JACOBS, 1983. Functional organization of the second cortical visual area in primates. *Science* 220:737–739.

TS'O, D. Y., and C. D. GILBERT, 1988. The organization of chromatic and spatial interactions in the primate striate cortex. *J. Neurosci.* 8:1712–1727.

TS'O, D. Y., A. W. ROE, and C. D. GILBERT, 2001. A hierarchy of the functional organization for color, form and disparity in primate visual area V2. *Vision Res.* 41:1333–1349.

UNGERLEIDER, L. G., and M. MISHKIN, 1982. Two cortical visual systems. In *Analysis of Visual Behaviour*, D. J. Ingle, M. A. Goodale, and R. J. W. Mansfield, eds. Cambridge, Mass.: MIT Press, pp. 549–586.

VAN ESSEN, D. C., 1985. Functional organization of primate visual cortex. In *Cerebral Cortex*, A. Peters, and E. Jones, eds. pp. 259–329. New York: Plenum Press.

VAN ESSEN, D. C., and J. L. GALLANT, 1994. Neural mechanisms of form and motion processing in the primate visual system. *Neuron* 13:1–10.

VAN ESSEN, D. C., W. T. NEWSOME, J. H. MAUNSELL, and J. L. BIXBY, 1986. The projections from striate cortex (V1) to areas V2 and V3 in the macaque monkey: Asymmetries, areal boundaries, and patchy connections. *J. Comp. Neurol.* 244:451–480.

WONG-RILEY, M. T., 1989. Cytochrome oxidase: An endogenous metabolic marker for neuronal activity. *Trends Neurosci.* 12: 94–101.

XIAO, Y., and D. J. FELLEMAN, 2004. Projections from primary visual cortex to cytochrome oxidase thin stripes and interstripes of macaque visual area 2. *Proc. Natl. Acad. Sci. U.S.A.* 101:7147–7151.

XIAO, Y., Y. WANG, and D. J. FELLEMAN, 2003. A spatially organized representation of colour in macaque cortical area V2. *Nature* 421:535–539.

XU, X, W. BOSKING, G. SARY, J. BOYD, M. JONES, I. KHAYTIN, J. STEFANSIC, D. SHIMA, D. FITZPATRICK, and V. A. CASAGRANDE, 2002. Orientation preference domains and their relation to cytochrome oxidase modules in owl monkey visual cortex. *Soc. Neurosci. Abstr.* 32:325.13.

YABUTA, N. H., and E. M. CALLAWAY, 1998. Functional streams and local connections of layer 4C neurons in primary visual cortex of the macaque monkey. *J. Neurosci.* 18:9489–9499.

YABUTA, N. H., A. SAWATARI, and E. M. CALLAWAY, 2001. Two functional channels from primary visual cortex to dorsal visual cortical areas. *Science* 292:297–300.

YOSHIOKA, T, J. B. LEVITT, and J. S. LUND, 1994. Independence and merger of thalamocortical channels within macaque monkey primary visual cortex: Anatomy of interlaminar projections. *Vis. Neurosci.* 11:467–489.

ZEKI, S., 1980. The representation of colours in the cerebral cortex. *Nature* 284:412–418.

ZEKI, S., and S. SHIPP, 1988. The functional logic of cortical connections. *Nature* 335:311–317.

18 Birdsong: Hearing in the Service of Vocal Learning

ALLISON J. DOUPE, MICHELE M. SOLIS,
CHARLOTTE A. BOETTIGER, AND NEAL A. HESSLER

ABSTRACT Hearing is required for localization and recognition of sounds, but also, in a subset of animals, for learning to produce sounds. Songbirds, much like humans, learn their vocal behavior, and must be able to hear both themselves and others to do so. They first must memorize an adult "tutor's" song. Then, both as juveniles, while they learn to sing, and later, as adults, songbirds use auditory feedback to compare their own vocalizations with an internal representation of the memorized tutor song. Studies of the brain areas involved in singing and song learning could reveal the underlying neural mechanisms. Here we describe experiments that explore the properties of the songbird anterior forebrain pathway (AFP), a basal ganglia–forebrain circuit known to be critical for song learning and for adult modification of vocal output, but not for normal adult singing. First, neural recordings in anesthetized, juvenile birds show that auditory AFP neurons become selectively responsive to the song stimuli that are compared during sensorimotor learning. Individual AFP neurons develop tuning to the bird's own song, and in many cases to the tutor song as well, even when these stimuli are manipulated to be very different from each other. Second, neural recordings from adult, singing birds reveal robust singing-related activity in the AFP that is present even in deaf birds. This activity is likely to originate from premotor areas and could represent an efference copy of motor commands for song, predicting the sensory consequences of those commands. Third, in vitro studies of the AFP show that recurrent synapses between neurons in the AFP outflow nucleus can undergo activity-dependent and timing-sensitive strengthening that appears to be restricted to young birds. Overall, these studies illustrate that this circuit is not simply a sensory pathway but contains highly interrelated sensory and motor signals that reflect the bird's acquisition of song. Such sensorimotor mixing seems to be true for brain areas involved in speech as well, and may be a critical feature of vocal motor learning. The AFP also contains synaptic mechanisms well-suited to represent the temporal pattern of activation of its inputs, consistent with a role in tutor song memorization and/or early refinement of song. Because the AFP includes a basal ganglia circuit focused on one specific behavior, it may be a tractable system for understanding how basal ganglia circuits function in guiding motor learning using sensory feedback signals, at both cellular and circuit levels.

ALLISON J. DOUPE Keck Center for Integrative Neuroscience, and Departments of Physiology and Psychiatry, University of California, San Francisco, Calif.

MICHELE M. SOLIS Keck Center for Integrative Neuroscience, and Departments of Physiology and Psychiatry, University of California, San Francisco, Calif., and Department of Otolaryngology, University of Washington, Seattle, Wash.

CHARLOTTE A. BOETTIGER Keck Center for Integrative Neuroscience, and Departments of Physiology and Psychiatry, University of California, San Francisco, and Helen Wills Neuroscience Institute, University of California, Berkeley.

NEAL A. HESSLER RIKEN Brain Science Institute, Lab for Vocal Behavior Mechanisms, Wako-Shi, Japan.

Hearing is important to most animals for localization and recognition of sounds, including behaviorally important communication sounds of other individuals of the same species, such as mating and warning calls. For a subset of animals known as vocal learners, another critical function of hearing is to learn to produce sounds imitated from others. Humans are consummate vocal learners: human speech is a fantastically complex and variable communication sound, and we depend critically on hearing both of self and of others for normal speech development. Much is being learned about brain areas associated with speech recognition and production, especially as imaging and electrophysiological techniques for studying the human brain evolve. To understand basic brain mechanisms of vocal learning and its disorders, however, it is important to be able to study animals with related behaviors. Surprisingly, there are relatively few other vocal learners besides humans. Although the vocalizations of nonhuman primates can be complex, none of them has as yet been shown to be learned. Among mammals, there is evidence for vocal learning only in cetaceans (whales and dolphins; Rendell and Whitehead, 2001) and some bats (Boughman, 1998). In contrast to this paucity of mammalian vocal learners, the many thousands of songbird species as well as the parrot and hummingbird groups must learn to make complex vocal sounds. Songbirds have provided a particularly useful model system. There is a wealth of information on their vocal behavior and the underlying brain substrates, with some striking parallels to human speech learning that will be outlined in this chapter.

Human speech and birdsong share numerous features (Doupe and Kuhl, 1999). Both are complex acoustic sequences generated by the coordinated actions of the vocal apparatus and the muscles of respiration. Most important, both speech and song are learned, and are highly dependent

245

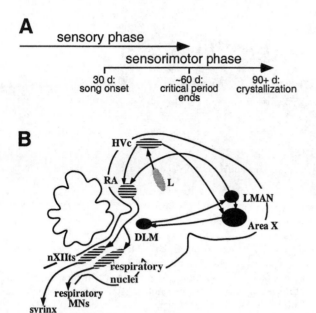

FIGURE 18.1   (A) Song learning occurs in two phases. For zebra finches, the sensory phase ends at approximately 60 days of age and the sensorimotor phase begins when birds are approximately 30 days old and continues until they are ≥90 days of age; thus, the phases of learning overlap in this species. (B) Anatomy of the song system, which consists of two major pathways. Motor pathway nuclei are striped, and AFP nuclei are in black. The motor pathway, necessary for normal song production throughout life, includes HVc, the robust nucleus of the archistriatum (RA), and the tracheosyringeal portion of the hypoglossal nucleus (nXIIts). RA also projects to nuclei involved in control of respiration. The AFP comprises area X (X), the medial nucleus of the dorsolateral thalamus (DLM), and the lateral magnocellular nucleus of the anterior neostriatum (LMAN). The field L complex and related areas (stippled) provide auditory input to the song system.

on hearing in early life and in adulthood: neither birds nor humans learn to vocalize normally in the absence of hearing, and, as adults, both show deterioration of vocal output after hearing loss (Konishi, 1965; Price, 1979; Waldstein, 1989; Cowie and Douglas-Cowie, 1992; Nordeen and Nordeen, 1992). Songbirds thus provide a promising model system for elucidating general neural mechanisms involved in vocal learning, including how the brain may evaluate auditory feedback and use it to modify vocal output, and what synaptic mechanisms could underlie this.

Experiments to investigate the neural basis of vocal learning in songbirds are aided by a wealth of information on the behavioral time course of learning (Immelmann, 1969; Marler, 1970; Eales, 1985) and its dependence on hearing (Konishi, 1965; Price, 1979). Song learning occurs in two stages, called the sensory and sensorimotor phases (figure 18.1A). During the sensory phase, a young bird listens to and memorizes the song of an adult tutor, usually the bird's father. This memory is often called the "template." The sensorimotor phase begins later, when the young bird begins to

sing; during sensorimotor learning the juvenile uses auditory feedback to compare its own immature vocalizations ("plastic song") to its memory of the tutor's song, and gradually refines and adapts its vocal output until it matches the tutor's song. Thus, auditory experience of both the tutor's song and the bird's own song (BOS) is required during learning. In adulthood, elimination or alteration of auditory feedback of BOS induces gradual deterioration of adult song structure (Nordeen and Nordeen, 1992; Leonardo and Konishi, 1999). These behavioral observations suggest that there must be neural circuitry involved in memorization and evaluation of song. Specifically, after the initial storage of a song template, there must be mechanisms that compare auditory feedback from vocal output with the internal song template, and that generate signals to guide changes in vocal output.

One candidate circuit for processing and evaluating these song experiences is the anterior forebrain pathway (AFP), a basal ganglia–forebrain circuit found within a system of interconnected nuclei dedicated to song learning and production (figure 18.1B, nuclei shown in black) (Nottebohm, Stokes, and Leonard, 1976). The AFP plays a special role during learning and song modification. Lesions of the AFP severely disrupt song learning in juveniles, whereas the same lesions do not affect song in normal adult zebra finches (Bottjer, Miesner, and Arnold, 1987; Sohrabji, Nordeen, and Nordeen, 1990; Scharff and Nottebohm, 1991). However, lesions in adults prevent the degradation of adult song normally caused by perturbations of song production or feedback (Williams and Mehta, 1999; Brainard and Doupe, 2000a). Both juvenile and adult results are consistent with the idea that the AFP participates in evaluating song feedback and computing or conveying instructive signals about the quality of song, which then drive adaptive (or in case of adult deafening, nonadaptive) changes in song (Brainard and Doupe, 2000b). The output of the AFP, the lateral magnocellular nucleus of the anterior neostriatum (LMAN), projects to the motor pathway for song, which is necessary for normal song production throughout life (Nottebohm, Stokes, and Leonard, 1976). Thus, the AFP is well positioned to influence activity in the motor pathway, and could drive changes in vocal output. We review here experiments that implicate AFP function in the sensory and sensorimotor phases of learning, as well as in sensorimotor processing in adulthood, and describe synaptic mechanisms well-suited to allow shaping of neural properties by song learning.

Song learning in juveniles

As might be expected of neural circuits involved in mediating song learning, neurons in the AFP are responsive to song stimuli. In adult, anesthetized zebra finches, these neurons respond more strongly to BOS than to acoustically similar songs of other zebra finches (conspecific songs; figure 18.2A)

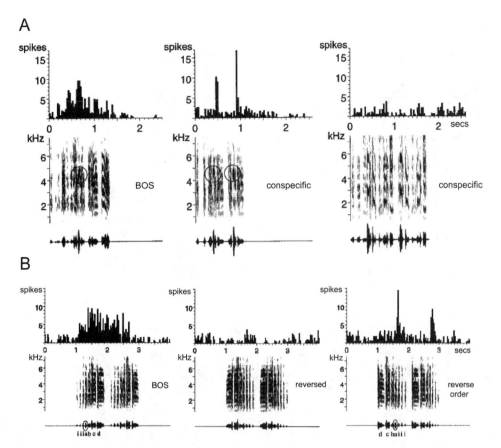

FIGURE 18.2   AFP neurons are song-selective. (A) A song-selective neuron from LMAN of an adult zebra finch. Peristimulus time histograms (PSTHs) show the greater response of a single LMAN neuron to bird's own song (BOS) than to two other conspecific songs. Song is shown underneath each PSTH as a sonogram (plot of frequency vs. time, with the energy of each frequency band shown by the darkness of the trace). Song-selective neurons respond to multiple acoustic features of the BOS: the circles in the sonograms identify a feature that is shared between BOS and the first conspecific song shown here and appears to elicit a response, but the figure also illustrates that many other features of BOS must contribute to the overall response of this neuron to BOS. (B) Song-selective neurons are also sensitive to temporal features of song. This single LMAN neuron responds strongly to BOS, especially the first phrase (also called motif), and very little to the fully reversed (mirror-image) song. The introductory notes (i) and syllables (a–d) of the first of the two repeated motifs of the song are labeled with lowercase letters. The BOS played in reverse order, which maintains the order within each syllable while reversing the sequence, is also a much less effective stimulus than the normal BOS, but elicits a phasic response after each occurrence of syllable a.

or BOS played completely in reverse or with the sequence reversed (figure 18.2B; Doupe, 1997). In addition, many of these neurons are "combination-sensitive" (figure 18.3): that is, they show a highly nonlinear increase in firing when the component sounds of song are combined and played in the correct sequence, compared to those sounds played alone. The properties of song neurons in the AFP are very similar to those of song-selective neurons first described in the song motor control nucleus HVc (figure 18.1B; McCasland and Konishi, 1981; Margoliash, 1983). Neurons that are sensitive to the complex spectral and temporal properties of song could be useful for processing song stimuli during learning. Song-selective neurons from the AFP in particular could provide feedback to the motor pathway, in the form of their firing rate or pattern, about how well sounds match the bird's goal, and when the correct sequence has been sung.

This "song selectivity" is not present in young birds but emerges during the course of song learning: AFP neurons from birds early in the sensory learning phase (30 days of age) respond equally well to all song stimuli (figure 18.4A). Over time, these neurons increase their response to BOS while losing responsiveness to other stimuli (Doupe, 1997; Solis and Doupe, 1997; figure 18.4B). There is a striking parallel to this result in human speech development: human infants initially show sensory discrimination of phonemes from all human languages tested, but gradually lose their capacity to accurately discriminate sounds that they are not experiencing, and improve their discrimination of the sounds of the language spoken around them (Eimas, Miller, and Jusczyk, 1987; Kuhl, 1994; Werker and Tees, 1994). In both cases, the initial broad sensitivity endows the young organism with the capacity to learn any language or

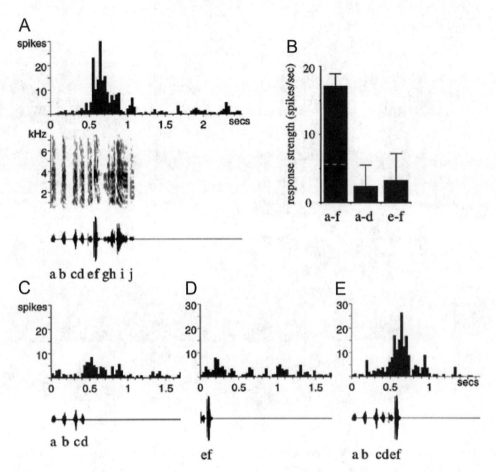

FIGURE 18.3   A combination-sensitive neuron in adult LMAN. (*A*) The response of the neuron to the entire BOS, whose syllables are indicated by lowercase letters below the oscillogram (plots of amplitude vs. time). (*B*) The mean response strength (response above background; error bars indicate SEM) to each of the indicated syllable combinations. The dashed white line in the first bar represents the linear sum of responses to a–d and e–f. (*C–E*)

PSTHs of the neuron's response to the indicated combinations of syllables. Presentation of the first four syllables alone elicits little response; the following two syllables in isolation also elicit only a weak response. In combination, however, these two stimuli (a–f) elicit a strong response that not only exceeds the sum of responses to stimuli a–d and e–f, but is as strong as the response to the entire song.

species-specific song, but this sensitivity is then narrowed and shaped by experience.

Song selectivity develops rapidly, since it is found in the AFP of zebra finches that have completed the sensory phase of learning (60 days of age: figure 18.1*A*, 18.4*B*; Solis and Doupe, 1997). At this time zebra finches are also in the middle of the sensorimotor phase and have been producing plastic song for about a month. Thus, experience of either the bird's own or the tutor song could have shaped the selectivity of these neurons. Knowing which experience is responsible for selectivity would inform our hypotheses about AFP function during song learning. For example, neurons tuned by BOS experience could provide information about the current state of BOS, whereas those tuned by tutor song could encode the tutor song memory. When we compared the neural responses to BOS and tutor song in 60-day-old birds, we found a range of preferences for one song over the other (figure 18.5*A*). Many neurons preferred BOS to tutor

song, supporting a role for BOS experience in shaping selectivity. A few neurons preferred tutor song to BOS, suggesting that they were tuned by tutor song experience. Finally, many neurons responded equally well to both songs. These neurons were clearly selective, because they did not respond as well to conspecific or reversed song stimuli. Thus, such neurons might reflect experiences of both BOS and tutor song.

Two important caveats exist with respect to the apparent shaping of AFP neurons by these two sensory experiences. First, although BOS selectivity might initially seem to reflect the bird's experience of its own song, it is also possible that it actually represents the template. If a bird memorized the tutor song poorly during sensory learning, then modeled its own song after this inaccurate template (figure 18.4*C*), BOS selectivity would be a better representation of the template than the tutor song. The question of whether BOS indeed reflects the bird's own vocalizations could be solved if the

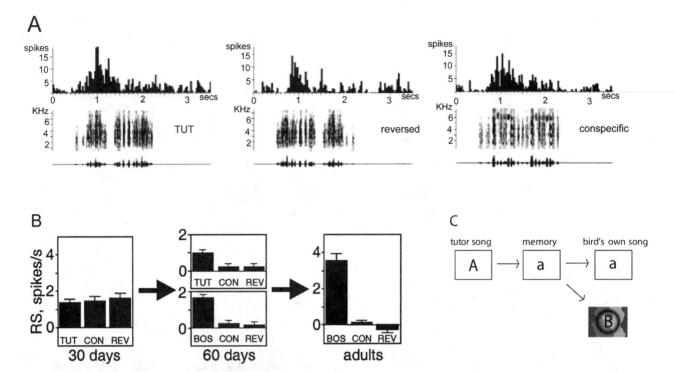

FIGURE 18.4 AFP neurons develop selectivity for song during development. (*A*) PSTHs of auditory responses of a single LMAN neuron from a young, presinging (approximately 30 day old) zebra finch. The neuron responds to the tutor song (TUT) played in normal forward order, but also to the tutor song fully reversed, and to a conspecific song that the bird has never heard. (*B*) In zebra finches 30 days of age, LMAN neurons exhibit equivalent response strengths (RS; mean stimulus-evoked response minus background) to tutor song (TUT), conspecific song (CON), and reverse tutor song (REV). By 60 days of age, these neurons respond significantly more to TUT than to CON or to REV. In addition, BOS also elicits a much stronger response than CON and reverse BOS (REV). In adults, LMAN neurons are extremely selective for BOS. (*C*) When a juvenile stores a good copy of the tutor song (A) as its template (a), and accurately models its own song after the template, the resulting BOS (a) will strongly resemble the tutor song. Thus, if a neuron is tuned by BOS experience only, it could also respond well to tutor song when the two songs are similar enough. This ambiguity could be resolved by making the BOS very different (B) from the tutor song, by interfering with vocal production mechanisms. In the experiments described here, this was done by cutting the tracheosyringeal (ts) nerves to the vocal muscles.

bird were made to sing something very different from its tutor by a manipulation of its peripheral vocal system (figure 18.4*C*). Since the bird would hear the highly abnormal BOS only as a result of its own singing, neurons tuned to the abnormal song would verify that it was the experience of BOS that was critical. Second, neurons tuned to both BOS and the tutor song might not reflect the experience of both of these songs, but simply reflect acoustic similarities between these two stimuli: the bird is trying to model its own song after the tutor song, and by 60 days of age, plastic song often resembles the tutor song. This question could also be addressed if the acoustic similarity that normally develops between BOS and tutor song were minimized, by inducing juvenile zebra finches to sing abnormal songs (figure 18.4*C*; Solis and Doupe, 1999). If the neurons that respond equally well to BOS and tutor song are actually shaped by the experience of the bird's voice but respond to both stimuli because of acoustic similarities between these songs, then this kind of neuron should not exist in birds with song unlike their tutor song (figure 18.5*B*, left panel). Alternatively, if

these neurons reflect independent contributions of both BOS and tutor song experience to selectivity, then they should persist in birds with song unlike their tutor song, perhaps as separate neural populations (figure 18.5*B*, right panel).

To induce abnormal song, we bilaterally transected the tracheosyringeal portion of the hypoglossal nerve (NXIIts) prior to song onset (~25 days of age in zebra finches; figure 18.1*A*), thus denervating the muscles of the avian vocal organ (the syrinx). These juveniles therefore experienced a normal sensory phase with their tutor, but their entire experience of BOS was of the abnormal, nerve cut ("ts cut") song. Song analyses demonstrated that this manipulation successfully minimized both the spectral and temporal similarity between BOS and tutor song.

Using ts cut song and tutor song as stimuli, we characterized neuronal selectivity in the AFP of ts cut birds at 60 days of age. Some neurons responded more strongly to the unique ts cut BOS ("tsBOS") than to tutor song, clearly demonstrating a role for BOS experience in shaping neural

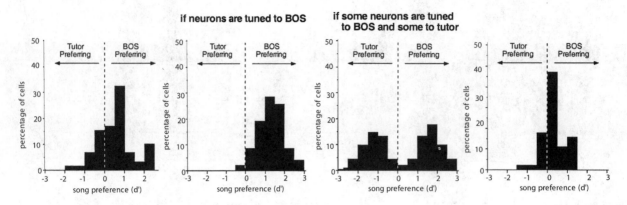

A: normal 60 d birds   B: some predictions of creating mismatch   C: nerve cut 60 d birds

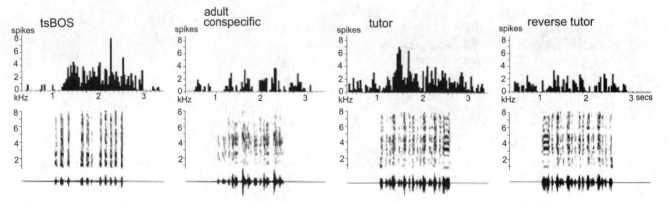

D: dually-responsive song neuron in 60 d nerve cut bird

tsBOS   adult conspecific   tutor   reverse tutor

FIGURE 18.5   Preferences for BOS versus tutor song by single AFP neurons. (*A*) Histograms show that in 60-day-old zebra finches, there is a range of preferences among LMAN neurons. The preference for each neuron is quantified with a d' value (Solis and Doupe, 1997; Theunissen and Doupe, 1998). When $d' \geq 0.5$, this indicates a strong preference for BOS over tutor song; when $d' \leq -0.5$, this indicates a strong preference for tutor song over BOS. Neurons with d' values in between were considered to have equivalent responses to both song stimuli. (*B*) Predicted results of the manipulation of BOS. *Left panel:* If neurons with equivalent responses to BOS and tutor song are shaped by BOS during development but respond to both stimuli as a result of acoustic similarities between these two songs, this type of dually responsive neuron is not expected in birds with songs unlike their tutor song, and the distribution should reveal only BOS-tuned neurons. *Right panel:* If

both BOS and tutor song independently shape different neurons in the AFP, the distribution in birds with songs very different from their tutor songs is predicted to be bimodal, as shown by the histogram. (*C*) The observed distribution of song preferences from ts cut birds at 60 days of age. Neurons with equivalent responses to BOS and tutor song were maintained, even though these birds' songs did not resemble the tutor song. (*D*) Equivalent responses to tsBOS (BOS of birds with ts nerve cuts) and tutor song. PSTHs show the responses of a single LMAN neuron to 13 presentations of each song. Although this neuron responded equally well to tsBOS and tutor song, it did not respond well to other adult conspecific songs, and it had developed order selectivity for the tutor song: reversed tutor song was a less effective stimulus than BOS or tutor.

selectivity. Strikingly, a sizable proportion of neurons still responded equally well to both tsBOS and tutor song, despite the acoustic differences between these two songs (figure 18.5*C*). These neurons were not simply immature, because they exhibited selectivity for tsBOS and tutor song over conspecific and reverse song (figure 18.5*D*). Thus, the presence of neurons with equivalent responses to tsBOS and tutor song in these ts cut birds suggests that *both* song experiences can shape the selectivity of single neurons.

How might these different types of song selectivity func-

tion in song learning? Since BOS selectivity reflects the bird's current vocal output, it might provide information about the state of plastic song to a neural circuit involved in comparing BOS to a tutor song template stored in sensory coordinates. The high selectivity for BOS might also provide a kind of filter or gating function, aiding the bird in distinguishing its own vocalizations from those of others. It may also reflect in some way the pattern of motor activation during singing, as has been seen in the robust nucleus of the archistriatum RA (Dave and Margoliash, 2000). The function of this selectivity could be further investigated with experiments in which AFP selectivity was broadened during song learning, perhaps with pharmacological agents.

Tutor song selectivity could encode information about the tutor song, and function during sensorimotor learning as the neural reference of tutor song. That is, this selectivity would result from experience of the tutor song during the sensory phase of learning. During the sensorimotor phase, the level or pattern of firing of these neurons in response to BOS would then reflect the degree to which BOS resembles the tutor song. A role for the AFP in sensory learning of the template is also supported by behavioral experiments that demonstrate a need for normal LMAN activity specifically during tutor song exposure (Basham, Nordeen, and Nordeen, 1996).

In addition, these experiments found that BOS selectivity often coexists with tutor song selectivity in the same individual AFP neurons. This "dual selectivity" may reflect a function for AFP neurons in the actual comparison of BOS and tutor song that is essential to learning. For example, auditory feedback from the bird's own vocalizations would elicit activity from BOS-selective cells. If this auditory feedback of the bird's own voice also matches the tutor song, then this might elicit greater or different activity in neurons that are also tuned to the tutor song than in neurons tuned to BOS or tutor song alone. Thus, the extent to which BOS resembles the tutor might be reflected in the activity of dually tuned neurons, which could then participate in the reinforcement of the motor pathway.

A further suggestion that song selectivity not only might be linked to evaluation of auditory feedback but is actually sensitive to how well that feedback matches the target comes from studies of adult birds that were experimentally prevented from ever producing a good copy of their tutor template. When birds with NXIIts transections prior to song onset were allowed to grow to adulthood, they had abnormally low song selectivity in the AFP (Solis and Doupe, 2000). Neurons were selective enough to discriminate BOS and tutor song from conspecific and reverse songs, but the degree of selectivity was less than that found in normal adults. This result suggests that selectivity is compromised by a chronic inability of birds to match their tutor song model. If true, then these neurons are not simply reflecting sensory experience but are influenced by the degree of matching during sensorimotor learning.

Despite the joint representation of BOS and tutor song in many AFP neurons, it seems likely that a pure sensory representation of tutor song is present somewhere in the brain. Although this could be encoded by an unidentified subset of neurons lying within other song system nuclei or even within the AFP, it seems equally plausible that such a representation lies elsewhere in the brain, perhaps in the earlier high-level auditory areas that also process songs of conspecifics (Mello, Vicario, and Clayton, 1992; Bolhuis et al., 2000; Gentner and Margoliash, 2003).

Singing-related activity in the AFP

Since the auditory feedback most relevant to song learning and maintenance occurs when the bird actually sings, it was clearly critical to record AFP activity during singing. To characterize signals present in the AFP of normal adult birds, we recorded single- and multi-unit activity in LMAN during singing in adult zebra finches (Hessler and Doupe, 1999a,b). LMAN neurons fired vigorously throughout singing in adult birds (figure 18.6), despite the fact that this nucleus is not required for normal song production. Moreover, excitation began prior to song output, indicating that at least some of the activity is independent of auditory feedback of the bird's own voice. On average there was a consistent pattern of activity related to individual song elements, and peaks of activity tended to precede syllables. This activity resembles that reported in previous studies of singing-related premotor activity in the song control nucleus HVc (McCasland, 1987; Yu and Margoliash, 1996). This raises the possibility that much of the AFP activity during singing originates from the song motor circuit, and may represent, in part, a version of the premotor signals also sent to the motor output pathway.

The properties of this singing-related activity raised the question of whether any of it is related to sensory feedback. In playback experiments, song-selective responses to auditory stimuli like those studied in anesthetized birds were apparent in LMAN of awake birds, although they were variable from trial to trial and between birds (Hessler and Doupe, 1999b), and it remains to be determined whether they are present in the same neurons that show singing-related activity. Moreover, the level of activity elicited by playback of auditory stimuli was low relative to singing-related activity, making it possible that small auditory feedback signals are embedded within the robust singing-related AFP activity. As an initial step to see whether AFP activity during singing contains both sensory and motor activity, we recorded multi-unit activity from LMAN before and 1–3 days after deafening. Neural activity during singing was very similar before and after deafening, indicating that much of the activity during singing is not dramatically altered by an acute loss of auditory feedback (Hessler and Doupe, 1999b).

Although selective responses to playback of BOS had suggested that sensorimotor learning influences the AFP, the marked AFP activity during singing demonstrates very directly that this circuit is not a pure sensory pathway but instead a sensorimotor circuit. Its function during singing may be clarified with studies that determine whether activity in individual neurons or across a population of neurons is a mixture of motor and sensory signals, and if so, how

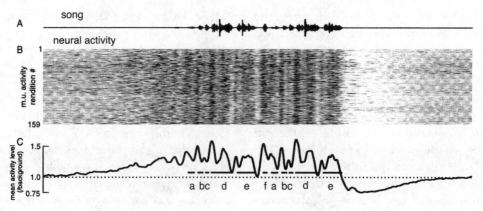

A   song

B   neural activity

m.u. activity rendition #

C   1.5

mean activity level (background)   1.0

0.75

a bc d e f a bc d e

FIGURE 18.6   LMAN neurons exhibit strong, singing-related activity. The oscillogram shows the song produced by the bird. The mean level of LMAN multi-unit activity recorded in this bird before, during and after each of 159 renditions of the song is shown below, aligned to the song. Activity level is represented by a gray scale, where black indicates high neural activity and white indicates low activity (Hessler and Doupe, 1999b). The bottom trace shows the mean of activity during all the renditions above, illustrating the onset of AFP activity before sound, and the peaks of activity related to syllables, which are indicated by the black bars and identified with letters. The duration of the entire panel is 4.5 s.

these relate to each other. In addition, recording LMAN activity in response to altered rather than absent feedback could be an important approach to studying these neurons; this would allow multiple interleaved recordings of song-related activity with and without altered feedback, which could be useful for detecting small sensory feedback signals.

The singing-related activity in the AFP might represent an "efference copy," perhaps predicting the sensory consequences of motor commands. The properties of AFP neurons are consistent with this hypothesis. Because efference copy signals are triggered by motor commands, neurons with such signals would be expected to be active during singing, even in the absence of auditory feedback. Furthermore, if these neurons encode an internally generated prediction of the sensory outcome of a motor command to sing, then they might exhibit BOS selectivity when probed with song stimuli in playback experiments. Efference copies are often seen in sensorimotor systems (von Holst and Mittelstaedt, 1950; Bell, 1989; Bridgeman, 1995) and can be useful for providing information about intended motor activity to multiple areas of the brain, and for comparing motor instructions with the consequences of these instructions. The utility of an efference copy signal during sensorimotor learning has been explored in a computational model (Troyer and Doupe, 2000a,b). In this model, premotor activity in HVc gradually becomes associated with the resulting auditory feedback. This creates an internal prediction of the auditory feedback expected after a particular motor command is elicited. Thus, this efference copy is learned, and the role of auditory feedback is to maintain an accurate efference copy. The AFP then evaluates this sensory prediction rather than the actual feedback. One advantage of this scheme is that it greatly shortens the normal delay between motor activity and auditory feed-

back, which otherwise might cause feedback evaluation signals to arrive during the motor commands for the next vocal gesture.

If a sensory prediction is learned as described above, then the considerable time it takes for altered auditory feedback to result in vocal change in adult birds (Leonardo and Konishi, 1999; Brainard and Doupe, 2000a) might reflect the time necessary to revise the efference copy signal. An instructive signal for change would emerge only after consistently altered feedback changed the pattern of association of auditory feedback and motor commands in HVc. Alternatively, the time course for vocal change after deafening could reflect the time necessary for an instructive signal to take effect within the motor pathway. In this scheme, altered auditory feedback would immediately result in an instructive signal; however, a change in vocal output would not occur until the instructive signal was maintained over a certain period of time. Simultaneous recordings in the AFP and the motor pathway, during singing and especially during song learning, should help clarify the relationship of AFP activity to motor output and sensory feedback. Presentation of incorrect feedback might again be a useful manipulation, since altered feedback should provide a more potent signal for altering the association between motor commands and feedback in the putative efference copy than the complete absence of sound. In humans, delayed or altered auditory feedback changes vocal output much more rapidly than deafness (Lee, 1950; Cowie and Douglas-Cowie, 1992; Houde and Jordan, 1998).

Synaptic mechanisms that could underlie song learning

The above experiments implicate LMAN in processing sensory and sensorimotor information related to song, and demonstrate that the properties of LMAN neurons change during learning. Cellular properties of these neurons also change during learning: in particular, NMDA receptors (NMDARs) are strongly expressed in LMAN of young birds, and are significantly down-regulated by the end of the sensory critical period (Aamodt et al., 1992). Moreover, blockade of NMDARs in LMAN during tutoring has been shown to prevent birds from producing a good copy of the tutor song (Basham, Nordeen, and Nordeen, 1996), consistent with LMAN contributing to tutor song memorization. These results raise the possibility that NMDAR-dependent long-term plasticity is present in LMAN during sensory learning. Such plasticity could contribute to the experience-dependent shaping of auditory responses in LMAN and to the memorization of tutor song.

We investigated the hypothesis that LMAN synapses of young birds can undergo activity-dependent plasticity with an in vitro zebra finch brain slice preparation (figure 18.7A). Using slices from zebra finches early in sensory learning and not yet engaged in sensorimotor learning of song (20 days of age; figure 18.1A; Immelmann, 1969; Eales, 1989), we made intracellular voltage recordings from LMAN principal neurons. There are two known excitatory glutamatergic inputs to these cells: afferents from the medial portion of the dorsolateral thalamus (DLM), and the recurrent axon collateral inputs that interconnect neurons within the nucleus (LMAN$_R$; figure 18.7A). We focused on the LMAN$_R$ synapses, which can be activated by stimulating the LMAN outflow tract, because they have a significantly greater NMDAR-mediated component at the cell's resting potential (V$_{REST}$) at 20 days than do the DLM synapses (Livingston and Mooney, 1997; Boettiger and Doupe, 1998; Bottjer, Brady, and Walsh, 1998).

Plasticity was induced by repeated (40×) delivery of single brief (100-ms) pulses of postsynaptic depolarizing current in conjunction with LMAN$_R$ stimulation. Each current injection elicited a burst of six to ten action potentials (APs) whose duration approximated the duration of the current pulse. This pairing protocol produced a longlasting increase in the LMAN$_R$ EPSP slope. On average, the mean LMAN$_R$ EPSP slope 30 minutes after pairing onset was increased by 21% relative to baseline (figure 18.7B), and when stable recordings could be maintained to 60 minutes after pairing, EPSP slopes were increased by 33% relative to baseline. Consistent with many other forms of cortical and hippocampal potentiation, the induction of LMAN$_R$ LTP depended on NMDAR activation: the presence of the NMDAR blocker DL-2-amino-5-phosphonovaleric acid (APV) during pairing blocked the increase in LMAN$_R$ responses normally observed after pairing and instead produced a small but significant depression (Boettiger and Doupe, 2001).

The changes in the LMAN$_R$ EPSP elicited by the pairing protocol also depended on the timing of the first spike

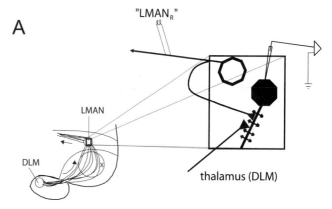

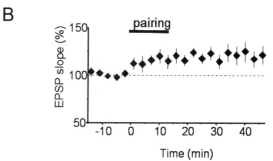

FIGURE 18.7   Synaptic plasticity in the LMAN slice. (A) Schematic of recording setup. Slices were cut oblique to the parasagittal plane. The thalamic inputs to LMAN (DLM) come in from below, while the recurrent collaterals between LMAN neurons (LMAN$_R$) interconnect LMAN neurons within the nucleus. The magnified view of LMAN and its inputs and outputs illustrates that the LMAN$_R$-stimulating electrode was placed in the LMAN outflow tract, thus activating these recurrent axon collaterals. Electrode placement was adjusted so that the individual neuron being recorded was not antidromically activated. The recording electrode used to investigate LMAN synapses was also used to inject current and elicit bursting. (B) Summary of LMAN$_R$ data from 12 birds of approximately 20 days of age. The slope of LMAN$_R$ extracellular synaptic potentials was significantly increased 30 minutes after pairing stimulation of LMAN$_R$ inputs with postsynaptic depolarizing bursts.

elicited by the current injection relative to the onset of the EPSP (figure 18.8A). When the first spike occurred after the LMAN$_R$ EPSP onset ("spike lags"; figure 18.8A, right inset), the LMAN$_R$ pathway was potentiated. In contrast, when the first spike in the burst preceded the EPSP onset ("spike leads"; figure 18.8A, left inset), potentiation did not occur, and in some cases the LMAN$_R$ EPSP was depressed. The pairing protocol induced significantly less potentiation of LMAN$_R$ responses in spike-leading versus spike-lagging experiments (figure 18.8A). Thus, LMAN$_R$ LTP in 20-day birds exhibits timing dependence, a computationally important feature (Roberts, 1999; Song, Miller, and Abbott, 2000) recently described in several systems (Bell et al., 1997; Magee and Johnston, 1997; Markram et al., 1997; Bi and Poo, 1998; Debanne, Gahwiler, and Thompson, 1998; Zhang et al.,

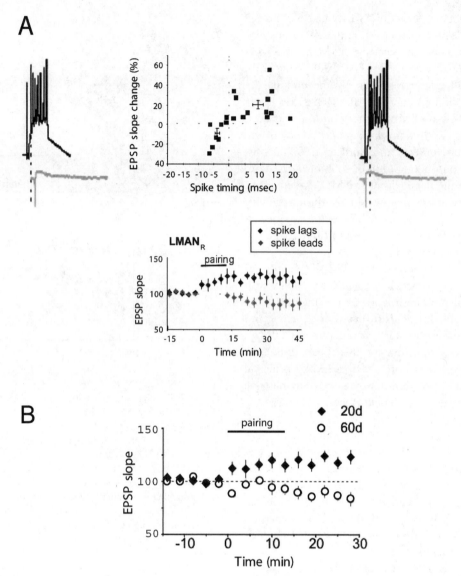

FIGURE 18.8 Timing and age dependence of LMAN_R LTP. (*A*) LMAN_R potentiation is dependent on the relative timing between the EPSP onset and the peak of the first spike elicited by the current injection; individual examples of postsynaptic spikes leading (left inset) and lagging (right inset) the LMAN_R EPSPs are shown. The upper graph plots the percent change of LMAN_R EPSP slope at 30 min versus spike timing relative to EPSP onset. Cross-hairs denote mean ± SEM for spike-lagging and spike-leading data. The lower graph plots group data showing the significant difference between LMAN_R EPSPs subjected to spike-lagging (♦, n = 12) versus spike-leading (♦, n = 8) pairing. (*B*) LMAN_R group data reveal the significant difference between the effects of the pairing protocol on slices from 20-day and 60-day birds. At 60 days, LMAN_R pairing induced no significant potentiation, instead eliciting depression.

1998; Egger, Feldmeyer, and Sakmann, 1999; Feldman, 2000). While the EPSP-AP burst pairing used in these experiments established this timing dependence, further experiments using a single AP will be necessary to provide a more complete description of the timing rule for LMAN_R synapses. Moreover, the lack of LTP induction when the first spike of a burst preceded the EPSP, despite subsequent spikes following the EPSP, suggests that the first spike plays a critical role in determining the sign of long-term plasticity in LMAN (see also Zhang et al., 1998).

Blockade of NMDARs in LMAN during tutoring, which impairs tutor learning (Basham, Nordeen, and Nordeen, 1996), would also have prevented the LMAN_R LTP described in 20-day finches. Lack of this LTP could thus be one factor preventing the incorporation of new tutor song information in young NMDAR-blocked birds. In addition, if LMAN_R LTP is critical to sensory learning, a decrease in LMAN_R LTP inducibility might also occur developmentally, contributing to the normal closure of the critical period for memorization of tutor song at approximately 60 days in zebra finches (figure 18.1*A*; Immelmann, 1969; Eales, 1985, 1987). To test this prediction, we paired postsynaptic bursts with LMAN_R synaptic stimulation in slices from birds 60 days of age.

The effect of the induction protocol on LMAN neurons' intrinsic synaptic inputs was strikingly different at this later age. Instead of inducing a potentiation of the $LMAN_R$ responses, a significant depression of $LMAN_R$ responses was observed at 30 minutes after spike-lagging pairing (average of −14%; figure 18.8*B*). This represented a significant decrease in the ability of the pairing protocol to induce $LMAN_R$ LTP at 60 days compared to that at 20 days. While these results do not rule out the possibility that potentiation of $LMAN_R$ responses could still be induced in older birds by a less physiological protocol, they indicate that the threshold for induction of this plasticity is substantially higher by the end of sensory learning. In addition, the change in sign of the plasticity at the $LMAN_R$ synapses suggests that functionally significant changes have taken place at these connections by 60 days.

Thus, long-term synaptic plasticity of intrinsic LMAN synapses can be induced by pairing stimulation of these synapses with postsynaptic bursts of APs, supporting the idea that excitatory feedback connections are key sites of synaptic plasticity within neural networks (Hua, Houk, and Mussa-Ivaldi, 1999). This $LMAN_R$ LTP, which depends on both NMDAR activation and the timing of the AP burst, is present at a time when sensory learning is occurring, and is no longer evident by the close of the sensory critical period. This timing suggests that LTP may play a role in tutor song memorization, and/or in the early stages of sensorimotor evaluation and refinement of song and of song-selective neurons. An advantage of the song system is that such correlations can be further tested in a straightforward manner by manipulating learning. For instance, raising zebra finches in isolation extends the normal critical period for tutor song learning (Eales, 1987, 1989). If $LMAN_R$ LTP is critical for song memorization, it should still be present in slices from 60 days finches raised in isolation. Alternatively, if $LMAN_R$ LTP is induced by early sensorimotor matching and development of song selectivity, it might still be inducible in 60-day birds that have memorized tutor song normally but have been prevented from hearing their own voice and refining their song (for instance, by muting or otherwise preventing audible auditory feedback). Given this ability to alter the behavior very specifically, circuitry in LMAN (and the song system as a whole) may prove to be particularly advantageous for pursuing a causal link between experience-dependent changes in synaptic strength and the learning of a complex behavior.

Finally, such spike timing–dependent $LMAN_R$ plasticity provides a simple and plausible mechanism for storage and recognition of a temporal pattern (Gerstner, Ritz, and van Hemmen, 1993; Abbott and Blum, 1996). This plasticity could be useful for generating connectivity within LMAN that reflects the temporal pattern of DLM afferent activity elicited by the tutor song, and thus comes to predict that

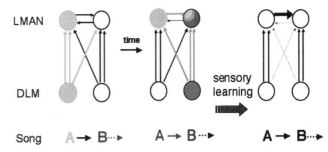

FIGURE 18.9 A simple model depicting a possible role for LMAN plasticity in song learning. During sensory learning, LMAN plasticity may establish a prediction within the recurrent circuitry of the temporal pattern of DLM afferent activation elicited by tutor song, as follows. A segment of tutor song A elicits firing in a subset of DLM projection neurons (left panel, shown in light gray), which in turn activate a subset of LMAN neurons (also in light gray), including their recurrent projections onto other LMAN neurons. Those LMAN neurons (shown in light and dark gray) activated by collateral inputs and simultaneously by DLM inputs responding to the next chunk of song B (middle panel, shown in dark gray), experience the conjunction required for $LMAN_R$ LTP. Because of spike timing dependence, the reciprocal collateral connection does not increase or even weakens: the postsynaptic cell spiking response to A will have begun before the collateral EPSP due to B arrives. Over the course of sensory learning, the spike timing–dependent strengthening of $LMAN_R$ synapses thus could come to reflect the temporal pattern of DLM afferent activation by tutor song (right panel). During subsequent sensorimotor learning, the production of the correct A-B sequence could lead to firing of strong $LMAN_R$ inputs driven by A coincident with spikes driven by B, leading to enhanced LMAN neuronal activity. This might represent an instructive signal for guiding vocal motor output at RA.

pattern. That is, if different subsets of DLM afferents fire at different time points in response to the sound of the tutor song, $LMAN_R$ LTP would cause LMAN neurons activated by DLM at one point in time to strengthen their connections onto LMAN neurons activated by DLM at a subsequent time point (figure 18.9). In contrast, because of the spike timing dependence of $LMAN_R$ LTP, the reciprocal $LMAN_R$ connections would weaken or remain static. These changes in synaptic strength over the course of sensory learning would come to represent the temporal pattern of DLM afferent activation in response to tutor song. Circuitry organized in this fashion could represent a memory of the tutor song, reminiscent of a proposed model for sequence prediction in the hippocampus (Abbott and Blum, 1996). During sensorimotor learning, such circuitry could then preferentially reinforce motor sequences produced by the bird that sound adequately similar to the tutor song (Troyer and Doupe, 2000).

Conclusions

The studies described in this chapter used a combination of neurophysiological studies and behavioral manipulations to investigate the function of the AFP, investigating not only normal birds at different stages of development but also animals in which the usual relationship between vocal motor output and sensory input had been in some way disrupted. The results reveal that AFP neurons develop auditory selectivity during learning for both BOS and tutor song, are strongly active during singing, even in deaf birds, and have synaptic mechanisms appropriate for developing temporal selectivity for song.

AFP neurons appear to reflect multiple sensory and motor aspects of song, suggesting that these processes are almost inextricably entangled, even at the level of single neurons. It seems likely that further understanding of AFP function will require learning how these auditory and motor signals relate to each other. In its intermixing of sensory and motor processing, birdsong is reminiscent of human speech (Doupe and Kuhl, 1999): electrical stimulation of a single language area can affect both the production and the perception of speech (Ojemann, 1991), and some cortical neurons respond differently to the same word, depending on whether it was spoken by the subject or by someone else (Creutzfeldt, Ojemann, and Lettich, 1989). Perhaps this entanglement indicates that the primary task assigned to the song system, and to many speech areas as well, is not sensory learning but rather the sensorimotor learning required to produce a vocal imitation. This difficult and protracted form of learning may alone have been sufficient to create the need for the song system, and to have specialized it for sensorimotor processing. Much of the initial, and more rapid, sensory processing and memorizing of songs could take place elsewhere in the brain, in areas afferent to the song system.

It is also relevant to the results here that the AFP is a cortical–basal ganglia circuit (Bottjer and Johnson, 1997; Luo and Perkel, 1999). Such basal ganglia circuits are well conserved evolutionarily and are generally implicated in motor and reinforcement learning (Graybiel et al., 1994; Knowlton, Mangels, and Squire, 1996), functions critical to sensorimotor learning of song. In primates, striatal neurons have predictive information related to movement and reward, and might participate in comparisons of motor output to internal models (Hikosaka, Sakamoto, and Usui, 1989; Hollerman, Tremblay, and Schultz, 1998; Tremblay, Hollerman, and Schultz, 1998). Spike timing–dependent plasticity similar to that observed here could be involved in generating such predictions. Like mammalian basal ganglia, AFP neurons could receive or even compute reinforcement signals and transfer them to the motor pathway. Because the AFP is a discrete basal ganglia–forebrain circuit specialized for one well-defined behavior, it may prove a particularly tractable system for elucidating the neural signals present in these structures, at both circuit and synaptic levels, and their function in the learning and modification of sequenced motor acts.

ACKNOWLEDGMENTS This work was supported by the National Institutes of Health (grant nos. MH55987 and NS34835 to A.J.D., MH11896 to C.A.B., and NS00913 to N.A.H.), a National Sciences Foundation graduate fellowship (M.M.S.), and the John Merck Fund and the EJLB Foundation (A.J.D.).

REFERENCES

AAMODT, S. M., M. R. KOZLOWSKI, E. J. NORDEEN, and K. W. NORDEEN, 1992. Distribution and developmental change in [³H]MK-801 binding within zebra finch song nuclei. *J. Neurobiol.* 23:997–1005.

ABBOTT, L. F., and K. I. BLUM, 1996. Functional significance of long-term potentiation for sequence learning and prediction. *Cereb. Cortex* 6:406–416.

AKUTAGAWA, E., and M. KONISHI, 1994. Two separate areas of the brain differentially guide the development of a song control nucleus in the zebra finch. *Proc. Natl. Acad. Sci. U.S.A.* 91:12413.

BASHAM, M. E., E. J. NORDEEN, and K. W. NORDEEN, 1996. Blockade of NMDA receptors in the anterior forebrain impairs sensory acquisition in the zebra finch (*Poephila guttata*). *Neurobiol. Learn. Mem.* 66:295–304.

BASHAM, M. E., F. SOHRABJI, T. D. SINGH, E. J. NORDEEN, and K. W. NORDEEN, 1999. Developmental regulation of NMDA receptor 2B subunit mRNA and ifenprodil binding in the zebra finch anterior forebrain. *J. Neurobiol.* 39:155–167.

BELL, C., 1989. Sensory coding and corollary discharge effects in mormyrid electric fish. *J. Exp. Biol.* 146:229–253.

BELL, C. C., V. Z. HAN, Y. SUGAWARA, and K. GRANT, 1997. Synaptic plasticity in a cerebellum-like structure depends on spike timing, synaptic strength and cell type. *Nature* 387:278–281.

BI, G., and M.-M. POO, 1998. Synaptic modifications in cultured hippocampal neurons: Dependence on spike timing, synaptic strength, and postsynaptic cell type. *J. Neurosci.* 18:10464–10472.

BOETTIGER, C. A., and A. J. DOUPE, 1998. Intrinsic and thalamic excitatory inputs onto songbird LMAN neurons differ in their pharmacological and temporal properties. *J. Neurophysiol.* 79:2615–2628.

BOETTIGER, C. A., and A. J. DOUPE, 2001. Developmentally restricted synaptic plasticity in a songbird nucleus required for song learning. *Neuron* 31:809–818.

BOLHUIS, J. J., G. G. O. ZIJLSTRA, A. M. DEN BOER-VISSER, and E. A. VAN DER ZEE, 2000. Localized neuronal activation in the zebra finch brain is related to the strength of song learning. *Proc. Natl. Acad. Sci. U.S.A.* 97:2282–2285.

BOTTJER, S. W., J. D. BRADY, and J. P. WALSH, 1998. Intrinsic and synaptic properties of neurons in the vocal-control nucleus lMAN from in vitro slice preparations of juvenile and adult zebra finches. *J. Neurobiol.* 37:642–658.

BOTTJER, S. W., and F. JOHNSON, 1997. Circuits, hormones, and learning: Vocal behavior in songbirds. *J. Neurobiol.* 33:602–618.

BOTTJER, S. W., E. A. MIESNER, and A. P. ARNOLD, 1984. Forebrain lesions disrupt development but not maintenance of song in passerine birds. *Science* 224:901–903.

BOUGHMAN, J. W., 1998. Vocal learning by greater spear-nosed bats. *Proc. R. Soc. Lond. B* 265:227–233.

BRAINARD, M. S., and A. J. DOUPE, 2000a. Interruption of a basal ganglia–forebrain circuit prevents plasticity of learned vocalizations. *Nature* 404:762–766.

BRAINARD, M. S., and A. J. DOUPE, 2000b. Auditory feedback in learning and maintenance of vocal behaviour. *Nat. Rev. Neurosci.* 1:31–38.

BRIDGEMAN, B., 1995. A review of the role of efference copy in sensory and oculomotor control systems. *Ann. Biomed. Eng.* 23: 409–422.

COWIE, R., and E. DOUGLAS-COWIE, 1992. *Postlingually Acquired Deafness: Speech Deterioration and the Wider Consequences*, W. Winter, ed. Berlin: Mouton de Gruyter.

CREUTZFELDT, O., G. OJEMANN, and E. LETTICH, 1989. Neuronal activity in the human lateral temporal lobe. II. Responses to the subject's own voice. *Exp. Brain Res.* 77:476–489.

DAVE, A., and D. MARGOLIASH, 2000. Song replay during sleep and computational rules for sensorimotor vocal learning. *Science* 270:812–816.

DEBANNE, D., B. H. GAHWILER, and S. M. THOMPSON, 1998. Long-term synaptic plasticity between pairs of individual CA3 pyramidal cells in rat hippocampus slice cultures. *J. Physiol.* 507:237–247.

DOUPE, A. J., 1997. Song- and order-selective neurons in the songbird anterior forebrain and their emergence during vocal development. *J. Neurosci.* 17:1147–1167.

DOUPE, A. J., and P. K. KUHL, 1999. Birdsong and human speech: Common themes and mechanisms. *Annu. Rev. Neurosci.* 22:567–631.

EALES, L. A., 1985. Song learning in zebra finches: Some effects of song model availability on what is learnt and when. *Anim. Behav.* 33:1293–1300.

EALES, L. A., 1987. Song learning in female-raised zebra finches: Another look at the sensitive phase. *Anim. Behav.* 35:1356–1365.

EALES, L. A., 1989. The influences of visual and vocal interaction on song learning in zebra finches. *Anim. Behav.* 37:507–508.

EGGER, V., D. FELDMEYER, and B. SAKMANN, 1999. Coincidence detection and changes of synaptic efficacy in spiny stellate neurons in rat barrel cortex. *Nat. Neurosci.* 2:1098–1105.

EIMAS, P. D., J. L. MILLER, and P. W. JUSCZYK, 1987. On infant speech perception and language acquisition. In *Categorical Perception*, S. Harnard, ed. New York: Cambridge University Press, pp. 161–195.

FELDMAN, D. E., 2000. Timing-based LTP and LTD at vertical inputs to layer II/III pyramidal cells in rat barrel cortex. *Neuron* 27:45–56.

GENTNER, T. Q., and D. MARGOLIASH, 2003. Neuronal populations and single cells representing learned auditory objects. *Nature* 424:669–674.

GERSTNER, W., R. RITZ, and J. L. VAN HEMMEN, 1993. Why spikes? Hebbian learning and retrieval of time-resolved excitation patterns. *Biol. Cybern.* 69:503–515.

GRAYBIEL, A. M., T. AOSAKI, A. W. FLAHERTY, and M. KIMURA, 1994. The basal ganglia and adaptive motor control. *Science* 265:1826–1831.

HESSLER, N. A., and A. J. DOUPE, 1999a. Social context modulates singing-related neural activity in the songbird forebrain. *Nat. Neurosci.* 2:209–211.

HESSLER, N. A., and A. J. DOUPE, 1999b. Singing-related neural activity in a dorsal forebrain–basal ganglia circuit of adult zebra finches. *J. Neurosci.* 19:10461–10481.

HIKOSAKA, O., M. SAKAMOTO, and S. USUI, 1989. Functional properties of monkey caudate neurons. III. Activities related to expectation of target and reward. *J. Neurophysiol.* 61:814–832.

HOLLERMAN, J. R., L. TREMBLAY, and W. SCHULTZ, 1998. Influence of reward expectation on behavior-related neuronal activity in primate striatum. *J. Neurophysiol.* 80:947–963.

HOUDE, J. F., and M. I. JORDAN, 1998. Sensorimotor adaptation in speech production. *Science* 36:1213–1216.

HUA, S. E., J. C. HOUK, and F. A. MUSSA-IVALDI, 1999. Emergence of symmetric, modular, and reciprocal connections in recurrent networks with Hebbian learning. *Biol. Cybern.* 81: 211–225.

IMMELMANN, K., 1969. Song development in the zebra finch and other estrildid finches. In *Bird Vocalizations*, R. A. Hinde, ed. London: Cambridge University Press, pp. 61–74.

JOHNSON, F., and S. W. BOTTJER, 1994. Afferent influences on cell death and birth during development of a cortical nucleus necessary for learned vocal behavior in zebra finches. *Development* 120:13–24.

KNOWLTON, B. J., J. A. MANGELS, and L. R. SQUIRE, 1996. A neostriatal habit learning system in humans. *Science* 6:1399–1402.

KONISHI, M., 1965. The role of auditory feedback in the control of vocalization in the white-crowned sparrow. *Z. Tierpsychol.* 22: 770–783.

KUHL, P. K., 1994. Learning and representation in speech and language. *Curr. Opin. Neurobiol* 4:812–822.

LEE, B. S., 1950. Effects of delayed speech feedback. *J. Acoust. Soc. Am.* 22:824–826.

LEONARDO, A., and M. KONISHI, 1999. Decrystallization of adult birdsong by perturbation of auditory feedback. *Nature* 399:466–470.

LIVINGSTON, F. S., and R. MOONEY, 1997. Development of intrinsic and synaptic properties in a forebrain nucleus essential to avian song learning. *J. Neurosci.* 17:8997–9009.

LUO, M., and D. J. PERKEL, 1999. A GABAergic, strongly inhibitory projection to a thalamic nucleus in the zebra finch song system. *J. Neurosci.* 19:6700–6711.

MAGEE, J. C., and D. JOHNSTON, 1997. A synaptically controlled, associative signal for Hebbian plasticity in hippocampal neurons. *Science* 275:209–213.

MARGOLIASH, D., 1983. Acoustic parameters underlying the responses of song-specific neurons in the white-crowned sparrow. *J. Neurosci.* 3:1039–1057.

MARKRAM, H., J. LÜBKE, M. FROTSCHER, and B. SAKMANN, 1997. Regulation of synaptic efficacy by coincidence of postsynaptic APs and EPSPs. *Science* 275:213–215.

MARLER, P., 1970. A comparative approach to vocal learning: Song development in white-crowned sparrows. *J. Comp. Physiol. Psychol.* 71:1–25.

McCASLAND, J. S., 1987. Neuronal control of bird song production. *J. Neurosci.* 7:23–39.

McCASLAND, J. S., and M. KONISHI, 1981. Interaction between auditory and motor activities in an avian song control nucleus. *Proc. Natl. Acad. Sci. U.S.A.* 78:7815–7819.

MELLO, C. V., D. S. VICARIO, and D. F. CLAYTON, 1992. Song presentation induces gene expression in the songbird forebrain. *Proc. Natl. Acad. Sci. U.S.A.* 89:6818–6822.

MORRISON, R. G., and F. NOTTEBOHM, 1993. Role of a telencephalic nucleus in the delayed song learning of socially isolated zebra finches. *J. Neurobiol.* 24:1045–1064.

NAKAMURA, K., K. SAKAI, and O. HIKOSAKA, 1999. Effects of local inactivation of monkey medial frontal cortex in learning of sequential procedures. *J. Neurophysiol.* 82:1063–1068.

NORDEEN, K. W., and E. J. NORDEEN, 1992. Auditory feedback is necessary for the maintenance of stereotyped song in adult zebra finches. *Behav. Neural. Biol.* 57:58–66.

NORDEEN, K. W., and E. J. NORDEEN, 1993. Long-term maintenance of song in adult zebra finches is not affected by lesions of a forebrain region involved in song learning. *Behav. Neural Biol.* 59:79–82.

NOTTEBOHM, F., T. M. STOKES, and C. M. LEONARD, 1976. Central control of song in the canary, *Serinus canarius*. *J. Comp. Neurol.* 165:457–486.

OJEMANN, G. A., 1991. Cortical organization of language. *J. Neurosci.* 11:2281–2287.

PETERS, S., P. MARLER, and S. NOWICKI, 1992. Song sparrows learn from limited exposure to song models. *Condor* 94:1016–1019.

PRICE, P. H., 1979. Developmental determinants of structure in zebra finch song. *J. Comp. Physiol. Psychol.* 93:260–277.

RENDELL, L., and H. WHITEHEAD, 2001. Culture in whales and dolphins. *Behav. Brain. Sci.* 24:309–324.

ROBERTS, P. D., 1999. Computational consequences of temporally asymmetric learning rules. I. Differential Hebbian learning. *J. Comput. Neurosci.* 7:235–246.

SCHARFF, C., and F. NOTTEBOHM, 1991. A comparative study of the behavioral deficits following lesions of the various parts of the zebra finch song system: Implications for vocal learning. *J. Neurosci.* 11:2896–2913.

SOHRABJI, F., E. J. NORDEEN, and K. W. NORDEEN, 1990. Selective impairment of song learning following lesions of a forebrain nucleus in the juvenile zebra finch. *Behav. Neural Biol.* 53:51–63.

SOLIS, M. M., and A. J. DOUPE, 1997. Anterior forebrain neurons develop selectivity by an intermediate stage of birdsong learning. *J. Neurosci.* 17:6447–6462.

SOLIS, M. M., and A. J. DOUPE, 1999. Contributions of tutor and bird's own song experience to neural selectivity in the songbird anterior forebrain. *J. Neurosci.* 19:4559–4584.

SOLIS, M. M., and A. J. DOUPE, 2000. Compromised neural selectivity for song in birds with impaired sensorimotor learning. *Neuron* 25:109–121.

SONG, S., K. D. MILLER, and L. F. ABBOTT, 2000. Competitive Hebbian learning through spike-timing-dependent synaptic plasticity. *Nat. Neurosci.* 3:919–923.

TCHERNICHOVSKI, O., T. LINTS, P. P. MITRA, and F. NOTTEBOHM, 1999. Vocal imitation in zebra finches is inversely related to model abundance. *Proc. Natl. Acad. Sci. U.S.A.* 96:12901–12904.

THEUNISSEN, F. E., and A. J. DOUPE, 1998. Temporal and spectral sensitivity of complex auditory neurons in the nucleus HVc of male zebra finches. *J. Neurosci.* 18:3786–3802.

TODT, D., H. HULTSCH, and D. HEIKE, 1979. Conditions affecting song acquisition in nightingales, *Luscinia megarhynchos*. *Z. Tierpsychol.* 51:23–35.

TREMBLAY, L., J. R. HOLLERMAN, and W. SCHULTZ, 1998. Modifications of reward expectation-related neuronal activity during learning in primate striatum. *J. Neurophysiol.* 80:964–977.

TROYER, T., and A. J. DOUPE, 2000a. An associational model of birdsong sensorimotor learning. I. Efference copy and the learning of song syllables. *J. Neurophysiol.* 84:1204–1223.

TROYER, T., and A. J. DOUPE, 2000b. An associational model of birdsong sensorimotor learning. II. Temporal hierarchies and the learning of song sequence. *J. Neurophysiol.* 84:1224–1239.

VON HOLST, E., and H. MITTELSTAEDT, 1950. Das Reafferenzprinzip. Wechselwirkungen zwischen Zentralnervensystem und Peripherie. *Naturwissenschaften* 37:464–476.

WALDSTEIN, R. S., 1989. Effects of postlingual deafness on speech production: Implications for the role of auditory feedback. *J. Acoust. Soc. Am.* 88:2099–2114.

WERKER, J. F., and R. C. TEES, 1992. The organization and reorganization of human speech perception. *Annu. Rev. Neurosci.* 15:377–402.

WILLIAMS, H., and N. MEHTA, 1999. Changes in adult zebra finch song require a forebrain nucleus that is not necessary for song production. *J. Neurobiol.* 39:14–28.

YU, A. C., and D. MARGOLIASH, 1996. Temporal hierarchical control of singing in birds. *Science* 273:1871–1875.

ZHANG, L. I., H. W. TAO, C. E. HOLT, W. A. HARRIS, and M.-M. POO, 1998. A critical window for cooperation and competition among developing retinotectal synapses. *Nature* 395:37–44.

19 Olfaction: From Sniff to Percept

MOUSTAFA BENSAFI, CHRISTINA ZELANO, BRAD JOHNSON, JOEL MAINLAND, REHAN KHAN, AND NOAM SOBEL

ABSTRACT All mammals have acute olfaction, and humans are no exception to this rule. Humans can detect and discriminate between a very large if still undetermined number of odorants. How this discrimination is achieved, and the metric of smell employed by the brain in this task, remain unknown. The olfactory percept is constructed within a hierarchical anatomy that starts with olfactory transduction at the olfactory epithelium, proceeds to initial processing in the olfactory bulb, and continues with further processing throughout a network of cortical structures, mostly in the ventral portion of the temporal lobe. Current evidence suggests that odor is encoded within this system as follows. There are about 1000 different mammalian olfactory receptor types. A given olfactory receptor type responds to a small number of odorants, and a given odorant will activate a number of different receptor types. All receptors of a particular type converge onto one or a few neuropil patches, termed glomeruli, within the olfactory bulb. Thus, a given odorant's identity may be encoded combinatorially through the particular spatiotemporal map of activated glomeruli. Olfactory cortex may then function as an associational system pairing different odor components of a single olfactory percept, or an olfactory percept with nonolfactory events. Like other distal senses, olfaction is subserved by a dedicated sensorimotor system, the olfactomotor system. This system produces sniffs that are rapidly modified by the odorant, and, more important, odorant content is reciprocally modified by the sniff. Different sniffs will better tune the olfactory system to different odorants. Furthermore, because sniff airflow rate is slightly different in each nostril, each nostril is better tuned to slightly different odorants within a given sniff. Thus, when a mammal takes a sniff, the sniff provides the brain with two simultaneous yet slightly disparate images of the olfactory world. How the brain combines these disparate images into a unified olfactory percept remains unknown.

Introduction

Oomvelt is a German term used in classic ethology to describe the primary perceptual space of an animal. A look at the table of contents of this book, or indeed the noun used at the beginning of this sentence, reveals the *oomvelt* of humans: vision. Humans' conscious perception of the world around them, and the language they use to describe it, are dominated by vision. This visual primacy, however, is far from the rule in vertebrates or mammals. Most animals, unlike humans, trust their sense of smell in the most important of behaviors. Mammals select a mate based on smell (Wysocki, 1979; Doty, 1986), females may choose to abort a pregnancy based on smell (Bruce, 1959), territories are marked (Mertl-Millhollen, 1979) and explored (Wallace, Gorny, and Whishaw, 2002) through smell, sharks may find their prey by smell (Hara, 1975), and pigeons may find their home through smell (Papi, 1991). Furthermore, intricate social hierarchy and behavioral intensions may all be conveyed through smell (Liebenauer and Slotnick, 1996). In sum, smell is a potent source of information about conspecifics, about other animals, and about the physical environment. There is an obvious selective advantage to gathering accurate environmental information from as many sources as possible. Thus, that humans would choose to ignore valuable information that may be contained in odor seems maladaptive at best. Indeed, extensive research suggests that human physiological state and behavior are in fact constantly affected by olfaction, but that humans are mostly unaware of this process (Kirk-Smith, Van Toller, and Dodd, 1983; Lorig, 1994; Stern and McClintock, 1998; Sobel, Prabhakaran, et al., 1999; Bensafi et al., 2002). This, however, will not be the major topic of this review. Because this is the only chapter on olfaction in this book, here we will offer the reader an overview of mammalian olfaction, focusing on the current view of how odor may be encoded within this system and on the significance of the olfactomotor system.

From molecule to percept

What is an odor? Any volatile (molecular weight <294 daltons) molecular species with surface activity, low polarity, some water solubility, a high vapor pressure, and a high lipophilicity will probably be detectable and discriminable by the mammalian olfactory system (Ohloff, 1986). Nobody knows exactly how many discrete odors this amounts to. Estimates have ranged from thousands to tens of thousands to hundreds of thousands, yet we know of no computed theoretical upper limit to this number. The human olfactory

MOUSTAFA BENSAFI Department of Neuroscience, University of California, Berkeley, Calif.

CHRISTINA ZELANO Department of Biophysics, University of California, Berkeley, Calif.

BRAD JOHNSON Department of Bioengineering, University of California, Berkeley, Calif.

JOEL MAINLAND and REHAN KHAN Department of Neuroscience, University of California, Berkeley, Calif.

NOAM SOBEL Departments of Neuroscience, Biophysics, Bioengineering, and Psychology, University of California, Berkeley, Calif.

system can detect these molecules with astonishing sensitivity, outperforming analytical instruments such as mass chromatographs (Cain, 1977) and performing on par with monkeys (Laska, Trolp, and Teubner, 1999), which themselves perform on par with rats (Laska, Seibt, and Weber, 2000), the latter being macrosmatic animals with a recognized outstanding sense of smell. The transformation from molecule to percept occurs along a hierarchically organized system that in mammals is summarized as follows: following transduction at olfactory receptor neurons in the olfactory epithelium, odor information is projected ipsilaterally via the olfactory nerve to the olfactory bulb. Following bulbar processing, the signal is projected ipsilaterally via the lateral olfactory tract to primary olfactory cortex within the ventral portions of the temporal lobe (figure 19.1). In this manner, olfaction differs from the distal senses of vision and audition, where peripheral input projects to cortex initially via a thalamic relay. In contrast, olfactory information projects to the thalamus from primary olfactory cortex. Additional primary olfactory cortex projections relay odor information to multiple brain regions, including what has been referred to as secondary olfactory cortex in the orbitofrontal region and flavor integration regions in the insula. Airborne chemicals are concurrently transduced by at least two additional mammalian neural subsystems, the vomeronasal system (Halpern, 1987; Meredith, 1991; Keverne, 1999; Dulac, 2000) and the trigeminal system (Doty, 1995; Hummel, 2000; Hummel and Livermore, 2002). However, in order to maintain a manageable scope, in this chapter we will focus on the main olfactory system only. We first briefly summarize the structure and events at each of the olfactory anatomical processing stages and then review the current understanding of how odor is encoded within this neuronal infrastructure.

Olfactory epithelium

For a molecule to be transduced into a neural signal it must reach olfactory receptors within the olfactory epithelia. The human epithelia are located bilaterally about 7 cm up the nasal passage, lining the cribriform plate and extending to the nasal turbinates (Clerico, To, and Lanza, 2003). These turbinates are convoluted to increase the surface area of the epithelium to about $1–2\,cm^2$ in humans (Moran et al., 1982), and $7\,m^2$ in some dogs (Moulton, 1977). An odorant molecule may reach the epithelium in three different ways. The first is by diffusion from an area of higher concentration (the environment) to an area of lower concentration (the nares). The second is by a process termed retronasal olfaction (Hornung and Enns, 1986), whereby an odorant enters the mouth in food or drink and propagates back up the throat into the nose. The third and most common route by which a molecule reaches the olfactory epithelium is transportation by either ongoing nasal inhalation or a sniff—a vigorous

contraction of the diaphragm leading to rapid nasal airflow (often exceeding $100\,L/min$ in humans) (figure 19.2).

The epithelium consists of many cell types (Carr et al., 1991; Huard et al., 1998), but most fall into four primary categories: olfactory receptor cells, sustentacular or supporting cells, basal cells, and duct cells of Bowman's glands. The latter are the secretory source of a mucous layer that lines the olfactory epithelium. This mucous layer plays a role in immune function (Getchell and Getchell, 1991) and various enzymatic processes (Lewis and Dahl, 1995), but it also directly affects olfaction by selectively modulating the passage of odorants to the receptors, and possibly by further modulating the later removal of odorants from the receptors (deactivation) (Lewis and Dahl, 1995). In addition to the passive mucosal effect on olfaction, the mucosa contains an odorant-binding protein (OBP) that assists in actively transferring hydrophobic odorants across the largely hydrophilic mucosa (Pevsner et al., 1985; Pelosi, 2001).

The olfactory receptor cells are bipolar neurons that are unique in at least two ways: (1) they constantly regenerate from the basal cell layer (Graziadei, Levine, and Monti-Graziadei, 1979; Graziadei and Monti Graziadei, 1983), with a typical life span in mammals ranging from a month to a year (Hinds, Hinds, and McNelly, 1984; Mackay-Sim and Kittel, 1991), and (2) they are in direct contact with the external environment. This direct link between the brain and the outside world has been postulated as a path of entry for pathogens from the environment directly to the brain (Roberts, 1986). Humans have about 6 million receptor cells in each epithelium (Moran et al., 1982). Each of these olfactory receptor neurons sends one dendrite into the mucous layer, terminating in an olfactory knob that contains between 3 and 50 nonmotile olfactory cilia, each about $5\,\mu m$ long (Morrison and Costanzo, 1990, 1992). It is these cilia that contain the site of olfactory transduction. Various lines of evidence suggested that this transduction was similar to transduction of light in retinal rods and cones. Doron Lancet and colleagues found that odorants induce activation of adenylate cyclase (Pace et al., 1985), and Nakamura and Gold (1987) found a cyclic nucleotide–gated conductance in olfactory receptor cilia. Randy Reed and colleagues later found this adenylate cyclase to be olfactory-specific (Bakalyar and Reed, 1990) and activated by an olfactory-specific G protein (Jones and Reed, 1989). In 1991, Linda Buck and Richard Axel brought this line of research to a culmination point by identifying a large multigene family that encodes the olfactory receptors. The olfactory receptors indeed belonged to the family of G-protein-coupled receptors of the 7-helix type that, surprisingly, contained around 1000 different olfactory receptor genes, the largest known gene family in the mammalian genome (Buck and Axel, 1991). This work has generated the following current view of olfactory transduction (figure 19.3): When an odorant

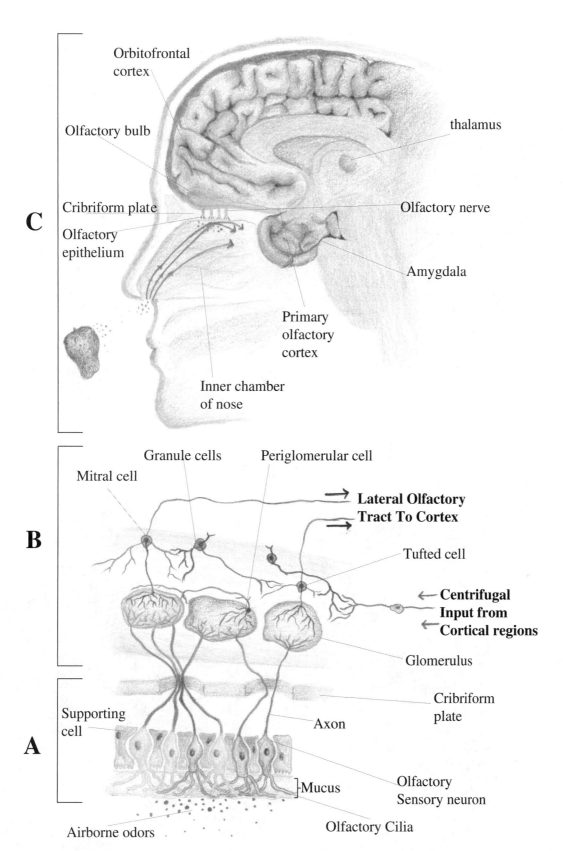

C

Orbitofrontal
cortex

Olfactory bulb

thalamus

Cribriform plate

Olfactory
epithelium

Olfactory nerve

Amygdala

Primary
olfactory
cortex

Inner chamber
of nose

B

Granule cells

Periglomerular cell

Mitral cell

**Lateral Olfactory
Tract To Cortex**

Tufted cell

← **Centrifugal
Input from
Cortical regions**

Glomerulus

Cribriform
plate

Supporting
cell

Axon

A

Mucus

Olfactory
Sensory neuron

Airborne odors

Olfactory Cilia

FIGURE 19.1 Structure of the human olfactory system. The human olfactory system can be segregated into three primary compartments: epithelium, bulb, and cortex. (*A*) Olfactory epithelium. Each olfactory sensory neuron expresses one olfactory receptor gene. Like receptors project to one or a small number of glomeruli. (*B*) Organization of the olfactory bulb. Glomeruli receive input from olfactory sensory neurons and cortical olfactory regions. Mitral and tufted cell dendrites contact receptor axons within glomeruli. The axons of the mitral and tufted cells project widely to higher brain structures, as labeled in *C*. Lateral processing in the olfactory bulb occurs across two types of interneurons, periglomerular cells and granule cells. (*C*) Sagittal view of the human head. The olfactory bulb and epithelium are highlighted in yellow. (See color plate 3.)

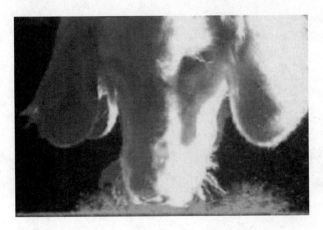

FIGURE 19.2 Airflow visualization using Schlieren imaging, from the work of Gary Settles (Settles, 2001; Settles et al., 2003). These visualizations revealed that before sniffing inward, dogs may also sniff outward in a lateral trajectory in order to distribute particles so that they can be inhaled and smelled. As this image clearly depicts, sensation is an active process, and olfaction is a good case in point. (See color plate 4.)

molecule binds to an olfactory receptor, it triggers the activation of the specific olfactory G protein, G_{olf}, which releases a subunit, $G_{\alpha olf}$, that stimulates production of adenylyl cyclase III. Adenylyl cyclase III increases intracellular cAMP, which opens a cyclic nucleotide–gated cation channel, depolarizing the cell and ultimately resulting in an action potential in the sensory neuron. John Ngai and colleagues demonstrated that blocking this cascade causes anosmia (Brunet, Gold, and Ngai, 1996).

A second transduction cascade has also been suggested whereby activation of the G protein and phospholipase C leads to the production of IP_3, which directly opens calcium channels that depolarize the cell (Boekhoff et al., 1990). Following transduction, odorant-induced action potentials propagate down the axons of olfactory receptor neurons, which join to form the olfactory nerve, pass through the cribriform plate, and synapse at the olfactory bulb.

Olfactory bulb

The mammalian olfactory bulb consists of six cellular layers. From superficial to deep, these are (1) the olfactory nerve

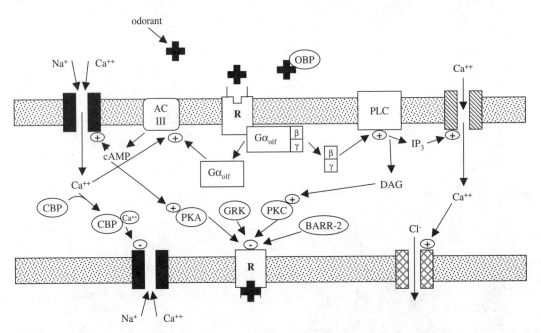

FIGURE 19.3 Odorant molecules bind to olfactory receptors (R) embedded within the olfactory epithelium. The binding causes the associated G-protein complex to release its two subunits (α and β). The α subunit stimulates the integral membrane protein adenylyl cyclase (AC III), which in turn increases the concentration of cAMP. Cyclic-gated nucleotide (CNG) channels open with cAMP, leading to membrane depolarization. If there is sufficient depolarization, an action potential is generated in the sensory axon. The $\beta\gamma$ complex released from the G protein stimulates phospholipase C (PLC), leading to higher intracellular inositol triphosphate (IP_3) and diacylglycerol (DAG). IP_3 opens Ca^{2+} channels, allowing Ca^{2+} to enter the neuron. The Ca^{2+} ions have multiple effector pathways.

Ca^{2+} stimulates Cl^- channels, allowing Cl^- ions to exit the cell (intracellular Cl^- concentration is greater than extracellular concentration). This ion exchange further depolarizes the membrane. Calcium also inhibits the transduction by combining with Ca^{2+}-binding protein (CBP), which closes the CNG channels, ending signal transduction. Signal termination is also mediated by a variety of protein kinases (PKA, GRK, PKC) that phosphorylate the olfactory receptor, and by β-arrestin-2 (BARR-2) interacting with the olfactory receptor. Odorant-binding proteins (OBP) in the nasal mucosa may increase odorant solubility and/or receptor-binding affinity, aiding transduction, or may assist in odorant clearance, aiding signal termination. (Image after Buck, 1996.)

layer, (2) the glumerular layer, (3) the external plexiform layer, (4) the mitral cell layer, (5) the internal plexiform layer, and (6) the granule cell layer (Kratskin and Belluzzi, 2003). These layers are arranged in a concentric manner reminiscent of an onion (Shepherd, 1972; Greer et al., 1981). The bulb contains functional elements, primarily consisting of an input neuron, an interneuron, and an output neuron. The inputs are from two sources: peripheral input from the olfactory receptors and centrifugal inputs from cortical olfactory regions (see figure 19.1). These centrifugal inputs are very extensive, are from various olfactory regions, and, although not yet fully understood, are thought to play a significant role in olfaction (Gray and Skinner, 1988). The peripheral input consists of axons of olfactory receptor neurons. These project unbranched from the epithelium to the olfactory nerve layer of the bulb, where they terminate in spherical neuropil structures, 50–200 μm in diameter, called glomeruli. The glomeruli form the glumerular layer, which is one or two glomeruli thick. In humans, each olfactory bulb contains approximately 8000 glomeruli, and, in a striking case of neural convergence, about 750 sensory axons converge onto one glomerulus (Meisami et al., 1998). Within the glomeruli, the receptor axons contact dendrites of either mitral or tufted output neurons and periglomerular interneurons. The bulb is the site of extensive olfactory processing modulated by interneurons consisting of short-axon cells, inhibitory periglomerular cells, and inhibitory axonless granule cells. Granule cells make inhibitory dendrodendritic reciprocal synaptic connections with mitral and tufted cells. Periglomerular cells project a primary dendrite into glomeruli, where they synapse with sensory axons, and additional dendrites make inhibitory dendrodendritic synapses with mitral and tufted cells. The mitral and tufted cell axons join to form the lateral olfactory tract, which is the output from the bulb to primary olfactory cortex in the ventral portions of the temporal lobe (see figure 19.1).

Olfactory cortex

By current definition, primary olfactory cortex consists of all brain regions that receive direct input from the mitral and tufted cell axons of the olfactory bulb (Allison, 1954; Price, 1973, 1987, 1990; de Olmos, Hardy, and Heimer, 1978; Carmichael, Clugnet, and Price, 1994; Shipley, 1995; Haberly, 2001). These compose most of the paleocortex, including (in order of occurrence along the olfactory tract) the anterior olfactory cortex (also referred to as the anterior olfactory nucleus), the ventral taenia tecta, anterior hippocampal continuation and indusium griseum, the olfactory tubercle, piriform cortex, the anterior cortical nucleus of the amygdala, the periamygdaloid cortex, and the rostral entorhinal cortex (Carmichael, Clugnet, and Price, 1994). In rodents, the anterior olfactory cortex may play a role in

interhemispheric communication between olfactory bulbs (Cleland and Linster, 2003), but in humans, both the anterior olfactory cortex and olfactory tubercle are poorly defined. Piriform cortex, the largest component of primary olfactory cortex in mammals, lies along the olfactory tract at the junction of temporal and frontal lobes, and continues onto the dorsomedial aspect of the temporal lobe. Piriform cortex is three-layered allocortex, with a superficial plexiform layer I and pyramidal cells densely packed in layer II and less so in layer III. Projections from the bulb synapse onto dendrites of pyramidal cells within layer I of piriform cortex. Caudally, piriform cortex fuses into the anterior cortical nucleus of the amygdala. Olfactory bulb projections terminate densely on the periamygdaloid cortex that inhabits the medial surface of the amygdala, and less so on the rostral portions of the entorhinal cortex. The entorhinal cortex is the only portion of primary olfactory cortex that is six-layered, and so is considered transitional between olfactory allocortex and isocortex. The entire cortical complex that forms primary olfactory cortex is extensively interconnected by association fibers projecting across regions to synapse at layer I, and within regions traversing the three cortical layers (Shipley, 1995). Furthermore, the primary olfactory cortical regions project extensive centrifugal input back to the olfactory bulb (Carmichael, Clugnet, and Price, 1994). Beyond these primary regions, olfactory information is projected throughout the brain, most prominently to orbitofrontal gyri and the insular cortex.

As can be appreciated from both the sheer area and diversity of cortical real estate that is considered primary olfactory cortex, this definition is far from functional. There is not one aspect of olfaction that can be functionally attributed to primary olfactory cortex as defined, since, as one can imagine, piriform cortex, the amygdala, and the entorhinal cortex each may contribute uniquely to olfactory processing. It is for this reason that this definition is nearing abandonment (Haberly, 2001; Sobel et al., 2003). Indeed, in a recent thorough review of central olfactory structures, Cleland and Linster (2003) simply shifted the definition by referring to the classic primary olfactory structures as secondary olfactory structures, noting that, as suggested by Haberly (2001), the definition of mammalian primary olfactory cortex may better fit the olfactory bulb than piriform cortex.

Odor encoding

Anatomically, the human olfactory system consists of three primary compartments: epithelium, bulb, and cortex (see figure 19.1). Some aspect of odor encoding occurs at each of these processing stages, and it is the combination of activity across these regions that gives rise to the complex percept of odor.

The number of discrete odorants that mammals can discriminate is unknown. That said, there is uniform agreement that it is more than 1000 (the estimated upper limit to the number of mammalian olfactory receptor types), and therefore odorants are probably not encoded in a simple, one-receptor-to-odorant scheme. Several lines of evidence suggest that each olfactory receptor neuron expresses only one type of olfactory receptor (Nef et al., 1992; Strotmann et al., 1992; Ressler, Sullivan, and Buck, 1993; Vassar, Ngai, and Axel, 1993; Chess et al., 1994). Furthermore, each individual receptor neuron responds to multiple odorants, and a given odorant activates several different olfactory receptor types (Sicard and Holley 1984; Firestein, Pico, and Menini, 1993; Raming et al., 1993; Sato et al., 1994; Krautwurst, Yau, and Reed, 1998; Zhao et al., 1998; Malnic et al., 1999). Thus, odor encoding may be the result of a combinatorial scheme in which different receptors respond to different molecular aspects of an odorant, and a given odorant is then represented by the subset of receptors that it activates (Axel, 1995; Buck, 1996; Mombaerts, 1999; Firestein, 2001). Such a scheme would enable the encoding of a very large number of different odorants within what is potentially a 1000-dimensional space.

Under the assumption that this is indeed the manner in which the peripheral olfactory system initially transduces odorants, one may ask how this high-dimensional information is organized by the brain to enable odor discrimination. Some unique principles may apply to odor encoding. First, odor coding appears to be synthetic. Most environmentally relevant odorants are complex mixtures of molecules, yet are processed as a whole. Indeed, the identification of specific odorant molecules or molecular features is far less behaviorally relevant than the ability to distinguish the complex odor of a ripened fruit or of a predator from background odors. Accordingly, mammals are quite bad at determining the composition of mixtures when the number of components reaches four or higher (Livermore and Laing, 1996; Linster and Smith, 1997). Second, in comparison to vision and audition, odor transduction is slow, because molecules must sorb across the mucosa, a process that takes about 150 ms (Firestein and Werblin, 1989). That the neural substrates of olfaction do not have to fire continuously to keep up with peripheral transduction (in contrast to vision and audition) may enable the system to use the temporal domain to encode complex odorant features. The brain can then combine temporal with spatial encoding in the construction of odor space.

Spatial encoding

Several lines of evidence point to spatial encoding in odor discrimination. This spatial coding may take form at the level of the epithelium, at the level of the bulb, and perhaps at the level of cortex. The olfactory epithelium is spatially segregated into four zones, roughly along the longitudinal axis of the cribriform plate (Buck, 1996). Although some olfactory receptors are randomly represented across these four zones (Strotmann et al., 1992, 2000; Sullivan et al., 1996), most neurons expressing a given olfactory receptor type are restricted to one of the four zones, where they are interspersed with other receptors in a seemingly unordered manner (Ressler, Sullivan, and Buck, 1993; Vassar, Ngai, and Axel, 1993; Strotmann et al., 1994). Thus, a rudimentary spatial map of odor identity is generated across these four zones of the epithelium (Mustaparta, 1971; Moulton, 1976; Thommesen and Doving, 1977; Mackay-Sim, Shaman, and Moulton, 1982; Edwards, Mather, and Dodd, 1988; Kent and Mozell, 1992; Scott et al., 1997; Scott and Brierley, 1999) (more on this later). Whereas the epithelium may offer crude spatial ordering, the nature of convergence from epithelium to bulb enables a much more detailed spatial map of odor at the bulbar level to be constructed. Receptor neurons expressing the same type of receptor typically converge onto two individual glomeruli in the bulb, one on the lateral and one on the medial surface, in a manner that is symmetrical between bulbs and similar across individuals within a species (Ressler, Sullivan, and Buck, 1994; Vassar et al., 1994; Mombaerts et al., 1996; Tsuboi et al., 1999). Thus, a strict relationship is maintained whereby a single receptor type is represented by a single glomerulus. Because different receptors may be sensitive to different aspects of odor molecules (termed *odotopes* or *pharmacophores*), a given odorant may then be represented by a spatial pattern of glumerular activity (Lancet et al., 1982; Shepherd, 1985). Furthermore, lateral inhibition between glomeruli may further sharpen this glumerular spatial map of odor (Mori and Shepherd, 1994; Yokoi, Mori, and Nakanishi, 1995). Several lines of evidence support this notion of odor maps on the olfactory bulb, including 2-deoxyglucose uptake (Stewart, Kauer, and Shepherd, 1979; Jourdan et al., 1980; Johnson, Woo, and Leon, 1998; Johnson et al., 1999; Johnson and Leon, 2000a,b), electrophysiology (Shepherd, 1985; Mori and Yoshihara, 1995), gene expression (Guthrie et al., 1993; Guthrie and Gall, 1995; Johnson et al., 1995; Sallaz and Jourdan, 1996; Inaki et al., 2002), and most recently optical imaging (Kauer, 1988; Rubin and Katz, 1999; Uchida et al., 2000; Meister and Bonhoeffer, 2001) (figure 19.4).

If a rudimentary spatial map of odorant identity is formed at the level of the epithelium and then sharpened at the level of bulb, one may ask whether this map is maintained at the level of cortex. Several lines of evidence point to a spatial axis of representation in primary olfactory cortex. Optical recording of activity in the rat cortex suggests that the piriform region is divided into several functionally heterogeneous regions (Litaudon, Datiche, and Cattarelli, 1997). Electrophysiological recordings suggest

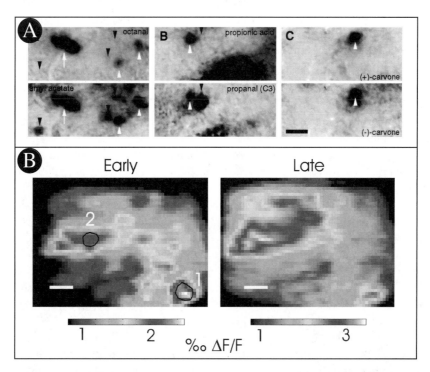

FIGURE 19.4 Odorant-specific spatial patterns of activity in the olfactory bulb. (*A*) Images from Rubin and Katz (1999) showing distinct patterns induced by different odorants. The black and white arrowheads point to glomeruli that are common or unique to each odorant. Although several glomeruli are activated by multiple odorants, each odorant is reflected by a unique glumerular map. (Reprinted from *Neuron*, vol. 23, B. D. Rubin and L. C. Katz, Optical imaging of odorant representations in the mammalian olfactory bulb, pp. 499–511, copyright 1999, with permission from Elsevier.) (*B*) Images from Spors and Grinvald (2002) showing the temporal development of the bulbar response to the odorant ethylbutyrate. Early response denotes data obtained 150–300 ms following stimulus onset, and late response denotes data obtained 300–500 ms following stimulation. The spatial pattern of response is clearly modified over time. (Reprinted from *Neuron*, vol. 34, H. Spors and A. Grinvald, Spatio-temporal dynamics of odor representations in the mammalian olfactory bulb, pp. 301–315, copyright 2002, with permission from Elsevier.)

that piriform cortex has at least four spatial receptive fields, specialized for odors delivered to the ipsilateral nostril, contralateral nostril, either nostril, or both nostrils (Wilson, 1997, 2001). Although these findings suggest some relation between the spatial organization of piriform cortex and odor input, until recently it was largely thought that the topography of projections from bulb to cortex was disordered, and that cortical representation did not maintain the spatial ordering of bulbar representation (Price and Sprich, 1975). However, recent developments in molecular methods have enabled Zou and colleagues (2001), working in the laboratory of Linda Buck, to use a transneuronal tracer to follow neurons expressing a single olfactory receptor type, starting at the olfactory epithelium, then onto their representation in the bulb, and then onto cortex. Zou and colleagues (2001) found, in contrast to previous notions, that the stereotyped map on the bulb is retained to some extent in cortex, where signals from a particular olfactory receptor type targeted specific clusters of neurons. Older work using single-cell recordings in monkeys found a high degree of odorant-specific responses in an even later stage of olfactory processing, namely, prefrontal cortex (Tanabe et al., 1974). Taken together, these findings suggest that odor identity may be spatially encoded at the level of cortex, but additional studies are needed in order to fully address this question.

Under the assumption of spatial mapping of odor at the olfactory epithelium, bulb, and cortex, the holy grail of olfactory research has shifted to identifying the metric of smell that governs olfactory perception, and hence this map. To date, scientists have been probing for this metric by systematically varying known structural aspects of molecular odorant structure while imaging the glumerular layer of the bulb. Based on work on the I7 receptor in mice and rats (Ivic et al., 2002), the most commonly probed structural axis is that of carbon chain length. For example, Johnson and colleagues (1999), using 2-deoxyglucose uptake, and Rubin and Katz (1999), Uchida and colleagues (2000), and Meister and Bonhoeffer (2001), using optical imaging, all stimulated with a homologous series of *n*-aliphatic aldehydes varying in carbon chain length as a possible odor metric. They found that each individual odorant could be represented by a unique spatial distribution of glomerular activity, and that the difference between these unique distributions or maps was greater for odorants that differed by increased length of carbon chain. In other words, odorants that differed by one carbon in chain length produced similar glomerular maps, and odorants that differed by several carbons produced increasingly different glomerular maps. Johnson and Leon (2000a,b) called clusters of glomeruli with similar response specificities *glomerular modules*, and found that in addition to carbon chain length, modular glomerular maps also encode for hydrocarbon branch structure and oxygen-containing functional group. These glomerular module maps were sufficiently consistent to allow Johnson and colleagues (2002) to predict both odorant structure based on patterns of glumerular activity and patterns of glomerular activity in response to novel odorants. The optical imaging studies also found that higher odorant intensities activated increased overall numbers of glomeruli, thus producing a somewhat smeared, yet retained, odorant identity map. This increased recruitment of glomeruli with increased odorant concentration was not always seen with 2-deoxyglucose uptake (discussed later).

Although the emerging picture of spatial odor encoding at all levels of the olfactory system is quite convincing, this view does have some significant caveats. First, as noted by Laurent (2002), even if the current view of encoding at the bulb is correct, this is not spatial encoding per se. In audition and vision, spatial ordering in the neural system represents spatial ordering in the physical world. For example, neighboring locations on the basilar membrane encode for neighboring frequencies. This is not the case as far as we know for spatial ordering of odorants in the bulb. Furthermore, extensive lesions at the level of olfactory bulb (Hudson and Distel, 1987; Lu and Slotnick, 1998; Slotnick and Bodyak, 2002) and olfactory cortex (Slotnick and Berman, 1980; Slotnick and Risser, 1990; Slotnick and Schoonover, 1993) do little to distort olfactory perception. If this perception were strongly linked to spatial representation within this neural architecture, one would expect these lesions to have far greater impact. Finally, patterns of activity throughout the olfactory system in general, and specifically in the olfactory bulb, are constantly modified through experience (Kauer, 1974; Meredith and Moulton, 1978; Di Prisco and Freeman, 1985; Harrison and Scott, 1986; Wellis, Scott, and Harrison, 1989; Eeckman and Freeman, 1990). Pure spatial mapping is an encoding scheme that would probably not lend itself to rearrangement within short time frames. By contrast, temporal encoding of information, namely encoding of odor within the temporal order of neural activity, may be far more plastic on short time scales, and conceivably less susceptible to anatomically restricted lesions.

Temporal coding

Olfactory behavior, and therefore neural activity within the olfactory system, are marked by rhythmic events. Since the pioneering work of Adrian (1942) and Freeman (1960), it has been known that two particular frequency domains domi-nate activity throughout the olfactory system. The first is the slow theta rhythm (typically 3–12 Hz) related to respiration or sniffing, and the second is the gamma rhythm (typically 30–100 Hz), an odor-related oscillation that rides on the respiratory wave. These oscillations occur in both the olfactory bulb and primary olfactory cortex in a correlated manner (Eeckman and Freeman, 1990), and are present in rodents (Adrian, 1942; Ueki and Domino, 1961; Bressler and Freeman, 1980; Ketchum and Haberly, 1993) and perhaps in humans (Hughes et al., 1969). Although it is clear that these oscillations are key to the process of olfaction, the exact functional significance of these patterns remains unclear. Several researchers have suggested that the gamma frequencies, coupled with the exceedingly large number of backprojecting pyramidal axons from anterior piriform cortex to the bulb, categorize olfactory stimuli in an increasingly specific fashion over successive sniff cycles (Bressler, 1990; Freeman and Barrie, 1994; Bhalla and Bower, 1997). Although temporal ordering of neural activity is a well-described encoding strategy in the olfactory system of insects (reviewed in Laurent, 2002), the suggestion of temporal coding in the mammalian system was met with hesitation by a field that has been dominated by the notion of spatial encoding. That said, a recent study by Spors and Grinvald (2002) begins to bridge the gap between these two schools (Friedrich, 2002). Spors and Grinvald combined optical imaging with voltage-sensitive dyes to obtain high spatial (10–20 μm) and temporal (50–200 Hz) resolution measurements from the olfactory bulbs of rodents. Using these methods, the authors found odorant-specific glomerular modules of activity similar to those previously described with optical imaging. However, the added temporal resolution revealed a highly dynamic spatial representation across the glomeruli that was constantly modified both within a sniff and across consecutive sniffs. In other words, odor was represented by a combined spatiotemporal pattern of activity. The brain may then read this spatiotemporal pattern as a sequence of discrete spatiotemporal events, like frames in a movie (Hopfield and Brody, 2001; Friedrich, 2002). By contrast, these successive representations may represent stages of an ongoing computation in the bulb, in which case "time" is a computational variable in the construction of the odor representation at the bulbar level (Bhalla and Bower, 1997; Friedrich and Laurent, 2001). In both cases, the temporal information on odor may be carried by the intrinsic oscillations, whereby it would alter the phase of activity in a specific manner (Hopfield, 1995).

In addition to directly participating in encoding of odorant content, the rapid oscillations may reflect the organization of network activity (Wilson and Bower, 1992; Protopapas and Bower, 2001). Specifically, current source density analysis suggests that each gamma oscillation decomposes each inspiratory cycle into temporal bins of about

20 ms duration (Ketchum and Haberly, 1993). Haberly (1998) suggested that the olfactory system uses these temporal bins to pair afferent input from the olfactory bulb with intrinsically generated associational activity and inhibition in piriform cortex in order to subserve this region's primary function as odor association cortex (Haberly, 1985, 2001).

Although it is quite clear that odor is reflected in unique spatial and temporal patterns of neural activity in the olfactory system, odor encoding is far from fully understood. In the study of vision, a large body of psychophysics links the space of color to its principal stimulus (wavelength), which led to elucidation of the neural encoding that subserves color vision. By contrast, little psychophysical effort has been made to elucidate the space of odor complete with a notion of a metric. It is our notion that only such a psychophysical understanding of odor space will enable thorough elucidation of odor coding. It is unlikely in our view that the olfactory system evolved to decipher carbon chain length. By contrast, psychophysical characterization of a behaviorally realistic metric of smell is likely to lead to a complete understanding of the neurobiology of smell.

Some efforts have recently been made in this respect by Christine Chee-Ruiter and colleagues, working in the laboratory of Jim Bower (Chee-Ruiter and Bower, 1998). They analyzed odor quality descriptors found in two published data sets of odorous monomolecular stimuli. First, using a cross-entropy analysis of the co-occurrence of pairs of descriptors associated with different molecules, they found that both data sets generated similar descriptors for the same odorants. Their analysis of these descriptors pointed to an organizational principle that segregated pleasant from unpleasant odor descriptors, and also segregated three types of odor families corresponding to descriptors elicited by molecules containing carbon, nitrogen, and sulfur. They interpreted this relationship to suggest that human olfactory perception is not organized around abstract chemical principles exemplified by structural homology but instead reflects an olfactory stimulus space organized by the principle of biogenetic pathways. This work is a first step that, in conjunction with efforts to look at classic psychophysical keys to perceptual space (such as cross-adaptation; Wise, Olsson, and Cain, 2000), as well as considerations of radically different possibilities such as molecular vibration (Turin, 2002) may create a much needed new conceptual framework for odor space.

The sniff as part of the olfactory percept

The recent advent of functional imaging enables one to address questions of neural coding in humans. Humans are an ideal animal model for odor encoding because their percept is readily obtainable. Although one can devise clever psychophysical experiments with animals, one can never be totally sure what aspect of the task the animal is in fact using to produce its symbolized answer. With humans there are no such doubts, and complex aspects of the percept can be obtained. For example, a human subject in an olfaction experiment can tell you that a given odor smells more "almondy" (like almonds) than a different odor. This type of information on perceptual similarities may be key to the formulation of a metric of odor space, and it is precisely this type of information that is hard to obtain from animals.

In order to probe odor coding in humans, we first asked whether neural activity in the human olfactory system is temporally linked to respiration, as it is in other mammals. We used functional magnetic resonance imaging (fMRI) to measure neural activity in primary olfactory cortex during sniffing of clean charcoal-filtered air. As in hedgehogs and rats, in humans, too, sniffing clean air induced pronounced patterns of activity in primary olfactory cortex, presumably a reflection of the slow theta rhythm (Sobel et al., 1998, 2000). However, as with previous work in rodents, it was unclear what this activity represented. Was this activity related to the motor action of sniffing, the somatosensory stimulation of sniff airflow in the nostrils, attentional mechanisms, or the process of analyzing the odor content of a sniff even when no odorant was present? We conducted a series of experiments to probe these possibilities and found that it was the somatosensory component of the sniff, namely, airflow in the nostrils, that primarily drives this activity. Using fMRI we found that (1) sniffing clean air will induce this activity in primary olfactory cortex, (2) the motor effort alone of trying to sniff with the nostrils occluded will not induce this activity, (3) artificially blowing air at the nostrils of otherwise passive subjects will induce this activity, (4) topical anesthesia of the nostril will reduce this activity while not hampering olfaction, and (5) when the airflow and resistance of sniffs are systematically varied, activity in primary olfactory cortex increases with increased airflow (figure 19.5) (Sobel et al., 1998).

These results instigated two main questions: (1) Under the assumption that primary olfactory cortex is more than a mere airflow rate–encoding device, how is odor represented in this region? and (2) Why is the rate of nasal airflow represented in primary olfactory cortex at all in the first place? The answer to the first question was related to the temporal patterns of activity in primary olfactory cortex. Electrophysiological and optical recordings show prolonged habituation patterns in piriform cortex neurons following an initial excitatory response (habituation here refers to a reduction in physiological response that may or may not alter behavioral performance) (Haberly, 1973; Scholfield, 1978; Litaudon, Datiche, and Cattarelli, 1997; Wilson, 1998). In rats, a 50-s continuous odorant stimulation led to a strong multi-unit increase in piriform cortex activity that decreased to baseline within 25–35 s (Wilson, 1998). Because this

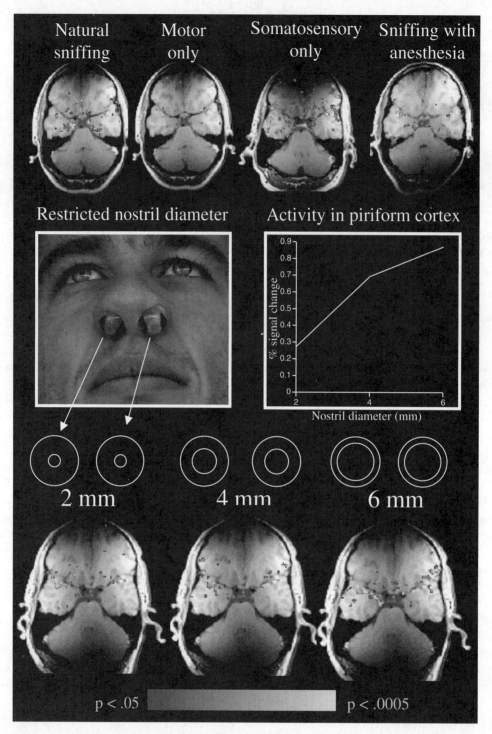

FIGURE 19.5   fMRI results obtained in humans. Top row, from left to right: MR activity induced by natural sniffing, by trying to sniff with the nostrils occluded, by artificial airflows directed at the nostrils, and by sniffing with topical anesthesia in the nostrils. Middle row, from left to right: The implants used to restrict nasal flow and the effect of this on fMRI signal in piriform cortex. Bottom row: The corresponding activation patterns. Taken together, these results demonstrate that activity in primary olfactory cortex is strongly affected by the somatosensory stimulation of sniffing. (Reprinted from N. Sobel, V. Prabhakaran, J. E. Desmond, et al., 1998. Sniffing and smelling: Separate subsystems in the human olfactory cortex. *Nature* 392:282–286. Copyright 1998, with permission from the Nature Publishing Group.) (See color plate 5.)

habituation was not considered in our initial modeling of hemodynamic responses, the odorant-induced activity was obscured in our analysis of the MR data. However, once we took this habituation into consideration, pronounced odorant-induced MR signal was measured in piriform cortex, within an 11% subset of the sniff-activated region (figure 19.6) (Sobel et al., 2000).

Although we could now measure odorant-induced MR activity in primary olfactory cortex, the primary driver of activity in this region was still airflow in the nose, and the question of why primary olfactory cortex was encoding this airflow was still open. An answer to this question was implicated in the elegant yet mostly unknown work of Teghtsoonian and colleagues (Teghtsoonian et al., 1978; Teghtsoonian and Teghtsoonian, 1982, 1984), and can be summed up in the term *olfactory constancy*. This term can be vividly explained through example. Imagine being presented with two jars of odor, one very concentrated and one very diluted. Further imagine that you are instructed to take a vigorous sniff of the diluted odorant and a mild sniff of the concentrated odorant. This procedure may result in an equal amount of odorant molecules activating olfactory receptors in each case (you took a lot of the diluted stimulus and a bit of the concentrated one). Yet if asked to choose which was the diluted and which the concentrated stimulus, you would have no problem doing so. Under the assumption that in both cases a similar number of molecules reached the epithelium, one must ask how the olfactory system could distinguish between these two stimuli. The simple answer is that the olfactory system also had to know the sniff. If the olfactory system knew that a vigorous sniff was employed in one sampling and a mild sniff in the second, the olfactory system could incorporate this information in its final assessment of odor concentration. In other words, the sniff itself is part of the olfactory percept, and it is for this reason that sniff airflow is represented in primary olfactory cortex.

That humans and rodents maintain olfactory constancy has been well documented. Laing first showed that sniff volume is inversely related to odorant concentration (1983). Using high-end olfactometry (devices that generate odorants with precise temporal and spatial resolution), Brad Johnson and Joel Mainland in our laboratory recently probed the time course of this mechanism and found that sniffs are odorant concentration invariant for about the first 150 ms of the sniff, after which sniffs are rapidly modulated to account for odorant intensity, so that intense odorants are sampled at lower airflow rates (figure 19.7A) (Johnson, Mainland, and Sobel, 2003). Overlooking this rapid olfactomotor modulation may have significant implications on our view of olfactory coding, a case in point being intensity coding. In most studies of mammalian odor intensity coding, odorants of different concentrations were artificially delivered in identical

quanta to the olfactory epithelium of an anesthetized animal. Such increases in concentration resulted in increased spatial extent of activity on the surface of the olfactory bulb, initially in 2-deoxyglucose studies (Stewart, Kauer, and Shepherd, 1979) and later with optical imaging (figure 19.7B) (Rubin and Katz, 1999; Uchida et al., 2000; Meister and Bonhoeffer, 2001; Spors and Grinvald, 2002). From these studies one might conclude that increased concentration was encoded through recruitment of additional glomeruli. In awake behaving mammals, however, the olfactomotor system would have prevented continued equal-flow-rate sampling of a high-concentration odorant. In the awake animal, an odorant would be sampled (sniffed) for a long duration with a high maximum flow rate when at low concentrations, but for a short duration with a low maximum flow rate when at high concentrations. Therefore, the increased glomeruli recruitment with increased odor concentration shown in these imaging studies might have resulted from negation of the olfactomotor system through anesthesia rather than representing a realistic mammalian encoding strategy. Indeed, the few studies that directly recorded neural activity in the olfactory system of behaving mammals revealed patterns of activity very different from those in the anesthetized preparation (Schoenbaum and Eichenbaum, 1995; Bhalla and Bower, 1997). Most pertinently, increasing odor concentration did not necessarily induce higher rates of activity in the olfactory bulb, but rather modulated complex patterns of excitation and suppression in awake behaving rabbits (Chaput and Lankheet, 1987), and temporally shifted the peak of activity to coincide with an earlier respiratory cycle following odor onset in awake behaving rats (Chalansonnet and Chaput, 1998). Although it is possible that the differences between results from the anesthetized and unanesthetized animals reflected direct effects of anesthesia on neural activity, we suggest they reflected anesthetic negation of the olfactomotor system and sniffing. Indeed, when unanesthetized sniffing rats were studied with 2-deoxyglucose, for three of five odorants in one study (Johnson and Leon, 2000a) and for all of nine odorants in a later study (Johnson et al., 2002), increasing concentration did not induce different spatial patterns of activity in the olfactory bulb (figure 19.7B).

It is clear from these studies and others (e.g., Youngentob et al., 1986) that the sniff is part of the intensity percept, but might the sniff contribute to additional aspects of the odor percept beyond intensity? The framework for such a possibility was set by the pioneering work of Mozell and colleagues (Mozell and Jagodowicz, 1973; Mozell, Kent, and Murphy, 1991). Mozell and colleagues demonstrated that odorants sorb to, and cross, the olfactory mucosa at different rates (Mozell and Jagodowicz, 1973). They established this phenomenon by measuring the relative sorption rates of 15 odorants across the mucosa of the frog (figure 19.8).

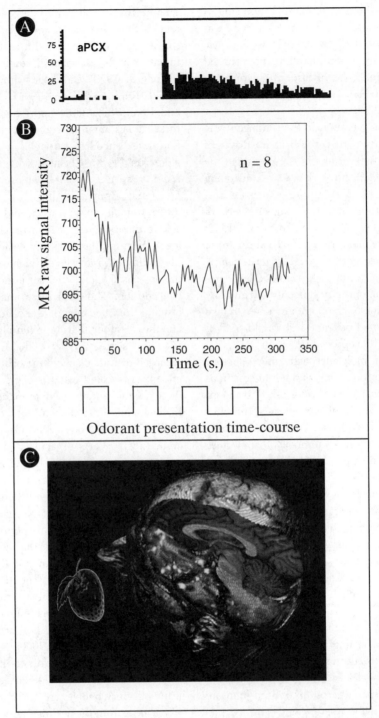

Figure 19.6 Habituation in olfactory cortex. (*A*) Data from Wilson (1998) showing a multi-unit recording in piriform cortex of the rat in response to a 50 s continuous odor pulse (denoted by bar above data). (Reprinted with permission from D. A. Wilson, Habituation of odor responses in the rat anterior piriform cortex. *J. Neurophysiol.* 79:1425–1440. Copyright 1998 by the American Physiological Society.) (*B*) Mean time course of fMRI signal from the piriform cortex of eight human subjects. Note the striking similarity between the time course in *A* (from rat) and the first 50 s in *B* (from human). (*C*) Once this habituation was taken into consideration in models of the expected hemodynamic response, odorant-induced activity was readily measurable in human piriform cortex. Here data from eight subjects smelling vanillin are overlaid on the three-dimensional image. (See color plate 6.)

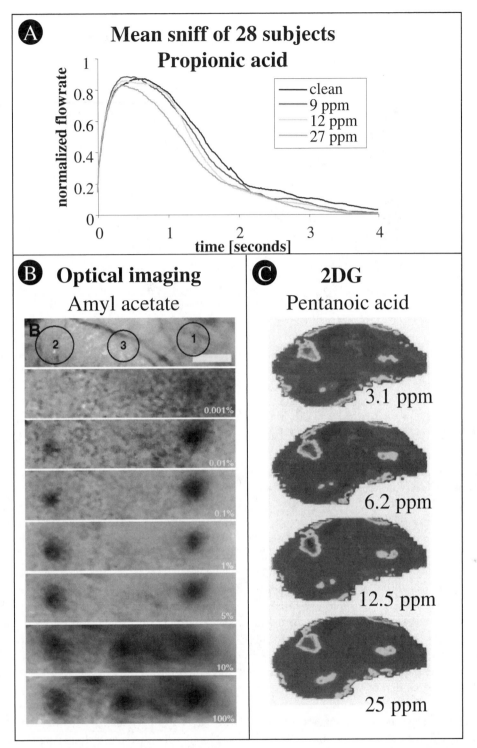

A **Mean sniff of 28 subjects**
Propionic acid

normalized flowrate / time [seconds]

— clean
— 9 ppm
— 12 ppm
— 27 ppm

B **Optical imaging**
Amyl acetate

0.001%
0.01%
0.1%
1%
5%
10%
100%

C **2DG**
Pentanoic acid

3.1 ppm

6.2 ppm

12.5 ppm

25 ppm

FIGURE 19.7 Coding intensity. (*A*) The mean sniffs of 28 subjects in response to three concentrations of propionic acid and clean air. Higher concentrations of odor were sampled at lower airflow rates. Airflow rate was adjusted to meet odorant concentration within 160 ms. (Reprinted from B. N. Johnson, J. D. Mainland, N. Sobel, 2003. Rapid olfactory processing implicates subcortical control of an olfactomotor system. *J. Neurophysiol.* 90:1084–1094. Copyright 2003 the American Physiological Society. Used by permission.) (*B*) Effects of increasing odorant concentration on the optical image obtained in the anesthetized rodent. Increased concentration was reflected in increased spatial extent of glomerular response. (Reprinted from *Neuron*, vol. 23, B. D. Rubin and L. C. Katz, Optical imaging of odorant representations in the mammalian olfactory bulb, pp. 499–511, copyright 1999, with permission from Elsevier.) (*C*) Effects of increasing odorant concentration on the 2DG image obtained in the awake behaving rodent. Increased concentration had no impact on spatial patterns of glomerular response. As implicated in panel *A*, awake behaving animals would not sample high- and low-intensity odorants with equal vigor. Data obtained from the anesthetized animal will fail to reflect this essential olfactory mechanism. (Reprinted with permission from B. A. Johnson and M. Leon, Modular representations of odorants in the glomerular layer of the rat olfactory bulb and the effects of stimulus concentration. *J. Comp. Neural.* 422:496–509. Copyright 2000, used by permission of Wiley-Liss, Inc., a subsidiary of John Wiley & Sons, Inc.) (See color plate 7.)

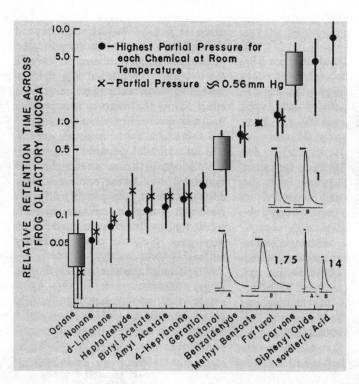

FIGURE 19.8 Sorption rates of 15 different odorants across the mucosa of the frog. The odorants used in our studies are indicated with rectangles. (Reprinted with permission from M. M. Mozell and M. Jagodowicz, Chromatographic separation of odorants by the nose: Retention times measured across in vivo olfactory mucosa. *Science* 181:1247–1249. Copyright 1973 by the American Association for the Advancement of Science.)

Structurally, the more an odorant was both water- and lipid-soluble, the higher was its sorption rate (Mozell, Kent, and Murphy, 1991).

Mozell and colleagues later found that the effect of an odorant on the magnitude of response in the olfactory nerve of the frog is the result of an interaction between the particular sorption rate of that odorant and the flow rate at which it flows across the olfactory mucosa (figure 19.9): A high-sorption-rate odorant flowing at a high flow rate will induce a large response and at a lower flow rate a smaller response. In contrast, a low-sorption-rate odorant flowing at a high flow rate will induce a small response and at a lower flow rate a larger response. A theoretical explanation of this is as follows: When a quantum of low-sorption odorant enters the nostril at a slow flow rate, there is a weak vector along the epithelium (slow flow) and a weak vector across the mucus (low sorption). This results in an even distribution of odorant molecules along the epithelium whereby a large epithelial surface area is affected, and the resulting response is large. In turn, when the same quantum of low-sorption odorant is flown rapidly across the mucosa, there is a strong vector along the epithelium (fast flow) and a weak vector across the mucus (low sorption). This results in a proportion of the molecules never sorbing before they are cleared into the respiratory system, and an uneven distribution of odorant molecules along the epithelium whereby only the posterior end of the epithelial surface area is affected, and the resulting response is small. In contrast, when a quantum of high-sorption odorant enters the nostril at a slow flow rate, there is a weak vector along the epithelium (slow flow) and a strong vector across the mucus (high sorption). This results in an uneven distribution of odorant molecules along the epithelium whereby the full quantum saturates the anterior portion of the epithelium, a small epithelial surface area is affected, and the resulting response is small. In turn, when the same quantum of high-sorption odorant is flown rapidly across the mucosa, there is a strong vector along the epithelium (fast flow) and a strong vector across the mucus (high sorption). This results in an even distribution of odorant molecules along the epithelium whereby a large epithelial surface area is affected, and the resulting response is large (figure 19.9). This interaction may be the driving force behind the odorant-specific spatial patterns of activity across the olfactory epithelium (Mustaparta, 1971; Moulton, 1976; Thommesen and Doving, 1977; Mackay-Sim, Shaman, and Moulton, 1982; Edwards, Mather, and Dodd, 1988; Kent and Mozell, 1992; Scott and Brierley, 1999), and is an additional aspect beyond intensity coding where the nature of the sniff strongly modulates, and is part of, the olfactory percept.

These findings suggest that particular airflows will optimize perception for particular odorants. High airflows will

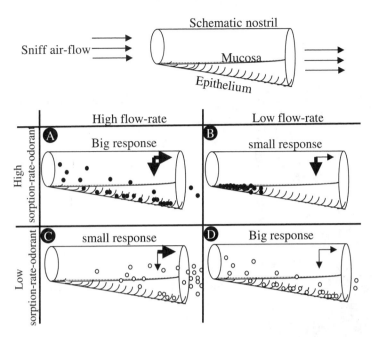

FIGURE 19.9 Schematic of theoretical framework for the results of Mozell et al. (1991). *Top*: Schematic of simplified nostril. Direction of airflow is from left to right. Thickness of the paired arrows in upper right corner of each nostril denotes the strength of the two vectors relevant to that condition: sorption toward the mucosa and flow out of the nostril. (*A*) A given quantity of a high-sorption-rate odorant passes over the mucosa at a high flow rate, involving a large portion of the epithelium and inducing a big response in the nerve. (*B*) The same quantity of the same high-sorption-rate odorant passes over the mucosa at a low flow rate, sorption occurs before flowing far down the mucosa, and a smaller portion of the epithelium is involved in the response, inducing only a small response in the nerve. (*C*) A given quantity of a low-sorption-rate odorant passes over the mucosa at a high flow rate. It will clear the nasal passage into the respiratory passage without sufficient time to sorb extensively, and thus only a small portion of the epithelium will be involved in the response, inducing only a small response in the nerve. (*D*) The same quantity of the same low-sorption-rate odorant passes over the mucosa at a low flow rate. It will have time to sorb and so will involve a large portion of the epithelium in the response, inducing a big response in the nerve. Note that (1) these combinations may differ not only in the size of epithelial surface involved in the response, but also in the specific spatial pattern (on the anterior-posterior axes) of the epithelium involved, (2) some sorption occurs at the preepithelial portion of the mucosa, and (3) this is a cartoon of a nostril, which is in fact a very complex structure with complex patterns of airflow (Keyhani, Scherer, and Mozell, 1997).

optimize perception of higher sorption rate odorants and low airflows will optimize perception of lower sorption rate odorants.

In mammals, the rate of airflow is usually higher in one nostril than in the other. This occurs because a bilateral, highly vascularized structure, the nasal turbinate, swells with blood flow in either one nostril or the other, increasing the resistance to airflow in one nostril in comparison to the other (figure 19.10) (Principato and Ozenberger, 1970; Bojsen-Moller and Fahrenkrug, 1971; Hasegawa and Kern, 1977). The nostril with higher airflow rate, left or right, alternates on an ultradian rhythm of uncertain periodicity (Gilbert and Rosenwasser, 1987; Mirza, Kroger, and Doty, 1997).

Considering the previously described findings in the frog, one may predict that the difference in airflow rate between the nostrils in the human will result in a different olfactory percept in each nostril as a function of the interaction between airflow and odorant sorption rates. Accordingly, we hypothesized that the high-flow-rate nostril is more sensitive to high-sorption-rate odorants and the low-flow-rate nostril is more sensitive to low-sorption-rate odorants.

To test this, we first used anterior rhinomanometry to determine which was the high-flow-rate nostril and which was the low-flow-rate nostril in 20 subjects. Airflow rate was higher in the right nostril in 11 subjects and in the left nostril in 9 subjects. Although there was no significant overall difference across subjects in flow rate between the left and right nostrils (left mean = 37 L/min, range = 13–60 L/min; right mean = 45 L/min, range = 10–77 L/min; $t(19)$ = 1.7, P = 0.1), the high-flow-rate nostril had an overall significantly higher flow rate than the low-flow-rate nostril (high mean = 51 L/min, low mean = 31 L/min; $t(19)$ = 5.6, P < 0.0001). All subjects then performed a task in which on each trial, an olfactometer produced an equally proportioned mixture of the low-sorption-rate odorant octane and the high-sorption-rate odorant l-carvone (figure 19.8). Although subjects were told that the mixtures would be slightly different on every trial, they were actually identical mixtures. The subject then (1) smelled the mixture with either the high-flow-rate nostril

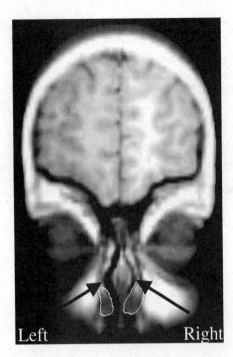

FIGURE 19.10 A coronal image of the nasal passage. The turbinates are traced in white. In this subject the right turbinate is expanded, largely blocking the right nostril. Thus, this subject has an open left nostril with a high airflow rate (green) and an occluded right nostril with a low airflow rate (red). (See color plate 8.)

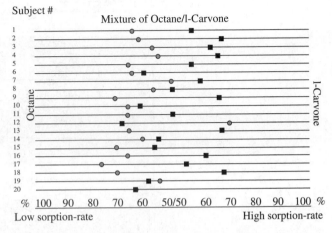

FIGURE 19.11 Mean judgment of 10 trials made by each of 20 subjects using the high-flow-rate nostril (square) and the low-flow-rate nostril (circle) separately to estimate the contents of the same mixture. The mixture was composed of 50% octane and 50% l-carvone. Using the high-flow-rate nostril, the average judgment was that the mixture was composed of 55% l-carvone and 45% octane. Using the low-flow-rate nostril, the average judgment was that the same mixture was composed of 61% octane and 39% l-carvone ($t(19) = 3.74$, $P = 0.001$). (Reprinted from N. Sobel, R. M. Khan, A. Saltman, et al., 1999. The world smells different to each nostril. *Nature* 402:35. Copyright 1999, with permission from the Nature Publishing Group.)

or low-flow-rate nostril, (2) smelled each component odorant individually, and (3) judged the composition of the mixture on a proportion scale (ranging from 100% octane to 50/50 octane/l-carvone to 100% l-carvone in 10% increments, as illustrated at bottom of figure 19.11). Each subject performed 20 trials. All experimental components were counterbalanced to prevent confounds of cross-adaptation and learning.

Although the mixture was always the same, we predicted that when the mixture was sniffed with the high-flow-rate nostril, the high-sorption-rate odorant would seem more prominent in the mixture, and when the same mixture was sniffed with the low-flow-rate nostril, the low-sorption-rate odorant would seem more prominent. As predicted, 17 of the 20 subjects judged the same mixture to have a higher l-carvone content (high-sorption-rate odorant) when sniffing with the high-flow-rate nostril and a higher octane content (low-sorption-rate odorant) when sniffing with the low-flow-rate nostril (binomial, $P < 0.002$) (figure 19.11). This finding demonstrated that the olfactory content obtained from each nostril in a given sniff was different. Each nostril was slightly better tuned to odorants that optimally sorb to the mucosa at the current flow rate in that nostril (Sobel, Khan, et al., 1999).

Because airflow rates oscillate between nostrils over time, we expected subjects' perception to oscillate as well. To test this, 8 subjects repeated the experiment, once when their right nostril had higher flow rate than their left and once

when their left nostril had higher flow rate than their right. The average time between test and retest was 2 days. As predicted, in 7 of the 8 subjects ($P < 0.04$), perception of the mixture changed with the change in nasal airflow. Using the high-flow-rate nostril, subjects judged the mixture to have a higher l-carvone (high-sorption-rate odorant) relative to octane (low-sorption-rate odorant) content. Using the low-flow-rate nostril, subjects judged the same mixture to have a higher octane (low-sorption-rate odorant) relative to l-carvone (high-sorption-rate odorant) content. This finding showed that not only is each nostril individually tuned, but that this tuning alternates between nostrils in synchrony with nasal airflow alterations.

To test whether the effect persists with different odorants, we repeated the experiment using the odorant butanol, which has a sorption rate between that of octane and l-carvone (see figure 19.8). Each of 10 subjects performed two experiments. One experiment was performed with a mixture of octane and butanol; in this mixture butanol was the higher-sorption-rate odorant. The second experiment was performed with a mixture of l-carvone and butanol; in this mixture butanol was the lower-sorption-rate odorant. Therefore, we expected subjects to report a relatively higher butanol content when using the high-flow-rate nostril during the first experiment and when using the low-flow-rate nostril in the second experiment.

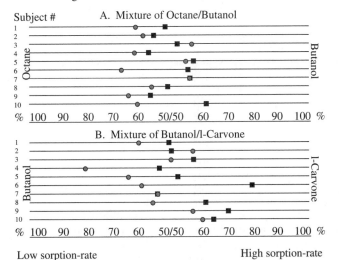

FIGURE 19.12 Mean judgment of 10 trials made by each of 10 subjects using the high-flow-rate nostril (square) and the low-flow-rate nostril (circle) separately to estimate the contents of the same mixture. (*A*) The mixture was composed of 50% octane and 50% butanol. The high-flow-rate nostril consistently perceived more butanol (mean 51% butanol, 49% octane) than the low-flow-rate nostril (mean 45% butanol, 55% octane) ($t(9) = 2.5$, $P = 0.03$). (*B*) The mixture was composed of 50% butanol and 50% l-carvone. The low-flow-rate nostril consistently perceived more butanol (mean 46% butanol, 54% l-carvone) than the high-flow-rate nostril (mean 42% butanol, 58% l-carvone) ($t(9) = 2.87$, $P = 0.02$).

As predicted, 8 of 10 subjects reported a relatively higher butanol content when using the high-flow-rate nostril during the first experiment and when using the low-flow-rate nostril in the second experiment (binomial, $P = 0.05$). The magnitude of the effects was smaller for butanol relative to the octane/l-carvone mixture, in agreement with the smaller differences in sorption rate between the components tested (figure 19.12).

These findings have recently been independently replicated by others (DePay and Hornung, 2002), demonstrating that (1) during each sniff, each nostril conveys to the brain a slightly different olfactory percept, and (2) this percept depends on airflow. This mechanism may contribute to olfaction in many ways. To smell an odorant, it first must be sniffed. The optimal rate of inhalation, however, is different for different odorants. The olfactory system partially overcomes this limiting factor by adopting two different simultaneous inhalation rates, one in each nostril, thus increasing the range of optimum olfactory sensitivity. In other words, the persistence of disparate airflows improves olfactory acuity by enlarging the olfactory repertoire that is within the window of optimum sensitivity within a given sniff. This mechanism holds not only for mammalian olfaction but also for machine olfaction. Recently Shawn Briglin

and colleagues, working in the laboratory of Nate Lewis at Caltech, have fashioned a simultaneous dual flow rate sampling mechanism in their electronic noses in a manner that emulates our findings in the human, and have found that this sampling strategy similarly increases the olfactory range of their device (Briglin et al., 2002). Finally, these findings show that with each sniff, each nostril conveys to the brain a slightly different image of the olfactory world. In vision and audition, the disparity of input from the two sensors gives rise to an additional dimension (depth in vision, spatial localization in audition). Further experimentation will reveal if and how the brain combines these different images of the olfactory world to form an additional dimension in olfaction.

Final words

The pioneering work of Linda Buck and Richard Axel, who identified the genes encoding for olfactory receptors, has brought about an explosion in olfaction research. Their findings led the way for researchers already in olfaction and for new researchers entering the field. Nevertheless, we still do not know how the mammalian nervous system encodes odors. It is our notion that the primary missing key for this puzzle can best be obtained with psychophysics. Careful psychophysical studies can reveal the metric of odor space, and it is this missing component that is necessary for further probing the physiological and molecular aspects of olfaction. We would argue that humans are the best animal in which to conduct such a psychophysical effort, and we see this as the major goal in the study of human olfaction.

REFERENCES

ADRIAN, E. D., 1942. Olfactory reactions in the brain of the hedgehog. *J. Physiol.* 100:459–473.

ALLISON, A., 1954. The secondary olfactory areas in the human brain. *J. Anat.* 88:481–488.

AXEL, R., 1995. The molecular logic of smell. *Sci. Am.* 273:154–159.

BAKALYAR, H. A., and R. R. REED, 1990. Identification of a specialized adenylyl cyclase that may mediate odorant detection. *Science* 250:1403–1406.

BENSAFI, M., A. PIERSON, C. ROUBY, et al., 2002. Modulation of visual event-related potentials by emotional olfactory stimuli. *Neurophysiol. Clin.* 32:335–342.

BHALLA, U. S., and J. M. BOWER, 1997. Multiday recordings from olfactory bulb neurons in awake freely moving rats: Spatially and temporally organized variability in odorant response properties. *J. Comput. Neurosci.* 4:221–256.

BOEKHOFF, I., E. TAREILUS, J. STROTMANN, and H. BREER, 1990. Rapid activation of alternative second messenger pathways in olfactory cilia from rats by different odorants. *Embo. J.* 9: 2453–2458.

BOJSEN-MOLLER, F., and J. FAHRENKRUG, 1971. Nasal swell-bodies and cyclic changes in the air passage of the rat and rabbit nose. *J. Anat.* 110:25–37.

BRESSLER, S. L., 1990. The gamma wave: A cortical information carrier? *Trends Neurosci.* 13:161–162.

BRESSLER, S. L., and W. J. FREEMAN, 1980. Frequency analysis of olfactory system EEG in cat, rabbit, and rat. *Electroencephalogr. Clin. Neurophysiol.* 50:19–24.

BRIGLIN, S. M., M. S. FREUND, P. TOKUMARU, and N. S. LEWIS, 2002. Exploitation of spatiotemporal information and geometric optimization of signal/noise performance using arrays of carbon black-polymer composite detectors. *Sensor Actuat. B-Chem.* 82:54–74.

BRUCE, H., 1959. An exteroreceptive block to pregnancy in the mouse. *Nature* 184:105.

BRUNET, L. J., G. H. GOLD, and J. NGAI, 1996. General anosmia caused by a targeted disruption of the mouse olfactory cyclic nucleotide–gated cation channel. *Neuron* 17:681–693.

BUCK, L., and R. AXEL, 1991. A novel multigene family may encode odorant receptors: A molecular basis for odor recognition. *Cell* 65:175–187.

BUCK, L. B., 1996. Information coding in the vertebrate olfactory system. *Annu. Rev. Neurosci.* 19:517–544.

CAIN, W. S., 1977. Differential sensitivity for smell: "Noise" at the nose. *Science* 195:796–798.

CARMICHAEL, S. T., M. C. CLUGNET, and J. L. PRICE, 1994. Central olfactory connections in the macaque monkey. *J. Comp. Neurol.* 346:403–434.

CARR, V. M., A. I. FARBMAN, L. M. COLLETTI, and J. I. MORGAN, 1991. Identification of a new nonneuronal cell type in rat olfactory epithelium. *Neuroscience* 45:433–449.

CHALANSONNET, M., and M. A. CHAPUT, 1998. Olfactory bulb output cell temporal response patterns to increasing odor concentrations in freely breathing rats. *Chem. Senses* 23:1–9.

CHAPUT, M. A., and M. J. LANKHEET, 1987. Influence of stimulus intensity on the categories of single-unit responses recorded from olfactory bulb neurons in awake freely-breathing rabbits. *Physiol. Behav.* 40:453–462.

CHEE-RUITER, C., and J. M. BOWER, 1998. Representing odor quality space: A perceptual framework for olfactory processing. In *Computational Neuroscience: Trends in Research*, J. M. Bower, ed. New York: Plenum Press, pp. 591–598.

CHESS, A., I. SIMON, H. CEDAR, and R. AXEL, 1994. Allelic inactivation regulates olfactory receptor gene expression. *Cell* 78:823–834.

CLELAND, T. A., and C. LINSTER, 2003. Central olfactory structures. In *Handbook of Olfaction and Gustation*, 2nd ed., R. L. Doty, ed. New York: Marcel Dekker, pp. 165–180.

CLERICO, D. M., W. C. TO, and D. C. LANZA, 2003. Anatomy of the human nasal passages. In *Handbook of Olfaction and Human Gustation*, 2nd ed., R. L. Doty, ed. New York: Marcel Dekker, pp. 1–16.

DE OLMOS, J., H. HARDY, and L. HEIMER, 1978. The afferent connections of the main and the accessory olfactory bulb formations in the rat: An experimental HRP study. *J. Comp. Neurol.* 15: 213–244.

DEPAY, K. S., and D. E. HORNUNG, 2002. *The contribution each nostril makes to olfactory perception.* Presented at the Association for Chemoreception Sciences 24th Annual Conference, Sarasota, Fla.

DI PRISCO, G., and W. FREEMAN, 1985. Odor-related bulbar EEG spatial pattern analysis during appetitive conditioning in rabbits. *Behav. Neurosci.* 99:964–978.

DOTY, R. L., 1986. Odor-guided behavior in mammals. *Experientia* 42:257–271.

DOTY, R. L., 1995. Intranasal trigeminal chemoreception: anatomy, physiology, and psychophysics. In *Handbook of Olfaction and Gustation*, R. L. Doty, ed. New York: Marcel Dekker, pp. 821–834.

DULAC, C., 2000. Sensory coding of pheromone signals in mammals. *Curr. Opin. Neurobiol.* 10:511–518.

EDWARDS, D. A., R. A. MATHER, and G. H. DODD, 1988. Spatial variation in response to odorants on the rat olfactory epithelium. *Experientia* 44:208–211.

EECKMAN, F., and W. FREEMAN, 1990. Correlations between unit firing and EEG in the rat olfactory system. *Brain Res.* 528:238–244.

FIRESTEIN, S., 2001. How the olfactory system makes sense of scents. *Nature* 413:211–218.

FIRESTEIN, S., C. PICCO, and A. MENINI, 1993. The relation between stimulus and response in olfactory receptor-cells of the tiger salamander. *J. Physiol. (Lond.)* 468:1–10.

FIRESTEIN, S., and F. WERBLIN, 1989. Odor-induced membrane currents in vertebrate-olfactory receptor neurons. *Science* 244:79–82.

FREEMAN, W. J., 1960. Correlations of electrical activity of prepyriform cortex and behavior in cat. *J. Neurophysiol.* 23:111–131.

FREEMAN, W. J., and J. BARRIE, 1994. Chaotic oscillations and the genesis of meaning in cerebral cortex. In *Temporal Coding in the Brain*, G. Buzsaki, R. Llinas, W. Singer, A. Berthoz, and C. Y. Berlin, eds. Berlin: Springer-Verlag, pp. 13–37.

FRIEDRICH, R. W., 2002. Real time odor representations. *Trends Neurosci.* 25:487–489.

FRIEDRICH, R. W., and G. LAURENT, 2001. Dynamic optimization of odor representations by slow temporal patterning of mitral cell activity. *Science* 291:889–894.

GETCHELL, M. L., and T. V. GETCHELL, 1991. Immunohistochemical localization of components of the immune barrier in the olfactory mucosae of salamanders and rats. *Anat. Rec.* 231: 358–374.

GILBERT, A. N., and A. M. ROSENWASSER, 1987. Biological rhythmicity of nasal airway patency: A re-examination of the "nasal cycle." *Acta Otolaryngol.* 104:180–186.

GRAY, C. M., and J. E. SKINNER, 1988. Centrifugal regulation of neuronal activity in the olfactory bulb of the waking rabbit as revealed by reversible cryogenic blockade. *Exp. Brain Res.* 69:378–386.

GRAZIADEI, P. P., R. R. LEVINE, and G. A. MONTI GRAZIADEI, 1979. Plasticity of connections of the olfactory sensory neuron: Regeneration into the forebrain following bulbectomy in the neonatal mouse. *Neuroscience* 4:713–727.

GRAZIADEI, P. P., and A. G. MONTI GRAZIADEI, 1983. Regeneration in the olfactory system of vertebrates. *Am. J. Otolaryngol.* 4: 228–233.

GREER, C. A., W. B. STEWART, J. S. KAUER, and G. M. SHEPHERD, 1981. Topographical and laminar localization of 2-deoxyglucose uptake in rat olfactory bulb induced by electrical stimulation of olfactory nerves. *Brain Res.* 217:279–293.

GUTHRIE, K. M., A. J. ANDERSON, M. LEON, and C. GALL, 1993. Odor-induced increases in c-fos mRNA expression reveal an anatomical "unit" for odor processing in olfactory bulb. *Proc. Natl. Acad. Sci. U.S.A.* 90:3329–3333.

GUTHRIE, K. M., and C. M. GALL, 1995. Functional mapping of odor-activated neurons in the olfactory bulb. *Chem. Senses* 20:271–282.

HABERLY, L. B., 1973. Unitary analysis of opossum prepyriform cortex. *J. Neurophysiol.* 36:762–774.

Haberly, L. B., 1985. Neuronal circuitry in olfactory cortex: Anatomy and functional implications. *Chem. Senses* 10:219–238.

Haberly, L. B., 1998. Olfactory cortex. In *The Synaptic Organization of the Brain*, G. M. Shepherd, ed. New York: Oxford University Press, pp. 317–345.

Haberly, L. B., 2001. Parallel-distributed processing in olfactory cortex: New insights from morphological and physiological analysis of neuronal circuitry. *Chem. Senses* 26:551–576.

Halpern, M., 1987. The organization and function of the vomeronasal system. *Annu. Rev. Neurosci.* 10:325–362.

Hara, T. J., 1975. Olfaction in fish. *Prog. Neurobiol.* 5:271–335.

Harrison, T., and J. Scott, 1986. Olfactory bulb responses to odor stimulation: Analysis of response pattern and intensity relationships. *J. Neurophysiol.* 56:1571–1589.

Hasegawa, M., and E. B. Kern, 1977. The human nasal cycle. *Mayo Clin. Proc.* 52:28–34.

Hinds, J. W., P. L. Hinds, and N. A. McNelly, 1984. An autoradiographic study of the mouse olfactory epithelium: Evidence for long-lived receptors. *Anat. Rec.* 210:375–383.

Hopfield, J. J., 1995. Pattern-recognition computation using action-potential timing for stimulus representation. *Nature* 376:33–36.

Hopfield, J. J., and C. D. Brody, 2001. What is a moment? Transient synchrony as a collective mechanism for spatiotemporal integration. *Proc. Natl. Acad. Sci. U.S.A.* 98:1282–1287.

Hornung, D. E., and M. P. Enns, 1986. Possible mechanisms for the processes of referred taste and retronasal olfaction. *Chem. Senses* 11:616.

Huard, J. M. T., S. L. Youngentob, B. J. Goldstein, M. B. Luskin, and J. E. Schwob, 1998. Adult olfactory epithelium contains multipotent progenitors that give rise to neurons and non-neural cells. *J. Comp. Neurol.* 400:469–486.

Hudson, R., and H. Distel, 1987. Regional autonomy in the peripheral processing of odor signals in newborn rabbits. *Brain Res.* 22:85–94.

Hughes, J., D. Hendrix, N. Wetzel, and J. Johnston, 1969. Correlations between electrophysiological activity from the human olfactory bulb and the subjective response to odoriferous stimuli. In *Olfaction and Taste III*, C. Pfaffmann, ed., New York: Academic Press, pp. 172–191.

Hummel, T., 2000. Assessment of intranasal trigeminal function. *Int. J. Psychophysiol.* 36:147–155.

Hummel, T., and A. Livermore, 2002. Intranasal chemosensory function of the trigeminal nerve and aspects of its relation to olfaction. *Int. Arch. Occup. Environ. Health* 75:305–313.

Inaki, K., Y. Takahashi, S. Nagayama, and K. Mori, 2002. Molecular-feature domains with posterodorsal-anteroventral polarity in the symmetrical sensory maps of the mouse olfactory bulb: Mapping of odourant-induced Zif268 expression. *Eur. J. Neurosci.* 15:1563–1574.

Ivic, L., C. Zhang, X. Zhang, S. O. Yoon, and S. Firestein, 2002. Intracellular trafficking of a tagged and functional mammalian olfactory receptor. *J. Neurobiol.* 50:56–68.

Johnson, B. A., S. L. Ho, Z. Xu, et al., 2002. Functional mapping of the rat olfactory bulb using diverse odorants reveals modular responses to functional groups and hydrocarbon structural features. *J. Comp. Neurol.* 449:180–194.

Johnson, B. A., and M. Leon, 2000a. Modular representations of odorants in the glomerular layer of the rat olfactory bulb and the effects of stimulus concentration. *J. Comp. Neurol.* 422:496–509.

Johnson, B. A., and M. Leon, 2000b. Odorant molecular length: One aspect of the olfactory code. *J. Comp. Neurol.* 426:330–338.

Johnson, B. A., C. C. Woo, H. C. Duong, V. Nguyen, and M. Leon, 1995. A learned odor evokes an enhanced Fos-like glomerular response in the olfactory bulb of young rats. *Brain Res.* 699:192–200.

Johnson, B. A., C. C. Woo, E. E. Hingco, K. L. Pham, and M. Leon, 1999. Multidimensional chemotopic responses to *n*-aliphatic acid odorants in the rat olfactory bulb. *J. Comp. Neurol.* 409:529–548.

Johnson, B. N., J. D. Mainland, and N. Sobel, 2003. Rapid olfactory processing implicates subcortical control of an olfactomotor system. *J. Neurophysiol.* 90:1084–1094.

Johnson, B. A., C. C. Woo, and M. Leon, 1998. Spatial coding of odorant features in the glomerular layer of the rat olfactory bulb. *J. Comp. Neurol.* 393:457–471.

Jones, D. T., and R. R. Reed, 1989. Golf: An olfactory neuron specific G protein involved in odorant signal transduction. *Science* 244:790–795.

Jourdan, F., A. Duveau, L. Astic, and A. Holley, 1980. Spatial distribution of [^{14}C]2-deoxyglucose uptake in the olfactory bulbs of rats stimulated with two different odours. *Brain Res.* 188:139–154.

Kauer, J. S., 1974. Response patterns of amphibian olfactory bulb neurones to odour stimulation. *J. Neurophysiol.* 243:695–715.

Kauer, J. S., 1988. Real-time imaging of evoked activity in local circuits of the salamander olfactory bulb. *Nature* 331:166–168.

Kent, P. F., and M. M. Mozell, 1992. The recording of odorant-induced mucosal activity patterns with a voltage-sensitive dye. *J. Neurophysiol.* 68:1804–1819.

Ketchum, K. L., and L. B. Haberly, 1993. Synaptic events that generate fast oscillations in piriform cortex. *J. Neurosci.* 13:3980–3985.

Keverne, E. B., 1999. The vomeronasal organ. *Science* 286:716–720.

Keyhani, K., P. W. Scherer, and M. M. Mozell, 1997. A numerical model of nasal odorant transport for the analysis of human olfaction. *J. Theor. Biol.* 186:279–301.

Kirk-Smith, M. D., C. Van Toller, and G. H. Dodd, 1983. Unconscious odour conditioning in human subjects. *Biol. Psychol.* 17:221–231.

Kratskin, I. L., and O. Belluzzi, 2003. Anatomy and neurochemistry of the olfactory bulb. In *Handbook of Olfaction and Gustation*, 2nd ed., R. L. Doty, ed. New York: Marcel Dekker, pp. 139–164.

Krautwurst, D., K. W. Yau, and R. R. Reed, 1998. Identification of ligands for olfactory receptors by functional expression of a receptor library. *Cell* 95:917–926.

Laing, D. G., 1983. Natural sniffing gives optimum odour perception for humans. *Perception* 12:99–117.

Lancet, D., C. A. Greer, J. S. Kauer, and G. M. Shepherd, 1982. Mapping of odor-related neuronal activity in the olfactory bulb by high-resolution 2-deoxyglucose autoradiography. *Proc. Natl. Acad. Sci. U.S.A.* 79:670–674.

Laska, M., A. Seibt, and A. Weber, 2000. "Microsmatic" primates revisited: Olfactory sensitivity in the squirrel monkey. *Chem. Senses* 25:47–53.

Laska, M., S. Trolp, and P. Teubner, 1999. Odor structure-activity relationships compared in human and nonhuman primates. *Behav. Neurosci.* 113:998–1007.

Laurent, G., 2002. Olfactory network dynamics and the coding of multidimensional signals. *Nat. Rev. Neurosci.* 11:884–895.

Leon, M., and B. A. Johnson, 2003. Olfactory coding in the mammalian olfactory bulb. *Brain Res. Brain Res. Rev.* 42:23–32.

LEWIS, J. E., and A. R. DAHL, 1995. Olfactory mucosa: Composition, enzymatic localization, and metabolism. In *Handbook of Olfaction and Gustation*, 1st ed., R. L. Doty, ed. New York: Marcel Dekker, pp. 33–52.

LIEBENAUER, L. L., and B. M. SLOTNICK, 1996. Social organization and aggression in a group of olfactory bulbectomized male mice. *Physiol. Behav.* 60:403–409.

LINSTER, C., and B. H. SMITH, 1997. A computational model of the response of honey bee antennal lobe circuitry to odor mixtures: Overshadowing, blocking and unblocking can arise from lateral inhibition. *Behav. Brain Res.* 87:1–14.

LITAUDON, P., F. DATICHE, and M. CATTARELLI, 1997. Optical recording of the rat piriform cortex activity. *Prog. Neurobiol.* 52:485–510.

LIVERMORE, A., and D. G. LAING, 1996. Influence of training and experience on the perception of multicomponent odor mixtures. *J. Exp. Psychol. Hum. Percept. Perform.* 22:267–277.

LORIG, T. S., 1994. EEG and ERP studies of low-level odor exposure in normal subjects. *Toxicol. Ind. Health* 10:579–586.

LU, X., and B. SLOTNICK, 1998. Olfaction in rats with extensive lesions of the olfactory bulbs: Implications for odor coding. *Neuroscience* 84:849–866.

MEREDITH, M., and D. MOULTON, 1978. Patterned response to odor in single neurones of goldfish olfactory bulb: Influence of odor quality and other stimulus parameters. *J. Gen. Physiol.* 71: 615–643.

MACKAY-SIM, A., and P. W. KITTEL, 1991. On the life span of olfactory receptor neurons. *Eur. J. Neurosci.* 3:209–215.

MACKAY-SIM, A., P. SHAMAN, and D. G. MOULTON, 1982. Topographic coding of olfactory quality: Odorant-specific patterns of epithelial responsivity in the salamander. *J. Neurophysiol.* 48:584–596.

MALNIC, B., J. HIRONO, T. SATO, and L. B. BUCK, 1999. Combinatorial receptor codes for odors. *Cell* 96:713–723.

MEISAMI, E., L. MIKHAIL, D. BAIM, and K. P. BHATNAGAR, 1998. Human olfactory bulb: Aging of glomeruli and mitral cells and a search for the accessory olfactory bulb. *Ann. N.Y. Acad. Sci.* 855:708–715.

MEISTER, M., and T. BONHOEFFER, 2001. Tuning and topography in an odor map on the rat olfactory bulb. *J. Neurosci.* 21:1351–1360.

MEREDITH, M., 1991. Sensory processing in the main and accessory olfactory systems: Comparisons and contrasts. *J. Steroid Biochem. Mol. Biol.* 39:601–614.

MERTL-MILLHOLLEN, A. S., 1979. Olfactory demarcation of territorial boundaries by a primate—*Propithecus verreauxi. Folia Primatol (Basel)* 32:35–42.

MIRZA, N., H. KROGER, and R. DOTY, 1997. Influence of age on the "nasal cycle." *Laryngoscope* 107:62–66.

MOMBAERTS, P., 1999. Molecular biology of odorant receptors in vertebrates. *Annu. Rev. Neurosci.* 22:487–509.

MOMBAERTS, P., F. WANG, C. DULAC, et al., 1996. Visualizing an olfactory sensory map. *Cell* 87:675–686.

MORAN, D. T., J. C. ROWLEY, B. W. JAFEK, and M. A. LOVELL, 1982. The fine structure of the olfactory mucosa in man. *J. Neurocytol.* 11:721–746.

MORI, K., and G. M. SHEPHERD, 1994. Emerging principles of molecular signal processing by mitral/tufted cells in the olfactory bulb. *Semin. Cell Biol.* 5:65–74.

MORI, K., and Y. YOSHIHARA, 1995. Molecular recognition and olfactory processing in the mammalian olfactory system. *Prog. Neurobiol.* 45:585–619.

MORRISON, E. E., and R. M. COSTANZO, 1990. Morphology of the human olfactory epithelium. *J. Comp. Neurol.* 297:1–13.

MORRISON, E. E., and R. M. COSTANZO, 1992. Morphology of olfactory epithelium in humans and other vertebrates. *Microsc. Res. Tech.* 23:49–61.

MOULTON, D. G., 1976. Spatial patterning of response to odors in peripheral olfactory system. *Physiol. Rev.* 56:578–593.

MOULTON, D. G., 1977. Minimum odorant concentrations detectable by the dog and their implications for olfactory receptor sensitivity. In *Chemical Senses in Vertebrates*, D. Muller-Schwarze and M. M. Mozell, eds. New York: Plenum Press, pp. 455–464.

MOZELL, M., P. KENT, and S. MURPHY, 1991. The effect of flow rate upon the magnitude of the olfactory response differs for different odorants. *Chem. Senses* 16:631–649.

MOZELL, M. M., and M. JAGODOWICZ, 1973. Chromatographic separation of odorants by the nose: Retention times measured across in vivo olfactory mucosa. *Science* 181:1247–1249.

MUSTAPARTA, H., 1971. Spatial distribution of receptor responses to stimulation with different odours. *Acta Physiol. Scand.* 82:154.

NAKAMURA, T., and G. H. GOLD, 1987. A cyclic nucleotide-gated conductance in olfactory receptor cilia. *Nature* 325:442–444.

NEF, P., I. HERMANSBORGMEYER, H. ARTIERESPIN, L. BEASLEY, V. E. DIONNE, and S. F. HEINEMANN, 1992. Spatial pattern of receptor expression in the olfactory epithelium. *Proc. Natl. Acad. Sci. U.S.A.* 89:8948–8952.

OHLOFF, G., 1986. Chemistry of odor stimuli. *Experientia* 42: 271–279.

PACE, U., E. HANSKI, Y. SALOMON, and D. LANCET, 1985. Odorant-sensitive adenylate cyclase may mediate olfactory reception. *Nature* 316:255–258.

PAPI, F., 1991. Orientation in birds: Olfactory navigation. *EXS* 60:52–85.

PELOSI, P., 2001. The role of perireceptor events in vertebrate olfaction. *Cell. Mol. Life Sci.* 58:503–509.

PEVSNER, J., R. R. TRIFILETTI, S. M. STRITTMATTER, P. B. SKLAR, and S. H. SNYDER, 1985. Purification and characterization of a pyrazine odorant binding protein. *Chem. Senses* 10:397.

PRICE, J. L., 1973. An autoradiographic study of complementary laminar patterns of termination of afferent fibers to the olfactory cortex. *J. Comp. Neurol.* 150:87–108.

PRICE, J. L., 1987. The central and accessory olfactory systems. In *Neurobiology of Taste and Smell*, T. E. Finger and W. L. Silver, ed. New York: Wiley, pp. 179–203.

PRICE, J. L., 1990. Olfactory system. In *The Human Nervous System*, G. Paxinos, ed. San Diego, Calif.: Academic Press, pp. 979–1001.

PRICE, J. L., and W. W. SPRICH, 1975. Observations on the lateral olfactory tract of the rat. *J. Comp. Neurol.* 162:321–336.

PRINCIPATO, J. J., and J. M. OZENBERGER, 1970. Cyclical changes in nasal resistance. *Arch. Otolaryngol.* 91:71–77.

PROTOPAPAS, A. D., and J. M. BOWER, 2001. Spike coding in pyramidal cells of the piriform cortex of rat. *J. Neurophysiol.* 86:1504–1510.

RAMING, K., J. KRIEGER, J. STROTMANN, et al., 1993. Cloning and expression of odorant receptors. *Nature* 361:353–356.

RESSLER, K. J., S. L. SULLIVAN, and L. B. BUCK, 1993. A zonal organization of odorant receptor gene expression in the olfactory epithelium. *Cell* 73:597–609.

RESSLER, K. J., S. L. SULLIVAN, and L. B. BUCK, 1994. Information coding in the olfactory system: Evidence for a stereotyped and highly organized epitope map in the olfactory bulb. *Cell* 79:1245–1255.

ROBERTS, E., 1986. Alzheimer's disease may begin in the nose and may be caused by aluminosilicates. *Neurobiol. Aging* 7:561–567.

RUBIN, B. D., and L. C. KATZ, 1999. Optical imaging of odorant representations in the mammalian olfactory bulb. *Neuron* 23: 499–511.

SALLAZ, M., and F. JOURDAN, 1996. Odour-induced c-fos expression in the rat olfactory bulb: Involvement of centrifugal afferents. *Brain Res.* 20:66–75.

SATO, T., J. HIRONO, M. TONOIKE, and M. TAKEBAYASHI, 1994. Tuning specificities to aliphatic odorants in mouse olfactory receptor neurons and their local distribution. *J. Neurophysiol.* 72: 2980–2989.

SCHOENBAUM, G., and H. EICHENBAUM, 1995. Information coding in the rodent prefrontal cortex. II. Ensemble activity in orbitofrontal cortex. *J. Neurophysiol.* 74:751–762.

SCHOLFIELD, C., 1978. Electrical properties of neurons in the olfactory cortex slice in vitro. *J. Physiol. (Lond.)* 275:535–546.

SCOTT, J. W., and T. BRIERLEY, 1999. A functional map in rat olfactory epithelium. *Chem. Senses* 24:679–690.

SCOTT, J. W., D. E. SHANNON, J. CHARPENTIER, L. M. DAVIS, and C. KAPLAN, 1997. Spatially organized response zones in rat olfactory epithelium. *J. Neurophysiol.* 77:1950–1962.

SETTLES, G. S., 2001. *Schlieren and Shadowgraph Techniques.* New York: Springer.

SETTLES, G. S., D. A. KESTER, and L. J. DODSON-DREIBELBIS, 2003. The external aerodynamics of canine olfaction. In *Sensors and Sensing in Biology and Engineering*, F. G. Barth, ed. New York: Springer Verlag, pp. 323–335.

SHEPHERD, G. M., 1972. Synaptic organization of the mammalian olfactory bulb. *Physiol. Rev.* 52:864–917.

SHEPHERD, G. M., 1985. The olfactory system: The uses of neural space for a non-spatial modality. *Prog. Clin. Biol. Res.* 176:99–114.

SHIPLEY, M. T., 1995. Olfactory System. In *The Rat Nervous System*, 2nd ed., G. Paxinos, ed. San Diego: Academic Press, pp. 899–928.

SICARD, G., and A. HOLLEY, 1984. Receptor cell responses to odorants: Similarities and differences among odorants. *Brain Res.* 292:283–296.

SLOTNICK, B., and E. BERMAN, 1980. Transection of the lateral olfactory tract does not produce anosmia. *Brain Res. Bull.* 5: 141–145.

SLOTNICK, B., and N. BODYAK, 2002. Odor discrimination and odor quality perception in rats with disruption of connections between the olfactory epithelium and olfactory bulbs. *J. Neurosci.* 15:4205–4216.

SLOTNICK, B., and J. RISSER, 1990. Odor memory and odor learning in rats with lesions of the lateral olfactory tract and mediodorsal thalamic nucleus. *Brain Res.* 529:23–29.

SLOTNICK, B., and F. SCHOONOVER, 1993. Olfactory sensitivity of rats with transection of the lateral olfactory tract. *Brain Res.* 616:132–137.

SOBEL, N., B. N. JOHNSON, J. MAINLAND, and D. M. YOUSEM, 2003. Functional neuroimaging of human olfaction. In *Handbook of Olfaction and Gustation*, 2nd ed., R. L. Doty, ed. New York: Marcel Dekker, pp. 251–273.

SOBEL, N., R. M. KHAN, A. SALTMAN, E. V. SULLIVAN, and J. D. GABRIELI, 1999. The world smells different to each nostril. *Nature* 402:35.

SOBEL, N., V. PRABHAKARAN, J. E. DESMOND, et al., 1998. Sniffing and smelling: Separate subsystems in the human olfactory cortex. *Nature* 392:282–286.

SOBEL, N., V. PRABHAKARAN, C. A. HARTLEY, et al., 1999. Blind smell: Brain activation induced by an undetected air-borne chemical. *Brain* 122(Pt. 2):209–217.

SOBEL, N., V. PRABHAKARAN, Z. ZHAO, et al., 2000. Time course of odorant-induced activation in the human primary olfactory cortex. *J. Neurophysiol.* 83:537–551.

SPORS, H., and A. GRINVALD, 2002. Spatio-temporal dynamics of odor representations in the mammalian olfactory bulb. *Neuron* 34:301–315.

STERN, K., and M. K. MCCLINTOCK, 1998. Regulation of ovulation by human pheromones. *Nature* 392:177–179.

STEWART, W. B., J. S. KAUER, and G. M. SHEPHERD, 1979. Functional organization of rat olfactory bulb analysed by the 2-deoxyglucose method. *J. Comp. Neurol.* 185:715–734.

STROTMANN, J., S. CONZELMANN, A. BECK, P. FEINSTEIN, H. BREER, and P. MOMBAERTS, 2000. Local permutations in the glomerular array of the mouse olfactory bulb. *J. Neurosci.* 20:6927–6938.

STROTMANN, J., I. WANNER, T. HELFRICH, et al., 1994. Olfactory neurons expressing distinct odorant receptor subtypes are spatially segregated in the nasal neuroepithelium. *Cell Tissue Res.* 276:429–438.

STROTMANN, J., I. WANNER, J. KRIEGER, K. RAMING, and H. BREER, 1992. Expression of odorant receptors in spatially restricted subsets of chemosensory neurons. *Neuroreport* 3:1053–1056.

SULLIVAN, S. L., M. C. ADAMSON, K. J. RESSLER, C. A. KOZAK, and L. B. BUCK, 1996. The chromosomal distribution of mouse odorant receptor genes. *Proc. Natl. Acad. Sci. U.S.A.* 93:884–888.

TANABE, T., M. IINO, Y. OOSHIMA, and S. F. TAKAGI, 1974. Olfactory area in prefrontal lobe. *Brain Res.* 80:127–130.

TEGHTSOONIAN, R., and M. TEGHTSOONIAN, 1982. Perceived effort in sniffing: The effects of sniff pressure and resistance. *Percept. Psychophys.* 31:324–329.

TEGHTSOONIAN, R., and M. TEGHTSOONIAN, 1984. Testing a perceptual constancy model for odor strength: The effects of sniff pressure and resistance to sniffing. *Perception* 13:743–752.

TEGHTSOONIAN, R., M. TEGHTSOONIAN, B. BERGLUND, and U. BERGLUND, 1978. Invariance of odor strength with sniff vigor: An olfactory analogue to size constancy. *J. Exp. Psychol. Hum. Percept. Perform.* 4:144–152.

THOMMESEN, G., and K. B. DOVING, 1977. Spatial distribution of Eog in rat: Variation with odor quality. *Acta Physiol. Scand.* 99:270–280.

TSUBOI, A., S. YOSHIHARA, N. YAMAZAKI, et al., 1999. Olfactory neurons expressing closely linked and homologous odorant receptor genes tend to project their axons to neighboring glomeruli on the olfactory bulb. *J. Neurosci.* 19:8409–8418.

TURIN, L., 2002. A method for the calculation of odor character from molecular structure. *J. Theor. Biol.* 216:367–385.

UCHIDA, N., Y. K. TAKAHASHI, M. TANIFUJI, and K. MORI, 2000. Odor maps in the mammalian olfactory bulb: Domain organization and odorant structural features. *Nat. Neurosci.* 3:1035–1043.

UEKI, S., and E. F. DOMINO, 1961. Some evidence for a mechanical receptor in olfactory function. *J. Neurophysiol.* 24:12–25.

VASSAR, R., S. K. CHAO, R. SITCHERAN, J. M. NUNEZ, L. B. VOSSHALL, and R. AXEL, 1994. Topographic organization of sensory projections to the olfactory bulb. *Cell* 79:981–991.

VASSAR, R., J. NGAI, and R. AXEL, 1993. Spatial segregation of odorant receptor expression in the mammalian olfactory epithelium. *Cell* 74:309–318.

WALLACE, D. G., B. GORNY, and I. Q. WHISHAW, 2002. Rats can track odors, other rats, and themselves: Implications for the study of spatial behavior. *Behav. Brain Res.* 131:185–192.

WELLIS, D., J. SCOTT, and T. HARRISON, 1989. Discrimination among odorants by single neurons of the rat olfactory bulb. *J. Neurophysiol.* 61:1161–1177.

WILSON, D. A., 1997. Binaral interactions in the rat piriform cortex. *J. Neurophysiol.* 78:160–169.

WILSON, D., 1998. Synaptic correlates of odor habituation in the rat anterior piriform cortex. *J. Neurophysiol.* 80:998–1001.

WILSON, D. A., 2001. Receptive fields in the rat piriform cortex. *Chem. Senses* 26:577–584.

WILSON, M., and J. M. BOWER, 1992. Cortical oscillations and temporal interactions in a computer simulation of piriform cortex. *J. Neurophysiol.* 67:981–995.

WISE, P., M. OLSSON, and W. CAIN, 2000. Quantification of odor quality. *Chem. Senses* 25:429–443.

WYSOCKI, C. J., 1979. Neurobehavioral evidence for the involvement of the vomeronasal system in mammalian reproduction. *Neurosci. Biobehav. Rev.* 3:301–341.

YOKOI, M., K. MORI, and S. NAKANISHI, 1995. Refinement of odor molecule tuning by dendrodendritic synaptic inhibition in the olfactory bulb. *Proc. Natl. Acad. Sci. U.S.A.* 92:3371–3375.

YOUNGENTOB, S. L., N. M. STERN, M. M. MOZELL, D. A. LEOPOLD, and D. E. HORNUNG, 1986. Effect of airway resistance on perceived odor intensity. *Am. J. Otolaryngol.* 7:187–193.

ZHAO, H. Q., L. IVIC, J. M. OTAKI, M. HASHIMOTO, K. MIKOSHIBA, and S. FIRESTEIN, 1998. Functional expression of a mammalian odorant receptor. *Science* 279:237–242.

ZOU, Z., L. F. HOROWITZ, J. P. MONTMAYEUR, S. SNAPPER, and L. B. BUCK, 2001. Genetic tracing reveals a stereotyped sensory map in the olfactory cortex. *Nature* 414:173–179.

20 Origins of Perception: Retinal Ganglion Cell Diversity and the Creation of Parallel Visual Pathways

DENNIS DACEY

ABSTRACT Visual pathways originate in the retina with approximately 20 ganglion cell populations that project in parallel to diverse brainstem targets. In primates, previously recognized cell groups—the midget, parasol and small bistratified cells—together make up about 65% of the total ganglion cells. The remaining ganglion cells are divided into a dozen or more novel populations, each present at relatively low spatial densities ranging from about 1%–3% of the ganglion cells. All of these low-density types can be retrogradely labeled from tracer injections into the lateral geniculate nucleus (LGN) or the superior colliculus or both. The novel ganglion cell types likely play significant roles in color and motion processing, although their physiological properties remain to be characterized in detail.

Extreme retinal cell type diversity creates parallel visual pathways

The vertebrate retina is a fascinating paradox. On the one hand, it is an elegantly simple structure at the periphery of the visual system. Mosaics of receptor cells sample the retinal image and transduce light to graded neural signals. Photoreceptor output is transmitted to a circuit of interneurons and an output neuron, the retinal ganglion cell, whose axon projects a representation of the visual world to the brain. On the other hand, the retina is an amazingly complex central nervous system (CNS) structure that continues to challenge neurobiologists (Masland and Raviola, 2000). It is now well understood that the retina contains on the order of 80 anatomically and physiologically distinct neural cell populations (Sterling, 1998; Masland, 2001). The interactions among most of these cell types are precisely arranged in a microlaminated sheet that provides the architecture for about 20 separate visual pathways (Wässle and Boycott, 1991; Rodieck, 1998; Roska and Werblin, 2001; Rockhill et al., 2002).

Each visual pathway originates from an anatomically distinct ganglion cell population and its associated retinal circuitry. The result is a unitary neural structure that gives rise to diverse output pathways with a broad range of distinct visual response properties, from neurons selective for the direction of image motion on the retina (Vaney et al., 2000) to cells with complex wavelength-coding properties used for color vision (Dacey, 1996). Thus, with about 80 cell types used to build 20 visual pathways, the retina represents a major processing stage for the central visual system, and the key to understanding the nature of parallel visual processing.

The retina, then, is a puzzle whose ultimate solution lies on the other side of the optic nerve in its connection with the brain. What is the impact of recognizing diverse pathways on the rest of the visual system? Specifically, how does each ganglion cell population contribute to the key properties of central visual structures, and ultimately to visual perception and performance? This chapter addresses these questions for the primate visual pathway, focusing on current understanding of the ganglion cell types of the macaque monkey retina and their central connections, physiological properties, and possible functional roles.

The reasons for focusing on the primate are related to a growing awareness that, perhaps more than any other part of the visual system, the retina of an Old World monkey, such as a macaque or a baboon, provides a near perfect stand-in for its human counterpart. For example, both human and Old World monkey share trichromatic color vision provided by long- (L), middle- (M), and short- (S) wavelength—sensitive cone types with virtually the same spectral tuning (Baylor, Nunn, and Schnapf, 1987; Schnapf, Kraft, and Baylor, 1987), anatomical organization (Roorda and Williams, 1999; Roorda et al., 2001), and postreceptoral

DENNIS DACEY Department of Biological Structure and the National Primate Research Center, University of Washington, Seattle, Wash.

circuitry (Kolb and Dekorver, 1991; Calkins et al., 1994). As far as has been measured, the color vision of macaques and humans is virtually identical (Jacobs, 1993; Jacobs and Deegan, 1997). Thus, psychophysical paradigms that define fundamental processes of human vision can be applied to primate retinal neurons to explore underlying cellular mechanisms (e.g., Lee, 1991; Kremers et al., 1993). Both monkey and man uniquely possess a fovea, the central specialization of the primate retina, where the neural circuitry for high visual acuity resides. Moreover, the many retinal cell types of macaque and human show a close correspondence, even at the level of fine anatomical detail, indicating that the circuitry and physiological properties of macaque retina are surely mirrored in the human (Rodieck et al., 1985; Dacey and Petersen, 1992; Kolb, Linberg, and Fisher, 1992; Dacey, 1993a,b; Peterson and Dacey, 1998, 1999, 2000). Finally, the recent development of new methods to probe the molecular biology and anatomy of cone photoreceptors (Roorda and Williams, 1999; Neitz and Neitz, 2003) as well as the anatomy and physiology of retinal circuitry (Dacey, 1999) has opened the door to rapid advances in the understanding of primate retinal organization.

Linking diverse ganglion cell types to diverse central targets

At least superficially, the diversity of retinal output pathways appears well matched to the diversity of retinal targets in the thalamus and midbrain. Seven main targets, further divisible into at least 24 nuclei or layers, receive direct retinal input (Kaas and Huerta, 1988; O'Brien, Abel, and Olavarria, 2001; figure 20.1). Most of these subdivisions of the visual system in the brainstem have been at least tentatively associated with distinct, diverse physiological processes. For example, the suprachiasmatic nucleus of the hypothalamus (figure 20.1; SCN) uses retinal input to photically entrain the endogenous circadian rhythm (Berson, Dunn, and Takao, 2002), while some pathways to the lateral geniculate nucleus (LGN) provide signals required for color perception (Merigan, 1989). So, a simple hypothesis is that each distinctive ganglion cell population projects in parallel to one or more of the many retinal targets in the brainstem. Previous work suggests that this is largely not the case, because the great majority, if not all, ganglion cells project to the superior colliculus (SC) and/or the LGN (e.g., Vaney et al., 1981). In macaque monkey, for example, it has been estimated that approximately 90% of the ganglion cells project to the LGN (Perry, Oehler, and Cowey, 1984). Does this mean that most ganglion cell *types* project to the LGN? The answer now emerging is yes, most if not all ganglion cell types in primate project to the LGN and/or the SC. In consequence, the many other smaller targets shown in figure 20.1 must therefore receive collateral projections from pathways that also project to these two major structures. In the sections that follow, I will review the evidence for these conclusions by dividing the ganglion cells into two broad groups. The first group is a classically recognized and intensively studied population that exists at relatively high densities. These cells—the midgets and parasols—comprise four distinct types and more than half of the total ganglion cells. The second group contains more recently identified populations, each population present in relatively low densities. Detailed characterization of this group is only just beginning, but it comprises at least 13 distinct types and accounts for the remaining 30%–40% of the total ganglion cells.

Classic high-density pathways to the LGN: Midget and parasol cells

The names *midget* and *parasol* refer to two anatomically distinct groups of ganglion cells that project respectively to the parvocellular and magnocellular sectors of the LGN (Leventhal, Rodieck, and Dreher, 1981; Perry, Oehler, and Cowey, 1984) (figure 20.2A). These two groups share the common feature of a high to moderate overall spatial density relative to all other ganglion cell types. Indeed, their relative numerosity is the reason why these cells are the only ganglion cells that were significantly sampled with classic anatomical and physiological methods and thus have driven most thinking about the functional organization of the primate retinogeniculate pathway (e.g., Kaplan and Shapley, 1986; Merigan and Maunsell, 1993). For this reason, midget ganglion cells are often referred to as P cells and parasol ganglion cells as M cells, to denote their central projection and, by implication, their visual function.

Many detailed reviews have considered the visual roles of midget and parasol ganglion cells (e.g., Shapley and Perry, 1986; Kaplan, Lee, and Shapley, 1990; Shapley, 1995). Because the LGN is the major thalamic relay for conscious visual perception of form, color, and motion, it is not surprising that all of these functional roles have been attributed to the midget and parasol ganglion cell types. With the recognition that other ganglion cell types project to the LGN, however, hypotheses about the functional roles of these pathways must be modified (e.g., Dacey, 1996). Here I briefly review some of the basic properties of the midget and parasol cells and summarize the limits of our understanding concerning the function of these major pathways. I will then argue, in the final section of the chapter, that the identification of novel visual pathways has the potential to solve some long-standing retinal puzzles.

Midget and parasol ganglion cells each compose two distinct populations whose dendrites stratify in either the inner or outer portion of the inner plexiform layer (IPL) (Watanabe and Rodieck, 1989; Silveira and Perry, 1991; Dacey, 1993b). This inner-outer dichotomy is a major

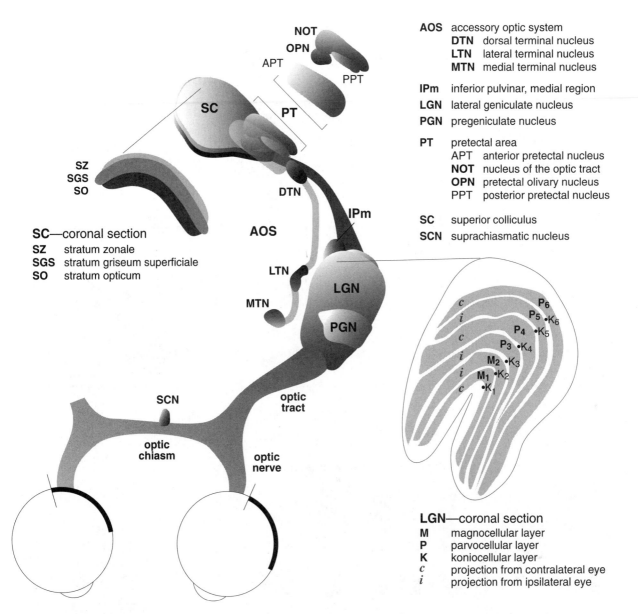

FIGURE 20.1 Primate visual pathways. The primate retina projects to at least 15 histologically distinct brainstem sites (Kaas and Huerta, 1988; O'Brien, Abel, and Olavarria, 2001). Retinorecipient nuclei in the hypothalamus, dorsal and ventral thalamus, and the midbrain are illustrated here semischematically, reconstructed from Nissl-stained coronal sections through the macaque brain (Paxinos, Huang, and Toga, 2000). The optic tract projects the contralateral visual hemifield via crossed nasal and uncrossed temporal ganglion cell axons to seven major brainstem targets: the suprachiasmatic nucleus (SCN) of the hypothalamus at the level of the optic chiasm; the lateral geniculate nucleus (LGN) of the dorsal thalamus; the pregeniculate nucleus (PGN) of the ventral thalamus, forming a thin dorsal "cap" over the rostral pole of the LGN; a component of the inferior pulvinar, medial subdivision (IPm), situated at the caudomedial pole of the LGN; the pretectal area (PT) at the thalamic–midbrain juncture; and the superior colliculus (SC)

and accessory optic system (AOS) of the midbrain. The AOS and PT are further subdivided into distinctive nuclei. The dorsal (DTN), lateral (LTN), and medial (MTN) terminal nuclei of the AOS are retinorecipient outposts linked by a separate optic fascicle that courses around the lateral surface of the midbrain. The nucleus of the optic tract (NOT) and the anterior pretectal (APT), olivary pretectal (OPN), and posterior pretectal (PPT) nuclei of the pretectal area are spatially intimate but histologically distinct nuclei situated along the course of the optic fibers at the rostrolateral pole of the SC. In addition, the LGN is a complex, laminated structure subdivided into magnocellular (M), parvocellular (P), and koniocellular retinorecipient layers. The retinorecipient zone of the SC is also a complex, layered structure: the stratum zonale (SZ), superficial gray layer (SGS), and the stratum opticum (SO) are all potential zones of input from distinct ganglion cell populations.

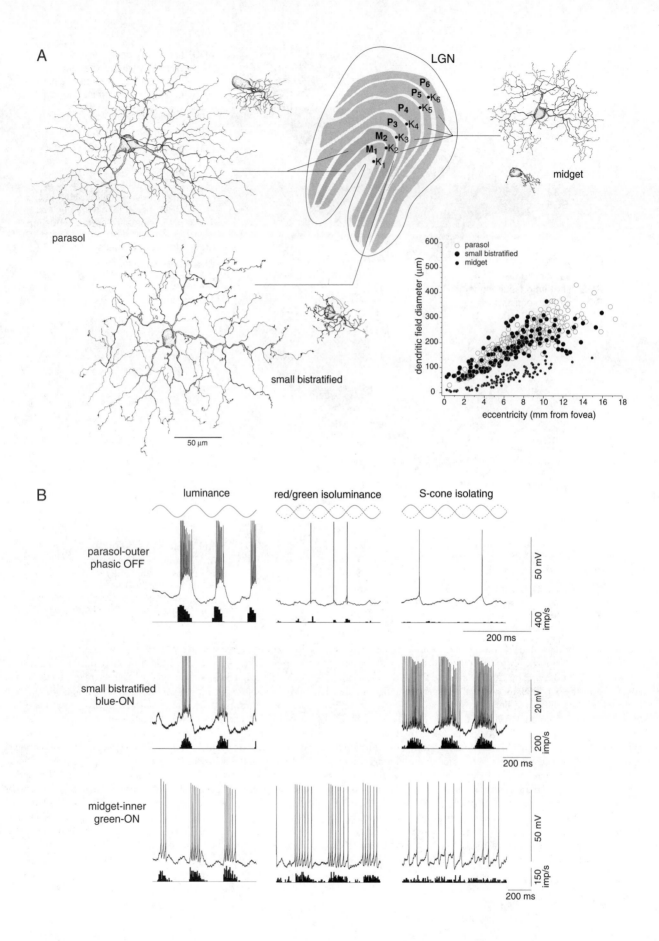

FIGURE 20.2   High- to moderate-density ganglion cell populations that project to the LGN. (*A*) Tracings of HRP-stained parasol, small bistratified, and midget cells illustrate dendritic morphology and the difference in dendritic field size of cells near the fovea (small tracings) and peripheral cells (larger tracings). Parasol cells project to the magnocellular layers of the LGN. This ganglion cell class comprises two populations with compact, highly branched trees, narrowly monostratified at ~35% (outer, OFF-center type) and ~65% (inner, ON-center type) depth of the inner plexiform layer (IPL); parasol cells also project to the SC. Each parasol type is estimated to make up 5%–8% of the total ganglion cell population. The small bistratified ganglion cell type composes a single population estimated at ~6% of the total and has a dendritic field diameter range similar to that of the parasol ganglion cells. The precise LGN terminus for this cell group is not well established, but current evidence suggests a projection to ventral P3 and/or to neighboring koniocellular layer K3. Small bistratified ganglion cells have a more sparsely branching dendritic tree that occupies two narrow strata at 25% and 80% depth in the IPL. Midget ganglion cells project to the parvocellular LGN layers and also comprise two populations with densely branched dendritic trees that stratify broadly at ~10%–25% (outer, OFF-center type) and ~75%–90% (inner, ON-center type) depth of the IPL. Midget ganglion cells are present at a relatively high density, with each type composing ~25% of the total ganglion cells. Schematic cross-section of the LGN shows the target lamina of these three cell types. Dendritic field size increases with increasing distance from the fovea, as shown in the plot on the right. (*B*) Intracellular responses of a parasol, small bistratified, and midget cell to red and green lights modulated in phase (luminance; L and M cones modulated in phase, L cones modulated at ~twice the depth of M cones; traces on the left), red and green lights modulated in counterphase (isoluminance; L cones modulated at ~twice the depth of M cones, middle traces), and to an S-cone-isolating stimulus (~80% S-cone contrast). Stimulus time course is shown above each column. Stimulus frequency was 10 Hz for the parasol cell, 4 Hz for the small bistratified cell, and 3.3 Hz for the midget cell. Spike histograms (impulses per second) are shown beneath each voltage trace. This parasol cell showed summed excitatory L- and M-cone input and had a response minimum at isoluminance, with no significant response to S-cone modulation. The midget ganglion responded to both luminance modulation and at isoluminance, with no response to S-cone modulation. Both parasol and midget ganglion cells, at least in retinal periphery, show variable responses to chromatic stimuli; the variability is likely related to variability in the relative weights of L- and M-cone input to an individual receptive field (see text for further discussion). The small bistratified cell shows a strong ON response to S-cone modulation and an OFF response to luminance modulation.

organizing principle that subdivides much of vertebrate retinal circuitry into ON- and OFF-center pathways (Famiglietti, Kaneko, and Tachibana, 1977). "Inner" cells receive excitatory input from depolarizing-ON cone bipolar cells and thus show ON-center receptive fields, and "outer" cells are driven by hyperpolarizing-OFF bipolar cells, which confer an OFF-center light response (Dacey et al., 2000). Thus, at any given retinal location there are two midget and two parasol cells that respond with opposite polarity to incremental versus decremental visual stimuli.

The midget and parasol ganglion cell populations show other anatomical features typical of many mammalian ganglion cells. The inner-ON and outer-OFF cells independently and uniformly tile the retinal surface with their dendritic trees and thereby create separate maps of the visual field with a characteristic central-to-peripheral gradient in cell density. Thus the density of the dendritic "tiles" composing these two maps changes systematically as a function of retinal eccentricity: in central retina, dendritic trees are small and cell density is high; with increasing distance from the fovea the dendritic tree enlarges and cell density decreases (figure 20.2*A*). A consequence of this inverse relationship between dendritic field size and density is that the visual map remains seamless but the spatial grain, and thus the spatial resolving power, of that map declines in the retinal periphery (Dacey and Brace, 1992; Dacey and Peterson, 1992; Dacey, 1993).

Beyond these similarities, midgets and parasols differ anatomically in two major ways that have been well documented. First, the dendritic field diameters of midget cells are significantly smaller than the dendritic field diameter of the parasol cells at any given eccentricity (figure 20.2*A*). Second, the two groups stratify at different depths in the inner and outer IPL (see figure 20.4). The difference in stratification depth reflects input from distinct cone bipolar-cell populations (Wässle, 1999). Thus, the parallel nature of these pathways begins at the level of the bipolar cell and its pattern of connections to the L-, M-, and S-cone photoreceptors. The degree to which these differences create functionally distinct pathways is considered for the midget and parasol cells in turn in the next section.

THE MIDGET PATHWAY: HIGH DENSITY FOR COLOR OPPONENCY, VISUAL ACUITY, OR BOTH?   It is well established that in the central 10° of visual angle, the midget dendritic arbor is barely 5 μm in diameter and receives virtually all of its excitatory input from a single, equally small midget bipolar cell, which in turn connects to a single cone photoreceptor (Polyak, 1941; Kolb and Dekorver, 1991; Calkins et al., 1994).

Because of this "private-line" circuit, the midget ganglion cells are present in very high density relative to all other ganglion cell types. In central retina, where cone density peaks, the midget pathway follows the cone density gradient, and there are two midget ganglion cells for every cone (Ahmad et al., 2003). Here the midget populations together constitute up to 70% of the total ganglion cell population (Calkins et al., 1995). In foveal retina, the peak density of cones sets the limit on achromatic spatial resolution (Packer and Williams, 2003), and the private-line midget circuit is capable of preserving and transmitting this information to the brain (Wässle et al., 1990; McMahon et al., 2000). As already mentioned, the midget ganglion cells project selectively to the parvocellular division of the LGN, and lesions of the parvocellular layers reduce visual acuity (Merigan, Byrne, and Maunsell, 1991; Merigan, Katz, and Maunsell, 1991; Lynch et al., 1992; Merigan, 1996). The conclusion thus seems inescapable that the midget cell signal functions to preserve the visual acuity afforded by the sampling density of the cone mosaic. Surprisingly, however, physiological studies of the visual responses of midget ganglion cells and parvocellular LGN relay cells have strongly emphasized not a primary role for midget cells in achromatic spatial vision but the major role that these cells play in color vision.

Wiesel and Hubel (1966) recognized that the single-cone midget pathway might be critical for trichromatic color vision in primates. To extract information about wavelength that can be used for color discrimination, the circuits of the visual system must compare the outputs of cone types with maximal sensitivities at different points along the visible spectrum. In trichromatic primates, the S, M, and L cones have sensitivity peaks at short, medium, and long wavelengths, respectively. The midget cell, via its dedicated excitatory connection to a single cone, thus has the potential to compare the excitatory input from one cone type with the inhibitory input from another cone type. Recordings from presumed foveal and parafoveal midget cells and their parvocellular LGN counterparts support this "midget hypothesis" of wavelength coding (figure 20.2B). Cells that are excited by input from L cones tend to be selectively inhibited by M cones, and this L- versus M-cone signal is referred to as cone opponency (e.g., DeValois, Abramov, and Jacobs, 1966; DeMonasterio and Gouras, 1975; Derrington, Krauskopf, and Lennie, 1984; Reid and Shapley, 2002). Such cone-signal opponency at the level of the retina has an important psychophysical correlate, where cone-opponent transformations are a critical step in the perception of color (e.g., Abramov and Gordon, 1994; Gegenfurtner and Kiper, 2003).

The apparently straightforward anatomy and physiology linking the midget pathway to both achromatic visual acuity and color vision has led to the suggestion that the midget pathway must do double duty (Lennie and D'Zmura, 1988). This hypothesis rests on a center-surround receptive field model in which chromatic stimuli at low spatial frequency engage center and surround and give rise to a strong response, while stimuli at high spatial frequencies engage primarily the receptive field center and transmit an achromatic signal (see, e.g., Gegenfurtner and Kiper, 2003, for a recent description of this view). The double-duty hypothesis has not gained universal acceptance, however, and views about the overall functional role of the midget pathway remain surprisingly contentious. Thus, it has been shown that the cone-

opponent, L-versus-M signal in the midget pathway can seriously degrade the achromatic contrast sensitivity, making these cells poor candidates for any significant role in achromatic vision (Kaplan and Shapley, 1986). To a luminance-modulated, achromatic stimulus, such as a drifting black-and-white grating, L and M cones are modulated in phase, so that a cell in which these two cone types are antagonistic responds poorly to such a stimulus due to cancellation of the cone signals. In essence, the color properties appear to be in direct conflict with the achromatic properties, and the mechanism by which both a robust achromatic signal and a chromatic signal could be extracted at higher processing levels remains unclear (Kaplan, Lee, and Shapley, 1990; Shapley, 1995). Consequently it has been proposed that the specialized, private-line midget pathway has evolved specifically to generate a specialized circuit needed to generate L-versus-M cone opponency for the purpose of color vision (Shapley and Perry, 1986; Lee, 1999).

At the same time, the fundamental role of the midget pathway in color coding has also been challenged (Rodieck, 1991; Calkins and Sterling, 1999). Although recent results argue that midget ganglion cells receive cone-type selective inputs to both the excitatory center and the inhibitory surround, just as might be predicted for a specialized color-coding circuit (Martin et al., 2001; Reid and Shapley, 2002), other results find the chromatic properties of midget cells more variable (Lankheet, Lennie, and Krauskopf, 1998; Diller et al., 2004). Moreover, both physiological and anatomical studies of the retinal circuits that create the inhibitory surround have not been able to uncover any cone-type specificity in retinal inhibitory pathways (Calkins and Sterling, 1996; Dacey et al., 1996). Finally, the discovery of another nonmidget ganglion cell type that transmits highly specific S-cone-opponent signals (Dacey and Lee, 1994) has focused attention on the role that other novel ganglion cell types might play in color vision.

In summary, it is quite remarkable that three distinct hypotheses—covering the complete range of possibilities for the function of the midget pathway—have all been forcefully argued: first, that the midget pathway is uniquely specialized for color vision (e.g., Reid and Shapley, 2002); second, that the midget cells are uniquely specialized for achromatic spatial vision and set the limit on peak visual resolution (e.g., Calkins and Sterling, 1999); and third, a middle ground, namely, that the midget pathway does "double duty" and is a critical component of both achromatic and chromatic vision (Lennie, 2000). Although this last hypothesis in principle is parsimonious, it remains to be shown that the midget ganglion cell receptive field consistently functions in this manner.

PARASOL PATHWAYS: MODERATE DENSITY AND HIGH ACHROMATIC SENSITIVITY   By contrast with the midget ganglion cells, the parasol ganglion cells show larger dendritic fields and are narrowly stratified near the center of the IPL. Each parasol population constitutes 5%–8% of the total number of ganglion cells in midperipheral retina. Unlike the midget pathway, the parasol cells receive input from multiple cone bipolar cells with larger dendritic fields that receive synergistic input from multiple L and M cones (Calkins, 1999; Jacoby and Marshak, 2000; Jacoby et al., 2000; Marshak et al., 2002). As a result, parasol cells respond strongly to achromatic or "luminance" stimuli in which L and M cones are modulated in phase, and more weakly to "chromatic" stimuli in which L and M cones are modulated in counterphase (figure 20.2B). Because parasol cells project to the magnocellular layers of the LGN, they are considered to be the major if not the sole source of the achromatic signal that is relayed from the magnocellular layers to primary visual cortex. However, it is important to note that parasol ganglion cells also project to the SC (Leventhal, Rodieck, and Dreher, 1981; Perry and Cowey, 1984; D. Dacey, unpublished observations). Parasol cells consistently show a very high sensitivity to achromatic contrast, much higher than that of midget cells to the same stimuli (Kaplan and Shapley, 1986). For this reason it has been argued that the parasol-magnocellular pathway may be the main signal for achromatic spatial vision (Lee, 1999). This role for the parasol cells would be consistent with the proposal that the midget system is uniquely specialized for color vision. The relatively low density of these cells relative to the density of midget cells in foveal retina seems to argue against such a primary role, however. More strikingly, lesions of the magnocellular layers of the LGN give rise to deficits in achromatic vision at low spatial frequencies but not at the high spatial frequencies presumably supported by the midget pathway (Merigan and Maunsell, 1990).

Parasol cells, by virtue of their projection to the magnocellular layers of the LGN, have also been implicated as the retinal origin of signals used to create direction selectivity at the level of visual cortex that reflect the first stage in a parallel pathway for motion perception (Chichilnisky and Kalmar, 2003). However, lesions of the magnocellular pathway, while reducing visual capacity, do not affect motion perception specifically (Merigan, Byrne, and Maunsell, 1991). In this regard, it is important to recognize that direction selectivity is a well-established property of certain mammalian retinal ganglion cells, and before reaching any strong conclusions about the role of the parasol cells in motion processing it will be necessary to fully assess the physiology and central projections of the remaining primate ganglion cell types.

In sum, parasol ganglion cells are clearly implicated as an important achromatic pathway, but the precise visual role these cells play relative to the midget ganglion cells and other ganglion cell types remains to be established.

Novel pathways to LGN and SC: Thirteen low-density types

Although the specific functional roles of both the midget and the parasol pathways remain unsettled, the recognition of ganglion cell diversity raises a number of new and relevant questions. How many other ganglion cell types contribute to the retinogeniculate pathway? How many participate in chromatic signaling? How many other types are clearly achromatic? Are there any types that are explicitly implicated in motion processing—that is, that show direction selectivity?

The midget and parasol ganglion cells together constitute over half the total ganglion cells but are only a fraction of the total ganglion cell types. Outside of the fovea, where relative densities can be easily calculated, these cell groups account for about 50%–65% of the total, depending on retinal location and estimates of local cell density (table 20.1). The number of remaining ganglion cell populations depends entirely on the relative density of each distinct group.

As will be discussed below, the majority of mammalian ganglion cell types exist at relatively low densities, ranging from less than 1% to about 5% of the total. Because of this basic feature of retinal organization, these low-density types have been extremely difficult to identify and characterize with standard physiological and anatomical methods. Low-density cells are rarely if ever sampled by the "blind" electrode of the physiologist or by anatomical labeling methods. However, the use of techniques directed at overcoming this natural bias has quickly revealed the true extent of retinal cell diversity. The emerging picture for primate retinal ganglion cells is summarized below; recent results for rodent (Sun, Li, and He, 2002), rabbit (Rockhill et al., 2002), and cat (Isayama, Berson, and Pu, 2000) reveal the same basic picture.

SMALL BISTRATIFIED GANGLION CELLS: A NONMIDGET PATHWAY FOR COLOR VISION The first quantitative picture of ganglion cell diversity in the primate came from experiments using an intact in vitro preparation of the human or macaque retina in which either vital staining or retrograde labeling from central tracer injections was used to target individual ganglion cells for intracellular staining (Watanabe and Rodieck, 1989; Dacey, 1989, 1993a,b; Rodieck and Watanabe, 1993; Peterson and Dacey, 1998, 1999, 2000). The results of these studies illustrated several morphologically distinct groups whose physiological properties were unknown. Among these cells was a distinctive bistratified ganglion cell population that was retrogradely labeled from tracer injections in the LGN and showed a dendritic tree size comparable to that of the parasol ganglion cell (Dacey, 1993; Rodieck and Watanabe, 1993) (figure 20.2A). Estimates of the density of the small bistratified cells suggested that they composed about 5% of the total ganglion cell population

TABLE 20.1

Summary of ganglion cell types in macaque retina

Ganglion Cell Morphological Type	Percent of Total Ganglion Cell Population*	Central Projections	Some Physiological Properties
1 Midget, inner	26	LGN parvo 5, 6	ON-center; OFF-surround Achromatic/chromatic L vs. M cone opponent
2 Midget, outer	26	LGN parvo 3, 4	OFF-center; ON-surround Achromatic/chromatic L vs. M cone opponent S cone OFF opponent group?
3 Parasol, inner	8.0	LGN magno 1, 2	ON-center; OFF-surround Achromatic L+M cone input S cone input controversial
4 Parasol, outer	8.0	LGN magno 1, 2	OFF-center; ON-surround Achromatic L+M cone input S cone input controversial
5 Small bistratified	6.2	LGN konio 3, 4	S-ON; L+M-OFF opponent
6 Large bistratified	2.7	LGN	S-ON opponent, details unknown
7 Thorny monostratified, inner	1.2	LGN	Unknown
8 Thorny monostratified, outer	1.2	LGN	Unknown
9 Broad thorny monostratified	1.2	LGN SC	Unknown
10 Recursive bistratified	4.2	SC	Possible correlate of ON-OFF direction selective
11 Recursive monostratified	1.9	SC LGN? Pretectal area (NOT?)	Possible correlate of ON direction selective
12 Moderate monostratified, inner	1.3	SC	Unknown
13 Moderate monostratified, outer	1.3	SC	Unknown
14 Sparse monostratified, inner	2.0	LGN	L+M-ON; S-OFF opponent
15 Sparse monostratified, outer	1.2	LGN	Unknown
16 Giant monostratified melanopsin-containing, inner/outer, weakly bistratified	1.0	LGN Pretectal area, PON Hypothalamus (SCN)	Sustained ON response S-OFF; L+M-ON opponent Strong rod input Intrinsically photosensitive via novel photopigment
17 Giant monostratified intrinsic axon-collaterals	1.0	Unknown	Unknown

Note: Low-density ganglion cell types dominate the retinal landscape. The majority of ganglion cell types that have been identified morphologically are present in relatively low densities of 1%–3% of the total population. Moderate-density cell populations (reaching 5%–6% of the total) include the inner and outer parasol and small bistratified types. The midget ganglion cells are an exception, with both inner and outer populations at ~25% at 7–8 mm from the fovea. Beyond the midget, parasol, and small bistratified populations, very little is currently known about the key physiological properties of the remaining types, though most if not all of these types project to the LGN and/or the SC, the two major relays for ascending visual pathways to visual cortical areas.

* Total ganglion cell density is from Wässle et al., 1989, for temporal retina ~8 mm from the fovea. Individual cell type densities were determined from cell density at ~8 mm (parasol cells; Perry and Cowey, 1985) or from dendritic field area at ~8 mm and coverage factor where known (thorny and giant monostratified cells, D. Dacey, unpublished; midget cells, Dacey, 1993). All other cell type densities were determined from measured dendritic field area at ~8 mm and estimated coverage.

(Dacey, 1994). The dendritic tree, stratified narrowly in both the inner and outer part of the IPL, suggested that these cells would receive input from both ON and OFF cone bipolar pathways. These results stimulated the further development of the macaque in vitro preparation to enable intracellular recording and staining methods to be used to directly link the bistratified morphology to visual receptive field properties (Dacey and Lee, 1994).

Recordings from the small bistratified cells in vitro revealed a strong excitatory ON input from the short-wavelength-sensitive S cones that was opposed to an inhibitory input from L and M cones (figure 20.2B). This type of S-cone-opponent response had been classically observed by extracellular recording methods at both the level of the retina and the LGN as part of the midget-parvocellular pathway and recognized as one of the major axes of opponent color space that is utilized for higher-order color processing (e.g., Derrington, Krauskopf, and Lennie, 1984). Using the same stimuli, it was also shown that such S-cone input was apparently lacking from identified midget and parasol ganglion cells that were also recorded from the in vitro preparation (figure 20.2B). The small bistratified cells may project to a restricted locus at the border between the magnocellular and parvocellular layers in or near koniocellular layer 3 (Martin et al., 1997; Hendry and Reid, 2000). The small bistratified ganglion cells thus represent a parallel pathway for S-cone-related color signals that is completely independent of the midget pathway.

Detailed study of the synaptic organization of this pathway reveals a distinct circuitry in which S-cone signals are transmitted to the inner dendritic tier of the small bistratified cell by a cone bipolar cell that makes selective connections with S cones (Calkins, Tsukamoto, and Sterling, 1998). The precise mechanism for the strong S versus L+M cone opponency remains to be fully worked out, but is likely to arise in the center-surround organization of the S-cone bipolar cell (Dacey, 2000) and by antagonistic L+M-cone input via OFF cone bipolar cell connections to the bistratified dendritic tree (Calkins, Tsukamoto, and Sterling, 1998).

Our understanding of S-cone pathways and their full role in color vision remains incomplete. As discussed in the next section, other novel ganglion cell types transmit S-cone opponent signals to the LGN. It has also been shown that OFF midget bipolar cells contact S cones, providing a potential midget pathway for S-OFF signals in the foveal retina (Klug et al., 1993, 2003).

RETINAL FIREWORKS DISPLAY REMAINING LOW-DENSITY GANGLION CELL TYPES The identification of the small bistratified cell as a previously unrecognized color-coding pathway initiated the systematic investigation of the remaining ganglion cell populations with the goal of making the link between central connections, morphology, and physiology

for novel retinal ganglion cell types using the in vitro preparation of the macaque retina. To achieve such a goal, retrogradely labeled ganglion cells can be successfully targeted for intracellular recording and staining in vitro. Reliably targeting a specific cell, especially a low-density type, is extremely difficult with this method, however. This is because little morphology is revealed after retrograde labeling to permit specific cell types to be consistently identified and studied both anatomically and physiologically; progress is therefore extremely slow. Recently, however, a tracing method, discovered by serendipity, has revealed the complete morphology of large numbers of retrogradely labeled cells in vitro and has quickly and efficiently revealed a more complete picture of primate ganglion cell morphology (Dacey, Peterson, et al., 2003). The method, termed retrograde photodynamics, relies on the tracer rhodamine-dextran. When ganglion cells retrogradely labeled with this tracer are observed in vitro, they show the typical granular accumulation of tracer in the cell body. However, when these cells are observed with epifluorescent illumination, the sequestered tracer is liberated into the cytoplasm, in a striking fireworks-like display. The tracer quickly diffuses throughout the dendritic tree, revealing the complete dendritic morphology of the retrogradely labeled cell (figure 20.3). The exact mechanism by which light leads to the release of the sequestered fluorophore is not known, though it is likely that rhodamine acts as a photosensitizing molecule in which excitation of the fluorophore by light leads to the creation of reactive oxygen species, which in turn damage the cellular structure that is locally concentrating the fluorophore (Georgakoudi and Foster, 1998).

The anatomical picture now emerging from retrograde photostaining after rhodamine-dextran injections placed in LGN and SC illustrates the characteristic mammalian pattern of extreme cell type diversity. Including the small bistratified cell, a total of 13 novel types have been clearly identified, and with further analysis this number may grow to at least 17. Two views of the morphological details are shown in figures 20.4 and 20.5. For discussion purposes, the retrogradely labeled cells can be divided into six new groups based on one or two shared, basic features of dendritic morphology. Each ganglion cell population within the group can be further distinguished by stratification pattern in the IPL (figure 20.4B).

THORNY CELLS The *thorny cell* group is characterized by a moderately large field of densely branching, fine-caliber dendrites that are studded with small thornlike extensions (figure 20.5). These thorny cells can be further divided into three types by depth of stratification in the IPL: the broad thorny type, with a thicker dendritic tree, in the center of the IPL, and two other types, narrowly monostratified near the inner and outer borders of the IPL (figure 20.4A, B).

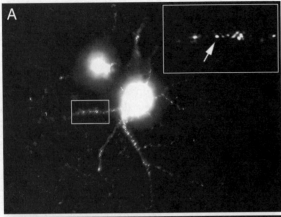

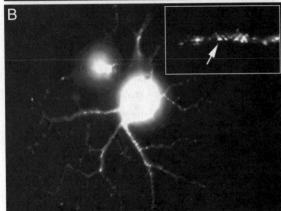

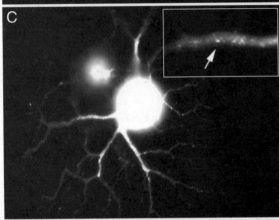

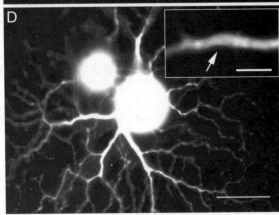

FIGURE 20.3 In vitro photodynamic staining reveals the detailed dendritic morphology of ganglion cells after retrograde labeling from tracer injections into retinorecipient structures. (*A–D*) Sequence of photomicrographs showing the progress of photostaining in vitro that was initiated by a brief light exposure. Plane of focus is in the IPL on the dendritic tree of a parasol ganglion cell retrogradely labeled from injections of rhodamine-dextran into the LGN. (*A*) Tracer initially appears as small bright granules in the soma and dendrites. On exposure to light, the granules burst and release the fluorescent tracer, which diffuses throughout the cytoplasm. Here photostaining has already begun in the soma, which is brightly and uniformly labeled; tracer in the dendrites still appears as small bright granules. Area indicated by the box is enlarged in the inset, and a single granule is indicated by the arrow. (*B*) Photostaining has begun in the dendrites; some granules have burst, and tracer is beginning to diffuse through the dendrites. The tracer granule indicated by the arrow in the inset has not yet burst. (*C*) Photostaining continues as more granules burst and release tracer into the dendrites. (*D*) Photostaining is complete. Note that the granule indicated by the arrow in the insets has now burst. The entire dendritic tree is uniformly tracer labeled. Photostaining can be used to efficiently characterize the morphology of a large number of retrogradely labeled ganglion cells and also to selectively target individual morphological types in vitro for physiological analysis (Dacey, Peterson, et al., 2003). Scale bar = 50 μm; inset scale bar = 10 μm. (See color plate 9.)

◄

Both the broad thorny and narrow thorny cells have been retrogradely labeled from the SC and the LGN (Rodieck and Watanabe, 1993b; Dacey, Peterson, et al., 2003). Complete cell counts of the thorny populations are not yet possible, but the relative spatial density of each type can be estimated from measurements of dendritic field diameter and observations of the local spacing of neighboring cells of the same morphological type from photostained retinas. At any given eccentricity, the thorny cell types show a dendritic field overlap characteristic of most ganglion cell types (coverage of about 1–2) but show about twice the dendritic field diameter as neighboring parasol ganglion cells. Based on total ganglion cell counts, each thorny population would account for about 1% of the total ganglion cell population in midperipheral retina (table 20.1).

The thorny cells have not yet been physiologically characterized in detail, but initial recordings of these cells in vitro suggest that these cells give transient light responses and are not direction selective. The broad thorny cells, as would be expected from a dendritic morphology that straddles the ON-OFF border at the center of the IPL, show a transient ON-OFF response, but also without the direction selectivity that is present in certain transient ON-OFF cells of other mammalian retinas. Nothing is currently known about the cone inputs to these cells or their possible roles in chromatic or achromatic visual pathways that reach the level of visual cortex or extrastriate cortex.

RECURSIVE CELLS: DIRECTION-SELECTIVE CIRCUITS IN PRIMATE RETINA? The *recursive* cell group shows moderately

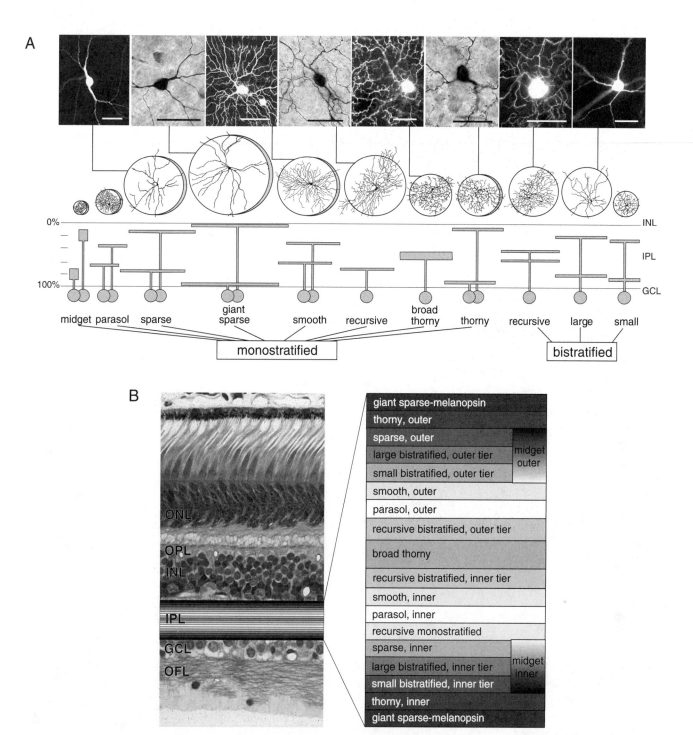

FIGURE 20.4 Diverse ganglion cell types with large dendritic field diameters and low to very low relative densities, as revealed by retrograde photostaining (Dacey et al., 2003). Thus far 12 distinctive dendritic morphologies composing up to 18 distinct ganglion cell populations have been identified by retrograde labeling from rhodamine-dextran tracer injections made into LGN, SC, and pretectum. (A) Photomicrographs at top illustrate morphological detail observed after retrograde tracer transport that permits cell type identification. Relative dendritic field sizes in retinal periphery are indicated by the disk that surrounds drawings of dendritic morphology observed in retinal flat-mounts. Tracer injections suggest that midget cells and small and large bistratified ganglion cells project exclusively to the LGN; parasol, thorny, smooth, sparse, and giant sparse cells are retrogradely labeled from tracer injection in LGN and SC. Thus far the recursive monostratified and recursive bistratified groups have been labeled only after tracer injection into the SC. The depth of dendritic stratification in the IPL is estimated

as percentage depth, with the ganglion cell layer (GCL) as 100%. Stratification of giant sparse cells was determined from melanopsin-labeled cells in vertical sections through the retina. Stratification of all other cell types was determined from HRP-stained cells in whole-mount retina by measuring the relative stratification of neighboring cells of different types with overlapping dendrites. Scale bars = 50 μm. (B) Photomicrograph on the left shows a cross-section of the retina. The IPL has been magnified on the right to show the relative dendritic stratification of the cells shown in A. The dendritic trees of most ganglion cell types occupy unique, narrow strata in the IPL. The IPL appears to be subdivided into at least 18 narrow bands; each band is 1–2 μm thick, and most ganglion-cell dendritic trees, with the exception of the midget and broad thorny types, are restricted to these narrow bands. GCL, ganglion cell layer; IPL, inner plexiform layer; INL, inner nuclear layer; OPL, outer plexiform layer; ONL, outer nuclear layer.

291

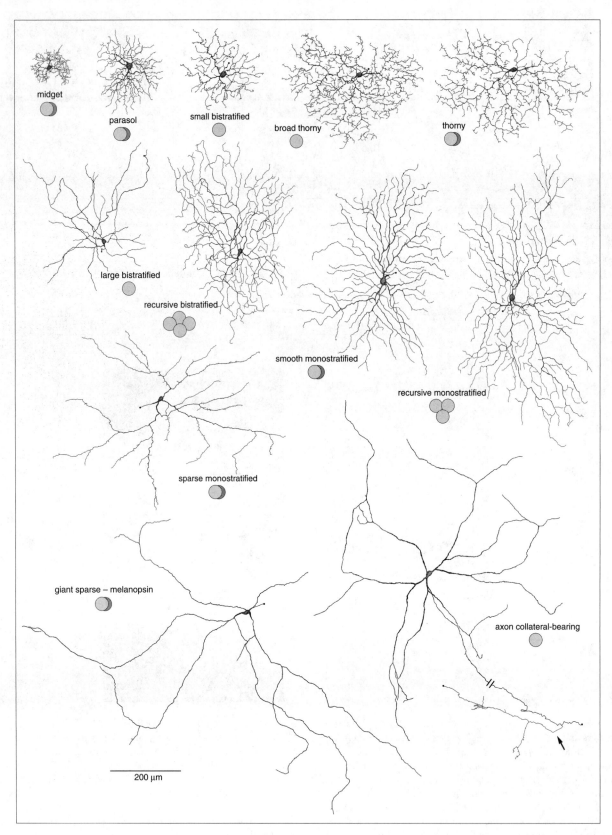

FIGURE 20.5 Morphology and relative dendritic field sizes for the ganglion cell types recognized thus far. Tracings were made from HRP-stained cells in peripheral retina. The axon collateral–bearing cell was HRP-stained following in vitro intracellular injection of Neurobiotin. An axon collateral (arrow) arises from the axon ~1 mm from the soma. The giant sparse cell was also HRP-stained following in vitro intracellular injection of Neurobiotin. All other cells were tracer-labeled by retrograde transport of biotinylated rhodamine-dextran injections placed in the LGN or SC. Shaded circles indicate the number of populations for each morphological group. For example, midget and parasol cells each comprise distinct inner and outer cell populations that are represented here by two overlapping circles. The recursive bistratified and recursive monostratified cells are possible correlates of ON-OFF direction-selective and ON direction-selective cells, respectively (see table 20.1). As in rabbit retina, they are represented here as composing four (recursive bistratified) and three (recursive monostratified) distinct populations.

densely branched trees in which many secondary dendritic branches have a strong tendency to curve back toward the cell body and in some instances form closed loops of apposing, recursive dendrites (figure 20.5). Another feature of these cells is that even though the dendritic fields are large, neighboring cells are very closely spaced, giving rise to a high degree of dendritic overlap; moreover, the overlapping dendrites of neighboring cells have a tendency to entwine and run together in dendritic fascicles. The recursive cells can be divided into a bistratified group, with separate strata near the center of the IPL and a single monostratified group with stratification in the inner portion of the IPL, where ON-center cells are expected to stratify (figure 20.4A, B). Both groups of recursive cells have been retrogradely labeled from tracer injections into the SC; in one instance, the monostratified group was labeled from injections placed into the LGN.

The recursive cells have not yet been recorded from, but their anatomical profile nicely fits the picture for the two major groups studied in great detail in rabbit retina—the ON and ON-OFF direction-selective (DS) cells (Vaney et al., 2000). First, the recursive branching is a characteristic feature of both ON and ON-OFF cells. Second, the high dendritic overlap and dendritic cofasciculation are also observed for rabbit DS cells; in rabbit, this reflects the subdivision of this group into several distinct types. Each type tiles the retina independently with little dendritic overlap and shows a characteristic directional preference (Vaney, 1994; Amthor and Oyster, 1995). Thus, in rabbit there are three ON DS types and four ON-OFF DS types. If this picture ultimately holds true for macaque the recursive ganglion cell group may provide an early, previously unrecognized stage for motion processing in the primate visual system.

LARGE BISTRATIFIED CELLS: A NEW S-ON CHROMATIC PATHWAY The *large bistratified cells* are present as a single population that is consistently labeled after tracer injections into the LGN (Dacey, Peterson, et al., 2003) (figure 20.5). These cells, like the small bistratified cells, show two strata near the inner and outer IPL borders, with the inner dendritic tier in the vicinity of the known stratification of the axon terminal of the S-cone-selective cone bipolar cell type (figure 20.4A, B). The large bistratified cell shows a more sparse branching pattern and larger dendritic field diameter than the small bistratified cells (figure 20.5). Dendritic field diameter and observed overlap suggest that these cells compose about 3% of the total ganglion cell population in the midperipheral retina (table 20.1). However, in foveal retina the large and small bistratified cells appear similar in size, so, like the midget ganglion cells, the relative density of this cell group may increase in central retina.

Strikingly, the first recordings from large bistratified cells revealed a clear excitatory input from S cones together with inhibitory input from L and/or M cones, and thus provide a second anatomically distinct S-ON opponent pathway to the LGN (figure 20.6B). At first glance, the light response of these cells appears much like that of the small bistratified cells, but detailed information about the relative signs and strengths of the L-, M-, and S-cone inputs to the receptive field and an overall understanding of the spectral sensitivity of this cell type will be needed before any conclusions can be drawn about the role of this pathway in chromatic processing.

SPARSE MONOSTRATIFIED CELLS: AN S-OFF CHROMATIC PATHWAY The group of *sparse monostratified cells* shows large and narrowly stratified dendritic trees like the smooth monostratified cells, but much more sparsely branching (figure 20.5). Two populations are stratified close to the outer and inner border of the IPL (figure 20.4). These cells are also consistently labeled from tracer injections into the LGN, and initial recording from this type revealed yet another S-cone opponent type in which the S-cone input is inhibitory and opposed by an excitatory input from combined L- and M-cone input (Dacey, Gamlin, et al., 2003) (figure 20.6A).

S-OFF opponent responses have been recorded at the level of the LGN and primary visual cortex, and an S-OFF signal is a well-established, psychophysically characterized component of opponent processing in human color vision (e.g., DeValois et al., 2000; DeValois, DeValois, and Mahon, 2000; Knoblauch and Shevell, 2001; Monnier and Shevell, 2003). However, since all known S-cone-related circuitry derives from an excitatory ON pathway to the inner part of the IPL, S-OFF responses recorded at higher levels are usually assumed to reflect more central processing of the S-cone signal (DeValois, DeValois, and Mahon, 2000; DeValois et al., 2000). Our current understanding of this pathway in relation to the S-ON circuitry is limited, and the source of the S-OFF signal is unclear. No S-cone-selective OFF-bipolar cells have been identified as a counterpart of the S-ON bipolar cells, and the large sparsely branching dendritic trees of the S-OFF ganglion cells are stratified in the inner portion of the IPL, where S-ON pathway signals are transmitted. Either the inhibitory S signal reaches this cell by a sign inversion of the S-ON bipolar signal or the S-cone signal is in some way introduced to the inhibitory surround of this cell. Future measurements of receptive field structure, together with pharmacological manipulations of ON and OFF signals, will be needed to address this question.

SMOOTH MONOSTRATIFIED CELLS: ALPHA-LIKE CELLS OF THE PRIMATE? In contrast to the thorny group, the *smooth monostratified* types are larger in dendritic field diameter, show thicker-caliber radiate and thornless dendrites, and form an inner and outer cell pair that are narrowly stratified near the center of the IPL, very close to but not overlapping the

A

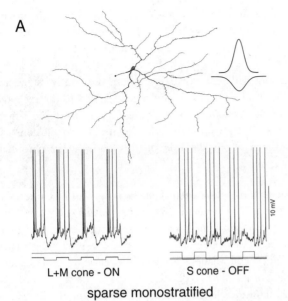

L+M cone - ON   S cone - OFF

10 mV

sparse monostratified

B

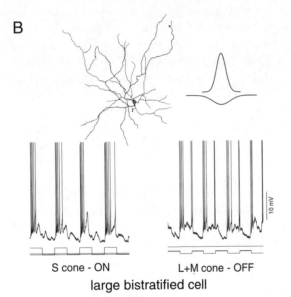

S cone - ON   L+M cone - OFF

10 mV

large bistratified cell

C

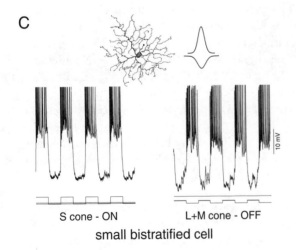

S cone - ON   L+M cone - OFF

10 mV

small bistratified cell

FIGURE 20.6   S-cone spectral opponency is present in a number of distinct ganglion cell populations. For each type, ganglion cell morphology is shown in relation to voltage recording in response to modulation of either the S cones or the L+M cones in isolation. To the right of each morphological drawing are shown best-fitting difference-of-Gaussian spatial profiles derived from mapping the sign, strength, and spatial extent of the S-versus-L+M cone input to the receptive field. *(A)* Large sparse monostratified ganglion cells show L+M ON, S OFF opponent receptive fields; these cells are stratified in the inner, ON portion of the IPL. The source of the inhibitory S-cone signal has not been determined. *(B)* Large bistratified ganglion cells show S ON responses much like that of the S ON small bistratified ganglion cell illustrated in *C*, and are likely also to receive direct excitatory input from the S-cone bipolar cell. *(C)* Small bistratified ganglion cells show S ON, L+M OFF opponent receptive fields. (A fourth S-cone-opponent type is shown in Figure 20.7.) Stimulus was a 2-Hz square wave modulation shown below each trace; red, green, and blue lights are varied in amplitude to create cone-isolating conditions. Receptive field structure shown in the difference-of-Gaussians model was measured by the spatial frequency response to drifting gratings that modulated either the S cones or the L+M cones in isolation.

stratification of the parasol cells (figures 20.4 and 20.5). Also like the parasol cells, the smooth monostratified cells have relatively large cell bodies and are retrogradely labeled from both the SC and LGN. Together the inner and outer populations probably account for about 2%–3% of the ganglion cells in the midretinal periphery (table 20.1).

This cell group has not yet been recorded from, but anatomically it is comparable to the intensively studied alpha cell of cat retina (Peichl, Ott, and Boycott, 1987). It is therefore possible that these cells are comparable to the alpha-Y-cell pathway. Previous studies have offered conflicting opinions about the primate correlate of the Y-cell system. If the primate retina is considered as giving rise to just two major functional retinogeniculate pathways, then the parasol-magnocellular projecting ganglion cells appear to correspond to the cat alpha-Y cells as the origin of signals that contribute to early motion processing (Rodieck, Brening, and Watanabe, 1993). At the same time it has been shown that the magnocellular layers contain cells that show both linear (X cells) and nonlinear spatial summation (Y cells), suggesting that multiple functional pathways project via the magnocellular layers (Shapley and Perry, 1986; Kaplan, Lee, and Shapley, 1990). The existence of some number of novel ganglion cell types projecting to the LGN now makes it necessary to reexamine this question.

GIANT MONOSTRATIFIED CELLS: A PUPILLOMOTOR, IRRADIANCE-CODING PATHWAY   *Giant monostratified cells* have been consistently labeled from tracer injections into the LGN and the pretectal olivary nucleus (PON) (Gamlin, Peterson, and Dacey, 2001; Dacey, Peterson, et al., 2003). They show extremely large and very sparsely branching dendritic trees that easily distinguish these cells from all other anatomical groups (figures 20.4 and 20.5). The PON is the well-established central relay for visual signals that drive the pupillary light reflex, and small tracer injections made into the PON can label the giant monostratified ganglion cells selectively, implicating these cells as the pupillomotor retinal output pathway. The unusual physiological properties of these cells are consistent with this role.

Intracellular recordings from giant monostratified ganglion cells reveal an extremely regular, maintained discharge that increases monotonically with increasing background illuminance (Gamlin, Peterson, and Dacey, 2001). The ability of these cells to uniquely code for irradiance is transmitted to the PON (Gamlin, Zhang, and Clarke, 1995; Zhang, Clarke, and Gamlin, 1996) and is a key physiological property required to link a fixed pupil diameter to a given irradiance level (Gamlin et al., 1998).

Intrinsic photosensitivity is the basis for irradiance coding by the giant monostratified ganglion cells The unique irradiance coding by the giant monostratified ganglion cells was paradoxical, given that a fundamental property of retinal physiology, beginning with the cone photoreceptors themselves, is the converse: a rapid reduction in sensitivity to increasing background levels that permits retinal cells to adapt to a wide range of irradiance levels (Shapley and Enroth-Cugell, 1984). However, recent results have now revealed that the basis for this irradiance-coding property lies in a novel photopigment present exclusively in the giant monostratified ganglion cells themselves. Characterization of this property in the giant cells has led to a more detailed picture of the anatomy, physiology, and central connections of this pathway. It is thus worth considering these results in some detail as an example of the first low-density ganglion cell type in primate to be characterized in detail.

First discovered in rat retina, photoreceptive ganglion cells quite surprisingly responded to light in the absence of all input from rods and cones (Berson, Dunn, and Takao, 2002). These intrinsically photosensitive ganglion cells provided a neural basis for previous observations that a novel photopigment residing in the mammalian eye was capable of entraining the circadian pacemaker of the hypothalamus and also of driving the pupillary light reflex. Thus, mice lacking all rods and cones retain circadian rhythms and residual pupil reflex driven by a novel photopigment with a peak sensitivity at about 480 nm (Lucas et al., 1999; Lucas, Douglas, and Foster, 2001). The light response of intrinsically photosensitive rat ganglion cells is also mediated by a novel photopigment with a peak sensitivity at about 480 nm. These cells contain melanopsin, an opsin-like protein, that has become the candidate photopigment, and they project to the suprachiasmatic nucleus and to the pupillomotor pretectum (Hattar et al., 2002). The intrinsic light response is

extremely slow and sustained and permits coding of gross changes in light intensity.

The link between the rat melanopsin-containing, photoreceptive ganglion cells and the giant monostratified pupillomotor ganglion cells occurred with the development of an antibody to human melanopsin. The melanopsin-containing cells were targeted for intracellular recording in vitro by retrograde photostaining from tracer injections into either the LGN or pretectum. Ganglion cells that were retrogradely stained and also melanopsin immunoreactive corresponded to the giant monostratified ganglion cell group that stratified at the extreme IPL borders (figure 20.4A, B). There are about 3000 melanopsin-containing ganglion cells in macaque and human retina, which is only about two-tenths of 1% of the total ganglion cell population (figure 20.7A). These cells peak in density around the fovea (about 25 cells/mm^2), where extremely large dendritic trees spiral around the foveal pit. In the periphery there are only a few cells/mm^2, but a loose meshwork of completely stained dendritic processes carpets the retina (Peterson et al., 2003) (figure 20.7A).

Melanopsin-containing cell bodies are present in both amacrine and ganglion cell layers and give rise to a distinctive bistratified dendritic plexus situated at the extreme inner and outer borders of the IPL (figure 20.7A). Macaque melanopsin-containing ganglion cells show a robust ON sustained cone-driven response to long-wavelength stimuli (figure 20.7B). But the use of cone-isolating stimuli shows that these cells are also a second type of S-OFF color opponent ganglion cell with large, coextensive S-cone inhibitory and L+M-cone excitatory receptive field components (Dacey, Gamlin, et al., 2003) (figure 20.7C). Not surprisingly, given the cone-driven light response, these cells also show an equally large rod-driven ON input under dark-adapted conditions.

Because of the strong cone input to these ganglion cells, the intrinsic light response could only be observed in isolation after the application of L-AP4 and CNQX to block glutamate transmission from outer to inner retina. When isolated in this way, the intrinsic light response shows the same surprisingly long response latency and slow turnoff observed in rat (figure 20.7D). As in the rat, the spectral tuning of the intrinsic light response is best described by a retinal-based pigment nomogram with a peak at 483 nm (figure 20.7E). These ganglion cells thus contain a single novel photopigment, possibly melanopsin, that binds retinal and shows a spectral peak situated between the S cone and the rods (Smith, Pokorny, and Dacey, 2003).

Other experiments show that in macaque, the intrinsic response is present at photopic levels and combines with the cone response. Adding the intrinsic response to the cone response achieves higher spike rates, which increase with increasing irradiance. The ability of these cells to show a

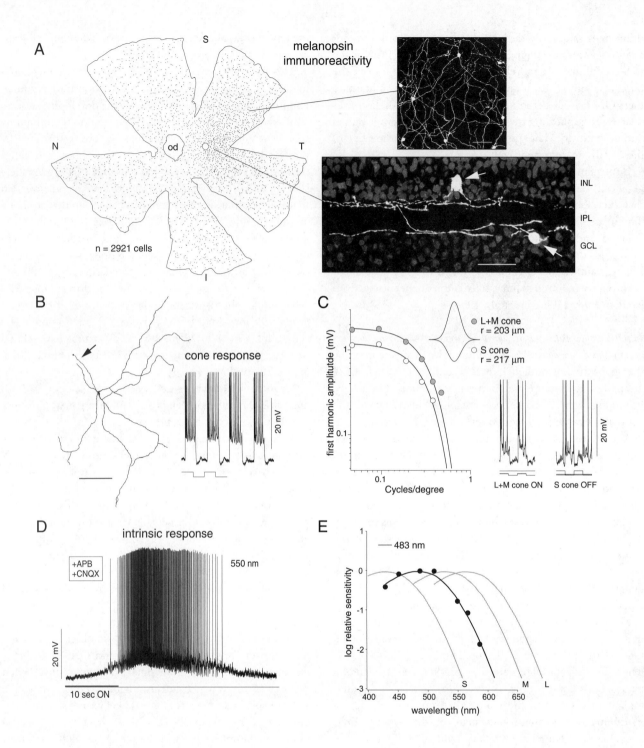

FIGURE 20.7 Spatial density, morphology, dendritic stratification, and physiology of the melanopsin-containing, photoreceptive ganglion cell type. (*A*) A tracing of a whole-mount retina reacted with an antibody against melanopsin is shown on the left. Each dot represents the location of an immunoreactive ganglion cell; both macaque and human retina contain ~3000 melansopsin-containing cells. Cell density is highest near the fovea and drops off sharply toward peripheral retina (T, N, S, I: temporal, nasal, superior, and inferior retina; od, optic disk). Confocal images of melanopsin-containing ganglion cells are shown on the right. Top micrograph shows a patch of peripheral melanopsin-labeled cells in a flat-mount retina (scale bar = 100 µm). Lower micrograph is a reconstruction of the dendritic arbors of two neighboring Alexa Fluor–labeled melanopsin-reactive cells (arrows) from confocal images taken in five consecutive vertical sections (25 µm thick) through temporal retina approximately 2 mm from the fovea. Retina was counterstained with a nuclear dye (propidium iodide) to visualize the nuclear layers. The dendrites of these cells can be seen to form two narrow strata located at the extreme inner and outer borders of the IPL (scale bar = 50 µm; GCL, ganglion cell layer; IPL, inner plexiform layer; INL, inner nuclear layer.) (*B*) Tracing of the complete dendritic tree of a photoreceptive ganglion cell recorded from in the in vitro retina, then intracellularly filled with Neurobiotin and processed for HRP histochemistry following tissue fixation. These cells correspond to the giant, sparse monostratified ganglion cells that can be retrogradely labeled from tracer injections into the SC. Arrow indicates axon. Scale bar = 200 µm. Voltage response at the right shows a sustained ON response to a 550-nm, 2-Hz modulation. Time course of the stimulus is shown below the voltage trace. (*C*) The cell had an L+M− ON, S-OFF opponent receptive field. The plot on the left gives the spatial frequency response to drifting gratings used to measure the receptive field. Drifting grating stimuli modulated either the L+M− cones (gray circles) or S cones (white circles) in isolation. The data were fitted with a difference-of-Gaussian receptive field model (solid lines); the two-dimensional Gaussian profile for these fits is shown to the right of the plot (r = Gaussian radius). Traces on the right show the voltage responses to L+M− and S-cone isolating stimuli. (*D*) Application of LAP4 and CNQX blocked excitatory glutamatergic transmission and revealed a very slow, sustained, intrinsic photoresponse. Stimulus was a 10-s, 550-nm monochromatic light step. (*E*) Measurements of the intrinsic photoresponse (solid circles) to a series of monochromatic lights over a 3 log unit range of illumination were used to determine spectral sensitivity of the intrinsic light response. The solid black line is the retinal-based pigment nomogram fit to the data, giving a spectral peak at 483 nm. The spectral sensitivities of S cones, M cones, and L cones (Baylor, Nunn, and Schnapf, 1987) are plotted for comparison (solid gray lines).

spike rate that is monotonically related to irradiance is thus created in the normal physiological situation by the combined cone and intrinsic signal over much of the photopic range.

In sum, melanopsin-containing cells in macaque show sustained light responses driven by rods and cones over the full scotopic-photopic range. The cone-mediated response shows an S-OFF type of color opponency. The cone response is summed with the intrinsic response over most of the photopic range. The significance of the S-cone opponency is not clear. Since these ganglion cells can be retrogradely labeled from the LGN, it is possible that they transmit a cone-opponent signal that participates in color processing. A second possibility is that color opponency may contribute to circadian regulation by providing information about large spectral changes at dusk. Thus, Foster and Helfrich-Forster (2001) have speculated, "If the circadian system was capable of using multiple photopigments to ratio changes in the relative amounts of short and long wavelength radiation and of coupling this information with irradiance levels, then the phase of twilight could be determined very accurately."

REMAINING TYPES: GANGLION CELLS WITH AXON COLLATERALS, AND OTHERS Based on estimates of the total number of macaque ganglion cells and estimates of the relative densities for each ganglion cell type identified thus far, the great majority, certainly at least 90%, of the ganglion cells have been accounted for. It is likely, however, that other low-density ganglion cell populations are present that will be revealed by further tracer injections into central targets. One example is a distinct cell type that shows intraretinal axon collaterals that terminate in the IPL (see figure 20.5). Such intraretinal axon collaterals are not a typical feature of retinal ganglion cells, and the functional significance of such ganglion cell feedback to the inner retina is not clear. These axon-collateral-bearing ganglion cells have been intracellularly stained in both human and macaque retina, and a correlate of this cell type has also been observed in both cat and turtle retina (Dacey, 1985; Peterson and Dacey, 1998).

Summary and conclusions

A broad picture of the primate ganglion cell population can now be sketched, although many critical details of structure and function remain to be added. Diverse ganglion cell populations create many parallel pathways, but it appears that virtually all of these pathways converge on the two major visual structures of the brainstem, the LGN and SC, with many ganglion cell types likely projecting to both of these targets. Thus, even though there are on the order of a dozen distinctive smaller retinal targets, it must be concluded that most, if not all, of these smaller structures receive collateral input from ganglion cell types that project to LGN and SC; a major question for the future concerns the roles that this complex set of inputs plays in the function of the geniculo-cortical and collicular pathways.

The diverse low-density ganglion cell populations sacrifice spatial grain to represent fine detail in the visual image but gain the advantage of a large number of functionally distinct pathways at little cost to the bottleneck of the optic nerve. Put simply, the retina can do a lot with a little. This is especially true if we consider that the ganglion cell axons, once projected into the brain, can easily collateralize to multiple targets, and their signals can be greatly amplified by mechanisms as simple as anatomical variation in the number and density of synaptic boutons in the terminal arbor of the axon. In other words, a low density of ganglion cells in the retina need not be an indication of the strength of the signal centrally. The strategy of doing a lot with little is beautifully demonstrated in the characterization of the giant monostratified ganglion cells, which make up less than one percent of the total ganglion cells yet project to multiple central targets and transmit unique signals appropriate to entrain circadian rhythms, drive the pupillary light reflex, and perhaps contribute to color processing.

Finally, table 20.1 clearly reveals the gaps in the current picture of the morphology, physiology, and central projections of macaque ganglion cell types. Surprisingly, it seems to be more the rule than the exception that distinct ganglion cell populations exist at very low densities—1%–5% of the total. The fundamental goal must be to complete the identification and description of the ganglion cell populations by making tracer injections into remaining retinal target structures and to characterize ganglion cell morphology and ultimately their detailed light-evoked responses. From what has been learned so far about the existence of multiple cone-opponent pathways and the melanopsin-containing photoreceptive pathway, these low-density cell populations will prove to reveal much about the way the retina contributes to the visual process.

ACKNOWLEDGMENTS   This work was supported by Public Health Service grants EY01730 (Vision Res Ctr), EY06678, and EY09625 to the National Eye Institute and RR0166 to the National Primate Research Center at the University of Washington. I thank Beth Peterson and Toni Haun for preparing the illustrations.

REFERENCES

ABRAMOV, I., and J. GORDON, 1994. Color appearance: On seeing red—or yellow, or green, or blue. *Annu. Rev. Psychol.* 45:451–485.

AHMAD, K. M., K. KLUG, S. HERR, P. STERLING, and S. SCHEIN, 2003. Cell density ratios in a foveal patch in macaque retina. *Vis. Neurosci.* 20:189–209.

AMTHOR, F. R., and C. W. OYSTER, 1995. Spatial organization of retinal information about the direction of image motion. *Proc. Natl. Acad. Sci. U.S.A.* 92:4002–4005.

BAYLOR, D. A., B. J. NUNN, and J. L. SCHNAPF, 1987. Spectral sensitivity of cones of the monkey *Macaca fascicularis*. *J. Physiol. (Lond.)* 390:145–160.

BERSON, D. M., F. A. DUNN, and M. TAKAO, 2002. Phototransduction by retinal ganglion cells that set the circadian clock. *Science* 295:1070–1073.

CALKINS, D. J., 1999. Synaptic organization of cone pathways in the primate retina. In *Color Vision: From Genes to Perception*, K. R. Gegenfurtner and L. T. Sharpe, eds. New York: Cambridge University Press, pp. 163–180.

CALKINS, D. J., S. J. SCHEIN, Y. TSUKAMOTO, and P. STERLING, 1994. M and L cones in macaque fovea connect to midget ganglion cells by different numbers of excitatory synapses. *Nature* 371:70–72.

CALKINS, D. J., S. J. SCHEIN, Y. TSUKAMOTO, and P. STERLING, 1995. Density of midget and nonmidget ganglion cells in macaque fovea. *Soc. Neurosci. Abstr.* 23:1257.

CALKINS, D. J., and P. STERLING, 1996. Absence of spectrally specific lateral inputs to midget ganglion cells in primate retina. *Nature* 381:613–615.

CALKINS, D. J., and P. STERLING, 1999. Evidence that circuits for spatial and color vision segregate at the first retinal synapse. *Neuron* 24:313–321.

CALKINS, D. J., Y. TSUKAMOTO, and P. STERLING, 1998. Microcircuitry and mosaic of a blue-yellow ganglion cell in the primate retina. *J. Neurosci.* 18:3373–3385.

CHICHILNISKY, E. J., and R. S. KALMAR, 2003. Temporal resolution of ensemble visual motion signals in primate retina. *J. Neurosci.* 23:6681–6689.

DACEY, D. M., 1985. Wide-spreading terminal axons in the inner plexiform layer of the cat's retina: Evidence for intrinsic axon collaterals of ganglion cells. *J. Comp. Neurol.* 242:247–262.

DACEY, D. M., 1989. Axon-bearing amacrine cells of the macaque monkey retina. *J. Comp. Neurol.* 284:275–293.

DACEY, D. M., 1993a. Morphology of a small-field bistratified ganglion cell type in the macaque and human retina. *Vis. Neurosci.* 10:1081–1098.

DACEY, D. M., 1993b. The mosaic of midget ganglion cells in the human retina. *J. Neurosci.* 13:5334–5355.

DACEY, D. M., 1994. Physiology, morphology and spatial densities of identified ganglion cell types in primate retina. In *Higher Order Processes in the Visual System*. London: Ciba Foundation, pp. 12–34.

DACEY, D. M., 1996. Circuitry for color coding in the primate retina. *Proc. Natl. Acad. Sci. U.S.A.* 93:582–588.

DACEY, D. M., 1999. Primate retina: Cell types, circuits and color opponency. *Prog. Retina Eye Res.* 18:737–763.

DACEY, D. M., 2000. Parallel pathways for spectral coding in primate retina. *Annu. Rev. Neurosci.* 23:743–775.

DACEY, D. M., and S. BRACE, 1992. A coupled network for parasol but not midget ganglion cells in the primate retina. *Vis. Neurosci.* 9:279–290.

DACEY, D. M., P. D. GAMLIN, V. C. SMITH, J. POKORNY, O. S. PACKER, B. B. PETERSON, F. R. ROBINSON, and K.-W. YAU, 2003. *Functional architecture of the photoreceptive ganglion cell in primate retina: intrinsic photosensitivity, S-cone spectral opponency and irradiance coding.* ARVO Abstract #3231. Available from www.arvo.org.

DACEY, D. M., and B. B. LEE, 1994. The blue-ON opponent pathway in primate retina originates from a distinct bistratified ganglion cell type. *Nature* 367:731–735.

DACEY, D. M., B. B. LEE, D. K. STAFFORD, J. POKORNY, and V. C. SMITH, 1996. Horizontal cells of the primate retina: Cone specificity without spectral opponency. *Science* 271:656–659.

DACEY, D. M., O. S. PACKER, L. C. DILLER, D. H. BRAINARD, B. B. PETERSON, and B. B. LEE, 2000. Center surround receptive field structure of cone bipolar cells in primate retina. *Vision Res.* 40:1801–1811.

DACEY, D. M., and M. R. PETERSEN, 1992. Dendritic field size and morphology of midget and parasol ganglion cells of the human retina. *Proc. Natl. Acad. Sci. U.S.A.* 89:9666–9670.

DACEY, D. M., B. B. PETERSON, F. R. ROBINSON, and P. D. GAMLIN, 2003. Fireworks in the primate retina: In vitro photodynamics reveals diverse LGN-projecting ganglion cell types. *Neuron* 37:15–27.

DEMONASTERIO, F. M., and P. GOURAS, 1975. Functional properties of ganglion cells of the rhesus monkey retina. *J. Physiol. (Lond.)* 251:167–195.

DERRINGTON, A. M., J. KRAUSKOPF, and P. LENNIE, 1984. Chromatic mechanisms in lateral geniculate nucleus of macaque. *J. Physiol. (Lond.)* 357:219–240.

DEVALOIS, R. L., I. ABRAMOV, and G. H. JACOBS, 1966. Analysis of response patterns of LGN cells. *J. Opt. Soc. Am. A* 56:966–977.

DEVALOIS, R. L., N. P. COTTARIS, S. D. ELFAR, L. E. MAHON, and J. A. WILSON, 2000. Some transformations of color information from lateral geniculate nucleus to striate cortex. *Proc. Natl. Acad. Sci. U.S.A.* 97:4997–5002.

DEVALOIS, R. L., K. K. DEVALOIS, and L. E. MAHON, 2000. Contribution of S opponent cells to color appearance. *Proc. Natl. Acad. Sci. U.S.A.* 97:512–517.

DILLER, L. C., O. S. PACKER, J. VERWEIJ, M. J. MCMAHON, D. R. WILLIAMS, and D. M. DACEY, 2004. L- and M-cone contributions to the midget and parasol ganglion cell receptive fields of macaque monkey retina. *J. Neurosci.* 24:1079–1088.

FAMIGLIETTI, E. V., A. KANEKO, and M. TACHIBANA, 1977. Neuronal architecture of on and off pathways to ganglion cells in carp retina. *Science* 198:1267–1269.

FOSTER, R. G., and C. HELFRICH-FORSTER, 2001. The regulation of circadian clocks by light in fruitflies and mice. *Philos. Trans. R. Soc. Lond. B Biol. Sci.* 356:1779–1789.

GAMLIN, P. D. R., B. B. PETERSON, and D. M. DACEY, 2001. Physiology and morphology of retinal ganglion cells projecting to the pretectal olivary nucleus of the rhesus monkey. *Invest. Ophthalmol. Visual Sci.* Suppl. 42:S676.

GAMLIN, P. D., H. Y. ZHANG, and R. J. CLARKE, 1995. Luminance neurons in the pretectal olivary nucleus mediate the pupillary light reflex in the rhesus monkey. *Exp. Brain Res.* 106:177–180.

GAMLIN, P. D., H. ZHANG, A. HARLOW, and J. L. BARBUR, 1998. Pupil responses to stimulus color, structure and light flux increments in the rhesus monkey. *Vision Res.* 38:3353–3358.

GEGENFURTNER, K. R., and D. C. KIPER, 2003. Color vision. *Annu. Rev. Neurosci.* 26:181–206.

GEORGAKOUDI, D., and T. H. FOSTER, 1998. Effects of the subcellular redistribution of two Nile Blue derivatives on photodynamic oxygen consumption. *Photochem. Photobiol.* 68:115–122.

HATTAR, S., H. W. LIAO, M. TAKAO, D. M. BERSON, and K.-W. YAU, 2002. Melanopsin-containing retinal ganglion cells: Architecture, projections, and intrinsic photosensitivity. *Science* 295:1065–1070.

HENDRY, S. H. C., and R. C. REID, 2000. The koniocellular pathway in primate vision. *Annu. Rev. Neurosci.* 23:127–153.

ISAYAMA, T., D. M. BERSON, and M. PU, 2000. Theta ganglion cell type of cat retina. *J. Comp. Neurol.* 417:32–48.

JACOBS, G. H., 1993. The distribution and nature of colour vision among the mammals. *Biol. Rev. Camb. Philos. Soc.* 68:413–471.

JACOBS, G. H., and J. F. DEEGAN II, 1997. Spectral sensitivity of macaque monkeys measured with ERG flicker photometry. *Vis. Neurosci.* 14:921–928.

JACOBY, R. A., and D. W. MARSHAK, 2000. Synaptic connections of DB3 diffuse bipolar cell axons in macaque retina. *J. Comp. Neurol.* 416:19–29.

JACOBY, R. A., A. F. WIECHMANN, S. G. AMARA, B. H. LEIGHTON, and D. W. MARSHAK, 2000. Diffuse bipolar cells provide input to OFF parasol ganglion cells in the macaque retina. *J. Comp. Neurol.* 416:6–18.

KAAS, J. H., and M. F. HUERTA, 1988. The subcortical visual system of primates. In *Comparative Primate Biology*, vol. 4, *Neurosciences.* New York: Alan R. Liss, pp. 327–391.

KAPLAN, E., B. B. LEE, and R. M. SHAPLEY, 1990. New views of primate retinal function. *Prog. Retina Eye Res.* 9:273–336.

KAPLAN, E., and R. M. SHAPLEY, 1982. X and Y cells in the lateral geniculate nucleus of macaque monkeys. *J. Physiol. (Lond.)* 330:125–143.

KAPLAN, E., and R. M. SHAPLEY, 1986. The primate retina contains two types of ganglion cells, with high and low contrast sensitivity. *Proc. Natl. Acad. Sci. U.S.A.* 83:2755–2757.

KLUG, K., S. HERR, I. T. NGO, P. STERLING, and S. SCHEIN, 2003. Macaque retina contains an S-cone OFF midget pathway. *J. Neurosci.* 23:9881–9887.

KLUG, K., Y. TSUKAMOTO, P. STERLING, and S. SCHEIN, 1993. Blue cone off-midget ganglion cells in macaque. *Invest. Ophthalmol. Visual Sci.* Suppl. 34:S986.

KNOBLAUCH, K., and S. K. SHEVELL, 2001. Relating cone signals to color appearance: Failure of monotonicity in yellow/blue. *Vis. Neurosci.* 18:901–906.

KOLB, H., and L. DEKORVER, 1991. Midget ganglion cells of the parafovea of the human retina: A study by electron microscopy and serial section reconstructions. *J. Comp. Neurol.* 303:617–636.

KOLB, H., K. A. LINBERG, and S. K. FISHER, 1992. Neurons of the human retina: A Golgi study. *J. Comp. Neurol.* 318:147–187.

KREMERS, J., B. B. LEE, J. POKORNY, and V. C. SMITH, 1993. Responses of macaque ganglion cells and human observers to compound periodic waveforms. *Vision Res.* 33:1997–2011.

LANKHEET, M. J. M., P. LENNIE, and J. KRAUSKOPF, 1998. Distinctive characteristics of subclasses of red-green P-cells in LGN of macaque. *Vis. Neurosci.* 15:37–46.

LEE, B. B., 1991. On the relation between cellular sensitivity and psychophysical detection. In *From Pigments to Perception*, A. Valberg and B. B. Lee, eds. New York: Plenum Press, pp. 105–113.

LEE, B. B., 1999. Receptor inputs to primate ganglion cells. In *Color Vision: From Genes to Perception*, K. R. Gegenfurtner and L. T. Sharpe, eds. New York: Cambridge University Press, pp. 203–218.

LENNIE, P., 2000. Color vision: putting it together. *Curr. Biol.* 10:R589–R591.

LENNIE, P., and M. D'ZMURA, 1988. Mechanisms of color vision. *Crit. Rev. Neurobiol.* 3:333–400.

LEVENTHAL, A. G., R. W. RODIECK, and B. DREHER, 1981. Retinal ganglion cell classes in the Old World monkey: Morphology and central projections. *Science* 213:1139–1142.

LUCAS, R. J., R. H. DOUGLAS, and R. G. FOSTER, 2001. Characterization of an ocular photopigment capable of driving pupillary constriction in mice. *Nat. Neurosci.* 4:621–626.

LUCAS, R. J., M. S. FREEDMAN, M. MUÑOZ, J. M. GARCIA-FERNÁNDEZ, and R. G. FOSTER, 1999. Regulation of the mammalian pineal by non-rod, non-cone, ocular photoreceptors. *Science* 284:505–507.

LYNCH, J. J. I., L. C. L. SILVEIRA, V. H. PERRY, and W. H. MERIGAN, 1992. Visual effects of damage to P ganglion cells in macaques. *Vis. Neurosci.* 8:575–583.

MARSHAK, D. W., E. S. YAMADA, A. S. BORDT, and W. C. PERRYMAN, 2002. Synaptic input to an ON parasol ganglion cell in the macaque retina: A serial section analysis. *Vis. Neurosci.* 19:299–305.

MARTIN, P. R., B. B. LEE, A. J. WHITE, S. G. SOLOMON, and L. RUTTIGER, 2001. Chromatic sensitivity of ganglion cells in the peripheral primate retina. *Nature* 410:933–936.

MARTIN, P. R., A. K. WHITE, H. D. WILDER, and A. E. SEFTON, 1997. Evidence that blue-on cells are part of the third geniculocortical pathway in primates. *Eur. J. Neurosci.* 9:1536–1541.

MASLAND, R. H., 2001. Neuronal diversity in the retina. *Curr. Opin. Neurobiol.* 11:431–436.

MASLAND, R. H., and E. RAVIOLA, 2000. Confronting complexity: Strategies for understanding the microcircuitry of the retina. *Annu. Rev. Neurosci.* 23:249–284.

McMAHON, M. J., M. J. M. LANKHEET, P. LENNIE, and D. R. WILLIAMS, 2000. Fine structure of parvocellular receptive fields in the primate fovea revealed by laser interferometry. *J. Neurosci.* 20:2043–2053.

MERIGAN, W. H., 1989. Chromatic and achromatic vision of macaques: Role of the P pathway. *J. Neurosci.* 9:776–783.

MERIGAN, W. H., 1996. Basic visual capacities and shape discrimination after lesions of extrastriate area V4 in macaques. *Vis. Neurosci.* 13:51–60.

MERIGAN, W. H., C. E. BYRNE, and J. H. R. MAUNSELL, 1991. Does primate motion perception depend on the magnocellular pathway? *J. Neurosci.* 11:3422–3429.

MERIGAN, W. H., L. M. KATZ, and J. H. MAUNSELL, 1991. The effects of parvocellular lateral geniculate lesions on the acuity and contrast sensitivity of macaque monkeys. *J. Neurosci.* 11:994–1001.

MERIGAN, W. H., and J. H. MAUNSELL, 1990. Macaque vision after magnocellular lateral geniculate lesions. *Vis. Neurosci.* 5:347–352.

MERIGAN, W. H., and J. H. R. MAUNSELL, 1993. How parallel are the primate visual pathways? *Annu. Rev. Neurosci.* 16:369–402.

MONNIER, P., and S. K. SHEVELL, 2003. Large shifts in color appearance from patterned chromatic backgrounds. *Nat. Neurosci.* 6: 801–802.

NEITZ, M., and J. NEITZ, 2003. Molecular genetics of human color vision and color vision defects. In *The Visual Neurosciences*, L. M. Chalupa and J. S. Werner, eds. Cambridge, Mass.: MIT, pp. 974–988.

O'BRIEN, B. J., P. L. ABEL, and J. F. OLAVARRIA, 2001. The retinal input to calbindin-D28k-defined subdivisions in macaque inferior pulvinar. *Neurosci. Lett.* 312:145–148.

PACKER, O. S., and D. R. WILLIAMS, 2003. Light, retinal imagery and photoreceptors. In *The Science of Color*, 2nd Edition. S. Shevell, ed. Amsterdam: Elsevier, pp. 41–102.

PAXINOS, G., X.-F. HUANG, and A. W. TOGA, 2000. *The Rhesus Monkey Brain in Stereotaxic Coordinates*. San Diego, Calif.: Academic Press.

PEICHL, L., H. OTT, and B. B. BOYCOTT, 1987. Alpha ganglion cells in mammalian retina. *Proc. R. Soc. Lond. B Biol. Sci.* 231:169–197.

PERRY, V. H., and A. COWEY, 1984. Retinal ganglion cells that project to the superior colliculus and pretectum in the macaque monkey. *Neuroscience* 12:1125–1137.

PERRY, V. H., R. OEHLER, and A. COWEY, 1984. Retinal ganglion cells that project to the dorsal lateral geniculate nucleus in the macaque monkey. *Neuroscience* 12:1101–1123.

PETERSON, B. B., and D. M. DACEY, 1998. Morphology of human retinal ganglion cells with intraretinal axon collaterals. *Vis. Neurosci.* 15:377–387.

PETERSON, B. B., and D. M. DACEY, 1999. Morphology of widefield, monostratified ganglion cells of the human retina. *Vis. Neurosci.* 16:107–120.

PETERSON, B. B., and D. M. DACEY, 2000. Morphology of widefield bistratified and diffuse human retinal ganglion cells. *Vis. Neurosci.* 17:567–578.

PETERSON, B. B., H.-W. LIAO, D. M. DACEY, K.-W. YAU, P. D. GAMLIN, and F. R. ROBINSON, 2003. *Functional architecture of the photoreceptive ganglion cell in primate retina: morphology, mosaic organization and central targets of melanopsin immunostained cells*. Association for Research in Vision and Ophthalmology Abstract #5182.

POLYAK, S. L., 1941. *The Retina*. Chicago: University of Chicago Press.

REID, R. C., and R. M. SHAPLEY, 2002. Space and time maps of cone photoreceptor signals in macaque lateral geniculate nucleus. *J. Neurosci.* 22:6158–6175.

ROCKHILL, R. L., F. J. DALY, M. A. MacNEIL, S. P. BROWN, and R. H. MASLAND, 2002. The diversity of ganglion cells in a mammalian retina. *J. Neurosci.* 22:3831–3843.

RODIECK, R. W., 1991. Which cells code for color? In *From Pigments to Perception*, A. Valberg and B. B. Lee, eds. New York: Plenum Press, pp. 83–93.

RODIECK, R. W., 1998. *The First Steps in Seeing*. Sunderland Mass.: Sinauer Associates.

RODIECK, R. W., K. F. BINMOELLER, and J. DINEEN, 1985. Parasol and midget ganglion cells of the human retina. *J. Comp. Neurol.* 233:115–132.

RODIECK, R. W., R. K. BRENING, and M. WATANABE, 1993. The origin of parallel visual pathways. In *Contrast Sensitivity*, R. Shapley and D. M.-K. Lam, eds. Cambridge, Mass.: MIT Press, pp. 117–144.

RODIECK, R. W., and M. WATANABE, 1993. Survey of the morphology of macaque retinal ganglion cells that project to the pretectum, superior colliculus, and parvicellular laminae of the lateral geniculate nucleus. *J. Comp. Neurol.* 338:289–303.

ROORDA, A., A. B. METHA, P. LENNIE, and D. R. WILLIAMS, 2001. Packing arrangement of the three cone classes in primate retina. *Vision Res.* 41:1291–1306.

ROORDA, A., and D. R. WILLIAMS, 1999. The arrangement of the three cone classes in the living human eye. *Nature* 397:520–522.

ROSKA, B., and F. WERBLIN, 2001. Vertical interactions across ten parallel, stacked representations in the mammalian retina. *Nature* 410:583–587.

SCHNAPF, J. L., T. W. KRAFT, and D. A. BAYLOR, 1987. Spectral sensitivity of human cone photoreceptors. *Nature* 325:439–441.

SHAPLEY, R., 1995. Parallel neural pathways and visual function. In *The Cognitive Neurosciences*, 1st ed., M. S. Gazzaniga, ed. Cambridge, Mass.: MIT Press, pp. 315–324.

SHAPLEY, R., and C. ENROTH-CUGELL, 1984. Visual adaptation and retinal gain controls. *Prog. Retin. Eye. Res.* 4:263–346.

SHAPLEY, R., and V. H. PERRY, 1986. Cat and monkey retinal ganglion cells and their visual functional roles. *Trends Neurosci.* 9:229–235.

SILVEIRA, L. C. L., and V. H. PERRY, 1991. The topography of magnocellular projecting ganglion cells (M-ganglion cells) in the primate retina. *Neuroscience* 40:217–237.

SMITH, V. C., J. POKORNY, and D. M. DACEY, 2003. *Functional architecture of the photoreceptive ganglion cell in primate retina: response dynamics and spectral sensitivity of a novel photopigment*. Association for Research in Vision and Ophthalmology Abstract #5185. Available from www.arvo.org.

STERLING, P., 1998. Retina. In *The Synaptic Organization of the Brain*, 4th ed., G. M. Shepherd, ed. New York: Oxford University Press, pp. 205–253.

SUN, W., N. LI, and S. HE, 2002. Large scale morphological survey of mouse retinal ganglion cells. *J. Comp. Neurol.* 451:115–126.

VANEY, D. I., 1994. Territorial organization of direction-selective ganglion cells in rabbit retina. *J. Neurosci.* 14:6301–6316.

VANEY, D., S. HE, W. TAYLOR, and W. LEVICK, 2001. Direction-selective ganglion cells in the retina. In *Motion Vision: Computational, Neural and Ecological Constraints*, J. Zanker and J. Zeil, eds. Berlin: Springer-Verlag, pp. 13–56.

VANEY, D. I., L. PEICHL, H. WASSLE, and R. B. ILLING, 1981. Almost all ganglion cells in the rabbit retina project to the superior colliculus. *Brain Res.* 212:447–453.

WÄSSLE, H., 1999. Parallel pathways from the outer to the inner retina in primates. In *Color Vision: From Genes to Perception*, K. R. Gegenfurtner and L. T. Sharpe, eds. New York: Cambridge University Press, pp. 145–162.

WÄSSLE, H., and B. B. BOYCOTT, 1991. Functional architecture of the mammalian retina. *Physiol. Rev.* 71:447–480.

WÄSSLE, H., U. GRÜNERT, J. RÖHRENBECK, and B. B. BOYCOTT, 1990. Retinal ganglion cell density and cortical magnification factor in the primate. *Vision Res.* 30:1897–1911.

WATANABE, M., and R. W. RODIECK, 1989. Parasol and midget ganglion cells of the primate retina. *J. Comp. Neurol.* 289:434–454.

WIESEL, T. N., and D. H. HUBEL, 1966. Spatial and chromatic interactions in the lateral geniculate body of the rhesus monkey. *J. Neurophysiol.* 29:1115–1156.

ZHANG, H. Y., R. J. CLARKE, and P. D. R. GAMLIN, 1996. Behavior of luminance neurons in the pretectal olivary nucleus during the pupillary near response. *Exp. Brain Res.* 112:158–162.

21 Mechanisms of Image Processing in the Visual Cortex

C. ELIZABETH BOUDREAU AND DAVID FERSTER

ABSTRACT Orientation selectivity in primary visual cortex represents a crucial step in the transformation of patterns of light incident on the retina into features that define recognizable objects in the visual world. Orientation-selective responses in cortical cells can be explained well by the pattern of inputs onto the cells, indicating that the design of the network, rather than highly specialized computational abilities of individual cells, may be responsible for creating and refining their very varied and precise response properties. In addition, most properties of cells in primary visual cortex can be accounted for by a model that is largely linear and processes information primarily in one direction. These findings also indicate that the elaboration of complex feature selectivity in the visual cortex results from the careful organization of simple mathematical units.

The visual cortex dramatically transforms the neuronal representation of the visual image. The neurons of the retina and lateral geniculate nucleus (LGN) encode the contrast of the image at each point, more or less independently of the shape of the image elements that give rise to local contrast. And yet the neurons of the primary visual cortex (V1), which receive the bulk of their information about the visual image directly from the LGN, encode information about the size, orientation, direction of motion, and depth of image features that fall within their receptive fields. None of this information is contained explicitly in the activity of single geniculate cells, so the cortical neurons are clearly integrating information they receive, either directly or indirectly, from a large number of geniculate inputs. In the cat, this transformation emerges almost fully articulated at the first cortical synapse, between the axons of geniculate relay neurons and the cortical recipient cells in layer 4.

The description of the cortical transformation raises many questions about its purpose. How does it benefit an organism to parse the visual image into elements of different orientation? What new abilities or limitations in visual perceptions arise from such an organization? But the visual transformation that occurs in V1 is also a compelling model of cortical information processing. The image transformation that occurs there is at once complex, and yet mathematically tractable and easily described, unlike the more mysterious processes that underlie higher cognitive tasks such as object recognition, speech, or intelligence. For those interested in how the cortex performs neuronal computations, then, V1, and in particular the way in which cortical circuitry gives rise to orientation selectivity, has been of intense and prolonged interest. The 40 years following Hubel and Wiesel's first description of cortical receptive fields have seen a remarkable and productive interaction between theory and experiment. The process has refined our understanding of the function of a fascinating and complex piece of neuronal circuitry.

Most cells in V1 are orientation selective, meaning that they are most active (produce the most action potentials) in response to the presentation of a contrast edge at a particular orientation (e.g., vertical), while edges of other orientations produce a smaller response. The relationship between response size and stimulus orientation for individual cells can be well described by Gaussian or bell-shaped mathematical functions. In cat V1, tilting a stimulus 10° away from the optimal orientation reduces a cell's response by 50% on average. As Hubel and Wiesel first demonstrated, cells within a single vertical column of the cortex all have the same preferred orientation, and the preferred orientation of each point in cortex forms an orderly map.

Although orientation selectivity is a property common to the primary visual cortices of many animal species, it is not always implemented in exactly the same way. In the cat, orientation selectivity is prevalent in all layers of primary visual cortex, and the narrowness of this selectivity does not change significantly as a function of laminar position. In the monkey, orientation selectivity is weakest in layer 4Cβ, where axons of LGN neurons terminate (Callaway, 1998; but see Ringach et al., 2002). In the ferret, as in the cat, cells receiving direct input from the LGN are very selective for orientation, on average (Usrey et al., 2003), while in the tree shrew orientation selectivity is largely absent in layer 4, emerging more strongly in layers to which layer 4 neurons project (Chisum et al., 2003). Whether these interspecies differences point to substantial variation in the mechanisms for producing orientation-selective responses is not known.

LGN relay cells exhibit weak or no selectivity for orientation, responding optimally instead to a light (ON-center

C. ELIZABETH BOUDREAU and DAVID FERSTER   Department of Neurobiology and Physiology, Northwestern University, Evanston, Ill.

cells) or dark (OFF-center cells) spot of the appropriate size presented in the center of their receptive fields, which are circularly symmetrical. In addition to the ON or OFF center, the receptive fields invariably have antagonistic surrounds (OFF surrounds for ON-center cells and ON surrounds for OFF-center cells), which serve to limit the relay cells' responses to large or diffuse stimuli. The surround is less sensitive per unit area then the surround, but because it is larger it tends to balance the center in total input, such that uniform illumination of the entire receptive field gives no response. In the absence of visual stimulation, most LGN cells fire action potentials spontaneously at about 15 Hz. Presentation of stimuli of the inappropriate polarity (dark in an ON-center or surround, or light in an OFF-center or surround) reduces the firing of a relay cell below its spontaneous rate, and when strong enough can completely silence the cell for brief periods.

Receptive field structure in primary visual cortex

Most neurons in primary visual cortex can be classified as either simple or complex, according to the structure of their spatial receptive fields (Hubel and Wiesel, 1962). Simple cells, similar to LGN relay cells, have distinct ON and OFF regions, but unlike relay cells, in which the ON and OFF regions are concentrically arranged, simple-cell ON and OFF regions are elongated and lie adjacent to one another. The axis of elongation is invariably the axis of the preferred orientation in simple cells. The arrangement of the subfields predicts the response of the cell to a moving bar or grating, with the cell responding as a bright bar enters an ON region or leaves on OFF region. The cells also respond vigorously to a grating of the appropriate orientation and size when the bright bar of the grating falls in the ON region simultaneously with a dark bar falling in the OFF region. As such a grating drifts across the receptive field, the firing rate or membrane potential of the cell is modulated at the drift rate of the grating. Many simple cells are located in the layers of the cortex where the axons of geniculate relay cells terminate (layers 4 and 6), and they have been shown to receive monosynaptic input from relay cells (Ferster and Lindström, 1983). Complex cells, in contrast to simple cells, have no distinct subregions in their receptive fields, responding uniformly to flashing stimuli, often with both ON and OFF responses. Nor can the spatial distribution of the flashing responses predict the response to moving stimuli, which usually consists of a single peak of activity centered on the receptive field. In response to a drifting grating, complex cells usually produce an unmodulated increase in membrane potential and firing rate. Compared to complex cells, then, simple cells behave more linearly (Movshon et al., 1978; Tolhurst and Dean, 1987; DeAngelis et al., 1993); their response to a stimulus approximates the sum of their responses to the components of the stimulus. Complex cells are preferentially (though not exclusively) located in layers 2, 3, and 5 and do not as often receive direct input from geniculate relay cells (Ferster and Lindström, 1983).

Feedforward models for orientation selectivity

The first theoretical description of how orientation-selective cortical simple cells are created from nonselective geniculate input was proposed by Hubel and Wiesel (1962), and it survives today as the basis for many modern models. Because in their model orientation selectivity arises from the spatial pattern of inputs from the LGN onto individual simple cells, it is known as a feedforward model of orientation selectivity. The distinguishing feature of this and other feedforward models is that a simple cell acts as a passive filter whose response is monotonically related to the spatial correlation between the actual stimulus and the cell's receptive field.

Hubel and Wiesel proposed that simple cell ON and OFF subregions arise directly from synaptic input from LGN ON- and OFF-center cells. An ON region, for example (figure 21.1), is generated by the combined input from several ON-center relay cells that have their receptive fields aligned in a row. Given this arrangement, a light bar aligned along the centers of the ON-center cells will maximally stimulate these cells and therefore maximally excite the simple cells. Conversely, when the orientation of the bar or grating is perpendicular to the long axis, only a small fraction of the ON-center inputs will be excited, and at the same time spontaneous activity in some OFF-center cells will be reduced. The resulting excitation to the simple cells will therefore be insufficient to bring the simple cell to threshold. It is important to note, however, that for a bar or grating that sweeps across the entire simple cell's receptive field, the *total* or integrated amount of excitation that reaches the simple cells is identical. Since each individual geniculate relay cell is insensitive to orientation, it will fire the same number of spikes in response to a stimulus of any orientation moving across its receptive field. What is different at different orientations is the relative timing of the relay cell inputs. At the preferred orientation, all the inputs from a single subfield are

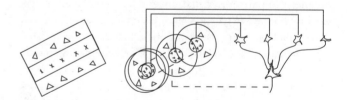

FIGURE 21.1 Hubel and Wiesel's (1962) model of orientation selectivity in cortical cells. The receptive field of a simple cell (left) is built up from input geniculate relay cells that have their receptive fields arranged in rows that correspond to the elongated ON and OFF subregions of the simple-cell receptive field.

simultaneous; at a nonpreferred orientation they are distributed in time.

Experimental evidence that supports the existence of Hubel and Wiesel's proposed connectivity scheme comes from simultaneous recordings of LGN and layer 4 simple cells (Reid and Alonso, 1995). These authors examined pairs of synaptically connected cells, where an action potential in the geniculate neuron had a high probability of evoking a spike in the cortical neuron. For such pairs, the LGN receptive field always overlapped simple-cell subregions of the same polarity, just as the Hubel–Wiesel model predicted.

Refinement of the feedforward model

Even though it is likely that the arrangement of relay-cell inputs to simple cells accounts for the spatial arrangement of their ON and OFF subregions, it does not directly follow that the elongated shape of the subregions can account for a simple cell's orientation selectivity in quantitative detail. In fact, just the opposite appeared to be true. Given the map of the receptive field of a simple cell, it is possible to predict the orientation selectivity of the cell using linear summation. The longer and narrower the subfields, the more selective or more sharply tuned for orientation one would expect the simple cell to be. But in most cases the cells were even more sharply tuned than the map of the receptive field would predict (Jones and Palmer, 1987; Gardner et al., 1999). This prompted suggestions that the generation of orientation selectivity is much more complex than can be explained by the simple feedforward model and might involve intracortical inhibitory interactions or excitatory feedback.

A simpler explanation for the failure of receptive field maps to predict orientation tuining may be found in one important nonlinear property of simple cells: the action potential threshold. Calculations of the orientation selectivity of a cell derived from the receptive field map predict the orientation tuning of the *excitatory synaptic input* to a simple cell, not the orientation tuning of the spike output. Because threshold in simple cells is considerably higher than the resting membrane potential, the flanks of the tuning curve for the synaptic input will invariably lie below threshold, so that the spike responses of the cell cover a smaller range of orientations than do the synaptic inputs (figure 21.2A, B). This "iceberg effect" was shown by Carandini and Ferster (2000) and by Eysel and colleagues (1998) to narrow the orientation tuning measured from the action potential firing rate relative to the orientation tuning measured from a cell's synaptic input. In considering whether the synaptic input from relay cells can account quantitatively for orientation selectivity, then, it is important to compare predictions made from receptive field maps with measurements made from membrane potential fluctuations, not from spike rate, as

was done by Jones and Palmer and by Gardner and colleagues. If orientation selectivity for intracellularly recorded stimulus-evoked changes in membrane potential is compared with the receptive field structure also derived from membrane potential, agreement between the two can be quite high (Lampl et al., 2001; see also Volgushev et al., 1996).

Contrast invariance of orientation tuning

A related difficulty with the Hubel–Wiesel model concerns the effect of stimulus contrast on orientation tuning of simple cells. The responses of LGN cells become stronger in proportion to increasing stimulus contrast, so their input to cortical cells will become greater as well (figure 21.2A). Because the responses of LGN cells are not selective for orientation, the synaptic input to the simple cell will increase at all orientations, and the orientation tuning curve will therefore be scaled up with increasing contrast. The problem arises when one considers how this scaling of input will affect the orientation tuning of the spike output of the cell. Because of the threshold-linear relationship between membrane potential and spike rate, a proportional increase in membrane potential response at all orientations will result in a disproportionately larger increase in responses at orientations away from the preferred. So the feedforward model appears to predict that at higher contrast, the orientation tuning of the spike responses of a simple cell should broaden. In real cortical cells, however, orientation tuning is invariant with contrast (Sclar and Freeman, 1982; Anderson, Lampl, et al., 2000). Neurons remain equally selective for orientation at all contrasts, and never respond to stimuli of orientations orthogonal to the preferred orientation (figure 21.2C). This is true of responses measured both intracellularly and extracellularly.

To account for this discrepancy, modelers have invoked inhibition in a variety of forms to reduce unwanted responses to the orthogonal orientation. Because there is no direct inhibitory input from the LGN to V1, all inhibitory mechanisms are understood to be cortical. One possibility is a feedforward form of inhibition that is exactly the inverse of the receptive field map of the cortical cell it inhibits, called push-pull or antiphase inhibition (Tolhurst and Dean, 1990; Troyer et al., 1998). ON-excitation is balanced or dominated by OFF-inhibition, and the reverse, at all points in the receptive field map. In this model, presentation of a grating at the preferred orientation will result in maximal excitation and minimal inhibition when the stimulus is in phase with the receptive field structure, and minimal excitation and maximal inhibition when it is opposite in phase. An orthogonally oriented stimulus will evoke an approximately equal (or even greater) amount of inhibition and excitation at all times as it crosses the receptive field, and increasing the contrast will increase the excitation and inhibition

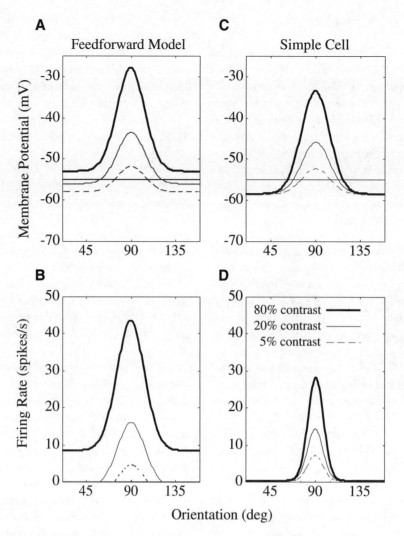

FIGURE 21.2   The problem of contrast invariance of orientation tuning. (*A*) The orientation tuning curves of membrane potential generated in a simple cells by synaptic input from geniculate relay cells arranged according to Hubel and Wiesel's feedforward model. The amplitude of the curves grows equally at all orientations as contrast increases, since the activity in geniculate relay cells also increases with increasing stimulus contrast. (*B*) The orientation tuning of the cell's spike output at different contrast, as predicted from applying a fixed threshold to the tuning curves in *A*. (*C* and *D*) A schematic of the orientation tuning recorded in cortical simple cells (*C*, membrane potential; *D*, spike rate).

proportionally, so that they continue to balance each other and result in no net excitation of the cortical cell. Because there is no physiological evidence for direct inhibition from the LGN to V1 (Freund et al., 1989; Callaway, 1998), antiphase inhibition would be mediated by inhibitory connections between cortical cells with complementary receptive field structures.

Push-pull inhibition in response to the preferred stimulus orientation is well demonstrated by intracellular recordings of membrane potential and conductance (Ferster, 1988; Hirsch et al., 1998). In these studies, receptive fields were mapped with light and dark spots, and then responses to stimuli of the nonpreferred polarity were tested at different locations within the receptive field. The results showed that, when a light stimulus was placed in an OFF subregion, for example, the total synaptic input to the cortical cell increased and the cell membrane hyperpolarized, implying that the increase was due to greater inhibitory input. Although a reduction in excitation would also cause a hyperpolarization of the membrane, this would be associated with a decrease, not an increase, in total synaptic input. Evidence for strong or dominant inhibition at the null orientation is more equivocal. Monier and colleagues (2003) see strong cross-oriented inhibition in a subset of cortical cells. Ferster (1986) and Anderson, Carandini, and colleagues (2000) found that inhibitory and excitatory input to cortical cells are tuned to the same orientation and have similar orientation tuning width. Although there was some inhibition evoked at nonpreferred orientations, it is not clear that the observed inhibition was strong enough to explain the lack of a depolarizing response at high contrasts and nonpreferred orientations.

Voltage-to-action potential transformation

The importance of the action potential threshold in converting membrane potential responses into the output of cortical cells has been highlighted already in this chapter. As mentioned earlier, an important consequence of antiphase inhibition, supported by the data, is that the orientation tuning of the synaptic input to cortical neurons should be contrast invariant. However, the orientation tuning of extracellularly measured action potentials is also contrast invariant. The application of a single threshold to the contrast-dependent tuning curves in figure 21.2*C* will result in an iceberg effect that appears to broaden orientation tuning with increasing contrast. It is unlikely that the action potential threshold of neurons changes in response to stimuli of different contrasts.

There is, however, a physiological reason why a flat threshold is not an accurate picture of the relationship between membrane voltage and action potential generation. This is simply the trial-to-trial variability of the responses of neurons (Anderson, Carandini, et al., 2000). The tuning curves of figure 21.2 are constructed from the average responses to many repeats of the same stimulus. For example, the spike threshold is often near or above the largest *average* response to a stimulus at the optimal orientation and the highest contrast. But such a stimulus, and many less effective ones as well, can evoke spikes, because on some individual trials the membrane potential exceeds threshold. The major difference between a high-contrast and low-contrast stimulus is not so much the size of the responses evoked but on how many trials a suprathreshold response occurs. The effect of this variability in response is shown in figure 21.3. A single threshold value can be represented as a linear function with a non-zero *x*-intercept (figure 21.3*A*). When the noise has depolarized the cell, it is as if the threshold were shifted down slightly for that trial; that is, the stimulus has to depolarize the membrane potential less in order to evoke spikes. When the noise hyperpolarizes the cell, the reverse is true. The average input-output function of the cell can be derived by averaging together the threshold functions for all trials (figure 21.3*B*). This average is no longer a threshold linear function but rather can be well approximated by a power law (Hansel and van Vreeswijk, 2002; Miller and Troyer, 2002). This smoothed curve, when applied to the Gaussian-like orientation tuning curves at different contrasts, narrows each one equally and thereby maintains contrast invariance both in membrane voltage and in action potential rate. The power law input-output function and the Gaussian-shaped tuning curves are the only such curves that show this property.

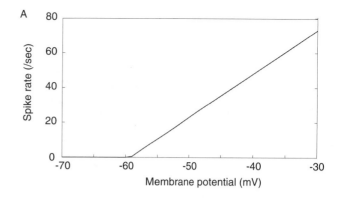

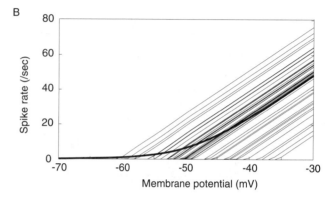

FIGURE 21.3   The effect of noise on the input-output relationship of a neuron. (*A*) The standard threshold-linear relationship between membrane potential and spike rate observed in most cells. (*B*) In the presence of noise, the curve is effectively shifted left or right on different stimulus trials. That is, when noise depolarizes the cell, a stimulus can be that much smaller and still evoke action potentials. When the noise is evenly distributed around the resting potential, then the average input-output curve over many trials can be approximated by a power law (thick curve).

Feedback models of orientation selectivity

Another explanation for the generation of orientation selectivity relies heavily on the organization, both laminar and columnar, of cortex. This class of models is known as feedback models, and their orientation tuning derives from recurrent excitatory connections that amplify responses to the preferred orientation and lateral interactions among neurons with different orientation preferences that damp down unwanted responses to the null orientation (Ben-Yishai, Bar-Or, and Sompolinsky, 1995; Somers, Nelson, and Sur, 1995). A generalized schematic of feedback model connectivity is shown in figure 21.4.

Feedback models have the advantage of requiring very simple rules for the connections between neurons. They can be implemented in networks in which cells are excited by and inhibited by all of their neighbors, with the strength of these connections declining uniformly with increasing distance between cells (McLaughlin et al., 2000). Others propose excitatory connections between cells of like

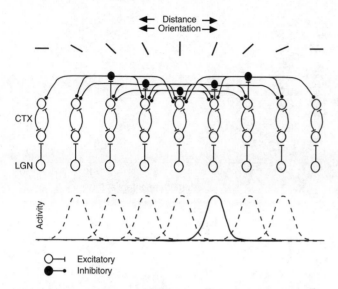

FIGURE 21.4   A schematic of feedback models of orientation selectivity. The horizontal axis represents distance along the cortical surface, and by virtue of the orientation maps on the surface of the cortex, orientation as well. Neurons within a column excite one another; neurons in adjacent columns inhibit one another. Such a circuit can take up any one of a number of stable states (multistable attractor) in which activity is confined to a single column. Each state is a winner-take-all outcome in which the maximally active column is suppressing activity in neighboring columns.

orientation preference and inhibition between cells that prefer opposite orientations. This results in a winner-take-all behavior in which stimulation that only weakly activates cells of one orientation preference will eventually result in a strong and stable representation of that orientation in the cortical network. Such models are very stable and resistant to noise in the visual stimulus, but it has important implications for the role of cortex in representing the visual world. Instead of passively filtering visual input, feedback models can actually impose their internal representation of the world on incoming visual images.

Because the width of orientation tuning in these models is dependent on cortical architecture, it is independent of stimulus parameters and contrast invariance of cortical responses is achieved automatically. However, this also means that these models are incapable of explaining observed changes in the width of orientation tuning with stimulus parameters such as spatial frequency (Webster and DeValois, 1985; Hammond and Pomfrett, 1990; discussed in Troyer et al., 1998).

Evidence for the lateral inhibition between neurons of different orientation preference comes from pharmacological experiments. Suppressing inhibition by the applications of GABA$_A$ antagonist such as bicuculline, for example, result in a nonspecific elevation of cortical excitability (Sato et al., 1996; Eysel et al., 1998; Sillito, 1975; Pfleger and Bonds, 1995). These manipulations cause a loss of orientation selec-

tivity measured extracellularly, but this effect can potentially be ascribed to a nonspecific increase in excitability, effectively raising previously subthreshold responses above the action potential threshold in a reverse iceberg effect. The bicuculline will affect not only the recorded cell but also any synaptic inputs from nearby cells, thus amplifying any nonspecific effects on loss of tuning. Intracellular application of the GABA antagonist muscimol in individual cells (Nelson et al., 1994) did not alter orientation selectivity. Inactivation of layer 6 cells (Allison and Bonds, 1994) or of layer 2/3 of cortical columns with different orientation preference (Eysel et al., 1992) by extracellular application of GABA has also been reported to broaden orientation tuning in upper cortical layers.

Estimating the contribution of cortical inputs to orientation selectivity

How can one determine whether feedforward input or feedback reverberation is more important in the generation of orientation selectivity? One critical prediction of the feedback models is that orientation tuning depends critically on synaptic interactions among cortical neurons. In feedforward models, orientation tuning depends only on the spatial organization of the input from geniculate relay cells. When spiking activity in cortical neurons is suppressed, therefore, the feedback models predict that orientation selectivity of the remaining synaptic input should be severely degraded, whereas feedback models predict that orientation selectivity of the remaining synaptic input should be nearly unchanged. To test these predictions, Ferster, Chung, and Wheat (1996) used cooling to reversibly inactivate the cortical network. This procedure reliably silenced most cortical layers, and drastically reduced activity in the deepest layers (farthest from the cooling element). Input from the LGN was also reduced in amplitude because of the direct effect of cooling on the terminals of the geniculate axons, but was otherwise unaffected. Intracellular recordings of individual layer 4 simple cells during cooling revealed that visually evoked responses were greatly reduced, but the orientation tuning of those responses was not changed.

The effects of cooling on a cortical simple cell are shown in figure 21.5A and B show the effects of cooling (at two different horizontal gains) on the responses of the neuron to electrical stimulation of the LGN. These records are important for demonstrating that the cooling has suppressed intracortical inhibition (note the lack of hyperpolarization in the 9°C traces) and the cooling has suppressed the responses of excitatory cortical neurons (note the lack of postinhibitory rebound in the second trace compared to the top trace). In addition, the cooling has noticeably slowed the responses. Figure 21.5C and D contain the responses of the cell to drifting sinusoidal gratings of different orientations. The

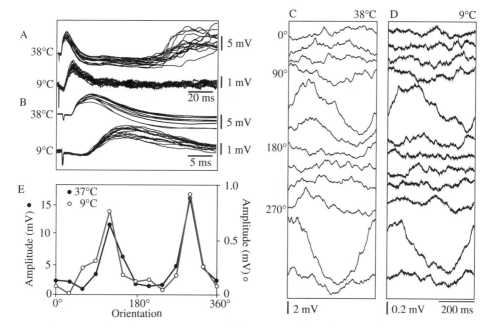

FIGURE 21.5 (*A*) The responses of a cortical simple cell to electrical stimulation of the LGN with the cortex at normal and cooled temperatures. During cooling, the initial evoked EPSP is reduced in size by fivefold and increased in latency. The longlasting inhibition that follows the EPSP is completely suppressed, as is the postinhibitory rebound excitation. (*B*) The traces in *A* at a higher horizontal gain. (*C*) The response of the cell to drifting sinusoidal gratings at different orientations. Each response shown is the average of 20 stimulus cycles. (*D*) Same as *C* but with the cortex cooled. Note the difference in vertical scale from *C*. (*E*) Orientation tuning curves drawn from the traces of *C* and *E*. Each point is the peak-to-peak amplitude of the first harmonic of the Fourier transform of the corresponding record. Cooling was done by a Peltier device attached to a copper plate, the end of which (4 × 4 mm) was placed on the surface of the brain. Intracellular recording electrode were inserted into the cortex through a small hole in the plate.

responses are reduced 10-fold in amplitude by the cooling (compare the vertical scale bars in *B* and *C*), and yet the orientation tuning is affected little. That the shape of the orientation tuning has hardly changed can be seen quantitatively from the tuning curves drawn from the two sets of traces (figure 21.5*E*). These results were typical for the 10 cells studied. They suggest that about 30% of the input to simple cells arises from the LGN, with the other 70% of the input coming from other cortical neurons. But there was little evidence that this cortical input was required to make cortical cells orientation selective, since the geniculate input remaining during cooling is fully orientation selective on its own.

In a second experiment (Chung and Ferster, 1998), electrical stimulation rather than cooling was used to inhibit cortical activity. The stimulation induces a strong, longlasting (100–200 ms) inhibition in all nearby cortical cells, during which visual stimulation fails to evoke cortical spikes. Again, geniculate activity is left intact. Any excitatory synaptic inputs recorded during the inhibition should therefore arise not from cortical cells but almost purely from geniculate input. The responses of two cortical simple cells to flashed gratings of different orientation are shown in figure 21.6*A* and *C*, with and without a preceding shock in the cortex nearby (thick and thin traces). The responses to the

gratings preceded by cortical stimulation are reduced in amplitude, both because the shock evokes a shunt in the recorded cell and because the components of the response mediated by other cortical cells are suppressed by the shock. The relative size of the responses to different orientations, however, is largely unaffected, so that orientation selectivity is not much changed. Figure 21.6*B* and *D* show three tuning curves: one taken from drifting gratings at 12 orientations, one taken from the responses to flashed grating of *A* and *C* recorded without cortical shock, and one taken from the responses to flashed gratings with cortical shock. The tuning curves all have comparable widths after being normalized to their peak amplitudes. A comparison of the width of tuning with and without cortical shock for nine cells is shown in figure 21.6*E*. Since orientation tuning of synaptic potentials was found to be unchanged during the suppression of cortical activity, it seems likely that the aggregate input from geniculate relay cells is by itself as well tuned for orientation as the total input from cortex and geniculate combined. These results strongly support a dominant role for feedforward input in determining orientation tuning of simple cells. Although the cortical circuit clearly has role in amplifying visual responses, these experiments show that orientation selectivity can be maintained even when the cortical network is disrupted.

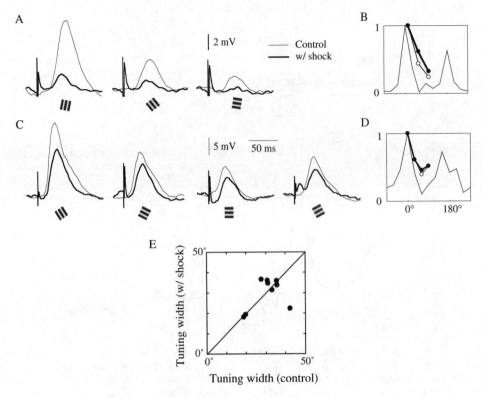

FIGURE 21.6 (A) The response of a simple cell to briefly (20 ms) flashed gratings confined to the classic receptive field. Grating orientation is indicated below each set of traces. Thin traces are control data. For the thick traces, an electrical stimulus to nearby cortex was delivered at the end of the flash. The shock reduces the amplitude of the response by introducing a shunt into the recorded cell and by suppressing the spike response of other cortical cells. What remains is therefore likely to arise almost exclusively from synaptic excitation from the LGN. (B) Orientation tuning curves derived from the responses in A (open and closed circles) and from drifting gratings at 12 different orientations. Each of the three curves is normalized to its own peak. (C and D) Similar data to A and B for a second simple cell. (E) A comparison of the width of tuning for control and shock data for nine cells. To obtain the tuning widths, curves similar to those in B and D were fitted to a Gaussian.

Dynamics of orientation tuning

Another experimentally testable difference between feedforward and feedback models of orientation tuning concerns the time course of orientation-tuned responses to brief stimuli. Feedback models, which propose that initial excitatory input to the cortex is largely untuned, also predict that as the initial responses are propagated through the cortical circuitry and fed back as orientation-selective signals to the cells, the orientation tuning of the response will be seen to sharpen. Such an effect has been reported in extracellular recordings in monkey visual cortex (Ringach et al., 1997; Shapley et al., 2003). Although most cells in the input layer 4β were not found to sharpen, some cells in other layers showed a change in their tuning characteristics over time, consistent with feedback models. Another extracellular study (Mazer et al., 2002) failed to find a change in the shape of orientation tuning over time, but the time sampling of their data may have been too coarse to resolve such changes. A study performed intracellularly in the cat (Gillespie et al., 2001) found no sharpening of orientation tuning over time

in cells of any layer. However, about 50% of cells in the sample showed a subtractive reduction in membrane potential over time, consistent with an increase in inhibition. As discussed earlier, shifting the membrane potential relative to the action potential threshold will narrow the orientation tuning of the extracellularly measured response without altering the selectivity of the synaptic inputs. These recent studies had the advantage of using stimulus presentation methods in which orientation was changed without large contrast changes. Earlier attempts to measure the time course of orientation selectivity of the membrane potential (Pei et al., 1994) were complicated by orientation-nonspecific contrast responses to the sudden onset of the flashed bar stimuli that were used.

Conclusions

Although there is not universal agreement on this point, there is a great deal of evidence that orientation selectivity in simple cells of the cat visual cortex is determined largely by the spatial organization of geniculate input, just as Hubel and Wiesel (1962) proposed. Inactivation of the cortical circuit does not cause a collapse of the orientation tuning of synaptic inputs to simple cells. And orientation tuning of simple cells can be linearly predicted from the receptive field map. Both inhibition and excitation may be involved in amplifying the geniculate input, removing its nonspecific or untuned component, and perhaps normalizing the cortical output (Troyer et al., 1998). But these operations can be accomplished with nonspecific or orientation-independent inputs that do not fundamentally alter the response properties or receptive field structure laid down by geniculate excitation.

At same time, the distribution of orientation selectivity in cortical cells is very broad, indicating that not all cells need share the same mechanism for its generation. There is the possibility that complex cells, or cells outside layer 4, may derive their orientation selectivity by different means. In addition, cortical mechanisms in primate visual cortex may differ from those in the cat.

Despite questions that remain unanswered about the specific implementation of orientation tuning in primary visual cortex, the general lessons of the study of this transformation of sensory information may provide guidelines for the understanding of other aspects of sensory processing. That new properties can be conferred upon neurons by the specific pattern of their excitatory connections, that inhibition is important for counteracting the development of unwanted nonspecific responses, and that the noisiness of neurons can be used constructively to enhance their representation of certain stimulus attributes are ideas that may eventually help to explain much more complex and varied aspects of visual processing.

REFERENCES

ALLISON, J. D., and A. B. BONDS, 1994. Inactivation of the infragranular striate cortex broadens orientation tuning of supragranular visual neurons in the cat. *Exp. Brain. Res.* 101:415–426.

ANDERSON, J. S., M. CARANDINI, et al., 2000. Orientation tuning of input conductance, excitation, and inhibition in cat primary visual cortex. *J. Neurophysiol.* 84:909–926.

ANDERSON, J. S., I. LAMPL, et al., 2000. The contribution of noise to contrast invariance of orientation tuning in cat visual cortex. *Science* 290:1968–1972.

BEN-YISHAI, R., R. L. BAR-OR, and H. SOMPOLINSKY, 1995. Theory of orientation tuning in visual cortex. *Proc. Natl. Acad. Sci. U.S.A.* 92:3844–3848.

CALLAWAY, E. M., 1998. Local circuits in primary visual cortex of the macaque monkey. *Annu. Rev. Neurosci.* 21:47–74.

CARANDINI, M., and D. FERSTER, 2000. Membrane potential and firing rate in cat primary visual cortex. *J. Neurosci.* 20:470–484.

CHISUM, H. J., F. MOOSER, et al., 2003. Emergent properties of layer 2/3 neurons reflect the collinear arrangement of horizontal connections in tree shrew visual cortex. *J. Neurosci.* 23:2947–2960.

CHUNG, S., and D. FERSTER, 1998. Strength and orientation tuning of the thalamic input to simple cells revealed by electrically evoked cortical suppression. *Neuron* 20:1177–1189.

DEANGELIS, G. C., I. OHZAWA, et al., 1993. Spatiotemporal organization of simple-cell receptive fields in the cat's striate cortex. II. Linearity of temporal and spatial summation. *J. Neurophysiol.* 69:1118–1135.

EYSEL, U. T., 1992. Lateral inhibitory interactions in areas 17 and 18 of the cat visual cortex. *Prog. Brain. Res.* 90:407–422.

EYSEL, U. T., J. M. CROOK, et al., 1990. GABA-induced remote inactivation reveals cross-orientation inhibition in the cat striate cortex. *Exp. Brain Res.* 80:626–630.

EYSEL, U. T., I. A. SHEVELEV, et al., 1998. Orientation tuning and receptive field structure in cat striate neurons during local blockade of intracortical inhibition. *Neuroscience* 84:25–36.

FERSTER, D., 1986. Orientation selectivity of synaptic potentials in neurons of cat primary visual cortex. *J. Neurosci.* 6:1284–1301.

FERSTER, D., 1988. Spatially opponent excitation and inhibition in simple cells of the cat visual cortex. *J. Neurosci.* 8:1172–1180.

FERSTER, D., S. CHUNG, and H. WHEAT, 1996. Orientation selectivity of thalamic input to simple cells of cat visual cortex. *Nature* 380:249–252.

FERSTER, D., and S. LINDSTRÖM, 1983. An intracellular analysis of geniculo-cortical connectivity in area 17 of the cat. *J. Physiol.* 342:181–215.

FREUND, T. F., K. A. MARTIN, et al., 1989. Arborisation pattern and postsynaptic targets of physiologically identified thalamocortical afferents in striate cortex of the macaque monkey. *J. Comp. Neurol.* 289:315–336.

GARDNER, J. L., A. ANZAI, et al., 1999. Linear and nonlinear contributions to orientation tuning of simple cells in the cat's striate cortex. *Vis. Neurosci.* 16:1115–1121.

GILLESPIE, D. C., I. LAMPL, et al., 2001. Dynamics of the orientation-tuned membrane potential response in cat primary visual cortex. *Nat. Neurosci.* 4:1014–1019.

HAMMOND, P., and C. J. POMFRETT, 1990. Influence of spatial frequency on tuning and bias for orientation and direction in the cat's striate cortex. *Vision Res.* 30:359–369.

HANSEL, D., and C. VAN VREESWIJK, 2002. How noise contributes to contrast invariance of orientation tuning in cat visual cortex. *J. Neurosci.* 22:5118–5128.

HIRSCH, J. A., J. M. ALONSO, et al., 1998. Synaptic integration in striate cortical simple cells. *J. Neurosci.* 18:9517–9528.

HUBEL, D. H., and T. N. WIESEL, 1962. Receptive fields, binocular interaction and functional architecture in the cat's visual cortex. *J. Physiol. (Lond.)* 160:106–154.

HUBEL, D. H., and T. N. WIESEL, 1972. Laminar and columnar distribution of geniculo-cortical fibers in the macaque monkey. *J. Comp. Neurol.* 146:421–450.

JONES, J. P., and L. A. PALMER, 1987. The two-dimensional spatial structure of simple receptive fields in cat striate cortex. *J. Neurophysiol.* 58:1187–1211.

LAMPL, I., J. S. ANDERSON, et al., 2001. Prediction of orientation selectivity from receptive field architecture in simple cells of cat visual cortex. *Neuron* 30:263–274.

MAZER, J. A., W. E. VINJE, et al., 2002. Spatial frequency and orientation tuning dynamics in area V1. *Proc. Natl. Acad. Sci. U.S.A.* 99:1645–1650.

MCLAUGHLIN, D., R. SHAPLEY, et al., 2000. A neuronal network model of macaque primary visual cortex (V1): Orientation selectivity and dynamics in the input layer 4Calpha. *Proc. Natl. Acad. Sci. U.S.A.* 97:8087–8092.

MILLER, K. D., and T. W. TROYER, 2002. Neural noise can explain expansive, power-law nonlinearities in neural response functions. *J. Neurophysiol.* 87:653–659.

MONIER, C., F. CHAVANE, et al., 2003. Orientation and direction selectivity of synaptic inputs in visual cortical neurons: a diversity of combinations produces spike tuning. *Neuron* 37:663–680.

MOVSHON, J. A., I. D. THOMPSON, et al., 1978. Spatial summation in the receptive fields of simple cells in the cat's striate cortex. *J. Physiol.* 283:53–77.

NELSON, S., L. TOTH, B. SHETH, and M. SUR, 1994. Orientation selectivity of cortical neurons during intracellular blockade of inhibition. *Science* 265:774–777.

PEI, X., T. R. VIDYASAGAR, M. VOLGUSHEV, and O. CREUTZFELDT, 1994. Receptive field analysis and orientation selectivity of postsynaptic potentials of simple cells in cat visual cortex. *J. Neurosci.* 14:7130–7140.

PFLEGER, B., and A. B. BONDS, 1995. Dynamic differentiation of GABAA-sensitive influences on orientation selectivity of complex cells in the cat striate cortex. *Exp. Brain Res.* 104:81–88.

REID, R. C., and J. M. ALONSO, 1995. Specificity of monosynaptic connections from thalamus to visual cortex. *Nature* 378:281–284.

RINGACH, D. L., M. J. HAWKEN, and R. SHAPLEY, 1997. Dynamics of orientation tuning in macaque primary visual cortex. *Nature* 387:281–284.

RINGACH, D. L., R. M. SHAPLEY, et al., 2002. Orientation selectivity in macaque V1: Diversity and laminar dependence. *J. Neurosci.* 22:5639–5651.

SATO, H., N. KATSUYAMA, et al., 1996. Mechanisms underlying orientation selectivity of neurons in the primary visual cortex of the macaque. *J. Physiol.* 494:757–771.

SCLAR, G., and R. D. FREEMAN, 1982. Orientation selectivity in the cat's striate cortex is invariant with stimulus contrast. *Exp. Brain Res.* 46:457–461.

SHAPLEY, R., M. HAWKEN, et al., 2003. Dynamics of orientation selectivity in the primary visual cortex and the importance of cortical inhibition. *Neuron* 38:689–699.

SILLITO, A. M., 1975. The contribution of inhibitory mechanisms to the receptive field properties of neurones in the striate cortex of the cat. *J. Physiol.* 250:305–329.

SOMERS, D. C., S. B. NELSON, and M. SUR, 1995. An emergent model of orientation selectivity in cat visual cortical simple cells. *J. Neurosci.* 15:5448–5465.

TOLHURST, D. J., and A. F. DEAN, 1987. Spatial summation by simple cells in the striate cortex of the cat. *Exp. Brain Res.* 66:607–620.

TOLHURST, D. J., and A. F. DEAN, 1990. The effects of contrast on the linearity of spatial summation of simple cells in the cat's striate cortex. *Exp. Brain Res.* 79:582–588.

TROYER, T. W., A. E. KRUKOWSKI, et al., 1998. Contrast-invariant orientation tuning in cat visual cortex: Thalamocortical input tuning and correlation-based intracortical connectivity. *J. Neurosci.* 18:5908–5927.

USREY, W. M., M. P. SCENIAK, et al., 2003. Receptive fields and response properties of neurons in layer 4 of ferret visual cortex. *J. Neurophysiol.* 89:1003–1015.

VOLGUSHEV, M., T. R. VIDYASAGAR, et al., 1996. A linear model fails to predict orientation selectivity of cells in the cat visual cortex. *J. Physiol.* 496(Pt 3):597–606.

WEBSTER, M. A., and R. L. DE VALOIS, 1985. Relationship between spatial-frequency and orientation tuning of striate-cortex cells. *J. Opt. Soc. Am. A* 2:1124–1132.

22 Receptive Fields and Suppressive Fields in the Early Visual System

MATTEO CARANDINI

ABSTRACT Powerful models are available to describe the responses of neurons in the early visual system, which includes the lateral geniculate nucleus (LGN) and the primary visual cortex (V1). According to these models, neurons perform image processing through simple arithmetic operations. Initial models proposed that these operations are weighted sums, with weights given by a neuron's classical receptive field. These models were later extended to include a nonclassical suppressive field, whose output divides the response of the receptive field, thus controlling the neuron's input-output gain. Both receptive fields and suppressive fields become more elaborate as one progresses from LGN to V1. Suppressive fields are likely to rely on more than one biophysical underpinning, and seem to confer to neurons in early visual system a number of computational advantages. Recent evidence in higher cortical areas suggests that the modulation of divisive suppression is the primary means of operation of visual attention.

Fifty years of research have yielded powerful models of the responses of neurons in the mammalian early visual system. According to these models, neurons process the intensity values in visual images by performing simple arithmetic operations. Initial models proposed that these operations are weighted sums, with weights given by a neuron's receptive field. These models explain the basic features of response selectivity. They were later extended to explain a number of suppressive effects originating within and outside the region of the receptive field. The resulting models rely on division. In this division, the receptive field feeds into the numerator, and the denominator is provided by a larger, nonclassical suppressive field.

While the receptive field confers on a neuron the basic selectivity for stimulus properties, the suppressive field modulates responsiveness. A divisive suppressive field confers on neurons in the early visual system a number of computational advantages. Recent evidence from higher cortical areas suggests that the modulation of divisive suppression is the primary means of operation of visual attention.

This chapter summarizes research on receptive fields and suppressive fields in lateral geniculate nucleus (LGN) and in primary visual cortex (V1). In the following discussion, the term *suppressive field* is used as though it had wide acceptance.

In reality, the concept was proposed only for LGN neurons (Levick, Cleland, and Dubin, 1972), and lay forgotten for 30 years.

Receptive fields in LGN

The traditional model for responses of LGN neurons (figure 22.1A) is based on a center-surround receptive field (Kuffler, 1953; Rodieck, 1965). The model takes as input a map of stimulus intensities $c(x, y, t)$ that is output by the retina. Neurons operate on this map and perform weighted sums, with weights determined by the receptive field: positive in ON regions and negative in OFF regions (Fig. 22.2A, B). Finally, to account for the encoding of intracellular signals (which can be negative) into firing rates (which have to be positive), the model is endowed with an additional stage following summation. At its simplest, this stage performs simple rectification; that is, it outputs zero for signals below a threshold and is linear above this threshold (Granit, Kernell, and Shortess, 1963; Carandini and Ferster, 2000).

To illustrate the behavior of LGN neurons and compare it with model predictions, I will show data from X cells of cat LGN. Most of the arguments, however, could be extended to other LGN neurons, including Y cells in cat and M and P cells in monkey.

The model based on the receptive field explains the basic features of spatial and temporal summation in LGN. For example, it explains size and the timing of the responses to drifting gratings varying in spatial frequency (figure 22.2C) and in temporal frequency (figure 22.2D) (Dawis et al., 1984; Cai, DeAngelis, and Freeman, 1997). Similar results, with a similar model, have been obtained in retinal ganglion cells (Enroth-Cugell et al., 1983; Enroth-Cugell and Robson, 1984). The model also predicts responses to full-field stimuli with rich temporal dynamics (Keat et al., 2001), and even captures the main aspects of responses to complex video sequences (Dan, Atick, and Reid, 1996).

Suppression in LGN

In addition to these behaviors, however, LGN neurons also exhibit response properties that cannot be explained by the

MATTEO CARANDINI Smith-Kettlewell Eye Research Institute, San Francisco, Calif.

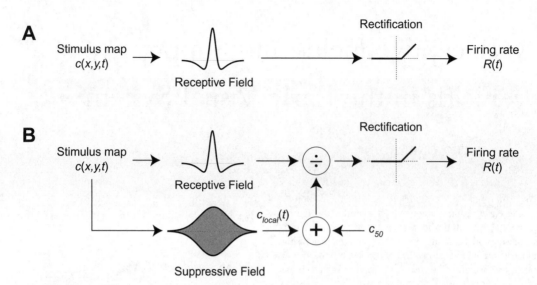

FIGURE 22.1   Two models of LGN responses. (*A*) Model based on the receptive field. The model includes a rectification stage that converts intracellular signals into a firing rate. (*B*) Model incorporating a suppressive field and divisive gain control.

receptive field alone. In particular, a number of phenomena indicate that the responses are affected by suppression originating both within and around the region of the receptive field.

A first phenomenon of suppression in LGN is contrast saturation, which can be observed with a single test drifting grating: as the contrast of the grating increases, responses grow much less than proportionally (figure 22.3*A*) (Maffei and Fiorentini, 1973; Sclar, Maunsell, and Lennie, 1990). For example, the responses to 100% contrast are only about twice as large as the responses to 10% contrast, not 10 times larger, as predicted by the linear model based on the receptive field.

A second phenomenon of suppression in LGN is masking, which can be observed by measuring responses to the test grating in the presence of a superimposed mask grating. Both test and mask provide stimulation to the receptive field, but because their temporal frequencies are incommensurate, they elicit responses with different periodicities (Victor and Shapley, 1980; Bonds, 1989). By measuring responses synchronized to the test, one can ignore the mask's effect in driving the cell and study its effect in suppressing responses. The latter effect is illustrated in figure 22.3*B* and *C*: the mask reduces the responses to the test, and this suppression increases with increasing

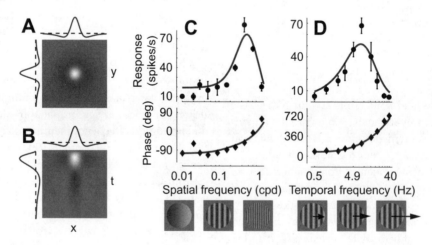

FIGURE 22.2   The receptive field of an LGN neuron explains selectivity for spatial and temporal frequency. (*A*) Profile in space (*x, y*) of the receptive field of an LGN neuron (an X cell in cat LGN), described using the model of Cai, DeAngelis, and Freeman (1997). (*B*) Profile in space-time (*x, t*) of the same receptive field. Curves illustrate corresponding one-dimensional profiles. (*C*) Responses of the cell to drifting gratings varying in spatial fre-

quency. Stimuli were presented in a large window and drifted at 16 Hz. Ordinates show amplitude (top) and phase (bottom) of responses measured at the stimulus frequency. Curves are predictions based on the receptive field. (*D*) Same for stimuli varying in temporal frequency tuning (presented at 0.7 cycles/deg.). (Modified from Mante, Bonin, and Carandini, 2002.)

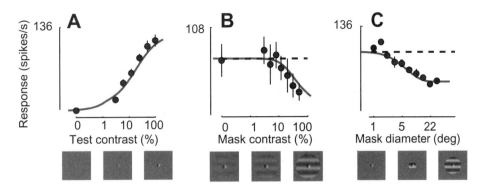

FIGURE 22.3   Saturation and suppression in an X cell in cat LGN. (*A*) Responses to an optimal-sized test grating of varying contrast. The window enclosing the grating has a diameter slightly larger than the receptive field center. Responses (in this panel and the others) are measured at the test frequency (7.8 Hz). (*B*) Effects of a superimposed orthogonal mask grating as a function of mask contrast. Mask temporal frequency is 12.0 Hz, incommensurate with test temporal frequency. Test contrast is 50% (dashed line is response to test alone). (*C*) Same for different mask diameters. (Modified from Bonin, Mante, and Carandini, 2003b.)

mask contrast (figure 22.3*B*) and mask diameter (figure 22.3*C*).

A third phenomenon of suppression in LGN is size tuning, which can be observed with a drifting grating of increasing size (figure 22.4). If the grating has low contrast, increasing its size leads to an increase in responses followed by a plateau (figure 22.4, ○). This is exactly the behavior that would be expected on the basis of the cell's receptive field. If the grating has high contrast, however, increasing its size beyond an optimal value leads to dramatic decreases in response (figure 22.4, ▼). This behavior is not explained by the receptive field, which would predict a scaled version of the responses to low contrast. LGN neurons thus are selective for size (Jones and Sillito, 1991; Walker, Ohzawa, and Freeman, 1999; Jones et al., 2000), but only at high contrast (Bonin, Mante, and Carandini, 2002, 2003a,b; Solomon, White, and Martin, 2002).

The initial wave of interest in these suppressive phenomena dates back to the 1960s. At this time it became clear that there are in LGN strong mechanisms of response reduction, as enlarging the size of disks used as visual stimuli reduced responses (e.g., Hubel and Wiesel, 1961). Disks and bars (Cleland, Lee, and Vidyasagar, 1983; Murphy and Sillito, 1987; Jones and Sillito, 1991), however, were inadequate stimuli to study this reduction; with such stimuli it is not clear if response reduction could be simply explained by the antagonistic surround of the receptive field or if it constituted an unexplained suppressive phenomenon. Nonetheless, these results led to fruitful studies of intrageniculate inhibition (e.g., Singer, Poppel, and Creutzfeldt, 1972) and to the description of previously unknown suppressive effects (Levick, Cleland, and Dubin, 1972). A key feature of these effects is that they can be caused equally by light increases and by light decreases, a behavior incompatible with a receptive field acting alone (Levick, Cleland, and Dubin, 1972).

More recently, there has been renewed interest in suppressive phenomena in LGN. Experiments with drifting gratings have made it clear that selectivity for stimulus size and other suppressive phenomena arising around the region of the receptive field would not be explained by a receptive field alone (Walker, Ohzawa, and Freeman, 1999; Jones et al., 2000; Solomon, White, and Martin, 2002). Moreover, experiments with sums of gratings (test and mask) (figure 22.5*B*, *C*) have allowed one to distinguish suppressive effects from effects due to the receptive field (Bonin, Mante, and Carandini, 2002, 2003a,b). These experiments allow the development of a quantitative model of suppression in LGN.

Suppressive fields in LGN

To explain the suppressive effects observed in LGN, it helps to go back to an elegant paper by Levick, Cleland, and

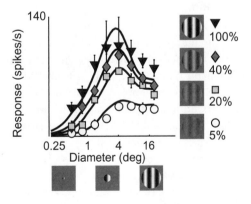

FIGURE 22.4   Selectivity for stimulus size in LGN, and its dependence on grating contrast. Responses of an X cell to drifting gratings varying in size and contrast as indicated. Curves are fits of the divisive model, with parameters held fixed as obtained in figure 22.3. One parameter, a responsiveness factor, was allowed to vary between data sets. (Modified from Bonin, Mante, and Carandini, 2003b.)

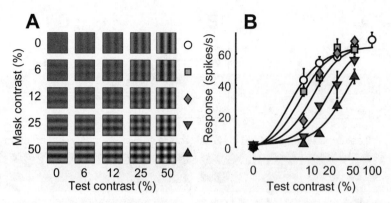

FIGURE 22.5 Cross-orientation suppression in cat V1. (*A*) Stimuli are plaids obtained by summing orthogonal drifting gratings, the test (top row) and the mask (left column). Test and mask have the same temporal frequency. (*B*) Mean response of a simple cell as a function of test contrast. Symbols correspond to mask contrasts, from zero (○) to 50% (▲). Curves indicate fits by the divisive model. (Modified from Freeman et al., 2002b.)

Dubin (1972). These authors proposed that neurons in LGN have not only a receptive field but also a *suppressive field*. The suppressive field is superimposed on the receptive field, and, as the term implies, its effect is suppressive. The suppressive field differs from the receptive field in two ways. First, it acts by modulating the responsiveness of the neuron, not by driving responses (for a distinction between driving inputs and modulating inputs to neurons, see Sherman and Guillery, 1998). Second, it responds to the absolute contrast of visual stimuli, regardless of their sign. Whereas for the receptive field reversing the sign of a stimulus from dark to light would reverse the sign of the response, for the suppressive field the response is equal in both circumstances (Levick, Cleland, and Dubin, 1972).

Another concept that helps us understand suppressive effects is that of mechanisms of gain control (Freeman et al., 2002b; Solomon, White, and Martin, 2002). These mechanisms control neuronal responsiveness, or gain, by performing division. In this division the numerator is given by the output of the receptive field, and a broader range of signals contributes to the denominator. This idea originated in earlier work aimed at explaining the responses of retinal ganglion cells (Shapley and Victor, 1978; Victor, 1987; Keat et al., 2001) and of V1 neurons (Albrecht and Geisler, 1991; Heeger, 1992; Carandini, Heeger, and Movshon, 1999; Chen et al., 2001; Sceniak, Hawken, and Shapley, 2001; Cavanaugh, Bair, and Movshon, 2002a).

We have recently advocated a model of LGN responses that joins these disparate elements—receptive field, suppressive field, and divisive gain control (Bonin, Mante, and Carandini, 2002, 2003a,b). In the model (figure 22.1*B*), processing takes place not only in the receptive field but also, in parallel, in a suppressive field. The outputs of receptive field and suppressive field feed into the numerator and denominator of a division stage. Before feeding into the denominator, however, the output of the suppressive field is added to

a constant, c_{50}; this sum ensures that even at zero contrast the denominator will be larger than zero. Following the intuition of Levick, Cleland, and Dubin, (1972), and building on research on retinal contrast gain control (Shapley and Victor, 1978; Victor, 1987), we define the output of the suppressive field to be a measure of local contrast $c_{local}(t)$, the standard deviation of the contrast map $c(x, y, t)$ in a local region weighted by the suppressive field profile. For stimuli such as gratings and sums of gratings, local contrast is simply the square root of the sum of the square contrasts of each component grating.

This model makes excellent predictions of the responses of LGN neurons to gratings and sums of gratings (Bonin, Mante, and Carandini, 2002, 2003a,b).In particular, it predicts the behaviors shown in figure 22.3. The model predicts contrast saturation (figure 22.3*A*, curve) because the denominator is dominated by c_{50} at low contrast and becomes noticeable at high contrast. The model explains masking because mask contrast appears in the denominator, reducing the responses to the test. In particular, the model captures how suppression increases with increasing mask contrast (figure 22.3*B*, curve) and with increasing mask diameter (figure 22.3*C*, curve). Some of these nonlinear effects had been previously explained with divisive models, but each effect was modeled and fitted individually (Freeman et al., 2002b; Solomon, White, and Martin, 2002). Data like those in figure 22.3 indicate that a divisive model can explain them all at once with a fixed set of parameters. Once these parameters are found they can be fixed, and used to predict novel data. For example, they explain the phenomenon of size tuning illustrated in figure 22.4. The model correctly predicts that, as shown by Solomon, White, and Martin, (2002) in macaque, cat LGN neurons are selective for size only at high contrast. Indeed, at high contrast, increasing stimulus size provides a powerful signal to the denominator, substantially suppressing the responses (figure 22.4, ▼). At low contrast, instead, signals in the denominator are dwarfed by the constant c_{50}, so they do not suppress responses to large stimuli (figure 22.4, ○).

ORIGINS OF LGN SUPPRESSIVE FIELDS   What are the origins of the suppressive field of LGN neurons? These origins certainly include retinal mechanisms of contrast gain control (Shapley and Victor, 1978, 1981; Victor, 1987). In addition, they might include thalamic circuitry (Singer and Creutzfeldt, 1970; Levick, Cleland, and Dubin, 1972; Singer, Poppel, and Creutzfeldt, 1972; Kaplan, Purpura, and Shapley, 1987) and feedback from primary visual cortex (Murphy and Sillito, 1987; Sillito, Cudeiro, and Murphy, 1993; Cudeiro and Sillito, 1996; Alitto and Usrey, 2003).

A clue to the origin of suppressive signals lies in their preferences for visual attributes. A prime visual attribute in this respect is stimulus orientation, as selectivity for this attribute would strongly suggest a cortical origin. However, opinions on the matter are not unanimous: some reports indicate that suppressive signals in LGN are selective for orientation (Cudeiro and Sillito, 1996; Sillito et al., 1993), but others suggest the opposite (Solomon, White, and Martin, 2002; Bonin, Mante, and Carandini, 2003b). Additional visual attributes that have been studied include spatial frequency and temporal frequency. Signals contributing to suppression are particularly responsive to low spatial frequencies and high temporal frequencies. Because V1 neurons barely respond to low spatial frequencies (Maffei and Fiorentini, 1973; De Valois and De Valois, 1988) and high temporal frequencies (see Freeman et al., 2002b, for references), this finding is suggestive of a retinal and/or thalamic origin of the suppressive signals.

Receptive fields in V1

We now turn to primary visual cortex. We examine models that are similar to those described for LGN (figure 22.1), based on receptive fields, suppressive fields, divisive gain control, and rectification. As in LGN, we find that these models go a long way toward explaining the visual responses of V1 neurons.

Just as in LGN, the simplest model for V1 responses is one in which neurons perform weighted sums, with weights determined by the receptive field (Hubel and Wiesel, 1959; Movshon, Thompson, and Tolhurst, 1978a). For V1 simple cells, this model is identical to the one depicted in figure 22.4A, with the difference that the receptive field would typically consist of a number of elongated ON and OFF subfields (Jones and Palmer, 1987). For V1 complex cells, moreover, the positive outputs of more than one receptive field would be summed together to yield an overall response that is insensitive to spatial position and stimulus sign (Hubel and Wiesel, 1962; Movshon, Thompson, and Tolhurst,

1978b; Spitzer and Hochstein, 1988; Szulborski and Palmer, 1990; Emerson, Bergen, and Adelson, 1992; Chance, Nelson, and Abbott, 1999; Lau, Stanley, and Dan, 2002; Touryan, Lau, and Dan, 2002). This model based on receptive field and a rectification stage explains successfully the basic features of V1 selectivity for stimulus attributes, including position, spatial frequency, orientation, temporal frequency, and direction of motion (reviewed in De Valois and De Valois, 1988; Carandini, Heeger, and Movshon, 1999).

Suppression in V1

As with LGN neurons, responses of V1 neurons reveal nonlinearities that require a revision of the receptive field model. In particular, these neurons exhibit clear phenomena of suppression.

First, V1 neurons receive suppression from within the receptive field (reviewed in Heeger, 1992; Carandini, Heeger, and Movshon, 1999). Responses can be reduced by adding to a test stimulus a mask stimulus that might elicit little if any response when presented alone. An example of this phenomenon is cross-orientation suppression (Morrone, Burr, and Maffei, 1982), which is observed by superimposing test bars at one orientation on mask bars at a different orientation. Effective masks can have a broad range of orientations, spatial frequencies, and temporal frequencies (Morrone, Burr, and Maffei, 1982; Bonds, 1989; Bauman and Bonds, 1991; DeAngelis et al., 1992; Allison, Smith, and Bonds, 2001; Freeman et al., 2002b). Cross-orientation suppression originates in a small central region within the receptive field (DeAngelis et al., 1992).

An example of cross-orientation suppression is illustrated in figure 22.5. An optimal test grating evokes a large response when presented on its own (figure 22.5B, ○), whereas an orthogonal mask typically evokes no response (figure 22.5B, leftmost data points). Adding the mask to the test, however, substantially reduces responses: the mask shifts the curves relating response to test contrast to the right, as if it reduced the test contrast seen by the cell (figure 22.5B). Because the scale of the abscissa is logarithmic, this reduction is divisive. Divisive effects of this kind have been measured in V1 in both cat (Bonds, 1989; Freeman et al., 2002b) and monkey (Carandini, Heeger, and Movshon, 1997). Although a similar effect is present in LGN (e.g., figure 22.3B), in most LGN neurons it is weaker than in V1 (Freeman et al., 2002b). This observation is consistent with the widely held view that cross-orientation suppression is a cortical phenomenon, that is, it is not inherited from LGN.

Second, V1 neurons receive suppression from an area wider than the receptive field (reviewed in Fitzpatrick, 2000). Responses often decrease once a stimulus extends beyond the receptive field, and can be greatly suppressed by a mask stimulus outside the receptive field (Hubel and Wiesel, 1965;

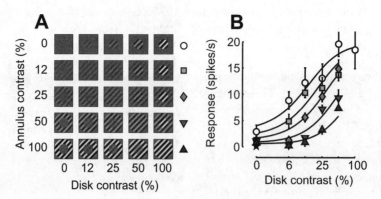

FIGURE 22.6   Surround suppression in cat V1. (*A*) Stimuli are drifting gratings enclosed in a disk (top row) and in a mask (left column). (*B*) Mean response of a complex cell as a function of disk contrast.

Symbols correspond to annulus contrasts, from zero (○) to 50% (▲). Curves indicate fits by the divisive model. (Modified from Freeman et al., 2002a.)

Blakemore and Tobin, 1972; Maffei and Fiorentini, 1976; Gilbert, 1977; Gulyas et al., 1987; Knierim and Van Essen, 1992; Li and Li, 1994; Cavanaugh, Bair, and Movshon, 2002a). The origins of this phenomenon might lie partially in LGN, as responses of LGN neurons are themselves subject to it (figures 22.3 and 22.4), but the effects in V1, are much stronger (Jones et al., 2000). Crucially, in V1, suppression originating from the surround is selective for orientation, being strongest when test and mask have the same orientation (Blakemore and Tobin, 1972; DeAngelis, Freeman, and Ohzawa, 1994) and absent when they have orthogonal orientation (DeAngelis et al., 1992).

An example of surround suppression is illustrated in figure 22.6. An optimal grating enclosed in a central disk evokes a large response when presented on its own (figure 22.6*B*, ○), whereas the same grating enclosed in a surrounding annulus evokes no response (figure 22.6*B*, leftmost data points). Adding the annulus to the disk substantially reduces the responses. This effect is similar to that of cross-orientation suppression (figure 22.6*B*).

Suppressive fields in V1

Just as with LGN neurons, suppressive effects in V1 neurons can be explained by a suppressive field that operates divisively (figure 22.5*B*). Such divisive models of V1 responses show great promise of explaining suppressive effects, both in the receptive field and in the surrounding region (Albrecht and Geisler, 1991; Heeger, 1992; Carandini, Heeger, Movshon, 1997, 1999; Chen et al., 2001; Sceniak, Hawken, and Shapley, 2001; Cavanaugh, Bair, and Movshon, 2002a). In fact, the divisive model including receptive field and suppressive field explains a number of suppression phenomena.

First, the model explains cross-orientation suppression (Albrecht and Geisler, 1991; Heeger, 1992; Carandini, Heeger, and Movshon, 1999; Freeman et al., 2002b). Consider, for example, the data in figure 22.5*B*. This example

involves an orthogonal mask, which provides little drive to the receptive field. The mask thus contributes only to the denominator and not to the numerator of the division operation (figure 22.1*B*), and its effect is to shift rightward the curves relating response to test contrast (Heeger, 1992). In a more general situation both gratings elicit responses when presented alone, and c_{test} and c_{mask} play a role both in the numerator and in the denominator. In this case, even though the responses are more complicated than a simple rightward shift, a divisive model similar to the one presented here predicts them closely (Carandini, Heeger, and Movshon, 1997).

Second, the model explains surround suppression (Chen et al., 2001; Sceniak, Hawken, and Shapley, 2001; Schwartz and Simoncelli, 2001; Cavanaugh, Bair, and Movshon, 2002a; Solomon, White, and Martin, 2002). This behavior is illustrated in figure 22.6*B* (curves). Because the annulus stimulates only the fringes of the receptive field, it contributes little to the numerator. Nonetheless, it does contribute to the denominator, because it stimulates the suppressive field extensively.

The model also accounts for a number of additional phenomena that, like cross-orientation suppression and surround suppression, would not be explained by the receptive field alone.

One of these phenomena is contrast saturation (Albrecht and Geisler, 1991; Heeger, 1992): At high contrasts responses grow much less than proportionally with contrast (figure 22.5*B*, ○; figure 22.6*B*, ○; figure 22.7*A*, ■). The model explains this behavior (curves) because as contrast increases, the output of the suppressive field goes beyond the constant c_{50} and divides the output of the receptive field by a progressively larger number. Without the suppressive field, the output of the model would have grown proportionally with contrast once above threshold.

Another of these otherwise unexplained phenomena is the selectivity for stimulus size that is observed at high contrast (Kapadia, Westheimer, and Gilbert, 1999; Sceniak

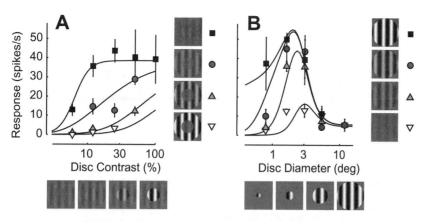

FIGURE 22.7 Responses to disks and annuli in a complex cell in cat V1. An optimal drifting grating is enclosed in a disk and an abutting annulus. Disk and annulus are abutting and centered on the receptive field. Their contrast and relative size are varied. Curves are predictions of the divisive model. (*A*) Dependence of response on disk contrast for four annulus contrasts (disk diameter = 3 deg.). (*B*) Dependence of response on disk diameter for four disk contrasts (annulus contrast = 0). The disk was centered 0.7 degrees away from the center of the receptive field, so that for small diameters, responses grow with disk diameter particularly steeply. The model was fitted to 180 responses obtained in a three-dimensional space of disk contrast, annulus contrast, and disk diameter, not just to the few illustrated here. (Data from V. Bonin, V. Mante, and M. Carandini, unpublished observations.)

et al., 1999; Sceniak, Hawken, and Shapley, 2001; Cavanaugh, Bair, and Movshon, 2002a). We have already seen this behavior in LGN neurons (figure 22.4) and noted how it is explained by the divisive suppressive field. In V1 neurons, however, selectivity for size can be much more pronounced than in LGN (Jones et al., 2000). An example of this behavior is illustrated in figure 22.7*B*, for a V1 neuron that is practically silenced by stimuli that extend beyond a critical size. For this neuron, selectivity for size appears to be present at all contrasts, but in more typical examples it is present only at high contrast, with the preferred size becoming smaller at higher contrasts (as in the LGN neuron of figure 22.4). As we have already noted, the divisive model explains this behavior: responses grow with size until the denominator becomes equal to the numerator, then responses decrease. At higher contrasts, this point of equality—the preferred size—is achieved with smaller stimuli.

These considerations suggest that commonly used methods are likely to lead to severe underestimation of receptive field size. Receptive field size is commonly estimated with high-contrast stimuli. Because they engage the suppressive field, these stimuli make the receptive field appear smaller than it really is. To come close to mapping the receptive field faithfully, one would want to use small, low-contrast stimuli. However, these stimuli elicit responses that are below threshold for spike generation, so they also lead to an underestimation of receptive field size. Only by considering the contribution of the suppressive field can one correctly estimate the size of the receptive field.

Underestimation of receptive field size might contribute to an explanation of phenomena of response enhancement resulting from remote stimulation. Indeed, there are numerous reports that regions surrounding the center of the recep-

tive field can enhance responses (Allman, Miezin, and McGuinness, 1985; Nelson and Frost, 1985; Kapadia et al., 1995; Sillito et al., 1995) or cause a combination of suppression and enhancement (Levitt and Lund, 1996; Polat et al., 1998; Kapadia, Westheimer, and Gilbert, 1999, 2000; Sceniak et al., 1999; Jones et al., 2001). These reports might become easier to understand if one considers that receptive field size is commonly three times larger than estimated with simple forms of stimulation (Cavanaugh, Bair, and Movshon, 2002a), so that these studies might have underestimated the area over which V1 neurons summate their inputs.

Indeed, the suppressive field explains many properties of surround suppression and enhancement, from the preference shown by surround enhancement for collinear stimuli (Polat et al., 1998) to the dependence of suppression effects on mask contrast (e.g., Levitt and Lund, 1996). The model might not explain complicated aspects of surround stimulation exhibited by some cells (e.g., Sillito et al., 1995; Jones, Wang, and Sillito, 2002), but such phenomena are not shared by a majority of cells (Cavanaugh, Bair, and Movshon, 2002b).

Finally, a contribution to response enhancement observed with remote stimulation might lie in disinhibition, that is, the effect of suppressing the responses of mechanisms that would otherwise cause suppression (Jones, Wang, and Sillito, 2002; Walker, Ohzawa, and Freeman, 2002). This effect is not captured by our model as it stands (figure 22.7*B*), because in the model the suppressive field's response cannot in turn be suppressed. A feedback implementation of the model in which the very same mechanisms that compute the suppressive field suppress each other (e.g., Carandini, Heeger, and Movshon, 1997) would likely capture these effects.

ORIGINS OF V1 SUPPRESSIVE FIELDS Given that LGN neurons exhibit a suppressive field, the origin of V1 suppressive fields is likely to lie at least partially in LGN. Mechanisms of suppression in V1, however, appear to be stronger than in LGN (e.g., Bonds, 1989; Sclar, Maunsell, and Lennie, 1990; Jones et al., 2000; Freeman et al., 2002b). Moreover, there are clear differences between suppressive fields in LGN and V1.

A first difference between suppressive fields in LGN and V1 is that the extent of the latter depends on stimulus orientation. For stimuli that are orthogonal to the preferred orientation of a V1 neuron, the suppressive field is small, smaller than the receptive field. For stimuli parallel to the preferred orientation of the neuron, the suppressive field is large and extends well beyond the receptive field. Indeed, suppressive signals originating in a small central region within the receptive field weigh all orientations equally (DeAngelis et al., 1992), whereas those from the surrounding region weigh orientations close to the neuron's preferred orientation more than others (Blakemore and Tobin, 1972; DeAngelis, Freeman, and Ohzawa, 1994; Li and Li, 1994). The peak strength of the suppressive field, however, should not depend on orientation: a small mask elicits about equal suppression at all orientations (DeAngelis et al., 1992).

A second difference between suppressive fields in V1 and in LGN lies in the spatial configuration. Suppressive fields in LGN are well described by a Gaussian envelope concentric to the receptive field (V. Bonin, Mante, and M. Carandini, unpublished observations). Suppressive fields of V1 neurons instead are asymmetrical, and contain clear "hot spots" not necessarily concentric with the receptive field (DeAngelis, Freeman, and Ohzawa, 1994; Walker, Ohzawa, and Freeman, 1999; Cavanaugh, Bair, and Movshon, 2002b).

In summary, the suppressive field of V1 neurons is likely to be inherited from LGN only in part. Mechanisms that could contribute to suppression within V1 include feedback connections from within V1 (e.g., Carandini, Heeger, and Movshon, 1997) or from higher cortical areas (e.g., Angelucci et al., 2002; Levitt and Lund, 2002).

In fact, the very first interpretation of suppression phenomena in V1 has been based on intracortical inhibition (figure 22.8). According to this view, cross-orientation suppression would be explained by inhibition between from V1 neurons with overlapping receptive fields and different preferred orientations (figure 22.8A). Likewise, surround suppression might be explained by inhibition from V1 neurons with displaced receptive fields and similar preferred orientations (figure 22.8B). This intracortical explanation of suppression has been criticized (Freeman et al., 2002b), but is ingrained in current thinking about suppressive phenomena. Indeed, cross-orientation suppression was initially termed cross-orientation inhibition (Morrone, Burr, and Maffei, 1982).

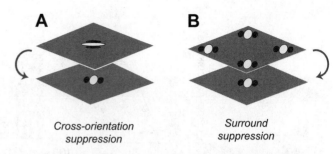

FIGURE 22.8 Interpretation of suppression phenomena in V1 in terms of intracortical inhibition. (*A*) Cross-orientation suppression might be explained by inhibition between from V1 neurons with overlapping receptive fields and different preferred orientations. (*B*) Surround suppression might be explained by inhibition from V1 neurons with displaced receptive fields and similar preferred orientations. (Modified from Durand et al., 2003.)

Limitations of current models

Although they promise to explain a large variety of phenomena both within and around the receptive field, current models based on suppressive fields and divisive gain control are limited in a number of ways.

First, current models are typically defined to account for suppressive effects individually. For example, a model designed to predict suppression within the receptive field is not specified to predict selectivity for size, and vice versa. Even when models are used to fit more than one data set from a given neuron, their parameters are usually not held fixed. It is thus hard to establish if a single model can explain a wide array of behaviors.

This limitation can be addressed by constraining a model with a set of measurements (as we did in figure 22.3) and then freezing the parameters to test responses to other stimuli (as we did in figure 22.4). Or it can be addressed by acquiring large data sets and fitting a model to the whole data set at once (as we did in figure 22.7, where responses to most of the 180 stimuli are not shown for reasons of space).

Second, current models are defined only for simple, spatially localized or homogeneous, repetitive visual stimuli. Simplified visual stimuli such as bars, gratings, and sums of two gratings were invaluable in allowing the development of much of our knowledge on the early visual system. They were designed to isolate particular response mechanisms and not engage others, and to simplify (or just enable) data analysis. Thus, an essential question about current models of LGN and V1 remains open: Can they predict responses to the complex, rapidly varying visual scenes that occur outside the laboratory?

Addressing this limitation is not trivial. Visual stimuli encountered outside the laboratory tend to violate two important constraints. First, complex stimuli do not necessarily have constant mean luminance. Current models take as input a map of contrast that is output by the retina as a result of processes of light adaptation (reviewed in Shapley and Enroth-Cugell, 1984; Walraven et al., 1990). In simple stimuli such as gratings and plaids, mean luminance is constant, so the retina is in an approximately constant state of adaptation, and light adaptation can be effectively ignored (Troy and Enroth-Cugell, 1993; Troy, Bohnsack, and Diller, 1999). In more complex stimuli, however, mean luminance can vary in space or in time, often abruptly. One must then ask, how fast is the computation of contrast? How is it influenced by luminances in recent past and local space? Second, complex stimuli are not necessarily constant for a few seconds. Divisive models of LGN and V1 are defined only for temporally stationary stimuli. In particular, the dynamics of the suppressive field contributing to the denominator have been only partially characterized.

Mechanisms of suppression

The divisive models, which I so strongly advocate, have the virtue and the fault of being abstract: with the exception of the rectification stage, which is related to spike threshold, their components do not map directly into biophysical mechanisms. In essence, these are models of the neural computations performed on images, not of the biophysical implementations of such computations. A compact description of computations performed by a neuron can then in turn guide research on the underlying biophysics.

For example, one may wonder how neurons or networks can perform an arithmetic division. There are at least two mechanisms that would yield division: shunting inhibition (Carandini and Heeger, 1994) and synaptic depression (Carandini, Heeger, and Senn, 2002). I will now describe these mechanisms, but it should be kept in mind that additional mechanisms could be at play. For example, it is possible to obtain divisive effects from subtractive inhibition from neurons whose responses grow steeply with contrast (Somers et al., 1998).

A first proposal for how division might be implemented in V1 was based on membrane conductance (figure 22.9). We proposed that cells suppress each other's response through shunting inhibition, that is, by increasing each other's conductance (Carandini and Heeger, 1994; Carandini, Heeger, and Movshon, 1997). We argued that increasing conductance divides the contrast that is effectively seen by a neuron. Initially, this proposal was criticized on the grounds that an increase in conductance per se does not necessarily have a divisive effect on firing rates (Holt and Koch, 1997). Recently, however, our view has been supported by the discovery of a role for membrane potential noise: increased inhibition would increase both conductance

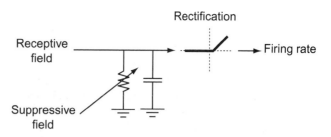

FIGURE 22.9   Divisive model based on conductance increases. The response of the receptive field is input to a simplified model of the cell membrane, a circuit composed of a resistor and a capacitor in parallel. The signals from the suppressive field control the conductance of the resistor. A rectification stage encodes the resulting signals into firing rate. (Modified from Carandini and Heeger, 1994; Carandini et al., 1997.)

and noise, and the overall effect would be divisive (Chance, Abbott, and Reyes, 2002).

We tested this model with intracellular in vivo measurements (Anderson, Carandini, and Ferster, 2000) and found its predictions to be only partially correct. To explain cross-orientation suppression, we expected that conductance would increase markedly with contrast, and that it would not depend on orientation (Carandini, Heeger, and Movshon, 1997). In a few neurons conductance did increase markedly, by about 300% (see also Borg-Graham, Monier, and Frégnac, 1998; Hirsch et al., 1998; Martinez et al., 2002). Conductance increases of this magnitude, however, were only obtained with stimuli of optimal orientation, and not in all cells. If our measurements are correct (we might have been blind to conductance increases occurring in the dendrites), our proposal of conductance increases to explain cross-orientation suppression and other divisive effects will need to be revised or refined.

In fact, we recently argued that cross-orientation suppression does not result from intracortical inhibition at all (Freeman et al., 2002b). The view that cross-orientation suppression originates from inhibition is widely held (Morrone, Burr, and Maffei, 1982; Bonds, 1989; Bauman and Bonds, 1991; DeAngelis et al., 1992; Heeger, 1992; Sengpiel and Blakemore, 1994; Sengpiel, Blakemore, and Harrad, 1995; Sengpiel et al., 1998; Walker, Ohzawa, and Freeman, 1998; Allison, Smith, and Bonds, 2001). However, the signals underlying cross-orientation suppression exhibit visual preferences that are hardly consistent with an intracortical origin: (1) suppression can be elicited by masks that barely evoke cortical responses, such as gratings drifting faster than about 20 Hz (Freeman et al., 2002b); and (2) unlike the responses of V1 neurons, the signals responsible for suppression are immune to pattern adaptation, the substantial reduction in V1 responses that follows prolonged stimulation (Freeman et al., 2002b). These observations suggest that to explain cross-orientation suppression, the signals providing input to the denominator in the divisive model should originate in LGN and not in cortex.

We searched for another mechanism that causes division, one that would carry signals from LGN to the denominator of V1 neurons. We found a promising candidate in synaptic depression (Carandini, Heeger, and Senn, 2002; Freeman et al., 2002b).

Depression is a promising candidate because a single depressing synapse displays both saturation and divisive suppression (figure 22.10*A*). Consider the responses to injection of a sinusoidal current. Depression causes a substantial saturation in response amplitude (figure 22.10*A*, ●) (Abbott et al., 1997; Tsodyks and Markram, 1997; Kayser, Priebe, and Miller, 2001). Adding noise to the injected current (figure 22.10*A*, ○) increases synaptic depression. The noise partially suppresses the responses to the sinusoidal current, and this suppression is divisive (figure 22.10*A*, ○, rightward shift on the logarithmic scale), as if the noise had divided the amplitudes of the injected sinusoidal current (Carandini, Heeger, and Senn, 2002).

To explore the degree to which depression can explain visual properties of V1 neurons, we included it in a classic model of a simple cell (Hubel and Wiesel, 1962). In the model, orientation selectivity (figure 22.10*D, E*) is determined by the spatial pattern of LGN inputs, with ON and OFF subregions of the receptive field (figure 22.10*B*) being driven by excitation from ON-center and OFF-center LGN neurons (Reid and Alonso, 1995; Alonso, Usrey, and Reid, 2001) (figure 22.10*C*). Excitation by ON-center neurons is matched by inhibition by OFF-center neurons, and vice versa (reviewed in Hirsch, 2003). Synaptic depression, in turn, produces cross-orientation suppression: the response to the plaid (figure 22.10*F*) is smaller than the response to the

test alone (figure 22.10*D*). The model correctly predicts that the effects of suppression are divisive: increasing the mask contrast shifts to the right curves relating response to test contrast (figure 22.10*G*). This behavior resembles that shown by real V1 neurons (figure 22.10*C*). We have studied model predictions for a variety of stimuli, and we have found them to capture a wide variety of effects (Carandini, Heeger, and Senn, 2002).

Synaptic depression would not explain suppression originating from outside the receptive field. In fact, even though both suppression within and around the receptive field are explained by a divisive model, they might not share a single biophysical mechanism. For one, these two forms of suppression have very distinct visual preferences. For example, cross-orientation suppression can be obtained with masks of all orientations (DeAngelis et al., 1992), whereas surround suppression is strongest when the mask has the preferred orientation of the neuron (DeAngelis, Freeman, and Ohzawa, 1994). So it is possible that the two forms of suppression originate from distinct biophysical mechanisms (Sengpiel et al., 1998; Carandini, Heeger, and Senn, 2002).

Advantages of suppression

In summary, even though their biophysical implementation is not clear, divisive models including a suppressive field represent a major improvement over models based on the receptive field alone. These models have the potential to explain a wide variety of suppressive phenomena.

We expect these phenomena to play an important role in responses to complex visual scenes. We have seen that a model that ignored suppression would fare badly in predicting responses, both in LGN (figures 22.3 and 22.4) and

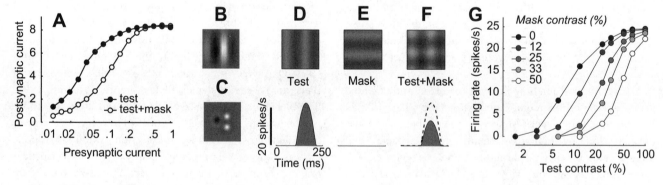

Figure 22.10 Modeling suppression with synaptic depression. (*A*) Saturation and suppression in a model depressing synapse. A 2-Hz sinusoidal test current is injected into the presynaptic neuron, and the response is measured by the 2-Hz component of the postsynaptic potential (●). This response is reduced (○) when a mask current (white noise) is added to the test current. (*B–G*) Cross-orientation suppression explained by thalamocortical synaptic depression. (*B*) Receptive field of a model V1 neuron. (*C*) Recep-tive fields of three model LGN neurons. (*D–F*) Firing rate in response to gratings and plaids drifting at 4 Hz. Average response to a stimulus cycle. Stimuli are a vertical grating (*D*), a horizontal grating (*E*), and the plaid obtained by summing the two (*F*). Dashed curve is response to plaid in the absence of synaptic depression. (*G*) First harmonic (4 Hz) of firing rate as a function of test contrast, for different mask contrasts. (Modified from Carandini et al., 2002; Freeman et al., 2002b.)

in V1 (figures 22.5, 22.6, and 22.7). It is hard to imagine that it would fare much better in predicting responses to more natural stimuli. Indeed, in natural images similar stimuli arise often, as the overlap of different orientations is extremely common (Schwartz and Simoncelli, 2001).

This brings us to a final question: What are the advantages conferred by a divisive suppressive field? It is difficult to answer to this question, because we know little of how signals in LGN and V1 are used in subsequent stages of visual processing to yield sensation and perception. As a result, we know little of how any computation in LGN and V1 can be advantageous to later stages. There are, nonetheless, a few suggestions that have been made and might be of relevance.

A first suggestion is that a divisive suppressive field would be needed to compress the range of responses without compromising the basic output of the receptive field (Heeger, 1992). In particular, a divisive suppressive field maintains a desirable property of receptive field outputs: that the ratio of the outputs of two neurons is largely independent of stimulus contrast (Heeger, 1992).

A second suggestion relies on a principle of optimality that has been suggested for neurons of the cerebral cortex: that they should strive to maintain statistical independence in their responses (Barlow and Földiák, 1989). It has been argued that divisive suppression of the kind shown by V1 neurons would maximize this independence (Schwartz and Simoncelli, 2001). If this is the case, evidence for divisive suppression being active already at the level of retina and LGN would suggest that the principles of statistical independence inform the responses of these subcortical structures as well.

Finally, and perhaps most interestingly to the readers of this volume, the mechanisms of divisive suppression might serve also in an eminently cognitive process, the deployment of visual attention. Considerable recent evidence suggests that visual attention enhances neuronal responses by changing neuronal gain (e.g., Reynolds, Pasternak, and Desimone, 2000; Fallah and Reynolds, 2001; Reynolds and Desimone, 2003; Maunsell and Ghose, this volume). It is thus conceivable that suppression and attention might engage the same mechanisms, one to obtain division, the other to obtain multiplication.

My hope is that the concept of a divisive suppressive field that has evolved from research on the visual responses of LGN and V1 neurons will prove useful to understanding this and other cognitive effects of neural responses to visual stimuli.

REFERENCES

ABBOTT, L. F., J. A. VARELA, K. SEN, and S. B. NELSON, 1997. Synaptic depression and cortical gain control. *Science* 275:220–224.

ALBRECHT, D. G., and W. S. GEISLER, 1991. Motion sensitivity and the contrast-response function of simple cells in the visual cortex. *Vis. Neurosci.* 7:531–546.

ALITTO, H. J., and W. M. USREY, 2003. Corticothalamic feedback and sensory processing. *Curr. Opin. Neurobiol.* 13:440–445.

ALLISON, J. D., K. R. SMITH, and A. B. BONDS, 2001. Temporal-frequency tuning of cross-orientation suppression in the cat striate cortex. *Vis. Neurosci.* 18:941–948.

ALLMAN, J., F. MIEZIN, and E. McGUINNESS, 1985. Stimulus specific responses from beyond the classical receptive field: Neurophysiological mechanisms for local-global comparisons in visual neurons. *Annu. Rev. Neurosci.* 8:407–430.

ALONSO, J. M., W. M. USREY, and R. C. REID, 2001. Rules of connectivity between geniculate cells and simple cells in cat primary visual cortex. *J. Neurosci.* 21:4002–4015.

ANDERSON, J., M. CARANDINI, and D. FERSTER, 2000. Orientation tuning of input conductance, excitation and inhibition in cat primary visual cortex. *J. Neurophysiol.* 84:909–931.

ANGELUCCI, A., J. B. LEVITT, E. J. WALTON, J. M. HUPE, J. BULLIER, and J. S. LUND, 2002. Circuits for local and global signal integration in primary visual cortex. *J. Neurosci.* 22:8633–8646.

BARLOW, H. B., and P. FÖLDIÁK, 1989. Adaptation and decorrelation in the cortex. In *The Computing Neuron*, R. Durbin, C. Miall, and C. Mitchison, eds. Workingham, England, Addison-Wesley, pp. 54–72.

BAUMAN, L. A., and A. B. BONDS, 1991. Inhibitory refinement of spatial frequency selectivity in single cells of the cat striate cortex. *Vision Res.* 31:933–944.

BLAKEMORE, C., and E. A. TOBIN, 1972. Lateral inhibition between orientation detectors in the cat's visual cortex. *Exp. Brain. Res.* 15:439–440.

BONDS, A. B., 1989. Role of inhibition in the specification of orientation selectivity of cells in the cat striate cortex. *Vis. Neurosci.* 2:41–55.

BONIN, V., V. MANTE, and M. CARANDINI, 2002. The contrast integration field of cat LGN neurons. In *Online Abstract Viewer*, Program No. 352.16. Washington, D.C.: Society for Neuroscience.

BONIN, V., V. MANTE, and M. CARANDINI, 2003. Origins of size tuning in LGN neurons. *J. Vision* 3:19a.

BONIN, V., V. MANTE, and M. CARANDINI, 2004. Nonlinear processing in LGN neurons. In *Advances in Neural Information Processing Systems*, 16, S. Thrun I. Saul, and B. Schölkopf, eds. Cambridge, MA: MIT Press.

BORG-GRAHAM, L. J., C. MONIER, and Y. FRÉGNAC, 1998. Visual input evokes transient and strong shunting inhibition in visual cortical neurons. *Nature* 393:369–373.

CAI, D., G. C. DEANGELIS, and R. D. FREEMAN, 1997. Spatiotemporal receptive field organization in the lateral geniculate nucleus of cats and kittens. *J. Neurophysiol.* 78:1045–1061.

CARANDINI, M., and D. FERSTER, 2000. Membrane potential and firing rate in cat primary visual cortex. *J. Neurosci.* 20:470–484.

CARANDINI, M., and D. J. HEEGER, 1994. Summation and division by neurons in visual cortex. *Science* 264:1333–1336.

CARANDINI, M., D. J. HEEGER, and J. A. MOVSHON, 1997. Linearity and normalization in simple cells of the macaque primary visual cortex. *J. Neurosci.* 17:8621–8644.

CARANDINI, M., D. J. HEEGER, and J. A. MOVSHON, 1999. Linearity and gain control in V1 simple cells. *Cereb. Cortex* 13:401–443.

CARANDINI, M., D. J. HEEGER, and W. SENN, 2002. A synaptic explanation of suppression in visual cortex. *J. Neurosci.* 22:10053–10065.

CAVANAUGH, J. R., W. BAIR, and J. A. MOVSHON, 2002a. Nature and interaction of signals from the receptive field center and surround in macaque V1 neurons. *J. Neurophysiol.* 88:2530–2546.

CAVANAUGH J. R., W. BAIR, and J. A. MOVSHON, 2002b. Selectivity and spatial distribution of signals from the receptive field surround in macaque V1 neurons. *J. Neurophysiol.* 88:2547–2556.

CHANCE, F. S., L. F. ABBOTT, and A. D. REYES, 2002. Gain modulation from background synaptic input. *Neuron* 35:773–782.

CHANCE, F. S., S. B. NELSON, and L. F. ABBOTT, 1999. Complex cells as cortically amplified simple cells. *Nat. Neurosci.* 2:277–282.

CHEN, C. C., T. KASAMATSU, U. POLAT, and A. M. NORCIA, 2001. Contrast response characteristics of long-range lateral interactions in cat striate cortex. *Neuroreport* 12:655–661.

CLELAND, B. G., B. B. LEE, and T. R. VIDYASAGAR, 1983. Response of neurons in the cat's lateral geniculate nucleus to moving bars of different length. *J. Neurosci.* 3:108–116.

CUDEIRO, J., and A. M. SILLITO, 1996. Spatial frequency tuning of orientation-discontinuity-sensitive corticofugal feedback to the cat lateral geniculate nucleus. *J. Physiol.* 490(Pt. 2):481–492.

DAN, Y., J. J. ATICK, and R. C. REID, 1996. Efficient coding of natural scenes in the lateral geniculate nucleus: Experimental test of a computational theory. *J. Neurosci.* 16:3351–3362.

DAWIS, S., R. SHAPLEY, E. KAPLAN, and D. TRANCHINA, 1984. The receptive field organization of X cells in the cat: Spatiotemporal coupling and asymmetry. *Vision Res.* 24:549–564.

DE VALOIS, R. L., and K. DE VALOIS, 1988. *Spatial Vision.* Oxford, England: Oxford University Press.

DEANGELIS, G. C., R. D. FREEMAN, and I. OHZAWA, 1994. Length and width tuning of neurons in the cat's primary visual cortex. *J. Neurophysiol.* 71:347–374.

DEANGELIS, G. C., J. G. ROBSON, I. OHZAWA, and R. D. FREEMAN, 1992. The organization of supression in receptive fields of neurons in cat visual cortex. *J. Neurophysiol.* 68:144–163.

DURAND, S., V. MANTE, T. C. B. FREEMAN, and M. CARANDINI, 2003. *Temporal resolution of suppression in cat primary visual cortex.* Unpublished manuscript.

EMERSON, R. C., J. R. BERGEN, and E. H. ADELSON, 1992. Directionally selective complex cells and the computation of motion energy in cat visual cortex. *Vision Res.* 32:203–218.

ENROTH-CUGELL, C., and J. G. ROBSON, 1984. Functional characteristics and diversity of cat retinal ganglion cells. *Invest. Ophthalmol Vis. Sci.* 25:250–267.

ENROTH-CUGELL, C., J. G. ROBSON, D. E. SCHWEITZER-TONG, and A. B. WATSON, 1983. Spatio-temporal interactions in cat retinal ganglion cells showing linear spatial summation. *J. Physiol. (Lond.)* 341:279–307.

FALLAH, M., and J. H. REYNOLDS, 2001. Attention! V1 neurons lining up for inspection. *Neuron* 31:674–675.

FITZPATRICK, D., 2000. Seeing beyond the receptive field in primary visual cortex. *Curr. Opin. Neurobiol.* 10:438–443.

FREEMAN, T. C. B., S. DURAND, D. KIPER, and M. CARANDINI, 2002a. Lateral inhibition and surround suppression in primary visual cortex. *FENS Abstr.* 1:A051.10.

FREEMAN, T. C. B., S. DURAND, D. C. KIPER, and M. CARANDINI, 2002b. Suppression without inhibition in visual cortex. *Neuron* 35:759–771.

GILBERT, C. D., 1977. Laminar differences in receptive properties of cells in cat primary visual cortex. *J. Physiol. (Lond.)* 268:391–421.

GRANIT, R., D. KERNELL, and G. K. SHORTESS, 1963. Quantitative aspects of repetitive firing of mammalian motoneurons, caused by injected currents. *J. Physiol. (Lond.)* 168:911–931.

GULYAS, B., G. A. ORBAN, J. DUYSENS, and H. MAES, 1987. The suppressive influence of moving textured backgrounds on responses of cat striate neurons to moving bars. *J. Neurophysiol.* 57:1767–1791.

HEEGER, D. J., 1992. Normalization of cell responses in cat striate cortex. *Vis. Neurosci.* 9:181–197.

HIRSCH, J. A., 2003. Synaptic physiology and receptive field structure in the early visual pathway of the cat. *Cereb. Cortex* 13:63–69.

HIRSCH, J. A., J. M. ALONSO, R. C. REID, and L. M. MARTINEZ, 1998. Synaptic integration in striate cortical simple cells. *J. Physiol.* 18:9517–9528.

HOLT, G. R., and C. KOCH, 1997. Shunting inhibition does not have a divisive effect on firing rates. *Neural Comput.* 9:1001–1013.

HUBEL, D. H., and T. N. WIESEL, 1959. Receptive fields of single neurones in the cat's striate cortex. *J. Physiol. (Lond.)* 148:574–591.

HUBEL, D., and T. N. WIESEL, 1961. Integrative action in the cat's lateral geniculate body. *J. Physiol. (Lond.)* 155:385–398.

HUBEL, D. H., and T. N. WIESEL, 1962. Receptive fields, binocular interaction and functional architecture in the cat's visual cortex. *J. Physiol. (Lond.)* 160:106–154.

HUBEL, D. H., and T. WIESEL, 1965. Receptive fields and functional architecture in two nonstriate visual areas (18–19) of the cat. *J. Neurophysiol.* 28:229–289.

JONES, H. E., I. M. ANDOLINA, N. M. OAKELY, P. C. MURPHY, and A. M. SILLITO, 2000. Spatial summation in lateral geniculate nucleus and visual cortex. *Exp. Brain. Res.* 135:279–284.

JONES, H. E., K. L. GRIEVE, W. WANG, and A. M. SILLITO, 2001. Surround suppression in primate V1. *J. Neurophysiol.* 86:2011–2028.

JONES, H. E., and A. M. SILLITO, 1991. The length-response properties of cells in the feline dorsal lateral geniculate nucleus. *J. Physiol. (Lond.)* 444:329–348.

JONES, H. E., W. WANG, and A. M. SILLITO, 2002. Spatial organization and magnitude of orientation contrast interactions in primate V1. *J. Neurophysiol.* 88:2796–2808.

JONES, J. P., and L. A. PALMER, 1987. The two-dimensional spatial structure of simple receptive fields in cat striate cortex. *J. Neurophysiol.* 58:1187–1211.

KAPADIA, M. K., M. ITO, C. D. GILBERT, and G. WESTHEIMER, 1995. Improvement in visual sensitivity by changes in local context: Parallel studies in human observers and in V1 of alert monkeys. *Neuron* 15:843–856.

KAPADIA, M. K., G. WESTHEIMER, and C. D. GILBERT, 1999. Dynamics of spatial summation in primary visual cortex of alert monkeys. *Proc. Natl. Acad. Sci. U.S.A.* 96:12073–12078.

KAPADIA, M. K., G. WESTHEIMER, and C. D. GILBERT, 2000. Spatial distribution of contextual interactions in primary visual cortex and in visual perception. *J. Neurophysiol.* 84:2048–2062.

KAPLAN, E., K. PURPURA, and R. SHAPLEY, 1987. Contrast affects the transmission of visual information through the mammalian lateral geniculate nucleus. *J. Physiol. (Lond.)* 391:267–288.

KAYSER, A., N. J. PRIEBE, and K. D. MILLER, 2001. Contrast-dependent nonlinearities arise locally in a model of contrast-invariant orientation tuning. *J. Neurophysiol.* 85:2130–2149.

KEAT, J., P. REINAGEL, R. C. REID, and M. MEISTER, 2001. Predicting every spike: A model for the responses of visual neurons. *Neuron* 30:803–817.

KNIERIM, J. J., and D. C. VAN ESSEN, 1992. Neural responses to static texture patterns in area V1 of the alert macaque monkey. *J. Neurophysiol.* 67:961–980.

KUFFLER, S. W., 1953. Discharge patterns and functional organization of mammalian retina. *J. Neurophysiol.* 16:37–68.

LAU, B., G. B. STANLEY, and Y. DAN, 2002. Computational subunits of visual cortical neurons revealed by artificial neural networks. *Proc. Natl. Acad. Sci. U.S.A.* 99:8974–8979.

LEVICK, W. R., B. G. CLELAND, and M. W. DUBIN, 1972. Lateral geniculate neurons of cat: Retinal inputs and physiology. *Invest. Ophthalmol.* 11:302–311.

LEVITT, J. B., and J. S. LUND, 1996. Contrast dependence of contextual effects in primate visual cortex. *Nature* 387:73–76.

LEVITT, J. B., and J. S. LUND, 2002. The spatial extent over which neurons in macaque striate cortex pool visual signals. *Vis. Neurosci.* 19:439–452.

LI, C.-Y., and W. LI, 1994. Extensive integration beyond the classical receptive field of cat's striate cortical neurons: Classification and tuning properties. *Vision Res.* 34:2337–2356.

MAFFEI, L., and A. FIORENTINI, 1973. The visual cortex as a spatial frequency analyzer. *Vision Res.* 13:1255–1267.

MAFFEI, L., and A. FIORENTINI, 1976. The unresponsive regions of visual cortical receptive fields. *Vision Res.* 13:1255–1267.

MANTE, V., V. BONIN, and M. CARANDINI, 2002. Responses of cat LGN neurons to plaids and movies. In *Online Abstract Viewer*, Program No. 352.15. Washington, D.C.: Society for Neuroscience.

MARTINEZ, L. M., J. M. ALONSO, R. C. REID, and J. A. HIRSCH, 2002. Laminar processing of stimulus orientation in cat visual cortex. *J. Physiol.* 540:321–333.

MORRONE, M. C., D. C. BURR, and L. MAFFEI, 1982. Functional implications of cross-orientation inhibition of cortical visual cells. I. Neurophysiological evidence. *Proc. R. Soc. Lond. B.* 216: 335–354.

MOVSHON, J. A., I. D. THOMPSON, and D. J. TOLHURST, 1978a. Spatial summation in the receptive fields of simple cells in the cat's striate cortex. *J. Physiol. (Lond.)* 283:53–77.

MOVSHON, J. A., I. D. THOMPSON, and D. J. TOLHURST, 1978b. Nonlinear spatial summation in the receptive fields of complex cells in the cat striate cortex. *J. Physiol. (Lond.)* 283:78–100.

MURPHY, P. C., and A. M. SILLITO, 1987. Corticofugal feedback influences the generation of length tuning in the visual pathway. *Nature* 329:727–729.

NELSON, J. I., and B. FROST, 1985. Intracortical facilitation among co-oriented, co-axially aligned simple cells in cat striate cortex. *Exp. Brain Res.* 6:54–61.

POLAT, U., K. MIZOBE, M. W. PETTET, T. KASAMATSU, and A. M. NORCIA, 1998. Collinear stimuli regulate visual responses depending on cell's contrast threshold. *Nature* 391:580–584.

REID, R. C., and J. M. ALONSO, 1995. Specificity of monosynaptic connections from thalamus to visual cortex. *Nature* 378:281–284.

REYNOLDS, J. H., and R. DESIMONE, 2003. Interacting roles of attention and visual salience in V4. *Neuron* 37:853–863.

REYNOLDS, J. H., T. PASTERNAK, and R. DESIMONE, 2000. Attention increases sensitivity of V4 neurons. *Neuron* 26:703–714.

RODIECK, R. W., 1965. Quantitative analysis of cat retina ganglion cell response to visual stimuli. *Vision Res.* 5:583–601.

SCENIAK, M. P., M. J. HAWKEN, and R. SHAPLEY, 2001. Visual spatial characterization of macaque V1 neurons. *J. Neurophysiol.* 85:1873–1887.

SCENIAK, M. P., D. L. RINGACH, M. J. HAWKEN, and R. SHAPLEY, 1999. Contrast's effect on spatial summation by macaque V1 neurons. *Nat. Neurosci.* 2:733–739.

SCHWARTZ, O., and E. P. SIMONCELLI, 2001. Natural signal statistics and sensory gain control. *Nat. Neurosci.* 4:819–825.

SCLAR, G., J. H. R. MAUNSELL, and P. LENNIE, 1990. Coding of image contrast in central visual pathways of the macaque monkey. *Vision Res.* 30:1–10.

SENGPIEL, F., R. J. BADDELEY, T. C. FREEMAN, R. HARRAD, and C. BLAKEMORE, 1998. Different mechanisms underlie three inhibitory phenomena in cat area 17. *Vision Res.* 38:2067–2080.

SENGPIEL, F., and C. BLAKEMORE, 1994. Interocular control of neuronal responsiveness in cat visual cortex. *Nature* 368:847–850.

SENGPIEL, F., C. BLAKEMORE, and R. HARRAD, 1995. Interocular suppression in the primary visual cortex: A possible neural basis of binocular rivalry. *Vision Res.* 35:179–196.

SHAPLEY, R. M., and C. ENROTH-CUGELL, 1984. Visual adaptation and retinal gain controls. *Prog. Ret. Res.* 3:263–346.

SHAPLEY, R. M., and J. D. VICTOR, 1978. The effect of contrast on the transfer properties of cat retinal ganglion cells. *J. Physiol.* 285:275–298.

SHAPLEY, R. M., and J. VICTOR, 1981. How the contrast gain modifies the frequency responses of cat retinal ganglion cells. *J. Physiol. (Lond.)* 318:161–179.

SHERMAN, S. M., and R. W. GUILLERY, 1998. On the actions that one nerve cell can have on another: Distinguishing "drivers" from "modulators." *Proc. Natl. Acad. Sci. U.S.A.* 95:7121–7126.

SILLITO, A. M., J. CUDEIRO, and P. C. MURPHY, 1993. Orientation sensitive elements in the corticofugal influence on centre-surround interactions in the dorsal lateral geniculate nucleus. *Exp. Brain Res.* 93:6–16.

SILLITO, A. M., K. L. GRIEVE, H. E. JONES, J. CUDEIRO, and J. DAVIS, 1995. Visual cortical mechanisms detecting focal orientation discontinuities. *Nature* 378:492–496.

SINGER, W., and O. D. CREUTZFELDT, 1970. Reciprocal lateral inhibition of on- and off-center neurones in the lateral geniculate body of the cat. *Exp. Brain Res.* 10:311–330.

SINGER, W., E. POPPEL, and O. CREUTZFELDT, 1972. Inhibitory interaction in the cat's lateral geniculate nucleus. *Exp. Brain Res.* 14:210–226.

SOLOMON, S. G., A. J. WHITE, and P. R. MARTIN, 2002. Extraclassical receptive field properties of parvocellular, magnocellular, and koniocellular cells in the primate lateral geniculate nucleus. *J. Neurosci.* 22:338–349.

SOMERS, D. C., E. V. TODOROV, A. G. SIAPAS, L. J. TOTH, D. S. KIM, and M. SUR, 1998. A local circuit approach to understanding integration of long-range inputs in primary visual cortex. *Cereb. Cortex* 8:204–217.

SPITZER, H., and S. HOCHSTEIN, 1988. Complex-cell receptive field models. *Prog. Neurobiol.* 31:285–309.

SZULBORSKI, R. G., and L. A. PALMER, 1990. The two-dimensional spatial structure of nonlinear subunits in the receptive fields of complex cells. *Vision Res.* 30:249–254.

TOURYAN, J., B. LAU, and Y. DAN, 2002. Isolation of relevant visual features from random stimuli for cortical complex cells. *J. Neurosci.* 22:10811–10818.

TROY, J. B., D. L. BOHNSACK, and L. C. DILLER, 1999. Spatial properties of the cat X-cell receptive field as a function of mean light level. *Vis. Neurosci.* 16:1089–1104.

TROY, J. B., and C. ENROTH-CUGELL, 1993. X and Y ganglion cells inform the cat's brain about contrast in the retinal image. *Exp. Brain Res.* 93:383–390.

TSODYKS, M. V., and H. MARKRAM, 1997. The neural code between neocortical pyramidal neurons depends on neurotransmitter release probability. *Proc. Natl. Acad. Sci. U.S.A.* 94:719–723.

VICTOR, J., 1987. The dynamics of the cat retinal X cell centre. *J. Physiol. (Lond.)* 386:219–246.

VICTOR, J., and R. SHAPLEY, 1980. A method of nonlinear analysis in the frequency domain. *Biophys. J.* 29:459–484.

WALKER, G. A., I. OHZAWA, and R. D. FREEMAN, 1998. Binocular cross-orientation suppression in the cat's striate cortex. *J. Neurophysiol.* 79:227–239.

WALKER, G. A., I. OHZAWA, and R. D. FREEMAN, 1999. Asymmetric suppression outside the classical receptive field of the visual cortex. *J. Neurosci.* 19:10536–10553.

WALKER, G. A., I. OHZAWA, and R. D. FREEMAN, 2002. Disinhibition outside receptive fields in the visual cortex. *J. Neurosci.* 22:5659–5668.

WALRAVEN, J., C. ENROTH-CUGELL, D. C. HOOD, D. I. A. MACLEOD, and J. SCHNAPF, 1990. The control of visual sensitivity. In *Visual Perception: The Neurophysiological Foundations*, L. Spillman and J. S. Werner, eds. San Diego, Calif.: Academic Press.

23 Characterization of Neural Responses with Stochastic Stimuli

EERO P. SIMONCELLI, LIAM PANINSKI, JONATHAN PILLOW, AND
ODELIA SCHWARTZ

ABSTRACT We provide a conceptual overview of two recently developed methodologies for quantitative characterization of sensory neural response properties from extracellular spiking data. Both rely on the use of stochastic stimuli, and both assume a response model with an initial linear stage that serves to reduce the dimensionality of the stimulus space. They differ primarily in their description of spike generation: One family of methods assumes an inhomogeneous Poisson model for spike generation, and the other assumes a generalized form of integrate-and-fire model. We show simulated examples to illustrate procedures for estimation of model parameters from data and discuss the constraints on stimulus design and convergence as a function of the amount of data collected.

A fundamental goal of sensory systems neuroscience is the characterization of the functional relationship between environmental stimuli and neural response. The purpose of such a characterization is to elucidate the computation being performed by the system. Qualitatively, this notion is exemplified by the concept of the receptive field, a quasi-linear description of a neuron's response properties that has dominated sensory neuroscience for the past 50 years. Receptive fields are typically determined by measuring responses to a highly restricted set of stimuli, parameterized by one or a few parameters. These stimuli are typically chosen both because they are known to produce strong responses and because they are easy to generate using available technology.

Although such experiments are responsible for much of what we know about the tuning properties of sensory neurons, they usually do not provide a complete characterization of neural response. The fact that a cell is tuned for a particular parameter or selective for a particular input feature does not necessarily tell us how it will respond to an arbitrary stimulus. Furthermore, we have no systematic method of knowing which particular stimulus parameters are likely to govern the response of a given cell, and thus it is difficult to design an experiment to probe neurons whose response properties are not at least partially known in advance.

This chapter provides an overview of some recently developed characterization methods. In general, the ingredients of the problem are (1) the selection of a set of experimental stimuli, (2) the selection of a model of response, and (3) identifying a procedure for fitting (estimation) of the model. We discuss solutions to this problem that combine stochastic stimuli with models based on an initial linear filtering stage that serves to reduce the dimensionality of the stimulus space. We begin by describing classic reverse correlation in this context, and then discuss several recent generalizations that increase the power and flexibility of this basic method.

Reverse correlation

More than 30 years ago, a number of authors applied techniques generally known as white noise analysis to the characterization of neural systems (e.g., deBoer and Kuyper, 1968; Marmarelis and Naka, 1972). There has been a resurgence of interest in these techniques, partly due to the development of computer hardware and software capable of both real-time random stimulus generation and computationally intensive statistical analysis. In the most commonly used form of this analysis, known as reverse correlation, one computes the spike-triggered average (STA) by averaging stimulus blocks preceding a spike:

$$\hat{s} = \frac{1}{N} \sum_{i=1}^{N} \vec{s}_i$$

where the vector $\vec{s}_i$ represents the stimulus block preceding the ith spike. The procedure is illustrated for discretized stimuli in figure 23.1. The STA is generally interpreted as a representation of the receptive field in that it represents the "preferred" stimulus of the cell. White noise analysis has been widely used in studying auditory neurons (e.g., Eggermont, Johannesma, and Aertsen, 1983). In the visual system, spike-triggered averaging has been used to characterize retinal ganglion cells (e.g., Sakai and Naka, 1987;

EERO P. SIMONCELLI, LIAM PANINSKI, and JONATHAN PILLOW Center for Neural Science and Courant Institute of Mathematical Sciences, New York University, N.Y.
ODELIA SCHWARTZ The Salk Institute for Biological Studies, La Jolla, Calif.

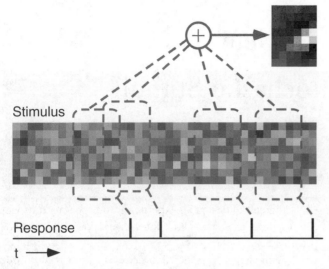

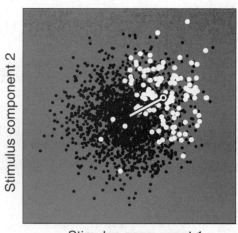

FIGURE 23.1 Two alternative illustrations of the reverse correlation procedure. *Left:* Discretized stimulus sequence and observed neural response (spike train). On each time step, the stimulus consists of an array of randomly chosen values (eight, for this example), corresponding to the intensities of a set of individual pixels, bars, or any other fixed spatial patterns. The neural response at any particular moment in time is assumed to be completely determined by the stimulus segment that occurred during a prespecified interval in the past. In this figure, the segment covers six time steps, and lags three time steps behind the current time (to account for response latency). The spike-triggered ensemble consists of the set of segments associated with spikes. The spike-triggered average (STA) is constructed by averaging these stimulus segments (and subtracting off the average over the full set of stimulus segments).

Right: Geometric (vector space) interpretation of the STA. Each stimulus segment corresponds to a point in a d-dimensional space (in this example, $d = 48$) whose axes correspond to stimulus values (e.g., pixel intensities) during the interval. For illustration purposes, the scatter plot shows only two of the 48 axes. The spike-triggered stimulus segments (white points) constitute a subset of all stimulus segments presented (black points). The STA, indicated by the line in the diagram, corresponds to the difference between the mean (center of mass) of the spike-triggered ensemble and the mean of the raw stimulus ensemble. Note that the interpretation of this representation of the stimuli is only sensible under Poisson spike generation; the scatter plot depiction implies that the probability of spiking depends only on the position in the stimulus space. (See color plate 10.)

Meister, Pine, and Baylor, 1994), lateral geniculate neurons (e.g., Reid and Alonso, 1995), and simple cells in primary visual cortex (V1) (e.g., Jones and Palmer, 1987; McLean and Palmer, 1989; DeAngelis, Ohzawa, and Freeman, 1993).

MODEL CHARACTERIZATION WITH SPIKE-TRIGGERED AVERAGING In order to interpret the STA more precisely, we can ask what model it can be used to characterize. The classic answer to this question comes from nonlinear systems analysis[1]: The STA provides an estimate of the first (linear) term in a polynomial series expansion of the system response function. If the system is truly linear, then the STA provides a complete characterization. It is well known, however, that neural responses are not linear. Even if one describes the neural response in terms of mean spike rate, this typically exhibits nonlinear behavior with respect to the input signal, such as thresholding and saturation. Thus, the first term of a Wiener–Volterra series, as estimated with the STA, will typically not provide a full description of neural response. One can, of course, include higher-order terms in the series expansion. But each successive term in the expansion requires a substantial increase in the amount of experimental data. And limiting the analysis only to the first- and second-order terms, for example, still may not be sufficient

to characterize nonlinear behaviors common to neural responses.

Fortunately, it is possible to use the STA as a first step in fitting a model that can describe neural response more parsimoniously than a series expansion. Specifically, suppose that the response is generated in a cascade of three stages: (1) a linear function of the stimulus over a recent period of time, (2) an instantaneous (also known as static or memoryless) nonlinear transformation, and (3) a Poisson spike generation process whose instantaneous firing rate comes from the output of the previous stage. That is, the probability of observing a spike during any small time window is a nonlinear function of a linear-filtered version of the stimulus. This model is illustrated in figure 23.2, and we will refer to it as a linear-nonlinear-Poisson (LNP) model. The third stage, which essentially amounts to an assumption that the generation of spikes depends only on the recent stimulus, and not on the history of previous spike times, often is not stated explicitly but is critical to the analysis.

Under suitable conditions on the stimulus distribution and the nonlinearity, the STA produces an estimate of the linear filter in the first stage of the LNP model (see Chichilnisky, 2001, for overview and additional references). The result is most easily understood geometrically, as depicted in figure

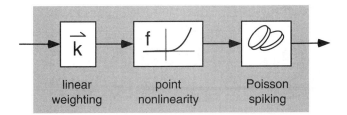

| linear | point | Poisson |
| weighting | nonlinearity | spiking |

FIGURE 23.2 Block diagram of the linear-nonlinear-Poisson (LNP) model. On each time step, the components of the stimulus vector are linearly combined using a weight vector, $\vec{k}$. This response of this linear filter is then passed through a nonlinear function $f()$, whose output determines the instantaneous firing rate of a Poisson spike generator.

23.1. Assume the stimulus is discretized, and that the response of the cell at any moment in time depends only on the values within a fixed-length time interval preceding that time. A typical stimulus would be the intensities of a set of pixels covering some spatial region of a video display, for every temporal video frame over the time interval (left panel in figure 23.1). In this case the stimulus segment presented over the interval preceding a spike corresponds to a vector containing d components, one for the intensity of each pixel in each frame. The vectors of all stimulus segments presented during an experiment may be represented as a set of points in a d-dimensional stimulus space, as illustrated in figure 23.1. We will refer to this as the *raw stimulus ensemble*. This ensemble is under the control of the experimenter, and the samples are typically chosen randomly according to some probability distribution. A statistically *white* ensemble corresponds to the situation in which the components of the stimulus vector are uncorrelated. If in addition the density of each component is Gaussian, and all have the same variance, then the full d-dimensional distribution will be spherically symmetrical.

In a model with Poisson spike generation, the probability of a spike occurring after a given stimulus block depends only on the content of that block, or equivalently, on the position of the corresponding vector in d-dimensional space. From an experimental perspective, this means that the distribution of the spike-triggered stimulus ensemble indicates which regions of the stimulus space are more likely (or less likely) to elicit spikes. More specifically, for each region of the stimulus space, the ratio of the frequency of occurrence of spike-triggered stimuli to that of raw stimuli gives the instantaneous firing rate. From this description, it might seem that one could simply count the number of spikes and stimuli in each region (i.e., compute multidimensional histograms of the binned raw and spike-triggered stimuli), and take the quotient to compute the firing rate. But this course is impractical, due to the so-called "curse of dimensionality": the amount of data needed to sufficiently fill the histogram bins in a d-dimensional space grows exponentially

with d. Thus, one cannot hope to compute such a firing rate function for a space of more than a few dimensions.

The assumption of an LNP model allows us to avoid this severe data requirement. In particular, the linear stage of the model effectively collapses the entire d-dimensional space onto a single axis, as illustrated in figure 23.3. The STA provides an estimate of this axis, under the assumption that the raw stimulus distribution is spherically symmetrical[2] (e.g., Chichilnisky, 2001; Theunissen et al., 2001). Once the linear filter has been estimated, we may compute its response and then examine the relationship between the histograms of the raw and spike-triggered ensembles within this one-dimensional space. Specifically, for each value of the linear response, the nonlinear function in the LNP model may be estimated as the quotient of the frequency of spike occurrences to that of stimulus occurrences (see figure 23.3). Because this quotient is taken between two one-dimensional histograms (as opposed to d-dimensional histograms), the data requirements for accurate estimation are greatly reduced. Note also that the nonlinearity can be arbitrarily complicated (even discontinuous). The only constraint is that it must produce a change in the mean of the spike-triggered ensemble, as compared with the original stimulus ensemble. Thus, the interpretation of reverse correlation in the context of the LNP model is a significant departure from the Wiener–Volterra series expansion, in which even a simple sigmoidal nonlinearity would require the estimation of many terms for accurate characterization.

The reverse correlation approach relies less on prior knowledge of the neural response properties in that it explores a wide range of visual input stimuli in a relatively short amount of time, and it can produce a complete characterization in the form of the LNP model (see Chichilnisky, 2001, for further discussion). But clearly, the method can fail if the neural response does not fit the assumptions of the model. For example, if the neural nonlinearity and the stimulus distribution interact in such a way that the mean of the raw stimuli and the mean of the spike-triggered stimuli do not differ, the STA will be zero, thus failing to provide an estimate of the linear stage of the model. Even if the reverse correlation procedure succeeds in estimating the model parameters, the model might not provide a good characterization. Specifically, the true neural response may not be restricted to a single direction in the stimulus space, or the spike generation may not be well described as a Poisson process. In the following sections, we describe some extensions of reverse correlation to handle these two types of model failure.

Extension to multiple dimensions with STC

The STA analysis relies on changes in the mean of the spike-triggered stimulus ensemble to estimate the linear stage of

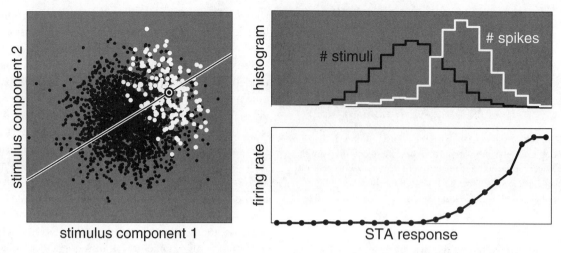

FIGURE 23.3 Simulated characterization of an LNP model using reverse correlation. The simulation is based on a sequence of 20,000 stimuli, with a response containing 950 spikes. *Left:* The STA (black-and-white "target") provides an estimate of the linear weighting vector, $\vec{k}$ (see also figure 23.1). The linear response to any particular stimulus corresponds to the position of that stimulus along the axis defined by $\vec{k}$ (line). *Right, top:* Raw (black) and spike-triggered (white) histograms of the linear (STA) responses. *Right, bottom:* The quotient of the spike-triggered and raw histograms gives an estimate of the nonlinearity that generates the firing rate.

an LNP model. This linear stage corresponds to a single filter that responds to a single direction in the stimulus space. But many neurons exhibit behaviors that are not well described by this model. For example, the "energy model" of complex cells in primary visual cortex posits the existence of two linear filters (an even- and odd-symmetrical pair), whose rectified responses are then combined (Adelson and Bergen, 1985). Not only does this model use two linear filters, but the symmetry of the rectifying nonlinearity means that the STA will be zero, thus providing no information about the linear stage of the model. In this particular case, a variety of second-order interaction analyses have been developed to recover the two filters (e.g., Emerson et al., 1987; Szulborski and Palmer, 1990; Emerson, Bergen, and Adelson, 1992).

We would like to be able to characterize this type of multiple filter model. Specifically, we would like to recover the filters, as well as the nonlinear function by which their responses are combined. The classic nonlinear systems analysis approach to this problem (Marmarelis and Marmarelis, 1978; Korenberg, Sakai, and Naka, 1989) proceeds by estimating the second-order term in the Wiener series expansion, which describes the response as a weighted sum over all pairwise products of components in the stimulus vector. The weights of this sum (the second-order Wiener kernel) may be estimated from the spike-triggered *covariance* (STC) matrix, computed as a sum of outer products of the spike-triggered stimulus vectors with the STA subtracted:[3]

$$C = \frac{1}{\mathcal{N}-1} \sum_{i=1}^{N} (\vec{s}_i - \hat{s}) \cdot (\vec{s}_i - \hat{s})^T$$

This second-order Wiener series gives a quadratic model for neural responses, and thus remains ill-equipped to accurately model sharply asymmetrical or saturating nonlinear-

ities. As in the case of the STA, however, the STC may be used as a starting point for estimation of another model that may be more relevant in describing some neural responses. In particular, one can assume that the neural response is again determined by an LNP cascade model (see figure 23.2), but that the initial linear stage now is multidimensional. That is, the response comes from applying a small set of linear filters, followed by Poisson spike generation, with firing rate determined by some nonlinear combination of the filter outputs.

Under suitable conditions on the stimulus distribution and the nonlinear stage, the STC may be used to estimate the linear stage (de Ruyter van Steveninck and Bialek, 1988; Brenner, Bialek, and de Ruyter van Steveninck, 2000; Paninski, 2003). Again, the idea is most directly explained geometrically: we seek those directions in the stimulus space along which the *variance* of the spike-triggered ensemble differs from that of the raw ensemble. Loosely speaking, an increase in variance (with no change in the mean) indicates a stimulus dimension that is excitatory, and a decrease in variance indicates suppression. The advantage of this description is that variance analysis in multiple dimensions is very well understood mathematically. The surface representing the variance (standard deviation) of the spike-triggered stimulus ensemble consists of those vectors $\vec{v}$ satisfying $\vec{v}^T C^{-1} \vec{v} = 1$. This surface is an ellipsoid, and the principal axes of this ellipsoid may be recovered using standard eigenvector techniques (i.e., principal component analysis). Specifically, the eigenvectors of C represent the principal axes of the ellipsoid, and the corresponding eigenvalues represent the variances along each of these axes.[4]

Thus, by determining which variances are significantly different from those of the underlying raw stimulus ensemble, the STC may be used to estimate the set of axes (i.e., linear filters) from which the neural response is derived. As with the STA, the second nonlinear stage of the model may then be estimated by looking at the spiking response as a function of the responses of these linear filters. The correctness of the STC-based estimator can be guaranteed if (but only if) the stimuli are drawn from a Gaussian distribution (Paninski, 2003), a stronger condition than the spherical symmetry required for the STA. Spike-triggered covariance analysis has been used to determine both excitatory (de Ruyter van Steveninck and Bialek, 1988; Brenner, Bialek, and de Ruyter van Steveninck, 2000; Touryan, Lau, and Dan, 2002; Rust et al., 2004) as well as suppressive (Schwartz, Chichilnisky, and Simoncelli, 2002; Rust et al., 2004) response properties of visual neurons. Here we will consider two simulation examples to illustrate the concept, and to provide some idea of the type of nonlinear behaviors that can be revealed using this analysis.

The first example, shown in figure 23.4, is a simulation of a standard V1 complex cell model (see also simulations in Sakai and Tanaka, 2000). The model is constructed from two space-time-oriented linear receptive fields, one symmetrical and the other antisymmetrical (Adelson and Bergen, 1985). The linear responses of these two filters are squared and summed, and the resulting signal then determines the instantaneous firing rate:

$$g(\vec{s}) = r\left[\left(\vec{k}_1 \cdot \vec{s}\right)^2 + \left(\vec{k}_2 \cdot \vec{s}\right)^2\right]$$

The recovered eigenvalues indicate that two directions within this space have substantially higher variance than the others. The eigenvectors associated with these two eigenvalues correspond to the two filters in the model.[5] The raw- and spike-triggered stimulus ensembles may then be filtered with these two eigenvectors, and the two-dimensional nonlinear function that governs firing rate corresponds to the quotient of the two histograms, analogous to the one-dimensional example shown in figure 23.1. Similar pairs of excitatory axes have been obtained from STC analysis of V1 cells in cat (Touryan, Lau, and Dan, 2002) and monkey (Rust et al., 2004).

As a second example, we chose a simplified version of a divisive gain control model, as has been used to describe nonlinear properties of neurons in primary visual cortex (Albrecht and Geisler, 1991; Heeger, 1992). Specifically, our model neuron's instantaneous firing rate is governed by one excitatory filter and one divisively suppressive filter:

$$g(\vec{s}) = r \frac{1 + \left(\vec{k}_1 \cdot \vec{s}\right)^2}{1 + \left(\vec{k}_1 \cdot \vec{s}\right)^2 \Big/ 2 + \left(\vec{k}_2 \cdot \vec{s}\right)^2}$$

The simulation results are shown in figure 23.5. The recovered eigenvalue distribution reveals one large-variance axis and one small-variance axis, corresponding to the two filters $\vec{k}_1$ and $\vec{k}_2$, respectively. After projecting the stimuli onto these

two axes, the two-dimensional nonlinearity is estimated, and reveals an approximately saddle-shaped function, indicating the interaction between the excitatory and suppressive signals. Similar suppressive filters have been obtained from STC analysis of retinal ganglion cells (both salamander and monkey) (Schwartz, Chichilnisky, and Simoncelli, 2002) and simple and complex cells in monkey V1 (Rust et al., 2004). In these cases, a combined STA/STC analysis was used to recover multiple linear filters. The number of recovered filters was typically large enough that direct estimation of the nonlinearity (i.e., by dividing the spike-triggered histogram by the raw histogram) was not feasible. As such, the nonlinear stage was estimated by fitting specific parametric models on top of the output of the linear filters.

Experimental caveats

In addition to the limitations of the LNP model, it is important to understand the tradeoffs and potential problems that may arise in using STA/STC characterization procedures. We provide a brief overview of these issues, which can be quite complex. (see Rieke et al., 1997; Chichilnisky, 2001; and Paninski, 2003, for further description).

The accuracy of STA/STC filter estimates depends on three elements: (1) the dimensionality of the stimulus space, (2) the number of spikes collected, and (3) the strength of the response signal, relative to the standard deviation of the raw stimulus ensemble.[6] The first two of these interact in a simple way: the quality of estimates increases as a function of the ratio of the number of spikes to the number of stimulus dimensions. Thus, the pursuit of more accurate estimates leads to a simultaneous demand for more spikes and reduced stimulus dimensionality.

These demands must be balanced against several opposing constraints. The collection of a large number of spikes is limited by the realities of single-cell electrophysiology. Experimental recordings are restricted in duration, especially since the response properties need to remain stable and consistent throughout the recording. On the other hand, reducing the stimulus dimensionality is also problematic. One of the most widely touted advantages of white noise characterization over traditional experiments is that the stimuli can cover a broader range of visual input stimuli, and these randomly selected stimuli are less likely to induce artifacts or experimental bias than a set that is hand-selected by the experimenter.

In practice, however, white noise characterization still requires the experimenter to place restrictions on the stimulus set. For visual neurons, even with stimuli composed in the typical fashion from individual pixels, one must choose the spatial size and temporal duration of these pixels. If the pixels are too small, then not only will the stimulus dimensionality be large (in order to fully cover the spatial and

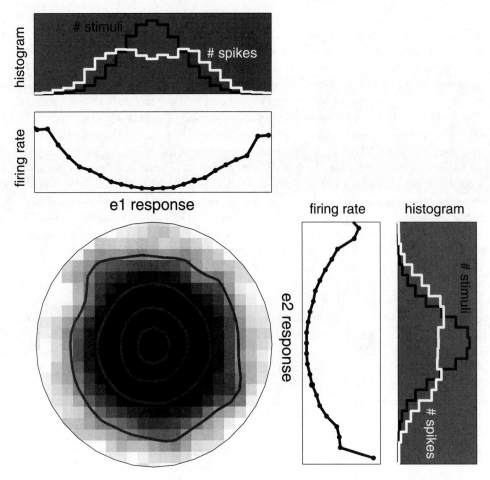

FIGURE 23.4 Simulated characterization of a particular LNP model using spike-triggered covariance (STC). In this model, the Poisson spike generator is driven by the sum of the squares of two oriented linear filter responses. As in figure 23.1, filters are 6 × 8, and thus live in a 48-dimensional space. The simulation is based on a sequence of 50,000 raw stimuli, with a response containing 4500 spikes. *Top left:* Simulated raw and spike-triggered stimulus ensembles, viewed in a two-dimensional subspace that illustrates the model behavior. The covariance of these ensembles within this two-dimensional space is represented geometrically by an ellipse that is 3 SD from the origin in all directions. The raw stimulus ensemble has equal variance in all directions, as indicated by the black circle. The spike-triggered ensemble is elongated in one direction, as represented by the white ellipse. *Top right:* Eigenvalue analysis of the simulated data. The principal axes of the covariance ellipse correspond to the eigenvectors of the spike-triggered covari-ance matrix, and the associated eigenvalues indicate the variance of the spike-triggered stimulus ensemble along each of these axes. The plot shows the full set of 48 eigenvalues, sorted in descending order. Two of these are substantially larger than the others and indicate the presences of two axes in the stimulus space along which the model responds. The others correspond to stimulus directions that the model ignores. Also shown are three example eigenvectors (6 × 8 linear filters). *Bottom, one-dimensional plots:* Spike-triggered and raw histograms of responses of the two high-variance linear filters, along with the nonlinear firing rate functions estimated from their quotient (see figure 23.3). *Bottom, two-dimensional plot:* The quotient of the two-dimensional spike-triggered and raw histograms pro-vides an estimate of the two-dimensional nonlinear firing rate func-tion. This is shown as a circular-cropped gray-scale image, where intensity is proportional to firing rate. Superimposed contours indicate four different response levels. (See color plate 11.)

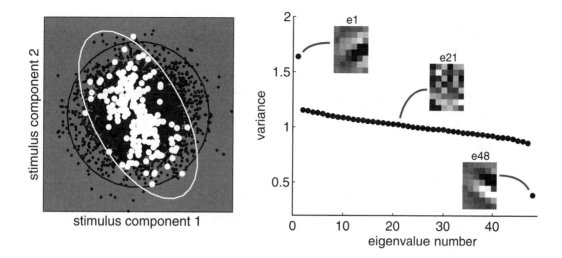

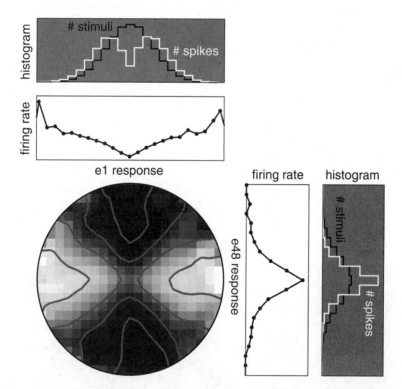

FIGURE 23.5 Characterization of a simulated LNP model, constructed from the squared response of one linear filter divided by the sum of the squares of its own response and the response of another filter. The simulation is based on a sequence of 200,000 raw stimuli, with a response containing 8000 spikes. See text and caption of figure 23.4 for details. (See color plate 12.)

temporal "receptive field"), but the effective stimulus contrast that reaches the neuron will be quite low, resulting in a low spike rate. Both of these effects will reduce the accuracy of the estimated filters. On the other hand, if the pixels are too large, then the recovered linear filters will be quite coarse (since they are constructed from blocks that are the size of the pixels). More generally, one can use stimuli that provide a better basis for receptive field description, and that are more likely to elicit strong neural responses, by defining them in terms of parameters that are more relevant than pixel intensities. Examples include stimuli restricted in spatial frequency (Ringach, Sapiro, and Shapley, 1997) and stimuli defined in terms of velocity (de Ruyter van Steveninck and Bialek, 1988; Bair, Cavanaugh, and Movshon, 1997; Brenner, Bialek, and de Ruyter van Steveninck, 2000).

Although the choice of stimuli plays a critical role in controlling the accuracy (variance) of the filter estimates, the probability distribution from which the stimuli are drawn must be chosen carefully to avoid bias in the estimates. For example, with the single-filter LNP model, the stimulus distribution must be spherically symmetrical in order to guarantee that the STA gives an unbiased estimate of the linear filter (e.g., Chichilnisky, 2001). Figure 23.6 shows two simulations of an LNP model with a simple sigmoidal nonlinearity, each demonstrating that the use of nonspherical stimulus distributions can lead to poor estimates of the linear stage. The first example shows a "sparse noise" experiment, in which the stimulus at each time step lies along one of the axes. For example, many authors have characterized visual neurons using images with only a single white or black pixel among a background of gray pixels in each frame (e.g., Jones

and Palmer, 1987). As shown in the figure, even a simple nonlinearity (in this case, a sigmoid) can result in an STA that is heavily biased.[7] The second example uses stimuli in which each component is drawn from a uniform distribution, which produces an estimate biased toward the "corner" of the space. The use of non-Gaussian distributions (e.g., uniform or binary) for white noise stimuli is quite common, as the samples are easy to generate and the resulting stimuli can have higher contrast and thus produce higher average spike rates. In practice, their use has been justified by assuming that the linear filter is smooth relative to the pixel size/duration (e.g., Chichilnisky, 2001).

Although the generalization of the LNP model to the multidimensional case substantially increases its power and flexibility, the STC method can fail in a manner analogous to that described for the STA. Specifically, if the neural response varies in a particular direction within the stimulus space, but the variance of the spike-triggered ensemble does not differ from the raw ensemble in that direction, then the method will not be able to recover that direction. In addition, the STC method is more susceptible to biases caused by statistical idiosyncrasies in the stimulus distribution than is the STA. These concerns have motivated the development of estimators that are guaranteed to converge to the correct linear axes under much more general conditions (Paninski, 2003; Sharpee, Rust, and Bialek, 2003). The basic idea is quite simple: instead of relying on a particular statistical moment (e.g., mean or variance) for comparison of the spike-triggered and raw stimulus distributions, one can use a more general comparison function that can identify virtually any difference between the two distributions. A natural

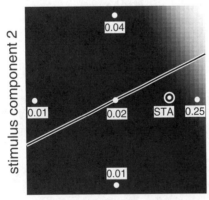 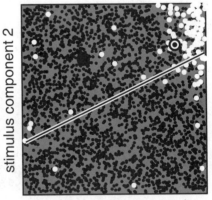

FIGURE 23.6 Simulations of an LNP model demonstrating bias in the STA for two different nonspherical stimulus distributions. The linear stage of the model neuron corresponds to an oblique axis (line in both panels), and the firing rate function is a sigmoidal nonlinearity (firing rate corresponds to intensity of the underlying grayscale image in the left panel). In both panels, the black-and-white target indicates the recovered STA. *Left:* Simulated response to sparse noise. The plot shows a two-dimensional subspace of a

10-dimensional stimulus space. Each stimulus vector contains a single element with a value of ±1, while all other elements are zero. Numbers indicate the firing rate for each of the possible stimulus vectors. The STA is strongly biased toward the horizontal axis. *Right:* Simulated response of the same model to uniformly distributed noise. The STA is now biased toward the corner. Note that in both examples, the estimate will not converge to the correct answer, regardless of the amount of data collected.

choice for such a function is information theoretic: one can compare the *mutual information* between a set of filter responses and the probability of a spike occurring. The resulting estimator is more computationally expensive, but has been shown to be more accurate in several different simulation examples (Paninski, 2003; Sharpee, Rust, and Bialek, 2003).

Non-Poisson spike generation

The LNP models described in the preceding sections provide an alternative to the classic Wiener series expansion, but they still assume that the information a neuron carries about the stimulus is contained in its instantaneous firing rate. These models thus ignore any history dependence in the spike train that might result from the dynamics underlying spike generation, such as the refractory period. A number of authors have demonstrated that these Poisson assumptions do not accurately capture the statistics of neural spike trains (Berry and Meister, 1998; Reich, Victor, and Knight, 1998; Keat et al., 2001). It is therefore important to ask: (1) How do realistic spiking mechanisms affect the LNP characterization of a neuron? and (2) Is it possible to extend the characterization methods described above to incorporate more realistic spiking dynamics?

The first of these questions has been addressed using simulations and mathematical analysis of neural models with both Hodgkin–Huxley and leaky integrate-and-fire spike generation (Agüera y Arcas, Fairhall, and Bialek, 2001; Paninski, Lau, and Reyes, 2003; Pillow and Simoncelli, 2003; Agüera y Arcas and Fairhall, 2003). In these cases, spike generation nonlinearities can interfere with the tem-

poral properties of the linear filters estimated with STA or STC analysis. Figure 23.7 shows an example, using a model in which a single linear filter drives a non-Poisson spike generator. In this case, the STA provides a biased estimate of the true linear filter. Moreover, the history-dependent effects of spike generation are not confined to a single direction of the stimulus space. Even though the model response is generated from the output of a single linear filter, STC analysis reveals additional relevant directions in the stimulus space. Thus, describing non-Poisson responses with an LNP model results in a high-dimensional characterization, when a low-dimensional model with a more appropriate spike generator would suffice.

A recently proposed approach to the problem of spike-history dependence is to perform STA/STC analysis using only isolated spikes, or those that are widely separated in time from other spikes (Agüera y Arcas, Fairhall, and Bialek, 2001; Agüera y Arcas and Fairhall, 2003). This has the advantageous effect of eliminating refractory and other short-term effects from the responses being analyzed, but as a consequence it does not characterize the history dependence of the spikes. Furthermore, the discarded spikes, which may constitute a substantial proportion of the total, correspond to periods of rapid firing and thus seem likely to carry potent information about a neuron's selectivity.

An alternative is to modify the LNP description to incorporate more realistic spike generation effects, and to develop characterization procedures for this model. One proposed technique incorporates a "recovery function" that modulates the spike probability following the occurrence of each spike (Miller, 1985; Berry and Meister, 1998; Kass and Ventura, 2001). Specifically, the instantaneous Poisson firing rate is set

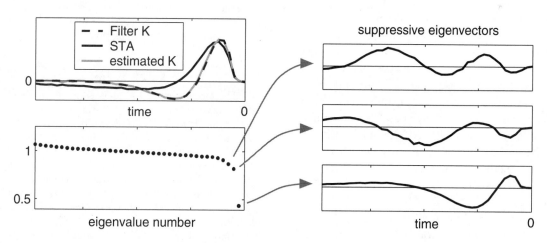

FIGURE 23.7 Simulated spike-triggered analysis of a neuron with noisy, leaky integrate-and-fire (NLIF) spike generation. Input is filtered with a single linear filter (K), followed by NLIF spiking. A purely temporal filter was selected because the effects of non-Poisson spike generation manifest themselves in the temporal domain. *Upper left:* Linear filter of the model (dashed line), a 32-sample function chosen to resemble the temporal impulse response of a macaque retinal ganglion cell. Also shown are the STA computed from a simulated spike train (solid), and the linear filter estimated using maximum likelihood (Pillow, Paninski, and Simoncelli, 2004). *Lower left:* Eigenvalues computed from the spike-triggered covariance of the simulated spike train. *Right:* Linear filters (eigenvectors) associated with the three smallest eigenvalues.

by the product of the output of an LN stage and this recovery function. The resulting model can produce both absolute and relative refractory effects.

Another alternative is to use an explicit parametric model of spike generation and to develop estimation techniques for front-end stimulus selectivity in conjunction with the parameters of the spike generator (e.g., Keat et al., 2001; Pillow, Paninski, and Simoncelli, 2004). As an example, consider the estimation of a two-stage model consisting of a linear filter followed by a noisy, leaky integrate-and-fire (NLIF) spike generator. The stimulus dependence of this model is determined by the linear filter, but the N and P stages of the LNP model are replaced by the NLIF mechanism. Although direct STA analysis cannot recover the linear filter in this model, it is possible to use a maximum likelihood estimator to recover both the linear filter and the parameters of the spike generator (threshold voltage, reset voltage, leak conductance, and noise variance) (Pillow, Paninski, and Simoncelli, 2004). The estimation procedure can start from the STA as an initial guess for the true filter, and ascend the likelihood function to obtain optimal estimates of the filter and the NLIF parameters. This procedure is computationally efficient and is guaranteed to converge to the correct answer. A simulated example is shown in figure 23.7. The method provides a characterization of both the spatiotemporal filter that drives neural response and the nonlinear biophysical response properties that transform this drive into spike trains.

Discussion

We have described a set of techniques for characterizing the functional response properties of neurons using stochastic stimuli. We have relied throughout on an assumption that the response of the neuron is governed by an initial linear stage that serves to reduce the dimensionality of the stimulus space. Although this assumption may seem overly restrictive, it is important to realize that it is the fundamental ingredient that allows one to infer general response properties from measured responses to a relatively small number of stimuli. The linear stage is followed by a nonlinearity upon which we place fairly minimal constraints. We described two moment-based methods of estimating the linear stage, STA and STC, which are both conceptually elegant and efficient to calculate.

In addition to the assumption of an initial low-dimensional linear stage, there are two well-known potential drawbacks of these approaches. First, the techniques place fairly strong constraints on the set of stimuli that must be used in an experiment. There has been an increased interest in recent years in presenting naturalistic stimuli to neurons, so as to assess their behavior under normal operating conditions (e.g., Dan, Attick, and Reid, 1996;

Baddeley et al., 1998; Theunissen et al., 2001; Ringach, Hawken, and Shapley, 2002; Smyth et al., 2003). Analysis of such data is tricky, since naturalistic images are highly non-Gaussian (Field, 1987; Daugman, 1989), and, as described earlier, the basic STA/STC technique relies on a Gaussian stimulus distribution. Estimators based on information-theoretic measures, as described under Experimental Caveats, seem promising in this context because they place essentially no restriction on the stimulus ensemble.

A second drawback is that the assumption of Poisson spike generation provides a poor account of the spiking behavior of many neurons (Berry and Meister, 1998; Reich, Victor, and Knight, 1998; Keat et al., 2001). As discussed under Non-Poisson Spike Generation, STA/STC analysis of an LN model driving a more realistic spiking mechanism (e.g., integrate-and-fire or Hodgkin–Huxley) can lead to significant biases in the estimate of the linear stage. A number of techniques currently in development are attempting to address these issues.

Finally, we mention two interesting directions for future research. First, the techniques described here can be adapted for the analysis of multineuronal interactions (e.g., Nykamp, 2003). Such methods have been applied, for example, in visual cortex (Tsodyks et al., 1999), motor cortex (Paninski et al., 2004), and hippocampus (Harris et al., 2003). Second, it would be desirable to develop techniques that can be applied to a cascaded series of LNP stages. This will be essential for modeling responses in higher-order sensory areas, which are presumably constructed from more peripheral responses.

ACKNOWLEDGMENTS This work was funded by the Howard Hughes Medical Institute and the Sloan-Swartz Center for Theoretical Visual Neuroscience at New York University. Thanks to Brian Lau, Dario Ringach, Nicole Rust, and Brian Wandell for helpful comments on the manuscript.

NOTES

1. The formulation is due to Wiener (1958), based on earlier results by Volterra (1913). See Rieke and colleagues (1997) or Dayan and Abbott (2001) for reviews of application to neurons.

2. Technically, an elliptically symmetrical distribution is also acceptable. The stimuli are first transformed to a spherical distribution using a whitening operation, the STA is computed, and the result is transformed back to the original stimulus space.

3. An alternative method is to project, rather than subtract, the STA from the stimulus set (Schwartz, Chichilnisky, and Simoncelli, 2002; Rust et al., 2004).

4. More precisely, the *relative* variance between the spike-triggered and raw stimulus ensembles can be computed either by performing the eigenvector decomposition on the difference of the two covariance matrices (de Ruyter van Steveninck and Bialek, 1988; Brenner, Bialek, and de Ruyter van Steveninck, 2000), or by applying an initial whitening transformation to the raw stimuli before computing the STC (Schwartz, Chichilnisky, and Simoncelli, 2002; Rust et al., 2004). The latter is equivalent to solving for principal

axes of an ellipse that represents the ratio of spike-triggered and raw variances.

5. Technically, the recovered eigenvectors represent two orthogonal axes that span a subspace containing the two filters.

6. Technically, the response signal strength is defined as the STA magnitude, or in the case of STC to the square root of the difference between the eigenvalue and σ^2, the variance of the raw stimuli (Paninski, 2003).

7. Note, however, that the estimate will be unbiased in the case of a purely linear neuron, or of a halfwave-rectified linear neuron (Ringach, Sapiro, and Shapley, 1997).

REFERENCES

ADELSON, E. H., and J. R. BERGEN, 1985. Spatiotemporal energy models for the perception of motion. *J. Opt. Soc. Am. A* 2:284–299.

AGÜERA Y ARCAS, B., and A. L. FAIRHALL, 2003. What causes a neuron to spike? *Neural Comput.* 15:1789–1807.

AGÜERA Y ARCAS, B., A. L. FAIRHALL, and W. BIALEK, 2001. What can a single neuron compute? In *Advances in Neural Information Processing Systems (NIPS*00)*, vol. 13, T. K. Lean, T. G. Dietterich, and V. Tresp, eds. Cambridge, Mass.: MIT Press, pp. 75–81.

ALBRECHT, D. G., and W. S. GEISLER, 1991. Motion sensitivity and the contrast-response function of simple cells in the visual cortex. *Vis. Neurosci.* 7:531–546.

BADDELEY, R., L. F. ABBOTT, M. C. BOOTH, F. SENGPIEL, T. FREEMAN, E. A. WAKEMAN, and E. T. ROLLS, 1998. Responses of neurons in primary and inferior temporal visual cortices to natural scenes. *Proc. R. Soc. (Lond.) B* 264:1775–1783.

BAIR, W., J. R. CAVANAUGH, and J. A. MOVSHON, 1997. Reconstructing stimulus velocity from neuronal responses in area MT. In *Advances in Neural Information Processing Systems (NIPS*96)*, vol. 9, M. C. Mozer, M. I. Jordan, and T. Petsche, eds. Cambridge, Mass.: MIT Press, pp. 34–46.

BERRY, M., and M. MEISTER, 1998. Refractoriness and neural precision. *J. Neurosci.* 18:2200–2211.

BRENNER, N., W. BIALEK, and R. R. DE RUYTER VAN STEVENINCK, 2000. Adaptive rescaling maximizes information transmission. *Neuron* 26:695–702.

CHICHILNISKY, E. J., 2001. A simple white noise analysis of neuronal light responses. *Netw. Comput. Neural Systems* 12:199–213.

DAN, Y., J. J. ATICK, and R. C. REID, 1996. Efficient coding of natural scenes in the lateral geniculate nucleus: Experimental test of a computational theory. *J. Neurosci.* 16:3351–3362.

DAUGMAN, J. G., 1989. Entropy reduction and decorrelation in visual coding by oriented neural receptive fields. *IEEE Trans. Biomed. Eng.* 36:107–114.

DAYAN, P., and L. F. ABBOTT, 2001. *Theoretical Neuroscience.* Cambridge, Mass.: MIT Press.

DE RUYTER VAN STEVENINCK, R., and W. BIALEK, 1988. Coding and information transfer in short spike sequences. *Proc. R. Soc. (Lond.) B Biol. Sci.* 234:379–414.

DEANGELIS, G. C., I. OHZAWA, and R. D. FREEMAN, 1993. The spatiotemporal organization of simple cell receptive fields in the cat's striate cortex. II. Linearity of temporal and spatial summation. *J. Neurophysiol.* 69:1118–1135.

DEBOER, E., and P. KUYPER, 1968. Triggered correlation. *IEEE Trans. Biomed. Eng.* 15:169–179.

EGGERMONT, J. J., P. I. M. JOHANNESMA, and A. M. H. J. AERTSEN, 1983. Reverse-correlation methods in auditory research. *Q. Rev. Biophys.* 16:341–414.

EMERSON, R. C., J. R. BERGEN, and E. H. ADELSON, 1992. Directionally selective complex cells and the computation of motion energy in cat visual cortex. *Vision Res.* 32:203–218.

EMERSON, R. C., M. C. CITRON, W. J. VAUGHN, and S. A. KLEIN, 1987. Nonlinear directionally selective subunits in complex cells of cat striate cortex. *J. Neurophysiol.* 58:33–65.

FIELD, D. J., 1987. Relations between the statistics of natural images and the response properties of cortical cells. *J. Opt. Soc. Am. A* 4:2379–2394.

HARRIS, K. D., J. CSICSVARI, H. HIRASE, G. DRAGOI, and G. BUZSÁKI, 2003. Organization of cell assemblies in the hippocampus. *Nature* 424:552–556.

HEEGER, D. J., 1992. Normalization of cell responses in cat striate cortex. *Vis. Neurosci.* 9:181–198.

JONES, J. P., and L. A. PALMER, 1987. The two-dimensional spatial structure of simple receptive fields in cat striate cortex. *J. Neurophysiol.* 58:1187–1211.

KASS, R. E., and V. VENTURA, 2001. A spike-train probability model. *Neural Comput.* 13:1713–1720.

KEAT, J., P. REINAGEL, R. C. REID, and M. MEISTER, 2001. Predicting every spike: A model for the responses of visual neurons. *Neuron* 30:803–817.

KORENBERG, M. J., H. M. SAKAI, and K. I. NAKA, 1989. Dissection of neuron network in the catfish inner retina. III. Interpretation of spike kernels. *J. Neurophysiol.* 61:1110–1120.

MARMARELIS, P. Z., and V. Z. MARMARELIS, 1978. *Analysis of Physiological Systems: The White Noise Approach.* London: Plenum Press.

MARMARELIS, P. Z., and K. NAKA, 1972. White-noise analysis of a neuron chain: An application of the Wiener theory. *Science* 175:1276–1278.

MCLEAN, J., and L. A. PALMER, 1989. Contribution of linear spatiotemporal receptive field structure to velocity selectivity of simple cells in area 17 of cat. *Vision Res.* 29:675–679.

MEISTER, M., J. PINE, and D. A. BAYLOR, 1994. Multi-neuronal signals from the retina: Acquisition and analysis. *J. Neurosci. Meth.* 51:95–106.

MILLER, M. I., 1985. Algorithms for removing recovery-related distortion from auditory-nerve discharge patterns. *J. Acoust. Soc. Am.* 77:1452–1464.

NYKAMP, D., 2003. White noise analysis of coupled linear-nonlinear systems. *Siam J. Appl. Math.* 63:1208–1230.

PANINSKI, L., 2003. Convergence properties of some spike-triggered analysis techniques. *Netw. Comput. Neural Systems* 14:437–464.

PANINSKI, L., M. FELLOWS, S. SHOHAM, N. HATSOPOULOS, and J. DONOGHUE, 2004. Nonlinear population models for the encoding of dynamic hand position signals in MI. In *Neurocomputing.* Proceedings of a conference, Computational Neuroscience, Alicante, Spain, July 2003.

PANINSKI, L., B. LAU, and A. REYES, 2003. Noise-driven adaptation: In vitro and mathematical analysis. In *Neurocomputing*, vol. 52, pp. 877–883. Proceedings of a conference, Computational Neuroscience, Alicante, Spain, July 2002. Elsevier.

PILLOW, J. W., L. PANINSKI, and E. P. SIMONCELLI, 2004. Maximum likelihood estimation of a stochastic integrate-and-fire neural model. In *Advances in Neural Information Processing Systems (NIPS*03)*, vol. 16, S. Thrun, L. Saul, and B. Schökopf, eds. Cambridge, Mass.: MIT Press.

PILLOW, J. W., and E. P. SIMONCELLI, 2003. Biases in white noise analysis due to non-Poisson spike generation. In *Neurocomputing*, vols. 52–54, pp. 109–115. Proceeding of a conference, Computational Neuroscience, Chicago, July 21–25, 2002. Elsevier.

REICH, D., J. VICTOR, and B. KNIGHT, 1998. The power ratio and the interval map: Spiking models and extracellular recordings. *J. Neurosci.* 18:10090–10104.

REID, R. C., and J. M. ALONSO, 1995. Specificity of monosynaptic connections from thalamus to visual cortex. *Nature* 378:281–284.

RIEKE, F., D. WARLAND, R. R. DE RUYTER VAN STEVENINCK, and W. BIALEK, 1997. *Spikes: Exploring the Neural Code.* Cambridge, Mass.: MIT Press.

RINGACH, D., M. HAWKEN, and R. SHAPLEY, 2002. Receptive field structure of neurons in monkey primary visual cortex revealed by stimulation with natural image sequences. *J. Vision.* 2:12–24.

RINGACH, D. L., G. SAPIRO, and R. SHAPLEY, 1997. A subspace reverse-correlation technique for the study of visual neurons. *Vision Res.* 37:2455–2464.

RUST, N. C., O. SCHWARTZ, J. A. MOVSHON, and E. P. SIMONCELLI, 2004. Spike-triggered characterization of excitatory and suppressive stimulus dimensions in monkey V1. In *Neurocomputing*, vols. 58–60, pp. 793–799. Proceedings of a conference, Computational Neuroscience, Alicante, Spain, July 2003.

SAKAI, H. M., and K. NAKA, 1987. Signal transmission in the catfish retina. V. Sensitivity and circuit. *J. Neurophysiol.* 58:1329–1350.

SAKAI, K., and S. TANAKA, 2000. Spatial pooling in the second-order spatial structure of cortical complex cells. *Vision Res.* 40:855–871.

SCHWARTZ, O., E. J. CHICHILNISKY, and E. P. SIMONCELLI, 2002. Characterizing neural gain control using spike-triggered covariance. In *Advances in Neural Information Processing Systems (NIPS*01)*, vol. 14, T. G. Dietterich, S. Becker, and Z. Ghahramani, eds. Cambridge, Mass.: MIT Press, pp. 269–276.

SHARPEE, T., N. C. RUST, and W. BIALEK, 2003. Maximizing informative dimensions: Analyzing neural responses to natural signals. In *Advances in Neural Information Processing Systems (NIPS*02)*, vol. 15, S. Becker, S. Thrun, and K. Obermayer, eds. Cambridge, Mass.: MIT Press.

SMYTH, D., B. WILLMORE, G. E. BAKER, I. D. THOMPSON, and D. J. TOLHURST, 2003. The receptive-field organization of simple cells in primary visual cortex of ferrets under natural scene stimulation. *J. Neurosci.* 23:4746–4759.

SZULBORSKI, R. G., and L. A. PALMER, 1990. The two-dimensional spatial structure of nonlinear subunits in the receptive fields of complex cells. *Vision Res.* 30:249–254.

THEUNISSEN, F. E., S. V. DAVID, N. C. SINGH, A. HSU, W. E. VINJE, and J. L. GALLANT, 2001. Estimating spatio-temporal receptive fields of auditory and visual neurons from their responses to natural stimuli. *Network* 12:289–316.

TOURYAN, J., B. LAU, and Y. DAN, 2002. Isolation of relevant visual features from random stimuli for cortical complex cells. *J. Neurosci.* 22:10811–10818.

TSODYKS, M., T. KENET, A. GRINVALD, and A. ARIELI, 1999. Linking spontaneous activity of single cortical neurons and the underlying functional architecture. *Science* 286:1943–1946.

VOLTERRA, V., 1913. *Leçons sur les fonctions de lignes.* Paris: Gauthier-Villars.

WIENER, N., 1958. *Nonlinear Problems in Random Theory.* New York: Wiley.

24 Neuronal Correlates of Visual Attention and Perception

DAVID J. HEEGER AND DAVID RESS

ABSTRACT   This chapter reviews results from a series of experiments using functional magnetic resonance imaging (fMRI) to reveal nonsensory signals in early visual cortex. These studies demonstrate that early visual areas do more than encode raw sensory signals: they also participate in processing activities that correspond to visual attention and perception.

Over the past few years, we have come to learn that early visual cortex does not act as a passive image-processing machine simply devoted to representing bottom-up sensory signals. Rather, the bottom-up sensory signals in visual cortex interact with top-down signals related to attention, so that the neural substrates of visual perception involve recurrent interactions among early visual areas (including primary visual cortex, V1) and a number of widely separated cortical areas in the temporal, parietal, and frontal lobes. In the experiments described in this chapter, we found that these top-down signals can affect or even dominate measurements of activity in early human visual cortex.

This interaction between bottom-up and top-down signals raises a puzzling question. How does attention improve performance by affecting the activity in early visual cortex, but without evoking a percept? As a possible solution to this puzzle, it will be helpful to keep in mind a simple theoretical framework to distinguish between the encoding of sensory signals and the encoding of attentional signals in visual cortex. Consider a vertical sine wave grating target, like that depicted in figure 24.3a. When the target is presented, it will evoke activity in a subpopulation of V1 neurons, those with vertical (or near vertical) orientation preferences and receptive fields overlapping the target annulus. Other V1 neurons (e.g., with horizontal orientation preferences) will not respond to the target. It is this difference (or, more likely, this ratio) between the responses of subpopulations of neurons that encodes the vertical orientation of the target. Perception, therefore, is hypothesized to depend on the relative activity of appropriate subpopulations of neurons, those that are and those that are not selec-

tive for the features of the stimulus. Attention, on the other hand, is hypothesized to boost the activity of neurons whose receptive fields overlap the attended location, regardless of the neurons' stimulus preferences. This top-down attentional boost can improve the reliability (the neuronal signal-to-noise ratio) of the bottom-up sensory signals, consequently improving performance accuracy. Attention does not evoke a percept, however, because percepts depend on a differential response, and the attentional boost does not evoke a differential response.

In this chapter, we summarize the results of two experiments performed using functional magnetic resonance imaging (fMRI) to measure sensory/perceptual signals and attentional signals in early visual cortex. We focus on measurements of activity in V1, although we observed similar results in each of several early visual cortical areas (V1, V2, and V3). The two experiments described here are nearly identical to one another, yet one of them reveals primarily the trial-to-trial variability in the attentional signals and the other reveals primarily the percept-related signals. We hypothesize that these two components of neuronal activity are superimposed, and hence summed in physiological measurements (single- or multi-unit firing rates, as well as fMRI), but that the two experimental protocols (in spite of their similarity) allow us to measure the attention- and percept-related signals separately.

Methodological note

The uncertain relationship between neuronal activity and hemodynamics is a major concern in interpreting fMRI data (Logothetis et al., 2001; Heeger and Ress, 2002; Logothetis, 2002). Accumulating evidence suggests that the fMRI signal may not be directly tied to the spiking activity that is typically measured with single-unit electrophysiological studies. It is widely believed that increased blood flow follows from increased synaptic activity, not uniquely from spiking activity (Fox et al., 1988; Mathiesen et al., 1998; Magistretti and Pellerin, 1999; Logothetis, 2002).

The interpretation of fMRI data depends crucially, therefore, on the extent to which the spiking activity in a patch of cortical tissue might be decoupled from the synaptic activity

DAVID J. HEEGER   Department of Psychology and Center for Neural Science, New York University, N.Y.
DAVID RESS   Department of Psychology, Stanford University, Stanford, Calif.

within that tissue. For example, the fMRI signal might reflect not only the firing rates of the local neuronal population but also subthreshold activity, simultaneous excitation and inhibition, or modulatory inputs (such as feedback from distant, higher-level areas of visual cortex) that might not evoke spikes. In addition, the fMRI signal might reflect changes in neuronal synchrony without a concomitant increase in mean firing rate (Fries et al., 2001). A further complication is that fMRI signals reflect the pooled activity of a very large number of neurons; modulations in the fMRI responses could be caused by either large changes in the firing rates in a small subpopulation of neurons or small changes in the firing rates in a much larger subpopulation of neurons (Scannell and Young, 1999).

In our experiments, we have largely circumvented these concerns by using visual contrast as the primary independent variable. In each of the early visual areas, the input, intracortical, and output firing rates all increase monotonically with stimulus contrast. Consequently, we expect that various different kinds of measurements (single-unit firing rates, multi-unit activity, local field potentials, and fMRI responses) are highly correlated with one another.

To verify this, we compared human fMRI and monkey single-unit data and found that fMRI and neuronal responses show a strikingly similar dependence on contrast (figure 24.1). In the fMRI experiment (Boynton et al., 1999), activity was measured in human V1 as a function of stimulus contrast for a plaid pattern composed of the sum of two contrast-reversing sine wave gratings. The data were ana-

lyzed in predetermined subregions of V1 gray matter that corresponded retintopically to the location of the stimulus in the visual field. As discussed further below, it is critical to control the subject's attention when attempting to measure stimulus-evoked responses in visual cortex. Several studies have shown that the attentional state of the observer can have dramatic effects on fMRI signals in visual cortex (Brefczynski and DeYoe, 1999; Gandhi, Heeger, and Boynton, 1999; Gardner et al., 1999; Martinez et al., 1999; Ress, Backus, and Heeger, 2000; Huk, Ress, and Heeger, 2001). Moreover, trial-to-trial variability in attention is correlated with trial-to-trial variability in the amplitude of the fMRI responses (Ress, Backus, and Heeger, 2000). To control attention, the subjects in our experiment performed a rapid series of trials of a difficult contrast discrimination task. We dynamically adjusted the task difficulty to control performance accuracy on the task and used this control of performance as a proxy for controlling attention.

In the electrophysiological experiments (Geisler and Albrecht, 1997), the responses of a population of V1 neurons were measured as a function of contrast, using drifting sine wave gratings of the optimal spatiotemporal frequency, orientation, and direction of motion. The responses for each neuron were fitted with a model and the resulting smooth curves were summed across the population. After subtracting the total maintained activity and dividing by the number of neurons, the average response was then scaled, based on the measured distributions of selectivity of V1 neurons for spatial frequency, temporal frequency, orientation, and direction of motion (Geisler and Albrecht, 1997). The relatively low average firing rates in figure 24.1 are the result of the high degree of selectivity of V1 neurons. That is, the contrast-reversing plaid pattern used in the fMRI experiments produces a response in only a small minority of V1 neurons; because most of the cells are not responding, the average spike rate per neuron for the population as a whole is correspondingly low.

Measuring fMRI response amplitudes in predetermined patches of cortical tissue is an attractive complement to the conventional statistical parameter mapping analysis of neuroimaging data. Figure 24.2 shows an analysis of the same data as in figure 24.1, but as a series of pictures rather than as a graph with error bars. In the statistical parameter map (figure 24.2), increasing contrast appears to "recruit" additional areas of activity. But in fact, that is not the case. Rather, the larger area of activation is just an artifact of the statistical threshold used in producing the pictures. As the response amplitudes increase with increasing contrast, a greater percentage of the voxels exceed the statistical threshold. These pictures, therefore, confound a fundamental property of the physiology (responses increase with contrast) with a limitation of the experimental method (noise in the fMRI measurements).

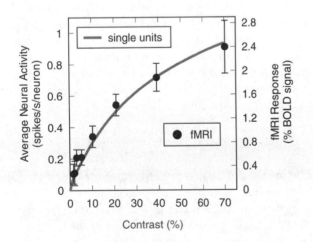

FIGURE 24.1 fMRI responses proportional to average firing rates. Data points indicate human V1 activity (Boynton et al., 1999). Error bars indicate SEM. Solid curve indicates the average firing rate in monkey V1, estimated from a large database (333 neurons) of microelectrode recordings (Geisler and Albrecht, 1997). Ordinates were scaled to obtain the best match between the two data sets. (Reprinted with permission from D. J. Heeger et al., Spikes versus BOLD: what does neuroimaging tell us about neuronal activity *Nat. Neurosci.* 3:631–633. © 2000 by Nature Publishing Group.)

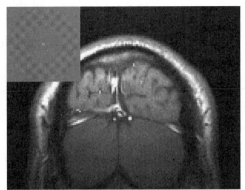

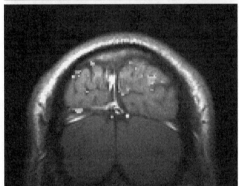

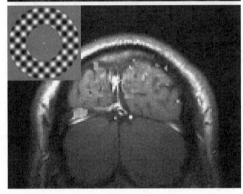

FIGURE 24.2 Statistical parameter maps of cortical activity as a function of stimulus contrast. Gray scale image is an obliquely oriented anatomical slice passing through the posterior occipital lobe and cerebellum. Colors indicate regions that achieve a criterion statistical threshold. (See color plate 13.)

Perception

For more than 30 years, psychophysical studies of visual pattern discrimination have paralleled research on the neurophysiological response properties of neurons in the visual cortex (Graham, 1989). The prevailing view has been that psychophysical judgments about visual patterns are limited by neuronal signals in the early stages of visual processing (i.e., retina, lateral geniculate nucleus, and primary visual cortex). Signal detection theory has provided the theoretical framework for linking the psychophysics and physiology.

The relationship between psychophysics and neurophysiology, as predicted by signal detection theory, can be illustrated in the context of the contrast detection task that we used in the experiments described next. On each trial, subjects were presented with one of two stimuli, either a background presented alone or the same background with a low-contrast target pattern superimposed (figure 24.3a). Subjects pressed one of two buttons to indicate whether they believed the target was present or absent. Logically, there are four possible outcomes on a given trial: hits, when the observer correctly responds yes on a target-present trial; correct rejects, when the observer correctly responds no on a target-absent trial; false alarms, when the observer erroneously responds yes on a target-absent trial; and misses, when the observer erroneously responds no on a target-present trial. Nearly all neurons in early visual cortex increase their activity monotonically with contrast (e.g., Carandini, Heeger, and Moushon, 1997; Geisler and Albrecht, 1997). Hence, the target-present stimulus will, on average, evoke slightly greater neuronal activity than the target-absent stimulus. Neuronal responses, however, are variable from one trial to the next, even when the physical stimuli are essentially identical (Dean, 1981; Softky and Koch, 1993; Geisler and Albrecht, 1997; Shadlen and Newsome, 1998). That is, under most stimulus conditions (except, for example, at very low light levels) the neuronal variability far exceeds the physical variability in the stimulus caused by factors such as instrument noise and photon variability. This neuronal variability implies that the target-present stimulus can sometimes evoke less activity than the target-absent stimulus (figure 24.3b, overlap between the two probability distributions).

A simple model of the decision process is that observers respond yes when the neuronal activity exceeds a fixed criterion (figure 24.3b, the vertical line), and otherwise respond no. This criterion divides the two response distributions into four parts corresponding to the four possible outcomes (figure 24.3b). According to this model, we would expect the cortical activity averaged over many neurons and many trials of each trial type to rank as follows: responses to hits > false alarms > misses > correct rejects. This prediction is intuitive for the trials when the subject responds correctly (hits > correct rejects): cortical activity should be greater when the target contrast pattern is physically present in the stimulus. The prediction is counterintuitive for the error trials (false alarms > misses): cortical activity should now follow the subject's percept, the opposite of what is physically presented in the stimulus. We used fMRI to measure activity in human visual cortex during a challenging contrast detection task to test the hypothesis that activity in early visual cortex is correlated with subjects' percepts even when those percepts are inaccurate (Ress and Heeger, 2003).

Subjects viewed a uniform gray field and continuously fixated a small, high-contrast mark at its center while lying in the bore of the MRI scanner. Once every 2 s, a visual

(a) Stimuli

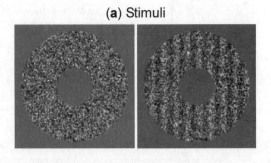

(b) Signal detection theory

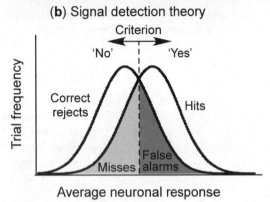

(c) Time series, subject AJN

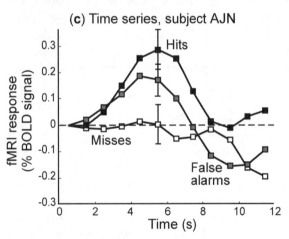

(d) Average response amplitudes

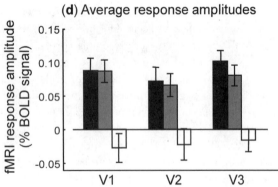

stimulus was displayed in an annulus around the fixation mark (figure 24.3a) for 1 s, followed by a response period. On most of the trials only a background pattern was presented; on the remaining (approximately one in six, randomly interleaved) trials a low-contrast target grating was added to the background. Subjects pressed one of two buttons to indicate whether they believed the target was present or absent. fMRI data were collected in visual cortex during several hundred trials for each of four subjects. The large number of trials was required to reliably measure the small fMRI signal changes (~0.2%) associated with the threshold-level stimulus contrast increments.

Data were analyzed separately in each of several predefined areas of visual cortex, but we focus here on the data from V1. These visual areas were identified using routine methods for mapping the retinotopic organization of visual cortex (Engel et al., 1994; Sereno et al., 1995; DeYoe et al., 1996; Engel, Glover, and Wandell, 1997). The analysis was restricted to the subregion of each visual area that corresponded retinotopically to the visual field location of the stimulus annulus. The trials were sorted into the four signal detection categories: hits, false alarms, misses, and correct rejects. Because the target pattern was presented infrequently, most of the trials (~70%) corresponded to correct rejects, and fMRI responses associated with correct-reject trials were taken as a baseline. We calculated the differential activity associated with hits, misses, and false alarms with respect to this baseline.

The observed ranking of cortical activity was hits ≈ false alarms > correct rejects ≈ misses. This was evident in the fMRI time series acquired from individual visual cortical areas in individual subjects (figure 24.3c). We infer that the underlying neuronal activity associated with each trial was largely confined to the first 1 or 2 s, and that the slow time

FIGURE 24.3 Activity in V1 corresponds to subjects' percepts. (a) Visual stimuli. On the left is shown a noise background; on the right, a noise background and vertical grating target. (b) Ideal observers make their decision on each trial by comparing a noisy internal response (e.g., the average firing rate of an appropriate subpopulation of neurons) with a fixed criterion. The mean responses (across trials) for the four trial types rank as follows: hits > false alarms > misses > correct rejects. (c) Average time courses of the fMRI signals from one typical subject, averaged across many trials and averaged throughout cortical gray matter corresponding to the V1 representation of the stimulus. Dashed line indicates baseline activity on correct reject trials. Error bars indicate typical SEM across trials at one time point. (d) fMRI response amplitudes averaged across subjects. Response amplitudes were computed for each trial type and each visual area as the average response during a time window in the vicinity of the peak activity. (Reprinted with permission from D. Ress and D. J. Heeger, Neuronal correlates of perception in early visual cortex. *Nat. Neurosci.* 6:414–420. © 2003 by Nature Publishing Group.)

(a) Stimulus pattern

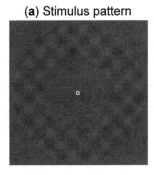

(b) Time series

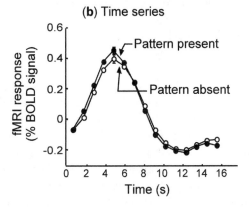

(c) Behavior

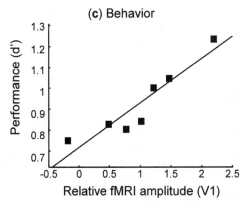

FIGURE 24.4 Attentional signals in V1 predict performance accuracy. (*a*) Visual stimulus, target pattern. (*b*) Average time courses of the fMRI signals from one typical subject, averaged across many trials and averaged throughout cortical gray matter corresponding to the V1 representation of the stimulus. Solid symbols indicate target present; open symbols, target absent. Error bar corresponds to typical SEM measured across trials at one time point. (*c*) Trial-to-trial variability in V1 activity was predictive of performance accuracy on the task. Performance (*d'*) is highly correlated with the amplitude of V1 activity ($r = 0.92$; $P < 0.001$). Solid line is the linear regression. (Reprinted with permission from D. Ress et al., Activity in primary visual cortex predicts performance in a visual detection task. *Nat. Neurosci.* 3:940–945, © 2000 by Nature Publishing Group.)

course of the fMRI measurements reflected a sluggish change in local cerebral blood flow and oxygenation. When the data were then combined across all subjects, the same ranking (hits ≈ false alarms > correct rejects ≈ misses) was again clearly evident (figure 24.3*d*). The differences between hits/false alarms and misses/correct rejects were highly statistically significant ($P \ll 0.001$). These effects were retinotopically specific, suggesting that they are related to the percepts themselves as opposed to a nonspecific effect (e.g., arousal) associated with yes responses. Of particular interest are the responses to the error trials (false alarms and misses) because they dissociate the percept from the physical presence or absence of the target. Critically, we found that activity was larger on average for false alarm trials than for misses. In other words, the activity in early visual cortex corresponded to the subjects' percepts even when that percept was opposite to what was physically presented in the stimulus, consistent with observers making perceptual decisions based on activity in these early visual areas.

These results are largely but not entirely consistent with the predictions of signal detection theory. There was little difference between the response amplitudes to hits and false alarms, and likewise between misses and correct rejects, as would be expected from the purely bottom-up interpretation based on signal detection theory. It is possible that our measurements of both cortical activity and behavioral performance may have been dominated by trial-to-trial variability in top-down signals, or by a combination of bottom-up and top-down processes. Specifically, cortical activity during our task may have consisted of an immediate response to the stimulus and a later signal associated with the percept (as reported in some single-unit electrophysiology experiments cited later). Because of the sluggishness of the hemodynamic response, our fMRI measurements would have yielded a superposition of the bottom-up sensory inputs and top-down percept-related signals. This may have obscured the difference between responses to hits and false alarms (and likewise between misses and correct rejects).

Signal detection in humans has been previously studied with event-related potentials. Some of these experiments used stimuli analogous to ours, either auditory or visual targets masked by a distracter stimulus or noise. Particular attention has been paid to a transient evoked potential called the P3 or P300 (Hillyard et al., 1971; K. C. Squires, Squires, and Hillyard, 1975a,b; N. K. Squires, Squires, and Hillyard, 1975; K. C. Squires et al., 1976; Parasuraman and Beatty, 1980; Polich and Kok, 1995; Hunter, Turner, and Fulham, 2001). Under auditory stimulus conditions analogous to those of our experiments, the magnitude of the P3 exhibited a dependence on trial type similar to what we have observed with fMRI (K. C. Squires, Squires, and Hillyard, 1975b). One interpretation of the P3 is that it reflects a working memory representation used in the process of stimulus discrimination. Another common interpretation of the P3 is that it reflects an oddball effect, a response to the detection of infrequent targets. Support for the "oddball" interpretation was provided by studies in which a key manipulation was to vary the prior probability of target presentation. Further experiments will have to be performed to elucidate the relationship between the P3 and our fMRI measurements.

Previous fMRI experiments have found that a number of brain areas show greater responses during correct target detection (hits > misses, hits > correct rejects) (Shulman et al., 1999, 2001; Clark et al., 2000; Corbetta et al., 2000; Grill-Spector et al., 2000). Studies of memory have yielded analogous results: the ability to later remember an experience is predicted by the magnitude of activity in particular brain structures during encoding (Brewer et al., 1998; Wagner et al., 1998; Davachi and Wagner, 2002; Davachi, Mitchell, and Wagner, 2003). However, none of those experiments was designed to measure the responses to false alarms, making a meaningful comparison to our results difficult. One recent fMRI study reported a result (including false alarms) that is similar to our own, but measured in an area of visual cortex that is believed to subserve object recognition (Grill-Spector and Kanwisher, 2001).

Threshold-level signal detection has also been studied previously by measuring single- and multi-unit activity in monkey cortex (for review, see Parker and Newsome, 1998). One series of experiments demonstrated that threshold-level visual motion signals are coded by the firing rates of neurons in cortical area MT, an area specialized for visual motion (Newsome, Britten, and Moushon, 1989; Britten et al., 1992; Shadlen et al., 1996). A second series of experiments demonstrated that threshold-level somatosensory signals are likewise coded by the firing rates of neurons in primary and secondary somatosensory cortex (Romo et al., 1998, 1999, 2000; Romo and Salinas, 1999, 2001, 2003; Hernández, Zainos, and Romo, 2000; Brody et al., 2002; Romo, Hernández, Zainos, Brody, et al., 2002; Romo, Hernández, Zainos, Lemus, et al., 2002; see also Romo, de Lafuente, and Hernández, this volume). Our results suggest an analogous process in human visual cortex, as early as V1, for threshold-level visual contrast signals. A third line of research used backward masking to affect the detection of a visual target while recording from macaque frontal eye-field neurons (Thompson and Schall, 1999, 2000). The initial responses of these neurons (<100 ms after stimulus onset) corresponded to the actual presence or absence of the target, while later activity (100–300 ms after stimulus onset) corresponded to the monkey's behavioral report, such that responses to false alarms were greater than responses to misses. A fourth series of experiments recorded multi-unit activity in V1 while monkeys performed a figure–ground discrimination task (Super, Spekreijse, and Lamme, 2001a).

Once again, two phases of responses were evident, an early response (<90 ms) that was directly related to the stimulus, and a later response (100–240 ms) that was stronger when the monkey correctly performed the task (hits > misses). The late-time activity was attributed to feedback mechanisms. Indeed, there is accumulating evidence that visual signals propagate rapidly from early visual cortex to other regions of the brain and back to visual cortex (Hupe et al., 1998, 2001; Lamme, Super, and Spekreijse, 1998; Schmolesky et al., 1998; Bullier et al., 2001; Super, Spekreijse, and Lamme, 2001a). As mentioned earlier, cortical activity during our task may have likewise consisted of an immediate response to the stimulus and a later signal associated with the percept.

Attention

Our ability to perform a visual discrimination task improves when we are cued to attend, without moving our eyes, to the relevant stimulus (e.g., Posner, 1980; Pashler, 1998). Shifts in attention are correlated with systematic changes in cortical activity that have been measured in a number of cortical areas using a variety of methods (for reviews see Desimone and Duncan, 1995; Colby and Goldberg, 1999; Kanwisher and Wojciulik, 2000; Kastner and Ungerleider, 2000; Kusunoki, Gottlieb, and Goldberg, 2000; Corbetta and Shulman, 2002; Goldberg et al., 2002). It is widely believed that top-down projections from prefrontal or parietal areas provide the attentional control signals that modulate visual processing (Mesulam, 1981; Posner et al., 1984; Corbetta et al., 1993, 2000; Nobre et al., 1997; Coull and Nobre, 1998; Shulman et al., 1999; Wojciulik and Kanwisher, 1999; Hopfinger, Buonocore, and Mangun, 2000; Moore and Fallah, 2001; Rushworth, Paus, and Sipila, 2001; Corbetta and Shulman, 2002; Yantis et al., 2002; Moore and Armstrong, 2003). These top-down control signals modulate activity in early visual cortical areas including V1 (Luck et al., 1997; Hillyard and Anllo-Vento, 1998; Tootell et al., 1998; Brefczynski and DeYoe, 1999; Chawla, Rees, and Friston, 1999; Gandhi, Heeger, and Boynton, 1999; Kastner et al., 1999; Martinez et al., 1999; McAdams and Maunsell, 1999; Reynolds, Chelazzi, and Desimone, 1999; Treue and Trujillo, 1999; Ress, Backus, and Heeger, 2000). These neuronal correlates of attention are spatially selective (Tootell et al., 1998; Brefczynski and DeYoe, 1999; Gandhi, Heeger, and Boynton, 1999; Ress, Backus, and Heeger, 2000) and depend on task difficulty (Spitzer, Desimone, and Moran, 1988). Notably, baseline firing rates of neurons in monkey visual cortex are elevated by attention, even in the absence of visual stimulation (Luck et al., 1997; Reynolds, Pasternak, and Desimone, 2000), and analogous phenomena have been observed in humans (Chawla, Rees, and Friston, 1999; Kastner et al., 1999; Martinez et al., 1999; Ress, Backus, and Heeger, 2000).

Although there is considerable evidence that attention modulates activity in visual cortex, only recently have there been any demonstrations of a link between attention-related increases in neural activity and improvements in behavioral performance (Ress, Backus, and Heeger, 2000; Moore and Fallah, 2001; Bisley and Goldberg, 2003). In one of these recent studies, we used fMRI to measure activity in human visual cortex during a challenging contrast detection task, to demonstrate a contingency between attentional signals in early visual cortex and performance accuracy (Ress, Backus, and Heeger, 2000).

Subjects viewed a uniformly gray field and continuously fixated a small high-contrast mark at its center (figure 24.4a) while lying in the bore of the MR scanner. Once every 20 s, a short auditory tone cued subjects that a new trial was beginning. On half the trials (randomly interleaved), a low-contrast pattern was presented briefly in a peripheral annulus around the fixation mark; on the other trials, no pattern was presented and the display remained uniformly gray. Subjects pressed one of two buttons to indicate whether they believed the pattern was present. fMRI data were collected during several hundred trials for each of three subjects. The trials were categorized according to whether the stimulus pattern was present or absent and whether the subject responded correctly or incorrectly. Although this experiment was very similar to the one described earlier, the results were rather different, for reasons discussed below.

We observed a large response in early visual cortex on every trial, even in the absence of a visual stimulus (figure 24.4b), evoked by the presentation of the auditory cue at the beginning of each trial. This cue-related *base response* was very similar for pattern-present and pattern-absent trials. The base response exhibited the signature characteristics of visual attention: it depended on task difficulty, and it was retinotopically selective, that is, evident only in the subregion of visual cortex corresponding to the representation of the stimulus aperture. Most important, the cue-related base response quantitatively predicted the subjects pattern detection performance. When activity was greater, the subject was more likely to correctly discern the presence or absence of the pattern (figure 24.4c).

The cue-related base response raised a number of puzzling questions for which we can now suggest only tentative answers.

Why is the base response so large? A number of electrophysiological studies have reported that baseline firing rates do not increase with attention (e.g., McAdams and Maunsell, 1999). Moreover, the studies that did find baseline increases in extrastriate cortex failed to find them in V1 (e.g., Luck et al., 1997). There is quite a large number of possible explanations for the discrepancy between those results and our results (along with those of Kastner et al., 1999) that do indicate baseline increases in V1. First, because cortical

neurons generally have low baseline firing rates, the responses of many neurons must be recorded to obtain statistically significant results. Therefore, these effects may be better revealed by fMRI measurements that reflect the activity of a large population of neurons. Second, the fMRI measurement may reflect subthreshold activity (e.g., due to excitation from distant inputs in the frontal or parietal lobes) that would be invisible to extracellular electrodes. Third, our data suggest that reliable and robust increases in baseline firing rates may be evident only when performing a particularly demanding task. Our task, in particular, included considerable spatial uncertainty because the location of the target annulus was not indicated on the otherwise blank (uniformly gray) background. The studies that failed to find baseline increases may have been insufficiently demanding of spatial attention, perhaps because they used tasks for which there was little or no spatial uncertainty. Fourth, the monkeys in those experiments may have been so highly trained that the usual attentional mechanisms were no longer needed to perform the task; training can have a critical effect on attentional signals (Ito and Gilbert, 1999). Fifth, small shifts in eye position, equal in size to the V1 receptive fields, present a difficulty for electrophysiology experiments. If eye position is systematically correlated with shifts in spatial attention, then the responses of individual V1 neurons will modulate as the receptive fields are shifted toward and away from the stimulus. These biases can be avoided by carefully accounting for eye position, but perhaps at the cost of underestimating the magnitude of the attentional effects. Small shifts in eye position do not present a difficulty in the fMRI experiments because they have a negligible effect on measurements of pooled neuronal activity. A small shift in gaze will cause the stimulus to move out of the receptive fields of one subpopulation of neurons and into the receptive fields of a neighboring subpopulation of neurons, hence causing a decrease in the responses of the first subpopulation simultaneous with an increase in the responses of the second subpopulation. Sixth, there may be a genuine species difference.

Why doesn't the base response itself evoke the percept of the target pattern? Subjects did not report seeing the target more frequently on trials for which the base response was larger. Rather, a larger base response improved performance accuracy (correct hits and correct rejects). To address this question, we refer back to the theoretical framework posed in the introduction to this chapter. Percepts depend on relative responses, not overall net increases in activity. We hypothesize that subjects' behavioral responses (answering yes or no) on this task depend on a response difference from successive intervals over time or from different subpopulations of neurons (i.e., with one subpopulation tuned for the orientation and spatial frequency components of the stimulus and the other not). These response differences, which ride

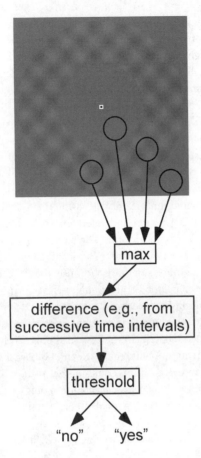

FIGURE 24.5   Model linking the cue-related base response with performance accuracy. A hypothetical decision process pools the responses of sensory neurons. The pooling rule is nonlinear, e.g., computing the maximum of the inputs and then comparing that maximum to a criterion. Boosting the amplitude of the inputs providing relevant information will result in those signals dominating the decision process, hence improving performance.

on top of the base response, are likely to be small in amplitude but selective in comparison to the base response.

How does the base response lead to improved performance? The base response might serve to reduce spatial uncertainty by boosting the relevant information coming from neurons whose receptive fields overlap the stimulus aperture (figure 24.5). Subjects detected a low-contrast target on an otherwise blank (uniformly gray) background, so that there was uncertainty about the precise spatial location of the target, even after extensive practice. The trial-to-trial variability in the base response might reflect this uncertainty. Signal detection theory offers a framework for understanding how a boost in the relevant neuronal signals can lead to improved performance (e.g., Palmer, Verghese, and Pavel, 2000), hence linking the trial-to-trial variability in performance accuracy with the trial-to-trial variability in the base response. Accuracy is improved by boosting the relevant neuronal signals (e.g., from neurons with receptive fields that overlap the stimulus aperture) relative to other signals (e.g.,

from neurons with receptive fields outside the stimulus aperture), which contribute only noise. Boosting the responses of the relevant sensory neurons, therefore, makes the decision process easier. The decision stage can adopt a simple pooling rule that does not have to keep track of where each input came from, while still optimizing performance.

In this context, we can address another puzzling question about attention: Why not deploy attention everywhere all the time? According to the model in figure 24.5, boosting the activity of all of the sensory neurons would make performance on this task worse. It is a good thing, making the job of the decision process easier, to enhance only the relevant neural signals, not the irrelevant ones.

Discussion

There is an apparent discrepancy between the results of the two experiments that we have presented in this chapter. One experiment found that the measured cortical activity was correlated with the reported percept (figure 24.3) and the other found that the measured activity was instead correlated with performance accuracy (figure 24.4). In contrast to the results of the second (attention) experiment, the data from the first (perception) experiment showed only a weak correlation between behavioral performance and cortical activity. The protocol in the first (perception) experiment had two features designed to control the effects of attention that dominated the results in the second (attention) experiment. First, in the perception experiment, we used a rapid trial sequence that engaged subjects nearly continuously in the task. In the attention experiment, subjects were permitted to completely disengage their attention during the long intertrial intervals. Second, in the perception experiment, we used an easily visible background pattern to minimize spatial uncertainty. In the attention experiment, subjects detected a low-contrast target on an otherwise blank (uniformly gray) background, so that there was uncertainty about the precise spatial location of the target, even after practice. There was, in addition, a third (inadvertent) difference between the two experiments: the target was presented on half the trials in the attention study but on only one-sixth of the trials in perception study. This may have had the side effect of confounding stimulus- and percept-related activity with an oddball effect (see earlier discussion of P3). Further experiments will have to be performed to determine which of the differences (rapid trial sequence, spatial uncertainty, oddball) between the two experimental protocols was critical. According to the model presented in figure 24.5, we would expect spatial uncertainty to be a contributing factor.

Together, the two experiments summarized in this chapter (figures 24.3, 24.4) demonstrate that there are both attention- and percept-related signals in early visual cortex.

By altering the experimental protocol, we have emphasized one or the other of these two signals in our measurements. We believe, of course, that both types of signals contribute to perception and behavior on all trials in both experiments. The different experimental protocols merely emphasized one over the other in our measurements. Both attention and perception are hypothesized to depend on the pooled activity of large numbers of neurons. Perception depends on the relative activity of selective subpopulations of neurons. Attention, on the other hand, improves performance without evoking a percept, by boosting the responses nonselectively at the attended location.

Single-unit electrophysiology studies provide support for the hypothesis that attention improves performance by boosting neural responses but without evoking differential responses among subpopulations of neurons with different stimulus preferences. First, baseline firing rates are elevated by attention even in the absence of visual stimulation (Luck et al., 1997; Reynolds, Pasternak, and Desimone, 2000). Second, attention boosts the gain of neural responses, such that responses increase without affecting neural selectivity (McAdams and Maunsell, 1999; Treue and Trujillo, 1999; Maunsell and Ghose, this volume). Hence, after subtracting the baseline firing rates, relative neuronal responses (i.e., the ratio of the responses of two neurons with the same receptive field location but different stimulus preferences) are independent of attention.

In addition to its impact on improving behavioral performance at an attended location, attention has a further role in visual processing. Attention has been shown to bias competitive interactions among neuronal signals corresponding to nearby spatial locations, causing neurons to respond primarily to the attended stimulus location (Reynolds, Chelazzi, and Desimone, 1999). This process of spatial selection does, of course, affect our conscious percepts. More than a century of behavioral research has shown that we are aware of only a small part of our visual environment at any instant in time, and that attention is involved in controlling what we are aware of from one moment to the next. Spatial selection may be a result of the very same underlying neural mechanisms discussed above. Consider a V4 neuron that pools a large number of V1 inputs, and consider boosting the baseline firing rates and the gain of a subset of those V1 inputs, all with the same receptive field location, but including every possible stimulus preference within that receptive field location. When coupled with competitive, mutually suppressive interactions between neurons with nearby receptive fields, this will have the effect of biasing the V4 neuron to respond to a subpart of its receptive field, "shrinking" the V4 receptive field around the selected spatial location (Reynolds, Chelazzi, and Desimone, 1999).

A final comment concerns the possible role of working memory in our experiments. An alternative explanation for

the results of both of the experiments described in this chapter involves working memory. The base response might correspond to the processing of a visual working memory representation of the target as it is compared with the incoming visual signals to perform the detection task. Errors would then occur on trials when the working memory processing within the retinotopic representation of the stimulus aperture was weak. The working memory hypothesis also provides a possible explanation for the signals observed in the perception experiments. While performing the discrimination task of the perception experiments, an excess of working memory processing might lead to false alarms, biasing the bottom-up sensory signals upward, while a lapse of processing could be responsible for misses, biasing the sensory signals downward. However, experiments investigating the role of early visual cortex in working memory have given mixed results. Some have reported activity in early visual areas (including V1) during visual working memory/ mental imagery (Le Bihan et al., 1993; Kosslyn et al., 1995, 1999; Chen et al., 1998; Gratton et al., 1998; Kosslyn, Ganis, and Thompson, 2001; Super, Spekreijse, and Lamme, 2001b), whereas others have failed to find delay-period activity in early visual areas during mental imagery (Roland and Gulyas, 1994; D'Esposito et al., 1997; Mellet et al., 1998; Ishai, Ungerleider, and Haxby, 2000). Thus, although it provides an attractive unification of the observed phenomena, the working memory hypothesis remains speculative.

REFERENCES

Bisley, J. W., and M. E. Goldberg, 2003. Neuronal activity in the lateral intraparietal area and spatial attention. *Science* 299:81–86.

Boynton, G. M., J. B. Demb, G. H. Glover, and D. J. Heeger, 1999. Neuronal basis of contrast discrimination. *Vision Res.* 39:257–269.

Brefczynski, J. A., and E. A. DeYoe, 1999. A physiological correlate of the "spotlight" of visual attention. *Nat. Neurosci.* 2:370–374.

Brewer, J. B., Z. Zhao, J. E. Desmond, G. H. Glover, and J. D. Gabrieli, 1998. Making memories: Brain activity that predicts how well visual experience will be remembered. *Science* 281: 1185–1187.

Britten, K. H., M. N. Shadlen, W. T. Newsome, and J. A. Movshon, 1992. The analysis of visual motion: A comparison of neuronal and psychophysical performance. *J. Neurosci.* 12: 4745–4765.

Brody, C. D., A. Hernandez, A. Zainos, L. Lemus, and R. Romo, 2002. Analysing neuronal correlates of the comparison of two sequentially presented sensory stimuli. *Philos. Trans. R. Soc. Lond. B Biol. Sci.* 357:1843–1850.

Bullier, J., J. M. Hupe, A. C. James, and P. Girard, 2001. The role of feedback connections in shaping the responses of visual cortical neurons. *Prog. Brain. Res.* 134:193–204.

Carandini, M., D. J. Heeger, and J. A. Movshon, 1997. Linearity and normalization in simple cells of the macaque primary visual cortex. *J. Neurosci.* 17:8621–8644.

CHAWLA, D., G. REES, and K. J. FRISTON, 1999. The physiological basis of attentional modulation in extrastriate visual areas. *Nat. Neurosci.* 2:671–676.

CHEN, W., T. KATO, X. H. ZHU, S. OGAWA, D. W. TANK, and K. UGURBIL, 1998. Human primary visual cortex and lateral geniculate nucleus activation during visual imagery. *Neuroreport* 9:3669–3674.

CLARK, V. P., S. FANNON, S. LAI, R. BENSON, and L. BAUER, 2000. Responses to rare visual target and distractor stimuli using event-related fMRI. *J. Neurophysiol.* 83:3133–3139.

COLBY, C. L., and M. E. GOLDBERG, 1999. Space and attention in parietal cortex. *Annu. Rev. Neurosci.* 22:319–349.

CORBETTA, M., J. M. KINCADE, J. M. OLLINGER, M. P. MCAVOY, and G. L. SHULMAN, 2000. Voluntary orienting is dissociated from target detection in human posterior parietal cortex [published erratum appears in *Nat. Neurosci.* 3(5):521, 2000]. *Nat. Neurosci.* 3:292–297.

CORBETTA, M., F. M. MIEZIN, G. L. SHULMAN, and S. E. PETERSEN, 1993. A PET study of visuospatial attention. *J. Neurosci.* 13:1202–1226.

CORBETTA, M., and G. L. SHULMAN, 2002. Control of goal-directed and stimulus-driven attention in the brain. *Nat. Rev. Neurosci.* 3:201–215.

COULL, J. T., and A. C. NOBRE, 1998. Where and when to pay attention: The neural systems for directing attention to spatial locations and to time intervals as revealed by both PET and fMRI. *J. Neurosci.* 18:7426–7435.

DAVACHI, L., J. P. MITCHELL, and A. D. WAGNER, 2003. Multiple routes to memory: Distinct medial temporal lobe processes build item and source memories. *Proc. Natl. Acad. Sci. U.S.A.* 100:2157–2162.

DAVACHI, L., and A. D. WAGNER, 2002. Hippocampal contributions to episodic encoding: Insights from relational and item-based learning. *J. Neurophysiol.* 88:982–990.

DEAN, A. F., 1981. The variability of discharge of simple cells in the cat striate cortex. *Exp. Brain Res.* 44:437–440.

DESIMONE, R., and J. DUNCAN, 1995. Neural mechanisms of selective visual attention. *Annu. Rev. Neurosci.* 18:193–222.

D'ESPOSITO, M., J. A. DETRE, G. K. AGUIRRE, M. STALLCUP, D. C. ALSOP, L. J. TIPPET, and M. J. FARAH, 1997. A functional MRI study of mental image generation. *Neuropsychologia* 35:725–730.

DEYOE, E. A., G. J. CARMAN, P. BANDETTINI, S. GLICKMAN, J. WIESER, R. COX, D. MILLER, and J. NEITZ, 1996. Mapping striate and extrastriate visual areas in human cerebral cortex. *Proc. Natl. Acad. Sci. U.S.A.* 93:2382–2386.

ENGEL, S. A., G. H. GLOVER, and B. A. WANDELL, 1997. Retinotopic organization in human visual cortex and the spatial precision of functional MRI. *Cereb. Cortex* 7:181–192.

ENGEL, S. A., D. E. RUMELHART, B. A. WANDELL, A. T. LEE, G. H. GLOVER, E. J. CHICHILNISKY, and M. N. SHADLEN, 1994. fMRI of human visual cortex. *Nature* 369:525.

FOX, P. T., M. E. RAICHLE, M. A. MINTUN, and C. DENCE, 1988. Nonoxidative glucose consumption during focal physiologic neural activity. *Science* 241:462–464.

FRIES, P., J. H. REYNOLDS, A. E. RORIE, and R. DESIMONE, 2001. Modulation of oscillatory neuronal synchronization by selective visual attention. *Science* 291:1560–1563.

GANDHI, S. P., D. J. HEEGER, and G. M. BOYNTON, 1999. Spatial attention affects brain activity in human primary visual cortex. *Proc. Natl. Acad. Sci. U.S.A.* 96:3314–3319.

GARDNER, J. L., A. ANZAI, I. OHZAWA, and R. D. FREEMAN, 1999. Linear and nonlinear contributions to orientation tuning of simple cells in the cat's striate cortex. *Vis. Neurosci.* 16:1115–1121.

GEISLER, W. S., and D. G. ALBRECHT, 1997. Visual cortex neurons in monkeys and cats: Detection, discrimination, and identification. *Vis. Neurosci.* 14:897–919.

GOLDBERG, M. E., J. BISLEY, K. D. POWELL, J. GOTTLIEB, and M. KUSUNOKI, 2002. The role of the lateral intraparietal area of the monkey in the generation of saccades and visuospatial attention. *Ann. N.Y. Acad. Sci.* 956:205–215.

GRAHAM, N., 1989. *Visual Pattern Analyzers*. New York: Oxford University Press.

GRATTON, G., M. FABIANI, M. R. GOODMAN-WOOD, and M. C. DESOTO, 1998. Memory-driven processing in human medial occipital cortex: An event-related optical signal (EROS) study. *Psychophysiology* 35:348–351.

GRILL-SPECTOR, K., and N. KANWISHER, 2001. *The functional organization of human ventral temporal cortex is based on stimulus selectivity not recognition task*. Presented at the Society for Neuroscience 31st Annual Meeting.

GRILL-SPECTOR, K., T. KUSHNIR, T. HENDLER, and R. MALACH, 2000. The dynamics of object-selective activation correlate with recognition performance in humans. *Nat. Neurosci.* 3:837–843.

HEEGER, D. J., A. C. HUK, W. S. GEISLER, and D. G. ALBRECHT, 2000. Spikes versus BOLD: What does neuroimaging tell us about neuronal activity? *Nat. Neurosci.* 3:631–633.

HEEGER, D. J., and D. RESS, 2002. What does fMRI tell us about neuronal activity? *Nat. Rev. Neurosci.* 3:142–151.

HERNÁNDEZ, A., A. ZAINOS, and R. ROMO, 2000. Neuronal correlates of sensory discrimination in the somatosensory cortex. *Proc. Natl. Acad. Sci. U.S.A.* 97:6191–6196.

HILLYARD, S. A., and L. ANLLO-VENTO, 1998. Event-related brain potentials in the study of visual selective attention. *Proc. Natl. Acad. Sci. U.S.A.* 95:781–787.

HILLYARD, S. A., K. C. SQUIRES, J. W. BAUER, and P. H. LINDSAY, 1971. Evoked potential correlates of auditory signal detection. *Science* 172:1357–1360.

HOPFINGER, J. B., M. H. BUONOCORE, and G. R. MANGUN, 2000. The neural mechanisms of top-down attentional control. *Nat. Neurosci.* 3:284–291.

HUK, A. C., D. RESS, and D. J. HEEGER, 2001. Neuronal basis of the motion aftereffect reconsidered. *Neuron* 32:161–172.

HUNTER, M., A. TURNER, and W. R. FULHAM, 2001. Visual signal detection measured by event-related potentials. *Brain Cogn.* 46:342–356.

HUPE, J. M., A. C. JAMES, P. GIRARD, S. G. LOMBER, B. R. PAYNE, and J. BULLIER, 2001. Feedback connections act on the early part of the responses in monkey visual cortex. *J. Neurophysiol.* 85:134–145.

HUPE, J. M., A. C. JAMES, B. R. PAYNE, S. G. LOMBER, P. GIRARD, and J. BULLIER, 1998. Cortical feedback improves discrimination between figure and background by V1, V2 and V3 neurons. *Nature* 394:784–787.

ISHAI, A., L. G. UNGERLEIDER, and J. V. HAXBY, 2000. Distributed neural systems for the generation of visual images. *Neuron* 28:979–990.

ITO, M., and C. D. GILBERT, 1999. Attention modulates contextual influences in the primary visual cortex of alert monkeys. *Neuron* 22:593–604.

KANWISHER, N., and E. WOJCIULIK, 2000. Visual attention: Insights from brain imaging. *Nat. Rev. Neurosci.* 1:91–100.

KASTNER, S., M. A. PINSK, P. DE WEERD, R. DESIMONE, and L. G. UNGERLEIDER, 1999. Increased activity in human visual cortex during directed attention in the absence of visual stimulation. *Neuron* 22:751–761.

KASTNER, S., and L. G. UNGERLEIDER, 2000. Mechanisms of visual attention in the human cortex. *Annu. Rev. Neurosci.* 23:315–341.

KOSSLYN, S. M., G. GANIS, and W. L. THOMPSON, 2001. Neural foundations of imagery. *Nat. Rev. Neurosci.* 2:635–642.

KOSSLYN, S. M., A. PASCUAL-LEONE, O. FELICIAN, S. CAMPOSANO, J. P. KEENAN, W. L. THOMPSON, G. GANIS, K. E. SUKEL, and N. M. ALPERT, 1999. The role of area 17 in visual imagery: Convergent evidence from PET and rTMS. *Science* 284:167–170.

KOSSLYN, S. M., W. L. THOMPSON, I. J. KIM, and N. M. ALPERT, 1995. Topographical representations of mental images in primary visual cortex. *Nature* 378:496–498.

KUSUNOKI, M., J. GOTTLIEB, and M. E. GOLDBERG, 2000. The lateral intraparietal area as a salience map: The representation of abrupt onset, stimulus motion, and task relevance. *Vision Res.* 40:1459–1468.

LAMME, V. A., H. SUPER, and H. SPEKREIJSE, 1998. Feedforward, horizontal, and feedback processing in the visual cortex. *Curr. Opin. Neurobiol.* 8:529–535.

LE BIHAN, D., R. TURNER, T. A. ZEFFIRO, C. A. CUENOD, P. JEZZARD, and V. BONNEROT, 1993. Activation of human primary visual cortex during visual recall: A magnetic resonance imaging study. *Proc. Natl. Acad. Sci. U.S.A.* 90:11802–11805.

LOGOTHETIS, N. K., 2002. The neural basis of the blood-oxygen-level-dependent functional magnetic resonance imaging signal. *Philos. Trans. R. Soc. Lond. B Biol. Sci.* 357:1003–1037.

LOGOTHETIS, N. K., J. PAULS, M. AUGATH, T. TRINATH, and A. OELTERMANN, 2001. Neurophysiological investigation of the basis of the fMRI signal. *Nature* 412:150–157.

LUCK, S. J., L. CHELAZZI, S. A. HILLYARD, and R. DESIMONE, 1997. Neural mechanisms of spatial selective attention in areas V1, V2, and V4 of macaque visual cortex. *J. Neurophysiol.* 77:24–42.

MAGISTRETTI, P. J., and L. PELLERIN, 1999. Cellular mechanisms of brain energy metabolism and their relevance to functional brain imaging. *Philos. Trans. R. Soc. Lond. B Biol. Sci.* 354:1155–1163.

MARTINEZ, A., L. ANLLO-VENTO, M. I. SERENO, L. R. FRANK, R. B. BUXTON, D. J. DUBOWITZ, E. C. WONG, H. HINRICHS, H. J. HEINZE, and S. A. HILLYARD, 1999. Involvement of striate and extrastriate visual cortical areas in spatial attention. *Nat. Neurosci.* 2:364–369.

MATHIESEN, C., K. CAESAR, N. AKGOREN, and M. LAURITZEN, 1998. Modification of activity-dependent increases of cerebral blood flow by excitatory synaptic activity and spikes in rat cerebellar cortex. *J. Physiol.* 512:555–566.

MCADAMS, C. J., and J. H. R. MAUNSELL, 1999. Effects of attention on orientation-tuning functions of single neurons in macaque cortical area V4. *J. Neurosci.* 19:431–441.

MELLET, E., L. PETIT, B. MAZOYER, M. DENIS, and N. TZOURIO, 1998. Reopening the mental imagery debate: Lessons from functional anatomy. *NeuroImage* 8:129–139.

MESULAM, M. M., 1981. A cortical network for directed attention and unilateral neglect. *Ann. Neurol.* 10:309–325.

MOORE, T., and K. M. ARMSTRONG, 2003. Selective gating of visual signals by microstimulation of frontal cortex. *Nature* 421:370–373.

MOORE, T., and M. FALLAH, 2001. Control of eye movements and spatial attention. *Proc. Natl. Acad. Sci. U.S.A.* 98:1273–1276.

NEWSOME, W. T., K. H. BRITTEN, and J. A. MOVSHON, 1989. Neuronal correlates of a perceptual decision. *Nature* 341:52–54.

NOBRE, A. C., G. N. SEBESTYEN, D. R. GITELMAN, M. M. MESULAM, R. S. FRACKOWIAK, and C. D. FRITH, 1997. Functional localization of the system for visuospatial attention using positron emission tomography. *Brain* 120:515–533.

PALMER, J., P. VERGHESE, and M. PAVEL, 2000. The psychophysics of visual search. *Vision Res.* 40:1227–1268.

PARASURAMAN, R., and J. BEATTY, 1980. Brain events underlying detection and recognition of weak sensory signals. *Science* 210:80–83.

PARKER, A. J., and W. T. NEWSOME, 1998. Sense and the single neuron: Probing the physiology of perception. *Annu. Rev. Neurosci.* 21:227–277.

PASHLER, H. E., 1998. *The Psychology of Attention.* Cambridge, Mass.: MIT Press.

POLICH, J., and A. KOK, 1995. Cognitive and biological determinants of P300: An integrative review. *Biol. Psychol.* 41:103–146.

POSNER, M. I., 1980. Orienting of attention. *Q. J. Exp. Psychol.* 32:3–25.

POSNER, M. I., J. A. WALKER, F. J. FRIEDRICH, and R. D. RAFAL, 1984. Effects of parietal injury on covert orienting of attention. *J. Neurosci.* 4:1863–1874.

RESS, D., B. T. BACKUS, and D. J. HEEGER, 2000. Activity in primary visual cortex predicts performance in a visual detection task. *Nat. Neurosci.* 3:940–945.

RESS, D., and D. J. HEEGER, 2003. Neuronal correlates of perception in early visual cortex. *Nat. Neurosci.* 6:414–420.

REYNOLDS, J. H., L. CHELAZZI, and R. DESIMONE, 1999. Competitive mechanisms subserve attention in macaque areas V2 and V4. *J. Neurosci.* 19:1736–1753.

REYNOLDS, J. H., T. PASTERNAK, and R. DESIMONE, 2000. Attention increases sensitivity of V4 neurons. *Neuron* 26:703–714.

ROLAND, P. E., and B. GULYAS, 1994. Visual imagery and visual representation. *Trends Neurosci.* 17:281–287.

ROMO, R., C. D. BRODY, A. HERNÁNDEZ, and L. LEMUS, 1999. Neuronal correlates of parametric working memory in the prefrontal cortex. *Nature* 399:470–473.

ROMO, R., A. HERNÁNDEZ, A. ZAINOS, C. D. BRODY, and L. LEMUS, 2000. Sensing without touching: Psychophysical performance based on cortical microstimulation. *Neuron* 26:273–278.

ROMO, R., A. HERNÁNDEZ, A. ZAINOS, C. BRODY, and E. SALINAS, 2002. Exploring the cortical evidence of a sensory-discrimination process. *Philos. Trans. R. Soc. Lond. B Biol. Sci.* 357:1039–1051.

ROMO, R., A. HERNÁNDEZ, A. ZAINOS, L. LEMUS, and C. D. BRODY, 2002. Neuronal correlates of decision-making in secondary somatosensory cortex. *Nat. Neurosci.* 5:1217–1225.

ROMO, R., A. HERNÁNDEZ, A. ZAINOS, and E. SALINAS, 1998. Somatosensory discrimination based on cortical microstimulation. *Nature* 392:387–390.

ROMO, R., and E. SALINAS, 1999. Sensing and deciding in the somatosensory system. *Curr. Opin. Neurobiol.* 9:487–493.

ROMO, R., and E. SALINAS, 2001. Touch and go: Decision-making mechanisms in somatosensation. *Annu. Rev. Neurosci.* 24:107–137.

ROMO, R., and E. SALINAS, 2003. Flutter discrimination: Neural codes, perception, memory and decision making. *Nat. Rev. Neurosci.* 4:203–218.

RUSHWORTH, M. F., T. PAUS, and P. K. SIPILA, 2001. Attention systems and the organization of the human parietal cortex. *J. Neurosci.* 21:5262–5271.

SCANNELL, J. W., and M. P. YOUNG, 1999. Neuronal population activity and functional imaging. *Proc. R. Soc. Lond. B Biol. Sci.* 266:875–881.

SCHMOLESKY, M. T., Y. WANG, D. P. HANES, K. G. THOMPSON, S. LEUTGEB, J. D. SCHALL, and A. G. LEVENTHAL, 1998. Signal timing across the macaque visual system. *J. Neurophysiol.* 79: 3272–3278.

SERENO, M. I., A. M. DALE, J. B. REPPAS, K. K. KWONG, J. W. BELLIVEAU, T. J. BRADY, B. R. ROSEN, and R. B. TOOTELL, 1995.

Borders of multiple visual areas in humans revealed by functional magnetic resonance imaging. *Science* 268:889–893.

SHADLEN, M. N., K. H. BRITTEN, W. T. NEWSOME, and J. A. MOVSHON, 1996. A computational analysis of the relationship between neuronal and behavioral responses to visual motion. *J. Neurosci.* 16:1486–1510.

SHADLEN, M. N., and W. T. NEWSOME, 1998. The variable discharge of cortical neurons: Implications for connectivity, computation, and information coding. *J. Neurosci.* 18:3870–3896.

SHULMAN, G. L., J. M. OLLINGER, E. AKBUDAK, T. E. CONTURO, A. Z. SNYDER, S. E. PETERSEN, and M. CORBETTA, 1999. Areas involved in encoding and applying directional expectations to moving objects. *J. Neurosci.* 19:9480–9496.

SHULMAN, G. L., J. M. OLLINGER, M. LINENWEBER, S. E. PETERSEN, and M. CORBETTA, 2001. Multiple neural correlates of detection in the human brain. *Proc. Natl. Acad. Sci. U.S.A.* 98:313–318.

SOFTKY, W. R., and C. KOCH, 1993. The highly irregular firing of cortical cells is inconsistent with temporal integration of random EPSPs. *J. Neurosci.* 13:334–350.

SPITZER, H., R. DESIMONE, and J. MORAN, 1988. Increased attention enhances both behavioral and neuronal performance. *Science* 240:338–340.

SQUIRES, K. C., N. K. SQUIRES, and S. A. HILLYARD, 1975a. Decision-related cortical potentials during an auditory signal detection task with cued observation intervals. *J. Exp. Psychol. Hum. Percept. Perform.* 1:268–279.

SQUIRES, K. C., N. K. SQUIRES, and S. A. HILLYARD, 1975b. Vertex evoked potentials in a rating-scale detection task: Relation to signal probability. *Behav. Biol.* 13:21–34.

SQUIRES, K. C., C. WICKENS, N. K. SQUIRES, and E. DONCHIN, 1976. The effect of stimulus sequence on the waveform of the cortical event-related potential. *Science* 193:1142–1146.

SQUIRES, N. K., K. C. SQUIRES, and S. A. HILLYARD, 1975. Two varieties of long-latency positive waves evoked by unpredictable auditory stimuli in man. *Electroencephalogr. Clin. Neurophysiol.* 38: 387–401.

SUPER, H., H. SPEKREIJSE, and V. A. LAMME, 2001a. Two distinct modes of sensory processing observed in monkey primary visual cortex (V1). *Nat. Neurosci.* 4:304–310.

SUPER, H., H. SPEKREIJSE, and V. A. LAMME, 2001b. A neural correlate of working memory in the monkey primary visual cortex. *Science* 293:120–124.

THOMPSON, K. G., and J. D. SCHALL, 1999. The detection of visual signals by macaque frontal eye field during masking. *Nat. Neurosci.* 2:283–288.

THOMPSON, K. G., and J. D. SCHALL, 2000. Antecedents and correlates of visual detection and awareness in macaque prefrontal cortex. *Vision Res.* 40:1523–1538.

TOOTELL, R. B., N. HADJIKHANI, E. K. HALL, S. MARRETT, W. VANDUFFEL, J. T. VAUGHAN, and A. M. DALE, 1998. The retinotopy of visual spatial attention. *Neuron* 21:1409–1422.

TREUE, S., and J. C. M. TRUJILLO, 1999. Feature-based attention influences motion processing gain in macaque visual cortex. *Nature* 399:575–579.

WAGNER, A. D., D. L. SCHACTER, M. ROTTE, W. KOUTSTAAL, A. MARIL, A. M. DALE, B. R. ROSEN, and R. L. BUCKNER, 1998. Building memories: Remembering and forgetting of verbal experiences as predicted by brain activity. *Science* 281:1188–1191.

WOJCIULIK, E., and N. KANWISHER, 1999. The generality of parietal involvement in visual attention. *Neuron* 23:747–764.

YANTIS, S., J. SCHWARZBACH, J. T. SERENCES, R. L. CARLSON, M. A. STEINMETZ, J. J. PEKAR, and S. M. COURTNEY, 2002. Transient neural activity in human parietal cortex during spatial attention shifts. *Nat. Neurosci.* 5:995–1002.

25 Dynamics of Attentional Modulation in Visual Cerebral Cortex

JOHN H. R. MAUNSELL AND GEOFFREY M. GHOSE

ABSTRACT Many studies have shown that attention to a visual stimulus can enhance the responses of cortical neurons that represent that stimulus, but few have examined the dynamics of these enhancements. Recent studies have shown that the strength of attentional modulation depends on the difficult of the task being performed: A shift in attention affects neuronal responses more when the subject does a more challenging task. Other studies have shown that attentional modulation of neuronal responses can vary rapidly over the course of a task, following the subject's expectations about when interesting events are likely to occur. Collectively, these studies show that attention depends on flexible and highly dynamic neuronal mechanisms.

We live in a constantly changing environment. Our brains must be able both to detect and to respond to these changes. A large body of work has described how neurons in different sensory systems can precisely signal the dynamics of sensory information. Some neurons near the sensory periphery can faithfully represent stimulus fluctuations with the precision of a millisecond or better (e.g., Rose et al., 1966; Talbot et al., 1968; Alonso, Usrey, and Reid, 1996), and some sensory representations in the cerebral cortex have a precision of 10 ms or better (see Bair and Koch, 1996; Buracas et al., 1998; Shadlen and Newsome, 1998; Bair, 1999). Although not all sensory neurons are likely to achieve such high levels of temporal precision, virtually all sensory systems must follow stimulus changes that occur over hundreds of milliseconds.

Studies using a variety of neurophysiological methods have shown that behavioral context can affect these sensory signals. For example, attention to a stimulus can increase the responses of cortical neurons that represent it (see Desimone and Duncan, 1995; Leon and Shadlen, 1998; Maunsell and Cook, 2002). The majority of these studies have not considered the possibility that the behavioral context and relevance of sensory stimuli might change rapidly.

JOHN H. R. MAUNSELL Howard Hughes Medical Institute and Division of Neuroscience, Baylor College of Medicine, Houston, Tex.
GEOFFREY M. GHOSE Division of Neuroscience, Baylor College of Medicine, Houston, Tex.

Neurophysiological studies of attention typical manipulate behavioral state by presenting two or more task conditions that encourage different allocations of attention and assume that attention is constant during task conditions that may span many trials. Relatively few studies have attempted to monitor or control changes in attention that occur over shorter periods.

Although neurophysiological experiments have given relatively little consideration to the dynamics of attention, the ability to change over time is the very essence of attention. The utility of spatial attention, for example, depends on its capacity to target different locations according to behavioral demands. Here we consider the dynamic aspects of attention and their correlates in the activity of individual neurons in visual cortex. Because virtually all of the relevant investigations have been done in behaving monkeys, the discussion will focus on those studies.

Vigilance: Changes in the amount of attention

Changes in attention take different forms. One is a change in the overall level of arousal, alertness, or vigilance, which can occur independently of how attention is allocated across space or sensory modalities. It is not clear that all changes in vigilance depend on the same neuronal mechanisms. For example, the brain systems that underlie variations in sleep and wakefulness may be different than those that underlie more subtle changes in effort while performing a complex task. For the current discussion we will not distinguish among different forms of alertness, and will refer to them collectively as vigilance.

Although overt sleepiness obviously has profound effects on behavioral performance, more subtle changes in vigilance also contribute to performance. Overall vigilance may vary as a subject is confronted with slightly different task demands. For example, human subjects are better able to discriminate a moderate change in orientation when this change occurs among other trials with a small, difficult-to-detect change than when the same moderate change occurs

351

among trials with a large, easily detected change (Urbach and Spitzer, 1995).

Some of the earliest recordings from cortex in unanesthetized subjects showed that vigilance affects not just behavior but also the responses of sensory neurons (Hubel et al., 1959). Since then, many neurophysiological studies have shown that neurons in visual cortex respond differently in situations that are likely to produce different levels of vigilance. Mountcastle, Andersen, and Motter (1981) provided a striking demonstration that a subject's level of effort can influence neuronal responses in parietal visual cortex. For each neuron recorded, they compared responses to a visual stimulus in two conditions. In one, the stimulus appeared while the animal was performing a visual task in which it had to fixate a small target and respond when it dimmed. In the other, the stimulus was presented in the same retinal location while the animal was not performing any task but instead sitting idle while waiting for the next trial to begin. About two-thirds of the neurons they recorded in area 7a had significantly stronger responses to stimulus presentations made while the animal was performing the visual task. The effect was substantial: among cells with significant increases, the median change was more than a factor of three.

Similar effects of varying attentional effort have been described in areas in ventral visual cortex. For example, neurons in area V4 respond more strongly when monkeys perform a more difficult version of a matching task. Spitzer, Desimone, and Moran (1988) recorded from monkeys performing color or orientation match-to-sample tasks. On some sets of trials, stimulus differences were large (90° of orientation or 77 nm of wavelength) and the task was very easy. On other sets of trials, the stimulus differences were smaller (22.5° or 19 nm), making the task more difficult. Figure 25.1 summarizes the effects of task difficulty. Responses to an optimal stimulus were 18% stronger (median) when that stimulus appeared while animals were performing the more difficult version of the task, compared to responses to the same stimulus when it appeared while animals were performing the easy version. The animal attended to the stimulus in both cases, so this change in neuronal response is presumably the effect of increased vigilance when the animal performed the difficult discrimination. Consistent with these results, Spitzer and Richmond (1991) found that the responses of inferotemporal neurons to a given stimulus were progressively stronger when they were presented during a fixation task, a dimming detection task, and a pattern discrimination task.

The effects of increased vigilance are not restricted to an overall increase in excitability. In at least some circumstances vigilance can modulate the effects of spatial attention. Boudreau and Maunsell (2001) trained monkeys to do an orientation-change detection task in which attention was directed to one of two stimuli, and the orientation change

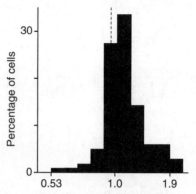

FIGURE 25.1 Effect of task difficult on the responses of V4 neurons. Each neuron's response to its preferred stimulus was measured in two conditions: once when it appeared during a set of difficult discriminations, and again when it appeared during a set of easy discriminations. This histogram plots the ratio of the responses to the optimal stimulus in the two conditions. Most neurons responded more strongly when the animal was performing the difficult task. (Reprinted with permission from H. Spitzer et al., Increased attention enhances both behavioral and neuronal performance. *Science* 240:338–346. © 1988 American Association for the Advancement of Science.)

was either easy to detect or difficult to detect on different sets of trials. In either condition, directing attention toward one stimulus increased neuronal responses to that stimulus relative to the other. However, the difference in responses to attended and unattended stimuli depended on task difficulty. During the difficult version, the difference between the responses to the attended and unattended stimuli was even larger. Thus, not only can vigilance increase the responses of visual neurons, it can also increase the modulation associated with shifts in spatial attention.

Rapid dynamics in attentional allocation

The experiments described in the preceding section show that attention can differ between task conditions. Those studies and most other neurophysiological studies of the effects of attention have implicitly assumed that such effects are constant over the duration of an individual behavioral trial. Consequently, relatively little is known about the dynamics of extraretinal signals over periods of a few seconds. Nevertheless, there is ample reason to believe that attention has dynamics that operate over brief periods.

Many psychophysical studies have shown rapid and transient shifts in spatial attention when a salient stimulus appears in the visual field (reviewed by Kinchla, 1992; Egeth and Yantis, 1997). For example, introducing a cue at an eccentric location causes a rapid and short-lived increase in perceptual performance at that site. Stimuli rapidly flashed at different locations can cause attention to shift within 50 ms (Saarinen and Julesz, 1991). Performance peaks at the location of a flashed stimulus about 100–200 ms after it appears, and then declines (Nakayama and Mackeben, 1989). Other experiments have shown that the appearance of a target stimulus leads to rapid changes in perceptual performance that differ in sign and magnitude across the visual field (Kristjánsson and Nakayama, 2002). On a slower time scale, studies of the effects of priming have shown transient changes in perceptual performance that occur over periods of seconds (Maljkovic and Nakayama, 1994).

Although it is well established from psychophysical studies that the allocation of attention can vary rapidly, relatively few neurophysiological studies have examined the time course of extraretinal signals in monkey visual cortex. These studies typically have found that attentional effects vary over periods from 500 ms to several seconds. The effects of spatial or featural attention on neuronal activity in several visual areas have been seen to increase monotonically over stimulus presentations of this duration (Motter, 1994a; McAdams and Maunsell, 1999; Seidemann and Newsome, 1999; Treue and Maunsell, 1999; Fries et al., 2001). With briefer stimulus presentations the progress of extraretinal modulation is more difficult to gauge, but in most cases more modulation is seen later in the response (Luck et al., 1997; Vidyasagar, 1998; Reynolds, Pasternak, and Desimone, 2000).

Although the consistent observation of an increase in attentional modulation during stimulus presentations suggests this might be a fundamental property of attention, there are reasons to doubt that such is the case. The time course of the changes in attentional modulation and the magnitude of modulation achieved vary between studies.

Furthermore, virtually all studies with long stimulus presentations entailed designs in which animals would have been motivated to attend more to later portions of the stimulus presentation, because those periods were closer to the time when a discrimination or response would be required. Thus, it is likely that attentional modulation grew over time in these studies not because attention always increases over time, but because the task design encouraged the animals to attend more to the stimulus as time progressed.

It has been shown that the neurophysiological effects of attention can vary more rapidly than the gradual increases just described. The speed with which shifts in attention can alter neuronal responses was examined directly by Motter (1994b). He trained monkeys to do a task in which a cue stimulus instructed them to pay attention to a subset of the stimuli within an array. On some trials the cue changed part way through the trial, instructing the animal to shift its attention to a different subset in the array. Motter recorded from individual neurons in V4 while the animals performed this task, and examined responses in the period after the animals were instructed to shift their attention. Figure 25.2 plots the average activity of a sample of V4 neurons on trials in which the cue initially instructed the animals to ignore the stimulus in the cell's receptive field, and then changed to instruct the animals to attend to the receptive field stimulus. The vertical line marks the time of the instruction change. The average response increased abruptly starting about 150 ms after the instruction changed. These data show that the effects of attention on neuronal response can change markedly over a period of a few hundred milliseconds.

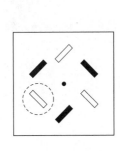
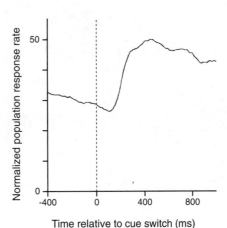

FIGURE 25.2 Change in neuronal response following a signal to shift attention. The diagram on the left shows the configuration of the stimulus array and receptive field (dashed line). The color of the central fixation point cued the animal about which subset of stimuli was behaviorally relevant. The color of the cue sometimes changed partway through a trial, requiring the animal to shift its attention to the other stimuli. The plot shows the average normalized response of 30 V4 neurons before and after monkeys were instructed to shift their attention from the set of stimuli that did not include the receptive field stimulus to the set of stimuli that did. The instruction occurred at time zero (dashed line). Neurons began to respond more strongly within a few hundred milliseconds after the instruction was given. (Modified with permission from B. C. Motter, Neural correlates of feature selective memory and pop-out in extrastriate area V4. *J. Neurosci.* 14:2190–2199. © 1994 by the Society for Neuroscience.)

Bisley and Goldberg (2003) provided another demonstration of rapid changes in neuronal responses associated with shifts in attention. They examined the effects of flashed stimuli on perceptual performance and neuronal responses in the lateral intraparietal area (LIP) of monkeys. Consistent with results of studies in humans, they showed that the abrupt onset of a distracter stimulus could capture a monkey's attention for a period of a few hundred milliseconds. The duration of the behavioral effect corresponded with the period during which the representation of the distracter location in LIP was more robust than the representation of the location to which the animal had been directing its attention before the distracter appeared.

Dynamics of spatial attention associated with task statistics

The neurophysiological data described in the previous section show that attentional effects can change over periods of a few hundred milliseconds. Although these changes were caused by an external cue stimulus, spontaneous shifts in attention might produce comparably rapid changes. We were interested in exploring whether subjects naturally change their attention over short periods when they are faced with tasks in which the probability of events varies in a predictable way. Platt and Glimcher (1999) showed that the responses of neurons in monkey LIP vary between blocks of

trials in a way that is correlated with the animal's expectation of receiving a reward. We wanted to see if neuronal effects related to expectation could be seen over the more rapid time course suggested by behavioral experiments.

We examined the dynamics of attentional modulation in visual cortex by recording from area V4 in monkeys while they preformed a task in which the probability that a behaviorally relevant event would occur varied with time (Ghose and Maunsell, 2002). Two monkeys were trained to do an orientation-change detection task while holding their gaze on a small fixation point in the center of a video monitor. On each trial, stimuli were presented in two or more positions on a screen in front of the animal (figure 25.3a). During a block of 12–15 trials, the animal was cued to attend to one stimulus location and release a lever when the stimulus in that location changed its orientation. Stimuli in other locations might change orientation as well, but the trial ended without reward if the animal responded to an orientation change at an uncued location. When a block of trials was completed, another stimulus location was cued, and the animal had to release the lever when changes occurred there.

The stimuli were positioned so that one or two stimuli were inside the receptive field of the neuron being recorded and one or two were outside the receptive field. Because all trials were completed with the animal holding its gaze on the central fixation point, cuing different stimulus locations allowed us to see how shifting attention toward or away from

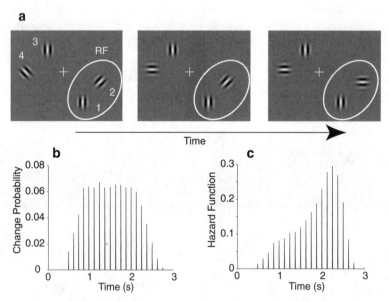

FIGURE 25.3 Orientation change detection task. (a) Typical stimulus configuration. Monkeys fixated a central cross while two or four stimuli were presented. One or two stimuli were within the receptive field (oval), and one or two were in the opposite hemifield. The animal had to release a lever when that stimulus changed orientation at the cued location, ignoring changes at other stimulus locations. (b) Orientation changes occurred at random times after stimulus onset according to the probability distribution shown.

(c) The probability that a change would occur at a given point in time given that one had not yet occurred (hazard function). The hazard function was zero for the first 500 ms (no changes occurred) and then rose to a maximum 2.25 s after stimulus onset. (Reproduced with permission from G. M. Ghose and J. H. R. Maunsell, Attentional modulation in visual cortex depends on task timing. *Nature* 419:616–620. © 2002 by Nature Publishing Group.)

a stimulus in the receptive field affected the response of the neuron. We measured the neurophysiological effects of attention by comparing responses to identical stimulus sets on trials when attention was directed toward the receptive field with responses from trials when attention was directed away from the receptive field.

To study the dynamics of attentional modulation, the probability of a change occurring was not kept constant throughout the trial. Although orientation changed at a random time during each trial, the probability that a change would occur varied in a predictable way as each trial progressed. Figure 25.3*b* shows the probability of a change occurring as a function of time within trials. Orientation changes never occurred during the first 500 ms of a trial. After that, the probability of a change rose rapidly to a relatively fixed level, and the stimulus almost always had changed orientation by 2.5 s after the start of the trial. The behaviorally relevant probability for the monkey was the probability that a change would occur at a given point in time, given that no changes had occurred up to that point (figure 25.3*c*). This conditional probability is called the hazard function, and in this case it increased steadily toward the time of the longest trial, then plunged to zero. That is, if no change had occurred by 2 s into a trial, it was extremely likely that the change would occur in the next few intervals.

We recorded responses from 80 individual neurons in V4 after monkeys had become familiar with this change detection task. The position, orientation and spatial frequency of the stimuli were optimized for each neuron recorded. We measured the effects of attention using an index that compared the responses to the receptive field stimulus when it was the cued stimulus to responses to the same stimulus when the animal's attention was directed away from the receptive field (see caption to figure 25.4). This index was zero if responses were identical in the two conditions (no effect of attention), and positive if responses were stronger when the animal was attending to the receptive field location. Because we wanted to compare identical stimulus conditions, responses from each trial were used only up to the first orientation change, regardless of where that change occurred.

Figure 25.4*A* plots the average attentional modulation index for the sample of neurons as a function of time. Attentional modulation was slightly negative before the trial start and for the first 200 ms, indicating that cuing the receptive field location actually reduced responses to stimuli within it. (The cause of this negative modulation is not clear. It is not a direct effect of a cuing stimulus, because a cue was not presented at the start of the trials that contributed to these data.) After a few hundred milliseconds the attentional modulation became positive, and it grew steadily throughout most of the trial. Figure 25.4*A* also plots a smoothed version

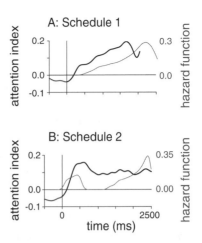

FIGURE 25.4 Attentional dynamics change according to task timing. The plot for each training schedule shows the average attentional modulation (heavy line) and the corresponding hazard function (light line). Each neuron's attentional modulation was computed as a function of time using the following index: (A − I) / (A + I), where A represents the response when the receptive field stimulus was attended, and I represents the response when the receptive field stimulus was not attended. A value of zero corresponds to no difference between the conditions, and a value of 0.2 corresponds to responses that are 50% stronger when the receptive fields stimulus is attended. The lines in both plots have been smoothed with a Gaussian filter ($\sigma = 75$ ms). In both cases the attentional modulation reflects the task statistics with which the animals were trained. (Reproduced with permission from G. M. Ghose and J. H. R. Maunsell, Attentional modulation in visual cortex depends on task timing. *Nature* 419:616–620. © 2002 by Nature Publishing Group.)

of the hazard function, and it can be seen that the attentional modulation has a similar shape.

The results in figure 25.4*A* suggest that the animals had captured the statistical structure of the task and adjusted their level of attention accordingly. However, as described earlier, a rising attentional modulation has been seen in other studies, including some in which there was no overt change in the behavioral significance of the stimulus with time. It is therefore possible that this change in attentional modulation represents a fundamental characteristic of neuronal responses to attended stimuli. To further examine the dependence of attentional modulation on task statistics, we retrained the same monkeys on the same task with a different hazard function (figure 25.4*B*). Although the original task had an initial period of 500 ms in which there were no orientation changes, in the modified task there was a relatively high probability of change during this period and a period of zero probability in the subsequent 500 ms. The new hazard function was the only change made to the task. After retraining for three weeks with this new probability schedule, we recorded from an additional 83 neurons in V4. Figure 25.4*B* shows the neurophysiological effects of this retraining. With the modified timing, there was a sharp rise in the attentional modulation shortly after stimulus onset that was not seen with the original schedule. Moreover, in contrast to the smoothly rising modulation seen in the first design, and in most previous reports, attentional modulation did not rise monotonically. Instead, it decreased shortly after the hazard function went to zero.

These results can be interpreted as showing the combined effects of spatial attention and vigilance. Attending to one stimulus or the other enhanced neuronal responses to that stimulus (positive attention index values in figure 25.4), reflecting the effects of spatial attention. However, the magnitude of the spatial attention effects varied with time, presumably reflecting fluctuations in the subject's vigilance as the stimulus changes it was trying to detect became more or less probable. These variations in the effects of spatial attention over time show that subjects form an internal representation of task timing acquired during the course of training, and then use this representation to temporally modulate behaviorally relevant visual responses. Unlike the spatial cues, there was no explicit requirement for the animals to monitor task timing and modulate their attention. Task timing was changed without any explicit instruction to alert the animals to the change. The results were consistent between the two animals, suggesting that temporal strategies that reflect expectations about a task are commonly adopted. Thus, just as task difficulty can affect the magnitude of attentional modulations, so can task timing affect the time course of such modulations.

Concluding comments

Collectively, the experiments discussed here make it clear that the effects of attention on neuronal responses can be highly dynamic. Attention can vary in a nonselective way as changes in the level of arousal or vigilance, and in a more selective form associated with shifts of attention to particular spatial locations or features. The data described here suggest that both forms vary over periods shorter than typical behavioral trials. Nevertheless, most neurophysiological studies have treated them as constant during the course of individual trials.

Differences in neuronal responses associated with attentional effort may explain why stronger or weaker attentional modulations have been reported by different studies. Although modulation by attention is widely observed, the magnitude of the modulation described for given areas in different studies can vary considerably. For example, the amount of attentional modulation report for neurons in MT tested with different tasks ranges from small (Ferrera, Rudolph, and Maunsell, 1994; Seidemann and Newsome, 1999) to moderate (Cook and Maunsell, 2002) or large (Treue and Maunsell, 1999). Some of this range is attributable to differences in stimuli and analyses, but some is likely

to arise from tasks that are more or less challenging. The potential effect of task difficulty raises problems for comparisons of the effects of attention from different studies or even different tasks within one study. Different magnitudes for the effects of attention may depend more on differences in task demands than on differences between stimuli, task structure, or the visual areas studied. Although some reports have carefully acknowledged this uncertainty (e.g., Richmond and Sato, 1987), others have not.

Similarly, the dynamics of attention may also explain why some studies have reported that attention alters spontaneous activity (Luck et al., 1997; Chelazzi et al., 1998; Reynolds, Pasternak, and Desimone, 2000), but others have not (McAdams and Maunsell, 1999; Jagadeesh et al., 2001). For example, McAdams and Maunsell (1999) found that cuing an animal to attend toward or away from the receptive fields of V4 neurons did not affect neuronal activity in the period immediately before the stimulus presentation. In that task, however, the stimulus appeared at a fixed delay after the animal had acquired the fixation spot, and it was always presented for a relatively long time (500 ms). There was no reason for the animal to direct its attention to the receptive field location before the stimulus was going to appear. Although the animal knew where it would need to direct its attention, it may not have shifted its attention to the peripheral location until after the stimulus appeared. In contrast, others have found that spatial attention affects spontaneous activity when stimuli are presented only briefly at somewhat unpredictable times (Luck et al., 1997; Reynolds, Pasternak, and Desimone, 2000). While direct tests will be needed to confirm that attentional dynamics are the source of the differences seen in spontaneous activity, it seems clear that intervals before the onset of a stimulus are not optimal for assessing attentional modulation of spontaneous activity. The most reliable measurements would be those made during periods embedded in a sequence of stimuli with timing sufficiently irregular to demand sustained attention.

Differences in effort may also explain differences seen between subjects in individual studies. It is frequently observed that attentional modulation differs between subjects within a study (e.g., Huk and Heeger, 2000; Cook and Maunsell, 2002). These differences might arise from innate differences between subjects or from individual applying more effort or adopting different strategies. Differences of this sort are difficult to bring under tight experimental control.

The dynamics of attention may have effects beyond quantitative differences in the measurements of attentional modulation. For example, fluctuations in attention can add variance (noise) to a neuron's response to a particular stimulus. As a result, measurements of a neuron's ability to discriminate sensory stimuli when attention is kept relatively constant will appear superior to measurements made when attention is allowed to fluctuate, even if the time-averaged level of attention is the same in both conditions. The dynamics of attention would similarly affect models that examine the advantages of combining signals from different neurons. Because the observed attentional modulations are relatively consistent between individual neurons, attention introduces covariance between pairs of neurons. This covariance will adversely affect the performance of models that discriminate sensory stimuli based on the pooled spikes from different neurons, but may improve the performance in models in which spikes are assigned to neurons that have different, known stimulus selectivities (Abbott and Dayan, 1999).

Attentional dynamics could also affect measurements of correlation between neurophysiological signals and behavioral responses. If a suprathreshold stimulus is presented for long periods, then an animal might attend only to an epoch sufficiently long to perform the task. The average of activity over the entire stimulus presentation could therefore dilute the behaviorally relevant signal and lead to underestimates of the correlations between behavior and physiological measurements. This is a particular concern for tasks in which there is no behavioral requirement to react quickly.

We currently have no information about the limits of how rapidly attention can be reallocated. Our results show that the modulation of neuronal responses by spatial attention can vary within behavioral trials over periods as brief as a few hundred milliseconds. However, our manipulations of task statistics probably did not provide a strong incentive to the animals to shift their attention rapidly, because excellent performance could have been achieved with constant attention to the cued stimulus. It is likely that attention can shift rapidly and frequently. Indeed, attention has frequently been closely linked to saccade eye movements (e.g., Kowler et al., 1995; Sheliga, Riggio, and Rizzolatti, 1995; Deubel and Schneider, 1996; Kustov and Robinson, 1996; Hafed and Clark, 2002; McFadden, Khan, and Wallman, 2002), which typically move gaze several times a second. It seems reasonable to expect that the dynamics of at least some neuronal effects of attention may approach those for saccadic eye movements. Neurophysiological recordings in animals performing tasks that are designed to encourage rapid shifts in attention may reveal faster dynamics than those described here.

We are likely to learn more as more studies move beyond studying behavioral state as a static entity. For example, it is possible that the modulations observed would be larger and more consistent in situations that more closely approximate brief fixation periods that occur during most natural viewing situations, rather than the less natural sustained inspections of peripheral targets are used in most studies. This change in perspective may also help lead to a better appreciation of the role of attentional modulation in coupling sensory responses to the initiation of behavioral responses.

ACKNOWLEDGMENTS   This work was supported by National Institutes of Health grant R01 EY05911. J.H.R.M. is an Investigator with the Howard Hughes Medical Institute.

REFERENCES

ABBOTT, L. F., and P. DAYAN, 1999. The effect of correlated variability on the accuracy of a population code. *Neural Comput.* 11:91–101.

ALONSO, J. M., W. M. USREY, and R. C. REID, 1996. Precisely correlated firing in cells of the lateral geniculate nucleus. *Nature* 383:815–819.

BAIR, W., 1999. Spike timing in the mammalian visual system. *Curr. Opin. Neurobiol.* 9:447–453.

BAIR, W., and C. KOCH, 1996. Temporal precision of spike trains in extrastriate cortex of the behaving monkey. *Neural Comput.* 8:44–66.

BISLEY, J. W., and M. E. GOLDBERG, 2003. Neuronal activity in the lateral intraparietal area and spatial attention. *Science* 299:81–86.

BOUDREAU, C. E., and J. H. R. MAUNSELL, 2001. Is spatial attention a limited resource for V4 neurons? *Soc. Neurosci. Abstr.* 27:574.3.

BURACAS, G. T., A. M. ZADOR, M. R. DEWEESE, and T. D. ALBRIGHT, 1998. Efficient discrimination of temporal patterns by motion-sensitive neurons in primate visual cortex. *Neuron* 20:959–969.

CHELAZZI, L., J. DUNCAN, E. K. MILLER, and R. DESIMONE, 1998. Responses of neurons in inferotemporal cortex during memory-guided visual search. *J. Neurophysiol.* 80:2918–2940.

COOK, E. P., and J. H. R. MAUNSELL, 2002. Attentional modulation of behavioral performance and neuronal responses in middle temporal and ventral intraparietal areas of macaque monkey. *J. Neurosci.* 22:1994–2004.

DESIMONE, R., and J. DUNCAN, 1995. Neural mechanisms of selective visual attention. *Annu. Rev. Neurosci.* 18:193–222.

DEUBEL, H., and W. X. SCHNEIDER, 1996. Saccade target selection and object recognition: Evidence for a common attentional mechanism. *Vision Res.* 36:1827–1837.

EGETH, H. E., and S. YANTIS, 1997. Visual attention: Control, representation, and time course. *Annu. Rev. Psychol.* 48:269–297.

FERRERA, V. P., K. K. RUDOLPH, and J. H. R. MAUNSELL, 1994. Responses of neurons in the parietal and temporal visual pathways during a motion task. *J. Neurosci.* 14:6171–6186.

FRIES, P., J. H. REYNOLDS, A. E. RORIE, and R. DESIMONE, 2001. Modulation of oscillatory neuronal synchronization by selective visual attention. *Science* 291:1560–1563.

GHOSE, G. M., and J. H. R. MAUNSELL, 2002. Attentional modulation in visual cortex depends on task timing. *Nature* 419:616–620.

HAFED, Z. M., and J. J. CLARK, 2002. Microsaccades as an overt measure of covert attentional shifts. *Vision Res.* 42:2533–2545.

HUBEL, D. H., C. O. HENSON, A. RUBERT, and R. GALAMBOS, 1959. "Attention" units in the auditory cortex. *Science* 129:1279–1280.

HUK, A. C., and D. J. HEEGER, 2000. Task-related modulations of visual cortex. *J. Neurophysiol.* 83:3524–3536.

JAGADEESH, B., L. CHELAZZI, M. MISHKIN, and R. DESIMONE, 2001. Learning increases stimulus salience in anterior inferior temporal cortex of the macaque. *J. Neurophysiol.* 86:290–303.

KINCHLA, R. A., 1992. Attention. *Annu. Rev. Psychol.* 43:711–742.

KOWLER, E., E. ANDERSON, B. A. DOSHER, and E. BLASER, 1995. The role of attention in the programming of saccades. *Vision Res.* 35:1897–1916.

KRISTJÁNSSON, A., and K. NAKAYAMA, 2002. The attentional blink in space and time. *Vision Res.* 42:2039–2050.

KUSTOV, A. A., and D. L. ROBINSON, 1996. Shared neural control of attentional shifts and eye movements. *Nature* 384:74–77.

LEON, M. I., and M. N. SHADLEN, 1998. Exploring the neurophysiology of decisions. *Neuron* 21:669–672.

LUCK, S. J., L. CHELAZZI, S. A. HILLYARD, and R. DESIMONE, 1997. Neural mechanisms of spatial selective attention in areas V1, V2, and V4 of macaque visual cortex. *J. Neurophysiol.* 77:24–42.

MALJKOVIC, V., and K. NAKAYAMA, 1994. Priming of pop-out: I. Role of features. *Mem. Cognit.* 22:657–672.

MAUNSELL, J. H. R., and E. P. COOK, 2002. The role of attention in visual processing. *Philos. Trans. R. Soc. Lond. B* 357:1063–1072.

MCADAMS, C. J., and J. H. R. MAUNSELL, 1999. Effects of attention on orientation-tuning functions of single neurons in macaque cortical area V4. *J. Neurosci.* 19:431–441.

MCFADDEN, S. A., A. KHAN, and J. WALLMAN, 2002. Gain adaptation of exogenous shifts in visual attention. *Vision Res.* 42:2709–2726.

MOTTER, B. C., 1994a. Neural correlates of attentive selection for color or luminance in extrastriate area V4. *J. Neurosci.* 14:2178–2189.

MOTTER, B. C., 1994b. Neural correlates of feature selective memory, and pop-out in extrastriate area V4. *J. Neurosci.* 14:2190–2199.

MOUNTCASTLE, V. B., R. A. ANDERSEN, and B. C. MOTTER, 1981. The influence of attentive fixation upon the excitability of the light-sensitive neurons of the posterior parietal cortex. *J. Neurosci.* 1:1218–1235.

NAKAYAMA, K., and M. MACKEBEN, 1989. Sustained and transient components of focal visual attention. *Vision Res.* 29:1631–1647.

PLATT, M. L., and P. W. GLIMCHER, 1999. Neural correlates of decision variables in parietal cortex. *Nature* 400:233–238.

REYNOLDS, J. H., T. PASTERNAK, and R. DESIMONE, 2000. Attention increases sensitivity of V4 neurons. *Neuron* 26:703–714.

RICHMOND, B. J., and T. SATO, 1987. Enhancement of inferior temporal neurons during visual discrimination. *J. Neurophysiol.* 58:1292–1306.

ROSE, J. E., N. B. GROSS, C. D. GIEISLER, and J. E. HIND, 1966. Some neural mechanisms in the inferior colliculus of the cat which may be relevant to localization of a sound source. *J. Neurophysiol.* 29:288–314.

SAARINEN, J., and B. JULESZ, 1991. The speed of attentional shifts in the visual field. *Proc. Natl. Acad. Sci. U.S.A.* 88:1812–1814.

SEIDEMANN, E., and W. T. NEWSOME, 1999. Effect of spatial attention on the responses of area MT neurons. *J. Neurophysiol.* 81:1783–1794.

SHADLEN, M. N., and W. T. NEWSOME, 1998. The variable discharge of cortical neurons: Implications for connectivity, computation, and information coding. *J. Neurosci.* 18:3870–3896.

SHELIGA, B. M., L. RIGGIO, and G. RIZZOLATTI, 1995. Spatial attention and eye movements. *Exp. Brain Res.* 105:261–275.

SPITZER, H., R. DESIMONE, and J. MORAN, 1988. Increased attention enhances both behavioral and neuronal performance. *Science* 240:338–340.

SPITZER, H., and B. J. RICHMOND, 1991. Task difficulty: Ignoring, attending to, and discriminating a visual stimulus yield progressively more activity in inferior temporal neurons. *Exp. Brain Res.* 83:340–348.

TALBOT, W. H., I. DARIAN-SMITH, H. H. KORNHUBER, and V. B. MOUNTCASTLE, 1968. The sense of flutter-vibration: Comparison of the human capacity with response patterns of mechanoreceptor afferents from the monkey hand. *J. Neurophysiol.* 31:301–334.

TREUE, S., and J. H. R. MAUNSELL, 1999. Effects of attention on the processing of motion in macaque middle temporal and medial superior temporal visual cortical areas. *J. Neurosci.* 19:7591–7602.

URBACH, D., and H. SPITZER, 1995. Attentional effort modulated by task difficulty. *Vision Res.* 35:2169–2177.

VIDYASAGAR, T. R., 1998. Gating of neuronal responses in macaque primary visual cortex by an attentional spotlight. *Neuroreport* 9:1947–1952.

26 Acoustic Stimulus Processing and Multimodal Interactions in Primates

GREGG H. RECANZONE

ABSTRACT This chapter focuses on recent studies of auditory cortical processes in humans and nonhuman primates. The primate auditory cortex consists of multiple cortical fields with a core-belt-parabelt organization. Recent anatomical and physiological experiments in nonhuman primates indicate that acoustic space is preferentially processed in the caudal cortical areas, and nonspatial information, such as the temporal and spectral components of acoustic stimuli, is processed in the more rostral cortical areas. Visual stimuli also influence our auditory perceptions in the spatial domain, giving rise to phenomena such as the ventriloquism effect. Similarly, auditory stimuli influence our perception of visual stimuli in the temporal domain, giving rise to illusions such as "seeing" visual stimuli that are consistent with simultaneously presented auditory stimuli. The cortical areas giving rise to these perceptions are still unknown and may be the result of feed-forward and feedback projections within a network of both multimodal and unimodal cortical areas.

The natural auditory environment is commonly rich, with multiple sound sources emitting a variety of different acoustic energies simultaneously. The auditory system must identify what the different sounds are (a bird singing, running water, conspecific vocalization), as well as where they are coming from. These two main functions of the auditory system are similar to those of the visual and somatosensory systems, and, like all sensory systems, the auditory system must integrate information from different sources in order to form unified percepts of objects in the environment. Thus, the auditory system must be able to extract not only what is being said but who is saying it, and from where. The nervous system as a whole combines this information with information from other sensory systems, such as the visual system, to form a more salient percept of who is talking and where that person is. Of key interest to auditory physiologists, and to sensory neuroscientists in general, is understanding what aspects of neuronal activity give rise to these seemingly effortless perceptions.

GREGG H. RECANZONE Center for Neuroscience and Section of Neurobiology, Physiology and Behavior, University of California at Davis, Davis, Calif.

As a first step in understanding these processes, it is important to recognize that the organization of the auditory system differs in several unique ways from the organization of the visual and somatosensory systems. The first difference is that auditory information is processed in multiple stations before reaching the cerebral cortex. Information from the cochlea arrives first at the cochlear nucleus and is then processed in the superior olivary nuclei, nucleus of the lateral lemniscus, inferior colliculus, and medial geniculate nucleus of the thalamus before reaching the auditory cortex (see Kelly et al., 2003, for a review). By contrast, retinal ganglion cells from the retina synapse directly onto thalamic neurons, and the primary afferents from the skin conveying cutaneous information synapse onto neurons in the dorsal column nuclei, which in turn project to thalamic neurons.

The second major difference is that information from both ears is combined early in the system. Inputs from each ear converge onto single neurons in the superior olivary nucleus in the brainstem. Both visual and somatosensory information from the two sides of the visual field and from the midline, respectively, are almost completely segregated until well beyond the primary sensory cortex.

The third difference is that the cells in the sensory epithelium, the hair cells in the cochlea, have no way of independently encoding the spatial location of the stimulus. Thus, the sound source location is necessarily computed from the inputs of many hair cells by the central nervous system (CNS). In contrast, both the retina and the skin can encode the spatial location of the stimulus by which receptors are activated, and therefore spatial information can be represented by a "labeled line" from the periphery.

Despite these unique aspects of organization of the central auditory nervous system, one key commonality among the auditory, visual, and somatosensory systems is a requisite role for the cerebral cortex in stimulus perception. How this transformation from sensory detection to perception occurs, however, remains a mystery. Although we do have a good understanding of the physical cues that can be used to extract stimulus location and, to a lesser extent of how these cues are processed by central auditory neurons, it is much less clear what stimulus parameters are selectively processed to identify and characterize different acoustic inputs. Thus, the neural processing relating to the perception of what is making sounds within the bombardment of acoustic input one experiences at any given time is almost completely unknown. This chapter reviews representative studies of stimulus processing in the auditory cortex of primates, as well as psychophysical studies of how visual and auditory stimuli influence the perception of both modalities. The chapter focuses on the responses of single neurons in the macaque monkey and on psychophysical studies in humans, with a lesser emphasis on how the results of these studies relate to results of studies in other primates, including functional imaging studies of auditory cortical function in humans.

The macaque monkey auditory cortex

The macaque monkey auditory cortex is made up of multiple cortical fields that are organized in a core–belt–parabelt fashion (figure 26.1) (for reviews, see Kaas and Hackett, 2000; Rauschecker and Tian, 2000). These different cortical fields can be defined using both anatomical (see Hackett and Kaas, this volume) and physiological criteria (e.g. figure 26.1) (Recanzone, Guard, and Phan, 2000). For example, both the primary auditory cortex (A1) and the rostral area (R) have koniocortical cytoarchitecture and sharp frequency tuning, but there is a frequency reversal at the A1—R border. In contrast, the belt fields have different cytoarchitecture than the core, and neurons in the belt fields tend to respond to a greater frequency range than those in the core fields.

A key question is how these different fields contribute to our perception of the acoustical world. It has been hypothesized that the auditory cortex processes different aspects of the acoustic signal into two major, parallel streams. In analogy with the primate visual cortex (Ungerleider and Mishkin, 1982; Ungerleider and Haxby, 1994), one stream processes "where" information, pertaining to the location of the sound in space. The other stream processes "what" information, pertaining to other spectral or temporal characteristics of the stimulus that would allow for the identification of what the stimulus is (e.g., alarm clock, car horn). The where pathway has been hypothesized to originate in the core and progress through the caudal belt (CM and CL) and caudal parabelt. The what pathway is also believed to originate in the core and to progress through the rostral belt (ML and AL) and rostral parabelt (Rauschecker, 1998; Rauschecker and Tian, 2000).

This is an attractive hypothesis in that the visual and auditory systems could be considered to be organized by the same general principles, with caudal auditory and dorsal

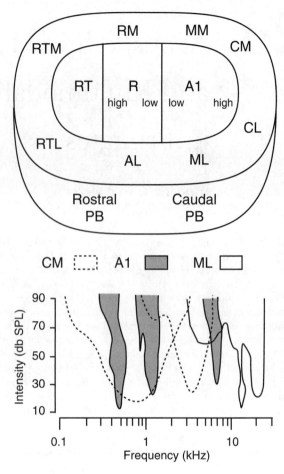

FIGURE 26.1   Schematic representation of macaque auditory cortical fields. *Top*: The core area includes the primary auditory cortex (A1), the rostral area (R), and the rostrotemporal area (RT). Areas A1 and R have an isofrequency representation, so that neurons responsive to high frequencies (high) are located at the caudal end of A1 and the rostral end of R. Neurons responsive to low frequencies are located at the A1/R border. The belt areas are comprised of the caudomedial (CM), caudolateral (CL), middle lateral (ML), anterolateral (AL), rostrotemporal lateral (RTL), rostrotemporal medial (RTM), rostromedial (RM), and middle medial (MM) areas. Lateral to the belt are the rostral and caudal divisions of the parabelt (PB). *Bottom*: Representative frequency response areas (FRAs) for single neurons from three different cortical areas. Each FRA was defined using 50-ms duration tone pips at 31 frequencies, each presented at 16 intensities. Outlined regions denote regions with more than 50% of the maximum response. Shaded FRAs correspond to neurons from A1 (three example cells), dashed FRAs are from neurons in CM (two cells), and the open FRA is from a neuron in ML. See Recanzone, Guard, and Phan (2000) for details.

visual areas processing where information and rostral auditory and ventral visual areas processing what information. This hypothesis is currently being tested by several laboratories; however, it is necessarily a complex enterprise, and definitive experiments have yet to be conducted. Those results that are available generally support this overall view. Perhaps some of the strongest data come from anatomical studies (see Hackett and Kaas, this volume). For example, the ultimate targets of caudal and rostral belt and parabelt areas in the frontal and parietal lobes are consistent with those from the dorsal and ventral streams of extrastriate cortex, respectively (for reviews, see Kaas and Hackett, 2000; Rauschecker and Tian, 2000).

This chapter reviews representative physiological and psychophysical studies on the primate auditory cortex. The first part explores how acoustic space is represented, and the second part explores how nonspatial parameters may be encoded. In each section, the influence of auditory-visual interactions on perception will be discussed.

Cortical processing of acoustic space

The ability to localize sounds in space is a fundamental perception shared by all hearing terrestrial chordates. The ability to locate a sound source is based on three classes of cues. Cues of the first two kinds compare the sounds processed by the two ears and are termed interaural difference cues or binaural cues. Sounds originating off the midline will reach the near ear sooner than the far ear, giving rise to interaural time and phase cues. In primates, these cues are effective only at low frequencies (below a few kilohertz). The head and to a lesser extent the body will also attenuate the sound, making it quieter at the far ear relative to the near ear. In primates, these interaural intensity cues are effective only at higher frequencies. The third cue is monaural (spectral) and arises as a result of the reflections of sound off the torso, head, and particularly the pinnae. These are the primary cues available for localization in elevation. As with interaural intensity cues, spectral cues are effective only at high frequencies.

Given these different sets of cues, sound localization ability is well predicted by the availability of each cue to the listener. For example, a tone stimulus contains only one set of cues and activates a limited population of auditory neurons. In contrast, a band-passed noise or broadband noise provides multiple cues and activates a larger number of auditory neurons. It is therefore not surprising that localization improves with increasing spectral bandwidth (e.g., humans: Recanzone, Makhamra, and Guard, 1998; monkeys: Recanzone, Guard, Phan, and Su, 2000). Similarly, auditory stimuli that do not contain multiple high frequencies, such as tones or low-frequency band-passed noises, are extremely difficult if not impossible to localize in elevation (Recanzone, Guard, Phan, and Su, 2000). Finally, low-intensity sounds, which fall below threshold for many CNS neurons, are more difficult to localize than higher-intensity sounds (e.g., Comalli and Alshuler, 1976; Su and Recanzone, 2001).

The processing of these localization cues begins in the brainstem and continues on throughout the ascending auditory nervous system (see Kelly et al., 2003, for review).

Although subcortical auditory nuclei are critical in processing sound location, lesion studies across a number of species have shown that the auditory cortex plays a key role in acoustic space processing (primate examples include humans: Sanchez-Longo and Forster, 1958; squirrel monkeys: Thompson and Cortez, 1983; and macaque monkeys: Heffner and Heffner, 1990).

NONHUMAN PRIMATES The sound localization ability of macaque monkeys is very similar to that of humans (Brown et al., 1978, 1980, 1982; May et al., 1986; Recanzone, Guard, Phan, and Su, 2000), indicating that the macaque is a good animal model of human auditory spatial acuity. Studies that have investigated the spatial sensitivity of auditory cortical neurons in the macaque (Benson, Hienz, and Goldstein, 1981; Ahissar et al., 1992; Recanzone, Guard, Phan, and Su, 2000; Tian et al., 2001) have found that most auditory cortical neurons respond to most locations tested, although there is some modulation in the response across acoustic space.

Recently, the spatial tuning profiles of neurons in the core (A1) and belt (CM) of the behaving macaque monkey have been directly compared (Recanzone, Guard, Phan, and Su, 2000). In this study, locations were tested at 0°, 15°, and 30° of eccentricity along the horizontal, vertical, and both diagonal axes. Monkeys were trained to make a response when they detected a change in the location of sequentially presented stimuli. For each cell, two different stimuli were presented on randomly interleaved trials. The first was a tone near the best frequency of the neuron. The second was either one of six different one-octave band-passed noises ranging from low (500–1000 Hz) to high (5000–10,000 Hz) frequencies, or broadband noise. Most neurons responded to many, if not all, of the locations tested. However, there was a substantial population of neurons, termed spatially sensitive neurons, that showed significant differences in their firing rate, depending on where the stimulus was located. Figure 26.2 shows the responses from two such single neurons. In these cells, there was a more robust response for stimuli in the contralateral field (in this case to the right of the midline) than in the ipsilateral field. In addition, most spatially sensitive neurons had spatial tuning that was consistent with the monkey's ability to localize the stimulus. Neurons had no change in the response rate as a function of the stimulus elevation for stimuli that the monkeys could not localize in elevation, such as pure tones. Similarly, the greatest rate of change in the response as a function of elevation was seen when the neurons were tested with broadband noise, which the monkeys localized most accurately. However, most spatially sensitive neurons were not able to differentiate between different locations in space as well as the monkey was able to. This implies that the activity across the population of neurons is pooled in order to generate the

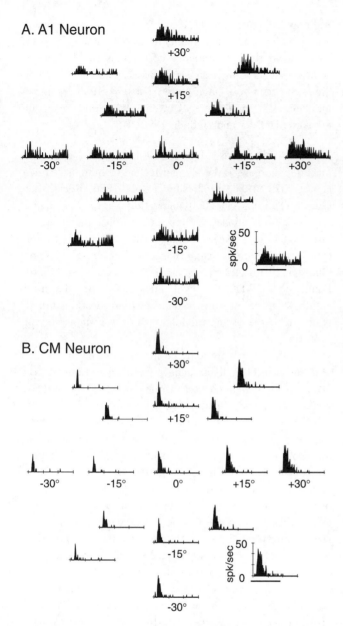

A. A1 Neuron

+30°

+15°

-30°   -15°   0°   +15°   +30°

-15°

spk/sec 50

0

-30°

B. CM Neuron

+30°

+15°

-30°   -15°   0°   +15°   +30°

-15°

spk/sec 50

0

-30°

C. Population Summary

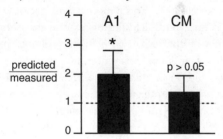

percept of the sound source location. To test this idea, the responses of the spatially sensitive neurons to the central location for each stimulus tested were compared with those at different eccentricities along the horizontal and vertical axes. The differences in the response between these pairs of locations were then compared with the ability of the monkey to detect that the sound had changed from the center to these same locations. Neurons pooled from A1 were again not able to account for the performance of the monkeys (figure 26.2C). However, the sensitivity of neurons pooled from CM was not significantly different from the sensitivity of the monkey. This was true in both azimuth and elevation for acoustic stimuli that were difficult to localize (such as tones) and for stimuli that were easy to localize (such as broadband noise), indicating that these pooled responses could account for sound localization ability across different spectral bandwidths.

Thus, whereas single neurons have very poor spatial localization ability, it appears that the population response in caudal auditory cortical areas does contain enough information in the neuronal firing rate to account for localization behavior. Similar results have recently been obtained in this laboratory. Neurons were tested across 360° of space at four different intensity levels (Woods, Su, and Recanzone, 2001). Again, neurons in the caudal areas (CM and CL) had sharper spatial tuning than neurons in the core (A1 and R) or more rostral belt areas (MM and ML).

Finally, the difference in processing spatial and nonspatial aspects of acoustic stimuli was explicitly tested in the lateral belt areas CL, ML, and AL in anesthetized monkeys (Tian et al., 2001). This study presented monkey vocalizations from different locations spanning ±60° in front of the animal. Overall, neurons in CL responded best to particular areas of space, regardless of which vocalization was pre-

◄————————————————

FIGURE 26.2   Comparison of spatial tuning between A1 and CM. (*A*) Neural responses from a single A1 neuron at each of 17 different locations in an alert macaque monkey. Speakers were located along the vertical, horizontal, and both diagonal axes at eccentricities of 0°, 15°, and 30°. Each PSTH represents the responses to 12 randomly interleaved presentations of a 200-ms broadband noise stimulus. The neuron responded to all tested locations but had a greater response to rightward (contralateral) locations. (*B*) Representative CM neuron from the same monkey. For this neuron, there was a clear increase in the response to rightward locations compared with the A1 neuron shown in *A*. (*C*) Summary of the ratio of the discrimination performance predicted by the pooled neurons divided by the measured behavioral performance of that monkey. Ratios were taken for both tone and noise stimuli in azimuth, and noise stimuli in elevation (21 total comparisons). A value of 1.0 indicates no difference. A1 neurons could on average discriminate between locations about half as well as the monkey. There was no statistically significant different between the predicted and measured responses when CM neurons were pooled. (Adapted from Recanzone, Guard, Phan, and Su, 2000.)

sented. Neurons in AL showed the opposite result: they had a greater modulation in their response depending on which vocalization was presented, and were less modulated by the location of the stimulus. Taken together, the limited data available are converging on the notion that acoustic space is preferentially processed in the caudal belt areas, consistent with the dual processing stream hypothesis of Rauschecker (1998).

CORTICAL SPATIAL PROCESSING IN HUMANS The recent explosion of functional imaging studies in normal human subjects has indicated that the auditory cortex in humans and macaques has similar organization (e.g., Weeks et al., 1999; Binder et al., 2000; Alain et al., 2001; Warren et al., 2002). Functional magnetic resonance imaging (fMRI) studies of sound localization are particularly difficult to perform because of the loud noise and confined space of the device. However, if the acoustic signals are recorded near each eardrum while sounds are played from loudspeakers a meter or so away from the subject, those signals will contain all of the interaural and spectral cues normally available (Wightman and Kistler, 1989a). By playing those same stimuli back to the subject via headphones, one can effectively mimic the natural environment (Wightman and Kistler, 1989b). Such a strategy is now being utilized, and the results indicate that the caudal areas of the lateral belt are selectively activated during sound localization tasks (e.g., Warren et al., 2002).

AUDITORY-VISUAL INTERACTIONS There is a well-established interaction between auditory and visual stimuli in spatial perception. If a visual stimulus is presented simultaneously with an auditory stimulus at a nearby (but not spatially overlapping) location, both stimuli are perceived to originate from the location of the visual stimulus. This phenomenon has been called the ventriloquism effect (Howard and Templeton, 1966) and is robust across a wide range of stimulus types, from synchronized video images of human speech (Warren, Welch, and McCarthy, 1981) to the use of simple tones and spots of light (Radeau, 1985; Slutsky and Recanzone, 2001). This illusion is influenced by both the spatial and temporal disparity between the two stimuli. The ventriloquism effect is greatest at small spatial disparities and decreases as the disparity increases, but this effect can be reduced by introducing a temporal disparity between the two stimuli (Slutsky and Recanzone, 2001). This temporal disparity is not symmetrical, as the two stimuli are more often erroneously perceived to occur at the same time if the visual stimulus leads the auditory stimulus (figure 26.3). This is exactly what occurs in nature due to the faster travel time of light compared to sound, and the nervous system is apparently well tuned to this discrepancy. For example, the perception of whether an auditory and visual stimulus occurs

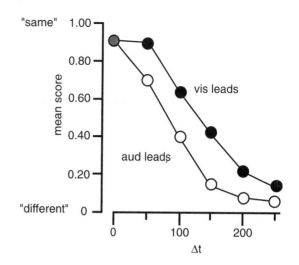

FIGURE 26.3 Temporal disparity functions in normal human subjects. Subjects were presented with a 200-ms 1-kHz tone and 200-ms light flash, and asked whether the two stimuli occurred at exactly the same time or at different times (y-axis). Stimulus onset times varied between 0 and 250 ms (x-axis). Subjects were better able to tell that the two stimuli were not presented at the same time when the auditory stimulus was presented before the visual stimulus (aud leads; open circles) than when the visual stimulus was presented before the auditory stimulus (vis leads; solid circles). This resulted in an offset between the two curves of about 50 ms. See Slutsky and Recanzone (2001) for details.

at the same time depends on how far away the visual stimulus appears to be (Sugita and Suzuki, 2003). This is likely a key parameter in parsing auditory and visual stimuli as belonging to the same or different objects or events.

Although the ventriloquism effect could be an ideal tool in understanding the neuronal mechanisms of integrating visual and acoustic stimuli, it is still unclear even what neural structures are involved in generating these illusions. Multimodal cortical areas are prime candidates for such interactions. In the parietal lobe, neurons respond to both auditory and visual stimuli (e.g., Mazzoni et al., 1996; Cohen, Batista, and Andersen, 2001), although previous training experience (Grunewald, Linden, and Andersen, 1999) and the behavioral task being performed (Linden, Grunewald, and Andersen, 1999) strongly influence the responses of parietal neurons to auditory stimuli. In a study of one patient with bilateral parietal lobe lesions, auditory-visual interactions still occurred, although in the opposite direction (Phan et al., 2000). This patient's visual spatial acuity was poorer than his auditory spatial acuity, and auditory stimuli had a strong influence on his ability to localize visual stimuli.

Other cortical areas that could be involved include the frontal lobe and cortical areas within the superior temporal sulcus, where neurons respond to both visual and auditory stimuli (e.g., Bruce, Desimone, and Gross, 1986; Russo and Bruce, 1994). In principle, either feedback connections from multimodal cortical areas or nonlemniscal inputs from the thalamus could also influence unimodal cortical areas. For example, somatosensory responses have been reported in CM (Schroeder et al., 2001), and eye position, but not visual stimuli, has been shown to influence the responses of neurons in the primary auditory cortex (Werner-Reiss et al., 2003) of the alert macaque. Thus, the question remains wide open as to both the neural structures and neuronal mechanisms that underlie the ventriloquism effect.

Nonspatial processing

NONHUMAN PRIMATE STUDIES The auditory system must resolve not only where a stimulus originated from, but also what the stimulus is. In humans this is a seemingly trivial task, yet very subtle differences in the acoustic signal can generate large perceptual differences. For example, different vowels are identified by changes in the frequency of different harmonics (see Kuhl, 2000). Complex acoustic stimuli can be broken down into two basic components: the spectral component, which corresponds to the frequencies within the signal, and the temporal component, which corresponds to the changes in overall energy with time.

Spectral processing. Processing spectral information appears to predominate in the belt areas of auditory cortex. Early studies noted that neurons in the lateral belt areas are more responsive to broadband stimuli than to tonal stimuli (Merzenich and Brugge, 1973). More recent studies in the alert macaque have confirmed this observation, with neurons in A1 and R having much sharper frequency tuning than neurons in the belt areas (CM and ML; Recanzone, Guard, and Phan, 2000; see figure 26.1). In the anesthetized macaque, neurons in the lateral belt areas (CL, ML, and AL) are more responsive to band-passed noise or broadband noise than to tones (Rauschecker, Tian, and Hauser, 1995).

Several studies have used primate conspecific vocalizations as stimuli to probe how auditory cortical neurons may encode spectrally and temporally complex stimuli. Results from early studies conducted in the 1970s investigating A1 were mixed. Although some neurons were found that seemed to be selective for certain vocalizations, it was not clear whether they were indeed vocalization-specific or were simply responding to a restricted portion of the spectral energy within the call (see Wang, 2000, for review). More recently, a comparison of forward versus reversed calls in the marmoset has shown that many neurons are indeed selective for forward calls (Wang et al., 1995). In addition, vocalizations could also be encoded by the population responses, where neurons with different spectral tuning contribute to the overall representation of the vocalizations across the extent of A1.

A study in anesthetized macaque monkeys explored the sensitivity to exemplar vocalizations in the lateral belt areas AL, ML, and CL (Rauschecker, Tian, and Hauser, 1995). The percentage of neurons that responded selectively to one or only a few of the vocalizations tested was greatest in area AL, decreased in area ML, and decreased further in area CL. This finding indicates that complex spectral processing increases in the rostral regions of the lateral belt. Preliminary studies using four exemplar vocalizations and comparing the responses when the vocalization were presented in the forward versus reversed direction showed a slightly different result in alert macaque monkeys (Su, Woods, and Recanzone, 2001). In this case, approximately 30% of the neurons in the rostral field (R) showed statistically significantly different responses to at least one call presented in the forward versus reversed direction. This was approximately two times the percentage of neurons showing such selectivity in the other fields studied (10%–15% in CL, ML, A1, CM, and MM). What is curious about this finding is that there was no particular selectivity in any of these areas for forward over reversed vocalizations: approximately the same number of neurons responded better to reversed vocalizations as responded better to forward vocalizations. One possibility is that the monkeys in our study heard the same forward and reversed vocalizations literally thousands of times over the course of these experiments, and therefore the novelty of a reversed vocalization was lost, and neither the forward nor the reversed vocalizations had any particular behavioral relevance. Neuroplasticity in the primate auditory cortex has been clearly documented (e.g., Recanzone, Merzenich, and Schreiner, 1993; see also Wang, 2000), and this may be yet another example of such a phenomenon. A second possibility is that the feature extraction of exemplar vocalizations does not occur in the core and belt areas of the auditory cortex in macaques, indicating that further processing in higher cortical areas is necessary for such feature specificity to occur.

Temporal processing. A variety of studies have explored the ability of single neurons to encode fast temporal events, commonly by testing the responses to click trains with different interclick intervals. Trains with large interclick intervals are perceived as distinct clicks, but as the interclick interval decreases, the sound is perceived as a continuous "buzz" with increasing pitch. There are fundamentally two ways in which a neuron can encode the temporal characteristics of a stimulus. The first is to faithfully represent each temporal change, or phase locking. Such temporally sensitive neurons are schematized in figure 26.4 (T neuron). In this case, each click in the train is encoded by the timing of the action potentials. At high click rates, this coding scheme breaks down, as cortical neurons do not follow each stimulus above a few tens of Hertz.

An alternative coding scheme is to represent the click rate by the number of action potentials, also known as a rate

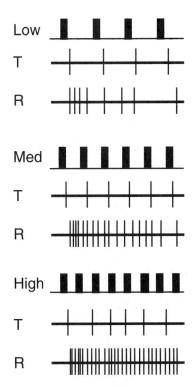

FIGURE 26.4 Schematic representation of a click-train stimulus and response properties of two hypothetical neurons. Each click is represented by the solid rectangle, each action potential is represented by a vertical line. For low click rates (Low), a hypothetical temporal neuron (T) will respond to each phase of the modulation. For higher click rates (Med) the firing rate of such a neuron would increase as it encodes each click in the train. At higher rates (High), the neuron can no longer follow each click in the train, but could in principle still encode the temporal rate by responding only during a particular phase of the stimulus (not shown). In contrast, a rate-coding neuron (R) would not respond to each click in the train, but could increase in firing rate as the click rate increased.

code. In this case, a neuron would increase firing as the click rate increased (R neuron of figure 26.4), and could in principle even be "tuned" to specific rates, similar to how neurons are tuned to specific spectral frequencies (as in figure 26.1).

Lu and colleagues found examples of both coding schemes in the responses of A1 neurons in alert marmoset monkeys (Lu, Liang, and Wang, 2001). One population of neurons responded to each individual click at low presentation rates (similar to the T neurons of figure 26.4) but the firing rate diminished at higher modulation rates. The second population responded to higher presentation rates with an increase in the firing rate that was not in phase with the stimulus (similar to the R neurons in figure 26.4). Further, these neurons showed the same coding strategy if the click trains were randomized, that is, there was not a continuous presentation of the same rate over time. These results indicate that temporal rates from 10 to up to 300 Hz can be represented by the population of A1 neurons.

AUDITORY-VISUAL INTERACTIONS   As in the spatial domain, there are also auditory-visual interactions in the spectral and temporal domains. A classic illusion demonstrating this interaction is the McGurk effect (McGurk and MacDonald, 1976). In this illusion, if one views a person pronouncing one phoneme (e.g., /ga/) but hears a different phoneme (e.g., /ba/), the percept is that the person is pronouncing a third phoneme (in this case, /da/). Thus, what one expects to hear from the visual input and what one expects to see from the auditory input somehow are melded in the nervous system to form an intermediate percept.

Auditory stimuli can have an even stronger influence on visual perception and come to almost completely dominate what one believes one sees. To a subject viewing two moving visual objects presented in silence that intersect each other, the stimuli appear to pass through each other and continue on their trajectories. However, if an auditory stimulus is presented when the two visual stimuli come in contact, the percept is that the two visual objects "bounce" off each other and change their trajectory (Sekuler, Sekuler, and Lau, 1997; Watanabe and Shimojo, 2001). In a second illusion, the number of times a subject perceives a visual flash is influenced by the number of auditory stimuli presented at the same time (Shamms, Kamitani, and Shimojo, 2000, 2002). This effect is very strong when a single light flash is paired with two auditory stimuli, giving rise to the percept of two visual flashes. This effect is reduced, but still apparent, when one visual stimulus is presented in the presence of up to four auditory stimuli.

A similar finding was noted when subjects were asked to discriminate changes in the temporal rate of auditory, visual, or combined auditory and visual stimuli (Recanzone, 2003). Using a 4-Hz comparison temporal rate, subjects were much better at detecting changes in the temporal rate of auditory stimuli compared to visual stimuli. When asked to discriminate the temporal rate of visual stimuli, subjects perceived the lights to flash at a higher or lower rate if a higher or lower rate auditory stimulus was simultaneously presented, respectively. In contrast, the presence of a visual stimulus had no influence on the perception of auditory temporal rates.

These results in human subjects indicate that there are clear nonspatial interactions between auditory and visual stimuli. As with the ventriloquism effect, the locations in the brain where such interactions could occur remain unknown. Bushara, Grafman, and Hallett (2001) found that the posterior parietal lobe, the frontal lobe, cortical areas within the superior temporal sulcus, and the insula were activated to combined auditory and visual stimuli. More recently, Bushara and colleagues (2003) explored the fMRI signals recorded while subjects viewed two bars of light that passed through each other, but on some trials an auditory stimulus was also introduced when the bars of light intersected (similar to the stimuli of Sekuler, Sekuler, and Lau, 1997). In this case, in the visual-only condition, the bars were perceived to pass through each other ("pass" condition). When the auditory stimulus was introduced, the two bars were perceived to bounce off each other ("collide" condition). The results showed again that the frontal and parietal lobes, insula, the superior and inferior temporal gyri, and locations within the occipital lobe were differentially activated on pass and on collide trials. Interestingly, the investigators also noted decreased activity in unimodal visual and auditory areas on collide trials. Again, these data indicate that multimodal processing may well be represented by a network of interconnected areas throughout many of the multisensory areas interconnected by both feedforward and feedback connections with unimodal cortical areas.

Summary

Data from a variety of laboratories studying the neuronal mechanisms of auditory perception in primates are slowly converging on the idea that different aspects of acoustic signals are processed in at least two parallel pathways. Unfortunately, there are still more questions than answers. A major question that remains is how nonspatial properties of acoustic stimuli are processed. The answer to this question should provide valuable clues to how complex stimuli, such as human speech, are processed. Psychophysical studies using combined auditory and visual stimuli indicate that there are strong interactions between these two modalities, with visual stimuli dominating spatial perceptions and auditory stimuli dominating temporal perceptions. Future experiments should be able to address the neural mechanisms of these interactions and provide important insights into how multiple stimulus attributes are integrated to form a unified perception of real-world objects.

ACKNOWLEDGMENTS   This work was supported in part by National Institutes of Health grants EY-013458 and DC-02371, the M.I.N.D. Institute, and a core grant from National Eye Institute to the University of California at Davis.

REFERENCES

AHISSAR, M., E. AHISSAR, H. BERGMAN, and E. VAADIA, 1992. Encoding of sound-source location and movement: Activity of single neurons and interactions between adjacent neurons in the monkey auditory cortex. *J. Neurophysiol.* 67:203–215.

ALAIN, C., S. R. ARNOTT, S. HEVENOR, S. GRAHAM, and C. L. GRADY, 2001. "What" and "where" in the human auditory system. *Proc. Natl. Acad. Sci. U.S.A.* 98:12301–12306.

BENSON, D. A., R. D. HIENZ, and M. H. GOLDSTEIN, JR., 1981. Single-unit activity in the auditory cortex of monkeys actively localizing sound sources: Spatial tuning and behavioral dependency. *Brain Res.* 219:249–267.

BINDER, J. R., J. A. FROST, T. A. HAMMEKE, P. S. F. BELLGOWAN, J. A. SPRINGER, J. N. KAUFMAN, and E. T. POSSING, 2000. Human temporal lobe activation by speech and nonspeech sounds. *Cereb. Cortex* 10:512–528.

BROWN, C. H., M. D. BEECHER, D. B. MOODY, and W. C. STEBBINS, 1978. Localization of primate calls by Old World monkeys. *Science* 201:753–754.

BROWN, C. H., M. D. BEECHER, D. B. MOODY, and W. C. STEBBINS, 1980. Localization of noise bands by Old World monkeys. *J. Acoust. Soc. Am.* 68:127–132.

BROWN, C. H., T. SCHESSLER, D. MOODY, and W. STEBBINS, 1982. Vertical and horizontal sound localization in primates. *J. Acoust. Soc. Am.* 72:1804–1811.

BRUCE, C. J., R. DESIMONE, and C. G. GROSS, 1986. Both striate cortex and superior colliculus contribute to visual properties of neurons in superior temporal polysensory area of macaque monkey. *J. Neurophysiol.* 55:1057–1075.

BUSHARA, K. O., J. GRAFMAN, and M. HALLETT, 2001. Neural correlates of auditory-visual stimulus onset asynchrony detection. *J. Neurosci.* 21:300–304.

BUSHARA, K. O., T. HANAKAWA, I. IMMISCH, K. TOMA, K. KANSAKU, and M. HALLETT, 2003. Neural correlates of cross-modal binding. *Nat. Neurosci.* 6:190–195.

COHEN, Y. E., A. P. BATISTA, and R. A. ANDERSEN, 2001. Comparison of neural activity preceding reaches to auditory and visual stimuli in the parietal reach region. *Neuroreport* 13:891–894.

COMALLI, P. E., and M. W. ALSHULER, 1976. Effect of stimulus intensity, frequency, and unilateral hearing loss on sound localization. *J. Aud. Res.* 16:275–279.

GRUNEWALD, A., J. F. LINDEN, and R. A. ANDERSEN, 1999. Responses to auditory stimuli in macaque lateral intraparietal area. I. Effects of training. *J. Neurophysiol.* 82:330–342.

HEFFNER, H. E., and R. S. HEFFNER, 1990. Effect of bilateral auditory cortex lesions on sound localization in Japanese macaques. *J. Neurophysiol.* 64:915–931.

HOWARD, I. P., and W. B. TEMPLETON, 1966. *Human Spatial Orientation.* New York: Wiley.

KAAS, J. H., and T. A. HACKETT, 2000. Subdivisions of auditory cortex and processing streams in primates. *Proc. Natl. Acad. Sci. U.S.A.* 97:11793–11799.

KELLY, K. A., R. METZGER, O. A. MULLETTE-GILLMAN, U. WERNER-REISS, and J. M. GROH, 2003. Representation of sound location in the brain. In *Primate Audition: Ethology and Neurobiology*, A. A. Ghazanfar, ed. Boca Raton Fla.: CRC Press, pp. 177–197.

KUHL, P. K., 2000. A new view of language acquisition. *Proc. Natl. Acad. Sci. U.S.A.* 97:11850–11857.

LINDEN, J. F., A. GRUNEWALD, and R. A. ANDERSEN, 1999. Responses to auditory stimuli in macaque lateral intraparietal area. II. Behavioral modulation. *J. Neurophysiol.* 82:343–358.

LU, T., L. LIANG, and X. WANG, 2001. Temporal and rate representations of time-varying signals in the auditory cortex of awake primates. *Nat. Neurosci.* 4:1131–1138.

MAY, B., D. B. MOODY, W. C. STEBBINS, and M. A. NORAT, 1986. Sound localization of frequency-modulated sinusoids by Old World monkeys. *J. Acoust. Soc. Am.* 80:776–782.

MAZZONI, P., R. M. BRACEWELL, S. BARASH, and R. A. ANDERSEN, 1996. Spatially tuned auditory responses in area LIP of macaques performing delayed memory saccades to acoustic targets. *J. Neurophysiol.* 75:1233–1241.

McGURK, H., and J. W. MacDONALD, 1976. Hearing lips and seeing voices. *Nature* 264:746–748.

MERZENICH, M. M., and J. F. BRUGGE, 1973. Representation of the cochlear partition on the superior temporal plane of the macaque monkey. *Brain Res.* 50:275–296.

PHAN, M. L., K. L. SCHENDEL, G. H. RECANZONE, and L. R. ROBERTSON, 2000. Auditory and visual spatial localization deficits following bilateral parietal lobe lesions in a patient with Balint's syndrome. *J. Cog. Neurosci.* 12:583–600.

RADEAU, M., 1985. Signal intensity, task context, and auditory-visual interactions. *Perception* 14:571–577.

RAUSCHECKER, J. P., 1998. Parallel processing in the auditory cortex of primates. *Audiol. Neurootol.* 3:86–103.

RAUSCHECKER, J. P., and B. TIAN, 2000. Mechanisms and streams for processing of "what" and "where" in auditory cortex. *Proc. Natl. Acad. Sci. U.S.A.* 97:11800–11806.

RAUSCHECKER, J. P., B. TIAN, and M. HAUSER, 1995. Processing of complex sounds in the macaque nonprimary auditory cortex. *Science* 268:111–114.

RECANZONE, G. H., 2003. Auditory influences on visual temporal rate perception. *J. Neurophysiol.* 89:1078–1093.

RECANZONE, G. H., D. C. GUARD, and M. L. PHAN, 2000. Frequency and intensity response properties of single neurons in the auditory cortex of the behaving macaque monkey. *J. Neurophysiol.* 83:2315–2331.

RECANZONE, G. H., D. C. GUARD, M. L. PHAN, and T. K. SU, 2000. Correlation between the activity of single auditory cortical neurons and sound-localization behavior in the macaque monkey. *J. Neurophysiol.* 83:2723–2739.

RECANZONE, G. H., S. D. D. R. MAKHAMRA, and D. C. GUARD, 1998. Comparison of relative and absolute sound localization ability in humans. *J. Acoust. Soc. Am.* 103:1085–1097.

RECANZONE, G. H., M. M. MERZENICH, and C. E. SCHREINER, 1993. Plasticity in the frequency representation of primary auditory cortex following discrimination training in adult owl monkeys. *J. Neurosci.* 13:87–103.

RUSSO, G. S., and C. J. BRUCE, 1994. Frontal eye field activity preceding aurally guided saccades. *J. Neurophysiol.* 71:1250–1253.

SANCHEZ-LONGO, L. P., and F. M. FORSTER, 1958. Clinical significance of impairment of sound localization. *Neurology* 8:119–125.

SCHROEDER, C. E., R. W. LINDSLEY, C. SPECHT, A. MARCOVICI, J. F. SMILEY, and D. C. JAVITT, 2001. Somatosensory input to auditory association cortex in the macaque monkey. *J. Neurophysiol.* 85:1322–1327.

SEKULER, R., A. B. SEKULER, and R. LAU, 1997. Sound alters visual motion perception. *Nature* 385:308.

SHAMS, L., Y. KAMITANI, and S. SHIMOJO, 2000. What you see is what you hear. *Nature* 408:788.

SHAMS, L., Y. KAMITANI, and S. SHIMOJO, 2002. Visual illusion induced by sound. *Cogn. Brain Res.* 14:147–152.

SLUTSKY, D. A., and G. H. RECANZONE, 2001. Temporal and spatial dependency of the ventriloquism effect. *Neuroreport* 12:7–10.

SU, T. K., and G. H. RECANZONE, 2001. Differential effect of near-threshold stimulus intensities on sound localization performance in azimuth and elevation in normal human subjects. *J. Assoc. Res. Otolaryngol.* 2:246–256.

SU, T. K., T. M. WOODS, and G. H. RECANZONE, 2001. Responses of auditory cortical neurons to frequency modulated sweeps and conspecific vocalizations in the macaque monkey. *Soc. Neurosci. Abstr.* 27.

SUGITA, Y., and Y. SUZUKI, 2003. Implicit estimation of sound arrival time. *Nature* 421:911.

THOMPSON, G. C., and A. M. CORTEZ, 1983. The inability of squirrel monkeys to localize sound after unilateral ablation of auditory cortex. *Behav. Brain Res.* 8:11–216.

TIAN, B., D. RESER, A. DURHAM, A. KUSTOV, and J. P. RAUSCHECKER, 2001. Functional specialization in rhesus monkey auditory cortex. *Science* 292:290–293.

UNGERLEIDER, L. G., and J. V. HAXBY, 1994. "What" and "where" in the human brain. *Curr. Opin. Neurobiol.* 4:157–165.

UNGERLEIDER, L. G., and M. MISHKIN, 1982. Two cortical visual systems. In *Analysis of Visual Behavior*, D. J. Ingle, M. A. Goodale, and R. J. W. Mansfield, eds. Cambridge, Mass: MIT Press, pp. 549–586.

WANG, X., 2000. On cortical coding of vocal communication sounds in primates. *Proc. Natl. Acad. Sci. U.S.A.* 97:1843–1849.

WANG, X., M. M. MERZENICH, R. BEITEL, and C. E. SCHREINER, 1995. Representation of a species-specific vocalization in the primary auditory cortex of the common marmoset: Temporal and spectral characteristics. *J. Neurophysiol.* 74:2685–2706.

WARREN, D. H., R. B. WELCH, and T. J. McCARTHY, 1981. The role of visual-auditory "compellingness" in the ventriloquism effect: Implications for transitivity among the spatial senses. *Percept. Psychophys.* 30:557–564.

WARREN, J. D., B. A. ZIELINSKI, G. G. R. GREEN, J. P. RAUSCHECKER, and T. D. GRIFFITHS, 2002. Perception of sound-source motion by the human brain. *Neuron* 34:139–148.

WATANABE, K., and S. SHIMOJO, 2001. When sound affects vision: Effects of auditory grouping on visual motion perception. *Psychol. Sci.* 12:109–116.

WEEKS, R. A., A. AZIZ-SULTAN, K. O. BUSHARA, B. TIAN, C. M. WESSINGER, N. DANG, J. P. RAUSCHECKER, and M. HALLETT, 1999. A PET study of human auditory spatial processing. *Neurosci. Lett.* 262:155–158.

WERNER-REISS, U., K. A. KELLY, A. S., TRAUSE, A. M. UNDERHILL, and J. M. GROH, 2003. Eye position affects activity in primary auditory cortex of primates. *Curr. Biol.* 13:554–562.

WIGHTMAN, F. L., and D. J. KISTLER, 1989a. Headphone simulation of free-field listening. I. Stimulus synthesis. *J. Acoust. Soc. Am.* 85:858–867.

WIGHTMAN, F. L., and D. J. KISTLER, 1989b. Headphone simulation of free-field listening. II. Psychophysical validation. *J. Acoust. Soc. Am.* 85:868–878.

WOODS, T. M., T. K. SU, and G. H. RECANZONE, 2001. Spatial tuning as a function of stimulus intensity of single neurons in awake macaque monkey auditory cortex. *Soc. Neurosci. Abstr.* 27.

27 Motion Perception and Midlevel Vision

JOSH McDERMOTT AND EDWARD H. ADELSON

ABSTRACT Motion, form, occlusion, and perceptual organization are closely related, and ambiguous moving stimuli provide a tool with which to study their relationship. Such stimuli reveal that form information about occlusion can exert a powerful influence on how motion is interpreted. In this chapter we review our studies of these interactions between form and motion; please see http://web.mit.edu/persci/demos/Motion&Form/Gazz.html. The simplest story one could tell about such interactions, involving local processes based on junctions, bears surprisingly little resemblance to the actual story that emerges from the experiments. Two general sorts of explanations are suggested by our results, process-based and optimization-based. In some cases the phenomena are best explained with reference to processes acting on local features, such as the convexity of the occluding contour. In other cases the simplest explanation is in terms of a cost function that is minimized, for instance one that penalizes illusory edges. In all cases isolated junctions have little explanatory power on their own, and we must appeal to more complex and interesting interactions between form and motion.

Like many aspects of vision, motion perception begins with a massive array of local measurements performed by neurons in area V1. Each receptive field covers a small piece of the visual world, and as a result suffers from an ambiguity known as the aperture problem, illustrated in figure 27.1. A moving contour, locally observed, is consistent with a family of possible motions (Wallach, 1935; Adelson and Movshon, 1982). This ambiguity is geometric in origin: motion parallel to the contour cannot be detected, as changes to this component of the motion do not change the images observed through the aperture. Only the component of the velocity orthogonal to the contour orientation can be measured, and as a result, the actual velocity could be any of an infinite family of motions lying along a line in velocity space, as indicated in figure 27.1. This ambiguity depends on the contour in question being straight, but smoothly curved contours are approximately straight when viewed locally, and the aperture problem is thus widespread. The upshot is that most local measurements made in the early stages of vision constrain object velocities but do not narrow them down to a single value; further analysis is necessary to yield the motions that we perceive.

JOSH McDERMOTT and EDWARD H. ADELSON   Department of Brain and Cognitive Science, MIT, Cambridge, Mass.

It is possible to resolve the ambiguity of local measurements by combining information across space, as shown in figure 27.2. The motion of two-dimensional (2D) features, such as the corner marked 2, is unambiguous and can be combined with the contour information to provide a consistent velocity estimate. On the other hand, some 2D features are the result of occlusion, such as the T-junction (marked 3) that occurs where the two squares of figure 27.2a overlap. The motion of such features is spurious and does not correspond to the motion of any single physical object; in figure 27.2 the two squares move left and right, but the T-junction moves down. (The phenomena described in this chapter are very difficult to understand without viewing the moving stimuli. The reader is urged to view the demos when reading the chapter, at http://web.mit.edu/persci/demos/Motion&Form/Gazz.html.) Distinguishing spurious features from real ones requires the use of form information, because the motion generated by such features does not in itself distinguish them.

An alternative way of extracting 2D motion is to combine the ambiguous information from different contours of the same object, as shown in figure 27.2b, c. In velocity space, the constraints from contours 4 and 5 intersect in a single point (Adelson and Movshon, 1982), which represents the correct leftward motion of the diamond on the left. Similarly, contours 6 and 7, when combined, signal the rightward motion of the other diamond. However, it is important that the constraints that are combined originate from the same object. If the constraints from contours 5 and 6 are combined, for instance, they will lead to a spurious upward motion estimate. Thus, it is critical to combine information across space, but it is also critical to do so correctly. In the motion domain, however, it is not obvious that contours 4 and 5 belong together but 5 and 6 do not. This again means that motion perception is inextricably bound up with form perception and perceptual organization.

In this chapter we review some of our work on the relationship between form, motion, occlusion, and grouping. We will consider these issues from two points of view. Sometimes it is most helpful to discuss them in terms of processes that act on local features, while in other cases explanations in

369

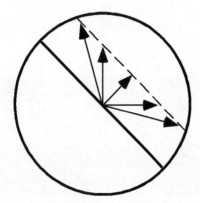

FIGURE 27.1 The aperture problem. Each of the motions (designated with arrows) on the depicted line in velocity space is physically consistent with the edge motion, because only the orthogonal component of its velocity can be detected.

terms of cost functions and optimization principles are most natural.

Motion interpretation: Features

The most well-known consequence of the aperture problem is the barber pole illusion, which was studied by Wallach and many others since (Wallach, 1935; Wuerger, Shapley, and Rubin, 1996). A tilted grating moves behind a rectangular aperture, as shown in figure 27.3. In the version shown in figure 27.3a, the aperture is the same color as the grating background, so there is no visible frame. Because of the aperture problem, the grating is consistent with various motions, including rightward or downward or diagonal motion. When the aperture is wider than it is high, as in this example, the grating will generally be seen as moving to the right. One way of explaining this effect is as follows. The grating is ambiguous, but the line terminators (the endpoints) are unambiguous 2D features. There are more rightward terminators than downward ones, and so the rightward interpretation wins.

An interesting variant of the barber pole illusion is shown in figure 27.3b. Visible occluders are added to the top and bottom. Now the same grating frequently appears to move downward. This could be explained as follows. The terminators along the top are now T-junctions, which could be the result of one contour being occluded by another. Since T-junctions can be created this way, their 2D motions are often the spurious product of occlusion and therefore should be ignored. This means that the only reliable moving features in figure 27.3b are the terminators along the left and right edges of the grating, and these are moving downward. Thus downward motion is seen.

The idea of junctions being detected, labeled, and possibly discounted is well established in the motion literature (e.g., Stoner, Albright, and Ramachandran, 1990;

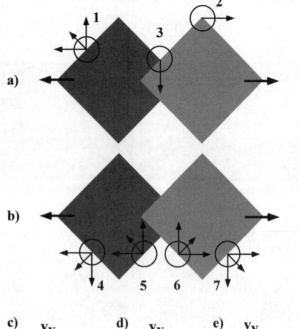

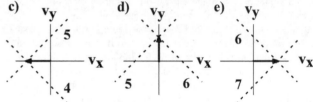

FIGURE 27.2 Example illustrating two problems that occur when integrating motion across space. In a and b, two squares translate horizontally. The edge motions (e.g., 1) are ambiguous, whereas the corner motions (e.g., 2) are unambiguous. The T-junction motions (e.g., 3) are also unambiguous, but their motion is spurious and must somehow be discounted. Integration also poses a problem: c, d, and e show the velocity-space representations of the motion constraints provided by edges 4 and 5, 5 and 6, and 6 and 7, respectively. If the motion constraints from two edges of the same object are combined via intersection of constraints, as in c and e, the correct horizontal motions result. If, however, motion constraints from edges of different objects are combined, as in d, an erroneous upward motion is obtained. Note that the three pairs of local motions are separated by approximately the same distance, and are not distinguished on the basis of their motion. Form information is apparently needed to determine which measurements originate from the same object.

Lorenceau and Shiffrar, 1992; Trueswell and Hayhoe, 1993; Stoner and Albright, 1998; Rubin, 2000). Shimojo, Silverman, and Nakayama (1989) distinguished intrinsic features, which really belong to an object, from extrinsic features, such as the T-junctions, which are side effects of occlusion. Nowlan and Sejnowski (1995), Liden and Pack (1999), and Grossberg, Mingolla, and Viswanathan (2001) have all discussed models in which T-junctions are detected and discounted. Indeed, it can be said that this is the standard view of how many motion phenomena work. However, our research shows that the actual rules governing form influ-

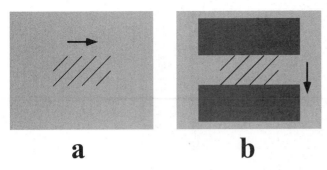

FIGURE 27.3 The barber pole illusion. (*a*) A grating drifts behind an invisible rectangular aperture and appears to move horizontally, along the long axis of the aperture. (*b*) When occluders are added at the top and bottom of the barber pole, vertical motion is often seen, even though the image motion is unchanged. Arrows denote perceived direction of motion.

ences on motion are subtle and complex, and, more surprisingly, that junction categories may have very little explanatory power. Before getting to the experimental results, we will consider the representational issues that arise in these displays.

Motion interpretation: Layers

The percepts associated with overlapping diamonds and moving barber poles involve much more than motion. The diamonds of figure 27.2 are seen as two opaque objects, one occluding the other and both occluding the background. Even if we cannot tell the exact depth of the various parts of this scene, we can tell their depth ordering and their opacity. A representation with motion, depth ordering, and opacity is known as a layered representation (Wang and Adelson, 1994), and it offers a basic tool for discussing the motion phenomena in this chapter.

Let us consider some layered decompositions associated with the barber poles of figure 27.4*a* and *b*. Figure 27.4*a* shows a decomposition corresponding to rightward motion. First there is a background layer, then a moving strip in the next layer, and then a pair of occluders in the top layer. (The moving strip is shown as extended beyond the occluders for illustrative purposes.) The main colors of all three layers are the same, so that only the black lines are visible in the actual

display. This is referred to as a case of invisible occluders, because the bounding contours that would normally demarcate the occluders cannot be seen. Figure 27.4*b* shows a decomposition corresponding to vertical motion. Now the invisible occluders are horizontal. Figure 27.4*c* shows a case in which the occluders are visible because they are a different color.

How can we connect these decompositions to what is observed perceptually? For the basic barber pole of figure 27.3*a*, there are two interpretations that involve invisible occluders, shown in figure 27.4*a* and *b*. The one with the shorter invisible occluders is preferred by the visual system. We believe that this reflects a widespread principle of avoiding interpretations that involve illusory edges. Because an accidental match between an occluder and its background (such as occurs when an illusory edge is perceived) is a rare event, the visual system prefers not to assume it has occurred. Given the choice of a longer or shorter stretch of invisible occluder, it will prefer the shorter stretch, leading it to choose the decomposition of figure 27.4*a*. In the case of figure 27.3*b* and the dark rectangles, however, there is no need to posit invisible occluders, since visible rectangles are clearly present, with their boundaries indicating possible points of occlusion. There is little cost to placing the rectangles in a separate layer, leading to the preferred decomposition of figure 27.4*c*, and therefore leading to the downward motion percept.

Complementary approaches to understanding perception

We have just walked through two very different explanations of the same barber pole phenomena. The first time through, we spoke of identifying, tracking, and discounting local features such as terminators and T-junctions. The second time through, we spoke of layered decompositions and accidental matches, but made no mention of terminators or T-junctions. The first, feature-based explanation could be used in developing a bottom-up model, in which various local image operations are combined in successive steps to build up a motion percept. The second, layer-based explanation could be used in a top-down model that sought an optimal solution to a stated problem, such as finding the most prob-

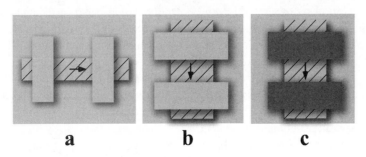

FIGURE 27.4 Layered interpretations of the barber pole stimuli of figure 27.3.

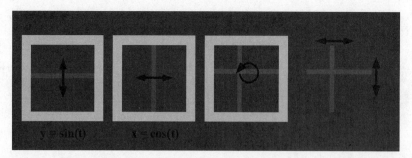

FIGURE 27.5 The cross stimulus. Two bars translate sinusoidally, 90° out of phase, such that their point of intersection executes a circular trajectory. When viewed within an occluding aperture, the bars perceptually cohere and appear to move together with this circular trajectory. When the occluding aperture is removed, coherence breaks down and the bars are seen to move separately, even though the image motion is unchanged.

able interpretation of motion given some assumptions about the statistics of the world. We have found both of these approaches to be useful in our thinking about motion phenomena.

The bottom-up approach is more popular in motion modeling. This is understandable, since modelers are often trying to determine the stages of neural processing that underlie the motion percepts, and these stages are usually conceived of as primarily feedforward. Optimization is also commonly considered to be difficult to implement, because it is often necessary to search through a large space to find the optimum. However, the optimization approach has many advantages. The idea of minimizing a cost function has a long history in perception. Helmholtz advocated the idea of finding the most likely interpretation of the sensory data, and others (e.g., Hochberg and McAlister, 1953; Attneave, 1954; Leeuwenberg, 1969) have proposed that humans seek to minimize the complexity of image descriptions. In motion perception, Restle (1979), Hildreth (1984), Grzywacz and Yuille (1991), and others have had success with various minimization rules. Recently, Weiss, Simoncelli, and Adelson (2002) have shown that many phenomena related to the aperture problem can be understood in terms of a Bayesian framework that finds the most likely single motion consistent with image data. Their results are noteworthy because they do not depend on the usual explicit mechanisms such as feature tracking, intersection of constraints, or vector averaging. Rather, they apply a unified principle that automatically captures the uncertainty associated with the aperture problem and with noise. In another paper, Weiss and Adelson (2000) show that similar minimization principles, when coupled with a layered decomposition, can account for a wide range of phenemona associated with rotating and distorting ellipses.

In this chapter we discuss a range of phenomena involving moving figures and occlusion. We cannot offer a single minimization principle to explain all phenomena, and some of the phenomena are indeed suggestive of feature-based processes. However, we feel that cost functions provide a

promising approach, and we hope that it will be possible to blend the feature-based descriptions with minimization principles in the future. In the present discussion we will use both ways of thinking, as seems appropriate.

The cross stimulus

Our explorations of junction-based rules began with the cross stimulus (figure 27.5). The cross, derived from Anstis's chopsticks illusion (Anstis, 1990), consists of two bars that move sinusoidally, 90° out of phase with each other (McDermott and Adelson, 2004a). When the bars are combined to form a cross, their intersection point traces out a circle, and if the cross is viewed within an occluding frame, as in figure 27.5c, the cross bars appear to cohere and move together in a circle. Without the frame in place, as in figure 27.5d, the bars appear to move separately, in the linear direction orthogonal to their orientation, even though the image motion is unchanged.

What accounts for the effect of the frame? As discussed earlier for the barber pole stimulus, the usual explanation involves tagging and discounting certain kinds of junctions. The bar endpoints provide unambiguous 2D motion signals, and without the frame, these signals are believed to determine the motion percept. The endpoints move linearly, and each bar follows along. When the frame is present, however, T-junctions are formed at the bar endpoints. These junctions provide a cue that the endpoint motions are the spurious result of occlusion. Accordingly, standard models discount motions that occur at T-junctions (Nowlan and Sejnowski, 1995; Liden and Pack, 1999; Grossberg, Mingolla, and Viswanathan, 2001). With the T-junctions in the cross stimulus discounted, the circular motion of the bar intersection determines the motion percept, as all the local motions in the stimulus apart from those of the endpoints are consistent with such a circular motion.

Elements of this story may be on the right track, but the reality is more complex and more interesting, as we learned when we took a closer look at the influence of junctions. We were surprised to find that the feature-based descriptions are of limited value, and in particular that the notion of tagging and discounting T-junctions can explain surprisingly little. Although certain other features may be important, we have also found that the optimization approach has the potential to explain quite a bit, although it does not offer a process-based explanation of the percepts.

Junctions and cost functions

To test for the presence of junction-dependent form constraints, we examined the effects of changing T-junctions to L-junctions in the cross stimulus by matching the luminance of the occluders with that of the moving bars. If the T-junctions that are formed where the bars and occluders overlap played any role in the interpretation of motion in the display, one would expect a change to the junctions to alter perceived motion. As shown in figure 27.6, we held either the bar contrast or the occluder contrast fixed, and swept the other through the point of accidental match (the point where the bars and occluders have the same luminance), observing the effect on coherence. Given that L-junctions are thought to be weaker cues to occlusion than T-junctions, we expected to see a dip in coherence when the bars and occluders matched in luminance.

In the first experiment the bar contrast was fixed and nine different occluder contrasts were tested (figure 27.6a), running through the point of accidental match. In the second experiment the occluder contrast was fixed and eight different bar contrasts were tested (figure 27.6b), again running through the point of accidental match. Observers were shown short clips of each stimulus and were asked to judge whether it was coherent, incoherent, or somewhere in between (for other details of the methods, see McDermott, Weiss, and Adelson, 2001). These ratings were converted into a coherence index, plotted in figure 27.7.

As shown in figure 27.7a and b, the dominant effect was an overall shift in coherence with contrast: coherence increased with occluder contrast and decreased with bar contrast. Shapley and colleagues (1995) obtained similar results with the barber pole stimulus; these contrast effects appear to be a general property of occlusion/motion interactions. We believe the effects are in part due to the role that contrast plays as a depth cue (O'Shea, Blackburn, and Ono, 1994; Stoner and Albright, 1998; Rohaly and Wilson, 1999), but we will not discuss it further in this chapter; we simply accept that the contrast effect is present.

The important point for our purposes is that there was no obvious drop in coherence at the point where L-junctions were generated at the bar endpoints. The curves passed smoothly through the match point, and the category of the junction generated at the bar endpoints had little to no effect on the coherence of the cross.

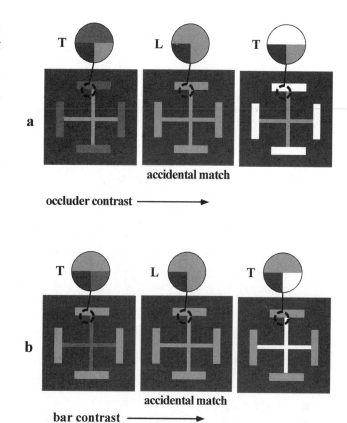

FIGURE 27.6 The effect of junction category was tested by varying bar (a) and occluder (b) contrast and examining the effect of a match in contrast between bars and occluders.

We also tested the role of the junctions at the center of the cross rather than at the bar endpoints. By changing the luminance of one of the bars we could change the L-junctions to T-junctions, as shown in figure 27.8. In this situation one would expect the L-junctions at the match point to produce an *increase* in coherence relative to stimuli with T-junctions at the center, since the L-junctions increase the likelihood that the two bars are a single, coherently moving object. We varied the luminance of one of the two moving bars while holding the luminance of everything else fixed, looking for an effect at the match point.

Curiously, in this case the match point did produce an obvious effect: coherence was highest where the bars matched in luminance, producing a blip in the graph in figure 27.8. We again observed the expected effect of bar contrast: coherence decreased with increasing bar contrast (although here the contrast varied for only one of the bars). But superimposed on this decreasing curve was a pronounced effect of the match point, consistent with what one would expect if junctions were important.

This effect of junction categories at the center intersection seems difficult to reconcile with the previous experiment, in which the category of the junctions at the bar endpoints apparently had little to no effect on the extent to

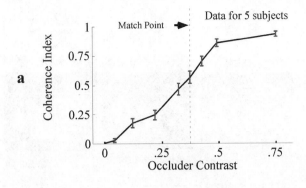

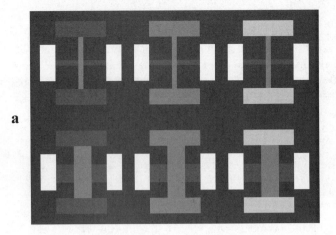

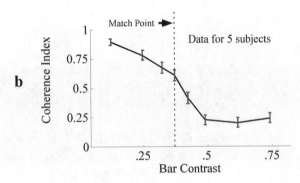

FIGURE 27.7 (*a* and *b*) Results of the experiment schematized in figure 27.6. Error bars in this and all other graphs denote standard errors.

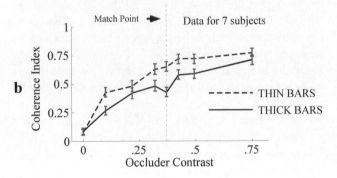

FIGURE 27.9 To control for resolution issues, we repeated the first experiment with bars that were 3.5 times as thick. Changing the junctions at the bar endpoints again has little to no effect.

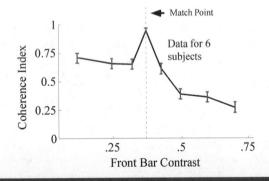

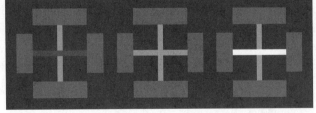

FIGURE 27.8 A match between the luminance of the two bars results in a pronounced peak in coherence.

which the endpoint motions were discounted. What could explain this pattern of results?

One possibility is that the junctions we varied at the bar endpoints were too small for the relevant visual processes to

resolve. Although these junctions were clearly visible in our stimuli (it was easy to distinguish Ts from Ls), it is conceivable that the mechanisms that analyze them for motion interpretation operate at coarse resolution. To test this idea, we made the cross bars thicker, effectively enlarging the pair of junctions formed where the cross bars meet the occluders.

The problem with simply thickening the bars of the cross is that the intersection of the crossbars is also altered. When the crossbars are the same luminance, as in our original stimulus, the length of the contours that have to be completed when the bars are incoherent increases as the bar width is increased. Presumably because of this, the bars are much less likely to appear fully incoherent when they are thick. To avoid ceiling effects, we used a version of the stimulus in which one of the bars was lower or higher in luminance than the other, which was fixed at the match point luminance (figure 27.9*a*). As we saw in the previous experiment, this results in somewhat lower overall coherence, but the stimulus otherwise behaves like the original cross. As a result of the luminance difference between the bars, however, the width of the bars can be changed without obviously changing basic aspects of the stimulus percept.

We varied the contrast of one pair of the occluders in this stimulus for two different bar thicknesses, again looking for

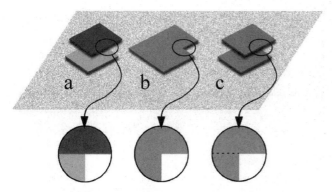

FIGURE 27.10   (*a* and *c*) T-junctions are generically associated with occlusion, L-junctions are not. Interpreting an L-junction in terms of occlusion requires postulating an illusory edge—a surface discontinuity that does not correspond to a luminance edge in the image.

an effect at the point where the occluders matched the bar in luminance and generated L-junctions instead of T-junctions. In the thin bar conditions, the bars were the same thickness as before; in the thick bar conditions the bars were 3.5 times as wide.

For the thin bars, there was again no apparent effect of junction category, as shown in figure 27.9*b*. With thick bars, there was a slight drop in coherence at the match point, but it was quite small. The dominant effect was that of bar contrast, as before. Even when the junctions were separated by large distances and were thus easy to resolve, their category was of little consequence.

Illusory edges

To understand this apparently puzzling set of results, we must consider how different types of junctions are associated with occlusion in the first place. As shown in figure 27.10*a*, T-junctions are produced whenever an occluder's color is different from that of the surface it occludes. We can say that

occlusion *generically* produces T-junctions because almost all combinations of surface colors produce the T. In contrast, an L-junction can result from occlusion only when the two surfaces involved accidentally match in color, as in figure 27.10*c*. Because an accidental match is involved, this interpretation involves postulating an illusory edge—an edge in the world (part of the occluding contour) where there is none in the image.

On grounds of parsimony alone, one would expect the visual system to minimize the number of surface edges in its perceptual interpretation that do not project to intensity edges in the image. If this were the case, then the visual system ought to be biased to interpret L-junctions as corners (figure 27.10*b*) rather than occlusion points, and T-junctions, which do not require postulating such edges, would clearly be the stronger occlusion cue.

Since the coherence of the cross seems to depend on evidence for occlusion, we had expected lower coherence at the point of accidental match, where L-junctions are generated at the bar endpoints. Upon inspection, however, both the coherent and incoherent percepts of the cross necessitate a discontinuity between the occluders and bars. As shown in figure 27.11*a*, this is because the occluders are static and the bars are moving, so regardless of whether the bars cohere and move under the occluders, there must be a surface discontinuity where they meet. When the bars are the same luminance at the match point, this discontinuity takes the form of an illusory edge. If the visual system is attempting to minimize such illusory edges, the coherent interpretation of the cross should in fact be no less likely at the match point despite the presence of L-junctions.

At the bar intersection, in contrast, the situation is different. When coherent, the bars are stuck together as one surface, and there is no discontinuity at their intersection. Thus, illusory edge minimization makes a different prediction, again correct, for the junctions at the bar intersection: coherence should be more likely when the bars match in

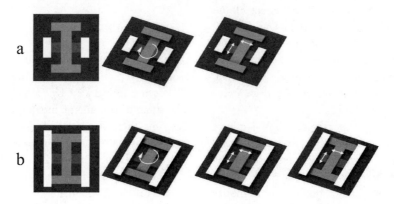

FIGURE 27.11   (*a* and *b*) Two variants of the cross stimulus with their perceptual interpretations at the bar-occluder match point. The long occluders in the new configuration allow the horizontal occluders to slide back and forth with the bars, giving rise to a novel third interpretation in which the bars and occluders translate together as a single I-shape.

luminance and generate L-junctions than when they differ in luminance and produce T-junctions. What appeared to be incompatible results actually provide evidence for a single, sensible computation based on the notion of optimization discussed earlier.

To put this notion to the test, we altered the cross stimulus once more. Our aim was to take the stimulus with matching bar and occluder luminances, shown in figure 27.11a, and selectively remove the endpoint discontinuity in the incoherent motion interpretation, to see if this might then produce a match point effect at the bar endpoints. In the stimulus of figure 27.11b, the white occluders have been extended to cover the horizontal occluders (whose luminance is varied in the experiment). As a result, the horizontal occluders need not be stationary, and can be seen to move with the vertical bar as a single I-shape. Thus, in addition to the two standard cross percepts, this new stimulus has a third perceptual interpretation, depicted in figure 27.11b (far right), in which the I-shape is seen to move back and forth without any discontinuity between the bar and the occluders. (This percept is difficult to imagine from the static figures but is readily experienced when viewing our online demos.) The incoherent interpretation thus does not necessitate an illusory edge at the match point, because the bar and its occluders can be seen as part of the same surface. When coherent, in contrast, the bars still must move under the occluders, generating the illusory discontinuity. Illusory edge constraints might therefore predict a drop in coherence at the match point, since there would be reason to prefer the incoherent interpretation. We therefore conducted another match point experiment with both configurations of figure 27.11, varying the luminance of one pair of the occluders and looking for an effect where they matched the bar luminance.

As shown in figure 27.12, the new configuration indeed resulted in a pronounced effect of the match point; there was a large decrease in coherence, comparable to the increase in coherence observed in figure 27.8, for the match at the bar intersection. We again observed a very small effect of the match point in our original configuration, but it was dwarfed by the big effect in the new configuration. This result is just that predicted by a computation minimizing the number of illusory edges in the perceptual interpretation. The visual system seems to try to avoid postulating surface discontinuities in the absence of visible edges.

The upshot of this series of experiments is that we have no evidence that there are form constraints on motion interpretation that are specifically tied to junctions. Instead, the behavior of the visual system seems well characterized by an optimization-based form computation that tries to minimize the presence of illusory edges in the perceptual representation. This explanation is much the same as that suggested earlier for the barber pole illusion. As before, the cost func-

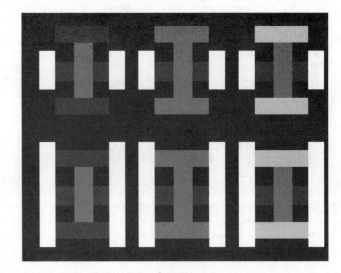

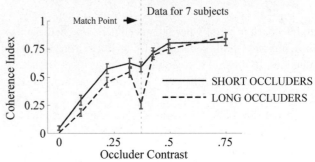

FIGURE 27.12   The match point produces a dip in coherence for the new configuration.

tion is easy to describe qualitatively, but its implementation is probably quite complex. It is not obvious how one could account for these effects with processes acting on local features. However, our description says nothing about what is involved mechanistically, and it is possible that junctions play a role at this level. But there is no simple account of the results that is based on junction categories, whereas there is a simple account based on the minimization of illusory edges.

Amodal completion

Illusory edges are not the only things that figure into the cost function for motion. Consider the square stimulus of figure 27.13, first introduced by Lorenceau and Shiffrar (1992). The stimulus is made of moving bars, just as before, except this time there are two pairs of bars. Each pair oscillates sinusoidally, 90° out of phase with the other pair. When viewed alone, as in figure 27.13a, the pairs of bars appear to move independently, translating horizontally and vertically. However, when static occluders are added to the display, as in figure 27.13b, the percept is quite different: the two pairs of bars appear to move together in a circle, as a single solid square. As before, we can ask what is driving the

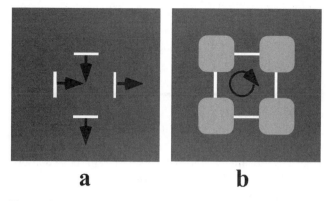

FIGURE 27.13 The basic diamond stimulus, generated by moving a diamond in a circle behind occluders, which can be either invisible (*a*) or visible (*b*). Arrows denote the perceived direction of motion (the image motion is identical in the two stimuli).

percept, and whether it is fruitful to think of the computations involved as minimizing some cost function.

In the case of the square, observers commonly report that when the four bars of the diamond appear to move coherently in a circle, the diamond corners perceptually complete behind the occluders. We wondered if amodal completion was merely an incidental feature of the percept or whether it might play some more fundamental role in determining perceived motion. To address this issue we manipulated the shape of the occluders, in a series of experiments more fully described elsewhere (McDermott, Weiss, and Adelson, 2001). We first compared the coherence obtained with full occluders, shown in figure 27.14*a*, to that produced by the L-shaped occluders of figure 27.14*b*. If the coherence of the fully occluded diamond is closely related to the amodal

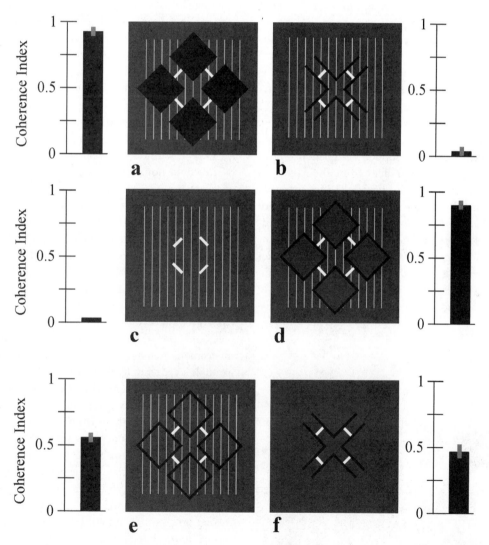

FIGURE 27.14 The influence of amodal completion on motion interpretation. (*a*) Diamond with thick occluders, supporting amodal completion. (*b*) Diamond with thin occluders, preventing amodal completion. (*c*) Diamond contours without occluders or T-junctions. (*d*) Diamond with outline occluders, restoring amodal completion and coherence. (*e*) Diamond with hollow outline occlud-

ers. Coherence is lower than for the solid outline occluders (*d*), presumably because there is less evidence for an extended occluding surface. (*f*) Diamond with thin occluders without background lines. Coherence is higher than when background lines are present (*b*), presumably because it is easier to interpret the Ls as borders of extended occluding surfaces. The results are for eight naive subjects.

completion of the diamond contours, one might expect coherence to be lower with the L-shaped occluders, as they do not provide room for the contours to complete. The thin gray lines in the background help to ensure that the entire background is seen as a single surface, leaving no room for the diamond contours to complete.

Even though the L-shaped occluders have the same occluding contour as the full occluders and produce similar T-junctions, they produce much lower levels of coherence. The stimulus of figure 27.14b was almost always incoherent, almost as often as when the bars were presented alone on the background (figure 27.14c). We were able to restore coherence by closing the L-shapes as shown in figure 27.14d, so that the Ls were seen as the borders of extended surfaces that provide room for the diamond contours to complete. The results are consistent with an important role for amodal completion in motion interpretation, and again underscore the conclusion that there is much more to the form computations than mere junction detection.

The sophistication of the form constraints is further shown with two manipulations of the background lines. As shown in figure 27.14e, coherence is reduced when the background lines are extended through the occluder outlines, presumably because they are inconsistent with the presence of extended surfaces that could support completion. Moreover, removing the background lines from the L-shaped occluder stimulus, as shown in figure 27.14f, increases coherence, presumably because without the lines the Ls are more likely to form the borders of extended surfaces. Gradually closing the L-shapes, as shown in figure 27.15, further increases coherence, again consistent with the increased likelihood of an extended surface. Motion interpretation again seems to be privy to rather subtle aspects of spatial form, and junctions by themselves seem to have little predictive value.

To further test the importance of completion, we manipulated the position of the diamond contours in ways that affected their ability to amodally complete. As with many of the other effects described in this chapter, the manipulations much easier to understand if one views the moving demos, for which we refer the reader to our demo Web page. Consider the contours of figure 27.16, in which the line segments are shown through apertures. In figure 27.16a, the line segments can be connected with a smooth contour to form a square. Kellman and Shipley have referred to such contours as "relatable" (1991). Relatability depends on the geometric relationships between the contours. In figure 27.16b, the horizontal segments have been moved inward so that a simple completion with the vertical segments is impossible; these contours are nonrelatable. When the line segments were set in motion and shown to observers, we found dramatic differences in how the motion was interpreted: although the relatable contours almost always cohered, the nonrelatable ones virtually never did. Note that proximity biases on motion integration (e.g., Nakayama and Silverman, 1988) would, if anything, predict that the nonrelatable stimulus should cohere more, because the segments are somewhat closer to each other than in the relatable stimulus. Evidently any proximity biases are swamped by the effect of relatability. One might nonetheless object that it is simply impossible to see the nonrelatable configuration as a single object in coherent motion. This is not the case. As shown in figure 27.16c, we added dots to the nonrelatable line segments and moved them with the same circular trajectory seen when the line segments cohered in figure 27.16a. With the addition of the dots, the line segments appeared to cohere, moving together as a single object. Apparently the moving dots captured the motion of each line segment, and the segments were then grouped together in accord with the *Gestalt* principle of common fate. Nonrelatability thus does not prevent coherence per se but rather the specific process of motion integration across contours. We suggest this is another example of a completion constraint: local motions seem to be preferentially integrated when the contours that give rise to them can amodally complete.

We can think of these completion-related effects as the product of a cost function as well. Motion interpretations appear to be penalized when they involve integrating the motion of contours that are separated in space but do not amodally complete.

However, a third example of the role of completion-related processes in motion interpretation is less conducive to such an explanation. Inspired by an experiment done by Shimojo, Silverman, and Nakayama (1989), we compared the motion seen with the single barber pole to that seen when identical barber poles are added to the top and bottom of the original one. The top and bottom barber poles tend to amodally complete with the middle one, and we thought

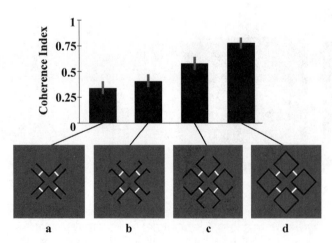

FIGURE 27.15 Closure. (*a*) Diamond with L-shaped occluders, preventing amodal completion. (*b–d*) Increasing closure increases coherence. The results are for five naive subjects.

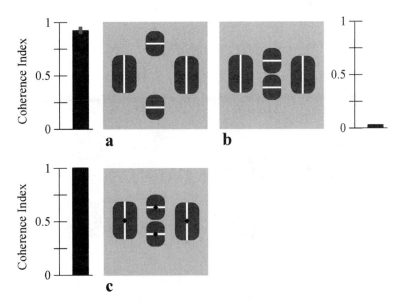

FIGURE 27.16   Relatability. (*a*) Relatable configuration, which generates high coherence. (*b*) Nonrelatable configuration, which never coheres. (*c*) Nonrelatable configuration with dots superimposed on the contours. The dots move in the direction of coherent motion, and with their addition the stimulus coheres. The results are for six naive subjects.

this might increase the tendency of the visual system to discount the horizontal line endings, because amodal completion occurs only between occluded contours. Indeed, as shown in figure 27.17, the triple barber pole was roughly twice as likely to be seen moving vertically than the single barber pole, suggesting that the presence of relatable contours in the adjacent gratings causes the occluded line endings to be discounted to a greater extent. Note that the relative proportion of different motion signals (horizontal line endings, vertical line endings, and line segments) is constant across the two stimuli, as the top and bottom barber poles are identical to the middle. Thus, it is not clear how to account for the result other than by supposing that the horizontal motion signals are discounted to a greater extent in the triple configuration. Completion-related constraints again seem to be exerting their influence, but in this case the most intuitive explanation is process-based, related to the weight given to particular motion signals as a function of the stimulus configuration.

Border ownership

As a further test of the importance of nonlocal cues to occlusion, we devised stimuli such as those in figure 27.18 (McDermott, Weiss, and Adelson, 2001). The stimuli of figure 27.18*a* and *b* have identical junctions at the bar endpoints, but differ globally in the extent to which the bars appear to be occluded. As shown in figure 27.18*c*, observers reported the second stimulus to be far less coherent than the first, consistent with the weaker impression of occlusion that it conveys. Again, the T-junctions alone do a poor job of predicting motion interpretation, since the same T-junctions are

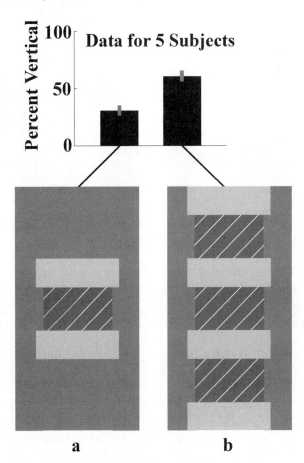

FIGURE 27.17   (*a* and *b*) Triple barber pole experiment. The single barber pole appears to move vertically some of the time, but this tendency is enhanced in the triple barber pole.

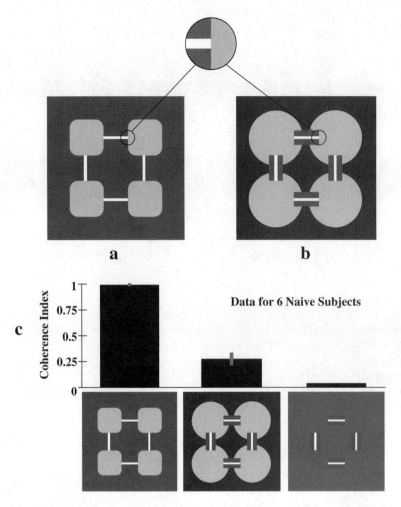

FIGURE 27.18 Influence of border ownership on motion interpretation. (*a, b*) Experimental stimuli that are identical in the local vicinity of the diamond contours but differ globally in the extent to which they support occlusion. (*c*) Observed coherence levels for each stimulus, for six naive subjects.

present in both cases. What is the nature of the process or computation that is responsible for this effect?

The stimuli of figure 27.18 differ in a number of ways, but we wondered whether the geometry of the occluding contour might be important. Note that in the stimulus of figure 27.18*a*, the occluding contour abutting each moving bar is convex, whereas in figure 27.18*b* it is concave. Contour convexity is a well-known cue to border ownership (Stevens and Brookes, 1988; Pao, Geiger, and Rubin, 1999), so it seemed possible that this might have something to do with the different motion seen in the two displays. To probe the role of convexity we conducted some experiments with outline stimuli, shown in figure 27.19, which allow for some interesting manipulations (McDermott and Adelson, 2004b). Figure 27.19*a* shows the diamond with outline occluders; this stimulus cohered most of the time as one would expect. In the stimulus of figure 27.19*b*, we removed most of the occluding contour, leaving just the T-junctions at the bar endpoints. This stimulus generated intermediate levels of coherence. In the stimuli of figure 27.19*c* and *d*, we added short line segments to the T-junctions to produce local convexities and concavities, respectively. The convexities increased the level of coherence relative to the T-junctions alone, while the concavities decreased it. Note that no occluders are visible in these stimuli; there are just isolated pieces of contour. Nonetheless, manipulating the local concavity produced a sizable effect.

Can convexity predict perceived coherence in other stimuli as well? We compared the coherence obtained for the occluded diamond with that for an identical square viewed through apertures with the same occluding contours as the occluders, as shown in figure 27.20. The apertures produced substantially lower levels of coherence than did the occluders, consistent with the notion that the degree of coherence is determined in part by the local convexity, and perhaps by the strength of occlusion, which may derive from the convexity.

We also wondered whether additional T-junctions along the occluding contour might influence border ownership and hence motion interpretation. The stimuli of figure

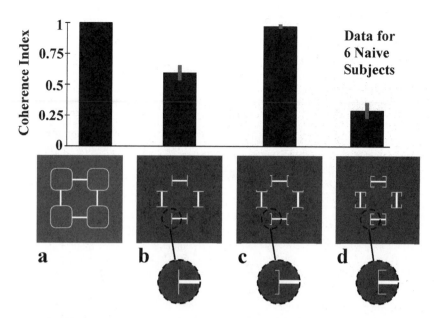

FIGURE 27.19 Contour convexity. (*a*) Outline occluders produce high levels of coherence. (*b*) T-junctions alone produce intermedi- ate levels of coherence, which is increased by adding convexities (*c*) and decreased by adding concavities (*d*).

27.21 were designed to address this issue. The round aper- tures of figure 27.21*a* alone produced moderate levels of coherence, as did the oddly shaped occluders of figure 27.21*b*. But when combined in the stimulus of figure 27.21*c*, coherence was substantially lower than in either stimulus alone, consistent with the weak percept of occlusion that most observers report. Here the weak coherence cannot be attributed merely to the shape of the occluding contour.

Something happens specifically when the two contours are combined. One appealing explanation is that the T- junctions of figure 27.21*c* modulate the strength of border ownership, which in turn influences motion interpretation. The control of figure 27.21*d* is further consistent with this notion.

These last examples of the effects of border ownership cues are most suggestive of processes acting on sets of local features. By themselves, the T-junctions at the bar endpoints seem to predict very little, but if we consider the junctions along with the geometry of the occluding contour in a region surrounding the junction, we can account for much more.

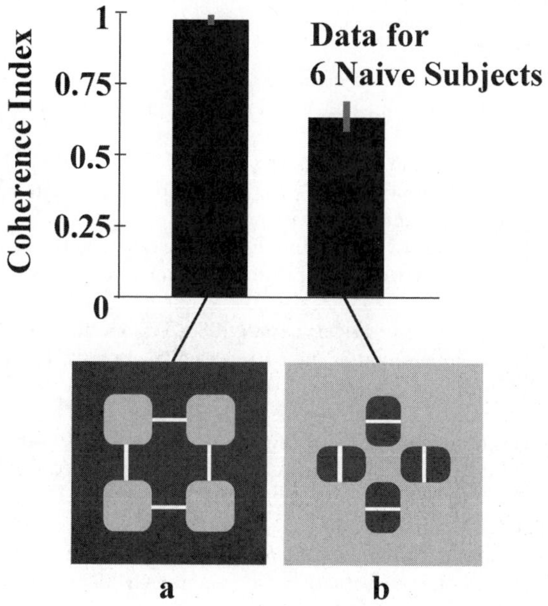

FIGURE 27.20 Occluders versus apertures. (*a*) With occluders the square is highly coherent. (*b*) Apertures with the same occluding contour produce lower coherence, perhaps because the occluding contour is concave.

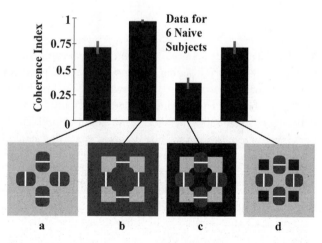

FIGURE 27.21 The role of static T-junctions along the occluding contour. When the round apertures of *a* and the occluders of *b* are combined in *c*, coherence is lower than it is for either stimulus alone. The control condition in *d* suggests the T-junctions created in *c* are key.

The results suggest that local cues such as contour convexity and junctions are combined to yield an estimate of the likelihood of occlusion, which then may be used to determine the motion interpretation. This explanation has a very different flavor from the explanation we offered of the cross experiments, in which we proposed a cost function that could be applied to each of the candidate perceptual interpretations. The cost function did not involve local image features, being a function only of the layered representation derived from the image data. Here, in contrast, it is hard to explain the phenomena without direct reference to particular critical image features. It remains a challenge for future research to show if and how these phenomena related to border ownership may be described as minimizing some cost function on perceptual interpretations.

Regardless of the kind of explanation adopted for the various phenomena in this chapter, certain general conclusions emerge. First, the form influences on motion serve to solve fundamental computational problems in motion interpretation introduced by occlusion. Feature motions are discounted when they are likely to be the spurious product of occlusion, and distant motions are integrated only if they are likely to be due to the same object. Second, the popular view that the form constraints on motion can be accounted for with isolated processes operating on junctions has little merit in the phenomena we have examined. Motion interpretation is influenced by a variety of nonlocal form computations, and the effect of these computations is quite powerful. They can effectively switch between different motion interpretations depending on the stimulus configuration, even when the junctions are unchanged. The complexity of these interactions would appear to implicate substantial cross-talk between the motion and form pathways, which may be another fruitful avenue for future investigation.

Summary

Motion, form, occlusion, and perceptual organization are intimately related, and ambiguous moving stimuli provide powerful tools to investigate their relationship. We have described phenomena involving moving crosses and squares that suggest a number of subtle and sophisticated links between motion and form. The simplest story one could tell about motion and form interactions, involving local processes based on junctions, bears surprisingly little resemblance to the various form processes that we find to be at work. Two general sorts of explanations are suggested by our phenomena, process-based and optimization-based. In some cases the phenomena are best explained with reference to processes that act on local features, such as the convexity of the occluding contour. In other cases the simplest explanation is in terms of a cost function that is minimized, for instance, one that penalizes illusory edges. In all cases, iso-lated junctions have little explanatory power, and we must appeal to more complex and interesting form computations to account for the ease and accuracy with which we perceive motion in real-world scenes.

REFERENCES

Adelson, E. H., and J. A. Movshon, 1982. Phenomenal coherence of moving visual patterns. *Nature* 300:523–525.

Anstis, S., 1990. Imperceptible intersections: The chopstick illusion. In *AI and the Eye*, A. Blake and T. Troscianko, eds. New York: John Wiley.

Attneave, F., 1954. Some informational aspects of visual perception. *Psychol. Rev.* 61:183–193.

Grossberg, S., E. Mingolla, and L. Viswanathan, 2001. Neural dynamics of motion integration and segmentation within and across apertures. *Vision Res.* 41:2521–2553.

Grzywacz, N. M., and A. L. Yuille, 1991. Theories for the visual perception of local velocity and coherent motion. In *Computational Models of Visual Processing*, J. Landy and J. Movshon, eds. Cambridge, Mass.: MIT Press.

Hildreth, E. C., 1984. *The Measurement of Visual Motion*. Cambridge, Mass: MIT Press.

Hochberg, J., and E. McAlister, 1953. A quantitative approach to figural "goodness." *J. Exp. Psychol.* 46:362–364.

Kellman, P., and T. Shipley, 1991. A theory of visual interpolation in object perception. *Cogn. Psychol.* 23:141–221.

Leeuwenberg, E., 1969. Quantitative specification of information in sequential patterns. *Psychol. Rev.* 76:216–220.

Liden, L., and C. Pack, 1999. The role of terminators and occlusion cues in motion integration and segmentation: A neural network model. *Vision Res.* 39:3301–3320.

Lorenceau, J., and M. Shiffrar, 1992. The influence of terminators on motion integration across space. *Vision Res.* 32: 263–273.

Lorenceau, J., and L. Zago, 1999. Cooperative and competitive spatial interactions in motion integration. *Vis. Neurosci.* 16:755–770.

McDermott, J., and E. H. Adelson, 2004a. Junctions and cost functions in motion interpretation. To appear in the *Journal of Vision*.

McDermott, J., and E. H. Adelson, 2004b. The geometry of the occluding contour and its effect on motion interpretation. To appear in the *Journal of Vision*.

McDermott, J., Y. Weiss, and E. H. Adelson, 2001. Beyond junctions: Nonlocal form constraints on motion interpretation. *Perception* 30:905–923.

Nakayama, K., and G. H. Silverman, 1988. The aperture problem. II. Spatial integration of information along contours. *Vision Res.* 28:747–753.

Nowlan, S., and T. Sejnowski, 1995. A selection model for motion processing in area MT of primates. *J. Neurosci.* 15:1195–1214.

O'Shea, R. P., S. G. Blackburn, and H. Ono, 1994. Contrast as a depth cue. *Vision Res.* 34:1595–1604.

Pao, H., D. Geiger, and N. Rubin, 1999. Measuring convexity for figure/ground separation. In *Proceedings of the 7th IEEE International Conference on Computing and Vision*, pp. 948–955.

Restle, F., 1979. Coding theory and the perception of motion configurations. *Psychol. Rev.* 86:1–24.

Rohaly, A. M., and H. R. Wilson, 1999. The effects of contrast on perceived depth and depth discrimination. *Vision Res.* 39: 9–18.

RUBIN, N., 2000. The role of junctions in surface completion and contour matching. To appear in *Perception*.

RUBIN, N., 2001. The role of junctions in surface completion and contour matching. *Perception* 30:339–366.

SHAPLEY, R., J. GORDON, C. TRUONG, and N. RUBIN, 1995. Effect of contrast on perceived direction of motion in the barberpole illusion. *Invest. Ophthalmol Vis. Sci.* 36:1845.

SHIMOJO, S., G. H. SILVERMAN, and K. NAKAYAMA, 1989. Occlusion and the solution to the aperture problem for motion. *Vision Res.* 29:619–626.

SHIMOJO, S., G. H. SILVERMAN, and K. NAKAYAMA, 1989. Occlusion and the solution to the aperture problem for motion. *Vision Res.* 29:619–626.

SHIPLEY, T. F., and P. J. KELLMAN, 1992. Strength of visual interpolation depends on the ratio of physically specified to total edge length. *Percept. Psychophys.* 52:97–106.

STEVENS, K. A., and A. BROOKES, 1988. The convex cusp as a determiner of figure-ground. *Perception* 17:35–42.

STONER, G. R., and T. D. ALBRIGHT, 1998. Luminance contrast affects motion coherency in plaid patterns by acting as a depth-from occlusion cue. *Vision Res.* 38:387–401.

STONER, G. R., T. D. ALBRIGHT, and V. S. RAMACHANDRAN, 1990. Transparency and coherence in human motion perception. *Nature* 344:153–155.

TRUESWELL, J. C., and M. M. HAYHOE, 1993. Surface segmentation mechanisms and motion perception. *Vision Res.* 33:313–328.

WALLACH, H., 1935. Uber visuell wahrgenommene Bewegungrichtung. *Psychol. Forsch.* 20:325–380.

WANG, J. Y. A., and E. H. ADELSON, 1994. Representing moving images with layers. *IEEE Trans. Image Proc.* 3(5):625–638.

WEISS, Y., and E. H. ADELSON, 2000. Adventures with gelatinous ellipses: Constraints on models of human motion analysis. *Perception* 29:543–566.

WEISS, Y., E. P. SIMONCELLI, and E. H. ADELSON, 2002. Motion illusions as optimal percepts. *Nat. Neurosci.* 5:598–604.

WUERGER, S., R. SHAPLEY, and N. RUBIN, 1996. On the visually perceived direction of motion by Hans Wallach: 60 years later. *Perception* 25:1317–1367.

28 Determining an Auditory Scene

WILLIAM A. YOST

ABSTRACT The sources of sound that constantly surround us provide a complex auditory scene that informs us about the objects and events in our world. Determining that auditory scene is the major task confronting the auditory system. The sounds from all of the sources in the auditory scene that arrive at the ears of a listener as one complex sound field are first coded at the auditory periphery as a spectral-temporal pattern of neural information flowing from the inner ear to the brainstem via the auditory nerve. The neural centers and circuits of the auditory brainstem and central nervous system parse this spectral-temporal code into neural substrates that allow for the determination of the sources of the originating sounds. Auditory models of the auditory periphery suggest that the pattern of the spectral-temporal code contains information that may form the basis for the central nervous systems ability to determine the auditory scene. This central nervous system processing involves a form of temporal integration that provides a stabilized auditory image. The stabilized auditory image contains several features that are probably used by the central auditory system for sound source determination: spectral separation, temporal separation, spatial separation, harmonicity and temporal regularity, intensity profile, differing onsets and offsets, and common modulation. Models of auditory scene analysis include computational models and perceptual models based on Gestalt principals. These models require a form of auditory processing that spans a wide range of the auditory spectrum and time in order to extract the features in the stabilized auditory image that determine the auditory scene. To understand better how the auditory system determines the auditory scene, auditory science will need to overcome several challenges.

Pause for a moment and reflect on what you are hearing. In all likelihood you will refer to what you are hearing in terms of the sound sources that surround you. You might "hear" the whine of a fan, the screeching of a car tire, the voice of a colleague, the rustling of blowing leaves on a tree, and so on. In the words of Bregman (1990), you are analyzing an auditory scene in which the images of this scene are your perceptions of the sources of the sounds that generated the scene. This chapter is about how the auditory system might determine auditory scenes.

Figure 28.1 places auditory scene analysis into a crude evolutionary context (de Cheveigne, 2001). The most primitive auditory function might be detection. A simple primordial fish might have evolved with a sound detector (an "ear") on each side of the body (upper panel). When a sound

WILLIAM A. YOST Parmly Hearing Institute, Loyola University, Chicago, Ill.

source (from a prey) appears on one side of the fish, the detector on that side transduces sound into a neural signal that is sent to a fin on the opposite side of the body, propelling the fish toward its prey. Such a system would be effective if the only sound sources were prey. If there were predators, such a detection system would be deadly for our simple detection system. To handle both prey and predators requires a discrimination system (middle panel). In this case, the peripheral sensor would have to discriminate the sound of a prey from that of a predator. If the sensing discriminator indicated a predator, a neural signal would be sent to a fin on the same side of the fish as the ear receiving the sound, thus sending the fish away from the predator. Such a nervous system wired for discrimination would work reasonably well if the fish encountered either prey or predator. However, if both prey and predator were simultaneously present, a more complicated "segregation" nervous system (bottom panel) would be required to ensure the fish's survival. This chapter describes some of what is known about the auditory segregation problem.

This way (figure 28.1) of formulating auditory perception reflects to some degree the history of the study of audition. Although the philosophers-physiologists-psychologists of the early nineteenth century wrote about "object perception," the history of audition since that time has been dominated by the study of the detection and discrimination of the physical attributes of sound (frequency, intensity, and timing) and the subjective correlates of these attributes (e.g., pitch, loudness, timbre). Such detection and discrimination research often has focused on simple sounds rather than on the complex sounds emanating from real-world sound sources. The studies of speech and music are notable exceptions to this trend. The 1990s saw the reintroduction of an interest in auditory perception of complex, real-world sounds (Hartmann, 1988; Bregman, 1990; Yost, 1992a, 1992b; Yost and Sheft, 1993; Moore, 1997).

While figure 28.1 implies that a segregation machine would be more complex than a detection or discrimination machine, the challenge for the auditory system is probably even more daunting than that implied by figure 28.1. First, the sounds from different sources are not physically segregated. The sound pressure waveforms from all of the sound sources are mixed into one complex sound field that arrives at the listener's ears. Second, the peripheral auditory system codes for the physical attributes (frequency, intensity, timing)

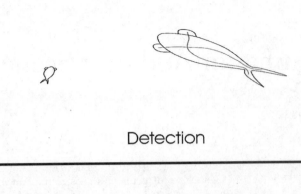

Detection

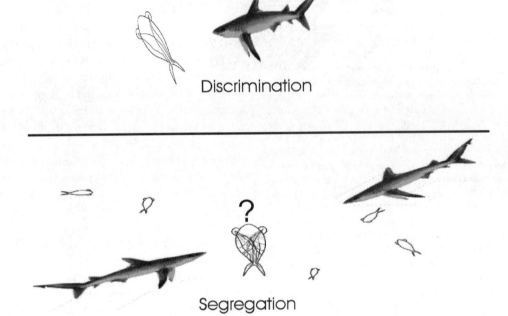

Discrimination

Segregation

FIGURE 28.1   Examples of a simple detection, discrimination, and segregation problem for a primordial fish dealing with prey and predators.

of this complex sound field, not for sound sources. Thus, it is up to the brainstem and cortex to "decode" the spectral-temporal code of the sound field provided by the peripheral auditory system in order to determine an auditory scene.

In real-life situations, the segregation challenge depicted in the bottom of figure 28.1 probably involves many components. The animal must segregate the sound sources and attend to the relevant source, with attention probably based on experience and motivation. While all these processes probably interact in allowing an animal to process sound sources, this chapter will deal primarily with issues related to the segregation problem.

The peripheral auditory system processes the vibrations associated with sound in both the time and frequency domain. The inner hair cell/auditory nerve complex sends neural impulses to the brainstem that are time (phase)-locked to the temporal pattern of vibrations received by the inner ear (figure 28.2). Thus, the patterns of neural discharges in the auditory nerve reflect the temporal fluctuations of sound. However, the accuracy of such temporal coding is limited to vibratory frequencies less than approximately 5000 Hz, because of several properties of neuronal functioning. The biomechanical properties of the inner ear (e.g., the traveling wave) also provide a spectral analysis of the incoming sound field that is relayed to the brainstem by the auditory nerve. The traveling wave motion of the inner ear responds in a frequency-specific manner such that the region of maximal vibratory displacement is frequency dependent (see Dallos, Popper, and Fay, 1996). The hair cells respond to this vibratory displacement and in turn stimulate fibers in the auditory nerve. Figure 28.3 shows the tuning curves of different auditory nerve fibers, indicating that each nerve fiber is tuned to a particular narrow spectral region, and in this sense would provide information to the central nervous system (CNS) about the existence of energy in the sound field in this particular spectral region. The tuning is proportional to the center frequency of the tuning curve. As a

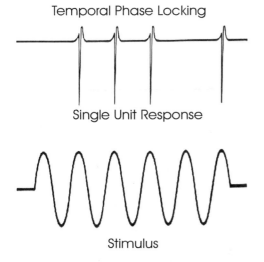

FIGURE 28.2 Neural phase-locking of neural discharges in the auditory nerve synchronized to the periodic peaks of a sound wave.

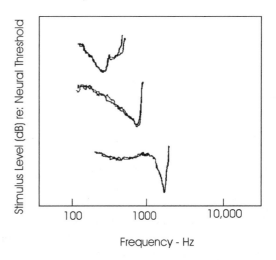

FIGURE 28.3 Tuning curves of three auditory nerve fibers. Figure shows the relative level (in dB) of a tonal stimulus, whose frequency (in Hz) is shown on the horizontal axis, required to increase the firing rate of an auditory nerve fiber above its spontaneous rate (a threshold response). Each fiber is "tuned" to a narrow region of frequencies near the frequency that yields the lowest threshold. (Adapted with permission from Yost, *Fundamentals of Hearing: An Introduction*, 4th ed. © 2000 by Springer-Verlag. Based on data from Liberman and Kiang, 1978).

result, the tuning curves for high-frequency sounds are wide, meaning that small differences in high-frequency sounds are not resolved by the auditory periphery.

As suggested from figures 28.2 and 28.3, the auditory peripheral apparatus provides a spectral-temporal code of the incoming sound field. Figure 28.4 displays the output of a computational model (Patterson, Allerhand, and Giguere, 1995) of the spectral-temporal code provided by the peripheral auditory system to a 100-ms segment of a vowel. This model simulates the middle ear transfer function (spectral changes that occur as sound travels from the source to the inner ear), the biomechanical filtering action of the inner ear (e.g., traveling wave), and the hair cell/neural transduction of the biomechanical output into neural discharges. Each horizontal line of figure 28.4 represents the histogram of neural discharges (neural activation pattern, NAP) from a small set of auditory nerve fibers tuned to the same narrow region of the spectrum indicated on the ordinate (i.e., each line is the neural output of a spectrally tuned auditory channel, as is measured by a post-stimulus time histogram). Low frequencies, which are transduced slightly later than high frequencies (e.g., the traveling wave takes time to reach the apex of the cochlea where low frequencies are transduced; see Dallos, Popper, and Fay, 1996), are indicated at the bottom of the display. Figure 28.4 is a simulation of the spectral-temporal code that the central auditory system uses to determine the sources of sounds.

In determining the auditory scene, the physical properties of the sound produced by sources can provide features in the spectral-temporal code that might be used by the central auditory system for auditory scene analysis. Then, one needs to understand what form of analysis is used by the central auditory system to extract the relevant information from these spectral-temporal features. For instance, there are at

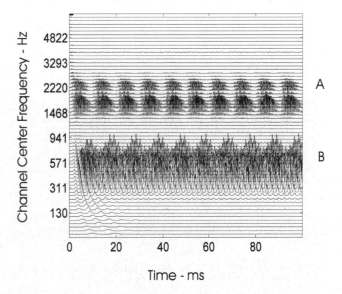

FIGURE 28.4 The model of Patterson et al. 1995 used to show the neural activation pattern to a vowel sound. Time is plotted along the abscissa, and the center frequency (Hz) of each tuned auditory channel is shown along the ordinate. At the locations labeled A, the amplitude modulation associated with the voicing of the vowel can be seen. The concentration of neural activity in certain channels (e.g., at B) indicates the formant frequencies of the vowel, as further indicated in figure 28.5.

least two features in the NAP of figure 28.4 that correspond to the physical properties of voiced speech and could be of interest to a central processor. In the horizontal or temporal dimension, a clear amplitude modulation of the neural discharges occurs (A in figure 28.4), corresponding to the vocal cords opening and closing during the production of the vowel (representing the fundamental frequency and, hence, the pitch of voicing). There are also clear indications that certain frequency channels are firing at higher rates than other channels (B in figure 28.4). This feature indicates that there are concentrations of energy in certain frequency regions during the production of the vowel, that is, the vocal tract formants associated with the production of the vowel. This spectral feature can be further analyzed by computing an excitation pattern representing an auditory spectrum (figure 28.5) by integrating the number of neural discharges over time in each frequency channel as a function of the channel's center frequency. The location of the spectral peaks as a function of channel center frequency in the auditory spectrum indicates the formant frequencies, and the height of these peaks corresponds to the relative intensity levels of these formats. Thus, this spectral-temporal code at the output of the auditory periphery contains features that represent the key physical attributes of vowel production by the human vocal cord and tract. Analyses such as computing the auditory spectrum are forms of processing that might be implemented by the CNS to extract information about these features.

Looking for features and analysis mechanisms that assist auditory scene analysis implies forms of processing across a broad range of frequency channels and over considerable time periods. Most of the auditory literature dealing with detection and discrimination has taken an almost opposite approach, concentrating on narrow regions of the spectrum and very short periods of time. For instance, in measuring the detection of masked tonal signals, the concept of a critical band filter is crucial for providing an account of such masking data (Moore, 1986). That is, in order for the auditory system to detect weak signals in the background of intense maskers, the auditory system must analyze the sound in a narrow frequency region centered on the frequency of the signal (the critical band). Similarly, the detection of brief transient signals requires a very short temporal window for analysis (Viemeister and Plack, 1993). Such narrow bandwidths and short-duration processing would not make auditory scene analysis possible, and wideband and long-duration processing would render the auditory system very insensitive to detecting and discriminating the physical attributes of sound. Thus, the auditory system probably evolved to process sound in narrow *and* wide frequency regions as well as over very short *and* long periods of time. Clearly, several compromises in processing strategies must have evolved to accomplish what at times would be

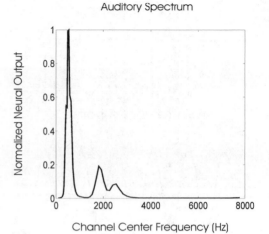

FIGURE 28.5 The auditory spectrum, showing the excitation pattern of the vowel shown in figure 28.4. The auditory spectrum indicates the amount of neural activity in each frequency-tuned auditory channel. The peaks in the Auditory Spectrum indicate the vowel formants.

contradictory tasks. Far less is known about wideband and long-duration processing than about the critical-band and short-duration auditory processing.

The auditory system faces another challenge that probably involves a form of temporal integration if the perceptions of everyday sounds are to be explained. Let us consider the following demonstration of the presentation of a single, very brief acoustic transient (e.g., a transient lasting $25\,\mu s$), which would be perceived as a single click. If this transient is then repeated at a slow rate, such as twice per second, it would be perceived as series of individual clicks appearing once every 500 ms. As the rate of presentation of the transients increases, so will the perceived rate of clicks, but as long as the rate is less than about 20 per second, the subject will perceive each individual transient as an independent click. When the rate exceeds approximately 20 per second, there is an important change in perception. The image stabilizes into a single percept that has a "rattle" quality, and the individual transients are no longer perceived as separate clicks. When the rate increases to approximately 35 transients per second, the stable percept takes on a pitch quality, with further increases in rate being perceived as a higher and higher pitch (Pressnitzer, Patterson, and Krumbholz, 2001).

Figure 28.6 shows the simulated spectral-temporal pattern for a single transient (top) and for a train of transients presented at a rate of 40 transients per second (bottom). If the information in the bottom panel were shown in real time, the information would flow from left to right, with the transient events occurring 40 times per second. That is, without some form of temporal integration, there would be no evidence of stabilization. Several forms of integration have been proposed (see Patterson, Allerhand, and Giguere, 1995) to produce a stabilized pattern. For the purposes of expla-

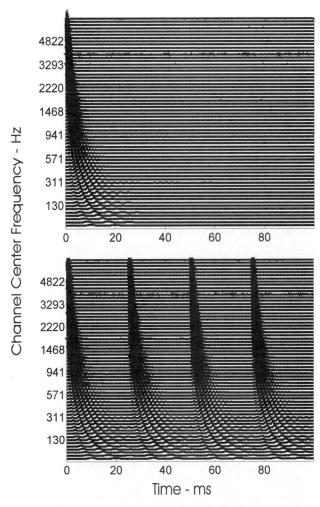

FIGURE 28.6 Neural activation patterns (NAP) for a single transient (top) and a train of transients presented 40 times per second (bottom). The individual transients would occur as single events in time within the NAP.

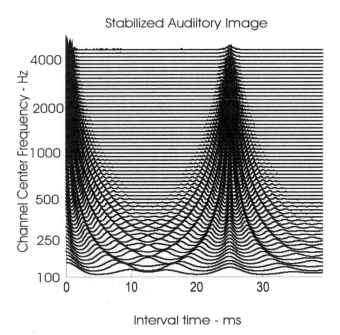

Stabilized Auditory Image

FIGURE 28.7 Stabilized auditory image for the train of transients presented at a 40-per-second rate. The image is produced by performing a channel-by-channel autocorrelation analysis to produce a stabilized image of the temporal intervals within the 40-Hz train of transients.

nation, figure 28.7 shows the result of subjecting the NAP of the lower panel of figure 28.6 to a channel-by-channel autocorrelation process (see Patterson, Allerhand, and Giguere, 1995). Autocorrelation offers certain advantages for temporal integration (e.g., it can also account for the pitch of most complex sounds; Meddis and Hewitt, 1991; but see Kaernbach and Demany, 1998, for criticisms of autocorrelation models), and there is no accepted theory of auditory temporal integration (see Viemeister and Plack, 1993).

Autocorrelation produces a display of time intervals as opposed to time per se, suggesting a stabilized estimate of the intervals in the pattern of information flowing to higher auditory centers. Autocorrelation also "normalizes" the NAP by "taking out" the time delay associated with the travel time of the traveling wave (i.e., the latency shift shown in figure 28.4 through 28.6 in the low-frequency channels). This allows for an alignment of the time intervals across

frequency. Although there is no physiological evidence of a neural autocorrelator, recent work by Meddis (2002) suggests that a similar process might be carried out by onset or choppers cells in the first auditory brainstem structure, the cochlear nucleus.

There are two additional aspects of real-world sounds and the function of the peripheral auditory system that should be considered. This chapter will not provide any details on these additional points, but they are crucial for auditory processing. First, in most acoustic environments the auditory system receives the sound from a source *and* the sound reflected from nearby surfaces (even outdoors, the ground provides a significant reflective surface). Study of the "effects of precedence" (see Litovsky et al., 1999) suggests ways in which the auditory system deals with sound from sources and their many reflections. Second, the auditory peripheral system is nonlinear. The biomechanics, aided by the function of the outer hair cells, produce a compressed nonlinear relationship between stimulus amplitude and neural output such that high-stimulus levels are neurally compressed more than low-stimulus levels (Moore, 1995). One consequence of this and other forms of peripheral nonlinearity is the production of spectral distortion products. These distortion products produce neural information in frequency channels for which there is no energy in the incoming sound field. Again, in many contexts one must consider the nonlinear aspects of peripheral processing to fully describe the information flowing to the central auditory system.

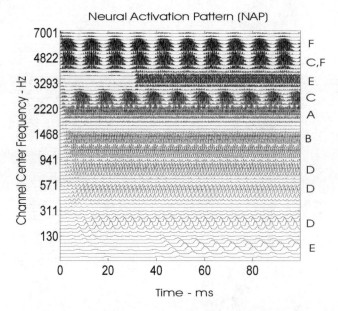

Neural Activation Pattern (NAP)

FIGURE 28.8   The neural activation pattern (NAP) to a complex auditory scene. The letters beside the different channels refer to different patterns in the NAP that may provide cues to auditory scene analysis, as explained in the text.

Figure 28.8 shows an NAP containing many of the features that have been suggested as possible cues for auditory scene analysis. These features include spectral separation, temporal separation, harmonicity (temporal regularity), intensity profile, differing onsets (and offsets), and common modulation. In addition, spatial separation of sound sources could aid sound source segregation (Yost, 1992a). The next section of this chapter introduces examples from the psychoacoustic literature that indicate how these various cues might aid in auditory scene analysis.

Auditary scene analysis

SPECTRAL SEPARATION   The frequency-resolving capabilities of the auditory periphery means those sound sources that have energy in different spectral regions (A in figure 28.8) produce different regions of neural excitation that could be used by the central auditory system to determine the existence of different sound sources. The challenge for the auditory system arises when the spectral components overlap within a frequency channel or in close proximity to a single frequency channel. In this case, features in addition to spectral separation would be required for the central auditory system to determine different sound sources.

TEMPORAL SEPARATION   If two sound sources occur at different times, any features in the auditory image will also occur at different times, making it possible for the CNS to segregate the sounds based on temporal differences. C in figure 28.8 shows a different form of temporal separation.

The information at one frequency is on, while that for the other frequency is off, and vice versa. This might indicate a single sound source with an alternating pitch, or there might be two sound sources, each with a different pulsating pitch.

The situation in C of figure 28.8 is similar to that used in experiments on auditory streaming (Bregman, 1990). In an auditory streaming task, two different sounds are each presented as trains of short-duration bursts. When one sound is on, the other is off, as indicated in C of figure 28.8. Listeners adjust a parameter of the sounds (e.g., the burst duration or the frequency difference) until they perceive the two sounds as two separate sources, that is, two separate auditory streams. The stimulus parameters that yield this "stream segregation" indicate the parameter values that might promote sound source segregation. Bregman (1990) and others have used all of the major features mentioned so far to explore stream segregation (perceiving two different "streams" or sound sources) and stream fusion (hearing a single "stream" or sound source). In general, spectral differences among the stimuli in a potential auditory scene provide the most potent means for generating stream segregation.

Stream segregation points to another issue related to auditory scene analysis. Often the sound from one source goes on and off, yet the hearer still perceives the sound as representing a single source and not the introduction of a new source with each repetition of the pulsating sound. That is, there is perception of continuity for pulsating sounds from a single source. A simple example of such continuity is the determination of "pulsation threshold" (Warren, 1999). In these tasks a masker such as a noise is presented continuously while a signal, a tone, is pulsed on and off. As the level of the tonal signal is lowered, the perception of a soft pulsating tone gives way to the perception of a very soft, steady tone in the presence of a steady masking noise. Further decreases in tonal level will eventually lower the tonal signal level below a signal-detection threshold. Thus, the "pulsation threshold" is that signal-to-noise ratio required to perceive a pulsating sound masked by a steady masker as also being steady.

A more complicated version of continuity has been studied by investigators such as Warren (1999). One example of these experiments involves the recognition of a sentence masked by a noise. The waveform of the sentence is "chopped" into temporal pieces, by deleting short segments of the sentence so that the sentence "waveform" is pulsed on and off. A noise is pulsed on when the sentence is pulsed off. When the level of the pulsating sentence is high relative to the noise level, the sentence is unintelligible, owing to the missing "pieces" of the sentence. However, as the level of the sentence is lowered (or the noise is increased) there is a range of the level of the sentence (relative to that of the noise) that yields a highly intelligible sentence. It is as if the noise fills in the missing parts of the sentence, allowing the sentence to be understood. Such evidence of continuity ("phonemic restoration," Warren, 1999) suggests an auditory system that has been designed to process pulsating sounds as a perceptually continuous single sound source.

HARMONICITY/TEMPORAL REGULARITY Many sound sources (e.g., the human voice, instruments, sounds from sources that have motors) consist of spectral components that are integer multiples (harmonics) of a fundamental frequency (D in figure 28.8). These harmonic sounds also have a temporal waveform that has a temporal regularity whose period of regularity is inversely proportional to the fundamental frequency. Thus, either harmonicity or the correlated temporal regularity of a sound is a potentially usable cue for auditory scene analysis. Quite often such harmonic complex sounds are perceived as having a salient pitch associated with the fundamental. It is this pitch that may signify the existence of a sound source.

Many complex sounds can produce a salient pitch even when there is no energy in the sound's spectrum at the reported pitch. We can consider a harmonic tonal sequence of 400 Hz, 600 Hz, 800 Hz, 1000 Hz, . . . This sound produces a strong pitch of 200 Hz, even though there is no frequency component at or near 200 Hz. In this case, the fundamental of the complex harmonic sound is 200 Hz, and therefore this type of pitch is referred to as the "missing fundamental pitch" (see Moore, 1992, for a review). Figure 28.9 shows the NAP for this sound. In the lower frequencies of the NAP the individual harmonics of 200 Hz are delineated, and in the upper-frequency regions there is also a 200-Hz amplitude modulation (amplitude changing every 5 ms). Both the harmonic relationship among the low-frequency resolved spectral components and the temporal modulation in the high-frequency region where the sound's spectrum is not resolved by the auditory system have been used to model the pitch of such complex sounds (see Moore, 1992).

Figure 28.10 represents the NAP of a sound referred to as iterated rippled noise (Yost, 1996). The NAP reveals neither clear resolvable spectral components in the low frequencies nor clear amplitude modulation in the higher frequencies, yet this sound also has a distinct 200-Hz pitch. If the NAP is subjected to an autocorrelation analysis (lower panel of figure 28.10) as was done for figure 28.7, a clear pattern of intervals of 5 ms and 10 ms is revealed. This autocorrelation pattern shows that there is a 200-Hz (reciprocal of 5 ms), fine-structure temporal pattern to this complex noisy waveform that could be the basis of its 200-Hz pitch. Thus, complex sounds with a harmonic structure, periodic amplitude modulation, and/or a regular waveform fine-structure pattern can produce a salient pitch, and this pitch can aid in the determination of an auditory scene.

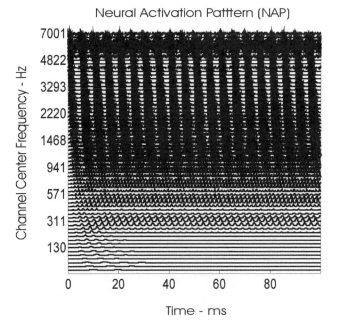

FIGURE 28.9   The neural activation pattern (NAP) to the "missing fundamental" pitch complex, as explained in the text. The harmonic structure can be seen in the lower-frequency channels and the amplitude modulation associated with the missing fundamental (5-Hz modulation for the 200-Hz missing fundamental) can be seen in the high-frequency channels.

An interesting example of sound source segregation occurs if a sound such as the 200-Hz harmonic sound cited above is played, but one of its harmonics is mistuned by more than approximately 8% (e.g, tonal components of 400, 600, 864 [8% change from 800 Hz], 1000, 1200 Hz . . .). In this case the 864-Hz tone perceptually "pops out" of the background complex pitch as a separate sound source (Moore, Peters, and Glasburg, 1985; Hartmann, McAdams, and Smith, 1990). The pitch of the missing fundamental complex is also slightly shifted to 205 Hz or so, but two "sources" are perceived: a complex pitch of about 205 Hz and a tonal pitch of 875 Hz. Examples of such "mistuned harmonics" reinforce the saliency of harmonic relationship in determining the pitch of complex sounds, and when such pitches may aid in determining the auditory scene.

If two different vowels (see figure 28.7) are computer generated such that they have the same fundamental frequency (as if the same vocal cords generated the vowels), the vowels are difficult to identify. However, as the fundamental frequencies of the two vowels differ, it is easier to identify each vowel. Both this two-vowel identification task and variations of fundamental voicing frequency are often used to study the role of harmonicity in determining the auditory scene (see Summerfield and Assmann, 1991; see Yost and Sheft, 1993, for a review).

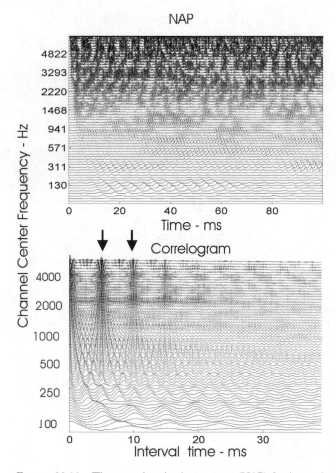

NAP

Correlogram

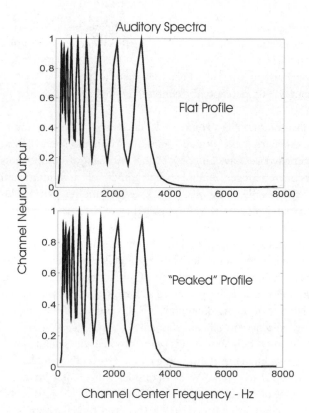

Auditory Spectra

Flat Profile

"Peaked" Profile

Channel Center Frequency - Hz

FIGURE 28.11 The auditory spectrum (see figure 28.5) for two spectra used in studies of profile analysis as explained in the text. The top panel shows the auditory spectrum for a "flat profile," where all tonal components were presented with the same amplitude. The bottom panel shows the auditory spectrum for a "peaked profile," in which the center tonal component was presented at a greater level than the other, equal-amplitude components.

FIGURE 28.10 The neural activation pattern (NAP) for iterated rippled noise that produces a salient 200-Hz pitch is shown at top. There is little evidence of a spectral or temporal structure to the NAP for this sound. The correlogram (generated in the same way as the stabilized auditory image in figure 28.7 in terms of a channel-by-channel autocorrelation) is shown at bottom and reveals a fine-structure temporal regularity at 5 and 10 ms (arrows) that may be the physiological basis for the perceived 200-Hz pitch.

INTENSITY PROFILE The spectra of different sound sources differ. Work on what has been referred to as profile analysis suggests the sensitivity of the auditory system in using such spectral differences to discriminate one potential sound source from another. Figure 28.11 shows the auditory spectra (see figure 28.5) of two sounds (Green, 1989). Each sound consists of the same nine frequency components, which are spaced logarithmically in frequency (thus avoiding cues associated with harmonically related spectral components). In the top panel, all of the spectral components have approximately the same amplitude (the small-amplitude variations are due to the random nature of neural transduction), whereas in the bottom panel, the middle spectral component is slightly more intense. Thus, the spectral profile on top is flat, but it peaks in the bottom panel. Subjects can detect a difference between the flat and peaked spectral profile when the spectral peak is at 1–2 dB,

even when the overall level of both complexes is randomly varied from trial to trial over a large range (e.g., a 40-dB range). Such acuity in spectral profile analysis in the face of this large random amplitude variation implies that the listener is attending to the spectral intensity profile rather than either an intensity change in a local spectral region near the incremented component (e.g., using a critical-band analysis) or the small overall loudness increases of the peaked spectral profile over that of the flat profile. As such, these profile analysis experiments indicate the ability of the auditory system to use across-spectral comparisons to determine the spectral profile of a sound and, thus, use differences in spectral profiles as one basis for sound source segregation.

ONSETS AND OFFSETS Sounds from different sources come on and go off at different times. Thus, components in the NAP (E in figure 28.8) that all come on together (or go off together) might provide a cue to determining the existence of a particular sound source. Common onsets have been shown to be powerful cues in auditory scene analysis in many contexts.

We can consider the case of two harmonic tonal complexes that are added together (e.g., 400, 600, 800, and 1000 Hz harmonic complex producing a 200-Hz complex pitch when presented alone; added to a 500, 750, 1000, and 1250 Hz harmonic complex, which would produce a 250-Hz complex pitch if presented alone). If these two harmonic series were added together simultaneously, it is unlikely that the two pitches of 200 and 250 Hz would be perceived. The auditory system in this case appears to behave synthetically rather than analytically, in that no clear pitch emerges. However, if the 200-Hz complex is turned on first and remains on when the 250-Hz complex is added 50 or so ms later, then two pitches can be perceived when both sounds are on together. That is, the separate onset times aid the auditory system in segregating the two complex sounds according to the pitches emanating from their unique harmonic relationships (Darwin, 1981).

COMMON MODULATION   Most sound sources impart a slow change to amplitude (amplitude modulation, e.g., voice jitter in speaking) or frequency (frequency modulation, e.g., vibrato in singing). Amplitude modulation, but not frequency modulation, appears to be a cue that the auditory system uses in sound source determination (see the common amplitude modulation in F of figure 28.8). Carlyon (1991) has argued that frequency modulation per se is probably not a cue used by the auditory system for determining an auditory scene. Frequency modulation can lead to a change in the sound's fundamental frequency, and frequency modulation can also result in amplitude modulation within the narrow spectral tuning of auditory nerve fibers. Thus, the resulting fundamental frequency change or amplitude modulation that may covary when sounds are frequency modulated are the likely cues used for segregating sound sources, rather than frequency modulation itself.

There are two areas of study that reveal aspects of amplitude modulation that might support auditory scene analysis. In a comodulation masking release (CMR) experiment (Hall, Haggard, and Fernandes, 1984), tonal detection is measured for two narrow-band maskers that are each amplitude modulated. The tone is centered in one of the narrow-band, amplitude-modulated maskers. If the pattern of amplitude modulation is the same for both maskers (i.e., they are comodulated), then the masked threshold is lower than when the two maskers are not comodulated. Most theories of CMR assume that when the two bands are comodulated, the auditory system "sees" them as a single sound source based on their common pattern of amplitude modulation, making it easier to detect the tonal source. When the two maskers have different envelopes, they are not fused as a single sound source, since a single sound source would not produce different envelopes in different spectral regions, and as a result there is no release from masking (i.e., no CMR).

Studies of modulation detection interference (MDI) also suggest that the auditory system uses common patterns of amplitude modulation in processing modulation (Yost, Stanley, and Opie, 1989). The task in an MDI experiment (Yost, Stanley, and Opie, 1989) is for the listener to detect a change in the depth of a sinusoidally amplitude-modulated carrier-probe tone when another tonal carrier (the masker) is also present. If the masker is not amplitude modulated, the threshold for detecting a change in modulation depth is low (e.g., 3%). If the masker is modulated at the same rate as the probe, then the threshold for detecting a change in modulation depth of the probe increases significantly (e.g., to 30%). It is argued that the common modulation caused the two carrier tones to form a single sound source, making it difficult for the auditory system to attend to the individual components of this complex source. One test of this idea is to make the rate of modulation for the masker carrier different from that of the probe carrier. In this case, there is not a common modulation, and the auditory system might process the two carriers as different sound sources, making it possible to attend to the modulation of the probe carrier by itself. If so, the threshold for detecting a change in the depth of modulation of the probe should improve, and this is what happens in studies of MDI (Yost, Stanley, and Opie, 1989).

SPATIAL SEPARATION   The auditory system can determine the location of sound sources in all three spatial dimensions based on the sound produced by these sources, even though sound has no spatial dimensions (Blauert, 1997). The auditory system computes the location of the sound source based on cues provided by the sound from the source. A different set of cues is used to spatially localize sound sources in each of the three spatial dimensions. The best understood cues are those used for sound localization in the azimuth, or horizontal, plane. Azimuthal localization is based on interaural differences of time and level (Blauert, 1997). Given that sounds are spatially localized, the perceived spatial separation of sound sources could be a basis for auditory scene analysis. Colin Cherry (1953) suggested spatial separation as the primary cue that would solve the "cocktail party problem," an earlier version of auditory scene analysis.

While spatial separation can be a cue for sound source segregation, it is unlikely that it is the only cue. All of the instruments (sound sources) of an orchestra can be identified when the sound is recorded by a single microphone and played back over a single loudspeaker. As such, there are no cues that can be used to determine the spatial position of the instruments in this recording (e.g., there are no interaural differences). Thus, cues in addition to those used to determine the spatial location of sound sources are most likely responsible for our ability to determine the various instruments of the orchestra in this case.

There is a large literature suggesting that the detection of a signal that is at one horizontal location based on one set of interaural differences of time and/or level masked by a masker at a different spatial location is improved over conditions when the signal and masker are at the same spatial location. (For masking-level difference literature, see Green and Yost, 1975.) However, there is less evidence that spatial separation by itself is a powerful cue for sound source segregation (Yost, 1997). Darwin and colleagues (Darwin and Hukin, 1999), using the two-vowel recognition task, argue that there may be "where" and "what" channels for processing sound sources. Darwin and colleagues showed that using interaural differences of time and level to attempt to improve vowel perception based on simulating horizontal spatial processing in the two-vowel task did not lead to much improvement in vowel recognition. However, if other cues such as changing the harmonic structure of each vowel (by using a different fundamental frequency for each vowel) were added, vowel recognition was improved, and when both fundamental frequency and interaural differences of time were introduced, there was an additional improvement in vowel recognition. These types of experiments lead to the suggestion of auditory channels dedicated to determining what a sound source is and then where it is.

Models and theories of auditory scene analysis

Modeling of and theorizing about auditory scene analysis can be divided into three categories: perceptual models and theories, computational and pattern recognition models, and models of how the different cues that may be used for auditory scene analysis are processed by the auditory system.

Bregman's (1990) application of Gestalt principles represents a major perceptual approach to theorizing about auditory scene analysis. He argued that auditory scene analysis is both a bottom-up process (based on auditory primitives) and a top-down process (a schema-based operation). The cues mentioned in this chapter form the primitives that allow for sequential integration of neural information that aids auditory scene analysis. Schemas are determined by experience and help govern auditory attention. Several rules are employed by the auditory system in analyzing the auditory scene. As an example, there is the principle of exclusive allocation, according to which one set of primitives can be assigned to only one sound source at one time. Bregman wove these processes and rules into a perceptual theory of auditory scene analysis.

Almost all computational and pattern recognition models (e.g., Hawkins et al., 1996) have "front ends" that simulate processing by the auditory periphery, as indicated in many of the figures provided in this chapter (e.g., figure 28.4). Most of the pattern recognition models then hypothesize some

form of a pattern matching process, often using prior knowledge about the stimulus context to extract information about sound sources in the spectral-temporal patterns that could be used to parse the NAP into a subset of neural patterns, where the subsets correspond to the spectral-temporal pattern of individual sound sources (see Meddis and Hewitt, 1992).

Shamma and colleagues (Shamma, Versnel, and Kowalski, 1995) offer a unique possibility for pattern recognition that is borrowed from visual pattern recognition. This linear system's approach views the auditory spectrum as a function relating neural output to frequency (on a logarithmic scale). Frequency is assumed to be mapped tonotopically to neural space, so that the function is viewed as neural output (e.g., spikes per second) related the neural space. If this function is subjected to a Fourier analysis, then the Fourier transform is in terms of the magnitude and phase of different spatial frequencies. One could also assume that there are channels tuned to spatial frequency (e.g., a channel tuned to a spectrum whose amplitudes change in a sinusoidal manner on a log-frequency axis with a period of, say, one-third of an octave). Such channels and their Fourier analysis using this approach have revealed spectral patterns that may suggest different sound sources in the auditory scene.

There are several models and theories of how many of the cues discussed in this chapter are processed by the auditory system. One that has been applied to both modulation processing and pitch processing is the set of models based on a modulation filter bank (Dau, Kollmeier, and Kohlraush, 1997). These models assume that there are processes tuned to amplitude modulation that can process the temporal structure in the peripheral spectral-temporal code. There is physiological evidence that there may be channels tuned to amplitude modulation in both the inferior colliculus and auditory cortex (Langner, 1992). Each modulation channel is tuned to a particular modulation rate, and then an ideal detector provides information about that rate for processing the auditory scene. The modulation filter bank models have had success in predicting a great deal of the data involving amplitude modulation, including CMR and MDI, and the models have had some success in handling some of the data from the complex pitch literature.

Although a great deal is beginning to be known about auditory scene analysis, there is still no overarching theory to explain perception of the many sound sources that make up a listener's acoustical environment. There are several possible reasons why such theories have not evolved. As already mentioned, most of the history of the study of hearing has involved detection and discrimination of simple sounds rather than complex sounds of auditory scenes. These studies of detection and discrimination have been best understood using theories based on narrow-band and short-duration processing, whereas determining the auditory scene requires wideband and long-duration processing. It is not easy to generate "arbitrary" sound sources that are perceptually relevant, meaning that actual sound sources must often be used. As such, the experience the listener might have with these natural sound sources can be a confound in determining the degree to which sound source segregation is based on segregation as opposed to the listener's experience. That is, if a set of arbitrary sound sources is generated by adding tonal components together in different spectral and temporal relationships, listeners often require considerable training to identify these arbitrary sound sources when they are presented one at a time (Kidd et al., 1998). Part of the difficulty in processing arbitrary sounds is that different sounds cannot be presented independently at the same time for comparison. Thus, sound identification requires auditory memory, which is aided by experience. Finally, the development of theories of auditory scene analysis is hindered by a lack of understanding of the function of the central auditory nervous system. Since the CNS is responsible for determining the auditory scene, it would help theory development if more were known about the function of the various neural centers and pathways in the ascending auditory system and cortex. Despite these limitations, there is little doubt that the study of the auditory scene is one of the liveliest areas of auditory science.

REFERENCES

BLAUERT, J., 1997. *Spatial Hearing*. Cambridge, Mass.: MIT Press.

BREGMAN, A. S., 1990. *Auditory Scene Analysis: The Perceptual Organization of Sound*. Cambridge, Mass.: MIT Press.

CARLYON, R. P., 1991. Discriminating between coherent and incoherent frequency modulation of complex tones. *Hear. Res.* 41:223–236.

CHERRY, C., 1953. Some experiments on the recognition of speech with one and with two ears. *J. Acoust. Soc. Am.* 25:975–981.

DALLOS, P., A. N. POPPER, and R. R. FAY, (eds.) 1996. *The Cochlea*. New York: Springer-Verlag.

DARWIN, C. J., 1981. Perceptual grouping of speech components differing in fundamental frequency and onset time. *Q. J. Exp. Psychol.* 33A:185–207.

DARWIN, C. J., and R. W. HUKIN, 1999. Auditory objects of attention: The role of interaural time differences. *J. Exp. Psychol. Percept. Perform.* 25:617–629.

DAU, T., B. KOLLMEIER, and A. KOHLRAUSH, 1997. Modeling auditory processing of amplitude modulation: II. Spectral and temporal integration in modulation detection. *J. Acoust. Soc. Am.* 102:2906–2919.

DE CHEVEIGNE, A., 2001. The auditory system as a "separation machine." In *Physiological and Psychophysical Bases of Auditory Function*, A. J. M. Houtsma, A. Kohlrausch, V. F. Prijs, and R. Schoonhoven, eds. Maastricht, The Netherlands: Shaker Publishers.

GREEN, D. M., 1989. *Profile Analysis*. New York: Oxford University Press.

GREEN, D. M., and W. A. YOST, 1975. Binaural Analysis. In *Handbook of Sensory Physiology*, vol. 5, W. D. Keidel and W. D. Neff, eds. New York: Springer-Verlag.

HALL, J. W., III, M. HAGGARD, and M. A. FERNANDES, 1984. Detection in noise by spectro-temporal pattern analysis. *J. Acoust. Soc. Am.* 76:50–60.

HARTMANN, W. M., 1988. Pitch perception and the organization and integration of auditory entities. In *Auditory Function: Neurobiological Bases of Hearing*, G. W. Edelman, W. E. Gall, and W. M. Cowan, eds. New York: Wiley.

HARTMANN, W. M., S. MCADAMS, and B. K. SMITH, 1990. Hearing a mistuned harmonic in an otherwise periodic complex tone. *J. Acoust. Soc. Am.* 88:1712–1724.

HAWKINS, H., T., MCMULLEN, A. N. POPPER, and R. R. FAY, eds., 1996. *Auditory Computation*. New York: Springer-Verlag.

KAERNBACH, K., and L. DEMANY, 1998. Psychophysical evidence against the autocorrelation theory of auditory temporal processing. *J. Acoust. Soc. Am.* 104:2298–2306.

KIDD, G., Jr., C. R. MASON, T. L. ROHTLA, and P. S. DELIWALA, 1998. Release from masking due to spatial separation of sources in the identification of non-speech auditory patterns. *J. Acoust. Soc. Am.* 104:422–431.

LANGNER, G., 1992. Periodicity coding in the auditory system. *Hear. Res.* 60:115–143.

LIBERMAN, M. C., and N. Y.-S. KIANG, 1978. Acoustic trauma in cats. *Acta Otolaryngol.* 358:1–63.

LITOVSKY, R., S. COLBURN, W. A. YOST, and S. GUZMAN, 1999. The precedence effect. *J. Acoust. Soc. Am.* 106:1633–1654.

MEDDIS, R., 2002. Computational model of pitch extraction in the auditory brainstem. In proceedings, *International Workshop: Pitch: Neural Coding and Perception*, Delmenhortz, Germany.

MEDDIS, R., and M. J. HEWITT, 1991. Virtual pitch and phase sensitivity of a computer model of the auditory periphery. I. Pitch identification. *J. Acoust. Soc. Am.* 89:2866–2882.

MEDDIS, R., and M. J. HEWITT, 1992. Modeling the identification of concurrent vowels with different fundamental frequencies. *J. Acoust. Soc. Am.* 91:233–245.

MOORE, B. C. J., 1986. *Frequency Selectivity in Hearing*. London, England: Academic Press.

MOORE, B. C. J., 1992. Frequency processing. In *Human Psychoacoustics*, W. A. Yost, A. N. Popper, and R. R. Fay, eds. New York: Springer-Verlag.

MOORE, B. C. J., 1995. *Perceptual Consequences of Cochlear Damage*. Oxford, England: Oxford University Press.

MOORE, B. C. J., 1997. *An Introduction to the Psychology of Hearing*, 3rd ed. London, England: Academic Press.

MOORE, B. C. J., R. W. PETERS, and B. R. GLASBURG, 1985. Thresholds for the detection of inharmonicity in complex tones. *J. Acoust. Soc. Am.* 77:1861–1867.

PATTERSON, R. D., M. ALLERHAND, and C. GIGUERE, 1995. Time-domain modeling of peripheral auditory processing: A modular architecture and a software platform. *J. Acoust. Soc. Am.* 98:1890–1895.

PRESSNITZER, D., R. D. PATTERSON, and K. KRUMBHOLZ, 2001. The lower limit of melodic pitch. *J. Acoust. Soc. Am.* 109:2074–2084.

SHAMMA, S. A., H. VERSNEL, and N. KOWALSKI, 1995. Ripple analysis to feret primary auditory cortex. I. Response characteristics of single units to sinusoidally rippled spectra. *Auditory Neurosci.* 1:233–254.

SUMMERFIELD, Q., and P. F. ASSMANN, 1991. Perception of concurrent vowel: Effects of harmonic misalignment and pitch-period asynchrony. *J. Acoust. Soc. Am.* 89:1364–1377.

VIEMEISTER, N. V., and C. PLACK, 1993. Temporal processing. In *Human Psychoacoustics*, W. A. Yost, A. N. Popper, and R. R. Fay, eds. New York: Springer-Verlag, pp. 116–154.

WARREN, R. M., 1999. *Auditory Perception: A New Analysis and Synthesis*. Cambridge, England: Cambridge University Press.

YOST, W. A., 1992a. Auditory image perception and analysis. *Hear. Res.* 56:8–19.

YOST, W. A., 1992b. Auditory perception and sound source determination. *Curr. Direct. Psychol. Sci.* 1:12–15.

YOST, W. A., 1996. Pitch of iterated rippled noise. *J. Acoust. Soc. Am.* 100:511–519.

YOST, W. A., 1997. The cocktail party effect: 40 years later. In *Localization and Spatial Hearing in Real and Virtual Environments*, R. Gilkey and T. Anderson, eds. Mahwah, N.J.: Erlbaum.

YOST, W. A., 2000. *Fundamentals of Hearing: An Introduction*, 4th ed. New York: Academic Press.

YOST, W. A., and S. SHEFT, 1993. Auditory processing. In *Human Psychoacoustics*, W. A. Yost, A. N. Popper, and R. R. Fay, eds. New York: Springer-Verlag, pp. 193–236.

YOST, W. A., S. STANLEY, and J. OPIE, 1989. Modulation detection interference: Effect of modulation frequency. *J. Acoust. Soc. Am.* 86:2138–2148.

29

Short-Term Memory for the Rapid Deployment of Visual Attention

KEN NAKAYAMA, VERA MALJKOVIC, AND ARNI KRISTJANSSON

ABSTRACT We describe a short-term memory system useful for the rapid deployment of focal visual attention. The memory system is primitive, temporary, cumulative, and efficacious. It automatically links separable features of objects to the act of attentional deployment so that visual perception and performance are greatly enhanced. The effects of the memory cannot be overridden by higher level knowledge. Its properties can account for those aspects of searching and foraging behavior currently attributed to "search images." The learning described here is likely to be general, not confined to the rapid deployment of focal visual attention.

Blindness as we commonly understand it is caused by damage to the eye or to some part of the visual pathway. This definition encompasses diseases of the retina as well as strokes affecting the visual cortex. There is another form of blindness that is not due to specific peripheral mechanisms but occurs in the absence of visual attention (McConkie and Zola, 1979). Grimes (1996) showed that if we look at a complex natural scene on a computer display and make a saccadic eye movement, we are highly insensitive to experimenter-induced changes during the very short interval of the saccade. Buildings and individuals can disappear from the screen or move large distances, yet subjects often report that they see no change. This phenomenon, known as *change blindness*, dispels the naive belief that we "see" all or most things in our visual world (Simons and Levin, 1997; O'Regan, Rensink, and Clark, 1999). Further confirmation of change blindness came from Rensink and colleagues (1997), who showed that if two, almost identical scenes are alternated sequentially with a short time gap between presentations, observers sometimes have great difficulty picking out prominent differences between the two pictures. Mack and Rock (1998) have dubbed this inability to see without

attention *inattentional blindness*. Their inescapable conclusion is that for humans to see an object, we must deploy our attention to it. Thus, it has been argued that vision is an active sense with greater similarities to the exploring hand than to a picture (Gibson, 1966). We must visually grasp an object with our attention in order to perceive it consciously (Nakayama, 1990).

If vision is active and attention is important for seeing, how is it that we do not notice this striking characteristic of vision in our everyday lives? Such "blindness" might suggest that we should often miss very important things. There are many reports of lapsed attention causing industrial and vehicular accidents. Such mishaps are very rare, however, and we do pretty well at staying out of trouble, even if research shows that we are blind to unattended objects. We must have a set of mechanisms that guide our attention effectively. This chapter examines one such mechanism in detail, a short-term memory mechanism that helps deploy attention to features of objects recently attended.

First we will review some current ideas on how visual attention might be appropriately deployed. Much of our everyday world is fairly predictable, and we can learn to direct our attention strategically in accordance with our knowledge and goals. In the case of driving, for example, experienced drivers pay attention to the roadway and the car they are following, but they also attend to cars farther ahead, to driveways, and to upcoming intersections. The full range of such attentional deployments is reached only after extended practice, along with an understanding of the driving environment.

Even when confronting less ordered or less well understood scenes, we are often assisted by low-level mechanisms that ensure that we pay attention to relevant things. The phenomenon of pop-out is one example. In pop-out, an odd feature among a homogeneous array of other elements attracts our attention (Treisman and Gelade, 1980). Most useful in everyday life is the motion of an object. In a large crowd, you can get a friend's attention by waving your arms. Related to motion are sensory transients; the

KEN NAKAYAMA Department of Psychology, Harvard University, Cambridge, Mass.

VERA MALJKOVIC Department of Psychology, University of Chicago, Chicago, Ill.

ARNI KRISTJANSSON Institute of Cognitive Neuroscience, London, U.K.

appearance or blinking of a light hardly ever fails to grab our attention.

Functional role of attention for survival

If attention determines whether or not we see, it should not be surprising that attention is consequential in life-or-death situations. Much has been written on the sensory capacities of animals and their role in determining whether the animal will survive or not (Lythgoe, 1979). The eagle has very good visual acuity, which it uses to detect and identify small prey at large distances. Cats are nocturnal animals and have an abundance of rods, so that they can see under very low illumination. Thus, basic visual capacities are important, and the ecology of animals is clearly related to sensory performance.

Less has been said about the role of attention and other cognitive capacities of animals in determining their population numbers, generally manifested in whether they will catch prey or avoid predation (but see Dukas, 1998). L. Tinbergen (1960), in accounting for the distribution of birds and insects in a Dutch woodland, suggested that the ecological balance between predator and prey depended critically on the cognitive capacities of the predator, in particular its ability to allocate attention effectively. In a much cited article, he suggested that

The intensity of predation depends . . . on the use of specific search images. This implies that the birds perform a highly selective sieving operation on the visual stimuli that reach their retina . . . birds can only use a limited number of different search images at the same time. (Tinbergen, 1960, pp. 332–333)

In support of the search image hypothesis, Dawkins (1971) found that newly hatched chicks, when presented with two different colors of grain, would peck for long runs of one color and then another, almost as if the bird were looking for one color for long stretches at a time, then for another. The search image hypothesis has been a key concept in the study of foraging, explaining the patterns by which animals obtain food successfully. Reid and Shettleworth (1992) demonstrated the power of the search image construct in successfully predicting that pigeons would overselect more frequently presented color grains. As such, the notion of the search image is explicitly mentalistic, a cognitive top-down process invoked to explain behavior. In this chapter we describe a short-term memory phenomenon, more akin to priming, that is well suited to serve the same purpose: to direct attention to features in scenes that have been recently attended to.

Transient attention and its flexible deployment

Before we describe the memory phenomenon, we first need to describe the properties of focal attention itself, in partic-

ular, a fast, transient attentional system that briefly enhances perception and performance (Reeves and Sperling, 1986). In a series of experiments (Nakayama and Mackeben, 1989), subjects were asked to report on the shape and color of a briefly presented probe target in a multiple-element array that appeared within a cue object. The cue appeared at various times (cue lead time) before the target and distracter array. The brief target array was immediately followed by a large, long-duration mask. The cue, the target array, and the mask are shown in figure 29.1A, which also shows the time relations of the various sequentially presented frames. Figure 29.1B shows performance on the discrimination task as a function of cue lead time. Subjects were instructed to fixate the central cross. The targets always fell within peripheral vision, requiring subjects to direct attention away from fixation without moving the eye. Subjects could maintain fixation easily, but just to make sure they did, we monitored eye movements using an infrared detector system. The data indicated by the open circles are from a session during which eye movements were monitored and were found to be negligible. The solid circles represent data from a session in which eye movements were not monitored. The lack of any eye movement and the same basic form of the function in each case indicate that the pattern of results is reproducible within and between subjects (Nakayama and Mackeben, 1989). The function invariably showed a rapid rise in performance from zero to about 100 ms, which we interpret as the time that attention needs to go to a location away from fixation.

Most surprising and unexpected, however, was the finding of a very reliable drop in performance as cue lead time increased beyond about 100 ms. Performance beyond about 200 ms is well below the peak performance seen for shorter cue lead times. Even though the position of the target location was fully specified for these longer cue lead times and the cue remained on when the target was visible, performance still declined. This finding suggests that something more is at play than the subject's knowledge of the target location, because the strongest manifestation of attention occurred early and then dropped, whereas knowledge of cue location rose quickly and remained high. Supporting this view, Nakayama and Mackeben (1989) found just as large a transient boost in performance when the cued location was the same from trial to trial and thus was always known.

Nakayama and Mackeben interpreted a rapid rise and noticeable fall in performance as a combination of two attentional processes, a weak, sustained component, which is related to the subject's knowledge of the target location, and a stronger transient component, which rises and quickly falls. The magnitude of transient attention is approximately twice that of the sustained component. At first glance, it might seem that this transient component is a reflex, because it is very fast and has a finite duration, and does not correspond to the subject's knowledge of the target location.

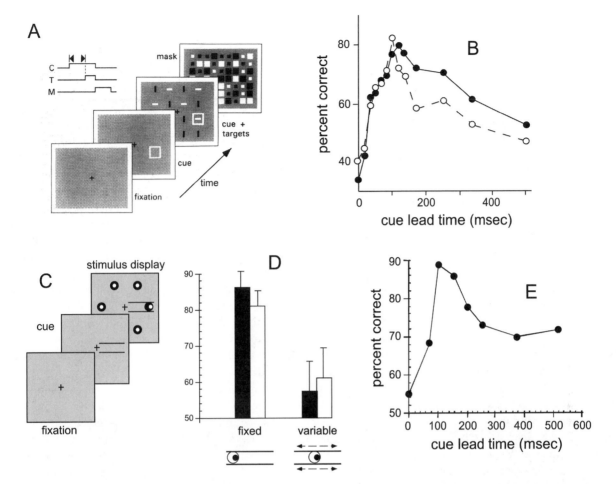

FIGURE 29.1 Transient attention and its flexible deployment. (A) The cuing paradigm originally used to characterize transient attention. A series of frames, fixation, cue, target (with cue and distracters), followed by a mask, is depicted. (B) Performance (percent correct) plotted as a function of cue lead time. Open circles represent data for sessions which eye movements were monitored, solid circles represent data from sessions in which eye movements were not monitored (C) stimulus situation to show the learning of transient attention. Note that the cue object is larger than the target. (D) Performance as a function of whether the target has a fixed or variable relation to the cue object, that is, whether it is on the same side or varies from trial to trial. (E) Performance in the fixed condition as a function of cue lead time. (Reprinted from Nakayama and Mackeben, 1989; Kristjansson, Mackeben, and Nakayama, 2001.)

Although the transient component does have these characteristics, it is much more flexible and can learn very simple relations. It can show dramatic changes in accordance with past experience.

To document this flexibility, we used an array very similar to the one just described, but with a few changes (Kristjansson, Mackeben, and Nakayama, 2001). First, the target and distracter array were arranged to form a circle (figure 29.1C). The target probe was an "eye" that could look in four possible directions. Most important, the cue was much larger than the target itself, consisting of two parallel horizontal lines within which the eye could be displayed (figure 29.1C). The subject's task was to report in which direction the eye was pointing. If the process of summoning transient attention were a simple reflex, we might expect that the benefits of attention to be bestowed equally within the cue object. There should be no preferred location where the

eye target would be the most visible. To examine this issue, we ran the experiment under two conditions. In the fixed condition, we ran a block of trials during which the target always appeared at one end of the cue (either right or left). In the variable condition, the probe target could move from trial to trial within the cue object on a random basis. A schematic of the fixed and variable conditions is shown below the horizontal axis of the graph in figure 29.1D. In this experiment, the cue lead time was fixed at 100 ms, where it was expected to capture the peak of the transient attention function (as depicted in figure 29.1B).

Again, if the summoning of transient attention were a simple reflex, one might expect the results of the two conditions to be the same. The results shown in figure 29.1D do not support this view. For both observers (one designated by black bars, the other by white bars), there is a large difference in performance between the fixed target case and the variable target case. With the target fixed, performance is approximately 80%–85% correct, whereas for a variable target, performance is very poor, approximately 50%–60% correct. The poor showing in the variable condition suggests that attention is diluted over the extent of a cue and that only when there is a consistent relation between a specific location within the cue object is there much benefit. We concluded that the difference between the two conditions is the result of experience. It is as if the system responsible for the deployment of transient attention has learned to go to a particular position within the cue object. This result is quite surprising, because the rapid deployment of attention and its transient nature suggest that deployment of transient attention might be a reflex, summoned by an exogenous cue, yet our results suggest that transient attention shows unsuspected flexibility and that it could adapt by going to just one portion of an object on the basis of past experience.

The existence of this unsuspected learning raises many questions that we sought to answer. First, we needed to establish whether the benefit seen for a consistent location within a larger cue (the fixed condition) reflected the learning capacity of transient attention, not sustained attention. Would the flexible deployment of attention (to go to a particular portion of a larger object) show the transient peak? To determine whether this was the case, we used the paradigm described in figure 29.1C and varied cue lead time. If transient attention were operative, we would expect to see a similar function, a fast rise followed by a fall in performance with increasing cue lead times. Figure 29.1E shows that this is the case. Performance is highest for intermediate lead times and shows a discernible falloff for durations greater than a few hundred milliseconds. This indicates it is the very rapid process of transient, seemingly reflexive, attention that can learn to go to a specific position within a larger object.

The learning curve

To examine the learning systematically, we conducted experiments to characterize its time course. First, we asked how rapidly the learning might take place. Would it grow slowly and incrementally, or would it occur more suddenly? To characterize how attention might learn to go to a specific place within a larger object, we used the paradigm shown in figure 29.1C, modifying it slightly. The probe target "eye" could be located on the left or the right end of the cue object, always remaining within the two parallel lines. The position of the target varied from trial to trial but was biased so that on average, there were more repetitions than changes of target location within the cue. Thus, there were streaks of random length where for a number of trials, the target would be on the left side of the cue, followed by a sequence of trials in which the target would be on the right. If learning occurred, we would expect to see some change in per-

formance as the position within a "same-position" streak was taken into account.

To document the hypothesized build-up of learning, we plotted the performance (percent correct) as a function of a trial's position within a streak of same target locations. If learning were taking place, we would expect that as the position within a same-position streak increased, performance would improve. Figure 29.2A shows that this was the case. As we look at the position within the streak, performance (percent correct) rises dramatically. For the first position within a streak (where the preceding trials had a different target position), performance is very poor, hovering around 50% for the two subjects. Note, however, as the position within the streak increases, there is a conspicuous rise in performance such that by the third repetition, performance has reached asymptote (at about 80% correct). This indicates that the presumed learning did indeed occur, and it occurred very quickly. Therefore, we have shown that the difference seen in figure 29.1D is very likely the product of rapid learning. In a very few trials, attention can learn to go to a particular part of an object (left or right), boosting performance dramatically.

It seems that we have discovered a malleable process for the directing of focal attention. We have shown that it can be flexibly and rapidly deployed to either end of a larger object. It is an object-relative phenomenon of learning, as the cue object can appear in many places around the circle, as depicted in figure 29.1C. At this point, it seems natural to determine whether this system can learn something else about objects. Could it learn to go to a portion of an object designated by some other property besides its relative left versus right position? For example, could attention learn to go to a distinctly colored region of an object even if the object changed its orientation, such as being flipped horizontally, as in a right-left reversal? For this purpose, we employed two kinds of distinctions within an object, color and shape. For the color case, the object was a pair of horizontal lines that were colored red at one end and green on the other. For the case of shape, the object had a keyhole form, so that one end was round and the other was angular. Most important for the experiments was the fact that these two features, color and shape, could vary randomly in position, left versus right. Thus, the green end of the cue could be on the left or on the right of the object in a streak of color-constant locations. The insets of figure 29.2B and C show two possible relations between the cue and target location, where the target is at the green or red end for the color experiment and at the round or angular end for the shape experiment.

The results, shown in figure 29.2B and C, indicate a dramatic increase in percent correct for the case where the target relation to color or shape repeats. This observation indicates that the transient attentional system can learn to

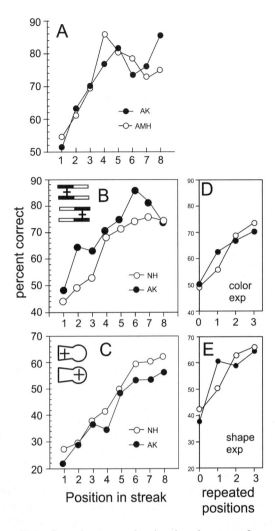

FIGURE 29.2 Learning curves showing the advantage of repeated positions, local colors, and local shapes on learning of mobe objects. (*A*) Effect of repeated position (left or right) as a function of the ordinal position in a streak length. (*B*) Similar effects were obtained for repeated color. Schematic at top left shows the repeated linkage of the target to a specific local color within the larger cue object even as the relation of local colors flips, left to right. (*C*) Similar effects were obtained for repeated local shape. Schematic at top left shows repeated linkage of target to a specific local shape (round vs. angular) over a series. (*D*) Evidence that during color learning, learning of relative position was also occurring. (*E*) Evidence that during shape learning, position learning was also occurring.

go quickly and efficiently to a given color or shape within an object, even for an object that flips horizontally.

Equally important, many of these learning processes can coexist and operate independently and simultaneously. Just as transient attention shows a learning curve for repeated shapes or colors, it also exhibits a simultaneous learning curve for position. Recall that to plot the learning curves for color or shape (as shown in figure 29.2*B*, *C*), we manipulated the sequence, to ensure long streaks of the same shape or color. At the same time, we arranged that probe target position (right or left) would flip randomly as a Bernoulli series, with no intertrial dependencies. By chance, however, such sequences have short runs of repeated target positions. Thus the target can appear on the right for a few trials, then on the left, even as we probe for the effects of longer streaks of color and shape. To show the learning of position, we used the exact same data sets and plotted performance in terms of the number of repeats of the same positions (right or left). These scores are plotted to the right of the color and position learning curves (figure 29.2*E* and *F*, respectively), showing that the experiments originally designed to get the learning curves for color and position also furnish learning curves for repeated position. Each shows the data from the same subject from the exact same series of trials, plotted as a function of number of repeats of the same position (left or right). Although we were only able to obtain reliable data from short streaks with a maximum of three repeats, the same rapid rate of learning is apparent. From this, we conclude that the learning of position, color, and shape occur independently and simultaneously.

It should be pointed out that this very rapid and robust learning takes place without any effort on the subject's part. Subjects are simply instructed to do the best they can in identifying the probe target when it appears within the cue. They are not told that there are streaks of trials during which the target will appear at one end or another, and they are not obviously aware of this relation.

Transient attention cannot learn simple contingent relations

Because learning occurs so easily and automatically, it might represent part of a specialized, dedicated system that lacks the flexibility of more general learning systems. To address this issue, we made the learning requirements slightly more complex. We ask whether attention could go to opposite ends of objects that are obviously distinct. Would it be possible for attention to go quickly to the left end of object A and to the right end of object B? We conducted two experiments using object properties (color and shape) that have already been shown to be used by this learning system (as demonstrated in figure 29.2*B*, *C*). For the shape experiment there were two objects, one rounded, one rectangular. In the

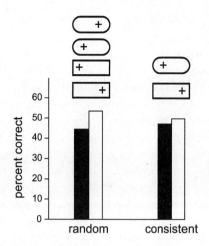

FIGURE 29.3   Demonstration that transient attention cannot learn to go to the left of one object and the right of another. Two very distinguishable cue objects, one rounded and the other rectangular, have either random or consistent cue-target relations. There is no advantage to consistent presentations, indicating the lack of learning of this relation. (From Kristjansson and Nakayama, 2003.)

experimental condition, which we call "consistent," the target was always on the left side if the object was rounded and on the right side if the object was rectangular. Schematics of these objects and this contingency relation are shown in figure 29.3. For comparison we had a random control condition in which there was no specific assignment of the target to the ends of particular objects. If transient attention could learn to go to a specific place within a given object, then we should expect to see improved performance in the consistent condition. The results as depicted in figure 29.3 show no difference in performance between the two conditions. Even though the two shapes are highly discriminable, there is no sign of learning. The attentional system, or at least this fast transient system, cannot learn this simple relation. We also found that there was no learning when we used color to distinguish the objects (Kristjansson and Nakayama, 2003). Transient attention could not learn to go the right of a red object and to the left of a green one.

At this point we should pause and reflect on the nature of the learning that we have characterized so far. The learning is very rapid, taking place over very few trials, but surprisingly powerful, going from near chance to reliable performance and doing so hundreds of milliseconds faster. Yet the suprising lack of the ability to learn contigent relations suggests that the learning is not registering information about the nature of the objects, but something more primitive. The learning is only concerned with the recurring features of objects, not with the objects themselves.

Learning to deploy attention in a visual search array

At the beginning of this chapter we reviewed the concept of a search image, according to which construct an animal

searching for food possesses a top-down template specific to the items sought. This construct could explain otherwise puzzling findings of Dawkins (1971), indicating that animals have runs of grain types in a free choice situation and often overselect for the more prevalent food type (Reid and Shettleworth, 1992).

Our experimental findings on cued attention in humans (Nakayama and Mackeben, 1989; Kristjansson, Mackeben, and Nakayama, 2001; Kristjansson and Nakayama, 2003) might seem only distantly related to these issues of search and foraging, yet the learning mechanism that we have delineated provides an alternative explanation, replacing the notion of the search image. To make this view more plausible, we will now describe the results obtained with a visual search paradigm in which the learning of attentional deployment is also evident. This paradigm also allows us to more readily make the case that the learning mechanism we have outlined might apply to searching and foraging. As originally derived from the work of Bravo and Nakayama (1992), the goal of the visual search paradigm was to develop a visual search task that would require the subject to deploy focal attention to an item in an array. For this purpose, we devised a task in which the subject had to discriminate a subtle shape difference of an oddly colored singleton that was presented along with two other colored distracters (Maljkovic and Nakayama, 1994). Thus, the subject's task was to report the shape of the odd-colored target while maintaining fixation on a central cross (figure 29.4A).

Maljkovic and Nakayama (1994) manipulated the length of runs of same-color odd targets and found a dramatic decrease in reaction time as the target's position within a streak increased. Figure 29.4B shows the results obtained in a representative observer. The reaction time fell systematically as the number of repetitions within a streak of same-color targets increased. So, just as in the attentional cuing experiments shown in figure 29.2, there is a strong benefit derived from repeating the color of the object of attention. This observation confirms the existence of a comparably rapid learning process in a very different paradigm and suggests that the results obtained with our cued attention experiments can be more widely generalized.

Because the experiment is more like a visual search task, we can now ask whether the results might be accounted for by a process akin to that involved in the search image. Does the subject form a mental template that aids the perception of targets that fit this template or search image? The implication in the search image literature is that a search image is adopted as a formed and structured template (corresponding to the desired target), which would explain the long streaks of trials of a given food selected (Dawkins, 1971) and the overselection for common colored foods (Reid and Shettleworth, 1992). A search image also suggests an active process, one that reflects the expectancy of the upcoming

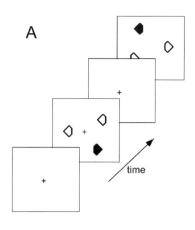

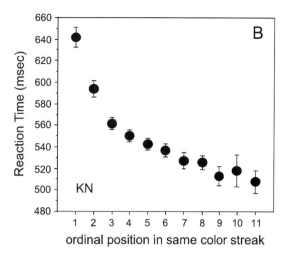

FIGURE 29.4 The learning of attentional deployment in a visual search task. (*A*) In a sequence of trials, the observer's task was to identify the shape of an odd-colored target. The color of the target could either remain the same or change, as could the target's position. (*B*) Reaction time as a function of target position in a same-color target streak. (From Maljkovic and Nakayama, 1994.)

target color. After a long run of same-color trials, expectancy for yet another similar trial would be high. Such a notion could plausibly explain our data, at least those shown in figure 29.4*B*.

Our aim, however, is to formulate a more mechanistic alternative to the search image hypothesis. We argue that the learning could consist of a passive association of isolated characteristics of previously attended sites and the "response" of attentional deployment, explicitly adopting the active hand metaphor for attention. In this scheme, expectancy plays no role. Attention is driven by its association with simple features. This accords with the piecemeal quality of the learning described for cued attention, where the learning of position (left or right), color, and shape occur independently and in parallel. The effects of learning are not overcome by knowledge, expectancy, or intention.

To evaluate these two different notions, we devised an experiment in which the predicted results from an expectancy hypothesis would be very different from those based on passive association. We used a deterministic sequence of trials that provided ample opportunity for both expectancy and passive learning to be evident. The sequence consisted of one pair of a set of "same" color trials, followed by the other pair of "same" color trials. Thus, all sequences had run lengths of two: targets were presented as two greens, two reds, two greens, and so on. The experiment was run under two sets of instructions. In the first set, we asked the subjects simply to do the experiment and not think about the pairs of same-color trials. We called this the passive condition. In the second case, we asked subjects to be fully aware of the completely predictable nature of this sequence and asked that they actively anticipate the color of each upcoming trial by subvocally voicing the upcoming color prior to each trial. We called this the active and expectant condition.

The results are shown in figure 29.5. In the case of the passive condition, with no conscious effort on the part of subjects to anticipate the color of the upcoming trial, there was clear evidence of learning. Reaction times were significantly shorter for the second trial of the sequence, confirming the same sequence of effects as shown in figures 29.2 and 29.4. Most critical are the results of the active condition. Expectancy is plainly evident, because the sequence is both simple and deterministic. Furthermore, expectancy should be the same for all positions within the sequences. Thus, we predict that the difference between the first and second trial of the sequence should be abolished. The lower curves in Figure 29.5 shows that this is not the case; the difference between trial 1 and trial 2 for the active condition is as great as that in the passive condition, even though the expectancies for trial 1 and trial 2 of the sequence should be identical.[1] This experiment shows that performance cannot be influenced by prior knowledge or expectancy. Whether a subject knows, pays attention to, or completely ignores the sequence of target colors is irrelevant. The process of learning proceeds independently of these higher-order cognitive factors. As such, the process of rapid attentional deployment is autonomous and machine-like, impervious to other mental processes and reflecting only passive repetition.

An elemental memory event

These results suggest that with each attentional deployment to a given feature (color, in this case), there is a primitive

---

[1] The overall reaction times are consistently faster for this active condition, perhaps reflecting the higher motivation of the subject, given the additional task of anticipating the color of the upcoming trial.

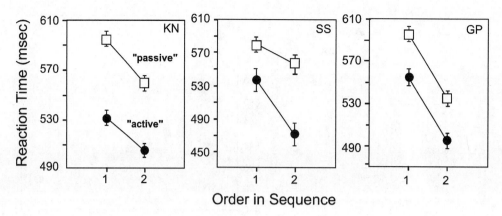

FIGURE 29.5 Irrelevance of expectancy, knowledge, and intention. Using the same stimulus display as shown in figure 29.4, a deterministic series of trials was presented, doubly alternating red and green so that the streak length was always two. Subjects could either passively just do the task (passive) or could consciously anticipate each trial (active). The learning was the same in each case. (From Maljkovic and Nakayama, 1994.)

process that effectively associates the deployment of attention with this feature and this process can be incremented over long sequences to boost performance significantly. How might such performance enhancement occur? One way to examine this is to ascertain the influence of a single episode of attentional allocation, to see how it, by itself, might influence future allocations. To explore such a hypothesized associative process in isolation, we devised a method to measure the influence of a single trial in the past, and thus to determine its influence on the future. We used the same search task schematized in figure 29.4A. As mentioned earlier, if the learning of attentional deployment is the result of the simple association of a feature to a past attentional deployment, we might be able to isolate this process and track its time course. Thus, our goal was to measure the influence of arbitrarily distant trials in the past. In the simplest case, we would expect to see an influence from the immediately preceding trial. If the previous trial's target color was the same, we would expect reaction times to be shorter than if the previous color was different. We can generalize this question beyond the consideration of a previous trial and consider the influence of any trial in the past. Because we used a Bernoulli sequence of target colors, such that each trial's target color was independent of all others, such performance differences can provide unbiased estimates for any given trial's influence. Computing this difference for up to 15 trials in the past and for a smaller number in the future (to gain a sense of noise of our measurements), we obtained a memory kernel function, the influence of such a single trial (Maljkovic and Nakayama, 1994). Figure 29.6 shows this function for two observers. The vertical dashed line separates past from future. It is apparent that the immediate previous trial has the largest influence on the current trial, such that reaction times are approximately 40–50 ms faster for same versus different color targets. But there is also is considerable residual influ-

ence from single trials much more distant in the past, as indicated by the extent to which this function deviates from the baseline of zero difference. This means that any given trial will have a lasting influence up to about six to eight trials into the future. Yet this influence, while very strong, does ultimately decay, and after a dozen or more trials it is effectively abolished.

Subsequent research has found that this decay is event driven: it is the intervening allocations of focal attention, not

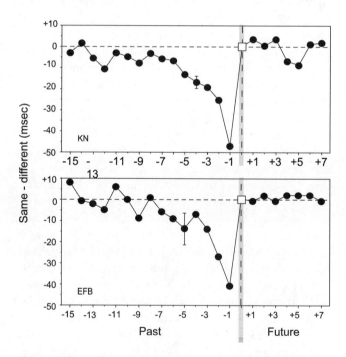

FIGURE 29.6 Influence of a single trial or event for two observers. Using the same stimulus display as shown in figure 29.4A, and with a series of random colored targets presented over time (a Bernoulli sequence), we showed the influence of past (or future) trials on the present. (From Maljkovic and Nakayama, 1994.)

simply time, that cause the memory to decay (Maljkovic and Nakayama, 2000). In addition, we also found that any deployments of focal attention to unrelated targets (neither red nor green) would also deplete the memory.

Summary of findings

We have demonstrated the existence of a very powerful attentional system that we have called transient attention, a brief heightening of visual processing that seems to require an exogenous cue. Its benefits are much stronger than those of sustained attention, and it seems curiously uncoupled from higher-order knowledge of a target's upcoming location. As such, it seems to have characteristics very similar to a reflex. Yet it is a flexible reflex. It can learn to go to a specific portion of a larger object, identified by color, shape, or position, and the associations formed are piecemeal, each is independent, and all occur simultaneously. But the piecemeal nature of learning has inherent bounds. Transient attention cannot learn to go to the left end of one identifiable object and to the right end of another. Thus the learning has a nonintegrative quality: it can learn the simplest first-order associations, but no more. Within these bounds, the learning is very strong, and its effects cannot be overcome by conscious knowledge of upcoming target properties. Finally the memory kernel functions (see figure 29.6) show that the learning from a single trial is temporary, decaying over a variable period up to six to eight trials.

The basic findings described here have been replicated by others (Hillstrom, 2000; Goolsby and Suzuki, 2001; Olivers and Humphreys, 2003). They have also been extended to eye movements and to manual pointing. McPeek, Maljkovic, and Nakayama (1999) showed the phenomenon in human saccadic latencies, and the same phenomenon has also been demonstrated for monkey saccades (McPeek and Keller, 2001; Bichot and Schall, 2002). Song and Nakayama (2003) showed that manual pointing with the finger exhibited the same benefit of feature repetition.

Discussion: Comparison with other forms of learning and possible neural substrates

Our findings indicate that with each allocation of attention, there is an increase in the association to those features that were at the site of attentional deployment. The influence from a single allocation of attention can summate, so that after a few repetitions of deployment of attention to particular features, performance is greatly enhanced. The diagram in figure 29.7 is a pictorial representation of the process suggested. After each attentional allocation to a given feature on an object, there is a transient boost in memory that will gradually fall off with increasing deployments of attention (figure 29.7A). With repeated deployments of attention to

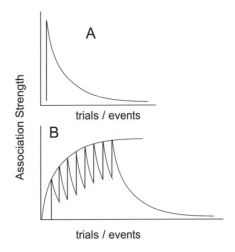

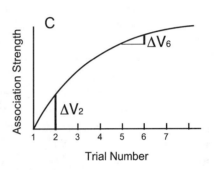

FIGURE 29.7 Contrasting of the learning of transient attention with other types of learning processes. *A* reproduces the memory kernel function in schematic form, while *B* shows how it is constant and summates. In *C*, we contrast this the with acquisition of more conventional learning, where each increment in learning decreases as learning proceeds. *B* and *C* show the negatively accelerating learning curves common to both transient attention and other forms of learning, respectively.

the same feature in a streak, such effects combine, so that effects can be quite large (figure 29.7B), accounting for the improved performance.

Superficially, there seems to be some similarity to all other forms of learning, including classical conditioning. In particular, the graded and incremental nature of the learning seems identical. With repeated deployment of attention to the same features over time, this system displays the familiar negatively accelerating learning curve (see figures 29.2, 29.4B) seen in most studies of learning and conditioning (figure 29.7C). Yet from our results, it is evident that the underlying process is likely to be very different.

Current theories of associative learning, such as Rescorla and Wagner's (1972) model, predict similar negatively accelerating learning functions. These formulations are based on a delta rule, according to which the increment of learning at any instant is variable, decreasing during the course of learning. This occurs as the amount of unused associative capacity is exhausted. The reduced increment in learning strength for such types of learning is depicted in figure 29.7*C*, which shows incremental reductions on later trials. This situation is to be contrasted to the learning of attentional deployment, where it is likely that the memory increment is constant for each attentional deployment and the negatively accelerating function is due to quick decay of the elementary memory event, which precludes summation beyond its own, very limited duration (figure 29.7*B*). Thus, the very temporary nature of the learning and its inevitable decay mark it as very different from more traditional forms of learning.

Another difference is the piecemeal nature of the learning. This was evident with the independent influence of position, color, and shape associations in facilitating speeded attentional cuing. They combine similarly for the visual search task (Maljkovic and Nakayama, 1996) and add linearly with separable effects (Norton and Maljkovic, 2001). To provide a framework to understand the independent nature of the underlying components, we suggest that the memory system is a distributed one, with separate associations to many simple features. In keeping with the analogy of attention being like a mobile hand, we depict the association to features as either positive or negative. For example, studies by Maljkovic and Nakayama (1994, 1996) show that there are equally strong inhibitory effects, such that colors and positions not attended to on a given trial are more slowly attended to in the future. Because the associations are to separate features, it is thus not surprising that the learning cannot be extended to anything of higher complexity. Thus it cannot learn, for example, to go to the right end of object A and the left end of object B.

We have described the rapid learning of transient attention as associative because from a behavioral perspective, stronger associations between particular features and the act of attentional deployment are evident. Yet if we are to think of possible neural mechanisms underlying such learning, we need to be cautious in drawing on known mechanisms of associative learning and memory. Most obvious is the very temporary nature of the learning. Being temporary, it does not require the cellular mechanisms of memory storage that are longer lasting. Consequently, the mechanisms of conditioning and other forms of permanent learning are unlikely to be applicable. The learning described here is also very automatic and noneffortful. This suggests that the learning is very different from the concept of working memory, and Maljkovic and Nakayama (2000) showed that indeed it is, that the properties of working memory cannot account for our results.

A very different type of process is required to explain the flexibility seen here. We suggest that phenomenon described should be regarded as modulatory, activating or suppressing the specific neural circuits that have been activated very recently. As such, those processes that enabled attention to go to particular portions of an object are facilitated or inhibited temporarily. Seen in this light, the learning can be considered more as a form of priming of existing associations. It is not a full-blown learning system by itself but a process that can modulate existing associations.

Where in the nervous system might such learning or modulation of associations occur? We suggest it occurs at some level removed from the early retinotopic stages of the visual system. This is mandated by the object-relative nature of the learning, that is, the fact that attention can learn to go to the left or right part of an object no matter where it appears in the visual field (see figures 29.1, 29.2; also Maljkovic and Nakayama, 1996).

That the learning is nonintegrative, piecemeal, and distributed suggests that at any given instant, the learning could occur across many different objects, and is not linked to specific stored object representations. This situation would suggest that the learning we have described is not found in parts of the cortex that represent specific objects. It argues against the inferotemporal cortex as the site of this particular type of learning.

Parts of the brain subserving the allocation of attention and eye movements are of particular interest, including frontal, parietal, and midline cortical areas (Posner and Raichle, 1994). Olson and colleagues (Olson, Olson, and Gettner, 1995; Olson, 2003) have shown that there are neurons in the supplementary area of the frontal cortex that fire before a monkey makes an eye movement to a specific position within an object, independent of its visual field position. Neurons in these frontal regions are specialized, so that some fire just before the monkey looks to the left part of an object, whereas other neurons fire preferentially just before a monkey looks to the right part. Because eye movements are preceded by shifts in focal attention (Kowler et al., 1995), the very specific properties of these object-relative neurons suggest that they could be the possible mediators of the learning effects described here.

More direct evidence regarding the likely locus of learning comes from the work of Bichot and Schall (2002). They characterized the same temporary learning of repeated target colors measuring saccadic eye movement latencies in the monkey. Most important, they showed the expected changes in frontal eye field movement neuronal firing. Such cells are strong candidates to mediate the effects that we have described here. It remains for future research to delineate the exact locus of learning, whether it is confined to these neurons themselves or to their specific inputs.

We now consider other types of learning that could be related. Of interest is the phenomenon of worsened performance when a subject changes from one task to another (task switching). The decrement in performance associated with task switching could be the flip side of short-term temporary learning. For example, Allport and Wylie (2000) report large costs of task switching, with performance restored to optimum asymptotic values only after three to eight repetitions. They found this under a very wide range of tasks and interpreted the phenomenon as a form of temporary associative learning between particular stimuli and responses. With these diverse tasks and task changes, it is not evident that all of these examples fall in the same category of learning that we have outlined. All are unlikely to be so easily explained by the learning of attentional deployment. In fact, it is clear that sequence effects can occur that are not directly tied to the learning of attentional deployment but are more related to surface formation or perceptual grouping (McCarley and He, 2001; Kristjansson, Wang, and Nakayama, 2002). As such, rapidly acquired temporary learning may be a very widespread phenomenon, not confined to the deployment of attention. We argue that it deserves much more investigation with respect to its scope and possible cellular mechanisms.

Short-term memory and priming as an alternative to search imagery

What advantages does our phenomenon have for the situation described earlier in the chapter, that of foraging? The short-term memory system could provide a more mechanistic replacement for the more cognitive couse of the search image. The properties of the temporary learning we have described are not those of the search image posited by Tinbergen (1960), but the two constructs may serve the same purpose. Rather than calling for a "highly selective sieving operation," we suggest a collection of passive features associatively linked to the act of attentional deployment. As soon as attention is deployed somewhere, it becomes more probable that it will be deployed to objects that share the same features or positions. This could explain much of the data supporting the the search image concept, especially the long runs of selecting foods with a certain feature (Dawkins, 1971) and the overselection of certain features with greater than base probability (Reid and Shettleworth, 1992). All of these behaviors could be explained by the more piecemeal temporary associations seen here. And because the learning is very temporary, there is no risk that the animal will be caught perserverating on a feature that was attended to a while back.

In a similar vein, the passive and piecemeal modulatory process that we have described might also supplant, at least in part, theories postulating top-down processes for visual search. For example, the guided search theory of Wolfe and colleagues (1989) has similarities to the notion of the search image by employing a top-down process to explain a variety of observations about a visual search, many of which observations could also be accounted for by the more mechanistic processes described here.

REFERENCES

ALLPORT, A., and G. WYLIE, 2000. Task switching, stimulus-response bindings and negative priming. In *Attention and Performance*, S. Monsell and J. Driver, eds. Cambridge, Mass.: MIT Press.

BICHOT, N. P., and J. D. SCHALL, 2002. Priming in macaque frontal cortex during popout visual search: Feature-based facilitation and location based inhibition of return. *J. Neurosci.* 22:4675–4685.

BRAVO, M., and K. NAKAYAMA, 1992. The role of attention in different visual search tasks. *Percept. Psychophys.* 51:465–472.

DAWKINS, M., 1971. Shifts of "attention" in chicks during feeding. *Anim. Behav.* 19:575–582.

DUKAS, R., 1998. Constraints on information processing and their effects on behavior. In *Cognitive Ecology*, R. Dukas, ed. Chicago: University of Chicago Press, pp. 89–127.

GIBSON, J. J., 1966. *The Senses Considered as Perceptual Systems*. Boston: Houghton Mifflin.

GOOLSBY, B. A., and S. SUZUKI, 2001. Understanding priming of color-singleton search: Roles of attention at encoding and "retrieval." *Percept. Psychophys.* 63:929–944.

GRIMES, J., 1996. On the failure to detect changes in scenes across saccades. In *Perception. Vancouver Studies in Cognitive Science*, vol. 5, K. Akins, ed. New York: Oxford University Press, pp. 89–109.

HILLSTROM, A. P., 2000. Repetition effects in visual search. *Percept. Psychophys.* 62:800–817.

KOWLER, E., E. ANDERSON, B. DOSHER, and E. BLASER, 1995. The role of attention in the programming of saccades. *Vision Res.* 35:1897–1916.

KRISTJANSSON, A., M. MACKEBEN, and K. NAKAYAMA, 2001. Rapid, object-based learning in the deployment of transient attention. *Perception* 30:1375–1387.

KRISTJÁNSSON, Á., and K. NAKAYAMA, 2003. A primitive memory system for the deployment of transient attention. *Percept. Psychophys.* 65:711–724.

KRISTJANSSON, A., D. WANG, and K. NAKAYAMA, 2002. The role of priming in conjunctive visual search. *Cognition* 85:37–52.

LYTHGOE, J. N., 1979. *Ecology of Vision*. New York: Oxford University Press.

MACK, A., and I. ROCK, 1998. *Inattentional Blindness*. Cambridge, Mass.: MIT Press.

MALJKOVIC, V., and K. NAKAYAMA, 1994. Priming of popout. I. Role of features. *Mem. Cogn.* 22:657–672.

MALJKOVIC, V., and K. NAKAYAMA, 1996. Priming of pop-out. II. The role of position. *Percept. Psychophys.* 58:977–991.

MALJKOVIC, V., and K. NAKAYAMA, 2000. Priming of popout. III. A short term implicit memory system beneficial for rapid target selection. *Vis. Cogn.* 7:571–595.

McCARLEY, J. S., and Z. J. HE, 2001. Repetition priming of 3-D perceptual organization. *Percept. Psychophys.* 63:195–208.

McCONKIE, G. W., and D. ZOLA, 1979. Is visual information integrated across successive fixations in reading? *Percept. Psychophys.* 25:221–224.

McPEEK, R. M., and E. L. KELLER, 2001. Short-term priming, concurrent processing, and saccade curvature during a target selection task in the monkey. *Vision Res.* 41:785–800.

McPEEK, R. M., V. MALJKOVIC, and K. NAKAYAMA, 1999. Saccades require focal attention and are facilitated by a short-term memory system. *Vision Res.* 39:1555–1566.

NAKAYAMA, K., 1990. The iconic bottleneck and the tenuous link between early visual processing and perception. In *Vision: Coding and Efficiency*, C. Blakemore, ed. Cambridge, Engl.: Cambridge University Press, pp. 411–422.

NAKAYAMA, K., and M. MACKEBEN, 1989. Sustained and transient components of focal visual attention. *Vision Res.* 29:1631–1647.

NORTON, J., and V. MALJKOVIC, 2001. Accumulation and decay properties of implicit short-term memory suggest separate mechanisms code object features and position. *Soc. Neurosci. Abstr.* 27,76.5.

OLIVERS, C. N. L., and G. W. HUMPHREYS, 2003. Attentional guidance by salient feature singletons depends on intertrial contingencies. *J. Exp. Psychol. Hum. Percept. Perform.* 29:650–657.

OLSON, C. R., 2003. Brain representation of object-centered space in monkeys and humans. *Annu. Rev. Neurosci.* 26:331–354.

OLSON, C. R., and S. N. GETTNER, 1995. Object-centered direction selectivity in the supplementary eye field of the macaque monkey. *Science* 269:985–988.

O'REGAN, J. K., R. A. RENSINK, and J. J. CLARK, 1999. Change-blindness as a result of "mudsplashes." *Nature* 398:34.

POSNER, M. I., and M. E. RAICHLE, 1994. *Images of Mind.* New York: Scientific American Library.

REEVES, A., and G. SPERLING, 1986. Attention gating in short term visual memory. *Psychol. Rev.* 93:180–206

REID, P. J., and S. J. SHETTLEWORTH, 1992. Detection of cryptic prey: Search image or search rate? *J. Exp. Psychol. Anim. Behav. Proc.* 18:273–286.

RESCORLA, R. A., and A. R. WAGNER, 1972. A theory of Pavlovian conditioning: Variations in the effectiveness of reinforcement and non-reinforcement. In *Classical conditioning*. Part II, *Current research and theory*, A. Black and W.F. Prokasy, eds. New York: Appleton-Century-Crofts, pp. 64–99.

RENSINK, R. A., J. K. O'REGAN, and J. J. CLARK, 1997. To see or not to see: The need for attention to perceive changes in scenes. *Psycholog. Sci.* 8:368–373.

SIMONS, D. J., and D. T. LEVIN, 1997. Change blindness. *Trends Cogn. Sci.* 1:261–267.

SONG, J.-H., and K. NAKAYAMA, 2003. The role of focal visual attention in a manual pointing task [Abstract]. *J. Vision* 3:264a.

TINBERGEN, L., 1960. The natural control of insects on pinewoods. I. Factors influencing the intensity of predation by songbirds. *Arch. Neerland. Zool.* 13:265–343.

TREISMAN, A. M., and G. GELADE, 1980. A feature-integration theory of attention. *Cogn. Psychol.* 12:97–136.

WOLFE, J. M., K. R. CAVE, et al., 1989. Guided search: An alternative to the feature integration model for visual search. *J. Exp. Psychol. Hum. Percept. Perform.* 15:419–433.

IV MOTOR SYSTEMS

Introduction

EMILIO BIZZI AND SCOTT GRAFTON

HUMAN BEHAVIOR is centered on our physical interactions with the environment. Physical interactions require control at multiple levels, ranging from cognitive models of action representation to the selection and implementation of appropriate motor commands. The chapters in this section take up three major issues in motor control: (1) how movements are represented in the brain, (2) how the perception of a stimulus translates into a detailed motor implementation, and (3) the neural mechanisms of motor learning.

The question of how action is represented in the brain remains a fundamental problem. At the output level there is emerging evidence that movements are formed from combinations of motor primitives. Bizzi and Mussa-Ivaldi demonstrate that patterns of cortical and spinal output lead to specific combinations of muscle synergies that can generate a broad repertoire of movement patterns. At a more abstract level, Rizzolatti and colleagues review evidence for canonical and mirror neurons, or cells within ventral premotor areas that respond to a visual stimulus denoting a goal-oriented action and also during the generation of a similar action. Together, these cells may be part of a representational structure for goal-oriented action vocabularies. Grafton and Ivry review several cognitive models of action representation. A major challenge is to understand the link between action knowledge and other cognitive domains. Strick examines recent anatomical data that provide insight into the separate cortical-basal ganglia and cerebellar circuits that subserve motor and cognitive processing.

The second theme of the section has to do with the problem of sensorimotor transformation. Drawing on the results of electrophysiological studies of neurons in subregions of the posterior parietal cortex, Andersen and colleagues demonstrate that neurons in the parietal reach region are essential to planning a reach response. The problem of coding arm movements to a location in space is addressed by Georgopoulos. Wolpert and Ghahramani provide an update of computational modeling of sensorimotor control. Using optimality theory, they provide strategies for dealing with many core problems in motor control, including delayed sensory information, perpetual noise, a nonlinear muscular system, and excessive degrees of freedom.

The third theme has to do with skill acquisition. Graybiel and Saka review the functional anatomy of the basal ganglia and provide evidence that neurons in the basal ganglia code whether a stimulus is aversive or rewarding, and therefore what the outcome of a behavioral response to that stimulus will be. These authors also show that there are changes in striatal neuron activity during maze learning. Shadmehr

and Wise present evidence from studies requiring participants (primate and human) to adapt their movements in the presence of an external force field. Electrophysiological studies using this paradigm have demonstrated that there are motor neurons that remain tuned to the force field even after the field is not present. Similarly, these studies illustrate that the motor system, which can adjust to a change in parameters during the execution of a movement, also can adapt to maximize effective behavior in routine and transient situations.

Motor behavior is our bridge between thought and action and is central to understanding cognitive neuroscience. The contributions to the third edition of this work underscore the remarkable progress that has been made in understanding the mechanisms underlying action.

30 Toward a Neurobiology of Coordinate Transformations

EMILIO BIZZI AND FERDINANDO A. MUSSA-IVALDI

ABSTRACT A broad variety of motor plans and concomitant control actions can be expressed by the superposition of force fields representing the mechanical effects of motor synergies. This principle of superposition may lead to the execution of motor plans by controlling the nonlinear dynamics of the body in the presence of redundant muscles and degrees of freedom.

In this chapter we discuss a number of issues related to the way in which the central nervous system (CNS) plans and executes movements. We begin by summarizing the evidence for explicit planning of trajectories, and we then consider the various hypotheses that have been put forward to explain the processes by which a motor plan is transformed into the appropriate pattern of muscle activation. We review experimental findings which suggest that the transformations leading to the execution of a motor plan are implemented by a small number of control modules. Finally, we show that a wide variety of movements can be obtained from a simple linear combination of these control modules.

From movement planning to execution

A critical issue in the generation of motor behavior concerns the hierarchical organization of movement planning and movement execution. This concept is derived from engineering notions of modular control, by which the problem of movement is decomposed into subproblems that can be addressed separately. One of the great complications of the movement control problem is that a given goal can be reached by a multiplicity of means. If the goal is to move the hand from point A to point B, a variety of paths can be plotted; a variety of trajectories in joint space can be utilized to realize the path. An example is the simple task of reaching for a glass of water on a table. In order to reach for it, our brain must generate a temporal sequence of activations of the arm muscles. The pattern of neural impulses that

controls the contraction of each muscle can be thought of as "coordinates" in an abstract geometrical space (Holdefer and Miller, 2002). In this space, the goal of reaching the glass can be represented as a point whose coordinates are the muscle activations needed to perform the appropriate reach. What happens to these motor coordinates—and to the goal of reaching the glass in the space of muscle activities—if our body moves to another position, such as from standing to sitting? To reach the glass, the arm must now move in a different way and the muscles must be driven by different commands. As a consequence, the coordinates of the goal of reaching the glass in the space of muscle activities are changed. This is what mathematicians call a *coordinate transformation*, a computation that can be of quite considerable complexity, given the many different ways in which the muscles may have to be activated in order to reach the same point in space.

A basic concept in many fields of science, including systems-level neuroscience, is the concept of a coordinate system (Bishop and Goldberg, 1980). A coordinate system is a system of numbers that, taken together, identify the location of a point in space. The space could be the ordinary three-dimensional (3D) space in which we move, or it could be an abstract space with a larger or even infinite number of dimensions that may be placed in correspondence with a physical system. For example, the posture of a marionette may be represented by specifying each of its joint angles on a separate axis. Thus, the joint angles provide a coordinate system for the marionette. The state of a biological system, such as the human arm, is described within the nervous system by the collection of neural activities that constitute incoming sensory signals and outgoing motor commands. Although there are several possible coordinate systems—actually, an infinite number—to describe different sensory and motor signals, these coordinate systems fall quite naturally into three classes: muscle coordinates, joint coordinates, and endpoint coordinates.

ENDPOINT COORDINATES Endpoint coordinates are appropriate for describing the goal of an action and the interaction with the environment. These coordinates may capture the highly regular properties of reaching behavior when the

EMILIO BIZZI McGovern Institute for Brain Research, Department of Brain and Cognitive Science, Massachusetts Institute of Technology, Cambridge, Mass.

FERDINANDO A. MUSSA-IVALDI Department of Physiology and Sensory Motor Performance Program, Northwestern University Medical School, Chicago, Ill.

413

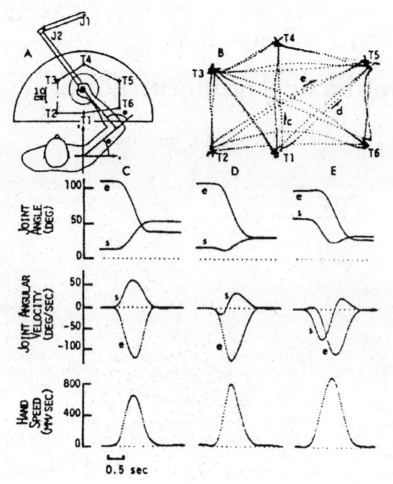

FIGURE 30.1 (A) Plan view of a seated subject grasping the handle of the two-joint hand-position transducer (designed by N. Hogan). The right arm was elevated to shoulder level and moved in a horizontal workspace. Movement of the handle was measured with potentiometers located at the two mechanical joints of the apparatus (J1, J2). A horizontal semicircular plate located just above the handle carried the visual targets. Six visual target locations (T1–T6) are represented by crosses. (B) A series of digitized handle paths (sampling rate, 100 Hz) performed by one subject in different parts of the movement space. The subject moved his hand to the illu-minated target and then waited for the appearance of a new target. Targets were presented in random order. Arrows show the direction of some of the hand movements. (C–E) Kinematic data for three of the movements, the paths of which are shown in B. Letters show correspondence, for example, data under C are the path c in B. Abbreviations: e, elbow joint; s, shoulder. Angles were measured as indicated in A. (From Bizzi and Abend, 1983, *Motor Control Mechanisms in Health and Disease*, J. E. Desmedt, ed. New York: Raven Press.)

location of the hand is rendered in Cartesian space. (Morasso, 1981). Morasso instructed human subjects to point with one hand to different visual targets that were randomly activated (figure 30.1). His analysis of the movements showed two kinematic invariances: (1) the hand trajectories were approximately straight segments, and (2) the tangential hand velocity for different movements always appeared to have a bell-shaped configuration, as the time needed to accelerate the hand was approximately equal to the time needed to bring it back to rest. Because these simple and invariant features were detected at different shoulder and elbow angles, these results suggest that planning by the CNS takes place in terms of hand motion in space. Here, the hand is almost regarded as a "disembodied object," whose movements are planned by the CNS independently of the geometrical and mechanical properties of the arm and its muscles. Morasso's observations were extended to more complex curved movements performed by human subjects in an obstacle avoidance task (Abend, Bizzi, and Morasso, 1982). Again, kinematic invariances were present in the hand and not in the joint motion. Later, Flash and Hogan (1985) showed that the kinematic behavior described by Morasso (1981) and Abend and colleagues (1982) could be derived from a single organizing principle based on optimizing endpoint smoothness.

MUSCLE COORDINATES Muscle coordinates (Holdefer and Miller, 2002) afford the most direct representation for the motor output of the CNS. A *position* in this coordinate system may be expressed, for example, as a collection of muscle lengths. Accordingly, a force in the same coordinate system is a collection of muscle tensions. The number of actuator coordinates depends on how detailed is the model of control under consideration. Unlike generalized coordinates, actuator coordinates do not constitute a system of mechanically independent variables; one cannot set arbitrary values to l_i without eventually violating a kinematic constraint.

At the most detailed level, individual motor units may be considered actuator elements. In that case, the order of magnitude of the actuator space can be of the order of tens or hundred thousands.

JOINT COORDINATES AND THE GENERATION OF FORCES   A different way of describing body motions is to provide the set of joint angles that define the orientation of each skeletal segment either with respect to fixed axes in space or with respect to the neighboring segments. Joint angles are a particular instance of *generalized coordinates*. Generalized coordinates are independent variables that are suitable for describing the dynamics of a system (Goldstein, 1980; Jose and Saletan, 1998). In particular, the dynamics of limbs such as the human arm are described by systems of coupled differential equations relating the generalized coordinates to their first and second time derivatives and to the generalized forces.

In vector notation, the dynamics equations for a multijointed limb can be succinctly written as:

$$I(q)\ddot{q} + G(q, \dot{q}) + E(q, \dot{q}, t) = C(q, \dot{q}, u(t)) \quad (1)$$

where $q = (q_1, q_2, \ldots, q_n)$ is the limb configuration in joint angle coordinates, $\dot{q}$ and $\ddot{q}$ are, respectively, the first (velocity) and second (acceleration) time derivatives of q, I is an $N \times N$ matrix of inertia (that is configuration dependent), $G(q, \ddot{q})$ is a vector of centripetal and Coriolis torques (Sciavicco and Siciliano, 2000), and $E(q, \dot{q}, t)$ is a vector of external torques that in general depends on the state of motion of the limb and on time. The whole left-hand side of Equation 1 represents the torque due to the inertial properties of the arm and to the action of the environment (part of which may be considered noise). The term $C(\cdot)$ on the right-hand side stands for the net torque generated nonlinearly by the muscles, by the environment (e.g., the gravitational torque), and by other dissipative elements, such as friction. The time function $u(t)$ is a control vector, for example, a set of neural signals directed to the motor neurons or a representation of a desired limb position at time t. The left side of Equation 1 represents the passive dynamics associated with limb inertia. The right side is the applied force, which in this case is the output of a control process. An additional term, to be added on the right side of Equation 1, is the noise associated with the control signal.

The way in which the CNS implements the dynamic Equation 1 has been the focus of a number of investigations in the last 20 years. Through work in humans and monkeys, a number of investigators have put forward the hypothesis that the CNS may generate forces by using forward internal models (Shadmehr and Mussa-Ivaldi, 1994; Flanagan and Wing, 1997; Kawato and Wolpert, 1998; Wolpert, Miall, and Kawato, 1998; Krakauer, Ghilardi, and Ghez, 1999).

Alternative proposals have been made that do not depend on the solution of complicated inverse dynamics problems. Specifically, it has been proposed that the CNS may transform the desired hand motion into a series of equilibrium positions (Bizzi et al., 1984). The forces needed to track the equilibrium trajectory result from the intrinsic elastic properties of the muscles and from local feedback loops (Feldman, 1966; Bizzi, Polit, and Morasso, 1976; Hogan, 1984).

Another view on solving the dynamic equations to execute a motor plan is the hypothesis that the motor behavior of vertebrates is based on simple units (motor primitives) that can be flexibly combined to accomplish a variety of motor tasks. Here is an apt and succinct quotation by Cvitanovic (2000) concerning the general problems posed by complex nonlinear dynamics:

Armed with a computer and a great deal of skill, one can obtain a numerical solution to a nonlinear partial differential equation. The real question is; once a solution is found, what is to be done with it? . . . Dynamics drives a given spatially extended system through a repertoire of unstable patterns; as we watch a "turbulent" system evolve, every so often we catch a glimpse of a familiar pattern. For any finite spatial resolution, the system follows approximately for a finite time a pattern belonging to a finite alphabet of admissible patterns, and the long-term dynamics can be thought of as a walk through the space of such patterns, just as chaotic dynamics with a low-dimensional attractor can be thought of as a succession of nearly periodic (but unstable) motions.

The key concept here is that complex behavior may be analyzed by a combination of patterns.

Building blocks for computation of dynamics: Compositionality

In the natural world, some complex systems are discrete combinatorial systems: they utilize a finite number of discrete elements to create larger structures. The genetic code and language phenomena are examples of systems in which discrete elements and a set of rules can generate a large number of meaningful entities that are quite distinct from those of their elements. A question of considerable importance is whether this fundamental characteristic of language and genetics is also a feature of other biological systems. In particular, we want to know whether the activity of the vertebrate motor system, with its impressive capacity to find original motor solutions to an infinite set of ever changing circumstances, results from combinations of discrete elements.

The ease with which we move hides the complexity inherent in the execution of even the simplest tasks. Even movements we make effortlessly, such as reaching for an object, involve the activation of many thousands of motor units in numerous muscles. Given this large number of degrees of freedom of the motor system, a number of investigators have put forward the hypothesis that the CNS handles this large space with a hierarchical architecture based on the utilization of discrete building blocks whose combinations result in the construction of a variety of different movements (Tsetlin, 1973; Arbib, 1981). In particular, investigators influenced by the artificial intelligence perspective on the control of complex systems have argued for a hierarchical decomposition with modules, or building blocks, as the most effective way to select a control signal from a large search space (Russell and Norvig, 1995).

Along similar lines, Arbib, Conklin, and Hill (1987) have argued that internal models of the world must be built of units called *schemas*, which in Arbib's view are both a process and a representation. Schemas may serve as units in the analysis of perceptual structures and in motor control (Arbib, 1981). In particular, a plan of action is considered by Arbib, Conklin, and Hill (1987) as "a program composed of motor schemas, each viewed as an adaptive controller that uses an identification procedure to updated its representation of the object being controlled." A motor schema would be a unit of behavior that directs, for example, the hand to grasp an object.

A possible neurophysiological instance of a grasping schema are the neurons in the premotor area F5 of the monkey, which have been described by Matelli and colleagues (1994) and inferred in humans by Grafton, Fagg, and Arbib (1998). These neurons, probably in conjunction with the grasping neurons described by Sakata and Taira (1994) in the parietal lobe, represent a "module" or schema that belongs to the higher level of the motor system; they represent the elements of a top-down modular organization.

We do not know how the CNS translates these high-level schemas into activation of the motor neurons. However, recent investigations focused on spinal cord interneurons have revealed that the spinal interneuronal system is also organized into a number of distinct units.

The idea of a modular organization of spinally produced movements is not a new one (Grillner, 1981; Gossard and Hultborn, 1991; Rossignol, 1996; Stein and Smith, 1997). The first formulation of this hypothesis was proposed by Brown (1911) to explain the production of locomotion in the cat. Grillner subsequently suggested the locomotor pattern consisted in the combination of several different "unit bursters." Each unit was assumed to control the activation of a small set of synergistic muscles acting around a single joint. Different motor behaviors could then be produced by flexibly coupling these different units. Evidence in support of such a modular organization of spinally generated motor behaviors has come from experiments performed in different preparations, such as the turtle (Stein, Mortin, and Robertson, 1986; Stein and Smith, 1997; Stein, McCullough, and Currie, 1998), mudpuppy (Wheatley and Stein, 1992; Cheng et al., 1998), frog (Bizzi, Giszter, and Mussa-Ivaldi, 1991; Giszter, Mussa-Ivaldi, and Bizzi, 1993; Bizzi et al., 2000), rat (Tresch, Saltiel, and Bizzi, 1999), and cat (Grillner and Zangger, 1979).

Building blocks for computation of dynamics: Spinal force fields

Modular organization of the frog and rat spinal motor system was first established by experiments examining the organization of motor outputs evoked by electrical microstimulation of the spinal interneuronal regions (Bizzi et al., 1991; Giszter and Kargo, 2000). Focal microstimulation of the lumbar spinal cord has revealed that the lumbar gray matter contains a number of circuits that are organized to produce muscle synergies. Whenever different circuits are activated, they produce precisely balanced contractions in different groups of muscles. The mechanical consequence of these balanced contractions is a force that can be measured at the ankle and that directs the leg toward an equilibrium point in space. Because of the changes in joint angles and muscle lever-arm at different locations of the leg's workspace, the amplitude and direction of this force depend on the position of the leg. Neural and biomechanical factors cooperate in the determination of a vector field that captures the dependence of the force on the leg's location (figure 30.2). Hence a vector field is a functional unit of the spinal cord circuitry that generates a motor output by producing a muscle synergy (a synergy is group of muscles in which both the activation level and the time of activation of individual muscles are specified together). Mapping of the interneuronal areas of the lumbar spinal cord revealed a limited number of discrete force fields (figure 30.3) (Bizzi, Giszter, and Mussa-Ivaldi, 1991).

Another observation derived from microstimulation of frog and rat spinal cord is that the fields induced by the focal activation of the cord follow the principle of vector summation. Mussa-Ivaldi, Giszter, and Bizzi (1994) and more recently Lemay and colleagues (2001) have shown that the simultaneous stimulation of two sites, each generating a different force field, results in the vector sum of the two fields in most instances. When the pattern of forces recorded at the ankle following costimulation was compared with the pattern computed by summation of the two individual fields, Mussa-Ivaldi and colleagues (1994) found that the

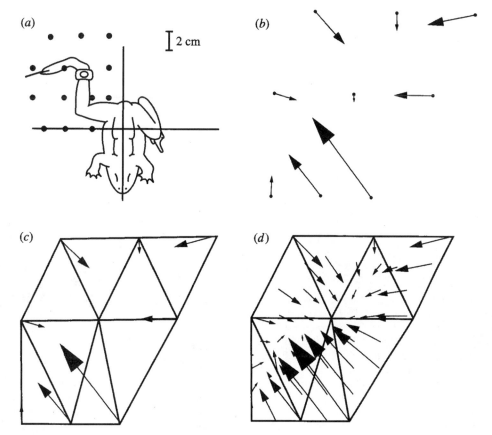

FIGURE 30.2   Force fields induced by microstimulation of the spinal cord in spinalized frogs. (*a*) The hindlimb was placed at a number of locations on the horizontal plane (indicated by the dots). At each location a stimulus was derived at a fixed site in the lumbar spinal cord. The ensuing force was measured by a six-axis force transducer. (*b*) Peak force vectors recorded at the nine locations shown in *a*. (*c*) The workspace of the hindlimb was partitioned into a set of nonoverlapping triangles. Each vertex is a tested point. The force vectors recorded on the three vertices are used to estimate, by linear interpolation, the forces in the interior of the triangle. (*d*) Interpolated force field. (From Bizzi, Giszter, and Mussa-Ivaldi, 1991.)

"costimulation fields" and the "summation fields" were equivalent in more than 87% of cases (figure 30.4). Similar results have been obtained by Tresch and Bizzi (1999) by stimulating the spinal cord of the rat. Recently, Giszter and Kargo (2000) showed that force field summation underlies the control of limb trajectories in the frog.

Vector summation of force fields implies that the complex nonlinearities that characterize the interactions both among neurons and between neurons and muscles are in some way suppressed or made irrelevant. This result has led to a novel hypothesis for explaining movement and posture based on combinations of few modules. These modules may be viewed as representing an elementary alphabet from which, through superimposition, a vast number of actions could be fashioned by impulses conveyed by supraspinal pathways or by the reflex pathways (or by both). Through computational analysis, Mussa-Ivaldi and Giszter (1992) and Mussa-Ivaldi (1997) verified that this view of generation of movement and posture has the competence for controlling a wide repertoire of movements of a multijoint limb.

SPINAL MODULARITY AND NATURAL BEHAVIOR   The force vectors that characterize the fields described by Bizzi and colleagues (1991), Mussa-Ivaldi and colleagues (1994), and Giszter and colleagues (1993) are the expression of specific groups of synergistically active muscles evoked either by the microinjection of NMDA or by the electrical stimulation of the interneuronal areas of the spinal cord. Recently, a method to identify muscle synergies with the help of a computational analysis was developed. This method was first used by Tresch, Saltiel, and Bizzi (1999), who described the muscle activation patterns evoked from cutaneous stimulation of the hindlimb in spinalized frogs. Tresch and colleagues (1999) applied a computational analysis to the muscle activation patterns evoked by cutaneous stimulation of different regions of the skin surface of the hindlimb. The results of this study showed that the muscle activation patterns involved in hindlimb withdrawal reflexes could be explained in terms of the combination of a small number of muscle synergies, consistent with the hypothesis of modular organization of the spinal motor system. Also of

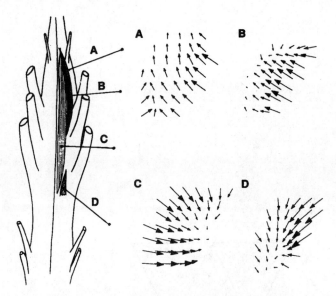

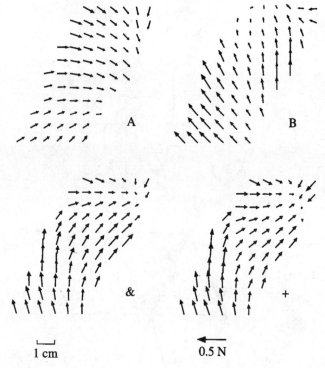

FIGURE 30.3 *Left*: Regions of the lumbar spinal cord containing the neural circuitry that specifies the force fields (*A–D*). Within each region, similar sets of CFFs are produced. The diagram is based on 40 CFFs elicited by microstimulation of premotor regions in three frogs with transected spinal cords. *Right*: Four types of CFFs. To facilitate comparison among CFFs recorded in different animals, we subtracted the passive force field from the force field obtained at steady state. The passive field is the mechanical behavior generated by the frog's leg (recorded at the ankle) in the absence of any stimulation. The force field is at steady state when the forces induced by the stimulation of the spinal cord have reached their maximal amplitude.

particular interest is the fact that Tresch and colleagues (1999) compared the distinct muscle synergies derived from cutaneous stimulation with the patterns of muscle activation evoked by microstimulation of the frog spinal cord (the force fields discussed earlier), and found that the two sets of EMG responses were very similar to one another.

Additional evidence in support of the hypothesis that behaviors can be produced by a combination of a small set of muscle synergies has come from recent experiments by Kargo and Giszter (2000), again in a spinal cord preparation.

The construction of natural motor behavior with muscle synergies

One of the basic questions in motor performance is whether the cortical motor areas control individual muscles or make use of synergistically linked groups of muscles (Macpherson, 1991). Insofar as no natural movement involves just one muscle, any motor act a fortiori involves a "muscle synergy," the question then becomes whether the synergistic activation of muscles derives from a fixed common neural drive or is merely a phenomenological event of a given motor coordination.

Paradoxically, the vast literature on this question indicates little consensus either for fixed synergies or for individual

FIGURE 30.4 Spinal force fields add vectorially. Fields *A* and *B* were obtained in response to stimulations delivered to two different spinal sites. The *&* field was obtained by stimulating simultaneously the same two sites. It matches closely (correlation coefficient > 0.9) the force field in *+*, which was derived by adding pairwise the vectors in *A* and *B*. This highly linear behavior was found to apply to more than 87% of dual stimulation experiments. (From Mussa-Ivaldi, Gisztor, and Bizzi, 1994.)

control of muscles. For instance, Howard and colleagues (1986) showed that the synergies around the elbow joint do not covary under all conditions because the relationship between the muscles varies with the nature of the task. Along similar lines, Hepp-Reymond and Diener (1983) found that muscles that appeared correlated at one level of force were not necessarily so at higher force levels. This observation was interpreted as reflecting a lack of amplitude scaling and not in keeping with idea of synergies.

In contrast to those conclusions, other reports have claimed that human postural responses are indeed organized synergistically (Nashner, 1977; McCollum, Horak, and Nashner, 1984; Nashner and McCollum, 1985; Crenna et al., 1987). However, the synergies described by these investigators were present only in restricted sets of movements, such as postural sways.

Various alternative mechanisms have been suggested, such as hierarchical control (Saltzman, 1979; Bullock and Grossberg, 1988; Das and McCollum, 1988). According to these experimenters there is a hierarchy of parameters or strategies that are controlled in any motor act. Once the strategy is chosen a coordinated pattern of muscle activity is selected, but the muscle groupings are not considered to be fixed; rather, they are formed and reformed each time.

Summing up, there is little doubt that the issue of muscle synergies remains unsettled. However, there is a reason for this predicament. The approaches that have been used to investigate this issue have been based on correlation methods, which are less than ideal for settling the muscle synergy question. To explain why the correlation method provides a distorted perspective, let us assume that a given muscle belongs to more than one synergy. According to the correlation method, two muscles, say, X and Y, are considered part of a same synergy, A, if they both scale in amplitude when more force output is required during a task. A potential problem with this approach may surface if, for example, muscle Y is also found in synergy B. Then, when synergies A and B are recruited together in different contexts, the amplitude scaling for X and Y might be different, and then the false conclusion could be reached that no synergy between X and Y exists.

The recent introduction of novel computational procedures to extract synergies from large sets of EMG signals in intact behaving animals has opened a different way to approach the issue of synergies (Soechting and Lacquaniti, 1989; Saltiel et al., 2001; d'Avella and Tresch, 2002; Tresch et al., 2002).

Recently, d'Avella, Saltiel, and Bizzi (2003) have tested the hypothesis that linear combinations of muscle synergies represent a general mechanism for the construction of motor behavior. To this end they examined several motor behaviors in intact, freely moving frogs and recorded simultaneously from a large number of hindlimb muscles during locomotion, swimming, jumping, and defensive reflexes (kicks). They extracted a set of time-varying synergies from the pooled, rectified, and integrated EMG records of 13 leg muscles using a new computational analysis (d'Avella and Tresch, 2002).

Because of this analysis, d'Avella and colleagues (2003) were able to describe the differences across the patterns observed during individual trials of kicking simply as differences in the amplitude scaling and time delaying of three time-varying synergies (figure 30.5). d'Avella and colleagues (2003) found that the level and time of recruitment of two of the three synergies were systematically modulated in relation to the movement kinematics (figure 30.6). This result represents a remarkable simplification, in view of the high dimensionality of the space of all possible time-varying muscle patterns. One possible explanation for this observed low dimensionality might be the existence of constraints on the muscle patterns deriving from the specific movements required by the task. However, it is unlikely that the observed dimensionality reduction arose simply from task-dependent constraints. First, even for a simple behavior described by a single parameter (e.g., kick direction), the set of muscle patterns capable of generating the entire movement repertoire need not be embedded in a low-dimensional space. Given the redundancy of the musculoskeletal system, the same goal can be achieved by different movements and the same movement can be generated by different muscle combinations, for example with different levels of cocontraction around a joint. Therefore, already the set of muscle patterns associated to a single value of the parameter describing the task could have high dimensionality.

Second, if the low dimensionality resulted purely from task-dependent constraints, one would not expect to observe many similarities between synergies across different tasks. However, many similarities among the synergies extracted from different behaviors were found.

A relevant and important question is whether the synergies extracted by this computational procedure correspond to those generated by the CNS. Criteria for validating the synergies are important because it is possible that the synergies identified with a computational procedure may simply represent the outcome of a statistical fitting technique. To answer this question, a set of procedures has been developed (d'Avella and Tresch, 2002). First, a criterion is the ability of the extracted synergies to predict the structure of novel muscle patterns, that is, muscle patterns observed in new tasks or in task conditions not used for the extraction. Second, it is important to ascertain whether the same synergy, with the timing between its muscles preserved, is present in two or more behaviors. And third, evidence is needed of amplitude scaling of individual synergies when the demands for force output increase.

Muscle synergies have long been recognized as a means to deal with the apparent redundancy of the motor system (Bernstein, 1967). The term *redundancy* indicates the abundance of muscles and joints with respect to the number of endpoint variables that are normally associated with the description of a motor task. By organizing the muscle into groups driven by the same input, the nervous system simplifies the problem of coordinating a large number of control signals. However, the presence of a fixed set of synergies could also remove the most important virtue of redundancy: the presence of multiple equivalent ways for carrying out a task. The possibility of reconfiguring synergies in different contexts (Loeb, 1985) and through mechanisms of adaptive learning would therefore simplify some of the computational problems associated with redundancy while not compromising the possibility of generating a wide range of mechanical behaviors.

Motor control as force field approximation

The microstimulation studies described in the previous section have revealed that the mechanical effect of a synergy is captured by a field of forces that vary both with space and

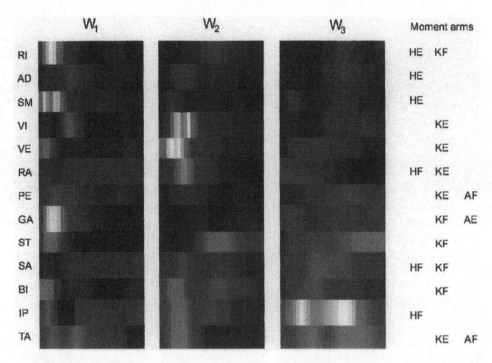

FIGURE 30.5 Three time-varying synergies extracted from the entire kicking data set. The first three columns (W₁–W₃) represent the three extracted synergies as a color-coded activation time course of 13 muscles over 30 samples (300 ms total duration) normalized to the maximum sample. The three synergies capture different features of the kicking muscle patterns: W_1 and W_2 show a high level of activation, especially in extensors muscles (in particular the hip extensors RI and SM for the first synergy and the knee

extensors VI and VE for the second). Mostly flexor muscles (IP, ST, TA, SA, BI) are recruited in W_3. The fourth column indicates the sign (flexion or extension) of the moment arms around hip, knee, and ankle joints of the 13 muscles included in each synergy. Abbreviations: HE, hip extension; HF, hip flexion; KE, knee extension; KF, knee flexion; AE, ankle extension; AF, ankle flexion. (See color plate 14.)

in time. In this section we show how the combination of force fields generated by multiple synergies offers the CNS a way to solve the problem of dynamics (Equation 1) in the presence of multiple forms of motor redundancy. This is a common situation in the control of multijoint limbs, such as the human arm, where there are more joint angles than endpoint variables and more muscles than joint angles. Many of the computational problems associated with redundancy are removed by expressing a motor plan as a force field in endpoint coordinates and by approximating this field with a superposition of force fields corresponding to muscle synergies. This is examined in more detail in the following argument.

The graph in figure 30.7A highlights the main challenge associated with redundancy of the musculoskeletal apparatus: the transformations between actuator, generalized, and endpoint variables are not invertible and are well defined only in the direction of the arrows. For example, given the angular configuration of the arm, q, it is possible to derive the position of the hand, r. However, the same position of the hand can be reached with different joint angles. Similarly, given the forces exerted by all the muscle on a joint, one derives the net torque, while any value of torque can be obtained with an infinite number of muscle force combina-

tions. How is it possible for the CNS to map a desired movement plan, in terms of endpoint behavior, into a corresponding command for the muscles? As shown in figure 30.7B, force fields provide additional pathways that map motions into forces. Thus, for example, a muscle synergy determines the force generated by the muscles in response to a stretch applied at any operating length. When multiple synergies are induced by a pattern of motor commands (u in figure 30.7B), their net effect is a field of torque vectors: for each configuration and state of motion of the joints there is one and only one corresponding torque vector.

The planning of a desired behavior can in turn be expressed as a force field that maps a state of the endpoint into a corrective force. For example, a field of forces that converge on the target and that vanish there provides a detailed specification for the task of reaching a target with the hand. If an obstacle is interposed along the hand path, the concurrent task of avoiding a collision can be represented as a field of forces that diverge from the obstacle. This mathematical representation has proved successful in dealing with problems of robot motion planning (Kathib, 1986; Rimon and Koditschek, 1989). Although a literal implementation of this approach within the CNS may seem unlikely, one should observe that when we plan an action,

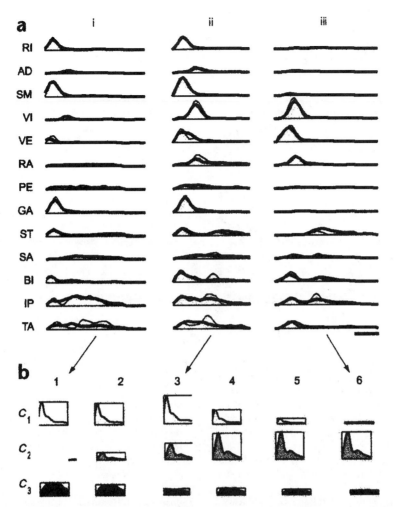

FIGURE 30.6 Reconstruction of kick muscle patterns as combinations of time-varying synergies. (*a*) Three different patterns (rectified, filtered, and integrated EMGs i to iii, thin line and shaded area) are reconstructed by scaling in amplitude, shifting in time, and summing together the three synergies extracted from pooled data (thick line). Scale bar-100 ms. (*b*) The amplitude coefficients (C_1–C_3) for the three kicks in *a* (1, 3, and 6) and three other kicks are illustrated as the height of three rectangles, whereas the horizontal position of the rectangles represents the position in time of the synergies with respect to the extent of the muscle pattern (gray background). The profiles within each rectangle represent the time course of the synergies averaged over the 13 muscles. The three examples in *a* show how the first two synergies are independently combined to generate different kicks: the first synergy, and not the second, is recruited for a medially directed kick (i and 1), involving mainly hip extension; the second synergy, and not the first, is recruited for a lateral kick (iii and 6), obtained with a knee extension; a caudal kick (ii and 3), involving both a knee and a hip extension, is constructed by a combination of the two synergies. A systematic modulation of amplitude and timing of the recruitment of the first two synergies can be seen in the six examples shown in *b*.

such as reaching for a target, we are specifying not only a point of space but also additional requirements, such as those of remaining at rest at the target and avoiding collisions. Force fields provide a rigorous framework for expressing these concurrent demands by exploiting a mechanism of superposition. It is critical to observe that once a force field is given in endpoint coordinates, it is always possible to translate this field into joint coordinates despite the kinematic redundancy of the arm. The arrows on the right side of figure 30.7*B* provide a path for this transformation: (1) The joint angles and angular displacements are mapped via *direct kinematics* into a corresponding position and displacement of the hand, (2) the planned force field assigns a hand force to this position and displacement of the hand, and (3) the hand force is mapped into the corresponding joint torque by the (direct) Jacobian matrix of the arm.

It is apparent that the fields associated with muscle synergies and the fields associated with the description of a task find a common representation in joint coordinates (more generally, in generalized coordinates). In this common geometrical space, plans can be mapped into action by finding the combination of synergies that generates the best approximation of the planned field (dashed arrows in figure 30.7*B*). This is a process that does not require ill-posed inversions of

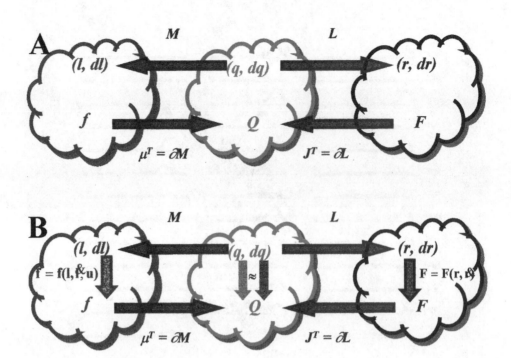

FIGURE 30.7 Coordinate transformations for planning and control of movement in a redundant limb. (*A*) Kinematic and force transformations for the human arm between muscle coordinates, joint coordinates, and endpoint coordinates. Arrows indicate the directions in which the transformations are well posed. Abbreviations: *l*, muscle lengths, *q*, joint angles; *r*, hand position; *F*, hand force; *Q*, joint torque; *f*, muscle force. *M* represent the transformation from joint angles to muscle lengths and *L* the transformation from joint angles to hand position. α*M* and α*L* are the respective Jacobian matrices. (*B*) The vertical arrows map motion variables (position and velocity) onto force variables. They represent force fields. On the left is the force field generated by the muscles. On the right is the force field in endpoint coordinates that represents a desired behavior. Both the endpoint field and the muscle field have a well-defined image in joint coordinates, and the implementation of a desired behavior can be represented as a problem of approximation.

redundant maps. Most important, force fields provide a way to compose building blocks of planning and building blocks of control through a single, straightforward rule of linear summation.

This view goes beyond the execution of a preplanned trajectory because it allows for uncertainty in the knowledge of the environment and of the limb's mechanical properties, and for a broader concept of motor planning that includes not only the generation of movements but also the exertion of contact forces. As for the first point, the uncertainty, a force field does not specify the accurate requirement of a position or of a trajectory but rather the tradeoff between a desired position (or trajectory) and the force that is exerted in response to a deviation from this desired trajectory.

Noise and uncertainty

The control of movements in uncertain and noisy environments is one of the most distinctive feature of biological control. Unlike industrial robots, biological systems have evolved to interact with environments that change in unpredictable ways. Muscles and sense organs are abundant but noisy and subject to variations in their transduction properties (van Beers, Baraduc, and Wolpert, 2002). Under these conditions, adaptability appears to be more valuable than precision. The external environment is not the only source of noise. The analysis of motor unit activities (Matthews, 1996) suggests a major role of synaptic noise in the excitation of motor neurons. Harris and Wolpert (1998) have proposed that the observed smoothness of natural motions observed in different motor behaviors (arm and eye movements, for example) may be accounted for by assuming that the biological controller minimizes the final error, while being subject to signal-dependent noise. This proposal is based on the idea that violations of smoothness, such as a large swing in a trajectory, are associated with large-amplitude control signals. Insofar as the signal variance accumulates additively along a movement, the net expected outcome of a jerky motion is a larger variance at the final point. Similar considerations are at the basis of a more general framework proposed recently by Todorov and Jordan (2002). They observed that in the presence of redundancy, one may identify within the space of control signals a lower-dimensional "task-relevant" manifold. This contains the combinations of motor commands that have a direct impact on the achievement of the established goal. Because of redundancy, at each point of this manifold there is a "null space" of control signals that do not affect the execution of the task. For example, when we place the index finger on a letter key, we may do so with an infinity of arm configurations. A common observation across a variety of behaviors is that variability tends to be higher in the task-irrelevant dimensions. Todorov and Jordan (2002) consider this to be a direct consequence of optimal feedback control. According to this scheme, the control system aims at minimizing the expected error on the final target, in the presence of signal-dependent noise. Although the outcomes of the optimization may depend on the specific distribution of variability among the system of actuators, the simulations presented by these authors indicate a general tendency of the control system to place the highest variance in the task-irrelevant dimensions, so as to achieve a higher degree of precision in the task-relevant dimensions. This view of the biological control system brings about two important (although yet to be proven valid) concepts:

1. that the control system is not necessarily concerned with the explicit planning of a trajectory but rather with the attainment of final goals with the least amount of variance; and

2. that the space spanned by the task-irrelevant dimensions plays the role of a "variance buffer," where the noise generated by the control signals has the largest effect so as to attain a higher performance in the space defined by the task.

Although this is a promising approach, with potentially important implications for the design of biomimetic controllers, the evidence for the explicit planning of trajectories remains rather strong (Flash, 1987; Shadmehr and Mussa-Ivaldi, 1994; Dingwell, Mah, and Mussa-Ivaldi, 2002). It is difficult to reconcile the observation of regularities observed in endpoint coordinates, such as the execution of smooth rectilinear motions of the hand, with properties such as signal-dependent noise, that concern the behavior of muscles and joints. To see this, let us consider a movement of the hand between two targets and suppose that the noise introduced by the shoulder muscles is greater than the noise introduced by the elbow muscles. If the only goal of the controller were to reduce the error on the final target, then the trajectory would be chosen to minimize the activity of the shoulder muscles. Obviously, a different trajectory would be chosen if the elbow muscles were the main source of noise. This framework appears difficult to reconcile with the observation of smooth and quasi-rectilinear hand paths. In conclusion, a system of muscle synergies together with one or more mechanisms of composition provides the means for translating any planned movement into an efficient pattern of control signals. This allows the motor system to take advantage of the mechanical properties of the muscles—and in particular of their built-in stability—without submitting to undesired features of musculoskeletal geometry.

REFERENCES

ABEND, W. K., E. BIZZI, and P. MORASSO, 1982. Human arm trajectory formation. *Brain* 105:331–348.

ARBIB, M. A., 1981. Perceptual structures and distributed motor control. In *Handbook of Physiology*, Sect. 2, *The nervous system*, vol. II, *Motor Control*, Part 1, V. B. Brooks, ed. Bethesda, Md.: American Physiological Society, pp. 1449–1480.

ARBIB, M. A., E. J. CONKLIN, and J. C. HILL, 1987. *From Schema Theory to Language*. Oxford, England: Oxford University Press.

BERNSTEIN, N., 1967. *The Coordination and Regulation of Movement*. Oxford, England: Pegamon Press.

BISHOP, R. L., and S. I. GOLDBERG, 1980. *Tensor Analysis on Manifolds*. New York: Dover.

BIZZI, E., N. ACCORNERO, W. CHAPPLE, and N. HOGAN, 1984. Posture control and trajectory formation during arm movement. *J. Neurosci.* 4:2738–2744.

BIZZI, E., S. GISZTER, and F. A. MUSSA-IVALDI, 1991. Computations underlying the execution of movement: A novel biological perspective. *Science* 253:287–291.

BIZZI, E., A. POLIT, and P. MORASSO, 1976. Mechanisms underlying achievement of final position. *J. Neurophysiol.* 39:435–444.

BIZZI, E., M. C. TRESCH, P. SALTIEL, and A. D'AVELLA, 2000. New perspectives on spinal motor systems. *Nat. Rev. Neurosci.* 1: 101–108.

BROWN, T. G., 1911. The intrinsic factors in the act of progression in the mammal. *Proc. R. Soc. (Lond.)* 84:308–319.

BULLOCK, D., and S. GROSSBERG, 1988. Neural dynamics of planned arm movements: Emergent invariants and speed-accuracy properties during trajectory formation. *Psychol. Rev.* 95: 46–90.

CHENG, J., R. B. STEIN, K. JOVANOVIC, K. YOSHIDA, D. J. BENNETT, and Y. HAN, 1998. Identification, localization, and modulation of neural networks for walking in the mudpuppy (*Necturus maculates*) spinal cord. *J. Neurosci.* 18:4295–4304.

CRENNA, P., C. FRIGO, J. MASSION, and A. PEDOTTI, 1987. Forward and backward axial synergies in man. *Exp. Brain Res.* 65:538–548.

CVITANOVIC, P., 2000. Chaotic field theory: A sketch. *Physica A* 288:61–89.

D'AVELLA, A., and M. C. TRESCH, 2002. Modularity in the motor system: Decomposition of muscle patterns as combinations of time-varying synergies. In *Advances in Neural Information Processing Systems*, vol. 14, T. G. Dietterich, S. Becker, and Z. Ghahramani, eds. Cambridge, Mass.: MIT Press.

D'AVELLA, A., P. SALTIEL, and E. BIZZI, 2003. Combinations of muscle synergies in the construction of a natural motor behavior. *Nat. Neurosci.* 6:300–308.

DAS, P., and G. MCCOLLUM, 1988. Invariant structure in locomotion. *Neuroscience* 25:1023–1034.

DINGWELL, J. B., C. D. MAH, and F. A. MUSSA-IVALDI, 2002. Manipulating objects with internal degrees of freedom: Evidence for model-based control. *J. Neurophysiol.* 88:222–235.

FELDMAN, A. G., 1966. Functional tuning of the nervous system with control of movement or maintenance of steady posture. II. Controllable parameters of the muscles. *Biophysics* 11:565–578.

FLANAGAN, J., and A. WING, 1997. The role of internal models in motion planning and control: Evidence from grip force adjustments during movements of hand-held loads. *J. Neurosci.* 17: 1519–1528.

FLASH, T., 1987. The control of hand equilibrium trajectories in multi-joint arm movements. *Biol. Cybern.* 57:257–274.

FLASH, T., and N. HOGAN, 1985. The coordination of arm movements: An experimentally confirmed mathematical model. *J. Neurosci.* 7:1688–1703.

GISZTER, S. F., and W. J. KARGO, 2000. Conserved temporal dynamics and vector superposition of primitives in frog wiping reflexes during spontaneous extensor deletions. *Neurocomputing* 32–33:775–783.

GISZTER, S., F. A. MUSSA-IVALDI, and E. BIZZI, 1993. Convergent force fields organized in the frog's spinal cord. *J. Neurosci.* 13:467–491.

GOLDSTEIN, H., 1980. *Classical Mechanics*, 2nd ed. Reading, Mass.: Addison-Wesley.

GOSSARD, J. P., and H. HULTBORN, 1991. The organization of spinal rhythm generation in locomotion. In *Plasticity of Motoneuronal Connections*, A. Wernig, ed. Amsterdam: Elsevier, pp. 385–404.

GRAFTON, S. T., A. H. FAGG, and M. A. ARBIB, 1998. Dorsal premotor cortex and conditional movement selection: A PET functional mapping study. *J. Neurophysiol.* 79:1092–1097.

GRILLNER, S., 1981. Control of locomotion in bipeds, tetrapods, and fish. In *Handbook of Physiology*, vol. 2, V. B. Brooks, ed. Bethesda, Md.: American Physiological Society, Sect. 1, pp. 1179–1236.

GRILLNER, S., and P. ZANGGER, 1979. On the central generation of locomotion in the low spinal cat. *Exp. Brain Res.* 34:241–261.

HARRIS, C. M., and D. M. WOLPERT, 1998. Signal-dependent noise determines motor planning. *Nature* 394:780–784.

HEPP-REYMOND, M. C., and R. DIENER, 1983. Neural coding of force and rate of force change in the precentral finger region of the monkey. *Exp. Brain Res. Supp.* 7:315–326.

HOGAN, N., 1984. An organizing principle for a class of voluntary movements. *J. Neurosci.* 4:2745–2754.

HOLDEFER, R. N., and L. E. MILLER, 2002. Primary motor cortical neurons encode functional muscle synergies. *Exp. Brain Res.* 146:233–243.

HOWARD, J. D., J. D. HOIT, R. M. ENOKA, and Z. HASAN, 1986. Relative activation of 2 human elbow flexors under isometric conditions: A cautionary note concerning flexor equivalence. *Exp. Brain Res.* 62:199–202.

JOSE, J. V., and E. J. SALETAN, 1998. *Classical Dynamics: A Contemporary Approach*. Cambridge, England: Cambridge University Press.

KARGO, W. J., and S. F. GISZTER, 2000. Rapid correction of aimed movements by summation of force-field primitives. *J. Neurosci.* 20:409–426.

KATHIB, O., 1986. Real-time obstacle avoidance for manipulators and mobile robots. *Int. J. Robotics Res.* 5:90–99.

KAWATO, M., 1999. International models for motor control and trajectory planning. *Curr. Opin. Neurobiol.* 9:718–727.

KAWATO, M., and D. WOLPERT, 1998. Internal models for motor control. *Novartis Found. Symp.* 218:291–304.

KRAKAUER, J., M. GHILARDI, and C. GHEZ, 1999. Independent learning of internal models for kinematic and dynamic control of reaching. *Nat. Neurosci.* 2:1026–1031.

LEMAY, M. A., J. E. GALAGAN, N. HOGAN, and E. BIZZI, 2001. Modulation and vectorial summation of the spinalized frog's hindlimb end-point force produced by intraspinal electrical stimulation of the cord. *IEEE Trans. Neural Syst. Rehab. Eng.* 9:12–23.

LOEB, G. E., 1985. Motoneurone task groups: Coping with kinematic heterogeneity. *J. Exp. Biol.* 115:137–146.

MACPHERSON, J. M., 1991. How flexible are muscle synergies? In *Motor Control: Concepts and Issues*, D. R. Humphryey and H. J. Freund, eds. New York: Wiley, pp. 33–47.

MATELLI, M., G. LUPPINO, A. MURATA, and H. SAKATA, 1994. Independent anatomical circuits for reaching and grasping linking and inferior parietal sulcus and inferior area 6 in macaque monkey (abstract). *Soc. Neurosci. Abstr.* 20:984.

MATTHEWS, P. B., 1996. Relationship of firing intervals of human motor units to the trajectory of post-spike after-hyperpolarization and synaptic noise. *J. Physiol.* 492:597–682.

McCOLLUM, G., F. B. HORAK, and L. M. NASHNER, 1984. Parsimony in neural calculations for postural movements. In *Cerebellar Functions*, J. Bloedel, J. Dichgans, and W. Precht, eds. Berlin: Springer-Verlag, pp. 52–66.

MORASSO, P., 1981. Spatial control of arm movements. *Exp. Brain Res.* 42:223–227.

MUSSA-IVALDI, F. A., 1997. Nonlinear force fields: A distributed system of control primitives for representing and learning movements. In *Proceedings of the 1997 IEEE International Symposium on Computation Intelligence in Robotics and Automation*. Los Alamitos, Calif.: IEEE Computer Society Press, pp. 84–90.

MUSSA-IVALDI, F., and S. GISZTER, 1992. Vector field approximation: A computational paradigm for motor control and learning. *Biol. Cybern.* 67:491–500.

MUSSA-IVALDI, F. A., S. F. GISZTER, and E. BIZZI, 1994. Motor learning through the combination of primitives, *Proc. Natl. Acad. Sci. U.S.A.* 91:7534–7538.

NASHNER, L. M., 1977. Fixed patterns of rapid postural responses among leg muscles during stance. *Exp. Brain Res.* 30:13–24.

NASHNER, L. M., and G. McCOLLUM, 1985. The organization of human postural movements: A formal basis and experimental synthesis. *Behav. Brain Sci.* 8:135–172.

RIMON, E., and D. E. KODITSCHEK, 1989. The construction of analytic diffeomorphisms for exact robot navigation on star worlds. In *Proceedings of the 1989 IEEE International Conference on Robotics and Automation*. Los Alamitos, Calif.: IEEE Computer Society Press, pp. 21–26.

ROSSIGNOL, S., 1996. Neural control of stereotypic movements. In *Handbook of Physiology*, L. B. Rowell and J. T. Sheperd, eds. Bethesda, Md.: American Physiological Society, Sect. 12, pp. 173–216.

RUSSELL, S., and P. NORVIG, 1995. *Artificial Intelligence: A Modern Approach*. Englewood Cliffs, N.J.: Prentice Hall.

SAKATA, H., and M. TAIRA, 1994. Parietal control of hand action. *Curr. Opin. Neurobiol.* 4:847–856.

SALTIEL, P., K. WYLER-DUDA, A. d'AVELLA, M. C. TRESCH, and E. BIZZI, 2001. Muscle synergies encoded within the spinal cord: Evidence from focal intraspinal NMDA iontophoresis in the frog. *J. Neurophysiol.* 85:605–619.

SALTZMAN, E., 1979. Levels of sensorimotor representation. *J. Math. Psychol.* 20:91–163.

SCIAVICCO, L., and B. SICILIANO, 2000. *Modeling and Control of Robot Manipulators*. New York: Springer-Verlag.

SHADMEHR, R., and F. A. MUSSA-IVALDI, 1994. Adaptive representation of dynamics during learning of a motor task. *J. Neurosci.* 14:3208–3224.

SOECHTING, J. F., and F. LACQUANITI, 1989. An assessment of the existence of muscle synergies during load perturbations and intentional movements of the human arm. *Exp. Brain Res.* 74:535–548.

STEIN, P. S., M. L. McCULLOUGH, and S. N. CURRIE, 1998. Spinal motor patterns in the turtle. *Ann. N.Y. Acad. Sci.* 16:142–154.

STEIN, P. S., L. I. MORTIN, and G. A. ROBERTSON, 1986. The forms of a task and their blends. In *Neurobiology of Vertebrate Locomotion*, S. Grillner, P. S. G. Stein, D. G. Stuart, H. Forssberg, and R. M. Herman, eds. London: Macmillan, pp. 201–216.

STEIN, P. S. G., and J. L. SMITH, 1997. Neural and biomechanical control strategies for different forms of vertebrate hindlimb motor tasks. In *Neurons, Networks, and Motor Behavior*, P. S. G. Stein, S. Grillner, A. I. Selverston, and D. G. Stuart, eds. Cambridge, Mass.: MIT Press, pp. 61–73.

TODOROV, E., and M. I. JORDAN, 2002. Optimal feedback control as a theory of motor coordination. *Nat. Neurosci.* 5:1226–1235.

TRESCH, M. C., and E. BIZZI, 1999. Responses from the spinal microstimulation in the chronically spinalized rats and their relationship to spinal systems activated by low threshold cutaneous stimulation. *Exp. Brain Res.* 129:401–416.

TRESCH, M. C., P. SALTIEL, and E. BIZZI, 1999. The construction of movement by the spinal cord. *Nat. Neurosci.* 2:162–167.

TRESCH, M. C., P. SALTIEL, A. D'AVELLA, and E. BIZZI, 2002. Coordination and localization in spinal motor systems. *Brain Res. Rev.* 40:66–79.

TSETLIN, M. L., 1973. *Automation Theory and Modeling of Biological Systems*. New York: Academic Press, pp. 160–196.

VAN BEERS, R. J., P. BARADUC, and D. M. WOLPERT, 2002. Role of uncertainty in sensorimotor control. *Philos. Trans. R. Soc. Lond. B Biol. Sci.* 357:1137–1145.

WHEATLEY, M., and R. B. STEIN, 1992. An in vitro preparation of the mudpuppy for simultaneous intracellular and electromyographic recording during locomotion. *J. Neurosci. Methods* 42:129–137.

WOLPERT, D. M., and Z. GHAHRAMANI, 2000. Computational principles of movement neuroscience. *Nat. Neurosci. Suppl.* 3:1212–1217.

WOLPERT, D., R. MIALL, and M. KAWATO, 1998. Internal models in the cerebellum. *Trends Cogn. Sci.* 2:338–347.

31 Cortical Mechanisms Subserving Object Grasping, Action Understanding, and Imitation

GIACOMO RIZZOLATTI, LEONARDO FOGASSI, AND VITTORIO GALLESE

ABSTRACT In this chapter we provide evidence that the cortical motor system, in addition to its role in action organization, is also involved in action understanding and imitation. In the first part of the chapter, we propose, on the basis of the functional properties of a monkey premotor area (area F5), that at the core of the cortical motor system there are vocabularies of motor actions. Neurons forming these vocabularies store both knowledge about actions and the description of how this knowledge has to be applied. When a specific population of these neurons becomes active, an internal representation of a specific action is generated. This action representation may be used for planning and executing goal-directed actions and for recognizing actions made by another individual. Action understanding is based on a match between an observed action and its internal motor representation (mirror system). In the second part of the chapter, we review data showing that a mirror system, similar to that of the monkey, exists also in humans. We present evidence that in humans this system is also involved in imitation.

A central problem in motor physiology is how sensory information is translated into movement. This problem is particularly difficult to resolve for visual information. The description of an action in the visual domain is radically different from its description in the motor domain, yet the nervous system is able to translate a seen action into a copy of it as it occurs in imitation. The translation of an object into movements may seem less problematic. Yet also in this case parameters that are visually extracted must correspond to parameters in the completely different motor domain.

The solution to the translation problem that we propose here is that at the core of the motor system is not movement but action. Action is defined by a goal and by an expectancy. In both the parietal lobe and the premotor areas, there are representations of actions. Furthermore, and most important, these representations may be addressed internally or may be triggered by appropriate sensory stimuli. When, because of internal motivations and external contingences, it is advantageous for the individual to act, these action representations become actual actions.

In addition to action generation, the motor system plays an important role in action recognition. The basic mechanism of this cognitive function is the same as that for sensorimotor translation. The visual description of the external reality is matched on action representations. The recognition occurs because the observed events evoke action representations whose outcome is known to the individual.

Although the notion of action representation is probably valid for the whole mosaic of areas forming the agranular frontal cortex and the inferior parietal lobule, evidence for it is particularly rich for those areas where hand actions are represented. This chapter discusses the functional properties of these areas. The first part of the chapter reviews their organization in the monkey; the second part discusses their organization in humans.

Action representation in monkeys

PREMOTOR AREA F5: MOTOR PROPERTIES Figure 31.1 shows a lateral view of the monkey brain. A premotor area that is involved in the control of distal hand actions is area F5. This area receives parietal input from areas PF and PFG, anterior intraparietal area (AIP), and SII. Other inputs arrive to it from prefrontal cortex (area 46) and the cingulate area 24c. F5 is directly connected with area F1 (primary motor cortex).

Evidence that F5 is involved in the control of hand movements comes from intracortical microstimulation studies and neuron recordings (Rizzolatti, Scandolara, Gentilucci, et al., 1981; Rizzolatti, Scandolara, Matelli, et al., 1981; Kurata and Tanji, 1986; Gentilucci et al., 1988; Rizzolatti et al., 1988; Hepp-Reymond et al., 1994). Particularly important for understanding the functions of F5 have been studies in which single neurons were recorded in a naturalistic context. These studies showed that, typically, the discharge of F5 neurons correlates much better with an action or with a fragment of an action (motor act) than with the movements forming it. Thus, many neurons discharge when an action

GIACOMO RIZZOLATTI, LEONARDO FOGASSI, and VITTORIO GALLESE Dipartimento di Neuroscienze, Sezione di Fisiologia, University of Parma, 39 via Volturno, I-43100 Parma, Italy.

427

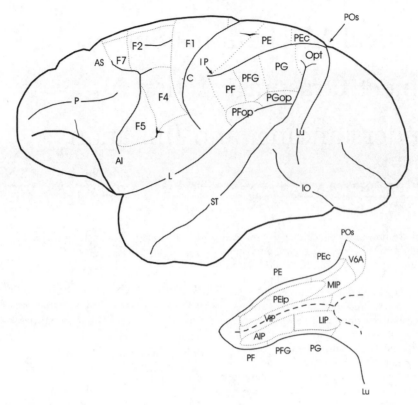

FIGURE 31.1 Lateral view of macaque monkey cerebral cortex with frontal and parietal areas indicated. The lower part of the figure shows an unfolded view of the areas located within the intraparietal sulcus. Frontal agranular cortical areas (F1–F7) are classified according to Matelli, Luppino, and Rizzolatti (1985). The cortical areas of the parietal convexity (PE, PEc, PF, PFG, PG, Opt, PFop, PGop) are classified according to Von Bonin and Bailey (1947) and Pandya and Seltzer (1982). Abbreviations: AIP, anterior intraparietal area; LIP, lateral intraparietal area; MIP, medial intraparietal area; PEip, PE intraparietal area; VIP, ventral intraparietal area.

(e.g., grasping) is performed with effectors as different as the right hand, the left hand, or the mouth (figure 31.2). Furthermore, for the vast majority of neurons, the same type of movement (e.g., an index finger flexion) effective in triggering a neuron during one action (e.g., grasping) is not effective during another action (e.g., scratching). For these cases the characterization of neuron activity in terms of individual movements is obviously not satisfactory.

When action was used as a classification criterion, F5 neurons could be subdivided into various categories, such as "grasping-with-the-hand-and-the-mouth" neurons, "grasping-with-the-hand" neurons, "holding" neurons, "tearing" neurons, and "manipulating" neurons.

In each class, many neurons (about 80%) code specific types of hand shaping, such as precision grip (the grip type most represented), whole hand prehension, and finger prehension. Regardless of whether they are specific or not for a certain type of prehension, neurons show a variety of temporal relations with the prehension phases. Some discharge during the whole action coded by them, sometimes starting to fire at stimulus presentation. Some are mostly active during the opening of the fingers, some during finger closure (see Jeannerod et al., 1995).

On the basis of these properties, it has been suggested that F5 contains a "vocabulary" (a storage) of *action representations*. This vocabulary is constituted by "words," each of which is represented by a set of F5 neurons. Some words indicate the general goal of an action (grasping, holding, tearing, etc.). Others indicate the way in which a specific action must be executed (e.g., precision grip or finger prehension). Finally, other words are concerned with the temporal segmentation of the action into smaller chunks, each coding a specific phase of the grip (e.g., hand opening, hand closure, etc.).

The concept of action representation is close to Arbib's (1981) notion of motor schemas. A motor schema is both a store of knowledge and the description of a process for applying that knowledge. The properties of F5 neurons fit this definition. These neurons store specific knowledge about an action and, when activated, provide the blueprint for implementing it.

This view has important functional implications. First, the existence of neurons that code specific motor schemas and are anatomically linked with primary motor cortex (F1) and subcortical motor centers facilitates the selection of the most appropriate combination of movements by reducing the

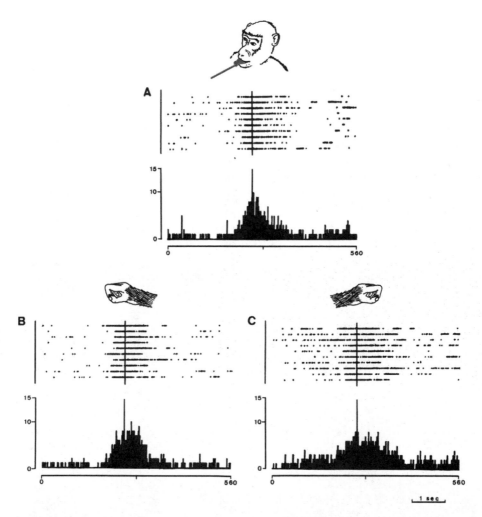

FIGURE 31.2 Example of a "grasping-with-the-hand-and-the-mouth" F5 neuron. (*A*) Neuron discharge during grasping with the mouth. (*B*) Neuron discharge during grasping with the hand contralateral to the recorded hemisphere. (*C*) Neuron discharge during grasping with the hand ipsilateral to the recorded hemisphere. Rasters and histograms are aligned with the moment in which the monkey touched the food. The histograms are the sum of 10 trials. Abscissae: time expressed in bins. Bin width: 10 ms. Ordinates: spikes/bin. (Modified from Rizzolatti et al., 1988.)

number of variables that the motor system has to control to achieve the action goal. Second, the concept of action representations simplifies the association between a given stimulus (i.e., a visually presented object) and the appropriate motor response toward it. Third, it gives the brain a storage of motor schemas (that is, a knowledge about actions) that provides the motor system with functions traditionally attributed to the sensory systems.

PREMOTOR AREA F5: CANONICAL NEURONS The motor properties of F5 described in the previous section are proper to all F5 neurons. Experiments in which F5 neurons were tested by presenting the monkey with visual stimuli, showed that many F5 neurons also respond to object presentation (Rizzolatti et al., 1988; Murata et al., 1997).

In the experiment of Murata and colleagues (1997), the monkey faced a dark box where geometric objects (cube, cylinder, sphere, ring, etc.) of different size and shape were located. The objects were presented one at the time. The trials started with the presentation of a colored spot of light on the object that remained invisible. At presentation of the spot of light, the monkey had to fixate it and press a bar. The pressing of the bar illuminated the box and made the object visible. After a variable delay, the spot of light changed color. This was the signal for the monkey to release the bar and reach for and grasp the object ("grasping-in-light" condition). In a second condition all the events were as before, but when the spot changed color, the monkey had only to release the bar. Object grasping was not allowed ("object fixation" condition). The two conditions were run in different blocks and the spot colors in them were different. In a third condition ("grasping-in-dark" condition) the same object was presented for many consecutive trials. The monkey saw the object before the beginning of the first experimental trial and therefore knew its characteristics, but had to perform the entire task without visual guidance.

The results showed that about half of the tested neurons responded to three-dimensional (3D) object presentation, and two-thirds of them were selective to one specific object or to a cluster of objects. A strict congruence between visual and motor selectivity was found in most recorded neurons. Figure 31.3 shows the responses of a visually selective neuron. Observation and grasping of the ring produced strong responses (figure 31.3, left). Responses to the other five objects were modest (sphere) or virtually absent.

The middle and right panels in figure 31.3 show the behavior of the same neuron in two other experimental conditions: object fixation and object grasping in dark. In the object fixation condition the objects were presented as before, but at the go signal the monkey, instead of grasping the object, had to release a key. Note that in this condition the object was totally irrelevant for task solution, which only required the detection of the go signal (spot color change).

Yet the neuron strongly discharged at the presentation of the preferred object (figure 31.3, middle).

How can these findings be explained? It is clear that the discharge to object presentation was not related to motor preparation because it was also present when no response to the object was required. Similarly, object specificity rules out factors such as attention to stimuli, or intention to act. These factors were identical for all presented objects. Thus, the most likely interpretation of the visual responses is that object presentation activated a specific stimulus-congruent action representation. This representation was automatically evoked at the stimulus presentation. It did not, however, necessarily lead to motor execution. The activation of premotor areas is under control of various systems such as the mesial cortical areas and the prefrontal areas. Only when these areas allow action execution does the activated action representation become actual action (see Rizzolatti and Luppino, 2001).

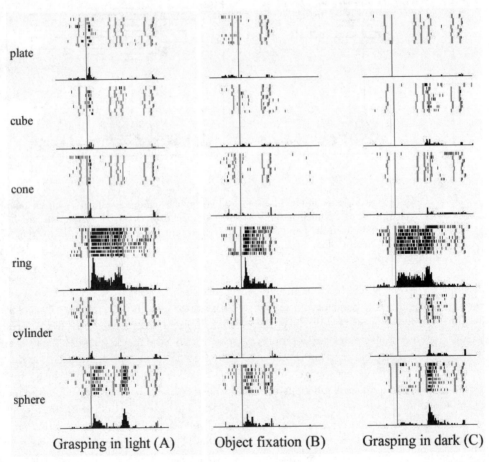

plate

cube

cone

ring

cylinder

sphere

Grasping in light (A)   Object fixation (B)   Grasping in dark (C)

FIGURE 31.3 Example of an F5 "grasping-with-the-hand" visuo-motor neuron. Panels show neural activity recorded during three different experimental conditions: grasping in light, object fixation, and grasping in dark. Rasters and histograms are aligned (vertical bar) with key press. In grasping-in-light and object fixation conditions, a key press determined the illumination of the object. Small gray bars in each raster of grasping-in-light and grasping-in-dark conditions indicate, from left to right, the appearance of a spot of light on the object; key press; change of color of the spot; key release; onset of object pulling; further change of color of the spot; onset of object release. Small gray bars in each raster of object fixation condition indicate, from left to right, the appearance of a spot of light on the object; key press; change of color of the spot; key release. Abscissae: time expressed in seconds. Ordinates: spikes/s. (Modified from Murata et al., 1997.)

THE AIP-F5 GRASPING CIRCUIT Anatomically, ventral premotor cortex is heavily connected with the inferior parietal lobule (Petrides and Pandya, 1984; Matelli et al., 1986; Cavada and Goldman-Rakic, 1989). Physiological experiments by Sakata and co-workers (Taira et al., 1990; Murata et al., 2000) showed that in the rostral half of the lateral bank of the intraparietal sulcus (IPS) there are neurons that become active during hand actions. They called this sector the anterior intraparietal area, or area AIP (see Sakata et al., 1995). Subsequent experiments showed that AIP and F5 are strongly reciprocally connected (Matelli et al., 1994; Matelli and Luppino, 1997).

AIP neurons fall into three main classes: motor-dominant neurons, visual and motor neurons, and visual-dominant neurons (Sakata et al., 1995). Two of them—motor-dominant neurons and visual and motor neurons—have discharge properties similar to those of motor and canonical F5 neurons, respectively, while the third class, visual-dominant neurons, is not present in F5. Visual-dominant neurons are active during object fixation and grasping movements executed under visual guidance, but they do not respond when the same movements are executed in darkness. Many of the AIP visually responsive neurons respond selectively to the presentation of one or a restricted group of visually similar objects (Murata et al., 2000). This indicates that AIP, although part of the dorsal stream, contains neurons that code 3D objects in visual terms.

INACTIVATION OF THE AIP-F5 CIRCUIT The functional properties of AIP and F5 neurons strongly suggest that the AIP-F5 circuit is involved in visuomotor transformations for grasping. This possibility was directly tested by inactivating the two areas and examining the consequent deficits.

Monkeys were trained to reach for and grasp geometric solids of different size and shape. A GABA agonist (muscimol) was then injected either in AIP (Gallese et al., 1994) or in F5 (Fogassi et al., 2001). Following AIP injection, the behavior of the hand contralateral to the injection side was markedly impaired. The deficit consisted in a mismatch between the intrinsic properties of the objects to be grasped, especially of the small ones, and the hand shaping necessary to grasp them. The consequence was an awkward object grasping or even a complete grasping failure. In the case of successful grasping the grip was very often achieved after several correction movements that relied on tactile exploration of the object. No deficit in reaching accuracy was observed.

Inactivation of F5 produced visuomotor deficits similar to those observed following AIP inactivation. The impairment was limited to precision grip of the hand contralateral to the lesion when small injections were made. Larger injections produced bilateral deficit concerning all grip types. Interestingly, a deficit in hand shaping, without any other type of

motor deficit, was also observed in the hand ipsilateral to the lesion. This deficit confirms the bilateral control of F5 over hand movements and, most important, shows that deficits following F5 lesion do not depend on hand paresis.

VISUOMOTOR TRANSFORMATION FOR GRASPING: A POSSIBLE NEURAL MODEL The functional properties of F5 and AIP just reviewed allow one to propose a model that can explain how the AIP-F5 circuit transforms visual information into action. Its main points are the following. The AIP visual-dominant neurons receive information about object properties from 3D object-sensitive neurons located in an area posterior to LIP, called caudal IPS (cIPS; see Shikata et al., 1996). AIP visuomotor neurons transform these visual object descriptions into a series of motor affordances. Among them one is chosen on the basis of the information concerning the object meaning and the contextual action goal. Given the strong connections linking AIP with the prefrontal cortex (Petrides and Pandya, 1984) and with IT cortex (Webster, Bachevalier, and Ungerleider, 1994; G. Luppino, personal communication), it is likely that this selection occurs within AIP. Information concerning the selected grip is sent then to F5, where the selected action remains a potential action until an appropriate go signal reaches it from the mesially located premotor area F6 (pre-SMA), recipient of strong prefrontal inputs and reciprocally connected to F5 (see Rizzolatti and Luppino, 2001). A computational model of the AIP-F5 circuit based on principles similar to those here described was recently proposed by Fagg and Arbib (1998).

Mirror neurons

Mirror neurons are a specific class of neurons that discharge both when the monkey performs an action and when it observes a similar action done by another monkey or by the experimenter. Mirror neurons were originally discovered in area F5 (Gallese et al., 1996; Rizzolatti, Fadiga, Fogasi, et al., 1996). More recently, mirror neurons were also found in the rostral part of the inferior parietal lobule (Fogassi et al., 1998; Gallese et al., 2002).

MIRROR NEURON PROPERTIES: EARLY STUDIES The visual stimuli effective in triggering mirror neurons are actions in which an agent (another monkey or an experimenter) interacts with an object using the hand or the mouth. Object presentation, including the presentation of interesting stimuli such as food items, faces, or body movements, is ineffective. Similarly, actions made using tools either did not activate the neurons or activated them only very weakly. An example of a mirror neuron is shown in figure 31.4.

The seen actions most effective in triggering the neurons are grasping, holding, manipulating, and tearing. More than half of neurons, among those activated by the observation

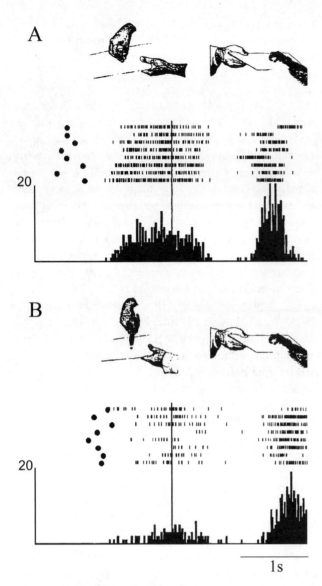

FIGURE 31.4 Example of the visual and motor responses of an F5 mirror neuron. The behavioral situations during which the neural activity was recorded are shown schematically above the rasters. (*A*) A tray with a piece of food placed on it was presented to the monkey and the experimenter grasped the food located on it. The tray with the food was then moved toward the monkey, which grasped it. The neural discharge was absent when the food was presented and moved toward the monkey. In contrast, a strong activation was present during the grasping of both the experimenter and the monkey. (*B*) As in *A*, except that the experimenter grasped the food with pliers. The response was much weaker when the observed grasping was performed with a tool. Rasters and histograms are aligned (vertical bar) with the moment in which the experimenter touched the food. Dots indicate the beginning of the trials (presentation of the tray with food). Abscissae: time. Ordinates: spikes/bin. Bin width: 20 ms. (From Gallese et al., 1996.)

of hand action, are active during the observation of one action only. Some neurons are selective not only to the general action aim (e.g., grasping) but also to how the action was performed, selectively firing during the observation of one particular type of grip (e.g., precision grip, but not whole hand prehension).

There is a large amount of generalization as far as the precise physical aspects of the effective agent are concerned. For many neurons the precise hand orientation is not crucial for activating them. Similarly, the distance from the monkey at which the action is executed in most cases does not influence the response. For the majority of neurons the effect is the same when the experimenter uses the right or the left hand. In one-third of tested neurons, however, the discharge is consistently stronger when the action is made by one hand instead of the other.

Mirror neurons discharge during active movements. A comparison between the actions they code and the actions that trigger them when seen show that for almost the totality of mirror neurons, there is a congruence between the observed and executed action. This congruence may be extremely strict, that is, the effective motor action (e.g., precision grip) coincided with the action that, when seen, triggered the neurons (e.g., precision grip). For the majority of neurons the congruence is rather broad. For them the motor requirements (e.g., precision grip) are usually stricter than the visual ones (any type of hand grasping).

MIRROR NEURON PROPERTIES: NEW STUDIES   Both humans and monkeys are able to understand an action even when the object target of the action is not visible, provided that there are clues sufficient to understand the observed action. A function that is frequently attributed to a mirror neuron is that of recognizing actions made by others. Mirror neurons, however, typically require, as the visual trigger feature, an interaction between the agent of the action and an object. There is here an apparent contradiction. If mirror neurons are indeed involved in action understanding, they should also become active during the observation of partially hidden actions.

This problem was recently addressed by Umiltà and colleagues (2001). They recorded the activity of mirror neurons while the monkey observed the experimenter reaching, grasping, and holding a piece of food located on a platform. There were two basic experimental conditions. In the first, the monkey saw the entire action made by the experimenter (full vision condition). In the second, the monkey saw only the beginning of the same action, its final part (the hand–object interaction) being hidden from the monkey's view by a screen (hidden condition). In the hidden condition the experimenter, before each trial, placed a piece of food on the platform in full view. Then the screen was moved and the food disappeared from the monkey's view. The meaning of the experimenter's action could therefore be inferred from the previous knowledge about food location and the vision of the initial arm movement.

The results showed that more than half of the recorded mirror neurons were also active in the hidden condition. The response was present not only in "grasping" but also in "holding" neurons. It should be noted that in the latter case the triggering feature of the neuron ("holding an object") was completely hidden from the view. These data show that action representations coded by mirror neurons may be evoked in the absence of the stimulus specifically triggering them if there are sufficient external clues.

Another evidence in favor of the notion that mirror neurons code the meaning of specific actions comes from experiments in which F5 mirror neurons were tested with the vision of an action normally accompanied by a characteristic sound, and by that sound alone (Kohler et al., 2002). Sounds produced by actions made by the experimenter in front of the monkey and sounds not related to hand actions were used.

About 15% of the tested neurons discharged both when the monkey performed a hand action and when it heard the action-related sound. An example of these "audiovisual" mirror neurons is shown in figure 31.5 (left side, neuron 1). This neuron responded to the vision (and sound) of a tearing action (paper ripping, V + S). The sound of the same action performed out of the monkey's sight was equally effective (S). To control for unspecific factors such as arousal or fear, non-action-related sounds (white noise, chimpanzee calls) were also presented. These stimuli did not evoke any excitatory response (CS1 and CS2). Another example of an audiovisual mirror neuron is presented in figure 31.5 (right side, neuron 2).

The capacity of the audiovisual mirror neurons to differentiate actions on the basis of action auditory and visual characteristics was also tested. The experimental design included two hand actions, randomly presented in vision-and-sound, sound only, vision only, and motor conditions (monkeys performing object-directed actions). The large majority of the tested audiovisual mirror neurons exhibited auditory selectivity. Taken together, these finding indicate that F5 neurons discharge when there are sensory cues sufficient to evoke in the monkey the meaning of an action. What these cues are is irrelevant. They could be visual or auditory. Once the action meaning is specified, the neuron fires.

POSSIBLE FUNCTIONS OF MIRROR NEURONS Macaque monkeys are social animals. They live in groups characterized by intense social interactions, such as parental care, mating, and grooming, that are disciplined by a well-delineated hierarchical organization. It is therefore crucial for each member of a given social group to recognize the actions of others and to "understand" the meaning of the observed action in order to appropriately react to it.

Action recognition may be achieved in various ways. The most ancient is probably the one based on the visual description of action and the association of this action with its consequences. No motor activation is needed here. This mechanism is similar to mechanisms allowing the comprehension of physical laws, but for the fact that it is mediated by a specific neural substrate (see Jellema et al., 2002).

The proposal put forward by several authors (e.g., Merleau-Ponty, 1962; Gordon, 1986; Goldman, 1989; see also Gallese and Goldman, 1998) that actions, in order to be understood, may require a re-acting of the observed action was exclusively based on theoretical considerations. The discovery of mirror neurons provided solid empirical grounding for this proposal. The observation of actions made by others activates action representations in the observer identical or similar to the observed ones. The way in which the mirror neurons are involved in action understanding is the following. When an individual acts, he selects an action representation whose motor consequences are known to him. The mirror neurons allow this knowledge to be extended to actions performed by others. Each time an individual observes an action done by another individual, neurons that represent that action are activated in his premotor cortex. Because the evoked motor representation corresponds to that internally generated during active action, it is recognized, and therefore implicitly understood, by the observer.

The observation of actions made by other individuals may have another important function, that of learning how to reproduce them. When we learn a new motor skill we observe and reproduce the action that the teacher is displaying in front of us. Eventually we learn it. However, the capacity to learn by imitation is absent in primates except humans and, possibly, apes (see Galef, 1988; Whiten and Ham, 1992; Tomasello, Kruger, and Ratner, 1993; Byrne, 1995; Visalberghi and Fragaszy, 2001). The link between mirrors neurons and imitation will be discussed after a review of the properties of the human mirror neuron system.

Action representation in humans

THE PARIETOFRONTAL HAND ACTION CIRCUIT The presence of a specific parietofrontal circuit for object-related hand actions in monkeys raised the issue of whether such a circuit is also present in humans. Initial results were rather ambiguous (Rizzolatti, Fadiga, Matelli, et al., 1996; Faillenot, Decety, and Jeannerod, 1999). Subsequent experiments showed, however, that an object-related hand action representation exists in humans and anatomically corresponds to that of the monkey.

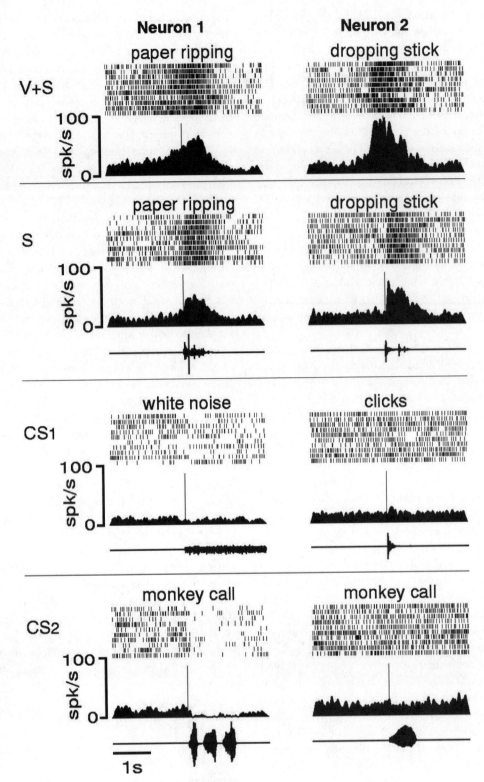

FIGURE 31.5   Two examples of neurons responding to the sound of actions. Histograms are shown together with spike density functions. Vertical lines indicate the time when the sound occurred. Traces under the spike density functions in S and CS conditions are oscillograms of the sounds used to test the neurons. The neuron responses are shown in four conditions: V + S = vision of the action and action-related sound; S = action-related sound, no vision; CS1 = control sound (white noise and clicks), CS2 = control sound (monkey calls).

Binkofski and colleagues (1999) asked normal human volunteers to manipulate multifaceted complex object. They compared this condition with another one in which volunteers manipulated a smooth sphere. The results showed that the complex manipulation activated the pars opercularis of the inferior frontal gyrus (IFG), roughly corresponding to Brodmann area 44 (Talairach coordinates −52, +8, +28), the adjacent ventral area 6, the cortex inside the anterior part of the intraparietal sulcus, and area SII. This cortical network closely corresponds to the monkey cortical circuit AIP-F5 plus area SII, which also in monkeys is connected with F5.

The functional homology between area 44 and F5 was further supported by a study by Ehrsson and colleagues (2000), in which they studied the cortical localization of different types of grip. The focus of the representation of the precision grip was found to be located in the pars opercularis of IFG (Talairach coordinates −56, +12, +32). This finding is in accord with monkey data showing that precision grip, in contrast to whole hand prehension, has a very rich representation in F5 (Rizzolatti et al., 1988).

Other studies showed that in humans also, simple finger and hand movements may activate the pars opercularis of IFG (Krams et al., 1998; Iacoboni et al., 1999). Finally, this sector of IFG was found to be active during hand action imaging (Decety et al., 1994; Grafton et al., 1996; Gerardin et al., 2000; Simon et al., 2002) and during hand mental rotation (Parsons et al., 1995).

THE CANONICAL NEURON SYSTEM IN HUMANS In addition to neurons coding hand actions, the IFG and the adjacent premotor cortex contain a system with properties similar to those of canonical neurons.

In an fMRI experiment, Chao and Martin (2000) presented volunteers with pictures of tools, animals, faces, and houses. The control stimuli were scrambled images of the same objects. In one experiment the task was to observe the stimuli, in a second to silently name pictures of tools and animals. In both experiments the presentation of tools produced a preferential response of the pars opercularis of the left IFG on the border with ventral premotor cortex, and of the left intraparietal cortex. These locations correspond to the location of canonical neurons and AIP neurons in the monkey.

More abstract objects, such as moving colored circles, also appear to be effective in triggering the human "prehension" circuit. Schubotz and von Cramon (2001) used these stimuli and asked volunteers to pay attention to object-specific, spatial, or temporal properties of the stimuli. The parietofrontal circuit was active in all conditions, but the intensity was maximal during object-related attention.

THE MIRROR NEURON SYSTEM IN HUMANS There is rich evidence that a mirror neuron system exists in humans. This

evidence comes from EEG, MEG, TMS, and brain imaging studies (e.g., Fadiga et al., 1995; Rizzolatti, Fadiga, Matelli, et al., 1996; Grafton et al., 1996; Grèzes, Costes, and Decety, 1998; Hari et al., 1998; Cochin et al., 1999; Iacoboni et al., 1999; Strafella and Paus, 2000; Gangitano, Mottaghy, and Pascal-Leone, 2001; Mantey, Schubotz, and von Cramon, 2003). The aim of this section is not to review this very rich literature but to discuss only some findings related to specific issues. For an exhaustive review on the mirror neuron system in humans, see Rizzolatti, Fogassi, and Gallese (2001); see also Stamenov and Gallese (2002).

Anatomy of the human mirror neuron system Early brain imaging studies showed that the observation of object-directed hand action activated the cortex of the superior temporal sulcus (STS), the rostral sector of the inferior parietal lobule, and the posterior part of the IFG (Rizzolatti, Fadiga, Matelli, et al., 1996; Grafton et al., 1996; Grèzes, Costes, and Decety, 1998). This circuit is very similar to that described in the monkey, where neurons sensitive to hand actions have been described in the cortex of STS (Perrett et al., 1989) and mirror neurons are present in areas PF and F5.

New experiments considered whether, beside hand actions, actions made by other effectors are also represented in the parietal and frontal areas. Buccino and colleagues (2001) addressed this issue using mouth, hand, and foot actions as stimuli. Transitive actions (actions directed toward an object) and intransitive (mimed) actions were used. Action observation was compared with the observation of a static face, hand, and foot, respectively.

Observation of object-related mouth movements determined activation of the pars opercularis of IFG bilaterally and of the adjacent ventral premotor cortex. In addition, two activation foci were present in the inferior parietal lobule. One focus was located in the rostral part of the inferior parietal lobule, the other in the gyrus angularis (figure 31.6, top). The observation of intransitive actions determined activation of the same premotor areas as the observation of transitive actions, but there was no parietal lobe activation.

Observation of object-related hand/arm actions (e.g., reaching to grasp a cup) determined two activation foci in the frontal lobe, one in the pars opercularis of IFG, and the other in the upper part of ventral area 6. Considering the motor organization of the region (see Rizzolatti, Fogassi, and Gallese, 2002), it is likely that the activation of area 44 was determined by the observation of grasping hand movements, while activation of area 6 was determined by the observation of reaching. As for mouth movements, there were two activation foci in the parietal lobe. The rostral focus was still in the rostral part of the inferior parietal lobule, but more posteriorly located than the one observed during mouth actions, while the caudal focus was essentially in the

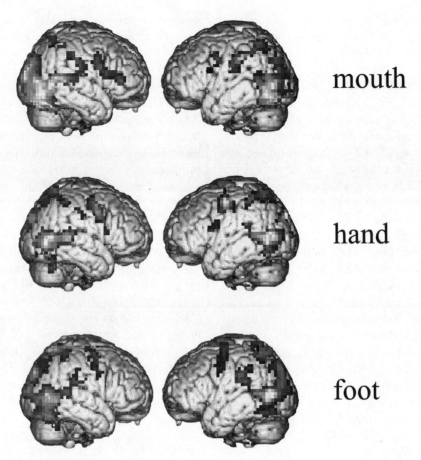

mouth

hand

foot

FIGURE 31.6 Activations of frontal and parietal cortical areas during observation of mouth, hand and foot actions, rendered on a standard brain schema (Montreal Neurological Institute): mouth, biting an apple; hand, grasping a cup or a ball; foot, kicking a ball or pushing a brake. All actions were compared with the observation of a static face, hand, and foot, respectively. (See color plate 15.)

same location as that for mouth actions (figure 31.6, middle). During the observation of intransitive movements the premotor activations were present, but not the parietal ones.

Finally, the observation of object-related foot actions determined an activation of a dorsal sector of area 6 and an activation of the posterior parietal lobule, in part overlapping with that seen during mouth and hand actions, in part extending more dorsally (figure 31.6, bottom). The observation of intransitive foot movements determined activation of area 6, as for transitive actions, but not the parietal activations.

The results of this study are important for several reasons. First, they demonstrate that the mirror system includes a large part of premotor cortex and of the inferior parietal lobule. Second, they show that the activation map obtained during observation of actions made with different effectors is similar to the motor map (the so-called homunculus) obtained with electrical stimulation of the same region (Penfield and Rasmussen, 1950). Finally, the results allow exclusion of the idea advanced by some authors (Grèzes and Decety, 2001; see also Heyes, 2001) that activation of area 44 is due to internal verbalization. It is unlikely that verbal-

ization is present during the observation of hand movements and then disappears during the observation of foot movements.

Mirror neuron system and imitation   Mirror neurons appear to be ideally suited for imitation (Jeannerod, 1994). The capacity to translate an observed action into a performed action, which for years was the stumbling block in the path toward understanding imitation, is easily explained by the properties of the mirror neuron system. Prompted by these considerations, investigators have carried out several brain imaging experiments with the aim of discovering the neural substrate specifically activated during imitation (Iacoboni et al., 1999, 2001; Nishitani and Hari, 2000, 2002; Tanaka et al., 2001; Tanaka and Inui, 2002; Koski et al., 2002, 2003).

Using fMRI, Iacoboni and colleagues (1999) studied normal human subjects in two basic conditions: observation-only and observation-execution. In the observation-only condition, subjects were shown a moving finger, a cross on a stationary finger, or a cross on empty background. The instruction was to observe the stimuli. In the observation-execution condition, the same stimuli were presented, but this time the instruction was to lift the right finger as fast as possible in response to them.

The fundamental comparison of the study was the one between the trials of the observation-execution condition, in which participants made the movement in response to an observed action ("imitation"), and the trials of the same condition, in which the movement was triggered by the cross projected on a finger or an empty background. The results showed that there were four areas in which the activity was stronger during imitation trials than during the other trials: the left pars opercularis of IFG, the right anterior parietal region, the right parietal operculum, and the right STS region (for this last activation, see Iacoboni et al., 2001).

In all trials, the motor action made by the subjects was identical. Thus, the stronger activation of the left pars opercularis of IFG during imitation than during the other two observation-execution conditions strongly suggests a direct mapping between the observed and the executed action in this area.

In a further study, Koski and colleagues (2002) used a rather similar paradigm, a major difference being that the participants had to imitate finger movements (finger downward movement) either in the absence or in the presence of a visible goal (a red dot). An interesting result of this study was that the presence of the goal increased bilaterally the activation of the pars opercularis of the IFG. This result fits the general organization of F5, where action goal rather than movements are coded.

Activation of the posterior part of the IFG during imitation was obtained also by Nishitani and Hari (2000), who used the event-related neuromagnetic technique. Nishitani and Hari asked volunteers to grasp a manipulandum, to observe the same movement performed by an experimenter, or to observe and replicate the observed action. The results showed that during active grasping, there was an early activation in the left inferior frontal cortex (the left pars opercularis of IFG), with a response peak appearing approximately 250 ms before the touching of the target. This activation was followed within 100–200 ms by activation of the left precentral motor area. During imitation, the pattern and sequence of frontal activations were similar to those found during grasping execution, but activation of the left pars opercularis of IFG was preceded by an occipital activation due to the visual stimulation present in the imitation condition.

More recently, Nishitani and Hari (2002) studied the dynamics of cortical activation while volunteers observed still pictures of verbal and nonverbal lip forms, imitated them while the model was present, or made similar lip forms without the model. In both visual conditions the activation started in the occipital lobe, moved progressively to the superior temporal region, the inferior parietal lobule, the

posterior part of IFG (Broca's area), and finally reached the primary motor cortex. These results beautifully confirm that the mirror circuit represents the core circuit for imitation.

It should be stressed that in the experiments reviewed to this point, as well as in others on the neural basis of imitation (Tanaka and Inui, 2002; Decety et al., 2002; Koski et al., 2003), the studied "imitation" was action execution in which the executed action was elicited by the observation of an identical action. According to its classic definition (Thorndyke, 1898), however, imitation includes learning. Imitation in this stricter sense has recently been studied (Buccino et al., 2004). The study confirmed the central role of the parietofrontal mirror circuits. It also showed, however, important contributions of prefrontal and rostral mesial areas.

The experiments on imitation without learning (see Iacoboni et al., 1999, 2001) also showed activations outside the mirror neuron circuit. One of them was the superior parietal lobule. This activation might reflect a mirror mechanism similar to that proposed for the left pars opercularis of IFG. This interpretation, however, is in contrast to the finding that superior parietal lobule activation is typically absent in experiments in which subjects are instructed only to observe actions. Furthermore, in the monkey, the superior parietal lobule, in contrast to the inferior one, does not receives input from STS, where visual templates of biological actions are coded (G. Luppino and M. Matelli, personal communication).

A possible alternative interpretation is that, during imitation, the mirror activation of motor representations also determines, through backward projections, sensory copies of the actions to be imitated. The superior parietal lobule is a higher-order center for proprioception (Mountcastle et al., 1975) involved in the representation of body schema (see Berlucchi and Aglioti, 1997), the parietal operculum contains various somatosensory areas (see Disbrow et al., 2000), and, finally, STS is a higher-order center for visual centers coding biological actions. On the basis of these properties, one may propose that activation of these areas represents not a mirror copy of the observed movements but internally generated kinesthetic, tactile, and visual copies of the intended movements.

Conclusions

We began this chapter by positing that at the core of the cortical motor system is not movement but action. The data reviewed showed the validity of this proposal. By putting the notion of action representation at the center of the functional organization of the cortical motor system we can achieve a unitary, coherent explanation of the classic motor properties of the cortical motor system and its recently discovered cognitive functions. Action representations, which are located in the inferior parietal lobule and in the agranular frontal cortex, are used, according to contingencies, to act, to understand others' actions, and, as far as humans are concerned, to imitate them.

It is likely that this conceptual framework might also account for another important cognitive function: the capacity to understand why an action has been done. Although this type of understanding may require symbolic functions, it is equally possible that the intentions of others may be understood simply by internally selecting the most likely actions that the observer would have done following the observed action. This motor mechanism may explain intention and is experimentally testable.

A further interesting aspect of the conceptualization of the cortical motor system presented in this chapter is that it indicates how action may become information. Your action activates my motor representation of that action, and thus visual and acoustical information becomes understandable. This semantic link between the sender and the receiver of a message is absent in the case of visual stimuli that do not activate an action representation because, unlike actions, they do not have a *intrinsic* semantic counterpart in the observer. It is important to stress that a common information code between the sender and the receiver of a message is at the basis of language. This and various anatomical and functional considerations (e.g., the homology between monkey F5 and human area 44) strongly suggest that the mirror system might be the system from which language derived (see Rizzolatti and Arbib, 1998). The capacity to imitate, which only later appeared in the evolution of primates, was probably one of the main factors that determined the transition from the mirror system as a system for understanding to the mirror system as a system for communicating.

ACKNOWLEDGMENTS   This work was supported by European grant IST-2000-29689 (Artesimit), European grant QLG3-CT-2002-00746 (Mirror), European Science Foundation OMLL, and the Ministero Istruzione Università e Ricerca.

REFERENCES

ARBIB, M. A., 1981. Perceptual structures and and distributed motor control. In *Handbook of Physiology—The Nervous System*, vol. II, part 1, V. B. Brooks, ed. Bethesda, Md.: American Physiological Society, pp. 1449–1480.

BERLUCCHI, G., and S. AGLIOTI, 1997. The body in the brain: Neural basis of corporal awareness. *Trends Neurosci.* 20:560–564.

BINKOFSKI, F., G. BUCCINO, S. POSSE, R. J. SEITZ, G. RIZZOLATTI, and H.-J. FREUND, 1999. A fronto-parietal circuit for object manipulation in man: Evidence from an fMRI study. *Eur. J. Neurosci.* 11:3276–3286.

BUCCINO G., F. BINKOFSKI, G. R. FINK, L. FADIGA, L. FOGASSI, V. GALLESE, R. J. SEITZ, K. ZILLES, G. RIZZOLATTI, and H.-J. FREUND, 2001. Action observation activates premotor and parietal areas in a somatotopic manner: An fMRI study. *Eur. J. Neurosci.* 13:400–404.

BUCCINO, G., S. VOGT, A. RITZL, G. R. FINK, K. ZILLES, H.-J. FREUND, and G. RIZZOLATTI, 2004. Neural circuits underlying imitation learning of hand actions: an event-related fMRI study. *Neuron* 42:323–334.

BYRNE, R. 1995. *The Thinking Ape. Evolutionary Origin of Intelligence.* Oxford, England: Oxford University Press.

CAVADA, C., and P. S. GOLDMAN-RAKIC, 1989. Posterior parietal cortex in rhesus monkey. II. Evidence for segregated corticocortical networks linking sensory and limbic areas with the frontal lobe. *J. Comp. Neurol.* 287:422–445.

CHAO, L. L., and A. MARTIN, 2000. Representation of manipulable man-made objects in the dorsal stream. *NeuroImage* 12: 478–484.

COCHIN, S., C. BARTHELEMY, S. ROUX, and J. MARTINEAU, 1999. Observation and execution of movement: Similarities demonstrated by quantified electroencephalography. *Eur. J. Neurosci.* 11:1839–1842.

DECETY, J., T. CHAMINADE, J. GRÈZES, and A. N. MELTZOFF, 2002. A PET exploration of the neural mechanisms involved in reciprocal imitation. *NeuroImage* 15:265–272.

DECETY, J., D. PERANI, M. JEANNEROD, V. BETTINARDI, B. TADARY, R. WOODS, J. C. MAZZIOTTA, and F. FAZIO, 1994. Mapping motor representations with PET. *Nature* 371:600–602.

DISBROW E., T. ROBERTS, and L. KRUBITZER, 2000. Somatotopic organization of cortical fields in the lateral sulcus of *Homo sapiens*: Evidence for SII and PV. *J. Comp. Neurol.* 418:1–21.

EHRSSON, H. H., A. FAGERGREN, T. JONSSON, G. WESTLING, R. S. JOHANSSON, and H. FORSSBERG, 2000. Cortical activity in precision-versus power-grip tasks: An fMRI study. *J. Neurophysiol.* 83: 528–536.

FADIGA, L., L. FOGASSI, G. PAVESI, and G. RIZZOLATTI, 1995. Motor facilitation during action observation: A magnetic stimulation study. *J Neurophysiol.* 73:2608–2611.

FAGG, A. H., and M. A. ARBIB, 1998. Modeling parietal-premotor interactions in primate control of grasping. *Neural Netw.* 11:1277–1303.

FAILLENOT, I., J. DECETY, and M. JEANNEROD, 1999. Human brain activity related to the perception of spatial features of objects. *NeuroImage* 10:114–124.

FOGASSI L., V. GALLESE, G. BUCCINO, L. CRAIGHERO, L. FADIGA, and G. RIZZOLATTI, 2001. Cortical mechanisms for the visual guidance of hand grasping movements in the monkey: A reversible inactivation study. *Brain* 124:571–586.

FOGASSI L., V. GALLESE, L. FADIGA, and G. RIZZOLATTI, 1998. Neurons responding to the sight of goal-directed hand/arm actions in the parietal area PF (7b) of the macaque monkey. *Soc. Neurosci. Abstr.* 24:654.

GALEF, B. G., Jr., 1988. Imitation in animals: History, definitions and interpretation of data from the psychological laboratory. In *Social Learning: Psychological and Biological Perspectives*, T. Zentall and B. G. Galef, Jr., eds. Hillsdale, N.J.: Lawrence Erlbaum, pp. 3–28.

GALLESE, V., L. FADIGA, L. FOGASSI, and G. RIZZOLATTI, 1996. Action recognition in the premotor cortex. *Brain* 119:593–609.

GALLESE V., L. FADIGA, L. FOGASSI, and G. RIZZOLATTI, 2002. Action representation and the inferior parietal lobule. In *Common Mechanisms in Perception and Action: Attention and Performance*, vol. XIX, W. Prinz and B. Hommel, eds. Oxford, England: Oxford University Press, pp. 334–355.

GALLESE, V., and A. GOLDMAN, 1998. Mirror neurons and the simulation theory of mind-reading. *Trends Cogn. Sci.* 12:493–502.

GALLESE, V., A. MURATA, M. KASEDA, N. NIKI, and H. SAKATA, 1994. Deficit of hand preshaping after muscimol injection in monkey parietal cortex. *Neuroreport* 5:1525–1529.

GANGITANO, M., F. M. MOTTAGHY, and A. PASCAL-LEONE, 2001. Phase-specific modulation of cortical motor output during movement observation. *Neuroreport* 12:1489–1492.

GENTILUCCI, M., L. FOGASSI, G. LUPPINO, M. MATELLI, R. CAMARDA, and G. RIZZOLATTI, 1988. Functional organization of inferior area 6 in the macaque monkey. I. Somatotopy and the control of proximal movements. *Exp. Brain Res.* 71:475–490.

GERARDIN, E., A. SIRIGU, S. LEHERICY, J.-B. POLINE, B. GAYMARD, C. MARSAULT, Y. AGID, and D. LE BIHAN, 2000. Partially overlapping neural networks for real and imagined hand movements. *Cereb. Cortex* 10:1093–1104.

GOLDMAN, A., 1989. Interpretation psychologized. *Mind Lang.* 4: 161–185.

GORDON, R., 1986. Folk psychology as simulation. *Mind Lang.* 1: 158–171.

GRAFTON S. T., M. A. ARBIB, L. FADIGA, and G. RIZZOLATTI, 1996. Localization of grasp representations in humans by PET. 2. Observation compared with imagination. *Exp. Brain Res.* 112: 103–111.

GRÈZES, J., N. COSTES, and J. DECETY, 1998. Top-down effect of strategy on the perception of human biological motion: A PET investigation. *Cogn. Neuropsychol.* 15:553–582.

GRÈZES, J., and J. DECETY, 2001. Functional anatomy of execution, mental simulation, observation, and verb generation of actions: A meta-analysis. *Hum. Brain Mapp.* 12:1–19.

HARI, R., N. FORSS, E. KIRVERSKARI, S. AVIKAINEN, S. SALENIUS, and G. RIZZOLATTI, 1998. Activation of human primary motor cortex during action observation: A neuromagnetic study. *Proc. Natl. Acad. Sci. U.S.A.* 95:15061–15065.

HEPP-REYMOND, M.-C., E. J. HUSLER, M. A. MAIER, and H.-X. QI, 1994. Force-related neuronal activity in two regions of the primate ventral premotor cortex. *Can. J. Physiol. Pharmacol.* 72: 571–579.

HEYES, C. M., 2001. Causes and consequences of imitation. *Trends Cogn. Sci.* 5:253–261.

IACOBONI, M., R. P. WOODS, M. BRASS, H. BEKKERING, J. C. MAZZIOTTA, and G. RIZZOLATTI, 1999. Cortical mechanisms of human imitation. *Science* 286:2526–2528.

IACOBONI, M., L. M. KOSKI, M. BRASS, H. BEKKERING, R. P. WOODS, M. C. DUBEAU, J. C. MAZZIOTTA, and G. RIZZOLATTI, 2001. Reafferent copies of imitated actions in the right superior temporal cortex. *Proc. Natl. Acad. Sci. U.S.A.* 98:13995–13999.

JEANNEROD, M., 1994. The representing brain: Neural correlates of motor intention and imagery. *Behav. Brain Sci.* 17:187–245.

JEANNEROD, M., M. A. ARBIB, G. RIZZOLATTI, and H. SAKATA, 1995. Grasping objects: The cortical mechanisms of visuomotor transformation. *Trends Neurosci.* 18:314–320.

JELLEMA, T., C. I. BAKER, M. W. ORAM, and D. I. PERRETT, 2002. Cell populations in the banks of the superior temporal sulcus of the macaque monkey and imitation. In *The Imitative Mind: Development, Evolution and Brain Bases*, A. N. Melzoff and W. Prinz, eds. Cambridge, England: Cambridge University Press, pp. 143–162.

KOHLER, E., C. KEYSERS, M. A. UMILTÀ, L. FOGASSI, V. GALLESE, and G. RIZZOLATTI, 2002. Hearing sounds, understanding actions: Action representation in mirror neurons. *Science* 297:846–848.

KOSKI, L., M. IACOBONI, M.-C. DUBEAU, R. P. WOODS, and J. C. MAZZIOTTA, 2003. Modulation of cortical activity during different imitative behaviors. *J. Neurophysiol.* 89:460–471.

KOSKI, L., A. WOHLSCHLAGER, H. BEKKERING, R. P. WOODS, M.-C. DUBEAU, J. C. MAZZIOTTA, and M. IACOBONI, 2002. Modulation of motor and premotor activity during imitation of target-directed actions. *Cereb. Cortex* 12:847–855.

KRAMS, M., M. F. S. RUSHWORTH, M.-P. DEIBER, R. S. J. FRACKOWIAK, and R. E. PASSINGHAM, 1998. The preparation, execution, and suppression of copied movements in the human brain. *Exp. Brain Res.* 120:386–398.

KURATA, K., and J. TANJI, 1986. Premotor cortex neurons in macaques: Activity before distal and proximal forelimb movements. *J. Neurosci.* 6:403–411.

MANTEY, S., R. I. SCHUBOTZ, and D. Y. VON CRAMON, 2003. Premotor cortex in observing erroneous action: An fMRI study. *Cogn. Brain Res.* 15:296–307.

MATELLI, M., R. CAMARDA, M. GLICKSTEIN, and G. RIZZOLATTI, 1986. Afferent and efferent projections of the inferior area 6 in the macaque monkey. *J. Comp. Neurol.* 251:281–298.

MATELLI, M., and G. LUPPINO, 1997. Functional anatomy of human motor cortical areas. In *Handbook of Neuropsychology*, vol. XI, F. Boller and J. Grafman, eds. Amsterdam: Elsevier, pp. 9–26.

MATELLI, M., G. LUPPINO, A. MURATA, and H. SAKATA, 1994. Independent anatomical circuits for reaching and grasping linking the inferior parietal sulcus and inferior area 6 in macaque monkey. *Soc. Neurosci. Abstr.* 20:404.4.

MATELLI, M., G. LUPPINO, and G. RIZZOLATTI, 1985. Patterns of cytochrome oxidase activity in the frontal agranular cortex of macaque monkey. *Behav. Brain Res.* 18:125–137.

MERLEAU-PONTY, M., 1962. *Phenomenology of Perception.* London: Routledge and Kegan Paul.

MOUNTCASTLE, V. B., J. C. LYNCH, A. GEORGOPOULOS, H. SAKATA, and C. ACUNA, 1975. Posterior parietal association cortex of the monkey: Command functions for operations within extrapersonal space. *J. Neurophysiol.* 38:871–908.

MURATA, A., L. FADIGA, L. FOGASSI, V. GALLESE, V. RAOS, and G. RIZZOLATTI, 1997. Object representation in the ventral premotor cortex (area F5) of the monkey. *J. Neurophysiol.* 78:2226–2230.

MURATA, A., V. GALLESE, G. LUPPINO, M. KASEDA, and H. SAKATA, 2000. Selectivity for the shape, size and orientation of objects for grasping in neurons of monkey parietal area AIP. *J. Neurophysiol.* 83:2580–2601.

NISHITANI, N., and R. HARI, 2000. Temporal dynamics of cortical representation for action. *Proc. Natl. Acad. Sci. U.S.A.* 97:913–918.

NISHITANI, N., and R. HARI, 2002. Viewing lip forms: Cortical dynamics. *Neuron* 36:1211–1220.

PANDYA, D. N., and B. SELTZER, 1982. Intrinsic connections and architectonics of posterior parietal cortex in the rhesus monkey. *J. Comp. Neurol.* 204:204–210.

PARSONS, L. M., P. T. FOX, J. HUNTER DOWN, T. GLASS, T. B. HIRSCH, C. C. MARTIN, P. A. JERABEK, and J. L. LANCASTER, 1995. Use of implicit motor imagery for visual shape discrimination as revealed by PET. *Nature* 375:54–58.

PENFIELD, W., and T. RASMUSSEN, 1950. *The Cerebral Cortex of Man: A Clinical Study of Localization of Function.* New York: Macmillan.

PERRETT, D. I., M. H. HARRIES, R. BEVAN, S. THOMAS, P. J. BENSON, A. J. MISTLIN, et al., 1989. Frameworks of analysis for the neural representation of animate objects and actions. *J. Exp. Biol.* 146: 87–113.

PETRIDES, M., and D. N. PANDYA, 1984. Projections to the frontal cortex from the posterior parietal region in the rhesus monkey. *J. Comp. Neurol.* 228:105–116.

PETRIDES, M., and D. N. PANDYA, 1994. Comparative architectonic analysis of the human and the macaque frontal cortex. In

Handbook of Neuropsychology, vol. IX, F. Boller and J. Grafman, eds. Amsterdam: Elsevier, pp. 17–58.

RIZZOLATTI, G., and M. A. ARBIB, 1998. Language within our grasp. *Trends Neurosci.* 21:188–194.

RIZZOLATTI, G., R. CAMARDA, L. FOGASSI, M. GENTILUCCI, G. LUPPINO, and M. MATELLI, 1988. Functional organization of inferior area 6 in the macaque monkey. II. Area F5 and the control of distal movements. *Exp. Brain Res.* 71:491–507.

RIZZOLATTI, G., L. FADIGA, L. FOGASSI, and V. GALLESE, 1996. Premotor cortex and the recognition of motor actions. *Cogn. Brain Res.* 3:131–141.

RIZZOLATTI, G., L. FADIGA, M. MATELLI, V. BETTINARDI, E. PAULESU, D. PERANI, and G. FAZIO, 1996. Localization of grasp representations in humans by PET: 1. Observation versus execution. *Exp. Brain Res.* 111:246–252.

RIZZOLATTI, G., L. FOGASSI, and V. GALLESE, 2001. Neurophysiological mechanisms underlying the understanding and imitation of action. *Nat. Rev. Neurosci.* 2:661–670.

RIZZOLATTI, G., L. FOGASSI, and V. GALLESE, 2002. Motor and cognitive functions of the ventral premotor cortex. *Curr. Opin. Neurobiol.* 12:149–154.

RIZZOLATTI, G., and G. LUPPINO, 2001. The cortical motor system. *Neuron* 31:889–901.

RIZZOLATTI, G., C. SCANDOLARA, M. GENTILUCCI, and M. MATELLI, 1981. Afferent properties of periarcuate neurons in macaque monkey. I. Somatosensory responses. *Behav. Brain Res.* 2:125–146.

RIZZOLATTI, G., C. SCANDOLARA, M. MATELLI, and M. GENTILUCCI, 1981. Afferent properties of periarcuate neurons in macaque monkey. II. Visual responses. *Behav. Brain Res.* 2:147–163.

SAKATA, H., M. TAIRA, A. MURATA, and S. MINE, 1995. Neural mechanisms of visual guidance of hand action in the parietal cortex of the monkey. *Cereb. Cortex* 5:429–438.

SCHUBOTZ, R. I., and D. Y. VON CRAMON, 2001. Functional organization of the lateral premotor cortex: fMRI reveals different regions activated by anticipation of object properties, location and speed. *Cogn. Brain Res.* 11:97–112.

SHIKATA, E., Y. TANAKA, H. NAKAMURA, M. TAIRA, and H. SAKATA, 1996. Selectivity of the parietal visual neurons in 3D orientation of surface of stereoscopic stimuli. *Neuroreport* 7:2389–2394.

SIMON, O., J. F. MANGIN, L. COHEN, D. LE BIHAN, and S. DEHAENE, 2002. Topographical layout of hand, eye, calculation, and language-related areas in the human parietal lobe. *Neuron* 33: 475–487.

STAMENOV, M. I., and V. GALLESE, eds., 2002. *Mirror Neurons and the Evolution of Brain and Language. Advances in Consciousness Research.* Amsterdam: John Benjamins Publishing Co.

STRAFELLA, A. P., and T. PAUS, 2000. Modulation of cortical excitability during action observation: A transcranial magnetic stimulation study. *Neuroreport* 11:2289–2292.

TAIRA, M., S. MINE, A. P. GEORGOPOULOS, A. MURATA, and H. SAKATA, 1990. Parietal cortex neurons of the monkey related to the visual guidance of hand movement. *Exp. Brain Res.* 83:29–36.

TANAKA, S., and T. INUI, 2002. Cortical involvement for action imitation of hand/arm postures versus finger configurations: An fMRI study. *Neuroreport* 13:1599–1602.

TANAKA, S., T. INUI, S. IWAKI, J. KONISHI, and T. NAKAI, 2001. Neural substrates involved in imitating finger configurations: An fMRI study. *Neuroreport* 12:1171–1174.

THORNDYKE, E. L., 1898. Animal intelligence: An experimental study of the associative process in animals. *Psychol. Rev. Monogr.* 2:551–553.

TOMASELLO, M., A. C. KRUGER, and H. H. RATNER, 1993. Cultural learning. *Behav. Brain Sci.* 16:495–552.

UMILTÀ, M. A., E. KOHLER, V. GALLESE, L. FOGASSI, L. FADIGA, C. KEYZERS, and G. RIZZOLATTI, 2001. I know what you are doing: A neurophysiological study. *Neuron* 31:155–165.

VISALBERGHI, E., and D. FRAGASZY, 2001. Do monkeys ape? Ten years after. In *Imitation in Animals and Artifacts*, K. Dautenhahn and C. Nehaniv, eds. Boston, Mass.: MIT Press.

VON BONIN, G., and P. BAILEY, 1947. *The Neocortex of Macaca mulatta*. Urbana, Ill.: University of Illinois Press.

WEBSTER, M. J., J. BACHEVALIER, and L. G. UNGERLEIDER, 1994. Connections of inferior temporal areas TEO and TE with parietal and frontal cortex in macaque monkeys. *Cereb. Cortex* 4:470–483.

WHITEN, A., and R. HAM, 1992. On the nature and evolution of imitation in the animal kingdom: Reappraisal of a century of research. *Adv. Study Behav.* 21:239–283.

32 The Representation of Action

SCOTT T. GRAFTON AND RICHARD B. IVRY

ABSTRACT This chapter examines how goal-directed actions are organized from a cognitive perspective. Actions are characterized at a behavioral, cognitive, and structural level within the central nervous system. Three broad approaches are reviewed: context-guided, ideomotor, and process models of action. Context-guided models are a generalization of stimulus-response mapping, embedded in a context that dictates task demands. Ideomotor models begin with a task goal that leads to the retrieval of action memory. Process models focus on constraints associated with action representation: how is information transformed, and how does that influence performance? Together, these approaches provide complementary insight into the organization of complex behavior.

Our ability to manipulate the environment with our hands is a remarkable evolutionary achievement. An everyday task such as tying one's shoes demands exquisite coordination between the hands. This action requires complex, integrative movements of the two hands. Moreover, there must be sufficient flexibility to allow for contextual variations, such as the stiffness of the laces, desired tightness of the shoes, or reorientation of the action, for example tying someone else's shoes. Dexterous behavior is readily accomplished with minimal thought of the procedures to perform the task or the eventual outcome of the action (Bernstein, 1967).

A fundamental problem in neuroscience is to understand goal-directed behavior in terms of the underlying cognitive structure and to link this to neural implementation. This remains a difficult problem because of the motor system's ability to create new motor combinations, to use varied implementations, and to adapt an action representation in response to a changing environment. To date there is no comprehensive model that adequately accounts for action representation. However, by examining a set of contemporary cognitive models for action representation, we can develop a perspective on the overall problem. In this chapter three broad cognitive approaches are reviewed: context-guided, ideomotor, and process models. The first two approaches provide basic insights into how actions are represented. Process models focus on constraints associated with these representations: how is information transformed, and

how does that influence performance? Although the chapter is organized around the different approaches, they overlap in substantial ways and therefore should be viewed as complementary.

Context-guided models

In context-guided models, action representations are linked to specific environmental stimuli. There is a long-standing tradition of viewing an action as a response to a stimulus. In this setting, action formation is a reaction to an external cause. This level of analysis can be traced to Descartes, who first defined actions in terms of perceptual events (Descartes, 1664). The subsequent emergence of experimental methods that largely relied on reaction time measurements allowed action to be explained in terms of the physical properties of stimuli (Donders, 1862 [1969]), and with the emergence of behaviorism this became the dominant paradigm in psychology. This approach facilitated the rapid advancement of theories of performance in which complex sets of stimuli and responses could be functionally linked by simple associative principles.

An important departure from strict behaviorism was to consider the stimulus-response pairing as more than a mapping or rule between input and output. This mapping, together with the context, could be considered as an action representation. Context-guided action-perception pairings are ubiquitous. We depress the brake pedal for a red light and the accelerator for a green light not because the colors demand these actions but because these arbitrary symbols have become associated with certain behavioral goals, such as avoiding collisions. In terms of implementation, at the cellular level there is clear evidence for neurons in the dorsal premotor cortex of nonhuman primate that map arbitrary stimuli to limb movements (Wise, Weinrich, and Mauritz, 1983) and more generally map body parts to objects and locations (Hoshi and Tanji, 2000). Premotor neurons in the monkey show learning-related changes in activity over time as a contextually guided association is acquired (Mitz, Godschalk, and Wise, 1991). Lesions of this area of premotor cortex in humans lead to an impairment in learning new visuomotor associations, such as making a gesture in response to a spatial or color cue (Halsband and Freund, 1990).

SCOTT T. GRAFTON Department of Psychological and Brain Sciences, Dartmouth College, Hanover, N.H.
RICHARD B. IVRY Department of Psychology, University of California at Berkeley, Berkeley, Calif.

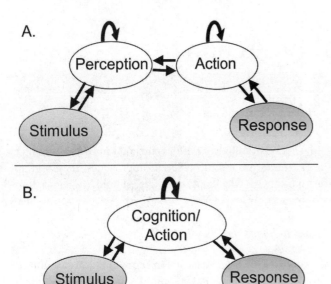

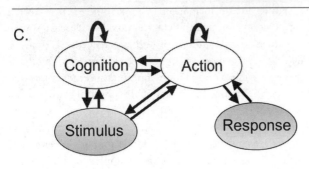

FIGURE 32.1. Different formulations of the perception-action interface. In *A*, perception and action are considered separable. In *B*, action and cognition are embodied in the same representational structure. In *C*, there is a direct path from stimuli to action and an indirect path via cognition, which is separable from action.

The notion of context-guided representation is important because it allows us to ask what is actually being represented (figure 32.1). Behavioral studies are inconclusive in determining if context-guided representations are formed with respect to the perceptual features of the task, the movements themselves, or some commonly coded representational structure. Physiological data also underscore the challenge of identifying specific representational structures. At the neuronal level there appears to be no evidence for a unitary representational structure for action. Within a single neuron it is possible to identify perceptual-based, response-based, and combined sensorimotor firing patterns. For example, when a monkey is trained to make pointing movements with a joystick in response to visual cues, many dorsal premotor neurons have increased firing rates to either the location of the instructional cue or the direction of the desired limb movement. However, there are also cells demonstrating both location and direction coding at different times within a single behavioral trial (Shen and Alexander, 1997).

An important aspect of context-guided actions is the reference frame used to define that representation. When we reach for our shoelaces, do we relate the location of the laces in allocentric or egocentric space? If egocentric, is the reference frame defined with respect to the eyes, the hand, the joints required to achieve the action, or some combination of these (see, e.g., Soechting and Flanders, 1992)? How are transformations achieved from one reference frame to another in the perception-action cycle? Physiological recordings suggest a multiplicity of reference frames within common regions of the parietal lobe (Colby, 1998). This proximity allows for the sharing and transformation of information across frames of reference. Anatomical projections from parietal to premotor areas provide information on the current state of the system and the external environment, represented in one or perhaps many frames of reference.

At the output level the limb must ultimately generate a useful movement. In terms of representation, we again need to consider whether movements are defined in an intrinsic or extrinsic coordinate system. Do we move the limb to achieve particular trajectories or final limb configurations, or at a level independent of kinematics in which we achieve a final goal location? Irrespective of the coordinate system used, how does the system accommodate changes of limb dynamics? Our ability to respond to contextual changes is evident when we succeed in tying our shoes even when wearing gloves on a wintry day, or in altering the force of our actions if we see that the lace is frayed.

By altering the dynamics in experimental settings, these problems become tangible. For example, when subjects learn to control the position of a cursor by moving a joystick that has a complex force field applied to it, learning, when assessed by altering the postural configuration of the limb, occurs in an intrinsic, muscle-centered coordinate frame (Shadmehr and Moussavi, 2000). However, after training with one arm, transfer is found only when the altered dynamics are preserved in terms of an extrinsic frame of reference (Criscimagna-Hemminger et al., 2003). Interestingly, there is no transfer if training is completed in the nondominant hand and transfer is to the dominant hand. This observation suggests that the representation accessed following intermanual transfer is generated in the dominant hemisphere and may be distinct from the representation that controls performance when the same limb is used but in another context.

Studies of sequence learning provide an impressive demonstration of the context dependency of stimulus-response associations. On the serial reaction time task (Nissen, Willingham, and Hartman, 1989), subjects press four individual keys with the fingers in response to spatially distinct visual cues. If the order of the cues is presented in a repeating pattern, for example a 12-element sequence, implicit learning is measured by the reduction in response times relative to blocks in which the stimulus sequence is set randomly. In this type of sequence learning there is typically good transfer across responses systems (Keele et al., 1995). If representational structures were strictly dichotomous, one would conclude that learning is perceptual. However, if the stimulus-response mapping used during training is incompatible, poor transfer is observed following a condition in which a compatible stimulus-response mapping is introduced and the transfer sequence involves a new response sequence but retains the original perceptual sequence (Willingham, 1999; Willingham et al., 2000). Under these conditions, transfer is observed when the response sequence remains invariant, even though this introduces a new stimulus sequence. Thus, the form of representation is likely dependent on task demands.

There is evidence that the level of representation in sequence learning changes over the time course of the training (Bapi and Doya, 1998; Bapi, Doya, and Harner, 2000; Koch and Hoffmann, 2000). For example, early in training, learning may be primarily related to the ordering of perceptual events and the formation of successive stimulus-response associations. With prolonged practice and repetition, learning appears to shift to a response-based level of representation (Karni et al., 1998; Rand et al., 2000). With enough practice we have the capacity to make highly specific, automated movements irrespective of perceptual instructions, and the degree of transfer to other response systems is reduced. Imaging studies of sequence learning demonstrate that retrieval of sequential structure at the response level of representation involves premotor areas in the medial wall of the superior frontal gyrus, including the supplementary motor area (SMA) and adjacent pre-SMA (Gerloff et al., 1997; Shima and Tanji, 2000; Bischoff-Grethe et al., 2003) (figure 32.2).

The preceding discussion suggests that the duration of training or context in which sequence acquisition takes place may constrain the level of representation. However, the form of representation is unlikely to simply reflect the level of expertise. Learning may be perceptual, effector-specific, or goal-based, related to the environmental consequences of the task (Hazeltine, 2002). Moreover, multiple forms of representation may emerge over the course of learning, reflecting constraints associated with different associative mechanisms. Context-dependent representations may require access to inputs from multiple sources, whereas more modular representations may be formed within stimulus-response channels (Keele et al., 2003).

Context-guided learning models are closely related to reinforcement learning algorithms where there is an iterative rule and some form of credit assignment leading to a change in the response (Sutton and Barto, 1998). The credit assignment need not be tied to a specific goal or distal effect. The flexibility of reinforcement learning allows for both supervised and unsupervised forms of learning and includes instrumental conditioning and paired associative learning. When we learn to tie our shoes, we perform thousands of iterations. Unlike reinforcement learning, however, the final goal is not experienced prior to its eventual achievement. Context-guided learning is insufficient for this sort of circumstance, in which there is (1) no predefined mapping or (2) the need to create an entirely new type of response. A comprehensive motor learning model would need to include generative processes for creating novel sensorimotor mapping rules and new forms of motor output.

Context-guided models allow one to consider how actions are selected in a world in which simultaneous inputs provide sources of convergence and competition for the selection of actions, suggesting a need for some form of control system, at least when performing in novel contexts or under conditions in which habitual behaviors are nonoptimal (Shallice et al., 1989). The importance of such control is demonstrated by certain clinical syndromes. Patients with inferior frontal lesions can develop pathological utilization behavior such that their actions are dictated completely by a salient

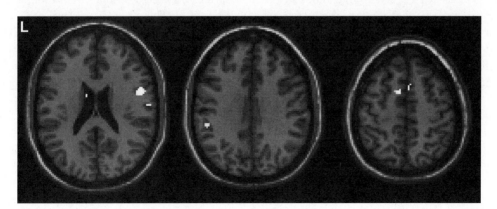

FIGURE 32.2. Functional localization of sequential action retrieval. As subjects perform an implicit sequential task, there is activation of the right ventral premotor cortex (left panel), left inferior parietal cortex (middle panel), and bilateral SMA (right panel) specific to the pattern of responses. Image left is left brain. (Adapted from Bischoff-Grethe et al., 2003.)

stimulus, even when highly inappropriate. For example, when three sets of eyeglasses were presented on the table, a patient proceeded to put them all on, one over the other (Lhermitte, 1983, 1986; Lhermitte, Pillon, and Serdaru, 1986). Slavery to stimulus-bound responses is also observed in the checking behavior exhibited by patients with obsessive-compulsive disorder (Ridley, 1994).

Ideomotor models

Ideomotor models seek to characterize the representation of action based on internal, volitional causes of action. In contrast to context-dependent models, they tend to ignore sensory causes. Actions emerge from internal mental operations rather than external triggers. A major advantage of the ideomotor approach is the formalization of a goal as a causal determinant. As such, ideomotor models work backward in time, with the goal defined initially, followed by a characterization of the implementation processes needed to achieve that goal. Early characterizations of the internal causes for actions were based in large part on self-introspection (James, 1890). Backward causation was first addressed by making a distinction between the goal state itself (a result of an action) and its cognitive representation (linked to the causal implementation).

Ideomotor models of action representation are historically based on findings in patients with apraxia. Apraxia is a disturbance of goal-directed motor behavior that is characterized by an inability to perform previously learned movements in the absence of weakness or sensory defects (Leiguarda and Marsden, 2000). For example, a patient asked to gesture how she would use a comb might fumble with her hand, tapping her head with a fist. Or she might use her fingers as a comb rather than miming gripping an imaginary comb. Success on tasks used to assess apraxia typically requires that the patient identify the action associated with a tool, access the appropriate movement representations, and implement the correct action. In addition, if the object is not presented or modeled, the patient must process linguistic stimuli in order to identify the test object.

Apraxia is more common and severe following left hemisphere lesions than following right hemisphere lesions (De Renzi, Motti, and Nichelli, 1980; Haaland, Harrington, and Knight, 2000). A left hemisphere specialization for action representation is supported by imaging studies showing activation of this hemisphere during action retrieval linked to tool use (figure 32.3). There is also greater left hemispheric involvement for sequential learning with either hand (Grafton, Hazeltine, and Ivry, 2002), as well as asymmetrical patterns of intermanual transfer following training in novel dynamic environments (Grafton, Hazeltine, and Ivry, 2002; Criscimagna-Hemminger et al., 2003).

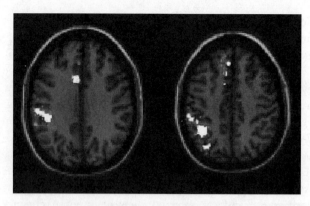

FIGURE 32.3. Common areas of activation among 12 right-handed subjects during gesture retrieval with either the right or left hand. Areas of activation are shown in white at two axial levels spanning the inferior parietal lobule (left section) and intraparietal sulcus (right section). Irrespective of hand, there is consistent activation of the left parietal cortex (image left is left brain).

A recent outgrowth of ideomotor models has been the development of simulation theory (Jeannerod, 2001). The central idea is that mental states of actions involve simulations of the processes associated with the execution of that action. In effect, action and cognition overlap, as shown in figure 32.1B. That is, conceptual knowledge of actions exists through reference to overt actions. Numerous studies have shown the tight linkage between imagined and real actions (e.g., Parsons, 1994; Johnson, 2000). This simulation idea is also supported by functional imaging studies of mental imagery that demonstrate overlap in activation patterns for real, observed, and imagined movements (Sirigu et al., 1995; Decety, 1996; Grafton et al., 1996; Johnson et al., 2001, 2002).

It should be noted that there is only partial overlap of brain areas for these different functions, and in some cases there is a clear distinction between the premotor areas engaged during action ideation and execution (Tyszka et al., 1994; Stephan et al., 1995). It is also not clear if the relationships between ideation, observation, and execution are symmetrical. There is good evidence for motor areas being recruited when we think about action-related concepts (Martin et al., 1995; Barsalou et al., 2003). However, it is not clear that the conceptual areas are recruited for action planning and implementation. Nor is there compelling evidence that lesions of areas associated with action implementation produce deficits in the conceptual knowledge of actions (Heilman, Rothi, and Valenstein, 1982). As will be discussed in the next section, there are many circumstances in which motor selection and control can occur with minimal or no conscious thought.

These patient and imaging studies provide evidence for the distinction between representations for a goal (a distal effect in the future) and the action (the actual implementation leading to the goal). However, goal states are elusive, unobservable entities and remain difficult to manipulate experimentally. As a result, a comprehensive conceptual framework for characterizing action goals based entirely on evidence from apraxia patients and imaging of simulated action is incomplete.

Process models

The emphasis in context-dependent and ideomotor models is on the form of action representation. Process models address the same question but through an analysis of the transformation of mental representations. By exploring constraints on actions, a characterization of the representations is possible. For example, in an overlearned task such as shoe tying, the relative timing for each step in the task, such as forming the loops with the laces, remains relatively constant across different contexts. This temporal structure suggests that the action consists of invariant properties that may be associated with invariance due to central mechanisms (Terzuolo and Viviani, 1980) once peripheral causes of invariance are also excluded (Gentner, 1987). Here we examine two process models that reveal insights into how actions are coupled in space and time.

REACH AND GRASP   When we reach and grasp the laces of our shoes, there is remarkable constancy in the timing between the peak acceleration of the reach and the opening of the fingers to match the size of the laces (Jeannerod, 1984). A key point is that the rate of transport is adjusted according to the size of the required hand aperture. This temporal invariance demonstrates the capacity for anticipation within the motor system and reveals that action representation for transport is formed with respect to the demands of the grasping component (Gentilluci et al., 1991). At a more abstract level, anticipation can also be seen in the grasp affordance, that is, the hand orientation and shaping used to grasp the object. The orientation will vary depending on whether we are picking up the laces to tie them or picking up the laces as a means of picking up the shoes (Rosenbaum et al., 1992). Behavioral evidence suggests that the processes associated with reaching and grasping are relatively distinct but interact in specific ways. This has been well-supported in neuropsychological and physiological studies. In both human and nonhuman primates, there is a circuit between the superior parietal lobule and dorsal premotor cortex that is critical for locating the hand in space and central for reaching (Andersen and Zipser, 1988; Caminiti et al., 1991; Andersen et al., 1997; Battaglia-Mayer et al., 2001; Marconi et al., 2001). Lesions of the superior parietal lobule lead to optic ataxia, an impairment of visually guided reaching (Perenin and Vighetto, 1988). Areas specific for grasping are located

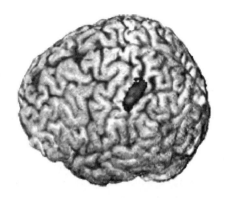

FIGURE 32.4.   Localization of anterior intraparietal activation during contralateral, right-hand grasping compared to pointing in a normal subject. Results are superimposed on a superior oblique view of the left hemisphere.

in the anterior intraparietal sulcus and ventral premotor cortex (Sakata et al., 1992; Jeannerod et al., 1995; Sakata et al., 1995; Murata et al., 2000). Circumscribed lesions of the anterior parietal cortex in humans can lead to deficits in hand shaping, with preservation of arm transport (Binkofski et al., 1998). Grasp-specific areas can also be identified with functional magnetic resonance imaging in normal subjects (figure 32.4). The neural substrates for both reach and grasp lie within the "where" or "how" visual processing stream (Ungerleider and Mishkin, 1982; Goodale et al., 1991).

Another important feature of process models is that motor output can be modified in real time as task goals change. Experimentally, this is demonstrated by perturbing the target during a reach and observing that corrections can occur without vision of the arm and prior to the availability of proprioceptive feedback. Such manipulations presumably mimic the fact that, although targets in a natural environment are usually stable, accurate reaching is impeded by the presence of noise in the motor system (Harris and Wolpert, 1998). To minimize the effects of this noise while sustaining fast, accurate movements, there must be an internal model estimating the current state of the motor system in real time that is available for revising ongoing motor activity. The intraparietal sulcus of the parietal lobe appears to be critical for maintaining and continuously updating an internal representation of the state of the body with respect to the world (Wolpert, Goodbody, and Hussain, 1998; Desmurget et al., 2001). This information would be used for generating error signals based on an efference copy of the motor commands and evolving sensory feedback (Desmurget and Grafton, 2000). Patients with bilateral parietal lesions have difficulty using such an online corrective mechanism, even though their initial reaching movements are relatively spared (Grea et al., 2002). Similarly, transcranial magnetic stimulation of parietal cortex in normal subjects at the onset of a reaching movement will block their ability to update a reaching movement to a target that has been displaced (Desmurget et al., 1999).

In prehension experiments, many features of the eye and hand movements are produced with minimal influence of cognitive control, and in fact may not be accessible to conscious control. This is evident when one plays sports—rapid body adjustments are executed without our awareness. Unwanted corrections can emerge in patients with parietal lobe lesions. Patients may make online adjustments during reaching movements even when these adjustments are counterproductive toward achieving a motor goal (Pisella et al., 2000). Conscious intervention can also contaminate learned skills under normal conditions. When we try to speed up or slow down a well-learned action such as shoe tying, performance often deteriorates.

Immediate action coding in these circumstances is likely not mediated by the same neural circuitry as action planning for distal effects such as goal selection. Patients may show an inability to consciously perceive or describe sensory information used to generate a motor behavior, but will perform the behavior well under natural conditions. For example, the visual agnosia patient D.F. could not perceive shape or orientation when tested with an explicit perceptual test. However, she could readily "post" an envelope through a slot with the proper hand orientation, a skill that required similar knowledge of orientation and target location (Goodale et al., 1991). This dissociation has been taken to imply that the intact dorsal how pathway allows for unconscious, automatic visually guided actions, including reach and grasp, whereas the damaged ventral what pathway is essential for object recognition and conscious recognition.

An alternative interpretation emphasizes differences in the representations and processes used to guide actions within the dorsal and ventral streams. When patient D.F. indicates the orientation of the object by reaching for the slot, the action is directly specified by the visual stimulus. In the test used to infer conscious knowledge, the action is more symbolic. D.F. observes the slot and attempts to match the orientation of her wrist and the slot without actually reaching. In this condition, the action requires a somewhat arbitrary translation between the stimulus and response, given the symbolic nature of the response.

BIMANUAL STUDIES   Recent studies on bimanual reaching suggest that there are qualitative differences between actions that are guided by either direct or symbolic representations (Diedrichsen et al., 2001). In these experiments, subjects make two pointing movements on each trial, one with the left hand and one with the right hand. The movement direction for each hand can be forward or sideways. Thus, the bimanual combination is classified as congruent (both forward or both sideways) or incongruent (one forward and one lateral). The critical manipulation centers on the manner in which the movements are cued (figure 32.5). In the symbolic cuing condition, the four possible target locations (two end locations for each hand) are visible at all times, and the letters F and S indicate the forward and sideways target locations, respectively. One letter is presented in the left visual field to indicate the left-hand movement and the other letter is presented in the right visual field to indicate the right-hand movement. In the direct cuing condition, the target locations are cued by the onset of the target circles, one appearing on each side.

In the symbolic condition, congruent responses are initiated faster than incongruent responses, consistent with previous findings that people show a strong preference for symmetrical bimanual movements. However, when the movements are directly cued, the subjects are much faster to initiate their movements overall, and, more important, congruency has no effect on reaction time. In fact, reaction times on bimanual trials are similar to those obtained on unimanual trials. Thus, the advantage for congruent bimanual actions cannot be attributed to motor programming or execution, as has been typically assumed in the motor control literature (Spijkers and Heuer, 1995; Andres et al., 1999; Cattaert, Semjen, and Summers, 1999; Kilner et al., 2003). These processes should be the same in the symbolic and direct cuing conditions, yet interference is observed only in the former.

The results suggest a distinction in the processes that constrain performance for actions that are symbolically or directly cued. One hypothesis centers on the idea that the two forms of cues result in the action goals being conceptualized in different ways. For symbolically cued actions, the goals are likely represented, at least initially, as abstract spatial codes specifying the desired movement trajectory or path. On congruent trials, these codes would be in correspondence; on incongruent trials, they would be a source of conflict. Not only are there conflicts between the component trajectories required for each hand, but the cues are presented on the left and right sides of the screen and must be assigned to the left and right hands (Diedrichsen et al., 2003). The costs observed on incongruent trials reflects interactions arising due to conflict between the various spatial codes defining the stimulus positions, the required trajectories, and the two hands (Kornblum, Hasbroucq, and Osman, 1990).

In contrast, action goals for directly cued movements are unlikely to be specified in terms of abstract trajectories or movement paths. Rather, the goals are related to the endpoint locations. For direct reaching the degree of conceptual overlap is similar for congruent and incongruent movements. Both require the representation of two distinct locations. The lack of a cost on direct bimanual relative to unimanual trials suggests that the representation of multiple locations can be generated and maintained as well as that of

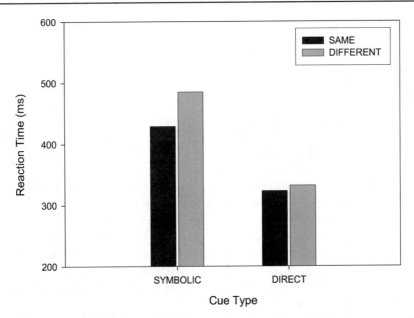

FIGURE 32.5   *Top:* Method to compare symbolic and direct cuing of reaching movements. Movements were either forward or sideways. In the symbolic condition, the letters F and S cued the required direction for each hand. In the direct condition, two circles appeared, with the location of the left and right circles indicating the target locations for the left and right hand movements, respectively. The movements of the two hands could either be in the same or different directions. The example shows a different direction trial with the arrows schematics of the movement paths. *Bottom:* Reaction times for the four conditions, averaged over the left and right hands. Directly cued movements were much faster and showed no cost on trials requiring movements of different directions. (Adapted from Diedrichsen et al., 2001.)

a single location. It should be noted that for either direct or symbolic actions, the resultant movement requires a translation into a signal that can be used to activate the required muscles. The point here is that the manner in which an action goal is represented, for example in terms of location- or trajectory-based codes, will help define constraints manifest during the performance of these actions.

We can consider an experiment in which three types of action cues were used to define multisegment bimanual movements (J. Diedrichsen, E. Hazeltine, and R. B. Ivry, unpublished observations). The segments formed a three-sided box and the orientation of the boxes for the two hands were either congruent (e.g., both U-shaped boxes) or incongruent (e.g., one U- and one C-shaped box). In the direct reaching condition, two target lights appeared on the table surface, one on the left and the other on the right. The subjects reached to these locations. As soon as their hands entered the target locations, new targets appeared indicating the next locations and the subjects were instructed to continue on to the next pair of targets. In this manner, the subjects produced the three-sided trajectories by moving from one direct cue to the next. In the symbolic condition, the four corners of the boxes were illuminated on the table surface at the beginning of the trial. The target shapes for a given trial were presented on a computer monitor, and the subjects reproduced the shapes on the table surface, moving from one corner to the next. In the third condition, the tracing condition, the four corners of the boxes were again illuminated at the start of the trial. The target shapes were then projected directly on the table, and the participants were asked to simply trace the two shapes simultaneously.

The time to initiate each segment was highly sensitive to the manner in which the actions were cued. The direct reaching condition was much easier than the other two conditions, with the onset times for successive segments on incongruent trials only slightly larger than for congruent trials (e.g., 30 ms increase on initial response time). At the other extreme, initiation times were slower by almost 500 ms in the incongruent condition for the symbolic cues. Of greatest interest was the tracing condition. One might suppose that tracing would be similar to the direct cuing condition, since participants simply had to move along the depicted contours from one target location to the next. However, the initiation times were more than 300 ms longer on incongruent trials than congruent trials. The manner in which the action was represented appears to have been radically changed by presenting the full shape prior to the initiation of the movements. We hypothesize that in the symbolic and tracing conditions, the participants represented the goals as target shapes composed of a series of directional vectors. When represented in this manner, interactions between varying spatial codes occurred and led to interference on incongruent trials.

The distinction between symbolic and directly cued actions suggests computational differences in how information is represented and processed within the dorsal and ventral visual streams. Processing models have emphasized the role of the dorsal stream in visually guided actions, including the representation of target locations and the coordinate transformations required for the translation of sensory information into reference frames useful for action (e.g., Flanders et al., 1992; Cohen and Andersen, 2002). With directly cued actions, the goals need not be abstract, and as such may be subject to the mediating effects of more symbolic representations. For example, it has been hypothesized that these representations are relatively immune to visual illusions associated with object recognition processes. Contrast effects are absent when perceived size is inferred from the aperture of a grasping action or the endpoint location of a pointing response (Goodale, 1998). Correspondingly, the lack of interference on incongruent trials in our bimanual reaching studies suggests that processing within the dorsal stream of each hemisphere is relatively immune to processing within the other hemisphere.

Although the dorsal stream may be sufficient for directly cued movements, symbolically cued movements likely require involvement of more ventral visual pathways. With symbolic cues, ventral areas may be necessary for stimulus identification and the mapping of these representations to appropriate motor output, perhaps in conjunction with premotor cortex. By this hypothesis, symbolically mediated actions entail an additional processing stage, one in which the abstract symbols are mapped onto action codes.

There are a number of reasons why the more abstract operations performed within the ventral pathway might lead to processing constraints not observed with direct actions. Psychologically, response selection processes required for linking abstract stimuli to intended actions have been shown to impose a prominent constraint on multitask performance (Pashler, 1994). This form of interference is especially pronounced for tasks involving overlapping representations, such as the abstract, trajectory-based codes we have associated with symbolically cued actions.

The interactions evident for symbolically cued bimanual movements in neurologically healthy subjects is abolished in split-brain patients (Franz et al., 1996; Eliassen, Baynes, and Gazzaniga, 1999). This suggests that the interactions involve callosal pathways. One possibility is that transcallosal interactions are more prominent for representations within the ventral pathway than for representations within the dorsal pathway. Physiological studies provide indirect support for this conjecture. Receptive field size increases as processing progresses along either the dorsal or ventral pathway. However, a prominent feature of inferotemporal cortex is that these neurons respond to stimuli from either visual field (Ito et al., 1995); thus, the input to these cells must come from either hemisphere. Alternatively, the lack of interference for directly cued bimanual movements may reflect reduced representational overlap between such actions. A location-based code entails two distinct target locations for both congruent and incongruent movements.

Recent elaborations of the two-visual-stream model offer a different account of why direct and symbolically cued actions exhibit different forms of constraint. It has been proposed that a third stream involving the inferior parietal cortex is sandwiched between the dorsal and ventral streams (Johnson-Frey, 2003). Moreover, this intermediate pathway is hypothesized to be highly lateralized and specialized for actions based on abstract representations and goals (Schluter et al., 1998, 2001). Damage to inferior parietal cortex in the left hemisphere in humans is associated with the most severe forms of apraxia (Heilman, Rothi, and Valenstein, 1982), and imaging studies show pronounced activation of this region for actions requiring the representation of complex object properties, such as when the actions involve the purposeful manipulation of tools (Johnson and Grafton, 2002).

Involvement of the left inferior parietal cortex may be essential for actions performed without the affordance of direct cues, that is, for actions planned on the basis of internal goals or symbolic cues. This hypothesis assumes that the computations performed within this region are required for symbolically cued movements produced by either hand. Interference would be expected when a single processor is trying to plan two incompatible actions. As such, interference during bimanual actions would be attributed to a functional hemispheric asymmetry for symbolically cued actions. Directly cued movements are not subject to this constraint because of a more symmetrical brain organization for regions involved in visually guided actions. An appealing feature of this laterality hypothesis is that it acknowledges the prominent role of the left hemisphere in the representation of complex, abstract actions.

Conclusion

By taking multiple conceptual approaches, it is possible to build a broad perspective on action representations and examine links between psychological constructs and probable neural mechanisms. A recurring observation is that there appears to be no evidence for a unitary frame of reference or representational structure that forms a comprehensive vocabulary for action representation. Action representations vary as a function of context, construct, and means.

REFERENCES

ANDERSEN, R. A., and D. ZIPSER, 1988. The role of the posterior parietal cortex in coordinate transformations for visual-motor integration. *Can. J. Physiol. Pharmacol.* 66:488–501.

ANDERSEN, R. A., L. H. SNYDER, D. C. BRADLEY, and J. XING, 1997. Multimodal representation of space in the posterior parietal cortex and its use in planning movements. *Annu. Rev. Neurosci.* 20:303–330.

ANDRES, F. G., T. MIMA, A. E. SCHULMAN, J. DICHGANS, M. HALLETT, and C. GERLOFF, 1999. Functional coupling of human cortical sensorimotor areas during bimanual skill acquisition. *Brain* 122:855–870.

BAPI, R. S., and K. DOYA, 1998. Evidence of effector independent and dependent components in motor sequence learning. *Soc. Neurosci. Abstr.* 24:167.

BAPI, R. S., K. DOYA, and A. M. HARNER, 2000. Evidence for effector independent and dependent representations and their differential time course of acquisition during motor sequence learning. *Exp. Brain Res.* 132:149–162.

BARSALOU, L. W., W. KYLE SIMMONS, A. K. BARBEY, and C. D. WILSON, 2003. Grounding conceptual knowledge in modality-specific systems. *Trends. Cogn Sci.* 7:84–91.

BATTAGLIA-MAYER, A., S. FERRAINA, A. GENOVESIO, B. MARCONI, S. SQUATRITO, M. MOLINARI, F. LACQUANITI, and R. CAMINITI, 2001. Eye-hand coordination during reaching. II. An analysis of the relationships between visuomanual signals in parietal cortex and parieto-frontal association projections. *Cereb. Cortex* 11: 528–544.

BERNSTEIN, N. A., 1967. *The Coordination and Regulation of Movements.* New York: Pergamon Press.

BINKOFSKI, F., C. DOHLE, S. POSSE, K. M. STEPHAN, H. HEFTER, R. J. SEITZ, and H. J. FREUND, 1998. Human anterior intra-parietal area subserves prehension: A combined lesion and functional MRI activation study. *Neurology* 50:1253–1259.

BISCHOFF-GRETHE A., K. M. GOEDERT, D. T. WILLINGHAM, and S. T. GRAFTON, 2003. Neural substrates of response-based sequence learning using fMRI. *J. Cogn. Neurosci.* (in press).

CAMINITI, R., P. B. JOHNSON, C. GALLI, S. FERRAINA, and Y. BURNOD, 1991. Making arm movements within different parts of space: The premotor and motor cortical representation of a coordinate system for reaching to visual targets. *J. Neurosci.* 11:1182–1197.

CATTAERT, D., A. SEMJEN, and J. J. SUMMERS, 1999. Simulating a neural cross-talk model for between-hand interference during bimanual circle drawing. *Biol. Cybern.* 81:343–358.

COHEN, Y. E., and R. A. ANDERSEN, 2002. A common reference frame for movement plans in the posterior parietal cortex. *Nat. Rev. Neurosci.* 3:553–562.

COLBY, C. L., 1998. Action oriented spatial reference frames in cortex. *Neuron* 20:15–30.

CRISCIMAGNA-HEMMINGER, S. E., O. DONCHIN, M. S. GAZZANIGA, and R. SHADMEHR, 2003. Learned dynamics of reaching movements generalize from dominant to nondominant arm. *J. Neurophysiol.* 89:168–176.

DE RENZI, E., F. MOTTI, and P. NICHELLI, 1980. Imitating gestures: A quantitative approach to ideomotor apraxia. *Arch. Neurol.* 37:6–10.

DECETY, J., 1996. Do imagined and executed actions share the same neural substrate? *Brain. Res. Cogn. Brain. Res.* 3:87–93.

DESCARTES, R., 1664. *L'homme.* Peris: Theodore Girard.

DESMURGET, M., C. M. EPSTEIN, R. S. TURNER, C. PRABLANC, G. E. ALEXANDER, and S. T. GRAFTON, 1999. Role of the posterior parietal cortex in updating reaching movements to a visual target. *Nat. Neurosci.* 2:563–567.

DESMURGET, M., and S. GRAFTON, 2000. Forward modeling allows feedback control for fast reaching movements. *Trends Cogn. Sci.* 4:423–431.

DESMURGET, M., H. GREA, J. S. GRETHE, C. PRABLANC, G. E. ALEXANDER, and S. T. GRAFTON, 2001. Functional anatomy of nonvisual feedback loops during reaching: A positron emission tomography study. *J. Neurosci.* 21:2919–2928.

DIEDRICHSEN, J., E. HAZELTINE, S. KENNERLEY, and R. B. IVRY, 2001. Moving to directly cued locations abolishes spatial interference during bimanual actions. *Psychol. Sci.* 12:493–498.

DIEDRICHSEN, J., R. B. IVRY, E. HAZELTINE, S. KENNERLEY, and A. COHEN, 2003. Bimanual interference associated with the selection of target locations. *J. Exp. Psychol. Hum. Percept. Perform.* 29:64–77.

DONDERS, F. C., 1862 (1969). On the speed of mental processes. *Acta Psychol.* 30:412–431.

ELIASSEN, J. C., K. BAYNES, and M. S. GAZZANIGA, 1999. Direction information coordinated via the posterior third of the corpus callosum during bimanual movements. *Exp. Brain Res.* 128:573–577.

FLANDERS, M., S. I. HELMS TILLERY, and J. F. SOECHTING, 1992. Early stages in a sensory motor transformation. *Behav. Brain Sci.* 15:309–362.

FRANZ, E. A., A. C. ELIASSON, R. B. IVRY, and M. S. GAZZANIGA, 1996. Dissociation of spatial and temporal coupling in the bimanual movements of callosotomy patients. *Psychol. Sci.* 7:306–310.

GENTILUCCI, M., U. CASTIELLO, M. L. CORRADINI, M. SCARPA, C. UMILTÁ, and G. RIZZOLATTI, 1991. Influence of different types of grasping on the transport component of prehension movements. *Neuropsychologia* 29:361–378.

GENTNER, D. R., 1987. Timing of skilled motor performance: Tests of the proportional duration model. *Psychol. Rev.* 94:255–276.

GERLOFF, C., B. CORWELL, R. CHEN, M. HALLETT, and L. G. COHEN, 1997. Stimulation over the human supplementary motor area interferes with the organization of future elements in complex motor sequences. *Brain* 120:1587–1602.

GOODALE, M. A., 1998. Vision for perception and vision for action in the primate brain. *Novartis. Found. Symp.* 218:21–34 [discussion 34–39].

GOODALE, M. A., A. D. MILNER, L. S. JAKOBSON, and D. P. CAREY, 1991. A neurological dissociation between perceiving objects and grasping them. *Nature* 349:154–156.

GRAFTON, S.T., M. A. ARBIB, L. FADIGA, and G. RIZZOLATTI, 1996. Localization of grasp representations in humans by positron emission tomography. 2. Observation compared with imagination. *Exp. Brain Res.* 112:103–111.

GRAFTON, S. T., E. HAZELTINE, and R. B. IVRY, 2002. Motor sequence learning with the nondominant left hand: A PET functional imaging study. *Exp. Brain Res.* 146:369–378.

GREA, H., L. PISELLA, Y. ROSSETTI, M. DESMURGET, C. TILIKETE, S. GRAFTON, C. PRABLANC, and A. VIGHETTO, 2002. A lesion of the posterior parietal cortex disrupts on-line adjustments during aiming movements. *Neuropsychologia* 40:2471–2480.

HAALAND, K. Y., D. L. HARRINGTON, and R. T. KNIGHT, 2000. Neural representations of skilled movement. *Brain* 123:2306–2313.

HALSBAND, U., and H. J. FREUND, 1990. Premotor cortex and conditional motor learning in man. *Brain* 113:207–222.

HARRIS, C. M., and D. M. WOLPERT, 1998. Signal-dependent noise determines motor planning. *Nature* 394:780–784.

HAZELTINE, E., 2002. The representational nature of sequence learning: evidence for goal-based codes. In *Common Mechanisms in Perception and Action: Attention and Performance*, XIX, W. Prinz and B. Hommel, eds. Oxford, England: Oxford University Press.

HEILMAN, K. M., L. J. ROTHI, and E. VALENSTEIN, 1982. Two forms of ideomotor apraxia. *Neurology* 32:342–346.

HOSHI, E., and J. TANJI, 2000. Integration of target and body-part information in the premotor cortex when planning action. *Nature* 408:466–470.

ITO, M., H. TAMURA, I. FUJITA, and K. TANAKA, 1995. Size and position invariance of neuronal responses in monkey inferotemporal cortex. *J. Neurophysiol.* 73:218–226.

JAMES, W., 1890. *Principles of Psychology.* New York: Holt.

JEANNEROD, M., 1984. The timing of natural prehension movements. *J. Mot. Behav.* 16:235–254.

JEANNEROD, M., 2001. Neural simulation of action: A unifying mechanism for motor cognition. *NeuroImage* 14:S103–S109.

JEANNEROD, M., M. A. ARBIB, G. RIZZOLATTI, and H. SAKATA, 1995. Grasping objects: The cortical mechanisms of visuomotor transformation. *Trends Neurosci.* 18:314–320.

JOHNSON, S. H., 2000. Thinking ahead: The case for motor imagery in prospective judgements of prehension. *Cognition* 74:33–70.

JOHNSON, S. H., P. M. CORBALLIS, and M. S. GAZZANIGA, 2001. Within grasp but out of reach: evidence for a double dissociation between imagined hand and arm movements in the left cerebral hemisphere. *Neuropsychologia* 39:36–50.

JOHNSON, S. H., and S. T. GRAFTON, 2002. From "acting on" to "acting with": The functional anatomy of object-oriented action schemata. In: *Neural control of space coding and action production. Progress in Brain Research*, Vol. 142. C. Prablanc, D. Pelisson, and Y. Rossetti, eds. Elsevier. New York: Elsevier. pp. 127–139.

JOHNSON, S. H., M. ROTTE, S. T. GRAFTON, H. HINRICHS, M. S. GAZZANIGA, and H. J. HEINZE, 2002. Selective activation of a parietofrontal circuit during implicitly imagined prehension. *NeuroImage* 17:1693–1704.

JOHNSON-FREY, S. H., 2003. Cortical mechanisms of human tool use. In *Taking Action: Cognitive Neuroscience Perspectives on the Problem of Intentional Acts*, S. H. Johnson-Frey, ed. Cambridge, Mass.: MIT Press.

KARNI, A., G. MEYER, C. REY-HIPOLITO, P. JEZZARD, M. M. ADAMS R. TURNER, and L. G. UNGERLEIDER, 1998. The acquisition of skilled motor performance: Fast and slow experience-driven changes in primary motor cortex. *Proc. Natl. Acad. Sci. U.S.A.* 95:861–868.

KEELE, S. W., R. IVRY, U. MAYR, E. HAZELTINE, and H. HEUER, 2003. The cognitive and neural architecture of sequence representation. *Psychol. Rev.* 110:316–339.

KEELE, S. W., P. JENNINGS, S. JONES, S. CAULTON, D. CAULTON, and A. COHEN, 1995. On the modularity of sequence representation. *J. Mot. Behav.* 27:17–30.

KILNER, J. M., S. SALENIUS, S. N. BAKER, A. JACKSON, R. HARI, and R. N. LEMON, 2003. Task-dependent modulations of cortical oscillatory activity in human subjects during a bimanual precision grip task. *NeuroImage* 18:67–73.

KOCH, I., and J. HOFFMANN, 2000. The role of stimulus-based and response-based spatial information in sequence learning. *J. Exp. Psychol. Learn. Mem. Cogn.* 26:863–882.

KORNBLUM, S., T. HASBROUCQ, and A. OSMAN, 1990. Dimensional overlap: Cognitive basis for stimulus response compatibility. A model and taxonomy. *Psychol. Rev.* 97:253–270.

LEIGUARDA, R. C., and C. D. MARSDEN, 2000. Limb apraxias: Higher-order disorders of sensorimotor integration. *Brain* 123:860–879.

LHERMITTE, F., 1983. "Utilization behaviour" and its relation to lesions of the frontal lobes. *Brain* 106:237–255.

LHERMITTE, F., 1986. Human autonomy and the frontal lobes. Part II. Patient behavior in complex and social situations: The "environmental dependency syndrome." *Ann. Neurol.* 19:335–343.

LHERMITTE, F., B. PILLON, and M. SERDARU, 1986. Human autonomy and the frontal lobes. Part I. Imitation and utilization behavior: A neuropsychological study of 75 patients. *Ann. Neurol.* 19:326–334.

MARCONI, B., A. GENOVESIO, A. BATTAGLIA-MAYER, S. FERRAINA, S. SQUATRITO, M. MOLINARI, F. LACQUANITI, and R. CAMINITI, 2001. Eye-hand coordination during reaching. I. Anatomical relationships between parietal and frontal cortex. *Cereb. Cortex* 11:513–527.

MARTIN, A., J. V. HAXBY, F. M. LALONDE, C. L. WIGGS, and L. G. UNGERLEIDER, 1995. Discrete cortical regions associated with knowledge of color and knowledge of action. *Science* 270:102–105.

MITZ, A. R., M. GODSCHALK, and S. P. WISE, 1991. Learning-dependent neuronal activity in the premotor cortex: Activity during the acquisition of conditional motor associations. *J. Neurosci.* 11:1155–1172.

MURATA, A., V. GALLESE, G. LUPPINO, M. KASEDA, and H. SAKATA, 2000. Selectivity for the shape, size, and orientation of objects for grasping in neurons of monkey parietal area AIP. *J. Neurophysiol.* 83:2580–2601.

NISSEN, M. J., D. WILLINGHAM, and M. HARTMAN, 1989. Explicit and implicit remembering: When is learning preserved in amnesia? *Neuropsychologia* 27:341–352.

PARSONS, L. M., 1994. Temporal and kinematic properties of motor behavior reflected in mentally simulated action. *J. Exp. Psychol. Hum. Percept. Perform.* 20:709–730.

PASHLER, H., 1994. Dual-task interference in simple tasks: Data and theory. *Psychol. Bull.* 116:220–244.

PERENIN, M. T., and A. VIGHETTO, 1988. Optic ataxia: A specific disruption in visuomotor mechanisms. I. Different aspects of the deficit in reaching for objects. *Brain* 111:643–674.

PISELLA, L., H. GREA, C. TILIKETE, A. VIGHETTO, M. DESMURGET, G. RODE, D. BOISSON, and Y. ROSSETTI, 2000. An "automatic pilot" for the hand in human posterior parietal cortex: Toward reinterpreting optic ataxia. *Nat. Neurosci.* 3:729–736.

RAND, M. K., O. HIKOSAKA, S. MIYACHI, X. LU, K. NAKAMURA, K. KITAGUCHI, and Y. SHIMO, 2000. Characteristics of sequential movements during early learning period in monkeys. *Exp. Brain Res.* 131:293–304.

RIDLEY, R. M., 1994. The psychology of perseverative and stereotyped behaviour. *Prog. Neurobiol.* 44:221–231.

ROSENBAUM, D. A., J. VAUGHAN, H. J. BARNES, and M. J. JORGENSEN, 1992. Time course of movement planning: selection of handgrips for object manipulation. *J. Exp. Psychol. Learn. Mem. Cogn.* 18:1058–1073.

SAKATA, H., M. TAIRA, S. MINE, and A. MURATA, 1992. Hand-movement related neurons of the posterior parietal cortex of the monkey: Their role in visual guidance of hand movements. In *Control of Arm Movement in Space: Neurophysiological and Computational Approaches*, R. Camaniti, P. B. Johnson, and Y. Burnod, eds. Berlin: Springer-Verlag, pp. 185–198.

SAKATA, H., M. TAIRA, A. MURATA, and S. MINE. 1995. Neural mechanisms of visual guidance of hand action in the parietal cortex of the monkey. *Cereb. Cortex* 5:429–438.

SCHLUTER, N. D., M. KRAMS, M. F. RUSHWORTH, and R. E. PASSINGHAM, 2001. Cerebral dominance for action in the human brain: The selection of actions. *Neuropsychologia* 39:105–113.

SCHLUTER, N. D., M. F. RUSHWORTH, R. E. PASSINGHAM, and K. R. MILLS, 1998. Temporary interference in human lateral premotor cortex suggests dominance for the selection of movements: A study using transcranial magnetic stimulation. *Brain* 121:785–799.

SHADMEHR, R., and Z. M. MOUSSAVI, 2000. Spatial generalization from learning dynamics of reaching movements. *J. Neurosci.* 20:7807–7815.

SHALLICE, T., P. W. BURGESS, F. SCHON, and D. M. BAXTER, 1989. The origins of utilization behaviour. *Brain* 112:1587–1598.

SHEN, L., and G. E. ALEXANDER, 1997. Preferential representation of instructed target location versus limb trajectory in dorsal premotor area. *J. Neurophysiol.* 77:1195–1212.

SHIMA, K., and J. TANJI, 2000. Neuronal activity in the supplementary and presupplementary motor areas for temporal organization of multiple movements. *J. Neurophysiol.* 84:2148–2160.

SIRIGU, A., L. COHEN, J. R. DUHAMEL, B. PILLON, B. DUBOIS, Y. AGID, and C. PIERROT-DESEILLIGNY, 1995. Congruent unilateral impairments for real and imagined hand movements. *Neuroreport* 6:997–1001.

SOECHTING, J. F., and M. FLANDERS, 1992. Moving in three-dimensional space: Frames of reference, vectors, and coordinate systems. *Annu. Rev. Neurosci.* 15:167–191.

SPIJKERS, W., and H. HEUER, 1995. Structural constraints on the performance of symmetrical bimanual movements with different amplitudes. *Q. J. Exp. Psychol. Hum. Exp. Psychol.* 48:716–740.

STEPHAN, K. M., G. R. FINK, R. E. PASSINGHAM, D. SILBERSWEIG, A. O. CEBALLOS-BAUMANN, C. D. FRITH, and R. S. FRACKOWIAK, 1995. Functional anatomy of the mental representation of upper extremity movements in healthy subjects. *J. Neurophysiol.* 73:373–386.

SUTTON, R. S., and A. G. BARTO, 1998. *Reinforcement Learning.* Cambridge, Mass.: MIT Press.

TERZUOLO, C. A., and P. VIVIANI, 1980. Determinants and characteristics of motor patterns used for typing. *Neuroscience* 5:1085–1103.

TYSZKA, J. M., S. T. GRAFTON, W. CHEW, R. P. WOODS, and P. M. COLLETTI, 1994. Parceling of mesial frontal motor areas during ideation and movement using functional magnetic resonance imaging at 1.5 tesla. *Ann. Neurol.* 35:746–749.

UNGERLEIDER, L. G., and M. MISHKIN, 1982. Two cortical visual systems. In *Analysis of Visual Behavior* D. J. Ingle, M. A. Goodale, and R. J. W. Mansfield, eds. Cambridge, Mass.: MIT Press, pp. 549–586.

WILLINGHAM, D. B., 1999. Implicit motor sequence learning is not purely perceptual. *Mem. Cogn.* 27:561–572.

WILLINGHAM, D. B., L. A. WELLS, J. M. FARRELL, and M. E. STEMWEDEL, 2000. Implicit motor sequence learning is represented in response locations. *Mem. Cogn.* 28:366–375.

WISE, S. P., M. WEINRICH, and K. H. MAURITZ, 1983. Motor aspects of cue-related neuronal activity in premotor cortex of the rhesus monkey. *Brain Res.* 260:301–305.

WOLPERT, D. M., S. J. GOODBODY, and M. HUSAIN, 1998. Maintaining internal representations: The role of the human superior parietal lobe. *Nat. Neurosci.* 1:529–533.

33 Basal Ganglia and Cerebellar Circuits with the Cerebral Cortex

PETER L. STRICK

ABSTRACT What do the basal ganglia and cerebellum do? The literature is filled with reports describing the motor deficits associated with damage to these subcortical structures. As a consequence, concepts about basal ganglia and cerebellar function have focused largely on their contributions to the generation and control of movement. We have taken an anatomical approach to this question and examined the macro-organization of basal ganglia and cerebellar connections with the cerebral cortex: Which cortical areas project to the basal ganglia and cerebellum and which cortical areas are the target of the outputs from these subcortical centers? The answers to these questions lead to some novel and important insights about basal ganglia and cerebellar function.

Classically, the macroorganization of basal ganglia and cerebellar circuitry is described using a relatively simple hierarchical model. The input layer of basal ganglia processing is represented by the striatum—the caudate, putamen, and ventral striatum. The functionally analogous level in cerebellar circuits is represented by specific pontine nuclei that send mossy fiber inputs to cerebellar cortex. A major source of afferents to the input layers of both circuits originates in widespread regions of the cerebral cortex, including motor, sensory, posterior parietal, prefrontal, cingulate, orbital frontal, and temporal cortical areas. The output layer of basal ganglia processing is represented by the internal segment of the globus pallidus (GPi), the pars reticulata of the substantia nigra (SNpr), and the ventral pallidum; comparable structures for cerebellar processing are the three deep cerebellar nuclei, the dentate, interpositus, and fastigial. Neurons in the output layers of both circuits send their axons to the thalamus, and by this route, project back upon the cortex. Thus, a major structural feature of basal ganglia and cerebellar circuits is their participation in multiple loops with the cerebral cortex (e.g., Evarts and Thach, 1969; Kemp and Powell, 1971; Allen and Tsukahara, 1974; Brooks and Thach, 1981; Alexander, DeLong, and Strick, 1986). These loops were believed to function largely in the domain of motor control. Indeed, basal ganglia and cerebellar efferents were thought

to terminate in a common region of the ventrolateral thalamus that projected to the primary motor cortex. Thus, these circuits were viewed as a neural substrate for enabling information from a diverse set of cortical areas to direct motor output at the level of the motor cortex. This view has been supported by the obvious motor symptoms that result from some basal ganglia and cerebellar lesions (for references and reviews, see Brooks and Thach, 1981; DeLong and Georgopoulos, 1981; Bhatia and Marsden, 1994).

Information that has accrued over the past 15 years on basal ganglia and cerebellar anatomy has led a number of investigators to challenge this view (e.g., Schell and Strick, 1984; Alexander, DeLong, and Strick, 1986; Goldman-Rakic and Selemon, 1990). It is now clear that basal ganglia and cerebellar efferents terminate in largely separate regions of the ventrolateral thalamus (for references and review, see Percheron et al., 1996). In addition, there is considerable evidence that basal ganglia and cerebellar efferents are directed to multiple subdivisions of the ventrolateral thalamus, which in turn project to myriad cortical areas. Thus, the outputs from the basal ganglia and cerebellum influence more widespread regions of the cerebral cortex than was previously recognized.

Based on these and other anatomical results, Alexander, DeLong, and Strick (1986) proposed that the basal ganglia participate in at least five separate loops with the cerebral cortex. These loops were designated the skeletomotor, oculomotor, dorsolateral prefrontal, lateral orbitofrontal, and anterior cingulate circuits, based in part on the cortical target of their output layer of processing. According to this scheme, the output of the basal ganglia has the potential to influence not only the control of movement but also higher-order cognitive and limbic functions subserved by prefrontal, orbitofrontal, and anterior cingulate cortex.

Similarly, Leiner, Leiner, and Dow (1986, 1991, 1993) suggested that cerebellar output is directed to prefrontal as well as to motor areas of the cerebral cortex. They noted that in the course of hominid evolution, the lateral output nucleus of the cerebellum, the dentate, underwent a marked expansion that paralleled the expansion of cerebral cortex in the frontal lobe. They argued that the increase in size of the dentate was accompanied by an increase in the extent of the cortical areas

PETER L. STRICK Department of Veterans Affairs Medical Center and Center for the Neural Basis of Cognition, Department of Neurobiology, University of Pittsburgh School of Medicine, Pittsburgh, Penna.

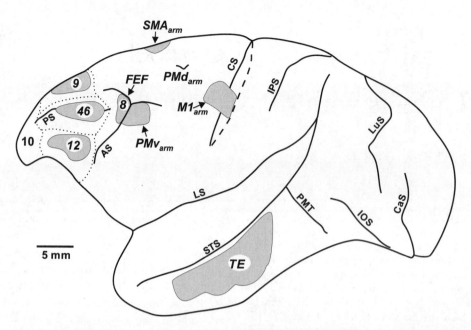

FIGURE 33.1 Location of virus injection sites in the cerebral cortex. Lateral view of a *Cebus* monkey brain. The shaded areas indicate the spread of virus from injections into each cortical area. The numbers 8, 9, 10, 12, and 46 refer to cytoarchitectonic areas of the frontal lobe. Dotted lines define the borders between several areas in prefrontal cortex. Abbreviations: AS, arcuate sulcus; CaS, calcarine sulcus; CS, central sulcus; FEF, frontal eye field; IOS, infe-rior occipital sulcus; IPS, intraparietal sulcus; LS, lateral sulcus; LuS, lunate sulcus; M1$_{arm}$, arm area of the primary motor cortex; PMT, posterior middle temporal sulcus; PMv$_{arm}$, arm area of the ventral premotor area; PS, principal sulcus; SMA$_{arm}$, arm area of the supplementary motor area; STS, superior temporal sulcus; TE, area of inferotemporal cortex. (Adapted from Middleton and Strick, 1996b.)

in the frontal lobe that are influenced by dentate output. As a consequence, Leiner and colleagues proposed that cerebellar function in humans has expanded to include involvement in certain language and cognitive tasks.

Attempts to test these proposals and to map cerebellar and basal ganglia projections to the cerebral cortex have been hindered by a number of technical limitations. Chief among these is the multisynaptic nature of these pathways and the general inability of conventional tracers to label more than the direct inputs and outputs of an area. To overcome these and other problems, we developed the use of neurotropic viruses (herpes simplex virus type 1 [HSV-1] and rabies virus) as transneuronal tracers in the central nervous system (CNS) of primates (for references and reviews, see Strick and Card, 1992; Kelly and Strick, 2000). This tracing method can effectively label a chain of up to three synaptically linked neurons in a single experiment (Kelly and Strick, 2003a,b). In this chapter, we review some of the new observations that have come from using viruses to trace basal ganglia and cerebellar loops with the cerebral cortex. These observations have led to important insights into the cortical targets of these circuits and the functional domains they influence.

Primary motor cortex

Our first experiments used retrograde transneuronal transport of HSV-1 to examine the organization of basal ganglia and cerebellar outputs to the primary motor cortex (M1; figure 33.1) (Hoover and Strick, 1993, 1999). In later experiments we used rabies virus as the transneuronal tracer. We injected virus into physiologically identified portions of M1 (i.e., regions where arm, face, or leg movements were evoked by intracortical stimulation with currents < 25 μA). Then we set the survival time to allow transneuronal transport of virus to label second-order neurons, which are the origin of basal ganglia and cerebellothalamocortical inputs to M1. The brain of each animal was processed using immuno-histochemical techniques to demonstrate the location of virus-specific antigen in infected neurons (for technical details see Strick and Card, 1992; Kelly and Strick, 2000).

Three major results came out of these experiments. First, we found that M1 is richly innervated by the output nuclei of the basal ganglia and cerebellum. The densest projections originate in the dentate nucleus (figure 33.2, M1$_{arm}$) and the GPi (figure 33.3, M1$_{arm}$). Less dense projections originate in portions of interpositus and the SNpr. Second, we found that both the dentate and the GPi contain separate face, arm, and leg areas that project via the thalamus to the face, arm, and leg areas of M1. Third, and perhaps most surprising, we discovered that projections to M1 originate in only 30% of the volume of the dentate and about 15% of the volume of the GPi. In particular, the ventral two-thirds of the dentate and the rostral and caudal thirds of the GPi did not contain labeled neurons after virus injections into either the

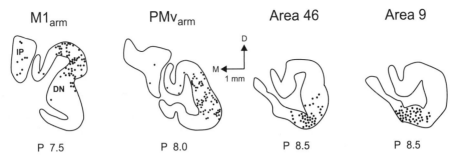

M1$_{arm}$	PMv$_{arm}$	Area 46	Area 9
P 7.5	P 8.0	P 8.5	P 8.5

FIGURE 33.2 Origin of cerebellar projections to M1, PMv, area 46, and area 9. Representative coronal sections through the dentate and interpositus nuclei of animals that received injections of virus into different cortical areas (see figure 33.1). Solid dots indicate the positions of neurons labeled by retrograde transneuronal transport of virus. Maps display labeled neurons found on two to three adjacent sections, whose approximate anteroposterior location is indicated at the bottom of each section outline. Abbreviations: D, dorsal; DN, dentate nucleus; IP, interpositus nucleus; M, medial. (Adapted from Middleton and Strick, 1996b.)

face, arm, or leg representations of M1. Thus, although the basal ganglia and cerebellum both project to M1, the output to M1 originates from restricted portions of each subcortical nucleus. Furthermore, the majority of the outputs from the basal ganglia and cerebellum are directed to other cortical areas. In subsequent studies we defined some of the additional cortical targets of GPi, SNpr, and dentate.

Premotor areas

Our next experiments used virus tracing to examine basal ganglia and cerebellar projections to the arm representations of two premotor areas in the frontal lobe, the ventral premotor area (PMv) and the supplementary motor area (SMA) (Hoover and Strick, 1993). Injections of HSV-1 into either the PMv or SMA consistently labeled GPi neurons in the middle of the nucleus rostrocaudally. Within this region, the dorsoventral location of labeled neurons varied, depending on the location of the cortical injection site. The SMA injections labeled neurons in a middorsal region of GPi (figure 33.3, SMA$_{arm}$). In contrast, PMv injections labeled neurons mainly in ventrolateral portions of GPi (figure 33.3, PMv$_{arm}$). Neurons labeled by virus injections into M1 were located between those labeled by the SMA and PMv injections (figure 33.3, M1$_{arm}$). In recent studies we have found evidence for additional output channels in GPi that project to the arm representation in the dorsal premotor area (PMd) and to the presupplementary motor area (PreSMA) (Dum and Strick, 1999; Akkal, Dum, and Strick, 2001, 2002). These observations indicate that pallidal output is not confined to M1 but projects via the thalamus to multiple premotor areas in the frontal lobe (see also Jinnai et al., 1993; Inase and Tanji, 1995; Sakai, Inase, and Tanji, 1999). Furthermore, the arm representation of each motor area receives input from a topographically distinct set of GPi neurons. We have proposed that this arrangement creates distinct output channels in the sensorimotor portion of GPi (Hoover and Strick, 1993).

We found a similar topographic organization of output neurons in the dentate. Injections of virus into the PMv labeled neurons in the middle of the dentate rostrocaudally (figure 33.2, PMv$_{arm}$). These labeled neurons were located ventral and lateral to the region of the dentate that contained labeled neurons after virus injections into the arm area of M1 (figure 33.2, M1$_{arm}$). In recent studies we have found that the arm areas of the SMA and PMd, as well as

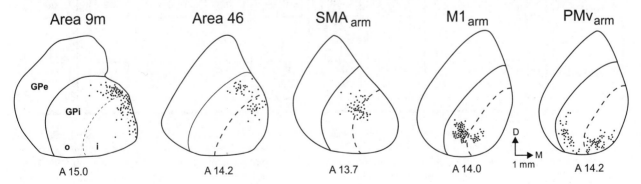

Area 9m	Area 46	SMA$_{arm}$	M1$_{arm}$	PMv$_{arm}$
A 15.0	A 14.2	A 13.7	A 14.0	A 14.2

FIGURE 33.3 Origin of pallidal projections to M1, PMv, SMA, area 46, and area 9. Representative coronal sections through the globus pallidus of animals that received injections of virus into different cortical areas (see figure 33.1). See figure 33.2 for conventions. Abbreviations: GPe, external segment of globus pallidus; o, outer portion of the internal segment of globus pallidus; i, inner portion of the internal segment of globus pallidus. (Adapted from Middleton and Strick, 1996b.)

the PreSMA, are the targets of separate output channels from the dentate. Thus, the dentate, like GPi, contains distinct output channels that innervate different cortical motor areas.

Results from single-neuron recording experiments in awake, trained monkeys provide physiological support for the existence of distinct output channels in GPi and dentate (Mushiake and Strick, 1993, 1995; Strick, Dum, and Picard, 1995). Specifically, these studies suggest that individual output channels are involved in different aspects of motor behavior. For example, some output channels appear to be especially concerned with movements that are internally generated, whereas others appear to be devoted to movements guided by exteroceptive cues. Taken together, these observations indicate that the basal ganglia and cerebellum have the capacity to influence a broad range of motor behavior using output channels that project to the premotor areas in the frontal lobe, as well as to M1. Thus, the skeletomotor circuit of Alexander, DeLong, and Strick (1986) is more accurately viewed as multiple discrete channels to each of the cortical motor areas (figure 33.4). A similar arrangement of output channels characterizes skeletal motor output from the dentate.

Frontal eye field

We have also used transneuronal transport of virus to examine subcortical inputs to the frontal eye field (FEF; figure 33.1) (Lynch, Hoover, and Strick, 1994). The results of prior studies with conventional tracers led to the proposal that the FEF receives input via the thalamus from three major subcortical nuclei: SNpr, the superior colliculus (SC), and the deep cerebellar nuclei. To test this proposal, we injected virus into physiologically identified portions of the FEF (i.e., regions where eye movements were evoked by intracortical stimulation with currents $< 50\,\mu A$). Neurons labeled by retrograde transneuronal transport were found in lateral portions of SNpr, the optic and intermediate gray layers of SC, and ventrally in posterior portions of the dentate nucleus. Within the dentate, the labeled neurons were found only in the most caudal third of the nucleus. Prior studies have shown that some neurons in this region display changes in activity that are correlated with saccadic eye movements (e.g., van Kan, Houk, and Gibson, 1993). Within the basal ganglia, FEF injections labeled neurons in a posterior and lateral region of SNpr (figure 33.5), where neurons display changes in activity related to saccadic eye

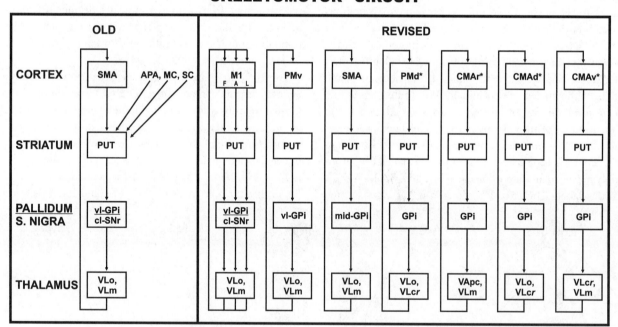

FIGURE 33.4 Original skeletomotor circuit proposed by Alexander, DeLong, and Strick (1986), and our revised scheme. Asterisks indicate loops whose existence is not yet proved. Cortical abbreviations: CMAd, dorsal cingulate motor area; CMAr, rostral cingulate motor area; CMAv, ventral cingulate motor area; M1, primary motor cortex; PMd, dorsal premotor area; PMv, ventral premotor area; SMA, supplementary motor area. Basal ganglia abbreviations: GPi, internal segment of globus pallidus; PUT, putamen, SNr, substantia nigra pars reticulata; cl, caudolateral; mid, middle; vl, ventrolateral. Thalamic abbreviations: VApc, nucleus ventralis anterior, parvocellular portion; VLcc, nucleus ventralis lateralis pars caudalis, caudal division; VLcr, nucleus ventralis lateralis pars caudalis, rostral division; VLm, nucleus ventralis lateralis pars medialis; VLo, nucleus ventralis lateralis pars oralis. (Adapted from Middleton and Strick, 2000.)

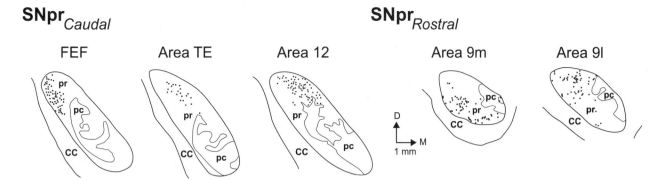

FIGURE 33.5   Origin of nigral projections to the FEF, area TE, area 12, area 9m, and area 9l. Coronal sections indicating the location of labeled neurons in caudal and rostral regions of SNpr following virus injections into five different cortical areas (see figure 33.1). Abbreviations: CC, crus cerebri; pc, pars compacta; pr, pars reticulata. (Adapted from Middleton and Strick, 1996b.)

movements (e.g., Hikosaka and Wurtz, 1983a,b). Overall, the regions of the basal ganglia and cerebellum that were labeled after injections of virus into FEF were strikingly different from those labeled after injections into any of the skeletomotor areas of the frontal lobe. Thus, the output channels in the basal ganglia and cerebellum that are concerned with oculomotor function are distinct from those concerned with skeletomotor function.

Prefrontal cortex

It is clear from the studies reviewed in the previous section that the output nuclei of the basal ganglia and cerebellum have well-organized projections to skeletomotor and oculomotor areas of cortex. However, it is also notable that substantial portions of these output nuclei do not project to the cortical motor areas. This observation raised the possibility that the remaining portions of these output nuclei target nonmotor areas of cortex. Because of prior suggestions that the basal ganglia and cerebellum influence some of the cognitive operations normally thought to be subserved by the frontal lobe (e.g., Alexander, DeLong, and Strick, 1986; Leiner, Leiner, and Dow, 1986, 1987, 1989, 1991, 1993) we used virus tracing to test whether basal ganglia and cerebellar projections to prefrontal cortex provide an anatomical substrate for this influence.

Our initial experiments focused on subfields within Walker's area 46 (Middleton and Strick, 1994). In more recent studies, we examined inputs to portions of areas 9 and 12 as well (Middleton and Strick, 2001, 2002). Each of these areas of prefrontal cortex appears to be involved in aspects of working memory and is thought to guide behavior based on transiently stored information rather than immediate external cues (for in-depth reviews, see Passingham, 1993; Goldman-Rakic, 1996; Fuster, 1997).

Virus injections into areas 9, 12, and 46 of prefrontal cortex labeled many neurons in the output nuclei of the basal ganglia (figures 33.3 and 33.5). Injections into area 12 labeled neurons in a localized portion of SNpr. In contrast, injections into area 46 labeled neurons largely in GPi. Injections into area 9 labeled neurons in both SNpr and GPi. The topographic nature of basal ganglia projections to prefrontal cortex is further emphasized by the finding that different regions within rostral SNpr project to medial and lateral portions of area 9 (figure 33.5, areas 9m and 9l). It is also important to note that, in all cases, the location of the neurons labeled in GPi and SNpr after injections into prefrontal areas of cortex was different from the location of neurons labeled after injections into motor areas of cortex.

Virus injections into areas 9 and 46 (but not area 12) also labeled neurons in ventral regions of the dentate nucleus (figure 33.2, areas 9 and 46). The neurons labeled after area 9 injections were found largely medial to those labeled by area 46 injections. The ventral regions of the dentate that project to areas 9 and 46 clearly differ from the more dorsal regions of this nucleus, which innervate motor areas of the cortex (figure 33.2, $M1_{arm}$ and PMv_{arm}). Thus, both the basal ganglia and the cerebellum project via the thalamus to multiple areas of prefrontal cortex. Furthermore, the output channels in the basal ganglia and cerebellum that influence prefrontal areas of cortex are separate from those that influence motor areas of cortex.

Inferotemporal cortex

In our studies of frontal cortex, each of the areas found to be a target of projections via the thalamus from the output stage of basal ganglia and/or cerebellar processing is known to send efferents to the input stage of these subcortical nuclei. This anatomical arrangement suggests that many cortical areas in the frontal lobe participate in "closed loop" circuits with the basal ganglia and cerebellum. To test whether this arrangement extends to areas outside the frontal lobe, we examined subcortical inputs to a region of inferotemporal cortex, area TE (Middleton and Strick, 1996a) (figure 33.1, area TE). Area TE is known to project to the input stage of basal ganglia processing (i.e., the tail of the caudate and ventral portions of the putamen) (Saint-Cyr, Ungerleider, and Desimone, 1990), but not to the input stage of cerebellar processing (Glickstein, May, and Mercier, 1985; Schmahmann and Pandya, 1997).

Virus injections into area TE did not result in any labeled neurons in the deep cerebellar nuclei. This suggests that TE neither projects to nor receives from the cerebellum. On the other hand, the same virus injections did result in a distinct cluster of labeled neurons in SNpr (figure 33.5, area TE). Most of these neurons were located dorsally in the caudal third of the nucleus. This portion of the SNpr appears to be separate from the regions of this nucleus that influence either the FEF or regions of prefrontal cortex. Thus, TE is both a source of input to, and a target of output from, a distinct portion of the basal ganglia.

TE is known to play a critical role in the visual recognition and discrimination of objects (e.g., Gross, 1972; Tanaka et al., 1991; Miyashita, 1993). Physiological studies have shown that the region of SNpr which influences TE contains some neurons that are responsive to the presentation of visual stimuli (e.g., Hikosaka and Wurtz, 1983a). These observations, together with our anatomical results, provide evidence that basal ganglia output is involved in higher order aspects of visual processing, as well as in motor and cognitive function.

Posterior parietal cortex

Areas 5 and 7 in posterior parietal cortex are known to project to the input stage of basal ganglia and cerebellar processing (e.g., Kemp and Powell, 1971; Glickstein, May, and Mercier, 1985; Cavada and Goldman-Rakic, 1991; Schmahmann and Pandya, 1997; Yeterian and Pandya, 1993). These connections led us to ask whether posterior parietal cortex is a target of basal ganglia and cerebellar output (Clower et al., 2001; Clower, Dum, and Strick, 2002). Although our studies are at an early stage, our initial results demonstrate that a portion of area 7b in the intraparietal sulcus is the target of output from the dentate nucleus, whereas a portion of area 7b on the cortical surface is the target of output from SNpr, as well as from the dentate nucleus. These results clearly extend the sphere of influence of basal ganglia and cerebellar output to include portions of the posterior parietal cortex. We have suggested that the cerebellar projection to posterior parietal cortex may provide signals that contribute to the sensory recalibration that occurs during some adaptation paradigms (Clower et al., 2001). The basal ganglia projection to the posterior parietal cortex may provide an anatomical basis for the visuospatial deficits observed in some patients with basal ganglia lesions (e.g., Karnath, Himmelbach, and Rorden, 2002). In any case, our observations on the posterior pari-

etal cortex provide further support for the concept that multiple closed-loop circuits represent a fundamental architectural feature of basal ganglia and cerebellar connections with the cerebral cortex.

Functional implications

Clearly, the outputs from the basal ganglia and cerebellum gain access to more widespread and diverse areas of cortex than previously imagined. To date our studies have shown that the output nuclei of the basal ganglia and cerebellum project (via the thalamus) to skeletomotor, oculomotor, prefrontal, and posterior parietal areas of cortex. In addition, a portion of SNpr projects to inferotemporal cortex. Thus, the anatomical substrate exists for the basal ganglia and cerebellum to influence higher-order aspects of cognition, such as planning, working memory, sequential behavior, visuospatial perception, and attention, as well as skeletomotor and oculomotor function. As a consequence, a sizable component of basal ganglia and cerebellar output operates outside the domain of motor control.

Some support for this conclusion comes from recent analyses of the consequences of cerebellar pathology in human subjects. In addition to the classic motor deficits, there is considerable evidence that cerebellar damage can lead to deficits in the performance of cognitive tasks that require rule-based learning, judgment of temporal intervals, visuospatial analysis, shifting attention between sensory modalities, as well as working memory and planning (see reviews by Leiner, Leiner, and Dow, 1986, 1987, 1989, 1991, 1993; Botez et al., 1989; Ivry and Keele, 1989; Schmahmann, 1991, 1997; Fiez et al., 1992; Akshoomoff and Courchesne, 1992; Grafman et al., 1992; Schmahmann and Sherman, 1998). Many of these deficits reflect functions normally thought to be subserved by areas of prefrontal cortex.

Based on our results, one interpretation of the origin of these deficits is that they result from an interruption of input to prefrontal cortex from the cerebellum. A study by Fiez and colleagues (1992) provides some support for this interpretation. They described a patient, designated RC1, who had circumscribed damage to the lateral portion of his right cerebellar cortex. This patient exhibited few of the classic signs of cerebellar damage but was impaired in the performance of specific types of rule-based language and memory tasks. The deficits appeared on tasks that in normal subjects activate lateral portions of the cerebellar hemispheres and areas 9 and 46 (Petersen et al., 1988; Raichle et al., 1994; Fiez et al., 1996). Recent anatomical studies suggest that the portions of the cerebellum damaged in RC1 are part of the cerebellar loop with the prefrontal cortex (Kelly and Strick, 1998, 2003). Thus, the cognitive deficits in RC1 may have been a consequence of interrupting this circuit.

In general, we found that basal ganglia and cerebellar projections to a cortical area originate from a localized cluster of neurons that we have termed an output channel. The output channels to different cortical areas display a surprising degree of topographic organization. For example, the output channels that influence dorsomedial regions of prefrontal cortex are located largely in GPi, whereas the output channels that influence ventrolateral regions of prefrontal cortex are located largely in SNpr. Both sets of output channels are separate from those that influence skeletomotor and oculomotor areas of cortex. Output channels within the dentate are as topographically organized as those in the basal ganglia, if not more so (Dum and Strick, 2003).

Evidence for a segregation of function in the human GPi comes from the observation that the cognitive and motor effects of pallidotomies, performed to ameliorate the symptoms of Parkinson's disease, depend significantly on the location of the lesion (Lombardi et al., 2000). Lesions located in the most anteromedial region of GPi, the likely origin of output channels to prefrontal cortex, produced the greatest degree of cognitive impairment. In contrast, lesions in the intermediate region of GPi, the likely origin of output channels to motor areas of cortex, led to maximal effects on motor performance, but produced little effect on cognition. Thus, the human GPi appears to have spatially separate motor and cognitive output channels.

Our current estimate is that the output channels to skeletomotor, oculomotor, prefrontal, and posterior parietal areas of cortex occupy approximately 70% of the volume of GPi, SNpr, and dentate. This means that the cortical targets for approximately 30% of the output from the basal ganglia and the dentate remain to be identified. The architecture of basal ganglia and cerebellar loops with the cerebral cortex allows us to make some predictions about the identity of these targets. As noted earlier, cingulate, orbital frontal, and posterior parietal cortex are known to be major sources of input to the basal ganglia and cerebellum. Our results suggest that cortical areas that project to the input stage of the basal ganglia and cerebellum processing are the targets of the output stage of processing in these circuits. In other words, multiple closed loops represent a major architectural unit of basal ganglia and cerebellar interconnections with the cerebral cortex. If this proposal is correct, then the remaining 30% of the basal ganglia and cerebellar output is directed at cingulate, orbital frontal, and posterior parietal areas of cortex. This prediction will be tested in future experiments.

The new insights gained from virus tracing have important implications for hypotheses about basal ganglia and cerebellar contributions to normal and abnormal behavior. Detailed discussions of this issue have been presented in recent publications (Middleton and Strick, 1996, 2001, 2002; Clower et al., 2001), and therefore only some examples will be presented here. It is known that abnormal activity in basal ganglia and cerebellar loops with motor areas of cortex results in striking disorders of movement. Likewise, abnormal activity in basal ganglia and cerebellar loops with nonmotor areas of the cerebral cortex could lead to a broad range of psychiatric and neurological symptoms such as those associated with depression, obsessive-compulsive disorder, Parkinson's disease, and Huntington's disease (for recent references and review, see Lichter and Cummings, 2000). For example, Courchesne and colleagues have suggested that alterations in the cerebellum and its projections to posterior parietal cortex may underlie some of the deficits seen in autistic patients (e.g., Courchesne et al., 1988, 1994). Rapoport and Wise (1988) have proposed that dysfunction in basal ganglia circuits with anterior cingulate and orbital frontal cortex may explain some of the features of obsessive-compulsive disorder. We have suggested that abnormal signals in the basal ganglia loop with area TE in inferotemporal cortex are responsible for the visual hallucinations seen in L-dopa toxicity (Middleton and Strick, 1996a). It is clear that additional studies aimed at unraveling these loops could lead to new insights into the pathophysiological basis of basal ganglia and cerebellar disorders.

In summary, virus tracing has revealed that the output of the basal ganglia and cerebellum targets motor, premotor, prefrontal, posterior parietal, and inferotemporal areas of cortex. These connections provide the basal ganglia and cerebellum with the anatomical substrate to influence not only the control of movement but also many aspects of cognitive behavior, such as planning, working memory, sequential behavior, visuospatial perception, and attention. Similarly, there is growing evidence that disorders such as schizophrenia, autism, attention-deficit disorder, and obsessive-compulsive disorder are associated with alterations in basal ganglia or cerebellar function. Thus, it is possible that abnormal activity in specific basal ganglia and cerebellar loops with the cerebral cortex results in identifiable sets of neuropsychiatric symptoms. Taken together, the recent findings about basal ganglia and cerebellar circuitry provide a new anatomical framework for understanding the contributions of these structures to diverse aspects of motor and nonmotor behavior.

ACKNOWLEDGMENTS This work was supported by funds from the Veterans Administration Medical Research Service and by U.S. Public Health Service grants R01 NS24328, MH56661, and NS44837.

REFERENCES

AKKAL, D., R. P. DUM, and P. L. STRICK, 2001. Cerebellar and pallidal inputs to the supplementary motor area (SMA). *Soc. Neurosci. Abstr.* 27:825.4.

AKKAL, D., R. P. DUM, and P. L. STRICK, 2002. Cerebellar and basal ganglia inputs to the presupplementary motor area (PreSMA).

2002 Abstract Viewer/Itinerary Planner, Program No. 462.14. Washington, D.C.: Society for Neuroscience.

AKSHOOMOFF, N. A., and E. COURCHESNE, 1992. A new role for the cerebellum in cognitive function. *Behav. Neurosci.* 106:731–738.

ALEXANDER, G. E., M. R. DELONG, and P. L. STRICK, 1986. Parallel organization of functionally segregated circuits linking basal ganglia and cortex. *Annu. Rev. Neurosci.* 9:357–381.

ALLEN, G. I., and N. TSUKAHARA, 1974. Cerebrocerebellar communication systems. *Physiol. Rev.* 54:957–1006.

BHATIA, K. P., and C. D. MARSDEN, 1994. The behavioural and motor consequences of focal lesions of the basal ganglia in man. *Brain* 117:859–876.

BOTEZ, M. I., T. BOTEZ, R. ELIE, and E. ATTIG, 1989. Role of the cerebellum in complex human behavior. *Ital. J. Neurol. Sci.* 10: 291–300.

BROOKS, V. B., and W. T. THACH, 1981. Cerebellar control of posture and movement. In *Handbook of Physiology*, Sect. 1. *The Nervous System*, vol. 2, *Motor Control*, Part II, V. B. Brooks, ed. Bethesda, Md.: American Physiological Society, pp. 877–946.

CAVADA, C., and P. S. GOLDMAN-RAKIC, 1991. Topographic segregation of corticostriatal projections from posterior parietal subdivisions in the macaque monkey. *Neuroscience* 42:683–696.

CLOWER, D. M., R. P. DUM, and P. L. STRICK, 2002. Substantia nigra pars reticulata provides input to area 7b of parietal cortex. *2002 Abstract Viewer/Itinerary Planner*, Program No. 460.1. Washington, D.C.: Society for Neuroscience.

CLOWER, D. M., R. A. WEST, J. C. LYNCH, and P. L. STRICK, 2001. The inferior parietal lobule is the target of output from the superior colliculus, hippocampus and cerebellum. *J. Neurosci.* 21: 6283–6291.

COURCHESNE, E., 1997. Brainstem, cerebellar and limbic neuroanatomical abnormalities in autism. *Curr. Opin. Neurobiol.* 7:269–278.

COURCHESNE, E., J. TOWNSEND, N. AKSHOOMOFF, O. SAITOH, R. YEUNG-COURCHESNE, A. LINCOLN, H. JAMES, R. HAAS, L. SCHREIBMAN, and L. LAU, 1994. Impairment in shifting attention in autistic and cerebellar patients. *Behav. Neurosci.* 108:848–865.

COURCHESNE, E., R. YEUNG-COURCHESNE, G. A. PRESS, J. R. HESSELINK, and T. L. JERNIGAN, 1988. Hypoplasia of cerebellar vermal lobules VI and VII in autism. *N. Engl. J. Med.* 318:1349–1354.

DELONG, M. R., and A. P. GEORGOPOULOS, 1981. Motor functions of the basal ganglia. In *Handbook of Physiology*, Sect. I, *The Nervous System*, vol. II, *Motor Control*, V. B. Brooks, ed. Bethesda, Md.: American Physiological Society, pp. 1017–1061.

DUM, R. P., and P. L. STRICK, 1999. Pallidal and cerebellar inputs to the digit representations of the lateral premotor areas. *Soc. Neurosci. Abstr.* 25:1925.

DUM, R. P., and P. L. STRICK, 2003. An unfolded map of the cerebellar dentate nucleus and its projections to the cerebral cortex. *J. Neurophysiol.* 89:634–639.

EVARTS, E. V., and W. T. THACH, 1969. Motor mechanisms of the CNS: Cerebrocerebellar interrelations. *Annu. Rev. Physiol.* 31: 451–498.

FIEZ, J. A., S. E. PETERSEN, M. K. CHENEY, and M. E. RAICHLE, 1992. Impaired non-motor learning and error detection associated with cerebellar damage. *Brain* 115:155–178.

FIEZ, J. A., E. A. RAIFE, D. A. BALOTA, J. P. SCHWARZ, M. E. RAICHLE, and S. E. PETERSEN, 1996. A positron emission tomography study of the short-term maintenance of verbal information. *J. Neurosci.* 16:808–822.

FUSTER, J. M., 1997. *The Prefrontal Cortex*. New York: Raven Press.

GLICKSTEIN, M., J. G. MAY, B. E. MERCIER, 1985. Corticopontine projection in the macaque: The distribution of labelled cortical cells after large injections of horseradish peroxidase in the pontine nuclei. *J. Comp. Neurol.* 235:343–359.

GOLDMAN-RAKIC, P. S., 1996. The prefrontal landscape: Implications of functional architecture for understanding human mentation and the central executive. *Philos. Trans. R. Soc. Lond. B Biol. Sci.* 351:1445–1453.

GOLDMAN-RAKIC, P. S., and L. D. SELEMON, 1990. New frontiers in basal ganglia research: Introduction. *Trends Neurosci.* 13:241–244.

GRAFMAN, J., I. LITVAN, S. MASSAQUOI, M. STEWART, A. SIRIGU, and M. HALLETT, 1992. Cognitive planning deficit in patients with cerebellar atrophy. *Neurology* 42:1493–1496.

GROSS, C. G., 1972. Visual functions of inferotemporal cortex. In *Handbook of Sensory Physiology*, R. Jung, ed. Berlin: Springer-Verlag, pp. 451–482.

HIKOSAKA, O., and R. H. WURTZ, 1983a. Visual and oculomotor functions of monkey substantia nigra pars reticulata. I. Relation of visual and auditory responses to saccades. *J. Neurophysiol.* 49:1230–1253.

HIKOSAKA, O., and R. H. WURTZ, 1983b. Visual and oculomotor functions of monkey substantia nigra pars reticulata. III. Memory-contingent visual and saccade responses. *J. Neurophysiol.* 49:1268–1284.

HOOVER, J. E., and P. L. STRICK, 1993. Multiple output channels in the basal ganglia. *Science* 259:819–821.

HOOVER, J. E., and P. L. STRICK, 1999. The organization of cerebello- and pallido-thalamic projections to primary motor cortex: An investigation employing retrograde transneuronal transport of herpes simplex virus type 1. *J. Neurosci.* 19:1446–1463.

INASE, M., and J. TANJI, 1995. Thalamic distribution of projection neurons to the primary motor cortex relative to afferent terminal fields from the globus pallidus in the macaque monkey. *J. Comp. Neurol.* 353:415–426.

IVRY, R. B., and S. W. KEELE, 1989. Timing functions of the cerebellum. *J. Cog. Neurosci.* 1:136–152.

JINNAI, K., A. NAMBU, I. TANIBUCH, and S. YOSHIDA, 1993. Cerebello- and pallido-thalamic pathways to areas 6 and 4 in the monkey. *Stereotactic Funct. Neurosurg.* 60:70–79.

KARNATH, H. O., M. HIMMELBACH, and C. RORDEN, 2002. The subcortical anatomy of human spatial neglect: Putamen, caudate nucleus and pulvinar. *Brain* 125:350–360.

KELLY, R. M., and P. L. STRICK, 1998. Cerebro-cerebellar "loops" are closed. *Soc. Neurosci. Abstr.* 24:1407.

KELLY, R. M., and P. L. STRICK, 2000. Rabies as a transneuronal tracer of circuits in the central nervous system. *J. Neurosci. Methods* 103:63–71.

KELLY, R. M., and P. L. STRICK, 2003. Cerebellar "loops" with motor cortex and prefrontal cortex of a non-human primate. *J. Neurosci.* 23:8432–8444.

KELLY, R. M., and P. L. STRICK, 2004. Macro-architecture of basal ganglia loops with the cerebral cortex: Use of rabies virus to reveal multisynaptic circuits. *Prog. Brain Res.* 143:449–459.

KEMP, J. M., and T. P. S. POWELL, 1971. The connexions of the striatum and globus pallidus: Synthesis and speculation. *Philos. Trans. R. Soc. Lond. B* 262:441–457

LEINER, H. C., A. L. LEINER, and R. S. DOW, 1986. Does the cerebellum contribute to mental skills? *Behav. Neurosci.* 100: 443–454.

LEINER, H. C., A. L. LEINER, and R. S. DOW, 1987. Cerebrocerebellar learning loops in apes and humans. *Ital. J. Neurol. Sci.* 8:425–436.

LEINER, H. C., A. L. LEINER, and R. S. DOW, 1989. Reappraising the cerebellum: What does the hindbrain contribute to the forebrain? *Behav. Neurosci.* 103:998–1008.

LEINER, H. C., A. L. LEINER, and R. S. DOW, 1991. The human cerebro-cerebellar system: Its computing, cognitive, and language skills. *Behav. Brain. Res.* 44:113–128.

LEINER, H. C., A. L. LEINER, and R. S. DOW, 1993. Cognitive and language functions of the human cerebellum. *Trends Neurosci.* 16:444–447.

LICHTER, D. G., and J. L. CUMMINGS, 2000. *Frontal-Subcortical Circuits in Psychiatry and Neurology.* New York: Guilford Press.

LOMBARDI, W. J., R. E. GROSS, L. L. TREPANIER, A. E. LANG, A. M. LOZANO, and J. A. SAINT-CYR, 2000. Relationship of lesion location to cognitive outcome following microelectrode-guided pallidotomy for Parkinson's disease: Support for the existence of cognitive circuits in the human pallidum. *Brain* 123:746–758.

LYNCH, J. C., J. E. HOOVER, and P. L. STRICK, 1994. Input to the primate frontal eye field from the substantia nigra, superior colliculus, and dentate nucleus demonstrated by transneuronal transport. *Exp. Brain Res.* 100:181–186.

MIDDLETON, F. A., and P. L. STRICK, 1994. Anatomical evidence for cerebellar and basal ganglia involvement in higher cognitive function. *Science* 266:458–461.

MIDDLETON, F. A., and P. L. STRICK, 1996a. The temporal lobe is a target of output from the basal ganglia. *Proc. Natl. Acad. Sci. U.S.A.* 93:8683–8687.

MIDDLETON, F. A., and P. L. STRICK, 1996b. New concepts regarding the organization of basal ganglia and cerebellar ouput. In *Integrative and Molecular Approach to Brain Function*, M. Ito and Y. Miyashita, eds. New York: Elsevier, pp. 253–271.

MIDDLETON, F. A., and P. L. STRICK, 2000. A revised neuroanatomy of frontal subcortical circuits. In *Frontal-Subcortical Circuits in Psychiatry and Neurology*, D. G. Lichter and J. L. Cummings, eds, New York: Guilford Press, pp. 44–58.

MIDDLETON, F. A., and P. L. STRICK, 2001. Cerebellar projections to the prefrontal cortex of the primate. *J. Neurosci.* 21:700–712.

MIDDLETON, F. A., and P. L. STRICK, 2002. Basal ganglia "projections" to the prefrontal cortex. *Cereb. Cortex* 12:926–935.

MIYASHITA, Y., 1993. Inferior temporal cortex: Where visual perception meets memory. *Annu. Rev. Neurosci.* 16:245–263.

MUSHIAKE, H., and P. L. STRICK, 1993. Preferential activity of dentate neurons during limb movements. *J. Neurophysiol.* 70:2660–2664.

MUSHIAKE, H., and P. L. STRICK, 1995. Pallidal neuron activity during sequential arm movements. *J. Neurophysiol.* 74:2754–2758.

PASSINGHAM, R., 1993. *The Frontal Lobes and Voluntary Action.* Oxford, England: Oxford University Press.

PERCHERON, G., C. FRANCOIS, B. TALBI, J. YELNIK, and G. FENCLON, 1996. The primate motor thalamus. *Brain Res. Rev.* 22:93–181.

PETERSEN, S. E., P. T. FOX, M. I. POSNER, M. MINTUN, and M. E. RAICHLE, 1988. Positron emission tomographic studies of the cortical anatomy of single-word processing. *Nature* 331:585–589.

RAICHLE, M. E., J. A. FIEZ, T. O. VIDEEN, A. M. MACLEOD, J. V. PARDO, P. T. FOX, and S. E. PETERSEN, 1994. Practice-related changes in human brain functional anatomy during nonmotor learning. *Cereb. Cortex* 4:8–26.

RAPOPORT, J. L., and S. P. WISE, 1988. Obsessive-compulsive disorder: Evidence for basal ganglia dysfunction. *Psychopharm. Bull.* 24:380–384.

SAINT-CYR, J. A., L. G. UNGERLEIDER, and R. DESIMONE, 1990. Organization of visual cortical inputs to the striatum and subsequent outputs to the pallido-nigral complex in the monkey. *J. Comp. Neurol.* 298:129–156.

SAKAI, S. T., M. INASE, and J. TANJI, 1999. Pallidal and cerebellar inputs to thalamocortical neurons projecting to the supplementary motor area in *Macaca fuscata*: A triple-labeling light microscopic study. *Anat. Embryol. (Berl).* 199:9–19.

SCHELL, G. R., and P. L. STRICK, 1984. The origin of thalamic inputs to the arcuate premotor and supplementary motor areas. *J. Neurosci.* 4:539–560.

SCHMAHMANN, J. D., 1991. An emerging concept: The cerebellar contribution to higher function. *Arch. Neurol.* 48:1178–1187.

SCHMAHMANN, J. D., 1997. Rediscovery of an early concept. *Int. Rev. Neurobiol.* 41:3–27.

SCHMAHMANN, J. D., and D. N. PANDYA, 1997. The cerebrocerebellar system. *Int. Rev. Neurobiol.* 41:31–60.

SCHMAHMANN, J. D., and J. C. SHERMAN, 1998. The cerebellar cognitive affective syndrome. *Brain* 121:561–579.

STRICK, P. L., and J. P. CARD, 1992. Transneuronal mapping of neural circuits with alpha herpesviruses. In *Experimental Neuroanatomy: A Practical Approach*, J. P. Bolam, ed. Oxford, England: Oxford University Press, pp. 81–101.

STRICK, P. L., R. P. DUM, and N. PICARD, 1995. Macro-organization of the circuits connecting the basal ganglia with the cortical motor areas. In *Models of Information Processing in the Basal Ganglia*, J. C. Houk, J. L. Davis, and D. G. Beiser, eds. Cambridge, Mass.: MIT Press, pp. 117–130.

TANAKA, K., H.-A. SAITO, Y. FUKUDA, and M. MORIYA, 1991. Coding visual images of objects in the inferotemporal cortex of the macaque monkey. *J. Neurophysiol.* 66:170–189.

VAN KAN, P. L. E., J. C. HOUK, and A. R. GIBSON, 1993. Output organization of intermediate cerebellum of the monkey. *J. Neurophysiol.* 69:57–73.

YETERIAN, E. H., and D. N. PANDYA, 1993. Striatal connections of the parietal association cortices in rhesus monkeys. *J. Comp. Neurol.* 332:175–197.

34 Sensorimotor Transformations in the Posterior Parietal Cortex

RICHARD ANDERSEN, DANIELLA MEEKER, BIJAN PESARAN,
BORIS BREZNEN, CHRISTOPHER BUNEO, AND HANS SCHERBERGER

ABSTRACT The posterior parietal cortex (PPC) sits at the interface between sensory and motor areas and performs sensorimotor transformations. Current research is beginning to unravel the details of this transformation process. The first part of this chapter focuses on planning signals found in the PPC. Experiments show that the thought to reach can be read out from the parietal reach region of monkeys and used to control the position of a computer cursor without any reach movements being made by the monkeys. The second section reviews recent studies of coordinate transformations, which are an important aspect of sensorimotor transformations and involve the PPC.

Early studies of the posterior parietal cortex (PPC) identified movement-related and sensory-related signals (Mountcastle et al., 1975; Robinson, 1978; Andersen et al., 1987). Although debate continues over whether responses in PPC during sensory-guided movements are sensory or movement related, control experiments indicate that both signals are present (Andersen et al., 1987). Moreover, there seems to be a dynamic evolution of activity, with sensory responses and responses related to movement plans occurring early in delayed-response tasks and movement-related activity occurring later (Zhang and Barash, 2000; Cohen, Batista, and Andersen, 2002; Sabes, Breznen, and Andersen, 2002).

Although visual responses in the lateral intraparietal (LIP) area have been well documented for a number of years, their significance has recently been reinterpreted by Goldberg and colleagues (Powell and Goldberg, 2000; Goldberg et al., 2002; Bisley and Goldberg, 2003). They have argued that the existence of visual responses means that the signals in LIP cannot be related to movement plans. It has been further argued that the nature of responses in LIP would make it difficult for other parts of the brain to determine whether activity is related to sensory responses or movement plans. Finally, they proposed that the signals must therefore be signaling salience.

One problem with the interpretation of Goldberg and colleagues is that the two kinds of responses can be distinguished. In LIP, activity related to eye movements can be distinguished from activity related to arm movements, even when the visual stimuli instructing these different movement types are similar (Snyder et al., 1997, 2000). The same is true in the parietal reach region (PRR). In LIP, when monkeys perform object-based saccades, the movement vector can be distinguished from the activity related to the object, even when the object is flashed on just prior to the eye movement. In antisaccade trials it has been claimed that there is activity related to the visual target and activity related to saccades, and thus they cannot be separated (Gottlieb and Goldberg, 1999). However, subsequent studies showed that the visual and movement activities exist in different populations of LIP cells and can in fact be easily distinguished (Zhang and Barash, 2000).

Although action-related activity is well established in PPC, a legitimate question is whether this activity is related to plans to make movements or instead reflects predicted changes in sensory input arising from the integration of efference copy. Probably both are in operation. The persistent activity in LIP and PRR on delay tasks has been shown not to reflect the sensory memory of targets or attention (Gnadt and Andersen, 1988; Mazzoni et al., 1996; Snyder et al., 1997, 1998; Batista and Andersen, 2001). Since it can precede the actual eye or arm movement by many seconds, it would appear to reflect the plan to move. However, there are additional changes in activity, both in the spiking and local field potentials that occur around the time of the movement, that likely reflect, among other possibilities, a prediction of the sensory consequences of movements (Andersen et al., 1987; Barash et al., 1991; Pesaran et al., 2002).

Reading out intended reaches

An interesting test of the idea that movement plans are conveyed in the activity of PPC neurons is to determine whether animals can use these plan-related signals to control external devices (Wessberg et al., 2000; Serruya et al., 2002;

RICHARD ANDERSEN, DANIELLA MEEKER, BIJAN PESARAN, BORIS BREZNEN, CHRISTOPHER BUNEO, and HANS SCHERBERGER Division of Biology, California Institute of Technology, Pasadena, Calif.

Taylor, Tillery, and Schwartz, 2002; Shenoy et al., 2003; Musallam et al., 2004). This research, while important from a purely scientific viewpoint, also serves the therapeutic application of developing a neural prosthetic that can be used for paralyzed patients.

PRR Signals   The PRR defined in early studies included the medial intraparietal area (MIP) and the dorsal aspect of the parietal occipital area (PO) (Snyder et al., 1997). It is similar to LIP in many aspects, the major difference being that it is active when monkeys plan arm movements, whereas LIP is most active when they plan eye movements. One of the most interesting similarities between these areas is that both code very different movement plans (reaches vs. saccades) in retinal coordinates (Stricanne et al., 1996; Batista et al., 1999; Cohen and Andersen, 2000a, b). Other similarities include shifts of activity within the retinotopic map to compensate for eye movements (Gnadt and Andersen, 1988; Duhamel et al., 1992; Batista et al., 1999), persistent activity for delayed movements (Gnadt and Andersen, 1988; Snyder et al., 1997), and activity for only the next movement in a sequence (Mazzoni et al., 1996; Batista and Andersen, 2001).

We reasoned that if PRR has activity related to the intention to make limb movements, then monkeys could use this plan signal to move a cursor on a computer screen by thinking about the movement but not executing it. In a recent study we examined whether we could decode where and when monkeys planned to make arm movements (Shenoy et al., 2003). We analyzed the activity of cells that had been recorded, one at a time, from PRR. In this task, the monkeys plan arm movements in different directions, but withhold their response until a go signal. If the target is within the response field of the cell being recorded, there is typically a visual response to the target, persistent "hold" activity related to the plan to move, and an additional increment above the hold activity just prior to and during the movement.

Figure 34.1 shows the computational architecture of a state machine that was designed to predict when an animal is planning a reach, where it intends to reach, and when it intends to execute the planned reach. Figure 34.1A shows the activity of one trial from each of 41 cells recorded from PRR of one monkey for a reach in a single direction. Two sliding window classifiers estimate the *direction* and *period* using maximum likelihood decoders (figure 34.1B). The classifier signals are fed to an *interpreter* (figure 34.1C) that determines when and where a reach should be generated. The interpreter transitions through different states and uses transition rules to improve performance. Using this decoder, performance for predicting reaches in any of eight directions exceeds 90% with as few as 40 neurons.

In the above experiments the analysis was performed off-line. In a recent study we have performed "closed-loop" experiments in real time (Meeker et al., 2002). In these studies single cells are recorded from PRR and their directional tuning is determined using the delayed-reach task. The two directions that give the statistically most distinguishable responses are chosen, and the experiments are performed again in those two directions. However, on this second set of trials the memory activity is used to predict the direction in which the monkey is planning to reach, even though no reach is actually performed. This prediction is based on the response of the cell, as well as on the data recorded during the previous set of trials using real reaches. In a subset of the trials, at the end of the delay period a cursor is placed in one of the two possible locations as predicted by the neural activity during that period. Overall, the animals were able to correctly position a cursor on about 70% of the trials, but for many cells they operated nearly perfectly. However, the most interesting finding was that during the cursor-control period of the task, when the monkey was not making reaches, about one third of the cells improved their direction tuning. This effect was fast, taking only tens of trials.

FIGURE 34.1   Computational architecture for generating high-level cognitive control signals from PRR premovement, plan activity. (A) Spike raster for each PRR neuron contributing to the control of the prosthetic device as a function of time in the delayed, center-out reach task. A single trial is illustrated. The visual target, specifying the eventual reach goal, occurs at 0 ms. The onset of arm movement occurs after 1100 ms (not shown). (B) *Classifiers* use neural activity from finite-duration sliding analysis windows to estimate the direction of arm movement (*direction classifier*) and the current neural/behavioral period (*period classifier*). Both classifiers first calculate the probability of each class, and then select the most probable class for subsequent use. (C) The *interpreter* receives the stream of period classifications (i.e., baseline, plan, or go) from the period classifier and the stream of real direction classifications (e.g., downward reach) from the direction classifier. The interpreter con-

sists of a finite-state machine that transitions among three states (baseline, plan, and reach) according to the period classification at each time step. Three different rules for transitioning from the plan state to the reach state (time, time consistency, and go) are considered. Once in the reach state, the interpreter always transitions back to the baseline state at the next time step in order to prepare for the next reach. During this transition, a high-level, cognitive control signal is issued stating that a reach should occur immediately to the location specified by the direction classifier's current estimate. More sophisticated interpreters may include additional states and may use additional signals (e.g., band-limited LFP power) to govern transitions. (Reprinted with permission from K. V. Shenoy et al., Neural prosthetic control signals from plan activity. *Neuroreport* 14:591–596. © 2003 by Lippincott Williams & Wilkins.)

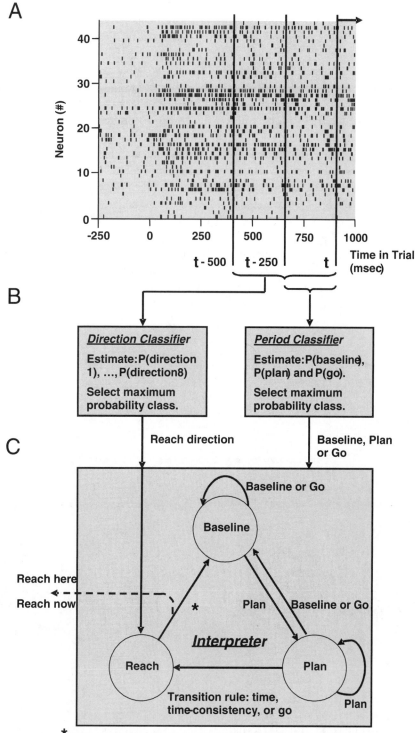

Since paralyzed patients cannot reach to calibrate a prosthetic system, the rapid plasticity seen in PRR is very promising and suggests that patients may be able to rapidly learn to control the prosthetic. This rapid plasticity may reflect the fact that PRR is at the interface between sensory and motor representations, and this adaptability may help to keep these representations in proper spatial register. Studies using prismatic adaptation paradigms suggest that PPC, along with the cerebellum, plays a major role in this calibration process. Recently, we have expanded this study to the examination of activity from many simultaneously recorded cells, with the animals positioning the cursor in more than two locations (Corneil, Mussallam, and Andersen, 2003; Musallam et al., 2003, 2004).

Local Field Potentials Figure 34.2 shows activity recorded from a neuron in area LIP, the eye movement area adjacent to PRR (Pesaran et al., 2002). The animal was performing a memory saccade task, the timing of events shown

in figure 34.2A. During the memory period the cell is very active when the monkey is planning to saccade into the response field of the neuron (upper panel of figure 34.2B). The lower panel shows part of the memory period expanded in time. Not only are spikes present during the delay, but there is also an oscillation in the local field potential (LFP). The spikes ride on top of the peaks in the LFP oscillations. The oscillation is generally in the range of 25–90 Hz, that is, in the so-called gamma band. It is produced by groups of cells around the electrode tip contributing to an averaged field potential. These oscillations are believed to be due primarily to excitatory postsynaptic potentials, which are synchronized in the local population of cells. The coherence of the spiking with the LFP is likely a result of this oscillating excitatory drive. Figure 34.2C shows traces for the same cell, but for saccades planned outside of the cell's response field. Of note, there are many fewer spikes during the delay period (upper panel), and the oscillatory LFP is also much reduced. The directional tuning of the LFPs is likely due to the colum-

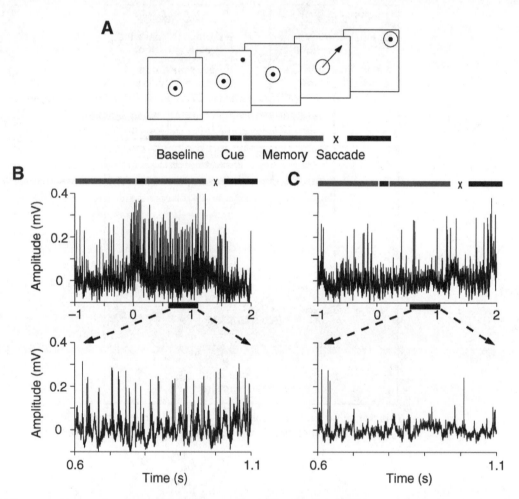

Figure 34.2 The memory saccade task. (A) The monkey performs a memory saccade in one of eight saccade directions. (B) Sample trace of extracellular potential for a trial during a saccade in the preferred direction. The polarity of the potential is reversed.

The data are viewed on an expanded time base during the memory period from 0.6 to 1.1 s—below. (C) Sample trace for a saccade in the antipreferred direction. (From Pesaran et al., 2002.)

nar organization for saccade direction that is known to exist in LIP (Pezaris et al., 1998).

The gamma band oscillation in LIP was found to be a good predictor of the direction in which monkeys planned to make saccades. Interestingly, another oscillation was also present in the beta band, centered at around 20 Hz. This oscillation was not direction tuned but rather indicated the behavioral state of the animal. When the animal was planning a saccade it slowly increased, while at the time of the eye movement it dramatically dropped to low amplitude (Pesaran et al., 2002).

From a neural coding point of view, these oscillations are of great interest. Their presence indicates that cells code the direction and state of the animals not only in the rate of action potentials, but also in the power of the local field oscillations. A similar temporal structure was also found in the spectrum of the spike trains. Thus, there are dynamic, temporal response fields that potentially could be "read out" by downstream structures, much like the rate. However, the functional role of these oscillations is not yet known.

From a practical point of view, these oscillations are extremely useful for neural prosthetics applications. A major challenge for cortical prosthetics is to acquire meaningful data from a large number of channels over a long period of time. This is particularly challenging if single spikes are used, since typically only a fraction of probes in an implant array will show the presence of spikes. Moreover, these spikes are difficult to hold over very long periods of time. However,

since local fields come from a less spatially restricted listening sphere, they should be easier to record and hold. In fact, it has been our experience that they can be recorded from most probes, and the recordings can last for at least as long as 2 years. Thus, it would be of great advantage to be able to use the LFPs for decoding when and where monkeys intend to make movements.

In recent experiments we directly compared decodes using spikes and LFPs obtained from LIP (Pesaran et al., 2002). A linear discriminant analysis was used to predict, from single trials, the direction of a planned movement (preferred vs. antipreferred direction, figure 34.3*A*). The performance for predicting direction was similar for spikes and LFPs. The correct prediction rate for the preferred direction was 87% for spikes and 87% for LFPs, and for the antipreferred direction 78% for spikes and 87% for LFPs. We also examined decoding the state (plan vs. execution state, figure 34.3*B*). The LFPs were better for this decode. The plan state was correctly identified 56% of the time for spikes and 71% for LFPs, and the execution state was correctly identified 57% of the time for spikes and 71% for LFPs. The better performance of the LFP state decodes may reflect the activity due to circuits within LIP or inputs to LIP from external sources. Further work will be required to distinguish between the two.

We have recently begun to characterize gamma band temporal structure in PRR as well (Scherberger et al., 2003). The gamma band temporal structure in PRR is also

A   Direction decode   **B**   State decode

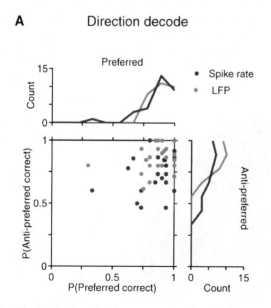
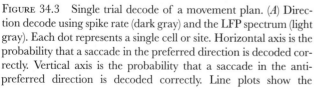
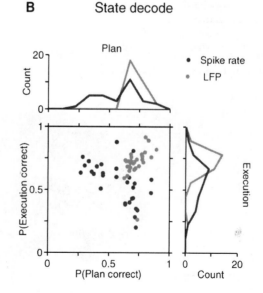

FIGURE 34.3   Single trial decode of a movement plan. (*A*) Direction decode using spike rate (dark gray) and the LFP spectrum (light gray). Each dot represents a single cell or site. Horizontal axis is the probability that a saccade in the preferred direction is decoded correctly. Vertical axis is the probability that a saccade in the antipreferred direction is decoded correctly. Line plots show the histograms for cell/site counts for each direction. (*B*) State decode. Horizontal axis is the probability that the activity from the plan state is decoded correctly. Vertical axis is the probability that the activity from the execution state is decoded correctly. Line plots show the histograms for cell/site counts for each state. (From Pesaran et al., 2002.)

direction tuned for the spikes and LFPs, but the peak power in the spatially tuned frequency band is 10–20 Hz lower in PRR than in LIP.

From both scientific and practical points of view, an important recent development was the identification of a homologue of PRR in the human (Connolly, Andersen, and Goodale, 2003; figure 34.4). In these experiments human subjects performed delayed saccades and delayed pointing, similar to delayed saccade and reach experiments that we have performed in monkeys. Using event-related functional magnetic resonance imaging, we were able to localize an area in parietal cortex that responded preferentially during the memory delay trials for planning pointing movements compared to saccades.

The PRR in humans has attributes that are different from motor cortex, which may be useful for deriving control signals for neural prosthetics. The main sensory feedback to motor cortex is from somatosensory inputs, whereas the major sensory feedback for PRR appears to be visual. Often, somatosensory feedback is lost with paralysis, whereas vision is not. Thus, feedback for evaluating terminal movement errors may be more naturally conveyed to PRR. In addition, the remarkable plasticity we have seen in PRR during cursor-control tasks bodes well for this region's ability to learn to control external devices. PRR is also more removed from motor areas, which undergo pathological changes with paralysis. Thus, it is possible that PRR will be more resilient to the changes that result from disuse following direct damage to corticospinal projections (as in spinal cord injury).

Coordinate transformations

Perceptually we have a good sense of where things are in the world, and behaviorally we can effortlessly use sensory stimuli to guide movements of a variety of body parts. These observations suggest that space is represented in many coordinate frames in the brain for perception and action. Interestingly, though, when neuroscientists have recorded from various sensory and motor representations in the brain, they have found that these representations are not simple maps containing receptive fields in a particular coordinate frame. For instance, areas in the sensorimotor pathway for visually guided movements often contain retinal response fields that are gain modulated by body position signals (Andersen et al., 1985; Salinas and Thier, 2000). Still other areas contain response fields that are partially shifted between retinotopic and other reference frames (Stricanne et al., 1996; Duhamel et al., 1997; Cohen and Andersen, 2000a, b; Buneo et al., 2002). One advantage of the "gain field" representation is that information in multiple reference frames can be represented simultaneously. Another is that information is not lost; for instance, cells that code head-centered locations using gain modulation still contain information about the retinal location of the target. Neural network models have demonstrated that this gain field mechanism can be used for coordinate transformations (Zipser and Andersen, 1988; Pouget and Sejnowski, 1995; Pouget and Snyder, 2000; Xing and Andersen, 2000a, b).

The fact that gain modulation is found in a variety of brain areas and seems to operate in a number of functional contexts suggests that its computational function may extend well beyond sensorimotor transformations and may be a general method for neural computation when transformations between brain representations are required (Salinas and Thier, 2000). Recently, we have examined whether gain modulation is reflected in human visual perception, and if it is psychophysically detectable (Nishida et al., 2003). In particular, we wished to determine the coordinate frames in

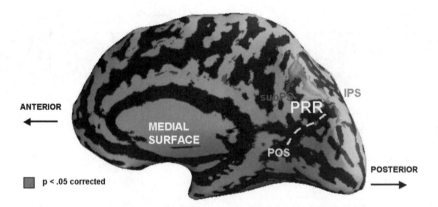

FIGURE 34.4   Medial view of an inflated cerebral cortex, showing unfolded sulci and gyri and the location of the fMRI delay interval activation, as determined using multiple regression analysis (ten subjects, P < 0.05). GLM signal timecourses that were subjected to further ANOVA analysis were situated anterior to the parieto-occipital sulcus, posterior to the subparietal sulcus, medial to the intraparietal sulcus. (Reprinted with permission from J. D. Connolly et al., fMRI evidence for a "parietal reach region" in the human brain. *Exp. Brain Res.* 153:140–145. © 2003 by Springer-Verlag.) (See color plate 16.)

which various perceptual phenomena may be represented in cortex.

To assess the effect of gaze on human visual perception, we examined gaze-dependent visual aftereffects. In these experiments subjects were adapted in one gaze direction and then tested in the same or a different gaze direction. In both same and different (opposite) gaze directions, the images of the test stimuli on the retinas were identical.

Figure 34.5*a* shows that small but significant differences were found for a wide variety of aftereffects, including the motion aftereffect (MAE), tilt aftereffect (TAE), and the size aftereffect (SAE). In all cases the aftereffect was greater for the same gaze direction compared to the opposite gaze direction by about 15% (figure 34.5*b*). The detection threshold elevation showed the same trend (see figure 34.5*b*) but did not reach statistical significance (see figure 34.5*a*), largely owing to greater variability of the effect.

These experiments suggest that gaze modulates visual activity in areas of striate and extrastriate cortex that are known to play a role in the percepts of motion, orientation, and size. In other experiments the aftereffects were tested for world- and object-centered effects. In the world-centered coordinate test, TAE magnitudes were compared between locations in space that were adapted by the test stimulus prior to testing at a different gaze direction. No aftereffect was found for retinally nonadapted loci that occupied the spatial location of the test stimulus after the gaze shift. Since the subjects did not shift their heads or bodies in this experiment, this study also indicates that head- or body-centered effects were not present. In the object-centered test, the test stimulus reappeared at the same world-centered location as the adaptation and then moved to a new location. No transfer of adaptation was found in this experiment.

The world- and object-centered tests were negative, which suggests that, at least for the TAE, the perception of orientation does not undergo a complete transformation from a retinotopic to a nonretinotopic representation anywhere in

the brain. Of course, there may be higher-level percepts that do undergo these transformations, particularly those more closely linked to motor systems. This question is an interesting topic for future research.

OBJECT-BASED SACCADES Lesions of the PPC in humans can produce object-fixed neglect, in which patients are unaware of the contralateral side of objects (Driver and Halligan, 1991; Behrmann and Moscovitch, 1994; Driver et al., 1994; Hillis and Caramazza, 1995). This result suggests that cells in PPC might code parts of an object in an object-based reference frame. In many experiments examining saccade-related neural structures, single spots of light are used to examine the response properties of neurons. This approach has been the case for area LIP, and it has been reported that the neurons in this area code visual targets, plans for eye movements, and saccade-related responses all in retinotopic coordinates (Andersen and Buneo, 2002). However, in natural situations, the pattern of eye movements is based on parts of objects and spatial relations between objects. Several studies have examined eye movement areas in the frontal and parietal cortex using tasks in which animals make eye movements to objects with particular features among groups of distracter objects (Bichot et al., 1996; Gottlieb et al., 1998; Bichot and Schall, 1999; Hasegawa, Matsumoto, and Mikami, 2000; Constantinidis and Steinmetz, 2001). In one experiment in the supplementary eye fields (SEF), target selection was studied within objects, and it was reported that the response fields of the neurons were in an object-fixed reference frame (Olson and Gettner, 1995).

Given the prevalence of object-fixed neglect in the PPC, we decided to examine the coordinate frame used to make object-based saccades by LIP (Sabes, Breznen, and Andersen, 2002). In this task, a filled polygon was used as the test object. On each trial, the monkey was presented with this polygon in one of a variety of possible orientations. One

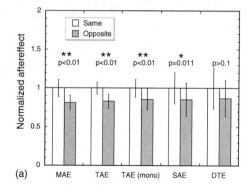

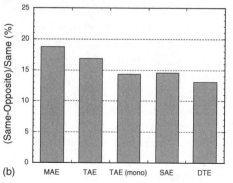

FIGURE 34.5 The graph shows the modulation ratio, defined as the contrast ratio of adaptation between the same and opposite directions of gaze. Gaze angle had a constant effect of around 15% for all types of adaptation tested. (Reprinted with permission from S. Nishida et al., Gaze modulation of visual aftereffects. *Vision Res.* 43:639–649. © 2003 by Elsevier.)

of four fingers on the object was indicated by a flashed cue, and the monkey memorized the location of the cue. The object then disappeared briefly and reappeared at a new orientation. At this point the animal was required to saccade to the end of the previously cued finger in order to receive a drop of juice reward.

We found that LIP neurons code the retinotopic location of the target and the retinotopic orientation of the object. No cells were specific for a finger, that is, for coded locations on the object in object-based coordinates. Individual cells were sensitive to target location, others to orientation, and some cells to both. Moreover, there was a dynamic evolution for tuning in the population, with about equal numbers of cells coding orientation and target location at the beginning of the task and many more cells coding the retinotopic location of the target later in the task, near the time of the saccade.

One possible explanation of the object-based neglect after parietal lesions is that it results from damage to a population of neurons, none of which carry explicit information about location in object coordinates but do so as an ensemble. Computational models have made exactly this point. Alternatively, it may be that the projection of PPC onto SEF and other frontal lobe structures results in the explicit representation of targets in object-fixed coordinates. We have begun examining this possibility by performing a variant of the object-based saccade task and recording from SEF neurons.

Cells with both orientation and target tuning could be separated using a general linear model (Sabes, Breznen, and Andersen, 2002). This was accomplished by probing cell activity using an object, or only a target for a saccade. When animals performed the object-based saccade task, it was found that, for cells with object orientation and target location sensitivity, the two components of activity added linearly. Interestingly, the target and orientation components could be easily separated even when the object reappeared at the new orientation. The go signal to make the saccade was given simultaneously with the reappearance of the object. Although the object's reappearance invoked a large visual response that indicated the orientation of the object, the direction of the planned movement could still be read out at all times. This readout of the two variables was demonstrated by computing population vectors for both variables (Breznen and Andersen, 2000). Thus, recent claims that movement plans cannot be distinguished from visual responses in LIP are incorrect (Powell and Goldberg, 2000; Goldberg et al., 2002; Bisley and Goldberg, 2003).

DIRECT COORDINATE TRANSFORMATIONS USING GAIN FIELDS
The coordinate transformation for visually guided reach movements requires that the eye-centered visual inputs be transformed to a limb-centered goal of the intended direc-

tion and amplitude of the movement. There are at least three ways in which this computation can be performed, as illustrated in figure 34.6. One is a sequential model (figure 34.6a), in which the transformation occurs in stages (Flanders et al., 1992; Henriques et al., 1998; McIntyre et al., 1998). The eye-centered location of the visual target is first combined with an eye position signal to form a representation of the target in head coordinates. Then head position information is added to form a representation in body-centered coordinates. Finally, the body-centered position of the hand is subtracted from the body position location of the target to generate a hand-centered representation of the target, indicating the motor error for acquiring the target. Psychophysical results suggest that such a sequential representation may be used for certain reach tasks (Flanders et al., 1992; McIntyre et al., 1998). However, this model requires a good deal of neural real estate, including intermediate representations of the reach targets in head- and body-centered coordinates. Recording experiments in the dorsal visual pathway associated with reaching movements have found only small numbers of cells in the ventral intraparietal area (VIP) and PO that use intervening stages such as head-centered representations (Battaglini et al., 1990; Duhamel et al., 1997).

A second, combinatorial model is shown in figure 34.6b (Battaglia-Mayer et al., 2000). In this model, all signals of retinal target location, eye position, head position, and limb position converge onto the same area, and the location of the target with respect to the hand is then read out of this high-dimensional representation. There is evidence for such a high degree of convergence within area PO. However, from a computational perspective this model suffers from the "curse of dimensionality," since at least three spatial dimensions of all the four variables must be encoded in this area. If only ten neurons were required along each dimension, even this sparse tiling would require a trillion neurons, about two orders of magnitude more neurons than are found in the cerebral cortex.

A third, direct model (Buneo et al., 2002) is shown in figure 34.6c and d. In this model the location of the target and the initial location of the hand are both represented in visual, that is, eye-centered, coordinates. The two are simply subtracted to produce a direct transformation of the target in hand coordinates. Such a method requires many fewer neurons, only 1 million by the above calculation, and thus does not suffer as much from the curse of dimensionality.

Recently, we have found evidence for this direct model in the PPC (Buneo et al., 2002). The PRR neurons code the location of reach targets in eye coordinates (Batista et al., 1999), and the initial position of the hand produces a gain modulation of the response. As indicated in the left part of figure 34.7, this gain modulation is also in eye coordinates. By converging inputs of cells with these gain fields onto cells

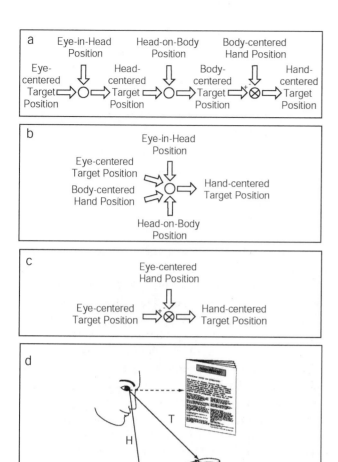

FIGURE 34.6 Schemes for transforming target position from eye-centered to hand-centered coordinates. (*a*) Sequential method. (*b*) Combinatorial method. (*c*) Direct method. (*d*) Illustration of reaching for a cup while fixating a newspaper, using the direct method. The position of the cup with respect to the hand (M) is obtained by directly subtracting hand position (H) from target position (T), both in eye coordinates. (Reprinted with permission from R. A. Andersen and C. A. Buneo, Sensorimotor integration in posterior cortex. In *The Parietal Lobes*, A. M. Siegel, R. A. Andersen, H.-J. Freund, and D. D. Spencer, eds. Baltimore: Lippincott Williams & Wilkins, pp. 159–177. © 2003 by Lippincott Williams & Wilkins.)

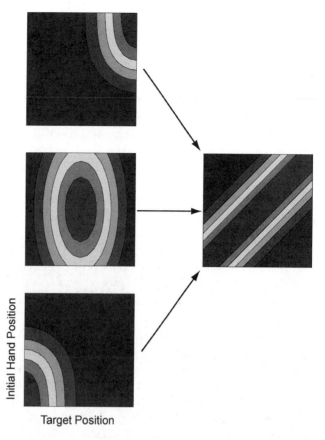

FIGURE 34.7 Schematic of how three PRR neurons, coding reach targets in eye coordinates and gain modulated by the initial hand position in eye coordinates, could converge onto another neuron to produce a receptive field in limb coordinates.

in other cortical areas, the subtraction of target- and hand-related signals can be accomplished (right part of figure 34.7). Thus, the convergence of inputs from PRR neurons onto premotor cortex could conceivably produce this transformation in one step. In area 5 we have found that cell response fields are partially shifted between eye and limb coordinates (Buneo et al., 1998). Again, this representation can be produced by a one-step convergence from PRR neurons. The reason for the partially shifted profile of area 5 cells may reflect the coordinate representation that is necessary for the computations performed by this area. Consis-

tent with this idea is the fact that area 5 receives visual signals, represented in eye coordinates, and efference copy signals and proprioceptive signals, represented in limb coordinates. Thus, the representation in area 5 may be optimal for making computations that use these different signals.

The use of coordinate transformation schemes may be context dependent. For instance, in the experiments of Buneo and colleagues, the initial position of the hand was visible to the animal, and thus a direct retinal subtraction may be the most parsimonious solution (Buneo et al., 1998). In other conditions where the hand is not visible a sequential model may be used (Flanders et al., 1992; McIntyre et al., 1998). We are currently performing experiments to distinguish between these possibilities.

SHARED BEHAVIORAL REFERENCE FRAME FOR TARGET SELECTION FOR REACHES AND SACCADES It would be parsimonious to represent arm and eye movements in the same coordinate frames, given the close coupling of these two types of action. The mere fact that so many eye movements are made compared with number of limb movements would suggest that an eye-centered reference frame be used. In fact, as reviewed above, PRR codes the locations of reach targets in eye coordinates (Batista et al., 1999). Also, the initial location of the hand is coded in eye coordinates in PRR and exerts its influence as a gain modulation of the target-related activity (Buneo et al., 2002).

Inspired by the above findings, we have recently examined the behavioral reference frame used by monkeys performing a hand/eye coordination task (Scherberger, Goodale, and Andersen, 2003). The influence of eye, head, and body position on target selection was examined for both eye and hand movements. We found that the initial position of the eyes in the orbits biased the monkey's choice. This finding was not surprising, insofar as the preferred direction was one that always tended to center the eyes in the orbits. This preference reduces the effort of maintaining the eyes at peripheral fixation angles, and also provides a more optimal operating range for subsequent eye movements. Also not surprising was the finding that the limb used also biased the decision, with rightward movement preferred for the right limb and leftward movement preferred for the left. What was counterintuitive was the finding that the positions of the eyes in the orbits influenced the selection of the reach direction, with the animals choosing to reach to targets that were closer to the fixation position. However, the orientation of the trunk showed much less effect on the selection. While the eye position had considerable effect on selection of reach targets, the arm position did not have an influence on the choice of saccade targets.

These experiments show behavioral evidence for a common reference frame for hand/eye coordination, at least for target selection. The results indicate that the eyes play a more dominant role, consistent with the eye-centered representations for reaches and saccades found in PPC. Technically, the reaches and saccades are chosen on the basis of head-centered coordinates; however, this decision can easily be accomplished by the eye position gain modulation of retinocentric representations that are found in parietofrontal cortical areas. Moreover, these decisions would bring targets more into the operating range of the cortical eye-centered representations. We are currently performing experiments to see where eye position signals exert their effect on the decisions made in this task.

Conclusion

This chapter has focused on two functions of PPC in sensorimotor transformations, the planning of movements and coordinate transformations. We have shown experimentally that parietal activity related to reach planning can be read out and used by monkeys to control a cursor on a monitor without reaching movements. These experiments are real-time and direct demonstrations that signals related to plan-

ning in the PPC can be used by the animals to control external devices. Moreover, the neural activity used for control is highly malleable by the animals, and they can rapidly adjust to increase their performance in closed-loop experiments. We also found that LFP activity can be used to decode the intentions of the monkeys. A practical advantage of using LFPs compared to spikes is the relative ease of recording and considerable stability over time. The demonstration of cursor control, the finding of rapid plasticity, and the ability to decode movement intentions with LFPs all bode well for the use of PPC as a source of control signals to assist paralyzed patients in neural prosthetics applications.

The PPC also plays an important role in coordinate transformations. The gain field mechanism proves to be a computationally efficient method for realizing these transformations. However, the gain field mechanism may also act more broadly in a variety of computations. New evidence for this broader applicability is the finding of eye position gain effects on a variety of visual percepts in humans.

In a new class of experiments, we examined whether object-centered coding is used by area LIP in a saccade task that requires the use of object-based information. We found that the orientation of the object and the target location on the object are both encoded in retinal, and not object-centered, coordinates. However, reminiscent of other gain field results, this information is all that is required to solve the task, and the explicit representation of the target in object-centered coordinates may not be required.

We have also found that the conversion from eye to limb coordinates for visually guided reach movements may occur in a direct fashion, one that can bypass intermediate head- and body-centered representations. Again, this transformation is accomplished with gain fields, but in this case the gain field is the target location, modulated by initial hand position, both represented in retinal coordinates. This type of gain field was found in PRR. We have also found behavioral results consistent with this eye-based coding of early reach plans. The selection of reach and saccade targets was found in monkeys to be highly biased by the position of the eyes, and reach targets were found to be much less affected by trunk position. Moreover, the position of the limb did not affect the choice of saccade targets.

Research in the PPC continues to be a fertile ground for studying how sensorimotor transformations are accomplished. The finding of possible human homologues of PRR, LIP, and AIP with fMRI experiments points to the use of fMRI in monkeys in the future as a powerful method to directly compare monkey and human results. Also, experiments that can read out and read in information to the PPC will be invaluable in providing direct tests of models of parietal lobe function. The future is bright for sensorimotor research.

ACKNOWLEDGMENTS   This work was supported by the National Eye Institute, the James G. Boswell Foundation, the McKnight Foundation, the Sloan-Swartz Center for Theoretical Neurobiology at Caltech, the Defense Advanced Research Projects Agency, and the Office of Naval Research.

REFERENCES

ANDERSEN, R. A., and C. A. BUNEO, 2002. Intentional maps in the posterior parietal cortex. *Annu. Rev. Neurosci.* 25:189–220.

ANDERSEN, R. A., and C. A. BUNEO, 2003. Sensorimotor integration in posterior parietal cortex. In *The Parietal Lobes*, A. M. Siegel, R. A. Andersen, H.-J. Freund, and D. D. Spencer, eds. Baltimore: Lippincott–Williams and Wilkins, pp. 159–177.

ANDERSEN, R. A., G. K. ESSICK, et al., 1985. Encoding of spatial location by posterior parietal neurons. *Science* 25:456–458.

ANDERSEN, R. A., G. K. ESSICK, et al., 1987. Neurons of area 7 activated by both visual stimuli and oculomotor behavior. *Exp. Brain Res.* 67:316–322.

BARASH, S., R. A. ANDERSEN, et al., 1991. Saccade-related activity in the lateral intraparietal area. I. Temporal properties. Comparison with area 7a. *J. Neurophysiol.* 66:1095–1108.

BATISTA, A. P., and R. A. ANDERSEN, 2001. The parietal reach region codes the next planned movement in a sequential reach task. *J. Neurophysiol.* 85:539–544.

BATISTA, A. P., C. A. BUNEO, et al., 1999. Reach plans in eye-centered coordinates. *Science* 285:257–260.

BATTAGLIA-MAYER, A., S. FERRAINA, T. MITSUDA, et al., 2000. Early coding of reaching in the parieto-occipital cortex. *J. Neurophysiol.* 83:2374–2391.

BATTAGLINI, P. P., P. FATTORI, et al., 1990. The physiology of area V6 in the awake, behaving monkey. *J. Physiol.* 423:100P.

BEHRMANN, M., and M. MOSCOVITCH, 1994. Object-centered neglect in patients with unilateral neglect: Effects of left-right coordinates of objects. *J. Cogn. Neurosci.* 6:1–16.

BICHOT, N. P., and J. D. SCHALL, 1999. Effects of similarity and history on neural mechanisms of visual selection. *Nat. Neurosci.* 2:549–554.

BICHOT, N. P., J. D. SCHALL, et al., 1996. Visual feature selectivity in frontal eye fields induced by experience in mature macaques. *Nature* 381:697–699.

BISLEY, J. W., and M. E. GOLDBERG, 2003. Neuronal activity in the lateral intraparietal area and spatial attention. *Science* 299:81–81.

BREZNEN, B., and R. A. ANDERSEN, 2000. Decoding of the population vector in LIP for object-based saccades. *Soc. Neurosci. Abstr.* 26:668.

BUNEO, C. A., A. P. BATISTA, et al., 1998. Frames of reference for reach-related activity in two parietal areas. *Soc. Neurosci. Abstr.* 24.

BUNEO, C. A., M. R. JARVIS, A. P. BATISTA, and R. A. ANDERSEN, 2002. Direct visuomotor transformations for reaching. *Nature* 416:632–636.

COHEN, Y. E., and R. A. ANDERSEN, 2000a. Eye position modulates reach activity to sounds. *Neuron* 27:647–652.

COHEN, Y. E., and R. A. ANDERSEN, 2000b. Reaches to sounds encoded in an eye-centered reference frame. *Neuron* 27:647–652.

COHEN, Y. E., A. P. BATISTA, and R. A. ANDERSEN, 2002. Comparison of neural activity preceding reaches to auditory and visual stimuli in the parietal reach region. *Neuroreport* 13:891–894.

CONNOLLY, J. D., R. A. ANDERSEN, and M. A. GOODALE, 2003. FMRI evidence for a "parietal reach region" in the human brain. *Exp. Brain Res.* 153:140–145.

CONSTANTINIDIS, C., and M. A. STEINMETZ, 2001. Neuronal responses in area 7a to multiple-stimulus displays. I. Neurons encode the location of the salient stimulus. *Cereb. Cortex* 11:581–591.

CORNEIL, B. D., S. MUSALLAM, and R. A. ANDERSEN, 2003. Representation of reward expectancy in the medial bank of the intraparietal sulcus: Implications for neural prosthetics. *Soc. Neurosci Abstr.* 29.

DRIVER, J., and P. W. HALLIGAN, 1991. Can visual neglect operate in object-centered coordinates? An affirmative single-case study. *Cogn. Neuropsychol.* 8:475–496.

DRIVER, J., G. C. BAYLIS, S. J. GOODRICH, and R. D. RAFAL, 1994. Axis-based neglect of visual shapes. *Neuropsychologia* 32:1353–1365.

DUHAMEL, J. R., F. BREMMER, et al., 1997. Spatial invariance of visual receptive fields in parietal cortex neurons. *Nature* 389:845–848.

DUHAMEL, J. R., C. L. COLBY, et al., 1992. The updating of the representation of visual space in parietal cortex by intended eye movements. *Science* 255:90–92.

FLANDERS, M., S. I. HELMS-TILLERY, et al., 1992. Early stages in a sensorimotor transformation. *Behav. Brain Sci.* 15:309–362.

GNADT, J. W., and R. A. ANDERSEN, 1988. Memory related motor planning activity in posterior parietal cortex of macaque. *Exp. Brain Res.* 70:216–220.

GOLDBERG, M. E., J. BISLEY, K. D. POWELL, J. GOTTLIEB, and M. KUSUNOKI, 2002. The role of the lateral intraparietal area of the monkey in the generation of saccades and visuospatial attention. *Ann. N.Y. Acad. Sci.* 956:205–215.

GOTTLIEB, J., and M. E. GOLDBERG, 1999. Activity of neurons in the lateral intraparietal area of the monkey during an anti-saccade task. *Nat. Neurosci.* 2:906–912.

GOTTLIEB, J. P., M. KUSUNOKI, et al., 1998. The representation of visual salience in monkey parietal cortex. *Nature* 391:481–484.

HASEGAWA, R. P., M. MATSUMOTO, and A. MIKAMI, 2000. Search target selection in monkey prefrontal cortex. *J. Neurophysiol.* 84:1692–1996.

HENRIQUES, D. Y., E. M. KLIER, et al., 1998. Gaze-centered remapping of remembered visual space in an open-loop pointing task. *J. Neurosci.* 18:1583–1594.

HILLIS, A. E., and A. A. CARAMAZZA, 1995. A framework for interpreting distinct patterns of hemispatial neglect. *Neurocase* 1:189–207.

MAZZONI, P., R. M. BRACEWELL, et al., 1996. Motor intention activity in the macaque's lateral intraparietal area. I. Dissociation of motor plan from sensory memory. *J. Neurophysiol.* 76:1439–1456.

MCINTYRE, J., F. STRATTA, et al., 1998. Short-term memory for reaching to visual targets: Psychophysical evidence for body-centered reference frames. *J. Neurosci.* 18: 8423–8435.

MEEKER, D., S. CAO, J. W. BURDICK, and R. A. ANDERSEN, 2002. Rapid plasticity in the parietal reach area demonstrated with a brain-computer interface. *Soc. Neurosci. Abstr.* 28.

MOUNTCASTLE, V. B., J. C. LYNCH, et al., 1975. Posterior parietal association cortex of the monkey: Command functions for operations within extrapersonal space. *J. Neurophysiol.* 38:871–908.

MUSALLAM, S., B. D. CORNEIL, R. BHATTACHARYYA, D. MEEKER, and R. A. ANDERSEN, 2003. Real time control of a cursor using multi-electrode arrays implanted in the medial bank of the intraparietal sulcus. *Soc. Neurosci. Abstr.* 29.

MUSALLAM, S., B. D. CORNEIL, B. GREGER, H. SCHERBERGER, and R. A. ANDERSEN, 2004. Cognitive control signals for neural prosthetics. *Science* 305:258–262.

NISHIDA, S., I. MOTOYOSHI, R. A. ANDERSEN, and S. SHIMOJO, 2003. Gaze modulation of visual aftereffects. *Vision Res.* 43:639–649.

OLSON, C. R., and S. N. GETTNER, 1995. Object-centered direction selectivity in the macaque supplementary eye field. *Science* 269: 985–988.

PESARAN, B., J. PEZARIS, M. SAHANI, P. M. MITRA, and R. A. ANDERSEN, 2002. Temporal structure in neuronal activity during working memory in macaque parietal cortex. *Nat. Neurosci.* 5:805–811.

PEZARIS, J. S., M. SAHANI, et al., 1998. Extracellular recording from multiple neighboring cells: Response properties in parietal cortex. *Computational Neuroscience: Trends in Research*, J. M. Bower, ed. New York: Plenum Press.

POUGET, A., and J. T. SEJNOWSKI, 1995. Spatial representations in the parietal cortex of the monkey: Command functions for operations within extra-personal space. *Adv. Neural Inform. Proc.* 7:157–164.

POUGET, A., and L. H. SNYDER, 2000. Computational approaches to sensorimotor transformations. *Nat. Neurosci.* 3:1193–1198.

POWELL, K. D., and M. E. GOLDBERG, 2000. Response of neurons in the lateral intraparietal area to a distractor flashed during the delay period of a memory-guided saccade. *J. Neurophysiol.* 84: 301–310.

ROBINSON, D. L., M. E. GOLDBERG, et al., 1978. Parietal association cortex in the primate: Sensory mechanisms and behavioral modulations. *J. Neurophysiol.* 41:910–932.

SABES, P. N., B. BREZNEN, and R. A. ANDERSEN, 2002. The parietal representation of object-based saccades. *J. Neurophysiol.* 88:1815–1829.

SALINAS, E., and P. THEIR, 2000. Gain modulation: A major computational principle of the central nervous system. *Neuron* 27:15–21.

SCHERBERGER, H., C.A. BUNEO, M. JARVIS, and R. A. ANDERSEN, 2003. Local field potential tuning in the macaque posterior parietal cortex during arm-reaching movements. *Soc. Neurosci. Abstr.* 29.

SCHERBERGER, H., M. A. GOODALE, and R. A. ANDERSEN, 2003. Target selection for reaching and saccades share a similar behavioral reference frame in the macaque. *J. Neurophysiol.* 89: 1456–1466.

SERRUYA, M. D., N. G. HATSOPOULOS, L. PANINSKI, M. R. Fellows, and J. P. Donoghue, 2002. Instant neural control of a movement signal. *Nature* 416:141–142.

SHENOY, K. V., D. MEEKER, S. Y. CAO, S. A. KURESHI, B. PESARAN, C. A. BUNEO, A. R. BATISTA, P. P. MITRA, J. W. BURDICK, and R. A. ANDERSEN, 2003. Neural prosthetic control signals from plan activity. *Neuroreport* 14:591–596.

SNYDER, L. H., A. P. BATISTA, et al., 1997. Coding of intention in the posterior parietal cortex. *Nature* 386:167–170.

SNYDER, L. H., A. P. BATISTA, et al., 1998. Change in motor plan, without a change in the spatial locus of attention, modulates activity in posterior parietal cortex. *J. Neurophysiol.* 79:2814–2819.

SNYDER, L. H., A. P. BATISTA, et al., 2000. Intention-related activity in the posterior parietal cortex: A review. *Vision Res.* 40:1433–1441.

STRICANNE, B., R. A. ANDERSEN, et al., 1996. Eye-centered, head-centered, and intermediate coding of remembered sound locations in area LIP. *J. Neurophysiol.* 76:2071–2076.

TAYLOR, D. M., S. I. H. TILLERY, and A. B. SCHWARTZ, 2002. Direct cortical control of 3D neuroprosthetic devices. *Science* 296:1829–1832.

WESSBERG, J., C. R. STAMBAUGH, et al., 2000. Real-time prediction of hand trajectory by ensembles of cortical neurons in primates. *Nature* 408:361–365.

XING, J., and R. A. ANDERSEN, 2000a. The memory activity of LIP neurons in sequential eye movements simulated with neural networks. *J. Neurophysiol.* 84:651–665.

XING, J., and R. A. ANDERSEN, 2000b. Models of the posterior parietal cortex which perform multimodal integration and represent space in several coordinate frames. *J. Cogn. Neurosci.* 12:601–614.

ZHANG, M., and S. BARASH, 2000. Neuronal switching of sensorimotor transformations for antisaccades. *Nature* 408:971–975.

ZIPSER, D., and R. A. ANDERSEN, 1988. A back-propagation programmed network that simulates response properties of a subset of posterior parietal neurons. *Nature* 331:679–684.

35 Brain Mechanisms of Praxis

APOSTOLOS P. GEORGOPOULOS

ABSTRACT This chapter deals with the neural mechanisms of *praxis*, that is, purposeful motor actions. Three typical praxis tasks were used: copy geometrical figures, find exit routes in mazes, and construct objects from component parts. These tasks are commonly used in clinical neurology to determine the presence, and evaluate the severity, of constructional apraxia. Brain mechanisms were investigated using various methods and in different species, including experimental psychology (in human subjects and monkeys), functional magnetic resonance imaging (in human subjects), and single cell recordings from multiple sites (in monkeys). The results obtained provided new insights into how the brain deals with dynamic visuomotor processes and carries out purposeful *eupractic* motor actions.

Apraxia and constructional praxis

Apraxia has been defined as the "inability to perform certain subjectively purposive movements or movement complexes with conservation of motility, of sensation and of coordination" (Wilson, 1909). Apraxia typically is the result of parietal lobe damage, and occurs in three main forms. In *ideational* apraxia (Liepmann, 1920) there is a failure to perform a complex series of actions (e.g., to fold a piece of paper and place it inside an envelope); in *ideomotor* apraxia (Liepmann, 1920), the subject cannot execute a familiar action (e.g., a gesture on command or by imitation); and in *constructional* apraxia there is a disturbance "in formative activities such as assembling, building and drawing, in which the spatial form of the product proves to be unsuccessful, without there being an apraxia for single movements" (Kleist, 1934), or the "inability to assemble component parts into a coherent whole" (Koski, Iacoboni, and Mazziotta, 2002). In the first two forms of apraxia affected individuals have difficulty reproducing previously well-learned motor tasks. Thus, the mechanisms thought to underlie ideomotor apraxia have been considered to be disconnections between language and frontal areas (Geschwind, 1975) or, in addition, damage to stored representations of learned movement engrams (Heilman and Rothi, 1985; Gonzalez Rothi, Ochipa, and Heilman, 1991; Poizner et al., 1995). In con-

trast, in constructional apraxia affected subjects have difficulty reproducing visual figures. Constructional apraxia is a fairly common neurological disorder (Gainotti, 1985; Förstl et al., 1993; Kirk and Kertesz, 1993). A crucial deficit in this disorder is the inability to copy a visual model (Benton, 1962, 1967; Gainotti, 1985) or assemble a two-dimensional or three-dimensional object from its component parts (Benton and Fogel, 1962). Although early studies pointed to a special role for the right cerebral hemisphere in constructional apraxia (Piercy, Hécaen, and Ajuriaguerra, 1960; Benton, 1967; Mack and Levine, 1981), more systematic later work (reviewed in De Renzi, 1982; Gainotti, 1985) supported the notion that this function is most probably subserved by both hemispheres.

Although constructional deficits are most often observed following damage to posterior parietal cortex, there is broad consensus that constructional deficits and other forms of apraxia also result from cortical damage that is confined to the prefrontal cortex (Luria and Tsvekova, 1964; Benton, 1968; Gainotti, 1985; Koski, Iacoboni, and Mazziotta, 2002). The fact that lesions in widespread cortical areas can cause constructional deficits led Benson and Barton (1970) to suggest that "drawing, by itself, is a reasonably good test for detecting brain damage." In fact, copying objects has been used as a probe to detect brain damage since early in the twentieth century (Poppelreuter, 1917). One possible reason why constructional ability is easily disturbed is that it is a complex task requiring the functional coordination of many different processes, including visuospatial perception and spatial motor planning. These factors are commonly tested in a different context, namely, route finding in simple drawings of mazes (Porteus Maze Test; Porteus, 1965). Interestingly, the performance of right-hemisphere-damaged patients in copying is highly correlated with their performance on route-finding tasks (Angelini, Frasca, and Grossi, 1992). These processes, then, collectively define *constructional praxis*.

Recently, we have studied the brain mechanisms underlying constructional praxis using three tasks, copying, mental maze solving, and mental object construction. The following discussion reviews our results and inferences that can be drawn from our studies.

COPYING Our first praxis task was copying shapes. To make a copy of a figure, one has to translate a visual pattern

APOSTOLOS P. GEORGOPOULOS Brain Sciences Center, Veterans Affairs Medical Center, and Departments of Neuroscience, Neurology, and Psychiatry, University of Minnesota Medical School, Minneapolis, Minn.

to a closely corresponding motor pattern. It is useful to contrast copying with tracing. In the case of tracing, the movement trajectory is *on* the visual template, whereas in the case of copying the movement trajectory is at a different spatial location. In tracing there is a close spatial proximity of the hand movement to the visual shape, and this enables the continuous visual guidance of the hand. In copying, on the other hand, the movement trajectory describes, ideally, the same figure as the visual shape, but is not superimposed on it. In other words, although there is a spatial correspondence between the visual figure and the movement, this correspondence is not immediately given but has to be imparted to the movement trajectory so that it conforms to the figure shown. Therefore, there are at least three key features of the function of copying: (1) the identification of the spatial characteristics of the figure, (2) the generation of a movement trajectory possessing the same spatial characteristics, and (3) in certain cases (e.g., handwriting) following a serial order in copying. Major theoretical contributions to these aspects were made by two great researchers of the twentieth century: N. Bernstein, on spatial aspects, and K. S. Lashley, on serial order.

Spatial aspects. In his article, "The Problem of the Interrelation of Co-ordination and Lateralization," Bernstein in 1935 drew attention to invariances in the shape of drawings made under very different conditions, such as using different effectors or different combinations of muscles and joints. He called these invariances "topological" and contrasted them with other, "metric" aspects of movement, such as size and location in space. He then speculated on the brain representation of motor topology, as follows:

. . . [T]here is the deeply seated inherent indifference of the motor control centre to the scale and position of the movement effected. . . . It is clear that each of the variations of a movement (for example, drawing a circle large or small . . .) demands a quite different muscular formula; and even more than this, involves a completely different set of muscles in the action. The almost equal facility and accuracy with which all these variations can be performed is evidence for the fact that they are ultimately determined by one and the same higher directional engram in relation to which dimensions and position play a secondary role. (Bernstein, 1984 [1935], p. 109)

Work in our laboratory over the past several years has addressed precisely these topics, namely, the neural coding of spatial motor parameters. Initial work on the motor cortex led to the discovery of directional tuning in space (Georgopoulos et al., 1982), which in turn made possible the neural construction of a motor trajectory in space (Georgopoulos, Kettner, and Schwartz, 1988; Schwartz, 1994). This "neural trajectory" proved to be an accurate and isomorphic representation of the actual motor trajectory. Remarkably, this was also predicted by Bernstein. He wrote,

"the higher engram . . . is extremely geometrical, representing a very abstract motor image of space" (Bernstein, 1984 [1935], p. 109). Indeed, space is pervasive in figure drawing. Unlike relatively pure temporal functions, such as tapping, figure drawing cannot be conceived apart from the spatial relations connecting the elements of the figure. Therefore, the geometric aspects of the shape become of fundamental importance for its drawing.

We recently studied the neural mechanisms of these more general spatial aspects in the prefrontal cortex of monkeys trained to copy simple geometric shapes using a joystick (Averbeck et al., 2002; Averbeck, Chafee, et al., 2003; Averbeck, Crowe, et al., 2003) (figure 35.1). The shapes were drawn as a series of oriented movement segments and therefore could be analyzed at different levels—for example, at the level of drawing single segments, at the level of the ordered sequence of segments, and at the level of the overall shape. The drawing trajectories that monkeys produced were divided into a series of discrete segments that varied in direction and length. We analyzed the neuronal activity of single cells by performing a stepwise multiple linear regression to identify those copy parameters that significantly influenced cell activity (Averbeck, Chafee, et al., 2003). We found that the copied shape (e.g., triangle, square) and the serial position of the segment within each trajectory were the most prevalent effects (in 46% and 43% of cells, respectively), followed by segment direction (32%) and length (16%). In contrast, significant effects of temporal factors (maximum segment speed and time to maximum segment speed) were less influential. These results demonstrate that prefrontal neurons encode global (i.e., shape), spatial (segment direction and amplitude), and serial order variables that define copy trajectories.

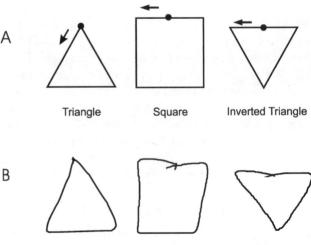

FIGURE 35.1 (*A*) Some shapes copied by monkeys. (*B*) Representative copies made by the monkeys. (Adapted from Averbeck et al., 2003a.)

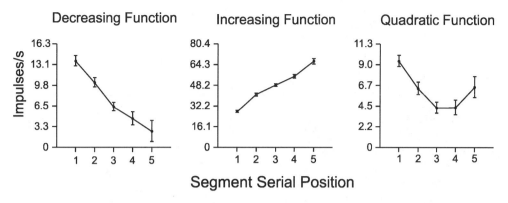

Decreasing Function   Increasing Function   Quadratic Function

Segment Serial Position

FIGURE 35.2 Typical curves of neural activity plotted against segment serial position. (Adapted from Averbeck, Chafee, et al., 2003.)

Serial order. In handwriting, letters and words are commonly written in an orderly, serial fashion similar to speech, where syllables and words are produced sequentially in time. Lashley (1951) pointed out that serial order is in fact fundamental to all forms of skilled action, from speech to reaching and grasping. He further believed that "[a]nalysis of the nervous mechanisms underlying order in the more primitive acts may contribute ultimately to the solution of the physiology of logic" (Lashley, 1951, p. 122). Speech is a prime example of elements organized serially at different levels: phonemes are uttered serially to make a syllable, syllables are strung together serially to form a word, words are uttered serially to make a sentence, sentences are combined serially to form a paragraph, and so on. In other motor actions, simple movements are executed serially to produce an integrated sequence (e.g., to reach for, grasp, and bring a cup to the mouth), a series of such sequences is performed to complete a task (e.g., get dressed), and so on.

One element common to all these examples is the serially ordered nesting of lower-order units of action (e.g., phonemes, simple movements) within higher-order units (e.g., syllables, integrated motor sequences such as drawing a shape). Lashley's major theoretical stance was the rejection of associative chaining theories and the suggestion of an alternative model based on parallel response activation. Much psychophysical evidence for this latter model has been gathered in speech and typing (MacNeilage, 1964; MacKay, 1970).

In the copying task we administered, monkeys copied the templates in a stereotypic order. Therefore, the serial order in copying consecutive figure segments was an integral aspect of the copying process. As noted earlier, the serial order in which the segment was presented and copied had a significant effect on prefrontal neural activity. In a subsequent analysis, we investigated whether this serial-order-related neural activity followed any systematic pattern. For this purpose we calculated adjusted means for the segments, that is, adjusted for the effects of all other main effects, except the serial position of the segment. This was done for

all cells whose activity was significantly related to segment serial position in the regression analysis. We discovered that in many cells there was a systematic variation of neural activity with the serial position of the segment, described by monotonically increasing and decreasing functions as well as by parabolic functions (figure 35.2). These findings indicate that, within the copying task, the serial segment position is a key factor for neural activity in the prefrontal cortex. Monotonically increasing and decreasing functions were found in 38/245 (16%) and 89/245 (36%) of cells, respectively. Other functions were observed in 118/245 (48%) of cells (Averbeck, Chafee, et al., 2003).

Neural coprocessing of spatial attributes and serial order. The multiple regression analysis we performed identified the factors that had a significant influence on cell activity. A major finding of this analysis was that single cell activity is influenced significantly by global (i.e., shape), spatial (segment direction and amplitude), and serial order variables that define copy trajectories. Therefore, we wanted to find out whether, and to what extent, these effects occurred together (for a single cell); that is, whether they occurred more frequently together than would happen by chance. For this purpose, we constructed a number of 2 × 2 tables containing data for a pair of factors (e.g., segment serial position and segment direction) and their binary attributes (significant effects present or absent). Chi-square statistics (two-tailed) were used to evaluate the level of statistical significance of association between the effects of a pair of factors. Because each factor could have an effect independently of the other factor, we also wanted to calculate the odds by which the co-occurrence of the two effects exceeded the level of independent occurrence. For this purpose we used the odds ratio. Finally, we were interested in testing the hypothesis that single cells might coprocess more than two of the four attributes—shape, segment serial position, direction, and length. We used loglinear analysis in this case to assess the statistical significance of higher-order associations.

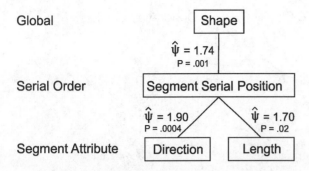

FIGURE 35.3 Systematic association in processing together various copying variables by single cells in the monkey prefrontal cortex. Numerical values are odds ratios. (Adapted from Averbeck, Chafee, et al., 2003.)

A major finding of this analysis was that specific groupings of significant effects tended to occur together in single neurons (Averbeck, Chafee, et al., 2003). Specifically, single neurons simultaneously processed the serial position of a segment within each trajectory along with the corresponding spatial (but not temporal) attributes of that segment (i.e., direction and length), as well as the overall shape to which the segments belong (figure 35.3). The effects were strong, as shown by the high values of the odds ratio. (In the absence of an effect, the odds ratio would equal 1.) For example, in the case of shape and segment serial position, the odds ratio of 1.74 means that the likelihood of these two factors being processed together was 74% higher than the likelihood of being processed separately.

Finally, the results of the loglinear analysis provided a clear result with respect to higher-order associations among the factors of shape, segment serial position, segment direction, and segment length. We found that the single four-way association among all of these factors was statistically significant ($P = 0.025$). This finding suggests that single cells also process all four factors concurrently. These findings underscore the central role of serial order, as well as the importance of global (shape) and specific spatial attributes (direction and length), for the neural mechanisms of copying in the prefrontal cortex.

Cotemporal representation of serial order. The results just described demonstrate the pervasive influence of serial order on neural activity at the single cell level. In a different analysis (Averbeck et al., 2002), we examined the simultaneously recorded activity in small neuronal ensembles to determine the time-varying representation of segment serial position. Specifically, we wanted to test Lashley's hypothesis that there is a cotemporal activation of serially ordered action units: "There are indications that, prior to the internal or overt enunciation of the sentence, an aggregate of word units is partially activated or readied" (Lashley, 1951, p. 119). Lashley also postulated a scanning mechanism by which these cotemporal representations would be translated into serial actions:

[I]ndications . . . that elements of the [sequence] are . . . partially activated before the order is imposed upon them in expression suggest that some scanning mechanism must be at play in regulating their temporal sequence. The real problem, however, is the nature of the selective mechanism by which the particular acts are picked out in this scanning process and to this problem I have no answer. (Lashley, 1951, p. 130)

In our experiments (Averbeck et al., 2002) we sought to (1) test Lashley's hypothesis on cotemporal activation of action representations, (2) seek a neural code for the serial order of these cotemporal representations, and (3) use this code to investigate several aspects of serial order behavior. For this purpose, we used a linear discriminant analysis to analyze the ensemble data recorded during copying and drawing of a sequence of segment, as follows. First, each trial was divided into a sequence of epochs, with each epoch spanning the drawing of a single segment of a shape. Then the average firing rate during the drawing of each segment was calculated for all the cells in an ensemble (these patterns of ensemble activity can be considered neural representations of the segments). Next, the ensemble pattern for each segment was averaged across correct trials and used to derive discriminant classification functions for that ensemble, namely, one classification function per segment. These functions were then used to classify particular ensemble activity patterns as belonging to a specific segment. For that purpose, we calculated the posterior probability that the pattern belonged to different segments, and the pattern was classified as belonging to the segment category with the highest posterior probability—that is, the "most probable" segment. We imposed the constraint that ensemble activity patterns in a given trial were classified only to those segments belonging to the shape drawn on that trial.

The results showed that the rank of the strength of representation of a segment in the neuronal population during this time predicted the serial position of the segment in the motor sequence. Moreover, an analysis of errors in copying and their neural correlates supplied additional evidence for this code and provided a neural basis for Lashley's hypothesis that errors in motor sequences would be most likely to occur when a subject was executing elements that had prior representations of nearly equal strength.

Mentally tracing a maze route

BEHAVIORAL AND NEUROPHYSIOLOGICAL STUDIES Our second praxis task involved maze solving. In this task neither copying nor construction is involved. Instead, the subject has to follow a route to exit a maze with blind alleys. Like copying and constructing, then, this task involves a dynamic spatial process.

In recent studies we investigated the behavioral (Crowe, Averbeck, et al., 2000; Chafee et al., 2002) and neural (Chafee et al., 1999; Crowe, Chafee, et al., 2000, 2003) mechanisms underlying this process in the absence of explicit tracing of the maze path. Subjects looked at mazes with orthogonal distracters and were required to indicate which of several possible routes exited the maze (Crowe, Averbeck, et al., 2000), or to indicate whether a given route exited or not (Chafee et al., 1999, 2002; Crowe, Chafee, et al., 2000, 2003). In both tasks, the response time increased as a linear function of the length of the path and the number of orthogonal turns in the path (figure 35.4). This finding

indicates that the postulated dynamic spatial process involves a mental tracing of the maze path. Direct neurophysiological evidence for that hypothesis was obtained from experiments in which neuronal activity was recorded in area 7a of the posterior parietal cortex of monkeys during mental maze solving (Crowe, Chafee, et al., 2000, 2003). In these experiments, monkeys were required to determine from a single point of fixation whether a critical path through the maze reached an exit or a blind ending. A delay period of 2–2.5 sec was imposed between the onset of the maze and the appearance of a go signal. We found that during the delay the activity of about 25% of neurons (N = 1200) in area 7a

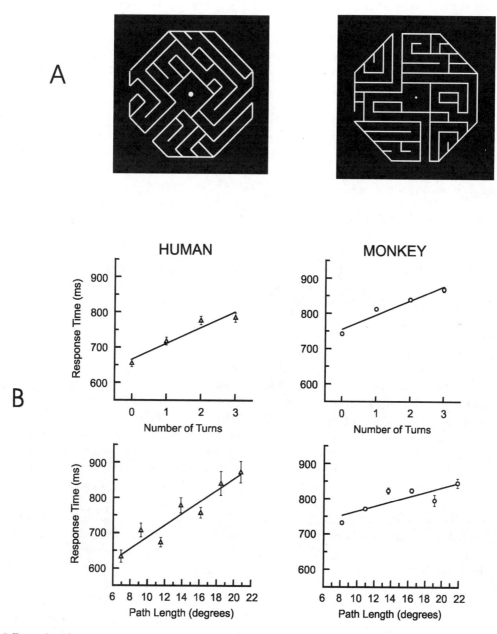

FIGURE 35.4   (A) Examples of mazes used. (B) Variation in response time with maze path length and number of turns in human subjects and monkeys. (Adapted from Chafee et al., 2002.)

was spatially tuned to maze path direction (Crowe et al., 2003). Clear evidence from control tasks indicated that the path tuning did not reflect a covert saccade plan, since the majority of neurons active during maze solution were not active on a delayed-saccade control task, and the minority that were active on both tasks did not exhibit congruent spatial tuning in the two conditions. We also obtained evidence that path tuning during maze solution was not due to the locations of visual receptive fields mapped outside the behavioral context of maze solution, in that receptive field centers and preferred path directions were not spatially aligned. Finally, neurons tuned to path direction were not present in area 7a when a naive animal viewed the same visual maze stimuli but did not solve them. These results support the hypothesis that path tuning in parietal cortex is not due to the lower-level visual features of the maze stimulus but rather is associated with maze solution, and as such reflects a cognitive process applied to a complex visual stimulus. Furthermore, an analysis of the ensemble activity using the neuronal population vector (Crowe, Chafee, et al., 2000) showed that time-varying population vectors traced the maze path, from the fixation point (at the center of the display) to the exit of the path. These findings are in accord with the behavioral evidence we obtained that mental maze solving is accomplished by mental tracing of the route.

FUNCTIONAL MAGNETIC RESONANCE IMAGING STUDIES The major and robust result of these neurophysiological studies was the finding of directional path tuning of single cells in the posterior parietal cortex. Prompted by this evidence, we carried out fMRI experiments in human subjects in which we focused on the superior parietal lobule during mental maze solving. Subjects solved the same kind of mazes that the monkeys solved. Octagonal mazes were shown for 300 ms. They had a straight main path that extended from the center to one of eight directions, every 45°; the rest of the maze was filled with random linear distracters. The main path was either open at the end ("exit maze") or closed by a line ("no-exit maze"); subjects had to indicate the exit status (present or absent) of the maze by pushing respectively the right or left buttons of a button press. High-spatial-resolution blood oxygen level-dependent (BOLD) activation images were acquired at high magnetic fields of 4 tesla (Tzagarakis et al., 2001, 2002, 2003; Gourtzelidis et al., 2003) and 7 tesla (Tzagarakis et al., 2003). In the 4-tesla experiments, the spatial resolution was $1.56 \times 1.56 \times 3 \,\text{mm}$, whereas in the 7-tesla experiment it was $1 \times 1 \times 1.5 \,\text{mm}$. On both experiments we found that the direction of the maze path had a significant effect on the BOLD signal in many voxels, and that a systematic variation of the pattern of activation with the direction of the maze path was also present. These results of the fMRI studies are in accord with those obtained from neurophysiological studies and, in

addition, provide evidence for an orderly representation of the direction of mental tracing in the human superior parietal lobule.

Mentally reconstructing an object

Our third praxis task involved the mental construction of an object out of its fragments. This task can be considered complementary to copying: in both tasks the same picture may be shown, but in copying, the component parts and the spatial relations among them are replicated, whereas in constructing, these relations are reproduced out of ready-made component parts.

We studied the process of object construction in its most abstract form, in dissociation from movements used to bring component parts together. Specifically, we used 25 geometric fragments of a square (figure 35.5) in two visual image-processing tasks requiring judgments on object construction (FIT task) or object sameness (SAME task). In initial behavioral studies (Whang, Crowe, and Georgopoulos, 1999), subjects rated the FIT-ness or SAME-ness of the pairs and also indicated (in a different session) whether the two fragments in a pair could make a complete square or whether they were the same. A multidimensional scaling analysis of the numerical subjective ratings and response times for these judgments showed that within the same set of geometric objects, different shape-related properties were emphasized under different task conditions. The similarity judgment depended most on a representational dimension related to enclosure of space, while the fit judgment depended to a greater extent on a dimension related to the symmetry properties of the fragments. This pattern of results was found in both the subjective ratings and the response times, as analyzed both by MDS and by confirmatory classic statistics. These findings suggested that mental representations of the same visual image—that is, a fragment pair—are task dependent.

Next, we investigated the neural mechanisms underlying these tasks in an fMRI study at 4 tesla (Georgopoulos et al., 2001). In the FIT task, subjects had to indicate, by pushing one of two buttons, whether the two fragments could match to form a perfect square, whereas in the SAME task they had to decide whether the fragments were the same or not. In a control task that preceded and followed each of these two tasks, a single square was presented at the same rate and subjects pushed any of the two keys at random. We found that the inferior temporal gyrus was activated exclusively during the FIT task, whereas all other areas showed activation during both tasks but to different extents. These results indicate that there are distributed, graded, and partially overlapping patterns of activation during performance of the two tasks. We attribute these overlapping patterns of activation to the engagement of partially shared processes, in accord with the results of neuropsychological studies, which

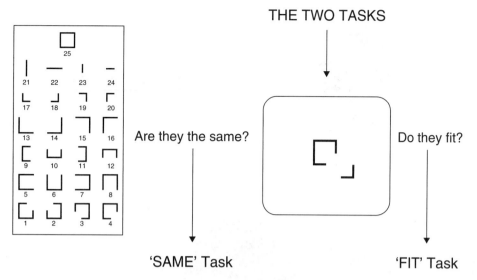

FIGURE 35.5 The 25 square fragments used in object discrimination and mental construction (left), and an example of the task (right). (From Georgopoulos et al., 2001.)

have shown that visuoperceptual, visuospatial, and visuoconstructive deficits can result from focal lesions in various cortical areas (Black and Bernard, 1984; Kertesz and Dubrowolski, 1981; Mehta, Newcombe, and Damasio, 1987).

A clustering analysis revealed three types of clusters with activated voxels: FIT-only (111 voxels), SAME-only (97 voxels), and FIT + SAME (115 voxels). Voxels contained in FIT-only and SAME-only clusters were distributed approximately equally between the left and right hemispheres, whereas voxels in the SAME + FIT clusters were located mostly in the left hemisphere (figure 35.6). With respect to gender, the left-right distribution of activated voxels was very similar in women and men for the SAME-only and FIT + SAME clusters but differed for the FIT-only case, in which there was a prominent right-sided preponderance for men (figure 35.7). Given that the two tasks involved the same visual stimuli (fragments of a square) as well as the same visual control stimuli (whole square), these results point to fundamental differences in the brain mechanisms underlying each task, as well as to basic differences between women and men in the visual object construction task. Specifically, we conclude that (1) cortical mechanisms common for processing visual object construction and discrimination involve mostly the left hemisphere, (2) cortical mechanisms specific for these tasks engage both hemispheres, and (3) in object construction only, men engage predominantly the right hemisphere, whereas women show a left-hemisphere preponderance.

Previous studies of the effects of sidedness and sex on the performance of visual tasks in people with brain damage focused on visuoconstructive abilities, best reflected in our FIT task, in addition to studies of language-related func-

tions. With respect to lateralization of visuoconstructive function, it is generally believed that the right hemisphere plays a crucial role in that function (Piercy, Hécaen, and Ajuriaguerra, 1960; Smith, 1969; Benton, 1967; Gott, 1973; Nebes, 1978; Mack and Levine, 1981). However, there is substantial controversy regarding this matter (see De Renzi, 1982; Gainotti, 1985). Part of this controversy stems from the fact that differences may exist between women and men such that the effects of right- or left-hemispheric lesions may depend on gender. In men, right-hemispheric lesions seem to be more effective in producing visuoconstructive deficits, as compared to either left-hemispheric lesions in men or right-hemispheric lesions in women (McGlone and Kertesz, 1973; Lewis and Kamptner, 1987). In women, on the other hand, the effects of left-hemispheric lesions on visuoconstructive functions are similar to those of right-hemispheric lesions in women (McGlone and Kertesz, 1973; Lewis and Kamptner, 1987) but similar (McGlone and Kertesz, 1973) or worse (Lewis and Kamptner, 1987) than the effects of left-hemispheric lesions in men. Assuming a preponderant role of the right and left hemispheres in visuoconstructive and language skills, respectively, it has been proposed that a given task may be performed using spatial or verbal procedures, and that women, being more expert in language skills (Hobson, 1947; Meyer and Bendig, 1961; Wechsler, 1958), may tend to use preferentially verbal strategies (Kimura, 1969), hence their smaller dependence on the right hemisphere. Then, the gender differences are explained by postulating that men and women employ fundamentally different strategies to perform these tasks, based on spatial or verbal operations, respectively. A variant of this idea makes use of the concept of "synthetic" (nonverbal) and "analytic" (verbal) functions for which the right and left

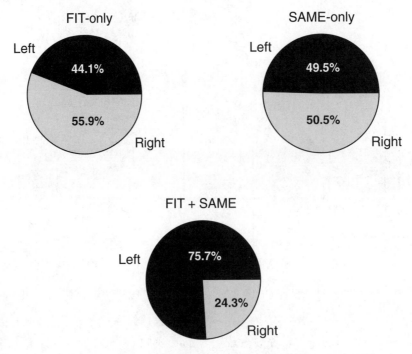

FIGURE 35.6   Percentages of activated voxels in the left and right hemisphere for the FIT-only, SAME-only, and FIT + SAME clusters. (Adapted from Georgopoulos et al., 2001.)

hemispheres are specialized, respectively (Levy, 1969). Specifically, it has been proposed that tasks involving perceptual synthesis rely on the right hemisphere in men, whereas tasks involving perceptual analysis or language skills rely on the left hemisphere in women (Tucker, 1976). The argument, then, can be formulated as follows: Men tend to use spatial/synthetic strategies, hence their right-hemisphere preponderance in solving visuoconstructive problems; in contrast, women tend to employ verbal/analytic strategies, hence their left-hemispheric preponderance. Although this is a plausible scheme with reasonable support, it includes a

fair amount of speculation. What seems to be especially weak is the supposed reliance of women on verbal strategies in solving visuoconstructive tasks. Although this could be the case for fairly complex tasks, it does not seem plausible for simple ones. And specifically, it is difficult to believe that a piecemeal, analytic, verbal strategy would be the strategy employed to perform our FIT task, in which the individual visual stimuli were simple line drawings and the whole figure was the highly common square. Therefore, it is hard to attribute the apparent left-hemispheric preponderance in women to the use of verbal strategies.

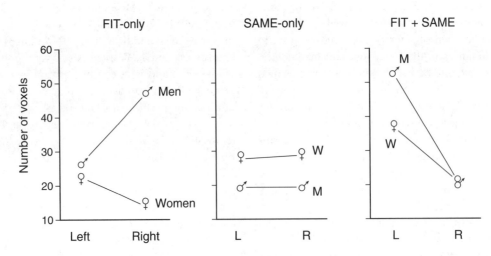

FIGURE 35.7   Number of activated voxels in women and in men for the FIT-only, SAME-only, and FIT + SAME clusters. (Adapted from Georgopoulos et al., 2001.)

We believe that, for our data, the crucial observation is not so much a preponderance of the left hemisphere as a substantial decrease in the involvement of the right hemisphere in women in performing the FIT task. Indeed, there was almost no difference between men and women with regard to *left*-hemispheric activation, whereas there was a major difference in the involvement of the *right* hemisphere, which was much more extensively activated in men than in women with regard to specific, FIT-only voxels (figure 35.7). Insofar as verbal strategies may not be plausible in our case, and assuming that right-hemispheric activation truly underlies visuoconstructive operations, it may be that women are much more efficient in using their right hemisphere than men, hence the reduced extent of activation of that hemisphere.

Concluding remarks

Constructional praxis tasks provide a rich behavioral set for probing the behavioral and neural mechanisms that underlie spatial cognition. They are nonsymbolic and therefore can be used in both human subjects and monkeys. In addition, they are suitable for studies using different technologies. In this chapter I have amplified on results obtained from behavioral, neurophysiological, and fMRI studies; studies using magnetoencephalography are ongoing (Georgopoulos et al., 2002). It is hoped that studying the same function across species and with a variety of complementary methods will lead to a better understanding of the brain mechanisms underlying such complex functions as constructional praxis.

ACKNOWLEDGMENTS   This study was supported by U.S. Public Health Service grants NS17413 and NS32919, the MIND Institute, the U.S. Department of Veterans Affairs, and the American Legion Chair in Brain Sciences.

REFERENCES

ANGELINI, R., R. FRASCA, and D. GROSSI, 1992. Are patients with constructional disorders different in visuo-spatial abilities? *Acta Neurol.* 14:595–604.

AVERBECK, B. B., M. V. CHAFEE, D. A. CROWE, and A. P. GEORGOPOULOS, 2002. Parallel processing of serial movements. *Proc. Natl. Acad. Sci. U.S.A.* 99:13172–13177.

AVERBECK, B. B., M. V. CHAFEE, D. A. CROWE, and A. P. GEORGOPOULOS, 2003. Neural activity in prefrontal cortex during copying geometrical shapes. I. Single cells encode shape, sequence and metric parameters. *Exp. Brain Res.* 150:127–141.

AVERBECK, B. B., D. A. CROWE, M. V. CHAFEE, and A. P. GEORGOPOULOS, 2003. Neural activity in prefrontal cortex during copying geometrical shapes. II. Decoding shape segments from neural ensembles. *Exp. Brain Res.* 150:142–153.

BENSON, D. F., and M. I. BARTON, 1970. Disturbances in constructional ability. *Cortex* 6:19–46.

BENTON, A. L., 1962. The visual retention test as a constructional praxis task. *Confin. Neurol.* 22:141–155.

BENTON, A. L., 1967. Constructional apraxia and the minor hemisphere. *Confin. Neurol.* 29:1–16.

BENTON, A. L., 1968. Differential behavioral effects in frontal lobe disease. *Neuropsychologia* 6:53–60.

BENTON, A. L., and M. L. FOGEL, 1962. Three-dimensional constructional praxis. *Arch. Neurol.* 7:347–354.

BERNSTEIN, N., 1984. The problem of interrelation of coordination and localization. In *Human Motor Actions*, H. T. A. Whiting, ed. Amsterdam: Elsevier/North-Holland, pp. 77–119. Originally published in *Archives of Biological Sciences*, 1935, vol. 38.

BLACK, F. W., and B. A. BERNARD, 1984. Constructional apraxia as a function of lesion locus and size in patients with focal brain damage. *Cortex* 20:111–120.

CHAFEE, M. V., B. B. AVERBECK, D. A. CROWE, and A. P. GEORGOPOULOS, 1999. Spatial selectivity of motor cortical activity during maze solution. *Soc. Neurosci. Abstr.* 25:1664.

CHAFEE, M. V., B. B. AVERBECK, D. A. CROWE, and A. P. GEORGOPOULOS, 2002. Impact of path parameters on maze solution time. *Arch. Ital. Biol.* 140:247–252.

CROWE, D. A., B. B. AVERBECK, M. V. CHAFEE, and A. P. GEORGOPOULOS, 2000. Mental maze solving. *J. Cogn. Neurosci.* 12:813–827.

CROWE, D. A., M. V. CHAFEE, B. B. AVERBECK, and A. P. GEORGOPOULOS, 2000. Dynamic spatial processing of maze stimuli in area 7a. *Soc. Neurosci. Abstr.* 26:2224.

CROWE, D. A., M. V. CHAFEE, B. B. AVERBECK, and A. P. GEORGOPOULOS, 2004. Neural activity in primate parietal area 7a related to a spatial analysis of visual mazes. *Cereb. Cortex* 14:23–34.

DE RENZI, E., 1982. *Disorders of Space Exploration and Cognition.* Baffins Lane, England: Wiley.

FÖRSTL, H., A. BURNS, R. LEVY, and N. CAIRNS, 1993. Neuropathological basis for drawing disability (constructional apraxia) in Alzheimer's disease. *Psychol. Med.* 23:623–629.

GAINOTTI, G., 1985. Constructional apraxia. In *Handbook of Clinical Neurology*, J. A. M. Frederiks, ed. Amsterdam: Elsevier, pp. 491–506.

GEORGOPOULOS, A. P., J. F. KALASKA, R. CAMINITI, and J. T. MASSEY, 1982. On the relations between the direction of two-dimensional arm movements and cell discharge in primate motor cortex. *J. Neurosci.* 2:1527–1537.

GEORGOPOULOS, A. P., R. E. KETTNER, and A. B. SCHWARTZ, 1988. Primate motor cortex and free arm movements to visual targets in three-dimensional space. II. Coding of the direction of movement by a neuronal population. *J. Neurosci.* 8:2928–2937.

GEORGOPOULOS, A. P., F. J. P. LANGHEIM, A. C. LEUTHOLD, and S. M. LEWIS, 2002. Mental maze solving: A MEG study. *Soc. Neurosc. Abstr.* 714.8.

GEORGOPOULOS, A. P., K. WHANG, M. A. GEORGOPOULOS, G. A. TAGARIS, B. AMIRIKIAN, W. RICHTER, S.-G. KIM, and K. UGURBIL, 2001. Functional magnetic resonance imaging of visual object construction and shape discrimination: Relations among task, hemispheric lateralization, and gender. *J. Cogn. Neurosci.* 13:72–89.

GESCHWIND, N., 1975. The apraxias: Neural mechanisms of disorders of learned movement. *Am. Scientist* 63:188–195.

GONZALEZ ROTHI, L. J., C. OCHIPA, and K. M. HEILMAN, 1991. A cognitive neuropsychological model of limb praxis. *Cogn. Neuropsychol.* 8:443–458.

GOTT, P. S., 1973. Cognitive abilities following right and left hemispherectomy. *Cortex* 9:266–274.

GOURTZELIDIS, P., C. TZAGARAKIS, S. M. LEWIS, T. A. JERDE, S.-G. KIM, K. UGURBIL, and A. P. GEORGOPOULOS, 2003. Relative spatial arrangement of directional preferences in the superior parietal lobule (SPL): An fMRI study of maze solving. *Soc. Neurosci. Abstr.* 823.1.

HEILMAN, K. M., and L. J. G. ROTHI, 1985. Apraxia. In *Clinical Neuropsychology*, K. M. Heilman and E. Velenstein, eds. New York: Oxford University Press, pp. 131–150.

HOBSON, J., 1947. Sex-differences in primary mental abilities. *J. Educ. Res.* 41:126–132.

KERTESZ, A., and S. DUBROWOLSKI, 1981. Right-hemisphere deficits, lesion size and location. *J. Clin. Neuropsychol.* 4, 283–299.

KIMURA, D., 1969. Spatial localization in the left and right visual fields. *Can. J. Psychol.* 23:445–458.

KIRK, A. and A. KERTESZ, 1993. Subcortical contributions to drawing. *Brain Cogn.* 21:57–70.

KLEIST, K., 1934. *Gehirnpathologie*. Leipzig: Barth.

KOSKI, L., M. IACOBONI, and J. C. MAZZIOTTA, 2002. Deconstructing apraxia: Understanding disorders of intentional movement after stroke. *Curr. Opin. Neurobiol.* 15:71–77.

LASHLEY, K., 1951. The problem of serial order in behavior. In *Cerebral Mechanisms in Behavior*, L. A. Jeffress, ed. New York: Wiley, pp. 112–136.

LEVY, J., 1969. Possible basis for the evolution of lateral specialization of the human brain. *Nature* 224:614–615.

LEWIS, R. S., and N. L. KAMPTNER, 1987. Sex differences in spatial task performance of patients with and without unilateral cerebral lesions. *Brain Cogn.* 6:142–152.

LIEPMANN, H., 1920. Apraxie. In *Real-Encyclopediae der gesamten Heilkunde, Ergebnisse der gesamten Medizin*, vol. 1, T. Brugsh and A. Eulenburg, eds. Berlin: Urban and Schwarzenberg, pp. 116–143.

LURIA, A. R., and L. S. TSVETKOVA, 1964. The programming of constructive ability in local brain injuries. *Neuropsychologia* 2:95–107.

MACK, J. L., and R. N. LEVINE, 1981. The basis of visual constructional disability in patients with unilateral cerebral lesions. *Cortex* 17:515–532.

MACKAY, D. G., 1970. Spoonerisms: The structure of errors in the serial order of speech. *Neuropsychologia* 8:323–350.

MACNEILAGE, P. F., 1964. Typing errors as clues to serial ordering mechanisms in language behaviour. *Langu. Speech* 7:144–159.

MCGLONE, J., and A. KERTESZ, 1973. Sex differences in cerebral processing of visuospatial tasks. *Cortex* 9:313–320.

MEHTA, Z., F. NEWCOMBE, and H. DAMASIO, 1987. A left hemisphere contribution to Nisuospatial processing. *Cortex* 23:417–461.

MEYER, W., and A. BENTIG, 1961. A longitudinal study of the primary mental abilities test. *J. Educ. Psychol.* 52:50–60.

NEBES, R. D., 1978. Direct examination of cognitive function in the right and left hemispheres. In *Asymmetrical Function of the Brain*, M. Kinsbourne, ed. Cambridge, England: Cambridge University Press, pp. 99–137.

PIERCY, M., H. HÉCAEN, and J. AJURIAGUERRA, 1960. Constructional apraxia associated with unilateral cerebral lesions: Left and right sided cases compared. *Brain* 83:225–242.

POIZNER, H., M. A. CLARK, A. S. MERIANS, B. MACAULEY, L. J. GONZALEZ ROTHI, and K. M. HEILMAN, 1995. Joint coordination deficits in limb apraxia. *Brain* 118:227–242.

POPPELREUTER, W., 1917. Die psychische Schädigungen durch Kopfschuss im Kriege, vol. 1. Leipzig: Voss.

PORTEUS, S. D., 1965. *The Porteus Maze Test: Fifty Years' Application*. Palo Alto, Calif.: Pacific Books.

SCHWARTZ, A. B., 1994. Direct cortical representation of drawing. *Science* 265:540–542.

SMITH, A., 1969. Nondominant hemispherectomy. *Neurology* 19:167–171.

TUCKER, D. M., 1976. Sex differences in hemispheric specialization for synthetic visuospatial functions. *Neuropsychologia* 14:447–454.

TZAGARAKIS, C., P. GOURTZELIDIS, S. M. LEWIS, T. A. JERDE, S.-G. KIM, K. UGURBIL, and A. P. GEORGOPOULOS, 2002. Spatial analysis of directional preference in superior parietal lobule during mental maze solving: An fMRI study. *Soc. Neurosci. Abstr.* 182.2.

TZAGARAKIS, C., S. M. LEWIS, T. A. JERDE, E. Auerbach, D. A. CROWE, S.-G. KIM, K. UGURBIL, and A. P. GEORGOPOULOS, 2001. High spatial resolution fMRI of parietal lobe activity during mental maze solving. *Soc. Neurosci. Abstr.* 80.7.

TZAGARAKIS, C., P. F. VAN DE MOORTELE, G. ADRIANY, S. M. LEWIS, P. GOURTZELIDIS, F. HUMBERT, K. UGURBIL, and A. P. GEORGOPOULOS, 2003. Functional imaging of superior parietal lobule (SPL) at ultra high magnetic field (7 Tesla) during performance of a maze task. *Soc. Neurosci. Abstr.* 182:2.

WECHSLER, D., 1958. *Measurement and Appraisal of Adult Intelligence*, 4th ed. Baltimore: Williams and Wilkins.

WHANG, K. C., D. A. CROWE, and A. P. GEORGOPOULOS, 1999. Multidimensional scaling analysis of two construction-related tasks. *Exp. Brain Res.* 125:231–238.

WILSON, S. A. K., 1909. A contribution to the study of apraxia with a review of the literature. *Brain* 31:164–216.

36 Computational Motor Control

DANIEL M. WOLPERT AND ZOUBIN GHAHRAMANI

ABSTRACT Unifying principles of movement have emerged from the computational study of motor control. We review several of these principles and show how they apply to processes such as motor planning, control, estimation, prediction, and learning. Our goal is to demonstrate how specific models emerging from the computational approach provide a theoretical framework for movement neuroscience.

From a computational perspective, the sensorimotor system allows us to take actions to achieve goals in an uncertain and varying world. We will consider a very general framework to phrase the computational problems of motor control and show how the main concepts of sensorimotor control arise from this framework. Consider a person who interacts with the environment by producing actions. The actions or motor outputs will cause muscle activations and, based on the physics of the musculoskeletal system and the outside world, will lead to a new state of both the person and environment. By *state* we refer to the set of time-varying parameters that, taken together with the fixed parameters of the system, the equations of motion of the body and world, and the motor output, allow a prediction of the consequences of the action. For example, to predict how a pendulum would respond to a torque acting on it, one would need to know the pendulum's angle and angular velocity, which together form its state. However, fixed parameters such as the length and mass of the pendulum do not form part of the state. In general, the state—for example, the set of activations of groups of muscles (synergies) or the position and velocity of the hand—changes rapidly and continuously within a movement. However, other key parameters change discretely, like the identity of a manipulated object, or on a slower time-scale, such as the mass of the limb. We refer to such discrete or slowly changing parameters as the *context* of the movement. Our ability to generate accurate and appropriate motor behavior relies on tailoring our motor commands to the prevailing movement context.

The central nervous system (CNS) does not have direct access to the state but receives as its input sensory feedback.

The sensory input provides information about the state of the world, such as the location of objects, as well as information about the state of our own body, such as the position and velocity of the hand. In addition to these sensory inputs, the CNS can monitor its own activity. For example, a copy of the motor output can be used to provide information about the ongoing movement. This signal is known as an *efference copy*, to reflect that it is a copy of the signal flowing out of the CNS to the muscles. We can also consider some sensory inputs as providing reward, such as the taste of chocolate or warmth on a cold day, or punishment, such as hunger or pain. Although some rewards or punishments are directly specified by the environments, others may be indirectly or internally generated.

Within this framework we can consider the goal of motor control as selecting actions to maximize future rewards (Sutton and Barto, 1998). For example, an infant may generate actions and receive reward if the actions bring food into its mouth, but punishment (negative rewards) if it bites its own fingers. Therefore, it has to choose actions to maximize food intake while minimizing the chance of biting itself. Often in computational motor control we specify a discount factor so that we regard an action that will lead to a reward tomorrow of less value than another action that will lead to the same reward immediately. Conversely, we choose an action that will achieve a reward at some distant time only if the reward greatly exceeds the immediate reward we would get for all other actions.

We will show how all the main themes of computational motor control, such as planning, control, and learning, arise from considering how *optimality* can be used to plan movements, *motor commands* are generated, *states* and *contexts* are estimated and predicted, and *internal models* are represented and learned. Recent progress in motor control has come both from more sophisticated theories and from the advent of virtual reality technologies and novel robotic interfaces. With the use of these technologies it has become possible, for the first time, to create sophisticated computer-controlled environments. Having such control over the physics of the world that subjects interact with has allowed detailed tests of computational models of planning, control, and learning (e.g., Shadmehr and Mussa-Ivaldi, 1994; Wolpert, Ghahramani, and Jordan, 1995; Gomi and Kawato, 1996; Ghahramani and Wolpert, 1997; Cohn, DiZio, and Lackner, 2000).

DANIEL M. WOLPERT Sobell Department of Motor Neuroscience, Institute of Neurology, University College London, London, U.K.
ZOUBIN GHAHRAMANI Gatsby Computational Neuroscience Unit, University College London, London, U.K.

Optimal control

Everyday tasks are generally specified at a high, often symbolic level, such as taking a drink of water from a glass. However, the motor system has to eventually work at a detailed level, specifying muscle activations leading to joint rotations and the path of the hand in space. There is clearly a gap between the high-level task and low-level control kinematics (Bernstein, 1967). In fact, almost any task can in principle be achieved in infinitely many different ways. Given all these possibilities, it is surprising that almost every study of the way the motor system solves a given task shows highly stereotyped movement patterns, both between repetitions of a task and between individuals on the same task location (e.g., Morasso, 1981; Flash and Hogan, 1985). The concept that some movements will lead to reward and others to punishment links naturally to the field of optimal motor control. Specifically, a cost (which can be thought of as punishment or reward) is specified as some function of the movement, and the movement with the lowest cost is executed. In the same way that being able to rank different routes from home to work allows us to select a particular route from those available, having a criterion with which to evaluate possible movements for a task would allow the CNS to select the best. Optimal control is therefore an elegant framework for dealing with just such a selection problem and can, therefore, translate from high-level tasks into detailed motor programs (Bryson and Ho, 1975). Although optimal control can be motivated from the point of view of reducing redundancy, we must always take into account the ultimate evolutionary role of behavior. From an evolutionary point of a view, the purpose of action is to maximize the chances of passing on genetic material. Clearly, some forms of action are more likely to lead to passing on genetic material, and the brain may have learned to indirectly represent this through costs functions ranking actions. The challenge has been to try to reverse engineer the cost function that is being optimized from observed movement patterns and perturbation studies.

Flash and Hogan (1985) and Uno, Kawato, and Suzuki (1989) proposed optimal control models of movement based on maximizing smoothness of the hand trajectory and of the torque commands, respectively. Although these models have been successful at reproducing a range of empirical data, it is unclear why smoothness is important, and how it is measured by the CNS over the movement. Moreover, these models are limited to a single motor system such as the arm. Harris and Wolpert (1998) have proposed an alternative cost model that provides a unifying model for goal-directed eye and arm movements. This model assumes that there is noise in the motor command and that the amount of noise scales with the magnitude of the motor command. In the presence of such signal-dependent noise, the same sequence of

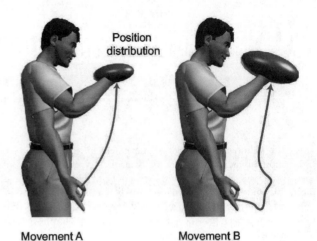

Position distribution

Movement A   **Movement B**

FIGURE 36.1 A schematic of the task optimization in the presence of signal-dependent noise (TOPS) model of Harris and Wolpert. Shown are average paths and expected final position distributions for two different motor sequences. Although the sequences bring the hand on average to the same final position, because of noise on the motor commands they have different final distributions. Movement A has a smaller spread than movement B and therefore has a lower cost than B. In general, the task determines the desired statistics of the movement, and the trajectory that optimizes the statistics is selected.

intended motor commands, if repeated many times, will lead to a probability distribution over movements. Aspects of this distribution, such as the spread of positions or velocities of the hand at the end of the movement, can be controlled by modifying the sequence of motor commands. In this model the task specifies the way aspects of the distribution are penalized, and it is this which forms the cost. For example, in a simple aiming movement, the task is to minimize the final error, as measured by the positional variance about the target. Figure 36.1 shows the consequences of two possible sequences of motor commands, one of which leads to higher endpoint variability (right ellipsoid) than the other. The aim of the optimal control strategy is to minimize the volume of the ellipsoid thereby being as accurate as possible. This model accurately predicts the trajectories of both saccadic eye movements and arm movements. Nonsmooth movements require large motor commands that generate increased noise; smoothness thereby leads to accuracy, but is not a goal in its own right. The cost, movement error, is behaviorally relevant and is simple for the CNS to measure. Recently, Todorov and Jordan (2002) have shown that optimal feedback control in the presence of signal-dependent noise may form a general strategy for movement production. This model suggests that parameters that are relevant to achieving the task are controlled at the expense of an increase in variance in task-irrelevant parameters. For example, in a tracking movement with the hand, the variability of the shoulder, elbow, and wrist joints may each be high, but by controlling correlations between them, the hand variability is kept low. Moreover, the optimal feedback control model shows that control can be achieved without the need for the CNS to specify a desired trajectory, such as a time series of desired hand positions or velocities.

State estimation and prediction

For the CNS to implement any form of control, it needs to know the current state of the body. However, the CNS faces two problems. First, considerable delays exist in the transduction and transport of sensory signal to the CNS. Second, the CNS must estimate the state of the system from the sensory signals, which may be contaminated by noise and may only provide partial information as to the state. As an example, we can consider a tennis ball we have just hit. If we simply used the retinal location of the ball to estimate its position, our estimate would be delayed by around 100 ms. A better estimate can be made by predicting where the ball actually is now using a predictive model. The relationship between our motor commands and the consequences is governed by the physics of musculoskeletal system and outside environment. Therefore, to make such a prediction requires a model of this transformation. Such a system is termed an *internal forward model* because it models the causal or forward relationship between actions and their consequences. The term *internal* is used to emphasize that this model is internal to the CNS. The primary role of these models is to predict the behavior of the body and world, so we use the terms predictors and forward models synonymously. In addition to delays, the system must cope with the fact that components of the ball's state, such as its spin, cannot be observed easily. However, the spin can be estimated using sensory information integrated over time, because the ball's spin will influence its path. By observing the position of the ball over time, we can obtain an estimate of its spin. The estimate from sensory feedback can be improved by incorporating information based on the forward model's predictions (even in a system with no delays).

This combination, using sensory feedback and forward models to estimate the current state, is known as an *observer* (Goodwin and Sin, 1984). The major objectives of the observer are to compensate for the delays in the sensorimotor system and to reduce the uncertainty in the state estimate that arises owing to noise inherent in both the sensory and motor signals. For a linear system, the Kalman filter is the optimal observer in that it produces estimates of the state with the least squared error (figure 36.2). Such a model has been supported by empirical studies examining estimation of hand position (Wolpert, Ghahramani, and Jordan, 1995), posture (Kuo, 1995), and head orientation (Merfeld, Zupan, and Peterka, 1999).

Using the observer framework, it is a simple computational step from estimating the current state to predicting future states and sensory feedback. Such predictions have many potential benefits (Wolpert and Flanagan, 2001). State prediction, by estimating the outcome of an action before sensory feedback is available, can reduce the effect of feedback delays in sensorimotor loops. Such a system is thought to underlie skilled manipulation. For example, when an object held in the hand is accelerated, the fingers tighten their grip in anticipation to prevent the object slipping, a process shown to rely on prediction (for a review, see Johansson and Cole, 1992). Modeling the performance of subjects who were asked to balance a pole on their fingertip has also provided evidence for predictive models. Examining a variety of control schemes, Mehta and Schaal (2002) concluded, through a process of elimination, that a forward predictive model was likely to be employed.

A sensory prediction can be derived from the state prediction and used to cancel the sensory effects of movement, that is reafference. By using such a system, it is possible to cancel out the effects of sensory changes induced by self-motion, thereby enhancing more relevant sensory information. In primates, neurophysiological studies by Duhamel, Colby, and Goldberg (1992) have shown predictive updating in parietal cortex anticipating the retinal consequences of an eye movement. In man, predictive mechanisms are believed to underlie the observation that the same tactile stimulus, such as a tickle or force, is felt less intensely when it is self-applied. It has been shown that the reduction in the felt intensity of self-applied tactile stimuli depends critically on the precise spatiotemporal alignment between the predicted and actual sensory consequences of the movement (Blakemore, Frith, and Wolpert, 1999).

Motor command generation

In general, the CNS can employ two distinct strategies to generate actions. One strategy is to represent the muscle activations or forces required to compensate for the dynamics of the body or an externally imposed perturbation. This compensation can be achieved by a system that can map desired behavior into the motor commands required to achieve the behavior. Such a system is termed an *inverse model*, because it inverts the relationship of the motor system that converts motor commands to the outcome of behavior. When a perfect inverse model is cascaded with the motor system, it should produce an identity mapping, in that the actual outcome should match the desired outcome. Therefore, to learn model-based compensations for the dynamics of objects we interact with, our CNS needs to learn *internal models* of these objects. An alternative to this model-based compensation is to use cocontraction of the muscles to increase the stiffness of the arm, thereby reducing the displacement caused by external or intersegmental forces (Fel'dman, 1966; Bizzi et al., 1984; Hogan, 1984).

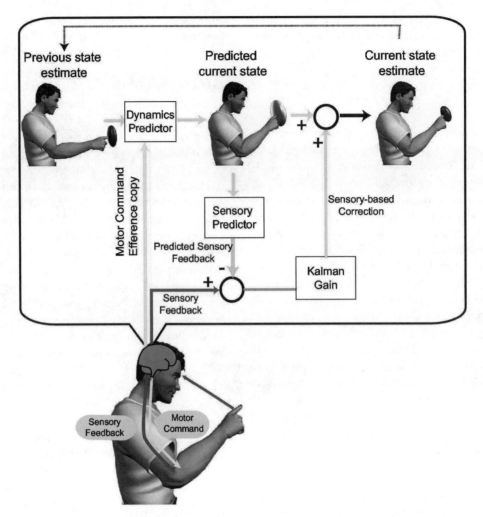

FIGURE 36.2 A schematic of one step of a Kalman filter model recursively estimating the finger's location during a movement. The current state is constructed from the previous state estimate (top left), which represents the distribution of possible finger positions, shown as a cloud of uncertainty. Using a copy of the motor command, that is, an efference copy, and a model of the dynamics, the current state distribution is predicted from this previous state. In general, the uncertainty is increased. This new estimate is then refined by using it to predict the current sensory feedback. The error between this prediction and the actual sensory feedback is used to correct the current estimate. The Kalman gain changes this sensory error into state errors and also determines the relative reliance placed on the efference copy and sensory feedback. The final state estimate (top right) now has a reduced uncertainty. Although there are delays in sensory feedback that must be compensated, they have been omitted from the diagram for clarity.

Both forms of compensation to perturbations are seen experimentally when subjects are exposed to novel force fields (figure 36.3). By force field we mean a force, usually generated by a robotic interface, that is related to the state of the hand, such as its position. During reaching in a predictable force field, the CNS tends to employ a low-stiffness strategy and learns to represent the compensatory forces. Early in learning, the stiffness of the arm reduces systematically as these compensatory responses are learned (Shadmehr and Mussa-Ivaldi, 1994; Nezafat, Shadmehr, and Holcomb, 2001; Wang, Dordevic, and Shadmehr, 2001). When manipulating an external object with internal degrees of freedom, like a mass-spring system, people also employ low-stiffness control (Dingwell, Mah, and Mussa-Ivaldi, 2002). However, in several situations it is not possible to reliably predict the forces the hand will experience, and therefore model-based compensation is difficult. In the example of drilling into a wall with a power drill, the aim is to maintain the drill bit perpendicular to the wall while an orthogonal force is applied. This situation is inherently unstable in that any deviations from orthogonality lead to forces that destabilize the posture (Rancourt and Hogan, 2001). In this situation the stiffness of the hand can be increased in all directions, thereby stabilizing the system. Burdet and colleagues (2001) have used an analogous task in which the instability was present in only one direction (shown schematically in figure 36.3, right). Subjects reached in a force field in which any deviation of the hand from a straight line between starting point and target was exacerbated by a force perpendicular to the line. They showed that

Model-based compensation

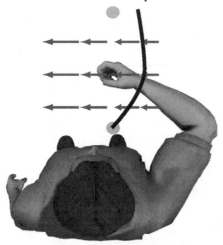

Task matched stiffness

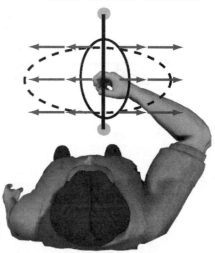

FIGURE 36.3   Schematic of two strategies for control when learning to move in a force field. Subjects reach between the two circular targets under a force field generated by a robot (not shown) that depends on the position of the hand. The force experienced for different positions is shown by the arrows. *Left:* Under a stable and predictable force field acting to the left, the subject will learn to produce a straight-line movement. If the field is unexpectedly turned off for a moment, subjects will show an aftereffect (black trajectory) reflecting the compensation they are producing in their

motor command to counteract the field. *Right:* The field is unstable, as any deviation from a straight hand path will generate force acting in the same direction. Subjects learn to move in a straight line but show no aftereffects when the force field is removed. The task is achieved by increasing the stiffness of the arm, but only in the direction of maximum instability. The stiffness ellipse represents restoring force to a step displacement of the hand in different directions (solid prior to learning and dotted after).

subjects tailored the stiffness of the hand to match the requirements of the task, stiffening the hand only in the perpendicular direction. This is the first demonstration that stiffness can be controlled independently in different directions. Therefore, it seems that the CNS employs both high- and low-stiffness control strategies, with the high-stiffness control reducing the effect of any perturbations that a compensation mechanism cannot represent.

Bayesian context estimation

When we interact with objects with different physical characteristics, the context of our movement changes in a discrete manner. Just as it is essential for the motor system to estimate the state, it must also estimate the changing context. One powerful formalism for such an estimation problem is the Bayesian approach, which can be used to estimate probabilities for each possible context. The probability of each context can be factored into two terms, the likelihood and the prior. The likelihood of a particular context is the probability of receiving the current sensory feedback given the hypothesized context. To estimate this likelihood, a sensory forward model of that context is used to predict the sensory feedback from the movement. The discrepancy between the predicted and actual sensory feedback is inversely related to the likelihood: the smaller the prediction error, the more likely the context. These computations can be carried out by

a modular neural architecture in which multiple predictive models operate in parallel (Wolpert and Kawato, 1998; Haruno, Wolpert, and Kawato, 2001). Each is tuned to one context and estimates the relative likelihood of its context. This array of models therefore acts as a set of hypothesis testers. The prior contains information about the structured way contexts change over time and how probable a context is prior to a movement. The likelihood and the prior can be optimally combined using *Bayes' rule*, which takes the product of these two probabilities and normalizes over all possible contexts to generate a probability for each context.

Figure 36.4 shows a schematic example of picking up what appears to be a full milk carton that in reality is empty. This sketch shows how the predictive models correct online for erroneous priors that initially weighted output of the controller for a full milk carton more than for an empty carton. Bayes' rule allows a quick correction to the appropriate control even though the initial strategy was incorrect. This example has two modules representing two contexts. However, the modular architecture can, in principle, scale to thousands of modules, that is, contexts. Although separate architectures have been proposed for state and context estimation (see figures 36.2 and 36.4), they both can be considered online ways of doing Bayesian inference in an uncertain environment.

The interpretation of the processes necessary for context estimation is consistent with recent neurophysiological

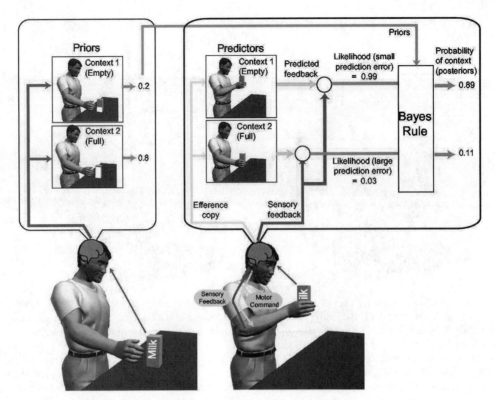

FIGURE 36.4 A schematic of Bayesian context estimation with just two contexts, that a milk carton is empty or that it is full. Initially sensory information from vision is used to set the prior probabilities of the two possible contexts, and in this case, the carton appears more likely to be full. When the motor commands appropriate for a full carton are generated, an efference copy of the motor command is used to simulate the sensory consequences under the two possible contexts. The predictions based on an empty carton suggest a large amount of movement compared to the full carton context. These predictions are compared with actual feedback. Because the carton is, in fact, empty, the sensory feedback matches the predictions of the empty carton context. This leads to a high likelihood of an empty carton and a low likelihood of a full carton. The likelihoods are combined with the priors using Bayes' rule to generate the final (posterior) probability of each context.

studies in primates showing that the CNS both models the expected sensory feedback for a particular context (Eskandar and Assad, 1999) and represents the likelihood of the sensory feedback, given the context (Kim and Shadlen, 1999). An elegant example of context estimation has been provided by Cohn, DiZio, and Lackner (2000). When subjects make a reaching movement while rotating their torso, they compensate for the velocity-dependent Coriolis forces arising from the rotation, which act on the arm. When subjects experience illusory self-rotation induced by a large moving visual image, they make movements as though they expect, based on the visual priors, the context of Coriolis force. This leads to misreaching, which over subsequent movements reduces as the sensory consequences of the expected Coriolis force are not experienced.

Motor learning

Internal models, both forward and inverse, capture information about the properties of the sensorimotor system. These properties are not static but change throughout life both on a short time scale, owing to interactions with the environment, and on a longer time scale, owing to growth. Internal models must therefore be adaptable to changes in the properties of the sensorimotor system. The environment readily provides an appropriate training signal to learn predictors of sensory feedback. The difference between the predicted and actual sensory feedback can be used as an error signal to update a predictive model. The neural mechanisms that lead to such predictive learning in the cerebellum-like structure of electric fish have recently been partially elucidated (Bell et al., 1997).

Acquiring an inverse internal model through motor learning is generally a difficult task. This is because the appropriate training signal, the error in the output of the inverse model, which is the motor command error, is not directly available. When we fail to sink a putt, no one tells us how our muscle activations should change to achieve the task. Instead, we receive error signals in sensory coordinates, and these sensory errors need to be converted to motor errors before they can be used to train an inverse model. An original proposal was to use direct inverse modeling (Widrow and Stearns, 1985; Miller, 1987; Kuperstein, 1988; Atkeson and Reinkensmeyer, 1988) in which an inverse model could be learned during a motor "babbling" stage. This controller would simply observe motor commands and sensory outcomes during babbling and try to learn how outcomes (as inputs to the inverse model) map to the motor commands that caused this outcome. For linear systems, such a process can be shown to usually converge to correct parameter estimates (Goodwin and Sin, 1984). However, there are several problems with such a system. First, it is not *goal-directed*; that is, it is not sensitive to particular output goals (Jordan and Rumelhart, 1992). The learning process samples randomly during babbling, and there is no guarantee that it will sample appropriately for a given task. Second, the controller is trained "off-line," that is, the input to the controller for the purposes of training is the actual sensory outcome, not the desired sensory outcome. For the controller to actually participate in the control process, it must receive the desired outcome as its input. The direct inverse modeling approach therefore requires a switching process: the desired plant output must be switched in for the purposes of control and the actual plant output must be switched in for the purposes of training. Finally, for nonlinear systems a difficulty arises that is related to the general degrees-of-freedom problem in motor control (Bernstein, 1967). The problem is due to a particular form of redundancy in nonlinear systems (Jordan, 1992). In such systems, the "optimal" parameter estimates in fact may yield an incorrect controller. Because of the redundancy in the motor system, there may be many motor commands that lead to the same outcome, and during direct inverse learning the system may see the same outcome many times, but caused by different motor commands. Most learning systems when trying to learn to map a single outcome into the multiple motor commands that lead to this outcome will finally map this outcome to the average of all these motor commands. However, for nonlinear systems it is rarely the case that the average of all these motor commands will lead to the desired outcome, and therefore direct inverse modeling fails for such nonlinear systems.

Two learning mechanism have been proposed to overcome these limitations (for a detailed review, see Jordan and Wolpert, 1999). Kawato, Forawaka, and Suzuki (1987) and Kawato and Gomi (1992) have proposed an ingenious solution to this problem, feedback error learning (figure 36.5). They suggest that a hard-wired, but not perfect, feedback controller exists that computes a motor command based on the discrepancy between desired and estimated state. The motor command is the sum of the feedback controller motor command and the output of an adaptive inverse model. They reasoned that if the feedback controller ended up producing no motor command, then there must be no discrepancy between desired and estimated state, that is, no error in performance, and the inverse model would be performing perfectly. Based on this reasoning, they regarded the output of the feedback controller as the error signal and

used it to train the inverse model—an approach that is highly successful. Therefore, feedback error learning makes use of a feedback controller to guide the learning of the feedforward controller. The feedforward controller is trained "online"; that is, it is used as a controller while it is being trained, and so is goal-directed. Neurophysiological evidence (Shidara et al., 1993) supports this learning mechanism within the cerebellum for the simple reflex eye movement called the ocular following response. The suggestion is that the cerebellum constructs an inverse model of the eye's dynamics.

Another solution is to use distal supervised learning (Jordan and Rumelhart, 1992). In distal supervised learning, the controller is learned indirectly, through the intermediary of a forward model of the motor apparatus. The forward model must itself be learned from observations of the inputs and outputs of the system. The distal supervised learning approach is therefore composed of two interacting processes, one process in which the forward model is learned, and another process in which the forward model is used in the training of the controller. The controller and the forward model are joined together and are treated as a single *composite learning system*. If the controller is to be an inverse model, then the composite learning system should be an identity transformation (i.e., a transformation whose output is the same as its input). This suggests that the controller can be trained indirectly by training the composite learning system to be an identity transformation. During this training process, the parameters in the forward model are held fixed. Thus the composite learning system is trained to be an identity transformation by a constrained learning process in which some of the parameters inside the system are held fixed. By allowing only the controller parameters to be altered, this process trains the controller indirectly.

Distal supervised learning and other models (Haruno, Wolpert, and Kawato, 2001) have suggested that we use a forward model to train a controller. In an experiment designed to simultaneously assess both forward and inverse model learning, subjects were required move an object along a straight line while the load on the object was varied during the trial (Flanagan et al., 2003). Over repeated trials, subjects learned to compensate for the load so that they could produce a straight trajectory. The hand trajectory was used to measure how quickly subjects learned to control the movement, whereas prediction was measured by looking at changes in grip force. In early trials, grip force was changed reflexively as the hand path (and therefore the load force) was perturbed, but subjects quickly learned to alter their grip force predictively. By contrast, it took many trials for them to learn to control the load. This suggests that we learn to predict the consequences of our actions before we learn to control them.

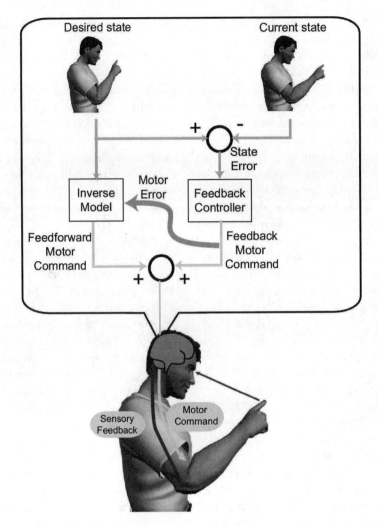

FIGURE 36.5   A schematic of feedback error learning. The aim is to learn an inverse model that can generate motor commands given a series of desired states. A hard-wired and low-gain feedback controller is used to correct for errors between desired and estimated states. This generates a feedback motor command, which is added to the feedforward motor command generated by the inverse model. If the feedback motor command goes to zero, then the state error will, in general, also be zero. Therefore, the feedback motor command is a measure of the error of the inverse model and is used as the error signal to train it.

Unifying principles

Computational approaches have started to provide unifying principles for motor control. Several common themes have already emerged in this review. First, internal models are fundamental for understanding a range of processes such as state estimation, prediction, context estimation, control, and learning. Second, optimality underlies many theories of movement planning, control, and estimation, and can account for a wide range of experimental findings. Third, the motor system has to cope with uncertainty about the world and noise in its sensory inputs and motor commands, and the Bayesian approach provides a powerful framework for optimal estimation in the face of such uncertainty. It is our belief that these and other unifying principles will be found to underlie the control of motor systems as diverse as the eye, arm, speech, posture, balance, and locomotion.

ACKNOWLEDGMENTS   This work was supported by grants from the Wellcome Trust, Gatsby Charitable Foundation, and the Human Frontiers Science Progamme.

REFERENCES

ATKESON, C. G., and D. J. REINKENSMEYER, 1988. Using associative content-addressable memories to control robots. Proceedings of the 27th IEEE Conference on Decision and Control, Vol. 1. pp. 792–797, Austin, Texas, Dec. 7–9.

BELL, C. C., V. Z. HAN, Y. SUGAWARA, and K. GRANT, 1997. Synaptic plasticity in a cerebellum-like structure depends on temporal order. Nature 387:278–281.

BERNSTEIN, N., 1967. The Coordination and Regulation of Movements. London: Pergamon Press.

BIZZI, E., N. ACCORNERRO, B. CHAPPLE, and N. HOGAN, 1984. Posture control and trajectory formation during arm movement J. Neurosci. 4:2738–2744.

BLAKEMORE, S. J., C. D. FRITH, and D. M. WOLPERT, 1999. Spatio-temporal prediction modulates the perception of self-produced stimuli. *J. Cogn. Neurosci.* 11:551–559.

BRYSON, A. E., and Y. C. HO, 1975. *Applied Optimal Control.* New York: Wiley.

BURDET, E., R. OSU, D. W. FRANKLIN, T. E. MILNER, and M. KAWATO, 2001. The central nervous system stabilizes unstable dynamics by learning optimal impedance. *Nature* 414:446–449.

COHN, J. V., P. DIZIO, and J. R. LACKNER, 2000. Reaching during virtual rotation: Context specific compensations for expected Coriolis forces. *J. Neurophysiol.* 83:3230–3240.

DINGWELL, J. B., C. D. MAH, and F. A. MUSSA-IVALDI, 2002. Manipulating objects with internal degrees of freedom: Evidence for model-based control. *J. Neurophysiol.* 88:222–235.

DUHAMEL, J. R., C. L. COLBY, and M. E. GOLDBERG, 1992. The updating of the representation of visual space in parietal cortex by intended eye movements. *Science* 255:90–92.

ESKANDAR, E. N., and J. A. ASSAD, 1999. Dissociation of visual, motor and predictive signals in parietal cortex during visual guidance. *Nat. Neurosci.* 2:88–93.

FEL'DMAN, A. G., 1966. Functional tuning of the nervous system with control of movement or maintenance of a steady posture. III. Mechanographic analysis of execution by arm of the simplest motor tasks. *Biophysics* 11:766–775.

FLANAGAN, J. R., P. VETTER, R. S. JOHANSSON, and D. M. WOLPERT, 2003. Prediction precedes control in motor learning. *Curr. Biol.* 13:146–150.

FLASH, T., and N. HOGAN, 1985. The co-ordination of arm movements: An experimentally confirmed mathematical model. *J. Neurosci.* 5:1688–1703.

GHAHRAMANI, Z., and D. M. WOLPERT, 1997. Modular decomposition in visuomotor learning. *Nature* 386:392–395.

GOMI, H., and M. KAWATO, 1996. Equilibrium-point control hypothesis examined by measured arm stiffness during multijoint movement. *Science* 272:117–120.

GOODWIN, G. C., and K. S. SIN, 1984. *Adaptive Filtering Prediction and Control.* Englewood Cliffs, N. J.: Prentice-Hall.

HARRIS, C. M., and D. M. WOLPERT, 1998. Signal-dependent noise determines motor planning. *Nature* 394:780–784.

HARUNO, M., D. M. WOLPERT, and M. KAWATO, 2001. Mosaic model for sensorimotor learning and control. *Neural Comput.* 13:2201–2220.

HOGAN, N., 1984. An organizing principle for a class of voluntary movements. *J. Neurosci.* 4:2745–2754.

JOHANSSON, R. S., and K. J. COLE, 1992. Sensory-motor coordination during grasping and manipulative actions. *Curr. Opin. Neurobiol.* 2:815–823.

JORDAN, M. I., 1992. Constrained supervised learning. *J. Math. Psychol.* 36:396–425.

JORDAN, M. I., and D. E. RUMELHART, 1992. Forward models: Supervised learning with a distal teacher. *Cogn. Sci.* 16:307–354.

JORDAN, M. I., and D. M. WOLPERT, 1999. Computational motor control. In *The New Cognitive Neurosciences*, M. Gazzaniga, ed. Cambridge, Mass.: MIT Press, pp. 601–620.

KAWATO, M., K. FURAWAKA, and R. SUZUKI, 1987. A hierarchical neural network model for the control and learning of voluntary movements. *Biol. Cybern.* 56:1–17.

KAWATO, M., and H. GOMI, 1992. The cerebellum and VOR/OKR learning models. *Trends Neurosci.* 15:445–453.

KIM, J., and M. N. SHADLEN, 1999. Neural correlates of a decision in the dorsolateral prefrontal cortex of the macaque. *Nat. Neurosci.* 2:176–185.

KUO, A. D., 1995. An optimal-control model for analyzing human postural balance. *IEEE Trans. Biomed. Eng.* 42:87–101.

KUPERSTEIN, M. 1988. Neural model of adaptive hand-eye coordination for single postures. *Science* 239:1308–1311.

MEHTA, B., and S. SCHAAL, 2002. Forward models in visuomotor control. *J. Neurophysiol.* 88:942–953.

MERFELD, D. M., L. ZUPAN, and R. J. PETERKA, 1999. Humans use internal model to estimate gravity and linear acceleration. *Nature* 398:615–618.

MILLER, W. T., 1987. Sensor-based control of robotic manipulators using a general learning algorithm. *IEEE J. Robot. Autom.* 3: 157–165.

MORASSO, P., 1981. Spatial control of arm movements. *Exp. Brain Res.* 42:223–227.

NEZAFAT, R., R. SHADMEHR, and H. H. HOLCOMB, 2001. Long-term adaptation to dynamics of reaching movements: A PET study. *Exp. Brain Res.* 140:66–76.

RANCOURT, D., and N. HOGAN, 2001. Stability in force-production tasks. *J. Mot. Behav.* 33:193–204.

SHADMEHR, R., and F. MUSSA-IVALDI, 1994. Adaptive representation of dynamics during learning of a motor task. *J. Neurosci.* 14:3208–3224.

SHIDARA, M., K. KAWANO, H. GOMI, and M. KAWATO, 1993. Inverse-dynamics encoding of eye movement by Purkinje cells in the cerebellum. *Nature* 365:50–52.

SUTTON, R., and A. G. BARTO, 1998. *Reinforcement Learning.* Cambridge, Mass.: MIT Press.

TODOROV, E., and M. I. JORDAN, 2002. Optimal feedback control as a theory of motor coordination. *Nat. Neurosci.* 5:1226–1235.

UNO, Y., M. KAWATO, and R. SUZUKI, 1989. Formation and control of optimal trajectory in human multijoint arm movement: Minimum torque-change model. *Biol. Cybern.* 61:89–101.

WANG, T., G. S. DORDEVIC, and R. SHADMEHR, 2001. Learning the dynamics of reaching movements results in the modification of arm impedance and long-latency perturbation responses. *Biol. Cybern.* 85:437–448.

WIDROW, B., and S. D. STEARNS, 1985. *Adaptive Signal Processing.* Englewood Cliffs, N. J.: Prentice-Hall.

WOLPERT, D. M., and J. R. FLANAGAN, 2001. Motor prediction. *Curr. Biol.* 11:R729–R732.

WOLPERT, D. M., Z. GHAHRAMANI, and M. I. JORDAN, 1995. An internal model for sensorimotor integration. *Science* 269: 1880–1882.

WOLPERT, D. M., and M. KAWATO, 1998. Multiple paired forward and inverse models for motor control. *Neural Netw.* 11: 1317–1329.

37 The Basal Ganglia and the Control of Action

ANN M. GRAYBIEL AND ESEN SAKA

ABSTRACT Clinical evidence, experimental studies in animals, and anatomical findings suggest that the basal ganglia act to influence both motor behavior and cognitive functions. We discuss the functions of the basal ganglia under four categories: (1) movement release and inhibition, (2) attention and assignment of salience, (3) response selection, and (4) learning and adaptive control of behavior. In the establishment of these functions, striatal output neurons lead into different output pathways: the direct, indirect, hyperdirect, and striosomal pathways. Divergence of cortical inputs to the striatum and reconvergence of these motor and cognitive signals in cortico-basal ganglia pathways is seen as essential in remapping forebrain representations of action and intrastriatal networks in the binding process. We propose that a crucial feature of this remapping is a learning-related recoding of sequential action representations so that they can be expressed as units. This chunking function of the striatum and associated cortico-basal ganglia loops may be a key mechanism operative across each of the functional categories of behavioral control attributed to the basal ganglia.

What the basal ganglia do has been a matter of interest to neurologists for over a century, but the basal ganglia have now also become a focus of interest for cognitive neuroscientists and for a range of others interested in brain and behavior. This change in perspective has come with evidence that the basal ganglia, either by themselves or, most probably, as parts of corticothalamo-basal ganglia loops, function not only in sensorimotor control but also in a wide range of cognitive processes ranging from attention to emotion, from response release and inhibition to response selection, and from online control to a primary function in learning and memory.

How could this system have such broad functions? A clue that the basal ganglia might contribute to cognitive processing is that the basal ganglia attain a very large size in the human brain. But a more telling clue is that a large part of the outflow of the basal ganglia in primates is directed via the thalamus toward executive areas of the frontal cortex—areas that are themselves associated with attention, planning, volitional decision, and selection among potential responses to external or internal cues (Miller and Cohen, 2001; Paus,

2001). Yet more evidence comes from imaging studies carried out in subjects engaged in cognitive tasks (Klein et al., 1994; Grafton, Hazeltine, and Ivry, 1995; Braver et al., 1997; Rao et al., 1997; Desmond, Gabrieli, and Glover, 1998; Poldrack et al., 1999; Peigneux et al., 2000; Poldrack and Gabrieli, 2001; Small et al., 2001; van den Heuvel et al., 2003) and from findings in patients with brain dysfunction due to disease or injury (Mendez, Adams, and Lewandowski, 1989; Bhatia and Marsden, 1994). Experiments on animals have also helped neuroscientists make working hypotheses about the neurobiology underlying basal ganglia function (Oberg and Divac, 1979; Graybiel, 1995, 1998; Miyashita, Hikosaka, and Kato, 1995; Bergman et al., 1998; Hikosaka et al., 1999; Jog et al., 1999; Brainard and Doupe, 2000; Mink, 2001; Packard and Knowlton, 2002). Together, these findings have brought the basal ganglia to the forefront of work on how the brain engages in interactions with the sensory and internal environment to form structured predictions about the world and, on this basis, to make and execute action plans (figures 37.1, and 37.2).

Perspective from anatomy: Substrates for basal ganglia functions

The basal ganglia have direct input not only from primary and higher-order sensory cortical areas and from motor and premotor cortical areas but also from the large areas of association cortex in the parietal, temporal, medial, and frontal association cortex (Webster, Bachevalier, and Ungerleider, 1993; Eblen and Graybiel, 1995; Yeterian and Pandya, 1998; Ferry et al., 2000; Leichnetz, 2001). There are other very large inputs from thalamic nuclei, especially the intralaminar nuclei (Parent et al., 1983; Haber and McFarland, 2001). If one includes, as should be done, the ventral striatum/ventral pallidum in the basal ganglia, cortical inputs to the system also come from the hippocampal formation and amygdala (Groenewegen, Wright, and Uylings, 1997; Fudge et al., 2002). When we add inputs from neuromodulatory systems, including the dopamine-containing nigrostriatal tract and serotonergic inputs, and inputs from the neocortex and elsewhere to other nuclei of the basal ganglia, the inputs to the basal ganglia system as a whole are

ANN M. GRAYBIEL and ESEN SAKA Department of Brain and Cognitive Sciences and the McGovern Institute for Brain Research, Massachusetts Institute of Technology, Cambridge, Mass.

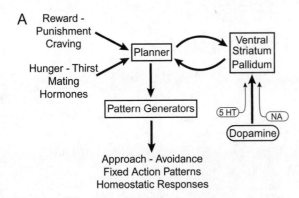

A

Reward -
Punishment
Craving

Hunger - Thirst
Mating
Hormones

Planner

Ventral
Striatum
Pallidum

Pattern Generators

5 HT   NA

Dopamine

Approach - Avoidance
Fixed Action Patterns
Homeostatic Responses

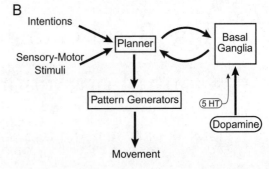

B

Intentions

Sensory-Motor
Stimuli

Planner

Basal
Ganglia

Pattern Generators

5 HT

Dopamine

Movement

FIGURE 37.1   Diagrams illustrating the postulated functions of the basal ganglia in relation to central pattern generators for eliciting goal-directed behavior (*A*) and movement (*B*). Planner circuits of the forebrain are influenced by motivation-related inputs (*A*) and sensorimotor stimuli (*B*). The basal ganglia are viewed as closely interacting with these planner mechanisms to shape activity in

behavioral pattern generators. Dopaminergic inputs to basal ganglia are essential in these interactions. The potential importance of serotonergic (5-HT) and noradrenergic (NA) inputs to the basal ganglia is also indicated. Implicit in the diagram is a possible evolutionary augmentation of limbic-based circuits in *A* by sensorimotor-based circuits in *B*. (Adapted from Graybiel, 1997.)

rich and diverse and by no means restricted to one functional domain.

It is also important to keep in mind that different regions within each nucleus of the basal ganglia are probably as different from one another functionally as different parts of the neocortex are from one another. When we think of behavior-related functions of the neocortex, we naturally think of the functions of individual cortical areas—for

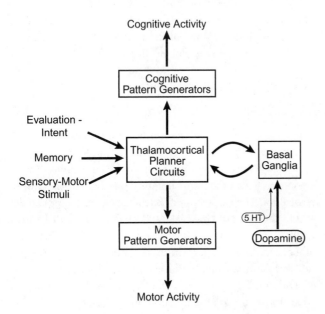

Cognitive Activity

Cognitive
Pattern Generators

Evaluation -
Intent

Memory

Sensory-Motor
Stimuli

Thalamocortical
Planner
Circuits

Basal
Ganglia

5 HT

Dopamine

Motor
Pattern Generators

Motor Activity

FIGURE 37.2   Schematic diagram illustrating potential influences of the basal ganglia not only on motor pattern generators but also on cognitive pattern generators. Evaluative and intention-related inputs, inputs related to remembered events, and ongoing sensorimotor inputs are illustrated to the left, and inputs from brainstem dopaminergic and serotonergic systems are illustrated to the right. (Adapted from Graybiel, 1997.)

example, the middle temporal area (MT) for visual motion, or parietal areas for reach and grasp, or prefrontal areas for working memory. We do not know as much about the regionally specialized subdivisions of the basal ganglia, but it is clear that there are different "families" of cortico-basal ganglia loops related to motor, associative, and limbic functions (Graybiel, 1984) and different cortico-basal ganglia loops defined by the cortical parts of the loops (Alexander, DeLong, and Strick, 1986). The behavioral evidence leading to this idea is important: lesion studies (Divac, Rosvold, and Szwarcbart, 1967; Goldman and Rosvold, 1972) have shown that localized lesions of the striatum produce symptoms very similar to those induced by lesions in the cortical areas projecting strongly to the particular parts of the striatum damaged. Somehow, the basal ganglia seem to mirror functionally what their cortical input sources do.

What the basal ganglia do, of course, depends not only on their inputs but also on their outputs. Here the story is interesting. Most current anatomical tract-tracing studies indicate that the largest ascending outflow of the basal ganglia is directed toward the frontal cortex via synaptic links in the thalamus. This puts the basal ganglia squarely in the "executive" realm of function. This view is consistent with the undoubted participation of these structures in motor control. But the frontal areas that receive basal ganglia outflow extend from the classic motor and premotor areas into the prefrontal cortex (Middleton and Strick, 2002). In fact, a large part of the neocortex in front of the central sulcus—including medial and lateral prefrontal, cingulate, and lateral and orbitofrontal cortex—is now thought to receive inputs (via thalamically processed routes) from the basal ganglia proper. Thanks to the ongoing anatomical work of Strick and colleagues based on viral transport methods, there is now evidence that at least part

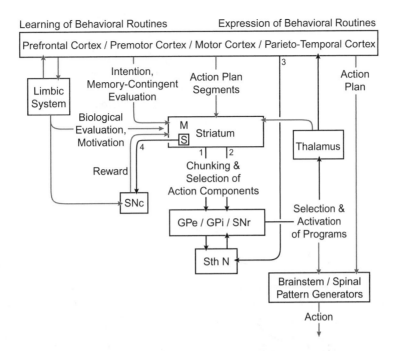

FIGURE 37.3 Schematic diagram of major basal ganglia circuits with highly schematized indications of component functions. The limbic system and association areas of the neocortex are shown as providing inputs for biological evaluation and memory-contingent evaluation. Inputs from motor and premotor cortical areas are related to action plan segments. The striatum with its matrix (M) and striosomal (S) compartments is centered in the diagram. Four major pathways are emphasized: the direct (1) and indirect (2) pathways, the hyperdirect pathway (3), and the striosomal pathway (4). Chunking and action-selection functions proposed for the striatum are shown, together with selection and activation of motor programs accomplished by interactions of the striatum, globus pallidus (GP), and subthalamic nucleus (Sth N) and the hyperdirect pathway. The outputs of the system lead to brainstem and spinal cord pattern generators, and also to the thalamus and cerebral cortex. The dopamine-containing substantia nigra pars compacta (SNc) is shown receiving limbic input and providing reward-related input to the system. Striosomes of the striatum, projecting to SNc, may modulate this dopamine-related function. (Adapted from Graybiel, 1997.)

of the inferotemporal cortex and at least part of the parietal cortex also receive inputs via basal ganglia-thalamocortical pathways (see Strick, this volume). These temporal and parietal areas are themselves linked to the executive network of the frontal lobes. Conceptually, then, the anatomy overwhelmingly favors the basal ganglia as poised to influence high-levels functions associated with activity in the frontal neocortex (figure 37.3).

This emphasis on the cortically directed pathways leading out from the basal ganglia is natural enough when thinking about the possible cognitive functions of the basal ganglia, but it is equally important to keep in mind that there are other robust outputs of the basal ganglia (Parent and Hazrati, 1995a,b). These outputs may also, directly or indirectly, influence potential cognitive functions of the basal ganglia. Such connections include strong projections to the reticular nucleus of the thalamus, a major controller of thalamocortical and corticothalamic state-dependent activity (McAlonan and Brown, 2002), and descending projections from the basal ganglia, among which are connections leading to the superior colliculus and brainstem reticular formation, and to the nuclei that are recurrently connected with the basal ganglia (Parent and Hazrati, 1995a,b).

The most studied of these recurrent pathway nuclei is the substantia nigra. The dopamine-containing subdivision of the substantia nigra degenerates in Parkinson's disease and in related parkinsonian disorders. Dopamine-containing neurons respond phasically to predictors of reward or to primary rewards themselves, and have tonic activity related to the probability of reward (uncertainty) (Schultz, 2002; Fiorillo, Tobler, and Schultz, 2003). A second key nucleus is the subthalamic nucleus. Lesions of this nucleus result in the hyperkinetic syndrome called ballism. Remarkably, it is now recognized that lesions or deep-brain stimulation in the subthalamic nucleus can relieve symptoms of Parkinson's disease (Bergman, Wichmann, and DeLong, 1990; Lang, 2000; Obeso et al., 2000; Benabid et al., 2003). The subthalamic nucleus is also now recognized as receiving strong input from the motor cortex (and some other cortical areas) and from the intralaminar thalamus, and is a key control nucleus for the basal ganglia (Feger, Bevan, and Crossman, 1994; Deschenes et al., 1996; Nambu, Tokuno, and Takada, 2002). A third nucleus related to the basal ganglia is the pedunculopontine nucleus, embedded in the reticular formation. The PPN, as it is known, sends outputs to motor control centers of the lower brainstem and is also a modulator of basal ganglia function by way of its recurrent upstream connections (Lavoie and Parent, 1994; Pahapill and Lozano, 2000).

Perspective from the clinic

In Parkinson's disease and Huntington's disease, classic basal ganglia disorders accompanied by motor abnormalities, patients frequently experience cognitive dysfunction, including memory deficiency, depression, and, most important, disordered executive functions (Brown and Marsden, 1990; Dubois, Pillon, and Agid, 1992; Bedard et al., 1998, 2003; Joel, 2001; Saint-Cyr, 2003). Moreover, dementia is frequent in these diseases and mostly exhibits the features of frontal dementia syndromes (Pillon et al., 1994; Saint-Cyr, 2003). These "additional" (i.e., nonmotor) symptoms are often taken to suggest that the basal ganglia proper have cognitive functions, but this view has been modified by the realization that both Parkinson's disease and Huntington's disease are neurodegenerative diseases with neuronal damage extending—and even starting—outside the basal ganglia (Sieradzan and Mann, 2001; Braak et al., 2003). It is thus not possible to attribute the cognitive signs and symptoms of these disorders to dysfunction of the basal ganglia alone.

There are other neurological disorders that at least appear to affect more selectively specific basal ganglia nuclei (e.g., certain cerebrovascular disorders). Dysfunction in multiple cognitive domains is reported with infarctions or hemorrhages apparently limited to the caudate nucleus (e.g., abulia, restlessness, disinhibition and impulsivity, executive dysfunction) or to the putamen (e.g., contralateral neglect, language abnormalities) (Mendez, Adams, and Lewandowski, 1989; Caplan et al., 1990; Bhatia and Marsden, 1994). Lesions in patient populations affecting the dorsolateral caudate nucleus are most closely associated with abulia. Lesions in the ventromedial caudate nucleus are associated with disinhibition and impulsivity. New work in the behaving primate supports such clinical findings and suggests detailed fractionation of behavioral control mechanisms within the basal ganglia (Francois et al., 2002; Tremblay et al., 2003).

Finally, imaging studies have demonstrated alterations of basal ganglia activity in disorders in which cognitive deficits are evident, for example, obsessive-compulsive (OC)-spectrum disorders such as Tourette's syndrome and obsessive-compulsive disorder (OCD), and attention-deficit/hyperactivity disorder (ADHD) (Graybiel and Rauch, 2000; Teicher et al., 2000; Rauch et al., 2001; Leckman, 2002). We will refer again to these disorders in what follows.

Favored hypotheses for basal ganglia function

We have grouped hypotheses about the functions of the basal ganglia into categories related to (1) movement release and inhibition, (2) attention and assignment of salience, (3) response selection, and (4) learning and adaptive control of behavior.

MOVEMENT RELEASE AND INHIBITION The main pathways that lead out from the basal ganglia are known as the direct and indirect pathways, the hyperdirect pathway, and the striosomal pathway (figure 37.3). These pathways are thought to influence motor control by release (direct pathway) or inhibition (indirect pathway and hyperdirect pathway) of motor behaviors (Albin, Young, and Penny, 1989; DeLong, 1990) and by control of the repetitiveness of behaviors, for the striosomal pathway (Graybiel, Canales, and Capper-Loup, 2000; Saka and Graybiel, 2003). The release-inhibit model suggests, in simplest form, that the neocortex excites the striatum, which inhibits the internal pallidum, which in turn inhibits the motor thalamus. The double inhibition suggests that cortical activation phasically "releases" the thalamus, which then can excite the neocortex. This movement-releasing pathway is, according to the release-inhibit model, in direct competition with the *indirect pathway*, which, due to its connecting link in the subthalamic nucleus, is thought to depress movement. The subthalamic nucleus is released by striatal excitation of its inhibitory input nucleus (the external pallidum), and the subthalamic nucleus then excites the internal pallidum, leading to less movement. Many current models of the basal ganglia focus on this winner-take-all model (Dominey, Arbib, and Joseph, 1995; Beiser and Houk, 1998; J. E. Brown, Bullock, and Grossberg, 1999; Gillies and Arbuthnott, 2000; Frank, Loughry, and O'Reilly, 2001; Kitano, Aoyagi, and Fukai, 2001).

The *hyperdirect pathway* consists of a fast, direct excitatory pathway from the motor cortex (and some other cortical areas) to the subthalamic nucleus, which can therefore rapidly excite the pallidum (Nambu, Tokuno, and Takada, 2002). This pathway bypasses the striatum, and could help to account for the efficacy of deep brain stimulation of the subthalamic nucleus to relieve symptoms of Parkinson's disease (Lang, 2000; Obeso et al., 2000; Benabid et al., 2003).

We emphasize that, if we extend the release-inhibit idea to the cognitive level, we can think of other actions—even thoughts or emotions—as being released through this mechanism (Swerdlow and Koob, 1987; Graybiel, 1997). This possibility is receiving potential support from the results of deep brain stimulation used as a therapeutic intervention for Parkinson's disease. For example, emotional distress and anguish, or irrepressible laughter and hilarity, can be evoked by stimulation in or near the substantia nigra and subthalamic nucleus (Bejjani et al., 1999; Krack et al., 2001).

The *striosomal pathway* is thought to lead from the anterior cingulate cortex and caudal orbitofrontal cortex to neurochemically defined compartments in the striatum that are called striosomes (striatal bodies). These in turn are interconnected with the dopamine-containing substantia nigra (Eblen and Graybiel, 1995; Prensa and Parent, 2001). These connections may serve to regulate the frequency and repetitiveness of behavior of actions.

ATTENTION AND ASSIGNMENT OF SALIENCE   The attention–salience assignment model suggests that the outputs of the basal ganglia are influential in modulating movement because they can influence attention to stimuli and because they have the capacity to assign salience to stimuli. This idea is strongly supported by work on the dopamine-containing inputs to the basal ganglia, which carry signals related to reinforcement probability, salience, and expectation of reinforcement (Schultz, Dayan, and Montague, 1997; Berridge and Robinson, 1998; Fiorillo, Tobler, and Schultz, 2003). We note, however, that several other systems that could have this function also project to the basal ganglia. These systems include the locus coeruleus/norepinephrine system (projecting especially strongly to the ventral striatum), the serotonergic raphe system, the intralaminar thalamic nuclei, and other structures such as the amygdala.

Clinical studies have repeatedly implicated the basal ganglia in attentional control (Mesulam, 2000), and, in modern formulations of this idea, the basal ganglia are particularly singled out as being important for attention to action (Jueptner, Stephan, et al., 1997). Imaging studies indicate that cortico-basal ganglia circuit dysfunction in Parkinson's disease may account for the marked attentional problems suffered by Parkinson's patients (see Saint-Cyr, 2003). There is, in addition, evidence for dysfunction of corticocortical connections linking the supplementary motor area and premotor areas (Rowe et al., 2002). This dysfunction at the cortical level could itself be related to abnormal basal ganglia influences on these cortical areas (Brooks, 1997; Samuel et al., 1997). It should be clear, however, that attention is a broad concept and, in the context of cortico-basal ganglia loops, includes functions ranging from saliency signals modulating signal-to-noise ratios to motor readiness (Denny-Brown and Yanagisawa, 1976; Robbins and Everitt, 1992; Aosaki, Graybiel, and Kimura, 1994; Brown, Schneider, and Lidsky, 1997; Jog et al., 1999). Considered in this way, attentional deficits in Parkinson's disease could lead to bradykinesia (slowness of movement), bradyphrenia (slowness of thought), and abulia (a cardinal sign of anterior striatal dysfunction in which a profound inertia of psychomotor response initiation occurs).

Studies of patients with Parkinson's disease and Huntington's disease have demonstrated deficiency in set shifting (Owen et al., 1993; Georgiou et al., 1996; Bedard et al., 1998), suggesting a particular function for the basal ganglia-based pathways in shifting of attention. Again, these deficits may be due to abnormalities in the basal ganglia proper, but they likely reflect cortico-basal ganglia-thalamocortical circuit dysfunction, or even neurodegeneration outside of these basal ganglia circuits. However, in normal persons there are significant and selective increases in regional cerebral blood flow in the putamen for tasks that measure shifting of attention in response to visual cues (Koski et al., 1999).

A dramatic deficiency in attentional control is present in ADHD, in which individuals exhibit hyperactive behavior, a lack of focusing ability and impulsivity. Functional imaging studies addressing the possible involvement of the basal ganglia in this disorder suggest that the capacity to inhibit motor activity and the capacity to sustain attention may be linked in ADHD individuals, and that these clinical measures of abnormal function are correlated with altered activity in the putamen (Teicher et al., 2000).

Electrophysiological studies in primates support the idea that the basal ganglia are part of forebrain attentional systems. Explicit tests of attentional shifting suggest that many striatal projection neurons fire for shifts in attention unaccompanied by overt movements (Kermadi and Boussaoud, 1995; Boussaoud and Kermadi, 1997). An instructive example comes from studies of striatal interneurons called tonically active neurons (TANs), which are broadly distributed through the caudate nucleus and putamen (figure 37.4). These neurons modify their responses to sensory stimuli depending on the saliency of the sensory stimuli. The salience can be unconditional (e.g., a loud, unexpected sound makes them respond) or can be built up through conditioning by pairing the sensory cues with positive or negative reinforcements (Aosaki, Kimura, and Graybiel, 1994; Apicella, 2002; Blazquez et al., 2002). The reward/saliency signals are partly dependent on inputs from the dopamine-containing neurons of the substantia nigra (Aosaki, Kimura, and Graybiel, 1994). But they depend also on inputs from the intralaminar nuclei of the thalamus (Matsumoto et al., 2001) and probably the neocortex as well. Because the TANs are widely distributed local network neurons and tend to have synchronous responses (Graybiel et al., 1994; Raz et al., 1996; Blazquez et al., 2002), they could coordinate together activity in functionally distinct cortico-basal ganglia loops to achieve sensorimotor and cognitive binding (figure 37.5) (see Graybiel et al., 1994; Graybiel, 1997).

This example gives an idea of how signals from many different brain regions could, ultimately, lead to salience signaling in basal ganglia networks and contribute to motor and cognitive attention. Remarkably, it has been estimated that the population activity of even a small number of these

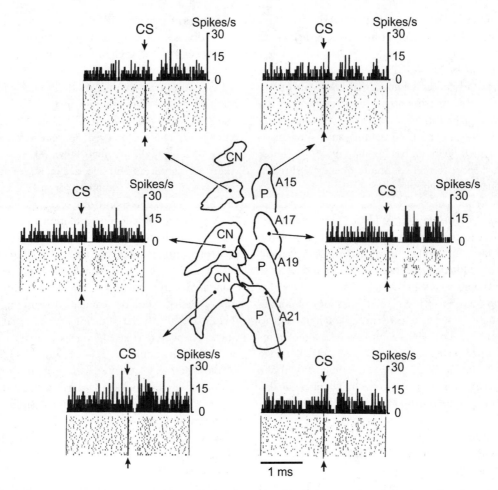

FIGURE 37.4   The responses of tonically active neurons (TANs) of the macaque monkey striatum in response to conditioned stimuli (CS: clicks or light-emitting diodes) in a simple behavioral conditioning paradigm in which the monkey received liquid rewards following delivery of the CS. The neurons acquired responses to the cues associated with the rewards (see pauses in activity). The responses of six representative TANs recorded at the illustrated sites (black dots or squares) are shown in raster plots and spike histograms, and the anteroposterior (AP) sites at which they were recorded are shown in diagrams with approximate AP coordinates. Note the widespread, coherent appearance of the response, suggesting that these interneurons might serve as a temporal binding mechanism across cortico-basal ganglia loops. (Adapted from Graybiel et al., 1994.)

interneurons can accurately predict ongoing behavioral events (Blazquez et al., 2002). This means that the intrinsic circuitry of the striatum has within it a signal proportional to behavioral outcome—exactly what is needed to develop a forward model for behavioral control (Blazquez et al., 2002).

RESPONSE SELECTION AND INHIBITION   Selection of which response to make is a huge job, probably engaging much of the neocortex and other brain regions, but the basal ganglia may strongly influence such selections if they do, as indicated in the preceding discussion, function to assign salience and to build up predictions, and if they do have the ability to release and inhibit motor and cognitive actions.

Disorders of response selection, cognitive and motor intrusions, inflexibility, repetitiveness, and overt cognitive and motor stereotypic responses occur in OC-spectrum disorders (Graybiel and Rauch, 2000; Leckman, 2002). Functional imaging studies of persons with OC-spectrum disorders indicate increased activity in the caudate nucleus combined with increased activity in the cingulate and orbitofrontal cortices (see Rauch et al., 2001). Moreover, symptom provocation in OCD patients further increases the activity of these regions (Breiter et al., 1996), and the increased activation can be lessened by treatment of the symptoms (Baxter et al., 1992; Schwartz et al., 1996). This dynamic modulation supports the idea that the basal ganglia and anterior cingulate/orbitofrontal cortical regions are important in response selection and attentional shifting.

There are two leading ideas about how such selection might be carried out by cortico-basal ganglia circuits. One is that the direct and indirect (and now also the hyperdirect)

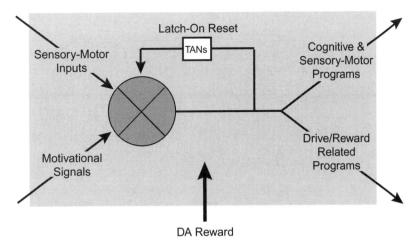

FIGURE 37.5 Diagram illustrating the hypothesis that the striatum acts as a dynamic modulator of cognitive and motor programs and that striatal interneurons, including tonically active neurons (TANs), function as part of the plastic neural mechanism underlying this dynamic modulation. Inputs to the striatum (circles) are combined to produce activity that is contingent both on reinforce-ment signals such as reward-related inputs from the dopaminergic nigrostriatal system (at bottom) and on the activity states of populations of striatal interneurons (TANs). As a result of the continuous modification of these circuits, cognitive and sensorimotor programs and drive/reward-related programs would be modified.

pathways compete in a winner-take-all fashion, with one dominating the level of activity in the output nuclei of the basal ganglia (the pallidum and substantia nigra). This is viewed not just as a battle between movement release and movement inhibition. Rather, the thought is that there is specific selection of a given motor response via the direct striatopallidal path and concurrent suppression of competing or unwanted responses via the indirect pathway (Filion, Tremblay, and Bédard, 1988; Mink, 2001). This view has been adapted to account for imaging data in OCD patients (Rauch et al., 2001) and some basal ganglia models (Beiser and Houk, 1998; J. E. Brown, Bullock, and Grossberg, 1999; Gillies and Arbuthnott, 2000), but remains controversial.

The second idea is that the striatum is important for selection of which behaviors to emit, and that this selection depends on a learning architecture set up in the striatum. In this view, most behavioral selections can be influenced by experience, and the striatum—and therefore the rest of the basal ganglia—participates strongly in the adaptive control of motor and cognitive behaviors. This idea originated with the recognition that corticostriatal inputs (and other inputs to the striatum) are modular, and that the cortical inputs show modular divergence but then can show reconvergence at the next stage of the basal ganglia circuit, within the pallidum (figure 37.6A) (Graybiel et al., 1994; Parthasarathy and Graybiel, 1997). This pattern resembles simple learning architectures (e.g., Jacobs et al., 1991), whereby information can be distributed divergently to an intermediate layer of the network, and then gated and recombined at an output layer (figure 37.6B). The dopaminergic input to the striatum could

be one strong gating mechanism. Thus, the modular architecture of the striatum could provide a mechanism for response selection through learning. This mechanism clearly could apply to cognitive actions, not only to motor actions (Graybiel, 1997).

Selecting which action to perform is critical for normal behavior. But when particular actions (or thoughts) are selected over and over again, the repetitiveness can signal the occurrence of syndromes such as OC-spectrum disorders or other disorders in which behavioral stereotypies occur. There is some evidence that the repetitiveness of action selection can be controlled independently of which action is selected. That is, different actions can be selected but, when selected, each is repetitively selected. In both rodents and primates, a specific modular pattern of neuronal activation in the striatum is highly predictive of the stereotypies induced by psychomotor stimulants: activity in striosomes is greater than activity in the surrounding matrix, regardless of which particular actions are being repeated—that is, regardless of which have been selected (figure 37.7) (see Canales and Graybiel, 2000; Saka and Graybiel, 2003). This is interesting, because anatomical work in the primate suggests that striosomes receive differentially strong input from parts of the anterior cingulate and orbitofrontal cortex (Eblen and Graybiel, 1995). In the human, these are cortical regions that are hyperactive in OCD patients (Graybiel and Rauch, 2000). Modular patterns of striatal activation have also been invoked to account for focal tics and repetitive actions in Tourette's syndrome (Mink, 2001). In this case, overactivity in particular modules (matrisomes) is thought to be involved

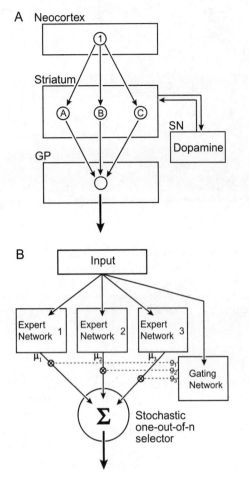

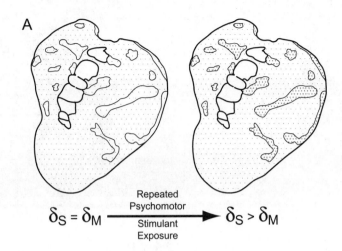

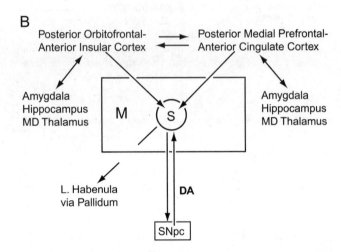

FIGURE 37.6 (*A*) Divergent-reconvergent processing of motor or cognitive signals through cortico-basal ganglia pathways. Divergence of cortical input to modules (matrisomes A, B, and C) occurs at the level of the striatum. In the globus pallidus (GP), information is reconverged, resulting in the remapping of the cortical output. Multiple interacting divergent-reconvergent networks can lead to recombinations of the original cortical inputs. The network is modulated by dopamine-containing inputs from the substantia nigra (SN) (modified from Graybiel et al., 1994). (*B*) Mixture-of-experts learning network model (modified from Jacobs et al., 1991). Note the similarity of the models in *A* and *B*.

in the "selection" of the repeated behavior (figure 37.6*A*). Thus, both striosomes and matrisomes could contribute to disorders of action selection and behavioral switching and could be important for the normal discharge of these complex functions.

LEARNING AND ADAPTIVE CONTROL OF BEHAVIOR   The idea that the basal ganglia are sites for learning has strong support from experimental work in animals, and increasing support from imaging and other work in humans. Commonly, attempts to formulate how the basal ganglia could contribute to learning involve comparing the basal ganglia to the hip-

FIGURE 37.7 (*A*) Schematization of neuronal activity mapped in the caudate nucleus and putamen of the squirrel monkey in response to either single (left) or repeated (right) exposure of the monkey to psychomotor stimulants. The activity measure is the average density of striatal neurons expressing early genes in response to the drug treatment, calculated separately for the striosome (δ_S) and matrix (δ_M) compartments. The single dose of the psychomotor stimulant induced only low levels of behavioral stereotypy and little predominance of striosomal activation. By contrast, with repeated exposure to the psychomotor stimulant, high levels of behavioral stereotypy were induced, accompanied by sharply increased striosome predominance. (*B*) Schematization of the major connections of the striosomes. The striatum is shown by the central rectangle, with its matrix (M) and striosomal (S) compartments. Inputs to striosomes come from limbic-related areas of the neocortex: posterior orbitofrontal, anterior cingulate, anterior insular, and posterior medial prefrontal cortex. These inputs are modulated by such limbic structures as the amygdala, hippocampus, and mediodorsal (MD) nucleus of the thalamus. Distinct outputs from striosomes are sent to the dopamine (DA)-containing substantia nigra pars compacta (SNpc) and to the lateral part of the habenular complex. (Part B adapted from Eblen and Graybiel, 1995, by permission of the Society for Neuroscience. Copyright 1995 by the Society for Neuroscience.)

pocampus, or comparing them to the cerebellum (Packard and Knowlton, 2002; Doyon, Penhune, and Ungerleider, 2003). Helpful as such comparisons may be, they are not enough to define the type of neural processing that occurs in basal ganglia networks and cortico-basal ganglia circuits during behavioral learning. New techniques are now beginning to let investigators approach this issue directly.

Studies in rat, monkey, and human suggest that, contrary to the hippocampal system, the basal ganglia mediate a particular type of learning and memory: stimulus-response (S-R) learning, in which learning proceeds by trial and error and performance improves according to the sensory feedback obtained as a result of the response (Packard and McGaugh, 1992; McDonald and White, 1994). Evidence for this has led to the notion that the basal ganglia are important for habit or skill learning (Graybiel, 1995; Packard and Knowlton, 2002). The function of the basal ganglia in feedback (S-R) learning may be highly conserved. In birds, the anterior forebrain pathway (AFP) is thought to be analogous to certain cortico-basal ganglia circuits in mammals, and it has been shown that this AFP pathway is critical to bird song learning (Brainard and Doupe, 2000).

Experimental psychologists working with rats have amassed strong evidence that the caudoputamen (dorsal striatum) is necessary for both the acquisition and the expression of S-R associations and memory and for "win-stay" learning, in which the animal repeats the behavior that led to reward (Packard, Hirsh, and White, 1989; Packard and McGaugh, 1992, 1996; McDonald and White, 1994). This behavior is contrasted to "win-shift" behavior, involving explicit memory of the context of the behavior. However, the situation may be more than one of different basal ganglia loops participating in different aspects of learning. For example, performance on S-R learning tasks suffers in rats with lateral (sensorimotor) striatal lesions, but in rats with medial striatal lesions, performance suffers on tasks similar to those requiring hippocampal function, for example, spatial navigation (Devan, McDonald, and White, 1999; Devan and White, 1999). Moreover, there is good reason to think that in most of the tasks used in such rodent experiments, explicit awareness of the associations (e.g., place learning) could occur, engaging the hippocampus. Some studies suggest that in such contexts, the hippocampus may operate during an early, explicit stage of learning, and that the striatum may then take over (or at least be more critical) when the task is repeated to the point at which the animal can perform the task without explicit knowledge (McDonald and White, 1994; Packard and McGaugh, 1996). Thus, even with damage to the striatum, habit learning could be partly intact, because learning strategies based on hippocampal function can partly compensate for the deficient recruitment of the basal ganglia (Packard and Knowlton, 2002). Interestingly, evidence in these rodent studies suggests that the

striatum and hippocampus can compete with each other, so that a lesion of one system may actually facilitate learning mediated by the other system. For example, a deficit in spatial learning strategy following hippocampal damage can improve performance of S-R learning (Packard, Hirsh, and White, 1989; McDonald and White, 1993; Schroeder, Wingard, and Packard, 2002).

In imaging studies of human performance, activation of the basal ganglia has been repeatedly found to accompany motor skill learning. Skill learning can be broken down into a number of phases but, as in learning a sport, requires practice, S-R (feedback) learning, and consolidation (Brashers-Krug, Shadmehr, and Bizzi, 1996; Karni et al., 1998; Hikosaka et al., 1999; Ungerleider, Doyon, and Karni, 2002; Saint-Cyr, 2003). Once learned, the sequence of movements can be carried out seemingly effortlessly with the same or similar effector groups used during practice. Many studies have employed the serial reaction time (SRT) task to study simple human motor skill learning (Grafton, Hazeltine, and Ivry, 1995; Willingham, Salidis, and Gabrieli, 2002). For example, subjects can be asked to press a series of buttons in an order instructed by target lights that appear either in a random sequence or in a predetermined, repeated sequence. With practice, the subjects become faster, especially with the repeated sequences. If the subject is told about the sequence beforehand, the reaction time advantage for the repeating sequence is thought to occur by virtue of declarative learning, but to involve nondeclarative, implicit learning if the subject does not know about the repeating sequence (or is distracted by a second task). Positron emission tomography and functional magnetic resonance imaging studies have demonstrated heightened activation in the putamen, along with a network of cortical areas, in the implicit condition (Grafton, Hazeltine, and Ivry, 1995; Hazeltine, Grafton, and Ivry, 1997; Willingham, Salidis, and Gabrieli, 2002), and in some explicit conditions as well (Willingham, Salidis, and Gabrieli, 2002).

Learning and performing a sequence of finger movements by trial and error with auditory feedback evokes activation of the striatum also, both in learning a new sequence and in the execution of a prelearned sequence (Jenkins et al., 1994). The acquisition phase favors more anterior activation (caudate nucleus, anterior putamen) by comparison with performance of a prelearned sequence (Jueptner, Frith, et al., 1997; Jueptner, Stephan, et al., 1997). Similar anterior-to-posterior shifts also occur in the frontal cortex during learning (Jueptner, Frith, et al., 1997). Attention to action may in part underlie the shift. When subjects attend to their next action in a prelearned (automized) sequence, the caudate nucleus, but not the (more posterior) putamen, exhibits differentiated activation (Jueptner, Stephan, et al., 1997). Such anteroposterior gradients have been found in primates: the anterior striatum and the pre-SMA (pre-supplementary motor area) are preferentially activated during acquisition of new sequences in trial and error (feedback) learning, but there is more predominant activation of the putamen during the execution of learned sequences (Miyachi et al., 1997; Nakamura, Sakai, and Hikosaka, 1998, 1999; Hikosaka et al., 1999).

If we think back to the anatomy of cortico-basal ganglia loops, we can see that these and other studies (Shadmehr and Brashers-Krug, 1997; Honda et al., 1998; Jueptner and Weiller, 1998; Karni et al., 1998; Peterson et al., 1998) suggest that the acquisition of motor skills probably engages the activity of a number of corticostriatal loop systems, and that which loops are engaged changes during different stages of learning, from the first learning of the basic structure of the task (its rules or constraints) to an eventual engagement of particular muscle groups in sequence without the conscious calling up of the single parts of the behavior. The early stages activate cortico-basal ganglia loops in which the caudate nucleus and anterior putamen participate, and later stages activate putamen-based loops. Interestingly, contrary to the activation of the putamen in motor skill learning, perceptual skill learning (e.g., mirror reading task) is linked to activation of the caudate nucleus (Poldrack and Gabrieli, 2001). The cerebellum is also activated in such tasks. One interesting idea is that different frames of reference (coordinate frames) are used for different phases of S-R sequential learning: early on, a spatial coordinate frame, and later a motor coordinate frame (Hikosaka et al., 1999).

More cognitive versions of S-R learning tasks, requiring implicit learning by feedback of probabilistic classifications, also differentially activate the caudate nucleus (Saint-Cyr, Taylor, and Lang, 1988; Knowlton, Squire, and Gluck, 1994; Poldrack et al., 1999). The medial part of the temporal lobe, by contrast, is activated when such tasks are acquired through observation (paired association tasks) rather than through guessing and learning by trial and error (Poldrack et al., 2001). Supporting the idea of antagonistic activity of striatal and hippocampal systems raised by studies in experimental animals, imaging studies in human subjects demonstrate deactivation of the MT lobe during acquisition of the feedback-based task. The activities of the caudate nucleus and of MT are negatively correlated (Poldrack et al., 2001). Patients with Parkinson's disease and Huntington's disease perform more poorly on the feedback-based probabilistic classification task than patients with localized frontal lobe lesions, suggesting that it is not only a dysfunction of the frontal part of the fronto-basal ganglia loop system but, more likely, deficits in neuronal processing in the striatum itself that lead to learning deficits in Parkinson's disease patients (Knowlton, Mangels, and Squire, 1996).

Impairments in motor and perceptual skill learning have been demonstrated in patients with Huntington's disease and Parkinson's disease (Martone et al., 1984; Heindel, Butters, and Salmon, 1988; M. A. Smith, Brandt, and Shadmehr, 2000). Patients with OCD have deficits in performing the implicit form of SRT tasks when a second task is introduced (Deckersbach et al., 2002), and they fail to exhibit activation of the striatum during the acquisition of SRT tasks (Rauch et al., 2001).

We have concentrated on the dorsal striatum (the caudate nucleus and putamen), but evidence suggests that the ventral striatum is also critical to reinforcement-based learning, together with its dopaminergic input from the ventral tegmental area. For example, neurons of the ventral striatum can apparently keep track of how close a monkey is to receiving reward (Bowman, Aigner, and Richmond, 1996; Shidara, Aigner, and Richmond, 1998; Rolls, 1999). Interestingly, the striosomes of the dorsal striatum, by virtue of their connections with many of the same brain structures as the ventral striatum, are likely also to be important in the learning and execution of rewarded tasks (Aosaki, Kimura, and Graybiel, 1995; White and Hiroi, 1998). Because the dorsal striatum and ventral striatum are believed to participate in different forms of learning (nondeclarative and declarative, respectively), it is possible that the reward evaluation function of the ventral striatum is taken over by striosomes in nondeclarative learning. As we noted earlier, activity in striosomes is correlated with maladaptive, perseverative responses following psychomotor stimulant exposure, raising the possibility that they could be active in relation to stereotypic behaviors in OC-spectrum disorders.

Chunking of action repertoires as a common theme for basal ganglia function

We have considered here four categories of hypotheses about the functions of the basal ganglia, ranging from the release of movements (or thoughts) to the assignment of saliences and attention to stimuli, to the selection of which responses to emit, and, finally, to a core function in behavioral learning, especially feedback-based learning. There are other behavioral categories that should also be considered, including sequencing of movements or cognitive acts, scaling or timing of these acts, or preparing for the next movement or thought. But regardless of the behavioral categorization, we must still remember that the basal ganglia are embedded in circuits that engage the thalamus and cerebral cortex, and other sites as well. How can we learn what part of any function to attribute to the basal ganglia, and what part to other structures in these basal ganglia-based circuits?

One important recent finding from primate physiology is that identified corticostriatal neurons in the motor cortex have quite different response properties than even very nearby motor cortex neurons projecting to the spinal cord (Turner and DeLong, 2000). In trained monkeys, at least, the responses of the neurons seem tuned to very discrete

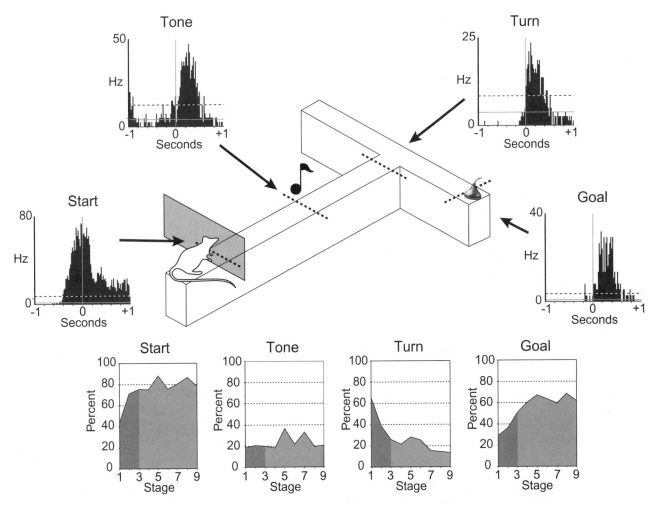

FIGURE 37.8 Event-related ensemble activity of neurons in the dorsolateral striatum of rats recorded during the acquisition and performance of an auditory conditional turning task in a T maze. A rat placed in the start arm of the maze starts behind a gate, and is trained to initiate a maze run when the gate is opened. A tone (1 or 8 kHz) instructs the rat that chocolate reward is located at the left or right arm of the T maze. With repeated trials, the rat associates the particular tone with the particular turning direction, and obtains the reward at the end of the correct goal arm. Perievent histograms displayed around the T maze show examples of the

activities of single striatal neurons in relation to start, tone, turn, and goal events. Plots below illustrate the reorganization of task-related activity patterns of the striatal neurons that occurs during the acquisition of the task (Jog et al., 1999). The behavioral criterion for acquisition (stage 3) was 72.5% correct performance ($P <$ 0.01 by χ^2 test). Note the large increase in the numbers of striatal neurons with start and goal responses, and the decrease in the numbers of striatal neurons with turn-related responses during learning. The stages following stage 3 represent the initial consolidation period. (Modified from Graybiel and Kubota, 2003.)

contexts, and they are nearly all direction-selective. This finding suggests that the information reaching the striatum is not an exact copy (efference copy or corollary discharge) of the motor command sent to the spinal cord. But it could be, for example, that cortical inputs to the subthalamic nucleus (hyperdirect pathway) are? This is not yet known. There is also suggestive evidence that inputs from the motor cortex tend to activate striatal neurons of the indirect pathway more than those of the direct pathway, and that the reverse is true for thalamostriatal inputs (Berretta, Parthasarathy, and Graybiel, 1997; Parthasarathy and Graybiel, 1997; Y. Smith et al., 1998). Even these two examples indicate that our understanding of cortico-basal ganglia networks is still primitive.

Another approach to the circuit issue has been to record in the striatum as animals undergo training in behaviors thought to require striatal function, such as procedural, S-R, habit, or win-stay learning. The results of such experiments are interesting. For example, in the experiment illustrated in figure 37.8, rats were trained to run down a simple T maze to obtain reward at one or the other of the end arms, and conditional auditory cues were given during the maze run to tell the animal which arm was baited (Jog et al., 1999). Each day during training, physiological recordings of the firing of ensembles of striatal neurons were made with tetrodes chronically implanted in the sensorimotor sector of the striatum. As shown in figure 37.8, there was a dramatic change in response patterns of striatal neurons during learning. Responses during the turn part of the task declined, but responses at the start and end of the task increased. In this experiment, at least, it seemed that the task boundaries became emphasized by ensemble activity in the striatum and in-between parts of the task became less prominently represented (Jog et al., 1999; Graybiel and Kubota, 2003). This start and end accentuation has now been found in corticostriatal loops in awake behaving primates, suggesting that the representation of action boundaries could be an important aspect of encoding for cortico-basal ganglia circuits (Fujii and Graybiel, 2003).

How could this work? One idea is that, through activity in cortico-basal ganglia loops, the representations of actions that are repeated over and over again get recoded: representations related to entire sequences of actions making up a behavior are built, so that each individual element of the behavior is no longer coded in detail in the loop in question. In this case, the basal ganglia could be viewed as structures that help remap action representations into expressible units. By analogy to memory units, these have been called chunks (Graybiel, 1998). This could, potentially, be a common theme tying together the apparently different categories of behavior attributed to the basal ganglia and discussed here. For example, the release-inhibition function, seen in these terms, would suggest that for automated behaviors, the behaviors are releasable (or repressible) as a whole, not necessarily element by element. For the attention and assignment of salience, cortico-basal ganglia circuits, through repetition, could be remapped so that particular salient sensory cues or "contexts" could trigger entire responses. This is, in fact, one definition of habit (James, 1890). Similarly, response selection, through repetition and learning, could be automated by such a chunking process. Finally, in this view, learning functions would be seen as critical and core functions of cortico-basal ganglia networks and, in particular, of corticostriatal networks.

REFERENCES

ALBIN, R. L., A. B. YOUNG, and J. B. PENNEY, 1989. The functional anatomy of basal ganglia disorders. *Trends Neurosci.* 12:366–375.

ALEXANDER, G. E., M. R. DeLONG, and P. L. STRICK, 1986. Parallel organization of functionally segregated circuits linking basal ganglia and cortex. *Annu. Rev. Neurosci.* 9:357–381.

AOSAKI, T., A. M. GRAYBIEL, and M. KIMURA, 1994. Effects of the nigrostriatal dopamine system on acquired neural responses in the striatum of behaving monkeys. *Science* 265:412–415.

AOSAKI, T., M. KIMURA, and A. M. GRAYBIEL, 1995. Temporal and spatial characteristics of tonically active neurons of the primate's striatum. *J. Neurophysiol.* 73:1234–1252.

AOSAKI, T., H. TSUBOKAWA, A. ISHIDA, K. WATANABE, A. M. GRAYBIEL, and M. KIMURA, 1994. Responses of tonically active neurons in the primate's striatum undergo systematic changes during behavioral sensorimotor conditioning. *J. Neurosci.* 14: 3969–3984.

APICELLA, P., 2002. Tonically active neurons in the primate striatum and their role in the processing of information about motivationally relevant events. *Eur. J. Neurosci.* 16:2017–2026.

BAXTER, L. R., JR., J. M. SCHWARTZ, K. S. BERGMAN, M. P. SZUBA, B. H. GUZE, J. C. MAZZIOTTA, A. ALAZRAKI, C. E. SELIN, H.-K. FERNG, and M. E. PHELPS, 1992. Caudate glucose metabolic rate changes with both drug and behavioral therapy of obsessive-compulsive disorder. *Arch. Gen. Psychiatry* 49:681–689.

BEDARD, M.-A., Y. AGID, S. CHOUINARD, S. FAHN, A. D. KORCZYN, and P. LESPERANCE, eds., 2003. *Mental and Behavioral Dysfunction in Movement Disorders.* Totowa, N.J.: Humana.

BEDARD, M. A., F. EL MASSIOUI, C. MALAPANI, B. DUBOIS, B. PILLON, B. RENAULT, and Y. AGID, 1998. Attentional deficits in Parkinson's disease: Partial reversibility with naphtoxazine (SDZ NVI-085), a selective noradrenergic alpha 1 agonist. *Clin. Neuropharmacol.* 21:108–117.

BEISER, D. G., and J. C. HOUK, 1998. Model of cortical-basal ganglionic processing: Encoding the serial order of sensory events. *J. Neurophysiol.* 79:3168–3188.

BEJJANI, B. P., P. DAMIER, I. ARNULF, L. THIVARD, A. M. BONNET, D. DORMONT, P. CORNU, B. PIDOUX, Y. SAMSON, and Y. AGID, 1999. Transient acute depression induced by high-frequency deep-brain stimulation. *N. Engl. J. Med.* 340:1476–1480.

BENABID, A. L., L. VERCUCIL, A. BENAZZOUZ, A. KOUDSIE, S. CHABARDES, L. MINOTTI, P. KAHANE, M. GENTIL, D. LENARTZ, C. ANDRESSEN, P. KRACK, and P. POLLAK, 2003. Deep brain stimulation: What does it offer? *Adv. Neurol.* 91:293–302.

BERGMAN, H., A. FEINGOLD, A. NINI, A. RAZ, H. SLOVIN, M. ABELES, and E. VAADIA, 1998. Physiological aspects of information processing in the basal ganglia of normal and parkinsonian primates. *Trends Neurosci.* 21:32–38.

BERGMAN, H., T. WICHMANN, and M. R. DeLONG, 1990. Reversal of experimental parkinsonism by lesions of the subthalamic nucleus. *Science* 249:1436–1438.

BERRETTA, S., H. B. PARTHASARATHY, and A. M. GRAYBIEL, 1997. Local release of GABAergic inhibition in the motor cortex induces immediate-early gene expression in indirect pathway neurons of the striatum. *J. Neurosci.* 17:4752–4763.

BERRIDGE, K. C., and T. E. ROBINSON, 1998. What is the role of dopamine in reward: Hedonic impact, reward learning, or incentive salience? *Brain Res. Brain Res. Rev.* 28:309–369.

BHATIA, K. P., and C. D. MARSDEN, 1994. The behavioural and motor consequences of focal lesions of the basal ganglia in man. *Brain* 117:859–876.

BLAZQUEZ, P., N. FUJII, J. KOJIMA, and A. M. GRAYBIEL, 2002. A network representation of response probability in the striatum. *Neuron* 33:973–982.

BOUSSAOUD, D., and I. KERMADI, 1997. The primate striatum: neuronal activity in relation to spatial attention versus motor preparation. *Eur. J. Neurosci.* 9:2152–2168.

BOWMAN, E. M., T. G. AIGNER, and B. J. RICHMOND, 1996. Neural signals in the monkey ventral striatum related to motivation for juice and cocaine rewards. *J. Neurophysiol.* 75:1061–1073.

BRAAK, H., K. DEL TREDICI, U. RUB, R. A. DE VOS, E. N. JANSEN STEUR, and E. BRAAK, 2003. Staging of brain pathology related to sporadic Parkinson's disease. *Neurobiol. Aging* 24:197–211.

BRAINARD, M. S., and A. J. DOUPE, 2000. Auditory feedback in learning and maintenance of vocal behaviour. *Nat. Rev. Neurosci.* 1:31–40.

BRASHERS-KRUG, T., R. SHADMEHR, and E. BIZZI, 1996. Consolidation in human motor memory. *Nature* 382:252–255.

BRAVER, T. S., J. D. COHEN, L. E. NYSTROM, J. JONIDES, E. E. SMITH, and D. C. NOLL, 1997. A parametric study of prefrontal cortex involvement in human working memory. *NeuroImage* 5:49–62.

BREITER, H. C., S. L. RAUCH, K. K. KWONG, J. R. BAKER, R. M. WEISSKOFF, D. N. KENNEDY, A. D. KENDRICK, T. L. DAVIS, A. JIANG, M. S. COHEN, C. E. STERN, J. W. BELLIVEAU, L. BAER, R. L. O'SULLIVAN, C. R. SAVAGE, M. A. JENIKE, and B. R. ROSEN, 1996. Functional magnetic resonance imaging of symptom provocation in obsessive-compulsive disorder. *Arch. Gen. Psychiatry* 53:595–606.

BROOKS, D. J., 1997. Advances in imaging Parkinson's disease. *Curr. Opin. Neurol.* 10:327–331.

BROWN, J. E., D. BULLOCK, and S. GROSSBERG, 1999. How the basal ganglia use parallel excitatory and inhibitory learning pathways to selectively respond to unexpected rewarding cues. *J. Neurosci.* 19:10502–10511.

BROWN, L. L., J. S. SCHNEIDER, and T. I. LIDSKY, 1997. Sensory and cognitive functions of the basal ganglia. *Curr. Opin. Neurobiol.* 7:157–163.

BROWN, R. G., and C. D. MARSDEN, 1990. Cognitive function in Parkinson's disease: From description to theory. *Trends Neurosci.* 13:21–29.

CANALES, J. J., and A. M. GRAYBIEL, 2000. A measure of striatal function predicts motor stereotypy. *Nat. Neurosci.* 3:377–383.

CAPLAN, L. R., J. D. SCHMAHMANN, C. S. KASE, E. FELDMANN, G. BAQUIS, J. P. GREENBERG, P. B. GORELICK, C. HELGASON, and D. B. HIER, 1990. Caudate infarcts. *Arch. Neurol.* 47:133–143.

DECKERSBACH, T., C. R. SAVAGE, T. CURRAN, A. BOHNE, S. WILHELM, L. BAER, M. A. JENIKE, and S. L. RAUCH, 2002. A study of parallel implicit and explicit information processing in patients with obsessive-compulsive disorder. *Am. J. Psychiatry* 159:1780–1782.

DELONG, M. R., 1990. Primate models of movement disorders of basal ganglia origin. *Trends Neurosci.* 13:281–289.

DENNY-BROWN, D., and N. YANAGISAWA, 1976. The role of the basal ganglia in the initiation of movement. *Res. Publ. Assoc. Res. Nerv. Ment. Dis.* 55:115–149.

DESCHENES, M., J. BOURASSA, V. D. DOAN, and A. PARENT, 1996. A single-cell study of the axonal projections arising from the posterior intralaminar thalamic nuclei in the rat. *Eur. J. Neurosci.* 8:329–343.

DESMOND, J. E., J. D. E. GABRIELI, and G. H. GLOVER, 1998. Dissociation of frontal and cerebellar activity in a cognitive task: Evidence for a distinction between selection and search. *NeuroImage* 7:368–376.

DEVAN, B. D., R. J. MCDONALD, and N. M. WHITE, 1999. Effects of medial and lateral caudate-putamen lesions on place- and cue-guided behaviors in the water maze: Relation to thigmotaxis. *Behav. Brain Res.* 100:5–14.

DEVAN, B. D., and N. M. WHITE, 1999. Parallel information processing in the dorsal striatum: Relation to hippocampal function. *J. Neurosci.* 19:2789–2798.

DIVAC, I., H. E. ROSVOLD, and M. K. SZWARCBART, 1967. Behavioural effects of selective ablation of the caudate nucleus. *J. Comp. Physiol. Psychol.* 63:184–190.

DOMINEY, P., M. ARBIB, and J. P. JOSEPH, 1995. A model of corticostriatal plasticity for learning oculomotor associations and sequences. *J. Cogn. Neurosci.* 7:311–336.

DOYON, J., V. PENHUNE, and L. G. UNGERLEIDER, 2003. Distinct contribution of the cortico-striatal and cortico-cerebellar systems to motor skill learning. *Neuropsychologia* 41:252–262.

DUBOIS, B., B. PILLON, and Y. AGID, 1992. Deterioration of dopaminergic pathways and alterations in cognition and motor functions. *J. Neurol.* 239(Suppl. 1):S9–S12.

EBLEN, F., and A. M. GRAYBIEL, 1995. Highly restricted origin of prefrontal cortical inputs to striosomes in the macaque monkey. *J. Neurosci.* 15:5999–6013.

FEGER, J., M. BEVAN, and A. R. CROSSMAN, 1994. The projections from the parafascicular thalamic nucleus to the subthalamic nucleus and the striatum arise from separate neuronal populations: A comparison with the corticostriatal and corticosubthalamic efferents in a retrograde fluorescent double-labeling study. *Neuroscience* 60:125–132.

FERRY, A. T., D. ONGUR, X. AN, and J. L. PRICE, 2000. Prefrontal cortical projections to the striatum in macaque monkeys: Evidence for an organization related to prefrontal networks. *J. Comp. Neurol.* 3:447–470.

FILION, M., L. TREMBLAY, and P. J. BÉDARD, 1988. Abnormal influences of passive limb movement on the activity of globus pallidus neurons in parkinsonian monkeys. *Brain Res.* 444:165–176.

FIORILLO, C. D., P. N. TOBLER, and W. SCHULTZ, 2003. Discrete coding of reward probability and uncertainty by dopamine neurons. *Science* 299:1898–1902.

FRANCOIS, C., C. JAN, K. MCCAIRN, D. GRABLI, E. C. HIRSCH, J. FEGER, and L. TREMBLAY, 2002. A primate model of Tourette's syndrome: Anatomical analysis of the basal ganglia territories involved in hyperactivity disorder with attention deficit (HD/AD) and stereotypy. *Soc. Neurosci. Abstr.* 23:663.6.

FRANK, M. J., B. LOUGHRY, and R. C. O'REILLY, 2001. Interactions between frontal cortex and basal ganglia in working memory: A computational model. *Cogn. Affect. Behav. Neurosci.* 1:137–160.

FUDGE, J. L., K. KUNISHIO, P. WALSH, C. RICHARD, and S. N. HABER, 2002. Amygdaloid projections to ventromedial striatal subterritories in the primate. *Neuroscience* 110:257–275.

FUJII, N., and A. GRAYBIEL, 2003. Representation of action sequence boundaries by macaque prefrontal cortical neurons. *Science* 301:1246–1249.

GEORGIOU, N., J. L. BRADSHAW, J. G. PHILLIPS, and E. CHIU, 1996. The effect of Huntington's disease and Gilles de la Tourette's syndrome on the ability to hold and shift attention. *Neuropsychologia* 34:843–851.

GILLIES, A., and G. ARBUTHNOTT, 2000. Computational models of the basal ganglia. *Mov. Disord.* 15:762–770.

GOLDMAN, P. S., and H. E. ROSVOLD, 1972. The effects of selective caudate lesions in infant and juvenile Rhesus monkeys. *Brain Res.* 43:53–66.

GRAFTON, S., E. HAZELTINE, and R. IVRY, 1995. Functional mapping of sequence learning in normal humans. *J. Cogn. Neurosci.* 7:497–510.

GRAYBIEL, A. M., 1984. Neurochemically specified subsystems in the basal ganglia. In *Functions of the Basal Ganglia. Ciba Found. Symp.* 107:114–149.

GRAYBIEL, A. M., 1995. Building action repertoires: Memory and learning functions of the basal ganglia. *Curr. Opin. Neurobiol.* 5:733–741.

GRAYBIEL, A. M., 1997. The basal ganglia and cognitive pattern generators. *Schizophr. Bull.* 23:459–469.

GRAYBIEL, A. M., 1998. The basal ganglia and chunking of action repertoires. *Neurobiol. Learn. Mem.* 70:119–136.

GRAYBIEL, A. M., T. AOSAKI, A. W. FLAHERTY, and M. KIMURA, 1994. The basal ganglia and adaptive motor control. *Science* 265:1826–1831.

GRAYBIEL, A. M., J. J. CANALES, and C. CAPPER-LOUP, 2000. Levodopa-induced dyskinesias and dopamine-dependent stereotypies: A new hypothesis. *Trends Neurosci.* 23:S71–S77.

GRAYBIEL, A. M., and M. KIMURA, 1995. Adaptive neural networks in the basal ganglia. In *Models of Information Processing in the Basal*

Ganglia, J. C. Houk, J. L. Davis, and D. G. Beiser, eds. Cambridge, Mass.: MIT Press, pp. 103–116.

GRAYBIEL, A. M., and Y. KUBOTA, 2003. Understanding basal ganglia function as part of a habit formation system. In *Mental and Behavioral Dysfunction in Movement Disorders*, M.-A. Bédard, Y. Agid, S. Chouinard, S. Fahn, A. Korczyn, and P. Lesperance, eds. Totowa, N.J.: Humana, pp. 51–57.

GRAYBIEL, A. M., and S. L. RAUCH, 2000. Toward a neurobiology of obsessive-compulsive disorder. *Neuron* 28:343–347.

GROENEWEGEN, H. J., C. I. WRIGHT, and H. B. UYLINGS, 1997. The anatomical relationships of the prefrontal cortex with limbic structures and the basal ganglia. *J. Psychopharmacol.* 11:99–106.

HABER, S., and N. R. MCFARLAND, 2001. The place of the thalamus in frontal cortical-basal ganglia circuits. *Neuroscientist* 7: 315–324.

HAZELTINE, E., S. T. GRAFTON, and R. IVRY, 1997. Attention and stimulus characteristics determine the locus of motor-sequence encoding: A PET study. *Brain* 120:123–140.

HEINDEL, W. C., N. BUTTERS, and D. P. SALMON, 1988. Impaired learning of a motor skill in patients with Huntington's disease. *Behav. Neurosci.* 102:141–147.

HIKOSAKA, O., H. NAKAHARA, M. K. RAND, K. SAKAI, X. LU, K. NAKAMURA, S. MIYACHI, and K. DOYA, 1999. Parallel neural networks for learning sequential procedures. *Trends Neurosci.* 22: 464–471.

HONDA, M., M. P. DEIBER, V. IBANEZ, A. PASCUAL-LEONE, P. ZHUANG, and M. HALLETT, 1998. Dynamic cortical involvement in implicit and explicit motor sequence learning: A PET study. *Brain* 121:2159–2173.

JACOBS, R. A., M. I. JORDAN, S. J. NOWLAN, and G. E. HINTON, 1991. Adaptive mixtures of local experts. *Neural Comput.* 3:79–87.

JAMES, W., 1890. *The Principles of Psychology.* New York: Dover.

JENKINS, I. H., D. J. BROOKS, P. D. NIXON, R. S. FRACKOWIAK, and R. E. PASSINGHAM, 1994. Motor sequence learning: A study with positron emission tomography. *J. Neurosci.* 14:3775–3790.

JOEL, D., 2001. Open interconnected model of basal ganglia-thalamocortical circuitry and its relevance to the clinical syndrome of Huntington's disease. *Mov. Disord.* 16:407–423.

JOG, M., Y. KUBOTA, C. I. CONNOLLY, V. HILLEGAART, and A. M. GRAYBIEL, 1999. Building neural representations of habits. *Science* 286:1745–1749.

JUEPTNER, M., C. D. FRITH, D. J. BROOKS, R. S. J. FRACKOWIAK, and R. E. PASSINGHAM, 1997. Anatomy of motor learning. II. Subcortical structures and learning by trial and error. *J. Neurophysiol.* 77:1325–1337.

JUEPTNER, M., K. M. STEPHAN, C. D. FRITH, D. J. BROOKS, R. S. J. FRACKOWIAK, and R. E. PASSINGHAM, 1997. Anatomy of motor learning. I. Frontal cortex and attention to action. *J. Neurophysiol.* 77:1313–1324.

JUEPTNER, M., and C. WEILLER, 1998. A review of differences between basal ganglia and cerebellar control of movements as revealed by functional imaging studies. *Brain* 121:1437–1449.

KARNI, A., G. MEYER, C. REY-HIPOLITO, P. JEZZARD, M. ADAMS, R. TURNER, and L. G. UNGERLEIDER, 1998. The acquisition of skilled motor performance: Fast and slow experience-driven changes in primary motor cortex. *Proc. Natl. Acad. Sci. U.S.A.* 95:861–868.

KERMADI, I., and D. BOUSSAOUD, 1995. Role of the primate striatum in attention and sensorimotor processes: Comparison with premotor cortex. *Neuroreport* 6:1177–1181.

KITANO, K., T. AOYAGI, and T. FUKAI, 2001. A possible functional organization of the corticostriatal input within the weakly-correlated striatal activity: A modeling study. *Neurosci. Res.* 40: 87–96.

KLEIN, D., R. J. ZATORRE, B. MILNER, E. MEYER, and A. C. EVANS, 1994. Left putaminal activation when speaking a second language: Evidence from PET. *Neuroreport* 5:2295–2297.

KNOWLTON, B. J., J. A. MANGELS, and L. R. SQUIRE, 1996. A neostriatal habit learning system in humans. *Science* 273:1399–1402.

KNOWLTON, B. J., L. R. SQUIRE, and M. A. GLUCK, 1994. Probabilistic classification learning in amnesia. *Learn. Mem.* 1:106–120.

KOSKI, L., T. PAUS, N. HOFLE, and M. PETRIDES, 1999. Increased blood flow in the basal ganglia when using cues to direct attention. *Exp. Brain Res.* 129:241–246.

KRACK, P., R. KUMAR, C. ARDOUIN, P. L. DOWSEY, J. M. MCVICKER, A. L. BENABID, and P. POLLAK, 2001. Mirthful laughter induced by subthalamic nucleus stimulation. *Mov. Disord.* 16:867–875.

LANG, A. E., 2000. Surgery for levodopa-induced dyskinesias. *Ann. Neurol.* 47:S193–S199 [discussion S199–S202].

LAVOIE, B., and A. PARENT, 1994. Pedunculopontine nucleus in the squirrel monkey: Distribution of cholinergic and monoaminergic neurons in the mesopontine tegmentum with evidence for the presence of glutamate in cholinergic neurons. *J. Comp. Neurol.* 344:190–209.

LECKMAN, J. F., 2002. Tourette's syndrome. *Lancet* 360:1577–1586.

LEICHNETZ, G. R., 2001. Connections of the medial posterior parietal cortex (area 7m) in the monkey. *Anat. Rec.* 263:215–236.

MARTONE, M., N. BUTTERS, M. PAYNE, J. T. BECKER, and D. S. SAX, 1984. Dissociations between skill learning and verbal recognition in amnesia and dementia. *Arch. Neurol.* 41:965–970.

MATSUMOTO, N., T. MINAMIMOTO, A. M. GRAYBIEL, and M. KIMURA, 2001. Neurons in the thalamic CM-Pf complex supply neurons in the striatum with information about behaviorally significant sensory events. *J. Neurophysiol.* 85:960–976.

MCALONAN, K., and V. J. BROWN, 2002. The thalamic reticular nucleus: More than a sensory nucleus? *Neuroscientist* 8:302–305.

MCDONALD, R. J., and N. M. WHITE, 1993. A triple dissociation of memory systems: Hippocampus, amygdala, and dorsal striatum. *Behav. Neurosci.* 107:3–22.

MCDONALD, R. J., and N. M. WHITE, 1994. Parallel information processing in the water maze: Evidence for independent memory systems involving dorsal striatum and hippocampus. *Behav. Neural Biol.* 61:260–270.

MENDEZ, M. F., N. L. ADAMS, and K. S. LEWANDOWSKI, 1989. Neurobehavioral changes associated with caudate lesions. *Neurology* 39:349–354.

MESULAM, M.-M., 2000. Attention, confusional states and neglect. In *Principles of Behavioral and Cognitive Neurology*, 2nd ed., M.-M. Mesulam, ed. New York: Oxford University Press, pp. 125–168.

MIDDLETON, F. A., and P. L. STRICK, 2002. Basal-ganglia "projections" to the prefrontal cortex of the primate. *Cereb. Cortex* 12: 926–935.

MILLER, E. K., and J. D. COHEN, 2001. An integrative theory of prefrontal cortex function. *Annu. Rev. Neurosci.* 24:167–202.

MINK, J. W., 2001. Neurobiology of basal ganglia circuits in Tourette syndrome: Faulty inhibition of unwanted motor patterns? *Adv. Neurol.* 85:113–122.

MIYACHI, S., O. HIKOSAKA, K. MIYASHITA, Z. KARADI, and M. K. RAND, 1997. Differential roles of monkey striatum in learning of sequential hand movement. *Exp. Brain Res.* 115:1–5.

MIYASHITA, N., O. HIKOSAKA, and M. KATO, 1995. Visual hemineglect induced by unilateral striatal dopamine deficiency in monkeys. *Neuroreport* 6:1257–1260.

NAKAMURA, K., K. SAKAI, and O. HIKOSAKA, 1998. Neuronal activity in medial frontal cortex during learning of sequential procedures. *J. Neurophysiol.* 80:2671–2687.

NAKAMURA, K., K. SAKAI, and O. HIKOSAKA, 1999. Effects of local inactivation of monkey medial frontal cortex in learning of sequential procedures. *J. Neurophysiol.* 82:1063–1068.

NAMBU, A., H. TOKUNO, and M. TAKADA, 2002. Functional significance of the cortico-subthalamo-pallidal "hyperdirect" pathway. *Neurosci. Res.* 43:111–117.

OBERG, R. G. E., and I. DIVAC, 1979. "Cognitive" functions of the neostriatum. In *The Neostriatum*, I. Divac and R. G. E. Öberg, eds. London: Pergamon, pp. 291–313.

OBESO, J. A., M. C. RODRIGUEZ-OROZ, M. RODRIGUEZ, R. MACIAS, L. ALVAREZ, J. GURIDI, J. VITEK, and M. R. DeLONG, 2000. Pathophysiologic basis of surgery for Parkinson's disease. *Neurology* 55:S7–S12.

OWEN, A. M., A. C. ROBERTS, J. R. HODGES, B. A. SUMMERS, C. E. POLKEY, and T. W. ROBBINS, 1993. Contrasting mechanisms of impaired attentional set-shifting in patients with frontal lobe damage or Parkinson's disease. *Brain* 116(Pt. 5):1159–1175.

PACKARD, M. G., and J. L. MCGAUGH, 1992. Double dissociation of fornix and caudate nucleus lesions on acquisition of two water maze tasks: Further evidence for multiple memory systems. *Behav. Neurosci.* 106:439–446.

PACKARD, M. G., and J. L. MCGAUGH, 1996. Inactivation of hippocampus or caudate nucleus with lidocaine differentially affects expression of place and response learning. *Neurobiol. Learn. Mem.* 65:65–72.

PACKARD, M. G., and B. J. KNOWLTON, 2002. Learning and memory functions of the basal ganglia. *Annu. Rev. Neurosci.* 25:563–593.

PACKARD, M. G., R. HIRSH, and N. M. WHITE, 1989. Differential effects of fornix and caudate nucleus lesions on two radial maze tasks: Evidence for multiple memory systems. *J. Neurosci.* 9:1465–1472.

PAHAPILL, P. A., and A. M. LOZANO, 2000. The pedunculopontine nucleus and Parkinson's disease. *Brain* 123(Pt. 9):1767–1783.

PARENT, A., and L. N. HAZRATI, 1995a. Functional anatomy of the basal ganglia. I. The cortico-basal ganglia-thalamo-cortical loop. *Brain Res. Brain Res. Rev.* 20:91–127.

PARENT, A., and L. N. HAZRATI, 1995b. Functional anatomy of the basal ganglia. II. The place of subthalamic nucleus and external pallidum in basal ganglia circuitry. *Brain Res. Brain Res. Rev.* 20:128–154.

PARENT, A., A. MACKEY, and L. DE BELLEFEUILLE, 1983. The subcortical afferents to caudate nucleus and putamen in primate: A fluorescence retrograde double labeling study. *Neuroscience* 10:1137–1150.

PARTHASARATHY, H. B., and A. M. GRAYBIEL, 1997. Cortically driven immediate-early gene expression reflects modular influence of sensorimotor cortex on identified striatal neurons in the squirrel monkey. *J. Neurosci.* 17:2477–2491.

PAUS, T., 2001. Primate anterior cingulate cortex: Where motor control, drive and cognition interface. *Nat. Rev. Neurosci.* 2:417–424.

PEIGNEUX, P., P. MAQUET, T. MEULEMANS, A. DESTREBECQZ, S. LAUREYS, C. DEGUELDRE, G. DELFIORE, J. AERTS, A. LUXEN, G. FRANCK, M. VAN DER LINDEN, and A. CLEEREMANS, 2000. Striatum forever, despite sequence learning variability: A random effect analysis of PET data. *Hum. Brain Mapp.* 10:179–194.

PETERSON, S. A., T. KLABUNDE, H. A. LASHUEL, H. PURKEY, J. C. SACCHETTINI, and J. W. KELLY, 1998. Inhibiting transthyretin conformational changes that lead to amyloid fibril formation. *Proc. Natl. Acad. Sci. U.S.A.* 95:12956–12960.

PILLON, B., B. DEWEER, A. MICHON, C. MALAPANI, Y. AGID, and B. DUBOIS, 1994. Are explicit memory disorders of progressive supranuclear palsy related to damage to striatofrontal circuits? Comparison with Alzheimer's, Parkinson's, and Huntington's diseases. *Neurology* 44:1264–1270.

POLDRACK, R. A., and J. D. E. GABRIELI, 2001. Characterizing the neural mechanisms of skill learning and repetition priming. *Brain* 124:67–82.

POLDRACK, R. A., V. PRABHAKARAN, C. A. SEGER, and J. D. GABRIELI, 1999. Striatal activation during acquisition of a cognitive skill. *Neuropsychology* 13:564–574.

POLDRACK, R. A., J. CLARK, E. J. PARE-BLAGOEV, D. SHOHAMY, J. CRESO MOYANO, C. MYERS, and M. A. GLUCK, 2001. Interactive memory systems in the human brain. *Nature* 414:546–550.

PRENSA, L., and A. PARENT, 2001. The nigrostriatal pathway in the rat: A single-axon study of the relationship between dorsal and ventral tier nigral neurons and the striosome/matrix striatal compartments. *J. Neurosci.* 21:7247–7260.

RAO, S. M., J. A. BOBHOLZ, T. A. HAMMEKE, A. C. ROSEN, S. J. WOODLEY, J. M. CUNNINGHAM, R. W. COX, E. A. STEIN, and J. R. BINDER, 1997. Functional MRI evidence for subcortical participation in conceptual reasoning skills. *Neuroreport* 8:1987–1993.

RAUCH, S. L., P. J. WHALEN, T. CURRAN, L. M. SHIN, B. J. COFFEY, C. R. SAVAGE, S. C. MCINERNEY, L. BAER, and M. A. JENIKE, 2001. Probing striato-thalamic function in obsessive-compulsive disorder and Tourette syndrome using neuroimaging methods. *Adv. Neurol.* 85:207–224.

RAZ, A., A. FEINGOLD, V. ZELANSKAYA, E. VAADIA, and H. BERGMAN, 1996. Neuronal synchronization of tonically active neurons in the striatum of normal and parkinsonian primates. *J. Neurophysiol.* 76:2083–2088.

ROBBINS, T. W., and B. J. EVERITT, 1992. Functions of dopamine in the dorsal and ventral striatum. *Semin. Neurosci.* 4:119–127.

ROLLS, E. T., ed. 1999. *The Brain and Emotion.* New York: Oxford University Press.

ROWE, J., K. E. STEPHAN, K. FRISTON, R. FRACKOWIAK, A. LEES, and R. PASSINGHAM, 2002. Attention to action in Parkinson's disease: Impaired effective connectivity among frontal cortical regions. *Brain* 125:276–289.

SAINT-CYR, J. A., 2003. Frontal-striatal circuit functions: Context, sequence, and consequence. *J. Int. Neuropsychol. Soc.* 9:103–127.

SAINT-CYR, J. A., A. E. TAYLOR, and A. E. LANG, 1988. Procedural learning and neostriatal dysfunction in man. *Brain* 111:941–959.

SAKA, E., and A. M. GRAYBIEL, 2003. Pathophysiology of Tourette's syndrome: striatal pathways revisited. *Brain Dev.* 25(Suppl 1):S15–S19.

SAMUEL, M., A. O. CEBALLOS-BAUMANN, N. TURJANSKI, H. BOECKER, A. GOROSPE, G. LINAZASORO, A. P. HOLMES, M. R. DeLONG, J. L. VITEK, D. G. THOMAS, N. P. QUINN, J. A. OBESO, and D. J. BROOKS, 1997. Pallidotomy in Parkinson's disease increases supplementary motor area and prefrontal activation during performance of volitional movements an H2(15)O PET study. *Brain* 120(Pt. 8):1301–1313.

SCHROEDER, J. P., J. C. WINGARD, and M. G. PACKARD, 2002. Posttraining reversible inactivation of hippocampus reveals interference between memory systems. *Hippocampus* 12:280–284.

SCHULTZ, W., 2002. Getting formal with dopamine and reward. *Neuron* 36:241–263.

SCHULTZ, W., P. DAYAN, and P. R. MONTAGUE, 1997. A neural substrate of prediction and reward. *Science* 275:1593–1599.

SCHWARTZ, J. M., P. W. STOESSEL, L. R. BAXTER, JR., K. M. MARTIN, and M. E. PHELPS, 1996. Systematic changes in cerebral glucose metabolic rate after successful behavior modification treatment of obsessive-compulsive disorder. *Arch. Gen. Psychiatry* 53:109–113.

SHADMEHR, R., and T. BRASHERS-KRUG, 1997. Functional stages in the formation of human long-term motor memory. *J. Neurosci.* 17:409–419.

SHIDARA, M., T. G. AIGNER, and B. J. RICHMOND, 1998. Neuronal signals in the monkey ventral striatum related to progress through a predictable series of trials. *J. Neurosci.* 18:2613–2625.

SIERADZAN, K. A., and D. M. MANN, 2001. The selective vulnerability of nerve cells in Huntington's disease. *Neuropathol. Appl. Neurobiol.* 27:1–21.

SMALL, D. M., R. J. ZATORRE, A. DAGHER, A. C. EVANS, and M. JONES-GOTMAN, 2001. Changes in brain activity related to eating chocolate: From pleasure to aversion. *Brain* 124:1720–1733.

SMITH, M. A., J. BRANDT, and R. SHADMEHR, 2000. Motor disorder in Huntington's disease begins as a dysfunction in error feedback control. *Nature* 403:544–549.

SMITH, Y., M. D. BEVAN, E. SHINK, and J. P. BOLAM, 1998. Microcircuitry of the direct and indirect pathways of the basal ganglia. *Neuroscience* 86:353–387.

SWERDLOW, N. R., and G. F. KOOB, 1987. Dopamine, schizophrenia, mania, and depression: Toward a unified hypothesis of cortico-striato-pallido-thalamic function. *Behav. Brain Res.* 10: 197–245.

TEICHER, M. H., C. M. ANDERSON, A. POLCARI, C. A. GLOD, L. C. MAAS, and P. F. RENSHAW, 2000. Functional deficits in basal ganglia of children with attention-deficit/hyperactivity disorder shown with functional magnetic resonance imaging relaxometry. *Nat. Med.* 6:470–473.

TREMBLAY, L., D. GRABLI, K. MCCAIRN, C. JAN, E. HIRSCH, J. FEGER, and C. FRANCOIS, 2003. A monkey model of Tourette's syndrome: Induction of hyperactivity disorder with attention deficit (HD/AD) and stereotypy by microinjections of biculline in the external segment of globus pallidus. *Soc. Neurosci. Abstr.* 23:663.7.

TURNER, R. S., and M. R. DELONG, 2000. Corticostriatal activity in primary motor cortex of the macaque. *J. Neurosci.* 20: 7096–7108.

UNGERLEIDER, L. G., J. DOYON, and A. KARNI, 2002. Imaging brain plasticity during motor skill learning. *Neurobiol. Learn. Mem.* 78: 553–564.

VAN DEN HEUVEL, O. A., H. J. GROENEWEGEN, F. BARKHOF, R. H. C. LAZERON, R. VAN DYCK, and D. J. VELTMAN, 2003. Frontostriatal system in planning complexity: A parametric functional magnetic resonance version of Tower of London task. *NeuroImage* 18:367–374.

WEBSTER, M. J., J. BACHEVALIER, and L. G. UNGERLEIDER, 1993. Subcortical connections of inferior temporal areas TE and TEO in macaque monkeys. *J. Comp. Neurol.* 335:73–91.

WHITE, N. M., and N. HIROI, 1998. Preferential localization of self-stimulation sites in striosomes/patches in the rat striatum. *Proc. Natl. Acad. Sci. U.S.A.* 95:6486–6491.

WILLINGHAM, D. B., J. SALIDIS, and J. D. GABRIELI, 2002. Direct comparison of neural systems mediating conscious and unconscious skill learning. *J. Neurophysiol.* 88:1451–1460.

YETERIAN, E. H., and D. N. PANDYA, 1998. Corticostriatal connections of the superior temporal region in rhesus monkeys. *J. Comp. Neurol.* 399:384–402.

38 Motor Learning and Memory for Reaching and Pointing

REZA SHADMEHR AND STEVEN P. WISE

ABSTRACT To control reaching and pointing movements, the primate motor system draws on vision, audition, and other sensory modalities to estimate hand and target locations. We argue that the motor system represents these variables in visual coordinates, relative to the fixation point. According to a computational theory presented here, neural networks in the parietal cortex align information about muscle lengths and joint angles with an estimate of hand location relative to the fixation point. Related networks in parietal and frontal cortex, together with the cerebellum and basal ganglia, align the desired hand displacements, also in visual coordinates, with the joint rotations and forces needed to reach the target. The motor system updates these estimates when the eye changes orientation and whenever the hand or target changes location. Each network learns an internal model (IM) of the relationships among these sensorimotor variables and, in so doing, computes coordinate transforms and predictions about the limb's future state. In motor learning, IMs adapt to distortions in visual feedback and altered limb dynamics. This process begins with adaptation of existing IMs and results, after extensive practice, in the formation of new ones: the motor system has acquired a new skill.

This chapter develops a computational theory of reaching and pointing in primates, one that owes much to previous ideas (Bullock and Grossberg, 1988; Cisek, Grossberg, and Bullock, 1998; Burnod et al., 1999; Andersen and Buneo, 2002).

Visually guided reaching in theory

We begin with a heuristic exercise in virtual robotics. Many robotic arms have a gripper, which serves as the *end effector*. End effectors include anything that biological or robotic arms control: hands, robotic grippers, sticks, laser pointers, and cursors controlled by a computer mouse. Robot engineers have devised many solutions to the problem of programming a robotic arm to move its end effector to a target. Some begin by determining the location of the target with respect to the location of the gripper. If the robot has a video camera, our imaginary engineer can use its signal to determine the location of both the end effector and the target (figure 38.1A). The end effector (*ee*) and target (*t*) locations, x_{ee} and x_t, respectively, define vectors in "camera-centered" coordinates, that is, a coordinate system that indicates the pixels occupied by both objects relative to some origin. The difference between these two vectors results in a third vector, x_{dv}, called the *difference vector*. It represents a high-order plan for movement.

Although our engineer has no choice but to use the camera to detect target location, he or she might use the lengths of each link of the robot's arm, together with the angle (θ) of each joint, to compute an estimate of the gripper's location. This computation is called *forward kinematics*.[1] The engineer could write a program to ensure that the gripper's location as estimated through forward kinematics always matches the location recorded by the camera. This program could be said to *align* inputs from the camera and joint angle sensors, and for the motor system, the analogous computation can be said to align an estimate of end effector location in *visual and proprioceptive coordinates*.

To align the robot's "proprioception" with its "vision," the engineer might use two neural networks with feedforward connections. One network would map proprioception to vision (i.e., it would compute forward kinematics, as described above) and another network would map vision to proprioception (called *inverse kinematics*). However, a better approach is to use a single neural network, one that finds the best alignment between the two sensory variables through feedback between the network's hidden layer and all of its input and output layers. This kind of network dynamics cleans up noise and can compute arbitrary transformations (Deneve, Latham, and Pouget, 2001). The neural network depicted in figure 38.1B has this architecture: it finds an alignment between an arm configuration $\hat{\theta}$ and an estimate

REZA SHADMEHR Department of Biomedical Engineering, Johns Hopkins School of Medicine, Baltimore, Md.
STEVEN P. WISE Laboratory of Systems Neuroscience, National Institute of Mental Health, Bethesda, Md.

---

[1] The term forward kinematics reflects the fact that this computation corresponds to the causal direction of information flow: in this example, the gripper's location changes because joint angles change, so computing end-effector location from joint angles corresponds to a forward computation.

511

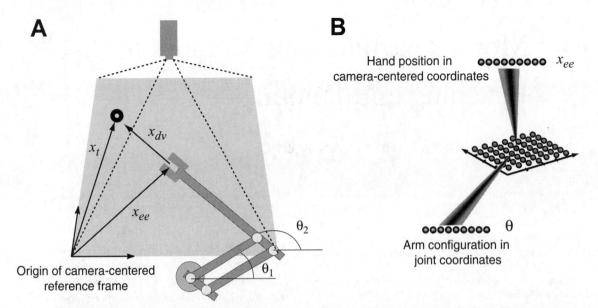

A

x_t

x_{dv}

x_{ee}

Origin of camera-centered
reference frame

θ_2

θ_1

B

Hand position in
camera-centered coordinates x_{ee}

Arm configuration in
joint coordinates θ

FIGURE 38.1   (*A*) A robotic arm that moves in two dimensions and a camera. The target *t* of the movement is the black ring. Gripper location and target locations are specified in camera-centered coordinates with vectors x_{ee} and x_t. The difference vector x_{dv}, also defined in camera-centered coordinates, is the distance and direction the gripper must move to reach the target. The joint-angle sensors on the robot measure joint angles θ_1 and θ_2. (*B*) Alignment of proprioception with vision. A recurrent neural network aligns estimate of end-effector location from the camera with the joint angle sensors with the camera. (*B* modified with permission from Deneve, Latham, and Pouget. Efficient computation and cue integration with noisy population codes. *Nat. Neurosci.* 4:826–831. © 2001 by the Nature Publishing Group.)

of gripper location $\hat{x}_{ee}$ (network 1 of figure 38.2).[2] We denote the network and its transformational mapping with the symbol $\hat{\theta} \leftrightarrow \hat{x}_{ee}$ and call it the *location map*. When this expression is viewed from left to right, this network appears to compute forward kinematics: $f(\hat{\theta}) = \hat{x}_{ee}$. Alternatively, viewed from right to left, it computes inverse kinematics: $f^{-1}(\hat{x}_{ee}) = \hat{\theta}$, that is, the network finds one of the several arm configurations for a given end effector location. In a sense, the network underlying the location map does not explicitly compute either forward or inverse kinematics but rather completes the "pattern" of whatever information it lacks, given the information it receives. Forward and inverse kinematics emerge as the product of this pattern completion network, and its computations correspond to an internal model (IM) of a relationship among the aligned variables.

The next step in planning a reaching movement involves comparing $\hat{x}_{ee}$ with $\hat{x}_t$ and computing a difference vector $x_{dv} = \hat{x}_t - \hat{x}_{ee}$. In the present model, another neural network with bidirectional connections performs this subtraction (network 3 in figure 38.2). It is important to note, however, that whereas the vector x_{dv} always points from the robot's gripper to the target, its coordinates system remain camera-centered.

Once this system has computed a difference vector in camera-centered coordinates, it can use the results of that computation to move the robot's arm. Thus, the final step in planning a movement involves associating the difference vector x_{dv} with joint rotations $\Delta\hat{\theta}$. Unlike network 1, which aligns the robot's vision and proprioception for locations, network 4 aligns information regarding end effector displacements. Thus, we call network 4 a *displacement map*. Later, we will argue that the distinction between location and displacement maps helps in understanding motor learning. For the present, it should be noted that, like the location map, the displacement map appears to compute either forward or inverse kinematics. Viewed from left to right, it performs the key inverse kinematics computation of traditional motor control theory. From right to left, it aligns movement commands with predicted end effector displacements.

For the desired displacement illustrated in figure 38.1*A*, the alignment between a gripper displacement x_{dv} and joint rotations $\Delta\hat{\theta}$ must depend on $\hat{\theta}$, which reflects the current arm configuration. The following symbolism denotes this dependence: $x_{dv} \overset{\hat{\theta}}{\leftrightarrow} \Delta\hat{\theta}$. As movement begins, the sensor readings will change. The joint and camera sensors update their estimate of arm configuration, which in turn leads to a new x_{dv} until $x_{dv} \to 0$. Reaching in biological systems involves an additional map, network 5 in figure 38.2, which involves the alignment of joint rotations and force commands. We denote this mapping as $\Delta\hat{\theta} \overset{\hat{\theta}}{\leftrightarrow} \hat{f}$ and call it a *dynamics map*.

---

[2] The "hat" diacritic $\wedge$ over a symbol indicates a computed estimate rather than a transduced value.

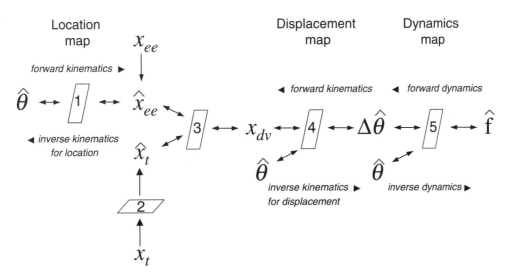

FIGURE 38.2 A schematic drawing of the computations involved in planning a reaching movement for the robotic arm illustrated in figure 38.1*A*. Each parallelogram represents a distributed neural network. Joint sensors provide a measure of arm configuration θ and a camera provides an estimate of hand and target location, x_{ee} and x_t, in camera-centered coordinates. A network with bidirectional connections associates joint- and camera-based estimate of hand location $\hat{\theta} \leftrightarrow \hat{x}_{ee}$. From the estimates of hand and target location, a difference vector x_{dv} is computed for the hand. This difference vector is then associated with a joint rotation needed to reach the target. Finally, these joint-angle changes need to be associated with the forces necessary to make the movement. Abbreviations: end effector, *ee*; difference vector, *dv*; target, *t*; force, *f*.

Learning location and displacement maps

One of the most important features of our imaginary robot is its adaptive element: the program that aligns the gripper location that the camera records with that based on joint angle transducers. If the alignment algorithm did not adapt, the robot would have trouble if the camera's optics or orientation changed. Primates can, however, adapt to radical distortions in visual inputs. In one study, a monkey was fitted with dove prisms, which invert images along the left–right plane (Sugita, 1996). For the first few weeks of continuous prism wearing, the monkeys could barely move, but after 4 weeks their movements improved markedly. Each day the monkeys attempted to reach to a sequence of targets. In 1–2 months the monkeys began to reach accurately to the targets, and similar results have been obtained by Sekiyama and colleagues (2000) in humans.

If the motor system uses location and displacement maps that align proprioceptive and visual signals (networks 1 and 4 of figure 38.2), then these maps must have changed during prism adaptation. What happened to the information that was contained in the maps for normal vision? After 2 months the prisms were removed, and for a day or so the monkeys again had trouble moving. They reached to the right when targets appeared to the left, a result of adaptation called an *aftereffect*. However, unlike the many weeks that it took the monkeys to adapt to the dove prisms, the aftereffects "washed out" by the third day. The slowness of initial adaptation and the rapidity of washout suggest that the prisms slowly changed the network in a way that accommodated the new alignment without losing the previous one. In the context of figure 38.2, we propose that some neural network gained an additional attractor state for its activity, and this attractor caused networks 1 and 4 to compute a different transform. Many neural networks have dynamics that converge when their internal states fall into an attractor, which corresponds to something like a "preferred activity state" of a network. According to this model, as a new attractor forms, the system gains a new capability, corresponding to a new motor skill. The networks' weight matrices have, at this point, been trained to solve both problems. According to this idea, some contextual input biases the networks collectively toward one or the other skill.

Adaptation to other kinds of prisms occurs much faster than for dove prisms. Typically, these prisms shift light by 5°–25° rather than inverting the visual field. Participants adapt to such prisms in 5 to 10 trials, suggesting a shift in existing attractors rather than the formation of new ones. Removal of the prisms requires the same number of de-adaptation trials as the original adaptation (Martin et al., 1996b). For this reason, adaptation with these prism glasses appears to result in the motor system regaining a former level of performance by shifting existing attractors. In contrast, perhaps skill acquisition leads to new capabilities by generating new attractors (Hallett, Pascual-Leone, and Topka, 1996).

The discussion to this point might lead to the conclusion that dove prisms induce new skills, but wedge prisms do not. However, with extensive experience, people can learn the "wedge prism" skill, as well. After several weeks of practice,

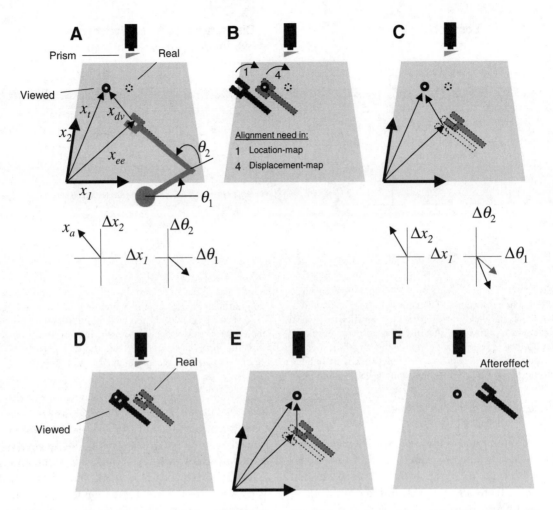

FIGURE 38.3   A prism that shifts the path of light to the left is inserted in front of the camera. (*A*) Before adaptation condition. Arm cannot be seen, and gripper location is estimated from proprioception. Target location in real space is at the dotted circle but is sensed by the camera at the semifilled circle. The subfigure below shows the desired hand displacement in camera-centered and joint-centered coordinates. (*B*) Result of the joint rotations. The camera sees the arm (black) miss the target to the left. Arm position in real space is drawn in gray. The curved arrows labeled 1 and 4 refer to adaptations of networks 1 and 4 in figure 38.2. (*C*) After adapta-

tion, both the estimated gripper location and the difference vector in joint coordinates have changed. The joint rotation vector prior to prism adaptation is shown as the gray arrow. Note that to reach the target after adaptation, θ_1 needs to increase less than before adaptation, whereas θ_2 needs to decrease more (more elbow extension). (*D*) Arm configuration at the end of the reaching movement after adaptation. (*E*) The prism is removed and the target is again presented. (*F*) The resulting reaching movement displays the aftereffect of adaptation.

experienced prism wearers eventually develop the ability to put on and remove the wedge prisms on demand, with minimal adaptation times and aftereffects (Martin et al., 1996b). Effectively, their motor system learns to switch between alignments appropriate for the prism and those appropriate for normal vision based on a context: the wearing of or freedom from prisms.

Our imaginary robot and its control networks can help explain prism adaptation. Imagine that a prism shifts the path of light so that, from the point of view of the camera, the visual world appears displaced to the left. Therefore, in figure 38.3*A* a target activates pixels on the camera to the left of the pixels that "should be" activated. The black ring indicates the viewed target location, as distorted by the

prisms; the dotted circle shows the target's actual location, often called "real" space. Before the prism appeared on the scene, the control system had adaptively aligned the location map $\hat{\theta} \leftrightarrow \hat{x}_{ee}$ and the displacement map $x_{dv} \overset{\hat{\theta}}{\leftrightarrow} \Delta\hat{\theta}$ in visual and proprioceptive coordinates.

Now assume that the camera cannot "see" the arm, and so the system must estimate its location $\hat{x}_{ee}$ in camera-centered coordinates from proprioception. Perhaps light must be conserved so that the camera only senses the light from a small light-emitting diode on the target and the room lights flash on briefly only at the end of the gripper's movement. The camera tells the central controller that the target is at x_t and the system computes a difference vector x_{dv} based on information from the joint angle sensors in the robot's arm, as converted into camera-centered coordinates $\hat{\theta} \leftrightarrow \hat{x}_{ee}$, $x_{dv} = \hat{x}_t - \hat{x}_{ee}$. Figure 38.3$A$ illustrates this difference vector, in camera-centered coordinates, beneath the drawing of the robot. Using the displacement map $x_{dv} \overset{\hat{\theta}}{\leftrightarrow} \Delta\hat{\theta}$, the controller computes a joint rotation vector. This vector flexes the robot's "shoulder" (increasing θ_1) and extends its "elbow" (decreasing θ_2), bringing the arm in to the location indicated by the gray arm in figure 38.3B. After the movement ends, the camera records the gripper at the location shown by the black arm. The gripper missed the target to the left.

Note that the prism induced two kinds of errors. First, for the displacement map (network 4 in figure 38.2), the desired difference vector produced joint rotations that moved the gripper too far to the left. Second, for the location map (network 1 in figure 38.2), the camera recorded the gripper's location further to the left than it "should have been," according to the robot's joint angles. Therefore, in planning the next movement, the robotic controller should reduce the amount of flexion for the shoulder computed by the displacement map, as well as adaptively realign the location map. The controller requires visual feedback for such recalibrations, which changes its IMs. After these two IMs—the displacement and location maps—adapt, the robot can again direct its gripper to the target without visual feedback: that is, it regains its former level of performance. Figure 38.3C shows the gripper's actual location in gray, and the dotted line shows its estimated location in camera-centered coordinates from proprioception. The system estimates the gripper's location to the left of its location in real space, but the system can compute a difference vector x_{dv} and map it to appropriate joint rotations. After adaptation to the prism, the displacement map estimates that target acquisition requires a smaller flexion in the shoulder angle along with a larger elbow extension. When the robot performs these joint rotations, the gripper moves to the gray location in figure 38.3D and the camera records it at the black location. In both real and camera-centered coordinates, the gripper reaches the target. After adaptation, targets at the illustrated location (away and to the left) map to joint rotations generating movements straight ahead (where the target actually is). Targets that appear straight ahead induce joint rotations that move the gripper away and to the right.

Figure 38.3E illustrates what happens when we remove the prism and require the robot to make another reaching movement from the same starting location. The camera senses the target position at x_t, which is now its actual location, straight ahead. However, when the robot's controller computes x_{dv} and maps it to joint rotations, the system now estimates that to move the gripper to a target appearing straight ahead, it needs to extend the elbow and flex the shoulder according to the mappings learned when the prisms distorted the camera's input: away and to the right.

This mapping causes the gripper to miss the target to the right: the negative aftereffect of adaptation.

The computations elaborated in our thought design have a number of interesting consequences, many of which have been tested in psychophysical experiments (Harris, 1965). For example, after participants in those experiments adapt to prisms, when they close their eyes and try to point straight ahead, they show aftereffects. These aftereffects arise because the imagined target $\hat{x}_t$ is the same as before the adaptation trials, but displacement map $x_{dv} \overset{\hat{\theta}}{\leftrightarrow} \Delta\hat{\theta}$ has changed. Further, when participants prism adapt for reaching to a spatial auditory stimulus, and later remove the prisms, their movements to visual targets show aftereffects for the same reason. Finally, if participants prism adapt with one hand, they show misreaching when they try to reach to that hand with their other hand. This aftereffect results from the change in $\hat{\theta} \leftrightarrow \hat{x}_{ee}$, the location map. The present model of prism adaptation resembles a previous three-factor model of prism adaptation (Welch, Choe, and Heinrich, 1974). It differs, however, in the present emphasis on extrinsic, vision-based coordinates for representing the target, end effector, and difference vector, as opposed to the body-centered coordinate frame assumed by that earlier model.

Updating the maps using efference copy

In the imaginary robot described so far, the camera never moves. Eyes are not like that, of course, and because the kinematic computations for reaching involve vision-based coordinates, eye movements pose a fundamental problem. Imagine that the target in figure 38.1A fell outside the camera's field of view. The robotic system described so far would be lost. Without a target activating some pixels in the camera's field of view, the controller could not compute a difference vector and could not move the gripper to the target. To alleviate this problem, the engineer might place the camera on a swivel that reorients the camera so that it covers more territory. This benefit, however, comes at a cost: the location of the target in real space is no longer a simple function of which camera pixels the target activates. The controller now has to keep track of the camera's orientation.

To illustrate these points, imagine someone reading this book at a coffee shop. As that person reads, he or she reaches to the left for a notepad, as illustrated in figure 38.4 (top left). Because the person continues to orient gaze toward the book, the notepad $\hat{x}_t$ lies in his or her peripheral field of view. Now imagine that someone approaches that person from the right as reaching begins. Both the reader's head and eyes orient toward the right, but reaching remains accurate. Note that the reader did not look at the target initially and looked even farther away from it when the other person approached.

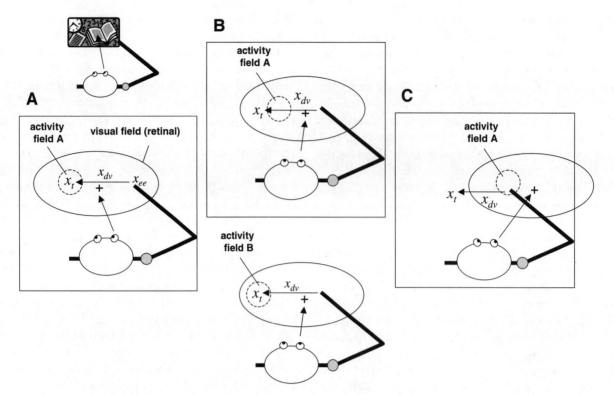

FIGURE 38.4 Need for updating target and end effector locations due to reorientation of the fovea. (*A*) The participant fixates the plus sign; the ellipse indicates the limits of the entire visual field (not to scale). The circle (dashed line) shows the activity field (in this case, a receptive field) of an imaginary neuron. (*B*) In diagram at top, the participant's fixation point shifts to the right, so the visual field as a whole and the cell's activity field in retinocentric coordi- nates shift by an equal amount. At bottom, the participant in the same situation as at top, but a cell with a different activity field is illustrated. Note that the target x_t has shifted out of the top cell's activity field and into that of the second cell's. (*C*) Another eye movement in the same direction shifts the target out of the visual field entirely.

When the reader's eyes and head moved, the location of the end effector and target changed in retinotopic coordinates, that is, the part of the retina on which the image of the target and end effector fell. Although eye movements resulted in a change in the location of $\hat{x}_t$ and x_{ee} in these retinotopic coordinates, the difference vector x_{dv} should have remained the same. According to the present model, changes in the orientation of the retina result in a recalculation of the difference vector because of the changes in the retino- topic location of the target and end effector. We call the coordinate frame that is based on the eye's orientation but is independent of the visual field fixation-centered, as opposed to retinotopic.

This fixation-centered frame corresponds to the camera- centered coordinates discussed for the imaginary robot but takes into account changes in the camera's orientation. A fixation-centered coordinate frame has two advantages over a retinotopic frame: fixation-centered coordinates can describe the location of the target and gripper beyond the retina's field of view, and they can do so in three dimensions. The same gain-field mechanisms that have been invoked to compute target location in head- or body-centered coor- dinates (Andersen et al., 1990; Bremmer, Distler, and Hoffmann, 1997; Salinas and Abbott, 2001; Andersen and Buneo, 2002) can also be used to compute target and end effector locations in fixation-centered coordinates as the eye's orientation changes. Gain-field networks essentially combine information about target location in retinotopic coordinates with information about the orientation of the eye to produce multiplicative computations that yield loca- tions in some other coordinate frame. In the present model, these computations yield locations with respect to the fixa- tion point.

Accordingly, the basic model sketched in figure 38.2 needs two augmentations: predictive *remapping* and the use of *effer- ence copy*. First, reorientation of the retina, through eye move- ments, requires the control system to update the kinematic maps to reflect the changes in target and end effector loca- tions relative to the fixation point. Movements of the hand and the target also lead to updating. For posterior parietal cortex, there is neurophysiological evidence that the remem- bered location of a visual target, $\hat{x}_t$, is updated in fixation- centered coordinates as the eyes move (Duhamel, Colby, and Goldberg, 1992). Neurons in the lateral intraparietal area discharge after a saccade brings a stimulus into the cell's activity field, as well as when a saccade brings the location

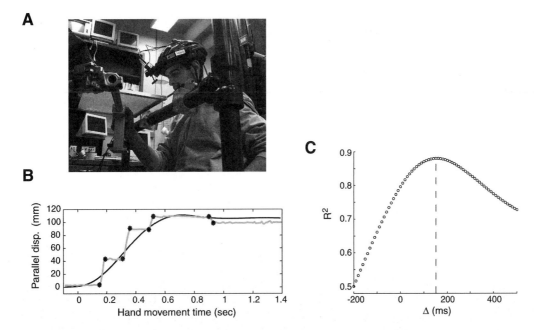

FIGURE 38.5 Estimating hand location during reaching movements. (A) Participants were asked to hold the handle of a robotic manipulandum while making reaching movements. They were instructed to look at their unseen hand as they reached to a remembered target location. The arm was not visible in the experiment but is shown uncovered here. (B) Hand location (black line) and eye orientation (gray line) are plotted for a typical movement. (C) Eye orientation at saccade endpoint correlates with end-effector location. Maximum correlation is at $\Delta = 150\,\text{ms}$, which means that participants fixate a location the hand will reach 150 ms later. (Reprinted with permission from G. Ariff et al., A real-time state predictor in motor control: Study of saccadic eye movements during reaching movements. *J. Neurosci.* 22:7721–7729. © 2002 by the *Journal of Neuroscience*.)

of a vanished stimulus into the cell's field (figure 38.4*B*, bottom). Thus, it seems reasonable that as the eyes or the head moves, the motor system remaps the representation of both $\hat{x}_t$ and $\hat{x}_{ee}$ in fixation-centered coordinates. If a movement is to be made with the hand, motion of the eye and head produce an updating of x_{dv}.

Let us return to our example of reaching for a notepad while reading a book. Now imagine that a breeze blows the notepad to the left as reaching begins (figure 38.4). The updating mechanism ensures that the end effector reaches the target: reaching movement terminates when the difference vector reaches zero. The motor system thus acts as an "autopilot," guiding the end effector to the target, and the posterior parietal cortex also has been implicated in this computation (Desmurget et al., 1998, 1999; Grea et al., 2002).

This remapping must rely in large part on a copy of motor commands sent to oculomotor and skeletomotor systems, known as efference copy. The finding that remapping occurs predictively—that is, in advance of a saccadic eye movement (Duhamel, Colby, and Goldberg, 1992)—suggests an efference copy-based mechanism, and direct evidence for this idea has recently been reported for eye movements (Sommer and Wurtz, 2002). Thus, in predictive updating, the kinematic IMs depicted in figure 38.2 not only align proprioception with vision but also predict changes in these

variables as a consequence of a planned and ongoing motor commands.

What might happen if the reader could not see the notepad in the first place? How could the motor system compute the location of an unseen target in visual coordinates? The answer is that the notepad had fallen in the reader's field of view in the past, perhaps even on the fovea, and the motor system retained that information in memory in the form of the notepad's location in fixation-centered coordinates, as illustrated in figure 38.4*C*. (Note that the target in figure 38.4*C* has fixation-centered, but not retinotopic, coordinates.) The motor system stores and updates the location of potential targets relative to the fixation point as eye, head, and body movements reorient gaze (Gaffan and Hornak, 1997), and this information remains valid even when the target lies outside the visual field. Regions of cortex posterior to the posterior parietal cortex need to interact with frontal areas for such remapping from memory to occur (Gaffan and Hornak, 1997).

This updating mechanism also subserves hand–eye coordination. Ariff and colleagues (2002) have shown that as the hand moves during a reach, the motor system updates its estimate $\hat{x}_{ee}$ based on efference copy. For a saccade at time t, the new fixation point best correlates with hand location 150 ms later (figure 38.5). This result suggests that the motor system updates $\hat{x}_{ee}$ as a reaching movement progresses.

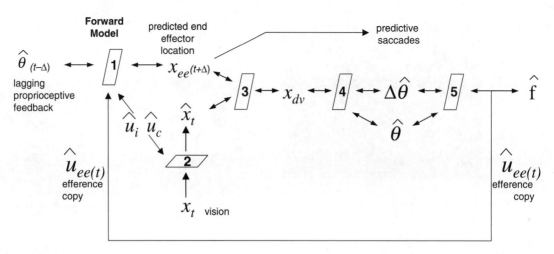

FIGURE 38.6 Predictive updating based on forward models and the influence of updating signals on the kinematic mappings depicted in figure 38.2. Abbreviations as in figure 38.2; efference copy, u; eye, i; head (cranium), c.

Because the estimate of hand location leads the actual hand location, the updating mechanism probably relies on efference copy.

If the motor system plans to move the eyes or the arm, it can update estimates of target and end effector locations through an IM of the mechanical dynamics of the arm. This idea is illustrated in figure 38.6. Such IMs are often called *forward models*. They describe how a physical object, such as an arm, should change state (e.g., location and velocity), given that it was acted upon by a force (Jordan and Rumelhart, 1992; Miall et al., 1993). The concept of forward models helps explain the oculomotor behavior illustrated in figure 38.5. As the motor system sends commands u_{ee} to the arm muscles to produce force, it also sends a copy of these commands $\hat{u}_{ee}$ to the forward model that estimates hand location $\hat{x}_{ee}$, presumably in the posterior parietal cortex. This IM also receives proprioceptive information $\hat{\theta}$ from the arm, but it arrives later. The "lagging" proprioceptive information $\hat{\theta}(t - \Delta)$ tells the network the arm's configuration a little while ago. The efference copy $\hat{u}_{ee}(t)$ tells it the commands that are about to act on the arm. Given the lagging proprioceptive information $\hat{\theta}(t - \Delta)$ and the current efference copy $\hat{u}_{ee}(t)$, the forward model of arm dynamics predicts end effector location at some future time $\hat{x}_{ee}(t + \Delta)$. As the movement unfolds, the accuracy of that prediction can be detected, and the forward model adjusted as necessary to produce accurate predictions in the future.

Learning the dynamics map

ADAPTING TO NOVEL FORCE FIELDS The primate arm has inertial dynamics that result in a complex relationship between motion and forces. In order to reliably make even the simplest movements, the motor system must predict the specific force requirements of a movement in generating the motor commands. We can think of this prediction as an alignment between a desired set of joint rotations and forces, or $\Delta\hat{\theta} \overset{\hat{\theta}}{\leftrightarrow} \hat{f}$, depicted as network 5 in figure 38.2.

The accuracy and adaptability of force prediction are particularly important for reaching because holding different objects can dramatically change the mechanical dynamics of the arm, and the motor system must accommodate this variability. In experiments aimed at studying this kind of adaptation, participants reach to a target while holding the handle of a robot that imposes forces of various kinds (Shadmehr and Mussa-Ivaldi, 1994). In a typical experiment, when the robot's motors are off (called the null field condition), participants make straight movements (figure 38.7*A*). When the robot applies a force field that depends on the velocity of the hand (figure 38.7*B*), these forces perturb the movement trajectory (figure 38.7*C*). With practice, however, participants learn to make smooth and nearly straight movements despite the force field. Catch trials—relatively rare, intermixed trials in which the robot does not impose the force field—reveal the motor system's ability to predict the initially novel forces and modify motor commands accordingly. Early in training with the novel forces, the participants make straight movements in catch trials. With further experience in the field, participants make straight movements in the force field, but their movements on catch trials resemble a negative image of the early, perturbed movements (figure 38.7*D*). Catch trials demonstrate the aftereffects of adaptation, the results of adapting the dynamics map.

The expression $\Delta\hat{\theta} \overset{\hat{\theta}}{\leftrightarrow} \hat{f}$ assumes that internal models of dynamics are maps that align a representation of limb state with forces. Conditt, Gandolfo, and Mussa-Ivaldi (1997) considered the merits of an alternative idea, according to which something analogous to a tape recorder might store the forces that were sensed in the previous movements. Movement direction and time provide the inputs to this imaginary tape-recorder system, which produces force as its output. Such a system would also adapt reaching movements

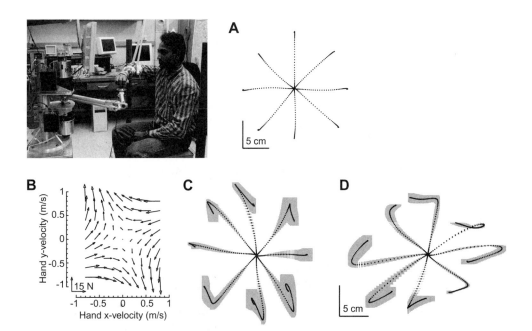

FIGURE 38.7 Experimental setup and typical data in a force field adaptation task. (*A*) Participants hold the handle of the robot and reach to a target. The plot shows hand trajectory (dots are 10 ms apart) for typical movements to eight targets. (*B*) The force field produced by the robot. Forces are plotted as a function of hand velocity. (*C*) Average hand trajectories (±SD) for movements during the initial trials in the force field. (*D*) Hand trajectories during catch trials. (Reprinted with permission from R. Shadmehr and F. A. Mussa-Ivaldi, Adaptive representation of dynamics during learning of a motor task. *J. Neurosci.* 14:3208–3224. © 1994 by the *Journal of Neuroscience*.)

to the force field without mapping joint displacement to force through an IM. To test this alternative, participants practiced reaching straight to a small number of targets while the novel force field was applied and later tried to draw a circle in the same field. If the motor system learned something like a tape recording of the forces encountered in reaching to each target, there should be little generalization to much longer, circular movements. However, Conditt and colleagues observed good performance for circular movements in the force field, and the subjects showed aftereffects when the robot ceased imposing the forces. This finding indicates that the neural system did not predict forces explicitly as a function of time. Rather, it learned to associate the states of the arm, primarily its location and velocity, with forces. The order in which those states were visited did not matter. What was important was the arm's velocity at locations traversed by the hand during reaching. These experiments indicate that with practice, participants adapted an IM of dynamics.

Consolidation of kinematics and dynamics maps

Behavioral measurements suggest that the IM of dynamics changed not only during the training session, but also in the hours that followed completion of training (Shadmehr and Brashers-Krug, 1997). The IM appeared to gradually

change from an initially fragile state to a more resistant one during a period of approximately 5 hours. Similarly, in a task that required participants to adapt to the dynamics of an inertial object, Krakauer and colleagues (2000) reported that the IM for one object could be disrupted if participants immediately practiced movements with a different object. Finally, disruptive transcranial magnetic stimulation (TMS) of primary motor cortex (M1) immediately after participants practiced a thumb flexion movement resulted in marked retention deficits, whereas stimulation 5 hours after practice did not (Muellbacher et al., 2002). Therefore, the passage of time alters the networks underlying the IMs in a way that consolidates their attractors.

Generalization of motor learning

To consider why adaptation to kinematic or dynamic perturbations produces a specific pattern of generalization, we need to go beyond a description of the variables that IMs align, to consider how the motor system might encode these variables. A population code provides one approach. Georgopoulos and colleagues (1982) first suggested one kind of population code, called the population vector, and although alternatives have been suggested subsequently, their ideas serve the present purposes. According to their idea, each cell has a preferred direction (PD), which can be represented as a vector of unit length $\mathbf{w}_i$. For movement direction α, each cell i discharges at a rate r_i, which can be decomposed into two terms: average activity $g_i(\alpha)$ for a variety of movement directions and noise:

$$r_i = g_i(\alpha) + n_i$$

Experiments show that the M1 tuning curves approximate Gaussian or cosine-like functions with half-widths at half-maximum values of approximately 56° (Amirikian and Georgopoulos, 2000). Experiments on neurons in visual cortex suggest that the noise term distributes normally with a variance proportional to the mean value of the tuning function (Tolhurst and Thompson, 1982). If cells did not have noise, a winner-take-all scheme might work well: to estimate which movement direction would move the end effector to the target, the motor system could simply determine that cell j discharged most during some movement, and estimate the appropriate movement direction $\hat{\alpha}$ to be the PD of that cell: $\hat{\alpha} = \mathbf{w}_j$. However, because cells are noisy, that estimate would have a large variance from trial to trial. A population code, employing the law of large numbers, avoids this problem because each cell's discharge is weighted by its PD vector: each cell in the population contributes to the network's output in its PD and does so in proportion to its activity for a given movement direction on a given trial. The sum of these vectors should vary less that a winner-take-all system in producing an estimate of movement direction:

$$\hat{\alpha} = \sum_i \mathbf{w}_i r_i = \sum_i (\mathbf{w}_i g_i(\alpha) + \mathbf{w}_i n_i) \qquad (1)$$

The success of this kind of population coding depends on computing with neurons that broadly encode the input variable (Seung and Sompolinsky, 1993).

The example of population coding described in Equation 1 provides an instance of identity mapping, or a mapping in which the output is an estimate of the input variable. Network 2 in our model provides another example. However, population codes can also map one input variable into another variable (Poggio, 1990; Pouget, Dayan, and Zemel, 2000):

$$\hat{y} = \sum_i (\mathbf{w}_i g_i(\alpha) + \mathbf{w}_i n_i) \qquad (2)$$

For the example of population coding described in Equation 2, the tuning curves of the neurons that participate in this computation become *basis functions* used to approximate output y. Basis functions are a set of functions that, when linearly combined, can approximate almost any linear or nonlinear function (Pouget and Sejnowski, 1997). Thus, population coding can be used to compute identity maps, as well as for the more general problem of computing linear and nonlinear functions. Note, however, that whereas in the population code for estimating movement direction (Equation 1), the weights were fixed vectors in a cell's PD, for learning alignment maps (Equation 2), the weight vectors change and have no specific relationship with the tuning function $g_i(\alpha)$.

Let us now return to the problem of how the motor system might compute an IM of dynamics, $\Delta\hat{\theta} \overset{\hat{\theta}}{\leftrightarrow} \hat{f}$. This mapping aligns a state of the arm (i.e., the desired displacement of the arm at a given position) with force $\mathbf{f}$. Assume (1) that the networks use a population code, (2) that each neuron has a tuning curve g_i that describes the average discharge of that cell as a function of hand location and velocity, and (3) that each cell also has a preferred force vector $\mathbf{w}_i$. The population vector for force can be estimated, as follows:

$$\hat{\mathbf{f}} = \sum_i \mathbf{w}_i g_i(\theta, \Delta\theta) + \mathbf{w}_i n_i$$

We now have a framework for relating tuning properties with behavioral generalization during adaptation to force fields. Consider the following experiment: participants experience force $\mathbf{f}_1$ as they move their arm in certain locations with certain velocities, which we call state $\mathbf{x}_1$. The error that they experience in a movement changes weights $\mathbf{w}$. Assuming Hebbian learning rules, the largest weight changes occur for those neurons that are most active when the arm was in or near state $\mathbf{x}_1$. Later, the participant makes reaching movements in other locations or with different velocities (state $\mathbf{x}_2$). If performance in state $\mathbf{x}_2$ after training differs from that in the naive condition, then the basis function g_i must be broad enough to be active in both $\mathbf{x}_1$ and $\mathbf{x}_2$. Therefore, if the IM is represented via a population code, the generalization function should correspond to the shape of the tuning curves—the basis functions—of the neural elements implementing its computation.

This prediction depends, of course, on the assumptions stated previously, which treat neurons in the motor system as spatial analyzers. Nevertheless, the theory predicts that if the neurons that subserve a given kind of motor learning have a given tuning property, then those properties affect the way in which motor learning generalizes.

GENERALIZING LOCATION MAPS   As described earlier (see figure 38.3), prism adaptation alters both the location and the displacement maps. To study how each map is constructed, and how adaptation of each mapping generalizes, it is important to devise experiments that require adaptation of one map but not the other.

In an experiment that isolated the location map (network 1), participants could view their hand only in one restricted location (Vetter, Goodbody, and Wolpert, 1999). At that location the visual information was altered so that the visual information regarding hand location did not match proprioception, and participants had to learn a new alignment $(\hat{\theta} + \varepsilon) \leftrightarrow \hat{x}_{ee}$. Adaptation of the location map at this single target location had global consequences, that is, it affected movements to distant targets. Thus, the map $\hat{\theta} \leftrightarrow \hat{x}_{ee}$ must be computed with spatial analyzers that broadly encode joint angle coordinates of the limb. In accord with this pattern of generalization, many neurons in the motor system encode static limb position with very broad, often linear functions (Georgopoulos, Caminiti, and Kalaska, 1984; Bosco, Rankin, and Poppele, 1996; Helms-Tillery, Soechting, and Ebner, 1996).

GENERALIZING DISPLACEMENT MAPS In order to isolate the displacement map, a different experimental design is needed. The goal is to leave the relationship between proprioception and vision for locations minimally changed, but dramatically change it for displacements. For normally viewed reaching movements, this goal is impossible to achieve, although it might be approximated for small differences in location. For cursors on a video monitor, however, this goal can be achieved easily: there should be no expectation that a cursor on a video monitor should match the proprioceptively sensed location of the hand. Cunningham (1989) pioneered this motor learning paradigm, often called "rotation experiments." These experiments vary the relationship between joint angle changes and end effector displacements. For example, in one condition, movements of the participant's hand to the left cause a movement of a cursor, the end effector, to the left, but in a "rotated" condition, the same hand movements cause the cursor to move downward, a −90° rotation. To move the cursor to a target, the motor system must learn to map the desired cursor displacement to a new set of joint rotations: $x_{dv} \overset{\hat{\theta}}{\leftrightarrow} (\Delta\hat{\theta} + \delta)$.

Rotation experiments study adaptation of displacement maps (Krakauer et al., 2000). Krakauer and colleagues (2000) observed that adaptation had only a local effect on reaching movements; movements trained in one location generalize only to neighboring directions, with little effect at movement angles, in polar coordinates, that differed by more than 45° from the trained movement direction. This finding implies that the displacement map is computed with elements that have more selective tuning functions than those involved in computing the location map. The angular distance over which adaptation generalized is consistent with spatial analyzers having tuning functions similar to those observed in M1 and the dorsal premotor cortex (PMd) (Caminiti et al., 1990; Kalaska et al., 1992), among other cortical and subcortical structures, such as the cerebellum (Johnson and Ebner, 2000; Fortier, Kalaska, and Smith, 1989) and basal ganglia (Turner and Anderson, 1997).

GENERALIZING DYNAMICS MAPS Shadmehr and Moussavi (2000) observed that adaptation to forces in one arm configuration generalized to another, very different arm configuration. Note that very different arm configurations imply

that the end effector, the hand, is in a very distant part of the workspace. The finding of Shadmehr and Moussavi means that the basis functions that compute $\Delta\hat{\theta} \overset{\hat{\theta}}{\leftrightarrow} \hat{f}$ must encode limb configuration quite broadly. As mentioned earlier, neurons in different parts of the motor system can be modulated globally and often linearly as a function of end effector location (Georgopoulos, Caminiti, and Kalaska, 1984; Bosco, Rankin, and Poppele, 1996; Helms-Tillery, Soechting, and Ebner, 1996; Sergio and Kalaska, 2003). Activity with that property occurs in M1, area 5d, and in cells giving rise to the dorsal spinocerebellar tract. These findings support the idea that cells with global, planar tuning functions play an important role in computing the dynamics map. Using this approach, generalization patterns have been used to make the following additional inferences about the nature of encoding in the internal model of dynamics:

• The basis functions encode hand velocity with spatial analyzers that have a PD but may be bimodally tuned (Donchin, Francis, and Shadmehr, 2003).
• The PDs of the basis functions rotate with the shoulder angle (Shadmehr and Moussavi, 2000).
• Basis functions have weak but distinct sensitivity to movements of the ipsilateral arm, and the PD of the basis functions remain arm-invariant if the workspace is near the midline (Criscimagna-Hemminger et al., 2003).

With the exception of bimodal tuning, neurons with all of these properties have been reported for M1, basal ganglia, and cerebellum (Georgopoulos, Caminiti, and Kalaska, 1984; Caminiti et al., 1991; Turner and Anderson, 1997; Johnson and Ebner, 2000). The invariance of the preferred direction with respect to movements of the contralateral and ipsilateral arms has been reported recently for M1 (Steinberg et al., 2002) and PMd (Cisek, Crammond, and Kalaska, 2003). Bimodal tuning in arm velocity space has been observed in the cerebellum (Coltz, Johnson, and Ebner, 1999), but not in M1 for the same task (Johnson and Ebner, 2000). We recognize the indirect nature of this argument, but these correlations remain intriguing and should lead to further testable predictions.

Neural basis of adapting internal models

NEURAL BASIS OF ADAPTING KINEMATICS Adaptation of maps that align kinematic variables (networks 1 and 4 in figure 38.2) appears to depend on three brain regions: the posterior parietal cortex, the premotor cortex, and the cerebellum. Patients (Weiner, Hallett, and Funkenstein, 1983; Martin et al., 1996a) and monkeys (Baizer, Kralj-Hans, and Glickstein, 1999) with cerebellar damage have deficits in adapting to prisms. One study employing a rotation experiment showed a deficit in adapting the displacement map after inactivating the dentate nucleus of the cerebellum (Robertson and Miall, 1999). Clower and colleagues (1996) presented neuroimaging support of a role of posterior parietal cortex in prism adaptation. And Kurata and Hoshi (1999) showed that temporary inactivation of PMv causes a deficit in prism adaptation in monkeys.

The most extensive analysis of neuronal activity during the adaptation of displacement maps has been for "rotation" experiments (Wise et al., 1998; Moody and Wise, 2001), although other transforms have also been used. As a population, cells in PMd, the supplementary motor area (SMA), and M1 showed dramatic changes in their properties during adaptation of displacement maps. These changes took the form of changes in the cells' PD, which were often very large, and changes in both the depth of tuning and the width of tuning. Approximately half of the sample of neurons in these areas showed significant changes in activity during adaptation, and as a population, this activity change appeared to lag the adaptation as measured behaviorally. This finding may be relevant to the time course of consolidation noted earlier, but remains poorly understood.

NEURAL BASIS OF ADAPTING DYNAMICS   Adaptation of the dynamics map also depends on cerebellar function (Smith, 2001; Maschke et al., 2004). Patients with cerebellar disease show a marked inability to adapt to the forces imposed by the robot, and little or no aftereffect. M1 probably also contributes to adapting the dynamics map, although the evidence for this idea is much less direct than for the cerebellum. A collection of muscles can substitute for the force variable as network 5's output (figure 38.2). Thoroughman and Shadmehr (1999) extended the figure 38.2 model in this way and noted that, for a particular class of force fields, adaptation produced a rotation in the preferred direction (PD) of arm muscles. M1 cells and muscles in monkeys show a median clockwise PD shift of comparable amounts as they adapt to the same force field (Li, Padoa-Schioppa, and Bizzi, 2001). In addition, Bizzi and his colleagues found that, whereas the EMG patterns returned to baseline conditions once the field was turned off (i.e., during washout trials), many cells in M1 retained their new PD. Other cells showed changes in PD specifically during the washout trials. As a population, these changes in PD balanced each other so that the population vector remained a good description of end effector's movement direction. Further analysis revealed similar phenomena in PMd and SMA, with an additional finding regarding SMA (Padoa-Schioppa, Li, and Bizzi, 2002). During an instructed-delay period, cells in SMA showed an increasing reflection of the forces needed to move the limb to the target. Thus, Padoa-Schioppa and colleagues concluded that SMA plays a role in the kinematics-to-dynamics transform $\Delta\hat{\theta} \overset{\hat{\theta}}{\leftrightarrow} \hat{f}$.

Summary

Reaching relies on computations that transform proprioceptive and exteroceptive information, in fixation-centered coordinates, into motor commands, and all of these mappings adapt. Altering vision with prisms, for example, changes the alignment between proprioception and hand location (mapping 1), as well as that between the difference vector and joint rotations (mapping 4). Altering the weight of the arm or imposing forces on it during movement changes the mapping of joint rotations onto force commands (mapping 5). With repeated adaptation, often consuming many weeks and hundreds of movements, new IMs form that can be recalled with contextual cues. For visually guided reaching in primates, motor learning begins with the adaptation of existing IMs and ends in formation of new ones. The motor system has acquired a new skill.

REFERENCES

AMIRIKIAN, B., and A. P. GEORGOPOULOS, 2000. Directional tuning profiles of motor cortical cells. *Neurosci. Res.* 36:73–79.

ANDERSEN, R. A., R. M. BRACEWELL, S. BARASH, J. W. GNADT, and L. FOGASSI, 1990. Eye position effects on visual, memory, and saccade-related activity in areas LIP and 7a of macaque. *J. Neurosci.* 10:1176–1196.

ANDERSEN, R. A., and C. A. BUNEO, 2002. Intentional maps in posterior parietal cortex. *Annu. Rev. Neurosci.* 25:189–220.

ARIFF, G., O. DONCHIN, T. NANAYAKKARA, and R. SHADMEHR, 2002. A real-time state predictor in motor control: Study of saccadic eye movements during unseen reaching movements. *J. Neurosci.* 22:7721–7729.

BAIZER, J. S., I. KRALJ-HANS, and M. GLICKSTEIN, 1999. Cerebellar lesions and prism adaptation in macaque monkeys. *J. Neurophysiol.* 81:1960–1965.

BOSCO, G., A. RANKIN, and R. E. POPPELE, 1996. Representation of passive hindlimb postures in cat spinocerebellar activity. *J. Neurophysiol.* 76:715–726.

BREMMER, F., C. DISTLER, and K. P. HOFFMANN, 1997. Eye position effects in monkey cortex. II. Pursuit- and fixation-related activity in posterior parietal areas LIP and 7A. *J. Neurophysiol.* 77: 962–977.

BULLOCK, D., and S. GROSSBERG, 1988. The VITE model: A neural command circuit for generating arm and articulator trajectories. In *Dynamic Patterns in Complex Systems*, J. A. S. Kelso, A. J. Mandell, and M. F. Shlesinger, eds. Singapore: World Scientific Publishers, pp. 305–326.

BURNOD, Y., P. BARADUC, A. BATTAGLIA-MAYER, E. GUIGON, E. KOECHLIN, S. FERRAINA, F. LACQUANITI, and R. CAMINITI, 1999. Parieto-frontal coding of reaching: An integrated framework. *Exp. Brain Res* 129:325–346.

CAMINITI, R., P. B. JOHNSON, Y. BURNOD, C. GALLI, and S. FERRAINA, 1990. Shift of preferred directions of premotor cortical cells with arm movements performed across the workspace. *Exp. Brain Res.* 83:228–232.

CAMINITI, R., P. B. JOHNSON, C. GALLI, S. FERRANINA, and Y. BURNOD, 1991. Making arm movements within different parts of space: The premotor and motor cortical representation of a coordinate system for reaching to visual targets. *J. Neurosci.* 11:1182–1197.

CISEK, P., D. J. CRAMMOND, and J. F. KALASKA, 2003. Neural activity in primary motor and dorsal premotor cortex in reaching tasks with the contralateral versus ipsilateral arm. *J. Neurophysiol.* 89:922–942.

CISEK, P., S. GROSSBERG, and D. BULLOCK, 1998. A cortico-spinal model of reaching and proprioception under multiple task constraints. *J. Cogn. Neurosci.* 10:425–444.

CLOWER, D. M., J. M. HOFFMAN, J. R. VOTAW, T. L. FABER, R. P. WOODS, and G. E. ALEXANDER, 1996. Role of posterior parietal cortex in the recalibration of visually guided reaching. *Nature.* 383:618–621.

COLTZ, J. D., M. T. V. JOHNSON, and T. J. EBNER, 1999. Cerebellar Purkinje cell simple spike discharge encodes movement velocity in primates during visuomotor arm tracking. *J. Neurosci.* 19:1782–1803.

CONDITT, M. A., F. GANDOLFO, and F. A. MUSSA-IVALDI, 1997. The motor system does not learn the dynamics of the arm by rote memorization of past experience. *J. Neurophysiol.* 78:554–560.

CRISCIMAGNA-HEMMINGER, S. E., O. DONCHIN, M. S. GAZZANIGA, and R. SHADMEHR, 2003. Learned dynamics of reaching movements generalize from dominant to nondominant arm. *J. Neurophysiol.* 90:4016–4021.

CUNNINGHAM, H. A, 1989. Aiming error under transformed spatial mappings suggests a structure for visual-motor maps. *J. Exp. Psychol.* 15:493–506.

DENEVE, S., P. E. LATHAM, and A. POUGET, 2001. Efficient computation and cue integration with noisy population codes. *Nat. Neurosci.* 4:826–831.

DESMURGET, M., C. M. EPSTEIN, R. S. TURNER, C. PRABLANC, G. E. ALEXANDER, and S. T. GRAFTON, 1999. Role of the posterior parietal cortex in updating reaching movements to a visual target. *Nat. Neurosci.* 2:563–567.

DESMURGET, M., D. PELISSON, Y. ROSSETTI, and C. PRABLANC, 1998. From eye to hand: Planning goal-directed movements. *Neurosci. Biobehav. Rev.* 22:761–788.

DONCHIN, O., J. T. FRANCIS, and R. SHADMEHR, 2003. Quantifying generalization from trial-by-trial behavior of adaptive systems that learn with basis functions: Theory and experiments in human motor control. *J. Neurosci.* 23:9032–9045.

DONCHIN, O., and R. SHADMEHR, 2002. Linking motor learning to function approximation: Learning in an unlearnable force field. *Adv. Neural Inform. Proc. Sys.* 14:197–203.

DUHAMEL, J.-D., C. L. COLBY, and M. E. GOLDBERG, 1992. The updating of the representation of visual space in parietal cortex by intended eye movements. *Science.* 255:90–92.

FORTIER, P. A., J. F. KALASKA, and A. M. SMITH, 1989. Cerebellar neuronal activity related to whole-arm reaching movements in the monkey. *J. Neurophysiol.* 62:198–211.

GAFFAN, D., and J. HORNAK, 1997. Visual neglect in the monkey: Representation and disconnection. *Brain.* 120:1647–1657.

GEORGOPOULOS, A. P., R. CAMINITI, and J. F. KALASKA, 1984. Static spatial effects in motor cortex and area 5: Quantitative relations in a two-dimensional space. *Exp. Brain Res.* 54:446–454.

GEORGOPOULOS, A. P., J. F. KALASKA, R. CAMINITI, and J. T. MASSEY, 1982. On the relations between the direction of two-dimensional arm movements and cell discharge in primate motor cortex. *J. Neurosci.* 2:1527–1537.

GREA, H., L. PISELLA, Y. ROSSETTI, M. DESMURGET, C. TILIKETE, S. GRAFTON, C. PRABLANC, and A. VIGHETTO, 2002. A lesion of the posterior parietal cortex disrupts on-line adjustments during aiming movements. *Neuropsychologia.* 40:2471–2480.

HALLETT, M., A. PASCUAL-LEONE, and H. TOPKA, 1996. Adaptation and skill learning: Evidence for different neural substrates. In *The Acquisition of Motor Behavior in Vertebrates,* J. R. Bloedel, T. J. Ebner, and S. P. Wise, eds. Cambridge, Mass.: MIT Press, pp. 289–301.

HARRIS, C. S., 1965. Perceptual adaptation to inverted, reversed, and displaced vision. *Psychol. Rev.* 72:419–444.

HELMS-TILLERY, S. I., J. F. SOECHTING, and T. J. EBNER, 1996. Somatosensory cortical activity in relation to arm posture: Nonuniform spatial tuning. *J. Neurophysiol.* 75:2423–2438.

JOHNSON, M. T. V., and T. J. EBNER, 2000. Processing of multiple kinematic signals in the cerebellum and motor cortices. *Brain Res. Rev.* 33:155–168.

JORDAN, M. I., and D. E. RUMELHART, 1992. Forward models: Supervised learning with a distal teacher. *Cogn. Sci.* 16:307–354.

KALASKA, J. F., D. J. CRAMMOND, D. A. D. COHEN, M. PRUD'HOMME, and M. L. HYDE, 1992. Comparison of cell discharge in motor, premotor, and parietal cortex during reaching. In *Control of Arm Movement in Space: Neurophysiological and Computational Approaches,* R. Caminiti and P. Johnson, eds. Berlin: Springer-Verlag, pp. 129–146.

KRAKAUER, J. W., Z. M. PINE, M. F. GHILARDI, and C. GHEZ, 2000. Learning of visuomotor transformations for vectorial planning of reaching trajectories. *J. Neurosci.* 20:8916–8924.

KURATA, K., and E. HOSHI, 1999. Reacquisition deficits in prism adaptation after muscimol microinjection into the ventral premotor cortex of monkeys. *J. Neurophysiol.* 81:1927–1938.

LI, C. S., C. PADOA-SCHIOPPA, and E. BIZZI, 2001. Neuronal correlates of motor performance and motor learning in the primary motor cortex of monkeys adapting to an external force field. *Neuron.* 30:593–607.

MARTIN, T. A., J. G. KEATING, H. P. GOODKIN, A. J. BASTIAN, and W. T. THACH, 1996a. Throwing while looking through prisms. I. Focal olivocerebellar lesions impair adaptation. *Brain.* 119:1183–1198.

MARTIN, T. A., J. G. KEATING, H. P. GOODKIN, A. J. BASTIAN, and W. T. THACH, 1996b. Throwing while looking through prisms. II. Specificity and storage of multiple gaze-throw calibrations. *Brain.* 119:1199–1211.

MASCHKE, M., C. M. GOMEZ, T. J. EBNER, and J. KONCZAK, 2004. Hereditary cerebellar ataxia progressively impairs force adaptation during goal directed arm movements. *J. Neurophysiol.* 91:230–238.

MIALL, R. C., D. J. WEIR, D. M. WOLPERT, and J. F. STEIN, 1993. Is the cerebellum a Smith predictor? *J. Motor Behav.* 25:203–216.

MOODY, S. L., and S. P. WISE, 2001. Connectionist contributions to population coding in the motor cortex. *Prog. Brain Res.* 130:245–266.

MUELLBACHER, W., U. ZIEMANN, J. WISSEL, N. DANG, M. KOFLER, S. FACCHINI, B. BOROOJERDI, W. POEWE, and M. HALLETT, 2002. Early consolidation in human primary motor cortex. *Nature.* 415:640–644.

PADOA-SCHIOPPA, C., C. S. LI, and E. BIZZI, 2002. Neuronal correlates of kinematics-to-dynamics transformation in the supplementary motor area. *Neuron.* 36:751–765.

POGGIO, T, 1990. A theory of how the brain might work. *Cold Spring Harbor Symp. Quant. Biol.* 55:899–910.

POUGET, A., P. DAYAN, and R. ZEMEL, 2000. Information processing with population codes. *Nat. Rev. Neurosci.* 1:125–132.

POUGET, A., and T. J. SEJNOWSKI, 1997. Spatial transformations in the parietal cortex using basis functions. *J. Cogn. Neurosci.* 9:222–237.

ROBERTSON, E. M., and R. C. MIALL, 1999. Visuomotor adaptation during inactivation of the dentate nucleus. *Neuroreport.* 10:1029–1034.

SALINAS, E., and L. F. ABBOTT, 2001. Coordinate transformations in the visual system: How to generate gain fields and what to compute with them. *Prog. Brain Res.* 130:175–190.

SEKIYAMA, K., S. MIYAUCHI, T. IMARUOKA, H. EGUSA, and T. TASHIRO, 2000. Body image as a visuomotor transformation device revealed in adaptation to reversed vision. *Nature.* 407: 374–377.

SERGIO, L. E., and J. F. KALASKA, 2003. Systematic changes in motor cortex cell activity with arm posture during directional isometric force generation. *J. Neurophysiol.* 89:212–228.

SEUNG, H. S., and H. SOMPOLINSKY, 1993. Simple models for reading neuronal population codes. *Proc. Natl. Acad. Sci. U.S.A.* 90:10749–10753.

SHADMEHR, R., and T. BRASHERS-KRUG, 1997. Functional stages in the formation of human long-term motor memory. *J. Neurosci.* 17:409–419.

SHADMEHR, R., and Z. M. K. MOUSSAVI, 2000. Spatial generalization from learning dynamics of reaching movements. *J. Neurosci.* 20:7807–7815.

SHADMEHR, R., and F. A. MUSSA-IVALDI, 1994. Adaptive representation of dynamics during learning of a motor task. *J. Neurosci.* 14:3208–3224.

SMITH, M. A, 2001. *Error correction, the basal ganglia, and the cerebellum.* Ph.D. Thesis, Johns Hopkins University.

SOMMER, M. A., and R. H. WURTZ, 2002. A pathway in primate brain for internal monitoring of movements. *Science.* 296: 1480–1482.

STEINBERG, O., O. DONCHIN, A. GRIBOVA, D. O. CARDOSA, H. BERGMAN, and E. VAADIA, 2002. Neuronal populations in primary motor cortex encode bimanual arm movements. *Eur. J. Neurosci.* 15:1371–1380.

SUGITA, Y, 1996. Global plasticity in adult visual cortex following reversal of visual input. *Nature.* 380:523–526.

THOROUGHMAN, K. A., and R. SHADMEHR, 1999. Electromyographic correlates of learning internal models of reaching movements. *J. Neurosci.* 19:8573–8588.

TOLHURST, D. J., and I. D. THOMPSON, 1982. Organization of neurones preferring similar spatial frequencies in cat striate cortex. *Exp. Brain Res.* 48:217–227.

TURNER, R. S., and M. E. ANDERSON, 1997. Pallidal discharge related to the kinematics of reaching movements in two dimensions. *J. Neurophysiol.* 77:1051–1074.

VETTER, P., S. J. GOODBODY, and D. M. WOLPERT, 1999. Evidence for an eye-centered spherical representation of the visuomotor map. *J. Neurophysiol.* 81:935–939.

WEINER, M. J., M. HALLETT, and H. H. FUNKENSTEIN, 1983. Adaptation to lateral displacement of vision in patients with lesions of the central nervous system. *Neurology.* 33:766–772.

WELCH, R. B., C. S. CHOE, and D. R. HEINRICH, 1974. Evidence for a three-component model of prism adaptation. *J. Exp. Psychol.* 103:700–705.

WISE, S. P., S. L. MOODY, K. J. BLOMSTROM, and A. R. MITZ, 1998. Changes in motor cortical activity during visuomotor adaptation. *Exp. Brain Res.* 121:285–299.

V ATTENTION

Introduction

ANNE TREISMAN

ATTENTION IS A fuzzy concept used in everyday language with a variety of different senses ranging from orienting to selection and to vigilance or sustained attention. Since the first edition of this book appeared, there has been tremendous progress in exploring the brain mechanisms underlying these different functions. This section begins with a review of the issues that historically prompted the most systematic exploration, showing both the progress that was made using behavioral and psychological data and the questions that remained open. The following chapters discuss in more detail different aspects of the neuroscience of attention. Klein reviews the simplest form of attention, orienting to a spatial cue, and its consequences for neural processing. Hopfinger, Luck, and Hillyard discuss the inferences obtained from evoked response potential (ERP) recording and magnetoencephalography (MEG), modalities that probe perceptual processing with fine temporal detail. Freiwald and Kanwisher review research on the underlying brain areas performed using single-unit recordings in animals and imaging techniques in humans. Driver, Vuilleumier, and Husain discuss the implications for normal functioning of findings in patients with brain damage to areas controlling attention and awareness. Humphreys and Samson describe the control systems of attention and how they break down. Tipper studies the interactions between attention and intention to act, showing how perception is affected by behavioral goals. Finally, Robertson and Garavan review the intensive dimensions of attention, namely, how arousal, alertness, and vigilance affect performance.

Although these varied manifestations of attention are all gathered under a single rubric, it seems doubtful that a single simple mechanism could be involved. However, we emerge with some sense of the complex interactive systems for selection that produce the smoothly integrated behavior observed and experienced in everyday life. These chapters help illuminate how the brain achieves a generally seamless control of action and mental function.

39 Psychological Issues in Selective Attention

ANNE TREISMAN

ABSTRACT This chapter reviews research on attention using behavioral and psychological methods. It attempts to illustrate what was learned through these tools alone and what is gained when methods from cognitive neuroscience are added. The psychological approaches defined many of the theoretical issues, such as the nature of the overloads that make attention necessary, the level of selection, the method of selection (enhancement of attended stimuli or suppression of unattended ones), the targets of selection (locations, objects, or attributes), the ways in which attention is controlled, and the role of attention in solving the feature binding problem. Psychology also developed many of the paradigms used to probe the underlying mechanisms, which are now being confirmed by converging evidence from brain imaging and from studies of brain damaged patients. Theories of attention have evolved from the early sequential "pipeline" model of processing to a more flexible and interactive model with parallel streams specializing in different forms of perceptual analysis, iterative cycles of processing, and reentry to earlier levels. Attentional selection takes many forms and applies at many levels. We learn as much from exploring the constraints on flexibility—what cannot be done—as from discovering what can.

Why should we still be interested in purely psychological studies? It would, of course, be foolish not to use the new tools from neuroscience. If, as Minsky said, the mind is what the brain does, then that is what, as psychologists, we are interested in, and it is almost bound to be helpful if we can watch the brain doing it. However, the designs of the behavioral tasks to be combined with brain imaging or to be tested with neurological patients are critical to the quality of the information we get. Psychological studies have sharpened and clarified the questions to be asked, and created a substantial number of experimental paradigms. Inferences are necessarily indirect, both in behavioral studies and in neuroscience. We can directly observe actions, or we can measure brain activation, but by putting them together we further constrain the theories we propose. Converging evidence is the key. We test hypotheses in a variety of different ways so that artifacts of one method are bypassed in others. Confidence in the conclusions grows with each potential disconfirmation that they survive. This chapter cannot attempt

to review the enormous field of relevant research. It is intended to set the scene, both historically and conceptually, for the subsequent chapters, which explore the neuroscientific approaches in more detail.

The traditional questions in attention research mostly started as di- or trichotomies, "Is it x, or y, or z?" The answer typically turns out to be, all of the above. Simplistic questions have evolved into attempts to specify when each answer applies, and why. I have selected seven such issues to discuss here, using mostly psychological methods and bringing in neural evidence where it can decide questions that could otherwise not be answered (see Freiwald and Kanwisher, this volume, for a more detailed look at the neural evidence about three of the same questions). In broaching the theoretical issues, I also introduce many experimental paradigms that have been used to study attention. These include dichotic listening, visual search, dual task performance, flanker tasks, rapid serial visual presentation, and negative priming. The goal here is to grasp the wide range of everyday phenomena encompassed by the label *attention* and bring them into the controlled conditions necessary for scientific study.

1. *What sets the limits: structural interference, general resources, or the need for behavioral coherence?*

One hypothesis is that limits arise only when two concurrent tasks depend on the same specialized system. Proponents of structural interference compared the competition between tasks that seemed likely to share common mechanisms and tasks that did not; for example, both were speech or one was speech shadowing and one was piano playing (Allport, Antonis, and Reynolds, 1972), both were visual or one was auditory and one visual (Treisman and Davies, 1973), or both used verbal rehearsal or one used imagery (Brooks, 1968). The results clearly showed more interference between tasks that were more similar. When the tasks were sufficiently different, they were sometimes combined without impairment.

There is evidence that different attributes such as color, motion, and shape are processed by at least partially separate systems (e.g., Corbetta et al., 1991). The structural

ANNE TREISMAN Psychology Department, Princeton University, Princeton, N.J.

interference view therefore predicts little difficulty in registering different properties of the same object, and this is what the evidence suggests. Interference can still arise at the response level if the different attributes evoke conflicting responses, as in the task of naming the colored inks in which different color names are written (Stroop, 1935). The reason why attention is so ineffective on tasks such as the Stroop task may be that the brain is forced to use whatever discriminative systems it has available *unless* these are fully occupied with other stimuli (Treisman, 1969). Early selection may be impossible when the perceptual load is low. Selection then has to be postperceptual, allowing conflict between incompatible responses (see Lavie, 1995).

The results described so far support the structural interference account. However, there are also more general effects of difficulty. Kahneman (1973) argued for a limited pool of resources or "effort." He showed that a secondary task (monitoring a stream of visual letters) was impaired when combined with a primary task of adding one to each of a string of auditory digits, although these two tasks are unlikely to share the same brain systems. Kahneman used the size of the pupil as an online index of effort, having previously shown that it correlates closely with difficulty across a wide range of tasks. Interference with visual letter detection was maximal when the memory load was highest and effort, as indexed by the pupil, was at a peak (figure 39.1).

Purely psychological studies are handicapped in determining how much information is processed about unattended messages by the fact that observable responses are needed as evidence. Brain imaging allows us to monitor the incidental and involuntary processing of unattended stimuli. Results have cast additional doubt on claims that only structural interference matters. Rees, Frith, and Lavie (1997) used functional magnetic resonance imaging (fMRI) to observe activity in area MT produced by irrelevant moving dots surrounding a central, task-relevant word. Two tasks differing in difficulty were used: case discrimination (easy) or detection of a bisyllabic word (more difficult). Thinking about the phonology of a word is unlikely to involve area MT. Yet fMRI activation to the irrelevant dots was reduced during the more difficult word task. Thus, attention limits generalize across very different types of processing.

Different sense modalities, however, do seem to have some independent capacity. When auditory words replaced the visual ones, task difficulty had no impact on MT activation by the moving dots. Psychological tests provided converging evidence: with visual words, the difficult task reduced the motion aftereffect generated by the irrelevant dots. However, with auditory words, the motion aftereffect was unaffected by the difficulty of the word task. The conclusion seems to be that resources are at least partly shared across very different tasks within vision, but may be separate across different

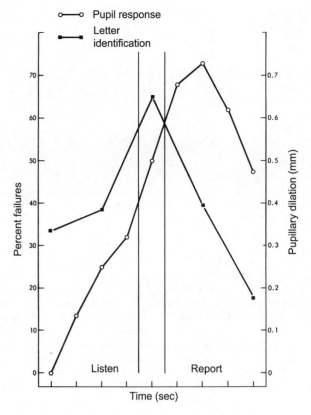

FIGURE 39.1 A measure of perceptual deficit and the pupillary response to a digit transformation task. Solid symbols indicate percentage of missed letters in a rapid visual sequence while participants listened to four digits, added one to each, and reported the results (at a rate of 1/s). Errors increased with each extra digit at intake and were greatest when participants were doing the mental addition. Errors decreased as each transformed digit was reported. Open symbols indicate the size of the pupil, reflecting the amount of effort or resources being used. Note that the pupil index lags behind the mental processing by about 2 s. (Modified from Kahneman, D., *Attention and Effort*, © 1972, p. 21. Reprinted by permission of Pearson Education, Inc., Upper Saddle River, New Jersey.)

ent modalities. An interesting exception to this conclusion concerns spatial coding, where a shared representation of space may create some overlap in resources (e.g., Spence and Driver, 1996).

In addition to the effects of attentional load, there are also constraints from the need for behavioral coherence. Both Tipper (this volume) and Humphreys and Samson (this volume) describe examples of attention being facilitated when the actions afforded by the stimulus are compatible with the response required (e.g., Tucker and Ellis, 1998; Craighero et al., 1999). The premotor theory of attention suggests that it is simply a preparation for response, selecting the goal of an intended action (Rizzolatti et al., 1987). The focus on response may explain why attentional systems seem to differ for space that is within reach and space that is beyond it. However, it seems unlikely that intended actions

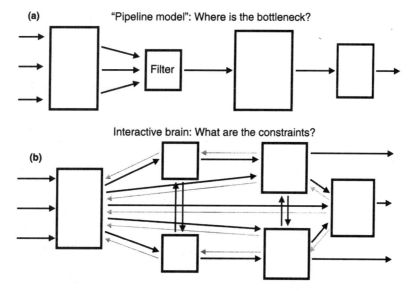

(a) "Pipeline model": Where is the bottleneck?

Filter

Interactive brain: What are the constraints?

(b)

FIGURE 39.2   (*a*) The early pipeline model of selection in attention tasks. (Modified from Broadbent, 1958.) (*b*) Schematic illustration of the more complex system more generally accepted now, with parallel pathways, top-down feedback, and lateral connections.

are the only source of capacity limits and attentional selection. Even when we have no intention to act and simply watch the scenes go by (e.g., at the movies), we select a subset of the information that reaches the senses.

Attention limits are typically found in unpracticed tasks, but most attention-demanding tasks can, with extensive practice, be automatized, or made independent of attention. Searching for a set of letters among other random letters initially demands attention and gives steep slopes of latencies against display size. But after weeks of practice with consistent target-distracter mapping, the slopes become flat (Schneider and Shiffrin, 1977). Two verbal tasks that are both similar and demanding (reading for comprehension and writing to dictation) could at first only be done in alternation, but after months of practice they were efficiently combined (Spelke, Hirst, and Neisser, 1976). The only remaining constraint was between tasks that required words to be combined in sentences. Theories of attention limits must also account for how these limits can, in many cases, be eliminated. When the connections are highly practiced, the bottlenecks seem to be bypassed and the correct action is automatically evoked.

2. *Does attention act early or late in processing?*

In the early days of attention research, information processing was seen as a pipeline of successive stages, the output of each becoming the input of the next, with information of increasing complexity abstracted at each level. Attention could potentially select between outputs at any level, to determine which should be passed on as inputs to the next. Largely through evidence from neuroscience, this model has been replaced by a more interactive system with reentry to

early levels and extensive lateral communication between separate parallel streams of analysis. The temporal sequence is no longer assumed simply to map onto the hierarchy of brain areas (figure 39.2).

The answer to the question of early or late will depend on how we interpret the word early—in terms of time, or of processing order, or of anatomy. Preattentive processing usually refers to processing that occurs before attentional selection. It need not be restricted to "early" visual areas. But preattentive processing is also sometimes used to refer to any processing that is not affected by attention. It may continue throughout an episode, guiding navigation (Neisser, 1967) and providing continuous information about the features present, even as attention scans the objects.

Advance information may affect the level of selection. When the relevant locations or features are known, we may preset the sensitivity of the appropriate receptors. Temporally preattentive processing is then ruled out. However, in many situations, the relevant locations or attributes are not known in advance, the window of attention cannot be preset, and selection is guided by preattentive organization.

EXPLICIT TESTS   The early–late dichotomy was actually always a "straw question," since proponents of early selection would not have denied that selection could and did also occur late. Obviously, conscious decisions can still be made and responses selected after perceptual processing is complete. The real question was, *can* attention act early (Broadbent, 1958), or is all perceptual processing automatic, with attention selecting only at the level of memory and response? (Deutsch and Deutsch, 1963). There are obvious links with the debate outlined earlier on the reason why we need attention at all.

Behavioral tests were designed to distinguish early from late selection by (1) contrasting the efficiency of selection based on properties that could be processed early (simple physical characteristics, such as location, color, and auditory pitch) with selection based on properties presumably processed only later (semantic content, abstract categories); (2) observing what information is lost for unattended messages and what remains available (the more complex the surviving material, the later the inferred selection); and (3) selecting the level of maximal load (e.g., by increasing the stimulus presentation rate to overload perception, or the complexity of response mapping to overload response) and seeing which most taxes performance.

Treisman and Riley (1969) used a dichotic listening experiment to test for early selection. We presented different speech messages to the two ears, asked participants to attend to and repeat back one of them, and compared detection of unattended targets defined by a simple physical feature (male voice) with those defined by category (digits in an unattended stream of letters). The perceptual load was high (two rapid speech messages) and response competition and memory load were minimized. The different voice was detected without difficulty, whereas the semantic category was not. So a simple physical feature was available without attention, but an equally simple semantic feature was not, suggesting that the limit arose somewhere between those two levels.

Proponents of late selection did not immediately surrender. Some argued that attention limits can be explained by decision effects alone: more stimuli lead to increased uncertainty and increased chances that noise alone will exceed a response criterion (e.g., Kinchla, 1974; Bundesen, 1990; Palmer, 1995). They showed that attention limits can and sometimes do arise at late stages, without, however, refuting the claim that they can also act early.

Attention limits that appear in the so-called psychological refractory period would seem to arise late. When separate speeded responses are required to two stimuli presented in close succession, the response to the second is typically delayed, reflecting an attentional bottleneck (Welford, 1952). Pashler (1993, 1994) used evidence of underadditivity of factors contributing to the two reaction times to locate the point at which overlap in the processing becomes impossible. He found convincing evidence that in this paradigm (though not necessarily in all attention-limited tasks), the bottleneck arises not in perception but in central decision and response selection (figure 39.3).

What seems to be critical is the level at which the potential overload occurs. If perception is demanding, selection needs to be early, whereas if the perceptual load is low, early selection may be not only unnecessary but actually impossible (Treisman, 1969). Lavie (1994, 1995) showed that interference from a flanking distracter decreased, and by inference early selection efficiency increased, as the attended

task became more difficult (figure 39.4). Earlier this chapter described her experiment with Rees and Frith showing that high perceptual load also decreased the amount of brain activation produced by irrelevant moving dots.

High perceptual load leads to early selection. But what if the load arises in the control systems that direct attention? Here high load might reduce the efficiency of early selection and increase the effects of irrelevant stimuli. With her colleagues, Lavie used a dual task in which participants were asked to remember the order of four digits, presented either in random order (high working memory load) or in a fixed, regular order (low load), while classifying famous names printed over irrelevant distracter faces (De Fockert et al., 2001). Incongruent faces this time produced more interference in the high-load condition, presumably because working memory involves the same frontal lobe executive system as attentional selection. Brain imaging in the same experiment provided converging evidence: activation in the fusiform face area was higher when working memory load was high, making selection inefficient.

IMPLICIT PROCESSING   In the 1960s and 1970s, it was often assumed that perceptual processing was fully reflected in conscious experience and that behavioral responses were a reliable guide to the information that was processed, either with or without attention. This probably contributed to the dominance of early selection accounts. The assumption was challenged by an early finding (Corteen and Dunn, 1974) that shock-associated words in an unattended message produced a galvanic skin response without also being consciously detected. Since then, other examples of implicit processing have been documented, using both indirect behavioral evidence such as priming, interference, or emotional responses and direct neural measures of responses to unattended stimuli.

Mack and Rock (1998) asked participants to judge the relative length of the arms of a cross, and showed that an additional unexpected stimulus often was simply not seen. Yet a subsequent word completion task showed priming from visual words to which the participant was "inattentionally blind" (figure 39.5). A smiling face and the participant's own name, both requiring detailed perceptual analysis, were among other stimuli that were also detected, presumably because of their subjective importance. Emotional stimuli may directly activate a separate pathway to the ventral prefrontal cortex and the amygdala (e.g., Yamasaki, Labar, and McCarthy, 2002), although, contrary to some prior claims, attentional resources do still appear to be needed for their detection (Pessoa et al., 2002).

Implicit processing of surprising complexity and persistence was shown in a negative priming experiment (DeSchepper and Treisman, 1996). We found a slight delay in responding to novel, previously unattended nonsense

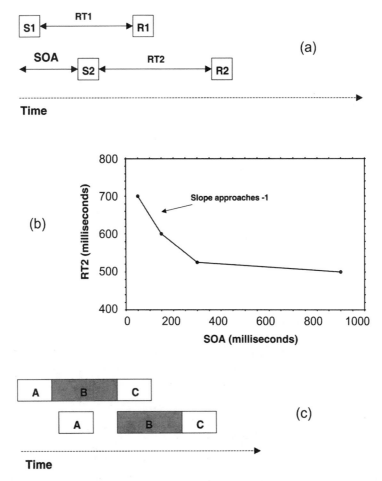

FIGURE 39.3   Psychological refractory period (from Pashler, 1994). (a) Objective sequence of events (S1 = stimulus 1; R1 = response 1; SOA = stimulus onset asynchrony). (b) Observed reaction time to second stimulus is delayed as the interval between the tasks is reduced. The slope approaches −1, indicating that, on average, the second response cannot be produced until a certain time after S1. (c) Hypothesized stages of mental processing: A = perceptual processing; B = central decision time; C = response programming time. Stage B forms a bottleneck where two separate decisions cannot overlap with each other. Other stages can operate in parallel.

shapes when they subsequently became relevant, even though explicit recognition memory was at chance (figure 39.6). This negative priming, which sometimes lasted for days or weeks, was established in a single trial and was specific enough to give at least partial discrimination among 260 different unfamiliar shapes.

Rapid serial visual presentation of two targets embedded in a string of distracters results in a reduced probability of detecting a second target when the first was identified within the few preceding items, as if the first occupies attention for several hundred milliseconds, blocking processing of the second (Shapiro and Raymond, 1994; figure 39.7). Yet unexpected words presented during this "attentional blink" triggered an N400 ERP component, implying that they were identified (Luck, Vogel, and Shapiro, 1996; see Hopfinger, Luck, and Hillyard, this volume).

Patients with unilateral neglect due to a right parietal lesion often show indirect evidence that they have identified stimuli that they are unable to report (e.g., McGlinchey-

Berroth, 1997; see Driver, Vuilleumier, and Husain, this volume, for other examples).

Implicit processing of unattended items complicates the attentional story, suggesting that attention can block access to consciousness without blocking all forms of perceptual processing. The fact that this can happen does not imply that it always must. The perceptual load was low in all the experiments that showed implicit effects, and when it was raised, the implicit effects often disappeared (Neumann and DeSchepper, 1992; Rees, Frith, and Lavie, 1997). But we still need to explain why attention should limit conscious access when the perceptual load is low. One possibility is that it takes more perceptual information to cross the threshold to consciousness than to generate implicit indices of priming and interference.

UNIQUE EVIDENCE FROM NEUROSCIENCE   Brain imaging may provide unique evidence on three issues in the early–late selection debate (see also Freiwald and Kanwisher, this volume).

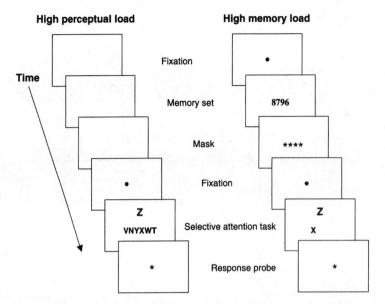

High perceptual load　　　　　**High memory load**

Time

	Fixation	•
	Memory set	8796
	Mask	****
•	Fixation	•
Z VNYXWT	Selective attention task	**Z** x
*	Response probe	*

FIGURE 39.4 Two forms of attention load with different effects on performance. The task is to find the X or Z in the foveal letter string or single letter. On the left, the irrelevant flanking Z causes more interference when the relevant task involves a single letter (low load) relative to a string. On the right, there is always just one central letter, but there is an additional memory task with either a high load (four random digits to remember) or a low load (four digits in sequential order, e.g., 6789). Interference from the irrelevant flanker is higher in this case when the load on working memory is high. The reason suggested is that the control of attention depends on the same areas as working memory.

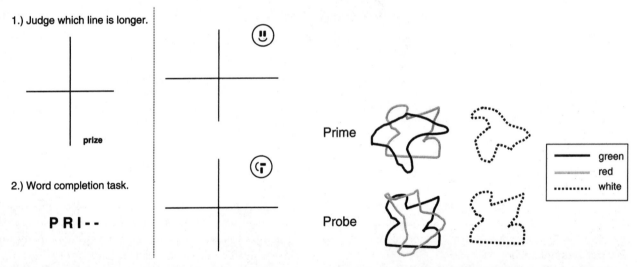

1.) Judge which line is longer.

prize

2.) Word completion task.

P R I - -

FIGURE 39.5 Inattentional blindness. On the left is illustrated an experiment showing implicit processing of unattended words. On the first three trials participants are shown only a plus sign and asked to judge which arm is longer. On the fourth trial a word appears in one of the quadrants and often is not seen. However, on a subsequent word completion task participants are more likely to respond with the unseen word, showing implicit priming from an unattended and undetected word. On the right side is a similar experiment in which the unexpected stimulus is a face. The smiling face is much more likely to be seen than the scrambled one or a sad face, showing the effects of meaning and emotion on implicit processing of unattended stimuli. (Modified from Mack and Rock, 1998.)

Prime

Probe

———	green
———	red
·········	white

FIGURE 39.6 Negative priming. Participants judge whether the green shape on the left matches the white shape on the right while ignoring the red shape on the left. They have no explicit memory for the unattended shapes, yet when one reappears as the shape to be attended, responses are slightly slowed, as though it had previously been inhibited or labeled irrelevant, and the label had to be cleared when the shape became relevant. This negative priming effect can last across hundreds of intervening trials and days' or weeks' delay. (Modified from DeSchepper, B., and A. M. Treisman, 1996. Visual memory for novel shapes: Implicit coding without attention. *J. Exp. Psychol. Learn. Mem. Cogn.* 22:27–47, Figure 1B. Copyright © 1996 by the American Psychological Association. Adapted with permission.)

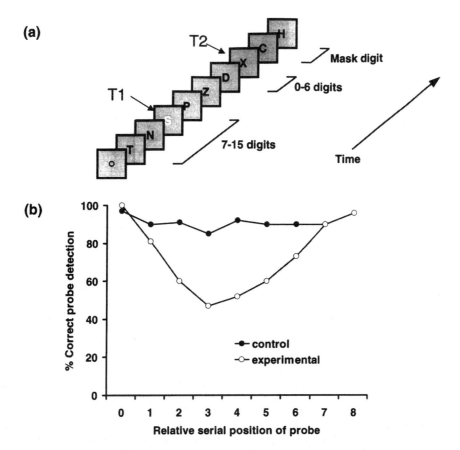

(a)

T2

T1

Mask digit

0–6 digits

7–15 digits

Time

(b)

% Correct probe detection

100
80
60
40
20
0

0 1 2 3 4 5 6 7 8

Relative serial position of probe

● control
○ experimental

FIGURE 39.7 The attentional blink. (*a*) Participants monitor a rapid visual sequence for two different targets. For example, T1 might be a white letter in a black string and T2 might be a letter X. (*b*) Open circles indicate the detection rates when participants do both tasks, and black circles show performance on T2 in the control condition in which they ignore the first target. In the combined tasks, T2 is very likely to be missed if it occurs within a few hundred milliseconds of T1, suggesting that detecting a first target makes the participant refractory to detecting a second for the next few hundred milliseconds. (Reprinted from K. L. Shapiro and J. E. Raymond, Temporal allocation of visual attention: Inhibition or interference? In *Inhibitory Processes in Attention, Memory, and Language,* D. Dagenbach and T. Carr, eds. Boston: Academic Press, 1994. Copyright 1994, with permission from Elsevier.)

1. Behavioral responses alone cannot distinguish selection before the stimulus appears (i.e., shifts in baseline activation) from gain control once it is present. fMRI activation and single unit changes occurring in anticipation of the stimulus have proved that attention can affect the baseline activity in specialized extrastriate areas even before the stimulus is presented—"early" indeed! (Chawla, Rees, and Friston, 1999; Hopfinger, Buonocore, and Mangun, 2000; Kastner and Ungerleider, 2000).

2. When baseline shifts are not present, divergence in ERPs or magnetoencephalograms between an attended and an unattended stimulus can define how soon after stimulus onset selection first occurs. The possibility of early attentional modulation was already confirmed in the 1970s by ERP effects that became evident as early as 70–100 ms after stimulus onset (e.g., Van Voorhis and Hillyard, 1977). It should be noted that the effect was to *attenuate* the response to unattended stimuli rather than to filter it out completely. Recent anatomical evidence from fMRI studies has shown that attention can act as peripherally as the lateral geniculate (O'Connor et al., 2002). Because of the multiple connections back from higher areas and the low temporal resolution of fMRI, it may be ambiguous whether attention affects a first pass through the visual hierarchy or acts only through reentrant connections. However combined with temporal evidence from ERPs (see Hopfinger, Luck, and Hillyard, this volume), the possibility of early attentional modulation, if not complete selection, is now clearly established.

3. On the other hand, differences in brain activation can also give online evidence of late selection by showing discrimination within an unattended message even when it has no effect on behavior. For example, Marois, Yi, and Chun (2004) presented a sequence of displays with faces in the center and places in the surround. While attempting to detect a one-back repetition of a face, participants failed to notice repetitions of the unattended places, suggesting early selection. However, fMRI showed decreased activation to the repeated scenes in the parahippocampal place area that responds only to places (Epstein and Kanwisher, 1998).

Adaptation to specific scenes implies that representations were formed and matched across trials without ever reaching conscious awareness. Again the fMRI effect was weaker than when the scenes received full attention, suggesting that there is some reduction in early processing when attention is focused elsewhere. These findings show that early selection is less complete than behavioral measures alone would suggest.

3. *Does attention select by enhancing relevant items, by inhibiting irrelevant items, or both?*

This is a difficult question to answer, either with behavioral tests or with brain imaging, because it is unclear what the baseline should be. We cannot be in a state of *no* attentional deployment. The alternatives to focused attention are inattention (i.e., focused attention to another object) or attention divided between two or more objects. Divided attention allocates some attention to the control objects or locations rather than none. One solution is to look only at the aftereffects of attention, comparing a previously attended or unattended stimulus with a new stimulus that was not present when attention was deployed (as in negative priming studies). But this does not probe the ongoing effects of attention. Most researchers have taken divided attention as the baseline with which to compare either full attention or rejection.

FACILITATION   In behavioral tasks, focused attention is generally found to facilitate the processing of selected signals relative to the divided attention baseline, improving the accuracy or the latency of response. But there is some disagreement about the form the facilitation takes—an increase in signal-to-noise ratio, a narrower tuning to sharpen discrimination, or a shift in criterion. Prinzmetal and colleagues (1998), exploring the phenomenology of attention, showed that the variance is reduced but the perceived intensity is unchanged. Signal detection theory can separate effects on sensitivity (d') and on decision criteria. For example, Shaw (1984) found that in detection of luminance increments, attention load affected only the decision criterion, but in a letter localization task it also affected d' measures (signal strength). Hawkins and colleagues (1990) differed with their conclusions on luminance detection: spatial cuing in their experiment affected both signal strength and criterion.

A related question, best answered with neural measures, is whether attention produces a multiplicative effect on the signal itself (a form of gain control) or simply changes the baseline activity on which the signal is superimposed. Hillyard, Vogel, and Luck (1998; see also Hopfinger, Luck, and Hillyard, this volume, and Freiwald and Kanwisher, this volume) reviewed the evidence and concluded that the gain control model fits best in early spatial selection, just as d' measures show attention effects in many behavioral studies.

But there is also evidence in some conditions for changes in baseline activity (Chawla, Rees, and Friston, 1999; Kastner et al., 1999).

INHIBITION   Some selective attention tasks suggest the use of active suppression of irrelevant stimuli in addition to facilitation of relevant signals. Whether inhibition is invoked may depend on how distracting the irrelevant stimuli would otherwise be. Thus, more active suppression may be needed when the target and distracters are superimposed rather than spatially separated. For example, in the negative priming paradigm, participants named one of two superimposed pictures more slowly when the currently relevant picture was the irrelevant one on the previous trial, as if it had been inhibited when it was irrelevant and the inhibition now had to be removed (Tipper, 1985; but see Neill et al., 1992, for an alternative account in terms of interference with episodic retrieval).

Inhibition may also be used to keep us from rechecking the same locations or stimuli that have already proved fruitless. Responses are slightly slower at locations that have previously received attention, an effect known as inhibition of return (IOR; Posner and Snyder, 1975; see also Klein, this volume). IOR has been shown both in detection tasks with a spatial cue and in visual search. Probe items get slightly slower responses when they appear in locations previously occupied by nontarget items (Cepeda et al., 1998; Klein and McInnes, 1999).

Improved search performance due to "marking" has also been attributed to inhibition (Watson and Humphreys, 1997). In the marking paradigm, a subset of distracters in a search display are shown in advance of the full display. This eliminates their contribution to search latencies. For example, we may observe an efficient feature search of just the items that appear in the final display instead of what would otherwise be a difficult conjunction search.

These behavioral findings suggest an inhibitory contribution to attentional control. Neuroscience offers more direct evidence of inhibition. fMRI measures suggest that attention to one spatial location, for example a stimulus at the fovea, strongly suppresses baseline activity in brain areas responding to other spatial locations (Smith, Singh, and Greenlee, 2000). Luck and colleagues (1994) explored ERP differences between attended and unattended items and suggested that both inhibition of irrelevant items (shown in the P1 ERP component) and facilitation of relevant ones (shown in the N1 component) can occur. When participants must *bind* features to identify the target, both a P1 and an N1 are shown, whereas when the presence of a color is sufficient, only the N1 (facilitation) effect remains (Luck and Hillyard, 1995). Thus again, inhibition is used when distracters would otherwise cause interference, and otherwise selective activation is enough.

4. *What does attention select?*

Traditionally the debate has centered on three possible goals of selection: locations, objects, and attributes. The answer seems yet again to be "all of the above," but in different circumstances. Spatial selection is implied when facilitation spreads to objects in the neighborhood of an attended target (Hoffman and Nelson, 1981). On the other hand, a number of findings also favor object selection. Attention appears to spread more easily within than between objects (Duncan, 1984; Egly, Driver, and Raful, 1994; Tipper and Behrmann, 1996; figure 39.8). Patients with neglect who are oblivious to the left side of space often also neglect the left side of objects (e.g., Halligan and Marshall, 1994; see also Driver, Vuilleumier, and Husain, this volume).

When overlapping objects share the same location, selective attention can still be very efficient—sufficient to make an unexpected gorilla invisible! (Neisser and Becklen, 1975;

Simons and Chabris, 1999). For selection to be by location here, location would have to be defined by the contours of the target object itself. Selection may be guided by properties of the target object, perhaps a color or a range of spatial frequencies, or simply by the colinearity and spatial continuity of its contours.

A dramatic demonstration of object-based selection with *no* distinguishing properties involves tracking a subset of identical moving dots (Pylyshyn and Storm, 1988). Participants are shown, for example, eight identical dots, of which four briefly brighten, indicating that they will be the targets. All eight dots then move on random independent paths, and participants attempt to keep track of the four targets. This pure case of selection must be based exclusively on spatiotemporal continuity, since after the initial cues, nothing else differentiates targets from distracters. Pylyshyn and Storm proposed that selection is maintained through preattentive indices attached to the cued targets. However, the

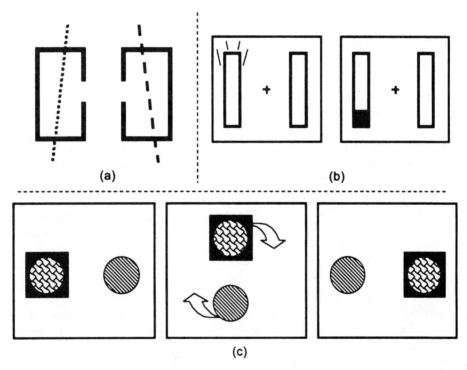

(a) (b)

(c)

FIGURE 39.8 Three experiments suggesting that attention is allocated to perceptual objects. (*a*) Participants were better at making two decisions on a single object (e.g., the orientation and texture of the line) than on two objects (e.g., the orientation of the line and the gap side of the rectangle), even though the two objects share the same location. (Reprinted from Duncan:1984, with permission.) (*b*) Two bars are presented and one end of one bar brightens temporarily. Then a target (indicated by the black area) is presented either at the cued end of the cued object, or at the opposite end (as in the example shown), or in the other object at the same spatial distance from the cue. Responses are fastest at the cued end, but they are also faster at the other end of the cued object than in the other object, indicating that a within-object shift of attention is faster than a between-objects shift. (Modified with permission from

Egly, Driver, and Rafal, 1994.) (*c*) Schematic illustration of the impact of left-sided neglect in the rotating objects experiment. When shown two objects, neglect patients with right parietal damage often see the one on the right and fail to see the one on the left. If they watch the objects rotate, however, they may continue to neglect the one that was originally on the left, even when it moves into the right field, suggesting that attention is allocated to the object rather than to its location. The shaded area reflects the part of the display neglected by the patients. (Modified from S. P. Tipper and M. Behrmann, Object-centered not scene-based visual neglect, *J. Exp. Psychol. Hum. Percept. Perform.* 22:1121–1278, 1996. Copyright © 1996 by the American Psychological Association. Adapted with permission.)

task is clearly subject to attention limits, showing a decrement in dual task conditions (Wilson and Treisman, unpublished; see Treisman, 1993).

Attributes may also be units of attentional selection. For example, we may attend to motion across the display and ignore color and shape (Corbetta et al., 1991). However, selection of an attribute within objects is less efficient than other forms of selection. There is a strong bias to attend to objects as wholes. The Stroop task illustrates failure to reject the word while attending to its color.

Can we further narrow attention to select a feature within an attribute (e.g., red within the attribute of color)? Blaser and colleagues (2000) tested people's ability to track one feature of an object as it changed over time and found this was possible so long as the changes were mostly gradual. Location was ruled out as a basis for selection because the target object was superimposed on an irrelevant object. However, it appears that feature selection was mediated by attention to the object as a whole: participants were able to track two changing features at once only if they characterized the same object.

When irrelevant attributes produce no behavioral interference with the relevant task, brain imaging may be needed to test whether they are truly suppressed (see Freiwald and Kanwisher, this volume). O'Craven, Downing, and Kanwisher (1999) used overlapping face and house stimuli and asked participants to report either the direction of the moving picture or the location (slightly shifted from center) of the static one. The picture with the relevant attribute also produced increased activation in the brain area specialized for its (irrelevant) category—PPA for houses and FFA for faces. Selection of one attribute here resulted in enhanced attention to the object as a whole.

On the other hand, Downing, Liu, and Kanwisher (2001) reported equally strong evidence that selecting the object in one location automatically enhances another object in the same location. Attending to one of two separately located colored ovals increased the activation produced by either the house or the face that shared the same location. The picture that emerges is that attention can be biased to select any of the three candidates, locations, objects, and attributes, depending on the requirements of the task, but that early selection is least effective for attributes.

One other form of attention should be mentioned: selection of scale with hierarchically organized stimuli (e.g., global letters made of local letters). Evidence for selection includes the finding that it can take time to reset attention from one level to another (Ward, 1982). Navon (1977) found faster responses to the global level ("global precedence"), although this preference can be modulated by the density and size of the local elements (Kimchi, 1992). Ivry and Robertson (1998) suggest that the attentional bias is relative rather than absolute, selecting the higher or the lower spatial

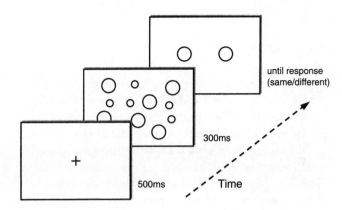

FIGURE 39.9 Implicit priming from the mean size of the previewed display. The task is to judge whether the two circles in the final display are the same size or different. Participants respond a little faster if one or both circles match the mean size of the preceding prime display, and faster even than when they match one of the presented sizes. It seems that participants automatically compute the mean size of an array of circles. (Experiment described in Chong and Treisman, 2001.)

frequencies in any given display. They link it to a cerebral asymmetry favoring higher frequencies in the left hemisphere and lower in the right. Robertson and Lamb (1991) describe data from neurological patients supporting this specialization.

Selection of scale may differ from other forms of attention in changing not only the scale but, with it, the nature of the processing: Chong and Treisman (2003) suggest that the global deployment of attention generates a statistical mode of processing. We confirmed a finding by Ariely (2001) that observers can accurately estimate the mean size of elements in a set, and showed that the mean is automatically registered when attention is distributed over a set of similar objects (figure 39.9).

5. *The role of attention in feature binding*

The visual system comprises many specialized areas coding different aspects of the scene. This poses the binding problem, namely, to specify how the information is put together in the correct conjunctions (e.g., red shirt and blue pants rather than an illusory pair of red pants). Behavioral results (Treisman and Gelade, 1980) suggest that we bind features by focusing attention on each object in turn. Evidence for this claim included (1) the finding that visual search depends on focused attention when the target is defined only by a conjunction of features (e.g., a green T among green Xs and brown Ts), whereas a search for either of two disjunctive features (e.g., blue *or* curved) among the same distracters resulted in target "popout," regardless of the number of items in the display. (2) When attention is prevented, binding errors or illusory conjunctions are frequently made. A blue circle might be seen with a brief presentation of a blue triangle and a yellow circle (Treisman and Schmidt, 1982). (3) A spatial precue helps detection of a conjunction much more than of a feature target (Treisman, 1988). (4) Boundaries between groups defined only by conjunctions are hard to detect, whereas those between features are easy (Treisman and Gelade, 1980).

Subsequent experiments showed that conjunction search for a known target with salient features could bypass the serial check, suggesting an additional mode of selection through feature grouping and guidance (Nakayama and Silverman, 1986; Wolfe, Cave, and Franzel, 1989; Treisman and Sato, 1990).

The theory was generally interpreted as predicting parallel search whenever a unique feature is available to mediate performance. This was correct, but the interpretation of "feature" as any unidimensional difference was not. When target and distracters differ only slightly on a single dimension, so that both activate the same detectors to different degrees, they can produce a wide range of search rates. Treisman and Gormican (1988) clarified the intended sense of feature as any property that activates neural detectors not also activated by surrounding elements. Thus, features are defined relative to a background. The claim that they are detected in parallel would be circular if there were no converging tests for featurehood, but some were in fact proposed: features are empirically defined as elements that can also migrate to form illusory conjunctions, that mediate effective grouping and boundary detection, and that can be separately attended. Neural evidence from single units may also be used to confirm candidates derived from behavioral criteria. There is evidence that new feature detectors can be set up through learning (e.g., Freedman et al., 2002).

Converging evidence for feature integration theory came from a patient, R.M., studied by Robertson and colleagues (1997). R.M. had bilateral parietal damage from two successive strokes. He showed the classic symptoms of Balint's syndrome: a failure to localize visual stimuli and an inability to see more than one or two objects at a time, or simultanagnosia. The theory predicts that he should also have difficulty binding features, since this requires focused attention to their shared location. Even with long exposures, R.M. frequently saw the shape of one letter in the color of another when two letters were present. He was unable to find a conjunction target, taking 2 or 3 s to search displays of three to five letters and making errors on at least 25% of trials. Interestingly, despite his severe simultanagnosia, R.M. had no difficulty with feature search. He could detect the presence of red in a display of blue letters, or a Q among Os, with very few errors. The unique color or the tail of the Q can be detected without localizing because each activates a unique population of feature detectors. On the other hand, search for an O in Qs was impossible because the target had no feature that was not shared by the distracters.

Brain imaging provides another logic for answering questions about functional mechanisms of binding. If binding requires spatial attention, and if we know that spatial attention always activates area A, we can see if area A also lights up when participants do a binding task. If it does not, we know that binding cannot require spatial attention. Corbetta and colleagues (1995), using positron emission tomography (PET), found that the same parietal areas were active both in spatial attention switching and in binding, but not in feature search. The result is consistent although not conclusive, since the parietal area might be active for different reasons in the two tasks. Further support for the role of parietal control in binding came from the finding that transcranial magnetic stimulation of the parietal lobes selectively disrupted conjunction but not feature search (Ashbridge et al., 1997). Luck and Hillyard (1995; see also Hopfinger, Luck, and Hillyard, this volume) showed ERP suppression effects specific to conjunction search. Some recent studies comparing conjunction search with difficult feature search gave mixed results. (Wojciulik and Kanwisher, 1999; Leonards et al., 2000; Donner et al., 2002). However, those that compared binding with difficult feature search are of questionable relevance, because the theory suggests that feature discrimination can also require focused attention when the differences are small (Treisman and Gormican, 1988).

6. *How is attention controlled?*

Attention can be "captured" by salient sensory events, though this may be compelling only when they signal the onset of a new object (Yantis and Jonides, 1996). It may be attracted by events that have been primed by the context, or by events with emotional significance whose threshold is low. But attention can also be endogenously controlled. Two general accounts have been proposed.

One proposes a specialized attention network that controls perceptual processing from the outside by amplifying relevant signals or attenuating irrelevant ones. (e.g., Mesulam, 1981; Posner and Dehaene, 1994). The existence of such an attentional control system is supported by several neural studies. For example, Corbetta et al. (1991) compared PET activation when attention was focused on one attribute and when it was divided between three. Selective attention produced more activation in the globus pallidus, caudate nucleus, posterior thalamus, inferior premotor cortex, insular cortex, and the lateral orbitofrontal cortex, whereas divided attention activated the anterior cingulate and right prefrontal cortex. D'Esposito and colleagues (1995) found that the dorsolateral prefrontal cortex and the anterior cingulate were activated only when two tasks (semantic classification of words and mental rotation of shapes) were performed concurrently, but not for either alone. They suggest that the dorsolateral prefrontal cortex is involved in the allocation of attentional resources.

An alternative account of attention sees selection as the emerging outcome of competition between neighboring objects, of which one or a few "attended" victors survive (Desimone and Duncan, 1995). In this "biased competition" account, different brain systems responding to the same object cooperate, ensuring that the same object becomes dominant across multiple areas. Top-down inputs can also bias the competition by adding to local activation or inhibition, allowing the possibility of an external control system as well as local competition.

It is not clear that purely behavioral evidence could distinguish the biased competition hypothesis from the structural interference view, which makes similar predictions about the specificity of interference. Thus, the supporting evidence is mainly neural. Reynolds, Chelazzi, and Desimone (1999) showed competitive interactions at the level of single units in monkey ventral areas. Kastner and Ungerleider (2000) found weaker fMRI activation when four pictures were shown together for 250 ms than when they were shown successively for 250 ms each. This was interpreted as evidence of mutual suppression between the concurrent pictures (although the increased number of onsets in the successive condition might contribute to the increased activation). In another study, Kastner and colleagues controlled for stimulus duration by presenting one picture in the upper visual field, either alone or together with three others in the lower field. The fMRI activation corresponding to the target location was again reduced by the added pictures, but when attention was directed to the upper picture in the combined presentation, the activation was restored.

Competition arises mainly within receptive fields, so the farther apart the stimuli, the higher the level of processing at which they should compete. This was strikingly confirmed by Kastner and colleagues (2001). However, there may also be competitive effects outside the classic receptive field, mediated by lateral connections. The early ERP effects of attention reflected selection between stimuli in different hemispheres, as do extinction effects in neglect patients. (Extinction is the loss of awareness of a stimulus in the field contralateral to the lesion that is induced by the presence of a concurrent stimulus in the ipsilateral field.) Thus, not all competition, even in early vision, arises within receptive fields. Another issue for the biased competition theory is to specify how local neurons "know" whether their activity is produced by parts of the same object, which should cooperate, or by different objects, which should compete. This may require substantial top-down control of local competition.

Biased competition could be a plausible implementation of earlier structural interference theories, with the added advantage of being neurally supported. In addition, it draws attention to phenomena that were less salient in the earlier context, such as distance effects, extinction, and dilution of priming.

7. *How does attention relate to consciousness?*

Some theories equate attention and consciousness. This suggestion is probably misleading. Not everything that has been attended to reaches awareness. We may attend to a spatial location and show implicit priming from what is presented there without becoming aware of what it was (Marcel, 1983a). We may look at an ambiguous figure and experience only one interpretation. It is even possible to show attention limits in unconscious perception: Kahneman and Chajczyk (1983) found "dilution" of priming and interference when a neutral word was presented together with the irrelevant color name in a Stroop color-naming task.

Thus, attention is not sufficient to ensure consciousness. Is it necessary? Can we be conscious of something that was not attended? There is an ambiguity here. I can be conscious of an unattended voice, but not of the words that are spoken. Am I conscious of the stimulus? In fact, we are probably never conscious of every property, even of fully attended stimuli—for example, that this cat is smaller than the Eiffel tower. We become explicitly aware of just a small fraction of the possible propositions that could be formulated about an object or event that we are observing, ranging from the belief that something is there (detection) to the way its features are bound, to its emotional valence, to the semantic interpretations it evokes. With unattended objects we are conscious of less than with attended ones; specifically, we lose those aspects for which capacity was overloaded and selection was made.

Attention seems to be neither necessary nor sufficient for conscious awareness, although the two are normally highly correlated. What, then, *is* necessary for conscious experience? The idea of reentry is much in the air these days. Several authors propose that the initial registration of stimuli consists of a rapid feedforward sweep through the visual areas without conscious awareness, then a possible return back to the early levels to check a tentative identification for selected elements against the sensory data (Marcel, 1983b; Damasio, 1989; Di Lollo, Enns, and Rensink, 2000; Lamme and Roelfsema, 2000; Hochstein and Ahissar, 2002). We become conscious of objects or events only if the match is confirmed.

Supporting evidence comes from the phenomenon of "object substitution" masking, in which a stimulus that begins at the same time as the target but outlasts it can mask it in a search array, even when there is no overlap of contours (Di Lollo, Enns, and Rensink 2000; figure 39.10). When the reentry check is made, only the mask remains, and it replaces the target in conscious experience. Related evidence is provided by Walsh and Cowey (1998), using transcranial magnetic stimulation to V1 to erase the stimuli before the reentry check can be made (around 80 ms after onset).

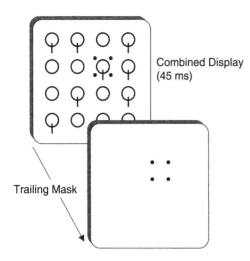

Combined Display
(45 ms)

Trailing Mask

FIGURE 39.10 Object substitution masking. The display contains up to 16 rings, half of which have a vertical bar across the bottom. The target is singled out by four dots, which also serve as the mask. Observers indicate whether the target contains the vertical bar. The sequence begins with a combined display of the target, mask, and distracters for 45 ms and continues with a display of the mask alone for durations of 0, 45, 90, 135 or 180 ms. The four dots produce no masking if they end with the display, but if they continue after it disappears, they render the stimulus that they surround invisible. The suggestion is that visual processing will not reach conscious awareness unless a reentry check confirms the information extracted on a first pass through the visual system. In the case illustrated, the dots remain alone in the location of one of the Qs and are substituted for it in conscious perception, whereas in the other locations there are no alternative stimuli to compete.

Hochstein and Ahissar (2002) suggest in their "reverse hierarchy" framework that awareness arises first at the highest levels, followed by a return to earlier areas if finer detail is needed from the smaller receptive fields in V1 and V2. Binding may also depend on reentry to early visual areas to ensure fine spatial resolution, controlled by a parietal scanning mechanism (Treisman, 1996).

Conclusions

Psychological studies posed many of the relevant questions, outlined possible mechanisms, and developed experimental paradigms to capture different aspects of what is meant by attention. The data provide constraints, ruling out many possible accounts. However, neuroscience has added powerful new tools to cast votes on issues that remained controversial, or sometimes to reframe the questions in ways that more closely match the way the brain functions.

The early information-processing view of the attention pipeline has been replaced by more complex models. Parallel processing streams in the brain deal with different types of information—"what" in the ventral areas versus "where" in the dorsal areas (Ungerleider and Mishkin, 1982), or objects and events for conscious representation in the ventral

pathway and the online control of actions in the dorsal pathway (Milner and Goodale, 1995). The pathways have many interconnections through which each can modulate others, and many recurrent loops through which higher-level hypotheses can be checked against sensory data.

Within each pathway, selection can occur at various levels, depending on the task, the load, and the degree to which concurrent tasks engage the same areas of the brain. Within this framework, some suggest that attention acts primarily through biases on intrinsic competitive local interactions. Others see it arising primarily or only at the decision level, following parallel perceptual processing. Still others (myself included) suggest that conscious perception, detailed localization, and perhaps binding of features may depend on focused attention through reentrant pathways. An initial rapid pass through the visual hierarchy provides the global framework and gist of the scene and primes competing identities through the features that are detected. Attention is then focused back to early areas to allow a serial check of the initial rough bindings and to form the representations of objects and events that are consciously experienced. The impact of cognitive neuroscience is obvious in these developments, but so is the ingenious and careful use of psychological paradigms to tease apart the mechanisms controlling our perception and action.

ACKNOWLEDGMENTS This work was supported by grant P50 MH62196 from the Conte Center, grant 1000274 from the Israeli Binational Science Foundation, and NIH grant R01 MH62331. Thanks also to Jon Driver for helpful suggestions.

REFERENCES

ALLPORT, D. A., B. ANTONIS, and P. REYNOLDS, 1972. On the division of attention: A disproof of the single-channel hypothesis. *Q. J. Exp. Psychol.* 24:225–235.

ARIELY, D., 2001. Seeing Sets: Representation by statistical properties. *Psychol. Sci.* 12:157–162.

ASHBRIDGE, E., V. WALSH, and A. COWEY, 1997. Temporal aspects of visual search studied by transcranial magnetic stimulation. *Neuropsychologia* 35:1121–1131.

BLASER, E., Z. W. PYLYSHYN, and A. HOLCOMBE, 2000. Tracking an object through feature-space. *Nature* 408:196–199.

BROADBENT, D. E., 1958. *Perception and Communication.* London: Pergamon Press.

BROOKS, L., 1968. Spatial and verbal components of the act of recall. *Can. J. Psychol.* 22:349.

BUNDESEN, C., 1990. A theory of visual attention. *Psychol. Rev.* 97:523–547.

CEPEDA, N. J., K. R. CAVE, N. P. BICHOT, and M.-S. KIM, 1998. Spatial selection via feature-driven inhibition of distractor locations. *Percept. Psychophys.* 60:727–746.

CHAWLA, D., G. REES, and K. J. FRISTON, 1999. The physiological basis of attentional modulation in extrastriate visual areas. *Nat. Neurosci.* 2:671–676.

CHONG, S. C., and A. TREISMAN, 2001. Representation of statistical properties (abstr. 54). *J. Vision 1.*

Chong, S., and A. Treisman, 2003. Representation of statistical properties. *Vision Res.* 43:393–404.

Corbetta, M., F. Miezin, S. Dobmeyer, G. Shulman, and S. Petersen, 1991. Selective and divided attention during visual discrimination of shape, color and speed: Functional anatomy by positron emission tomography. *J. Neurosci.* 11:2383–2402.

Corbetta, M., G. L. Shulman, F. M. Miezin, and S. E. Petersen, 1995. Superior parietal cortex activation during spatial attention shifts and visual feature conjunction. *Science* 270:802–805.

Corteen, R. S., and D. Dunn, 1974. Shock associated words in a nonattended message: A test for momentary awareness. *J. Exp. Psychol.* 102:1143–1144.

Corteen, R. S., and B. Wood, 1972. Autonomic responses to shock associated words in an unattended channel. *J. Exp. Psychol.* 94: 308–313.

Craighero, L., L. Fadiga, G. Rizzolatti, and C. Umiltà, 1999. Action for perception: A motor-visual attentional effect. *J. Exp. Psychol. Hum. Percept. Perform.* 25:1673–1692.

Damasio, A. R., 1989. Time-locked multiregional retroactivation: A systems-level proposal for the neural substrates of recall and recognition. *Cognition* 33:25–62.

De Fockert, J. W., G. Rees, C. D. Frith, and N. Lavie, 2001. The role of working memory in visual selective attention. *Science* 291:1803–1806.

DeSchepper, B., and A. Treisman, 1996. Visual memory for novel shapes: Implicit coding without attention. *J. Exp. Psychol. Learn. Mem. Cogni.* 22:27–47.

Desimone, R., and J. Duncan, 1995. Neural mechanisms of selective visual attention. *Annu. Rev. Neurosci.* 18:193–222.

D'Esposito, M., J. A. Detre, D. C. Alsop, R. K. Shin, S. Atlas, and M. Grossman, 1995. The neural basis of the central executive system of working memory. *Nature* 378:279–281.

Deutsch, A., and D. Deutsch, 1963. Attention: Some theoretical considerations. *Psychol. Rev.* 70:80–90.

Di Lollo, V., J. T. Enns, and R. A. Rensink, 2000. Competition for consciousness among visual events: The psychophysics of reentrant visual processes. *J. Exp. Psychol. Gen.* 129:481–507.

Donner, T., A. Kettermann, E. Diesch, F. Ostendorf, A. Villringer, and S. Brandt, 2002. Visual feature and conjunction searches of equal difficulty engage only partially overlapping frontoparietal networks. *Neuroimage* 15:16–25.

Downing, P., J. Liu, and N. Kanwisher, 2001. Testing cognitive models of visual attention with fMRI and MEG. *Neuropsychologia* 39:1329–1342.

Duncan, J., 1984. Selective attention and the organization of visual information. *J. Exp. Psychol. Gen.* 113:501–517.

Egly, R., J. Driver, and R. Rafal, 1994. Shifting visual attention between objects and locations: Evidence from normal and parietal lesion subjects. *J. Exp. Psychol. Gen.* 123:161–177.

Epstein, R., and N. Kanwisher, 1998. A cortical representation of the local visual environment. *Nature* 392:598–601.

Freedman, D., M. Riesenhuber, T. Poggio, and E. Miller, 2002. Visual categorization and the primate prefrontal cortex: Neurophysiology and behavior. *J. Neurophysiol.* 88:929–941.

Hawkins, H. L., S. A. Hillyard, S. J. Luck, M. Mouloula, C. Downing, and D. P. Woodward, 1990. Visual attention modulates signal detectability. *J. Exp. Psychol. Hum. Percept. Perform.* 16:802–811.

Heinze, H. J., H. Hinrichs, M. Scholz, W. Burchert, and G. R. Mangun, 1998. Neural mechanisms of global and local processing: A combined PET and ERP study. *J. Cogn. Neurosci.* 10:485–498.

Halligan, P. W., and J. C. Marshall, 1994. Towards a principled explanation of unilateral neglect. *Cogn. Neuropsychol.* 11:167–206.

Hillyard, S. A., E. K. Vogel, and S. J. Luck, 1998. Sensory gain control (amplification) as a mechanism of selective attention: Electrophysiological and neuroimaging evidence. *Philos. Trans. R. Soc. Lond. B* 353:1257–1270.

Hochstein, S., and M. Ahissar, 2002. View from the top: Hierarchies and reverse hierarchies in the visual system. *Neuron* 36:791–804.

Hoffman, J. E., and B. Nelson, 1981. Spatial selectivity in visual search. *Percept. Psychophys.* 30:283–290.

Hopfinger, J. B., M. H. Buonocore, and G. R. Mangun, 2000. The neural mechanisms of top-down attentional control. *Nat. Neurosci.* 3:284–291.

Ivry, R. B., and L. Robertson, 1998. *The Two Sides of Perception.* Cambridge, Mass: MIT Press.

Kahneman, D., 1973. *Attention and Effort.* Englewood Cliffs, N.J.: Prentice-Hall.

Kahneman, D., and D. Chajczyk, 1983. Tests of the automaticity of reading: dilution of Stroop effects by color-irrelevant stimuli. *J. Exp. Psychol. Hum. Percept. Perform.* 9:497–509.

Kastner, S., P. De Weerd, M. Pinsk, M. Elizondo, R. Desimone, and L. Ungerleider, 2001. Modulation of sensory suppression: Implications for receptive field sizes in the human visual cortex. *J. Neurophysiol.* 86:1398–1411.

Kastner, S., M. A. Pinsk, P. De Weerd, R. Desimone, and L. G. Ungerleider, 1999. Increased activity in human visual cortex during directed attention in the absence of visual stimulation. *Neuron* 22:751–761.

Kastner, S., and L. G. Ungerleider, 2000. Mechanisms of visual attention in the human cortex. *Annu. Rev. Neurosci.* 23:315–341.

Kimchi, R., 1992. Primacy of wholistic processing and global local paradigm: A critical review. *Psychol. Bull.* 112:24–38.

Kinchla, R., 1974. Detecting targets in multi-element arrays: A confusability model. *Percept. Psychophys.* 15:149–158.

Klein, R. M., 1988. Inhibitory tagging facilitates visual search. *Nature* 334:430–431.

Klein, R. M., and W. J. MacInnes, 1999. Inhibition of return is a foraging facilitator in visual search. *Psychol. Sci.* 10:346–362.

Lamme, V., and P. Roelfsema, 2000. The distinct modes of vision offered by feedforward and recurrent processing. *Trends Neurosci.* 23:571–579.

Lavie, N., 1994. Perceptual load as a major determinant of the locus of selection in visual attention. *Percept. Psychophys.* 56:183–197.

Lavie, N., 1995. Perceptual load as a necessary condition for selective attention. *J. Exp. Psychol. Hum. Percept. Perform.* 21:451–468.

Lavie, N., 2000. Selective attention and cognitive control: dissociating attentional functions through different types of load. In *Attention and Performance XVIII*, S. Monsell and J. Driver, eds. Cambridge, Mass.: MIT Press, pp. 175–194.

Lavie, N., A. Hirst, J. W. de Fockert, and E. Colledge, 2004 (in press). Load theory of selective attention. *J. Exp. Psychol. Gen.*

Leonards, U., S. Sunaert, P. Van Hecke, and G. Orban, 2000. Attention mechanisms in visual search: An fMRI study. *J. Cogn. Neurosci.* 12:61–75.

Luck, S. J., S. A. Hillyard, M. Mouloua, M. G. Woldorff, V. P. Clark, and H. L. Hawkins, 1994. Effects of spatial cuing on luminance detectability: Psychophysical and electrophysiological evidence for early selection. *J. Exp. Psychol. Hum. Percept. Perform.* 20:887–904.

Luck, S. J., and S. A. Hillyard, 1995. The role of attention in feature detection and conjunction discrimination: An electrophysiological analysis. *Int. J. Neurosci.* 80:281–297.

Luck, S., E. Vogel, and K. Shapiro, 1996. Word meanings can be accessed but not reported during the attentional blink. *Nature* 383:616–618.

Mack, A., and I. Rock, 1998. *Inattentional Blindness: Perception Without Attention*. Cambridge, Mass.: MIT Press.

Marcel, A., 1983a. Conscious and unconscious perception: Experiments on visual masking and word recognition. *Cogn. Psychol.* 15:238–270.

Marcel, A. J., 1983b. Conscious and unconscious perception: An approach to the relations between phenomenal experience and perceptual processes. *Cogn. Psychol.* 15:271–300.

Marois, R., D.-J. Yi, and M. M. Chun, 2004. The neural fate of consciously perceived and missed events in the attentional blink. *Neuron* 41:465–472.

McGlinchey-Berroth, R., 1997. Visual information -processing in hemispatial neglect. *Trends Cogn. Sci.* 1:91–97.

Mesulam, M.-M., 1981. A cortical network for directed attention and unilateral neglect. *Ann. Neurol.* 10:309–325.

Milner, A. D., and M. A. Goodale, 1995. *The Visual Brain in Action*. Oxford, England: Oxford University Press.

Nakayama, K., and G. H. Silverman, 1986. Serial and parallel processing of visual feature conjunctions. *Nature* 320:264–265.

Navon, D., 1977. Forest before trees: The precedence of global features in visual perception. *Cogn. Psychol.* 9:353–383.

Neill, W. T., L. A. Valdes, K. M. Terry, and D. S. Gorfein, 1992. The persistence of negative priming: II Evidence for episodic trace retrieval. *J. Exp. Psychol. Learn. Mem. Cognit.* 18:993–1000.

Neisser, U., 1967. *Cognitive Psychology*. New York: Appleton-Century-Crofts.

Neisser, U., and R. Becklen, 1975. Selective looking: Attending to visually specified events. *Cogn. Psychol.* 7:480–494.

Neumann, E., and B. G. DeSchepper, 1992. An inhibition-based fan effect: Evidence for an active suppression mechanism in selective attention. *Can. J. Psychol.* 46:1–40.

O'Connor, D., M. Fukui, M. Pinsk, and S. Kastner, 2002. Attention modulates responses in the human lateral geniculate nucleus. *Nat. Neurosci.* 5:1203–1209.

O'Craven, K., P. Downing, and N. Kanwisher, 1999. fMRI evidence for objects as the units of attentional selection. *Nature* 401:584–587.

Palmer, J., 1995. Attention in visual search: Distinguishing four causes of a set-size effect. *Curr. Direct. Psychol. Sci.* 4:118–123.

Pashler, H., 1993. Dual-task interference and elementary mental mechanisms. In *Attention and Performance* vol. 14, D. Meyer and S. Kornblum, eds. Cambridge, Mass.: MIT Press, pp. 245–264.

Pashler, H., 1994. Dual task interference in simple tasks: Data and theory. *Psychol. Bull.* 116:220–244.

Pessoa, L., S. Kastner, et al., 2002. Attentional control of the processing of neutral and emotional stimuli. *Cogn. Brain Res.* 15:31–45.

Posner, M. I., and S. Dehaene, 1994. Attentional networks. *Trends Neurosci.* 17:75–79.

Posner, M. I., and C. R. R. Snyder, 1975. Facilitation and inhibition in the processing of signals. In *Attention and Performance*, vol. 5, P. M. A. Rabbitt and S. Dornic, eds. New York: Academic Press, pp. 669–682.

Prinzmetal, W., H. Amiri, K. Allen, and T. Edwards, 1998. The phenomenology of attention. 1. Color, location, orientation and spatial frequency. *J. Exp. Psych. Hum. Percept. Perform.* 24:261–282.

Prinzmetal, W., I. Nwachuku, and L. Bodanski, 1997. The phenomenology of attention. 2. Brightness and contrast. *Consciousness Cognit.* 6:372–412.

Pylyshyn, Z. W., and R. W. Storm, 1988. Tracking multiple independent targets: Evidence for a parallel tracking mechanism. *Spat. Vision* 3:179–197.

Rees, G., C. D. Frith, and N. Lavie, 1997. Modulating irrelevant motion perception by varying attention load in an unrelated task. *Science* 278:1616–1619.

Reynolds, J., L. Chelazzi, and R. Desimone, 1999. Competitive mechanisms subserve attention in macaque areas V2 and V4. *J. Neurosci.* 19:1736–1753.

Rizzolatti, G., L. Riggio, I. Dascola, and C. Umilta, 1987. Reorienting attention across the horizontal and vertical meridians: Evidence in favor of a premotor theory of attention. *Neuropsychologia* 25:31–40.

Robertson, L., A. Treisman, S. Friedman-Hill, and M. Grabowecky, 1997. The interaction of spatial and object pathways: Evidence from Balint's syndrome. *J. Cogn. Neurosci.* 9:254–276.

Robertson, L. C., and M. R. Lamb, 1991. Neuropsychological contributions to theories of part-whole organization. *Cogn. Psychol.* 23:299–330.

Schneider, W., and R. M. Shiffrin, 1977. Controlled and automatic human information processing. I. Detection, search and attention. *Psychol. Rev.* 84:1–66.

Shapiro, K. L., and J. E. Raymond, 1994. Temporal allocation of visual attention: Inhibition or interference. In *Inhibitory Processes in Attention, Memory and Language*, D. Dagenbach and T. Carr, eds. New York: Academic Press.

Shaw, M., 1984. Division of attention among spatial locations: A fundamental difference between detection of letters and detection of luminance increments. In *Attention and Performance*, X, H. Bouma and D. Bouwhuis, eds. Hillsdale, NJ: Erlbaum, pp. 109–121.

Simons, D. J., and C. F. Chabris, 1999. Gorillas in our midst: Sustained inattentional blindness for dynamic events. *Perception* 28:1059–1074.

Smith, A. T., K. D. Singh, and M. W. Greenlee, 2000. Attentional suppression of activity in the human visual cortex. *Neuroreport* 11:271–277.

Spelke, E., W. Hirst, and U. Neisser, 1976. Skills of divided attention. *Cognition* 4:215–230.

Spence, C., and J. Driver, 1996. Audiovisual links in endogenous covert spatial attention. *J. Exp. Psychol. Hum. Percept. Perform.* 22:1005–1030.

Stroop, J. R., 1935. Studies of interference in serial verbal reactions. *J. Exp. Psychol.* 18:643–662.

Tipper, S. P., 1985. The negative priming effect: Inhibitory effects of ignored primes. *Q. J. Exp. Psychol.* 37A:571–590.

Tipper, S. P., and M. Behrmann, 1996. Object-centered not scene-based visual neglect. *J. Exp. Psychol. Hum. Percep. Perform.* 22:1261–1278.

Treisman, A., 1969. Strategies and models of selective attention. *Psychol. Rev.* 76:282–299.

Treisman, A., 1988. Features and objects: The Fourteenth Bartlett Memorial Lecture. *Q. J. Exp. Psychol.* 40A:201–237.

Treisman, A., 1993. The perception of features and objects. In *Attention: Selection, awareness and control: A tribute to Donald Broadbent*, A. Baddeley and L. Weiskrantz, eds. Oxford, England: Clarendon Press, pp. 5–35.

Treisman, A., 1996. The binding problem. *Curr. Opin. Neurobiol.* 6:171–178.

TREISMAN, A., and A. DAVIES, 1973. Divided attention to ear and eye. In *Attention and Performance, IV*, S. Kornblum, ed. New York: Academic Press, pp. 101–117.

TREISMAN, A., and G. GELADE, 1980. A feature integration theory of attention. *Cogn. Psychol.* 12:97–136.

TREISMAN, A., and S. GORMICAN, 1988. Feature analysis in early vision: Evidence from search asymmetries. *Psychol. Rev.* 95:15–48.

TREISMAN, A., and J. RILEY, 1969. Is selective attention selective perception or selective response? A further test. *J. Exp. Psychol.* 79:27–34.

TREISMAN, A., and S. SATO, 1990. Conjunction search revisited. *J. Exp. Psychol. Hum. Percept. Perform.* 16:459–478.

TREISMAN, A., and H. SCHMIDT, 1982. Illusory conjunctions in the perception of objects. *Cogn. Psychol.* 14:107–141.

TUCKER, M., and R. ELLIS, 1998. On the relations between seen objects and components of potential actions. *J. Exp. Psychol. Hum. Percept. Perform.* 24:830–846.

UNGERLEIDER, L. G., and M. MISHKIN, 1982. *Two Cortical Visual Systems.* Cambridge, Mass.: MIT Press.

VAN VOORHIS, S. T., and S. A. HILLYARD, 1977. Visual evoked potentials and selective attention to points in space. *Percept. Psychophys.* 22:54–62.

WALSH, V., and A. COWEY, 1998. Magnetic stimulation studies of visual cognition. *Trends Cogn. Sci.* 2:103–110.

WARD, L., 1982. Determinants of attention to local and global features of visual forms. *J. Exp. Psychol. Hum. Percept. Perform.* 8:562–581.

WATSON, D. G., and G. W. HUMPHREYS, 1997. Visual marking: Prioritizing selection for new objects by top-down attentional inhibition of old objects. *Psychol. Rev.* 104:90–122.

WELFORD, A., 1952. The "psychological refractory period" and the timing of high speed performance: A review and a theory. *B. J. Psychol.* 43:2–19.

WOJCIULIK, E., and N. KANWISHER, 1999. The generality of parietal involvement in visual attention. *Neuron* 23:747–764.

WOLFE, J. M., K. R. CAVE, and S. L. FRANZEL, 1989. Guided search: An alternative to the feature integration model for visual search. *J. Exp. Psychol. Hum. Percept. Perform.* 15:419–433.

YAMASAKI, H., K. LABAR, and G. MCCARTHY, 2002. Dissociable prefrontal brain systems for attention and emotion. *Proc. Nat. Acad. Sci. U.S.A.* 99:11447–11451.

40 Orienting and Inhibition of Return

RAYMOND KLEIN

ABSTRACT   The behavioral properties of an inhibitory aftermath of exogenous orienting, which has come to be called "inhibition of return," and then our growing understanding of its neural implementation are described. IOR is generated by oculomotor activity and it affects subsequent orienting and other spatial responding. The effect is local, graded, and coded in environmental or, when a cued object moves, in object-based, coordinates. Several locations or objects can be tagged simultaneously. By discouraging attention from returning to previously inspected objects or locations IOR serves as a search or foraging facilitator. Neuroscientific studies suggest that IOR, when generated using the model cuing task pioneered by Posner, begins with the presentation of the cue but is not seen in behavior until attention is disengaged from the cue, thus removing attention-related facilitation. Neuropsychological and developmental studies point to the superior colliculus as critical in the generation of IOR. Studies of human brain electrical activity suggest that the effects of IOR begin early in target processing, and single unit studies reveal a reduction in the strength of sensory signals reaching the superior colliculus, though the colliculus itself does not appear to be inhibited. Cortical circuits are necessary for object coding of IOR, and environmental coding of IOR depends on circuits in the right parietal lobe.

Orienting, a set of mechanisms that results in the selection of some input signals for preferential processing and the consequent deselection of others, can be overt or covert. Overt orienting is the alignment of a receptor toward an actual or future source of information. In vision, overt orienting is easily observed in the form of saccadic or pursuit eye movements that bring to or maintain on the fovea objects of interest. In contrast, in covert orienting internal adjustments (James, 1890; Broadbent, 1958) are brought to bear on the neural signals after those signals have been picked up by the sensory organs. Perhaps because these adjustments cannot be directly observed—they must be inferred through converging operations (Garner, Hake, and Eriksen, 1956)—we are only just beginning to understand how these internal selections and deselections are implemented by neural systems at a computational level of analysis. Whether overt or covert, orienting can be controlled from within, by the observer's expectations and intentions, or from without, by

RAYMOND KLEIN   Department of Psychology, Dalhousie University, Halifax, Nova Scotia, Canada.

external stimuli whose spatial coordinates reflexively activate orienting mechanisms. The top-down, strategic mode of control has been called endogenous; the bottom-up, automatic mode of control has been called exogenous (Posner, 1980; Klein, Kingstone, and Pontefract, 1992).

The creative use of model tasks (Posner, 1996) has played a pivotal role in generating a rich empirical foundation for a cognitive-level description of covert orienting and its relation to overt orienting. Some of these model tasks are sufficiently simple that they can be tailored for use with infants and nonhuman primates, enabling the generation of valuable data on the development of orienting and its neuroscientific implementation. Using such a model task, Posner and Cohen (1984) discovered inhibition of return (Posner et al., 1985), a consequence of orienting that has been conceptualized as an inhibition of subsequent orienting. By testing normal adults, patients with brain lesions, infants, and nonhuman primates, and using modalities other than vision, static and moving displays, and manual and oculomotor responses, researchers have explored the time course, frames of reference, causes, effects, functional significance, development, and neural implementation of inhibition of return (IOR).

Model and modal task

We begin by considering the model task whose sequence of displays is shown in figure 40.1a. Three boxes are displayed, one at the center of the display and one on either side of fixation. One of the peripheral boxes brightens briefly, and after various delays a target, which might be an asterisk appearing with equal probability in one of the peripheral boxes, calls for a simple detection response. When the target is presented in close temporal proximity to the onset of the cue, its simple detection is speeded at the cued location in relation to the uncued location leading to faster cued than uncued reaction times (RTs). This benefit for cued targets has been attributed to an exogenously elicited shift of attention to the cued location (Posner, 1980; Jonides, 1981). At longer intervals the cued and uncued RT functions cross over, and targets presented at the originally facilitated location appear to be inhibited (figures 40.1b, 40.2a).

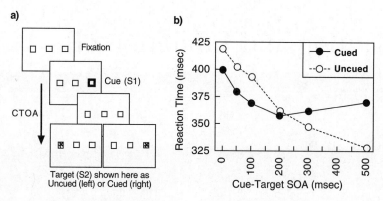

FIGURE 40.1 Inhibition of return: model task and prototypical data. (*a*) The sequence of events in a typical trial of the model task described in the text. A fixation display is followed by the first stimulus (S1, cue), shown here as the brightening of one of the two peripheral boxes. After varying intervals (cue–target onset asynchronies, CTOAs) from the onset of the cue, a target (S2), shown here as an asterisk, is presented at the cued or uncued location. The observer's task is to make a speeded response as soon as the asterisk is detected. (*b*) Reaction time data from Posner and Cohen (1984).

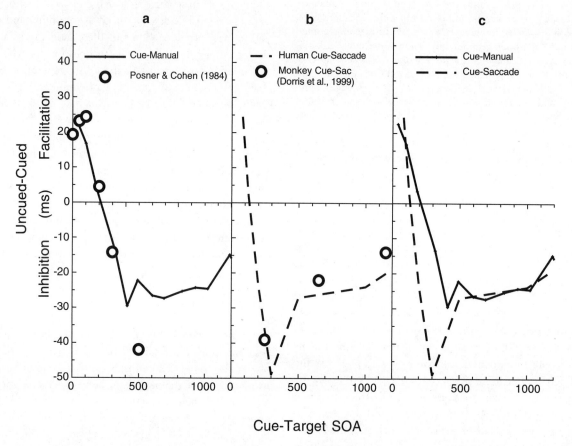

FIGURE 40.2 Time course of IOR with manual and saccadic responses. (*a*) Time course of facilitation and inhibition in studies using a cue–target task (as in figure 40.1*a*) with simple manual detection responses. The solid line summarizes the data from 27 studies reviewed by Samuel and Kat (2003) (from which redrawn). The open circles replot the data of Posner and Cohen (1984) in figure 40.1*b* as difference scores. (*b*) Time course of facilitation and inhibition in studies using a cue-target task with saccadic localization responses. The dashed line summarizes data from six studies of human performance (redrawn from Klein, 2000); the open circles show the data from nonhuman primates reported by Dorris and colleagues (1999). (*c*) The data from human subjects shown in *a* and *b* combined to illustrate the earlier appearance of IOR when the target task requires a prosaccade.

The studies whose findings are illustrated in figure 40.2a (Samuel and Kat, 2003) share certain methodological properties (a relatively brief, uninformative peripheral stimulus requiring no response, followed after one or more cue-target onset asynchronies [CTOAs] by a peripheral target requiring simple manual detection response) while differing in others. IOR has also been observed in studies using variants of this model task. The variants include responding to the first, IOR-causing stimulus; the use of more complex responses (choice or go/no go) to the second, IOR-measuring stimulus; the use of auditory and tactile stimuli, and stimulus pairs presented to different modalities; overt orienting, in the form of eye movements, occurs during the experiment, either incidentally or as a task requirement.

The cue–target procedure of the model task might be criticized for the possible contribution of inhibition of a response to the cue (Harvey, 1980). Yet this method can be used while minimizing the possibility of response inhibition through obvious physical differences between the cue and target or through a target task whose responses are orthogonal to (and hence would not be automatically activated by) the cue's location (Spence and Driver, 1997). Some investigators have explored IOR following responses to relevant targets. This target–target paradigm, with its consecutive orienting responses, seems more characteristic of real-world behavior (e.g., search of complex scenes), and when it is used there is no inhibition of possible responses to the IOR-generating stimulus, because responses are actually made to them. However, a response repetition heuristic ("when things are the same, repeat the previous response") might be used to bypass full processing of repeated targets in this situation (e.g., Christie and Klein, 2001). Such a bypass mechanism may make it appear that there is less (or no) IOR than there actually is (Tanaka and Shimojo, 1996; Taylor and Donnelly, 2002). In light of their different strengths and weaknesses, it is recommended that neither method (cue–target, target–target) be abandoned.

The extended model task has been useful in the effort to characterize IOR in normal adults, as well as explore it in infants, patients, and nonhuman primates. Nevertheless, researchers seeking to understand its function have found it fruitful to break out of the methodological mold of this model task by using dual tasks (Klein, 1988) and tasks with greater ecological validity (Gilchrist, North, and Hood, 2001).

Time course

When does IOR begin, and how long does it last? In most studies that vary the cue–target SOA, IOR has been observed at the longest SOAs tested. In a recent parametric exploration of this question, Samuel and Kat (2003) observed a robust IOR, that was relatively constant at about 25 ms, for over 3 s, after which IOR declined.

Two methodological features of Posner and Cohen's (1984) implementation of the model task underlie an important implicit assumption about whether and when IOR may be observed. To ensure that the observer's attention would be unlikely to linger at the location containing the uninformative precue, either (1) targets were more likely to be presented at fixation than at the peripheral locations, thus encouraging the endogenous allocation of attention back to fixation, or (2) following presentation of the peripheral cue, the center box was flashed (sometimes called a second cue), thus exogenously attracting attention back to fixation. Posner and Cohen assumed that if attention remained at the cued location, IOR would not be *observed*. Even if this were true, it would not necessarily mean that IOR was not *present* at the cued location.[1] Reaction time depends on the durations of a sequence of stages of processing, beginning with the encoding of the stimulus and ending with the execution of the response. Because facilitation of some of these stages might coexist with inhibition of others, IOR could be present while not being manifest in reaction time (RT). As highlighted by Klein (2000, Box 1), two fundamentally different construals of the timing of IOR have been proposed. One view holds that inhibition begins with the cue, and hence takes place in parallel with signal enhancements that are attributed to the capture of attention by the cue. To explain the early facilitation of RTs and the biphasic pattern, it is assumed that the initial facilitatory effect on RT is larger than the inhibitory effect, and that as facilitation decreases (with removal of attention from the cued location), the net effect on RT will be dominated by the inhibition. The other view holds that the biphasic pattern reflects a facilitation that lasts until attention is removed from the originally cued location and that the inhibition begins with this removal. It is noteworthy that under both views, the crossover from facilitation to inhibition depends on *when* attention is disengaged from the cue. Danziger and Kingstone's (1999) impressive finding of IOR within 50 ms of a peripheral cue that signaled that a target was likely to be presented elsewhere (90° clockwise from the cue) is equally consistent with both views, because the contingency likely elicited a very rapid removal of attention from the cued location. Distinguishing between these views may rest on a neuroscience-based approach.

When the return of attention following an uninformative peripheral cue is left to the devices of the observer (that is, there is no exogenous return via a cue at fixation), the time course of IOR has been shown to vary considerably with task demands (e.g., Lupianez et al., 1997; Khatoon, Briand, and Sereno, 2002) and subject variables (e.g., Larrison-Faucher, Briand, and Sereno, 2002; Macpherson, Klein, and Moore, 2003). Klein (2000) explains the variability due to task by assuming that the attentional control setting observers adopt to perform the target task will also apply to the cue, and therefore, the more attention that is required to perform the target task, the more difficult it will be to disengage attention from the cue, and the later IOR would be observed (see also Lupianez, Milliken, and Solano, 2001). This applies to difficulty of the stimulus-response mapping as well as to perceptual difficulty, as can be seen by comparing the time course of IOR with manual detection responses (figure 40.2a) and saccadic localization responses (figure 40.2b). For the former, the correct response is arbitrarily linked to the stimuli, whereas for the latter, the brain's overt orienting machinery provides a reflexive pathway. Because attention is particularly required to make arbitrary stimulus-response mappings, and by definition is not required for reflexive ones, Klein's attentional control setting principle predicts that IOR should appear sooner with the saccadic responses, a prediction confirmed in figure 40.2c. This principle can be extended to help explain why IOR appears to start later in schizophrenics than in healthy subjects (Larrison-Faucher, Briand, and Sereno, 2002) and in older than in younger adults (Castel et al., 2003), and why it may not be observed at all in children (Brodeur and Enns, 1997) unless a cue-back to fixation is used, as demonstrated by MacPherson and colleagues (2003) and suggested by the findings of Sapir and colleagues (2001) and Faust and Balota (1997). Once attention has been captured by the peripheral cue, some groups of individuals, perhaps those with diminished prefrontal executive control, may lack the strategy to return attention to a fovea-centric "neutral" position, or may have difficulty executing this strategy (for a review, see Klein, in press).

Cause and effect

For IOR to be observed in a behavioral study, two conditions must be satisfied (Taylor and Klein, 1998): a manipulation must cause IOR, and the target task must require a stage of processing that is affected by IOR. For example, when attention is controlled endogenously (and without an event in the periphery to guide it), its withdrawal from the cued location does not result in IOR (Posner and Cohen, 1984; Rafal et al., 1989). From this, Posner and Cohen inferred that stimulation of the periphery was necessary and sufficient to cause IOR. In a counter-demonstration, Rafal and colleagues (1989) found IOR following cancellation of an endogenously prepared saccade, a condition that activates the oculomotor system but does not entail asymmetrical peripheral stimulation. Of the full set of conditions tested by Rafal and colleagues (1989), the five that showed IOR (table 40.1) involve direct activation of the oculomotor system, whereas the one that did not show IOR (withdrawal of an endogenously shifted attention) either does not involve

TABLE 40.1

Do the following conditions elicit IOR?

Response to Cue	Type of Cue	
	Exogenous	Endogenous
Execute saccade	Yes	Yes
Prepare saccade	Yes	Yes
Attend	Yes	No

Note: Study by Rafal and colleagues (1989). A *yes* answer indicates the condition did elicit inhibition of return.

oculomotor programming (Klein and Pontefract, 1994) or involves active inhibition of oculomotor programming.

Whereas there is general agreement that oculomotor programming is involved in causing IOR, researches have debated whether IOR, once caused, directly affects input processes (e.g., Handy, Jha, and Mangun, 1999), attention (e.g., Reuter-Lorenz, Jha, and Rosenquist, 1996) or motor processes (Tassinari et al., 1987; Klein and Taylor, 1994; Ivanoff and Klein, 2001), with evidence in favor of one locus usually accepted as evidence against the others. Because there is strong evidence for effects of IOR on both early, stimulus-encoding and later, response-selection stages of processing, a more fruitful strategy might be to determine the boundary conditions for eliciting effects at these different loci. For example, when a go/no-go simple detection task is used (Ivanoff and Klein, 2001), a reluctance to respond to cued targets (as originally proposed by Klein and Taylor, 1994) seems to dominate performance. In contrast, when the target task emphasizes a nonspatial discrimination, input processing seems to be affected, either directly or through an IOR-mediated delay of orienting to the target (e.g., Cheal, Chastain, and Lyon, 1998; Handy, Jha, and Mangun, 1999; Klein and Dick, 2002).

Exploring 24 combinations for generating and measuring IOR, Taylor and Klein (2000) found that depending on whether or not the oculomotor machinery was tonically inhibited during the experiment, participants ignored or made manual or saccadic responses to a first stimulus (S1) that was a peripheral onset or central arrow, and then about a second later they made manual or saccadic responses to a second (S2) peripheral onset or central arrow, the spatial code (left/right) of which repeated or did not repeat that of the first stimulus. In all conditions that required a saccade (either to S1 or to S2), if IOR was obtained with peripheral targets, it was also obtained when subjects responded to central arrows (figure 40.3). Because there is no peripheral stimulus, the IOR caused in these conditions appears to be response-based or motoric. In contrast, when participants were not making saccades at all, IOR was confined to peripheral targets, consistent with inhibition of perception or attention (see also Abrams and Dobkin, 1994; Kingstone and Pratt, 1999; Hunt and Kingstone, 2003).

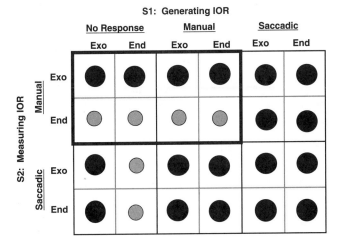

S1: Generating IOR

	No Response		Manual		Saccadic	
	Exo	End	Exo	End	Exo	End

S2: Measuring IOR

FIGURE 40.3 Results from Taylor and Klein (2000). Participants ignored or made manual or saccadic localization responses to the first stimulus (S1), and about a second later made manual or saccadic responses to the second stimulus. Stimuli were peripheral onsets (exogenous, Exo) or central arrows pointing left or right (endogenous, End). Black circles denote conditions for which significant IOR was obtained. Conditions enclosed by the thick black outline rectangle suggest an effect of IOR on input processing and/or attention. In the remaining conditions, whenever IOR was obtained with a peripheral S2 target, a similar magnitude of IOR was also obtained in response to an arrow.

Spatial coding and frame of reference

The effect of IOR is spatially local and graded, being maximal in the vicinity of the cue. For example, when there is more than one possible stimulus location on each side of fixation, it is generally observed that RT is slowest at the cued location (even when compared to noncued locations in the same field; e.g., Berlucchi, Chelazzi, and Tassinari, 2000) and decreases monotonically with distance from the cued location (Maylor and Hockey, 1985; Bennett and Pratt, 2001). Similarly, when cues and targets are placed on the circumference of a circle centered on fixation, RT decreases monotonically as the angular distance between the cue and the target increases, with most of this decrease taking place within 90° of the cued location (Maylor and Hockey, 1985; Snyder, Schmidt, and Kingstone, 2001), particularly at long cue–target SOAs (Samuel and Kat, 2003).

Second, IOR is neither retinal (Maylor, 1993, using dichoptic viewing, demonstrated complete interocular transfer; Tassinari and Berlucchi, 1993) nor merely oculocentric (see Abrams and Pratt, 2000, for a possible exception); rather, it is coded in an environmental (Posner and Cohen, 1984; Maylor and Hockey, 1985) or object-based (Tipper, Driver, and Weaver, 1991) frame of reference. The environmental and retinal locations, which are confounded in the model task (figure 40.1a) can be separated by interposing an eye movement between presentation of the cue and the target (figure 40.4a). Following a cue in one of two locations, Maylor and

Hockey (1985) required their participants to make a downward saccade, after which a target calling for a manual detection response was presented at the environmental or retinal location of the cue (or at the corresponding locations on the opposite side). IOR was observed only at the environmental location of the cue. By moving the stimuli after one of them had been cued (figure 40.4b), Tipper, Driver, and Weaver (1991) demonstrated that IOR could be tagged to objects. This finding has been replicated and extended in numerous ways (e.g., Abrams and Dobkin, 1994; Tipper et al., 1994). Tipper, Jordan, and Weaver (1999) found IOR at both the location of the cue and the location of the cued object after motion. The relative size of the object effect was enhanced when the elements in the scene were integrated rather than segregated, suggesting a flexible assignment of tags to different representational frames. Object-based IOR survives occlusion of the cued object when it moves behind a visual barrier (Yi, Kim, and Chun, 2003).

That IOR can be coded in an environmental or object-based frame of reference places the inhibition at some distance from the sensory machinery and is quite compatible with the idea that IOR is a mechanism that affects our actions (including covert orienting) toward objects in space. The compelling demonstration of IOR between all pairings of vision, touch, and audition (Spence et al., 2000), which implies that IOR is represented in a supramodal map of space, dovetails nicely with this "perception-for-action" interpretation of IOR.

Once IOR has been tagged to an object or location in a scene, is the inhibition maintained or lost in the face of subsequent orienting events? Although the tags begin to lose their strength as subsequent locations are cued, IOR can be maintained at multiple locations (Tipper, Weaver, and Watson, 1996; Snyder and Kingstone, 2000). Paul and Tipper (2003) recently demonstrated a greater capacity for storing inhibitory tags when objects, rather than locations in empty space, had been cued.

Functional significance

Posner and Cohen (1984) suggested that by discouraging orienting toward previously attended locations in a scene, IOR might serve as a novelty-seeking mechanism. Klein (1988) extended this suggestion, hypothesizing that by biasing orienting away from previously attended locations in the environment, IOR could serve to facilitate visual search when the target does not pop out. Indeed, the conventional view of serial self-terminating search implies the operation of just such a mechanism. Several of the properties reviewed in the previous discussion are necessary for IOR to serve this function: the inhibitory tags must be local; they must be coded in environmental (so that they are maintained when we move our eyes) and in object (so that they are maintained when

a)   b)

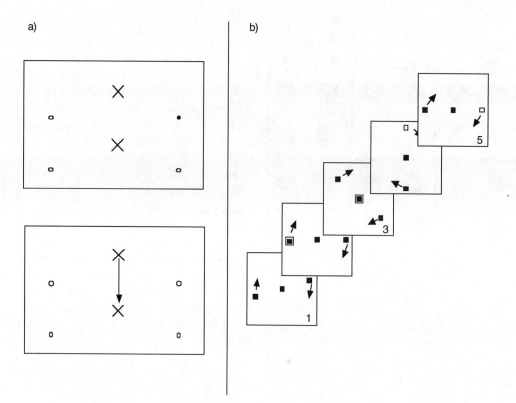

FIGURE 40.4 Methods for revealing environmental and object coding of IOR. (*a*) The method used by Maylor and Hockey (1985). At the start of a trial the participant fixated the upper fixation point (X), while four LEDs are positioned below at the corners of a 24° × 9° rectangle. One of the upper two LEDs was flashed briefly, and its offset was a signal for the participant to move his or her eyes down to the lower fixation point. Between 900 and 1300 ms after the onset of the cue, the target (any one of the four LEDs) was presented. Environmental IOR was tested when the target LED was the same as the cue LED. In this example, presenting the target at the bottom right LED would test for oculocentric IOR. (*b*) The method used by Tipper and colleagues (1991). An animated sequence was presented beginning with frame 1. One of the two peripheral boxes was cued when a horizontal arrangement was achieved. As the peripheral boxes continued to move, the central box was cued. The target (a white square superimposed on one of the black objects) was presented when the objects had rotated 90° from their originally cued position (panel 4) or 180° (panel 5) or 270° (not shown).

the objects we inspect move) coordinates; they must last long enough (several seconds) to operate during typical search episodes; and there must be several tags, so that multiple objects or regions can be inhibited at the same time.

Klein tested this hypothesis by presenting simple detection probes in the locations of search array items (on probes) or in previously empty locations (off probes) following efficient (popout) or inefficient (serial) search. If array items are inspected sequentially in the inefficient search task and if each inspection leaves behind an inhibitory tag, then at the time of a target-absent decision, there would be inhibitory tags at the location of each array item. If, however, as the flat search functions suggest, attention is not required in the efficient search task, then the display locations containing items should not be inhibited. The easy search task provides a control for forward masking from array items on the detection probe and for other effects of the array itself. Klein reasoned that if the foraging facilitator hypothesis is correct, then on-probe RT should exceed off-probe RT following serial search by more than it might following popout search,

which is precisely what was found. Although this pattern is not always obtained (Wolfe and Pokorny, 1990; Klein and Taylor, 1994), it has since been replicated in several other laboratories. As suggested by Tipper and colleagues (1994), a critical variable is whether the search array is removed before the probe is delivered (Müller and von Mühlenen, 2000; Takeda and Yagi, 2000). When a relatively rich scene is presented, the inhibition is more likely to be tagged to objects in the scene than to locations in space (Tipper, Jordan, and Weaver, 1999), and hence removal of the search array is likely to remove the inhibitory tags.

Klein and MacInnes (1999) monitored eye movements while participants searched complex scenes for a camouflaged target. Consistent with the operation of IOR in this difficult search task, when search was interrupted by the reappearance of the fixation disk, saccadic RT to foveate these probes was slower when they were presented in the region of a previous fixation. This dependence of saccadic RT on the angular distance between the probe and a previous fixation was absent if the scene was removed when the probe was presented, a finding that strongly supports the proposal that with complex scenes, the inhibition is scene-based rather than space-based. Freely made search saccades in this study were biased away from preceding fixations. This bias might be caused by IOR, or IOR might be caused by this oculomotor bias. Strongly favoring IOR as the causal agent, a similar pattern was obtained when MacInnes and Klein (2003) discouraged active oculomotor preparation at the time of the probe by asking their subjects to search for something interesting and stop there (see also McCarley et al., 2003).

If the foraging facilitator proposal is correct (see Horowitz and Wolfe, 2003, for a view of search in which it is unnecessary), then individuals who show greater IOR (reflecting a more efficacious inhibitory tagging system) should, all other things being equal, excel at serial visual search. Separate studies of search (O'Riordan et al., 2001) and IOR (Brian, 2000) in autistic individuals appear to confirm this expectation. O'Riordan and colleagues (2001) found that compared with controls, autistic subjects showed shallower search slopes (faster search) in difficult search, while Brian (2000) found larger magnitudes of IOR in autistic than in control participants. This relationship should be regarded cautiously until it is confirmed in a single study in which IOR and search efficiency are assessed in the same individuals.

Development

Johnson (1990) generated a remarkable set of observations about the development of orienting based on the relative rates of development of the neural systems involved. Subsequent behavioral studies of orienting in infants have, for the most part, confirmed Johnson's predictions. Two methods have been used to elicit orienting in infants: a covert method, in which a peripheral stimulus is presented briefly enough that a saccade is not initiated to foveate it, or an overt method, in which the peripheral stimulus onset is accompanied by offset of fixation and the subsequent saccade to the peripheral stimulus is followed by a return event to capture gaze back to fixation. Studies of orienting in infants have used overt orienting, or saccadic eye movements, to measure the effects of prior covert or overt orienting events. Following overt orienting, newborns show IOR in the form of slower saccades in the direction of the immediately preceding saccade (Simion et al., 1995; Valenza, Simion, and Umiltà, 1994). Since the superior colliculus (SC) is relatively fully operational in newborns, this observation is consistent with evidence suggesting that the SC is implicated in causing IOR (Rafal et al., 1989). SC activity is regulated by the basal ganglia and substantia nigra. Johnson suggests that this pathway, which comes into play at around 1 month of age, involves perseveration and obligatory attention (Johnson, Posner, and Rothbart, 1994). Perseveration tends to work against IOR; hence the IOR that is seen in newborns is absent in 1–2-month olds (Clohessy et al., 1991; Johnson, 1994; Johnson and Tucker, 1996; Butcher, Kalverboer, and Geuze, 1999). With the subsequent development of cortical systems, control is gained over the subcortical regulation of the SC by the basal ganglia/substantia nigra pathway, and overt IOR reappears (Clohessy et al., 1991; Harman, Posner, and Rothbart, 1994; Johnson and Tucker, 1996) and covert IOR emerges (Hood, 1993; Johnson, 1994; Butcher, Kalverboer, and Geuze, 1999).

Brain damage

Early observations on patients with subcortical damage due to progressive supranuclear palsy and cortical lesions involving the parietal and frontal lobes suggested that subcortical but not cortical systems were involved in the manifestation of IOR (e.g., Posner et al., 1985). More recent studies have confirmed a critical role for the SC in causing IOR and have begun to paint an interesting picture of cortical involvement. Sapir and colleagues (1999) tested a patient with a unilateral lesion of the right SC on the model task shown in figure 40.1a. Leftward eye movements are mediated by the right SC. Hence, the absence of IOR in the temporal visual field of the left eye and the nasal visual field of the right eye in this patient with preservation of IOR in the opposite direction provides compelling evidence that the neural machinery in the SC is necessary for the generation of IOR (see also Briand, Szapiel, and Sereno, 2003).

Because the SC represents space in oculocentric coordinates, the tags generated by it must be transferred to cortical structures able to preserve them as the eyes or the previously attended objects move through space. Providing strong support for such cortical involvement, Tipper and colleagues (1997) demonstrated that object-tagged IOR, which is preserved following object motion within the visual fields (hence hemispheres) of two split-brain patients, does not cross between them. The need for an intact corpus callosum to transfer inhibitory tags from one hemisphere to the other points to a cortical substrate for representing IOR in object-based coordinates, but it does not tell us what this substrate is.

Recently, Sapir and colleagues (2004) tested patients with damage to the intraparietal sulcus on a version of the cuing paradigm used by Maylor and Hockey (1985) to establish the environmental coding of IOR. Following a cue above or below fixation, participants maintained fixation or made a saccade left or right in response to a foveal arrow. Patients and normal subjects showed similar amounts of IOR in the stationary condition. In the movement conditions the target could be presented at the retinal or environmental location of the cue. Controls showed IOR for targets presented in both reference frames, but patients with right parietal damage only showed IOR at the retinal location of the cue.

This finding supports the suggestion (Klein, 2000) that the parietal lobes may be responsible for preserving inhibitory tags laid down by the SC and is consistent with evidence that regions of the parietal cortex mediate remapping of space in anticipation of saccades (Duhamel, Colby, and Goldberg, 1992). Whether the same brain structures will be shown to be involved in object-based coding of IOR remains to be determined.

Transcranial magnetic stimulation (TMS), which can be used to temporarily disable a region of cortex, is a powerful tool for cognitive neuroscience (Walsh and Pascual-Leone, 2003). Ro, Farnez, and Chang (2003) were the first to apply this technique to IOR. After localizing the right frontal eye field (FEF), TMS was applied at 200 ms and 600 ms following a peripheral cue. In separate blocks, TMS over the right superior parietal lobule was used as a control. The cue–target SOA was 750 ms, and the target called for a manual localization response. TMS decreased mean RT from 338 ms to 312 ms, no doubt because of the arousing effect of the sound of the TMS pulse. In the absence of TMS, IOR averaged about 18 ms. IOR was more or less unaffected by parietal lobe deactivation. FEF deactivation eliminated IOR when the pulse was delivered 600 ms after the cue (150 ms prior to a target), but only when the target was on the right (that is, ipsilateral to the disabled FEF). Ro and colleagues' (2003) interpretation is that to avoid foveating the cue, a saccade program is generated, via the FEF, that is opposite in direction from the saccade activated by the cue, and this FEF activity countermands overt orienting to the cue. It is critical to this proposal that the deleterious effect of ipsilateral FEF stimulation is seen only when this stimulation is delivered late, close to when the IOR will be measured. It is implicitly assumed from the biphasic pattern normally seen in performance (figure 40.1b) that IOR is not present during the earlier intervals, and therefore that the FEF's countermanding activity has not yet been activated.

Whereas Ro and colleagues' application of TMS to IOR is praiseworthy, there are a variety of weaknesses in this proposal. First, if the FEF's countermanding activity prevents overt orienting to the cue, should not a cue-directed saccade be a consequence of FEF disruption? Second, if, as suggested in the next section (see figure 40.8), IOR starts with the cue, then the earlier (200 ms) FEF stimulation should also eliminate ipsilateral IOR. Third, IOR is robustly obtained in a target–target paradigm when responses (whether manual localization, as used here, or saccades) are made successively (Maylor and Hockey, 1985; Taylor and Klein, 2000). In this situation the FEF would be working with the SC (not counteracting it), and therefore, according to Ro's countermanding FEF proposal, IOR should not be observed.

It is important to remember that the region targeted by TMS is part of a larger network, and that an effect on behavior from stimulation of one region could arise because modules not directly stimulated are nevertheless disrupted by virture of the anomalous signals received from the stimulated module. This possibility suggests the following explanation of Ro et al.'s findings. FEF stimulation transiently disrupts a brain structure where the effects of IOR are normally imposed on target processing. In contrast, the inhibitory tags are stored in a system that is unaffected by this stimulation. Hence, when all the transiently disrupted structures recover, which they have time to do when the pulse is early (550 ms before the target, 200 ms post-cue), the inhibitory effects on behavior are reinstated. According to this proposal, IOR was temporarily disrupted by the early TMS pulse, and had IOR been assessed 150 ms later, at 350 ms, its disruption would have been observed.

Neuroimaging

Three techniques, differing dramatically in their spatial and temporal precision, for imaging neural activity have begun to be used to explore the neural implementation and representation of IOR: event-related potentials (ERPs), functional magnetic resonance imaging (fMRI), and single-unit recording. Although one fMRI exploration has been directly aimed at IOR (Lepsien and Pollman, 2002), because of its low temporal resolution, this neuroimaging method is not particularly well-suited for drawing firm conclusions. Based on the typical finding that IOR is observed in target processing at long but not short cue–target SOAs, to isolate IOR, Lepsien and Pollman (2002) subtracted cued and uncued trials when there was a long cue–target SOA from cued and uncued trials when the SOA was short:

(valid/SOA 500 msec + invalid/SOA 500 msec)
   − (valid/SOA 100 msec + invalid/SOA 100 msec)

Because IOR may be present from cue onset and is just as likely to follow a target as to follow a cue (e.g., Taylor and Klein, 2000), there is little ground for thinking that the differences revealed by this subtraction reflect IOR. Since one difference between the long and short cue–target SOAs is the time following an exogenous cue during which it would be necessary to maintain fixation, it seems likely that the imaging results of this study reflect mechanisms used to suppress oculomotor behavior during this interval.

Several papers have recorded ERPs in versions of the model task described earlier (Hopfinger and Mangun, 1998, 2001; McDonald, Ward, and Kiehl, 1999; Prime and Ward, 2004). Whereas it is limited in its spatial resolution, this imaging modality's high temporal resolution makes it particularly valuable to shed light on the stages of processing that are affected by IOR. Because the methodological similarities among these studies are greater than their differences, their data have been combined and subjected to a meta-analysis (figure 40.5). An early ERP component, P1,

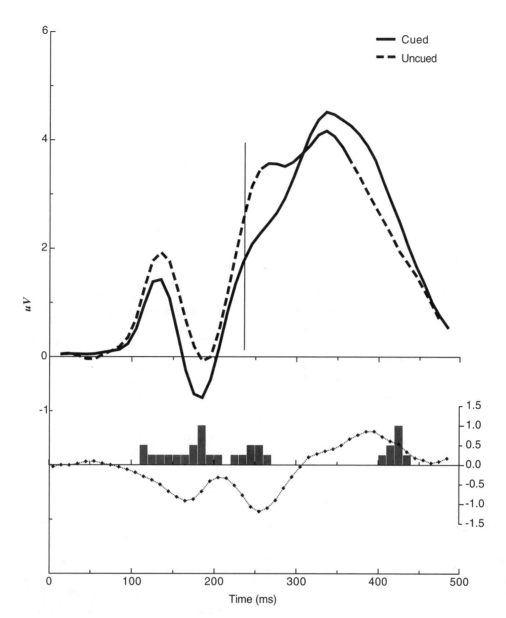

FIGURE 40.5   The data from the occipitally recorded ERP wave-forms from six conditions of four studies (Hopfinger and Mangun, 1998, 2001, long ISI; McDonald et al., 1999, Experiment 1, 500–700 SOAs; Experiment 1, 900–1100 ms SOAs, and Experiment 3; Prime and Ward, 2004) was extracted from the authors' figures. When separated by hemifield of target and/or hemisphere of recording electrode, the data were collapsed to yield two waveforms for each experiment, one for cued targets and one for uncued targets. The data in the upper plot show the grand average of these waveforms (with each experiment weighted equally). The vertical line shows the point in time beyond which the data are based on only five data sets (because one study did not report ERPs beyond this point). The curve in the lower plot is the difference waveform (cued minus uncued), and the histogram reveals where, based on *t*-tests with each study contributing one pair of values, the difference is significant. The heights of the bars represent *P* values of 0.01 (large), 0.025 (medium), and 0.05 (small). Note that for the grand average waveforms, positive is plotted upward.

thought to reflect sensory extraction processing stages was reduced at the cued location in all the experiments (although in one experiment the reduction was not significant). This difference, also describable as an increased negativity for cued targets, extends from about 125 ms to about 250 ms. Although the post-P1 increased negativity for cued targets is reminiscent of the N2pc component that reflects attentional selectivity (Hopfinger, Luck, and Hillyard, this volume), we must be cautious in the inferences we draw. First, the N2pc "signature" is contralateral, whereas the IOR effect shown in figure 40.5 was occasionally stronger when ipsilateral than when contralateral to target. Second, a confident source localization of this ERP reflection of IOR has not yet been achieved.

One of these ERP studies (Prime and Ward, 2004) was designed to test the idea that IOR involves inhibited responding (Tassinari et al., 1987) using the lateralized readiness potential that is linked to response activation (e.g., Miller, 1998). As for RT, the onset of the LRP was delayed for cued targets. When time-locked to the response, however, the LRP was unaffected by cuing, leading the authors to conclude that IOR in this task does not preactivate responding in the uncued direction (or delay responding in the cued direction).

Of the neuroimaging modalities that have focused on IOR, single-unit recording has yielded the most useful evidence for developing a computationally explicit model of how the inhibitory effects are caused and represented in the nervous system. The first study to explicitly examine single-unit responses in an effort to understand the neural implementation of IOR was conducted by Dorris and colleagues (1998, 2002). As illustrated in figure 40.6, recording from the superficial and intermediate layers of the SC, Dorris and colleagues (2002) observed a greatly reduced sensory response to targets presented at a previously cued as compared to a previously uncued location. This reduction was shown to be correlated, on a trial-by-trial basis, with saccadic reaction times to the targets. Importantly, residual activity following the cue was not suppressed, and when electrical stimulation was delivered through the recording electrode to elicit a saccade, the latency of these electrically evoked saccades was actually faster when the cued region was stimulated. These two findings demonstrate that after a cue, the cued region of the SC is not itself inhibited but rather is receiving inputs whose sensory responses are already reduced.

IOR has recently been observed in the response patterns of neurons in the FEFs (Bichot and Schall, 2002). Monkeys were trained to make a saccade to a singleton target appearing in evenly spaced arrays of four or six items centered about fixation. When the target on a trial happened to be in the same location as on the preceding trial, saccadic RT was 17.1 ms slower than when the location changed. Although

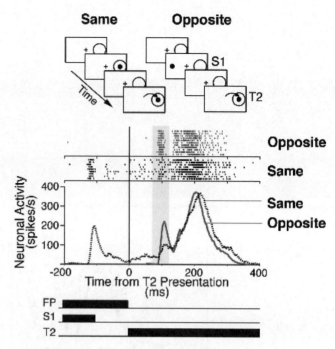

FIGURE 40.6 The sequence of events for same (or cued) and opposite (uncued) trials is shown on the top, where the open circle represents the receptive field of the cell being recorded from and the solid black circles represent the cue (S1) and target (T2). The arrow represents the saccadic response to the target. The timing of the events is shown at bottom. The results from a typical visuo-motor cell recorded from the intermediate layers of the SC is shown in the middle, with trial-by-trial data (rasters) plotted above the average firing rates. For both the individual trials and the average firing rates, data from the opposite condition are plotted in dark gray and data from the same condition are plotted in black (dotted line for the average activity). (From Dorris et al., 2002.)

the response of an FEF neuron to an item in its receptive field was not as greatly affected by the presence of IOR as was the case for SC neurons (figure 40.7a), the neuronal response rates discriminated targets from distracters in their receptive fields 16 ms later when the previous target had been in its receptive field (figure 40.7b). In other words, one effect of IOR is to cause a small delay in stimulus encoding by FEF neurons.

As noted earlier, behavioral data might not distinguish between two dramatically different interpretations of when, in relation to the eliciting event, signals begin to be inhibited: with onset of the eliciting event or when attention is withdrawn from it. A neuroscientific approach, wherein we examine time-locked activity in structures that are affected by IOR, can address this question. The behavioral (upper panel) and single-unit (lower panel) data from two studies of SC activity in a peripheral cuing task are combined in figure 40.8. Because of the differences between these studies,[2] a dedicated empirical attack on this question, without such differences, would be welcome. Nevertheless, none of the differences is particularly challenging to the conclusion these

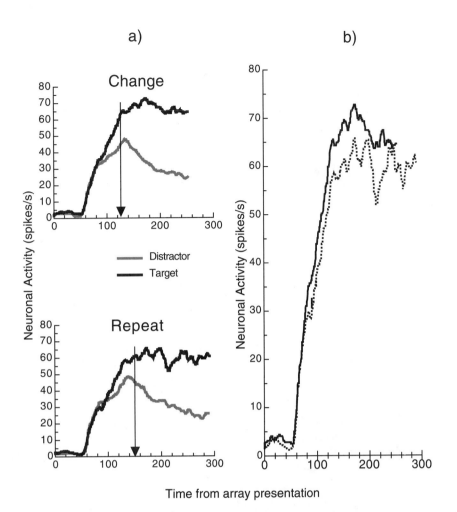

a) Change

b)

Distractor
Target

Repeat

Time from array presentation

FIGURE 40.7   Single-unit data recorded from the frontal eye fields of two monkeys performing a sequence of singleton search trials. (*a*) Neural activity when either the singleton target (black lines) or a distracter was presented in the cell's receptive field. The vertical arrows show that time at which the cell reliably distinguished between targets and distracters. The upper panel shows data from all trials when the preceding target was presented in a different location; in the lower panel the target location was repeated. (Redrawn from Bichot and Schall, 2002, figure 8.) (*b*) The target data from *a* were extracted and plotted as a function of whether the target was repeating or changing locations from the previous target.

data warrant: IOR begins with the cue. As can be seen in the behavioral data, early facilitation is followed by later IOR. Yet the sensory responses of colliculus neurons are reduced at a previously cued (as compared to uncued) location over most of the time period explored, and, most important, even at the shortest cue–target interval when facilitation was observed.

If search slopes in inefficient search reflect the time spent on each item in a self-terminating process, then the reinspection-discouraging tags would need to be in play sooner than illustrated in figures 40.1 and 40.2. Both the neuroscience data showing that IOR is present within 50 ms of an uninformative peripheral cue and Danziger and Kingstone's finding that IOR can be seen in behavior within 50 ms of a cue that elicits a rapid switch of attention (as in search) show that the time course seen in the model paradigm is not necessarily pertinent to search, and undermine any arguments against the foraging-facilitator proposal based on the relatively slow appearance of IOR derived from this paradigm (Horowitz and Wolfe, 2003).

Looking ahead

It has barely been 20 years since IOR was discovered. As our appreciation of the complexity of its behavioral manifestations has grown, so too have the range and power of the methods that have been aimed at revealing its neural implementation. What is most needed to advance our cognitive neuroscientific understanding are some comprehensive and computationally explicit theories of the inhibitory aftermath of orienting. If implemented as artificial neural network models (e.g., Deco and Schürmann, 2000; Trappenberg et al., 2001), such theories would be guided by single-unit recording data and, reciprocally, would guide single-unit

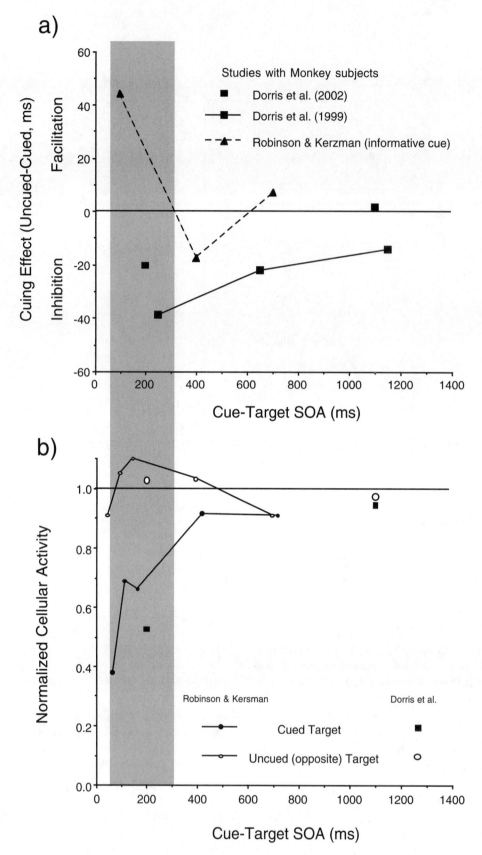

FIGURE 40.8 (a) The effect of a spatial precue on saccadic latencies (shown as SRT to cued targets minus SRT to uncued targets)
is plotted as a function of the SOA between cue and target. Data
from our studies in rhesus monkeys (solid squares) in a cue-saccade
paradigm that used uninformative peripheral cues are plotted
together with the data from Robinson and Kerzman (1995), who
used informative peripheral cues (solid triangles, dotted line). (b)
Activity of colliculus cells from these two studies as a function of
cue condition (cued = same; uncued = opposite) and cue–target
SOA. Data have been normalized to the mean activity in the
uncued condtion (= 1.0). (Redrawn from Klein and colleagues,
2001.)

explorations. It is clear that a viable model of this type must include a hierarchy of modules to implement the cause, representation, storage, and transformation of the inhibitory tags, as well as the multiplicity of effects they may have on subsequent processing. Guided by such neurocognitive models, studies of development, brain damage (including reversible neural disruption, neurochemical or magnetic), and neuroimaging will generate even more fruitful and exciting data than they have yielded to date.

NOTES

1. Some investigators have combined peripheral cuing with an instruction or incentive to attend endogenously. Berlucchi, Chelazzi, and Tassinari (2000), for example, presented uninformative peripheral cues at one of four locations arranged horizontally, and in different blocks instructed their participants to attend broadly, to attend the cued location, or to attend an uncued location with a certain relationship to the cued location. They found a remarkable additivity between the facilitatory effect of the instruction and the inhibitory effect of the cue, from which they concluded "a coexistence of attention and an undiminished IOR at the same location" (p. 658).

2. Like Dorris and colleagues (2002), Robinson and Kerzman (1995) observed attenuation of SC stimulus-related activity in a covert attention task. Their study differed in several important respects from ours. Their cues were informative about the likely location of the target. In the IOR literature, uninformative cues have been used because of the presumption that IOR will not be observed and may not even be generated until attention is removed from the cued location (this was implicit in Posner and Cohen's methods and has been demonstrated by Wright and Richard, 2000). Therefore, this methodological feature was, according to conventional wisdom, not well-suited for obtaining IOR behaviorally (this was not a problem for Robinson and Kerzman, who were not looking for IOR). Second, as reported in much of the attention and IOR literature on humans, Robinson and Kerzman's monkeys made a manual detection response to the target onset, whereas ours made saccades to the targets. Finally, whereas the shortest cue–target SOA we used was 200 ms, Robinson and Kerzman used SOAs as short as 100 ms for their behavioral observations and 50 ms in their assessment of neural activity.

REFERENCES

Abrams, R. A., and R. S. Dobkin, 1994. Inhibition of return: Effects of attentional cuing on eye movement latencies. *J. Exp. Psychol. Hum. Percept. Perform.* 20:467–477.

Abrams, R. A., and J. Pratt, 2000. Oculocentric coding of inhibited eye movements to recently attended locations. *J. Exp. Psychol. Hum. Percept. Perform.* 26:776–788.

Bennett, P. J., and J. Pratt, 2001. The spatial distribution of inhibition of return. *Psychol. Sci.* 12:76–80.

Berlucchi, G., L. Chelazzi, and G. Tassinari, 2000. Volitional covert orienting to a peripheral cue does not suppress cue-induced inhibition of return. *J. Cogn. Neurosci.* 12:648–663.

Bichot, M. P., and J. D. Schall, 2002. Priming in macaque frontal cortex during popout visual search: Feature-based facilitation and location-based inhibition of return. *J. Neurosci.* 22:4675–4685.

Brian, J., 2000. *Inhibition in Autism: Evidence of Excessive Inhibition-of-Return.* Doctoral diss., York University, Toronto, Ontario.

Briand, K. A., S. V. Szapiel, and A. B. Sereno, 2003. Disruption of reflexive visual orienting in an individual with a collicular lesion.

Broadbent, D. E., 1958. *Perception and Communication.* Oxford, England: Pergamon Press.

Brodeur, D. A., and J. T. Enns, 1997. Covert visual orienting across the lifespan. *Can. J. Exp. Psychol.* 51:20–35.

Butcher, P. R., A. F. Kalverboer, and R. H. Geuze, 1999. Inhibition of return in very young infants: A longitudinal study. *Infant Behav. Dev.* 22:303–319.

Castel, A. D., A. L. Chasteen, C. T. Scialfa, and J. Pratt, 2003. Adult age differences in the time course of inhibition of return. *J. Gerentol. Serres B: Psychol. Sci. Soc. Sci.* 58:256–259.

Cheal, M. L., G. Chastain, and D. R. Lyon, 1998. Inhibition of return in identification tasks. *Vis. Cogn.* 5:365–388.

Christie, J. J., and R. M. Klein, 2001. Negative priming for spatial location? *Can. J. Exp. Psychol.* 55:24–38.

Clohessy, A. B., M. I. Posner, M. K. Rothbart, and S. P. Vecera, 1991. The development of inhibition of return in early infancy. *J. Cogn. Neurosci.* 3:345–350.

Danziger, S., and A. Kingstone, 1999. Unmasking the inhibition of return phenomenon. *Percept. Psychophys.* 61:1024–1037.

Deco, G., and B. Schürmann, 2000. A hierarchical neural system with attentional top-down enhancement of the spatial resolution for object recognition. *Vision Res.* 40:2845–2859.

Dorris, M. C., S. Everling, R. M. Klein, and D. P. Munoz, 1998. Neuronal correlate of inhibition of return (IOR): Visual and motor preparatory signals in the monkey superior colliculus. Presented at a meeting of the Society for Neuroscience, Los Angeles, Calif.

Dorris, M. C., R. M. Klein, S. Everling, and D. P. Munoz, 2002. Contribution of the primate superior colliculus to inhibition of return. *J. Cogn. Neurosci.* 148:1256–1263.

Dorris, M. C., T. Taylor, R. M. Klein, and D. P. Munoz, 1999. Influence of previous visual stimulus or saccade on saccadic reaction times in monkey. *J. Neurophysiol.* 81:2429–2436.

Duhamel, J. R., C. L. Colby, and M. E. Goldberg, 1992. The updating of the representation of visual space in parietal cortex by intended eye movements. *Science* 255:90–92.

Faust, M. E., and D. A. Balota, 1997. Inhibition of return and visuospatial attention in healthy older adults and individuals with dementia of the Alzheimer type. *Neuropsychology* 11:13–29.

Garner, W. R., H. W. Hake, and C. W. Eriksen, 1956. Operationism and the concept of perception. *Psychol. Rev.* 63:149–159.

Gilchrist, I. D., A. North, and B. Hood, 2001. Is visual search really like foraging? *Perception* 30:1459–1464.

Handy, T. C., A. P. Jha, and G. R. Mangun, 1999. Promoting novelty in vision: Inhibition of return modulates perceptual-level processing. *Psychol. Sci.* 10:157–161.

Harman, C., M. I. Posner, and M. K. Rothbart, 1994. Development of orienting to locations and objects in human infants. *Can. J. Exp. Psychol.* 48:301–318.

Harvey, N., 1980. Non-informative effects of stimuli functioning as cues. *Q. J. Exp. Psychol.* 32:413–425.

Hood, B., 1993. Inhibition of return produced by covert shifts of visual attention in 6-month-old infants. *Infant Behav. Develop.* 16:245–254.

Hopfinger, J. B., and G. R. Mangun, 1998. Reflexive attention modulates processing of visual stimuli in human extrastriate cortex. *Psychol. Sci.* 9:441–447.

HOPFINGER, J. B., and G. R. MANGUN, 2001. Tracking the influence of reflexive attention on sensory and cognitive processing. *Cogn. Affect. Behav. Neurosci.* 1:56–65.

HOROWITZ, T. S., and J. M. WOLFE, 2003. Memory for rejected distractors in visual search? *Vis. Cogn.* 10:257–298.

HUNT, A. R., and A. KINGSTONE, 2003. Inhibition of return: Dissociating attentional and oculomotor components. *J. Exp. Psychol. Hum. Percept. Perform.* 29:1068–1074.

IVANOFF, J., and R. M. KLEIN, 2001. The presence of a nonresponding effector increases inhibition of return. *Psychonom. Bull. Rev.* 8:307–314.

JAMES, W., 1890. *The Principles of Psychology.* New York: Dover.

JOHNSON, M. H., 1990. Cortical maturation and the development of visual attention in early infancy. *J. Cogn. Neurosci.* 2:81–95.

JOHNSON, M. H., 1994. Visual attention and the control of eye movements in early infancy. In *Attention and Performance XV: Conscious and Unconscious Processing*, C. Umiltà and M. Moscovitch, eds. Cambridge, Mass.: MIT Press, pp. 291–310.

JOHNSON, M. H., M. I. POSNER, and M. K. ROTHBART, 1994. Facilitation of saccades toward a covertly attended location in early infancy. *Psychol. Sci.* 5:90–93.

JOHNSON, M. H., and L. A. TUCKER, 1996. The development and temporal dynamics of spatial orienting in infants. *J. Exp. Child Psychol.* 63:171–188.

JONIDES, J., 1981. Voluntary versus automatic control over the mind's eye's movements. In *Attention and Performance 9*, J. B. Long and A. D. Baddeley, eds. Hillsdale, N. J.: Erlbaum, pp. 187–203.

KHATOON, B., K. A. BRIAND, and A. B. SERENO, 2002. The role of response in spatial attention: Direct and indirect stimulus response mappings. *Vision Res.* 42:2963–2708.

KINGSTONE, A., and J. PRATT, 1999. Inhibition of return is composed of attentional and oculomotor processes. *Percept. Psychophys.* 61:1046–1054.

KLEIN, R. M., 1988. Inhibitory tagging system facilitates visual search. *Nature* 334:430–431.

KLEIN, R. M., 2000. Inhibition of return. *Trends Cogn. Sci.* 4:138–147.

KLEIN, R. M., in press. On the role of endogenous orienting in the inhibitory aftermath of exogenous orienting. In *Developing Individuality in the Human Brain: A Tribute to Michael Posner*, U. Mayr, E. Awh and S. Keele, eds. Washington, D. C.: APA Books.

KLEIN, R. M., and B. DICK, 2002. Temporal dynamics of reflexive attention shifts: A dual-stream rapid serial visual presentation exploration. *Psychol. Sci.* 13:176–179.

KLEIN, R. M., A. KINGSTONE, and A. PONTEFRACT, 1992. Orienting of visual attention. In *Eye Movements and Visual Cognition: Scene Perception and Reading*, K. Rayner, ed. New York: Springer-Verlag, pp. 46–67.

KLEIN, R. M., and W. J. MACINNES, 1999. Inhibition of return is a foraging facilitator in visual search. *Psychol. Sci.* 10:346–352.

KLEIN, R. M., D. P. MUNOZ, M. DORRIS, and T. TAYLOR, 2001. Inhibition of return in monkey and man. In *Attraction, Distraction, and Action: Multiple Perspectives on Attentional Capture*, C. Folk and B. Gibson, eds. Elsevier Science, pp. 27–47.

KLEIN, R. M., and A. PONTEFRACT, 1994. Does oculomotor readiness mediate cognitive control of visual attention? Revisited! In *Attention and Performance XV: Conscious and Unconscious Processing*, C. Umiltà and M. Moscovitch, eds. Cambridge, Mass.: MIT Press, pp. 333–350.

KLEIN, R. M., and T. L. TAYLOR, 1994. Categories of cognitive inhibition with reference to attention. In *Inhibitory Processes in Attention, Memory and Language*, D. Dagenbach and T. Carr, eds. San Diego, Calif.: Academic Press, pp. 113–150.

LARRISON-FAUCHER, A., K. A. BRIAND, and A. B. SERENO, 2002. Delayed onset of inhibition of return in schizophrenia. *Progr. Neuro-psychopharmacol. Biol. Psychiatry* 26:505–512.

LEPSIEN, J., and S. POLLMANN, 2002. Covert reorienting and inhibition of return: An event-related fMRI study. *J. Cogn. Neurosci.* 14:127–144.

LUPIANEZ, J., E. G. MILAN, F. J. TORNAY, E. MADRID, and P. TUDELA, 1997. Does IOR occur in discrimination tasks? Yes, it does, but later. *Percept. Psychophys.* 59:1241–1254.

LUPIANEZ, J., B. MILLIKEN, and C. SOLANO, 2001. On the strategic modulation of the time course of facilitation and inhibition of return. *Q. J. Exp. Psychol. Hum. Exp. Psychol.* 54A:753–773.

MACINNES, W. J., and R. M. KLEIN, 2003. Inhibition of return biases orienting during the search of complex scenes. *Sci. World J.* 3:75–86.

MACPHERSON, A. C., R. M. KLEIN, and C. M. MOORE, 2003. Inhibition of return in children and adolescents. *J. Exp. Child Psychol.* 85:337–351.

MAYLOR, E. A., and R. HOCKEY, 1985. Inhibitory component of externally controlled covert orienting in visual space. *J. Exp. Psychol. Hum. Percept. Perform.* 11:777–787.

McCARLEY, J. S., R. F. WANG, A. F. KRAMER, D. E. IRWIN, and M. S. PETERSON, 2003. How much memory does oculomotor search have? *Psychol. Sci.* 14:422–426.

McDONALD, J. J., L. M. WARD, and K. A. KIEHL, 1999. An event-related brain potential study of inhibition of return. *Percept. Psychophys.* 61:1411–1423.

MILLER, J., 1998. Effects of stimulus-response probability on choice reaction time: Evidence from the lateralized readiness potential. *J. Exp. Psychol. Hum. Percept. Perform.* 24:1521–1534.

MÜLLER, H., and A. VON MÜHLENEN, 2000. Probing distractor inhibition in visual search. *J. Exp. Psychol. Hum. Percept. Perform.* 26:1591–1605.

O'RIORDAN, M. A., K. C. PLAISTED, J. DRIVER, and S. BARON-COHEN, 2001. Superior visual search in autism. *J. Exp. Psychol. Hum. Percept. Perform.* 27:719–730.

PAUL, M. A., and S. P. TIPPER, 2003. Object-based representations facilitate memory for inhibitory processes. *Exp. Brain Res.* 148:283–289.

POSNER, M. I., 1980. Orienting of attention. *Q. J. Exp. Psychol.* 32:3–25.

POSNER, M. I. 1996. Interaction of arousal and selection in the posterior attention network. In *Attention: Selection, Awareness, and Control*, A. Baddeley and L. Weiskrantz, eds. Oxford, England: Clarendon Press, pp. 390–405.

POSNER, M. I., and Y. COHEN, 1984. Components of visual orienting. In *Attention and Performance X*, H. Bouma and D. G. Bouwhuis, eds. Hillsdale, N.J.: Erlbaum, pp. 531–556.

POSNER, M. I., R. D. RAFAL, L. S. CHOATE, and J. VAUGHAN, 1985. Inhibition of return: Neural basis and function. *Cogn. Neuropsychol.* 2:211–228.

PRIME, D. J., and L. M. WARD, 2004. Inhibition of return from stimulus to response. *Psychol. Sci.* 15:272–276.

RAFAL, R. D., P. A. CALABRESI, C. W. BRENNAN, and T. K. SCIOLTO, 1989. Saccade preparation inhibits reorienting to recently attended locations. *J. Exp. Psychol. Hum. Percept. Perform.* 15:673–685.

REUTER-LORENZ, P. A., A. P. JHA, and J. N. ROSENQUIST, 1996. What is inhibited in inhibition of return? *J. Exp. Psychol. Hum. Percept. Perform.* 22:367–378.

RO, T., A. FARNE, and E. CHANG, 2003. Inhibition of return and the human frontal eye fields. *Exp. Brain Res.* 150:290–296.

ROBINSON, D. L., and C. KERZMAN, 1995. Covert orienting of attention in macaques. III. Contributions of the superior colliculus. *J. Neurophysiol.* 74:713–721.

SAMUEL, A. G., and D. KAT, 2003. Inhibition of return: A graphical meta-analysis of its time course, and an empirical test of its temporal and spatial properties. *Psychonom. Bull. Rev.* 10: 897–906.

SAPIR, A., A. HAYES, A. HENIK, S. DANZIGER, and R. RAFAL, 2004. Parietal lobe lesions disrupt saccadic remapping of inhibitory location tagging. *J. Cogn. Neurosci.* 16:503–509.

SAPIR, A., A. HENIK, M. DOBRUSIN, and E. Y. HOCHMAN, 2001. Attentional asymmetry in schizophrenia: Disengagement and inhibition of return deficits. *Neuropsychology* 5:361–370.

SAPIR, A., N. SOROKER, A. BERGER, and A. HENIK, 1999. Inhibition of return in spatial attention: Direct evidence for collicular generation. *Nat. Neurosci.* 2:1053–1054.

SIMION, F., E. VALENZA, C. UMILTA, and B. DALLA, 1995. Inhibition of return in newborns is temporo-nasal asymmetrical. *Infant Behav. Dev.* 8:189–194.

SNYDER, J. J., and A. KINGSTONE, 2000. Inhibition of return and visual search: How many separate loci are inhibited. *Percept. Psychophys.* 62:452–458.

SNYDER, J. J., W. C. SCHMIDT, and A. KINGSTONE, 2001. Attentional momentum does not underlie the inhibition of return effect. *J. Exp. Psychol. Hum. Percept. Perform.* 27:1420–1432.

SPENCE, C., and J. DRIVER, 1997. On measuring selective attention to a specific sensory modality. *Percept. Psychophys.* 59:389–403.

SPENCE, C., D. LLOYD, F. McGLONE, M. E. R. NICHOLLS, and J. DRIVER, 2000. Inhibition of return is supramodal: A demonstration between all possible pairings of vision, touch, and audition. *Exp. Brain Res.* 134:42–48.

TAKEDA, Y., and A. YAGI, 2000. Inhibitory tagging in visual search can be found if search stimuli remain visible. *Percept. Psychophys.* 62:927–934.

TANAKA, T., and S. SHIMOJO, 1996. Location vs. feature: Reaction time reveals dissociation between two visual functions. *Vision Res.* 36:2125–2140.

TASSINARI, G., S. AGLIOTI, L. CHELAZZI, C. A. MARZI, and G. BERLUCCHI, 1987. Distribution in the visual field of the costs of voluntarily allocated attention and the inhibitory after-effects of covert orienting. *Neuropsychologia* 25:55–71.

TASSINARI, G., and G. BERLUCCHI, 1993. Sensory and attentional components of slowing of manual reaction time to non-fixated visual targets by ipsilateral primes. *Vision Res.* 33:1525–1534.

TAYLOR, T. L., and M. P. W. DONNELLY, 2002. Inhibition of return for target discriminations: The effect of repeating discriminated and irrelevant stimulus dimensions. *Percept. Psychophys.* 64: 292–317.

TAYLOR, T. L., and R. M. KLEIN, 1998. On the causes and effects of inhibition of return. *Psychonom. Bull. Rev.* 5:625–643.

TAYLOR, T. L., and R. M. KLEIN, 2000. Visual and motor effects in inhibition of return. *J. Exp. Psychol. Hum. Percept. Perform.* 26: 1639–1656.

TIPPER, S. P., J. DRIVER, and B. WEAVER, 1991. Object-centred inhibition of return of visual attention. *Q. J. Exp. Psychol. A* 43: 289–298.

TIPPER, S. P., H. JORDAN, and B. WEAVER, 1999. Scene-based and object centered inhibition of return: Evidence for dual orienting mechanisms. *Percept. Psychophys.* 61:50–60.

TIPPER, S. P., R. RAFAL, P. A. REUTER-LORENZ, Y. STARRVELDT, T. RO, R. EGLY, S. DANZIGER, and B. WEAVER, 1997. Object based facilitation and inhibition from visual orienting in the human split brain. *J. Exp. Psychol. Hum. Percept. Perform.* 23:1522–1532.

TIPPER, S. P., B. WEAVER, L. M. JERREAT, and A. L. BURAK, 1994. Object-based and environment-based inhibition of return of visual attention. *J. Exp. Psychol. Hum. Percept. Perform.* 20:478–499.

TIPPER, S. P., B. WEAVER, and F. L. WATSON, 1996. Inhibition of return to successively cued spatial locations: Commentary on Pratt and Abrams 1995. *J. Exp. Psychol. Hum. Percept. Perform.* 22:1289–1293.

TRAPPENBERG, T. P., M. C. DORRIS, D. P. MUNOZ, and R. M. KLEIN, 2001. A model of saccade initiation based on the competitive integration of exogenous and endogenous signals in the superior colliculus. *J. Cogn. Neurosci.* 13:256–271.

VALENZA, E. L., F. L. SIMION, and C. L. UMILTÀ, 1994. Inhibition of return in newborn infants. *Infant Behav. Dev.* 17:293–302.

WALSH, V., and A. PASCUAL-LEONE, 2003. *Transcranial Magnetic Stimulation: A Neurochronometrics of Mind.* Cambridge, Mass.: MIT Press.

WOLFE, J. M., and C. W. POKORNY, 1990. Inhibitory tagging in visual search: A failure to replicate. *Percept. Psychophys.* 48: 357–362.

WRIGHT R, D., and RICHARD, C. M. 2000. Location cue validity affects inhibition of return of visual processing. *Visi. Res.* 40: 2351–2358.

YI, D.-J., M-S. KIM, and M. M. CHUN, 2003. Inhibition of return to occluded objects. *Percept. Psychophys.* 65:122–130.

41 Selective Attention: Electrophysiological and Neuromagnetic Studies

JOSEPH B. HOPFINGER, STEVEN J. LUCK, AND STEVEN A. HILLYARD

ABSTRACT In order to manage the abundance of incoming sensory information from the natural world, the human visual system employs an array of attentional mechanisms capable of selecting relevant information at multiple stages of processing. Recent visual attention experiments using noninvasive recordings of brain activity have clarified the nature of the underlying mechanisms of selection. In particular, recordings of event-related brain potentials (ERPs) and event-related magnetic fields (ERFs) have provided timing information that is critical for understanding the dynamic operation of different attentional processes. In some cases, these ERP and ERF recording have been combined with parallel neuroimaging studies to yield a more complete spatiotemporal picture of the attentional operations under study. These approaches have shed light on the mechanisms underlying spatial attention, visual search, the automatic capture of attention, postperceptual selection, and the voluntary control of attention.

Visuospatial attention

Psychophysical studies show that allocating visual attention to a selected region of the visual field may enhance perception of stimuli at that location (Luck et al., 1994; Luck, Hillyard, et al., 1996; Yeshurun and Carrasco, 1998). The neural basis of this perceptual facilitation has been investigated extensively in both animal and human studies. Considerable progress has been made in identifying the specific cortical areas where spatial attention influences visual processing and in specifying the timing of those selection processes. This research has also led to new proposals about the controversial role of the primary visual cortex (area V1) in attention.

MULTIPLE VISUOCORTICAL AREAS ARE INFLUENCED BY VISUOSPATIAL ATTENTION Recordings of single-unit activity in monkeys have shown that neural responses evoked by attended-location stimuli are enhanced in extrastriate visual areas V2, V3a, V4, and MT, as well as in higher areas in inferotemporal cortex and the posterior parietal lobe (Maunsell and McAdams, 2000; Reynolds and Desimone, 2001). There is also evidence that spatial attention can modulate neural activity in the primary visual cortex (area V1) under certain conditions, such as when multiple competing stimuli are presented (Motter, 1993; Roelfsema, Lamme, and Spekreijse, 1998; Vidyasagar, 1999). These attention-related changes in V1 activity were often found to be delayed well beyond the initial geniculostriate evoked response in V1, however, which suggests that they may be mediated by delayed feedback projections from higher visual areas (Vidyasagar, 1999; Schroeder, Mehta, and Foxe, 2001).

Neuroimaging studies have confirmed the participation of both striate and extrastriate visual areas in spatial attention in humans. Using functional magnetic resonance imaging (fMRI), it was found that directing attention to a stimulus position results in increased neural activity in circumscribed zones of visual areas V1, V2, V3, V3a, and V4 that correspond to the retinotopic projection of the attended location (Tootell et al., 1998; reviewed in Martinez et al., 1999, 2001). Given the limited temporal resolution of fMRI, however, it has been difficult to determine whether these attention-related increases in activity represent an enhancement of early sensory-evoked responses, a delayed modulation of activity due to feedback from higher areas, or a sustained increase in activity associated with the spatial focusing of attention.

TIME COURSE OF ATTENTIONAL MODULATION The time course of these spatial attention effects in humans has been clarified by recordings of event-related potentials (ERPs) and event-related magnetic fields (ERFs). In the typical experimental design, stimuli are presented in randomized sequences to two (or more) locations in the visual field while the subject pays attention to only one location at a time (figure 41.1). Numerous studies of this type conducted over the past 25 years have shown that stimuli at attended locations typically elicit enlarged positive (P1 at 80–130 ms) and negative (N1 at 150–200 ms) components over the posterior

JOSEPH B. HOPFINGER Department of Psychology, University of North Carolina at Chapel Hill, Chapel Hill, N.C.
STEVEN J. LUCK Department of Psychology, University of Iowa, Iowa City, Iowa.
STEVEN A. HILLYARD Department of Neuroscience, University of California, San Diego, Calif.

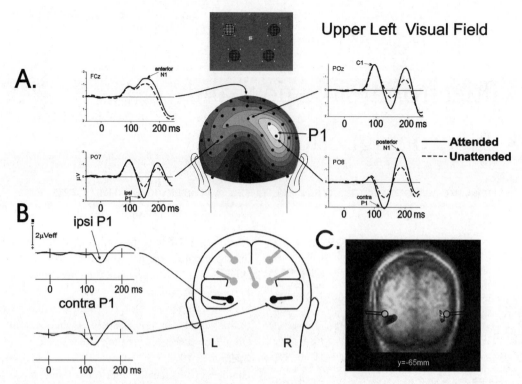

Upper Left Visual Field

— **Attended**
--- **Unattended**

FIGURE 41.1 (*A*) Averaged ERPs recorded from four scalp sites in response to stimuli in the upper left visual field in a spatial attention experiment by Di Russo, Martinez, and Hillyard (2003). Positive is plotted downward in all figures. Stimuli were small circular checkerboards flashed in random order to the upper left and right visual fields while subjects attended to one field at a time. Superimposed ERP waveforms compare conditions when the upper left stimuli were attended (solid lines) versus when stimuli in the opposite field were attended (dashed lines). Note that the P1 (80–130 ms) and N1 (140–200 ms) components are enhanced in amplitude by spatial attention. Head with voltage map shows the contralateral occipital scalp distribution of the late phase of the P1 (100–130 ms) that is enhanced by attention. (*B*) Dipole model of the neural sources of the enhanced contralateral and ipsilateral P1 components indicates neural generators in ventral occipital cortex. (*C*) Coregistration of dipolar sources of the enhanced P1 with fMRI activations (shaded spots) in the ventral fusiform gyrus obtained from the same subjects performing the same experiment in a different session.

scalp, relative to stimuli at unattended locations (reviewed in Hillyard and Anllo-Vento, 1998; Luck and Hillyard, 2000). As illustrated in figure 41.1, these amplitude modulations of the P1 and N1 components usually occur with little or no change in component latencies or scalp distributions (Mangun, 1995; Di Russo, Martinez, and Hillyard, 2003), suggesting that the voluntary focusing of attention involves a gain control or amplification mechanism within the early visual pathways (Hillyard, Vogel, and Luck, 1998). The general idea of a gain control mechanism is also supported by single-unit (Reynolds, Chelazzi, and Desimone, 1999) and psychophysical studies (Lu and Dosher, 1998). Increasing the sensory gain at a given location may enhance perception by increasing the size of small sensory signals relative to the brain's internal noise (Hawkins et al., 1990) or by giving the attended location a competitive advantage over ignored locations (Desimone and Duncan, 1995).

The neural generators of the attention-sensitive P1 and N1 components have been localized through dipole source modeling and coregistration with positron emission tomog-raphy (PET) and fMRI data to specific zones of extrastriate visuocortical areas (figures 41.1 and 41.2; Heinze et al., 1994; Mangun et al., 1997; Martinez et al., 1999, 2001; Di Russo et al., 2001; Di Russo, Martinez, and Hillyard, 2003). As illustrated in figure 41.2, the initial phase of the P1 (at 80–100 ms) appears to originate from mid-occipital regions in or near areas V3/V3a and the immediately anterior middle occipital gyrus, while the later phase of the P1 (at 100–130 ms) appears to arise from ventral occipital cortex in or near area V4 and the adjacent fusiform gyrus (DiRusso et al., 2001). The N1 was also found to arise from multiple generators, including an early posterior parietal phase (140–160 ms) and a later ventral occipital-temporal phase (160–200 ms). Thus, the earliest modulations of visual-evoked neural activity by the spatial focusing of attention were found to occur at multiple sites along the extrastriate visual pathways.

ROLE OF PRIMARY VISUAL CORTEX   ERP and ERF recordings have been informative about the way in which spatial

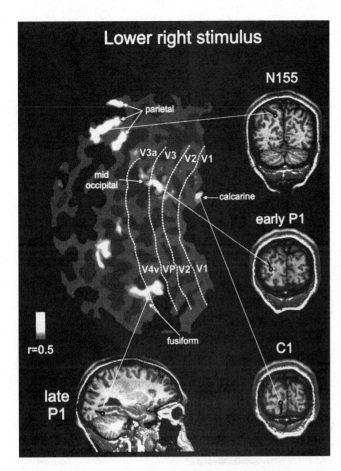

FIGURE 41.2 Spatial correspondence between calculated positions of dipoles accounting for different components of the visual ERP (based on grand average waveforms) and fMRI activations in response to the same stimuli in a single subject. fMRI activations in response to circular checkerboard stimuli flashed to the lower right visual field are projected onto a flattened cortical representation of the left hemisphere. Dashed white lines represent the boundaries between the different visual areas determined by visual field sign mapping. Coronal and saggital sections display those activations (before flattening) that correspond in position to the dipoles representing the different components. (Reprinted with permission from Di Russo et al., The cortical sources of the early components of the visual evoked potential. *Hum. Brain Mapp.* 15:95–111. © 2001 by John Wiley & Sons, Inc., Publisher.)

attention influences neural activity in area V1. There is good evidence that the earliest visual ERP component (the C1 wave, at 50–60 ms; figure 41.1) represents the initial stimulus-evoked response in area V1 (figure 41.2). The C1 wave inverts in polarity for stimuli in the upper versus lower visual fields, in accordance with the retinotopic organization of area V1 within the calcarine fissure, and dipole modeling has been consistent with a calcarine generator site (Martinez et al., 2001; Noesselt et al., 2002; Di Russo, Martinez, and Hillyard, 2003). In studies to date, the C1 has been found to be unaffected by spatial attention (reviewed in Di Russo, Martinez, and Hillyard, 2003) or by attention to other visual features such as spatial frequency (Martinez et al., 2001) or

color (Anllo-Vento, Luck, and Hillyard, 1998). These findings support the view that the initial feedforward geniculostriate response in area V1 is not subject to attentional control. Dipole modeling studies, however, have provided evidence of a delayed modulation of V1 activity during spatial attention that begins at around 130–160 ms after stimulus onset (Martinez et al., 2001; Noesselt et al., 2002; Di Russo, Martinez, and Hillyard, 2003). This suggests a mechanism whereby selection of attended-location stimuli first occurs in extrastriate cortical areas at a latency of 80–100 ms, as described above, and delayed feedback from these higher areas then modulates neural activity in V1. Support for such attention-related feedback signals comes from neurophysiological studies in monkeys (Lamme and Spekreijse, 2000; Schroeder, Mehta, and Foxe, 2001), and it has been proposed that delayed reentrant activity in area V1 may improve figure–ground segregation and enhance the salience of stimuli at attended locations (Lamme et al., 2000).

DISSOCIABLE MECHANISMS OF VISUOSPATIAL ATTENTION Although the P1 and N1 waves occur in close temporal proximity and are both affected by spatial attention, there are clear indications that these components reflect different aspects of spatial selection. Dissociations between the P1 and N1 components have been observed in trial-by-trial cuing experiments, in which each trial begins with a symbolic cue that directs the subject to attend to the indicated location for that trial. Mangun and Hillyard (1991) found that the N1 component was enhanced for valid targets, relative to invalid targets, only when a discrimination of the target's features was required, whereas the P1 component exhibited a robust attention effect (valid greater than invalid) during both difficult discrimination and simple detection tasks. A dissociation between the P1 and N1 was also obtained by Luck and colleagues (1994), who compared ERPs from stimuli at attended and ignored locations with ERPs on neutral (baseline) trials in which attention was diffusely distributed. Compared to baseline trials, the P1 was found to be suppressed at the ignored location but did not show an enhancement at the attended location. In contrast, the N1 was enhanced at the attended location but not suppressed at the ignored location relative to the baseline trials. To account for these effects, Luck (1995) proposed that the P1 effect reflects an early sensory gain control mechanism that suppresses noise at ignored locations, whereas the N1 effect reflects the addition of a limited-capacity discriminative process at the attended location. Subsequent studies have confirmed that the N1 wave, but not the P1 wave, is enhanced when subjects perform discrimination tasks on a stimulus compared to when they make simple detection responses (Vogel and Luck, 2000; for a similar dissociation see Handy and Mangun, 2000). A recent magnetoencephalographic (MEG) study (Hopf et al., 2002) provided evidence that the discriminative processing associated with the N1 component takes place in inferior occipitotemporal cortex of the ventral stream beginning approximately 150 ms after stimulus onset.

Visual search

In the studies described in the previous section, attention was directed to specific locations by explicit verbal instructions or symbolic cues. To study how attention operates when the target location is unknown, attention researchers have used visual search tasks in which subjects try to find a predefined target stimulus within an array of distracters. When the target contains a distinctive feature, it can be detected rapidly, even if many distracters are present. When the target does not contain a distinctive feature, however, search may be slow and effortful, and reaction times may increase as the number of distracters increases. In such cases, some researchers have proposed that attention shifts from object to object until the target is detected (Treisman and Gelade, 1980; Wolfe, 1994). ERP studies of visual search have sought to answer two major questions. First, are the attentional mechanisms that were described in the previous section also used when attention is focused onto an object during visual search? Second, does attention indeed shift serially from object to object in difficult search tasks?

To determine whether sensory processing is enhanced at the attended location in visual search, Luck, Fan, and Hillyard (1993) used visual search arrays containing 14 red items, one blue item, and one green item. Subjects were required to discriminate the form of either the blue item or the green item. To measure sensory processing at the attended location, a task-irrelevant probe square was flashed at the location of either the blue item or the green item shortly (250 ms) after the onset of the search array. By the time of the probe flash, subjects should have localized and focused attention onto the target item. The probe stimulus elicited larger P1 and N1 waves when it was presented at the location of the target item than when it was presented at the location of the nontarget item, just as stimuli presented at explicitly cued locations elicit larger P1 and N1 waves than stimuli presented at uncued locations. Moreover, a follow-up study showed that the P1 effect in visual search reflects suppressed processing at the nontarget location, whereas the N1 effect reflects enhanced processing at the target location (Luck and Hillyard, 1995), in line with the P1/N1 dissociation described earlier. These results suggest that the mechanisms of attention used spontaneously during visual search are basically the same as the mechanisms used when attention is directed by explicit instructions.

The allocation of attention during visual search may also be investigated by examining the ERP waveform elicited by the search array itself. In particular, when attention is directed to an item in a search array, a negative-going ERP component is elicited over the contralateral visual cortex. This ERP component is labeled N2pc (N2-posterior-contralateral) to indicate that it usually occurs in the time range of the N2 family of components (ca. 200–300 ms after the onset of the search array) with a posterior, contralateral scalp distribution. A typical paradigm for eliciting the N2pc component is shown in figure 41.3A. Each search array consists of 15 black distracter items and a white target item in either the left visual field (LVF) or the right visual field (RVF). Subjects make a button-press response to indicate whether the target item is an upright T or an inverted T. This paradigm is designed to allow subjects to shift attention to the target with minimal trial-by-trial variability in latency, which is important when stimulus-locked ERP averages are examined. The N2pc can be visualized by comparing the averaged waveforms calculated for contralateral targets (i.e., left-hemisphere/right-target waveforms averaged with right-hemisphere/left-target waveforms) and for ipsilateral targets (i.e., left-hemisphere/left-target waveforms averaged with right-hemisphere/right-target waveforms). This comparison is shown in figure 41.3B.

Several pieces of evidence indicate that the N2pc component reflects the allocation of attention (see Luck and Hillyard, 1994; Luck et al., 1997). The N2pc may be a human ERP homologue of single-unit attention effects from area V4 and inferotemporal cortex that have been observed in monkeys performing visual search tasks (Chelazzi, Duncan et al., 1998; Chelazzi, Miller et al., 1993, 2001); it has the same timing, and it is similarly influenced by factors such as target type and distracter density (Luck et al., 1997). Consistent with this proposal, a recent MEG study indicated that the N2pc component is generated primarily in occipital-temporal cortex, with a small contribution from posterior parietal cortex (Hopf et al., 2000).

Two major conclusions have emerged from studies of the N2pc component in visual search. First, consistent with Treisman's (1988) feature integration theory, these ERP studies have indicated that greater allocation of attention is required for targets defined by conjunctions of features than for single-feature targets. This conclusion was based on studies showing that the N2pc component was significantly larger in a variety of task situations when subjects performed conjunction discriminations than when they discriminated the presence or absence of a single feature (Luck and Hillyard, 1995; Luck et al., 1997; Luck and Ford, 1998).

The second major conclusion arising from studies of the N2pc component during visual search is that attention does indeed shift serially from object to object during some difficult search tasks. This was inferred from experiments in which the N2pc was found to switch from one hemisphere to the other as attention switched from one visual hemifield to the other (Woodman and Luck, 1999, 2003). The design of these experiments took advantage of the fact that subjects

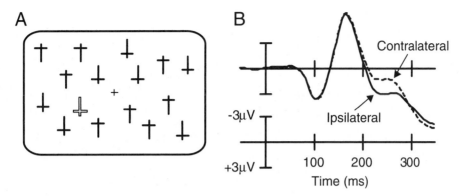

A   B

FIGURE 41.3 Example of typical stimuli (*A*) and ERP waveforms (*B*) in an N2pc experiment. In the task shown here, stimulus arrays consist of 16 upright and inverted T shapes, 15 drawn in black and one drawn in white. Subjects are instructed to attend to the white item and press one of two buttons for each array to indicate whether this item is an upright or inverted T. The ERP waveforms are averaged separately for trials on which the target is ipsilateral versus contralateral to a given electrode site. That is, the ipsilateral waveform consists of left visual field targets for left hemisphere elec-trodes averaged with right visual field targets for right hemisphere electrodes, and the contralateral waveform consists of right visual field targets for left hemisphere electrodes averaged with left visual field targets for right hemisphere electrodes. The contralateral waveform is typically more negative (less positive) from approximately 200–300 ms, and the difference in amplitude between the contralateral and ipsilateral waveforms is used to measure the N2pc component.

spontaneously tend to search items near fixation before searching items far from fixation, even when the objects are scaled according to the cortical magnification factor (Carrasco et al., 1995; Wolfe, O'Neill, and Bennett, 1998). Figure 41.4*A* illustrates one of these experiments, in which two red potential target items were presented among many distracter items; one of the red items was near fixation and the other was far from fixation, and they were equally likely to be the target (a square with a gap on the left). When the two items were in opposite hemifields, subjects should search the near item first and then the far item. Consistent with this, the N2pc was first negative contralateral to the near item, and then it became negative contralateral to the far item (figure 41.4*B*). Thus, attention first switched to the near item at approximately 200 ms post-stimulus and then switched to the far item approximately 100 ms later.

This experiment measured the relative allocation to the near and far items within a single set of ipsilateral and contralateral waveforms; it is therefore possible that subjects actually attended to both the near and far items at the same time, shifting only the relative allocation of attention over time. However, a follow-up study used a slightly different method that allowed the N2pc to be measured separately for the near and far items, and this study demonstrated that the allocation of attention was truly serial: only the near item was attended initially, and after a brief transition period, only the far item was attended (Woodman and Luck, 2003).

Automatic capture of attention

Behavioral research has long made a distinction between voluntary and automatic or reflexive attention systems (e.g., Posner, Nissen, and Ogden, 1978; Jonides, 1981). Voluntary attention refers to the effortful, top-down controlled process wherein one decides where to attend. Reflexive attention, on the other hand, refers to a bottom-up mechanism wherein attention is *captured*—in a rapid and involuntary fashion—by an object or location that has just undergone a salient change. Behavioral data have shown that reflexive attention is engaged more rapidly, is more resistant to interference, and dissipates more quickly than voluntary attention. Furthermore, reflexive attention produces a unique biphasic effect on reaction times. Specifically, attention-capturing cues initially result in faster and more accurate responses to stimuli at the captured location, but at slightly longer delays, subjects are actually slower to respond to stimuli at that location. This phenomenon has been termed *inhibition of return* (IOR; Posner and Cohen, 1984), as attention appears to be inhibited from returning to the location at which it was previously captured (see Klein, 2000, for a comprehensive review). Despite behavioral evidence for the distinction between these systems, studies of the neural mechanisms of attention have focused predominantly on the voluntary system.

Recently, however, ERPs have been used to investigate the mechanisms of reflexive attention. In studies of reflexive attention, the "cue" is typically an abrupt flash or change in the visual scene that is not predictive of the location or type of target stimulus that follows. At short cue-to-target intervals, Hopfinger and Mangun (1998) found that these nonpredictive reflexive cues result in enhanced processing for subsequent stimuli that occurred at the cued location relative to stimuli at uncued locations. Specifically, the P1 component was significantly larger for cued location targets

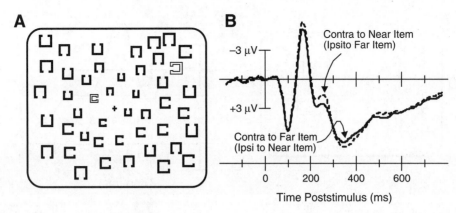

FIGURE 41.4 (A) Stimuli from the study of Woodman and Luck (1999). Subjects searched for a target (a square with a gap on the left side), which was present on 50% of trials. When present, the target was one of the two red items in the array (represented in the figure by white items outlined in black). One of the red items was near fixation and the other was far from fixation. Even though the target was equally likely to be near or far, subjects tend to search the near item first. (B) ERP waveforms from target-absent trials. When the near and far red items were in opposite hemifields, the N2pc first appeared as a negativity contralateral to the near item (ca. 200–300 ms) and then appeared as a negativity contralateral to the far item (ca. 300–400 ms). This pattern is consistent with a serial shifting of attention from nontarget to nontarget.

(figure 41.5A). Furthermore, the enhancement of the P1 component occurred whether subjects were performing a difficult discrimination task (Hopfinger and Mangun, 1998), were engaged in a simple detection task (Hopfinger and Mangun, 2001a), or were viewing task-irrelevant stimuli (Hopfinger, Maxwell, and Mangun, 2000). This pattern of results, combined with the fact that the cue stimuli were non-predictive of target location or target type, suggests that the P1 effect here is due to truly reflexive mechanisms. These results suggest that voluntary and reflexive attention may be able to affect processing at a similar neural locus. However, unlike voluntary attention, reflexive attention has not been found to enhance the N1 component, even in a difficult discrimination task.

Although the facilitatory effects of reflexive orienting on visual processing at short cue-to-target intervals appear to be robust across different task parameters, the conclusions are not yet as clear for the effects at longer interstimulus intervals (ISIs). Several studies have found the P1 amplitude to be reduced to stimuli at cued versus uncued locations at long ISIs (figure 41.5B), but this IOR-like pattern has not always been associated with the strongest behavioral inhibition (Hopfinger and Mangun, 1998, 2001a; McDonald, Ward, and Kiehl, 1999). These studies suggest that an early sensory modulation may not fully explain the IOR phenomenon, which may consist of a combination of sensory and response-related factors (see also Kingstone and Pratt, 1999). The results from ERP experiments, however, do suggest a specific perceptual-level locus at which the inhibitory effects may be manifest.

CROSS-MODAL CAPTURE OF ATTENTION In addition to the effects that visual transients have on subsequent visual pro-

cessing, visual processing can also be affected by attentional capture in other sensory modalities. Spence and Driver (1997) provided behavioral evidence for a cross-modal link in auditory and visual attention, finding that a nonpredictive auditory "cue" resulted in faster response times to a visual target stimulus that occurred at the same location as the auditory cue. More recent studies have shown that nonpredictive auditory events can enhance the perceptibility of a visual stimulus presented at the same location (Dufour, 1999; McDonald and Ward, 2000). ERP recordings have shown that this cross-modal effect on visual perception was associated with an enhanced negativity in the interval 120–180 ms following the visual target (McDonald et al., 2003). The early phase of this negativity (at 120–140 ms) was localized by dipole modeling to the multimodal region of the superior temporal cortex, while the later phase (at 140–180 ms) was attributed to generators in the ventral occipital cortex of the fusiform gyrus. These results provide support for proposals that cross-modal influences on visual perception are mediated by feedback from multimodal areas (such as the superior temporal cortex) to unimodal visual processing regions (Driver and Spence, 1998; Macaluso, Frith, and Driver, 2000; McDonald and Ward, 2000).

A nonpredictive tactile stimulus can also facilitate the processing of a subsequent visual stimulus presented at the same location (Spence et al., 1998). In an ERP study, Kennet and colleagues (2001) showed that a tactile cue produced enhancement of visual-evoked negativity in the 110–200 ms range, including a lateral occipital N1 component. This cross-modal facilitation was shown to depend on a common spatial location of the tactile and visual stimuli, when conditions of crossed and uncrossed arms were compared. Taken together, these studies show that abruptly onsetting

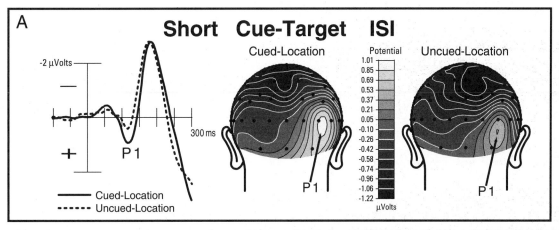

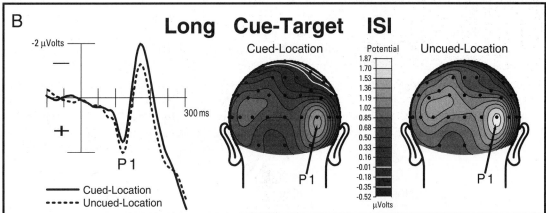

FIGURE 41.5 Averaged ERPs and scalp voltage topographies from a study of reflexive attention by Hopfinger and Mangun (1998). (*A*) ERPs to target stimuli at the short cue-to-target ISIs (34–234 ms), collapsed over contralateral scalp sites (data from the left hemisphere for right visual field targets combined with data from the right hemisphere for left visual field targets). ERP data are from lateral occipital electrodes OL and OR, which are located midway between T5 and O1, and T6 and O2, respectively, of the International 10–20 system of electrode placement (Jasper, 1958). Cued-location targets (solid lines) elicited a significantly enhanced P1 component compared to uncued-location targets (dashed lines). At middle and right are shown scalp topographic voltage maps, collapsed over contralateral and ipsilateral scalp sites. The left scalp hemisphere of each map represents the ipsilateral hemisphere (data from the left hemisphere for left visual field targets combined with data from the right hemisphere for right visual field targets), while the right scalp hemisphere of each map represents the contralateral hemisphere. The small black dots on each topographic map indicate the location of the electrodes. Voltage maps are shown from a back view of the head, for the time period corresponding to the P1 component (110–120 ms). At these short ISIs, the cued-location targets (left map) produced a significantly enhanced P1 component relative to uncued-location targets (right map). (*B*) ERPs to target bar stimuli at long cue-to-target ISIs (566–766 ms), collapsed over contralateral scalp sites. Cued-location targets (solid lines) elicited a significantly smaller P1 component than uncued-location targets (dashed lines). Scalp topographic voltage maps of the time period corresponding to the P1 component (110–120 ms) are shown at middle and right. At the long ISIs, the cued location targets (left map) produced a significantly *reduced* P1 component relative to uncued-location targets (right map). As with the short-ISI trials, the distribution of activity during this time period was highly similar, with the main difference being the strength of the P1. (Figure adapted with permission from J. B. Hopfinger and G. R. Mangun, 2001b, Electrophysiological studies of reflexive attention, in *Attraction, distraction, and action: Multiple perspectives on attentional capture* (C. Folk and B. Gibson, eds.), pp. 3–26. Copyright 2001 by Elsevier.)

stimuli in different modalities (visual, auditory, or tactile) can capture attention automatically and facilitate the processing of colocalized visual targets at an early stage of the extrastriate cortical pathways.

Postperceptual attention mechanisms

A great deal of research has been devoted to understanding the role of attention in perception, but attention also has large effects on postperceptual processes, such as working memory encoding and response selection[1]. ERPs have been very useful in isolating the specific postperceptual processes that are influenced by attention in a variety of paradigms. Here, we will focus on the attentional blink paradigm, which has been the focus of intense study over the past decade.

Potter (1976) showed observers rapid sequences of photographs of complex scenes and found that the observers could identify the photographs at very high presentation rates (e.g., 8/s) but could not store them in working memory at these high rates. This result implies that we can perceive much more than we can store in working memory. More recent studies using rapid sequences of simpler stimuli have shown that detecting one target (called T1) leads to a period

of approximately 500 ms during which a second target (called T2) is not detected. If, however, subjects ignore T1, they can accurately detect T2. This pattern of results, shown in figure 41.6, is called the attentional blink, because detecting T1 leads to a blink of attention during which T2 is not detected. Because Potter (1976) demonstrated that observers can perceive information at the high rates used in these experiments, it seems plausible that T2 is perceived during this blink of attention. However, the process of transforming a perceptual representation into a durable working memory representation may be slower than the process of forming a perceptual representation. Thus, during the period in which T1 is being consolidated into working memory, T2 may fail to be consolidated, and this may explain failures to detect T2 (see Shapiro, Arnell, and Raymond, 1997).

According to this explanation of the attentional blink, the detection of T1 does not impair perceptual processing of T2 but leads to a failure of working memory encoding. This hypothesis was tested in a series of ERP experiments (Luck, Vogel, and Shapiro, 1996; Vogel, Luck, and Shapiro, 1998; Vogel and Luck, 2002). In contrast to the spatial attention experiments described earlier, in which the P1 and N1 waves

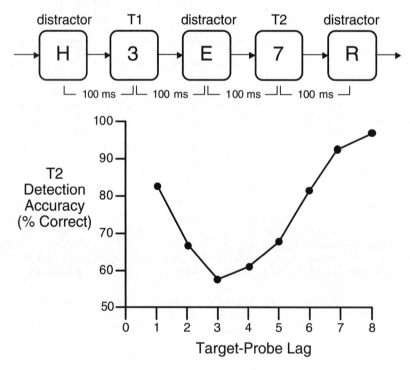

FIGURE 41.6 Typical attentional blink paradigm and behavioral results. In this version, alphanumeric characters are presented at fixation at a rate of 10/s, and a trial consists of a sequence of 30 stimuli. Of these, 28 are letters and two are numbers. The two numbers are the targets (T1 and T2) and must be reported at the end of the trial. The lag between T1 and T2 varies between 1 and 8 (e.g., at lag 1, T2 immediately follows T1; at lag 3, T2 is the third item after T1). In most experiments, accuracy is fairly high at lag

1, drops to a minimum at lag 3, and then recovers to asymptote by lag 5–8. Accuracy is thought to be relatively high at lag 1 because of temporal imprecision in the process of transferring perceptual representations into working memory. That is, when T1 is detected, both T1 and T2 are transferred into working memory, leading to fairly accurate performance when T2 is the item that immediately follows T1.

were found to be suppressed for ignored stimuli compared to attended stimuli, there was no suppression of the P1 and N1 waves elicited by a probe stimulus during the attention blink period (Vogel, Luck, and Shapiro, 1998, Experiment 1).

A second experiment used words as the target stimuli and examined the N400 component (Luck, Vogel, and Shapiro, 1996), which is elicited when a word mismatches a previously established semantic context. In this experiment, a semantic context was established at the beginning of each trial, and the T2 word either matched or mismatched this context. Before a mismatching word can elicit an N400 component, the word must be identified and compared with the semantic context. Thus, a larger N400 for mismatching words than for matching words provides strong evidence that the words were identified to a lexical or semantic level. In this experiment, the N400 was indeed larger for mismatching words than for matching words, and this effect was not reduced during the attentional blink period. This experiment thus provides strong evidence that the failure to detect T2 during the attentional blink period reflects an impairment in postperceptual processing.

A subsequent experiment examined the P3 wave (Vogel, Luck, and Shapiro, 1998, Experiment 4), which is thought to reflect processes associated with working memory encoding (Donchin, 1981; Donchin and Coles, 1988). Unlike the P1, N1, and N400 components, the P3 wave was completely eliminated when T2 was presented during the attentional blink period. This finding supports the hypothesis that the attentional blink occurs because of a failure to encode the perceptual representation of T2 into working memory.

When T2 is the last item in the sequence, however, the perceptual representation of T2 will not be masked by a subsequent item and may persist for a few hundred milliseconds. This fading perceptual representation may still be available when the consolidation of T1 has been completed, allowing T2 to be consolidated and available for report. Indeed, Giesbrecht and Di Lollo (1998) found that the attentional blink was eliminated when T2 was the last item in the sequence. In a related ERP study, Vogel and Luck (2002) found that the P3 wave was not eliminated when T2 was the last item in the sequence; instead, the P3 wave was delayed. This result supports the hypothesis that the processing of T1 leads to a delay in the consolidation of T2. When T2 is followed by another item, the following item masks T2 before it has been consolidated, impairing T2 detection performance and eliminating the T2-elicited P3 wave. When T2 is the final item, consolidation is delayed, leading to a delayed P3 wave but accurate T2 detection.

Attentional control

The preceding sections have described the effects that attention has on perceptual and postperceptual processing, after attention has been concentrated at a specific location or object. Another area of research concerns attentional control, or the processes and neural mechanisms that account for the movement and focusing of attentional resources. Recent hemodynamic neuroimaging and ERP studies have provided new insights into the neural structures and dynamics underlying attentional control processes.

In trial-by-trial cuing paradigms, it is possible to investigate not only the effects of attention on target processing but also the neural processes that occur in response to instructions (e.g., the cue) to orient attention to a specific location, *before* the target stimulus appears. In an ERP study of spatial cuing, Harter and colleagues (e.g., Harter et al., 1989) found that instructive cue stimuli produced two prominent components that were largest over the scalp contralateral to the attended visual hemifield. The first component was termed the "early directing attention negativity" (EDAN), a posterior parietal negativity occurring from approximately 200- to 400 ms after the instructive central cue. Following this component, at latencies of 500–700 ms after the cue, a positivity termed the "late directing attention positivity" (LDAP) was found over occipital scalp sites. The EDAN was interpreted as indexing a control process that acts on sensory areas to modulate the excitability of neurons representing attended regions of space. It was proposed that this latter modulation of excitability was reflected in the LDAP component.

Hopf and Mangun (2000) conducted a similar experiment using a higher-density montage of recording sites to provide a more precise localization of the processes underlying attentional control. The results replicated the basic EDAN and LDAP findings described above. However, Hopf and Mangun also found an additional effect occurring in the time interval between the EDAN and the LDAP that was maximal over frontal regions. Contrary to theories of attention that postulate that regions of the frontal lobe initiate attentional control mechanisms (e.g., Posner and Petersen, 1990; LaBerge, 1997), these findings provide new data suggesting that attentional control activity in parietal regions may actually precede the activity in frontal cortex. Another important result from this study was that the topography of the LDAP effect was highly similar to the topography of the P1 attention effect that was found to the subsequent target stimuli. This provides support for the hypothesis that attention acts to prime sensory processing regions, and that the LDAP reflects a biasing of neural activity that may be responsible for the later selective processing of stimuli occurring at attended locations.

Recent neuroimaging results are providing new evidence regarding the neural structures underlying these attentional control processes. Earlier neuroimaging and neuropsychological studies provided evidence that a widespread network of brain regions underlies attention mechanisms, including regions of posterior parietal cortex (Mesulam, 1981; Posner and Cohen, 1984; Corbetta et al., 1993; Gitelman et al., 1999), thalamus (Petersen, Robinson, and Morris, 1987; Heinze et al., 1994; LaBerge, 1997), superior temporal sulcus (Watson et al., 1994; Nobre et al., 1997), and regions of frontal cortex (Henik, Rafal, and Rhodes, 1994; Corbetta et al., 1998). However, because of limitations in analysis methods, early neuroimaging studies were not well-suited for separating control processes of attention from the selective processing of target stimuli that occur later.

More recently, however, the introduction of event-related fMRI analysis techniques (e.g., Buckner et al., 1996; Josephs, Turner, and Friston, 1997; McCarthy et al., 1997) has allowed researchers to analyze attentional control and preparatory processes separately from the subsequent effects of attention on the processing of target stimuli (Kastner et al., 1999; Corbetta et al., 2000; Hopfinger, Buonocore, and Mangun, 2000). Hopfinger, Buonocore, and Mangun (2000) revealed a dissociation between the brain regions active in response to the instructive cue versus the brain regions active in response to the subsequent target stimuli. For instance, the intraparietal sulcus was found to be active only in response to the instructive cue stimuli, consistent with a role in controlling shifts of spatial attention. The superior temporal cortex, regions of the frontal lobe near the frontal eye fields (FEF), and regions of the superior frontal gyrus anterior to the FEF also showed activity specific to processing of the instructive cue stimuli, suggesting that these regions are involved in attentional control, as opposed to being involved in later aspects of selective target processing. Target stimuli evoked activity in a highly distinct set of brain regions, including bilateral regions of the supplementary motor area, extending into the midcingulate gyrus, bilateral ventrolateral prefrontal regions, bilateral visual cortex, and the precentral and postcentral gyri. Giesbrecht and colleagues (2003) recently expanded upon these results, finding that portions of the attentional control network (including inferior and medial frontal gyri and posterior parietal regions) were common to both space- and feature-based attentional control (see also Wojciulik and Kanwisher, 1999; Shulman et al., 2002). However, this study also revealed specificity in parts of the control network, as activity in more superior frontal and parietal regions was significantly greater in spatial shifts of attention compared to feature-based attention.

As mentioned earlier, the LDAP component is thought to index a priming of visual processing regions in response to instructive cues that precedes and is highly similar in scalp distribution to the attention effects (e.g., P1) on target processing. Event-related fMRI techniques are now providing converging evidence. In the study by Hopfinger, Buonocore, and Mangun (2000), enhanced activity in response to the target stimuli was found contralateral to the attended hemi-

field in two visual processing regions, a ventral region within the lingual/fusiform gyri and a more dorsal region in the cuneus. Finding selective attention effects in extrastriate regions confirms numerous previous studies (e.g., Heinze et al., 1994; Mangun et al., 1997; Woldorff et al., 1997); however, this study was able to additionally isolate the processing in this region that occurred in response to the instructive cues, before the target stimuli appeared. This revealed increases in activity in the visual cortex of the hemisphere contralateral to the attended hemifield. Of note, these regions overlapped with the regions where attention effects were subsequently found in response to the target stimuli (figure 41.7). Because this differential activity was found in response to the cue and before target processing, it provides further support for models of attention that posit a preset gain-control mechanism that enhances the excitability of visual cortical neurons coding the attended regions of space (e.g., Hillyard and Mangun, 1986; Chawla, Rees, and Friston, 1999; Kastner et al., 1999).

Woldorff and colleagues (2004) have recently performed a rapid-event-related fMRI investigation of these mechanisms of attention. By applying techniques initially used for dissociating overlapping ERP components (e.g., Woldorff, 1993; Burock et al., 1998), they have identified fMRI activity for events occurring in relatively close succession, allowing a more direct comparison with previous behavioral and ERP studies of attention that used much shorter ISIs. This rapid-event-related fMRI study provided an important confirmation of the biasing in extrastriate regions in response to the cue stimuli, before the appearance of target stimuli. Although these analysis techniques are providing new possibilities for dissociating the sub-component processes of attention, fMRI techniques cannot alone provide the temporal resolution necessary to fully characterize the dynamics of attention processes in the brain. Combining these approaches with ERP and neuromagnetic measures of mental function, however, promises to provide exciting results that should significantly expand our understanding of the mechanisms and processes of attention.

Conclusion

In this chapter, we have reviewed electrophysiological, neuromagnetic, and neuroimaging studies that are informing theories of selective attention mechanisms and the neural underpinnings of attention processes. These studies have provided evidence that attention affects visual processing at both perceptual and postperceptual levels. Perceptual level processing has been found to be enhanced as early as 80–130 ms latency (i.e., the P1 component), and the studies reviewed in this chapter show that this effect can be generated either by explicit instructions, or by visual search processes, or by the involuntary capture of attention. The effects of

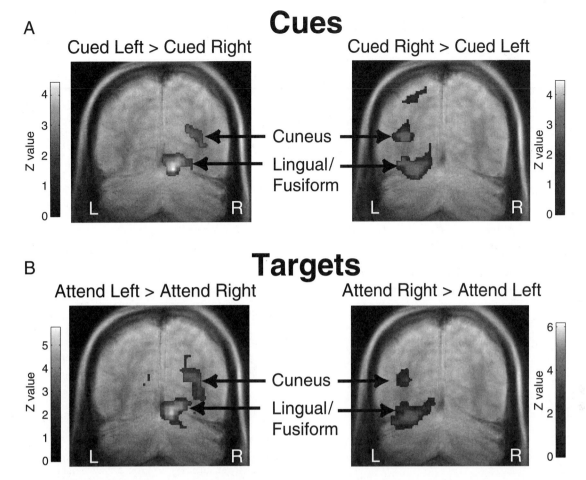

Cues

A

Cued Left > Cued Right

Cuneus

Lingual/
Fusiform

Cued Right > Cued Left

Targets

B

Attend Left > Attend Right

Cuneus

Lingual/
Fusiform

Attend Right > Attend Left

FIGURE 41.7   Results from Hopfinger, Buonocore, and Mangun (2000) showing selective attention effects in visual processing regions overlaid on an averaged proton density MRI scan (slice at $y = -64$). (*A*) Top panels show attention effects in response to the attention-directing *cue* stimuli. Left panels show regions showing greater cue-related activity for attend left than attend right conditions; right panels shows regions exhibiting greater activity for attend right cues then attend left cues. Cue-induced activity was greater contralateral to the direction of attention in ventral lingual/fusiform regions and in a more dorsal region of the cuneus. (*B*) Bottom panels show regions with differential activity for *target* processing as a function of where attention was focused. Target processing was significantly enhanced contralateral to the direction of attention, and the effects were in regions that closely overlapped with where the attention effects were seen in response to the cue stimuli (compare with upper panels). (Adapted with permission from Hopfinger, Buonocore, and Mangun, 2000.)

attention on perceptual level processing include longer latency effects as well (the N1, 140–200 ms), and this slightly later attention effect has been dissociated from the earlier P1 effect. Electrophysiological indices of postperceptual processing (e.g., the P3 component) provide further evidence that attention acts at multiple levels of processing. Finally, ERP and event-related fMRI studies are beginning to identify the neural systems and dynamic processes that underlie attentional control processes. These studies are providing converging evidence for the roles of frontal and parietal regions in the biasing of sensory processing regions that occurs prior to the selective processing of subsequent stimuli. Future studies aimed at further dissociating the subcomponent processes of attention promise to provide even greater precision in identifying the neural dynamics of selective attention.

NOTE

1. It should be noted that we are using the terms *perceptual* and *postperceptual* to distinguish between the processes that transform sensory inputs into abstract, amodal representations of object identities (perceptual processes) and the processes that that store, manipulate, and respond to these representations (postperceptual processes). The term *perception* is not meant to imply awareness or phenomenological experience (which would obviate concepts such as "perception without awareness").

REFERENCES

ANLLO-VENTO, L., S. J. LUCK, and S. A. HILLYARD, 1998. Spatiotemporal dynamics of attention to color: Evidence from human electrophysiology. *Hum. Brain Mapp.* 6:216–238.

BUCKNER, R. P., A. BANDETTINI, K. M. O'CRAVEN, R. L. SAVOY, S. E. PETERSEN, M. E. RAICHLE, and B. R. ROSEN, 1996.

Detection of cortical activation during averaged single trials of a cognitive task using functional magnetic resonance imaging. *Proc. Natl. Acad. Sci. U.S.A.* 93:14302–14303.

BUROCK, M. A., R. L. BUCKNER, M. G. WOLDORFF, B. R. ROSEN, and A. M. DALE, 1998. Randomized event-related experimental designs allow for extremely rapid presentation rates using functional MRI. *Neuroreport* 9:3735–3739.

CARRASCO, M., D. L. EVERT, I. CHANGE, and S. M. KATZ, 1995. The eccentricity effect: Target eccentricity affects performance on conjunction searches. *Percept. Psychophys.* 57:1241–1261.

CHAWLA, D., G. REES, and K. J. FRISTON, 1999. The physiological basis of attentional modulation in extrastriate visual areas. *Nat. Neurosci.* 2:671–676.

CHELAZZI, L., J. DUNCAN, E. K. MILLER, and R. DESIMONE, 1998. Responses of neurons in inferior temporal cortex during memory-guided visual search. *J. Neurophysiol.* 80:2918–2940.

CHELAZZI, L., E. K. MILLER, J. DUNCAN, and R. DESIMONE, 1993. A neural basis for visual search in inferior temporal cortex. *Nature* 363:345–347.

CHELAZZI, L., E. K. MILLER, J. DUNCAN, and R. DESIMONE, 2001. Responses of neurons in macaque area V4 during memory-guided visual search. *Cereb. Cortex* 11:761–772.

CORBETTA, M., E. AKBUDAK, T. E. CONTURO, A. Z. SNYDER, J. M. OLLINGER, H. A. DRURY, M. R. LINENWEBER, S. E. PETERSEN, M. E. RAICHLE, D. C. VAN ESSEN, and G. L. SHULMAN, 1998. A common network of functional areas for attention and eye movements. *Neuron* 21:761–1773.

CORBETTA, M., J. M. KINCADE, J. M. OLLINGER, M. P. McAVOY, and G. L. SHULMAN, 2000. Voluntary orienting is dissociated from target detection in human posterior parietal cortex. *Nat. Neurosci.* 3:292–297.

CORBETTA, M., F. MIEZIN, G. L. SHULMAN, and S. E. PETERSEN, 1993. A PET study of visuospatial attention. *J. Neurosci.* 13:1202–1226.

D'ESPOSITO, M., D. BALLARD, G. K. AGUIRRE, and E. ZARAHN, 1998. Human prefrontal cortex is not specific for working memory: A functional MRI study. *NeuroImage* 8:274–282.

DESIMONE, R., and J. DUNCAN, 1995. Neural mechanisms of selective visual attention. *Annu. Rev. Neurosci.* 18:193–222.

DI RUSSO, F., A. MARTINEZ, and S. A. HILLYARD, 2003. Source analysis of event-related cortical activity during visuo-spatial attention. *Cereb. Cortex* 13:486–499.

DI RUSSO, F., A. MARTINEZ, M. SERENO, S. PITZALIS, and S. A. HILLYARD, 2001. The cortical sources of the early components of the visual evoked potential. *Hum. Brain Mapp.* 15:95–111.

DONCHIN, E., 1981. Surprise! . . . Surprise? *Psychophysiology* 18:493–513.

DONCHIN, E., and M. G. H. COLES, 1988. Is the P300 component a manifestation of context updating? *Behav. Brain Sci.* 11:357–374.

DRIVER, J., and C. SPENCE, 1998. Attention and the crossmodal construction of space. *Trends Cogn. Sci.* 2:254–262.

DUFOUR, A., 1999. Importance of attentional mechanisms in audiovisual links. *Exp. Brain Res.* 126:215–222.

EIMER, M., 1994. "Sensory gating" as a mechanism for visuospatial orienting: Electrophysiological evidence from trial-by-trial cuing experiments. *Percept. Psychophys.* 55:667–675.

GIESBRECHT, B. L., and V. DI LOLLO, 1998. Beyond the attentional blink: Visual masking by object substitution. *J. Exp. Psychol. Hum. Percept. Perform.* 24:1454–1466.

GIESBRECHT, B. L., M. G. WOLDORFF, A. W. SONG, and G. R. MANGUN, 2003. Neural mechanisms of top-down control during spatial and feature attention. *NeuroImage* 19:496–512.

GITELMAN, D. R., A. C. NOBRE, T. B. PARRISH, K. S. LABAR, Y. H. KIM, J. R. MEYER, and M. M. MESULAM, 1999. A large-scale distributed network for covert spatial attention. *Brain* 122:1093–1106.

HANDY, T. C., and G. R. MANGUN, 2000. Attention and spatial selection: Electrophysiological evidence for modulation by perceptual load. *Percept. Psychophys.* 62:175–186.

HARTER, M. R., S. L. MILLER, N. J. PRICE, M. E. LALONDE, and A. L. KEYES, 1989. Neural processes involved in directing attention. *J. Cogn. Neurosci.* 1:223–237.

HAWKINS, H. L., S. A. HILLYARD, S. J. LUCK, M. MOULOUA, C. J. DOWNING, and D. P. WOODWARD, 1990. Visual attention modulates signal detectability. *J. Exp. Psychol. Hum. Percept. Perform.* 16:802–811.

HEINZE, H. J., G. R. MANGUN, W. BURCHERT, H. HINRICHS, M. SHOLZ, T. F. MUNTE, A. GOS, M. SCHERG, S. JOHANNES, H. HUNDESHAGEN, M. S. GAZZANIGA, and S. A. HILLYARD, 1994. Combined spatial and temporal imaging of brain activity during selective attention in humans. *Nature* 372:543–546.

HENIK, A., R. RAFAL, and D. RHODES, 1994. Endogenously generated and visually guided saccades after lesions of the human frontal eye fields. *J. Cogn. Neurosci.* 6:400–411.

HILLYARD, S. A., and L. ANLLO-VENTO, 1998. Event-related brain potentials in the study of visual selective attention. *Proc. Natl. Acad. Sci.* 95:781–787.

HILLYARD, S. A., and G. R. MANGUN, 1986. The neural basis of visual selective attention: A commentary on Harter and Aine. *Biol. Psychol.* 23:265–270.

HILLYARD, S. A., E. K. VOGEL, and S. J. LUCK, 1998. Sensory gain control (amplification) as a mechanism of selective attention: Electrophysiological and neuroimaging evidence. *Philos. Trans. R. Soc. Biol. Sci.* 353:1257–1270.

HOPF, J.-M., S. J. LUCK, M. GIRELLI, T. HAGNER, G. R. MANGUN, H. SCHEICH, and H. J. HEINZE, 2000. Neural sources of focused attention in visual search. *Cereb. Cortex* 10:1233–1241.

HOPF, J.-M., and G. R. MANGUN, 2000. Shifting visual attention in space: An electrophysiological analysis using high spatial resolution mapping. *Clin. Neurophysiol.* 111:1241–1257.

HOPF, J.-M., E. K. VOGEL, G. F. WOODMAN, H. J. HEINZE, and S. J. LUCK, 2002. Localizing visual discrimination processes in time and space. *J. Neurophysiol.* 88:2088–2095.

HOPFINGER, J. B., M. H. BUONOCORE, and G. R. MANGUN, 2000. The neural mechanisms of top-down attentional control. *Nat. Neurosci.* 3:284–291.

HOPFINGER, J. B., and G. R. MANGUN, 1998. Reflexive attention modulates processing of visual stimuli in human extrastriate cortex. *Psychol. Sci.* 9:441–447.

HOPFINGER, J. B., and G. R. MANGUN, 2001a. Tracking the influence of reflexive attention on sensory and cognitive processing. *Cogn. Affect. Behav. Neurosci.* 1:56–65.

HOPFINGER, J. B., and G. R. MANGUN, 2001b. Electrophysiological studies of reflexive attention. In *Attraction, distraction, and action: Multiple perspectives on attentional capture*, C. Folk and B. Gibson, eds. Amsterdam, Elsevier, pp. 3–26.

HOPFINGER, J. B., J. MAXWELL, and G. R. MANGUN, 2000. *Reflexive attention captured by the irrelevant appearance or disappearance of visual objects modulates early visual processing.* Poster presented at the 7th Annual Meeting of the Cognitive Neuroscience Society, San Francisco, Calif.

JASPER, H., 1958. The ten twenty electrode system of the International Federation. *Electroencephalogr. Clin. Neurophysiol.* 10:371–375.

JONIDES, J., 1981. Voluntary versus automatic control over the mind's eye movement. In *Attention and Performance IX*, J. B.

Long and A. D. Baddeley, eds. Hillsdale, N.J.: Erlbaum, pp. 187–203.

Josephs O., R. Turner, and K. Friston, 1997. Event-related fMRI. *Hum. Brain Mapp.* 5:243–248.

Karnath, H. O., S. Ferber, and M. Himmelbach, 2001. Spatial awareness is a function of the temporal not the posterior parietal lobe. *Nature* 411:951–953.

Kastner, S., M. A. Pinsk, P. De Weerd, R. Desimone, and L. G. Ungerleider, 1999. Increased activity in human visual cortex during directed attention in the absence of visual stimulation. *Neuron* 22:751–761.

Kennett, S., M. Eimer, C. Spence, and J. Driver, 2001. Tactile-visual links in exogenous spatial attention under different postures: Convergent evidence from psychophysics and ERPs. *J. Cogn. Neurosci.* 13:462–478.

Klein, R. M., 2000. Inhibition of return. *Trends Cogn. Sci.* 4: 138–147.

Kingstone, A., and J. Pratt, 1999. Inhibition of return is composed of attentional and oculomotor processes. *Percept. Psychophys.* 61:1046–1054.

Kojima, S., and P. S. Goldman-Rakic, 1982. Delay-related activity of prefrontal neurons in rhesus monkeys performing delayed response. *Brain Res.* 248:43–50.

LaBerge, D., 1997. Attention, awareness, and the triangular circuit. *Consciousness Cogn.* 6:149–181.

Lamme, V. A. F., and H. Spekreijse, 2000. Contextual modulation in primary visual cortex and scene perception. In *The New Cognitive Neurosciences*, M. S. Gazzaniga, ed. Cambridge, Mass.: MIT Press, pp. 279–296.

Lamme, V. A., H. Super, R. Landman, P. R. Roelfsema, and H. Spekreijse, 2000. The role of primary visual cortex (V1) in visual awareness. *Vision Res.* 40:1507–1521.

Lu, Z., and B. A. Dosher, 1998. External noise distinguishes attention mechanisms. *Vision Res.* 38:1183–1198.

Luck, S. J., 1995. Multiple mechanisms of visual-spatial attention: Recent evidence from human electrophysiology. *Behav. Brain Res.* 71:113–123.

Luck, S. J., S. Fan, and S. A. Hillyard, 1993. Attention-related modulation of sensory-evoked brain activity in a visual search task. *J. Cogn. Neurosci.* 5:188–195.

Luck, S. J., and M. A. Ford, 1998. On the role of selective attention in visual perception. *Proc. Natl. Acad. Sci. U.S.A.* 95:825–830.

Luck, S. J., M. Girelli, M. T. McDermott, and M. A. Ford, 1997. Bridging the gap between monkey neurophysiology and human perception: An ambiguity resolution theory of visual selective attention. *Cogn. Psychol.* 33:64–87.

Luck, S. J., and S. A. Hillyard, 1994. Spatial filtering during visual search: Evidence from human electrophysiology. *J. Exp. Psychol. Hum. Percept. Perform.* 20:1000–1014.

Luck, S. J., and S. A. Hillyard, 1995. The role of attention in feature detection and conjunction discrimination: An electrophysiological analysis. *Int. J. Neurosci.* 80:281–297.

Luck, S. J., and S. A. Hillyard, 2000. The operation of selective attention at multiple stages of processing: Evidence from human and monkey electrophysiology. In *The New Cognitive Neurosciences*, M. S. Gazzaniga, ed. Cambridge, Mass.: MIT Press, pp. 687–700.

Luck, S. J., S. A. Hillyard, M. Mouloua, and H. L. Hawkins, 1996. Mechanisms of visual-spatial attention: Resource allocation or uncertainty reduction? *J. Exp. Psychol. Hum. Percept. Perform.* 22:725–737.

Luck, S. J., S. A. Hillyard, M. Mouloua, M. G. Woldorff, V. P. Clark, and H. L. Hawkins, 1994. Effects of spatial cuing on luminance detectability: Psychophysical and electrophysiological evidence for early selection. *J. Exp. Psychol. Hum. Percept. Perform.* 20:887–904.

Luck, S. J., E. K. Vogel, and K. L. Shapiro, 1996. Word meanings can be accessed but not reported during the attentional blink. *Nature* 382:616–618.

Macaluso E., C. D. Frith, and J. Driver, 2000. Modulation of human visual cortex by crossmodal spatial attention. *Science* 289:1206–1208.

Mangun, G. R. 1995. Neural mechanisms of visual selective attention. *Psychophysiology* 32:4–18.

Mangun, G. R., and S. A. Hillyard, 1991. Modulations of sensory-evoked brain potentials indicate changes in perceptual processing during visual-spatial priming. *J. Exp. Psychol. Hum. Percept. Perform.* 17:1057–1074.

Mangun, G. R., J. B. Hopfinger, C. Kussmaul, E. Fletcher, and H. J. Heinze, 1997. Covariations in PET and ERP measures of spatial selective attention in human extrastriate visual cortex. *Hum. Brain Mapp.* 5:1–7.

Martinez, A., L. Anllo-Vento, M. I. Sereno, L. R. Frank, R. B. Buxton, D. J. Dubowitz, E. C. Wong, H. J. Heinze, and S. A. Hillyard, 1999. Involvement of striate and extrastriate visual cortical areas in spatial attention. *Nat. Neurosci.* 2:364–369.

Martinez, A., F. DiRusso, L. Anllo-Vento, M. I. Sereno, R. B. Buxton, and S. A. Hillyard, 2001. Putting spatial attention on the map: Timing and localization of stimulus selection processes in striate and extrastriate visual areas. *Vision Res.* 41:1437–1457.

Maunsell, J. H. R., and C. J. McAdams, 2000. Effects of attention on neuronal response properties in visual cerebral cortex. In *The New Cognitive Neurosciences*, M. S. Gazzaniga, ed. Cambridge, Mass.: MIT Press, pp. 290–305.

McCarthy, G., M. Luby, J. Gore, and P. Goldman-Rakic, 1997. Infrequent events transiently activate human prefrontal and parietal cortex as measured by functional MRI. *J. Neurophysiol.* 77:1630–1634.

McDonald, J. J., W. A. Teder-Sälejärvi, F. DiRusso, and S. A. Hillyard, 2003. Neural substrates of perceptual enhancement by crossmodal spatial attention. *J. Cogn. Neurosci.* 15:1–10.

McDonald, J. J., and L. M. Ward, 2000. Involuntary listening aids seeing: Evidence from human electrophysiology. *Psychol. Sci.* 11:167–171.

McDonald, J. J., L. M. Ward, and K. A. Kiehl, 1999. An event-related brain potential study of inhibition of return. *Percept. Psychophys.* 61:1411–1423.

Mesulam, M. M. 1981. A cortical network for directed attention and unilateral neglect. *Ann. Neurol.* 10:309–325.

Motter, B. C., 1993. Focal attention produces spatially selective processing in visual cortical areas V1, V2 and V4 in the presence of competing stimuli. *J. Neurophysiol.* 70:909–919.

Nobre, A. C., G. N. Sebestyen, D. R. Gitelman, M. M. Mesulam, R. S. Frackowiak, and C. D. Frith, 1997. Functional localization of the system for visuospatial attention using positron emission tomography. *Brain* 120:515–533.

Noesselt, T., S. A. Hillyard, M. G. Woldorff, T. Hagner, L. Jaencke, C. Tempelmann, H. Hinrichs, and H. J. Heinze. 2002. Delayed striate cortical activation during spatial attention. *Neuron* 35:575–587.

Petersen, S. E., D. L. Robinson, and J. D. Morris, 1987. Contributions of the pulvinar to visual spatial attention. *Neuropsychologia* 25:97–105.

Posner, M. I., and Y. Cohen, 1984. Components of visual orienting. In *Attention and Performance X*, H. Bouma and Bouwhis, eds. Hillsdale, N.J.: Erlbaum, pp. 531–556.

POSNER, M. I., M. J. NISSEN, and W. C.OGDEN, 1978. Attended and unattended processing models: The role of set for spatial locations. In *Modes of Perceiving and Processing Information*, H. L. Pick and F. J. Saltzman, eds. Hillsdale, N.J.: Erlbaum, pp. 137–157.

POSNER, M. I., and S. E. PETERSEN, 1990. The attention system of the human brain. *Ann. Rev. Neurosci.* 13:25–42.

POTTER, M. C., 1976. Short-term conceptual memory for pictures. *J. Exp. Psychol. Hum. Learn. Mem.* 2:509–522.

REYNOLDS, J. H., L. CHELAZZI, and R. DESIMONE, 1999. Competitive mechanisms subserve attention in macaque areas V2 and V4. *J. Neurosci.* 19:1736–1753.

REYNOLDS, J. H., and R. DESIMONE, 2001. Neural mechanisms of attentional selection. In *Visual Attention and Cortical Circuits*, J. Braun, C. Koch, and J. L. Davis, eds. Cambridge, Mass.: MIT Press, pp. 121–136.

ROELFSEMA, P. R., V. A. F. LAMME, and H. SPEKREIJSE, 1998. Object-based attention in the primary visual cortex of the macaque monkey. *Nature* 395:376–381.

SCHROEDER, C. E., A. D. MEHTA, and J. J. FOXE, 2001. Determinants and mechanisms of attentional modulation of neural processing. *Front. Biosci.* 6:672–684.

SHAPIRO, K. L., K. M. ARNELL, and J. E. RAYMOND, 1997. The attentional blink: A view on attention and a glimpse on consciousness. *Trends Cogn. Sci.* 1:291–296.

SPENCE, C., and J. DRIVER, 1997. Audiovisual links in exogenous covert spatial orienting. *Percept. Psychophys.* 59:1–22.

SPENCE, C., M. R. NICHOLLS, N. GILLESPIE, and J. DRIVER, 1998. Crossmodal links in exogenous covert spatial orienting between touch, audition, and vision. *Percept. Psychophys.* 60:544–557.

SHULMAN, G. L., G. D'AVOSSA, A. P. TANSY, and M. CORBETTA, 2002. Two attentional processes in the parietal lobe. *Cereb. Cortex* 12:1124–1131.

TOOTELL, R. B., N. HADJIKHANI, E. K. HALL, S. MARRETT, W. VANDUFFEL, J. T. VAUGHAN, and A. M. DALE, 1998. The retinotopy of visual spatial attention. *Neuron* 21:1409–1422.

TREISMAN, A., 1988. Features and objects: The Fourteenth Bartlett Memorial Lecture. *Q. J. Exp. Psychol.* 40:201–237.

TREISMAN, A. M., and G. GELADE, 1980. A feature-integration theory of attention. *Cogn. Psychol.* 12:97–136.

VIDYASAGAR, T. R., 1999. A neuronal model of attentional spotlight: Parietal guiding the temporal. *Dev. Brain Res.* 30:66–76.

VOGEL, E. K., and S. J. LUCK, 2000. The visual N1 component as an index of a discrimination process. *Psychophysiology* 37:190–123.

VOGEL, E. K., and S. J. LUCK, 2002. Delayed working memory consolidation during the attentional blink. *Psychonom. Bull. Rev.* 9:739–743.

VOGEL, E. K., S. J. LUCK, and K. L. SHAPIRO, 1998. Electrophysiological evidence for a postperceptual locus of suppression during the attentional blink. *J. Exp. Psychol. Hum. Percept. Perform.* 24:1656–1674.

WATSON, R. T., E. VALENSTEIN, A. DAY, and K. M. HEILMAN, 1994. Posterior neocortical systems subserving awareness and neglect. *Arch. Neurol.* 51:1014–1021.

WOJCIULIK, E., and N. KANWISHER, 1999. The generality of parietal involvement in visual attention. *Neuron* 23:747–764.

WOLDORFF, M. G., 1993. Distortion of ERP averages due to overlap from temporally adjacent ERPs: Analysis and correction. *Psychophysiology* 30:98–119.

WOLDORFF, M., P. T. FOX, M. MATZKE, J. L. LANCASTER, S. VEERASWAMY, F. ZAMARRIPA, M. SEABOLT, T. GLASS, J. H. GAO, C. C. MARTIN, and P. JERABEK, 1997. Retinotopic organization of early visual spatial attention effects as revealed by PET and ERPs. *Hum. Brain Mapp.* 5:280–286.

WOLDORFF, M. G., C. HAZLETT, H. M. FICHTENHOLTZ, D. WEISSMAN, A. DALE, and A. W. SONG, 2004. Functional parcellation of attentional control regions of the human brain. *J. Cogn. Neurosci.* 16:149–165.

WOLFE, J. M., 1994. Guided search 2.0: A revised model of visual search. *Psychonom. Bull. Rev.* 1:202–238.

WOLFE, J. M., P. O'NEILL, and S. C. BENNETT, 1998. Why are there eccentricity effects in visual search? Visual and attentional hypotheses. *Percept. Psychophys.* 60:140–156.

WOODMAN, G. F., and S. J. LUCK, 1999. Electrophysiological measurement of rapid shifts of attention during visual search. *Nature* 400:867–869.

WOODMAN, G. F., and S. J. LUCK, 2003. Serial deployment of attention during visual search. *J. Exp. Psychol. Hum. Percept. Perform.* 29:121–138.

YESHURUN, Y., and M. CARRASCO, 1998. Attention improves or impairs visual performance by enhancing spatial resolution. *Nature* 396:72–75.

42 Visual Selective Attention: Insights from Brain Imaging and Neurophysiology

WINRICH A. FREIWALD AND NANCY G. KANWISHER

ABSTRACT Attentional processes have been studied using all the methods of cognitive neuroscience. Brain imaging in humans and single-cell electrophysiology in macaque monkeys offer complementary perspectives, one providing a large scale view of brain activity, the other a close-up view with high spatial and temporal resolution. These methodologies have increasingly been used to answer the same questions about the mechanisms of visual selective attention. Here we review insights obtained into three longstanding questions in attention research: whether attention selects "early" or "late," the nature of the units of attentional selection, and the specific effects of attention on neural representations. The current literature indicates that attention can affect information processing even at the first stages of visual processing but that under some task conditions selection may be shifted to later processing stages. In terms of the units attention operates over, attention can select regions of space, stimulus features, and whole objects. Finally, attention has been shown to change neural representations in myriad ways, from changes in the mean firing rate of neurons representing target information and changes in neural selectivity to synchronization across neural populations.

The contents of our minds at any given moment are not rigidly determined by the stimuli that happen to be impinging on our senses. Instead, we perceivers actively select a subset of the available perceptual information for detailed processing, relegating other information to the shadows of consciousness. This active process of perceptual selection, *attention*, has been extensively studied for decades using all of the methods of cognitive neuroscience. Here we outline recent progress from brain imaging studies in humans and neurophysiological studies in monkeys. The research reviewed focuses on three longstanding and fundamental questions about visual attention: (1) What is the locus of attentional selection? (2) What are the units of information that are selected by attention? and (3) How exactly does neural processing differ for attended versus unattended information? In this chapter we will not review the recent imaging and electrophysiological literature on the sources of attentional signals in the frontal and parietal regions, a topic that is addressed elsewhere (see Humphreys and Samson, this volume; see also Colby and Goldberg, 1999; Kanwisher and Wojciulik, 2000; Gottlieb, 2002; Culham and Kanwisher, 2001; Kastner and Ungerleider, 2000; Corbetta and Shulman, 2002).

Does attention select early or late?

One of the classic questions in attention research concerns the locus of attentional selection (Broadbent, 1958; Deutsch and Deutsch, 1963). According to the late selection view, the entire visual array is perceptually analyzed preattentively to a high level, including identification of objects. Attention then selects a subset of this highly processed information for further analysis and response planning. In contrast, the early selection view holds that only rudimentary perceptual processing is carried out preattentively, and focused attention is necessary for object recognition and many other aspects of perceptual analysis.

To distinguish between these two views, two critical questions can be addressed with electrophysiological and imaging techniques. First, what is the earliest stage in the visual pathway where attentional effects can be observed? Second, what is the earliest latency after stimulus presentation when the response to that stimulus is affected by attention?

LATERAL GENICULATE NUCLEUS The primary visual pathway to the cortex, which we shall focus on here, connects the retina to the lateral geniculate nucleus (LGN) of the thalamus, and the LGN to the visual cortex. Within this pathway, the LGN is the first anatomical structure that receives feedback connections from higher centers, a prerequisite for attentional control. These corticogeniculate feedback projections (which outnumber retinogeniculate inputs by far) reach the LGN both directly and via a second thalamic nucleus, the reticular complex (TRC), which forms inhibitory connections with the LGN. Owing to their strategic location within this pathway, it has long been suspected

WINRICH A. FREIWALD Department of Neurobiology, Harvard Medical School, Boston, Mass.

NANCY G. KANWISHER Department of Cognitive and Brain Sciences, Massachusetts Institute of Technology, Cambridge, Mass.

that the TRC and LGN play a major role in attentional selection (Crick, 1984; Koch and Ullman, 1985).

Experimental evidence in support of this idea, however, has been slow to materialize. Few electrophysiological studies have been performed in the LGN during attention tasks (Mehta, Ulbert, and Schroeder, 2000; Bender and Youakim, 2001), and none of these has found effects of attention on neural activity. However, a metabolic mapping study, using a deoxyglucose double-labeling technique, demonstrated attention-dependent activity within macaque LGN (Vanduffel, Tootell, and Orban, 2000). Further, substantial effects of attention have been described recently in human LGN using functional magnetic resonance imaging (fMRI) (O'Connor et al., 2002). Guided by results of these two imaging studies, and using similar tasks and stimuli, future electrophysiological investigations may provide direct evidence for attentional effects in the LGN. Such electrophysiological evidence would both validate the fMRI results and determine whether the attentional modulation measured with blood oxygen level-dependent (BOLD) imaging, an indirect measure of neural activity, reflects input from cortex (Logothetis et al., 2001) or the spiking activity of LGN cells themselves.

PRIMARY VISUAL CORTEX   Early physiological studies found little evidence for attentional modulation of neural activity in primary visual cortex (V1) (Wurtz and Mohler, 1976) but substantial attention effects in the parietal (Wurtz, Goldberg, and Robinson, 1980; Mountcastle, Andersen, and Motter, 1981) and temporal lobes (Moran and Desimone, 1985). However, several more recent studies have demonstrated robust attentional effects in V1. Motter (1993) found that many cells produced a higher response when the animal's attention was directed to stimuli inside (compared to outside) their receptive fields (RFs). This attentional effect increased in magnitude as irrelevant information was added to the display. Using a stimulus array with multiple distracter items, Vidyasagar (1998) also found strong attentional modulation in V1. Direct evidence that the context of the stimulus is critical comes from a study by Ito and Gilbert (1999). They found that although the response of a single bar placed inside the RF was rarely modulated by attention, the contextual effect of neighboring bars placed just outside the RF was greatly modulated by attention. Such contextual effects may also be the source of the increased response strength of V1 neurons that Roelfsema, Lamme, and Spekreijse (1998) observed when monkeys attentionally traced a curve passing through the cell's RF. In sum, attention can exert a context-dependent influence on neural processing in V1.

The case for attentional modulation of neural responses in V1 has received independent support in recent years from fMRI (Watanabe, Harner et al., 1998; Watanabe, Sasaki, et al., 1998; Somers et al., 1999; Brefczynski and DeYoe, 1999; Gandhi, Heeger, and Boynton, 1999; Kastner et al., 1999; Martínez et al., 1999). In one experiment (Gandhi, Heeger, and Boynton, 1999), subjects maintained central fixation while judging the speed of one of two moving gratings displayed to the left and right of this point. To find the precise region within V1 that responded to each grating, retinotopic mapping was carried out in individual subjects. Attentional modulation of the V1 response was sizable, about 25% as great as the modulation in response to stimulus presence versus absence.

BEYOND PRIMARY VISUAL CORTEX   Attention effects have generally been found to increase in magnitude as one proceeds from V1 up the visual pathway into the parietal and temporal lobes. Within the same experiments, attentional modulation of response strength was found to be stronger in V4 than in V1 (Haenny and Schiller, 1988; McAdams and Maunsell, 1999a; Mehta, Ulbert, and Schroeder, 2000), stronger in V4 than in V2 (Mehta, Ulbert, and Schroeder, 2000) and stronger in MST than in MT (Treue and Maunsell, 1996). These findings are in agreement with hierarchical accounts of attentional function (Desimone and Duncan, 1995; Maunsell, 1995) that posit modulation of bottom-up processes by top-down attentional signals at all processing stages (see also Hochstein and Ahissar, 2002), with increasing magnitude from stage to stage.

LATENCIES OF ATTENTION EFFECTS   The evidence cited above indicates that attention can modulate visual processing at anatomically early stages of processing (the LGN and V1), leaving open the question of whether the modulation occurs at a temporally early stage of processing. It is possible that the first pass of visual information up the visual pathway is not modulated by attention, with attentional effects occurring only later, after feedback arrives from higher areas. Some evidence for this hypothesis comes from combined event-related potential (ERP) and fMRI studies (Martínez et al., 1999; Noesselt et al., 2002; Di Russo, Martínez, and Hillyard, 2003; see also Hopfinger, Luck, and Hillyard, this volume) that used the high spatial resolution of fMRI to demonstrate attention effects in V1, and the high temporal resolution of ERPs to show that the earliest visual cortical response is unmodulated by attention. Here we consider the evidence from electrophysiological studies in monkeys.

Two lines of physiological evidence support the idea of a top-down progression of attentional effects. In general agreement with the notion of a top-down spread of attentional control signals (Tsotsos et al., 1995), latencies of attention effects have been found to be of shorter duration at later stages of processing than at earlier ones (Mehta, Ulbert, and Schroeder, 2000; Miller, 2000). Furthermore, just as attention effects tend to grow stronger as one ascends the processing hierarchy, within each processing stage they grow stronger over time (Motter, 1994; McAdams and Maunsell, 1999a; Reynolds, Chelazzi, and Desimone, 1999; Seidemann and Newsome, 1999; Treue and Maunsell, 1999; Mehta, Ulbert, and Schroeder, 2000).

The latency after stimulus onset at which attention modulates responses within early cortical areas varies widely across studies. Some have reported modulation in V1 beginning as late as 200 ms after stimulus onset (Roelfsema et al., 1998; Mehta, Ulbert, and Schroeder, 2000), while others have described modulation of the very first wave of activity (Motter, 1993; Ito and Gilbert, 1999), or even of the spontaneous activity preceding stimulus onset (Luck et al., 1997; Reynolds, Pasternak, and Desimone, 2000). Such early response modulation occurs only when attention is cued in advance of stimulus onset, but even in this case, the first response transient induced by stimulus onset often remains unaltered by attention, or attentional modulation of this first response is difficult to reveal with the neuron reaching saturation (e.g., Seidemann and Newsome, 1999; Treue, 2001). A major determinant of the lag between response onset and onset of attentional modulation is stimulus contrast. When a high-contrast stimulus is turned on, stimulus response latency is relatively short and attentional modulation lags behind, while for relatively low-contrast stimuli, response onset and onset of attentional modulation can coincide. Reynolds, Pasternak, and Desimone (2000) demonstrated this pattern for cortical area V4, which is confirmed by a comparison of contrasts used in various other studies. Thus, a highly salient task-irrelevant stimulus may be processed to a high degree, in agreement with the late selection hypothesis, while a stimulus of low saliency may be filtered out early. Other factors, such as physical stimulus attributes and task requirements, may also influence the time of attentional selection.

SUMMARY Collectively, these electrophysiological and neuroimaging results provide an answer to one of the longstanding questions about visual attention: neural responses to visual stimuli can be modulated at early stages in the visual processing pathway, and even the first phase of a visual response can be modulated. It should be noted, however, that this is not proof for the generality of early selection, for several reasons. First, attention does not always affect the first processing stages, but does so to different extents in different tasks. According to one theory (Lavie and Tsal, 1994; Lavie, 1995), the stage of selection depends on the processing load of the primary task, with early selection occurring when the processing load is high and selection occurring at a later stage when the processing load is low. Consistent with this hypothesis, one imaging study (Rees, Frith, and Lavie, 1997) showed that the neural response to an irrelevant

moving stimulus measured in the motion-processing region MT/MST is weaker when the primary task is difficult than when it is easy (see also Handy and Mangun, 2000, and a related account by Luck and Hillyard, 2000). Second, the occurrence of response modulation does not necessarily imply the workings of a genuine selection, since the response to the nonattended distracter may still be substantial. Finally, the shortest-latency visual responses are not always modulated by attention, and therefore at least the first wave of activity traveling up the visual pathway may be largely attention-independent.

What are the units of attentional selection?

Does attention select spatial locations, feature dimensions, or whole objects or groups? To demonstrate location-based selection, for example, it is not sufficient to show that subjects can report visual information at a given location. The critical question is what other task-irrelevant visual information "comes along for the ride." That is, if a task requires subjects to direct their attention to the color of a red stimulus in a particular location, will they also automatically process (1) the features of other objects appearing at the same location (as predicted by location-based selection), (2) other features—say, shape—of the task-relevant object (as predicted by location-based and object-based selection), or (3) other red objects elsewhere in the visual field (as predicted by feature-based selection)? Neurophysiological and imaging studies have shed considerable light on this question.

LOCATION-BASED SELECTION In many studies, attention is directed to a specific spatial location while distracting information is present in other locations. Such spatial selection can be highly efficient, as implied by the "spotlight" metaphor of attention (Eriksen and Eriksen, 1974; Posner, 1980). Consistent with this metaphor, many neurophysiological and imaging studies have shown enhancement of the neural response to a stimulus when attention is directed to it versus to another spatial location (Moran and Desimone, 1985; Corbetta et al., 1993). However, such studies leave open the question of what exactly gets selected, the location, the feature dimension, or the object? These factors can be unconfounded by investigating the effects of attention on task-irrelevant information. Evidence that location often serves as the unit of attentional selection comes from behavioral studies showing greater interference from distracters appearing near a target stimulus compared to those appearing farther away (Eriksen and Eriksen, 1974). Similarly, both neurophysiological (Connor et al., 1996, 1997) and brain imaging (Downing, Liu, and Kanwisher, 2001) (figure 42.1B) studies have demonstrated enhancement of the response to task-irrelevant stimuli appearing near the target location. Because the task-irrelevant stimuli in these studies are

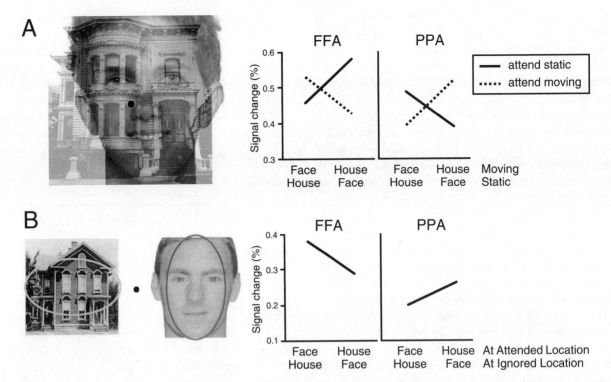

FIGURE 42.1 (*A*) Example stimulus (left) and main results (right) of the imaging study by O'Craven, Downing, and Kanwisher (1999) demonstrating object-based attention. BOLD response strength, expressed as percent signal change, was higher in the fusiform face area (FFA) when "faceness" was the irrelevant property of the attended object than when it was a property of the unattended object. The response pattern of the parahippocampal place area (PPA) was identical for "houseness."

(*B*) Example stimulus (left) and main results (right) of the study by Downing, Liu, and Kanwisher (2001). Here, attention was

drawn to the orientation of an oval of a given color while a second oval of different color and at a different location was ignored. When the attended oval was superimposed over a task-irrelevant picture of a face, FFA activity increased as compared to when the picture appeared at the task-irrelevant position. Results for PPA followed the same pattern for pictures of houses. Since task-relevant stimuli (ovals) and task-irrelevant stimuli (pictures) neither shared particular features nor appeared as parts of the same object, these results can only be accounted for in terms of location-based attention, not feature- or object-based attention.

neither part of nor share features with the attended target, these effects can only be accounted for in terms of spatial selection.

FEATURE-BASED SELECTION Behavioral studies in humans (Treisman, 1969; Wolfe, Cave, and Franzel, 1989; Chaudhuri, 1990) indicate that it is possible to select visual information by feature dimensions, such as color or motion, and imaging studies (Corbetta et al., 1990, 1991; Beauchamp, Cox, and DeYoe, 1997; O'Craven et al., 1997) suggest that such feature-based selection enhances activation of cortical areas specialized for processing that feature.

In the first physiological demonstration of feature-based attentional selection, Treue and Martínez Trujillo (1999) trained monkeys to report the occurrence of a speed or direction change in a moving random dot pattern, while responses in MT to a second (task-irrelevant, spatially separate) dot pattern were recorded. Activation by the task-irrelevant stimulus was higher when it moved in the same direction as the attended stimulus, as predicted by feature-based attention. Importantly, Treue and Martínez Trujillo

found these feature-based effects to be additive with space-based effects (i.e., when the strength of feature-based and space-based attention effects were determined independently in two separate experiments, their sum closely approximated the strength of a combined space- and feature-based attention effect determined in a third experiment), which may indicate that these two attentional mechanisms can act independently of each other, at least under some conditions. Similar results have been reported for area V4 (McAdams and Maunsell, 2000).

In an analogous experiment using imaging in humans, Saenz, Buracas, and Boynton (2002) showed that when subjects performed a speed judgment task on one of two spatially separate moving dot arrays, responses in areas V1, V2, V3, V3A, V4, and MT+ to the ignored dot array were higher when it moved in the same direction as the attended array; likewise, when subjects performed a color discrimination task on one of the dot arrays, the neural response in V4 to the task-irrelevant dot array was higher when it was the same color as the task-relevant array. All of these findings suggest feature-based selection (see also Beauchamp,

Cox, and DeYoe, 1997). However, an alternative account is possible. Common motion and common color are grouping cues (Köhler, 1930), so the observed attentional enhancement of the task-irrelevant stimulus may reflect attentional selection of the whole group. Such group-based selection is often considered a variant of object-based selection.

OBJECT-BASED SELECTION   Feature-based attentional selection is not always perfect, as illustrated by Stroop interference, in which subjects are unable to ignore a word when naming the color of the ink it is written in. Indeed, substantial behavioral evidence suggests that attention often selects whole objects or groups with all of their features (Duncan, 1984; Kanwisher and Driver, 1992; Valdés-Sosa et al., 1998; Blaser, Plyshyn, and Holcombe, 2000; Rodriguez, Valdés-Sosa, and Freiwald, 2002).

Evidence for both feature-based and object-based attention comes from a study (O'Craven, Downing, and Kanwisher, 1999) in which two stimuli, a face and a house, were transparently superimposed in the same location (figure 42.1). On each trial, either the face or the house oscillated back and forth along one of four axes; because the moving stimulus did not travel far, the face and house remained largely overlapping. Subjects' attention was directed in different conditions to the face, the house, motion direction, or the position of the stationary stimulus (which was displaced very slightly off-center). Consistent with feature-based selection, neural activity was higher in the face-selective fusiform face area, FFA (Kanwisher, McDermott, and Chun, 1997), when subjects attended to the face, in the place-selective parahippocampal place area, PPA (Epstein and Kanwisher, 1998), when subjects attended to the house, and in MT/MST when subjects attended to the direction of motion. Further, neural activity in each of the three cortical areas was higher when the visual attribute processed in that area was the irrelevant property of an attended object than when it was a property of the unattended object. For example, when subjects attended to the face, the signal was higher in MT/MST if it was the face that was moving than if the house moved, even though all features were present in the same location and even though motion was completely irrelevant to the task. These data indicate that objects function as the units of attentional selection over and above any tendency to select features or locations, even when the task requires only selection of a single visual attribute. Since two completely overlapping surfaces were used as stimuli in this experiment, the use of spatial mechanisms of selection was rendered difficult or impossible.

A similar display strategy was used in a study by Valdés-Sosa and colleagues (1998) to demonstrate the working of early non-space-based attentional selection. Two completely overlapping stimuli, a red and a green semitransparent random dot field, were presented, and one was cued as the target by the color of the fixation spot. Phases of counterphase rotations were interrupted by brief linear displacements of one of the surfaces on which subjects had to perform a direction discrimination task. Early components of motion-onset-related potentials, P1 and N1, were substantially suppressed when the moving surface was not attended. Thus, following scene segmentation and the grouping of information from two feature domains, color and motion, a nonspatial attentional selection occurred affecting the same early ERP components that space-based attention does in different paradigms (see Hopfinger, Luck, and Hillyard, this volume).

Stringent evidence at the single-cell level for object-based attention demonstrating enhancement of task-irrelevant feature information is still lacking. However, Roelfsema and colleagues (Roelfsema, Lamme, and Spekreijse, 1998; Roelfsema and Spekreijse, 2001) found attentional modulation of V1 responses to an entire curve along which the monkey was trained to trace his attention. This result could be explained by an object-based attention account or a hybrid model in which spatial attention conforms to the shape of stimulus objects (grouped array model; see Vecera and Farah, 1994; Kramer, Weber, and Watson, 1997).

SUMMARY   Task-irrelevant visual information that is in the same location, object, or feature dimension as an attended target feature may get selected together with the attended information, providing evidence for all three modes or units of attentional selection (location-based, feature-based, and object-based). These different modes of attentional selection are not mutually exclusive. Instead, each can be seen as a different way in which packets of visual attributes stick together preattentively, and hence get selected together all of a piece.

What aspect of neural activity is affected by attention?

How is attentional selection implemented at the neural level? In most general terms, the neural population representing the target must exert an increased effect on downstream neurons compared to the neural population representing the distracter. Such impact boosting by attention could in principle be achieved via at least two mechanisms: an increase in firing rate or an increase in the synchronization of neural activity (figure 42.2). Attention effects on firing rates have been studied extensively—in fact all, electrophysiology results presented in the preceding sections are based on firing rate measurements. We will first inspect several facets of attention effects on firing rates, then turn to evidence for the role of synchronization.

ATTENTIONAL EFFECTS ON FIRING RATE   First, are responses to attended stimuli increased or are responses to

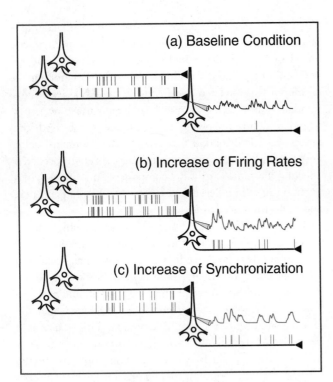

(a) Baseline Condition

(b) Increase of Firing Rates

(c) Increase of Synchronization

FIGURE 42.2 Schematic illustration of two potential ways in which the impact of a neuron's firing can be increased. In (b), an increase in firing rate of a group of presynaptic neurons will lead to increased firing of a postsynaptic neuron they connect to. In (c), an increase in the synchrony of a substantially lower number of presynaptic spikes will lead to a comparable increase in firing of the postsynaptic neuron. Note that an increase in synchronization at one processing stage can be translated into an increased firing rate at the next level. Thus, attentional modulation of synchrony and mean activity may be closely related.

nonattended stimuli suppressed, or do both mechanisms occur? Second, does attention act via a stimulus-independent top-down signal, adding a constant amount to activity in sensory cortical areas, or by modulating neural responses in a multiplicative way, or do both occur? The clearest example of the additive model is provided by attentional modulation of spontaneous activity. Support for the multiplicative or gain modulation model will be discussed in the context of the third question: How does attention affect the coding properties of a neural population? Fourth, is attentional modulation independent of physical stimulus attributes, or do they interact? An especially interesting case concerns stimulus contrast, which is closely correlated with stimulus saliency.

Response enhancement and suppression   A longstanding question regarding the effect of attention on neural activity has been whether it exerts its influence by strengthening the representation of the attended stimulus or by inhibiting the representation of the unattended stimulus, or both. On the basis of behavioral experiments (Posner, Snyder, and Davidson,

FIGURE 42.3   (*A*) Example of attentional enhancement and suppression. Responses of an MT neuron are shown in three attentional conditions (left to right). In all conditions, three moving dots (trajectories indicated by black bars) were presented, two moving up and down in counterphase with each other within the cell's receptive field (RF, gray ellipse, gray arrow to the right shows preferred motion direction), and one outside (horizontal arrows shown above the RF) moving left and right during stimulus phases 1 and 2. Left and center: When attention was drawn to one of the dots (marked by a Ⓣ, for target) inside the RF, the cell's response was dominated by this dot. Thus, when attention was switched from one dot to the other (left and center), the response pattern of the cell was almost completely inverted. A baseline is provided by the case in which attention was drawn outside the RF (right; dotted horizontal lines indicate average firing rate in the two stimulus phases of the baseline condition). Compared to this baseline, attention paid to the preferred stimulus direction leads to a genuine response enhancement and attention paid to the nonpreferred stimulus direction leads to response suppression (most clearly seen in the second stimulus phase). (Modified from S. Treue and J. H. R. Maunsell, Attentional modulation of visual motion processing in cortical areas MT and MST. *Nature* 399:539–541. Copyright 1996 by Nature Publishing Group.)

(*B*) Schematic of three potential effects that attention may exert on neural tuning curves, shown here as the firing rate as a function of stimulus motion direction, all of which could potentially occur in combination. Empirical support is strongest for "gain modulation" (Treue and Martínez Trujillo, 1999; McAdams and Maunsell, 1999a), in which firing rate is amplified in a multiplicative fashion, resulting in greater enhancement of responses to preferred than nonpreferred stimuli. Alternatively, attention may increase a cell's offset firing rate value, adding a constant amount of activity to every response. Finally, attention could alter the tuning function's width (e.g., render the neuron more selective for its preferred stimulus features). A narrowing of the tuning curve as well as an increase in gain can increase the slope of tuning functions, which would lend the neuron higher discriminative power (maximal around +45° and −45° motion direction in this example). This list of potential effects is neither exhaustive nor exclusive (see, e.g., an fMRI study [Murray and Wojeinlik, 2004] and a single-unit study [Wegener, Freiwald, and Kreiter, 2004] arguing for extensions of the multiplicative gain model).

(*C*) Schematic of two potential effects of attention on a neuron's contrast response function. According to the response gain model (right), attention produces a multiplicative increase of response magnitude for all contrast values—similar to the scaling of tuning curves. According to the contrast gain model (left), attention acts to shift this curve to the left, rendering the neuron more sensitive to lower contrast stimuli. Thus, in the contrast gain model, attention and contrast act interchangeably, such that an increase of attention can directly compensate for lower stimulus contrast. Data from areas V4 and MT support the contrast gain model (Martínez-Trujillo and Treue, 2002; Reynolds, Pasternak, and Desimone, 2000; Reynolds and Desimone, 2003).

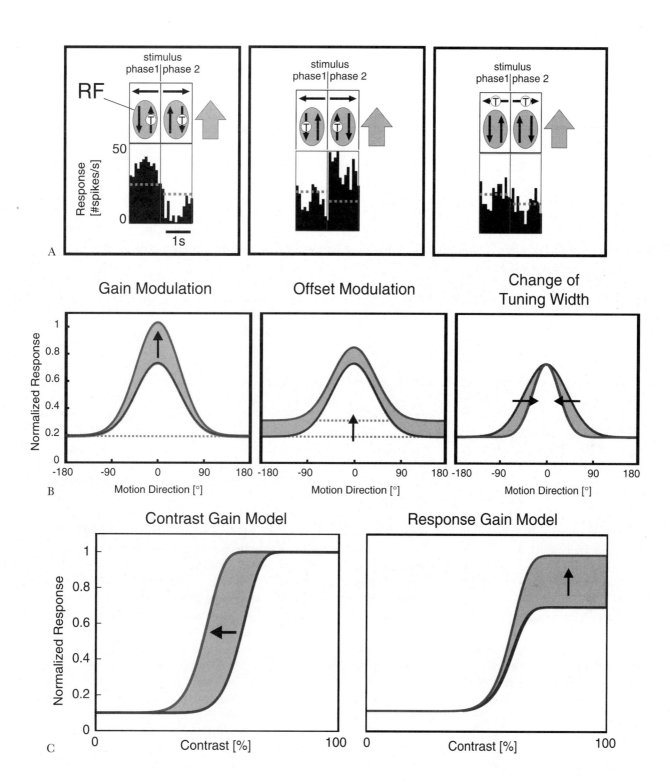

1980), it has been argued that both mechanisms are important, because performance is both enhanced by a valid location cue and disrupted by an invalid cue, in each case compared with a noninformative, "neutral" cue. In a similar vein, one fMRI study argued for the existence of suppressive (as well as enhancing) effects of attention (Smith, Singh, and Greenlee, 2000). These studies found that baseline activity was lower in peripheral retinotopic cortex when subjects attended to a foveal stimulus than when they passively viewed the same stimulus, even if no stimulus was present in the periphery in either condition. Although these data are consistent with suppression in the most general sense, they do not necessarily imply an active inhibitory process or indeed any process beyond enhancement. Instead, they can be explained if, first, during the passive condition attention is allocated diffusely over the entire field, and second, focusing attention entails not only increasing it at the target location but also withdrawing it (relative to the passive baseline) from all other locations. Therefore, current fMRI evidence does not resolve the question of whether attention involves two mechanisms, one enhancing and one suppressive.

In many single-unit studies it has been similarly difficult to identify genuine response increments and decrements because of the difficulty of identifying a neutral condition, especially in highly overtrained animals. What has been demonstrated in many investigations is a response enhancement when attention is directed to a cell's RF compared to when attention is directed elsewhere, an effect modulated by task difficulty (Spitzer, Desimone, and Moran, 1988; Spitzer and Richmond, 1991) and stimulus contrast (Reynolds, Pasternak, and Desimone, 2000). This effect has been found in many visual cortical areas of dorsal and ventral stream: V1 (Boch, 1986; Haenny and Schiller, 1988; Motter, 1993), V2 (Motter, 1993; Luck et al., 1997; Mehta, Ulbert, and Schroeder, 2000), V3A (Nakamura and Colby, 2000), V4 (Fischer and Boch, 1985; Haenny, Maunsell, and Shiller, 1988; Haenny and Schiller, 1988; Maunsell et al., 1991; Motter, 1993; Connor et al., 1996, 1997; McAdams and Maunsell, 1999a; Mehta, Ulbert, and Schroeder, 2000), IT (Richmond, Wurtz, and Sato, 1983; Richmond and Sato, 1987; Spitzer and Richmond, 1991; Mehta, Ulbert, and Schroeder, 2000), MT (Treue and Maunsell, 1996, 1999), MST (Treue and Maunsell, 1996, 1999), and LIP (Bushnell, Goldberg, and Robinson, 1981; Colby, Duhamel, and Goldberg, 1996; Gottlieb, Kusunoki, and Goldberg, 1998). Although these studies provide clear demonstrations of a modulatory influence of attention on firing rates, it is often unclear whether these effects reflect enhancement or suppression.

One proposed way to address this question uses an experimental paradigm introduced by Moran and Desimone for the ventral pathway (Moran and Desimone, 1985) and later adapted by Treue and Maunsell to the dorsal pathway (Treue and Maunsell, 1996) (figure 42.3A). In this paradigm, two stimuli are placed within a cell's RF, and attention is directed toward either one or the other of them. A much larger response is typically found when attention is directed toward the stimulus that matches the cell's preference than when it is directed toward the nonpreferred stimulus. It has been argued (Treue, 2001) that a third condition, in which attention is drawn to a stimulus outside the RF under study, can serve as a reference condition. Compared to this condition, attention does not generally enhance response magnitude when drawn to one of the stimuli inside the RF. Rather, attention toward the nonpreferred stimulus has a suppressive effect and attention toward the preferred stimulus has an enhancing effect (Treue and Maunsell, 1996, 1999a; Luck et al., 1997; Reynolds, Chelazzi, and Desimone, 1999). Thus, according to this logic, both mechanisms, enhancement and suppression, appear to exist. However, one might argue that even this case does not present a true neutral condition, since attention is after all directed somewhere, just not within the cell's RF.

The distinction of two mechanisms of attention, one enhancing and the other suppressive, becomes less important in one prominent view of attention, the biased competition model (Desimone and Duncan, 1995), supported by electrophysiological and imaging data (Kastner et al., 1998, 2001). According to this theory, competition takes place between objects for neural processing resources, leading to sensory suppression among multiple, simultaneously present stimuli. This competition can be biased by bottom-up saliency differences or by top-down attention signals favoring one stimulus over the other.

Attentional modulation of spontaneous activity Under some circumstances, attention can increase the baseline firing of neurons whose RFs are at the attended location or whose tuning profiles match the attended feature, even when no stimulus is present in the RF. That is, spontaneous firing rates of neurons in both the ventral and dorsal pathway are increased when attention is covertly shifted toward the location of an upcoming target stimulus, even before any stimulus is presented (Colby, Duhamel, and Goldberg, 1996; Luck et al., 1997). While other studies have not observed this baseline shift in retinotopic cortex (McAdams and Maunsell, 1999a; Mehta, Ulbert, and Schroeder, 2000), functional imaging studies have provided strong evidence for such stimulus-independent response modulation.

Kastner and colleagues (1999) found that during the 10 s interval when subjects were expecting a visual target to appear, neural activity increased in the retinotopically appropriate region within V2, V4, and TEO, as well as in parietal regions and, in two of the five subjects, in V1 (see also Greenlee, Magnussen, and Reinvang, 2000). This effect is unlikely to reflect working memory for the position of the upcoming target, as it occurred even when subjects did not have to keep the information in mind because the stimulus contained a small dot indicating the position of the expected target. In a related study (Ress, Backus, and Heeger, 2000), subjects were asked to detect the presence or absence of a low-contrast ring at a fixed 1 s interval after the presentation of an auditory tone. An event-related fMRI technique was used, enabling a separate analysis of target-present and target-absent trials. As expected, the MR signal from the retinotopically appropriate region of V1 showed the typical evoked hemodynamic response for trials in which the stimulus was present, peaking at about 6 s post-stimulus and decaying to baseline after about 20 s. Surprisingly, a very similar function was obtained for trials in which the stimulus was absent. This was not a response to the tone itself, as it was not found when subjects heard the auditory stimulus passively while not performing the visual task. Apparently, the tone cued subjects to attend to the location of the annulus, producing a large baseline response in V1 even when the stimulus did not appear. Furthermore, this effect was restricted to the region within V1 that responded to the location of the stimulus, so it cannot reflect a generalized increase in arousal in response to the tone. Finally, the baseline response was correlated with performance in the detection task, though this correlation was not found in another similar study (Ress and Heeger, 2003).

Attention-induced baseline increases are not restricted to retinotopic cortex. Shulman and colleagues (1999; see also Chawla, Rees, and Friston, 1999) found increases in neural activity in area MT/MST when subjects viewed a stationary cue that indicated the likely direction of motion for a subsequent test stimulus (compared with viewing a neutral cue that provided no directional information). Related results have been reported in studies of mental imagery. Goebel and colleagues (1998) reported activity in the human motion-processing area MT/MST when subjects imagined moving compared with stationary stimuli, and similarly, O'Craven and Kanwisher (2000) found selective activation of FFA and PPA during phases of imagery of faces and places (see also Kourtzi and Kanwisher, 2000; Hochstein and Ahissar, 2002). Although the mechanisms involved in attention and mental imagery may differ in important respects, the imagery results provide further evidence that extrastriate cortex can be strongly driven by pure top-down signals when no stimulus is present at all.

Thus, the evidence is now quite strong that attention (and other phenomena) can take the form of a top-down control signal to both retinotopic cortex and higher-level visual areas. How do these baseline increases in activity enhance perception of the attended item? Ress, Backus, and Heeger (2000) speculate that increasing baseline activity in the relevant neural population may bring these cells into a dynamic range where the same stimulus input will produce a larger response. In other words, the increase in baseline activity may result in an increase in the gain of the response to any stimulus that matches the expected target. However, Kastner and colleagues (1999) point out that, for most cortical areas, the magnitude of the baseline attentional increase when no stimulus was present was not strongly correlated with the magnitude of the attentional increase when a stimulus was present, indicating that the two effects may derive from different but partly overlapping populations of neurons (see also Rees, Frackowiak, and Frith, 1997).

Attention and stimulus coding As a result of attentional selection, performance on many tasks is enhanced. How can this behavioral effect be explained in terms of neural coding? First, as a result of multiplicative response increases (figure 42.3B, left), coding quality can be directly improved: due to an increased slope of the tuning curve, responses to two different features, such as 30° and 60° motion direction, are more distinct with attention than they are without attention.

However, this advantage of increased mean response magnitude (signal) will translate into improved coding quality only if noise is kept in check. Noise is presented by the variability of a neuron's response strength to the same stimulus from one instance of stimulus presentation to the next. The lower this variability, the more informative a neuron's response. Thus, a reduction of response variability (noise) presents a potential second mechanism by which attention could enhance coding quality. McAdams and Maunsell (1999b) studied this idea in area V4 but found no genuine effect of attention on response variability; in other words, response variability scaled with response magnitude with and without attention in quantitatively the same way. Because this scaling of noise with signal was sublinear, and because attention enhanced mean response magnitude, the neurons' signal-to-noise ratios still improved with attention.

Another way attention may improve stimulus representation is by a sharpening of neural tuning curves (figure 42.3B, right). A strong case for a close connection between enhanced discrimination performance and a change of neural tuning width was made in a recent combined quantitative psychophysical and computational study (Lee et al., 1999). Lee and colleagues found that attention lowered subjects' thresholds in demanding orientation and spatial frequency discrimination tasks. In order to quantitatively reproduce these behavioral results in a simple computational model, it was necessary to posit a sharpening of neural tuning for orientation and spatial frequency (figure 42.3B, right).

However, the picture from electrophysiology is not generally supportive of this idea. Although early investigations of color and orientation tuning curves in area V4 (Haenny and Schiller, 1988; Spitzer, Desimone, and Moran, 1988) had reported sharpened tuning, two recent systematic investigations of tuning properties in areas V4 and MT did not find any such change (McAdams and Maunsell, 1999a; Treue and Martínez Trujillo, 1999). Rather, attention effects were best described by a simple scaling of tuning functions in a multiplicative fashion: attention apparently enhanced the response strength for all stimulus orientations or motion directions by the same factor (see figure 42.2C, left). The conflicting findings in these studies might be explained if tuning curves are sharpened only for demanding tasks, as in the study of Spitzer and colleagues, but other explanations for these discrepancies exist (see, e.g., McAdams and Maunsell, 1999a; Treue, 2001).

From a theoretical point of view, though, improved coding properties of a neural population are not necessarily achieved by narrowed tuning curves (Pouget et al., 1999; Zhang and Sejnowski, 1999; Eurich and Wilke, 2000). Among the further factors that can affect the precision of a neural population code are variability of tuning widths across the population of cells (Wilke and Eurich, 2000), correlated responses between neurons, stimulus dependence of correlations (Oram et al., 1999), and distribution of correlation values within the population (Pouget, Deneve, and Latham, 2001; Nakahara and Amari, 2002; Wilke and Eurich, 2002). Most of these factors have not yet been studied experimentally.

Stimulus contrast and gain modulation Just as some experiments have investigated the effect of attention on neural tuning functions (figure 42.3B), other experiments have investigated the independent question of the effect of attention on contrast response functions (figure 42.3C). In principle, attention could affect contrast dependence in at least two ways. It could either shift the contrast response function to the left (figure 42.3C, left), thereby enhancing the neuron's sensitivity to the stimulus mostly at lower stimulus contrasts, or it could produce a multiplicative increase in responses at all contrasts (figure 42.3C, right).

Evidence that attention increases neural sensitivity (as in figure 42.3C, left) has been obtained in both areas V4 (Reynolds, Pasternak, and Desimone, 2000; Reynolds and Desimone, 2003) and MT (Martínez-Trujillo and Treue, 2002). Thus, attention shifts the dynamic range of neural responsiveness toward lower stimulus contrasts but has only a small effect at high contrasts. This finding indicates that attention acts on the gain of the inputs to the recorded neurons rather than on its output's gain. The strong dependence of the strength of attentional effects observed in these studies on stimulus contrast may also explain quantitative differences of attention effects reported across the literature, because a large variety of contrasts have been used in different experiments.

SYNCHRONIZATION AS A MECHANISM FOR ATTENTIONAL SELECTION Increasing the firing rate of a population of cells coding for an attended stimulus will increase the impact this population has on subsequent processing stages. A different way to enhance the impact of a neural population code on subsequent stages is to synchronize the activity in the population: postsynaptic cortical neurons are more likely to fire if EPSPs arrive simultaneously (Alonso, Usrey, and Reid, 1996; Larkum, Zhu, and Sakmann, 1999; Azouz and Gray, 2000; Usrey, Alonso, and Reid, 2000). If attention utilizes this mechanism, it would have the advantage of avoiding interference with rate coding (Niebur, Hsiao, and Johnson, 2002). Extending earlier theoretical work on the function of cortical cell assemblies (Milner, 1974; von der Malsburg and Schneider, 1986; Singer et al., 1990), Crick and Koch (1990a,b) proposed synchrony as a mechanism for attentional selection. More specific computational models demonstrated physiological plausibility and reproduced known attentional modulations of firing rates at subsequent stages (Niebur, Koch, and Rosin, 1993; Niebur and Koch, 1994).

The first direct evidence for a role of synchronization in attentional mechanisms was provided by Steinmetz and colleagues (2000) in macaque somatosensory cortex S2, while the animal was performing a visuotactile intermodal attention task. With a difficult version of the task, about a quarter of all pairs of neurons encountered showed increased synchronization when the animal paid attention to the tactile stimulus. Using a visual selective attention task, Fries and colleagues (2001) provided further support for a role of synchrony in attention. They measured synchronization between spikes and the local field potential (LFP), an EEG-like quantity. When attention was directed to the RFs of the neurons under study, Fries and colleagues observed not only very robust firing rate increases but also enhanced synchronization of spikes with the LFP. Modulation of synchrony and firing rates may thus offer two nonexclusive mechanisms for attentional selection. Interestingly, attentional effects on synchrony have been found in these two studies to occur specifically at high frequencies in the gamma range (35–90 Hz), reminiscent of earlier work on the role of synchrony in feature binding (Singer and Gray, 1995). Several EEG studies have also reported increased gamma power with attention (Gruber et al., 1999; Müller, Gruber, and Keil, 2000) or closely related cognitive functions, such as working memory (Tallon-Baudry et al., 1998, 1999). It is therefore tempting to speculate that these processes take advantage of similar neural mechanisms to enhance the impact of neural populations on subsequent processing stages.

Conclusions

Research based on neurophysiology in monkeys and neuroimaging in humans has provided answers to three long-standing questions about attention: the stage of selection, the units of selection, and the difference between neural representations of attended versus unattended objects.

ACKNOWLEDGMENTS This work was supported by a Human Frontiers grant to N. G. Kanwisher and Volkswagen Foundation and German Science Foundation (SFB 517) grants to W. A. Freiwald.

REFERENCES

ALONSO, J.-M., W. M. USREY, and R. C. REID, 1996. Precisely correlated firing in cells of the lateral geniculate nucleus. *Nature* 383:815–819.

AZOUZ, R., and C. M. GRAY, 2000. Dynamic spike threshold reveals a mechanism for synaptic coincidence detection in cortical neurons in vivo. *Proc. Natl. Acad. Sci. U.S.A.* 97:8110–8115.

BEAUCHAMP, M. S., R. W. COX, and E. A. DEYOE, 1997. Graded effects of spatial and featural attention on human area MT and associated motion processing areas. *J. Neurophysiol.* 78:516–520.

BENDER, D. B., and M. YOUAKIM, 2001. Effect of attentive fixation in macaque thalamus and cortex. *J. Neurophysiol.* 85:219–234.

BLASER, E., Z. W. PYLYSHYN, and A. O. HOLCOMBE, 2000. Tracking an object through feature space. *Nature* 408:196–199.

BOCH, R., 1986. Behavioral modulation of neuronal activity in monkey striate cortex: Excitation in the absence of active central fixation. *Exp. Brain Res.* 64:610–614.

BREFCZYNSKI, J. A., and E. A. DEYOE, 1999. A physiological correlate of the "spotlight" of visual attention. *Nat. Neurosci.* 2:370–374.

BROADBENT, D. E., 1958. *Perception and Communication*. London: Pergamon Press.

BUSHNELL, M. C., M. E. GOLDBERG, and D. L. ROBINSON, 1981. Behavioral enhancement of visual responses in monkey cerebral cortex. I. Modulation in posterior parietal cortex related to selective visual attention. *J. Neurophysiol.* 46:755–772.

CHAUDHURI, A., 1990. Modulation of the motion aftereffect by selective attention. *Nature* 344:60–62.

CHAWLA, D., G. REES, and K. FRISTON, 1999. The physiological basis of attentional modulation in extrastriate visual areas. *Nat. Neurosci.* 2:671–676.

COLBY, C. L., J. R. DUHAMEL, and M. E. GOLDBERG, 1996. Visual, presaccadic, and cognitive activation of single neurons in monkey lateral intraparietal area. *J. Neurophysiol.* 76:2841–2852.

COLBY, C. L., and M. E. GOLDBERG, 1999. Space and attention in parietal cortex. *Annu. Rev. Neurosci.* 22:319–349.

CONNOR, C. E., J. L. GALLANT, D. C. PREDDIE, and D. C. VAN ESSEN, 1996. Responses in area V4 depend on the spatial relationship between stimulus and attention. *J. Neurophysiol.* 75:1306–1308.

CONNOR, C. E., D. C. PREDDIE, J. L. GALLANT, and D. C. VAN ESSEN, 1997. Spatial attention effects in macaque area V4. *J. Neurosci.* 17:3201–3214.

CORBETTA, M., F. M. MIEZIN, S. DOBMEYER, G. L. SHULMAN, and S. E. PETERSEN, 1990. Attentional modulation of neural processing of shape, color, and velocity in humans. *Science* 248:1556–1559.

CORBETTA, M., F. M. MIEZIN, S. DOBMEYER, G. L. SHULMAN, and S. E. PETERSEN, 1991. Selective and divided attention during visual discrimination of shape, color, and speed: Functional anatomy by positron emssion tomograpy. *J. Neurosci.* 11:2383–2402.

CORBETTA, M., F. M. MIEZIN, G. L. SHULMAN, and S. E. PETERSEN, 1993. A PET study of visuospatial attention. *J. Neurosci.* 13:1226.

CORBETTA, M., and G. L. SHULMAN, 2002. Control of goal-directed and stimulus-driven attention in the brain. *Nat. Rev. Neurosci.* 3:201–215.

CRICK, F., 1984. Functions of the thalamic reticular complex: The searchlight hypothesis. *Proc. Natl. Acad. Sci. U.S.A.* 81:4586–4590.

CRICK, F., and C. KOCH, 1990a. Some reflections on visual awareness. *Symp. Quant. Biol.* 55:953–962.

CRICK, F., and C. KOCH, 1990b. Towards a neurobiological theory of consciousness. *Semin. Neurosci.* 2:263–275.

CULHAM, J. C., and N. G. KANWISHER, 2001. Neuroimaging of cognitive functions in human parietal cortex. *Curr. Opin. Neurobiol.* 11:157–163.

DESIMONE, R., and J. DUNCAN, 1995. Neural mechanisms of selective visual attention. *Annu. Rev. Neurosci.* 18:193–222.

DEUTSCH, J. A., and D. DEUTSCH, 1963. Attention: Some theoretical considerations. *Psychol. Rev.* 70:80–90.

DI RUSSO, F., A. MARTÍNEZ, and S. A. HILLYARD, 2003. Source analysis of event-related cortical activity during visuospatial attention. *Cerebral Cortex* 13:486–499.

DOWNING, P., J. LIU, and N. KANWISHER, 2001. Testing cognitive models of visual attention with fMRI and MEG. *Neuropsychologia* 39:1329–1342.

DUNCAN, J., 1984. Selective attention and organization of visual information. *J. Exp. Psychol. Gen.* 113:501–517.

EPSTEIN, R., and N. KANWISHER, 1998. A cortical representation of the local visual environment. *Nature* 392:598–601.

ERIKSEN, B. A., and C. W. ERIKSEN, 1974. Effects of noise letters upon the identification of a target letter in a non-search task. *Perception & Physchophysics* 16:143–149.

EURICH, C. W., and S. D. WILKE, 2000. Multi-dimensional encoding strategy of spiking neurons. *Neural Comp.* 12:1519–1529.

FISCHER, B., and R. BOCH, 1985. Peripheral attention versus central fixation: Modulation of the visual activity of prelunate cortical cells of the rhesus monkey. *Brain Res.* 345:111–123.

FRIES, P., J. H. REYNOLDS, A. E. RORIE, and R. DESIMONE, 2001. Modulation of oscillatory neuronal synchronization by selective visual attention. *Science* 291:1560–1563.

GANDHI, S. P., D. J. HEEGER, and G. M. BOYNTON, 1999. Spatial attention affects brain activity in human primary visual cortex. *Proc. Natl. Acad. Sci. U.S.A.* 96:3314–3319.

GOEBEL, R., D. KHORRAM-SEFAT, L. MUCKLI, H. HACKER, and W. SINGER, 1998. The constructive nature of vision: Direct evidence from functional magnetic resonance imaging studies of apparent motion and motion imagery. *Eur. J. Neurosci.* 10:1563–1573.

GOTTLIEB, J., 2002. Parietal mechanisms of target representation. *Curr. Opin. Neurobiol.* 12:134–140.

GOTTLIEB, J. P., M. KUSUNOKI, and M. E. GOLDBERG, 1998. The representation of visual salience in monkey parietal cortex. *Nature* 391:481–484.

GREENLEE, M. W., S. MAGNUSSEN, and I. REINVANG, 2000. Brain regions involved in spatial frequency discrimination: Evidence from MRI. *Exp. Brain Res.* 123(4):481–484.

GRUBER, T., M. M. MÜLLER, A. KEIL, and T. ELBERT, 1999. Selective visual-spatial attention alters induced gamma band responses in the human EEG. *Clin. Neurophysiol.* 110:2074–2085.

HAENNY, P. E., J. H. R. MAUNSELL, and P. H. SCHILLER, 1988. State dependent activity in monkey visual cortex. II. Retinal and extraretinal factors in V4. *Exp. Brain Res.* 69:245–259.

HAENNY, P. E., and P. H. SCHILLER, 1988. State dependent activity in monkey visual cortex. I. Single cell activity in V1 and V4 on visual task. *Exp. Brain Res.* 69:225–244.

HANDY, T. C., and G. R. MANGUN, 2000. Attention and spatial selection: Electrophysiological evidence for modulation by perceptual load. *Percept. Psychophys.* 62:175–186.

HOCHSTEIN, S., and M. AHISSAR, 2002. View from the top: Hierarchies and reverse hierarchies in the visual system. *Neuron* 36: 791–804.

ITO, M., and C. D. GILBERT, 1999. Attention modulates contextual influences in the primary visual cortex of alert monkeys. *Neuron* 22:593–604.

KANWISHER, N., and J. DRIVER, 1992. Objects, attributes, and visual attention: Which, what, and where. *Curr. Direct. Psychol. Sci.* 1:26–31.

KANWISHER, N., J. McDERMOTT, and M. M. CHUN, 1997. The fusiform face area: A module in human extrastriate cortex specialized for face perception. *J. Neurosci.* 17:4302–4311.

KANWISHER, N., and E. WOJCIULIK, 2000. Visual attention: Insights from brain imaging. *Nat. Rev. Neurosci.* 1:91–100.

KASTNER, S., P. DE WEERD, R. DESIMONE, and L. G. UNGERLEIDER, 1998. Mechanisms of directed attention in the human extrastriate cortex as revealed by functional MRI. *Science* 282: 108–111.

KASTNER, S., P. DE WEERD, M. A. PINSK, M. I. ELIZONDO, R. DESIMONE, and L. G. UNGERLEIDER, 2001. Modulation of sensory suppression: Implications for receptive field sizes in the human visual cortex. *J. Neurophysiol.* 86:1398–1411.

KASTNER, S., M. A. PINSK, P. DE WEERD, R. DESIMONE, and L. G. UNGERLEIDER, 1999. Increased activity in human visual cortex during directed attention in the absence of visual stimulation. *Neuron* 22:751–761.

KASTNER, S., and L. G. UNGERLEIDER, 2000. Mechanisms of visual attention in the human cortex. *Annu. Rev. Neurosci.* 23: 315–341.

KOCH, C., and S. ULLMAN, 1985. Shifts in selective visual attention: Towards the underlying neural circuitry. *Hum. Neurobiol.* 4:219–227.

KOURTZI, Z., and N. KANWISHER, 2000. Activation in human MT/MST by static images with implied motion. *J. Cogn. Neurosci.* 12:48–55.

KÖHLER, W., 1930. *Gestalt Psychology*. London: Bell and Sons.

KRAMER, A. F., T. A. WEBER, and S. E. WATSON, 1997. Object-based attentional selection: Grouped arrays or spatially invariant representations? Comment on Vecera and Farah (1994). *J. Exp. Psychol. Gen.* 126:3–13.

LARKUM, M. E., J. J. ZHU, and B. SAKMANN, 1999. A new cellular mechanism for coupling inputs arriving at different cortical layers. *Nature* 398:338–341.

LAVIE, N., 1995. Perceptual load as a necessary condition for selective attention. *J. Exp. Psychol. Hum. Percept. Perform.* 21:451–468.

LAVIE, N., and Y. TSAL, 1994. Perceptual load as a major determinant of the locus of visual selection in visual attention. *Percept. Psychophys.* 56:183–197.

LEE, D. K., L. ITTI, C. KOCH, and J. BRAUN, 1999. Attention activates winner-take-all competition among visual filters. *Nat. Neurosci.* 2:375–381.

LOGOTHETIS, N. K., J. PAULS, M. AUGATH, T. TRINATH, and A. OELTERMANN, 2001. Neurophysiological investigation of the basis of the fMRI signal. *Nature* 412:150–157.

LUCK, S. J., L. CHELAZZI, S. A. HILLYARD, and R. DESIMONE, 1997. Neural mechanisms of spatial selective attention in areas V1, V2, and V4 of macaque visual cortex. *J. Neurophysiol.* 77:24–42.

LUCK, S. J., and S. A. HILLYARD, 2000. The operation of selective attention at multiple stages of processing: Evidence from human and monkey electrophysiology. In *The New Cognitive Neurosciences*, M. S. Gazzaniga, ed. Cambridge, Mass.: MIT Press, pp. 687–710.

MARTÍNEZ-TRUJILLO, J. C., and S. TREUE, 2002. Attentional modulation strength in cortical area MT depends on stimulus contrast. *Neuron* 35:365–370.

MARTÍNEZ, A., L. ANLLO-VENTO, M. I. SERENO, L. R. FRANK, R. B. BUXTON, D. J. DUBOWITZ, E. C. WONG, H. J. HINRICHS, H. J. HEINZE, and S. A. HILLYARD, 1999. Involvement of striate and extrastriate visual cortical areas in spatial attention. *Nat. Neurosci.* 2:364–369.

MAUNSELL, J. H. R., 1995. The brain's visual world: Representation of visual targets in the cerebral cortex. *Science* 270:764–769.

MAUNSELL, J. H. R., G. SCALAR, T. A. NEALEY, and D. D. DEPRIEST, 1991. Extraretinal representations in area V4 in the macaque monkey. *Vis. Neurosci.* 7:561–573.

McADAMS, C. J., and J. H. R. MAUNSELL, 1999a. Effects of attention on orientation-tuning functions of single neurons in macaque cortical area V4. *J. Neurosci.* 19:431–441.

McADAMS, C. J., and J. H. R. MAUNSELL, 1999b. Effects of attention on the reliability of individual neurons in monkey visual cortex. *Neuron* 23:765–773.

McADAMS, C. J., and J. H. MAUNSELL, 2000. Attention to both space and feature modulates neuronal responses in macaque area V4. *J. Neurophysiol.* 83:1751–1755.

MEHTA, A. D., I. ULBERT, and C. E. SCHROEDER, 2000. Intermodal selective attention in monkeys. I. Distribution and timing of effects across visual areas. *Cerebral Cortex* 10:343–358.

MILLER, E. K., 2000. The neural basis of top-down control of visual attention in the prefrontal cortex. In *Attention and Performance 18: Control of Cognitive Processes*, S. Monsell and J. Driver, eds. Cambridge, Mass.: MIT Press, pp. 511–534.

MILNER, P. M., 1974. A model for visual shape recognition. *Psychol. Rev.* 81:521–535.

MORAN, J., and R. DESIMONE, 1985. Selective attention gates visual processing in the extrastriate cortex. *Science* 229:782–784.

MOTTER, B. C., 1993. Focal attention produces spatially selective processing in visual cortical areas V1, V2, and V4 in the presence of competing stimuli. *J. Neurosci.* 70:909–919.

MOTTER, B. C., 1994. Neural correlates of attentive selection for color or luminance in extrastriate area V4. *J. Neurosci.* 14:2178–2189.

MOUNTCASTLE, V. B., R. A. ANDERSEN, and B. C. MOTTER, 1981. The influence of attentive fixation upon the excitability of the light-sensititve neurons of the posterior parietal cortex. *J. Neurosci.* 1:1218–1235.

MÜLLER, M. M., T. GRUBER, and A. KEIL, 2000. Modulation of induced gamma band activity in the human EEG by attention and visual information processing. *Int. J. Psychophysiol.* 38:283–299.

MURRAY, S. O., and E. WOJCIULIK, 2004. Attention increases neural selectivity in the human lateral occipital complex. *Nat. Neurosci.* 7:70–74.

NAKAHARA, H., and S. AMARI, 2002. Attention modulation of neural tuning through peak and base rate in correlated firing. *Neural Netw.* 15:41–55.

NAKAMURA, K., and C. L. COLBY, 2000. Visual, saccade-related, and cognitive activation of single neurons in monkey extrastriate area V3A. *J. Neurophysiol.* 84:677–692.

NIEBUR, E., S. S. HSIAO, and K. O. JOHNSON, 2002. Synchrony: A neuronal mechanism for attentional selection? *Curr. Opin. Neurobiol.* 12:190–194.

NIEBUR, E., and C. KOCH, 1994. A model for the neuronal implementation of selective visual attention based on temporal correlation among neurons. *J. Comp. Neurosci.* 1:141–158.

NIEBUR, E., C. KOCH, and C. ROSIN, 1993. An oscillation-based model for the neuronal basis of attention. *Vision Res.* 333:2789–2802.

NOESSELT, T., S. A. HILLYARD, M. G. WOLDORFF, A. SCHOENFELD, T. HAGNER, L. JANCKE, C. TEMPELMANN, H. HINRICHS, and H. J. HEINZE, 2002. Delayed striate cortical activation during spatial attention. *Neuron* 35:575–587.

O'CONNOR, D. H., M. M. FUKUI, M. A. PINSK, and S. KASTNER, 2002. Attention modulates responses in the human lateral geniculate nucleus. *Nature Neurosci.* 5:1203–1209.

O'CRAVEN, K. M., B. R. ROSEN, K. K. KWONG, A. TREISMAN, and R. L. SAVOY, 1997. Voluntary attention modulates fMRI activity in human MT-MST. *Neuron* 18:591–598.

O'CRAVEN, K. M., P. E. DOWNING, and N. KANWISHER, 1999. fMRI evidence for objects as the units of attentional selection. *Nature* 401:584–587.

O'CRAVEN, K. M., and N. KANWISHER, 2000. Mental imagery of faces and places activates corresponding stiimulus-specific brain regions. *J. Cogn. Neurosci.* 12:1013–1023.

ORAM, M. W., P. FÖLDIÁK, D. I. PERRETT, and F. SENGPIEL, 1999. The "ideal homunculus": Decoding neural population signals. *Trends Cogn. Sci.* 21:259–265.

POSNER, M. I., 1980. Orienting of attention. The VIIth Sir Frederic Bartlett Lecture. *Q. J. Exp. Psychol.* 320:3–25.

POSNER, M. I., C. R. R. SNYDER, and B. J. DAVIDSON, 1980. Attention and the detection of signals. *J. Exp. Psychol. Gen.* 109:160–174.

POUGET, A., S. DENEVE, J.-C. DUCOM, and P. E. LATHAM, 1999. Narrow versus wide tuning curves: What's best for a population code? *Neural Comp.* 11:85–90.

POUGET, A., S. DENEVE, and P. E. LATHAM, 2001. The relevance of Fisher information for theories of cortical computation and attention. In *Visual Attention and Cortical Circuits*, J. Braun, C. Koch, and J. L. Davis, eds. Cambridge, Mass.: MIT Press, pp. 265–283.

REES, G., R. FRACKOWIAK, and C. FRITH, 1997. Two modulatory effects of attention that mediate object categorization in human cortex. *Science* 275:835–838.

REES, G., C. D. FRITH, and N. LAVIE, 1997. Modulating irrelevant motion perception by varying attentional load in an unrelated task. *Science* 278:1616–1619.

RESS, D., B. BACKUS, and D. J. HEEGER, 2000. Activity in primary visual cortex predicts performance in a visual detection task. *Nat. Neurosci.* 3:940–945.

RESS, D., and D. J. HEEGER, 2003. Neuronal correlates of perception in early visual cortex. *Nat. Neurosci.* 6:414–420.

REYNOLDS, J. H., L. CHELAZZI, and R. DESIMONE, 1999. Competitive mechanisms subserve attention in macaque areas V2 and V4. *J. Neurosci.* 19:1736–1753.

REYNOLDS, J. H., and R. DESIMONE, 2003. Interacting roles of attention and visual salience in V4. *Neuron* 37:853–863.

REYNOLDS, J. H., T. PASTERNAK, and R. DESIMONE, 2000. Attention increases sensitivity of V4 neurons. *Neuron* 26:703–714.

RICHMOND, B. J., and T. SATO, 1987. Enhancement of inferior temporal neurons during visual discrimination. *J. Neurophysiol.* 58:1292–1306.

RICHMOND, B. J., R. H. WURTZ, and T. SATO, 1983. Visual responses of inferior temporal neurons in awake rhesus monkey. *J. Neurophysiol.* 50:1415–1432.

RODRIGUEZ, V., M. VALDÉS-SOSA, and W. FREIWALD, 2002. Dividing attention between form and motion during transparent surface perception. *Cogn. Brain Res.* 13:187–193.

ROELFSEMA, P. R., V. A. F. LAMME, and H. SPEKREIJSE, 1998. Object based attention in the primary visual cortex of the macaque monkey. *Nature* 395:376–381.

ROELFSEMA, P. R., and H. SPEKREIJSE, 2001. The representation of erroneously perceived stimuli in the primary visual cortex. *Neuron* 32:853–863.

SAENZ, M., G. T. BURACAS, and G. M. BOYNTON, 2002. Global effects of feature-based attention in human visual cortex. *Nat. Neurosci.* 5:631–632.

SEIDEMANN, E., and W. T. NEWSOME, 1999. Effect of spatial attention on the responses of area MT neurons. *J. Neurophysiol.* 81:1783–1794.

SHULMAN, G. L., J. M. OLLINGER, E. AKBUDAK, T. E. CONTURO, A. Z. SNYDER, S. E. PETERSEN, and M. CORBETTA, 1999. Areas involved in encoding and applying directional expectations to moving objects. *J. Neurosci.* 19:9480–9496.

SINGER, W., and C. M. GRAY, 1995. Visual feature integration and the temporal correlation hypothesis. *Annu. Rev. Neurosci.* 18:555–586.

SINGER, W., C. GRAY, A. ENGEL, P. KÖNIG, A. ARTOLA, and S. BRÖCHER, 1990. Formation of cortical cell assemblies. *Symp. Quant. Biol.* 55:939–952.

SMITH, A. T., K. D. SINGH, and M. W. GREENLEE, 2000. Attentional suppression of activity in the human visual cortex. *Neuroreport* 11:271–277.

SOMERS, D. C., A. M. DALE, A. E. SEIFFERT, and R. B. H. TOOTELL, 1999. Functional MRI reveals spatially specific attentional modulation in human primary visual cortex. *Proc. Natl. Acad. Sci. U.S.A.* 96:1663–1668.

SPITZER, H., R. DESIMONE, and J. MORAN, 1988. Increased attention enhances both behavioral and neuronal performance. *Science* 240:338–340.

SPITZER, H., and B. J. RICHMOND, 1991. Task difficulty: Ignoring, attending to, and discriminating a visual stimulus yield progressively more activity in inferior temporal neurons. *Exp. Brain Res.* 83:340–348.

STEINMETZ, P. N., A. ROY, P. J. FITZGERALD, S. S. HSIAO, K. O. JOHNSON, and E. NIEBUR, 2000. Attention modulates synchronized neuronal firing in primate somatosensory cortex. *Nature* 404:187–190.

TALLON-BAUDRY, C., O. BERTRAND, F. PERONNET, and J. PERNIER, 1998. Induced gamma-band activity during the delay of a visual short-term memory task in humans. *J. Neurosci.* 18:4244–4254.

TALLON-BAUDRY, C., A. K. KREITER, and O. BERTRAND, 1999. Sustained and transient oscillatory responses in the gamma and beta bands in a visual short-term memory task in humans. *Vis. Neurosci.* 16:449–459.

TREISMAN, A. M., 1969. Strategies and models of selective attention. *Psychol. Rev.* 76:282–299.

TREUE, S., 2001. Neural correlates of attention in primate visual cortex. *Trends Neurosci.* 24:295–300.

TREUE, S., and J. C. MARTÍNEZ TRUJILLO, 1999. Feature-based attention influences motion processing gain in macaque visual cortex. *Nature* 399:575–579.

TREUE, S., and J. H. R. MAUNSELL, 1996. Attentional modulation of visual motion processing in cortical areas MT and MST. *Nature* 382:539–541.

TREUE, S., and J. H. R. MAUNSELL, 1999. Effects of attention on the processing of motion in macaque middle temporal and medial superior temporal visual cortical areas. *J. Neurosci.* 19:7591–7602.

TREUE, S., and J. C. TRUJILLO, 1999. Feature-based attention influences motion processing gain in macaque visual cortex. *Nature* 399:575–579.

TSOTSOS, J. K., S. CULHANE, W. WAI, Y. LAI, N. DAVIS, and F. NUFLO, 1995. Modeling visual attention via selective tuning. *Artif. Intel.* 78:135–160.

USREY, W. M., J. M. ALONSO, and R. C. REID, 2000. Synaptic interactions between thalamic inputs to simple cells in cat visual cortex. *J. Neurosci.* 20:5461–5467.

VALDÉS-SOSA, M., M. A. BOBES, V. RODRIGUEZ, and T. PINILLA, 1998. Switching attention without switching the spotlight: Object-based attentional modulation of brain potentials. *J. Cogn. Neurosci.* 10:137–151.

VANDUFFEL, W., R. B. H. TOOTELL, and G. A. ORBAN, 2000. Attention-dependent suppression of metabolic activity in the early stages of the macaque visual system. *Cerebral Cortex* 10: 109–126.

VECERA, S. P., and M. J. FARAH, 1994. Does visual attention select objects or locations? *J. Exp. Psychol. Gen.* 123:146–160.

VIDYASAGAR, T. R., 1998. Gating of neuronal responses in macaque primary visual cortex by an attentional spotlight. *Neuroreport* 9:1947–1952.

VON DER MALSBURG, C., and W. SCHNEIDER, 1986. A neural cocktail-party processor. *Biol. Cybern.* 54:29–40.

WATANABE, T., A. M. HARNER, S. MIYAUCHI, Y. SASAKI, M. NIELSEN, D. PALOMO, and I. MUKAI, 1998. Task-dependent influences of attention on the activation of human primary visual cortex. *Proc. Natl. Acad. Sci. U.S.A.* 95:11489–11492.

WATANABE, T., Y. SASAKI, S. MIYAUCHI, B. PUTZ, N. FUJIMAKI, M. NIELSEN, R. TAKINO, and S. MIYAKAWA, 1998. Attention-regulated activity in human primary visual cortex. *J. Neurophysiol.* 79:2218–2221.

WEGENER, D., W. A. FREIWALD, and A. K. KREITER, 2004. The influence of sustained selective attention on stimulus selectivity in macaque area MT. *J. Neurosci.* 24:6106–6114.

WILKE, S. D., and C. W. EURICH, 2000. Representational accuracy of stochastic neural populations. *Neural Comp.* 14:155–189.

WILKE, S. D., and C. W. EURICH, 2002. Representational accuracy of stochastic neural populations. *Neural. Comput.* 14:155–189.

WOLFE, J. M., K. R. CAVE, and S. L. FRANZEL, 1989. Guided search: An alternative to the feature integration model for visual search. *J. Exp. Psychol. Hum. Percept. Perform.* 15:419–433.

WURTZ, R. H., M. E. GOLDBERG, and D. L. ROBINSON, 1980. Behavioral modulation of visual responses in the monkey: Stimulus selection for attention and movement. *Prog. Biopsychobiol. Physiol. Psychol.* 9:43–83.

WURTZ, R. H., and C. W. MOHLER, 1976. Enhancement of visual responses in monkey striate cortex and frontal eye fields. *J. Neurophysiol.* 39:766–772.

ZHANG, K., and T. J. SEJNOWSKI, 1999. Neuronal tuning: To sharpen or broaden? *Neural Comp.* 11:75–84.

43 Spatial Neglect and Extinction

JON DRIVER, PATRIK VUILLEUMIER, AND MASUD HUSAIN

ABSTRACT Patients suffering from spatial neglect after right-hemisphere strokes exhibit striking disruptions of attention and spatial awareness, often behaving as if the left side of their world no longer exists. This syndrome often results from extensive brain damage and this can involve many component deficits, some of which do not only affect the left side of space. The various component deficits, including some that would not cause neglect on their own, can exacerbate neglect when combined. Much recent progress in understanding the neglect syndrome has come from relating the patients' deficits to issues arising from the study of normal attention and normal spatial representation, to physiological findings from animal work on the associated brain regions, and to functional neuroimaging results in both neurologically healthy people and in patients with neglect. This convergent approach has revealed how neglect can affect both conscious perception and spatial exploration while differing from primary sensory or motor deficits. The role of attention and other factors that influence whether or not a particular stimulus will reach the patients' awareness has also been highlighted. Extensive residual abilities have been revealed, along with their neural bases, giving some grounds for optimism about possible rehabilitation of this disabling syndrome and shedding new light on the role of frontoparietal circuits in awareness.

The clinical disorder of neglect

Neglect is a common and disabling syndrome following right hemisphere strokes (see Heilman, Watson, and Valenstein, 2003; Karnath, Milner, and Valnar, 2003). Studies of neglect have shed light on the neural basis of attention, awareness, spatial representation, multisensory integration, and sensorimotor transformation. Patients with spatial neglect often behave as if one side of their world no longer existed, appearing oblivious to stimuli falling toward the contralesional (usually left) side.

Recent research suggests that the neglect syndrome often reflects a combination of deficits, some of which do not only affect the contralesional side of space. The exact pattern of deficits varies from one patient to another, as does the asso-ciated lesion, but the following clinical signs can occur. Patients may ignore people, objects, and events toward the contralesional (left) side, in overt behavior or when describing a scene. Their eyes, head, and trunk may be oriented rightward. They may eat food from only the right side of a plate, shave or apply makeup to just the right side of their face, dress only the right side of their body, and overlook or forget left turns in routes. Even if their left hand is not paralyzed, they may not use it spontaneously.

Neglect may arise at different spatial scales within the same patient. As well as ignoring stimuli at the extreme left in their environment, patients may neglect, say, a left page when reading a small book, words to the left of the right page, and even letters at one end of each word. Both the stimuli presented and the task performed can modulate the extent of neglected space.

Many neglect patients do not realize they are missing information (a condition known as anosognosia). If their lesion also causes paralysis of contralesional limbs, some patients remain unaware even of this. The reason remains unclear (Vuilleumier, 2000a), but neglect itself may contribute, with contralesional losses going unnoticed partly because leftward space is no longer fully represented and attended.

Measuring neglect with standard clinical tests reveals symptoms but has limitations

Neglect can be demonstrated by pen-and-paper tests. In cancellation tasks, patients search for and mark target shapes on a page. Patients with neglect after right-hemisphere damage typically mark only some targets toward the right, missing leftward targets even with unlimited time (figure 43.1A). The extent of this neglect can depend on the search array (Grabowecky, Robertson, and Treisman, 1993) and the discrimination required (Eglin, Robertson, and Knight, 1989). Such tests presumably draw on processes similar to those recruited for visual search in studies of normal attention (Wolfe, 2003) but typically require marking of multiple targets, with saccadic and manual contributions.

In bisection tests, patients must mark the midpoint of horizontal lines or other stimuli. Some patients deviate ipsilesionally, as if ignoring or compressing (Bisiach et al., 1996) contralesional extent (figure 43.1B). Clinical test batteries also include drawing from memory, or copying. Omissions

JON DRIVER Institute of Cognitive Neuroscience, University College London, London, U.K.
PATRIK VUILLEUMIER Institute of Cognitive Neuroscience, University College London, London, U.K., and Department of Neuroscience, Medical Center, University of Geneva, Geneva, Switzerland.
MASUD HUSAIN Institute of Cognitive Neuroscience, University College London, London, U.K., and Division of Neuroscience and Psychological Medicine, Imperial College London, U.K.

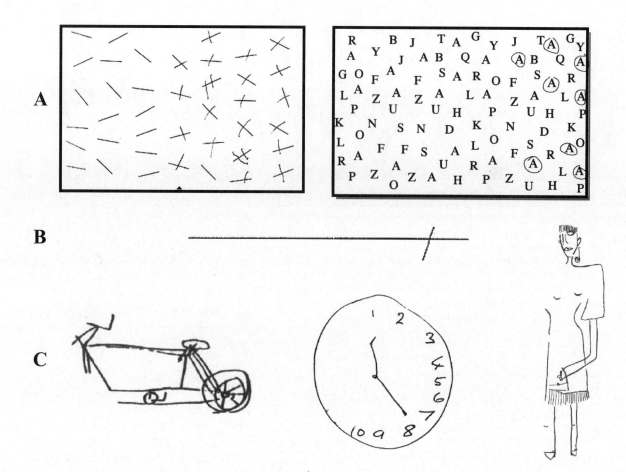

FIGURE 43.1 Examples of left-sided neglect after right hemisphere damage on clinical pen-and-paper tests. (*A*) Cancellation tests. Patient was asked either to mark all lines or just to mark target As among other nontarget letters. More severe left neglect is evident in a letter task requiring attention-demanding discrimination between intermingled targets and nontargets. (*B*) Line bisection biased toward ipsilesional end. (*C*) Drawings of a bicycle, a clock, and a woman, made from memory. Neglect is evident at multiple scales for the bicycle and the woman (e.g., not only the entire left wheel is missing but also the left pedal; not only the left arm of the woman but also the left side of the handbag strap, the left earring, etc.).

on the contralesional side can be observed (figure 43.1*C*), even for objects with prescribed layouts (e.g., a clockface).

Clinical pen-and-paper tests conducted within "free vision" may involve not only perceptual and attentional processes but also exploratory, motor, transaccadic, planning, and even memory processes. Deficits in these processes might be related or independent but nevertheless often joint contributors to the observed deficit when co-occurring. More specific experimental situations are therefore needed to dissect out potential components.

Neglect without vision can reveal its multimodal and representational nature

Even when neglect patients are blindfolded, haptic exploration can deviate toward the ipsilesional side (De Renzi, 1982) (figure 43.2*d, e*). When neglect patients search in darkness for an isolated spot of light (absent on critical trials measuring self-organized exploration, figure 43.2*b*), scan paths of the eyes and head can also show an ipsilesional bias

(Karnath, Niemeier, and Dichgans, 1998). Exploratory movements can be observed in both left and right directions (often with equal frequency; Niemeier and Karnath, 2000), but the "center of mass" of the scan path is shifted ipsilesionally (e.g., by 40° in figure 43.2*c*). Patients may also judge that their subjective midline is shifted correspondingly rightward (Karnath, Niemeier, and Dichgans, 1998).

Aspects of neglect can also be observed for perceptual judgments in tactile, proprioceptive, and auditory modalities (Vallar, 1998), even when spatial motor factors are held constant, suggesting that neglect can be multisensory. Auditory localization may be especially poor for free-field contralesional targets, and such auditory deficits can correlate with the severity of visual neglect on cancellation tasks (Pavani et al., 2004).

Remarkably, neglect can also arise in memory or imagery tasks testing for so-called representational aspects. Patients may fail to describe elements that would be situated toward the contralesional side for remembered settings or imagined situations, ranging from a large city scene (Bisiach and

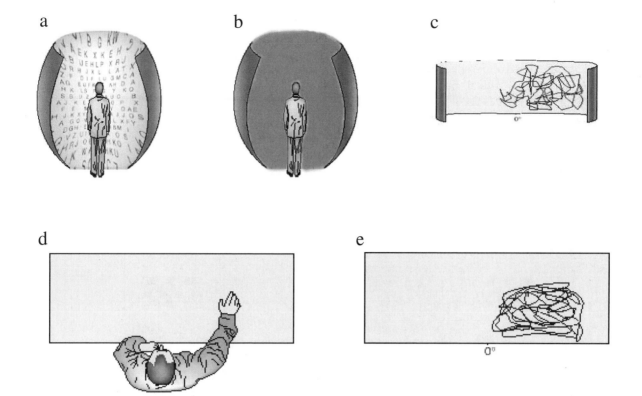

a   b   c

d   e

FIGURE 43.2 Exploratory biases in left neglect after right hemisphere damage, both with and without vision (adapted with author's permission from Karnath, 2002). (*A*) Patient searches for (missing) target letter in cabin, when surrounded by different non-target letters on all sides. Scan path is miscentered toward the right side, although movements can be observed in both directions (often equally). (*B*) Similar phenomenon is evident when patient searches

for a (missing) spot of light in total darkness. (*C*) Example scan path from one patient; search field is biased substantially (here 40°) to the right, but with movements in both directions. Normal subjects have a search field that is centered straight ahead, but otherwise quite similar. (*D*) Manual search for (missing) tactile target. Center of the search field (now manual) is again biased toward the right, as shown for one example in (*E*), even in the absence of vision.

Luzzatti, 1978) to an imagined clockface (Grossi et al., 1989). They may also fail to recall objects presented earlier on the contralesional side, even when they successfully named these at exposure (Denis et al., 2002). When neglect patients are asked to adopt a different perspective in their mind's eye (e.g., a viewpoint from the other side of a familiar city square), previously omitted details may now be reported and previously reported details may be missed (Bisiach and Luzzatti, 1978). Even neglect during imagery can thus depend on the spatial "viewpoint" adopted.

Differences from primary sensory loss reveal the spatial nature of neglect

Neglect cannot be explained solely by primary sensory or motor losses, an observation consistent with the finding that lesions often spare primary sensory or motor cortices. Many patients with primary losses only (e.g., visual field cuts) do not exhibit neglect. Conversely, other patients may exhibit spatial neglect but no sensory or motor loss (although primary deficits may exacerbate neglect when jointly present; Dorrichi and Angelelli, 1999). Patients with neglect

can fail to see despite not being literally blind. Understanding this aspect of neglect has benefited from analogies drawn with normal inattention, where the absence of appropriate attention to a stimulus can analogously lead to a normally sighted person failing to see (as in situations of "inattentional blindness" [Mack and Rock, 1998] or "change blindness" [Rensink, O'Regan, and Clark, 1997] in normal subjects).

GRADED NATURE OF DEFICITS IN NEGLECT Patients with primary sensory losses often show step functions in performance at anatomical midlines (e.g., blindness for one visual hemifield in hemianopic field cuts). This kind of loss differs from neglect, where deficits are more graded, with patients often showing increasingly worse performance for stimuli further in the contralesional direction, even within the ipsilesional hemifield (Smania et al., 1998). Such gradients may reflect the loss through lesion of correspondingly graded subpopulations of neurons (Pouget and Driver, 2000) that exist within one hemisphere for visually responsive regions remote from primary visual cortex, such as in posterior parietal cortex (Ben Hamed et al., 2001). This would imply a role for such neural populations in the normal generation of visual awareness.

MODULATION OF NEGLECT BY POSTURE   Visual field cuts are tied to a specific region of retinal space, moving with the eyes. Likewise, primary somatosensory losses are tied to specific regions of the skin, regardless of where in space that skin is placed. By contrast, in patients with neglect, visual abilities for specific retinal locations can depend on current posture, as may tactile abilities.

Visual performance can depend on both eye-in-orbit posture (Vuilleumier et al., 1999) and head-on-neck posture (Karnath, 1997), with less neglect for a given retinal location in the left visual field when the patient is gazing rightward, so that the same retinal location shifts further to the right of

head and body (figure 43.3a–c). If the patient's trunk is twisted instead (figure 43.3f, g), analogous modulation can be observed, with better performance for a fixed retinotopic—and now also craniotopic—visual location with the trunk twisted leftward (so that the retinal stimulus now falls further rightward relative to the trunk). Vibrating the neck muscles to simulate afferent inputs produced by such head-on-trunk realignment can induce analogous effects (Karnath, 1997). These effects arise not only in visuomotor tasks (e.g., saccades to a target) but also in perceptual/ attentional tasks in which spatial motor factors are held constant (e.g., detection or discrimination of peripheral visual targets with the gaze kept steady).

A potential explanation for these remarkable phenomena is suggested by physiological work in monkey parietal cortex

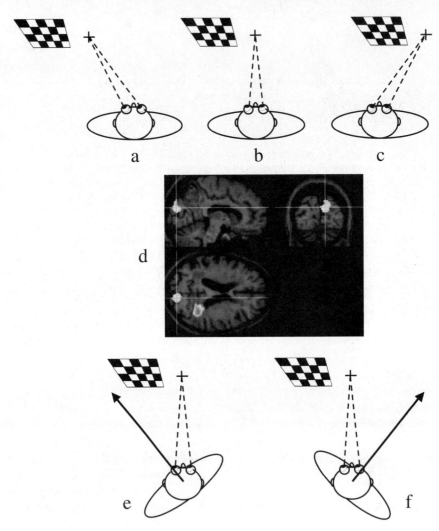

FIGURE 43.3   Postural modulation of left visual neglect after right hemisphere damage. A left retinal stimulus that is neglected when gazing leftward (a) or straight ahead (b) may be detected or judged better when gazing rightward (c). Region in right occipital cortex (d) for a single case of left neglect after right parietal damage (lesion visible in transverse section) that showed higher activation specifically when patient was gazing rightward for left-minus-right retinal

stimulation (see text for further details). Head-on-trunk posture can also modulate visual neglect (e and f). Performance for fixed retinotopic and craniotopic left visual stimulus can be improved with the trunk twisted leftward (e, arrow depicts straight-ahead direction from trunk) than with trunk straight or twisted rightward (f). (See color plate 17.)

and related areas, plus computational modeling. Neurons in parietal area 7a show retinotopic responses to visual stimuli that are gain-modulated by eye-in-orbit posture (Andersen, Essick, and Siegel, 1985), such that maximal response reflects a preferred combination of retinal location and eye posture. Further physiological studies show that various postural factors (and corresponding proprioceptive, vestibular, or efference copy inputs) can modulate sensory responses in several parietal and premotor areas (see Colby, Duhamel, and Goldberg, 1993; Andersen et al., 1997). Lesions to neural populations combining, say, retinal receptive fields with particular eye positions (or other postural factors) might leave an uneven subset of preferences overall. For instance, left retinal locations might then be strongly represented only when combined with rightward gaze (Pouget and Driver, 2000). Modulation of visual neglect by other posture-related factors (e.g., neck muscle vibration, or even caloric vestibular stimulation; Vallar, 1998) might similarly be explained in terms of the combined input preferences of surviving neural populations (Pouget and Driver, 2000). In addition to potentially explaining such aspects of neglect, accounts of this type also imply a role for these neuronal populations in normal visual awareness.

Accounts in these terms can now be related to residual brain activity in patients with neglect. Rees and colleagues (unpublished observations) used functional magnetic resonance imaging (fMRI) to examine modulation of visual responses by eye-in-orbit posture in a patient with a right parietal lesion showing left neglect. Behaviorally, he detected left visual field stimuli better when gazing rightward. In different blocks during fMRI, he maintained fixation centrally, leftward or rightward, while checkerboard stimuli were presented in the left or right retinal field. fMRI showed higher activation to left field checkerboards during rightward gaze, within one specific region of the right occipital lobe (probably V3A, closely connected with parietal cortex; see figure 43.3d). There was also stronger coupling ("effective connectivity") in this situation between that occipital cluster and parietal cortex, both surrounding the lesion and in symmetrical parietal areas of the intact left hemisphere. This finding accords with modulation of the occipital response by remaining parietal subpopulations combining left retinal inputs with rightward eye-in-orbit posture.

Postural factors can also modulate nonvisual neglect. Unlike primary somatosensory defects, neglect for touch on the contralesional hand can be ameliorated by placing that hand on the ipsilesional side of the body (Aglioti, Smania, and Peru, 1999) or by gazing toward it (Vaishnavi, Calhoun, and Chatterjee, 2001). The neural basis of these effects may relate to multisensory neurons found in parietal and premotor cortex, as well as the putamen, with spatially corresponding visual and tactile receptive fields that get updated when the corresponding body part is moved, or when gaze

shifts (Graziano and Gross, 1998). A recent study found that awareness of right hand touch was reduced when a neglect patient's right hand was placed on the left versus the right side of his body (Valenza et al., 2003). fMRI revealed a corresponding decreases of neural responses to tactile stimuli in contralateral somatosensory cortex (S1), as well as a decreased response bilaterally in premotor cortex (middle frontal gyri).

Extinction, biased competition, and attention

A further difference from primary sensory loss is illustrated by a component present in many (but not all) neglect patients: perceptual extinction. Patients with extinction can usually perceive a unilateral stimulus presented alone toward the affected side (at least under some postures) but miss the same stimulus under the same posture when it is presented concurrently with another stimulus further toward the ipsilesional side (figure 43.4a–c). The ipsilesional stimulus is said to extinguish awareness of a contralesional stimulus that would otherwise be detected. This deficit thus seems to arise only (or primarily) when two stimuli must compete for attention. It has often been suggested that extinction may reflect a pathological bias in spatial attention (favoring ipsilesional locations), possibly combined with some reduction in overall capacity (to explain why two salient stimuli cannot both be perceived, as discussed later under simultanagnosia; see Driver et al., 1997).

Extinction seems reminiscent of a normal attentional phenomenon: interference between two targets occurring at (or around) the same point in time that can lead normal observers to miss one or the other target (Duncan, 1980; Driver et al., 1997). However, extinction is pathological in at least two respects. First, it has a consistent spatial nature; that is, it usually affects contralesional targets (though see Robertson, 1989). Second, extinction can affect even a salient, unmasked contralesional target, whereas two-target costs in normal individuals may arise only with very brief masked displays. Nevertheless, much progress in understanding extinction has stemmed from relating it to constraints on attentional competition in the normal brain (including single-cell and functional neuroimaging evidence; see Driver and Vuilleumier, 2001a; Kastner and Ungerleider, 2001). Neural accounts of selective attention (Desimone and Duncan, 1995; see also Freiwald and Kanwisher, this volume) regard it increasingly as the emergent outcome of various biases in competitive sensory processing, encompassing both bottom-up and top-down influences. In neglect and extinction, the lesion might be viewed as a chronic bias disadvantaging some stimulus locations relative to others in competitive terms.

Like neglect, extinction can be multimodal, arising within vision, touch, audition, and even smell or motor action

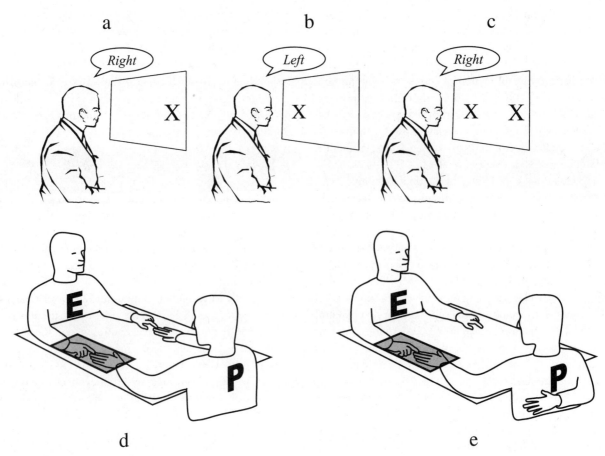

a   b   c

d   e

FIGURE 43.4 Perceptual extinction after right hemisphere damage. Patient can typically detect not only right unilateral visual stimulus (*a*) but also left unilateral stimulus on affected side (*b*), yet misses the latter in the presence (*c*) of an ipsilesional competitor during bilateral stimulation. Extinction can also be observed cross-modally, as when a right visual event extinguishes awareness of a left hand touch that would otherwise be felt. This is depicted here (*d*) for the clinical method of "confrontation," whereby the examiner (indicated by E) uses his or her own fingers to produce stimulation for the patient (indicated by P). Movement of examiner's finger in the patient's right visual field can extinguish concurrent unseen (obscured by cover) touch on the patient's left hand by the examiner. This can depend on the right visual event falling near the patient's right hand (even when this is not touched by the examiner's finger moving very close to it), being reduced if that event or the patient's right hand is moved away, as when the patient's right hand is placed behind the back (*e*). Similar results can be obtained with computerized stimuli.

(Driver et al., 1997; Heilman, Watson, and Valenstein, 2003). It can also be elicited cross-modally, as when a visual stimulus on the ipsilesional right side extinguishes awareness of a touch on the left hand that would otherwise have been felt (Di Pellegrino, Ladavas, and Farne, 1997). Interestingly, this may require right visual stimulation to fall near in space to the (unstimulated) right hand (see figure 43.4*d*, *e*). Visual stimulation near the left hand instead can actually boost detection of touch there (Ladavas et al., 1998). This may again relate to multisensory neurons whose visual receptive fields fall close to the body parts on which the tactile receptive fields lie (Graziano and Gross, 1998).

Extinction can provide useful measures of perceptual/ attentional performance in patients, without requiring overt exploratory behavior or spatially directed responses. Extinction tests do not tap all aspects of the neglect syndrome, but may unveil important components associated with spatial competition and perceptual awareness. Pathologically unequal spatial competition may play a role in other aspects of neglect also. Cancellation tests (figure 43.1*A*) involve multiple competing elements, as do most search tasks. Neglect in such tasks is typically reduced if each target is erased when found, rather than marked, so that competing stimuli are gradually removed (Mark, Kooistra, and Heilman, 1988).

Extinction may be reconciled with the graded deficits for single stimuli mentioned earlier if competition exaggerates the loss of saliency for events toward the contralesional side (Pouget and Driver, 2000). Extinction can also be modulated by postural factors (Aglioti, Smania, and Peru, 1999). Finally, extinction-like deficits can be induced in neurologically healthy subjects by transcranial magnetic stimulation (TMS) over parietal cortex and other sites (see Hilgetag, Theoret, and Pascual-Leone, 2001; Lomber et al., 2002). Further

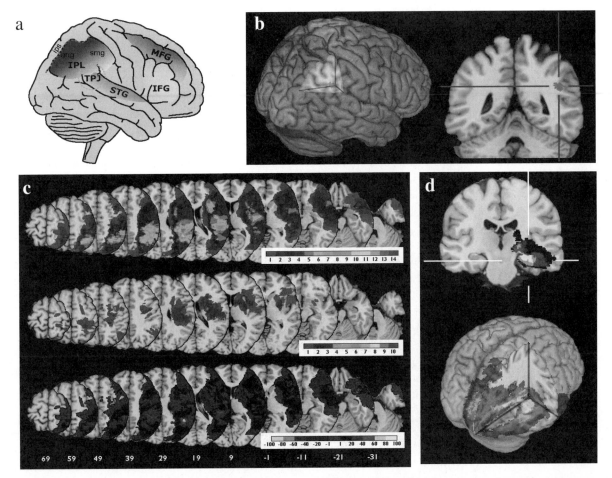

FIGURE 43.5   Anatomy of neglect syndrome. (*a*) Regions associated with lesions in neglect patients include the right inferior parietal lobe (IPL), the temporoparietal junction (TPJ), the middle and inferior frontal gyri (MFG and IFG, respectively), and the superior temporal gyrus (STG). Subcortical lesions or white matter damage may also play a role (see text). Lesions in individual patients with neglect can often be large. (*b*) Region of maximum overlap for damage in neglect patients found in angular gyrus by Mort and colleagues (in press). Coronal section's shown at right of panel, with the location shown by the cutout at the left of the panel. (*c*) Detailed lesion anatomy from this study. Top row shows anatomy in neglect patients with right middle cerebral artery (CA) infarctions, middle row shows anatomy in right middle CA controls without neglect, and bottom row shows subtraction. Note the presence of an angular gyrus hotspot in *c*, plus other areas. (*d*) Coronal section and cutout showing lesion overlap for right posterior CA neglect patients minus nonneglect right posterior CA controls (from Mort and colleagues, 2003). (See color plate 18.)

TMS work should clarify the anatomy of extinction and the critical points in time at which various brain sites can bias spatial attention and affect awareness for competing stimuli.

Other differences between neglect or extinction and sensory deficits have also been attributed to attentional factors. Whereas true visual field cuts (or other sensory losses) cannot be alleviated by directing attention to the affected region, performance for otherwise neglected stimuli can often be improved by cuing covert attention there (Posner et al., 1984). This can lead to difficulties in assessing the visual fields of neglect patients. Walker and colleagues (1991) described a patient with neglect who usually missed left visual stimuli during perimetric field testing, but not when the central fixation point was switched off just before onset. Whereas such modulation of elementary visual function was once viewed as puzzling, it now fits with evidence that attention can affect early sensory processing even in the normal brain (see, e.g., Freiwald and Kanwisher, this volume).

Anatomy of the neglect syndrome

Severe neglect is more common after right than left hemisphere damage, especially in enduring form (see, e.g., Vallar, 1993). Possible reasons for this may involve left hemisphere specialization for language in humans, the representation of both ipsilateral and contralateral space by some right hemisphere regions, and additional nonspatial deficits after right lesions, exacerbating the bias to one side. Many patients with neglect have large lesions.

A network of interconnected right hemisphere areas has been implicated in neglect (Mesulam, 1999; Heilman, Waston, and Valenstein, 2003) (figure 43.5*a*), as well as in various aspects of normal attention and spatial cognition, based on functional neuroimaging (e.g., Corbetta and Shulman, 2002; Husain and Rorden, 2003). Cortical damage involving the right inferior parietal lobe (IPL) or the nearby temporoparietal junction (TPJ) is classically associated with neglect (Vallar, 1993), possibly together with underlying white matter damage (Samuelsson et al., 1997). Focal inferior right frontal lesions can also produce neglect (Husain and Kennard, 1996), though usually more transiently. Most commonly, large middle cerebral artery (MCA) strokes associated with severe neglect span both posterior and anterior regions (Kumral and Evyapan, 1999).

Karnath, Ferber, and Himmelbach (2001) challenged the conventional view that IPL and TPJ are the main posterior sites associated with neglect. They mapped lesions in patients with neglect but without visual field cuts and concluded that maximal lesion overlap occurred in the mid-superior temporal gyrus (STG, see figure 43.5a), a result they replicated in a larger follow-up study (H.O. Karnath, personal communication). However, a recent anatomical study using high-resolution MRI (Mort et al., 2003) found that although the STG is involved in many neglect patients (50% in their sample), right STG damage is not always associated with neglect. In that study, every patient with neglect following MCA stroke had damage to the right angular gyrus (figure 43.5b, c). This parietal region may also be involved in Balint's syndrome, following bilateral damage.

Subcortical lesions in MCA territory, involving the right basal ganglia or thalamus, can also produce neglect (Vallar, 1993; Karnath, Himmelbach, and Rordan, 2002), but this may reflect diaschisis or hypoperfusion in overlying parietal and frontal regions, as demonstrated by single-proton emission computed tomography (SPECT) and MR perfusion studies (Perani et al., 1987; Demeurisse at al., 1997; Hillis et al., 2002). Parietal lesions themselves can cause remote dysfunction in frontal and cingulate areas, correlating with neglect severity (Leibovitch et al., 1998). Finally, some patients with posterior cerebral artery (PCA) territory stroke also suffer from neglect, although this has been less studied. Whereas occipital lesions typically produce hemianopia, larger PCA strokes extending into the posterior thalamus and/or medial temporal lobe may cause neglect. Recent data (Mort et al., 2003) suggest that damage to parahippocampal regions (closely interconnected with the parietal cortex) may be critical (figure 43.5d). It is unknown whether neglect differs qualitatively after PCA versus MCA damage.

Because neglect is likely to involve multiple deficits, the anatomy of individual components may be more revealing than localization of the whole syndrome. Studies of spatial neglect in animals can contribute to this (Wardack, Olivier, and Duhamel, 2003). It remains controversial whether brain lesions in monkeys can produce deficits closely mimicking human neglect. Extinction-like deficits have been demon-

strated, as have biases in search and exploration, following unilateral lesions to structures associated with human neglect, or after white matter damage isolating particular regions (Gaffan and Hornak, 1997). Temporary chemical lesions within specific subregions of the intraparietal sulcus can produce highly specific deficits (Li, Mazzoni, and Andersen, 1999). However, deficits in monkey appear less severe and short-lived compared with the human syndrome, even after extensive damage (see Marshall et al., 2000). Humans may exhibit hemispheric specialization that other species do not. Nevertheless, animal studies can shed important light on specific component deficits, even when a full-blown neglect syndrome is not induced. One approach is to consider all the component deficits that might contribute to the neglect syndrome, even if some of these components would not produce neglect for the contralesional side in isolation. We pursue this concept later, but first we consider evidence that neglect for the contralesional side can itself arise in different forms.

Putative dissociations between different forms of neglect for one side in humans

DISSOCIATIONS BETWEEN STANDARD CLINICAL TESTS FOR NEGLECT Clinical tests for neglect can dissociate in some cases (e.g., cancellation vs. bisection; Halligan and Marshall, 1992). This may partly relate to different lesions (Binder et al., 1992). As yet such dissociations have not been related unequivocally to specific cognitive processes, because the basic tests were devised for clinical screening, not to tap particular processes. fMRI data from normal subjects provide further evidence that various search tasks (e.g., Gitelman et al., 2002) or bisection tasks (e.g., Fink et al., 2000) may involve different neural substrates. Extinction may also dissociate from other aspects of neglect, which might again relate to lesion site (Karnath, Himmelbach, and Kuker, 2003).

NEGLECT FOR PRESENTED STIMULI VERSUS REPRESENTATIONAL NEGLECT IN IMAGERY Neglect for stimuli presented externally, versus represented mentally in imagery or memory, can also dissociate in some cases (Guariglia et al., 1991; Coslett, 1997). Representational neglect might reflect damage to right frontal rather than parietal regions, but this requires anatomical confirmation in further cases.

NEGLECT IN NEAR VERSUS FAR SPACE In monkeys, unilateral damage to different areas of premotor cortex can produce contralesional neglect or extinction-like phenomena for different spatial domains: within space close to the head following damage to premotor area 6, sparing behavior for more distant stimuli, but vice versa following damage to area 8 (Rizzolatti and Camarda, 1987). Patients have been reported whose neglect was more severe for stimuli in near than far space (Halligan and Marshall, 1991) or vice versa (Vuilleumier et al., 1998). Such dissociations suggest that neglect may affect different types of spatial representation independently, rather than disrupting only one single "master map". Neuroimaging in neurologically intact subjects provides further evidence of the substrates involved when subjects perform tasks in near versus far space (Weiss et al., 2000). Finally, one single-case study suggests that near and far space might dissociate even for neglect in imagery (Ortigue et al., 2001).

NEGLECT WITHIN VERSUS BETWEEN VISUAL OBJECTS   Right hemisphere patients who neglect entire objects at the extreme left of their environment may also neglect the left side of individual objects to which they respond (Driver, Baylis, and Rafal, 1993), but some patients with bilateral brain damage can show neglect for leftward parts of individual objects (e.g., missing initial letters in words), yet neglect whole objects on the opposite right side of space (e.g., missing whole words on the right side of the page; Humphreys and Riddoch, 1995). Such patterns again suggest deficits affecting separable spatial maps, now at different spatial scales or levels of segmentation.

PERCEPTUAL VERSUS MOTOR ASPECTS OF NEGLECT   Many tasks eliciting neglect involve not only perception or attention for the affected side but also require spatial motor responses there (as in cancellation tests). Failures to respond to contralesional targets might thus reflect not just perceptual/attentional biases but also intentional deficits in planning or executing movements toward the affected side, even with the ipsilesional limb.

Several studies have used ingenious methods to uncouple the direction of sensory information versus the required motor response (e.g., with pulley systems, videos, mirrors, etc; see Bisiach et al., 1990; Coslett et al., 1990; Tegner and Levander, 1991) and have suggested a distinction between perceptual neglect after posterior lesions of the IPL or TPJ and motor neglect after prefrontal lesions (Bisiach et al., 1990). But patients with anterior lesions often had larger lesions that involved posterior areas as well. Moreover, apparent frontal involvement in motor components might instead reflect the unusual requirement to move *away* from sensory targets (see Mattingley and Driver, 1997), in those studies that reversed the required motor direction for targets in a given sensory direction, because frontal damage often produces general impairments in such incompatible tasks.

More recent work separated perceptual and motor requirements by changing the hand start position for reaches toward the same visual target (Mattingley et al., 1998). Patients with right IPL (but not frontal) lesions were impaired not only at perceiving contralesional visual stimuli but also at initiating contralesional reaches with the ipsile-

sional arm, consistent with a combined perceptual-motor deficit. This finding may accord both with suggestions that parietal regions can serve as sensorimotor interfaces (Colby and Duhamel, 1996; Andersen et al., 1997), and also with some aspects of spatial attention arising at such interfaces (see Rizzolatti and Camarda, 1987; see also Tipper, this volume).

In contrast to a directional motor deficit, other intentional aspects of neglect may manifest as a lack of spontaneous use of the contralesional hand and arm, even when that arm can be skillfully used on prompting (Laplane and Degos, 1983). Motor extinction may be observed, with deficient contralesional movements only during bimanual actions (Valenstein and Heilman, 1981). This might reflect competitive aspects analogous to those for perceptual extinction, but possibly within different neural structures.

Putative additional components to neglect, including nonspatial deficits

Other common deficits after extensive right hemisphere damage may contribute to neglect, even though they may not lead to neglect if they arise alone. Some of these deficits might exacerbate spatial biases, despite being nonspatial deficits in the sense of affecting both sides of space (Robertson, 2001; Husain and Rorden, 2003).

BIASES TOWARD LOCAL VISUAL DETAILS   Using hierarchical local-global visual stimuli (e.g., large letters made up of small letters), Lynn Robertson and colleagues (1988) observed that whereas lesions of the left TPJ produced biases toward the global level, damage to the right TPJ (commonly included in neglect lesions) produced biases toward local details. These local biases can arise without neglect, but they may exacerbate neglect when combined with spatial deficits disadvantaging the contralesional side (with attention now locking onto ipsilesional details, to preclude perception of even more items in the contralesional direction). Several aspects of neglect may involve failure to direct attention at an appropriately global level (Marshall and Halligan, 1994). A local bias may also contribute to various "object-based" aspects of neglect (Driver, 1999), and may explain why spatial neglect can sometimes arise even within very small stimuli (Pavlovskaya et al., 1997).

SIMULTANAGNOSIA   Bilateral parietal-occipital damage, typically including angular gyri, is associated with Balint's syndrome (Balint, 1909). This syndrome is characterized by a triad of signs: spatial disorientation with misreaching, fixity of gaze, and simultanagnosia. The latter is a failure to perceive multiple concurrent stimuli, sometimes even for superimposed objects (e.g., seeing the examiner's face but not his or her glasses, or vice versa), with awareness shifting only slowly between distinct objects or object parts. Patients with right hemisphere neglect might also show some form of simultanagnosia (possibly relating to their local biases), but with this being overlooked, owing to their striking bias toward one side. Like visual extinction, simultanagnosia can be modulated by object-grouping mechanisms, and, like patients with right TPJ damage, patients with Balint's syndrome may show prominent local biases (Karnath et al., 2000).

NONSPATIAL DEFICITS IN SELECTIVE ATTENTION Husain et al. (1997) observed that patients with right hemisphere neglect showed a pathologically extended "attentional blink" (i.e., tendency to miss a second target shortly after detecting an initial target in a rapid series of items at fixation; see figure 43.6a–d). fMRI in normal subjects shows that regions often damaged in neglect patients (e.g., the right intraparietal sulcus and right frontal cortex) are activated during similar tasks (Wojciulik and Kanwisher, 1999; Marois, Chun, and Gore, 2000), even though only one constant location must be attended (figure 43.6e). These regions may thus play a broader role in attentional capacity than just mediating shifts of spatial attention. Attentional capacity restrictions have been observed in patients with neglect and extinction even for stimuli presented within the ipsilesional hemifield (Duncan et al., 1999; Vuilleumier and Rafal, 2000).

The three types of impairment listed above (i.e., local biases, simultanagnosia, and nonspatial capacity limits) might arguably be interrelated, because all involve difficulties in dealing with multiple stimuli around the same time. Moreover, restricted attentional capacity after right hemisphere lesions may interact with other deficits that disadvantage the contralesional side, to exacerbate spatial aspects of neglect. Increases in attentional load for a central visual stream can impair contralesional detection in parietal patients with neglect (Mattingley et al., 2003; Russell and Husain, 2003). Moreover, whereas in neurologically intact subjects central load typically reduces cortical responses to peripheral visual stimuli bilaterally and symmetrically (Schwartz et al., 2003), preliminary patient fMRI results from our group suggest greater reduction for contralesional than ipsilesional stimuli in neglect during high versus low attentional load in a task at central fixation.

DEFICITS IN ATTENTION SHIFTS TO UNEXPECTED OR DEVIANT STIMULI Posner and colleagues (1984) first reported that patients with right parietal damage are markedly impaired at detecting contralesional targets when their covert attention has been "invalidly" cued ipsilesionally. Although initially linked to superior parietal damage, this "disengage deficit" is more common in patients with right hemisphere TPJ lesions (Friedrich et al., 1998). Using event-related fMRI, Corbetta and colleagues (see Corbetta and Shulman, 2002) found activations of right TPJ in normals for invalidly

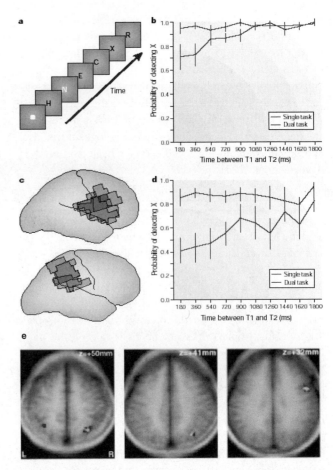

FIGURE 43.6 (a–d) Prolonged "attentional blink" in neglect patients for rapid sequence of visual stimuli at central fixation (figure adapted with authors' permission from Husain and Rorden, 2003; data from Husain et al., 1997). (a) Schematic stimulus sequence. Observer must name the white letter (first target, T1) and detect whether or not an X (second target, T2) is presented afterward, on each trial. (b) Normal results show performance for T2 is impaired if presented shortly after T1, under dual-task conditions (i.e., when monitoring for both targets rather than for just T2). (c) In neglect patients with right parietal or frontal damage, this impairment is pathologically extended (d). (e) Activation of related brain areas is found in normals subjects (data from Marois et al., 2000) in similar attentional tasks on rapid visual streams at fixation (see also Wojciulik and Kanwisher, 1999). (See color plate 19.)

cued minus validly cued targets, and argued that this inferior network operates as a circuit-breaker, interrupting existing attentional states (figure 43.7). These regions operate regardless of target modality (Macaluso, Frith, and Driver, 2002), consistent with supramodal aspects of neglect (Pavani et al., 2004). The right TPJ is also implicated in neural responses to "deviant" stimuli in sequences (Knight et al., 1989), and some of the associated ERP components can be disrupted in neglect (Deouell, Bentin, and Soroker, 2000).

DEFICITS IN SUSTAINED ATTENTION Robertson and Garavan (this volume) argue that right hemisphere lesions can disrupt networks involved in endogenously maintaining

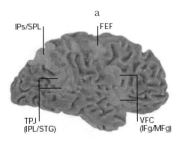
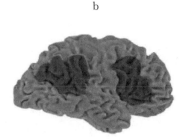
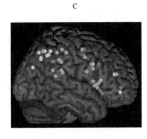

FIGURE 43.7 (*a*) Distinct superior (blue) and inferior (yellow) attention-related networks (adapted with authors' permission from review by Corbetta and Shulman, 2002, on functional neuroimaging results in normals). They suggest the superior network is activated by preparatory attention, often bilaterally, while the inferior network is more strongly right lateralized, and associated with interruption of preexisting attentional states (as when a target suddenly appears on an unexpected side for invalidly cued trials; see main text). They argue that damage to this inferior right lateralized network may play a role in neglect, consistent with their view (see *b*) of brain areas commonly lesioned in neglect (see also figure 43.5).

When reviewing neuroimaging results in normals that may relate to neglect, Husain and Rorden (2003) emphasized similar inferior regions (see *c*, adapted with authors' permission from their review paper), arguing these do not solely play a role in interrupting existing attentional states but also in sustained attention (red circles here, coordinates of activation maxima from several studies), in nonspatial selective attention (yellow; c.f. figure 43.5*e*) in transaccadic spatial working memory (green), and salience detection (blue). Processes related to all these functions might thus be disrupted in many patients with neglect, in addition to their spatial bias toward the right side. (See color plate 20.)

alertness, which may exacerbate the effects of any (separate) spatial biases in neglect. Patients with neglect exhibit fluctuations in performance during daily life, and show deficits on tests of sustained attention that correlate with neglect severity (Robertson, 2001). Phasically alerting patients (e.g., with abrupt warning sounds) can transiently ameliorate their perceptual and attentional deficits for contralesional stimuli (Robertson et al., 1998).

SPATIAL WORKING MEMORY DEFICITS fMRI studies of spatial working memory in normals (e.g., Jonides et al., 1993) reveal a primarily right-lateralized network resembling the brain areas often lesioned in neglect. Physiological and neuropsychological evidence suggests that some of these areas are involved in transaccadic updating of spatial information (e.g., Colby, Duhamel, and Goldberg, 1993). Taken together, this led to proposals that deficits in such spatial working memory processes might be a further component contributing to neglect during search (Husain et al., 2001; Wojciulik et al., 2001). When combined with attentional biases toward the ipsilesional side, this might explain why neglect patients show recursive search: they may revisit ipsilesional locations already inspected (figure 43.8) partly because they do not remember that these locations have been searched already. Neglect patients often respond as if a new target has been found when refixating an old rightward target in search (Husain et al., 2001). This may be linked to damage to the rostral intraparietal sulcus. Finally, patients with neglect can show deficits on spatial working memory tasks for locations in a purely vertical array (column), designed to eliminate any impact of ipsilesional attentional biases (Malhotra et al., in press). Although such a deficit in spatial working memory might be found without neglect, it correlates with more

severe neglect on clinical cancellation measures when found in association with neglect.

VISUAL FEATURE INTEGRATION Treisman's feature integration theory argued that spatial attention may act to solve the binding problem for separate visual features, within the window of currently attended space (see Treisman, this volume). Although neglect, extinction, and Balint's syndrome can abolish awareness even for stimulus presence (including all stimulus features), deficits in feature integration can be disproportionate to those for reporting individual features in some cases. Friedman-Hill, Robertson, and Treisman (1995) observed many "illusory conjunctions" in a patient with Balint's syndrome and bilateral lesions when the patient reported the shape and color of two concurrent items, although he rarely reported absent features (see also Humphreys et al., 2000). Patients with Balint's syndrome are very poor at explicitly locating each stimulus, which might contribute to feature miscombinations. Deficits in feature integration may also be apparent in some patients with unilateral neglect, provided that performance for individual features is sufficiently above chance to allow comparison (Cohen and Rafal, 1991). This agrees with some evidence in normal individuals and may relate to attentional influences on effective spatial resolution (Ashby et al., 1996).

Residual processing in neglect and extinction

Despite the dramatic loss of awareness in neglect, extinction, and Balint's syndrome, several findings suggest that substantial residual processing can arise unconsciously (for reviews, see Driver, 1996; Driver and Vuilleumier, 2001b; Berti, 2003). Behavioral findings indicate that various

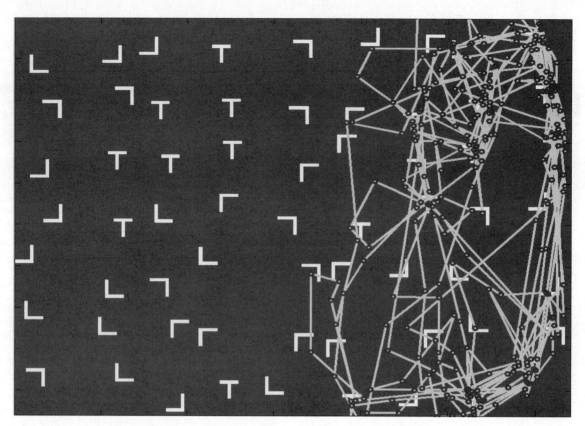

FIGURE 43.8   Deficits in retaining the locations of targets already found, due to impaired spatial working memory, may contribute to pathological search in neglect. Shown are example eye movement data from a patient with neglect after right parietal damage searching for Ts among Ls, with the instruction to click on a response button only when a "new" T has been found (adapted with authors' permission from Husain et al., 2001). The patient revisits previously discovered targets many times and erroneously treats them as new discoveries, indicating a failure to retain the locations of targets already found across saccades. Such mistakes increase with the load on spatial working memory (e.g., for displays with more items, even though the probability of returning by chance should decrease for these). (See color plate 21.)

stimulus properties can determine whether a contralesional stimulus will become reportable (e.g., its emotional valence [Vuilleumier, 2000b]; its color or shape in relation to an ipsilesional stimulus and the current task [Baylis, Rafal, and Driver, 1993], whether or not it can be grouped with the ipsilesional stimulus to form a single gestalt [Mattingley, Davis, and Driver, 1997], whether it gets segmented as figure or ground (Driver, Baylis, and Rafal, 1993), its action-related correspondence with an ipsilesional item [Riddoch et al., 2003], and its category [Vuilleumier, 2000b]). This has been taken to imply that the properties influencing whether or not a stimulus will reach awareness may be extracted even on trials where the stimulus escapes awareness.

Further evidence comes from effects produced by contralesional stimuli that do escape awareness but nevertheless influence responses to a concomitant ipsilesional or central stimulus. Several patient studies have used priming or congruency methods drawn from the literature on the fate of unattended or subliminal stimuli in normal individuals (where substantial implicit processing has also been shown; Driver, 1996). Congruency or priming effects have been

shown from neglected or extinguished stimuli based on their presence, shape, color, identity, and even semantics (see Driver, 1996; Driver and Vuilleumier, 2001b; Berti, 2003). Although such effects have been considered short-lived, Vuilleumier and colleagues (2002) observed longlasting priming (up to 50 minutes) for recognition of fragmented objects (figure 43.9) from a single extinguished presentation of the complete object in the contralesional field. These results imply that unconscious residual processing of extinguished stimuli may produce neural activation with lasting traces.

The basis of such residual processing can now be understood in terms of functional anatomy. Given that striate and extrastriate visual cortex often remain structurally intact in neglect and extinction patients (along with ventral pathways into temporal cortex), it seems plausible that residual visual processing might take place here. Recent studies addressed this directly using e-fMRI in patients with right hemisphere damage and left extinction (Rees et al., 2000, 2002; Driver et al., 2001; Vuilleumier et al., 2001, 2002). Striate and extrastriate cortex in the damaged right hemisphere can be

Phase 1: Naming of complete pictures   *Phase 2: Identification of fragmented pictures*

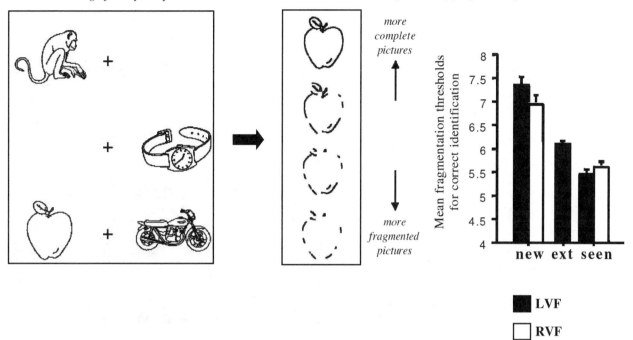

FIGURE 43.9 Extinguished contralesional visual stimuli can produce enduring implicit priming effects. (*a*) Left panel depicts example stimuli from Phase 1 of experiment. Complete objects were briefly shown unilaterally on the right or left or bilaterally for detection and identification. Extinction arose on those bilateral trials where patients with right hemisphere damage remained unaware of left object (c.f. figure 43.4*c*). In later Phase 2 (up to 50 min delay), single objects were shown on the left or right for un-limited time, in eight decreasingly fragmented steps (four such steps shown here for apple), until the subject indicated identity or failure to identify. Results (graph at right) showed priming of fragment identification (i.e., success at earlier step, reduced fragmentation threshold) for objects previously shown in complete form. This result was found not only for previously seen right objects (light bar at far right) relative to new object baseline but also for previous left objects, including not just those that had been consciously seen but also those extinguished at initial exposure (ext in graph). (Adapted with authors' permission from Vuilleumier et al., 2002.)

activated by extinguished left stimuli that escape awareness (figure 43.10*a*), while fusiform regions may still show some residual specificity for the category of extinguished stimuli (face vs. house; Rees et al., 2002), and limbic regions such as amygdala and orbitofrontal cortex can still respond to their emotional value (for fearful faces; Vuilleumier et al., 2002). Event-related potentials (ERPs) have also revealed some residual processing for extinguished stimuli (Marzi et al., 2000; Driver et al., 2001; Vuilleumier et al., 2001).

Such results raise the intriguing question of what is missing in the neural response to extinguished or neglected stimuli such that the patient remains unaware of, say, a face on the left, despite conventional visual pathways for object and face processing remaining structurally intact and demonstrably activatable. This question has also been addressed with fMRI (Driver et al., 2001; Vuilleumier et al., 2001, 2002; Rees et al., 2002) and ERPs (Marzi et al., 2000; Driver et al., 2001; Vuilleumier et al., 2001), by comparing bilateral trials where both stimuli are detected with those where extinction arises in patients who do not show extinction on every trial. Awareness versus extinction of a left face was associated with greater fMRI responses in occipital and

ventral temporal areas of the damaged hemisphere, plus parietal and frontal areas of the intact left hemisphere (figure 43.10*b*). Moreover, activity showed increased coupling (effective connectivity) between right visual cortex and left parietal-frontal regions when the left stimulus was con-sciously detected. Visual awareness may depend not solely on activity within visual cortex, as traditionally conceived, but on the interplay between posterior occipitotemporal cortex and parietofrontal regions in a broad network (or "global neuronal workspace"; Baars and Franklin, 2003) that normally makes sensory contents from specialized regions widely available for awareness but that is disrupted in neglect. We have argued elsewhere that parietofrontal cir-cuits may be particularly influential in determining selection for awareness owing to extreme winner-takes-all spatial com-petition within them (Driver and Vuilleumier, 2001a).

Evidence for unconscious residual processing in neglect and extinction has been taken to indicate that "preattentive" stages of sensory processing (e.g., initial image segmentation; Driver, 1996, 1999) can remain intact. In traditional accounts, such processing was considered to precede later, attentive processing in a strictly feedforward stream of

a Extinction (Bilateral extinguished > Unilateral right)

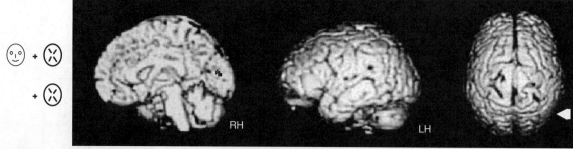

b Awareness (Bilateral seen > Bilateral extinguished)

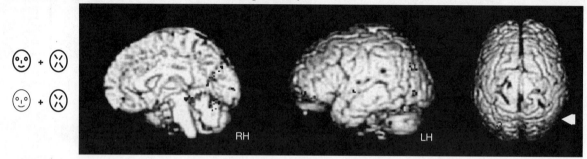

FIGURE 43.10 Neural correlates of unconscious residual processing (*a*) or visual awareness (*b*), as revealed by e-fMRI in a chronic patient who had sustained a right parietal stroke (lesion indicated schematically by arrowed region in superior view at far right). Similar results have been found in other cases (see text). When presented with bilateral stimuli (left face + right shape here), the patient often remained unaware of the left stimulus. (*a*) Comparing these bilateral extinction trials against unilateral trials (see schematic cartoons of these two trial types at far left) revealed residual activation in visual areas of the contralateral occipital and temporal cortex, despite unawareness (see medial view of right hemisphere). Such activation was restricted to visual cortex. (*b*) On some bilateral trials, the patient correctly detected both stimuli (i.e., left face as well as right shape). Comparing identical bilateral events with awareness versus extinction of the left side of the face (see cartoons at far left, with lack of awareness for extinguished face indicated by fainter lines) revealed increased activation in early visual areas of the right hemisphere, as well as bilateral fusiform cortex, left parietal cortex (homologous to the right damaged areas), and left frontal cortex. Note that this activation now extends to a more widespread neural network. (Figure adapted with authors' permission from Driver et al., 2001, data from Vuilleumier et al., 2001.)

processing. However, emerging neural perspectives on attention suggest major roles for feedback as well as feedforward influences (see Driver et al., 2004; Freiwald and Kanwisher, this volume), prompting the question of whether posterior visual cortex can function normally when deprived of feedback from lesioned structures in neglect (see Driver and Vuilleumier, 2001b). Further neuroimaging studies in patients should resolve this issue complemented by related animal models (e.g., Moore and Armstrong, 2003). Existing research on residual processing in neglect and extinction has concentrated mainly on the visual modality, but analogous work in other modalities has begun (Remy et al., 1999; Deouell, Bentin, and Soroker, 2000; Eimer et al., 2002; Valenza et al., 2003) and should determine the generality of the framework.

Comment

The findings reviewed in this chapter reveal many aspects of the neglect syndrome: how it can affect both conscious perception and exploration while differing from primary sensory and motor deficits; the involvement of attention and other factors that modulate whether a stimulus will be neglected or will reach awareness; some of the separate component deficits that also contribute; plus extensive residual abilities and their neural bases. The neglect syndrome is a complex disorder, with the combined deficits having a devastating impact on the patient's awareness and behavior and being highly disabling in daily life. The many recent scientific advances in understanding neglect may lead to more effective forms of rehabilitation, as promised by some recent innovations (see Rossetti et al., 1998).

REFERENCES

AGLIOTI, S., N. SMANIA, and A. PERU, 1999. Frames of reference for mapping tactile stimuli in brain-damaged patients. *J. Cogn. Neurosci.* 11:167–179.

ANDERSEN, R. A., G. K. ESSICK, and R. M. SIEGEL, 1985. Encoding of spatial location by posterior parietal neurons. *Science* 230:456–458.

ANDERSEN, R., L. H. SNYDER, D. C. BRADLEY, and J. XING, 1997. Multimodal representation of space in the posterior parietal cortex and its use in planning movement. *Annu. Rev. Neurosci.* 20:303–330.

ASHBY, F. G., W. PRINZMETAL, R. IVRY, and W. T. MADDOX, 1996. A formal theory of feature binding in object perception. *Psychol. Rev.* 103:165–192.

BAARS, B. J., and S. FRANKLIN, 2003. How conscious experience and working memory interact. *Trends Cogn. Sci.* 7:166–172.

BALINT, R., 1909. Seelenlaehmung des Schauens, optische Ataxie, raeumliche Stoerung der Aufmerksamkeit. *Monatsschr. Psychiatr. Neurol.* 25:51–81.

BAYLIS, G., R. RAFAL, and J. DRIVER, 1993. Visual extinction and stimulus repetition. *J. Cogn. Neurosci.* 5:453–466.

BEN HAMED, S., J. R. DUHAMEL, F. BREMMER, and W. GRAF, 2001. Representation of the visual field in the lateral intraparietal area of macaque monkeys: A quantitative receptive field analysis. *Exp. Brain Res.* 140:127–144.

BERTI, A., 2003. Unconscious processing in neglect. In *The Cognitive and Neural Bases of Spatial Neglect*, H. O. Karnath, A. D. Milner, and G. Vallar, eds. Oxford, England: Oxford University Press.

BINDER, J., R. MARSHALL, R. LAZAR, J. BENJAMIN, and J. P. MOHR, 1992. Distinct syndromes of hemineglect. *Arch. Neurol.* 49:1187–1194.

BISIACH, E., G. GEMINIANI, A. BERTI, and M. L. RUSCONI, 1990. Perceptual and premotor factors of unilateral neglect. *Neurology* 40:1278–1281.

BISIACH, E., and C. LUZZATTI, 1978. Unilateral neglect of representational space. *Cortex* 14:129–133.

BISIACH, E., L. PIZZAMIGLIO, D. NICO, and G. ANTONUCCI, 1996. Beyond unilateral neglect. *Brain* 119(Pt. 3):851–857.

COHEN, A., and R. RAFAL, 1991. Attention and feature integration: Illusory conjunction in a patient with a parietal lobe lesion. *Psychol. Sci.* 2:106–110.

COLBY, C. L., and J. R. DUHAMEL, 1996. Spatial representations for action in parietal cortex. *Brain Res. Cogn. Brain Res.* 5:105–115.

COLBY, C. L., J. R. DUHAMEL, and M. E. GOLDBERG, 1993. The analysis of visual space by the lateral intraparietal area of the monkey: The role of extraretinal signals. *Prog. Brain. Res.* 95:307–316.

CORBETTA, M., and G. L. SHULMAN, 2002. Control of goal-directed and stimulus-driven attention in the brain. *Nat. Rev. Neurosci.* 3:201–215.

COSLETT, H. B., 1997. Neglect in vision and visual imagery: A double dissociation. *Brain* 120:1163–1171.

COSLETT, H. B., D. BOWERS, E. FITZPATRICK, B. HAWS, and K. M. HEILMAN, 1990. Directional hypokinesia and hemispatial inattention in neglect. *Brain* 113:475–486.

DE RENZI, E., 1982. *Disorders of Space Exploration and Cognition.* New York: Wiley.

DEMEURISSE, G., C. HUBLET, J. PATERNOT, C. COLSON, and W. SERNICLAES, 1997. Pathogenesis of subcortical visuo-spatial neglect: A HMPAO SPECT study. *Neuropsychologia* 35:5731–5735.

DENIS, M., N. BESCHIN, R. H. LOGIE, and S. DELLA SALA, 2002. Visual perception and verbal descriptions as sources for generating mental representations: Evidence from representational neglect. *Cogn. Neuropsychol.* 19:97–112.

DEOUELL, L. Y., S. BENTIN, and N. SOROKER, 2000. Eletrophysiological evidence for an early (preattentive) information processing deficit in patients with right hemisphere damage and unilateral neglect. *Brain* 123:353–365.

DESIMONE, R., and J. DUNCAN, 1995. Neural mechanisms of selective visual attention. *Annu. Rev. Neurosc.* 18:193–222.

DI PELLEGRINO, G., E. LADAVAS, and A. FARNE, 1997. Seeing where your hands are. *Nature* 388:370.

DORICCHI, F., and P. ANGELELLI, 1999. Misrepresentation of horizontal space in left unilateral neglect: role of hemianopia. *Neurology* 52:1845–1852.

DRIVER, J., 1996. What can visual neglect and extinction reveal about the extent of "preattentive" processing? In *Convergent Operations in the Study of Visual Selective Attention*, A. F. Kramer, M. G. H. Cole, and G. D. Logan, eds. Washington, D. C.: APA Press, pp. 193–224.

DRIVER, J., 1999. Egocentric and object-based visual neglect. In *The Hippocampal and Parietal Foundations of Spatial Cognition*, N. K. Burgess and J. O'Keefe, eds. Oxford, England: Oxford University Press.

DRIVER, J., G. C. BAYLIS, and R. D. RAFAL, 1993. Preserved figure-ground segmentation and symmetry perception in a patient with neglect. *Nature* 360:73–75.

DRIVER, J., M. EIMER, E. MACALUSO, and V. VELZEN, 2004. Neurobiology of human spatial attention: Modulation, generation and integration. In *Attention and Performance XX: Functional Imaging of Visual Cognition*, N. Kanwisher and J. Duncan, eds. Oxford, England: Oxford University Press, pp. 267–300.

DRIVER, J., J. B. MATTINGLEY, C. RORDEN, and G. Davis, 1997. Extinction as a paradigm measure of attentional bias and restricted capacity following brain injury. In *Parietal Lobe Contributions to Orientation in 3D Space*, H.-O. Karnath and P. Thier, eds. Berlin: Springer, pp. 401–429.

DRIVER, J., and P. VUILLEUMIER, 2001a. Perceptual awareness and its loss in unilateral neglect and extinction. *Cognition* 79:39–88.

DRIVER, J., and P. VUILLEUMIER, 2001b. Unconscious processing in neglect and extinction. In *Out of mind: Varieties of Unconscious Processing*, B. DeGelder, E. H. F. DeHaan, and C. A. Heywood, eds. Oxford, England: Oxford University Press, pp. 107–139.

DRIVER, J., P. VUILLEUMIER, M. EIMER, and G. REES, 2001. Functional MRI and evoked potential correlates of conscious and unconscious vision in parietal extinction patients. *NeuroImage* 14:68–75.

DUNCAN, J., 1980. The locus of interference in the perception of simultaneous stimuli. *Psychol. Rev.* 87:272–300.

DUNCAN, J., C. BUNDESEN, A. OLSON, G. HUMPHREYS, S. CHAVDA, and H. SHIBUYA, 1999. Systematic analysis of deficits in visual attention. *J. Exp. Psychol. Gen.* 128:450–478.

EGLIN, M., L. C. ROBERTSON, and R. T. KNIGHT, 1989. Visual search performance in the neglect syndrome. *J. Cogn. Neurosci.* 1:372–385.

EIMER, M., A. MARAVITA, J. VAN VELZEN, M. HUSAIN, and J. DRIVER, 2002. The electrophysiology of tactile extinction: ERP correlates of unconscious somatosensory processing. *Neuropsychologia* 40:2438–2447.

FINK, G. R., J. C. MARSHALL, N. J. SHAH, P. H. WEISS, P. W. HALLIGAN, M. GROSSE-RUYKEN, et al., 2000. Line bisection judgments implicate right parietal cortex and cerebellum as assessed by fMRI. *Neurology* 54:1324–1331.

FRIEDMAN-HILL, S. R., L. C. ROBERTSON, and A. TREISMAN, 1995. Parietal contributions to visual feature binding: Evidence from a patient with bilateral lesions. *Science* 269:853–855.

FRIEDRICH, F. J., R. EGLY, R. D. RAFAL, and D. BECK, 1998. Spatial attention deficits in humans: A comparison of superior parietal and temporal-parietal junction lesions. *Neuropsychology* 12:193–207.

GAFFAN, D., and J. HORNAK, 1997. Visual neglect in the monkey: Representation and disconnection. *Brain* 120:1647–1657.

GITELMAN, D. R., T. B. PARRISH, K. J. FRISTON, and M. M. MESULAM, 2002. Functional anatomy of visual search: Regional segregations within the frontal eye fields and effective connectivity of the superior colliculus. *NeuroImage* 15:970–982.

GRABOWECKY, M., L. C. ROBERTSON, and A. TREISMAN, 1993. Preattentive processes guide visual search: Evidence from patients with unilateral visual neglect. *J. Cogn. Neurosci.* 5:283–302.

GRAZIANO, M. S., and C. G. GROSS, 1998. Spatial maps for the control of movement. *Curr. Opin. Neurobiol.* 8:2195–2201.

GROSSI, D., A. MODAFFERI, L. PELOSI, and L. TROJANO, 1989. On the different roles of the cerebral hemispheres in mental imagery: The "o'clock test" in two clinical cases. *Brain. Cogn.* 10:18–27.

GUARIGLIA, C., A. PADOVANI, P. PANTANO, and L. PIZZAMIGLIO, 1991. Unilateral neglect restricted to visual imagery. *Nature* 364:235–237.

HALLIGAN, P. W., and J. C. MARSHALL, 1991. Left neglect for near but not far space in man. *Nature* 350:498–500.

HALLIGAN, P. W., and J. C. MARSHALL, 1992. Left visuo-spatial neglect: a meaningless entity? *Cortex* 28:525–535.

HEILMAN, K. M., R. T. WATSON, and E. VALENSTEIN, 2003. Neglect and related disorders. In *Clinical neuropsychology*, 4th ed.; K. M. Heilman and E. Valenstein, eds. New York: Oxford University Press, pp. 279–336.

HILGETAG, C. C., H. THEORET, and A. PASCUAL-LEONE, 2001. Enhanced visual spatial attention ipsilateral to rTMS-induced "virtual lesions" of human parietal cortex. *Nat. Neurosci.* 4:953–957.

HILLIS, A. E., R. J. WITYK, P. B. BARKER, N. J. BEAUCHAMP, P. GAILLOUD, K. MURPHY, O. COOPER, and E. J. METTER, 2002. Subcortical aphasia and neglect in acute stroke: The role of cortical hypoperfusion. *Brain* 125:1094–1104.

HUMPHREYS, G. W., C. CINEL, J. WOLFE, A. OLSON, N. KLEMPEN, 2000. Fractionating the binding process: Neuropsychological evidence distinguishing binding of form from binding of surface features. *Vision Res.* 40:1569–1596.

HUMPHREYS, G. W., and M. J. RIDDOCH, 1995. Separate coding of space within and between perceptual objects: Evidence from unilateral visual neglect. *Cogn. Neuropsycho.* 12:283–311.

HUSAIN, M., and C. KENNARD, 1996. Visual neglect associated with frontal lobe infarction. *J. Neurol.* 243:652–657.

HUSAIN, M., S. MANNAN, T. HODGSON, E. WOJCIULIK, J. DRIVER, and C. KENNARD, 2001. Impaired spatial working memory across saccades contributes to abnormal search in parietal neglect. *Brain* 124(Pt. 5):941–952.

HUSAIN, M., and C. RORDEN, 2003. Non-spatially lateralized mechanisms in hemispatial neglect. *Nat. Rev. Neurosci.* 4:26–36.

HUSAIN, M., K. SHAPIRO, J. MARTIN, and C. KENNARD, 1997. Abnormal temporal dynamics of visual attention in spatial neglect patients. *Nature* 385:154–156.

JONIDES, J., E. SMITH, R. KOEPPE, E. AWH, S. MINOSHIMA, and M. MINTUN, 1993. Spatial working memory in humans as revealed by PET. *Nature* 363:623–625.

KARNATH, H.-O., 1997. Neural encoding of space in egocentric coordinates? Evidence for and limits of a hypothesis derived from patients with parietal lesions and neglect. In *Parietal Lobe Contributions to Orientation in 3D Space*, P. Thier and H. O. Karnath, eds. Berlin: Springer-Verlag, pp. 497–520.

KARNATH, H. O., S. FERBER, and M. HIMMELBACH, 2001. Spatial awareness is a function of the temporal not the posterior parietal lobe. *Nature* 411:950–953.

KARNATH, H. O., S. FERBER, C. RORDEN, and J. DRIVER, 2000. The fate of global information in dorsal simultanagnosia. *Neurocase* 6:295–306.

KARNATH, H. O., M. HIMMELBACH, and W. KUKER, 2003. The cortical substrate of visual extinction. *Neuroreport* 14:437–442.

KARNATH, H. O., M. HIMMELBACH, and C. RORDEN, 2002. The subcortical anatomy of human spatial neglect: Putamen, caudate nucleus and pulvinar. *Brain* 125(Pt. 2):350–360.

KARNATH, H. O., A. D. MILNER, and G. VALLAR, 2003. *The Cognitive and Neural Bases of Spatial Neglect*. Oxford, England: Oxford University Press.

KARNATH, H. O., M. NIEMEIER, and J. DICHGANS, 1998. Space exploration in neglect. *Brain* 121(Pt. 12):2357–2367.

KASTNER, S., and L. G. UNGERLEIDER, 2001. The neural basis of biased competition in human visual cortex. *Neuropsychologia* 39:1263–1276.

KNIGHT, R. T., D. SCABINI, D. L. WOODS, and C. C. CLAYWORTH, 1989. Contributions of temporal-parietal junction to the human auditory P3. *Brain Res.* 502:109–116.

KUMRAL, E., and D. EVYAPAN, 1999. Associated exploratory-motor and perceptual-sensory neglect without hemiparesis. *Neurology* 52:199–202.

LADAVAS, E., G. DI PELLEGRINO, A. FARNE, and G. ZELONI, 1998. Neuropsychological evidence of an integrated visuotactile representation of peripersonal space in humans. *J. Cogn. Neurosci.* 10:581–589.

LAPLANE, D., and J. D. DEGOS, 1983. Motor neglect. *J. Neuro. Neurosurg. Psychiatry* 46:152–158.

LEIBOVITCH, F. S., S. E. BLACK, C. B. CALDWELL, P. L. EBERT, L. E. EHRLICH, and J. P. SZALAI, 1998. Brain-behavior correlations in hemispatial neglect using CT and SPECT: The Sunnybrook Stroke Study. *Neurology* 50:901–908.

LI, C., P. MAZZONI, and R. ANDERSEN, 1999. Effect of reversible inactivation of macaque lateral intraparietal area on visual and memory saccades. *J. Neurophysiol.* 81:1827–1838.

LOMBER, S. G., B. R. PAYNE, C. C. HILGETAG, and J. RUSHMORE, 2002. Restoration of visual orienting into a cortically blind hemifield by reversible deactivation of posterior parietal cortex or the superior colliculus. *Exp. Brain Res.* 142:463–474.

MACALUSO, E., C. D. FRITH, and J. DRIVER, 2002. Supramodal effects of covert spatial orienting triggered by visual or tactile events. *J. Cogn. Neurosci.* 14:389–401.

MACK, A., and I. ROCK, 1998. *Inattentional Blindness*. Cambridge, Mass: MIT Press.

MALHOTRA, P., S. MANNAN, J. DRIVER, and M. HUSAIN, (in press). Impaired spatial working memory: One component of the visual neglect syndrome? *Cortex*.

MARK, V. W., C. A. KOOISTRA, and K. M. HEILMAN, 1988. Hemispatial neglect affected by non-neglected stimuli. *Neurology* 38:1207–1211.

MAROIS, R., M. M. CHUN, and J. C. GORE, 2000. Neural correlates of the attentional blink. *Neuron* 28:299–308.

MARSHALL, J. C., and P. W. HALLIGAN, 1994. Independent properties of normal hemispheric specialization predict some characteristics of visuo-spatial neglect. *Cortex* 30:509–517.

MARSHALL, J. W., A. J. CROSS, D. M. JACKSON, A. R. GREEN, H. F. BAKER, and R. M. RIDLEY, 2000. Clomethiazole protects against hemineglect in a primate model of stroke. *Brain Res. Bull.* 52:21–29.

MARZI, C., M. GIRELLI, C. MINIUSSI, N. SMANIA, and A. MARAVITA, 2000. Electrophysiological correlates of conscious vision: Evidence from unilateral extinction. *J. Cogn. Neurosci.* 12:869–877.

MATTINGLEY, J. B., G. DAVIS, and J. DRIVER, 1997. Preattentive filling-in of visual surfaces in parietal extinction. *Science* 275:671–674.

MATTINGLEY, J. B., and J. DRIVER, 1997. Distinguishing sensory and motor deficits after parietal damage: An evaluation of response selection biases in unilateral neglect. In *Parietal Lobe Contributions to Orientation in 3D Space*, P. Thier and H. O. Karnath, eds. Berlin: Springer, pp. 309–338.

MATTINGLEY, J., N. BERBEROVIC, C. RORDEN, and J. DRIVER, 2003. *Attentional load at fixation modulates the spatial gradient for detection of visual stimuli in extinction.* Paper presented at Cognitive Neuroscience Society Annual Meeting, New York.

MATTINGLEY, J. B., M. HUSAIN, C. RORDEN, C. KENNARD, and J. DRIVER, 1998. Motor role of human inferior parietal lobe revealed in unilateral neglect patients. *Nature* 392:179–182.

MESULAM, M. M., 1999. Spatial attention and neglect: parietal, frontal and cingulate contributions to the mental representation and attentional targeting of salient extrapersonal events. *Philos. Trans. R. Soc. Lond. B Biol. Sci.* 354:1325–1346.

MOORE, T., and K. M. ARMSTRONG, 2003. Selective gating of visual signals by microstimulation of frontal cortex. *Nature* 421:370–373.

MORT, D. J., P. MALHOTRA, S. K. MANNAN, C. RORDEN, A. PAMBAKIAN, C. KENNARD, and M. HUSAIN, 2003. The anatomy of visual neglect. *Brain* 126:1986–1997.

NIEMEIER, M., and H. O. KARNATH, 2000. Exploratory saccades show no direction-specific deficit in neglect. *Neurology* 54:515–518.

ORTIGUE, S., I. VIAUD-DELMON, J. M. ANNONI, T. LANDIS, C. MICHEL, O. BLANKE, et al., 2001. Pure representational neglect after right thalamic lesion. *Ann. Neurol.* 50:401–404.

PAVANI, F., M. HUSAIN, E. LADAVAS, and J. DRIVER, (in press). Auditory deficits in visual neglect patients. *Cortex*.

PAVLOVSKAYA, M., I. GLASS, N. SOROKER, N. BLUM, and Z. GROSWASSER, 1997. Coordinate frame for pattern recognition in unilateral spatial neglect. *J. Cogn. Neurosci.* 9:824–834.

PERANI, D., G. VALLAR, S. CAPPA, C. MESSA, and F. FAZIO, 1987. Aphasia and neglect after subcortical stroke. A clinical/cerebral perfusion correlation study. *Brain* 110:1211–1229.

POSNER, M. I., J. A. WALKER, F. J. FRIEDRICH, and R. RAFAL, 1984. Effects of parietal injury on covert orienting of visual attention. *J. Neurosci.* 4:1863–1874.

POUGET, A., and J. DRIVER, 2000. Relating unilateral neglect to the neural coding of space. *Curr. Opin. Neurobiol.* 10:242–249.

REES, G., E. WOJCIULIK, K. CLARKE, M. HUSAIN, C. D. FRITH, and J. DRIVER, 2000. Unconscious activation of visual cortex in the damaged right hemisphere of a parietal patient with extinction. *Brain* 123:1624–1633.

REES, G., E. WOJCIULIK, K. CLARKE, M. HUSAIN, C. FRITH, and J. DRIVER, 2002. Neural correlates of conscious and unconscious vision in parietal extinction. *Neurocase* 8:387–393.

REMY, P., M. ZILBOVICIUS, J. D. DEGOS, A. C. BACHOUD-LEVY, G. RANCUREL, P. CESARO, et al., 1999. Somatosensory cortical activations are suppressed in patients with tactile extinction: A PET study. *Neurology* 52:571–577.

RENSINK, R. A., J. K. O'REGAN, and J. J. CLARK, 1997. To see or not to see: The need for attention to perceive changes in visual scenes. *Psycho. Sci.* 8:368–373.

RIDDOCH, M. J., G. W. HUMPHREYS, S. EDWARDS, T. BAKER, and K. WILLSON, 2003. Seeing the action: Neuropsychological evidence for action-based effects on object selection. *Nat. Neurosci.* 6:82–89.

RIZZOLATTI, G., and R. CAMARDA, 1987. Neural circuits for spatial attention and unilateral neglect. In *Neurophysiological and Neuropsychological Aspects of Spatial Neglect*, vol. 45, M. Jeannerod, ed., Amsterdam: North-Holland, pp. 289–314.

ROBERTSON, I., 1989. Anomalies in the laterality of omissions in unilateral left visual neglect: implications for an attentional theory of neglect. *Neuropsychologia* 27:157–165.

ROBERTSON, I. H., 2001. Do we need the "lateral" in unilateral neglect? Spatially nonselective attention deficits in unilateral neglect and their implications for rehabilitation. *NeuroImage* 14:S85–S90.

ROBERTSON, I. H., J. B. MATTINGLEY, C. RORDEN, and J. DRIVER, 1998. Phasic alerting of neglect patients overcomes their spatial deficit in visual awareness. *Nature* 395:169–172.

ROBERTSON, L. C., M. R. LAMB, and R. T. KNIGHT, 1988. Effects of lesions of the temporal-parietal junction on perceptual and attentional processing in humans. *J. Neurosci.* 8:3757–3769.

ROSSETTI, Y., G. RODE, L. PISELLA, A. FARNE, L. LI, D. BOISSON, et al., 1998. Prism adaptation to a rightward optical deviation rehabilitates left hemispatial neglect. *Nature* 395:166–169.

RUSSELL, C., and M. HUSAIN, 2003. *Attentional perimetry: Simple detection of peripheral dots is dependent on attentional load of central task.* Paper presented at the Cognitive Neuroscience Society Annual Meeting, New York.

SAMUELSSON, H., C. JENSEN, S. EKHOLM, H. NAVER, and C. BLOMSTRAND, 1997. Anatomical and neurological correlates of acute and chronic visuospatial neglect following right hemisphere stroke. *Cortex* 33:271–285.

SCHWARTZ, S., P. VUILLEUMIER, C. HUTTON, A. MARAVITA, J. DRIVER, and R. J. DOLAN, 2003. *Effects of central attentional load on visual responses to irrelevant peripheral stimuli: An fMRI study.* Paper presented at the Cognitive Neuroscience Society Annual Meeting, New York.

SMANIA, N., M. MARTINI, G. GAMBINA, G. TOMELLERI, A. PALAMARA, E. NATALE, et al., 1998. The spatial distribution of visual attention in hemineglect and extinction patients. *Brain* 121:1759–1770.

TEGNER, R., and M. LEVANDER, 1991. Through a looking glass: A new technique to demonstrate directional hypokinesia in unilateral neglect. *Brain* 113:1943–1951.

VAISHNAVI, S., J. CALHOUN, and A. CHATTERJEE, 2001. Binding personal and peripersonal space: Evidence from tactile extinction. *J. Cogn. Neurosci.* 13:181–189.

VALENSTEIN, E., and K. M. HEILMAN, 1981. Unilateral hypokinesia and motor extinction. *Neurology* 31:445–448.

VALENZA, N., M. L. SEGHIER, S. SCHWARTZ, F. LAZEYRAS, and P. VUILLEUMIER, 2003. *Tactile awareness modulated by limb position: Behavioral and fMRI evidence in a right parietal patient with spatial neglect.* Paper presented at the Cognitive Neuroscience Society Annual Meeting, New York.

VALLAR, G., 1993. The anatomical basis of spatial neglect in humans. In *Unilateral Neglect: Clinical and Experimental Studies*, I. H. Robertson and J. C. Marshall, eds. Hillsdale, N.J.: Erlbaum, pp. 27–62.

VALLAR, G., 1998. Spatial hemineglect in humans. *Trends Cogn. Sci.* 2:87–97.

VUILLEUMIER, P., 2000a. Anosognosia. In *Behavior and Mood Disorders in Focal Brain Lesions*, J. Bogousslavsky and J. L. Cummings, eds. Cambridge, England: Cambrige University Press, pp. 465–519.

VUILLEUMIER, P., 2000b. Faces call for attention: Evidence from patients with visual extinction. *Neuropsychologia* 38:693–700.

VUILLEUMIER, P., J. ARMONY, K. CLARKE, M. HUSAIN, J. DRIVER, and R. DOLAN, 2002. Neural response to emotional faces with and without awareness: Event-related fMRI in a parietal patient with visual extinction and spatial neglect. *Neuropsychologia* 40:2156–2166.

VUILLEUMIER, P., and R. RAFAL, 2000. A systematic study of task-dependent visual extinction: Between and within-field deficits of attention in hemispatial neglect. *Brain* 123:1263–1279.

VUILLEUMIER, P., N. SAGIV, E. HAZELTINE, R. POLDRACK, D. SWICK, R. RAFAL, et al., 2001. Neural fate of seen and unseen faces in unilateral spatial neglect: A combined event-related fMRI and ERP study of visual extinction. *Proc. Natl. Acad. Sci. U.S.A.* 98:3495–3500.

VUILLEUMIER, P., S. SCHWARTZ, K. CLARKE, M. HUSAIN, and J. DRIVER, 2002. Testing memory for unseen visual stimuli in patients with spatial neglect and extinction. *J. Cogn. Neurosci.* 14:875–886.

VUILLEUMIER, P., N. VALENZA, E. MAYER, A. RÉVERDIN, and T. LANDIS, 1998. Near and far visual space in unilateral neglect. *Ann. Neurol.* 43:406–410.

VUILLEUMIER, P., N. VALENZA, S. PERRIG, E. MAYER, and T. LANDIS, 1999. To see better to the left when looking more to the right: Effects of gaze direction and frame of spatial coordinates in unilateral neglect. *J. Int. Neuropsychol. Soc.* 5:75–82.

WALKER, R., J. M. FINDLAY, A. W. YOUNG, and J. WELCH, 1991. Disentangling neglect and hemianopia. *Neuropsychologia* 29:1019–1027.

WARDACK, C., E. OLIVIER, and J. R. DUHAMEL, 2003. Neglect in monkeys: Effect of permanent and reversible lesions. In *The Cognitive and Neural Bases of Spatial Neglect*, H. O. Karnath, A. D. Milner, and G. Vallar, eds. Oxford, England: Oxford University Press.

WEISS, P. H., J. C. MARSHALL, G. WUNDERLICH, L. TELLMANN, P. W. HALLIGAN, H. J. FREUND, et al., 2000. Neural consequences of acting in near versus far space: A physiological basis for clinical dissociations. *Brain* 123(Pt. 12):2531–2541.

WOJCIULIK, E., M. HUSAIN, K. CLARKE, and J. DRIVER, 2001. Spatial working memory deficit in unilateral neglect. *Neuropsychologia* 39:390–396.

WOJCIULIK, E., and N. KANWISHER, 1999. The generality of parietal involvement in visual attention. *Neuron* 23:747–764.

WOLFE, J. M., 2003. Moving towards solutions to some enduring controversies in visual search. *Trends Cogn. Sci.* 7:70–76.

44 Attention and the Frontal Lobes

GLYN W. HUMPHREYS AND DANA SAMSON

ABSTRACT The frontal lobes play a critical part in the control of human behavior. We review evidence from neuropsychology and functional brain imaging on the cognitive functions subserved by the frontal lobes in working memory, in the endogenous control of attention, in response selection, inhibition and response monitoring, and in responding to affective signals and reward-related aspects of the environment. Finally, we consider developmental disorders of cognitive function that may be accounted for in terms of the abnormal control of attention mediated by the frontal lobes.

Damage to the frontal lobes of the brain can be extremely disabling for everyday life. Patients can exhibit poor generation and maintenance of goal-driven behavior, impulsive responding to stimuli, and abnormal responses to affective stimuli associated with prior rewards or punishments. Nevertheless, many core cognitive processes can remain intact, among them sensory and perceptual coding of stimuli from different modalities, language, memory, spatial coding, and motor programming. Frontal lobe deficits, sometimes sitting above a set of spared cognitive abilities, have been difficult to understand in terms of traditional "box-and-arrow" cognitive theories. These theories are built around functionally independent modules whose purpose is to map input to output through sets of derived and stored internal representations (e.g., Fodor, 1984). In patients with frontal lobe lesions, the modules may continue to operate, but there are problems in ensuring that their activation is constrained by the task at hand. In this chapter we examine the attentional functions subserved by the frontal lobes, particularly those functions that ensure that our behavior is goal-driven. We begin by reviewing behavioral evidence on four specific issues. In the first section, we evaluate whether there is a core process, concerned with holding task goals in working memory, that is crucial to understanding the role of the frontal lobes in behavioral control. In subsequent sections we discuss the involvement of the frontal lobes in imposing internal rather than external (stimulus-driven) control over behavior, and whether critical control processes fractionate, with frontal lobe functions being weighted toward the response end of task performance. In the fourth section, we review evidence on the role of frontal lobe processes in

GLYN W. HUMPHREYS and DANA SAMSON Behavioural Brain Sciences Centre, School of Psychology, University of Birmingham, Birmingham, U.K.

responding to affect, reward, and punishment. Our primary evidence in each section is drawn from studies in patients with impaired attentional control following damage to the frontal lobes, but we will also use evidence from functional brain imaging and single-cell recordings in nonhuman animals where relevant. In a final section, we discuss evidence for developmental deficits in attentional control. At least some of the problems found in adults with frontal lobe lesions can be observed in children with problems in controlling attention, and studies in adults may help us understand such developmental disorders.

Working memory and the frontal lobes

Normally, attentional control of behavior may be contingent on participants' generating and maintaining task goals in working memory. Working memory may be needed (1) to impose the appropriate task set by modulating activation in other systems (which respond to stimuli in a more automatic fashion), (2) to manipulate temporarily held representations (e.g., when formulating plans), and (3) to reconfigure task goals when another task must be performed (see Baddeley, 1986, 2002, for this view of working memory). It follows that a working memory deficit after frontal lobe damage could induce a wide range of problems in the control of attention, in planning, and in switching between tasks.

The link between the frontal lobes and working memory enjoys considerable support from studies using functional brain imaging (e.g., Petrides et al., 1993; D'Esposito et al., 1995; Cohen et al., 1997; LeBar et al., 1999) and from single-cell recordings in monkey (e.g., Goldman-Rakic, 1996; Goldman-Rakic and Leung, 2002). These studies have demonstrated activation in lateral frontal areas centered around the middle frontal gyrus (figure 44.1) when information must be temporarily held in memory as a task is being performed. Consistent with this observation, patients with lateral prefrontal lesions can show impairment on working memory tasks when there is a delayed response (Freedman and Oscar-Berman, 1986), when information may no longer be maintained by rehearsal (cf. Baddeley, 1986). Similarly, degrading effects of transcranial magnetic stimulation (TMS) over lateral prefrontal cortex have been reported for normal participants when they must hold information across a delay (Pascal-Leone and Hallett, 1994; Muri et al., 1996; Brandt et al., 1998). In humans there can be

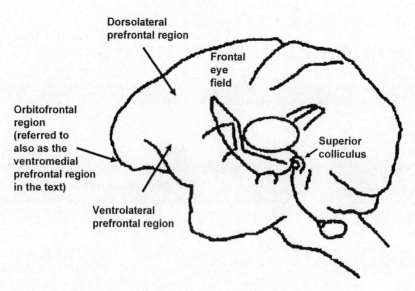

FIGURE 44.1   Brain areas involved in the frontal lobes concerned with the control of attention.

increased activation, particularly of the left prefrontal cortex, when verbal material is maintained across a delay (Postle and D'Esposito, 2000), while the right prefrontal cortex may be involved in maintaining spatial material (Smith et al., 1995; but see D'Esposito and Postle, 2002).

Those aspects of working memory supported by the frontal lobes appear crucial for representing task goals and not just particular stimuli. Wallis, Anderson, and Miller (2001) trained monkeys to switch between two tasks involving the same stimuli. On each trial a sample object was presented, followed by a test stimulus, which could be the same as or different from the sample object. The monkeys were cued either to respond if the stimuli matched or to withhold their response if the stimuli matched (and respond if they mismatched). Wallis and colleagues found that more than 40% of the neurons were selective to the rule (respond match vs. respond nonmatch) rather than the stimuli.

Task goals held in working memory may be necessary to impose attentional control over behavior. In humans, the working memory system involved can be abstracted from verbal representations held in an articulatory loop. Humphreys, Forde, and Francis (2000) had patients manipulate objects to verbal instructions that could violate the usual actions on the objects (e.g., "put the saucer on the cup," rather than vice versa). Frontal lobe patients made many "action reversals," performing the familiar action rather than the behavior instructed. These action reversals occurred even when the patients could repeat back the task instructions, presumably using information held in an articulatory loop (cf. Baddeley, 2002). Interestingly, the number of action reversals increased with the memory load, which was manipulated through the number of instructions presented. With a greater load, patients were less able to impose the novel task set on behavior, despite maintaining a verbal

memory in an articulatory loop. Here there may be problems with maintaining the task set (to follow the instructions, not the overlearned behavior) in an abstract working memory system as the load on this system increases.

MAINTAINING AND MANIPULATING INFORMATION IN WORKING MEMORY   Other investigators have attempted to distinguish the role of the frontal cortex in maintaining and actively manipulating information in working memory. For example, D'Esposito and colleagues (1999) used a delayed recognition task in which five letters were presented simultaneously in random order. Participants either maintained the letters as given (e.g., MJDFO) or they rearranged them mentally, in alphabetical order (DFJMO). Participants were subsequently cued with a letter and a number (F2) and had to verify if, in the memory representation, the letter was in the position indicated by the number (according to the task condition: in our example, respond no in the maintain condition, but yes in the manipulate condition). D'Esposito and colleagues reported activation of both dorso- and ventrolateral prefrontal cortex in both conditions, but only the dorsolateral prefrontal cortex showed increased activation when stimuli had to be manipulated and not just maintained (see also Postle et al., 2000). They suggest that both dorsal and ventrolateral prefrontal cortex are involved in maintaining stimulus information, but the dorsolateral region makes a greater contribution to manipulation processes. In humans with frontal lobe lesions, the ability to manipulate and order information can be markedly impaired even when the ability to maintain information in working memory without manipulating it is spared (e.g., Humphreys and Forde, 1998; Rumiati et al., 2001). However, such studies have not yet separated maintenance from manipulation problems by lesion site.

MANIPULATING INFORMATION AND SWITCHING TASK SETS
Being able to manipulate information in working memory may be a prerequisite for generating an appropriate strategy for a task, and for switching from one task to another (discarding processes set up for the old task and reconfiguring a new set of processes). Shallice (2002) proposes that the left dorsolateral prefrontal cortex is important for strategy generation, based on imaging studies that varied the difficulty of finding a strategy for memory performance. Consistent with this proposal, many patients with frontal lobe lesions show poor strategy generation when asked to carry out complex, multistep tasks (e.g., Burgess & Shallice, 1996).

There is also evidence linking frontal lobe damage to deficits in task switching. Clinical measures such as the Wisconsin Card Sort Test (WCST) are often taken as a measure of shifting attentional set, and deficits on this task are classically associated with frontal lesions (Milner, 1963). This fits with imaging data showing that the lateral prefrontal cortex is activated during category shifts in the WCST (Konishi et al., 1999). On the other hand, the WCST involves multiple abilities, including the control of perseverative responses, that could be affected by frontal lesions. The deficit may not be specific to task switching. In other studies explicitly requiring switching between tasks, performance has been reported not to be disrupted by frontal lesions (Mecklinger et al., 1999), while other investigators have reported task switching deficits (e.g., Rogers et al., 1998). However, the neuropsychological results may depend on subtle factors, such as the manner in which task switches are signaled. Duncan and colleagues (1996) had patients read out a letter on a particular side (left or right) of a pair of stimuli. At the beginning of each trial block, a direct cue indicated which side to respond to (e.g., "watch left"). Toward the end of the block, a second, indirect cue indicated which of the following items had to be responded to (the symbols + and − were used for the right and left sides). Duncan and colleagues found that patients with frontal lobe lesions regularly failed to respond to the correct side when the indirect cue required them to switch from the previously attended side. This behavior was observed even though the patients could repeat correctly the instructions after the task (as in Humphreys, Forde, and Francis, 2000). In this case, when the cue did not directly signal task switching, the patients appeared to show "goal neglect," or inattention to the task goals. Goal neglect may arise in such experiments because in order to induce switching behavior, the cues must be matched to the goal set held in working memory.

Problems also arise when a stimulus can be mapped onto the prior as well as the new response, as a result of the patient failing to discard a prior task set. Kumada and Humphreys (in press) compared task switching under two conditions in a patient with left lateral prefrontal damage. In one condition, the words LEFT or RIGHT appeared in the

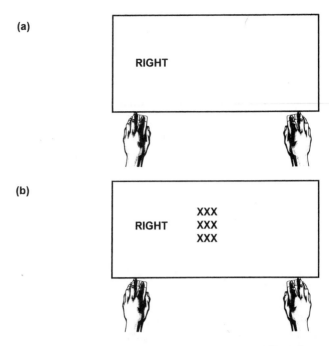

FIGURE 44.2 Example stimuli used by Kumada and Humphreys (2002). (*a*) In the low-load condition, a single word (LEFT or RIGHT) was shown on the left or right of the screen. The task was either to respond to the meaning of the word or to its location. (*b*) In the high-load condition, the same words were presented, but this time simultaneously with a matrix of Xs at the center. Now, interference from the word's meaning decreased when the task required responding to the location of the word.

left and right fields. The patient had to switch between blocks of trials in which he had to press buttons according to the meaning of the words while ignoring their location and blocks of trials in which he had to respond according to the location of the words while ignoring their meaning. In this condition there was a massive increase in switching costs, compared to the effects found in control participants, and these costs continued across a block of trials (figure 44.2a). In a second condition, the words LEFT or RIGHT were presented in different colors. This time the patient had to switch between blocks of trials in which he responded to the meaning of the words while ignoring their color, or to the color of the words while ignoring their meaning. Here, the critical dimensions of the stimulus (its color and its meaning) may be attended independently, perhaps unlike word location and meaning (in the first condition). In this second condition Kumada and Humphreys found that there was an abnormally large switching cost on the first trial after the switch, but costs were subsequently much reduced. Large costs on a first switching trial may be due to difficulty setting up the new task goal. However, continued interference (in the first condition) suggests that the patient failed to discard the initial task set. When the critical dimensions cannot be attended selectively, the prior (nondiscarded) stimulus-response mappings may continue to be activated, creating competition and slowed responding (see Keele and Rafal, 2000, for a further example).

Endogenous control of attention

The task set maintained within the frontal lobes may be necessary in order to impose endogenous, task-based control over performance. One example of impaired task-based control emerges from the Stroop task, where participants must name the hue of a color word. The Stroop task requires that attention be applied to the dimension of the stimulus deemed relevant by the task instructions (the hue rather than the name of the word), even though this may not be the most salient aspect of the stimulus; thus, it requires endogenous control. Problems on the Stroop task have been found after damage to both left (Perret, 1974; Corcoran and Upton, 1993) and right lateral areas (Vendrell et al., 1995), as well as after damage to the superior medial region (Holzt and Vilkki, 1988). Problems on incongruent Stroop trials (when the color word and hue are incompatible) are most marked after damage to the right, superior medial frontal cortex (Stuss et al., 2001). Similar problems on other tasks, where participants must filter out distracting information presented at the same time as a target, have been reported after unilateral right frontal damage (Chao and Knight, 1985), and patients with right frontal damage can have problems in keeping out from subsequent processing items that should previously have been filtered and rejected as irrelevant (negative priming, Tipper, 1985; see Stuss et al., 1999, for evidence). In each of these instances, it can be argued that patients have problems using the task instructions to select the appropriate stimulus or stimulus dimension (in the Stroop task) to minimize processing of irrelevant information. In some accounts of frontal lobe deficits (e.g., Braver, Cohen, and Barch, 2002), this deficit has been described as a problem in using contextual information in a top-down manner to override strong bottom-up cues for selection and action.

In addition to its role in stimulus selection, endogenous attention is also important for task-appropriate response selection. Striking examples of poor endogenous control of response selection can be observed in patients showing "utilization" behavior. Lhermitte (1986) described patients who made "automatic" responses to stimuli that were placed in front of them. For example, a pair of spectacles on a table would be grasped and placed on the patient's nose. This behavior would occur repeatedly if other spectacles were put on the table, even if it involved the spectacles being positioned one on top of another on the patient's face! Riddoch and colleagues (1998, 2000a) conducted experimental studies of patients with basal ganglia and frontal lobe damage to examine the factors that determine these utilization errors. Patients had to make a grasp response to a cup placed either to the right or left of their body, using the left hand if the cup was on the left and the right hand if the cup was on the right (figure 44.3a). Despite repeating back the instruction, patients made many errors when the handle of the cup was incompatible with the required response (e.g., using the right hand to grasp a cup on the left with its handle on the right). These utilization errors decreased if the cups

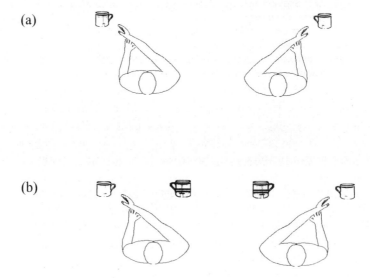

FIGURE 44.3   Conditions used in studies of grasp responses to cup stimuli. (*a*) A single cup was presented on the left or right of the patient's midline. The task was to grasp the cup using the hand on the same side as the cup. Here we illustrate conditions in which the handle of the cup was incongruent with the required response, and the patient erred by reaching to the cup with the wrong hand (after Riddoch et al., 1998). (*b*) Two cups were presented, and the task was to grasp the cup with the stripes. Errors occurred on occasions when the target cup was incongruent with the required response and the distracter cup (without stripes) was congruent (after Boutsen and Humphreys, 2003).

were inverted or if cuplike objects were used where a grasp response still had to be made to a small handle attached to a larger cylinder (now the patients were more likely to use their left hand to grasp a left-side cup with its handle turned to the right). Thus, the errors were determined by the familiarity of the objects (for cups vs. noncups) and their orientation with respect to the relevant effector. These factors likely influence the strength of any exogenous signal for action. In the face of the strong exogenous signal for one action, and with poor endogenous control of attention, patients selected the wrong (task-inappropriate) response.

INTERACTIONS BETWEEN ENDOGENOUS AND EXOGENOUS ATTENTION Behavioral studies with normal participants suggest that endogenous and exogenous mechanisms of attention interact, so that endogenous attention modulates the tendency for strong exogenous cues to capture attention. For example, the effects of a salient singleton distracter on visual search are contingent on participants' adopting a set to select a target based on its singleton value: a green singleton distracter presented among red distracters is likely to capture attention if participants search for an "odd one out" along a different dimension (e.g., when asked to find the odd shape). However, singleton distracter effects reduce when this odd-one-out search mode is not adopted (e.g., Bacon and Egeth, 1994). Similarly, the capture of attention by new objects can be overcome if a focused rather than a distributed mode of attending is adopted (e.g., if observers have to focus attention on each item in turn to find a target, rather than depending on the target "popping out," based on it being salient within a display; Yantis and Egeth, 1999). Single-cell studies in animals concur with these results and indicate that the prefrontal cortex (controlling endogenous attention) can modulate processing in earlier brain areas. For example, prefrontal lesions disrupt the ability of sensory association areas to hold information across temporal delays in match-to-sample tasks, consistent with the prefrontal areas' influencing activation in these other regions (Fuster et al., 1995; Desimone, 1996). Here we can think of prefrontal activity setting up "memory templates" that serve to bias attention in earlier brain regions in favor of goal-relevant targets (see, e.g., Chelazzi et al., 1993, for evidence on the biasing effects of such templates in the inferotemporal lobe). These memory templates form part of the set for the task. When endogenous, top-down effects are decreased by frontal lobe damage, then individuals may be overly directed to action by salient exogenous signals.

INTERNAL AND EXTERNAL CUING OF TASK SET So far we have discussed endogenous control of attention as if it were a unitary process, but there is also evidence that a set for a task can be established in a number of different ways, depending on the external properties of stimuli as well as the internal goals of the participant. Kumada and Humphreys (2002) described the performance of a patient with bilateral medial frontal damage on a task requiring responses to the locations of the words RIGHT and LEFT, presented in the right or left visual fields. When the words appeared alone, marked effects of congruency were found (see figure 44.2a). However, these congruency effects decreased when the perceptual load of the displays increased (see figure 44.2b). This fits with proposals made by Lavie (1995) concerning the effects of perceptual load on attentional selection. Lavie argued that, under conditions of high perceptual load, there was early selection of targets and minimal processing of distracters (or irrelevant attributes of stimuli). However, irrelevant information in displays was more likely to be processed under conditions of low perceptual load. In the study of Kumada and Humphreys, increasing the perceptual load may have helped the patient select targets at an early stage of processing, decreasing the effects of word meaning on a task requiring responses to a word's location. The study illustrates that task set can be induced in different ways, and that internal generation and maintenance of a task set may be separate from external cuing of a task set. The process of internal generation and maintenance of task set may be particularly dependent on medial frontal regions.

Deficits in response selection, response inhibition, and response monitoring

Although we have noted instances of patients exhibiting poor selection of which stimulus must be responded to in a task, several authors have argued that patients with frontal lobe lesions have particular difficulties in controlling their responses: in selecting a correct response, in inhibiting an incorrect response, or in monitoring any responses that are made. Here we ask whether frontal lobe lesions lead to isolated deficits in response control.

IMPAIRMENTS IN RESPONSE SELECTION A distinction between the processes involved in stimulus selection and response selection has been made in studies of utilization errors. Riddoch, Humphreys, and Edwards (2000b) used an extension of their cups experiments, where in two cups were presented in different colors and the patient was asked to grasp the cup in one color. The patients made no errors by grasping the incorrect cup, but they continued to make utilization errors in which the correct cup was grasped but with the wrong hand (i.e., with the hand congruent with the handle and not the location of the cup). Thus, the patients remained able to select the correct stimulus for action, but they were impaired in selecting the correct action to the stimulus (failing to override a familiar action that did not accord with the instructions). Here frontal damage seems to

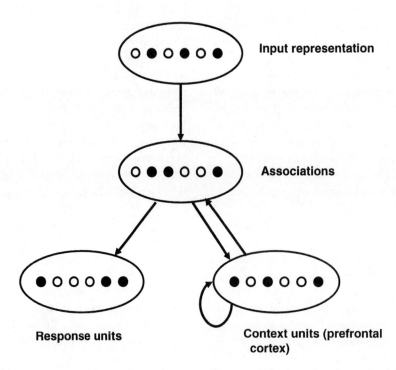

Input representation

Associations

Response units

Context units (prefrontal cortex)

FIGURE 44.4   Framework for the connectionist model proposed by Cohen and colleagues (1997). The model maps representations of an input through to a response by means of stored associations. The associative mapping, from stimulus to response, is modulated by activation of "context units" assumed to be represented in the prefrontal cortex.

have a selective effect on response but not on stimulus selection.

However, the situation is not so straightforward. Boutsen and Humphreys (2003) examined a cup task similar to that of Riddoch, Humphreys, and Edwards (2000b), but instead of having the target in a constant color they switched color across trials. Now errors were made in selecting the incorrect cup, particularly when the distracter was associated with a more familiar response than the target (see figure 44.3b). In the study reported by Riddoch, Humphreys, and Edwards, stimulus selection might have been good because it was based on a goal set that was constant across trials, while the goal set for response selection had to compete with an overlearned stimulus-response mapping ("pick up the cup using the hand congruent with the handle"). When the goal set for stimulus selection required reconfiguration across trials (and perhaps greater working memory involvement), problems were again apparent.

Poor stimulus selection may also contribute to other deficits frequently attributed to impaired response inhibition in patients with frontal lesions (e.g., abnormal interference from simultaneously presented distracters; Leimkuhler and Mesulam, 1985). Several interesting findings emerge from a brain imaging study by de Fockert and colleagues (2001). Participants had to hold a series of digits in working memory while performing a selective attention task that required them to ignore distracter faces. Higher memory loads increased activity in prefrontal regions, and they also pro-

duced greater distracter interference on behavior. Interestingly, there was also increased face-related activity in visual cortex under these conditions. Apparently, reduced frontally mediated attention to the central item (under load conditions) was linked to increased perceptual processing of distracters. It follows that abnormal sensitivity to irrelevant distracters in patients with frontal lobe lesions can reflect poor perceptual processing rather than poor response selection. This is also indicated by the study of Kumada and Humphreys (2002), in which an apparent problem in response selection (e.g., increased congruency effects in a reverse Simon task) was improved by increasing the perceptual load in the task. We have interpreted this result as due to facilitation of early perceptual selection under increased load conditions.

Although we have suggested that both stimulus and response selection are intimately linked to holding task goals in working memory, we may ask whether aspects of working memory can be separated from these selection processes. Rowe and colleagues (2000; see Passingham and Rowe, 2002, for a review) conducted an event-related functional magnetic resonance imaging (fMRI) study that attempted to separate maintenance and response selection processes. Participants had to memorize the positions of dots and then align a probe with the location of a dot after the dots had disappeared. During the maintenance period (before the probe), there was activation in area BA8, dorsal and anterior to the frontal eye fields. In contrast, the dorsolateral prefrontal region (area

BA46) was activated when the response was selected. They suggest that the dorsolateral prefrontal cortex is primarily involved in response selection, while the maintenance component of working memory depends on a more superior and posterior frontal area. However, from these results alone it remains unclear whether the dorsolateral prefrontal cortex is specifically recruited for response selection or whether its involvement was more tied to the manipulation of information in working memory (D'Esposito and Postle, 2002).

Other imaging data distinguish the process of maintaining a task set from processes involved in response inhibition, the latter being specifically recruited when competing responses must be resolved. MacDonald and colleagues (2000) used fMRI to study performance on a Stroop task, measuring activation separately during a period when the instructions were given and when the stimuli were presented. Activation of dorsolateral prefrontal cortex was increased during the instruction period when the task was to name the hue rather than the word, but not on response-congruent relative to response-incongruent trials (for scans following presentation of the stimulus). In contrast, activation of the more medial (anterior cingulated) region of frontal cortex did not vary with the task during the instruction period but increased following stimulus presentation for response-incongruent compared with response-congruent trials (see also Botvinick et al., 1999; Carter, Mintun, and Cohen, 1995; Carter et al., 1998). Also, individuals with greater dorsolateral prefrontal activation in the instruction period manifested lower Stroop interference. These results implicate the dorsolateral prefrontal cortex in setting up and maintaining the task goals and the anterior cingulate cortex in detecting and resolving response conflict. The stronger the representation of the task set, the lower the competition between the hue and word name responses on incongruent trials. This distinction between areas involved in maintaining the task set and areas involved in dealing with response conflict fits the neuropsychological data noted earlier, where problems on response-incongruent trials in the Stroop effect were associated with lesions of the superior and medial frontal cortex (Stuss et al., 2001). However, the precise role of the anterior cingulate cortex remains controversial. Jonides and colleagues (see Jonides et al., 2002, for a summary) conducted several imaging studies in which they varied the magnitude of response conflict and failed to find increased anterior cingulate activation. Jonides and colleagues (2002) propose that the anterior cingulate may not be specifically involved in resolving response conflicts (e.g., through inhibition of a task-incongruent response) but rather may be involved in detecting that a response conflict has arisen (see Bush, Liu, and Posner, 2000, for a more extended discussion).

IMPAIRMENTS IN RESPONSE MONITORING   Poor monitoring of behavior is a classic clinical symptom of frontal lobe damage that is expressed when patients make confabulations in memory (Moscovitch, 1995) or judge that they have completed a task successfully when in fact errors have occurred (Forde and Humphreys, 2002). Stuss and colleagues (1994) conducted a recall task with either unrelated words or words blocked by category. Although patients with left prefrontal lesions recalled relatively few items, those with right prefrontal lesions generated an abnormal number of repeated items in their protocols. This finding is consistent with imaging studies demonstrating activation of the right dorsolateral prefrontal cortex when participants need to check whether they have produced a response previously (Henson, Shallice, and Dolan, 1999; Shallice, 2002).

In behavioral studies, there are also indications that this monitoring operation can be dissociated from processes involved in implementing a task goal and inhibiting inappropriate responses. For instance, Humphreys and Forde (1998) studied errors in everyday life tasks in patients with frontal lobe lesions. They observed occasions on which patients continued to make action errors while verbally describing that an error was occurring. (One patient, when ask to wrap a gift, repetitively cut the wrapping paper with scissors until it was far too small to cover the gift. Concurrent with making the cutting actions, the patient remarked that "the paper is now too small for the gift," yet went on cutting the paper into even smaller pieces.) In such cases a process of response monitoring still seems to operate, but there is a failure in implementing the task goal in order to prevent repetitive responding. Response monitoring may require some forward running of a predictive model of behavior to know when an error occurs (when there is a mismatch of the model and behavior). It is possible that this forward model may be run even when patients lose the current goal in working memory for what they are doing, and so fail to correct their behavior.

Affect, reward, and punishment

In addition to having problems with cognitive tasks, patients with frontal damage can also produce a range of abnormal behaviors linked to the affective and reward values of stimuli. Bechera and colleagues (1994) first studied the performance of patients with ventromedial damage to the frontal lobes on a gambling task in which different rewards were given when participants turn over cards from any of four decks. After a card was selected, there was either a monetary reward or a reward along with a penalty. The task was rigged so that two decks received higher immediate rewards but higher longer-term penalties, whereas the other decks received lower immediate rewards but also lower long-term penalties. Patients with ventromedial damage failed to shift their pattern of responding as the task progressed, whereas control participants and patients with lesions of other brain regions gradually shifted their responses away from decks with higher immediate reward and higher longer-term penalties. In addition, control participants generated anticipatory changes in galvanic skin responses prior to card selection, suggesting some prediction of the reward value; this did not occur for patients with ventromedial damages even though sometimes they could report that some decks were disadvantageous (Bechera et al., 1996). Bechera and colleagues propose that there is a nonconscious signaling process, reflecting a prior record of rewards and possibly linked emotional states, that is disrupted by damage to ventromedial regions of the frontal lobes. Such nonconscious signals may generate covert biases in attention, influencing conscious decision making. This evidence also fits with imaging studies showing that activity in the ventromedial frontal cortex varies according to hedonic sensory experience and the magnitudes of rewards and punishments (Blair et al., 1999; Rolls, 2000). Reduced responsivity to rewards, punishments, and emotional valence may also contribute to the reports of personality change following frontal lobe lesions (Tranel, 2002).

It is of interest too that patients with ventromedial lesions do not necessarily show impairments on the Stroop color-word interference task (Stuss et al., 1981). Thus, the processes involved in establishing endogenous control of performance in emotionally neutral tasks may be distinct from processes that control behavior based on a history of reward, punishment, and emotional association (see also Bush, Liu, and Posner, 2000, for a distinction between inferior and more superior regions of anterior cingulate cortex activated respectively on emotional and neutral Stroop tasks).

Developmental disorders and frontal attentional systems

Although we have concentrated on disorders of attention following frontal lobe damage in adults, some developmental disorders of attention resemble the acquired disorders we have discussed. We will briefly mention one, attention-deficit hyperactivity disorder (ADHD). ADHD is one of the most common referrals for psychiatric treatment in children (Barkley, 1997), with the diagnosis based on difficulties in sustaining attention, difficulties in organizing tasks, being easily distracted and forgetful, and difficulty in waiting a turn. Many of these behaviors are characteristic of adults with frontal lobe lesions, and the deficits in adults may provide a means of understanding the developmental deficits in children with ADHD.

One major account is that ADHD children have problems in response inhibition (see Logan, Schachar, and Tannock, 2002), which can cascade through to generate the constellation of behavioral problems associated with the disorder. Evidence for a deficit in response inhibition comes from go/no-go and 'stop' response tasks (ADHD children are

poor at using stop signal to interrupt a programmed response; see Logan, Shachar, and Tannock, 2000; Manly et al., 2001). However, the deficits are not limited to cases where response inhibition is a prominent aspect of task performance. For example, there are impairments in so-called N-back working memory tasks (the children may be given a list of numbers and have to match whether a number presented after a tone is the same as the number preceding the tone, or even a number further back in the sequence; see Shallice et al., 2002), while deficits from distracter interference occur under conditions where normal subjects limit interference by early perceptual filtering rather than response inhibition (Jonkman et al., 1999; Brodeur and Pond, 2001). There is also evidence that some problems reflect a difficulty in generating and maintaining the set that can lead to early perceptual filtering. An example is a study that used an "attentional blink" procedure, in which observers show a deficit in identifying the second of two targets presented in a rapid stream of stimuli—the attentional blink (cf. Raymond, Shapiro, and Arnell, 1992). Mason, Humphreys, and Kent (in press) had ADHD and control children identify a red letter target among white letter distracters, but presented irrelevant asterisks around a letter preceding the target (cf. Folk, Leber, and Egeth, 2002). When the asterisks were red (i.e., the same color as the target), both the children with ADHD and the control children showed an attentional blink relative to when no asterisks were present. This observation suggests that the children selected the asterisks based on their matching the target-defining feature (its color), which then disrupted the identification of subsequent targets. However, although the control subjects showed no disruption when the asterisks were green, and did not match the target feature, the children with ADHD generated an attentional blink. The ADHD children were impaired in implementing the task set (select the red target), and hence were distracted by the presence of irrelevant distracters. This last pattern of performance cannot easily be attributed to a deficit in response inhibition, since no overt response was made to the asterisk.

Concluding remarks

The frontal lobes subserve a number of important attentional control functions, including maintaining, manipulating, and switching task sets, top-down (endogenous) modulation of both stimulus and response selection, and response monitoring. In light of these different functions, it is unlikely that a coherent frontal lobe syndrome exists; rather, patients with frontal lobe deficits may exhibit a number of contrasting deficits, which need to be understood in terms of detailed models of cognition. The same also likely holds for developmental disorders such as ADHD. We propose that models of adult frontal lobe function can provide a framework to help the diagnosis and (eventual) remediation of such cases.

ACKNOWLEDGMENTS This work was supported by grants from the Medical Research Council and the Stroke Association (U.K.).

REFERENCES

BADDELEY, A. D., 1986. *Working Memory.* Oxford, England: Oxford University Press.

BADDELEY, A. D., 2002. Fractionating the central executive. In *Principles of Frontal Lobe Function*, D. T. Stuss and R. T. Knight, eds. Oxford, England: Oxford University Press, pp. 246–260.

BACON, W. F., and H. E. EGETH, 1994. Overriding stimulus-driven attentional capture. *Percept. Psychophys.* 55:485–496.

BARKLEY, R. A., 1997. Behavioral inhibition, sustained attention and executive functions: Constructing a unifying theory of ADHD. *Psychol. Bull.* 121:65–94.

BECHERA, A., A. R. DAMASIO, H. DAMASIO, and S. W. ANDERSON, 1994. Insensitivity to future consequences following damage to human prefrontal cortex. *Cognition* 50:7–15.

BECHERA, A., D. TRANEL, H. DAMASIO, and A. R. DAMASIO, 1996. Failure to respond autonomically to anticipated future outcomes following damage to prefrontal cortex. *Cereb. Cortex* 6:215–225.

BLAIR, R. J. R., J. S. MORRIS, C. D. FRITH, D. I. PERRET, and R. J. DOLAN, 1999. Dissociable neural responses to facial expressions of sadness and anger. *Brain* 122:883–893.

BOTVINICK, M., L. E. NYSTROM, K. FISSELL, C. CARTER, and J. D. COHEN, 1999. Conflict monitoring versus selection-for-action in anterior congulate cortex. *Nature* 402:179–181.

BOUTSEN, L., and G. W. HUMPHREYS, 2003. On the interaction between perceptual and response selection: Neuropsychological evidence. *Neurocase* 9:239–250.

BRANDT, S. A., C. J. PLONER, B. U. MEYER, S. LEISTNER, and A. VILLRINGER, 1998. Effects of repetitive transcranial magnetic stimulation over dorsolateral prefrontal and posterior parietal cortex on memory-guided saccades. *Exp. Brain Res.* 118:197–204.

BRAVER, T. S., J. D. COHEN, and D. M. BARCH, 2002. The role of prefrontal cortex in normal and disordered cognitive control: A cognitive neuroscience perspective. In *Principles of Frontal Lobe Function*, D. T. Stuss and R. T. Knight, eds. Oxford, England: Oxford University Press, pp. 428–447.

BRODEUR, D. A., and M. POND, 2001. The development of selective attention in children with attention deficit hyperactivity disorder. *J. Abnorm. Child Psychol.* 29:229–239.

BURGESS, P. W., and T. SHALLICE, 1996. Response suppression, initiation and strategy use following frontal lobe lesion. *Neuropsychologia* 34:263–273.

BUSH, G., P. LIU, and M. I. POSNER, 2000. Cognitive and emotional influences in anterior cingulate cortex. *Trends Cogn. Sci.* 4:215–222.

CARTER, C. S., T. S. BRAVER, D. M. BARCH, M. M. BOTVINICK, D. NOLL, and J. D. COHEN, 1998. Anterior cingulated cortex, error detection and the online monitoring of performance. *Science* 280:747–749.

CARTER, C. S., M. MINTUN, and J. D. COHEN, 1995. Interference and facilitation effects during selective attention: An H_2O^{15} PET study of Stroop task performance. *NeuroImage* 2:264–272.

CHAO, L. L., and R. T. KNIGHT, 1995. Human prefrontal lesions increase distractability to irrelevant sensory inputs. *Neuroreport* 6:1605–1610.

CHELAZZI, L., E. K. MILLER, J. DUNCAN, and R. DESIMONE, 1993. A neural basis for visual search in inferior temporal cortex. *Nature* 363:345–347.

COHEN, J. D., W. M. PERISTEIN, T. S. BRAVER, L. E. NYSTROM, D. C. NOLL, J. JONIDES, and E. E. SMITH, 1997. Temporal dynamics of brain activation during a working memory task. *Nature* 386:604–606.

CORCORAN, R., and D. UPTON, 1993. A role for the hippocampus in card sorting? *Cortex* 29:293–304.

DE FOCKERT, J. W., G. REES, C. D. FRITH, and N. LAVIE, 2001. The role of working memory in visual selective attention. *Science* 291:1803–1806.

DESIMONE, R., 1986. Neural mechanisms for visual memory and their role in attention. *Proc. Nat. Acad. Sci. U.S.A.* 93:13494–13499.

D'ESPOSITO, M., G. K. AGUIRRE, E. ZARAHN, and D. BALLARD, 1998. Functional MRI studies of spatial and nonspatial working memory. *Cogn. Brain Res.* 7:1–13.

D'ESPOSITO, M., J. A. DETRE, D. C. ALSOP, R. K. SHIN, S. ATLAS, and M. GROSSMAN, 1995. The neural basis of the central executive system of working memory. *Nature* 378:279–281.

D'ESPOSITO, M., and B. R. POSTLE, 2002. The organization of working memory function in lateral prefrontal cortex: Evidence from event-related functional MRI. In *Principles of Frontal Lobe Function*, D. T. Stuss and R. T. Knight, eds. Oxford, England: Oxford University Press, pp. 168–187.

D'ESPOSITO, M., B. R. POSTLE, D. BALLARD, and J. LEASE, 1999. Maintenance versus manipulation of information held in working memory: An event-related fMRI study. *Brain Cogn.* 41:66–86.

DUNCAN, J., H. EMSLIE, P. WILLIAMS, R. JOHNSON, and C. FREER, 1996. Intelligence and the frontal lobe: The organisation of goal-directed behaviour. *Cogn. Psychol.* 30:257–303.

FODOR, J., 1984. *The Modularity of Mind.* Cambridge, Mass.: Bradford Books.

FORDE, E. M. E., and G. W. HUMPHREYS, 2002. Dissociations in routine behaviour across patients and everyday tasks. *Neurocase* 8:151–167.

FOLK, C. L., A. B. LEBER, and H. E. EGETH, 2002. Made you blink! Contingent attentional capture produces a spatial blink. *Percept. Psychophys.* 64:741–753.

FREEDMAN, M., and M. OSCAR-BERMAN, 1996. Bilateral frontal lobe disease and selective delayed response deficits in humans. *Behav. Neurosci.* 100:337–342.

FUSTER, J. M., R. H. BAUER, and J. P. JERVEY, 1985. Functional interactions between inferotemporal and prefrontal cortex in a cognitive task. *Brain Res.* 330:299–307.

GOLDMAN-RAKIC, P. S., 1996. The prefrontal landscape: Implications of functional architecture for understanding human mentation and the central executive. *Philos. Trans. R. Soc. B* 351:1445–1453.

GOLDMAN-RAKIC, P. S., and H.-C. LEUNG, 2002. Functional architecture of the dorsolateral prefrontal cortex in monkeys and humans. In *Principles of Frontal Lobe Function*, D. T. Stuss and R. T. Knight, eds. Oxford, England: Oxford University Press, pp. 85–95.

HENSON, R. N. A., T. SHALLICE, and R. J. DOLAN, 1999. Right prefrontal cortex and episodic memory retrieval: A functional MRI test of the monitoring hypothesis. *Brain* 122:1367–1381.

HOLZT, P., and J. VILKKI, 1988. Effect of frontomedial lesions on performance on the Stroop test and word fluency tests. *J. Clin. Exp. Neuropsychol.* 10:79–80.

Humphreys, G. W., and E. M. E. Forde, 1998. Disordered action schema and action disorganisation syndrome. *Cogn. Neuropsychol.* 15:771–812.

Humphreys, G. W., E. M. E. Forde, and D. Francis, 2000. The sequential organisation of action. In *Attention and Performance XVIII: Control of Cognitive Processes*, S. Monsell and J. Driver, eds. Cambridge, Mass.: MIT Press, pp. 427–442.

Jonides, J., D. Badre, C. Curtis, S. L. Thompson Schill, and E. E. Smith, 2002. Mechanisms of conflict resolution in prefrontal cortex. In *Principles of Frontal Lobe Function*, D. T. Stuss and R. T. Knight, eds. Oxford, England: Oxford University Press, pp. 233–245.

Jonides, J., C. Marshuetz, E. E. Smith, P. A. Reuter-Lorenz, R. A. Koeppe, and A. Hartley, 2000. Age differences in behavior and PET activation reveal differences in interference resolution in verbal working memory. *J. Cogn. Neurosci.* 12:188–196.

Jonkman, L. M., C. Kemner, M. N. Verbaten, H. van Engeland, J. L. Kenemans, G. Camfferman, J. K. Buitelaar, and H. S. Koelega, 1999. Perceptual and response interference in children with attention-deficit hyperactivity disorder and the effects of methylphenidate. *Psychophysiology* 36:419–429.

Keele, S. W., and R. D. Rafal, 2000. Deficits of task set in patients with left prefrontal cortex lesions. In S. Monsell and J. Driver, eds. *Attention and Performance XVIII: Control of Cognitive Processes.* London: Academic Press, pp. 627–651.

Kumada, T., and G. W. Humphreys 2002. Early selection influenced by perceptual load in a patient with frontal lobe damage: External vs. internal modulation of processing control. *Cogn. Neuropsychol.* 19:49–65.

Kumada, T., and G. W. Humphreys (in press). Dimensional weighting and task switching following frontal lobe damage: Fractionating the task switching deficit. *Cogn. Neuropsychol.*

Konishi, S., K. Nakajima, I. Uchida, H. Kikyo, M. Kameyama, and Y. Miyashita, 1999. Common inhibitory mechanism in human inferior prefrontal cortex revealed by event-related functional MRI. *Brain* 122:981–991.

Lavie, N., 1995. Perceptual load as a necessary condition for selective attention. *J. Exp. Psychol. Hum. Percept. Perform.* 21:451–468.

LeBar, K. S., D. R. Gitelman, T. D. Parrish, and M.-M. Mesulam, 1999. Neuroanatomic overlap of working memory and spatial attention networks: A functional fMRI comparison within subjects. *NeuroImage* 10:695–704.

Leimkuhler, M. E., and M.-M. Mesulam, 1985. Reversible go-no go deficits in a case of frontal lobe tumour. *Ann. Neurol.* 18: 617–619.

Lhermitte, F., 1986. Human autonomy and the frontal lobes. II. Patient behaviour in complex and social situations. The "environmental dependency syndrome." *Ann. Neurol.* 19:335–343.

Logan, G. D., R. J. Schachar, and R. Tannock, 2000. Executive control problems in childhood psychopathology: Stop signal studies of attention deficit hyperactivity disorder. In S. Monsell and J. Driver, eds., *Attention and Performance XVIII: Control of Cognitive Processes.* London: Academic Press, pp. 654–677.

Manly, T., V. Anderson, I. Nimmo-Smith, A. Turner, P. Watson, and I. Robertson, 2001. The differential assessment of children's attention: The Test of Every Attention for Children (TEA-Ch): Normative sample and ADHD performance. *J. Child Psychol. Psychiatry* 42:1065–1081.

Mason, D. J., G. W. Humphreys, and L. S. Kent (in press). Insights into the control of attentional set in ADHD using the attentional blink paradigm. *J. Child Psychiatry Psychol.*

MacDonald, A. W., J. D. Cohen, V. A. Stenger, and C. S. Carter, 2000. Dissociating the role of the dorsolateral pre-

frontal and anterior cingulated cortex in cognitive control. *Science* 288:1835–1838.

Mecklinger, A., D. Y. von Cramon, A. Springer, and M. von Cramon, 1999. Executive control functions in task switching: Evidence from brain injured patients. *J. Clini. Exp. Neuropsychol.* 21:606–619.

Milner, B., 1963. Some effects of different brain lesions on card sorting. *Arch. Neurol.* 9:90–100.

Moscovitch, M., 1995. Confabulation. In D. L. Schacter, J. T. Coyle, G. D. Fischbach, M.-M. Mesulam, and L. E. Sullivan, eds., *Memory Distortion.* Cambridge, Mass.: MIT Press, pp. 226–251.

Muri, R. M., A. I. Vermersch, S. Rivaud, B. Gaymard, and C. Pierrot-Deseilligny, 1996. Effects of single-pulse transcranial magnetic stimulation over the prefrontal and posterior parietal cortices during memory guided saccades in humans. *J. Neurophysiol.* 76:2102–2106.

Pascal-Leone, A., and M. Hallett, 1994. Induction of errors in a delayed response task by repetitive transcranial magnetic stimulation of the dorsolateral prefrontal cortex. *Neuroreport* 5:2517–2520.

Passingham, R. E., and J. B. Rowe, 2002. Dorsal prefrontal cortex: Maintenance in memory or attentional selection? In D. T. Stuss and R. T. Knight, eds., *Principles of Frontal Lobe Function.* Oxford, England: Oxford University Press, pp. 221–232.

Perret, E., 1974. The left frontal lobe of man and the suppression of habitual responses in verbal categorical behaviour. *Neuropsychologia* 12:323–330.

Petrides, M., B. Alivisatos, A. C. Evans, and E. Meyer, 1993. Dissociation of human mid-dorsolateral from posterior dorsolateral frontal cortex in memory processing. *Proc. Nat. Acad. Sci. U.S.A.* 90:873–877.

Postle, B. R., J. S. Berger, A. M. Taich, and M. D'Esposito, 2000. Activity in human frontal cortex associated with spatial working memory and saccadic behaviour. *J. Cogn. Neurosci.* 12: 2–14.

Postle, B. R., and M. D'Esposito, 2000. Evaluating models of the topographical organization of working memory function in frontal cortex with event-related fMRI. *Psychobiology* 28:132–145.

Raymond, J. E., K. L. Shapiro, and K. M. Arnell, 1992. Temporary suppression of visual processing in an RSVP task: An attentional blink? *J. Exp. Psychol. Hum. Percep. Perform.* 18:849–860.

Riddoch, M. J., M. G. Edwards, G. W. Humphreys, R. West, and T. Heafield, 1998. Visual affordances direct action. Neuropsychological evidence from manual interference. *Cogn. Neuropsychol.* 15:645–684.

Riddoch, M. J., G. W. Humphreys, and M. Edwards, 2000a. Visual affordances and object selection. In S. Monsell and J. Driver, eds., *Attention and Performance XVIII: Control of Cognitive Processes.* Cambridge, Mass.: MIT Press, pp. 603–626.

Riddoch, M. J., G. W. Humphreys, and M. G. Edwards, 2000b. Neuropsychological evidence distinguishing object selection from action (effector) selection. *Cogn. Neuropsychol.* 17:547–562.

Rogers, R. D., B. J. Sahakian, J. R. Hodges, C. E. Polkey, C. Kennard, and T. W. Robbins, 1998. Dissociating executive mechanisms of task control following frontal lobe damage and Parkinson's disease. *Brain* 121:815–842.

Rolls, E. T., 2000. The orbitofrontal cortex and reward. *Cereb. Cortex* 10:284–294.

Rowe, J. B., I. Toni, O. Josephs, R. S. J. Frackowiak, and R. E. Passingham, 2000. The prefrontal cortex: Response selection or maintenance within working memory? *Science* 288:1656–1660.

RUMIATI, R., S. ZANINI, L. VORANO, and T. SHALLICE, 2001. A form of ideational apraxia as a selective deficit of contention scheduling. *Cogn. Neuropsychol.* 18:617–642.

SHALLICE, T., 2002. Fractionation of the supervisory system. In *Principles of Frontal Lobe Function*, D. T. Stuss and R. T. Knight, eds. Oxford, England: Oxford University Press, pp. 261–277.

SHALLICE, T., G. M. MARZOCCHI, S. COSER, M. DEL SAVIO, R. F. MEUTER, and R. I. RUMIATI, 2002. Executive function profile of children with attention deficit hyperactivity disorder. *Dev. Neuropsychol.* 21:43–71.

SMITH, E. E., J. JONIDES, R. A. KOEPPE, E. H. SCHUMACHER, and M. SATOSHI, 1995. Spatial versus object working memory: PET investigations. *J. Cogn. Neurosci.* 7:337–356.

STUSS, D. T., M. P. ALEXANDER, C. L. PALUMBO, L. BUCKLE, L. SAYER, and J. POGUE, 1994. Organizational strategies of patients with unilateral or bilateral frontal lobe injury in word list learning tasks. *Neuropsychology* 8:355–373.

STUSS, D. T., D. F. BENSON, E. F. KAPLAN, W. S. WEIR, and C. DELLA MALVA, 1981. Leucotomized and nonleucotomized schizophrenics: Comparison on tests of attention. *Biol. Psychiatry* 16:1085–1100.

STUSS, D. T., D. FLODEN, M. P. ALEXANDER, B. LEVINE, and D. KATZ, 2001. Stroop performance in focal lesion patients: Dissociation of processes and frontal lobe lesion location. *Neuropsychologia* 39:771–786.

STUSS, D. T., J. P. TOTH, D. FRANCHI, M. P. ALEXANDER, S. TIPPER, and F. I. M. CRAIK, 1999. Dissociation of attentional processes in patients with focal frontal and posterior lesions. *Neuropsychologia* 37:1005–1027.

TIPPER, S. P., 1985. The negative priming effect: Inhibtory priming by ignored objects. *Q. J. Exp. Psychol.* 37A:571–590.

TRANEL, D., 2002. Emotion, decision making, and the ventromedial prefrontal cortex. In *Principles of Frontal Lobe Function*, D. T. Stuss and R. T. Knight, eds. Oxford, England: Oxford University Press, pp. 338–353.

VALLAR, G., and T. SHALLICE, 1990. (Eds.) *Neuropsychological Impairments of Short-Term Memory*. Cambridge, England: Cambridge University Press.

VENDRELL, P., C. JUNQUE, J. PUJOL, M. A. JURADO, J. MOLET, and J. GRAFMAN, 1995. The role of prefrontal regions in the Stroop task. *Neuropsychologia* 33:341–352.

WALLIS, J. D., K. C. ANDERSON, and E. K. MILLER, 2001. Single neurons in prefrontal cortex encode abstract rules. *Nature* 411:953–956.

YANTIS, S., and H. E. EGETH, 1999. On the distinction between visual salience and stimulus-driven attentional capture. *J. Exp. Psychol. Hum. Percept. Perform.* 25:661–676.

45 Attention and Action

STEVEN P. TIPPER

ABSTRACT Visual perception provides the information that allows an organism to act appropriately in its environment. Therefore, neural systems that can fluently convert visual inputs into action-based representations evolved. Such vision-to-action processes are rapid and appear to take place automatically, in the sense that the actions evoked by viewed objects are encoded even when a person has no intention to act toward the object. Two implications of such visuomotor processes are discussed. First, rapidly encoded action can influence visual attention such that the actions evoked by an object can guide search and ameliorate deficits of attention. Second, objects can evoke actions in parallel and interfere with goal-directed behavior, and inhibitory feedback processes that act on competing action-based representations have evolved to solve this selection-for-action problem.

It is apparent that vision and action systems evolved together to enable successful interactions with the environment (e.g., Gibson, 1979). The ability to extract information to guide goal-directed behavior, such as pursuit of prey or avoidance of predators, is fundamental to an organism's survival. Hence, massive evolutionary pressure has ensured that the most exquisitely efficient systems have evolved.

Perception and action (motor control) have often been studied as separate disciplines. Traditional models of perception and action describe a sequence of stages in which processes completed on perceptual inputs subsequently feed in to action systems (e.g., Sternberg, 1969); the opposite interaction of action influencing perceptual processes, is not allowed. However, a number of authors have stressed the close link between these systems, proposing that initially perception evolved purely to serve action, and hence in many circumstances perception and action cannot easily be considered separate and independent systems (e.g., James, 1890; Greenwald, 1970; Gibson, 1979; MacKay, 1987). The intimate relationship between perception and action is being carefully reconsidered. For example, the theory of event coding proposed by Hommel and colleagues (2001) offers a framework within which perceptual processes and action plans are coded in a common representational medium. Hence, notions that selective attention is embedded within and can only serve perceptual processes are also being questioned. There is increasing evidence that attention can interact with action-based representations.

Most early work studying links between attention and action has examined saccades. For example, the premotor theory (e.g., Rizzolatti et al., 1987) is based on two complementary ideas. The first is the notion that preparation of eye movements automatically involves shifts of attention. For example, Moore and Fallah (2001) required monkeys to detect subtle changes of a target stimulus presented among distracters. They also identified motor fields of neurons in frontal eye fields (FEFs). On some trials the target was presented in the motor field, and the cell was stimulated at levels below that evoking a saccade. Discrimination of the target was facilitated in this situation, demonstrating the influence of motor systems on the allocation of spatial attention. The second idea concerns the alternative relationship between attention and saccades. That is, orienting attention to a location automatically activates motor responses such as saccades to the location (even though no overt saccades need be produced). For example, Kustov and Robinson (1996) showed that the trajectory of saccades evoked by stimulation of cells in the superior colliculus was influenced by the spatial location of the monkey's covert attention. A substantial amount of evidence now supports a link between attention and saccades (e.g., Shepherd, Findlay, and Hockey, 1986; Kowler et al., 1995; Deubel and Schneider, 1996; but see Klein and Pontefract, 1984, for an alternative account). Evidence in support of the mandatory coupling of attention and eye movements is reviewed elsewhere (e.g., Hoffman, 1998; Craighero et al., 1999). This chapter concentrates on the link between prehension (reaching and grasping) and attention, as this is a less studied topic.

Attention and prehension

Arbib (1991), Jeannerod (1988), and others have argued that there are two components to prehension: reach, in which the hand is moved from one location to another location containing an object, and grasp, in which the fingers are formed into the appropriate shape prior to object contact. Thus, there appear to be body-centered frames guiding reaching through medial intraparietal cortex (Caminiti, Ferraina, and Johnson, 1996) to dorsal premotor cortex (Lacquaniti et al., 1995), and a second system based on object shape that

STEVEN P. TIPPER   Centre for Cognitive Neuroscience, School of Psychology, University of Wales, Bangor, Gwynedd, U.K.

encodes grasping information through anterior intraparietal cortex (Sakata et al., 1995) to ventral premotor cortex (F4/F5).

Primate visuomotor systems are capable of fluently translating two-dimensional (2D) visual information projected onto the retina into body-centered representations necessary for action. Such processes can be so rapid and automatic that subjects need not be consciously aware of these processes. Indeed, there is abundant evidence that visual processes can flow automatically into actions, such that the latter can be evoked with little or no conscious intention to act (e.g., Bridgeman et al., 1979; Reason, 1979; Norman, 1981; Lhermitte, 1983; Coles et al., 1985; Weiskrantz, 1986; Goldberg and Segraves, 1987; Miller and Hackley, 1992).

Following are three examples of automatic links between vision and actions involving the hands. The first example is what is known as the Simon effect (Simon, 1969). In this task subjects might be asked to report the color of a stimulus with a key press; for example, they are asked to press the right key with the right hand if the color is red and to press the left key with the left hand if the color is green. Importantly, the spatial location of the stimulus on the computer screen is totally irrelevant to the color identification task. Nevertheless, a clear compatibility effect is observed. When subjects are asked to report the red color with the right key press, reaction times (RTs) are faster when the stimulus is on the right side of the screen than when it is on the left. An intuitively obvious explanation for this result is that the right-sided stimulus is closer to the responding hand, and this reveals an automatic link between a stimulus and goal-directed reaching actions.

Such Simon-like effects have been widely investigated and are not restricted to the spatial visuomotor relationships that would guide reaching. Stürmer, Aschersleben, and Prinz (2000) demonstrated hand posture or grasp compatibility effects. Subjects were required to report the color of a hand stimulus with a grasp or spread finger response. Irrelevant to this color response was the shape of the hand on the screen, which could also be in a grasp or finger-spread form. Responses were faster when response and visual image of the hand shape were compatible. This automatic encoding of grasp information has been demonstrated in quite different procedures, such as in the studies of Tucker and Ellis (1998).

As this second example of the automatic encoding of vision into action, Tucker and Ellis (1998) required subjects to report, with right- and left-hand key presses, whether an object was in its normal orientation or inverted. They demonstrated that, even though irrelevant to the task demands, the grasp afforded by the object facilitated response if the hand producing the key press was compatible. For example, if a right key press was required, an object such as a frying pan with the handle oriented toward the right hand was classified faster than if the handle was oriented toward the left hand (see also Tucker and Ellis, 2001).

The third example of automatic visuomotor processing demonstrates important interactions between the ventral and the dorsal visual streams (e.g., Ungerleider and Mishkin, 1982). The ventral stream is specialized for consciously recognizing objects in the visual scene, whereas the dorsal route specializes in visual guidance for action, such as saccades or reach to grasp, which can be unavailable to conscious awareness (e.g., Goodale and Milner, 1992).

Schmidt (2002) has recently demonstrated that unconscious processing of information in the ventral stream, such as analysis of color, can automatically prime motor responses encoded in the dorsal stream, such as pointing. For example, when subjects are required to reach to a target of a particular color, a color prime briefly presented at the same location facilitates reaching if it is the same color as the target. When the prime and target are inconsistent, reach initially starts in the wrong direction and is corrected online. These path deviations are emergent properties of selection from population codes, as described later in the chapter. The priming effects described by Schmidt are robust even when subjects cannot consciously report the presence of the prime (see also Dehaene et al., 1998, and Leuthold and Kopp, 1998, for neural measures demonstrating that primes directly trigger the motor responses assigned to them).

These three examples show that the spatial relationship between a visual stimulus and responding hand, the grasp evoked by an object, and interactions between different stimulus and response properties such as color and reach trajectory, are automatically computed. Of course, one of the most striking features of the behavior of higher mammals is its selectivity. Selection for action (e.g., Allport, 1987; Neumann, 1987) ensures that the many actions that are automatically evoked by visual inputs are not necessarily released. We can consider an apparently trivial task, such as picking up a cup from a table holding several other cups (see Tipper, Lortie, and Baylis, 1992). How does the hand consistently reach one particular cup, given that each of the other cups evokes a similar action? Extremely efficient mechanisms to achieve goals such as these have had to evolve. These selection mechanisms have been associated with the subjective phenomenon of attention, in which the mind selects from a multitude of available perceptual inputs one for deeper contemplation and action (James, 1890).

The relationship between action and attention will be briefly discussed in two further sections: first, the effects of action on target identification and visual search processes will be discussed, and then the interference effects produced by distracters, and the mechanisms resolving such interference, will be described.

Action effects on target search and identification processes

A central question has concerned the role of selective attention in object identification. A number of models of attention assumed that spatial attention oriented toward an object was critical for recognition to occur (e.g., Broadbent, 1958; LaBerge and Brown, 1989). Similarly, to detect objects defined in terms of conjunctions of features in cluttered environments, the influential feature integration theory of Treisman and Gelade (1980) also assumed that spatial attention had to be oriented to each object in the scene. However, there is increasing evidence that action processes can directly influence these apparently purely visual attention processes.

It has been demonstrated that planned prehension (reach and grasp) influences visual object recognition (e.g., Müsseler and Hommel, 1997; Deubel, Schneider, and Paprotta, 1998). For instance, the intention to grasp an object influences visual processing of shape. That is, when a grasp is prepared, visual processing of a similar graspable object is facilitated (Craighero et al., 1999). The fact that such a coupling of perception and action took place even when the action did not predict subsequent visual stimuli suggests that these are obligatory processes (but see Bonfiglioni et al., 2002, for contrary data).

Other work has demonstrated that action affordances can influence visual search. That is, the action properties/affordances of a stimulus facilitate how easy it is to find it in cluttered environments. For example, Bekkering and Neggers (2002) presented a target of a particular orientation and color among distracters. Subjects were required to look at and point to, or to look at and grasp, the target. Bekkering and Neggers examined whether the type of action (point or grasp) could affect the early selection processes by recording the initial saccades. Errors to objects containing the wrong perceptual property of color were unaffected by the type of action. However, saccade errors to the action-related properties of orientation were influenced by the type of action. That is, fewer saccades to objects with the wrong orientation were made in the grasp than in the point condition. Thus, action intentions such as grasping can influence early perceptual and spatial attention processes (see also Brown, Moore, and Rosenbaum, 2002).

Similar conclusions concerning the effect of action on visual search have been drawn by Humphreys and Riddoch (2001). They described a patient with damage to the frontotemporoparietal region of the right hemisphere who had difficulty finding a target among distracters based on its name (e.g., "find the cup") or perceptual qualities such as color (e.g., "find the blue object"). However, this patient was able to find the target when it was defined by the action it afforded. For example, when asked to find the object that "you would drink from," he was much more efficient, and indeed, he reported adopting this strategy of thinking about

what to do with a searched-for object in everyday life. Similarly, Riddoch and colleagues (2003) have shown that the action affordances evoked by objects can reduce visual neglect in patients with lesions of the parietal lobe.

The studies of Humphreys and Riddoch (2001) and Bekkering and Neggers (2002) are important because they clearly demonstrate that attentional processes mediating visual search, such as maintaining a target template, can be based on intended actions. These are actions automatically evoked by objects that afford specific actions, such as grasping a handle. Thus, action-based search is not observed when objects are reoriented such that their handles point away from the patient, or when words naming the objects are searched. The standard view has been that attentional mechanisms access visual representations, such as color or shape. Clearly, however, in some circumstances the medium of attention can be based on the actions evoked by objects (see also Handy et al., 2003, for further evidence that implicit recognition of an object's motor affordance biases visual attention).

Distracter interference and selection mechanisms

It is evident that vision can be converted rapidly and without conscious effort into action, and that this conversion of vision to action can take place independently of an individual's intentions. One of the drawbacks to such efficient vision-action systems is that, unrestrained, they would result in chaotic behavior that is unrelated to behavioral goals. Under conditions of disinhibition, such as can occur with damage to the frontal lobes of the brain, the great propensity to respond to stimuli is released (e.g., Lhermitte, 1983). That is, the most dominant perceptual input captures action, and this varies haphazardly over time. Therefore, to exercise free choice and control, it is essential that organisms have the capacity to resist the strongest response of the moment (Diamond, 1990).

The experimental measures described here provide insights into the control of these automatically evoked responses. They throw light both on the medium of attention, which is the set of internal representations with which attention interacts, and on the mechanisms by which selection is achieved. Three kinds of dependent measure will be described: (1) The interference effects caused by the presence of a distracting, to-be-ignored object can be used to infer the kinds of internal representation achieved by the ignored object, and the medium or frame of reference within which selection takes place. (2) Negative priming measures enable us to infer the frame of reference of selection, and in addition reveal which of a distracter's representations are associated with inhibition during selection. (3) The influence of an ignored object on the path of the hand and eye as the subject reaches to a target can be used to infer mechanisms of selection, using ideas based on distributed neural representations for motor processes.

INTERFERENCE EFFECTS   During visuomotor processes, multiple internal representations are formed, reflecting various stages of processing. Furthermore, selective attention mechanisms can access various forms of these internal representations, such as retinotopic, environment-based, or object-centered frames of reference, depending on task demands (e.g., Tipper et al., 1994). Of most relevance here, when the behavioral goal is to reach for an object, the frame of reference in which the objects are represented and on which selective inhibition mechanisms act is hand-centered. This means that the location of an object is specified at the neuronal level in respect to the location of the hand and the movement required to apprehend the object from that location (e.g., Georgopoulos et al., 1984), or in terms of the final posture of the arm (e.g., Graziano, Taylor, and Moore, 2002).

Distracter interference effects have been widely used to infer the level of processing of irrelevant stimuli. For example, Stroop (1935) demonstrated that irrelevant color words interfered with color naming responses, and Eriksen and Eriksen (1974) showed that irrelevant letters interfered with the key press response to identify target letters. By examining such interference effects during a selective reaching task, it is possible to infer the form of internal representation accessed by stimuli and on which attention processes act.

In studies by Tipper and colleagues (e.g., Meegan and Tipper, 1998; Tipper, Lortie, and Baylis, 1992), subjects were required to reach for targets in the presence of distracters. Tipper and colleagues showed that the pattern of distracter interference was determined by the relationship between the distracter and the responding hand. Various control conditions ruled out other frames of reference. For example, as the starting position of the hand was changed so that the relationship between hand and distracter was altered, the pattern of interference effects changed. This was the case even though the visual information projected to the retina and to other body-centered frames, such as the head and shoulder, remained unchanged. Keulen and colleagues (2002; see also Pratt and Abrams, 1994; Lyons et al., 1999; Humphreys and Riddoch, 2000, Experiment 1; Buxbaum and Permaul, 2001) have confirmed the existence of such hand-centered frames in selective reaching tasks, and Chieffi, Allport, and Woodin (1999) have shown hand-centered frames of reference in visuospatial working memory.

Meegan and Tipper (1999) demonstrated further that it was the *relative* ease of response that determined distracter interference, rather than just some spatial relationship between the responding hand and distracter. That is, those distracters that produced more rapid responses than targets

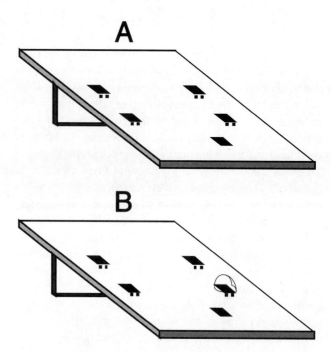

FIGURE 45.1   Subjects were required to reach for and depress keys that were illuminated red while ignoring green distracters. (*A*) The near-right distracter usually produced most interference because it was the easiest stimulus to reach for, hence winning the race for action against the other stimuli. (*B*) The near-right stimulus is occluded by a transparent plastic shield. This stimulus could be seen, but reach had to deviate around the obstacle.

interfered most, even when the spatial relationship between distracter and responding hand was held constant. Figure 45.1 demonstrates how this was revealed. Panel *A* shows the standard task with the various keys requiring response. Typically in this situation the near-right distracter produces most interference because it is near and ipsilateral to the responding right hand. This is an easier reach, and hence this distracter activates response rapidly and competes for the control of action. In a second condition (panel *B*), this near-right stimulus was occluded by a transparent obstacle. Subjects were able to see the stimulus normally but had to reach around the barrier to depress the key. This deviation around the obstacle makes the response much more difficult. Therefore it was predicted that in this latter situation, the distracter would produce significantly less interference, as it loses the race for the control of action. This pattern of interference effects was indeed observed.

In summary, interference effects support the idea that on selective reaching tasks, irrelevant, to-be-ignored stimuli are processed to the level of response. The form of action evoked by the stimulus, such as its spatial relationship with the reaching hand, or the complexity of the action, determine how much it competes with the target for the control of action. The mechanisms that resolve this competition are discussed next.

NEGATIVE PRIMING EFFECTS The mechanisms that enable action to be directed to one object in the presence of other objects that evoke competing responses have been extensively debated. Our account suggests that there are dual mechanisms of attention (e.g., Houghton and Tipper, 1994). That is, as well as excitatory feedback processes directed toward the target, there are also inhibitory feedback processes directed toward the distracter. Priming procedures have been developed as one means by which the inhibitory processes can be observed (e.g., Neill, 1977; Tipper, 1985). The logic of the procedure is as follows: If the internal representation of a distracter is associated with inhibition during selection of the target, then processing of subsequent stimuli that require the same inhibited representations will be impaired. For example, if a picture of a dog is ignored while the participant attends to a picture of a table, the representations activated by the picture of the dog are inhibited. Thus, processing of the picture of the dog shortly afterward will be impaired if the prior inhibitory processing is retrieved. This latter inhibitory priming effect has been termed negative priming (Tipper, 1985; see Tipper, 2001, and Tipper, Meegan, and Howard, 2002, for discussions concerning alternative accounts of negative priming effects such as perceptual mismatch [Park and Kanwisher, 1994] and response rebinding [Hommel et al., 2001]).

Houghton and Tipper (1994; Houghton et al., 1996) have argued that this inhibition mechanism is reactive, responding to the activation level of the distracter relative to the target. In the present reaching tasks, distracters close to the hand have greater levels of activation than those far from the hand, which is the reason for their greater interference with responses to the target. Negative priming reflects this pattern of salience. That is, those distracters closer to the hand are associated with greater inhibition. Furthermore, Tipper, Meegan, and Howard (2002) demonstrated that when distracters were occluded (see figure 45.1B), such that action was made more difficult, less inhibition was associated with such distracters.

There have been a couple of recent theoretical developments concerning this inhibitory selection mechanism. First, Houghton and Tipper (1999) proposed two aspects to inhibitory control. One was a form of lateral inhibition in a winner-take-all model. If the target stimulus was more salient than the distracter, then lateral inhibition between these stimuli would solve the selection problem, as the distracter would be suppressed. However, in situations where distracters were more salient (e.g., closer to the responding hand), the lateral inhibition mechanism was not sufficient for selection. In this latter situation the reactive feedback inhibition mechanism was activated. The level of inhibition was determined by the level of distracter activation via a negative feedback loop.

Recently Aron, Sahakian, and Robbins (2003) studied patients with either early Huntington's disease or prefrontal lobe damage. These patients participated in selective reaching tasks in which targets had to be selected from distracters. From the pattern of errors obtained, they concluded that the lateral inhibition mechanism was affected in Huntington's disease, and hence may be mediated by the basal ganglia. On the other hand, the reactive inhibition mechanism required when distracters are more salient was affected by lateral frontal damage. Furthermore, it is possible that this latter reactive inhibition mechanism is more specifically mediated by right frontal cortex (e.g., Stuss et al., 1999).

The second development concerns the form of inhibition associated with distracters during selective reaching tasks. In the work discussed so far, the reach component of prehension has been studied where subjects were simply required to depress a key. This has shown that the ease of reach to a distracter influences how much it interferes with ongoing behavior and how much it is inhibited. Other work has suggested that the grasp evoked by a distracter is also encoded and can interfere with response to a target (e.g., Kriticos et al., 2000; Pavese and Buxbaum, 2002; Weir et al., 2003), and furthermore that the competing grasp response is inhibited during selection (Humphreys and Riddoch, 2000; Ellis, Symes, and Tucker, 2004).

SELECTION FROM POPULATION CODES Most studies of attention have presented 2D images on computer screens and required indirect actions such as key-press responses on a keyboard in a location separate from that of the selected visual object. One of the central motivations behind the studies of selective reaching discussed in the previous section has been the greater ecological validity of the tasks. Unlike typical key-press tasks, reaching behavior is directed toward an object of interest, and hence it is played out through space as well as time. Consideration of the physiology mediating such reaching behavior enabled various predictions to be made concerning the path of the reach.

As noted by Kristan and Shaw (1997), evidence from neurophysiological recordings indicates that population codes are used widely throughout the brain. More specifically, directional vector coding for reaching responses has been observed in the cerebellum (Fortier, Kalaska, and Smith, 1989), area 2 and 5 of the parietal cortex (Kalaska, Caminiti, and Georgopoulos, 1983), dorsal premotor cortex (Caminiti et al., 1991), and primary motor cortex (Georgopoulos et al., 1984). In these areas a particular reach is represented by the activity of a population of cells. Each individual neuron's level of activity is broadly tuned to various reach directions, which are centred on its particular preferred direction of reach, in which highest activity is evoked. Accordingly, a given cell will contribute, to a greater or lesser extent, to reaching movements in various directions. The direction of

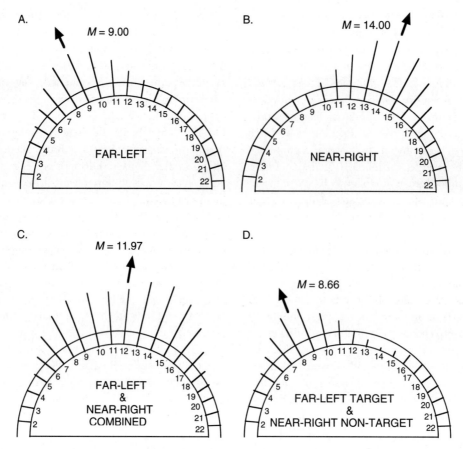

FIGURE 45.2 (A) The population code for a reach toward the target stimulus that is presented to the left of the reaching hand. (B) The population activated by the irrelevant, to-be-ignored distracter. This distracter is closer to the hand than the target, and hence the overall level of activity in population B is greater than that of the target population (A). (C) The actual neural activation state when both a target and distracter are encoded in parallel. (D) Neural activity after reactive inhibition mechanisms have acted on the distracter population in B. Note that the population vector in D is 8.66, slightly to the left of the population vector when target A is presented alone (M = 9.00). Thus the population vector in D would result in a reach veering away from the distracter.

the reach is determined by the sum of the single-cell contributions to the population vector.

There are two further features of population codes that are of importance here. First, a particular neuron can be activated in two populations coding for two similar stimuli, such as line orientations in visual cortex or reaching responses in motor cortex. Second, if two similar stimuli are encoded in parallel, then two population codes will be activated, and because particular cells can be activated by both stimuli, there can be overlap between the two neural populations.

As made clear so far, a number of actions can be simultaneously represented. For example, Cisek and Kalaska (2002) have shown that two populations of cells in rostral areas of dorsal premotor cortex are active simultaneously when two potential targets are viewed, and subsequent mechanisms (possibly inhibitory) select one population for response (see also Goldberg and Segraves, 1987; Kim and Shadlen, 1999; and Schall and Thompson, 1999, for some examples of parallel response activation in reach and

saccade systems). Therefore, Tipper, Howard, and Jackson (1997) wondered how such competing neural representations might influence reaches during selection for action. A schematic example is shown in figure 45.2. In panel A, the direction of reach to a target that is far and to the left of the reaching hand is represented by the population vector (M = 9 in this example). In panel B, the reach to a competing distracter, which is to the right and slightly closer to the hand and hence more potent, is represented (M = 14). In panel C, the overall neural activity when these two objects evoke action in parallel is shown. Two things are of note: first, a number of cells are common to both reaches (cells 10–13), and second, without some selection mechanism, reach will travel between the two objects (M = 11.97), as can saccades in center-of-gravity effects (Findlay, 1982).

The properties of such overlapping neural populations (panel C) have recently been investigated by Treue, Hol, and Rauber (2000) in MT motion cells. They have demonstrated that the underlying populations (panels A and B) that produce the complex population codes of panel C can be

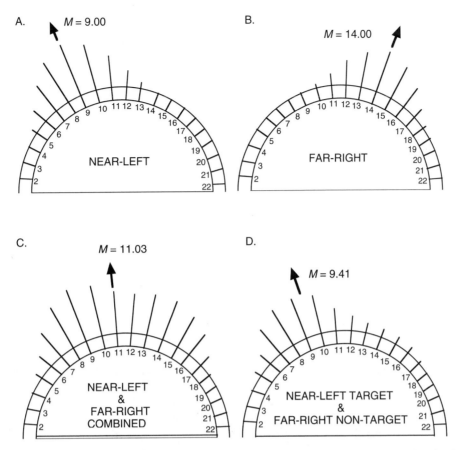

FIGURE 45.3 Similar to figure 45.2, except that the target (A) is closer to the responding hand than the distracter (B). Therefore, first, neural activity in A is greater than in B; second, selection is via lateral inhibition. Thus the population code associated with the distracter in B is not suppressed below background resting levels, resulting in trajectories toward the target that veer slightly toward the distracter (D).

recovered. We can apply their ideas to our model. Thus, the population Gaussian when reaching to a single target might have a width of approximately 8 units in our example (see figure 45.2A). The range of stimulus sensitivity of the individual neurons determines this width. However, the range of neural activity is far higher in panel C (approximately 13 units), and hence this must represent more than one reach. By subtracting Gaussians of approximately 8 units wide, the two underlying population codes activated by two objects can be recovered from the complex neural activity in the brain as represented by panel C (see Treue, Hol, and Rauber, 2000, for details).

A second way for the underlying population codes to be retrieved from the overall activity depicted in panel C might be via neural synchrony (e.g., Singer and Gray, 1995). Thus cells within a particular population (e.g., panel A) fire in a synchrony that is different from the synchrony of firing in the population depicted in panel B. The neurons activated in both populations (10–13) can be affected in one of two ways. First, if activity in population B is greater because this stimulus is closer to the hand, as in figure 45.2, then they will be captured by this population and will fire in synchrony

with the other cells of population B. Thus, when population B activity is actively suppressed, these cells will also be depressed, as shown in panel D. In contrast, if population A is more potent because it is closer to the responding hand, these ambiguous cells (10–13) will be captured within the synchronous firing rate of population A. Furthermore, because population B is not suppressed below resting levels in this situation (see figure 45.3), these cells still receive inputs from population B, and hence are slightly more active than usual, resulting in a population code for reach A skewed slightly toward reach B, as shown in panel D of figure 45.3.

Selection is achieved by inhibition of the population code activated by the distracter stimulus, shown in panel B (see Howard and Tipper, 1997; Tipper, Howard, and Jackson, 1997, for details). The level of inhibition is determined by the initial activation state of the distracter via a reactive feedback system (e.g., Houghton and Tipper, 1994). Thus, distracters that are more potent than the target (figure 45.2) receive greater levels of reactive self-inhibition feeding back onto themselves. The effect of such selection processes is to alter the path of the hand as it reaches to the target. This is because the inhibition of cells common to both reaches changes the overall population profile of the cells encoding the target reach. This is shown in figure 45.2*D*, in which severe levels of inhibition acting on the distracter population of panel *B* have resulted in a population vector that, although successfully approaching the target, veers slightly away from the direction of the distracter. In contrast, distracters that are less potent than the target (farther from the hand) can be selected against via lateral inhibition (see figure 45.3). Although suppressed, the population code of the distracter remains a little above background activity levels, resulting in slight skewing of population code A toward the distracter. Of course, in this latter situation the population vector veers slightly toward the distracter (see also Welsh, Elliott, and Weeks, 1999; Keulen et al., 2002; and Sailor et al., 2002, for distracter repulsion and attraction effects).

One of the advantages of linking behavior to the mediating physiology is that the emerging models have generality. Thus we have been able to apply the same selection mechanisms to the saccade system. Georgopolous (1990) argued that the specification of movement direction involves similar codes in both arm and eye movement systems. That is, occulomotor and manual behavior is distributed within neural assemblies in which direction of movement is uniquely specified only at the population level. Interestingly, as in arm reaches, saccade path is also affected by stimuli competing for action. More specifically, saccades also veer away from irrelevant stimuli (e.g., Sheliga, Riggio, and Rizzolatti, 1995; Tipper, Howard, and Houghton, 2000; Doyle and Walker, 2001; Tipper, Howard, and Paul, 2001), as a model describing selection from overlapping population codes might predict.

It is important to note that overlapping population codes are the core ideas that underlie these studies of reach and saccade path. We have based our ideas on the work of Georgopoulos and colleagues. However, these ideas could apply to alternative accounts of reaching behavior such as that proposed by Graziano, Taylor, and Moore (2002). In that account, neurons encode final arm posture. This posture is reached from a variety of different starting positions; hence the cells are not coding a particular reach direction. However, it is assumed that such final posture representations are encoded within a population of neural activity and that these postures are topographically mapped. Thus, two reasonably close targets that automatically activate final posture may well depend on overlapping neural populations. Hence, the movement of the arm through space to achieve the final posture will be influenced by the level of inhibition acting on the overlapping competing population codes. Therefore, the central idea is of population coding, and the possibility that in some circumstances two stimuli encoded in parallel may have overlapping populations. Selection for action from these representations remains a central problem, despite the specifics of the representation.

There has been debate concerning such effects, however, and alternative accounts have been proposed. For example, Tresilian (1999) argued that distracter interference effects in selective reaching tasks are caused by obstacle avoidance strategies. Clearly, in some circumstances this is possible, but in many studies (e.g., Tipper, Howard, and Jackson, 1997) an effort was made to avoid such confounds. As two other situations where obstacle avoidance cannot explain distracter interference effects, we can consider the following: first, in the experiments depicted in figure 45.1, obstacle avoidance accounts have to predict greater interference when distracters are larger obstacles (figure 45.1*B*); the opposite pattern was observed where less interference was produced by such distracters. Second, throughout evolution the saccade system has never had to avoid obstacles. Nevertheless, saccade deviations away from distracters, similar to reach deviations, have been demonstrated as predicted by the population coding account.

Development of attention and action

Only one research area will be commented on here. The A-not-B task developed by Piaget requires infants to select a target from a distracter. In this task the infant is initially trained to reach to container A to retrieve a hidden object. After a number of trials, the object is hidden in full view of the infant, in container B. After a short delay the display is moved closer to the infant, and she is allowed to reach. Infants between 7 and 12 months of age often make an error and reach for container A. Therefore, the irrelevant distracter A can win the competition for the control of action.

Thelen and colleagues (2001) have recently reviewed this area and proposed a field theory of perseverative reaching. In this account, the infant's performance reflects a number of the properties of the visuomotor systems described earlier in this chapter. For example, the activation state of the target B is influenced by attention: a hungry infant is more likely to attend to and successfully retrieve the object from container B if it is a cookie. Furthermore, the frame of reference appears to be action-based. Thus, after viewing the hiding of the object, if the infant is placed in a different location (e.g., lifted from her mother's lap and placed closer to the floor), errors are less likely. This suggests that the competing action evoked by container A is a specific reaching response. This latter action-centered representation is also reflected in the neural architecture described by Thelen and colleagues (2001). For instance, reaches are encoded in neural populations, and the distributed representations of the target (B) and distracter (A) can overlap to varying degrees, as discussed earlier.

The anatomical sites that might be developing, and the specific mechanisms mediating selective behavior in infants, are still debated. For example, Diamond (1990) has proposed that it is maturation of dorsolateral prefrontal cortex that enables the maintenance of target information and inhibition of prepotent distractors, whereas Thelen and colleagues question these ideas, proposing instead multiple parallel and integrated mechanisms, providing many avenues of change. Further study of the development of the mechanisms enabling selective visuomotor processing with this and other new methodologies should provide important new insights into these processes.

Comment

There appears to be a close relationship between attention and action. In particular, the intimate relationship between attention and saccades has been extensively studied. However, the discussion in this chapter has concentrated on the less well-established link between prehension (reach and grasp) and attention. Visual inputs can be converted fluently and automatically into reaching/grasping actions, and hence attention mechanisms have evolved to select from among competing motor responses. Furthermore, the intentions of a subject to reach toward or grasp an object can influence the processes required to identify a target, and attentional search processes necessary to detect targets in cluttered environments can also be determined by action intentions.

Finally, there are still many things we do not understand about the relationship between action and attention. There is little doubt that people cannot prevent activation of actions, even when those actions compete with and hence impair current task performance. However, automatically evoked actions do not necessarily require a strong late selection model in which actions are evoked prior to and independently of attention (e.g., Deutsch and Deutsch, 1963). In the selective reaching studies described in this chapter, for example, limited visual arrays were presented. Therefore a limited range of objects could simultaneously activate competing actions when target location is not known in advance because attention is diffusely spread across the array (e.g,. Castiello, 1999). Thus, attention toward objects may be necessary for action to be encoded, but this encoding is automatic, in the sense that the subject has no intention to act on the viewed object. On the other hand, intended actions seem to determine the processes of visual attention, such as search for a target. Further research investigating the dynamic interplay between attention and action is necessary.

REFERENCES

ALLPORT, D. A., 1987. Selection for action: Some behavioural and neurophysiological considerations of attention and action. In *Perspectives on Perception and Action*, H. Heuer and F. Sanders, eds. Hillsdale, N.J.: Erlbaum.

ARBIB, M. A., 1991. Interaction of multiple representations of space in the brain. In *Brain and Space*, J. Paillard, ed. Oxford, England: Oxford University Press.

ARON, A. R., B. J. SAHAKIAN, and T. W. ROBBINS, 2003. Distractability during selection-for-action: Differential deficits in Huntington's disease and following frontal lobe damage. *Neuropsychologia* 41:1137–1147.

BEKKERING, H., and S. F. W. NEGGERS, 2002. Visual search is modulated by action intentions. *Psychol. Sci.* 13:370–374.

BONFIGLIOLI, C., J. DUNCAN, C. RORDEN, and S. KENNET, 2002. Action and perception: Evidence against converging selection processes. *Vis. Cogn.* 9:458–476.

BRIDGEMAN, B., S. LEWIS, G. HEIT, and M. NAGLE, 1979. Relation between cognitive and motor-oriented systems of visual position perception. *J. Exp. Psychol. Hum. Percept. Perform.* 5:692–700.

BROADBENT, D. E., 1958. *Perception and Communication*. New York: Pergamon Press.

BROWN, L. E., C. M. MOORE, and D. A. ROSENBAUM, 2002. Feature-specific perceptual processing dissociates action from recognition. *J. Exp. Psychol. Hum. Percept. Perform.* 28:1330–1344.

BUXBAUM, L. J., and P. PERMAUL, 2001. Hand-centered attentional and motor asymmetries in unilateral neglect. *Neuropsychologia* 39:653–664.

CAMINITI, R., S. FERRAINA, and P. B. JOHNSON, 1996. The sources of visual information in the primate frontal lobe: A novel role for the superior parietal lobule. *Cereb. Cortex* 6:319–328.

CAMINITI, R., P. B. JOHNSON, C. GALLI, S. FERRAINA, and Y. BURNOD, 1991. Making arm movements within different parts of space: The premotor and motor cortical representation of a coordinated system for reaching to visual targets. *J. Neurosci.* 11:1182–1197.

CASTIELLO, U., 1999. Mechanism of selection for the control of hand action. *Trends Cogn. Sci.* 3:264–271.

CHIEFFI, S., D. A. ALLPORT, and M. WOODIN, 1999. Hand-centred coding of target location in visuo-spatial working memory. *Neuropsychologia* 37:495–502.

CISEK, P., and J. F. KALASKA, 2002. Simultaneous encoding of multiple reach direction in dorsal premotor cortex. *J. Neurophysiol.* 87:1149–1154.

COLES, M. G., G. GRATTON, T. R. BASHORE, C. W. ERIKSEN, and E. DONCHIN, 1985. A psychophysical investigation of the continuous flow model of human information processing. *J. Exp. Psychol. Hum. Percept. Perform.* 11:529–553.

CRAIGHERO, L., L. FADIGA, G. RIZZOLATTI, and C. UMILTÀ, 1999. Action for perception: A motor-visual attentional effect. *J. Exp. Psychol. Hum. Percept. Perform.* 25:1673–1692.

DEHAENE, S., L. NACCACHE, H. G. LE CLEC, E. KOECHLIN, M. MUELLER, G. DEHAENE-LAMBERTZ, P. F. VAN DE MOORTELE, and D. LE BIHAN, 1998. Imagining unconscious semantic priming. *Nature* 385:597–600.

DEUBEL, H., and W. X. SCHNEIDER, 1996. Saccade target selection and object recognition: Evidence for a common attentional mechanism. *Vision Res.* 36:1827–1837.

DEUBEL, H., W. X. SCHNEIDER, and I. PAPROTTA, 1998. Selective dorsal and ventral processing: Evidence for a common attentional mechanism in reaching and perception. *Vis. Cogn.* 5:81–107.

DEUTSCH, J. A., and D. DEUTSCH, 1963. Attention: Some theoretical considerations. *Psych. Rev.* 70:80–90.

DIAMOND, A., 1990. Developmental time course in human infants and infant monkeys, and the neural bases of inhibitory control in reaching. *Ann. N.Y. Acad. Sci.* 608:637–676.

DOYLE, M., and R. WALKER, 2001. Voluntary and reflexive saccades curve away from irrelevant distractors. *Exp. Brain Res.* 139:147–151.

ELLIS, R., M. TUCKER, and E. SYMES, 2004. *Micro-affordance in dual object scenes: Does ignoring an object entail inhibition of the actions associated with it?* Unpublished manuscript.

ERIKSEN, B. A., and C. W. ERIKSEN, 1974. Effects of noise letters upon the identification of a target letter in a non-search task. *Percept. Psychophys.* 16:143–149.

FINDLAY, J. M., 1982. Global visual processing for saccadic eye movements. *Vision Res.* 22:1033–1045.

FORTIER, P. A., J. F. KALASKA, and A. M. SMITH, 1989. Cerebellar neural activity related to whole-arm reaching movements in the monkey. *J. Neurophysiol.* 62:198–211.

GEORGOPOULOS, A. P., 1990. Neural coding of the direction of reaching and a comparison with saccadic eye movements. *Cold Spring Harbor Symp. Quant. Biol.* 55:849–859.

GEORGOPOULOS, A. P., J. F. KALASKA, M. D. CRUTCHER, R. CAMINITI, and J. T. MASSEY, 1984. The representation of movement direction in the motor cortex: Single cell and population studies. In *Dynamic Aspects of Neocortical Function*, G. M. Edelman, ed. New York: John Wiley, pp. 501–515.

GIBSON, J. J., 1979. *The Ecological Approach to Visual Perception*. Boston: Houghton-Mifflin.

GOLDBERG, M. E., and M. A. SEGRAVES, 1987. Visuospatial and motor attention in the monkey. *Neuropsychologia* 25:107–118.

GOODALE, M., and D. MILNER, 1992. Separate visual pathways for perception and action. *Trends Neurosci.* 15:20–25.

GRAZIANO, M. S. A., C. S. R. TAYLOR, and T. MOORE, 2002. Complex movements evoked by microstimulation of precentral cortex. *Neuron* 34:841–851.

GREENWALD, A., 1970. Sensory feedback mechanisms in performance control: With special reference to the ideomotor mechanism. *Psychol. Rev.* 77:73–99.

HANDY, T. C., S. T. GRAFTON, N. M. SHROFF, S. KETAY, and M. S. GAZZANIGA, 2003. Graspable objects grab attention when the potential for action is recognized. *Nat. Neurosci.* 6:421–427.

HOFFMAN, J. E., 1998. Visual attention and eye movements. In *Attention*, H. Pashler, ed. Sussex, U.K.: Psychology Press, pp. 119–154.

HOMMEL, B., J. MÜSSELER, G. ASCHERSLEBEN, and W. PRINZ, 2001. The theory of event coding: A framework for perception and planning. *Behav. Brain Sci.* 24:849–892.

HOMMEL, B., and W. X. SCHNEIDER, 2002. Visual attention and manual response selection: Distinct mechanisms operate on the same code. *Vis. Cogn.* 9:392–420.

HOUGHTON, G., and S. P. TIPPER, 1994. A model of inhibitory mechanisms in selective attention. In *Inhibitory Mechanisms of Attention, Memory and Language*, D. Dagenback and T. Carr, eds. Boca Raton, Fla.: Academic Press, pp. 53–112.

HOUGHTON, G., and S. P. TIPPER, 1999. Attention and the control of action: An investigation of the effects of selection on population coding of hand and eye movement. In *Connectionist Models in Cognitive Neuroscience*, D. Heinke, G. W. Humphreys, and A. Olson, eds. London: Springer-Verlag, pp. 283–298.

HOUGHTON, G, S. P. TIPPER, B. WEAVER, and D. I. SHORE, 1996. Inhibition and interference in selective attention: Some tests of a neural network model. *Vis. Cogn.* 3:119–164.

HOWARD, L., and S. P. TIPPER, 1997. Hand deviations away from visual cues: Indirect evidence for inhibition. *Exp. Brain Res.* 113:144–152.

HUMPHREYS, G. W., and M. J. RIDDOCH, 2000. One more cup of coffee for the road: Object-action assemblies, response blocking and response capture after frontal lobe damage. *Exp. Brain Res.* 133:81–93.

HUMPHREYS, G. W., and M. J. RIDDOCH, 2001. Detection by action: Neuropsychological evidence for action-defined templates in search. *Nat. Neurosci.* 4:84–88.

JAMES, W., 1890. *The Principles of Psychology*. New York: Holt.

JEANNEROD, M., 1988. *The Neural and Behavioural Organisation of Goal-Directed Movements*. Oxford, England: Clarendon Press.

KALASKA, J. F., 1988. The representation of arm movements in postcentral and parietal cortex. *Can. J. Physiol. Pharmacol.* 66:455–463.

KALASKA, J. F., R. CAMINITI, and A. P. GEORGOPOULOS, 1983. Cortical mechanisms related to the direction of two-dimensional arm movements: Relations in parietal area 5 and comparison with motor cortex. *Exp. Brain Res.* 51:247–260.

KEULEN, R. F., J. J. ADAM, M. H., FISCHER, H. KUIPERS, and J. JOLLES, 2002. Selective reaching: Evidence for multiple frames of reference. *J. Exp. Psychol. Hum. Percept. Perform.* 28:515–526.

KIM, J. N., and M. N. SHADLEN, 1999. Neural correlates of a decision in the dorsolateral prefrontal cortex of the macaque. *Nat. Neurosci.* 2:176–185.

KLEIN, R. M., and A. PONTEFRACT, 1994. Does occulomotor readiness mediate cognitive control of visual attention? Revisited! In *Attention and Performance XV*, C. Umiltà and M. Moscovitch, eds. Cambridge, Mass.: MIT Press, pp. 333–550.

KOWLER, E., E. ANDERSON, B. DOSHER, and E. BLASER, 1995. The role of attention in the programming of saccades. *Vision Res.* 35:1897–1916.

KRISTAN, W. B., and B. K. SHAW, 1997. Population coding and behavioural choice. *Curr. Opin. Neurobiol.* 7:826–831.

KRITICOS, A., K. M. B. BENNETT, J. DUNAI, and U. CASTIELLO, 2000. Interference from distractors in reach-to-grasp movements. *Q. J. Exp. Psychol.* 53A:131–151.

KUSTOV, A. A., and D. L. ROBINSON, 1996. Shared neural control of attentional shifts and eye movements. *Nature* 384:74–77.

LABERGE, D., and V. BROWN, 1989. Theory of attentional operations in shape identification. *Psychol. Rev.* 96:101–124.

LACQUANITI, F., E. GUIGON, L. BIANCHI, S. FERRAINA, and R. CAMINITI, 1995. Representing spatial information for limb movements: role of area 5 in the monkey. *Cereb. Cortex* 5:391–409.

LEUTHOLD, H., and B. KOPP, 1998. Mechanisms of priming by masked stimuli: Inferences from event-related brain potentials. *Psychol. Sci.* 9:263–269.

LHERMITTE, F., 1983. "Utilization behaviour" and its relation to lesions of the frontal lobes. *Brain* 106:237–255.

LYONS, J., D. ELLIOTT, K. L. RICKER, D. J. WEEKS, and R. CHUA, 1999. Action-centred attention in virtual environments. *Can. J. Exp. Psychol.* 53:176–187.

MACKAY, D., 1987. *The Organization of Perception and Action*. New York: Springer.

MEEGAN, D., and S. P. TIPPER, 1998. Reaching in to cluttered visual environments: Spatial and temporal influences of distracting objects. *Q. J. Exp. Psychol.* 51A:225–249.

MEEGAN, D., and S. P. TIPPER, 1999. Visual search and target directed action. *J. Exp. Psychol. Hum. Percept. Perform.* 25:1347–1362.

MILLER, J., and S. A. HACKLEY, 1992. Electrophysiological evidence for temporal overlap among contingent mental processes. *J. Exp. Psychol. Gen.* 121:195–209.

MOORE, T., and M. FALLAH, 2001. Control of eye movements and spatial attention. *Proc. Nat. Acad. Sci. U.S.A.* 98:1273–1276.

MUSSELER, J., and B. HOMMEL, 1997. Blindness to response-compatible stimuli. *J. Exp. Psychol. Hum. Percept. Perform.* 23:861–872.

NEIL, W. T. 1977. Inhibitory and facilitatory processes in selective attention. *J. Exp. Psychol. Hum. Percept. Perform.* 3:444–450.

NEUMANN, O., 1987. Beyond capacity: A functional view of attention. In *Perspectives on Perception and Action*, H. Heuer and F. Sanders, eds. Hillsdale, N.J.: Erlbaum.

NORMAN, D. A., 1981. Categorization of action slips. *Psychol. Rev.* 88:1–15.

PARK, J., and N. KANWISHER, 1994. Negative priming for spatial locations: Identity mismatching, not distractor inhibition. *J. Exp. Psychol. Hum. Percept. Perform.* 20:613–623.

PAVESE, A., and L. J. BUXBAUM, 2002. Action matters: The role of action plans and object affordances in selection for action. *Vis. Cogn.* 9:559–590.

PIAGET, J., 1954. *The Origins of Intelligence in Children.* New York: International Universities Press.

PRATT, J., and R. A. ABRAMS, 1994. Action-centred inhibition: Effects of distractors on movement planning and execution. *Hum. Movement Sci.* 13:245–254.

REASON, J. T., 1979. Actions not as planned. In *Aspects of Consciousness*, vol. 1, G. Underwood and R. Stevens, eds. London: Academic Press.

RIDDOCH, M. J., G. W. HUMPHREYS, S. EDWARDS, T. BAKER, and K. WILLSON, 2003. Seeing the action: Neuropsychological evidence for action-based effects on object selection. *Nat. Neurosci.* 6:82–89.

RIZZOLATTI, G., L. RIGGIO, I. DASCOLA, and C. UMILTA, 1987. Reorienting attention across the horizontal and vertical meridians: Evidence in favour of a premotor theory of attention. *Neuropsychologia* 25:31–40.

SAILOR, U., T. EGGERT, J. DITTERICH, and A. STRAUBE, 2002. Global effect of a nearby distractor on targeting eye and hand movements. *J. Exp. Psychol. Hum. Percept. Perform.* 28:1432–1446.

SAKATA, H., M. TAIRA, A. MURATA, and S. MILNE, 1995. Neural mechanisms of visual guidance of hand action in the parietal cortex of the monkey. *Cereb. Cortex* 5:429–438.

SCHALL, J. D., and K. G. THOMPSON, 1999. Neural selection and control of visually guided eye movements. *Annu. Rev. Neurosci.* 22:241–259.

SCHMIDT, T., 2002. The finger in flight: Real-time motor control by visually masked color stimuli. *Psychol. Sci.* 13:112–118.

SHELIGA, B. M., L. RIGGIO, and G. RIZZOLATTI, 1995. Spatial attention and eye movements. *Exp. Brain Res.* 105:261–275.

SHEPHERD, M., J. M. FINDLAY, and R. J. HOCKEY, 1986. The relationship between eye movements and spatial attention. *Q. J. Exp. Psychol.* 38A:475–491.

SIMON, J. R., 1969. Reaction towards the source of stimulation. *J. Exp. Psychol.* 81:174–176.

SINGER, W., and C. M. GRAY, 1995. Visual feature integration and the temporal correlation hypothesis. *Ann. Rev. Neurosci.* 18:555–586.

STERNBERG, S., 1969. The discovery of processing stages: Extension of Donder's method. In *Attention and Performance II*, W. G. Koster, ed. Amsterdam: Elsevier/North-Holland.

STROOP, J. R., 1935. Studies of interference in serial verbal reactions. *J. Exp. Psychol.* 18:643–662.

STUSS, D. T., J. P. TOTH, D. FRANCHI, M. P. ALEXANDER, S. P. TIPPER, and F. I. G. CRAIK, 1999. Dissociation of attentional processes in patients with focal frontal and posterior lesions. *Neuropsychologia* 37:1005–1027.

STÜRMER, B., G. ASCHERSLEBEN, and W. PRINZ, 2000. Correspondence effects with manual gestures and postures: A study on imitation. *J. Exp. Psychol. Hum. Percept. Perform.* 26:1746–1759.

THELEN, E., G. SCHONER, C. SCHEIER, and L. B. SMITH, 2001. The dynamics of embodiment: A field theory of infant perseverative reaching. *Behav. Brain Sci.* 24:1–86.

TIPPER, S. P., 1985. The negative priming effect: Inhibitory priming with to be ignored objects. *Q. J. Exp. Psychol.* 37A:571–590.

TIPPER, S. P., 2001. Does negative priming reflect inhibitory mechanisms? A review and integration of conflicting views. *Q. J. Exp. Psychol.* 54A:321–343.

TIPPER, S. P., L. A. HOWARD, and G. HOUGHTON, 1998. Action-based mechanisms of attention. *Philos. Trans. R. Soc. Lond. B* 353:1385–1393.

TIPPER, S. P., L. A. HOWARD, and G. HOUGHTON, 2000. Behavioural consequences of selection from population codes. In *Attention and Performance XVII*, S. Monsell and J. Driver, eds. Cambridge, Mass.: MIT Press, pp. 223–246.

TIPPER, S. P., L. A. HOWARD, and S. R. JACKSON, 1997. Selective reaching to grasp: Evidence for distractor interference effects. *Vis. Cogn.* 4:1–32.

TIPPER, S. P., L. A. HOWARD, and M. PAUL, 2001. Reaching affects saccade trajectories. *Exp. Brain Res.* 136:241–249.

TIPPER, S. P., C. LORTIE, and G. C. BAYLIS, 1992. Selective reaching: Evidence for action-centered attention. *J. Exp. Psychol. Hum. Percept. Perform.* 18:891–905.

TIPPER, S. P., D. MEEGAN, and L. A. HOWARD, 2002. Action-centred negative priming: Evidence for reactive inhibition. *Vis. Cogn.* 9:591–614.

TIPPER, S. P., B. WEAVER, L. JERREAT, and A. BURAK, 1994. Object and environment based inhibition of return. *J. Exp. Psychol. Hum. Percept. Perform.* 20:478–499.

TRESILIAN, J. R., 1999. Selective attention in reaching: When is an object not a distractor? *Trends Cogn. Sci.* 3:407–408.

TREISMAN, A., and G. GELADE, 1980. A feature-integration theory of attention. *Cogn. Psychol.* 12:97–136.

TREUE, S., K. HOL, and H.-J. RAUBER, 2000. Seeing multiple directions of motion-physiology and psychophysics. *Nat. Neurosci.* 3:270–276.

TUCKER, M., and R. ELLIS, 1998. On the relations between seen objects and components of actions. *J. Exp. Psychol. Hum. Percept. Perform.* 24:830–846.

TUCKER, M., and R. ELLIS, 2001. The potentiation of grasp types during visual object categorization. *Vis. Cogn.* 8:830–846.

UNGERLEIDER, L. G., and M. MISHKIN, 1982. Two cortical visual systems. In *Analysis of Visual Behavior*, D. J. Ingle, M. A. Goodale, and R. J. W. Mansfield, eds. Cambridge, Mass.: MIT Press, pp. 549–586.

WEIR, P. L., D. J. WEEKS, T. WELSH, D. ELLIOTT, R. CHUA, E. A. ROY, and J. LYONS, 2003. Influence of terminal action requirements on action-centred distractor effects. *Exp. Brain Res.* 149:207–213.

WEISKRANTZ, L., 1986. *Blindsight: A Case Study and Implications.* Oxford, England: Clarendon Press.

WELSH, T. N., D. ELLIOT, and D. J. WEEKS, 1999. Hand deviations toward distractors: Evidence for response competition. *Exp. Brain Res.* 127:207–212.

46 Vigilant Attention

IAN H. ROBERTSON AND HUGH GARAVAN

ABSTRACT When train drivers pass through warning or stop signals as they do many thousands of times per day throughout the world, this is an example, we argue, of an inefficiency in the functioning of a right hemispheric, frontoparietal attention system for "vigilant attention". Closely linked to Posner's notion of the "alerting" system, vigilant attention is distinct from Posner's other two functionally and anatomically distinct supramodal attentional systems—selection and control respectively. We review evidence for the validity of this three-factor typology of attention and clarify the frequently articulated misconception that "vigilance" and "sustained attention" are defined by time-on-task decrements over extended periods of test performance, as originally proposed by Mackworth. Rather, we show that vigilant attention involves a half-life measured in seconds rather than minutes, and is most sensitively measured in situations in which routine action cycles are underway. We further show evidence of how everyday action error propensities link to specific functional brain activation patterns and how Attention Deficit Disorder can be an excellent model system for malfunctioning of this system. We end by demonstrating the rehabilitation of this system.

A neglected dimension of attention

At 24 minutes past 5 P.M. on August 8, 1996, the 17.04 train from London's Euston Station to Milton Keynes passed through a red signal near Watford Junction and ploughed into an empty goods train, killing just one person, Ruth Holland, associate editor of the *British Medical Journal* and a close colleague of the first author of this chapter.

The driver of the train, Peter Afford, was later cleared of criminal charges for having passed the red signal; the court accepted his defense that trees and bushes had obscured the signal. He also told the court that he could not remember seeing two early warning signals that would have told him to expect a red light at the next signal point.

Signals passed at danger (SPAD) is the most common cause of accidents on railways (Edkins and Pollock, 1997), and imperfectly sustained attention is by far the major factor in these errors. Every day, thousands of signals are passed at danger by train drivers worldwide, but thankfully, only a small number result in tragedy—partly through good fortune and partly through the presence of other backup safety measures. This type of error is classified as a skill-based slip that typically occurs during routine action sequences (Reason, 1992). The job of driving a train is typically routine, entailing stopping at stations and traveling sections of track that the driver has passed many times before. Familiar surroundings and well-practiced sequences of actions minimize the need for effortful attention on the part of the driver.

This chapter focuses on the type of attentional control that is crucially required for error-free performance of this type of task. This type of attention is linked to a number of hitherto ambiguously defined concepts such as vigilance, alertness, sustained attention, and arousal. We will use the term *vigilant attention* to characterize it here. Among the first studies of vigilant attention to be carried out were those by Mackworth and his colleagues at the MRC Applied Psychology Unit in Cambridge, U.K. These studies were particularly inspired by the problems encountered by operators of the recently developed radar, who had to maintain attention to a small, dim, and mostly unchanging screen for rare but crucially important events—enemy sightings or about-to-collide aircraft. Mackworth concluded that it was often difficult to pull human observers off ceiling on this type of vigilance task and that errors, when they did occur, were observed only after relatively long time periods, usually more than 30 minutes (N. H. Mackworth, 1950; J. F. Mackworth, 1968).

The difficulty in finding sensitive measures of vigilant attention, as demonstrated by these contemporary measures, may have been one factor that led to its relative neglect for the next 30 years—in comparison, that is, to the burgeoning research in other major aspects of attention linked to selection, working memory, and switching. A second reason for its demise as a major subject of research may have been the loss of confidence in the unitary nature of its sister process, arousal. The classic studies of Moruzzi and Magoun (1949) suggesting the existence of a single arousal-modulating reticular formation gave way before evidence pointing to the existence of multiple ascending pathways from subcortical nuclei, each linked to different neurotransmitters and different cortical innervation paths (Olszewski and Baxter, 1982).

The resurrection of vigilant attention as an important dimension of attention is largely a result of the work of Michael Posner (Posner and Boies, 1971) and Raja Parasuraman (Parasuraman, 1983), with the onset of human

IAN H. ROBERTSON and HUGH GARAVAN   Department of Psychology and Institute of Neuroscience, Trinity College, Dublin, Ireland.

functional brain imaging providing a major boost to the validity of their typologies of attention (Posner and Peterson, 1990). Posner and colleagues suggested the existence of three main functionally and anatomically distinct types of supramodal attentional control systems, *selection, orientation,* and *alertness.* This was somewhat different from Posner and Boies's earlier typology of selection, capacity, and alertness but close to Parasuraman's typology of selection, control, and vigilance (Parasuraman, 1998). The important aspect of these typographies, however, is the clear distinction between attention as selection/management of goals in working memory, on the one hand, and attention as vigilant attention linked to alertness on the other. It is the latter of these two dimensions that is of interest here.

The restless brain: why doing little is so hard

If vigilance is such a fundamental dimension of attention, why is it relatively difficult to show decrements on standard vigilance tasks in normal human adults? Mackworth's would-be radar operators in a darkened room often performed normally for an hour or longer before they began to show the vigilance decrement that was seen to be the hallmark of this attentional system. Even in people with traumatic brain injury and consequently impaired frontal lobe/attentional deficits, marginal decrements in sustained attention could be observed only when the visual stimuli were heavily perceptually degraded (Parasuraman, Mutter, and Molloy, 1991).

RESPONDING TO INFREQUENT TARGET VERSUS INHIBITING ONGOING BEHAVIOR Why should train drivers frequently miss danger signals but participants in vigilance experiments show such good performance? A possible answer to this question may be that, unlike the radar operators, who must *make* a response to rare targets, train drivers must *inhibit* their ongoing behavior in the context of a rare target, namely, a red or warning signal. When a subject is required to make a response, presentation of a rare target can facilitate performance insofar as (1) the default response on a task such as this is not to respond, thereby providing time to detect the target and make the appropriate response, and (2) the presentation of the rare target can itself serve to orient attention to its presence. Contrast this to the circumstance in which people must inhibit responding to rare stimuli. Here, the ongoing default behavior (responding, or, in the case of the train driver, keep driving forward) is opposite to the desired response (interrupt the default behavior). Furthermore, the ongoing behavior that engages the person in well-practiced behaviors can create the illusion that the person is attentively engaged in the task at hand. However, the automatic quality of the behavior can be deceptive, because it in fact requires little vigilant attention. Consequently, the com-

mission error might be committed before the person can countermand it or, as in the case of the train driver, without the person even noticing that the countermand was required. This distinction between responding and inhibiting also rests on whether the vigilant attention for the task must be generated endogenously or is supported by exogenous task demands, an important issue that will be addressed later.

This distinction can be seen clearly when frontally and attentionally impaired traumatic brain injury patients are compared with control subjects on a task that requires detection of rare targets versus one that requires inhibition of response to rare targets, the latter being more closely analogous to the train driver situation. In a study by Robertson, Manly, and colleagues (1997), control subjects and patients with traumatic brain injury made statistically indistinguishable numbers of errors when they had to *detect* rare (11%) targets—ascending or descending trios of digits (e.g., 234 or 987 in an otherwise random stream of one-per-second digits). Yet the frontally impaired patients did show significant impairment—twice the error rate of controls—on a task on which they had to *withhold* a response to the number 3, also appearing 11% of the time in the same stream of randomly appearing digits (Sustained Attention to Response Task, or SART). We believe these deficits result from a dynamic interaction between inhibitory abilities and vigilant attention, as became apparent when we made the sequence of digits entirely predictable, such as 1, 2, 3, 4, 5, 6, 7, 8, 9, 1, 2, 3. . . . Whereas normal control subjects make only occasional errors on this task, patients with traumatic brain injury have considerable difficulty and in one study made errors in more than 7 out of 25 instances, or an error rate of 28%, despite there being a totally predictable sequence leading up to the target letter (Manly, Owen, et al., 2003) (figure 46.1). Here, the inability to withhold responding is likely due to an inability to maintain a sufficient level of arousal and a sufficiently strong representation of the task goals ("don't respond to 3"): when vigilant attention is poor, the patient defaults to the frequent response. Later we will expand on these two central components of vigilant attention, arousal and goal representation.

EXOGENOUS VERSUS ENDOGENOUS MODULATION OF VIGILANT ATTENTION As we will discuss later in the section on arousal, vigilant attention can be impaired through administration of drugs—for instance, clonidine—that inhibit noradrenaline release. One study, for example (Smith and Nutt, 1996), confirmed that noradrenaline suppression in humans led to vigilant attention lapses, but also showed that this effect was much attenuated when the participants were exposed to loud white noise while performing the task. This finding suggests that external stimuli can induce bottom-up or exogenous modulation of the cortical systems for vigilant

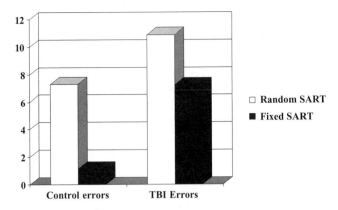

FIGURE 46.1 Commission errors on the random versus fixed SART for patients with traumatic brain injury versus controls (see text) (Manly, Owen, et al., 2003).

attention. Coull and her colleagues confirmed that this is indeed the case (Coull et al., 1995a,b), showing that clonidine-induced noradrenergic suppression impaired vigilant attention performance much more when the task was familiar than when it was unfamiliar. Furthermore, other research by Arnsten and Contant (1992) showed that the clonidine affected delayed response performance during a delay period *less* when a distracter was interpolated in the delay period than when the period was free of distracters. This apparently paradoxical effect, in which the deleterious effect of a drug is reduced by making the task more difficult, is a key finding in understanding how the vigilant attention system might function. What these findings suggest is that this system can be engaged by both endogenous and exogenous means; furthermore, when exogenous activation takes place, we argue, this considerably reduces the demands on the endogenous components of the system. But do exogenous and endogenous input activate the system in the same way? One of our recent studies suggests that this may not be the case.

In a recent functional magnetic resonance imaging (fMRI) study of the SART (O'Connor et al., 2004) we showed that, compared with a rest period, the standard SART (press to digits, except to randomly appearing, 11% frequency, 3 s) showed precisely the right frontoparietal activation that we would predict as being needed for a task that placed demands on the vigilant attention system. We had previously shown, however, that performance on SART and on other tasks requiring vigilant attention could be much enhanced by presenting noninformative auditory arousing tones randomly during task performance (Manly et al., 2002; Manly, Heutink et al., 2004). On the basis of these data, we predicted that these exogenous stimuli externally activated vigilant attention, hence reducing the demands on the endogenous components of that system that we argue are based in the right hemisphere frontoparietal system. What we in fact found was that presenting alerting tones during

SART did eliminate the right frontal activation, but did not eliminate the right parietal activation. In other words, it seems as if the parietal component of the right hemisphere vigilant attention system may be a common pathway for both endogenous and exogenous routes, while the right frontal element may be particularly linked to endogenous activation. We have also shown that increasing the task demand in the SART paradoxically reduces the proportional number of errors of commission. When the inhibit target is relatively rare, 11%, proportionately more errors are made than when the target is more common (25%) and the proportional error rate declines linearly as the target rate increases to 50% (Manly et al., 1999) (figure 46.2B). Furthermore, self-reported proneness to everyday attentional slips, such as forgetting why one has walked into a room (as measured by the Cognitive Failures Questionnaire; Broadbent et al., 1982), are significantly related to the proportion of errors made on the 11% target frequency SART, but not when the targets are more frequent (Manly et al., 1999) (figure 46.2A). We interpret these effects as being due to the repeated targets in the higher-frequency condition providing increased exogenous support for the task through repeated activation of the "inhibit response" motor action and goal representation. We believe that one feature of tasks sensitive to the vigilance system is that this type of exogenous support is absent or relatively weak, and consequently the vigilance system must be maintained endogenously, a function for which the right prefrontal areas appear especially important.

Attention and arousal

WHAT IS AROUSAL? Arousal has been defined as "some level of non-specific neuronal excitability deriving from the structures formerly known as the reticular formation but now generally referred to as specific chemically defined or thalamic systems that innervate the forebrain" (Robbins and Everitt, 1995). This definition rescues the concept of arousal from doubts about its unitary nature that followed the original identification of this function with the reticular formation (Moruzzi and Magoun, 1949). This identification was based in part on the finding that electrical stimulation of this subcortical region elicited behavioral arousal and electroencephalographic (EEG) desynchronization characteristic of the alert state. Furthermore, lesions of this region caused coma, and these and other findings led to the concept of the midbrain reticular formation and associated structures as a key system for regulating cortical arousal. Subsequent research, however, showed that a number of neuroanatomically and neurochemically distinct systems projected to various parts of the cortex from different subcortical nuclei, including the cholinergic basal forebrain, the noradrenergic locus coeruleus (LC), the dopaminergic median forebrain bundle, and the serotonergic dorsal raphe nucleus. Understandably,

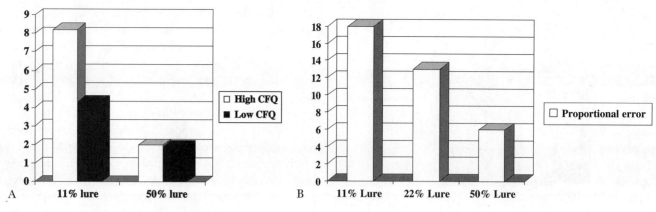

FIGURE 46.2 (*A*) On the SART, the proportion of omission errors increases as the no-go target probability decreases. (*B*) Commission errors on 11% no-go versus 50% no-go (SART) for high- and low-cognitive-failure-prone subjects (Manly, et al., 1999).

confidence in a single construct of "cortical arousal" was considerably weakened by these findings (Olszewski and Baxter, 1982).

Human functional brain imaging helped revive the flagging concept of arousal as a useful explanatory heuristic. Kinomura, Paus, and their colleagues identified the midbrain reticular formation and the intralaminar and other thalamic nuclei with arousal (Kinomura et al., 1996; Paus et al., 1997). Both Paus (Paus et al., 1997) and Critchley (Critchley et al., 2001, 2002) have proposed that the anterior cingulate plays a key role in regulating arousal in response to task demands, thereby providing neuroanatomical guidance on how the vigilant attention system might interface with subcortical arousal mechanisms. The extensive connectivity between frontoparietal areas and the cingulate may enable the communication between these two systems.

Electrophysiological measures have also continued to generate data that confirm the utility of (for heuristic purposes, at least) accepting the existence of arousal as a viable concept. In the study by Paus et al cited earlier, for instance, which used positron emission tomography, the decline in sustained attention over time was associated not only with a decline in metabolic activity in the right hemisphere cortical and subcortical regions already described, it was also correlated with an increase in low-frequency activity in the EEG spectrum. A further study (Makeig and Jung, 1995) showed that vigilance errors were linked to short-term changes in the EEG spectrum, and these changes correlated with concurrent changes in level of performance on a sustained auditory detection task. These authors concluded, "the one-dimensional relationship between detection performance and the EEG spectrum confirms quantitatively the intuitive assumption that minute-scale changes in behavioral alertness during drowsiness are predominantly linked to changes in global brain dynamics along a single dimension of psychophysiological arousal" (p. 213).

Although it is outside the scope of this chapter to review the neurochemistry of arousal, a number of authors (Posner and Peterson, 1990; Usher et al., 1999; Berridge and Waterhouse, 2003) make a strong case for a particularly close linkage between vigilant attention, on the one hand, and the activity of the noradrenergic system on the other. Animal research shows, for instance, that activity is higher when animals are observed as being behaviorally alert (Aston-Jones, Chiang, and Alexinsky, 1991). Furthermore, the appearance of a low-probability target among foils leads to increased LC activity and widespread noradrenergic release (Berridge and Waterhouse, 2003). The relationship is likely more complex than this, but the evidence of a close linkage between noradrenergic activity and vigilant behavior is strong. This is particularly true given the evidence that in humans, reducing noradrenaline release through clonidine administration results in the sorts of attentional lapses characteristic of states of poor alertness/sustained attention (Smith and Nutt, 1996). There is some evidence also that noradrenaline may have a stronger right than left hemisphere innervation (Oke et al., 1978; Robinson, 1979), giving further support to a particularly close relationship between the vigilant attention system and noradrenaline activity. Although the cholinergic system is also involved in vigilant attention (Sarter, Givens, and Bruno, 2001), it is the evidence for noradrenergic right hemispheric lateralization, combined with the clear right hemisphere dominance for vigilant attention, that led many authors to postulate a particular linkage between noradrenaline and vigilant attention.

LINKS BETWEEN ATTENTION AND AROUSAL In 1908, Robert Yerkes and John Dodson studied the effects of different degrees of arousal (by varying degree of shock) in mice on their ability to learn discriminations between the luminance of two compartments. They found that when lightness levels could be easily discriminated, the mice performed better at high levels of arousal, whereas difficult light discriminations were best learned at low levels of arousal. On the basis of these experiments, they formulated the Yerkes–Dodson law. This law proposes that any task will have an optimal level of arousal below and beyond which performance will decline, and that this optimal level is lower in challenging tasks than in routine tasks. Similarly, Donald Broadbent showed that stress can improve performance on routine, nondemanding tasks, but the same levels of stress can impair performance on more complex and demanding tasks (D. E. Broadbent, 1971). These classic psychological studies suggesting an interaction between arousal levels, optimal performance, and degree of challenge in a task mesh well with the notion of exogenous modulation of arousal. They also suggest, however, that the relationship between the system for vigilant attention and arousal may not be a simple one of mutual facilitation. A number of other, more recent studies support such a view.

Progress has been made in identifying the neuroanatomical basis for this attention–arousal coupling. For example, LC activity has been shown to correlate closely with behavioral performance when monkeys have to detect relatively rare (20% probability) visual targets among foils, but optimal performance was achieved not at maximum levels of LC activity but rather at intermediate levels (Usher et al., 1999). Increased tonic LC noradrenergic activity was linked to decreased reponsivity of LC neurons to target stimuli, as well as to poor behavioral performance. Usher and colleagues proposed that high tonic LC activity offers a mechanism for sampling new stimuli and behaviors by decreasing attentional selectivity and increasing the behavioral responsiveness to unexpected or novel stimuli. Intermediate levels of tonic LC activity, on the other hand, allow the optimizing of performance in a stable environment. In a comprehensive review of catecholamine modulation of prefrontal cognitive function, Arnsten showed that many studies have confirmed the findings of Usher and colleagues by showing a Yerkes–Dodson type of inverted-U relationship between levels of noradrenaline release, on the one hand, and behavioral performance on the other (Arnsten, 1998). Arnsten concluded that different neuropsychiatric conditions may reveal impairment in executive control of complex behaviors for reasons of either deficient or excessive levels of noradrenaline.

The study mentioned earlier, by Paus and colleagues (Paus et al., 1997), demonstrated the interrelatedness of attention and arousal. To recap, in this study healthy participants were asked to perform a simple vigilance task for around 60 minutes. Every 10 minutes, regional cerebral blood flow and EEG were measured. Significant reductions in blood flow were observed in subcortical structures, the thalamus, substantia innominata, and putamen, and in right hemisphere cortical areas, including frontal and parietal cortex. These reductions in blood flow were interpreted by the authors as indications of a subcortical arousal system and right cortical attentional system, respectively. Increases in low theta activity, associated with a reduction in arousal, were also observed on the EEG as the task progressed. Despite the reduction in blood flow in the right-hemisphere-based "attentional" and subcortical "arousal" networks, the number of successful target detections did not significantly decline over the hour of the task. This finding was interpreted as reflecting a need for active attentional engagement early on in the task, a need that declined as target detection became increasingly automatic. Results such as these suggest that the term sustained attention may be somewhat inappropriately applied to situations that clearly require sustained *performance* but may actually make relatively limited demands on what might be termed vigilant attention. This distinction is perhaps best captured by consideration of whether maintaining responsivity to an arbitrary but overlearned stimulus such as one's own name requires anything approaching active maintenance of attention at all.

Such a conclusion would be supported by Coull and colleagues (1996), who also found declines in thalamic and right frontoparietal perfusion over an 18-minute task period in which participants had to respond whenever any letter appeared on the screen (these stimuli appeared on average every 20, with a range of 10–30 s). However, when the task was made a relatively difficult selective attention task by requiring participants to respond only to red Bs interspersed among red and blue Bs and Gs, no significant decline in perfusion of the right frontal and parietal cortices was observed. This observation is in line with the earlier arguments about the effects of exogenous demand on vigilant attention and suggests that this right frontoparietal system for vigilant attention is at least in part a system needed to maintain alert and reasonably accurate responding in the absence of strong external demands or stimuli that otherwise support alert responding.

If this is the case, then a major role of the right frontoparietal system is to modulate arousal, particularly when that arousal is not externally generated by task demand or stimulus. As mentioned earlier, the anterior cingulate may serve as the interface between cognition and emotion and may serve as a conduit by which the right prefrontoparietal system modulates arousal levels.

This appearance of a functional wood out of the neurochemical trees allows us to begin to develop the concept of a broad mesencephalic arousal system operating in concert with a predominantly right hemisphere frontoparietal vigilant attention system. What distinct contributions the right prefrontal and right parietal structures might make to vigilant attention is the topic to which we turn next.

Frontoparietal interactions in vigilant attention

The right dorsolateral prefrontal and inferior parietal cortices of the right hemisphere have been widely implicated in vigilant attention. It is possible that the right prefrontal cortex plays a particular role in the endogenous components of this system, whereas the inferior parietal cortex may be commonly activated by both endogenous and exogenous pathways. We have shown that the effects of exogenous alerting stimuli on performance on the SART, described earlier (O'Connor et al., 2004) were to reduce neuronal activity in the right prefrontal cortex, but not in the right inferior parietal cortex. A recent meta-analysis of error-related activations (n = 44) from a number of our event-related go/no-go response inhibition tasks similar in structure to the SART has revealed robust right inferior parietal lobule activation that correlated negatively with the number of errors subjects committed. We have consistently seen this parietal area and right dorsolateral prefrontal cortex coactivated during response inhibition (Garavan, Ross, and Stein, 1999; Garavan et al., 2002). The presence of the parietal activation for both errors and successful inhibitions suggests that it has a more general attentional role in processing the salient no-go stimuli and not in response inhibition per se, while the negative correlation suggests that greater activation here is associated with better performance. The right prefrontal area is probably critical to the response selection process itself (Garavan, Ross, and Stein, 1999; Rowe et al., 2000; Garavan et al., 2002).

Combined, these disparate findings suggest that the right inferior parietal cortex has a role in the routine, semi-automatic maintenance of sustained vigilant responding, whereas the right dorsolateral prefrontal cortex has a more "executive" role in maintaining the vigilant state. One hypothesis for what this executive role involves might be to engage/initiate the vigilant state based on a dynamic assessment of the optimal arousal level to match performance to task demands. This implies that the monitoring of either one's endogenous arousal levels or of one's performance is information crucial for the functioning of the vigilant attention system. This monitoring function might be performed by the right prefrontal area itself with, for example, inputs from relevant midline structures that detect errors or response conflict (Dehaene, Posner, and Tucker, 1994; Botvinick et al., 2001). Alternatively, if these other structures perform the monitoring function themselves, then the role of the right prefrontal cortex would be to modulate arousal levels based on their outputs. Either way, it would seem to be the case that vigilant attention operates in an interactive way with other executive functions, a topic that we turn to next.

Relationship between vigilant attention and other executive systems

We conceive of the right parietal-prefrontal network and its interactions with the midbrain arousal systems as the circuitry by which vigilant attention is maintained. This circuitry can be "turned up" endogenously or with exogenous support. Within this system, we believe that the prefrontal cortex plays a central role in maintaining and monitoring optimal arousal levels to match current task demands. Although we can conceive of this system as somewhat independent and autonomous, in order to be responsive to changing tasks demands, changing performance levels, or changing physiological resources such as might be depleted by fatigue, monitoring processes must be tightly coupled with, or intrinsic to, its functioning. In addition, this system works in the service of current task goals, and close interaction between it and goal representations is to be expected. Consequently, the type of attentional control that has been the focus of this chapter need not be isolated from the other aspects of attention linked to selection, working memory, and switching that were mentioned at the beginning of the chapter.

The nature of the relationship between goal state representation and vigilance is, however, not very well understood. It may be the case that the goal state (e.g., take the train safely from station A to station B) may call on the vigilant attention system to ensure the goal is attained in the circumstances already described, in which exogenous support is minimal. If, however, the goal can be actively maintained in a focus of attention within working memory (Garavan, 1998), this may in fact reduce reliance on the vigilance system. For example, inhibiting a response to the number 3 in the SART task is quite easy if you have just refreshed that rule, perhaps by subvocally reiterating to yourself that you must not respond to 3s (indeed, we have demonstrated in patients with impaired frontoparietal function that precisely this type of verbal regulation can compensate for suboptimal vigilance; Robertson et al., 1995). Inhibiting to the 3 becomes difficult and reliant on the vigilant attention system if the "inhibit to 3" goal is no longer prominent but instead has been allowed to decay. A number of lines of evidence implicate left prefrontal areas in this type of goal maintenance (Frith and Dolan, 1996; Garavan, 1998; MacDonald et al., 2000; Brass and Cramon, 2002; Ruchsow et al., 2002), which implies interhemispheric interaction between goal representations and vigilant attention.

Combined, this conceptualization of vigilant attention and its interaction with goal representations provides a basis for different types of attentional impairment. First, the subcortical arousal or cortical vigilant attention systems—the "machinery" of attention—might be damaged, leading to gross vigilance impairments that may not be easily amenable to rehabilitation. Second, the functioning of the task goal system and/or its interaction with the vigilance systems may be compromised. That is, whereas the machinery (i.e., the ability to attend) may be intact, the mechanisms by which this machinery is mustered in the service of task goals might be compromised. Patients who can muster sufficient attentional resources with exogenous support (e.g., cuing, phasic alerting) but have difficulty doing so without this support may have this second type of dysfunction.

We can perhaps gain an insight into the interactions between vigilant attention and other executive functions by observing the processes involved in preparing for an attentionally demanding task. A predictive cue that warns of an impending task involves the endogenous activation of a vigilant state. We have recently shown that the areas activated in anticipation of a response inhibition include right prefrontal and parietal cortex (Hester et al., 2004). This may reflect either engagement of the vigilant attention system or, given that these areas were necessary for the subsequent inhibition, preparatory activation of task-specific areas. Left prefrontal cortex was also activated following the cue, which we believe reflects task set activation, as described earlier. Furthermore, what uniquely distinguished a successful preparation from an unsuccessful one (i.e., despite the cue, a commission error was made) was the deactivation of midline prefrontal areas that are thought to be involved in the monitoring of internal emotional states (Gusnard et al., 2001). The deactivation of task-inappropriate areas confirms a finding of similar deactivations underlying good performance in a rapid visual information processing task (Lawrence et al., in press). Together, these additional processes, the preparatory activation of task-relevant areas and the deactivation of task-inappropriate areas, may serve as additional attentional mechanisms that obviate reliance on the vigilant attentional system.

The notion that vigilant attention is linked to deactivation of inappropriate areas raises the question as to whether inhibition can be regarded as one means by which vigilant attention is maintained: in the case of the London train driver, for instance, the ability to detect the yellow warning signals may have been predicated on the ability to inhibit non-task-relevant cognitions, emotions, and perceptions. While not synonymous, vigilant attention and inhibition may be strongly overlapping functions both functionally and anatomically, which would explain the very strong similarity in activation patterns for vigilant attention and inhibitory tasks. Figure 46.3 shows activation associated with go/ no-go response inhibition based on a meta-analysis of 58 subjects (Garavan and Hester, 2004). Robust event-related activation in the right dorsolateral prefrontal and right inferior parietal lobule parallels tonic activation patterns observed for vigilance tasks. The speculation follows that vigilant attention might be conceptualized as a continuous inhibition of task irrelevances. Also shown in figure 46.3 is a more ventral activation of the right inferior frontal gyrus. Inhibition-related activation in this inferior region was significantly greater in those subjects scoring higher on the Cognitive Failures Questionnaire that we described earlier

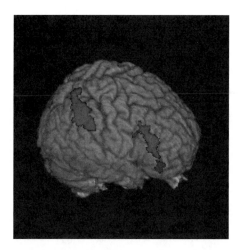

FIGURE 46.3   Extensive dorsolateral and parietal activation (in red) is shown for event-related response inhibition. Activation (in blue) of the right inferior frontal gyrus was correlated with the CFQ score, suggesting a greater reliance on this right prefrontal area in subjects scoring highest on everyday absentmindedness (Garavan and Hester, 2004). (See color plate 22.)

as correlating with SART performance. The region in question in figure 46.3 also shows a correlation between inhibition-related activation and age, suggesting that this structure is used more both by highly absentminded people and by older people (Garavan and Hester, 2004). Furthermore, older subjects also showed significantly greater left prefrontal activation than younger subjects, consistent with an age-relate increased in dependence on the left hemisphere task set reactivation mechanism. Although the relationship between vigilant attention and inhibition must be investigated further, these results offer encouragement in the search for the neuroanatomical bases for these executive functions and their relationship to normal individual variability and pathological disturbance.

Attention-deficit/hyperactivity disorder

Attention-deficit/hyperactivity disorder (ADHD) is a complex condition with a number of different subtypes and a range of associated cognitive and motivational impairments (Castellanos and Tannock, 2002). What is interesting about this disorder in the context of the current discussion is the fact that the inattentive subtype of the disorder includes a profile of impaired sustained attention, absentmindedness, distractibility, and action slips that are extremely close to the pattern of adult behavior we have described in this chapter as being linked to a deficient vigilant attention system. Bearing in mind this similarity in behavior patterns, and without wishing to ignore the abnormalities in other brain regions such as the caudate nucleus and the vermis of the cerebellum that have been identified in ADHD, it is of considerable interest that there are also abnormalities in the right frontal lobe, particularly in the underlying white matter (Castellanos et al., 1996), in ADHD. Furthermore, we have also shown that, compared with IQ-matched controls, children with ADHD are impaired on sustained but not selective attention performance (Manly et al., 2001).

The remarkable responsiveness of these attentional deficits in ADHD to methylphenidate or amphetamine (Solanto, Arnsten, and Castellanos, 2001), drugs that potentiate noradrenergic as well as dopaminergic release, also links the vigilant attention system and its arousal-modulating role to this clinical syndrome. This is particularly true in light of EEG evidence of low tonic arousal as manifested by high theta power in the EEG spectrum (Bresnahan and Barry, 2002). We have recently shown that the fixed sequence SART that discriminated patients with traumatic brain injury from controls so well also discriminates between ADHD and controls (O'Connell, Bellgrove, and Robertson, 2004). Furthermore, tests of vigilant attention in a children's battery of attention measures consistently discriminate ADHD participants from controls in a way that selective attention tests do not (Manly et al., 2001).

To summarize, important aspects of the ADHD syndrome may constitute an important manifestation of deficits of the vigilant attention system, and therefore progress that has been made toward rehabilitation of deficits in this system may potentially be applicable to ADHD. It is to this final question that we turn now.

Rehabilitation and vigilant attention

The ability to sustain vigilant attention seems to be an important factor in determining recovery of motor and other function following stroke (Ben-Yishay et al., 1968; Blanc-Garin, 1994). Furthermore, we have shown that motor recovery following stroke over a 2-year period was significantly predicted by measures of sustained attention taken 2 months after right hemisphere stroke. Specifically, the ability to sustain attention to a tone-counting task (a validated measure of sustained attention related to right frontal function; Wilkins, Shallice, and McCarthy, 1987) at 2 months after stroke predicted not only everyday life function 2 years later but also the functional dexterity of the left hand in a pegboard task (Robertson, Ridgeway, et al., 1997).

Impairment in sustained attention may also be a key factor in the development of the disabling condition of unilateral spatial neglect, a relatively common consequence of right-hemisphere stroke (Robertson, 2001; Husain and Rorden, 2003). Apart from the disabling consequences of impaired vigilant attention itself, it is likely that impairments in this system have more wide-ranging consequences for recovery from brain damage and the learning that underpins rehabilitation effects (Robertson and Murre, 1999).

It is possible to enhance vigilant attention both in the short term, through exogenous means (Manly et al., 2002; Manly, Heutink, et al., 2004), and also over longer periods, by training patients endogenously to implement metacognitive, verbally regulated strategies (Robertson et al., 1995). We have further shown that short-term exogenous activation of the vigilant attention and arousal systems can temporarily alleviate neglect-induced spatial bias (Robertson et al., 1998). Similar methods have now been incorporated as an element in a successful system of rehabilitation for executive problems following frontal lobe damage (Levine et al., 2000).

Comment

When a driver has driven a train a hundred times through a light that was always green, it is all too easy for the driver's brain to miss the yellow light that appears on the 101st journey and to let the train-driving motor program run on, unsupervised—occasionally to catastrophe. If that yellow light is detected, the accelerator handle released, and the train slowed down in preparation to stop at the next light, it is thanks to the right hemisphere of the brain, and in particular the right dorsolateral prefrontal and inferior parietal cortices, working in concert with thalamic and mesencephalic circuits. Repeated, unchallenging stimuli in the context of highly practiced actions diminish arousal, dull sensory responsiveness, and blunt vigilant oversight of one's actions and environment. The reciprocal action of a right hemisphere cortical network and a subcortical arousal network has evolved to protect against such a potentially dangerous diminution in awareness and monitoring. Because so much of what we do is practiced and automatic, this system is needed throughout our waking day. The next time you walk into a room, scratch your head, and wonder, now, why did I come in here? you are witnessing a minor inefficiency of this system.

REFERENCES

ARNSTEN, A. F. T., 1998. Catecholamine modulation of prefrontal cortical cognitive function. *Trends Cogn. Sci.* 2:436–447.

ARNSTEN, A. F. T., and T. A. CONTANT, 1992. Alpha-2 adrenergic agonists decrease distractibility in aged monkeys performing the delayed response task. *Psychopharmacology* 108:159–169.

ASTON-JONES, G., C. CHIANG, and T. ALEXINSKY, 1991. Discharge of noradrenergic locus coeruleus neurons in behaving rats and monkeys suggests a role in vigilance. *Prog. Brain Res.* 88:501–520.

BEN-YISHAY, Y., L. DILLER, L. GERSTMAN, and A. HAAS, 1968. The relationship between impersistence, intellectual function and outcome of rehabilitation in patients with left hemiplegia. *Neurology* 18:852–861.

BERRIDGE, C. W., and B. D. WATERHOUSE, 2003. The locus-coeruleus-noradrenergic system: Modulation of behavioral state and state-dependent cognitive processes. *Brain Res. Rev.* 42:33–84.

BLANC-GARIN, J., 1994. Patterns of recovery from hemiplegia following stroke. *Neuropsychol. Rehabil.* 4:359–385.

BOTVINICK, M. W., C. S. CARTER, T. S. BRAVER, D. M. BARCH, and J. D. COHEN, 2001. Conflict monitoring and cognitive control. *Psychol. Rev.* 108:624–652.

BRASS, M., and D. Y. V. CRAMON, 2002. The role of the frontal cortex in task preparation. *Cereb. Cortex* 12:908–914.

BRESNAHAN, S. M., and R. J. BARRY, 2002. Specificity of quantitative EEG analysis in adults with attention deficit hyperactivity disorder. *Psychiatry Res.* 112:133–144.

BROADBENT, D. B., P. F. COOPER, P. FITZGERALD, and K. R. PARKES, 1982. The Cognitive Failures Questionnaire (CFQ) and its correlates. *Br. J. Clin. Psychol.* 21:1–16.

BROADBENT, D. E., 1971. *Decision and Stress.* London: Academic Press.

CASTELLANOS, F. X., J. N. GIEDD, W. L. MARSH, S. D. HAMBURGER, A. C. VAITUZIS, D. P. DICKSTEIN, et al. 1996. Quantitative brain magnetic-resonance-imaging in attention-deficit hyperactivity disorder. *Arch. Gen. Psychiatry* 53:607–616.

CASTELLANOS, F. X., and R. TANNOCK, 2002. Neuroscience of attention-deficit/hyperactivity disorder: The search for endophenotypes. *Nat. Rev. Neurosci.* 3:617–628.

COULL, J. T., C. D. FRITH, R. S. J. FRACKOWIAK, and P. M. GRASBY, 1996. A fronto-parietal network for rapid visual information-processing: A PET study of sustained attention and working memory. *Neuropsychologia* 34:1085–1095.

COULL, J. T., H. C. MIDDLETON, T. W. ROBBINS, and B. J. SAHAKIAN, 1995a. Clonidine and diazepam have differential effects on tests of attention and learning. *Psychopharmacology* 120:322–332.

COULL, J. T., H. C. MIDDLETON, T. W. ROBBINS, and B. J. SAHAKIAN, 1995b. Differential effects of clonidine, haloperidol, diazepam and tryptophan depletion on focused attention and attentional search. *Psychopharmacology* 121:222–230.

CRITCHLEY, H. D., R. N. MELMED, E. FEATHERSTONE, C. J. MATHIAS, and R. J. DOLAN, 2001. Brain activity during biofeedback relaxation: A functional neuroimaging investigation. *Brain* 124:1003–1012.

CRITCHLEY, H. D., R. N. MELMED, R. N. FEATHERSTONE, C. J. MATHIAS, and R. J. DOLAN, 2002. Volitional control of autonomic arousal: A functional magnetic resonance study. *NeuroImage* 16:909–919.

DEHAENE, S., M. I. POSNER, and D. M. TUCKER, 1994. Localization of a neural system for error detection and compensation. *Psychol. Sci.* 5:303–305.

EDKINS, G., and C. POLLOCK, 1997. The influence of sustained attention on railway accidents. *Accident Anal. Prevent.* 29:533–539.

FRITH, C., and R. DOLAN, 1996. The role of the prefrontal cortex in higher cognitive functions. *Cogn. Brain Res.* 5:175–181.

GARAVAN, H., 1998. Serial attention within working memory. *Memo. Cogn.* 26:263–276.

GARAVAN, H., and R. HESTER, 2004. *Individual differences in executive control: A meta-analysis of four event-related fMRI studies using the GO/NOGO task.* Unpublished manuscript.

GARAVAN, H., T. J. ROSS, K. MURPHY, R. A. P. ROCHE, and E. A. STEIN, 2002. Dissociable executive functions in the dynamic control of behaviour: Inhibition, error detection and correction. *NeuroImage* 17:1820–1829.

GARAVAN, H., T. J. ROSS, and E. A. STEIN, 1999. Right hemispheric dominance of inhibitory control: An event-related fMRI study. *Proc. Nat. Acad. Sci. U.S.A.* 96:8301–8306.

GUSNARD, D. A., E. AKBUDAK, G. L. SHULMAN, and M. E. RAICHLE, 2001. Medial prefrontal cortex and self-referential mental activity: Relation to a default mode of brain function. *Proc. Nat. Acad. Sci. U.S.A.* 98:4259–4264.

HESTER, R., C. FASSBENDER, and H. GARAVAN, 2004. *Individual differences in error processing: A review and meta-analysis of three event-related fMRI studies using the GO/NOGO task.* Unpublished manuscript.

HESTER, R., K. MURPHY, D. M. FOXE, J. FOXE, and H. GARAVAN, 2004. *Predicting success: The effect of pre-target cueing on inhibition performance.* Unpublished manuscript.

HUSAIN, M., and C. RORDEN, 2003. Non-spatially lateralized mechanisms in hemispatial neglect. *Nat. Rev. Neurosci.* 4:26–36.

KINOMURA, S., J. LARSSON, B. GULYAS, and P. E. ROLAND, 1996. Activation by attention of the human reticular formation and thalamic intralaminar nuclei. *Science* 271:512–515.

LAWRENCE, N., T. ROSS, R. HOFFMAN, H. GARAVAN, and E. A. STEIN (in press). Activation and deactivation during the rapid visual information processing task: An fMRI study. *J. Cogn. Neurosci.*

LEVINE, B., I. ROBERTSON, L. CLARE, G. CARTER, J. HONG, B. A. WILSON, et al., 2000. Rehabilitation of executive functioning: An experimental-clinical validation of goal management training. *J. Int. Neuropsychol. Soc.* 6:299–312.

MACDONALD, A. W., J. D. COHEN, A. STENGER, and C. S. CARTER, 2000. Dissociating the role of the dorsolateral prefrontal and anterior cingulate cortex in cognitive control—1838. *Science* 288:1835–1838.

MACKWORTH, J. F., 1968. Vigilance, arousal and habituation. *Psychol. Rev.* 75:308–322.

MACKWORTH, N. H., 1950. Researches in the measurement of human performance. *Selected Papers on Human Factors in the Design and Use of Control Systems,* H. A. Sinaiko, ed. Dover: Dover Publications.

MAKEIG, S., and T.-P. JUNG, 1995. Changes in alertness are a principal component of variance in the EEG spectrum. *Neuroreport* 7:213–216.

MANLY, T., V. ANDERSON, I. NIMMO-SMITH, A. TURNER, P. WATSON, and I. H. ROBERTSON, 2001. The differential assessment of children's attention: The Test of Everyday Attention for Children (TEA-Ch), normative sample and ADHD performance. *J. Child Psychol. Psychiatry* 42:1–10.

MANLY, T., K. HAWKINS, J. EVANS, K. WOLDT, and I. H. ROBERTSON, 2002. Rehabilitation of executive function: Facilitation of effective goal management on complex tasks using periodic auditory alerts. *Neuropsychologia* 40:271–281.

MANLY, T., J. HEUTINK, B. DAVISON, B. GAYNORD, E. GREENFIELD, A. PARR, et al., 2004. An electronic knot in the handkerchief: "Content free cueing" and the maintenance of attentive control. *Neuropsychol. Rehabil.* 14:89–116.

MANLY, T., A. M. OWEN, L. MCAVINUE, A. DATTA, G. A. LEWIS, S. K. SCOTT, et al., 2003. Enhancing the sensitivity of a sustained attention task to frontal damage: Convergent clinical and functional imaging evidence. *Neurocase* 9:340–349.

MANLY, T., I. H. ROBERTSON, M. GALLOWAY, and K. HAWKINS, 1999. The absent mind: Further investigations of sustained attention to response. *Neuropsychologia* 37:661–670.

MORUZZI, G., and H. W. MAGOUN, 1949. Brainstem reticular formation and activation of the EEG. *Electroencephalogr. Clin. Neurophysiol.* 1:455–473.

O'CONNELL, R., M. BELLGROVE, and I. H. ROBERTSON, 2004. Vigilant attention in ADHD. Unpublished manuscript.

O'CONNOR, C., T. MANLY, I. H. ROBERTSON, S. J. HEVENOR, and B. LEVINE, 2004. Endogenous vs. exogenous engagement of sustained attention: An fMRI study. *Brain Cogn.* 54:133–135.

OKE, A., R. KELLER, I. MEFFORD, and R. ADAMS, 1978. Lateralization of norepinephrine in human thalamus. *Science* 200:1411–1413.

OLSZEWSKI, J., and D. BAXTER, 1982. *Cytoarchitecture of the Human Brainstem*, 2nd ed. New York: S. Karger.

PARASURAMAN, R., 1983. Vigilance, arousal and the brain. In *Physiological Correlates of Human Behaviour*. A. Gale and J. A. Edwards, eds. London: Academic Press, pp. 35–55.

PARASURAMAN, R., 1998. *The Attentive Brain*. Cambridge, Mass.: MIT Press.

PARASURAMAN, R., S. A. MUTTER, and R. MOLLOY, 1991. Sustained attention following mild closed-head injury. *J. Clin. Exp. Neuropsychol.* 13:789–811.

PARASURAMAN, R., J. WARM, and J. SEE, 1998. Brain systems of vigilance. In *Varieties of Attention*, R. Parasuraman, ed. Cambridge, Mass.: MIT Press, pp. 221–256.

PAUS, T., R. J. ZATORRE, N. HOFLE, Z. CARAMANOS, J. GOTMAN, M. PETRIDES, et al., 1997. Time-related changes in neural systems underlying attention and arousal during the performance of an auditory vigilance task. *J. Cogn. Neurosci.* 9:392–408.

POSNER, M. I., 1978. *Chronometric Explorations of Mind*. Hillsdale, N.J.: Erlbaum.

POSNER, M. I., and S. BOIES, 1971. Components of attention. *Psychol. Rev.* 78:391–408.

POSNER, M. I., A. W. INHOFF, and F. J. FRIEDRICH, 1987. Isolating attentional systems: A cognitive-anatomical analysis. *Psychobiology* 15:107–121.

POSNER, M. I., and S. E. PETERSON, 1990. The attention system of the human brain. *Annu. Rev. Neurosci.* 13:25–42.

REASON, J., 1992. *Human Error*. Cambridge, England: Cambridge University Press.

ROBBINS, T. W., and B. J. EVERITT, 1995. Arousal systems in attention. In *The Cognitive Neurosciences*, M. S. Gazzaniga, ed. Cambridge, Mass.: MIT Press, pp. 703–720.

ROBERTSON, I. H., 2001. Do we need the "lateral" in unilateral neglect? Spatially nonselective attention deficits in unilateral neglect and their implications for rehabilitation. *NeuroImage* 14:S85–S90.

ROBERTSON, I. H., T. MANLY, J. ANDRADE, B. T. BADDELEY, and J. YIEND 1997. Oops! Performance correlates of everyday attentional failures in traumatic brain injured and normal subjects: The Sustained Attention to Response Task (SART). *Neuropsychologia* 35:747–758.

ROBERTSON, I. H., J. B. MATTINGLEY, C. RORDEN, and J. DRIVER, 1998. Phasic alerting of neglect patients overcomes their spatial deficit in visual awareness. *Nature* 395:169–172.

ROBERTSON, I. H., and J. M. J. MURRE, 1999. Rehabilitation of brain damage: Brain plasticity and principles of guided recovery. *Psychol. Bull.* 125:544–575.

ROBERTSON, I. H., V. RIDGEWAY, E. GREENFIELD, and A. PARR, 1997. Motor recovery after stroke depends on intact sustained attention: A two-year follow-up study. *Neuropsychology* 11:290–295.

ROBERTSON, I. H., R. TEGNER, K. THAM, A. LO, and I. NIMMO-SMITH, 1995. Sustained attention training for unilateral neglect: Theoretical and rehabilitation implications. *J. Clin. Exp. Neuropsychol.* 17:416–430.

ROBINSON, R. G., 1979. Differential behavioral and biochemical effects of right and left hemispheric infarction in the rat. *Science* 205:707–710.

ROWE, J. B., I. TONI, O. JOSEPHS, R. S. J. FRACKOWIAK, and R. E. PASSINGHAM, 2000. The prefrontal cortex: Response selection or maintenance within working memory? *Science* 288:1656–1660.

RUCHSOW, M., J. GROTHE, M. SPITZER, and M. KIEFER, 2002. Human anterior cingulate coretx is activated by negative feedback: Evidence from event-related potentials in a guessing task. *Neurosci. Lett.* 325:203–206.

SARTER, M., B. GIVENS, and J. P. BRUNO, 2001. The cognitive neuroscience of sustained attention: Where top-down meets bottom-up. *Brain Res. Rev.* 35:146–160.

SMITH, A., and D. NUTT, 1996. Noradrenaline and attention lapses. *Nature* 380:291.

SOLANTO, M. V., A. F. T. ARNSTEN, and F. X. CASTELLANOS, 2001. *Stimulant Drugs and ADHD: Basic and Clinical Neuroscience*. Oxford, England: Oxford University Press.

USHER, M., J. D. COHEN, D. SERVAN-SCHREIBER, J. RAJKOWSKI, and G. ASTON-JONES, 1999. The role of locus coeruleus in the regulation of cognitive performance. *Science* 283:549–553.

WILKINS, A. J., T. SHALLICE, and R. MCCARTHY, 1987. Frontal lesions and sustained attention. *Neuropsychologia* 25:359–365.

YERKES, R. M., and J. D. DODSON, 1908. The relation of strength of stimulus to rapidity of habit-formation. *J. Comp. Neurol. Psychol.* 18:459–482.

VI MEMORY

Introduction

DANIEL L. SCHACTER

MEMORY IS A TOPIC that has engaged psychologists and neuroscientists for as long as they have been interested in the relationship between brain and mind. Memory is so fundamental to the operation of the brain/mind that students of memory could be forgiven if they felt that their object of study was among the most central—perhaps *the* most central—in all of cognitive neuroscience. But what is memory? Though we cannot yet provide a satisfactory answer to this question, we do know something worth knowing about what memory is not: it is not a single entity or concept. As Endel Tulving stated in the introduction to the memory chapters in the first edition of this book, "Memory is many things, even if not everything that has been labeled memory corresponds to what cognitive neuroscientists think of as memory. Memory is a gift of nature, the ability of living organisms to retain and to utilize acquired information. The term is closely related to *learning*, in that memory in biological systems always entails learning (the acquisition of information) and in that learning implies retention (memory) of such information." Tulving also characterized memory as a trick of evolution, a biological abstraction, and a convenient chapter heading for certain kinds of problems that scientists study.

Memory is all of these things, and it can also be thought of as a nonunitary entity in other senses, too. For many decades, neuroscientists searched for the brain location of the engram—a term for the persisting aftereffects of experience in the nervous system that was coined by the German biologist Richard Semon in the first decade of the twentieth century. Yet the search for a single location in the brain that corresponds to a memory never succeeded, as highlighted in Karl Lashley's famous paper, in which he described his failed search for the engram. Today, most memory researchers would agree that there is some sort of an engram—a stored representation of experience in the brain—but few would maintain that it is in a single location, or that there is any one place in the brain that one could point to as the site of a particular memory. Instead, there is a general consensus that engrams consist of multiple features that are likely distributed across several brain locations and are bound together by the hippocampus and related structures in the medial temporal lobe.

Memory is also a nonunitary entity at the level of processes and systems. The starting point for virtually any scientific analysis of memory involves a decomposition into processes of encoding, storage, and retrieval; it is difficult to imagine a contemporary approach that does not incorporate these basic distinctions. Furthermore, a prominent theme in cognitive neuroscience for the past two decades is that memory can be divided into multiple forms or systems—collections of processes that operate on different kinds of information and according to different rules. The distinction between short-term and long-term memory is perhaps the most venerable among memory distinctions of the modern era, dating at least to the 1950s and 1960s. Today, researchers often invoke a similar distinction between working memory, which maintains and allows the online manipulation of information over brief time periods to guide behavior, and a long-term memory that can retain information for years and decades. Contemporary theorists have put forward a variety of conceptual schemes to subdivide forms of long-term memory. Nonetheless, there is widespread agreement on a fundamental distinction between an explicit or declarative form of memory, which supports the conscious calling to mind of previous experiences and acquired facts, and an implicit or nondeclarative form of memory, which involves changes in behavior or performance as a result of past experiences, even when those experiences themselves cannot be consciously remembered. Within these broad outlines, forms of memory such as episodic, semantic, priming, and procedural memory are all familiar to contemporary researchers.

The idea that memory is not a single thing even extends to memory's imperfections. Memory is not a simple matter of success or failure. Memory can go awry because of either forgetting or distortion, and each of these types of error can be subdivided into several distinguishable forms. Though psychologists have long recognized that memory is prone to various kinds of errors that can reveal important principles of memory functioning, the idea is just now starting to gain momentum in cognitive neuroscience.

The seven chapters in this section highlight the nonunitary nature of memory at different levels of analysis. One of the keys to progress in the cognitive neuroscience of memory has been that researchers working at various levels, from the synapse to large-scale systems, have all embraced a number of fundamental ideas. Bailey and Kandel illustrate this point in their review of neurobiological evidence concerning the cellular bases of short-term and long-term memory, as well as implicit and explicit forms of memory. They summarize evidence indicating that short-term memory depends on alterations in the strength and effectiveness of already existing synapses, whereas long-term memory involves the synthesis of new proteins and growth of new synapses. Their chapter highlights the increasingly sophisticated and detailed understanding of molecular mechanisms of memory, including the role of genetic mechanisms that appear to be involved in several different forms of memory.

Davachi, Romanski, Chafee, and Goldman-Rakic focus on working memory. Tasks that engage working memory processes generally recruit a network of brain regions that include frontal and more posterior parietal or temporal regions. Studies using single-unit neuronal recordings in awake and behaving primates have allowed researchers to monitor event-related neuronal activity during these processes, and thus probe the underlying circuitry. Various tasks have demonstrated that neurons within frontal regions display sustained activation during delay periods when animals are required to hold the information in mind. There is also evidence from this research that working memory contains domain-specific processes: activity observed in posterior regions is linked with frontal cortex, such that regions of parietal cortex code for spatial information, whereas regions in temporal cortex code for object information.

There is perhaps no topic more central to the cognitive neuroscience of memory than the role of the hippocampus and related medial temporal lobe structures in various forms of memory. Ever since the groundbreaking observations of Scoville and Milner during the 1950s concerning the severe amnesia observed in patient H.M. after bilateral resection of the medial temporal lobes for relief of intractable epilepsy, attempting to understand this region's role in memory and learning has constituted a kind of holy grail for memory researchers.

Eichenbaum examines theoretical and empirical aspects of declarative memory, focusing mainly on experiments conducted with rodents. Eichenbaum amasses considerable evidence for the hypothesis that the hippocampus contributes to declarative memory through its role in relational processing, or the ability to link together previously unrelated bits of information in a manner that later allows for their flexible use in a variety of different contexts. Using elegant behavioral paradigms in conjunction with highly localized lesions, Eichenbaum elucidates the role of the hippocampus in such processes as inferential memory expression. Squire, Clark, and Bayley focus on work with human amnesic patients to examine spared and impaired functions after medial temporal lobe damage, and to delineate the contributions of specific components of the medial temporal region to declarative memory. They integrate their work on amnesic patients with studies in nonhuman animals, as well as functional imaging studies, to illuminate such diverse topics as recognition memory, retrograde amnesia, and classical conditioning. While acknowledging that it is likely that regions within the medial temporal lobe are associated with specific functions, they believe that each region contributes in important ways to components of declarative memory such as item recognition and associative or relational memory.

As in other areas of cognitive neuroscience, the advent of functional neuroimaging has had dramatic consequences for the study of memory. For the past decade and more, researchers have applied PET and fMRI techniques to an ever-increasing variety of topics in memory research. The chapters in this section by Wagner, Bunge, and Badre, Rugg, and Buckner and Schacter provide a broad overview of the progress and issues to date in this rapidly expanding and exciting enterprise. Wagner and his colleagues integrate fMRI studies of working memory, semantic memory, and priming, delineating their relationship to issues of executive function and cognitive control. Their discussion focuses heavily on contributions of the frontal lobe to memory, a topic that has been brought to the forefront of the field in part by the consistent finding of robust frontal activations during various types of memory tasks. Their detailed discussion of the theoretical implications of dissociations between anterior and posterior frontal regions in several task domains illustrates the ever-increasing specificity of neuroanatomical and functional conclusions that can be drawn on the basis of imaging studies.

Rugg combines a refined cognitive analysis of the components of retrieval processes in episodic memory with both electrophysiological and hemodynamic imaging approaches. Distinguishing among processes used to identify the targets of memory search (cue specification), the actual retrieval of target information (episodic recovery), and postretrieval operations involved in assessing retrieved contents (recollection monitoring), Rugg delineates the contrasting neural signature of these components using compelling task designs. Buckner and Schacter likewise examine neural correlates of episodic retrieval processes, and also provide an overview of the emerging cognitive neuroscience of memory errors and distortions. They emphasize and examine the contributions of various frontal regions to strategic components of retrieval, summarize a growing body of evidence indicating that regions within left parietal cortex are associated with the subjective conviction that an item or event has been experienced previously, and also discuss evidence for domain-specific reactivation of particular types of retrieved content. Buckner and Schacter's discussion of memory errors incorporates the idea that memory's imperfections can be divided into seven "sins" that involve various forms of forgetting and distortion. Recent research on the cognitive neuroscience of false memories, using both imaging techniques and behavioral studies of amnesic patients, is helping to unravel the constructive nature of memory retrieval.

Endel Tulving concluded his introduction to the memory chapters in the second edition of this book by observing, "These are exciting times in neurocognitive memory research. Happenings at the horizon point to the next 5 years being even more so." He was right, and there is more to come. Stay tuned.

47 Synaptic Growth and the Persistence of Long-Term Memory: A Molecular Perspective

CRAIG H. BAILEY AND ERIC R. KANDEL

ABSTRACT The elementary events that underlie synaptic plasticity, the ability of neurons to modulate the strength of their synapses in response to extra- or intracellular cues, are thought to be fundamental for both the fine-tuning of synaptic connections during development and behavioral learning and memory storage in the adult organism. Indeed, activity-dependent modulation of synaptic strength and structure is emerging as one of the key mechanisms by which information is processed and stored within the brain. Earlier behavioral studies in vertebrates and invertebrates have shown that the formation of both explicit (declarative) and implicit (nondeclarative) forms of memory consist of two temporally distinct stages: short-term memory lasting minutes to hours and long-term memory lasting days, weeks, or longer. This temporal distinction in behavior is reflected in specific forms of synaptic plasticity that underlie each form of behavioral memory, as well as specific molecular requirements for each of these two forms of synaptic plasticity. In each case, the short-term form involves the covalent modifications of preexisting proteins mediated in part by cAMP and cAMP-dependent protein kinase (PKA) and is expressed as an alteration in the effectiveness of preexisting connections. In contrast, the long-term forms require PKA, MAPK, and CREB-mediated gene expression, new mRNA and protein synthesis, and are often associated with the growth of new synaptic connections. For both implicit and explicit memory storage, the synaptic growth is thought to represent the final and self-sustaining change that stabilizes the long-term process. Here we focus on recent studies of the structural plasticity that accompanies long-term facilitation in *Aplysia* and consider some of the molecular insights provided by these studies into the mechanisms that underlie both the initiation and stabilization of learning-related synaptic growth and the functional role that these structural alterations may play in the different temporal phases of long-term memory storage.

Modern studies in cognitive neuroscience have shown that memory is not a single process but consists of several forms that can be grouped into at least two general categories, each with its own rules (Polster, Nadel, and Schachter, 1991;

CRAIG H. BAILEY Center for Neurobiology and Behavior, College of Physicians and Surgeons of Columbia University, New York, N.Y.

ERIC R. KANDEL Howard Hughes Medical Institute and Center for Neurobiology and Behavior, College of Physicians and Surgeons of Columbia University, New York, N.Y.

Squire and Zola-Morgan, 1991). Explicit or declarative memory is the conscious recall of knowledge about people, places, and things and is particularly well developed in the vertebrate brain. Implicit or procedural memory is memory for motor skills and other tasks and is expressed through performance, without conscious recall of past experience. Implicit memory includes simple associative forms, such as classic conditioning, and nonassociative forms, such as sensitization and habituation. These two forms of memory have been localized to different neural systems within the brain (Milner, 1985). As first shown by neuropsychological studies of a patient, H.M., explicit memory is critically dependent on structures in the temporal lobe of the cerebral cortex, including the hippocampal formation. Implicit memory involves the cerebellum, the striatum, the amygdala, and, in the simplest cases, only the sensory and motor pathways recruited for particular perceptual or motor skills utilized during the learning process. As a result, implicit memory can also be studied in a variety of simple reflex systems, including those of higher invertebrates, whereas explicit forms can best (and perhaps only) be studied in mammals.

Recent cellular and molecular studies of a variety of memory processes, ranging in complexity from simple forms of implicit memory in invertebrates to more complex forms of explicit memory in mammals, suggest that changes in the strength and structure of synaptic connections underlie these diverse forms of memory storage (Kandel, 2001). For both implicit and explicit memory, two types of storage mechanisms have been described. Short-term memory, lasting minutes to hours, involves an alteration in the effectiveness of preexisting synaptic connections as a result of the covalent modification of preexisting proteins. By contrast, long-term memory, lasting days, weeks, or years, is initiated by a program of cyclic adenosine monophosphate (cAMP)-induced and cAMP-responsible element binding protein (CREB)-mediated gene expression, accompanied by the synthesis of new proteins and the growth of new synaptic connections. Thus, at the level of both the nucleus and the synapse, the switch from short-term to long-term memory appears to be a switch from a process-based memory to a structure-based memory. For both implicit and explicit memory storage, the synaptic growth is thought to represent the final and self-sustaining change that leads to the persistence of the long-term memory process (Bailey, Bartsch, and Kandel, 1996).

Despite this association of synaptic remodeling and growth with different forms of learning and memory, surprisingly little is known about the mechanisms that give rise to these structural changes. In this chapter, we address this issue by focusing on recent molecular studies of learning-related structural plasticity in *Aplysia*. We begin by examining the growth of sensory neuron synapses that accompanies long-term sensitization—an elementary form of implicit memory in *Aplysia*. We then consider some of the recent molecular insights that have been provided by these neurobiological studies into the mechanisms responsible for both the initiation and stabilization of the synaptic growth associated with long-term facilitation. Finally, we briefly consider the degree to which the signaling pathways and transcriptional events for synaptic growth and synaptic maintenance are conserved in the two major forms of long-term memory storage.

Synaptic growth and the persistence of long-term sensitization: An implicit form of memory in Aplysia

The nervous system of the marine snail *Aplysia californica* has proved useful as a model system for studying the cellular and molecular bases of learning and memory. It contains only approximately 20,000 large, identifiable nerve cells, clustered into 10 major ganglia. The ability to identify individual neurons and record their activity has made it possible to define the major components of the neuronal circuits of specific behaviors and to delineate the critical sites and underlying mechanisms used to store memory-related representations.

The molecular mechanisms contributing to implicit memory storage have been most extensively studied for the gill withdrawal reflex of *Aplysia* (Kandel, 2001). As is true for other types of defensive reflexes, the gill withdrawal reflex can be modified by several different forms of implicit learning. We will focus here on sensitization, an elementary form of nonassociative learning by which an animal learns about the properties of a single noxious stimulus. The animal learns to strengthen its defensive reflexes and to respond vigorously to a variety of previously neutral stimuli after it has been exposed to a potentially threatening stimulus. In *Aplysia*, sensitization of the gill withdrawal reflex can be induced by a strong stimulus applied to the tail. This activates facilitatory interneurons that synapse on identified sensory neurons and strengthen the synaptic connection between the sensory neurons and their target motor neurons.

As is the case for other defensive withdrawal reflexes, the behavioral memory for sensitization of the gill withdrawal reflex is graded and retention is proportional to the number of training trials. A single stimulus to the tail gives rise to short-term sensitization lasting minutes to hours. Repetition of this stimulus produces long-term behavioral sensitization that can last for days or weeks (Frost et al., 1985; figure 47.1).

Short- and long-term sensitization lead to enhanced synaptic transmission at the monosynaptic connection between identified mechanoreceptor sensory neurons and motor neurons. Although this component accounts for only a part of the behavioral modification measured in the intact animal, its simplicity has facilitated the cellular and molecular analysis of both the short- and long-term forms of sensitization. The monosynaptic pathway can be reconstituted in dissociated cell culture in which serotonin (5-hydroxytryptamine, or 5-HT), a modulatory neurotransmitter normally released by sensitizing stimuli, can substitute for the tail shock used during behavioral training in the intact animal (Montarolo et al., 1986). In parallel to behavioral sensitization, a single application of 5-HT produces short-term changes in synaptic effectiveness, whereas five spaced applications given over a period of 1.5 hours produce long-term changes lasting 1 or more days. These findings of an elementary cellular representation of the short- and long-term memory for sensitization have allowed us to address directly the following question: What are the molecular substrates and regulatory mechanisms that underlie memory storage?

Biophysical and biochemical studies of the connections between sensory and motor neurons in both the intact animal and cells in culture indicate that the short-term and long-term changes share aspects of a common molecular mechanism. Both processes are initiated by 5-HT, and a component of the increase in synaptic strength observed during both the short and the long term is due to enhanced transmitter release by the sensory neuron. This presynaptic increase in excitability is due to the spike broadening that results from the modulation by 5-HT of potassium currents (Klein and Kandel, 1980; Frost et al., 1985; Montarolo et al., 1986; Dale, Kandel, and Schacher, 1987; Scholz and Byrne, 1987).

Despite these several similarities, the short-term cellular changes differ from the long-term modifications in two important ways. First, the short-term change involves only covalent modification of preexisting proteins and an alteration of preexisting connections. Both short-term behavioral sensitization in the animal and short-term facilitation in dissociated cell culture do not require ongoing macromolecular synthesis (Schwartz, Castellucci, and Kandel et al., 1971; Montarolo et al., 1986). In contrast, inhibitors of transcription or translation block the induction of the long-term changes in both the semi-intact preparation (Castellucci

Long-Term but not Short-Term Memory is Dependent on New Protein Synthesis

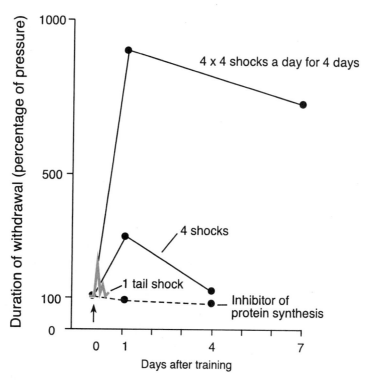

FIGURE 47.1 Behavioral long-term sensitization. A summary of the effects of long-term sensitization training on the duration of the gill and siphon withdrawal reflexes in *Aplysia californica*. The retention of the memory for sensitization is a graded function proportional to the number of training trials. Before sensitization, a weak touch to the siphon causes only a brief siphon and gill withdrawal reflex. Following a single noxious sensitizing shock to the tail, that same weak touch now elicits a much larger response that lasts about 1 hour. More tail shocks increase the size and duration of the response. Application of protein synthesis inhibitors blocks the long-term but not the short-term memory for sensitization (Modified with permission from W. N. Frost et al. Monosynaptic connections made by the sensory neurons of the gill- and siphon-withdrawal reflex in *Aplysia* participates in the storage of long-term memory for sensitization. *Proc. Natl. Acad. Sci. U.S.A.* 82:8266–8269, 1985.)

et al., 1989) and primary cell culture (Montarolo et al., 1986). Most striking is the finding that the induction of long-term facilitation at this single synapse in *Aplysia* exhibits a requirement for protein and RNA synthesis during a critical time window or consolidation period. A variety of forms of memory in both vertebrates and invertebrates share this requirement for macromolecular synthesis during the consolidation period. From a molecular perspective, these studies indicate that the long-term behavioral and cellular changes require the expression of genes and proteins not required for short-term processes. The identification of the gene products required for this consolidation remains a major goal of molecular research into memory processes.

Second, the long-term process, but not the short-term process, involves a structural change (Bailey and Kandel, 1993). Bailey and Chen (1983, 1988a) demonstrated that in *Aplysia*, long-term sensitization training is associated with the growth of new synaptic connections between the sensory neurons and their follower cells.

To study the morphological bases of the synaptic plasticity that underlies both short- and long-term memory, Bailey and Chen combined selective intracellular labeling techniques with the analysis of serial sections to study complete reconstructions of unequivocally identified sensory neuron synapses from both control and behaviorally modified animals (for a review, see Bailey and Kandel, 1993). They found that the memory for long-term sensitization is accompanied by a family of alterations that reflect structurally detectable modifications at two distinct levels of synaptic organization: (1) alterations in focal regions of membrane specialization of the synapse—the number, size and vesicle complement of sensory neuron transmitter release sites (active zones) are larger in sensitized animals than in control animals (Bailey and Chen, 1983, 1988b), and (2) a parallel and more widespread effect involving modulation of the total number of presynaptic varicosities per sensory neuron (Bailey and Chen, 1988a). Sensory neurons from long-term sensitized animals exhibited a twofold increase in the total number of synaptic varicosities, as well as an enlargement in the size of each neuron's axonal arbor (figure 47.2). The duration of the changes in the number of varicosities and active zones parallel the behavioral time course of memory, indicating that only the changes in the number of sensory neuron synapses contribute to the maintenance of long-term sensitization (Bailey and Chen, 1989). These findings suggest that the growth of new sensory neuron synapses may represent the final and perhaps most stable phase of long-term sensitization and provide evidence for an intriguing notion, namely, that the stability of the long-term memory process may be achieved, at least in part, because of the relative stability of synaptic structure.

The growth of new sensory neuron synapses that occurs in the behaving animal during long-term sensitization can be reconstituted in dissociated sensory to motor neuron cocultures by repeated applications of 5-HT (Glanzman, Kandel, and Schacher, 1990; Bailey, Montarolo, et al., 1992). In culture, the structural change can be correlated with the long-term (24-hour) enhancement in synaptic effectiveness and depends on the presence of an appropriate target cell similar to the synapse formation that occurs during development. The nature of this interaction between the presynaptic cell and its target is not known. The signal from the postsynaptic neuron may be cell-associated, such as a constituent of the motor cell's membrane, or diffusible, perhaps being released locally from the motor cell's processes. In both the ganglion and in culture, the long-term increase in the number of sensory neuron varicosities is dependent on new macromolecular synthesis (Bailey, Montarolo, et al., 1992).

Activation of silent synapses and the growth of new functional synapses: Two temporally and morphologically distinct presynaptic changes contribute to long-term facilitation of the Aplysia *sensory to motor neuron connection*

All of the studies of sensory to motor neuron connections mentioned thus far, during both long-term sensitization in the behaving animal (Bailey and Chen, 1983, 1988a,b, 1989) and long-term facilitation in culture (Glanzman, Kandel, and Schacher, 1990; Bailey, Montarolo, et al., 1992), were done on populations of sensory neuron varicosities. Thus, they could not follow structural changes at the same specific synaptic varicosities continuously over time. They also did not examine the functional contribution of presynaptic structural changes to the different temporal phases of long-term facilitation. As a result, these earlier studies could not determine whether the increase in synaptic strength resulted from the conversion of preexisting but nonfunctional (silent) synapses or from the addition of newly formed synapses, or both.

To examine these alternative possibilities, and as a first step in exploring the molecular mechanisms that contribute to learning-induced structural changes, Kim and associates (2003) have recently combined time-lapse confocal imaging of individual presynaptic varicosities of sensory neurons labeled with three different fluorescent markers: the whole cell marker, Alexa-594, and two presynaptic marker proteins, synaptophysin-eGFP, which monitors changes in the distribution of synaptic vesicles within individual varicosities, and synapto-PHluorin (synPH), a monitor of active transmitter release sites (Miesenbock, De Angelis, and Rothman, 1998). They found that repeated pulses of 5-HT induce two temporally, morphologically, and molecularly distinct presynaptic changes: (1) a rapid activation of silent presynaptic terminals through the filling of preexisting empty varicosities with synaptic vesicles, which requires translation but not transcription, and (2) a generation of new synaptic varicosities, which occurs more slowly and does require transcription. The enrichment of preexisting but empty varicosities with synaptophysin is completed within 3–6 hours, parallels intermediate-term facilitation, and accounts for approximately 32% of the newly activated synapses evident at 24 hours. Indeed, when intermediate-term facilitation is isolated from long-term facilitation (Ghirardi, Montarolo, and Kandel, 1995), only the enrichment of empty varicosities occurs, without the formation of new varicosities, suggesting that this redistribution of synaptic vesicles may represent a structural and mechanistic signature of the intermediate-term phase. By contrast, the new sensory neuron varicosities, which account for 68% of the newly activated synapses at 24 hours, do not form until 12–18 hours after exposure to five pulses of 5-HT. These results indicate, for the first time, the synaptic enhancement that underlies long-term facilitation consists of two temporally and morphologically distinct phases: the activation of preexisting silent synapses and the growth of new functional synapses (figure 47.3). The rapid activation of silent presynaptic terminals suggests that in addition to its role in long-term facilitation, this modification of preexisting synapses may also contribute to the intermediate phase of synaptic plasticity and memory storage (Ghirardi, Montarolo, and Kandel, 1995; Mauelshagen, Parker, and Carew, 1996; Sutton et al., 2001).

The redistribution of synaptic vesicle proteins in both preexisting and newly formed sensory neuron synapses is likely to involve cytoskeleton rearrangements (Benfenati, Onofri, and Giovedi, 1999). For example, structural remodeling of synapses in response to physiological activity requires the reorganization of actin (Colicos et al., 2001; Huntley, Benson, and Colman, 2002) and the inhibition of actin function blocks synapse formation and interferes with long-term synaptic plasticity (Hatada et al., 2000; Krucker, Siggins, and Halpain, 2000; Zhang and Benson, 2001). Furthermore, several synaptic proteins such as synapsin can bind to the

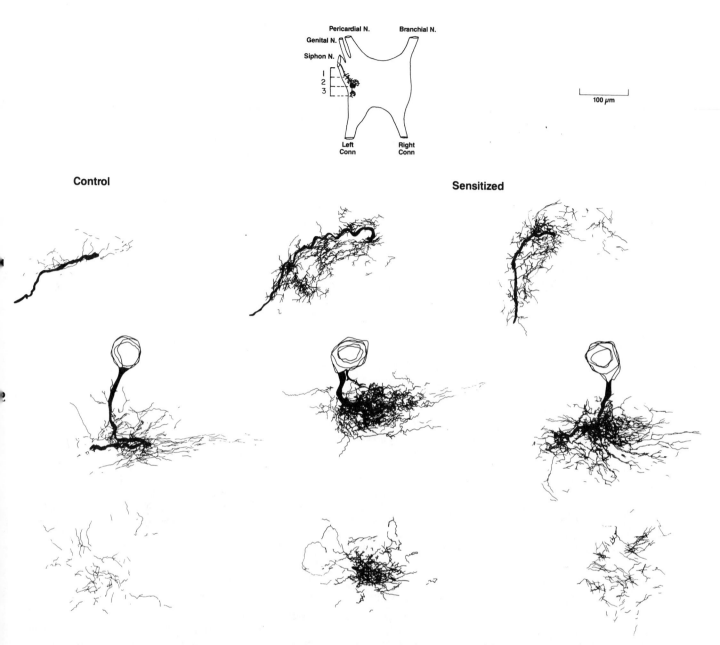

Figure 47.2 Serial reconstruction of sensory neurons from long-term sensitized and control animals. Total extent of the neuropil arbors of sensory neurons from one control and two long-term-sensitized animals are shown. In each case, the rostral (row 3) to caudal (row 1) extent of the arbor is divided roughly into thirds. Each panel was produced by the superimposition of camera lucida tracings of all horseradish peroxidase-labeled processes present in 17 consecutive slab-thick sections and represents a linear segment through the ganglion of roughly 340 μm. For each composite, ventral is up, dorsal is down, lateral is to the left, and medial is to the right. By examining images across each row (rows 1, 2, and 3), the viewer is able to compare similar regions of each sensory neuron. In all cases, the arbor of long-term-sensitized cells is markedly increased compared with the control preparation. (Reprinted with permission from C. H. Bailey and M. Chen, long-term memory in *Aplysia* modulates the total number of varicosities of single identified sensory neurons. *Proc. Natl. Acad. Sci. U.S.A.* 85:2373–2377. © 1988 by the National Academy of Sciences, Washington, D.C.)

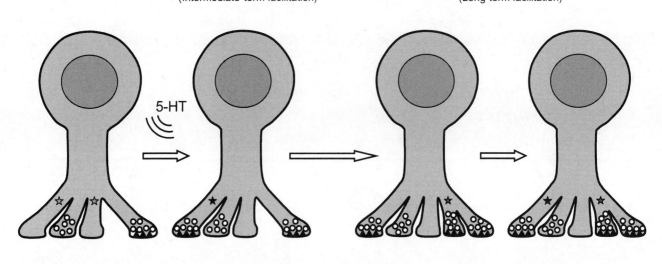

0 hr	3 - 6 hr	12 - 18 hr	24 hr
	(Intermediate-term facilitation)	(Long-term facilitation)	

☆ Empty Synapse   ★ Synapse Filling & Activation of Silent Presynaptic Terminals   ★ New Synapse Formation   ★★ Newly Activated Synapses

FIGURE 47.3   Model of time course and functional contribution of two distinct presynaptic structural changes associated with intermediate- and long-term facilitation. Five pulses of 10 μM 5-HT trigger the redistribution of synaptic vesicles to preexisting silent synapses (3–6 hours) and the formation of new synapses (12–18 hours). The resultant newly filled and newly formed synapses are competent for evoked transmitter release, which is likely to contribute to the synaptic enhancement that underlies long-term facilitation. The rapid activation of silent presynaptic terminals at 3 hours suggests that in addition to its role in long-term facilitation, this modification of preexisting synapses may also contribute to the intermediate phase of synaptic plasticity. Red triangles represent functionally competent release sites (active zones) and empty circles indicate synaptic vesicles. (Reprinted with permission from Kim et al., Activation of preexisting silent synapses and formation of new synapses: Two temporally and morphologically presynaptic changes contribute to intermediate- and long-term facilitation of the *Aplysia* sensory to motor connection. *Neuron* 40:151–165, 2003.)

actin cytoskeleton and participate in synaptic vesicle trafficking (Humeau et al., 2001).

One attractive molecule candidate that may participate in the organization of the cytoskeleton at the presynaptic active zone is the Rho family of small GTPases, which can modulate actin polymerization in response to extracellular signals (Hall, 1998; Luo, 2000) and can be regulated by neuronal activity in vivo (Li, Aizenman, and Cline, 2002). In *Aplysia*, the application of toxin B, a general inhibitor of the Rho family, blocks 5-HT-induced long-term facilitation, as well as growth of new synapses in sensory motor neuron cocultures (Udo et al., 2001). These molecules can be induced or activated by repeated presentations of 5-HT, and thus may promote the assembly, insertion, and functional maturation of active transmitter release sites. The relationship between these signaling pathways and the time course of activation of both preexisting and newly formed synaptic connections are likely to provide new insights into the molecular mechanisms that underlie each class of structural plasticity, as well as their specific contribution to the changes in synaptic function associated with the storage of long-term memory.

At present, it is not clear why more than a half of the sensory neuron varicosities enriched in either synaptophysin-eGFP or synPH were not functional. Perhaps the maturation of transmitter release sites is not yet complete in these varicosities. For example, it has been proposed that there are at least two kinds of preassembled presynaptic packets in developing neurons, one kind that contains synaptic vesicle proteins and another kind that contains active zone components (Friedman et al., 2000; Zhai et al., 2001). It is likely that those varicosities that are enriched in presynaptic vesicle proteins but lack a fully mature active zone would not be functionally competent.

Why do only a specific subset of varicosities become enriched and activated whereas others do not? Since repeated 5-HT treatment leads to a differential enrichment of synaptic vesicle proteins only in specific sensory neuron varicosities, proteins produced locally at each varicosity might contribute to this structural alteration. Alternatively, these proteins might not be synthesized within or nearby each varicosity but might be transported and captured at specific varicosities that have been "tagged" following 5-HT stimulation (Frey and Morris, 1997; Martin et al., 1997).

Thus, the 5-HT-induced enrichment of synaptic vesicle proteins at a specific subset of sensory neuron varicosities and the subsequent functional activation of these previously silent synapses may be one of the local structural consequences of long-term synapse-specific plasticity. Another possibility involves the potential role of the postsynaptic neuron in modulating the 5-HT-induced structural and functional changes observed in presynaptic terminals (Bailey and Chen, 1988a; Glanzman, Kandel, and Schacher, 1990; Bao, Kandel, and Hawkins, 1998; Schacher et al., 1999). This interaction between postsynaptic and presynaptic neurons is critical for the formation and maturation of synapses during development (Tao and Poo, 2001), and is likely to play a key role in both the pre- and postsynaptic expression of the structural plasticity associated with learning and memory storage.

Toward a molecular biology of learning-related synaptic growth in Aplysia

Since the functional and structural changes that accompany long-term sensitization in *Aplysia* require new protein synthesis, Barzilai and colleagues (1989) utilized quantitative two-dimensional gels and [^{35}S]-methionine incorporation to examine changes in specific proteins in the sensory neurons in response to 5-HT. They found that 5-HT initiates a large increase in overall protein synthesis during training and also produces three temporally discrete sets of changes in specific proteins that could be resolved on two-dimensional gels. First, 5-HT induces a rapid and transient increase at 30 minutes in the rate of synthesis of 10 proteins and a transient decrease in five proteins; the increase and decreases subside within 1 hour and are in all cases dependent on transcription. These early changes are followed by at least two further rounds of changes in the expression of specific proteins, some of which are transient and some of which persist for at least 24 hours. The 15 early proteins induced by repeated exposure to 5-HT can also be induced by cAMP. These features—rapid induction, transcriptional dependence, and second-messenger mediation—suggest the possibility that this control might involve a gene cascade whereby early regulatory proteins activate later effector genes. The early proteins induced by 5-HT and cAMP during the acquisition phase of long-term facilitation in *Aplysia* may therefore resemble the immediate-early gene products induced in vertebrate cells by growth factors.

Long-term facilitation requires the activation of cAMP-dependent gene expression and the recruitment of CREB-related transcription factors

Bacskai and associates (1993) first examined how protein kinase A (PKA) participates in this RNA- and protein synthesis-dependent long-term process. They found that with one pulse of serotonin, which produces only short-term facilitation, the free PKA catalytic subunit was restricted to the cytoplasm. However, following repeated pulses of serotonin, which induce long-term facilitation, the catalytic subunit translocated to the nucleus, where it is now spatially positioned to phosphorylate transcription factors and thereby regulate gene expression. Both cAMP and PKA are essential components of the signal transduction pathway for consolidating memories not only in *Aplysia*, but also for certain types of memory in *Drosophila* and mammals. Several olfactory learning mutants in *Drosophila* map to the cAMP pathway (Drain, Folkers, and Quinn, 1991; Davis et al., 1995; Davis, 1996), indicating that blocking PKA function blocks memory formation in flies. In parallel, the late but not the early phase of long-term potentiation (LTP) of the CA3 to CA1 synapse in the hippocampus is impaired by pharmacological or genetic interference of PKA (Frey, Huang, and Kandel, 1993; Huang, Li, and Kandel, 1994; Abel et al., 1997). This interference with PKA blocks longlasting spatial memory in mice without interfering with short-term memory.

The results of these studies in snails, flies, and mice indicate that the long-term modulation of transmitter release requires cAMP-related gene activation. Increasing the concentration of cAMP can induce gene expression by activating transcription factors that bind to the cAMP-responsive element (CRE) (Montminy et al., 1986). The CRE-binding protein CREB (Hoeffler et al., 1988) is a major target of PKA phosphorylation of a regulatory P box, which in turn activates transcription by recruiting the CREB-binding protein CBP (Gonzalez and Montminy, 1989). During long-term facilitation in *Aplysia* neurons, PKA appears to activate gene expression via an *Aplysia* CREB (Dash, Hochner, and Kandel, 1990). Dash and colleagues (1990) first tested the role of CREB in long-term facilitation by microinjecting CRE oligonucleotides into sensory neurons. The CRE oligonucleotide binds to the CREB protein within the cell and thereby prevents it from binding to CRE sites in the regulatory regions of cAMP-responsive genes. Although injection of the CRE oligonucleotide had no effect on short-term facilitation, it selectively blocked long-term facilitation. Kaang, Kandel, and Grant (1993) further explored the mechanisms of CREB activation in long-term facilitation by microinjecting two constructs into *Aplysia* sensory neurons: an expression plasmid containing a chimeric transacting factor made by fusing the GAL4 DNA-binding domain to the mammalian CRE-activation domain, and a reporter plasmid containing the chloramphenicol acetyltransferase (CAT) gene under the control of GAL4 binding sites. Following coinjection of these two plasmids into sensory neurons, exposure to 5-HT produced a 10-fold stimulation of CAT expression. Finally, Bartsch and colleagues (2000) directly demonstrated that CREB is essential for long-term facilitation. They cloned the *Aplysia* CREB gene and showed that blocking expression of one of the CREB1 gene products of the CREB1a protein in sensory neurons by microinjection of antisense oligonucleotides or antibodies blocks long-term but not short-term facilitation. Not only is CREB1a activator necessary for long-term facilitation, it is also sufficient to induce long-term facilitation, albeit in reduced form. Thus, sensory cell injection of recombinant CREB1a phosphorylated in vitro by PKA led to an increase in EPSP amplitude at 24 hours in the absence of any serotonin stimulation.

Initiation of long-term facilitation requires the coordinated regulation of both CREB1 and CREB2

During long-term facilitation, PKA appears to activate gene expression in *Aplysia* sensory neurons via an *Aplysia* homologue of CREB1. Does CREB1 act alone or in concert with other transcription factors? CREB1 belongs to a family of basic region leucine zipper (bZIP) transcription factors that function as homo- or heterodimers. The bZIP domain is bipartite, mediating both dimerization and DNA binding. Bartsch and colleagues (1995) used the dimerization capability of the bZIP domain in a two-hybrid screen in yeast to identify novel *Aplysia* bZIP transcription factors. One of these transcription factors, ApCREB2, has been studied in detail.

ApCREB2 is expressed in the basal state (without exposure to 5-HT) in *Aplysia* sensory neurons and is not induced by 5-HT. Although the sequence of this transcription factor contains a bZIP domain, it does not contain a CREB1-like consensus site for phosphorylation by PKA (the KID domain or P box). In overall primary structure, ApCREB2 is homologous to both human CREB2 and mouse ATF4, transcription factors that act as repressors of CREB1-mediated gene expression (Hai et al., 1989; Karpinski et al., 1992). Indeed, in cotransfection studies in F9 cells, ApCREB2 is a repressor of transcriptional activation by *Aplysia* and mammalian CREB1. Intriguingly, ApCREB2 can function as a PKA-dependent transcriptional activator in certain circumstances. Since ApCREB2 does not contain any consensus PKA phosphorylation sites, PKA may regulate the activity of CREB2 by modifying other bZIP transcription factors that interact with CREB2, including CREB1. Thus, the dimerization partner of CREB2 (and CREB1) may be critical in determining the resultant effect on transcriptional regulation.

To test directly the learning-related role of ApCREB2, Bartsch and colleagues (1995) generated specific antibodies against this transcription factor and injected them into the nucleus of sensory neurons in sensorimotor neuron cocultures. They found that injection of CREB2 antibodies into sensory neurons allowed a single pulse of 5-HT, which nor-

mally induces only short-term facilitation lasting minutes, to evoke facilitation lasting more than 1 day.

This facilitation has all the properties of long-term facilitation: it requires transcription and translation, induces the growth of new synaptic connections, and occludes further facilitation by five pulses of 5-HT. Thus, ApCREB2 is a functional repressor of long-term facilitation, and relief of this repression potentiates the activation process. cAMP-induced gene expression may therefore involve at least two related steps: the activation of CREB1 and relief of the repression of CREB2. The results in *Aplysia* point to the interesting possibility that removal of ApCREB2-mediated repression may be limiting in regulating the long-term increase in synaptic strength.

How might the repression of ApCREB1 by ApCREB2 be relieved? Insofar as there is no significant degradation of the ApCREB2 protein after exposure to 5-HT, covalent modification of ApCREB2 induced by the repeated pulses of 5-HT is likely involved. Indeed, there are changes in phosphorylation of ApCREB2 following repeated exposure to 5-HT. It is interesting that ApCREB2 shares protein kinase C and MAP kinase (MAPK) phosphorylation sites with its human and mouse homologues. Furthermore, MAPK is activated by 5-HT in *Aplysia* neurons, and, like PKA, MAPK translocates to the nucleus with prolonged 5-HT treatment (Martin and Michael, 1997; Michael and Martin, 1998). The translocation of both PKA and MAPK to the nucleus may provide some insight into why long-term facilitation requires repeated pulses of 5-HT. These may be needed to allow persistent activation of both PKA and MAPK so as to activate the activators (CREB1) and relieve the repressors (CREB2). In addition, the pathways regulating each of these processes may have distinct kinetics. Such differences in kinetics could define the optimal time window between training trials and account for the well-established difference between massed and spaced training in both *Aplysia* and *Drosophila*. Perhaps spaced training is more effective than massed training because only spaced training allows the coordinated activation of ApCREB1 and the derepression of ApCREB2. According to this view, the physiological role of ApCREB2 may be twofold. First, it may prevent the long-term process from being turned on adventitiously without repeated exposures to 5-HT. Second, it may regulate the amplitude of synaptic change by integrating the activation of ApCREB1 by PKA with signals from additional second-messenger pathways.

These studies reveal that long-term synaptic changes are governed by both positive and negative regulators, and that the transition from short-term facilitation to long-term facilitation thus requires the simultaneous removal of transcriptional repressors and activation of transcriptional activators. These transcriptional repressors and activators can interact with each other both physically and functionally. It is likely that the transition is a complex process involving temporally distinct phases of gene activation, repression, and regulation of signal transduction. The balance between CREB activator and repressor isoforms is also critically important in long-term behavioral memory, as first shown in *Drosophila*. Expression of an inhibitory form of CREB (dCREB-2b) blocks long-term olfactory memory but does not alter short-term memory (Yin et al., 1994). Overexpression of an activator form of CREB (dCREB-2a) increases the efficacy of massed training in long-term memory formation (Yin et al., 1995).

The CREB-mediated response to extracellular stimuli can be modulated by a number of kinases (PKA, CaMKII, CaMKIV, RSK2 MAPK, and PKC) and phosphatases (PP1 and calcineurin). The CREB regulatory unit may therefore serve to integrate signals from various signal transduction pathways. This ability to integrate signaling as well as mediate activation or repression may explain why CREB is so central to memory storage (Martin and Kandel, 1996; figure 47.4).

Consolidation of long-term facilitation requires induction of the immediate early gene ApC/EBP

The activation of adenylyl cyclase by 5-HT, the generation of cAMP, the activation of PKA, the translocation of the PKA catalytic subunit to the nucleus, and the phosphorylation of CREB1 are all unaffected by inhibitors of RNA or protein synthesis. Where, then, does the RNA and protein synthesis-dependent step that characterizes the consolidation phase appear? Clearly, it must require an additional step—the synthesis of proteins encoded by the genes whose expression is induced by CREB1 and repressed by CREB2.

To examine which genes are downstream from CREB1, Alberini and colleagues (1994) focused on cAMP-regulated transcription factors in order to identify genes expressed during the consolidation of long-term facilitation. Some of the transcription factors known to be activated by cAMP belong to a family known as CCAAT/enhancer-binding proteins (C/EBPs). A member of this family, C/EBP, is expressed in the rat pheochromocytoma PC12 cell line, where it has been shown to be activated by cAMP and to regulate the expression of the *c-fos* gene by binding to the enhancer response element (ERE) in the *c-fos* promoter. Since *Aplysia* neurons contain specific binding activity for ERE, Alberini and colleagues used the ERE binding sequence to isolate a clone encoding a protein that interacted specifically with C/EBP DNA binding sites. The *Aplysia* C/EBP mRNA is expressed at low levels in the basal state, but it is rapidly and transiently induced by 5-HT and cAMP. This cAMP-dependent regulation of ApC/EBP expression may be mediated directly by CREB1, since a CRE site is found upstream of the *ApC/EBP* gene.

Is activation of ApC/EBP critical for the conversion of short- to long-term facilitation? To address this question, Alberini and colleagues (1994) injected ERE oligonucleotides into sensory neurons in sensorimotor neuron cocultures. This selectively blocked the 5-HT-induced long-term facilitation without affecting short-term facilitation. Similar results were obtained by microinjection of either ApC/EBP antisense RNA or an antibody to ApC/EBP. These results suggest that *Aplysia* C/EBP, an immediate early gene activated during the consolidation phase of long-term facilitation, serves as part of a molecular switch for converting short-term to long-term memory.

How long does this transcription factor need to be active? Is the binding of ApC/EBP to its target sequences required throughout the entire maintenance period, or does the facilitation become self-perpetuating as a result of the subsequent expression of effector genes? By injecting ERE oligonucleotides into sensory cells at various times after 5-HT treatment, Alberini and colleagues (1994) demonstrated that ApC/EBP activity was required only during the first 12 hours following training. Therefore, the induction of ApC/EBP during the 5-HT treatment leads to the activation of a cascade of self-perpetuating events essential for the late phase of long-term facilitation.

The existence of C/EBP, a cAMP-regulated immediate early gene transcription factor that regulates other genes, leads to a model of sequential gene activation. CREB1a, CREB1b, CREB1c, and CREB2 represent the first level of control, since all are constitutively expressed. Stimuli that lead to long-term facilitation perturb the balance between CREB1-mediated activation and CREB2-mediated repression through the action of PKA, MAPK, and possibly other kinases. This leads to the up-regulation of a family of immediate early genes. Some of these immediate early genes are transcription factors, such as C/EBP; others are effectors, such as ubiquitin hydrolase, and contribute to consolidation by extending the inducing signal or by initiating the changes at the synapse that cause long-term facilitation.

Recent studies by Guan and colleagues (2002) have examined directly the role of CREB-mediated responses in long-term synaptic integration by studying the long-term interactions of two opposing modulatory transmitters important for behavioral sensitization in *Aplysia*. Toward that end, they utilized a single bifurcated sensory neuron that contacts two spatially separated postsynaptic neurons (Martin and Casadio, 1997). They found that when a neuron receives input—at one set of synapses from the facilitatory transmitter 5-HT—and at the same time receives input from the inhibitory transmitter FMRFamide at another set of synapses, the synapse-specific long-term facilitation normally induced by 5-HT is suppressed, and synapse-specific long-term depression produced by FMRFamide dominates. These opposing inputs are integrated in the neuron's

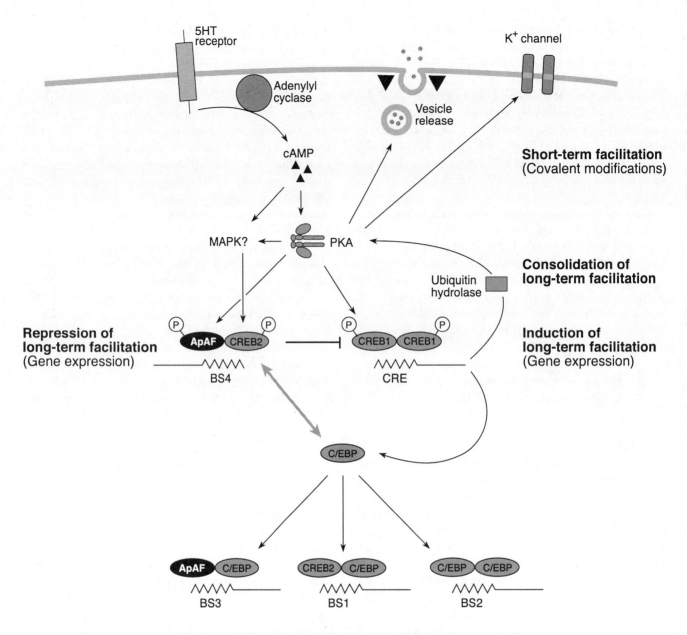

Short-term facilitation
(Covalent modifications)

Consolidation of
long-term facilitation

Repression of
long-term facilitation
(Gene expression)

Induction of
long-term facilitation
(Gene expression)

Stabilization of long-term facilitation
(Structural change)

FIGURE 47.4   Regulation of the transition from short- to long-term facilitation involves the cascade with cooperative action of CREB1, CREB2, ApC/EBP, and ApAF. ApAF is constitutively expressed in sensory neurons, and its level of expression is not affected by 5-HT. Although ApAF can form heterodimers with both ApCREB2 and ApC/EBP in vitro, the major functional role of ApAF for long-term facilitation appears to be downstream from both CREB1 and ApCREB2. On induction of ApC/EBP in sensory neurons by 5-HT, the ApC/EBP protein can interact with ApAF. Since each dimer (ApCREB2-ApC/EBP, ApC/EBP-ApC/EBP, ApAF-ApC/EBP) can bind different DNA motifs (BS1, BS2, and BS3, respectively), the dimerization may serve to broaden the number of genes that can be activated. The major role of ApAF is in the stabilization of long-term facilitation rather than its initiation. In contrast to CREB1a, ApAF alone, even when phosphorylated by PKA, is unable to induce long-term facilitation. In the basal state, the threshold for induction of long-term facilitation is maintained by the functional balance of the products of the CREB1 gene (CREB1a, CREB1b, and CREB1c) and the ApCREB2 repressor. Only when paired with one pulse of 5-HT, which activates PKA and induces CREB1a phosphorylation, does ApAF overexpression convert short-term into long-term facilitation. Once CREB1a is activated and the repression by ApCREB2 is removed, the expression of genes downstream from CREB1, including expression of ApC/EBP, is induced. Thus, ApAF is critical for enhancing and stabilizing gene expression changes induced by phosphorylated CREB1a and derepression of ApCREB2. (Reprinted with permission from Bartsch et al., Enhancement of memory-related long-term facilitation by ApAF, a novel transcription factor that acts downstream from both CREB1 and CREB2. *Cell* 103:595–608, 2000.)

nucleus and are evident in the repression of the CAAT-box-enhanced-binding protein (C/EBP), a transcription regulator critical for long-term facilitation. Whereas 5-HT induces C/EBP by activating CREB1 and recruiting CREB-binding protein to acetylate histones, FMRFamide displaces CREB1 with CREB2 and recruits histone deacetylase to deacetylate histones. When 5-HT and FMRFamide are given together, FMRFamide overrides 5-HT by recruiting CREB2 and the deacetylase to displace CREB1 and CBP, thereby inducing histone deacetylation and repression of C/EBP. Thus, the facilitatory and inhibitory modulatory transmitters that are important for long-term memory in *Aplysia* activate signal transduction pathways that alter nucleosome structure bidirectionally through acetylation and deacetylation.

Activity-dependent modulation of cell adhesion molecules and the initiation of synaptic growth

The products of this network of genes, only a few of which have been identified, ultimately lead to the growth of new synaptic connections between the sensory neurons and their follower cells, a structural change that appears to be required for the persistence of long-term facilitation in *Aplysia*. How might the gene induction contribute to synaptic growth? Of the 15 early proteins Barzilai and colleagues (1989) observed to be specifically altered in expression during the acquisition of long-term facilitation, six have now been identified. Two proteins that increase (clathrin and tubulin) and four proteins that decrease their level of expression (NCAM-related cell adhesion molecules) all seem to relate to structural changes.

Mayford and associates (1992) first focused on the four proteins, D1–D4, which decrease their expression in a transcriptionally dependent manner following the application of 5-HT or cAMP, and found that they encoded different isoforms of an immunoglobulin-related cell adhesion molecule, designated apCAM, which shows greatest homology to NCAM in vertebrates and Fasciclin II in *Drosophila*. Imaging of fluorescently labeled MAbs to apCAM shows that not only is there a decease in the level of expression but that even preexisting protein is lost from the surface membrane of the sensory neurons within one hour after the addition of 5-HT. This transient modulation by 5-HT of cell adhesion molecules, therefore, may represent one of the early molecular steps required for initiating learning-related growth of synaptic connections. Indeed, blocking the expression of the antigen by MAb causes defasciculation, a step that appears to precede synapse formation in *Aplysia* (Keller and Schacher, 1990).

To examine the subcellular mechanisms by which 5-HT modulates apCAM, and the significance this modulation might have for the synaptic growth that is induced by 5-HT, Bailey, Chen, and colleagues (1992) combined thin-section electron microscopy with immunolabeling using a gold-conjugated monoclonal antibody (MAb) specific to apCAM. They found that a 1-hour application of 5-HT led to a 50% decrease in the density of gold-labeled apCAM complexes at the surface membrane of the sensory neuron. This down-regulation was particularly prominent at adherent processes of the sensory neurons and was achieved by a heterologous, protein synthesis-dependent activation of the endosomal pathway, leading to internalization and apparent degradation of apCAM. As is the case for down-regulation at the level of expression, the 5-HT-induced internalization of apCAM can be simulated by cAMP.

The 5-HT-induced decrease in apCAM is thought to have at least two major structural consequences: (1) disassembly of homophilically associated fascicles of the sensory neurons (defasciculation), a process that may destabilize adhesive contacts normally inhibiting growth, and (2) endocytic activation that may lead to a redistribution of membrane components to sites where new synapses form. Thus, aspects of the initial steps in the learning-related growth of synaptic connections that is a hallmark of the long-term process may eventually be understood in the context of a novel and targeted form of receptor-mediated endocytosis.

To further define the molecular mechanisms whereby 5-HT leads to the down-regulation of apCAM, Bailey and colleagues (1997) used epitope tags to examine the fate of the two apCAM isoforms (membrane-bound and GPI-linked) and found that only the transmembrane form is internalized. This internalization was blocked by overexpression of transmembrane apCAM with a point mutation in the two MAPK phosphorylation consensus sites, as well as by injection of a specific MAPK antagonist into sensory neurons. These data suggest that activation of the MAPK pathway is important for the internalization of apCAMs and may represent one of the initial and perhaps permissive stages of learning-related synaptic growth in *Aplysia*. Furthermore, the combined actions of MAPK both in the cytoplasm and in the nucleus suggest that MAPK plays multiple roles in long-lasting synaptic plasticity and appears to regulate each of the two distinctive processes that characterize the long-term process: activation of transcription and growth of new synaptic connections. The differential down-regulation of the GPI-linked and transmembrane forms of apCAM raised the interesting possibility that learning-related synaptic growth in the adult may be initiated by an activity-dependent recruitment of specific isoforms of cell adhesion molecules. In conjunction with the recruitment of the family of CREB isoforms described previously, this may provide a regulatory unit capable of acting sequentially at multiple nuclear, cytoplasmic, and plasma membrane sites during the early, inductive phases of the long-term process.

Han and colleagues (2004) have recently overexpressed in *Aplysia* sensory neurons various HA-epitope tagged recombinant apCAM molecules to examine directly if the down-regulation of the transmembrane isoform of apCAM is required for the synaptic growth that accompanies 5-HT-induced long-term facilitation. They found that overexpression of the transmembrane isoforms, but not the GPI-linked isoform of apCAM, blocked both the long-term synaptic facilitation as well as the long-term enhancement of synaptic growth. This inhibition of long-term facilitation by the overexpression of transmembrane apCAM was restored by interrupting the adhesive function of apCAM with the anti-HA antibody. In addition, long-term facilitation was completely blocked by the overexpression of the cytoplasmic tail portion of apCAM fused with GFP, designed to bind proteins such as MAP kinase p4.2 that might normally bind to the cytoplasm of the sensory neuron. These studies indicate that the extracellular domain of transmembrane apCAM has an inhibitory function that needs to be neutralized by internalization to induce long-term facilitation and that the cytoplasmic tail provides an interactive platform for both signal transduction and the internalization machinery.

Local protein synthesis and the stabilization of synaptic growth

Since long-term synaptic plasticity requires transcription and therefore the nucleus, it raises the question of whether all long-term changes must necessarily be cellwide, or whether a long-term change be restricted to some synapses and not others. To address this question, Martin, Casadio, and colleagues (1997) developed a culture system in *Aplysia* in which a single bifurcated sensory neuron of the gill withdrawal reflex was plated in contact with two spatially separated gill motor neurons. In this culture system, application of a single pulse of 5-HT to one of the two sets of synapses results in a synapse-specific, short-term facilitation of pre-existing connections that lasts for minutes. Five pulses of 5-HT, designed to simulate the spaced training that leads to long-term memory, elicit a synapse-specific long-term facilitation that lasts for 3 or more days. Whereas the short-term form does not require new protein synthesis, the long-term form requires both CREB-dependent transcription and local protein synthesis at activated synapses, and is accompanied by the growth of new sensory neuron synapses. This long-term facilitation as well as the longlasting synaptic growth can be captured by a single pulse of 5-HT applied at the opposite sensory-to-motor-neuron synapse. By contrast to the synapse-specific forms, cellwide long-term facilitation generated by repeated pulses of 5-HT at the cell body is not associated with growth and does not persist beyond 48 hours. However, this cellwide facilitation also can be captured and growth can be induced in a synapse-specific manner by a single pulse of 5-HT applied to one of the peripheral synapses (Casadio et al., 1999).

Thus, CREB-mediated transcription appears to be necessary for the establishment of all four forms of long-term facilitation in *Aplysia* and for the initial maintenance of the synaptic plasticity at 24 hours. But CREB-mediated transcription is not sufficient for the self-maintained stabilization of the plastic changes. To obtain persistent facilitation and specifically to obtain the growth of new synaptic connections, one needs, in addition to CREB-mediated transcription, a marking signal produced by a single pulse of 5-HT applied to the synapse. This single pulse of 5-HT has at least two marking functions. First, it produces a PKA-mediated covalent modification that marks the captured synapse for growth. Second, it stimulates a rapamycin-sensitive component of local protein synthesis, which is required for the long-term maintenance of the plasticity and stabilization of the growth beyond 24 hours.

The finding of two distinct components for the marking signal first suggested that there is a mechanistic distinction between the initiation of long-term facilitation and synaptic growth that does not require local protein synthesis and the stable maintenance of the long-term functional and structural changes that are dependent on local protein synthesis. What might constitute the mark necessary for stabilizing long-term facilitation? Since mRNAs are made in the cell body, the need for the local translation of some mRNAs suggests that these mRNAs may be dormant before they reach the marked synapse. If that is true, then the synaptic mark for stabilization might be a regulator of translation capable of activating mRNAs that are translationally dormant.

In a search for components of the synaptic marking machinery required for stabilization of synapse-specific facilitation, Si and associates (2003) recently identified the *Aplysia* homologue of CPEB (cytoplasmic polyadenylation element binding protein), a protein capable of activating dormant mRNAs. This novel, neuron-specific isoform of CPEB is present in the processes of sensory neurons and is induced in the process by a single pulse of 5-HT. The induction of CPEB is independent of transcription but requires new protein synthesis, and is sensitive to rapamycin and to inhibitors of the P13 kinase. Moreover, the induction of CPEB coincides with the polyadenylation of neuronal actin, and blocking CPEB locally at the activated synapse blocks the long-term maintenance of synaptic facilitation but not its early expression at 24 hours. Thus, CPEB has all the properties required of the local protein synthesis-dependent component of marking and supports the idea that there are separate mechanisms for initiation of the long-term process and its stabilization.

How might ApCPEB stabilize the late phase of long-term facilitation? As outlined above, the stability of long-term facilitation seems to result from the persistence of the structural changes in the synapses between sensory and motor neurons, the decay of which parallels the decay of the behavioral memory. These structural changes include the remodeling of preexisting facilitated synapses as well as the growth and establishment of new synaptic connections. Reorganization and growth of new synapses has two broad requirements: (1) structural (changes in shape, size, and number) and (2) regulatory (where and when to grow). The genes involved in both of these aspects of synaptic growth might be potential targets of ApCPEB. The structure of the synapse is dynamically controlled by reorganization of the cytoskeleton, which can be achieved either by redistribution of preexisting cytoskeletal components or by their local synthesis. The observation that N-actin and Tα1 tubulin (K. C. Martin et al., unpublished observation) are present in the peripheral population of mRNAs at the synapse and can be polyadenylated in response to 5-HT suggests that at least some of the structural components required for synaptic growth can be controlled through CPEB-mediated local synthesis (Kim and Lisman, 1999). In addition, recently CPEB has been found to be involved in the regulation of local synthesis of EphA2 (Brittis, Lu, and Flanagan, 2002), a member of the family of receptor tyrosine kinases, which have been implicated in axonal pathfinding and the formation of excitatory synapses in the mammalian brain. Thus, CPEB might contribute to the stabilization of learning-related synaptic growth by controlling the synthesis of both the structural molecules such as tubulin and N-actin as well as the regulatory molecules such as CAMK11 and members of the ephrin family.

An overall view

One of the unifying principles emerging from the molecular studies of explicit and implicit processes is the unexpected realization that these distinct forms of memory share a common set of genetic mechanisms for long-term storage. In *Aplysia* these mechanisms include a sequence of three steps. First, the initiation step involves the PKA-mediated activation of CREB1 and the derepression of CREB2. Second, the consolidation step involves the induction by CREB1 of a set of immediate early genes, such as the C-terminal ubiquitin hydrolase and the transcription factor ApC/EBP. Third, the stabilization step involves the down-regulation of apCAMs and the growth of new synaptic connections (figure 47.5). Since many studies in the vertebrate brain have now shown that immediate early genes are induced in the hippocampus and certain regions of the neo-cortex by treatments that lead to LTP, it will be of particular interest to investigate whether genes induced by CREB, perhaps of the C/EBP family, are also required for long-term synaptic modifications in mammals.

The finding that long-term memory requires new macromolecular synthesis and is associated with synaptic remodeling and synaptic growth raises three important questions.

First, it raises the question of how the covalent modification of preexisting proteins and the alteration of the strength of preexisting connections during short-term memory become transformed into the growth of new functional synaptic connections. Are these structural changes dependent on, and perhaps induced by, the changes in gene and protein expression in the neurons involved? If so, what are the signaling pathways that trigger gene induction, and what are the downstream molecules and mechanisms that initiate the growth process? Second, the finding of synaptic growth provides a new way of thinking about the stability of long-term memory storage. Is the stability of long-term memory, which would seem to require some mechanism that can survive molecular turnover, achieved because of the relative stability of synaptic structure? If so, what are the cellular and molecular processes that serve to stabilize synaptic structure, and how does this structural reorganization lead to the persistence of memory storage? Finally, the finding that synaptic growth and the formation of new synaptic connections are hallmarks for the long-term process raises the question of how closely these mechanisms for learning-related structural plasticity are conserved in the storage of both implicit and explicit forms of long-term memory.

Beginning insights into some of these questions have come from recent molecular studies of the synaptic growth that accompanies long-term sensitization in *Aplysia*. These studies indicate that long-term memory involves the trafficking of information from receptors on the cell surface to the genome, as seen in other processes of cellular differentiation and growth. Such changes may reflect the recruitment by environmental stimuli of developmental processes that are inhibited in the fully differentiated neuron. A number of studies have shown that the growth changes accompanying long-term memory storage share features in common with synapse formation during neuronal development. In both cases, the structural change exhibits a requirement for new protein and mRNA synthesis. These alterations in transcriptional and translational state can be initiated in the long-term process by the repeated or prolonged exposure to modulatory transmitters that, in this respect, appear to mimic the effects of growth factors and hormones during the cell cycle and differentiation. Thus, modulatory transmitters important for learning and memory activate not only the cytoplasmic second-messenger cascades required for the short-term process but also a nuclear messenger system by which the transmitter can exert a long-term regulation over the excitability and, ultimately, the architecture of the neuron through changes in gene expression.

Studies in *Aplysia* further suggest that the initiation of the subcellular and molecular events that lead to the formation of long-term memory involves the activity-dependent modulation of an immunoglobulin-related cell adhesion

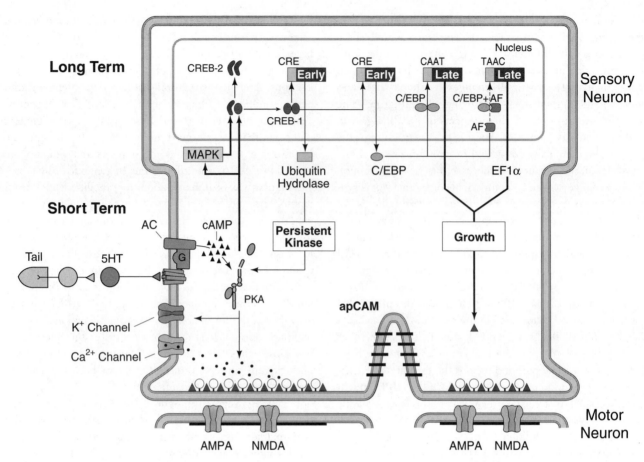

Long Term

Short Term

FIGURE 47.5   Effects of short- and long-term sensitization on the monosynaptic component of the gill withdrawal reflex of *Aplysia*. In short-term sensitization (lasting minutes to hours) a single tail shock causes a transient release of 5-HT that leads to covalent modification of preexisting proteins. 5-HT acts on a transmembrane 5-HT receptor to activate the enzyme adenylyl cyclase (AC), which converts ATP to the second messenger cyclic AMP. In turn, cAMP recruits the cAMP-dependent protein kinase A (PKA) by binding to the regulatory subunits (spindles), causing them to dissociate from and free the catalytic subunits (ovals). These subunits can then phosphorylate substrates (channels and exocytosis machinery) in the presynaptic terminals, leading to enhanced transmitter availability and release. In long-term sensitization, repeated stimulation causes the level of cAMP to rise and persist for several minutes. The catalytic subunits can then translocate to the nucleus,

and recruit the mitogen-activated protein kinase (MAPK). In the nucleus, PKA and MAPK phosphorylate and activate the cAMP response element-binding (CREB) protein and remove the repressive action of CREB2, an inhibitor of CREB1. CREB1 in turn activates several immediate-response genes, including a ubiquitin hydrolase necessary for regulated proteolysis of the regulatory subunit of PKA. Cleavage of the (inhibitory) regulatory subunit results in persistent activity of PKA, leading to persistent phosphorylation of the substrate proteins of PKA. A second immediate-response gene activated by CREB1 is C/EBP, which acts both as a homodimer and as a heterodimer with activating factor (AF) to activate downstream genes (including elongation factor la, EF1α) that ultimately lead to the growth of new synaptic connections between the sensory neurons and their follower cells. (From Kandel, 2001. Originally published in *Science* 294:1030–1038.)

molecule homologous to NCAM. The *Aplysia* NCAM is present in all cells of the developing embryo until the emergence of the nervous system, at which point it becomes expressed exclusively in neurons, and specifically enriched at synapses. These cell adhesion molecules are maintained into adulthood, when they can be down-regulated by 5-HT, a transmitter important for sensitization and classical conditioning in *Aplysia*, and by AMP, a second-messenger activated by 5-HT. This endocytically mediated down-regulation appears to serve as a preliminary and perhaps permissive step for the growth of synaptic connections that accompanies the long-term process. Thus, a molecule used

during development for cell adhesion and axon outgrowth is retained into adulthood, when it seems to restrain or inhibit growth until it is rapidly and transiently decreased at the cell surface by a modulatory transmitter important for learning.

Findings in other invertebrate systems and the mammalian brain suggest that the modulation of cell adhesion molecules is important for long-lasting forms of both developmental and learning-related synaptic plasticity (Martin and Kandel, 1996; Murase and Schuman, 1999; Benson et al., 2000). Indeed, a number of studies in vertebrates have now shown that at critical developmental stages, the refinement of synaptic connections, both their growth and regression, is determined by an activity-dependent process that seems related to LTP in the hippocampus (Constantine, Cline, and Debski, 1990; Antonini and Stryker, 1993; Goodman and Shatz, 1993).

The similarity in the cellular and molecular strategies that underlie enduring forms of learning-related synaptic plasticity appears to reflect the fact that the long-term storage component for both implicit and explicit memory is associated with structural changes and, in particular, the growth of new synaptic connections (Bailey and Kandel, 1993). This stable and self-sustaining long-term process is switched on by the activation of cAMP-responsive genes and the recruitment of CREB-related transcription factors. That the late phase of mossy fiber, Schaffer collateral, and perforant pathway LTP also involves cAMP raises the attractive possibility that, in the hippocampus as well, cAMP and PKA are recruited because they may be able to access the signaling pathways and transcriptional machinery required for synaptic growth and the persistence of memory storage.

ACKNOWLEDGMENTS This work was supported in part by National Institutes of Health grant MH37134 (C.H.B.) and by a grant from the Howard Hughes Medical Institute (E.R.K.).

REFERENCES

ABEL, T. P. V., V. NGUYEN, M. BARAD, T. A. DEUEL, E. R. KANDEL, and R. BOURTCHOULADZE, 1997. Genetic demonstration of a role for PKA in the late phase of LTP and in hippocampus-based long-term memory. *Cell* 88:615–626.

ALBERINI, C. M., M. GHIRARDI, R. METZ, and E. R. KANDEL, 1994. C/EBP is an immediate-early gene required for the consolidation of long-term facilitation in *Aplysia*. *Cell* 76:1099–1114.

ANTONINI, A., and M. P. STRYKER, 1993. Rapid remodeling of axonal arbors in the visual cortex. *Science* 260:1819–1821.

BACSKAI, B. J., B. HOCHNER, M. MAHAUT-SMITH, S. R. ADAMS, B. K. KAANG, E. R. KANDEL, and R. Y. TSIEN, 1993. Spatially resolved dynamics of cAMP and protein kinase A subunits in *Aplysia* sensory neurons. *Science* 260:222–226.

BAILEY, C. H., D. BARTSCH, and E. R. KANDEL, 1996. Toward a molecular definition of long-term memory storage. *Proc. Natl. Acad. Sci. U.S.A.* 93:13445–13452.

BAILEY, C. H., and M. CHEN, 1983. Morphological basis of long-term habituation and sensitization in *Aplysia*. *Science* 220:91–93.

BAILEY, C. H., and M. CHEN, 1988a. Long-term memory in *Aplysia* modulates the total number of varicosities of single identified sensory neurons. *Proc. Natl. Acad. Sci. U.S.A.* 85:2373–2377.

BAILEY, C. H., and M. CHEN, 1988b. Long-term sensitization in *Aplysia* increases the number of presynaptic contacts onto the identified gill motor neuron L7. *Proc. Natl. Acad. Sci. U.S.A.* 85:9356–9359.

BAILEY, C. H., and M. CHEN, 1989. Time course of structural changes at identified sensory neuron synapses during long-term in *Aplysia*. *J. Neurosci.* 9:1774–1780.

BAILEY, C. H., M. CHEN, F. KELLER, and E. R. KANDEL, 1992. Serotonin-mediated endocytosis of apCAM: An early step of learning-related synaptic growth in *Aplysia*. *Science* 256:645–649.

BAILEY, C. H., B. K. KAANG, M. CHEN, C. MARIN, C. S. LIM, A. CASADIO, and E. R. KANDEL, 1997. Mutation in the phosphorylation sites of MAP kinase blocks learning-related internalization of apCAM in *Aplysia* sensory neurons. *Neuron* 18:913–924.

BAILEY, C. H., and E. R. KANDEL, 1993. Structural changes accompanying memory storage. *Annu. Rev. Physiol.* 55:397–426.

BAILEY, C. H., P. G. MONTAROLO, M. CHEN, E. R. KANDEL, and S. SCHACHER, 1992. Inhibitors of protein and RNA synthesis block the structural changes that accompany long-term heterosynaptic plasticity in the sensory neurons of *Aplysia*. *Neuron* 9:749–758.

BAO, J. X., E. R. KANDEL, and R. D. HAWKINS, 1998. Involvement of presynaptic and postsynaptic mechanisms in a cellular analog of classical conditioning in *Aplysia* sensory-motor neuron synapses in isolated cell culture. *J. Neurosci.* 18:458–466.

BARTSCH, D., M. GHIRARDI, A. CASADIO, M. GIUSTETTO, K. A. KARL, H. ZHU, and E. R. KANDEL, 2000. Enhancement of memory-related long-term facilitation by ApAF, a novel transcription factor that acts downstream from both CREB1 and CREB2. *Cell* 103:595–608.

BARTSCH, D., M. GHIRARDI, P. A. SKEHEL, K. A. KARL, S. P. HERDER, A. CHEN, C. H. BAILEY, and E. R. KANDEL, 1995. *Aplysia* CREB2 represses long-term facilitation: Relief of repression converts transient facilitation into long-term functional and structural changes. *Cell* 83:979–992.

BARZILAI, A., T. E. KENNEDY, J. D. SWEATT, and E. R. KANDEL, 1989. 5-HT modulates protein synthesis and the expression of specific proteins during long-term facilitation in *Aplysia* sensory neurons. *Neuron* 2:1577–1586.

BENFENATI, F., F. ONOFRI, and S. GIOVEDI, 1999. Protein-protein interactions and protein modules in the control of neurotransmitter release. *Philos. Trans. R. Soc. Lond B Biol. Sci.* 354:243–257.

BENSON, D. L., L. M. SCHNAPP, L. SHAPIRO, and G. W. HUNTLEY, 2000. Making memories stick: Cell adhesive molecules in synaptic plasticity. *Trends Cell Biol.* 10:473–480.

BRITTIS, P. A., Q. LU, and J. G. FLANAGAN, 2002. Axonal protein synthesis provides a mechanism for localized regulation at an intermediate target. *Cell* 110:223–235.

CASADIO, A., K. C. MARTIN, M. GIUSTETTO, H. ZHU, M. CHEN, D. BARTSCH, C. H. BAILEY, and E. R. KANDEL, 1999. A transient, neuron-wide form of CREB-mediated long-term facilitation can be stabilized at specific synapses by local protein synthesis. *Cell* 99:221–237.

CASTELLUCCI, V. F., H. BLUMENFELD, P. GOELET, and E. R. KANDEL, 1989. Inhibitor of protein synthesis blocks long-term behavioral sensitization in the isolated gill-withdrawal reflex of *Aplysia*. *Science* 220:91–93.

COLICOS, M. A., B. E. COLLINS, M. J. SAILOR, and Y. GODA, 2001. Remodeling of synaptic actin induced by photoconductive stimulation. *Cell* 107:605–616.

CONSTANTINE-PATON, M., H. T. CLINE, and E. DEBSKI, 1990. Patterned activity, synaptic convergence, and the NMDA receptor in developing visual pathways. *Annu. Rev. Neurosci.* 13:129–154.

DALE, N., E. R. KANDEL, and S. SCHACHER, 1987. Serotonin produces long-term changes in the excitability of *Aplysia* sensory neurons in culture that depend on new protein synthesis. *J. Neurosci.* 7:2232–2238.

DASH, P. K., B. HOCHNER, and E. R. KANDEL, 1990. Injection of the cAMP-responsive element into the nucleus of *Aplysia* sensory neurons blocks long-term facilitation. *Nature* 345:718–721.

DAVIS, R. L., 1996. Physiology and biochemistry of *Drosophila* learning mutants. *Physiol. Rev.* 76:299–317.

Davis, R. L., J. Cherry, B. Dauwalder, P. L. Han, and E. Skoulakis, 1995. The cyclic AMP system and *Drosophila* learning. *Mol. Cell Biochem.* 149–150:271–278.

Drain, P., E. Folkers, and W. G. Quinn, 1991. cAMP-dependent protein kinase and the disruption of learning in transgenic flies. *Neuron* 6:71–82.

Frey, U., Y.-Y. Huang, and E. R. Kandel, 1993. Effects of cAMP simulate a late stage of LTP in hippocampal CA1 neurons. *Science* 260:1661–1664.

Frey, U., and R. G. Morris, 1997. Synaptic tagging and long-term potentiation. *Nature* 385:533–536.

Friedman, H. V., T. Bresler, C. C. Garner, and N. E. Ziv, 2000. Assembly of new individual excitatory synapses: Time course and temporal order of synaptic molecule recruitment. *Neuron* 27:57–69.

Frost, W. N., V. F. Castellucci, R. D. Hawkins, and E. R. Kandel, 1985. Monosynaptic connections made by the sensory neurons of the gill- and siphon-withdrawal reflex in *Aplysia* participates in the storage of long-term memory for sensitization. *Proc. Natl. Acad. Sci. U.S.A.* 82:8266–8269.

Ghirardi, M., P. G. Montarolo, and E. R. Kandel, 1995. A novel intermediate stage in the transition between short- and long-term facilitation in the sensory to motor neuron synapse of *Aplysia*. *Neuron* 14:413–420.

Glanzman, D. L., E. R. Kandel, and S. Schacher, 1990. Target-dependent structural changes accompanying long-term synaptic facilitation in *Aplysia* neurons. *Science* 249:779–802.

Gonzalez, G. A., and M. R. Montminy, 1989. Cyclic AMP stimulates somatostatin gene transcription by phosphorylation of CREB at serine 133. *Cell* 59:675–680.

Goodman, C. S., and C. J. Shatz, 1993. Development mechanisms that generate precise patterns of neuronal connectivity. *Cell* 72:77–98.

Guan, Z., M. Giustetto, S. Lomvardas, J.-H. Kim, M. D. Miniaci, J. H. Schwartz, D. Thanos, and E. R. Kandel, 2002. Integration of long-term memory related synaptic plasticity involves bi-directional regulation of gene expression and chromatin structure. *Cell* 111:483–493.

Hai, T. W., F. Liu, W. J. Coukos, and M. K. Green, 1989. Transcription factor ATF cDNA clones: An extensive family of leucine zipper proteins able to selectively form DNA-binding heterodimers [published erratum appears in *Genes Dev.* 1990 Apr. 4(4):682]. *Genes Dev.* 3:2083–2090.

Hall, A., 1998. Rho GTPases and the actin cytoskeleton. *Science* 279:509–514.

Han, J.-H., C.-S. Liu, E. R. Kandel, and B. K. Kaang, 2004. The down-regulation of the transmembrane apCAM isoform in *Aplysia* sensory neurons is necessary for long-term facilitation. *Learn. Mem.* (in press).

Hatada, Y., F. Wu, R. Silverman, S. Schacher, and D. J. Goldberg, 1999. En passant synaptic varicosities form directly from growth cones by transient cessation of growth cone advance but not of actin-based motility. *J. Neurobiol.* 41:242–251.

Hoeffler, J. P., T. E. Meyer, Y. Yun, J. L. Jameson, and J. F. Habener, 1988. Cyclic AMP-responsive DNA-binding protein: Structure based on a cloned placental cDNA. *Science* 242:1430–1433.

Huang, Y.-Y., X. C. Li, and E. R. Kandel, 1994. cAMP contributes to mossy fiber LTP by initiating both a covalently mediated early phase and macromolecular synthesis-dependent late phase. *Cell* 79:69–79.

Huntley, G. W., D. L. Benson, and D. R. Colman, 2002. Structural remodeling of the synapse in response to physiological activity. *Cell* 108:1–4.

Humeau, Y., F. Doussau, F. Vitiello, P. Greengard, F. Benfenati, and B. Poulain, 2001. Synapsin controls both reserve and releasable synaptic vesicle pools during neuronal activity and short-term plasticity in *Aplysia*. *J. Neurosci.* 21:4195–4206.

Kandel, E. R., 2001. The molecular biology of memory storage: A dialogue between genes and synapses. *Science* 294:1030–1038.

Kaang, B. K., E. R. Kandel, and S. G. Grant, 1993. Activation of cAMP-responsive genes by stimuli that produce long-term facilitation in *Aplysia* sensory neurons. *Neuron* 10:427–435.

Karpinski, B. A., G. D. Morle, J. Huggenvik, M. D. Uhler, and J. M. Leiden, 1992. Molecular cloning of human CREB-2: An ATF/CREB transcription factor that can negatively regulate transcription from the cAMP response element. *Proc. Natl. Acad. Sci. U.S.A.* 89:4820–4824.

Keller, Y., and S. Schacher, 1990. Neuron-specific membrane glycoproteins promoting neurite fasciculation in *Aplysia californica*. *J. Cell Biol.* 111:2637–2650.

Kim, C. H., and J. E. Lisman, 1999. A role of actin filaments in synaptic transmission and long-term potentiation. *J. Neurosci.* 19:4314–4321.

Kim, J.-H., H. Udo, H.-L. Li, T. Y. Youn, M. Chen, E. R. Kandel, and C. H. Bailey, 2003. Activation of preexisting silent synapses and formation of new synapses: Two temporally and morphologically presynaptic changes contribute to intermediate- and long-term facilitation of the *Aplysia* sensory to motor connection. *Neuron* 40:151–165.

Klein, M., and E. R. Kandel, 1980. Mechanism of calcium current modulation underlying presynaptic facilitation and behavioral sensitization in *Aplysia*. *Proc. Natl. Acad. Sci. U.S.A.* 77:6912–6916.

Krucker, T., G. R. Siggins, and S. Halpain, 2000. Dynamic actin filaments are required for stable long-term potentiation (LTP) in area CA1 of the hippocampus. *Proc. Natl. Acad. Sci. U.S.A.* 97:6856–6861.

Li, Z., C. D. Aizenman, and H. T. Cline, 2002. Regulation Rho GTPases by crosstalk and neuronal activity in vivo. *Neuron* 33:741–750.

Luo, L., 2000. Rho GTPases in neuronal morphogenesis. *Nat. Rev. Neurosci.* 1:173–180.

Martin, K. C., and E. R. Kandel, 1996. Cell adhesion molecules, CREB and the formation of new synaptic connections during development and learning. *Neuron* 17:567–570.

Martin, K. C., A. Casadio, H. Zhu, E. Yaping, J. Rose, M. Chen, C. H. Bailey, and E. R. Kandel, 1997. Synapse-specific long-term facilitation of *Aplysia* sensory somatic synapses: A function for local protein synthesis memory storage. *Cell* 91:927–938.

Martin, K. C., D. Michael, J. C. Rose, M. Barad, A. Casadio, H. Zhu, and E. R. Kandel, 1997. MAP kinase translocates into the nucleus of the presynaptic cell and is required for long-term facilitation in *Aplysia*. *Neuron* 18:899–912.

Mauelshagen, J., G. R. Parker, and T. J. Carew, 1996. Dynamics of induction and expression of long-term synaptic facilitation in *Aplysia*. *J. Neurosci.* 16:7099–7108.

Mayford, M., A. Barzilai, F. Keller, S. Schacher, and E. R. Kandel, 1992. Modulation of an NCAM-related adhesion molecule with long-term synaptic plasticity in *Aplysia*. *Science* 256:638–644.

Michael, D., and K. C. Martin, 1998. Repeated pulses of serotonin required for long-term facilitation activate mitogen-activated protein kinase in sensory neurons of *Aplysia*. *Proc. Natl. Acad. Sci. U.S.A.* 95:1864–1869.

MIESENBOCK, G., D. A. DE ANGELIS, and J. E. ROTHMAN, 1998. Visualizing secretion and synaptic transmission with pH-sensitive green fluorescent proteins. *Nature* 394:192–195.

MILNER, B., 1985. Memory and the human brain. In *How We Know*, M. Shafto, ed. San Francisco: Harper and Row.

MONTAROLO, P. G., P. GOELET, V. F. CASTELLUCCI, J. MORGAN, E. R. KANDEL, and S. SCHACHER, 1986. A critical period for macromolecular synthesis in long-term heterosynaptic facilitation in *Aplysia*. *Science* 234:1249–1254.

MONTMINY, M. R., K. A. SEVARINO, J. A. WAGNER, G. MANDEL, and R. H. GOODMAN, 1986. Identification of a cyclic-AMP-responsive element within the rat somatostatin gene. *Proc. Natl. Acad. Sci. U.S.A.* 83:6682–6686.

MURASE, S., and E. M. SCHUMAN, 1999. The role of cell adhesion molecules in synaptic plasticity and memory. *Curr. Opin. Cell Biol.* 11:549–553.

POLSTER, M. R., L. NADEL, and D. L. SCHACHTER, 1991. Cognitive neuroscience: An analysis of memory. A historical perspective. *J. Cogn. Neurosci.* 3:95–116.

SCHACHER, S., F. WU, J. D. PANYKO, Z. Y. SUN, and D. WANG, 1999. Expression and branch-specific export of mRNA are regulated by synapse formation and interaction with specific postsynaptic targets. *J. Neurosci.* 19:6338–6347.

SCHOLZ, K. P., and J. H. BYRNE, 1987. Long-term sensitization in *Aplysia*: Biophysical correlates in tail sensory neurons. *Science* 235:685–687.

SCHWARTZ, H., V. F. CASTELLUCCI, and E. R. KANDEL, 1971. Functions of identified neurons and synapses in abdominal ganglion of *Aplysia* in absence of protein synthesis. *J. Neurophysiol.* 34:9639–9653.

SI, K., M. GIUSTETTO, A. ETKIN, R. HSU, A. M. JANISIEWICZ, M. C. MINIACI, J. H. KIM, H. ZHU, and E. R. KANDEL, 2003. A neuronal isoform of CPEB regulates local protein synthesis and stabilizes synapse-specific long-term facilitation in *Aplysia*. *Cell* 115:893–904.

SQUIRE, L. R., and S. ZOLA-MORGAN, 1991. The medial temporal lobe memory system. *Science* 253:1380–1386.

SUTTON, M. A., S. E. MASTERS, M. W. BAGNALL, and T. J. CAREW, 2001. Molecular mechanisms underlying a unique intermediate phase of memory in *Aplysia*. *Neuron* 31:143–154.

TAO, H. W., and M. POO, 2001. Retrograde signaling at central synapses. *Proc. Natl. Acad. Sci. U.S.A.* 98:11009–11015.

UDO, H., H.-L. LI, C. H. BAILEY, E. R. KANDEL, and J. KIM, 2001. A role of rho family GTPases for long-term facilitation and structural change in *Aplysia* sensory-motor neuron co-culture system. *Soc. Neurosci. Abstr.* 27:390.8.

YIN, J. C., M. DEL VECCHIO, H. ZHOU, and T. TULLY, 1995. CREB as a memory modulator: Induced expression of a dCREB2 activator isoform enhances long-term memory in *Drosophila*. *Cell* 81:107–115.

YIN, J. C., J. S. WALLACH, M. DEL VECCHIO, E. L. WILDER, H. ZHOU, W. G. QUINN, and T. TULLY, 1994. Induction of a dominant negative CREB transgene specifically blocks long-term memory in *Drosophila*. *Cell* 79:49–58.

ZHAI, R. G., H. VARDINON-FRIEDMAN, C. CASES-LANGHOFF, B. BECKER, E. D. GUNDELFINGER, N. E. ZIV, and C. C. GARNER, 2001. Assembling the presynaptic active zone: A characterization of an active one precursor vesicle. *Neuron* 29:131–143.

ZHANG, W., and D. L. BENSON, 2001. Stages of synapse development defined by dependence on F-actin. *J. Neurosci.* 21:5169–5181.

48 Domain Specificity in Cognitive Systems

LILA DAVACHI, LIZABETH M. ROMANSKI, MATTHEW V. CHAFEE, AND PATRICIA S. GOLDMAN-RAKIC

ABSTRACT Humans have evolved an extraordinary ability to behave flexibly with respect to achieving desired goals. The cognitive processes that underlie this behavioral flexibility are likely supported by the prefrontal cortex, which has undergone a tremendous expansion coincident with these emerging cognitive capacities. How do regions within the prefrontal cortex relate to phylogenetically older sensory and motor areas? Are cognitive functions organized according to a different set of principles than those that govern sensory and motor areas? This chapter provides insight into how a cognitive process supported by the prefrontal cortex—working memory—is organized. The data summarized discuss the extent to which the prefrontal cortex is organized into domain specific regions based on anatomical connections with high-order sensory association areas. Evidence for a domain specific organization from electrophysiological, neuropsychological, and neuroimaging experiments emerging from both animal and human investigations will be presented.

The majority of species respond to their environment in a stereotypical fashion determined by their evolutionary history and current sensory input. For most organisms, the capacity for behavioral plasticity within the life span of the individual is limited, and adaptation is largely a matter of selection of genetic variation across generations. Change by this mechanism is slow, and the complex behavioral capacities that can result are nonetheless instinctual, reflexive, and comparatively fixed. In contrast to this broad array of stimulus-driven organisms, the human species evolved to acquire an unprecedented capacity for verbal intelligence and forethought. The range and rate of behavioral adaptation increased. Responses to the environment became increasingly flexible, reflecting greater ability to model and predict the external world. What corresponding step occurred in the phylogenetic development of the brain? The mechanisms

that enabled such an unparalleled capacity to behave adaptively with respect to future consequences coincided with the evolution of a greatly enlarged prefrontal cortex in primates in general, and particularly in humans.

The diverse anatomy of the prefrontal cortex gives rise to diverse function. Since both the cytoarchitecture and the connections of prefrontal areas differ, it is not surprising that function differs across these areas as well. However, fractionation of functions within the prefrontal cortex has recently become a hotly debated topic. Although a variety of investigators have long argued for a segregation of functions, based on lesion and electrophysiological data (Fulton, 1950; Mishkin, 1964; Fuster, 1980; Goldman-Rakic, 1987; Wilson, Scalaidhe, and Goldman-Rakic, 1993; Levy and Goldman-Rakic, 2000), some recent work has focused on the homogeneity of working memory processes within the prefrontal cortex (Rao, Rainer, and Miller, 1997; Owen et al., 1998).

One theoretical construct invoked to describe the diversity of frontal lobe organization that many have witnessed is that of domain specificity (Goldman-Rakic, 1987). This hypothesis argues for a segregation of frontal lobe regions based on information domains. It has been written that "the dorsolateral prefrontal cortex as a whole has a generic function—'on-line' processing . . . or working memory," with autonomous subdivisions that process different types of information (Goldman-Rakic, 1987). In this chapter, we discuss recent work from our laboratory that explores, at the level of proximal causation, the functional organization of prefrontal areas involved in working memory, a critical computational resource for neural systems that can sustain internal models of the external world. In particular, we show that prefrontal mechanisms are constrained by content at the cellular, circuit, and areal levels determined by circuit relationships with posterior association cortices. We begin with a review of the cellular underpinnings of these processes.

Cellular specificity of the dorsolateral prefrontal cortex: The neuron's memory field

The human prefrontal cortex accounts for approximately one-fourth of the cerebral surface and has been mapped by

LILA DAVACHI Department of Psychology, New York University, New York, N.Y.

LIZABETH M. ROMANSKI Department of Neurobiology and Anatomy and the Center for Navigation and Communication Sciences, University of Rochester, Rochester, N.Y.

MATTHEW V. CHAFEE Department of Neuroscience, Minnesota Medical School, Minneapolis, Minn.

PATRICIA S. GOLDMAN-RAKIC Section of Neurobiology, Yale University, New Haven, Conn.

a variety of methods, including single-unit recording in non-human primates and functional imaging in both monkeys and humans. Single-neuron recording, however, is the only method currently capable of dissecting the neuronal elements involved in working memory processes. We have applied this method in conjunction with performance on an oculomotor delayed-response (ODR) task, in which the location of a briefly presented visuospatial stimulus is maintained in working memory to provide guidance for subsequent saccadic eye movements (figure 48.1A). An essential feature of this task is that the item to be recalled has to be updated on every trial in an analogous fashion to the moment-to-moment process of human mentation. Similar tasks have become paradigmatic for probing working memory both in animals and in humans, by way of imaging studies (figure 48.1).

Following the seminal report that prefrontal neurons exhibit neuronal firing bridging a stimulus-absent delay period specifically in support of memory functions (Kojima

and Goldman-Rakic, 1984), much research has been conducted to further explore the role of the prefrontal cortex in working memory. In particular, prefrontal neurons with "memory fields" are particularly relevant to our discussion of cellular mechanisms. The concept of a memory field is based on the finding that a given prefrontal neuron increases its firing rate during the delay period of the ODR task only when specific spatial locations are stored in working memory, and this spatial preference is constant across trials. For example, the neuron shown in the upper portion of figure 48.2 is activated consistently on every occasion that the monkey must recall a particular location. Populations of prefrontal neurons similar to this neuron are tuned to a single preferred location, and their level of activity falls off as a function of the distance between that location and the one stored in working memory (Funahashi, Bruce, and Goldman-Rakic, 1989). In instances in which the firing of prefrontal neurons is not maintained through the delay and the activity falters, the animal is more likely to make an error

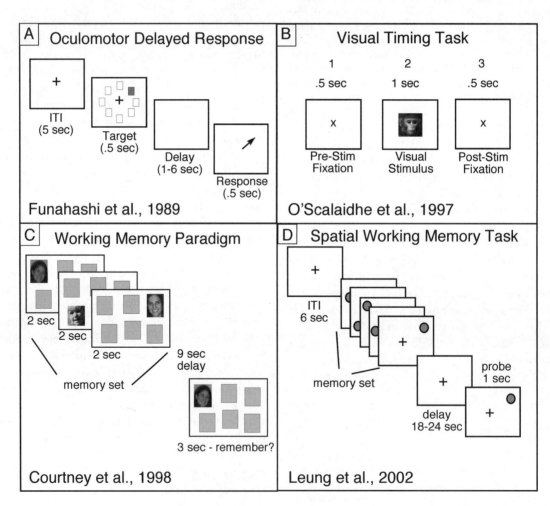

FIGURE 48.1   Common design of working memory paradigms as employed in studies of nonhuman primates (A and B) and humans (C and D). All tasks employ sequential presentation of the item or items to be recalled (in these examples, faces or markers of location), delay periods over which items must be maintained, and recall or response periods.

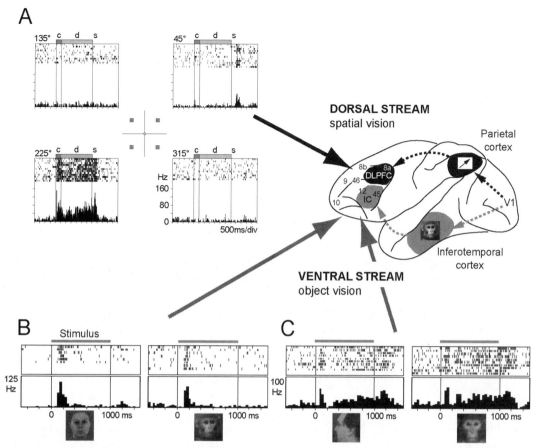

FIGURE 48.2 Spatial and object-processing domains of the primate prefrontal cortex. (*A*) A single neuron with a spatially selective response to a visual stimulus recorded from the dorsolateral prefrontal cortex (DLPFC) of a nonhuman primate while performing the oculomotor delayed-response task. This cell responded with an increase in firing during the cue and delay periods for visual stimuli presented only at 225° eccentricity. (*B, C*) Two cells with phasic (*B*) and sustained activity (*C*) to face stimuli recorded from the inferior convexity of the prefrontal cortex in a monkey while he performed a fixation task. The cell depicted in *B* had a selective response to face stimuli that lasted beyond the stimulus presentation. At top right is shown a schematic of the macaque brain,

depicting the locations in prefrontal cortex of the spatial and object or face domains. The visual spatial domain in DLPFC (black) receives a reciprocal projection from the posterior parietal cortex as part of the continuation of the dorsal visual stream. The inferior convexity (IC, gray), where object or face cells were recorded, receives projections from inferotemporal cortex as part of the ventral visual stream concerned with object and face processing. In the top histogram plots, onset of the visual stimuli is depicted by a colored bar located at the top of the graph. The first task epoch is labeled *c* to indicate the cue period and the second is labeled *d* to indicate the delay period. In the bottom panels, the stimulus period lasted 1000 ms, as indicated by the colored bar on top of the graph.

(Funahashi, Bruce, and Goldman-Rakic, 1989). The finding that neuronal firing is location-specific and directly associated with accurate recall is a dramatic example of a compartmentalized and constrained architecture for memory processing reminiscent of that observed in sensory systems. Highlighting this effect is the finding that, after the creation of small lesions within the dorsolateral prefrontal cortex, very specific mnemonic "scotomas," or memory deficits for particular hemifields or visual field locations, have been demonstrated (Funahashi, Bruce, and Goldman-Rakic, 1993).

Prefrontal neurons are adapted to and defined by the type of data they retain. In this case, single neurons store single spatial locations, and the brain solves the problem of working memory by breaking it down into a set of funda-

mental operations, each performed by a dedicated group of prefrontal neurons. This functional compartmentalization appears to map onto an anatomical one within prefrontal cortex. Individual neurons capable of holding specific visuospatial coordinates "online" have been observed predominantly within the dorsolateral prefrontal cortex, a region occupying the extent of the cortex from the principal sulcus at the lateral edge to the midline of the cerebral hemisphere. In this dorsal prefrontal region, retention of spatial information is the organizing principle: spatial tuning is a common cellular property (Chafee and Goldman-Rakic, 1998), and this spatial storage mechanism is elaborated into discrete neural populations coding the locations either of past stimuli (Chafee and Goldman-Rakic, 1998; Constantinidis,

Franowicz, and Goldman-Rakic, 2001b; Funahashi, Chafee, and Goldman-Rakic, 1993) or of future movements (Funahashi, Chafee, and Goldman-Rakic, 1993). This neural representation of space is influenced by the organization of local circuits within dorsolateral prefrontal cortex such that cells that code the same spatial locations are functionally linked. Neural activity is most strongly correlated when neurons share the same preferred direction and are active during the same epoch of the task (Constantinidis, Franowicz, and Goldman-Rakic, 2001a). The degree of this correlation further depends on whether pyramidal neurons or interneurons are involved (Constantinidis and Goldman-Rakic, 2002). Accordingly, if a volume of this cortical architecture is removed or its normal function is degraded, a circumscribed defect in spatial working memory results, such that monkeys lose online memory for some target locations while other locations are spared (Sawaguchi and Goldman-Rakic, 1991; Funahashi, Bruce, and Goldman-Rakic, 1993). These and other results provide strong evidence at a cellular level that neurons in dorsolateral area 46 and 8A compose a neural architecture for working memory that is dedicated by content, even at the level of specific visuospatial coordinates. The same neuron and local circuit are activated to store the same location and guide the same directional response, trial after trial. Conversely, each location in the visual field is represented by a distinct cohort of neurons in dorsolateral prefrontal cortex.

Although there are significant constraints on the information processing machinery of prefrontal cortex, this does not mean that a prefrontal neuron's sensory, mnemonic, or response-related activity is immutable. Within this modular architecture, mechanisms exist for plasticity in the neurons' responses to changing events. In particular, the memory fields of prefrontal cortex are subject to modulation by neurotransmitters, such as dopamine, serotonin, and the inhibitory neurotransmitter, γ-aminobutyric acid (GABA). Examination of the memory fields of neurons in vivo shows that the mnemonic process can be sculpted by a combination of actions at the soma of a pyramidal cell (Rao, Williams, and Goldman-Rakic, 1999), by serotonergic actions at the level of 5-HT_2 receptors on its proximal dendrites (Jakab and Goldman-Rakic, 1998), and by D_1 dopaminergic action on the spines, the portions of the neuron triggered by excitatory input (Williams and Goldman-Rakic, 1995). These studies show that physiologically realistic changes in the availability of dopamine or serotonin can dramatically alter the tuning of a "working memory" neuron and can either attenuate or enhance the response magnitude. By revealing basic mechanisms of neural plasticity, these findings have the potential to form the groundwork for a rational approach to drug design for cognitive enhancement in aging and in disease (Goldman-Rakic et al., 1996; Goldman-Rakic, 1997).

Network specificity: Neuronal activity patterns in macaque prefrontal and posterior parietal cortex during spatial working memory performance

The aforementioned data identify the dorsolateral prefrontal cortex as a critical element in a neural system that uses working memory to hold specific items of spatial information online. This spatial working memory "area" is coextensive with the projection field of the posterior parietal cortex (Cavada and Goldman-Rakic, 1989). The posterior parietal cortex and dorsolateral prefrontal cortex are joined functionally and anatomically, sharing a common specialization in spatial processing (Andersen, 1995), as well as direct anatomical projections. This functional-anatomical dovetailing provides compelling evidence that the working memory functions of the prefrontal cortex depend on a reciprocal exchange between prefrontal cortex and other areas of association cortex.

To investigate this possibility more directly, we recorded neural activity alternately in both prefrontal area 8a and posterior parietal area LIP of macaque monkeys as they stored spatial locations in working memory in the context of the ODR task. This recording enabled a direct comparison between the patterns of neural activity in the two cortical areas while they were recruited to meet a common behavioral demand. These two populations of cortical neurons are linked by a direct reciprocal projection and share a common, distributed set of physiological signals to encode spatial variables in the ODR task (Chafee and Goldman-Rakic, 1998). Three primary neural populations were distinguished on the basis of the timing of their activation relative to the events of the ODR task: neurons transiently activated by the visual stimulus (cue), others whose sustained discharge maintained the location of the stimulus during the working memory interval (delay), and, finally, neurons transiently activated around the time of the saccadic response (response). We found that each of these functional groups was represented by corresponding neural populations in both prefrontal and parietal cortex. Moreover, functionally corresponding neural populations in the two cortical areas had nearly identical spatial tuning characteristics and were matched in the temporal patterning of their activity (figure 48.3). To determine if neural signals observed within parietal and prefrontal cortex reflected an interaction between the two cortical areas, we reversibly inactivated one of them, in turn, and recorded neural activity in the other while monkeys performed the ODR task (Chafee and Goldman-Rakic, 2000). The results showed that all ODR task-defined patterns of neural activity in either prefrontal or posterior parietal cortex were equally disrupted by remote inactivation, including the activity during the spatial working memory delay period (Chafee and Goldman-Rakic, 2000). No "firewall" was evident in this cortical system to confine signals to one

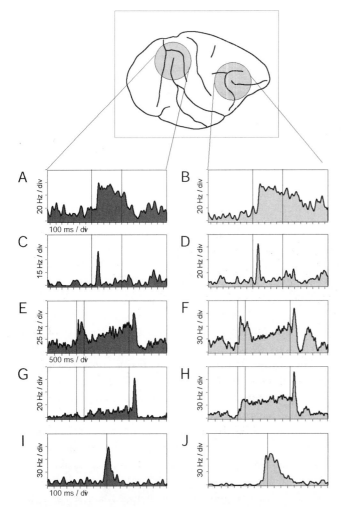

FIGURE 48.3   Prefrontal (area 8a) and parietal (area 7ip) neurons exhibit remarkably similar patterns of activity during spatial working memory tasks. Spike density functions in each panel represent the activity of a single parietal neuron (left column) or prefrontal neuron (right column) during an oculomotor delayed response task in which monkeys made saccades to remembered target locations. Neurons in both cortical areas exhibited (*A* and *B*) tonic cue period activity and (*C* and *D*) phasic cue period activity during the interval of visual stimulation (the two vertical lines in each panel indicate the onset and offset of the visual stimulus). (*E–H*) Neurons in both cortical areas exhibit sustained activity during the delay period intervening between the sensory cue and the motor response (the three vertical lines in each panel indicate, from left to right, cue stimulus onset, offset, and fixation target offset serving as the go-signal for the saccade). In both neural populations, sustained delay period activity is found in various combinations with greater phasic discharge at the time of the sensory and/or motor events. (*I* and *J*) Neurons in both cortical areas exhibited phasic neural activity preceding the onset of the saccadic response (the vertical line in the raster indicates the initiation of the saccade). Neural activity in each cell (*A–J*) varied with the spatial location of the remembered stimulus or pending movement (activity in the preferred direction is shown).

or the other cortical area, or limit the interaction to either feedforward or feedback directions. These data indicate that physiological signals in prefrontal and parietal neurons are system-level events, emerging from interactions between these two cortical areas and possibly others. They also suggest that the afferent innervation from posterior parietal cortex is a pivotal factor in delimiting the functions of the dorsolateral prefrontal cortex.

The interactive model of parietal-prefrontal engagement we have described is also supported by 2-deoxyglucose studies of cortical metabolism in primates during working memory tasks (Friedman and Goldman-Rakic, 1994). Coactivation of parietal and prefrontal neurons, along with their common dedication to the coding of spatial variables, attests to the principle that information shared by interconnected regions of prefrontal and association cortex is domain-specific.

Areal specificity: Multiple working memory domains, multiple modalities, in the prefrontal cortex

The wealth of afferent input from association cortices to the prefrontal cortex permits the processing of a wide variety of sensory information. An important tenet of the domain specificity hypothesis is that subregions of the prefrontal cortex may be organized according to informational domain, each with a specific set of anatomical connections that mediate online processing (Goldman-Rakic, 1987). We have already described evidence for the localization of spatial working memory function to dorsolateral prefrontal cortex. The next question is how the frontal lobe processes other, nonspatial aspects of information. To examine the issue of domain specificity, several studies have contrasted the visual selectivity of neurons in dorsolateral prefrontal cortex with that of more ventrolateral areas, including a region known as the inferior convexity (areas 12 and 45), which lies just below the principal sulcus and just anterior to the inferior limb of the arcuate sulcus (Wilson, O'Scalaidhe, and Goldman-Rakic, 1993; O'Scalaidhe, Wilson, and Goldman-Rakic, 1997, 1999). These studies have determined that neurons within the inferior convexity are selectively activated by object and face stimuli (see figure 48.2). The inferior convexity (or ventrolateral prefrontal cortex) is a likely candidate for processing nonspatial information—color and form—since lesions of this area produce deficits on tasks requiring memory for the color or patterns of stimuli (Passingham, 1975; Mishkin and Manning, 1978). In addition, the receptive fields of neurons in this area, unlike those in areas 46 and 8 on the dorsolateral cortex, represent the fovea (Suzuki and Azuma, 1983), the region of the retina specialized for the analysis of fine detail and color. In the physiological analysis of the inferior convexity, Wilson, O'Scalaidhe, and Goldman-Rakic (1993) used objects and

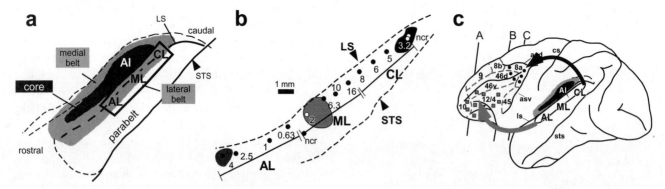

FIGURE 48.4   Connections of the auditory belt cortex with the prefrontal cortex. (*a*) A schematic of the core, belt auditory system, depicting the locations of belt cortical areas AL, ML, and CL. (*b*) Sites of injections of anterograde and retrograde tracers placed into these regions. These injections were physiologically guided, and the best frequencies (numbers in kilohertz) are shown adjacent to each electrode penetration (dots). (*c*) Analysis of the projections

of AL, ML, and CL indicate topographic innervation of rostral and ventral prefrontal cortex (gray squares) by anterior auditory cortex (gray arrow) and projections to caudal and dorsolateral prefrontal cortex (black circles) from caudal auditory cortical regions (black arrow). This dorsal-ventral segregation of auditory inputs is similar to the organization of dorsal and ventral visual streams that process spatial and object information.

faces as memoranda and presented them foveally while monkeys fixated a central point, both in a simple fixation task and in a delayed-response task. Neurons were also tested in a spatial task in order to determine if they had directional preferences. These studies demonstrated that the neurons in the inferior convexity are highly responsive to the sight of complex stimuli, such as pictures of faces or objects, but do not show evidence of directional or spatial selectivity (Wilson, O'Scalaidhe, and Goldman-Rakic, 1993; O'Scalaidhe, Wilson, and Goldman-Rakic, 1997, 1999). Furthermore, the response of object- or face-selective neurons often continues beyond the offset of the visual stimulus in both trained and naive subjects, suggesting that delay period activity reflects an intrinsic property of the neurons' responses. Thus, distinct prefrontal cortical regions process object or face features versus spatial features, with object-face-processing cells confined to the inferior convexity (areas 12 and 45) and spatially selective cells located in dorsolateral prefrontal cortex (areas 46 and 8a).

The anatomical connections of this ventrolateral prefrontal area are indicative of its role in object vision. The inferior convexity, known as Walker's areas 12 and 45 or as areas 12/47 and 45 (Petrides and Pandya, 1999), receives direct projections from areas TE and TEO in inferotemporal cortex (Webster, Bachevalier, and Ungerleider, 1994), both of which are relays in the ventral visual pathway for object vision (Ungerleider and Mishkin, 1982). Neurons in inferotemporal cortex respond selectively to the features of object and face stimuli (Gross, Rocha-Miranda, and Bender, 1972; Rolls and Baylis, 1986). Thus the ventral visual pathway may continue from the inferotemporal cortex to the ventrolateral prefrontal cortex, where neurons are specialized for maintaining the identity of objects and faces online in a manner analogous to the mechanism by which dorso-

lateral prefrontal cortex mediates working memory of visuospatial information.

This segregation of memory domains is not confined to the visual modality. Through a series of anatomical studies, a similar organization was demonstrated for prefrontal auditory processing. In one such study, the lateral belt auditory cortex, areas AL, ML, and CL, was physiologically characterized and injected with anatomical tracers in order to determine the frontal lobe targets (Romanski et al., 1999). These studies revealed that there are highly specific rostrocaudal, frontal–temporal connections, which suggests the existence of separate auditory streams targeting distinct regions of the frontal lobes (figure 48.4). One pathway, originating in the anterior auditory cortex, is reciprocally connected with the frontal pole (area 10), rostral principal sulcus (area 46), and ventral prefrontal regions, including the inferior convexity (areas 12 and 45), whereas the caudal belt is mainly connected with the caudal principal sulcus (area 46) and frontal eye fields (area 8a). Thus, auditory information processing is segregated, with one auditory pathway targeting caudal dorsolateral prefrontal cortex and the other pathway projecting to rostral and ventrolateral prefrontal cortex.

Accordingly, some evidence has surfaced that the dorsolateral and ventrolateral prefrontal regions may process spatial and nonspatial auditory information separately, in a manner that is analogous to the dorsal and ventral visual processing. For example, neurons in the periarcuate region that respond to auditory stimuli are affected by the location of the sound source (Benson, Hienz, and Goldstein, 1981; Azuma and Suzuki, 1984; Russo and Bruce, 1989; Kikuchi-Yorioka and Sawaguchi, 2000) and increase their firing during auditory localization tasks as compared with passive listening. These observations of dorsolateral prefrontal audiospatial function are complemented by the observation that neurons in the caudal belt region, which project to the dorsolateral prefrontal cortex, are sensitive to the location of auditory stimuli (Leinonen, Hyvarinen, and Sovijarvi, 1980; Benson, Hienz, and Goldstein, 1981; Tian et al., 2001). Thus, the caudal principalis and periarcuate regions are the targets of a dorsal, auditory-spatial processing stream, originating in the caudal belt and parabelt, similar to the dorsal visual stream, which terminates in the dorsolateral prefrontal cortex.

Although spatial localization of sounds has been examined physiologically in nonhuman primates, comparable efforts to study frontal auditory processing that mediates communication and nonspatial acoustic signaling are sparse. In previous physiology studies, auditory neurons responded weakly, were seen sporadically, or were not tested with complex acoustic stimuli (Newman and Lindsley, 1976; Benevento et al., 1977; Tanila et al., 1992), and none of these previous studies found a discrete locus for nonspatial auditory processing. Building on previous anatomical studies that predicted an auditory region in ventrolateral prefrontal cortex (Romanski, Bates, and Goldman-Rakic, 1999; Romanski et al., 1999), we have recently described an auditory responsive region in this region (Romanski and Goldman-Rakic, 2002). These experiments indicate that a discrete region of the frontal lobe that includes inferior convexity area 12 (both lateral and orbital) has neurons that respond to complex acoustic stimuli, including species-specific vocalizations. Of note, these neurons do not respond to visual stimuli or saccadic eye movements (figure 48.5). In these experiments, many cells responded to both vocalization and nonvocalization stimuli, but a subset of cells was selectively responsive to vocalizations. Furthermore, the localization of auditory responses to the inferior prefrontal convexity in the nonhuman primate is suggestive of some functional similarities between this region and the inferior frontal gyrus of the human brain (including Broca's area).

Involvement of the prefrontal cortex in auditory processing is further confirmed by clinical studies in humans showing deficits in auditory and language processing following lesions of frontal cortical areas. Large lesions of the lateral frontal cortex in nonhuman primates have been reported to disrupt performance on auditory discrimination tasks (Gross and Weiskrantz, 1962; Goldman and Rosvold, 1970). In many of these studies, ventrolateral prefrontal cortex (VLPFC) or the principal sulcus was included in the lesion.

Thus, separate auditory streams that originate in caudal and rostral auditory cortex and target spatial (dorsolateral) and nonspatial (ventrolateral) domains of the frontal lobe, respectively, may be analogous to the "what" and "where" streams of the visual system. This observation strengthens the domain specificity hypothesis by proving that infor-

mation domains—that is, spatial versus nonspatial—are processed in separate regions of dorsal and ventrolateral prefrontal cortex, respectively, while modality of the information being processed—auditory and visual—is conserved, and may even be integrated across these regions.

Domain specificity of working memory function in human cognition

The advent of noninvasive imaging techniques, such as functional magnetic resonance imaging (fMRI), has allowed investigation of the functional architecture of working memory within the human brain. In agreement with the findings from nonhuman primates, considerable evidence for a domain-specific organization of working memory processes within the human brain has been found. This section presents functional imaging and neuropsychological data supporting a neuroanatomical distinction between object and spatial working memory in the human prefrontal cortex. Evidence for the existence of other potential domain-specific regions within prefrontal cortex will also be introduced.

Considerable data have shown that the ventral prefrontal cortex (specifically, the inferior frontal gyrus) is engaged when subjects are asked to maintain feature or object information in mind in order to guide subsequent behavior. Interestingly, face stimuli seem to selectively activate the inferior frontal gyrus of the prefrontal cortex in humans in a region that is similar to the areas activated by object or face stimuli in single-unit studies of monkeys (Haxby et al., 1996; Courtney et al., 1997; Kelley et al., 1998; Allison et al., 1999). Furthermore, working memory for features of objects has also been shown to engage the same ventral regions of prefrontal cortex (Courtney et al., 1996; McCarthy et al., 1996; Belger et al., 1998; Kelley et al., 1998; Adcock et al., 2000).

A more controversial topic is whether dorsal regions of the prefrontal cortex of humans, homologous to regions within the dorsolateral prefrontal cortex of monkeys, are selectively engaged during spatial working memory. A highly consistent finding across studies of spatial working memory is that activation within the superior frontal sulcal region of the dorsal prefrontal cortex is seen during maintenance of spatial information (Jonides et al., 1993; Baker et al., 1996; Courtney et al., 1996; Owen, Evans, and Petrides, 1996; Carlson et al., 1998; Zarahn, Aguirre, and D'Esposito, 1999; Nystrom et al., 2000; Rowe et al., 2000; Glahn et al., 2002; Pessoa et al., 2002). In fact, Courtney and colleagues (1998) have argued that this more superior region may be analogous to the spatial working memory region within the principal sulcus (area 46) in monkeys, because both this region and the spatial working memory region in the monkey would then sit directly anterior to the frontal eye fields (Courtney et al., 1998). This observation suggests that with the tremendous

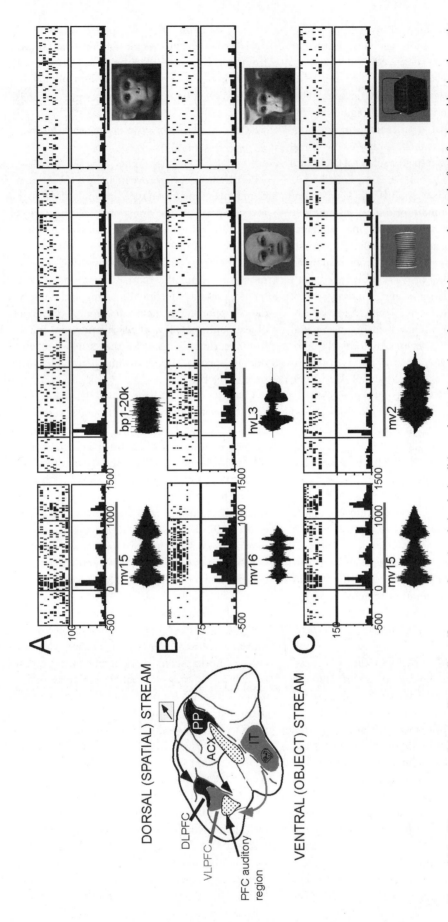

FIGURE 48.5   The responses of three cells to auditory (first two columns) and visual stimuli (second two columns) are shown as histogram plots. At the far left a lateral brain schematic indicates the locations of the visual spatial (black), visual object (gray), and their respective cortical relays. (A) The neuron here responded to both vocalization (first panel, mv15) and nonvocalization stimuli (bp1-20k) with an early phasic burst but did not respond to face or object stimuli. (B) This cell had a more sustained response that was best for both monkey (first panel, mv16) and human (second panel, hvL3) vocalizations. It did not respond to face or object stimuli. (C) Only macaque vocalizations elicited phasic bursts from this cell, while pictures of objects and faces did not evoke a response. The durations of the auditory and visual stimuli are depicted by solid gray (auditory) or black (visual) bars below each histogram. Onset of all stimuli is at time 0. The numbers at the far left for each row of plots indicates the scale in spikes per second. Abbreviations: ACX, auditory cortex, DLPFC, dorsolateral prefrontal cortex; VLPFC, ventrolateral prefrontal cortex; IT, inferotemporal cortex; PP, posterior parietal cortex.

expansion of the human prefrontal cortex during evolution, the putative spatial working memory area may have been pushed dorsally and posteriorly even as it maintained its position relative to other movement-related regions within the prefrontal cortex. However, the prefrontal brain region homologous to area 46 in the monkey, based on cytoarchitectonic criteria (Rajkowska and Goldman-Rakic, 1995), has been shown to lie in the middle frontal gyrus, not in the superior frontal sulcus. Although initial efforts to show activation in the middle frontal gyrus (BA 46) during maintenance of spatial information failed, there have been recent reports that activation here is load dependent and is seen only when the number of memoranda is increased to more than three or four locations (figure 48.6) (Leung, Gore, and Goldman-Rakic, 2002; Rypma, Berger, and D'Esposito, 2002). Furthermore, in addition to showing load-related increases in activation, the middle frontal gyrus has also been shown to be engaged when subjects are asked to retrieve visuo-

spatial information from long-term memory or immediate experience through representation-based action (McCarthy et al., 1994; Nichelli et al., 1994; Baker et al., 1996; Owen et al., 1996; Smith, Jonides, and Koeppe, 1996; Sweeney et al., 1996; Rowe et al., 2000; Stern et al., 2000). Thus, these data support the idea that dorsal and ventral prefrontal cortical regions differentially support working memory processes and are organized based on informational domain.

Other studies, however, have failed to show a strict neuroanatomical distinction between object memory and spatial working memory (Owen et al., 1998; Postle et al., 2000; Stern et al., 2000), with some showing overlapping middle frontal gyral activation during both object and spatial processing. A popular alternative hypothesis is that the prefrontal cortex is organized according to cognitive process and not informational domain, such that simple maintenance of objects and locations will activate ventral prefrontal regions, whereas additional manipulation of this information (such as updating and reordering) will require engagement of the dorsal prefrontal regions (Petrides, 1995; Owen et al., 1999; Curtis and D'Esposito, 2003).

It is possible, on the surface, to adjudicate between these two theories, and, accordingly, many experiments have been conducted manipulating either stimulus type (i.e., object or location) or cognitive process (i.e., maintenance or manipulation) (Owen, Evans, and Petrides, 1996; Owen et al., 1999; Rypma et al., 1999; D'Esposito, Postle, and Rypma, 2000; Rama et al., 2001; Glahn et al., 2002; Hautzel et al., 2002; Sala, Rama, and Courtney, 2003; Veltman, Rombouts, and Dolan, 2003). Disparate findings have emerged and might be attributable to difficulties in achieving process- or domain-pure manipulations. For example, one can imagine engaging in a spatial analysis of geometric objects in order to maintain them in mind over many seconds. Likewise, one might rely on a verbal strategy to label spatial locations (i.e., left quadrant, lower right quadrant) in order to maintain them over a delay period. It should also be kept in mind that the existence of domain specificity for simple maintenance of object and spatial information does not preclude additional neuroanatomical distinctions based on the cognitive operations that are performed.

Recently, an elegant study directly addressed these issues by using object stimuli with more or less spatial features (e.g., houses vs. faces) and compared the activation seen in prefrontal cortex during maintenance of these items with the activation seen during maintenance of spatial locations (Sala, Rama, and Courtney, 2003). The investigators found that the prefrontal activation during maintenance of houses overlapped with that seen during maintenance of spatial location, whereas the activity associated with face maintenance was more distinct from the activity associated with maintenance of both other stimuli and, in agreement with

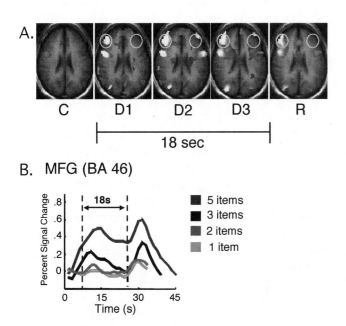

FIGURE 48.6 Activation within middle frontal gyrus (area 46) during spatial working memory tasks increases with increasing load. (*A*) Statistical maps superimposed on anatomical axial section showing significant activations (in hot colors) during maintenance of five spatial locations, compared with a control condition. The same effect was not seen when activation during maintenance of three spatial locations was compared with a control condition. Middle frontal gyrus is delineated by blue circles (C = cue period, D1–D3 = three segments of delay period, 6s each, R = response period). (*B*) Time course percent signal change in the middle frontal gyrus (area 46/9) during maintenance of one, two, three, and five locations. Dashed lines indicate beginning and end of delay period (18 s here). (Adapted from Leung, Gore, and Goldman-Rakic, 2002.) (See color plate 23.)

previous studies, was seen to lie in ventral prefrontal cortex. These data suggest that some objects (such as houses) are perceived in a more spatial fashion, whereas others, including faces, are processed more as a gestalt. In support of this claim, it was demonstrated that behavioral performance of a spatial working memory task is more affected by dual maintenance of house information than by face information (Sala, Rama, and Courtney, 2003), suggesting overlap between neural systems dedicated to spatial and house processing. Furthermore, these data suggest that the disparate findings across studies may be due to the use of different "object" stimuli, such as houses and faces. In addition, they provide support for a segregation of function based on informational domain. However, further work is clearly needed not only to adjudicate between the domain specificity and cognitive process accounts of human lateral prefrontal organization, but also to expand our knowledge of the role that other, more anterior, orbital and medial prefrontal regions play in cognition.

Human imaging has become a powerful means of understanding human cognition. One important caveat of imaging techniques (as well as of single-cell recordings), however, is that the data obtained in these studies cannot reveal whether regions within the prefrontal cortex are *necessary* for object and spatial working memory. However, there is evidence from patients with prefrontal cortical damage, as well as from healthy adults with temporary disruption of prefrontal cortex (e.g., via repetitive transcranial magnetic stimulation, or rTMS), to indicate that intact functioning of the dorsal and ventral prefrontal regions is indeed necessary for spatial and object working memory, respectively. Specifically, it has been reported that a patient with damage to the right superior frontal cortex displayed a selective deficit in spatial working memory without a corresponding deficit in the object or verbal domains (Carlesimo et al., 2001). Conversely, data have been presented suggesting that another patient with damage to left ventral prefrontal cortex was selectively impaired at object working memory (Bechara et al., 1998). Furthermore, attempts to transiently disrupt neural processing in intact humans using rTMS have also provided evidence for a neuroanatomical distinction between dorsal and ventral prefrontal cortex. Robertson and colleagues (2001) showed that rTMS of the dorsolateral prefrontal cortex specifically impaired sequence learning with spatial cues but not with color or combined color and spatial cues (Robertson et al., 2001). Likewise, Mottaghy and colleagues (2002) applied rTMS to dorsomedial, dorsolateral, and ventrolateral prefrontal cortex while subjects performed object and spatial delayed-response tasks. They showed that rTMS of dorsomedial prefrontal cortex disrupted performance on a spatial delayed-response task. Conversely, ventral prefrontal stimulation disrupted performance on a face version of the same task, while dorsolateral prefrontal

stimulation disrupted performance on both tasks (Mottaghy et al., 2002). Thus, these data complement and strengthen the neuroimaging results by showing that domain specificity within prefrontal cortex is fundamental to and underlies cognitive functioning.

Interestingly, in addition to dissociation of spatial and object working memory, other neuroanatomical distinctions that deserve mention have been shown to exist within the human prefrontal cortex. Perhaps the most undisputed and consistent finding that has emerged from the human imaging literature is a domain-specific distinction across prefrontal cortical hemispheres, with the left prefrontal cortex being consistently engaged when verbal material needs to be kept in mind (Paulesu, Frith, and Frackowiak, 1993; Awh et al., 1996; Smith et al., 1998; Chein and Fiez, 2001; Davachi, Maril, and Wagner, 2001; Gruber, 2001), while predominantly right prefrontal cortex is engaged during maintenance of visuospatial information (Brewer et al., 1998; Kelley et al., 1998; Rama et al., 2001). As to the remaining expanse of prefrontal areas, less is known. The evidence from recent studies of the medial wall and orbital surface indicate that these regions are compartmentalized similarly as to informational domain. Baylis and colleagues and others have mapped a taste area in the caudolateral orbitofrontal cortex near an area concerned with olfaction (Tanabe et al., 1974; Baylis, Rolls, and Baylis, 1995; Carmichael and Price, 1995). Studies of orbital lesions in humans have revealed an autonomic pattern of deficits (Damasio, Tramel, and Damasio, 1991), as well as deficits in real-world social contexts (Grattan et al., 1994; Eslinger, Grattan, and Geder, 1995). Interestingly, recent functional imaging experiments have revealed a selective engagement of medial prefrontal cortex when humans cogitate about social agents, including themselves (Kelley et al., 2002; Mitchell, Heatherton, and Macrae, 2002), perhaps representing another domain specific to social knowledge. Whether these prefrontal regions mediate online memory functions remains an issue for further investigation.

Comment

Neurophysiological, neuropsychological, and imaging studies in humans and in nonhuman primates demonstrate the organization of prefrontal cortex into domains, consonant with its anatomical connections. This observation suggests that organisms that primarily respond to sensory input and motor output may have developed the capacity to hold information online by extending sensory responses to persist after the termination of sensory stimulation, and thereby to flexibly instruct responses mediated by stored information, that is, information not available in the immediate stimulus environment. Ultimately, the elaboration of this process may have contributed to humans' ability to behave independently of their immediate stimulus milieu and thereby prepare for, and think about, future consequences of their actions.

ACKNOWLEDGMENT This chapter is dedicated to the memory of Patricia S. Goldman-Rakic, who died on July 31, 2003, and whose seminal contributions to neuroscience will forever affect how we think about the brain and cognition.

REFERENCES

ADCOCK, R. A., R. T. CONSTABLE, J. C. GORE, and P. S. GOLDMAN-RAKIC, 2000. Functional neuroanatomy of executive processes involved in dual-task performance. *Proc. Natl. Acad. Sci. U.S.A.* 97:3567–3572.

ALLISON, T., A. PUCE, D. D. SPENCER, and G. McCARTHY, 1999. Electrophysiological studies of human face perception. I. Potentials generated in occipitotemporal cortex by face and non-face stimuli. *Cereb. Cortex* 9:415–430.

ANDERSEN, R. A., 1995. Encoding of intention and spatial location in the posterior parietal cortex. *Cereb. Cortex* 5:457–469.

AWH, E., J. JONIDES, E. E. SMITH, and E. SCHUMACHER, 1996. Dissociation of storage and rehearsal in verbal working memory: Evidence from positron emission tomography. *Psychol. Sci.* 7: 25–31.

AZUMA, M., and H. SUZUKI, 1984. Properties and distribution of auditory neurons in the dorsolateral prefrontal cortex of the alert monkey. *Brain Res.* 298:343–346.

BAKER, S. C., C. D. FRITH, R. S. FRACKOWIAK, and R. J. DOLAN, 1996. Active representation of shape and spatial location in man. *Cereb. Cortex* 6:612–619.

BAYLIS, L. L., E. T. ROLLS, and G. C. BAYLIS, 1995. Afferent connections of the caudolateral orbitofrontal cortex taste area of the primate. *Neuroscience* 64:801–812.

BECHARA, A., H. DAMASIO, D. TRANEL, and S. W. ANDERSON, 1998. Dissociation of working memory from decision making within the human prefrontal cortex. *J. Neurosci.* 18:428–437.

BELGER, A., A. PUCE, J. H. KRYSTAL, J. C. GORE, P. GOLDMAN-RAKIC, and G. McCARTHY, 1998. Dissociation of mnemonic and perceptual processes during spatial and nonspatial working memory using fMRI. *Hum. Brain Mapp.* 6:14–32.

BENEVENTO, L. A., J. FALLON, B. J. DAVIS, and M. REZAK, 1977. Auditory–visual interaction in single cells in the cortex of the superior temporal sulcus and the orbital frontal cortex of the macaque monkey. *Exp. Neurol.* 57:849–872.

BENSON, D. A., R. D. HIENZ, and M. H. GOLDSTEIN, JR., 1981. Single-unit activity in the auditory cortex of monkeys actively localizing sound sources: Spatial tuning and behavioral dependency. *Brain Res.* 219:249–267.

BREWER, J. B., Z. ZHAO, J. E. DESMOND, G. H. GLOVER, and J. D. GABRIELI, 1998. Making memories: Brain activity that predicts how well visual experience will be remembered. *Science* 281: 1185–1187.

CARLESIMO, G. A., R. PERRI, P. TURRIZIANI, F. TOMAIUOLO, and C. CALTAGIRONE, 2001. Remembering what but not where: Independence of spatial and visual working memory in the human brain. *Cortex* 37:519–534.

CARLSON, S., S. MARTINKAUPPI, P. RAMA, E. SALLI, A. KORVENOJA, and H. J. ARONEN, 1998. Distribution of cortical activation during visuospatial n-back tasks as revealed by functional magnetic resonance imaging. *Cereb. Cortex* 8:743–752.

CARMICHAEL, S. T., and J. L. PRICE, 1995. Sensory and premotor connections of the orbital and medial prefrontal cortex of macaque monkeys. *J. Comp. Neurol.* 363:642–664.

CAVADA, C., and P. S. GOLDMAN-RAKIC, 1989. Posterior parietal cortex in rhesus monkey. II. Evidence for segregated corticocortical networks linking sensory and limbic areas with the frontal lobe. *J. Comp. Neurol.* 287:422–445.

CHAFEE, M. V., and P. S. GOLDMAN-RAKIC, 1998. Matching patterns of activity in primate prefrontal area 8a and parietal area 7ip neurons during a spatial working memory task. *J. Neurophysiol.* 79:2919–2940.

CHAFEE, M. V., and P. S. GOLDMAN-RAKIC, 2000. Inactivation of parietal and prefrontal cortex reveals interdependence of neural activity during memory-guided saccades. *J. Neurophysiol.* 83:1550–1566.

CHEIN, J. M., and J. A. FIEZ, 2001. Dissociation of verbal working memory system components using a delayed serial recall task. *Cereb. Cortex* 11:1003–1014.

CONSTANTINIDIS, C., M. N. FRANOWICZ, and P. S. GOLDMAN-RAKIC, 2001a. Coding specificity in cortical microcircuits: A multiple-electrode analysis of primate prefrontal cortex. *J. Neurosci.* 21: 3646–3655.

CONSTANTINIDIS, C., M. N. FRANOWICZ, and P. S. GOLDMAN-RAKIC, 2001b. The sensory nature of mnemonic representation in the primate prefrontal cortex. *Nat. Neurosci.* 4:311–316.

CONSTANTINIDIS, C., and P. S. GOLDMAN-RAKIC, 2002. Correlated discharges among putative pyramidal neurons and interneurons in the primate prefrontal cortex. *J. Neurophysiol.* 88:3487–3497.

COURTNEY, S. M., L. PETIT, J. M. MAISOG, L. G. UNGERLEIDER, and J. V. HAXBY, 1998. An area specialized for spatial working memory in human frontal cortex. *Science* 279:1347–1351.

COURTNEY, S. M., L. G. UNGERLEIDER, K. KEIL, and J. V. HAXBY, 1996. Object and spatial visual working memory activate separate neural systems in human cortex. *Cereb. Cortex* 6:39–49.

COURTNEY, S. M., L. G. UNGERLEIDER, K. KEIL, and J. V. HAXBY, 1997. Transient and sustained activity in a distributed neural system for human working memory [see comments]. *Nature* 386:608–611.

CURTIS, C. E., and M. D'ESPOSITO, 2003. Persistent activity in the prefrontal cortex during working memory. *Trends Cogn. Sci.* 7: 415–423.

DAMASIO, A. R., D. TRANEL, and H. DAMASIO, 1991. Somatic markers and guidance of behavior: Theory and preliminary testing. In *Frontal Lobe Function and Dysfunction*, H. S. Levin, H. M. Eisenberg, and A. L. Benton, eds. New York: Oxford University Press.

DAVACHI, L., A. MARIL, and A. D. WAGNER, 2001. When keeping in mind supports later bringing to mind: Neural markers of phonological rehearsal predict subsequent remembering. *J. Cogn. Neurosci.* 13:1059–1070.

D'ESPOSITO, M., B. R. POSTLE, and B. RYPMA, 2000. Prefrontal cortical contributions to working memory: Evidence from event-related fMRI studies. *Exp. Brain Res.* 133:3–11.

ESLINGER, P. J., L. M. GRATTAN, and L. GEDER, 1995. Impact of frontal lobe lesions on rehabilitation and recovery from acute brain injury. *NeuroRehabilitation* 5:161–182.

FRIEDMAN, H. R., and P. S. GOLDMAN-RAKIC, 1994. Coactivation of prefrontal cortex and inferior parietal cortex in working memory tasks revealed by 2DG functional mapping in the rhesus monkey. *J. Neurosci.* 14:2775–2788.

FULTON, J. F., 1950. *Frontal Lobotomy and Affective Behavior.* New York: Norton.

Funahashi, S., C. J. Bruce, and P. S. Goldman-Rakic, 1989. Mnemonic coding of visual space in the monkey's dorsolateral prefrontal cortex. *J. Neurophysiol.* 61:331–349.

Funahashi, S., C. J. Bruce, and P. S. Goldman-Rakic, 1993. Dorsolateral prefrontal lesions and oculomotor delayed-response performance: Evidence for mnemonic "scotomas." *J. Neurosci.* 13:1479–1497.

Funahashi, S., M. V. Chafee, and P. S. Goldman-Rakic, 1993. Prefrontal neuronal activity in rhesus monkeys performing a delayed anti-saccade task. *Nature* 365:753–756.

Fuster, J. M., 1980. *The Prefrontal Cortex.* New York: Raven Press.

Glahn, D. C., J. Kim, M. S. Cohen, V. P. Poutanen, S. Therman, S. Bava, T. G. Van Erp, M. Manninen, M. Huttunen, J. Lonnqvist, C. G. Standertskjold-Nordenstam, and T. D. Cannon, 2002. Maintenance and manipulation in spatial working memory: Dissociations in the prefrontal cortex. *NeuroImage* 17:201–213.

Goldman, P. S., and H. E. Rosvold, 1970. Localization of function within the dorsolateral prefrontal cortex of the rhesus monkey. *Exp. Neurol.* 27:291–304.

Goldman-Rakic, P. S., 1987. Circuitry of primate prefrontal cortex and regulation of behavior by representational memory. In *Handbook of Physiology: The Nervous System.* Bethesda, Md.: American Physiological Society, pp. 373–417.

Goldman-Rakic, P. S., 1997. Molecular mechanisms of neuronal communication in cognition. In *Molecular Mechanisms of Neuronal Communication*, K. Fuxe, T. Hokfelt, L. Olson, D. Ottoson, A. Dahlstrom, and A. Bjorklund, eds. Tarrytown, N.Y.: Elsevier Science.

Goldman-Rakic, P. S., L. Bergson, L. Mrzljak, and G. V. Williams, 1996. Dopamine receptors and cognitive function in nonhuman primates. In *The Dopamine Receptors*, K. A. Neve and R. L. Neve, eds. Totowa, N.J.: Humana Press.

Grattan, L. M., R. H. Bloomer, F. X. Archambault, and P. J. Eslinger, 1994. Cognitive flexibility and empathy after frontal lobe lesion. *Neuropsychiatry Neuropsychol. Behav. Neurol.* 7:251–259.

Gross, C. G., C. E. Rocha-Miranda, and D. B. Bender, 1972. Visual properties of neurons in inferotemporal cortex of the macaque. *J. Neurophysiol.* 35:96–111.

Gross, C. G., and L. Weiskrantz, 1962. Evidence for dissociation of impairment on auditory discrimination and delayed response following lateral frontal lesions in monkeys. *Exp. Neurol.* 5: 453–476.

Gruber, O., 2001. Effects of domain-specific interference on brain activation associated with verbal working memory task performance. *Cereb. Cortex* 11:1047–1055.

Hautzel, H., F. M. Mottaghy, D. Schmidt, M. Zemb, N. J. Shah, H. W. Muller-Gartner, and B. J. Krause, 2002. Topographic segregation and convergence of verbal, object, shape and spatial working memory in humans. *Neurosci. Lett.* 323:156–160.

Haxby, J. V., L. G. Ungerleider, B. Horwitz, J. M. Maisog, S. I. Rapoport, and C. L. Grady, 1996. Face encoding and recognition in the human brain. *Proc. Natl. Acad. Sci. U.S.A.* 93: 922–927.

Jakab, R. L., and P. S. Goldman-Rakic, 1998. 5-Hydroxytryptamine2A serotonin receptors in the primate cerebral cortex: Possible site of action of hallucinogenic and antipsychotic drugs in pyramidal cell apical dendrites. *Proc. Natl. Acad. Sci. U.S.A.* 95: 735–740.

Jonides, J., E. E. Smith, R. A. Koeppe, E. Awh, S. Minoshima, and M. A. Mintun, 1993. Spatial working memory in humans as revealed by PET [see comments]. *Nature* 363:623–625.

Kelley, W. M., C. N. Macrae, C. L. Wyland, S. Caglar, S. Inati, and T. F. Heatherton, 2002. Finding the self? An event-related fMRI study. *J. Cogn. Neurosci.* 14:785–794.

Kelley, W. M., F. M. Miezin, K. B. McDermott, R. L. Buckner, M. E. Raichle, N. J. Cohen, J. M. Ollinger, E. Akbudak, T. E. Conturo, A. Z. Snyder, and S. E. Petersen, 1998. Hemispheric specialization in human dorsal frontal cortex and medial temporal lobe for verbal and nonverbal memory encoding. *Neuron* 20:927–936.

Kikuchi-Yorioka, Y., and T. Sawaguchi, 2000. Parallel visuospatial and audiospatial working memory processes in the monkey dorsolateral prefrontal cortex. *Nat. Neurosci.* 3:1075–1076.

Kojima, S., and P. S. Goldman-Rakic, 1984. Functional analysis of spatially discriminative neurons in prefrontal cortex of rhesus monkey. *Brain Res.* 291:229–240.

Leinonen, L., J. Hyvarinen, and A. R. Sovijarvi, 1980. Functional properties of neurons in the temporo-parietal association cortex of awake monkey. *Exp. Brain Res.* 39:203–215.

Leung, H. C., J. C. Gore, and P. S. Goldman-Rakic, 2002. Sustained mnemonic response in the human middle frontal gyrus during on-line storage of spatial memoranda. *J. Cogn. Neurosci.* 14:659–671.

Levy, R., and P. S. Goldman-Rakic, 2000. Segregation of working memory functions within the dorsolateral prefrontal cortex. *Exp. Brain Res.* 133:23–32.

McCarthy, G., A. M. Blamire, A. Puce, A. C. Nobre, G. Bloch, F. Hyder, P. Goldman-Rakic, and R. G. Shulman, 1994. Functional magnetic resonance imaging of human prefrontal cortex activation during a spatial working memory task. *Proc. Natl. Acad. Sci. U.S.A.* 91:8690–8694.

McCarthy, G., A. Puce, R. T. Constable, J. H. Krystal, J. C. Gore, and P. Goldman-Rakic, 1996. Activation of human prefrontal cortex during spatial and nonspatial working memory tasks measured by functional MRI. *Cereb. Cortex* 6:600–611.

Mishkin, M., 1964. Perseveration of central sets after frontal lesions in monkeys. In *The Frontal Granular Cortex and Behavior*, J. K. Warren and K. Akert, eds. New York: McGraw-Hill.

Mishkin, M., and F. J. Manning, 1978. Non-spatial memory after selective prefrontal lesions in monkeys. *Brain Res.* 143:313–323.

Mitchell, J. P., T. F. Heatherton, and C. N. Macrae, 2002. Distinct neural systems subserve person and object knowledge. *Proc. Natl. Acad. Sci. U.S.A.* 99:15238–15243.

Mottaghy, F. M., M. Gangitano, R. Sparing, B. J. Krause, and A. Pascual-Leone, 2002. Segregation of areas related to visual working memory in the prefrontal cortex revealed by rTMS. *Cereb. Cortex* 12:369–375.

Newman, J. D., and D. F. Lindsley, 1976. Single unit analysis of auditory processing in squirrel monkey frontal cortex. *Exp. Brain Res.* 25:169–181.

Nichelli, P., J. Grafman, P. Pietrini, D. Alway, J. C. Carton, and R. Miletich, 1994. Brain activity in chess playing. *Nature* 369:191.

Nystrom, L. E., T. S. Braver, F. W. Sabb, M. R. Delgado, D. C. Noll, and J. D. Cohen, 2000. Working memory for letters, shapes, and locations: fMRI evidence against stimulus-based regional organization in human prefrontal cortex. *NeuroImage* 11: 424–446.

O'Scalaidhe, S. P., F. A. Wilson, and P. S. Goldman-Rakic, 1997. Areal segregation of face-processing neurons in prefrontal cortex. *Science* 278:1135–1138.

O'SCALAIDHE, S. P., F. A. WILSON, and P. S. GOLDMAN-RAKIC, 1999. Face-selective neurons during passive viewing and working memory performance of rhesus monkeys: Evidence for intrinsic specialization of neuronal coding. *Cereb. Cortex* 9:459–475.

OWEN, A. M., A. C. EVANS, and M. PETRIDES, 1996. Evidence for a two-stage model of spatial working memory processing within the lateral frontal cortex: A positron emission tomography study. *Cereb. Cortex* 6:31–38.

OWEN, A. M., N. J. HERROD, D. K. MENON, J. C. CLARK, S. P. DOWNEY, T. A. CARPENTER, P. S. MINHAS, F. E. TURKHEIMER, E. J. WILLIAMS, T. W. ROBBINS, B. J. SAHAKIAN, M. PETRIDES, and J. D. PICKARD, 1999. Redefining the functional organization of working memory processes within human lateral prefrontal cortex. *Eur. J. Neurosci.* 11:567–574.

OWEN, A. M., B. MILNER, M. PETRIDES, and A. C. EVANS, 1996. Memory for object features versus memory for object location: A positron-emission tomography study of encoding and retrieval processes. *Proc. Natl. Acad. Sci. U.S.A.* 93:9212–9217.

OWEN, A. M., C. E. STERN, R. B. LOOK, I. TRACEY, B. R. ROSEN, and M. PETRIDES, 1998. Functional organization of spatial and nonspatial working memory processing within the human lateral frontal cortex. *Proc. Natl. Acad. Sci. U.S.A.* 95:7721–7726.

PASSINGHAM, R., 1975. Delayed matching after selective prefrontal lesions in monkeys (*Macaca mulatta*). *Brain Res* 92:89–102.

PAULESU, E., C. D. FRITH, and R. S. FRACKOWIAK, 1993. The neural correlates of the verbal component of working memory. *Nature* 362:342–345.

PESSOA, L., E. GUTIERREZ, P. BANDETTINI, and L. UNGERLEIDER, 2002. Neural correlates of visual working memory: fMRI amplitude predicts task performance. *Neuron* 35:975–987.

PETRIDES, M., 1995. Impairments on nonspatial self-ordered and externally ordered working memory tasks after lesions of the mid-dorsal part of the lateral frontal cortex in the monkey. *J. Neurosci.* 15:359–375.

PETRIDES, M., and D. N. PANDYA, 1999. Dorsolateral prefrontal cortex: Comparative cytoarchitectonic analysis in the human and the macaque brain and corticocortical connection patterns. *Eur. J. Neurosci.* 11:1011–1036.

POSTLE, B. R., C. E. STERN, B. R. ROSEN, and S. CORKIN, 2000. An fMRI investigation of cortical contributions to spatial and nonspatial visual working memory. *NeuroImage* 11:409–423.

RAJKOWSKA, G., and P. S. GOLDMAN-RAKIC, 1995. Cytoarchitectonic definition of prefrontal areas in the normal human cortex. I. Remapping of areas 9 and 46 using quantitative criteria. *Cereb. Cortex* 5:307–322.

RAMA, P., J. B. SALA, J. S. GILLEN, J. J. PEKAR, and S. M. COURTNEY, 2001. Dissociation of the neural systems for working memory maintenance of verbal and nonspatial visual information. *Cogn. Affect. Behav. Neurosci.* 1:161–171.

RAO, S. C., G. RAINER, and E. K. MILLER, 1997. Integration of what and where in the primate prefrontal cortex. *Science* 276:821–824.

RAO, S. G., G. V. WILLIAMS, and P. S. GOLDMAN-RAKIC, 1999. Isodirectional tuning of adjacent interneurons and pyramidal cells during working memory: Evidence for microcolumnar organization in PFC. *J. Neurophysiol.* 81:1903–1916.

ROBERTSON, E. M., J. M. TORMOS, F. MAEDA, and A. PASCUAL-LEONE, 2001. The role of the dorsolateral prefrontal cortex during sequence learning is specific for spatial information. *Cereb. Cortex* 11:628–635.

ROLLS, E. T., and G. C. BAYLIS, 1986. Size and contrast have only small effects on the responses to faces of neurons in the cortex of the superior temporal sulcus of the monkey. *Exp. Brain Res.* 65:38–48.

ROMANSKI, L. M., J. F. BATES, and P. S. GOLDMAN-RAKIC, 1999. Auditory belt and parabelt projections to the prefrontal cortex in the rhesus monkey. *J. Comp. Neurol.* 403:141–157.

ROMANSKI, L. M., and P. S. GOLDMAN-RAKIC, 2002. An auditory domain in primate prefrontal cortex. *Nat. Neurosci.* 5:15–16.

ROMANSKI, L. M., B. TIAN, J. FRITZ, M. MISHKIN, P. S. GOLDMAN-RAKIC, and J. P. RAUSCHECKER, 1999. Dual streams of auditory afferents target multiple domains in the primate prefrontal cortex. *Nat. Neurosci.* 2:1131–1136.

ROWE, J. B., I. TONI, O. JOSEPHS, R. S. FRACKOWIAK, and R. E. PASSINGHAM, 2000. The prefrontal cortex: Response selection or maintenance within working memory? *Science* 288:1656–1660.

RUSSO, G. S., and C. J. BRUCE, 1989. Auditory receptive fields of neurons in frontal cortex of rhesus monkey shift with direction of gaze. *Soc. Neurosci. Abstr.* 15:1204.

RYPMA, B., J. S. BERGER, and M. D'ESPOSITO, 2002. The influence of working-memory demand and subject performance on prefrontal cortical activity. *J. Cogn. Neurosci.* 14:721–731.

RYPMA, B., V. PRABHAKARAN, J. E. DESMOND, G. H. GLOVER, and J. D. GABRIELI, 1999. Load-dependent roles of frontal brain regions in the maintenance of working memory. *NeuroImage* 9:216–226.

SALA, J. B., P. RAMA, and S. M. COURTNEY, 2003. Functional topography of a distributed neural system for spatial and nonspatial information maintenance in working memory. *Neuropsychologia* 41:341–356.

SAWAGUCHI, T., and P. S. GOLDMAN-RAKIC, 1991. D1 dopamine receptors in prefrontal cortex: Involvement in working memory. *Science* 251:947–950.

SMITH, E. E., J. JONIDES, and R. A. KOEPPE, 1996. Dissociating verbal and spatial working memory using PET. *Cereb. Cortex* 6:11–20.

SMITH, E. E., J. JONIDES, C. MARSHUETZ, and R. A. KOEPPE, 1998. Components of verbal working memory: Evidence from neuroimaging. *Proc. Natl. Acad. Sci. U.S.A.* 95:876–882.

STERN, C. E., A. M. OWEN, I. TRACEY, R. B. LOOK, B. R. ROSEN, and M. PETRIDES, 2000. Activity in ventrolateral and mid-dorsolateral prefrontal cortex during nonspatial visual working memory processing: Evidence from functional magnetic resonance imaging. *NeuroImage* 11:392–399.

SUZUKI, H., and M. AZUMA, 1983. Topographic studies on visual neurons in the dorsolateral prefrontal cortex of the monkey. *Exp. Brain Res.* 53:47–58.

SWEENEY, J. A., M. A. MINTUN, S. KWEE, M. B. WISEMAN, D. L. BROWN, D. R. ROSENBERG, and J. R. CARL, 1996. Positron emission tomography study of voluntary saccadic eye movements and spatial working memory. *J. Neurophysiol.* 75:454–468.

TANABE, T., M. IINO, Y. OOSHIMA, and S. F. TAKAGI, 1974. An olfactory area in the prefrontal lobe. *Brain Res.* 80:127–130.

TANILA, H., S. CARLSON, I. LINNANKOSKI, F. LINDROOS, and H. KAHILA, 1992. Functional properties of dorsolateral prefrontal cortical neurons in awake monkey. *Behav. Brain Res.* 47:169–180.

TIAN, B., D. RESER, A. DURHAM, A. KUSTOV, and J. P. RAUSCHECKER, 2001. Functional specialization in rhesus monkey auditory cortex. *Science* 292:290–293.

UNGERLEIDER, L. G., and M. MISHKIN, 1982. Two cortical visual systems. In *Analysis of Visual Behavior*, D. J. Ingle, M. A. Goodale, and R. J. W. Mansfield, eds. Cambridge, Mass.: MIT Press, pp. 549–586.

VELTMAN, D. J., S. A. ROMBOUTS, and R. J. DOLAN, 2003. Maintenance versus manipulation in verbal working memory revisited: An fMRI study. *NeuroImage* 18:247–256.

WEBSTER, M. J., J. BACHEVALIER, and L. G. UNGERLEIDER, 1994. Connections of inferior temporal areas TEO and TE with parietal and frontal cortex in macaque monkeys. *Cereb. Cortex* 4:470–483.

WILLIAMS, G. V., and P. S. GOLDMAN-RAKIC, 1995. Modulation of memory fields by dopamine D1 receptors in prefrontal cortex. *Nature* 376:572–575.

WILSON, F. A., S. P. O'SCALAIDHE, and P. S. GOLDMAN-RAKIC, 1993. Dissociation of object and spatial processing domains in primate prefrontal cortex. *Science* 260:1955–1958.

ZARAHN, E., G. K. AGUIRRE, and M. D'ESPOSITO, 1999. Temporal isolation of the neural correlates of spatial mnemonic processing with fMRI. *Brain Res. Cogn. Brain Res.* 7:255–268.

49 An Information Processing Framework for Memory Representation by the Hippocampus

HOWARD EICHENBAUM

ABSTRACT Declarative memory is composed of episodic memory, the capacity to recall unique experiences, and semantic memory, our body of general knowledge. This chapter outlines a simple model of information processing in the hippocampus that could mediate these two components of declarative memory. The model is based on biologically realistic properties of hippocampal circuitry and plasticity that support the representation of sequences of events and the linkage of sequence representations into relational networks that support inferential memory expression. In support of the model, neuropsychological evidence shows that the hippocampus is critical to the capacity to remember the order of events in unique experiences and to the creation of relational networks that support inferential memory expression. Complementary recording studies show that hippocampal neurons encode sequences of events, including both conjunctions of stimuli, actions, and places that compose events in unique experiences and features of events that are common across experiences and could link episodic representations. Furthermore, the hippocampus creates distinct and linked representations for experiences in both nonspatial and spatial tests of memory. Finally, while the hippocampus is critical to the creation and use of relational memory networks, it seems likely that detailed representations of experience are not stored in the hippocampus. Rather, it is likely that the hippocampus coordinates and organizes detailed memory representations stored in widespread areas of cortex.

There is general agreement that the hippocampus and related brain areas mediate declarative (or explicit) memory in humans. However, little is known about the fundamental cognitive mechanisms supported by the hippocampus. Nor is there a clear insight into the nature of the neural network representations within the hippocampus that underlie declarative memory. In this chapter, I outline a framework for information processing by the hippocampus and related cortical structures in declarative memory. This model is biologically realistic in that it is based on known circuitry and

plasticity properties of the hippocampus. It is cognitively robust in that it can account for the major features of declarative memory as observed in humans.

The chapter begins with an overview of the fundamental features of declarative memory. This discussion is followed by an outline of the qualitative model of hippocampal network representation built on known properties of its circuitry and plasticity. The model is supported with evidence from neuropsychological studies that identify memory performance dependent on the hippocampus, and from neurophysiological studies that characterize the nature of information encoded by hippocampal neurons. Finally, I will show how this framework can account for spatial as well as nonspatial memory in rodents and humans.

Declarative memory

One of the major breakthroughs in memory research was the demonstration that the hippocampal region is critical for declarative or explicit memory (Cohen and Squire, 1980; see Schacter and Tulving, 1994; Eichenbaum and Cohen, 2001). Declarative memory is generally conceived of as a combination of episodic memory, our record of unique personal experiences, and semantic memory, our general world knowledge. These two kinds of memory are typically distinguished by their contents and their organization. Tulving (1983, 2002) described episodic memory as the capacity to mentally travel back to a previous time in one's life and reexperience a particular event. The contents of episodic memory involve autobiographical information, and episodic memory is organized along temporal dimensions. By contrast, the contents of semantic memory involve an accumulation of time-independent factual information and semantic memory is organized by logical and abstract dimensions. In addition, declarative memory is distinct from other forms of memory in that declarative memories are subject to conscious recollection, the capacity to bring

HOWARD EICHENBAUM Center for Memory and Brain, Boston University, Boston, Mass.

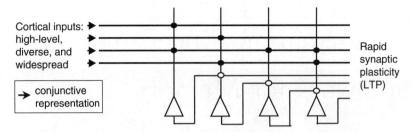

Recurrent connections: widespread, sparse-asymmetrical, mainly excitatory

→ sequential activation

FIGURE 49.1 Schematic diagram of circuitry of the principal cells in hippocampal area CA3 that could mediate properties of declarative memory. Two major pathways are shown, one pathway involving inputs from diverse neocortical association areas that send widespread projections to the dendrites of pyramidal cells and the other pathway involving recurrent, sparse projections from pyramidal cells to other pyramidal cells in the same network. Connections of both of these pathways are subject to activity-dependent rapid synaptic plasticity.

memories up to conscious experience and manipulation. Although declarative memories are typically subject to verbal expression, verbal expression per se is not a requisite feature. Indeed, declarative memory is characterized by its broad range of expression. As such, declarative memory expression is described as flexible in that the contents of memory can guide a variety of behaviors and in a variety of situations outside of repetition of the learning event.

Although these properties are common in descriptions of declarative memory, it is not obvious how they are integrated with one another. In particular, to the extent that we distinguish episodic and semantic memory by their fundamental organizing features (Tulving, 1983, 2002), it becomes difficult to conceive how they also share a common organization within the same memory system. It is also unclear how flexible expression emerges as a property of both episodic and semantic memory. In addition, explaining the generation of conscious experience in recollection remains a major challenge. It is not obvious what biologically realistic mechanisms could mediate high-level cognitive properties such as mental time travel, flexible expression, and conscious recollection. The model described in the next section, which is based on well-known properties of hippocampal network circuitry and plasticity, offers a framework for understanding the phenomena of declarative memory.

Information processing by the hippocampus

A few prominent features of hippocampal circuitry, particularly area CA3, can work in combination to support the properties of declarative memory (figure 49.1). First, the principal neurons of each subdivision of the hippocampus receive convergent afferents from virtually all cortical association areas via a confluence of inputs that pass through the parahippocampal region (Amaral and Witter, 1995; Burwell, Witter, and Amaral, 1995). These afferents contain highly preprocessed information from the final stages of all the hierarchical streams of sensory, motor, emotional, and cognitive processing. Thus, the information supplied to the hippocampus contains the final products of cortical analyses of perceptual events, one's actions, and one's location in the environment—indeed, the full range of attended experience. These inputs are widely distributed to the principal cell population in multiple subdivisions of the hippocampus, including CA3 (Amaral and Witter, 1995). Second, the principal neurons of area CA3 send considerable projections to other CA3 principal cells. These recurrent connections are broad across the CA3 population, sparse in that each cell connects with 5%–20% of the other cells, and involve mainly excitatory glutamatergic synapses. Third, the hippocampus is noted for the prevalence of a rapid form of synaptic plasticity known as long-term potentiation (LTP; Bliss and Collingridge, 1993). In particular, a form of hippocampal LTP that is dependent on N-methyl-D-aspartate (NMDA) receptors has been strongly linked to memory (Martin, Grimwood, and Morris, 2000) and to the memory-associated firing properties of hippocampal neurons (Shapiro and Eichenbaum, 1999).

A combination of widespread, high-level inputs converging on hippocampal principal cells and LTP can work together to support "conjunctive representations" (see figure 49.1). The simultaneous activation of multiple high-level afferents to CA3 principal cells could support rapid induction of associative LTP, such that the synapses at each of the active inputs are enhanced for an extended duration (Bliss and Collingridge, 1993). This associative LTP would support pattern completion, such that subsequent presentation of any element of the encoded conjunction would fire the cell, constituting retrieval of the pattern associated with all the high-level features. Thus, principal neurons in CA3 and other hippocampal subdivisions can each encode highly complex combinations of the stimuli, behavioral actions,

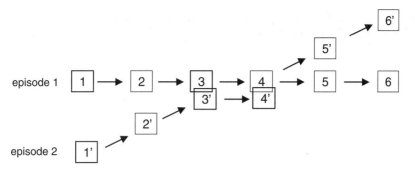

FIGURE 49.2 A diagram of a simple relational memory network. The representation of each of two episodes is conceived of as a sequence of neural elements (boxes) encoding sequential events (1–6 and 1′–6′). Events that are common between the episodes (3/3′ and 4/4′) are represented by overlapping neural elements.

and spatial cues that constitute an event and the place where it occurs (figure 49.2).

A combination of the recurrent pathways, conjunctive encoding, and LTP can support the temporal sequencing of the record of events in experience (see figure 49.1). Thus, when temporally patterned inputs reach the hippocampus, different sets of principal cells are activated for conjunctive coding, as described above. In addition, because the principal cells also connect to each other, an additional component of the conjunctive encoding is a rapid LTP mechanism that enhances connections between cells that fire in sequence. The likelihood of a reciprocal (backward) connection of forward-connected cells is very low, due to the overall sparse connectivity. Therefore the enhancement of recurrent connections is mostly unidirectional, leading to an asymmetry of the enhanced connectivity. Thus, when partial inputs are reproduced during retrieval, the network is more likely to complete the sequence of the full initial input pattern. In addition, when sequences are repeated (practiced) just a few times, cells representing neighboring sequential events converge on background cells that enhance sustained activity, providing a context that bridges the firings of neurons representing salient sequential events (Levy, 1989, 1996; Wallenstein, Eichenbaum, and Hasselmo, 1998). Although sequence storage and recall was initially proposed as characteristic of CA3, subsequent models (Lisman, 1999) have shown how more complex and reciprocally connected recurrent networks in the dentate gyrus and CA3 can coordinate to provide more faithful recall of sequences, leaving CA1 to decode the sequence signals back to the cortex and to compare predictions of the network for the next sequential item to actual information as it arrives. Although the details of the functional circuitry supporting sequencing are currently unclear, the capacity for sequence coding and retrieval appears to be a distinctive feature of hippocampal information processing that can support remembering the flow of events in experiences (see figure 49.2).

Few everyday episodes are truly unique. Instead, virtually all of our daily experiences share common elements with previous as well as future experiences. These common elements include a broad variety of features, for example, a common person with whom one speaks about many topics, a common topic that comes up in many conversations, and a common place where many discussions occur. When a feature of a current episode was also part of a previous experience, it is likely that the some of the same neurons that encoded that feature in the previous experience will also be activated during the current episode (see figure 49.2). There are two major consequences of this shared coding of common elements. One is that the common information becomes a regularity of experience that is not bound to a particular episode, and is therefore timeless and may be construed as semantic information. The other consequence is that memories that share neural representations are linked to one another. Therefore, when elements of one episodic representation are activated, elements of other linked representations may also become activated via the partially common recurrent paths (see figure 49.2). In this way the activation of one memory can generate the activation of multiple related memories, and the reactivated traces contain both episodic and shared semantic elements.

We call the organization of linked memory representations a relational memory network. This framework is simple. At the same time, it is potentially very powerful in its ability to support the properties of declarative memory. Thus, relational networks can encode and retrieve the flow of events in episodic memories, and can encode and retrieve predictable information that is common across experiences constituting semantic memory. This framework is consistent with the common view that episodic memory is the "gateway" through which we initially encode everyday events, and that semantic memories are composed of a synthesis of episodic memories. This perspective is consistent with the observation that the hippocampus is critical to episodic memory (Vargha-Khadem et al., 1997), and with findings indicating that the hippocampus plays a role in the networking of semantic information (Squire and Zola, 1998; Bayley and Squire, 2002).

In addition, our capacity for conscious recollection and flexible memory expression can be viewed as a natural product of linked memory networks. Thus, one can envision a capacity to "surf" a network of memories, bringing related memories to consciousness and allowing the opportunity to compare and contrast related memories. The capacity to relate memories obtained at different times in different venues has been highlighted as a central feature of declarative memory by Cohen (1984). A natural consequence of such a capacity is to make inferences and generalizations from memory, also highlighted in Cohen's characterization, and so to support flexible expression of memories across many situations and circumstances. The properties of episodic recall, systematic organization, and flexible expression of memories are accomplished to varying extents within several previously proposed models of associative networks (e.g., Ratcliff and McKoon, 2000; Schvaneveldt, 2003). The present proposal is unique in its biologically realistic basis derived from the combination of sequential and associative dimensions characteristic of the connectivity of hippocampal circuits.

How can the properties of declarative memory be assessed in animals?

Investigation of the relational memory hypothesis depends in part on the development of animal model systems. Only in animals can the background history of experience can be fully controlled and can detailed biological manipulations and recordings be accomplished. At the same time, the success of animal models depends crucially on the ability to identify the basic properties of declarative memory that must be incorporated into behavioral assays. Thus, although there are routine methods for assessing episodic and semantic memory, conscious recollection, and flexible memory expression in humans, none of these methods readily lends itself to traditional behavioral assays of memory in animals. In humans, episodic memory is typically evaluated by subjective reports and semantic memory is distinguished through tests that depend on linguistic competence. Measuring conscious recollection is also not possible in animals, and memory in animals is traditionally tested by repetition of the learning protocols, and not by evaluations of flexible memory expression.

The relational network hypothesis suggests specific novel ways in which fundamental properties of episodic and semantic memory and flexible memory expression should be assessed in animals. According to the relational network view, episodic memory relies on remembering the flow of events within a unique experience, a capacity that can be tested in animals. Also, in animals we cannot directly assess a capacity for conscious recollection. But we can create operational tests for the capacity to link distinct experiences in support of flexible, inferential memory expression. In addition, by recording the activity of principal neurons within the hippocampus of behaving animals, we can determine if information is organized as sequences of events, some of which are unique to particular episodes and some of which contain features that are common across related episodes. The finding of such a functional organization would strongly support the existence of relational memory networks in the hippocampus.

Testing the relational memory hypothesis

We have been pursuing experiments that test the relational memory hypothesis. Some of our studies examine whether the hippocampus is critical for remembering the flow of events in unique experiences and for the organization and flexible expression of related memories. Other experiments characterize the firing properties of hippocampal neurons, in an effort to determine whether hippocampal neurons encode sequential events during specific experiences and represent conjunctions of events and places that are unique to particular episodes and common features that could link related experiences.

In one line of studies, we have developed behavioral testing protocols that assess memory for the sequential order of a series of olfactory stimuli (Fortin, Agster, and Eichenbaum, 2002; see also Kesner et al., 2002). The stimuli consist of distinctive odorous spices added to clean playground sand through which rats dig to obtain buried cereal rewards. In addition, we directly compared memory for the sequential order of events with recognition of the prior occurrence of events independent of knowledge about their order. On each trial assessing memory for sequential order, rats were presented with a series of five odors randomly selected from a large pool of stimuli. Memory for each series was subsequently probed in a choice test where the animal was reinforced for selecting the earlier of two of the odors that had appeared in the series (figure 49.3). Sessions included six different types of probes. For example, the rat might be presented with odors A then B then C then D then E. Following a 5-minute delay, two nonadjacent odors, such as B and D, were presented, and the animal would be rewarded for selecting B. On each trial, any pair of nonadjacent odors might be presented as the probe, so the animal had to remember the entire sequence in order to perform well throughout the testing session.

Following acquisition of the task, rats then underwent an operation to create a selective lesion of the hippocampus or a sham procedure. On postoperative testing, control rats performed well on all types of probes, whereas animals with hippocampal lesions performed at near chance levels (see figure 49.3). In addition, whereas performance on probe trials was dependent on the separation (lag) between items

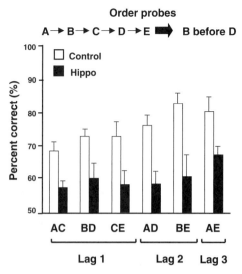

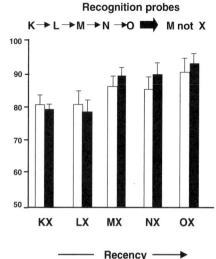

FIGURE 49.3 Tests of memory for the order of a unique series of odors, and recognition of the odors in the series. At the top of the left panel is a schematic of the order of odors (alphabetic letters) in a prototypical trial and one possible probe test. The graph itself shows the performance of sham control rats and rats with hippocampal lesions on probes that differed in the number of inter- vening items during presentation (the lag). At the top of the right panel is a schematic of the order of odors on a prototypical recognition trial and one possible probe test. The graph shows the performance of animals on probes that differed in their recency to the probe.

during presentation of the series for both groups, rats with hippocampal damage were impaired at all lags.

After completion of sequential order tests, the same rats were also tested on their ability to recognize the recent occurrence of odors presented in the series. On each trial, a series of five odors was presented in a format identical to that used in the sequential order task. Then recognition was probed using a choice test in which the animal was presented with one of the odors from the series and another odor from the pool that was not initially presented. Reinforcement was given for selecting the odor not presented in the series. For example, the rat might be presented with the series K then L then M then N then O. Then, following a 5-minute delay, one of the odors, randomly selected, and an odor not pre- sented in the sequence, such as M and X, were presented. The rat would be rewarded for choosing X.

Both control rats and rats with hippocampal lesions acquired the task rapidly, and there was no overall perfor- mance difference between the groups in acquisition rate (see figure 49.3). Subsequent analyses of performance on the individual probes showed that rats with hippocampal lesions performed as well as nonlesioned rats in recognition throughout the series. Furthermore, in both groups, recog- nition scores were consistently superior on probes involving odors that had appeared more recently, suggesting some for- getting of items that had to be remembered for a longer period and through more intervening items. Thus, we con- clude that animals with hippocampal damage had a fully intact capacity to recognize the odors, even though they could not remember the order of their appearance.

In other experiments, we have developed protocols for assessing whether rats link multiple experiences that share common elements and can use this organized representation for flexible, inferential memory expression. The simplest of these protocols involves a transitive inference task based on odor-guided paired associate learning (Bunsey and Eichen- baum, 1996). Rats are first trained on a two sets of odor- paired associates that shared overlapping items (figure 49.4). On each trial, initially the first odor of each initial pair is presented, followed by a choice between the two second odors of those pairs; the rat is required to associate each sample with a particular choice odor and not with the alter- native. After training on both sets of paired associates, the rats are tested for their capacity to identify associations between items that were only indirectly related. Additionally, the rats are tested for their ability to identify associations between items presented in the reverse order from presen- tations during training.

Rats with hippocampal lesions learned the sets of paired associates with as few errors as normal rats. In addition, normal rats showed transitive interference, as reflected in a positive preference index for indirectly associated stimuli (see figure 49.4). By contrast, rats with hippocampal damage did not show a preference significantly different from chance. In addition, normal rats showed strong symmetry of asso- ciations, reflected in a preference for a sample stimulus following presentation of its associate, whereas rats with hippocampal damage showed no capacity for symmetry of the associations. From this experiment, we concluded that other brain systems can support the acquisition of specific

Paired associate learning

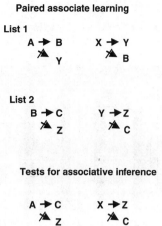

Associative transitivity

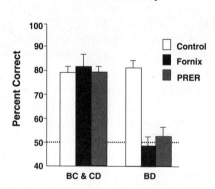

FIGURE 49.4 Tests of the organization of memory for paired associates that share an overlapping item. On the left is shown the training protocol for the pairs of odors (alphabetic letters). Each trial began with presentation of the first odor in a pair (e.g., A), followed by a choice between both possible second odors (B vs. Y) in that list, and the rat was rewarded for selecting the assigned associate (in this case, B and not Y). Following training on two lists, associate transitivity was tested by presentation of a first item from list 1, followed by a choice between second items on list 2. On the right is shown performance on associative transitivity measured by a preference index based on relative time digging at the appropriate odor versus the alternative.

habitual responses to stimulus combinations (if A then B, etc.), but the hippocampus is required to encode items within a larger organization that supports flexible and inferential memory expression.

Another protocol explored whether rats can be trained on a series of overlapping pairwise choice judgments, and then tested for the capacity to organize the distinct choice pairings into a larger framework that supports logical inferences among indirectly related items (figure 49.5). Animals were first presented with a series of blocks of trials involving four pairwise odor discrimination problems. Each problem was composed of two adjacent items in an arbitrarily assigned hierarchical ordering of odors. Thus, subjects were initially rewarded for selecting the appropriate item in overlapping premise pairs, A > B, B > C, C > D, and D > E, where A–E are different odors and > indicates "is selected over." In subsequent intermediate stages of training, the number of trials in training blocks was gradually reduced until each pair was presented only once in each sequence. Finally, all the premise pairs were presented intermixed in random order in the same session. Then, in the transitive inference testing sessions, all the premise problems were presented in random order, along with occasional probe trials that included the pair B > D as the critical test of transitive inference. Another probe involved the pair A > E. Like the transitive probe, this pairing is novel, but it can be solved without reference to the

Transitive Inference

Pemise pairs: A > B

                          B > C

                                  C > D

                                          D > E

Ordered
Representation: A > B > C > D > E

Test for
transitivity: B vs D

Test for Transitivity

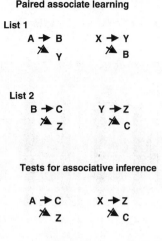

FIGURE 49.5 Test of the organization of choice judgments formulated as a hierarchical series. As shown on the left, initially, animals are trained on a series of pairwise odor choices, then tested for whether they have formed the hierarchical representation of those judgments by a test of transitive inference between two items never presented together. On the right is shown the performance of control rats and rats with the hippocampus disconnected either from subcortical areas via a fornix transection or from cortical areas via ablation of the perirhinal and entorhinal cortex (PRER).

orderly relations among the items because, during training, item A was always rewarded and item E was never rewarded. Thus, the animal could be expected to choose A over E without reference to knowledge about the intervening items in between them in the series.

Intact rats acquired each of the premise pairs rapidly and performed well during probe testing (see figure 49.5). In particular, normal rats made the appropriate transitive judgment between stimuli B and D about as accurately as their overall performance on the premise pairs. This finding indicates that rats have a robust capacity for transitive inference and therefore are capable of developing and flexibly expressing a relational organization of the odor items.

Animals with the hippocampus disconnected by fornix transection or ablation of the parahippocampal region acquired the premise pairs at the normal rate and continued to perform accurately on concurrent presentations of all the premise pairs. These observations indicate that the rats with hippocampal disconnections had somehow acquired appropriate responses to each repetitively stimulus pairing, and their performance was sensitive to consistent reinforcement contingencies. However, in contrast to their intact performance on the premise pairs, rats with either type of hippocampal disconnection showed no capacity for transitive inference (see figure 49.5). On the B > D transitive judgment task, they performed much worse than normal rats, and their performance was not better than would be expected by chance. In the A > E control probes, intact rats and rats with either type of hippocampal disconnection accurately selected A over E, which could be guided by biases about these individual stimuli. This finding indicates that the deficit in rats with hippocampal disconnections was not due merely to the novelty of the stimulus combination in a probe trial. In addition, none of the groups learned the new pairs when they were presented occasionally intermixed among presentations of premise pairs, indicating it was unlikely that performance on B > D was due to learning the correct choice across repetitions of that probe. Combining all of these findings, it is clear that some form of stimulus-stimulus representations can be acquired independent of the hippocampus itself. However, these representations are "hyperspecific," that is, they can be expressed only within the confined context of a reproduction of the learning event (Schacter, 1985). Only a hippocampally mediated representation can support the linkage and flexible expression of memories within a relational organization.

The nature of neural representations within the hippocampus

How does the hippocampus encode information? What is that nature of the neural representation that supports memory for the flow of events in distinct experiences and a linking of memories within a relational organization? Across a broad range of behavioral tests, many studies have shown that individual hippocampal neurons fire serially in relation to each and every sequential event (Eichenbaum et al., 1999). Also, a wealth of evidence indicates that hippocampal neurons respond to a large range of feature conjunctions, such as those defining spatial locations (O'Keefe, 1976), stimulus configurations (Fried, MacDonald, and Wilson, 1997), and task-relevant behaviors (Berger, Alger, and Thompson, 1976). Combining these two general observations, we have suggested that the hippocampus represents experiences as a series of encodings of sequential events and the places where they occur (Eichenbaum et al., 1999). In addition, these representations are proposed to contain two types of codings. Some involve episode-specific combinations of information, including the particular stimuli, behaviors, and places that define events unique to a particular experience. Other codings involve features of experiences that are shared across distinct episodes and therefore could serve to link them. Together, the coding of distinct experiences as sequences of events and places plus the codings of common features that connect related episodes would constitute the contents of a relational memory network in the hippocampus.

There is substantial evidence that hippocampal neurons exhibit firing properties that include the representation of entire experiences, and include both codings that are specific to distinct experiences and codings that reflect common features among distinct episodes (see Eichenbaum et al., 1999). Virtually all experiments that involve recording the activity of hippocampal neurons in behaving animals report that the hippocampal network is continuously active, with individual cells firing for punctuate periods in association with each sequential event. In addition, in virtually all situations in which the behavioral sequences can be identified, the activity of individual hippocampal neurons is found to reflect both the ongoing behavior of the animal and the place where it occurs. For example, it is commonly observed that when rats perform the radial maze task, most hippocampal cells fire as the animal moves through a particular place, either outward as it traverses a maze arm to obtain a reward or inbound as the rat returns to the center of the maze (McNaughton, Barnes, and O'Keefe, 1983; Muller et al., 1994). This combination of firing properties is not dependent on the physical structure of the maze but occurs even in situations other than the radial maze, for example, in open fields where the structure of the environment puts no physical constraint on the animal's movements (Wiener, Paul, and Eichenbaum, 1989; Markus et al., 1995).

In addition, there is an emerging body of evidence that hippocampal cells fire differentially in association with distinctive experiences within the same environment, such that largely different representations are constructed within the

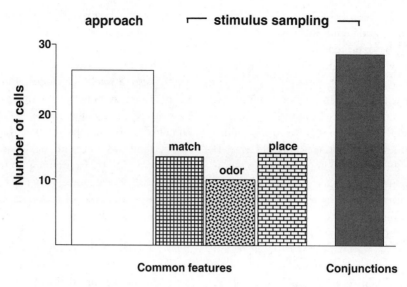

FIGURE 49.6   Incidence of hippocampal principal neurons that fire in association with distinct events during performance of a continuous delayed non-match-to-sample task. Some cells fired during a particular phase of the approach to the stimulus, whereas others fired during stimulus sampling. Some of those cells fired in associ- ation with either a particular feature of the task (a phase of the approach, the match/nonmatch status, odor, or place of the stim- ulus) that was common across different types of trials or a combi- nation of those features that was unique to a particular trial type.

hippocampus whenever the animal appears to perceive two experiences within the environment as distinct (Bostock, Muller, and Kubie, 1991; Markus et al., 1995; Gothard et al., 1996; Skaggs and McNaughton, 1998). Of note, in each of these situations, whereas many cells encode the events and places that are distinct to a particular type of experience, some cells encode features of the situation that are common between the experiences (Markus et al., 1995; Tanila, Shapiro, and Eichenbaum, 1997; Skaggs and McNaughton, 1998).

We explored these properties in detail using a protocol in which rats performed the same task at several different loca- tions in an environment (Wood, Dudchenko, and Eichen- baum, see also Kreiman, Kock, and Fried, 2000). Rats were trained on a recognition memory task in which cups with scented sand were the relevant cues. On each trial a cup was placed in any of nine locations. Regardless of its location, the cup contained a reward if the odor was different from that of the previous cup (a nonmatch). Because the location of the discriminative stimuli was varied systematically, cellu- lar activity related to the stimuli and behavior could be dis- sociated from activity related to the animal's location. We found that individual hippocampal cells were active during each event in a trial, consistent with the idea that the hip- pocampus was involved in the representation of entire trial episodes (figure 49.6). Some cells fired in association with highly specific combinations of stimuli, behavior, and loca- tion, consistent with the idea that the hippocampus encodes events that are unique to particular types of trial experi- ences. Other cells encoded a variety of the features that were

common among types of trials. For example, some cells fired at a particular phase in the approach to any stimulus cup. Still others fired as the rat sampled a particular odor, regard- less of its location (figure 49.7). Yet others distinguished the match and nonmatch relationship between successive stimuli, independent of the odor or its location. And some cells fired only when the rat performed the task at a partic- ular place, independent of the odor or its match/nonmatch status (see figure 49.7). Others have characterized hip- pocampal cells as firing exclusively or primarily associated with the animal's instantaneous location (e.g., O'Keefe, 1999). However, in this situation, in which the same events occurred at several locations, the majority of cells with iden- tifiable firing patterns showed specificity for nonspatial events equivalently across all locations. Furthermore, these nonspatial codings were as robust as spatial specificities observed in other cells. The combination of these observa- tions indicates that all salient regularities of experience are captured in hippocampal neural activity. Hippocampal net- works encode both complex actions and places that are unique to distinct experiences and features that are common among them.

Generalizing the relational memory hypothesis

Most of the experiments described so far involved tests of olfactory memory. However, it is proposed that relational memory networks support memory for all kinds of infor- mation. Therefore, demonstrations of the applicability of the model to other modalities of learned material are criti-

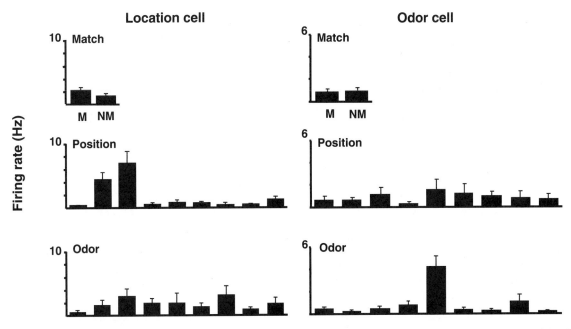

FIGURE 49.7 The selective firing patterns of two hippocampal principal neurons that were active in association with the location where the stimulus was sampled independent of the odor and other features (left) or were associated with the odor independently of the place or other features (right).

cal to generalizing the model. In particular, because of the prevalent alternative view that the hippocampus is dedicated to spatial information processing (O'Keefe and Nadel, 1978), it is important to show that relational memory networks can support the phenomena of spatial memory dependent on hippocampal function.

We suggest a common role for the hippocampal relational memory networks in spatial and nonspatial memory. Accordingly, we suggest that in spatial learning, the hippocampus initially forms a representation of sequential events in each journey that is taken in a novel environment. Each spatial episode consists of a series of views from places occupied, the subject's own movements through space, and any attended events witnessed along the way. The representation of these sequential places and events constitutes memory for the route of each journey. As the subject pursues additional journeys through the same environment, many of the routes are likely to intersect. Consistent with the relational network account, the common places among these routes are represented by overlapping hippocampal neuronal elements, such that representations of related routes become linked. As intersections are shared among many otherwise distinct journeys, some of the neurons would be expected to represent only the common places, and those cells would constitute true "place cells" as described by O'Keefe (1976). In addition, when the subject arrives at a location that is shared among different routes, the hippocampus may be able to generate many of the representations of routes that included the common location, mediating a capacity for navigation in novel directions, an

ability known to depend on the hippocampus (Eichenbaum, Stewart, and Morris, 1990).

Consistent with this perspective, recent studies have characterized the acquisition of spatial representations as embodied in the correlated activity among cells that are sequentially activated when an animal repeatedly traverses a route (McHugh et al., 1996). In addition, other studies have characterized off-line memory processing of repeated traversals of a route as the sequential activation of places traversed (Louie and Wilson, 2001; Lee and Wilson, 2002).

In an additional recent study we found strong evidence that hippocampal networks represent distinct experiences even when spatial and behavioral features of performance are tightly controlled (Wood et al., 2000; see also Frank, Brown, and Wilson, 2000). In this study rats performed a spatial alternation task in a T maze. Each trial began with the rat at the base of the stem of the T and commenced when the rat traversed the stem and then selected either the left- or the right-choice arm. Rewards were available at the end of each arm according to an alternation sequence. Thus, the rat was required to distinguish between its left-turn and right-turn experiences and to use its memory for the most recent experience to guide the current choice.

Individual hippocampal cells fired as the rats passed through each of a sequence of locations traversed within each trial. The key observation in this experiment was that the firing patterns of all the cells depended on whether the rat was performing a left- or right-turn episode (figure 49.8). That is, the cells fired differently on left-turn or right-turn trials, even when the rat traveled the same segments of the

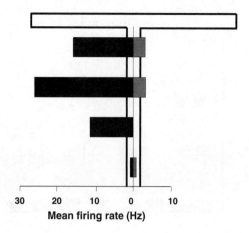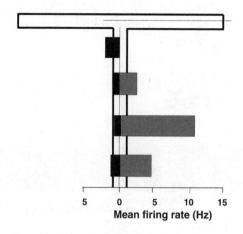

FIGURE 49.8   The selective firing patterns of two hippocampal principal neurons that were active associated with the animal traversing a particular portion of the stem of the T maze on one type of trial episode. The bars for left- and right-turn trials show firing rates associated with quadrants of the stem. The cell on the left fired when the rat was near the end of the stem selectively on left-turn trials. The cell on the right fired when the rats was near the beginning of the stem selectively on right-turn trials.

stem of the T and its overt behavior was identical on both types of trials. Indeed, detailed analyses indicated that minor variations in the animal's speed, direction of movement, or position within the relevant areas on the stem did not account for the different firing patterns on left-turn and right-turn trials for most of these cells. Although most cells showed a very strong differential activity (at least 10:1) on one trial type, some cells fired substantially when the rat was at the same point in the stem on either trial type, indicating a representation of the common spatial information between the two trial types (figure 49.9). Thus, the hippocampus encoded both the left-turn and right-turn experiences using distinct representations, and also encoded information that could link them though the common features (locations) of both experiences.

The hippocampal-cortical memory system

The present considerations have focused on the role of the hippocampus. However, a comprehensive understanding will require consideration of the large system of cortical (and other) areas with which the hippocampus is connected. Among these are neocortical association areas that play specific roles in episodic and semantic memory, and the parahippocampal cortical region that surrounds the hippocampus (figure 49.10). It is generally believed that the hippocampus has too few cells and a lack of topographic organization likely to support representation of details of events and places that compose the information in declarative memories. Rather, it seems likely that the details of information in memory are represented in widespread cortical areas and that the hippocampus mediates the organization of those cortical representations. Therefore, it is assumed that the specificity of firing patterns observed in hippocampal neurons is a consequence of the convergent

inputs from cortical areas, or is a reflection of activity that will regenerate those representations.

The combination of all these observations suggests that multiple neocortical areas, the parahippocampal region, and the hippocampus work in concert to mediate relational memory (Eichenbaum et al., 1999). According to this view, neocortical areas mediate the representation of stimulus details, and these converge in persistent representations of configural items in the parahippocampal region. The hippocampus records the flow of information arriving from the parahippocampal region and can use the persistent stimulus representations typical of this region in identifying common features along episodes by iterative interactions between these areas. Subsequently, the retrieval of hippocampal representations can direct the contents and timing of recovery

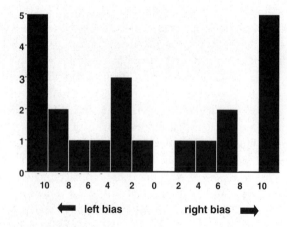

FIGURE 49.9   Incidence of hippocampal neurons with different selectivities of firing at some point on the stem of the T maze as rats performed left-turn and right-turn trials on the spatial alternation task.

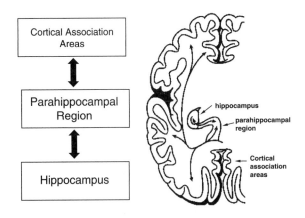

FIGURE 49.10 The hippocampal memory system. On the left is a schematic diagram and on the right a sketch of the same brain areas in a horizontal section of the human brain. Each diagram indicates bidirectional pathways between levels of the system.

of detailed cortical representations both for episodic and semantic information. Such a scheme could account for the full phenomena of declarative memory.

REFERENCES

AMARAL, D. G., and M. P. WITTER, 1995. Hippocampal formation. In *The Rat Nervous System*, 2nd ed., G. Pacinos, ed. San Diego, Calif. Academic Press, pp. 443–493.

BAYLEY, P. J., and L. R. SQUIRE, 2002. Medial temporal lobe amnesia: Gradual acquisition of factual information by nondeclarative memory. *J. Neurosci.* 22:5741–5748.

BERGER, T. W., B. E. ALGER, and R. F. THOMPSON, 1976. Neuronal substrates of classical conditioning in the hippocampus. *Science* 192:483–485.

BLISS, T. V. P., and G. L. COLLINGRIDGE, 1993. A synaptic model of memory: Long-term potentiation in the hippocampus. *Nature* 361:31–39.

BOSTOCK, E., R. U. MULLER, and J. L. KUBIE, 1991. Experience-dependent modifications of hippocampal place cell firing. *Hippocampus* 1:193–206.

BUNSEY, M., and H. EICHENBAUM, 1996. Conservation of hippocampal memory function in rats and humans. *Nature* 379:255–257.

BURWELL, R. D., M. P. WITTER, and D. G. AMARAL, 1995. Perirhinal and postrhinal cortices in the rat: A review of the neuroanatomical literature and comparison with findings from the monkey brain. *Hippocampus* 5:390–408.

COHEN, N. J., 1984. Preserved learning capacity in amnesia: Evidence for multiple memory systems. In *The Neuropsychology of Memory*, N. Butters and L. R. Squire, eds. New York: Guilford Press, pp. 83–103.

COHEN, N. J., and L. R. SQUIRE, 1980. Preserved learning and retention of a pattern-analyzing skill in amnesia: Dissociation of knowing how and knowing that. *Science* 210:207–210.

DUSEK, J. A., and H. EICHENBAUM, 1997. The hippocampus and memory for orderly stimulus relations. *Proc. Nat. Acad. Sci. U.S.A.* 94:7109–7114.

EICHENBAUM, H., and N. J. COHEN, 2001. *From Conditioning to Conscious Recollection: Memory Systems of the Brain.* Oxford, England: Oxford University Press.

EICHENBAUM, H., P. DUDCHENKO, E. WOOD, M. SHAPIRO, and H. TANILA, 1999. The hippocampus, memory, and place cells: Is it spatial memory or memory space? *Neuron* 23:1–20.

EICHENBAUM, H., C. STEWART, and R. G. M. MORRIS, 1990. Hippocampal representation in spatial learning. *J. Neurosci.* 10:331–339.

FORTIN, N. J., K. L. AGSTER, and H. EICHENBAUM, 2002. Critical role of the hippocampus in memory for sequences of events. *Nat. Neurosci.* 5:458–462.

FRANK, L. M., E. N. BROWN, and M. WILSON, 2000. Trajectory encoding in the hippocampus and entorhinal cortex. *Neuron* 27:169–178.

FRIED, I., K. A. MACDONALD, and C. L. WILSON, 1997. Single neuron activity in human hippocampus and amygdala during recognition of faces and objects. *Neuron* 18:753–765.

GOTHARD, K. M., W. E. SKAGGS, K. M. MOORE, and B. L. MCNAUGHTON, 1996. Binding of hippocampal CA1 neural activity to multiple reference frames in a landmark-based navigation task. *J. Neurosci.* 16:823–835.

KESNER, R. P., P. E. GILBERT, and L. A. BARUA, 2002. The role of the hippocampus in memory for the temporal order of a sequence of odors. *Behav. Neurosci.* 116:286–290.

KREIMAN, K., C. KOCK, and I. FRIED, 2000. Category specific visual responses of single neurons in the human medial temporal lobe. *Nat. Neurosci.* 3:946–953.

LEE, A. K., and M. A. WILSON, 2002. Memory of sequential experience in the hippocampus during slow wave sleep. *Neuron* 36:1183–1194.

LEVY, W. B., 1989. A computational approach to hippocampal function. In *Computational Models of Learning in Simple Systems*, R. D. Hawkins and G. H. Bower, eds. New York: Academic Press, pp. 243–305.

LEVY, W. B., 1996. A sequence predicting CA3 is a flexible associator that learns and uses context to solve hippocampal-like tasks. *Hippocampus* 6:579–590.

LISMAN, J. E., 1999. Relating hippocampal circuitry to function: Recall of memory sequences by reciprocal dentate-CA3 interactions. *Neuron* 22:233–242.

LOUIE, K., and M. A. WILSON, 2001. Temporally structured replay of awake hippocampal ensemble activity during rapid eye movement sleep. *Neuron* 29:145–156.

MARKUS, E. J., Y.-L. QIN, B. LEONARD, W. E. SKAGGS, B. L. MCNAUGHTON, and C. A. BARNES, 1995. Interactions between location and task affect the spatial and directional firing of hippocampal neurons. *J. Neurosci.* 15:7079–7094.

MARTIN, S. J., P. D. GRIMWOOD, and R. G. M. MORRIS, 2000. Synaptic plasticity and memory, an evaluation of the hypothesis. *Annu. Rev. Neurosci.* 23:649–711.

MCHUGH, T. J., K. I. BLUM, J. Z. TSIEN, S. TONEGAWA, and M. A. WILSON, 1996. Impaired hippocampal representation of space in CA1-specific NMDAR1 knockout mice. *Cell* 87:1339–1349.

MCNAUGHTON, B. L., C. A. BARNES, and J. O'KEEFE, 1983. The contributions of position, direction, and velocity to single unit activity in the hippocampus of freely-moving rats. *Exp. Brain Res.* 52:41–49.

MULLER, R. U., E. BOSTOCK, J. S. TAUBE, and J. L. KUBIE, 1994. On the directional firing properties of hippocampal place cells. *J. Neurosci.* 14:7235–7251.

O'KEEFE, J. A., 1976. Place units in the hippocampus of the freely moving rat. *Exp. Neurol.* 51:78–109.

O'KEEFE, J., and L. NADEL, 1978. *The Hippocampus as a Cognitive Map.* New York: Oxford University Press.

O'KEEFE, J., 1999. Do hippocampal pyramidal cells signal non-spatial as well as spatial information? *Hippocampus* 9: 352–364.

RATCLIFF, R., and G. McKOON, 2000. Memory models. In *The Oxford Handbook of Memory*, E. Tulving and F. I. M. Craik, eds. Oxford, England: Oxford University Press, pp. 571–581.

SCHACTER, D. L., 1985. Multiple forms of memory in humans and animals. In *Memory Systems of the Brain*, N. M. Weinberger, J. L. McGaugh, and G. Lynch, eds. New York: Guilford Press, pp. 351–380.

SCHACTER, D. L., and E. TULVING, eds., 1994. *Memory Systems 1994*. Cambridge, Mass.: MIT Press.

SCHVANEVELDT, R. W., 2003. Coding processes: Organization of memory. In *Learning and Memory*, 2nd ed., J. H. Byrne, ed. New York: Macmillan, pp. 82–84.

SHAPIRO, M. L., and H. EICHENBAUM, 1999. Hippocampus as a memory map, synaptic plasticity and memory encoding by hippocampal neurons. *Hippocampus* 9:365–384.

SKAGGS, W. E., and B. L. McNAUGHTON, 1998. Spatial firing properties of hippocampal CA1 populations in an environment containing two visually identical regions. *J. Neurosci.* 18:8455–8466.

SQUIRE, L. R., and S. M. ZOLA, 1998. Episodic memory, semantic memory and amnesia. *Hippocampus* 8:205–211.

TANILA, H., M. L. SHAPIRO, and H. E. EICHENBAUM, 1997. Discordance of spatial representation in ensembles of hippocampal place cells. *Hippocampus* 7:613–623.

TULVING, E., 1983. *Elements of Episodic Memory*. New York: Oxford University Press.

TULVING, E., 2002. Episodic memory: From mind to brain. *Annu. Rev. Psychol.* 53:1–25.

VARGHA-KHADEM, F., D. G. GADIN, K. E. WATKINS, A. CONNELLY, W. VAN PAESSCHEN, and M. MISHKIN, 1997. Differential effects of early hippocampal pathology on episodic and semantic memory. *Science* 277:376–380.

WALLENSTEIN, G. V., H. EICHENBAUM, and M. E. HASSELMO, 1998. The hippocampus as an associator of discontiguous events. *Trends Neurosci.* 21:315–365.

WIENER, S. I., C. A. PAUL, and H. EICHENBAUM, 1989. Spatial and behavioral correlates of hippocampal neuronal activity. *J. Neurosci.* 9:2737–2763.

WOOD, E. R., P. A. DUDCHENKO, H. EICHENBAUM, 1999. The global record of memory in hippocampal neuronal activity. *Nature* 397: 613–616.

WOOD, E., P. DUDCHENKO, J. R. ROBITSEK, and H. EICHENBAUM, 2000. Hippocampal neurons encode information about different types of memory episodes occurring in the same location. *Neuron* 27:623–633.

50 Medial Temporal Lobe Function and Memory

LARRY R. SQUIRE, ROBERT E. CLARK, AND PETER J. BAYLEY

ABSTRACT The hippocampus and anatomically related structures in the medial temporal lobe support the capacity for conscious recollection (declarative memory). This chapter considers a number of topics that have been prominent in recent discussions of medial temporal lobe function: the possibility that information ordinarily acquired by declarative memory can be supported by nondeclarative memory, the role of awareness in medial temporal lobe-dependent memory, the nature of recognition memory, memory for single items versus memory for conjunctions or associations, remote memory in experimental animals, remote spatial memory, remote autobiographical memory, semantic memory and the hippocampus, delay and trace classical eyeblink conditioning.

The profound effects of medial temporal lobe resection on memory were described in 1957 in a patient who became known as H.M. (Scoville and Milner, 1957). The successful development of an animal model of H.M.'s memory impairment in the nonhuman primate (Mishkin, 1978; Squire and Zola-Morgan, 1983) led eventually to the identification of the structures that compose the medial temporal lobe memory system: the hippocampal region (the CA fields, the dentate gyrus, and the subicular complex) and the adjacent perirhinal, entorhinal, and parahippocampal cortices (Squire and Zola-Morgan, 1991) (figure 50.1A).

During this same period, it became understood that only one kind of memory is impaired following medial temporal lobe damage (Squire, 1992; Schacter and Tulving, 1994; Squire, in press). The kind of memory impaired in H.M. and other amnesic patients is termed declarative memory. Declarative memory supports the capacity to recollect facts and events, and it supports the encoding of memories in terms of relationships among the elements being learned. The stored representations are flexible and can guide successful performance under a wide range of test conditions.

Declarative memory can be contrasted with a collection of nondeclarative memory abilities including skills and habits, simple forms of conditioning, the phenomenon of priming, and other ways in which experience can change how we interact with the world. Nondeclarative forms of memory occur as modifications within specialized performance systems, and what is learned is expressed through performance rather than recollection. The different forms of nondeclarative memory are supported by specific brain systems (Eichenbaum and Cohen, 2001) (figure 50.1B).

Acquisition of factual knowledge by nondeclarative memory

Memory-impaired patients with medial temporal lobe lesions often have some residual capacity for acquiring declarative knowledge (Tulving, Hayman, and MacDonald, 1991; Westmacott and Moscovitch, 2001). In these cases, the question of interest is, what kind of learning occurs? Is learning supported by a residual capacity for declarative memory, or is some other (nondeclarative) memory system able to support performance?

This question was addressed in a study of patient E.P., who became profoundly amnesic in 1992 at the age of 70 as the result of viral encephalitis (Bayley and Squire, 2002). E.P. sustained extensive, virtually complete bilateral damage to the hippocampus, amygdala, entorhinal cortex, and perirhinal cortex, as well as damage to the anterior parahippocampal cortex and anterior fusiform gyrus (Stefanacci et al., 2000). In the laboratory, E.P. has demonstrated no ability to form new declarative memories.

E.P.'s capacity to acquire new factlike information was tested using 48 novel three-word sentences (e.g., "venom caused fever"; Tulving, Hayman, and MacDonald, 1991). E.P. was given a total of 24 study sessions (two trials per session and two sessions per week for 12 weeks, for a total of 48 training trials). Control subjects were given a total of two study sessions (two trials per session and one session per week for 2 weeks, for a total of four training trials). E.P. performed much more poorly than control subjects but demonstrated unmistakable improvement across the sessions on both cued recall tests (e.g., "venom caused ???") and forced-choice tests (figure 50.2).

LARRY R. SQUIRE Veterans Affairs Healthcare System and the Departments of Psychiatry, Neurosciences, and Psychology, University of California, San Diego, La Jolla, Calif.

ROBERT E. CLARK Veterans Affairs Healthcare System and the Department of Psychiatry, University of California, San Diego, La Jolla, Calif.

PETER J. BAYLEY Veterans Affairs Healthcare System and the Department of Psychiatry, University of California, San Diego, La Jolla, Calif.

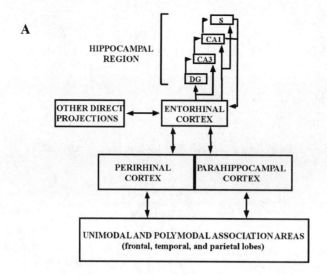

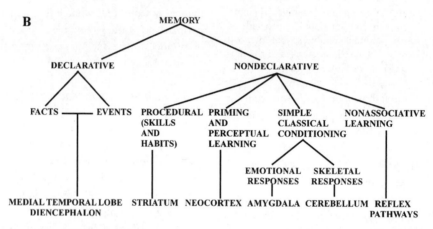

FIGURE 50.1 (*A*) A schematic view of the medial temporal lobe memory system for declarative memory, which is composed of the hippocampal region together with the perirhinal, entorhinal, and parahippocampal cortices. (From Manns and Squire, 2002.) The hippocampal region is composed of the dentate gyrus (DG), the CA fields, and the subiculum (S). (*B*) A taxonomy of mammalian long-term memory systems. The taxonomy lists the brain structures thought to be especially important for each form of declarative and nondeclarative memory. In addition to its central role in emotional learning, the amygdala is able to modulate the strength of both declarative and nondeclarative memory. (From Squire and Knowlton, 2000.)

The nature of E.P.'s acquired knowledge was illuminated by additional observations. First, unlike the control group, E.P. never indicated that he believed he was producing correct answers. Second, his confidence ratings were the same for his correct answers as for his incorrect answers. Third, on the forced-choice test, his response times were identical for correct and incorrect responses. Finally, he did poorly (1 of 48 correct) when the second word in each sentence was replaced by a synonym (e.g., "venom induced ???"). Thus, what E.P. learned was not factual knowledge in the ordinary sense. It was rigidly organized, unavailable as conscious knowledge, and in every respect exhibited the characteristics of nondeclarative memory, perhaps something akin to perceptual learning.

We propose that in those cases when memory-impaired patients do successfully acquire some factual information as declarative, conscious knowledge (e.g., Shimamura and Squire, 1988; Hamann and Squire, 1995; Westmacott and Moscovitch, 2001; O'Kane, Kensinger, and Corkin, 2004), then intact structures remaining within the medial temporal lobe are responsible for the learning. In contrast, when medial temporal lobe damage is more complete, then whatever learning occurs is acquired gradually as nondeclarative knowledge, outside of awareness, and directly in neocortex.

Awareness and the medial temporal lobe

The kind of learning dependent on the medial temporal lobe is typically accompanied by awareness of what is learned (Reed et al., 1997; Clark and Squire, 1998). A recent study questioned whether this is always true (Chun and Phelps, 1999). On each trial of a perceptual learning task, healthy volunteers searched for a 90°-rotated, colored T among colored right angles, and indicated the direction

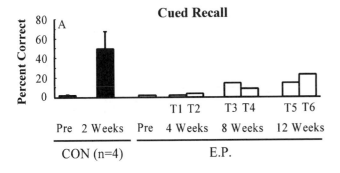

Cued Recall

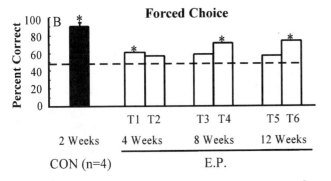

Forced Choice

FIGURE 50.2   Control subjects (CON) and amnesic patient E.P. studied 48 three-word sentences (e.g., "shark killed octopus"). Retention tests were given to control subjects after 2 weeks of training (four training trials) and to E.P. after 4, 8, and 12 weeks of training (16, 32, and 48 training trials, T1–T6). (*A*) Percent correct cued recall of target words in response to the first two words in each sentence. Performance is shown for the pretest (Pre, before study) and after each study period. (*B*) Percent correct forced-choice recognition when the first two words of each sentence were presented together with two possible target words. Performance is shown after each study period. The dashed line shows the score obtained by a group (n = 10) that received no study. Brackets indicate SEM. Asterisks indicate significant difference versus the no-study group (*P* < 0.05). (From Bayley and Squire, 2002.)

in which the base of the T was pointing. After practice, the participants were able to find the T in repeated displays faster than in new displays (perceptual learning). Four memory-impaired patients (two with both medial temporal and lateral temporal lobe damage and two others with less-well-identified damage) did not show this advantage for repeated displays. The interesting finding was that neither the control subjects nor the patients could recognize which displays were repeated. Thus, performance on the task was not accompanied by awareness, raising the possibility that tasks dependent on the medial temporal lobe might sometimes be learned without awareness. An important question is what damage was responsible for poor performance on this task.

A subsequent study of the same task involved five patients with damage thought to be limited to the hippocampal formation (Manns and Squire, 2001). These patients responded faster to repeated displays than to new displays, just as

matched controls did. In contrast, three other patients with large medial temporal lobe lesions and variable damage to lateral temporal cortex did not exhibit an advantage for repeated displays, like the patients in the earlier study (Chun and Phelps, 1999). Thus, damage limited to the hippocampal formation spared performance on this task. Accordingly, the available data do not contradict the idea that medial temporal lobe-dependent memory is accessible to conscious recollection. More extensive damage that includes the medial temporal cortex adjacent to the hippocampus, as well as lateral temporal cortex, may be necessary to impair performance.

An additional issue that deserves attention is the matter of how awareness is to be assessed and what kind of awareness should be evident when declarative (medial temporal lobe-dependent) memory has been acquired (Greene et al., 2001). We suggest that if a task is dependent on the integrity of the medial temporal lobe, then as learning occurs participants should develop measurable, conscious knowledge that their responses are correct and measurable, conscious knowledge about the structure of the task.

Recognition memory

Recognition memory refers to the capacity to judge a recently encountered item as familiar, and is one of the most widely studied examples of declarative memory. In humans, bilateral damage restricted to the hippocampal region (CA fields, dentate gyrus, and subicular complex) impaired performance on standard tasks of recognition memory (Reed and Squire, 1997; Manns et al., 2003). Performance is even more impaired when additional damage occurs to the medial temporal cortex adjacent to the hippocampus (e.g., patient E.P.; Reed et al., 1997). The same pattern of findings is observed in nonhuman primates (Zola-Morgan, Squire, and Ramus, 1994).

Tulving (1985) introduced the distinction between "remembering" and "knowing" to reflect two kinds of recognition, also termed recollection and familiarity, respectively. When a recently presented item evokes a recollection of the learning episode itself, one is said to "remember." By contrast, when a recently presented item is experienced simply as familiar, without evoking knowledge of the learning episode, one is said to experience "knowing." The question of interest is whether this distinction is useful in understanding the function of the hippocampal region and the function of adjacent cortex. There are three kinds of data potentially relevant to this issue.

First, recognition memory was found to be unusually good in a patient (Jon) with restricted hippocampal damage that occurred perinatally (Baddeley, Vargha-Khadem, and Mishkin, 2001). Jon's good performance was proposed to depend on a relatively preserved ability to make judgments based on familiarity. As the authors suggest, Jon's pattern of findings might be limited to cases of developmental amnesia, where there is the possibility of functional reorganization during development and the opportunity to acquire alternative learning strategies. Second, neuroimaging data have shown that in the hippocampus (as well as in adjacent cortex), retrieval associated with remembering is associated with more activation than retrieval associated with knowing (Eldridge et al., 2000). This difference could mean that the medial temporal lobe is more involved in recollective remembering than in making familiarity judgments. Alternatively, this observation could reflect differences in the amount of information being retrieved (that is, differences in information content) rather than differences in kinds of recognition memory.

The third kind of relevant data comes from studies of patients with lesions limited to the hippocampal region (figure 50.3). In one study of seven such patients (Manns et al., 2003), the capacity for familiarity (knowing) was unmistakably impaired, and this impairment was as severe as the impairment in recollection (remembering) (figure 50.4). One patient with adult-onset amnesia did perform well on recognition memory tasks (Holdstock et al., 2002; for additional discussion of this case, see Manns et al., 2003). Other data come from patients for whom anatomical information is unavailable (Yonelinas et al., 2002; for clarification of these data, see Wixted and Squire, 2004). Although a consensus has not been achieved, the lesion data for well-characterized patients suggest that both recollection and familiarity depend on the integrity of the hippocampal region, and that the distinction between recollection and familiarity does not adequately describe the division of labor between the hippocampus and adjacent cortex. One possibility is that familiarity depends on the integrity of structures within the medial temporal lobe, including the hippocampal region, and that episodic recollection depends on these same structures and also on the frontal lobes (Shimamura and Squire, 1987; Davidson and Glisky, 2002).

Recent studies of recognition memory in rodents make a similar point about the importance of the hippocampus. Specifically, hippocampal lesions markedly impair recognition memory when the lesions are sufficiently large and when the retention delay is sufficiently long. Thus, hippocampal lesions impaired performance on the delayed nonmatching-to-sample task (Clark et al., 2001) as well as on the visual paired-comparison task (also called the novel object recognition task; Clark, Zola, and Squire, 2000) (figure 50.5). Similar findings have been obtained after intrahippocampal injections of APV (Baker and Kim, 2002) and with mice lacking the NMDAR-1 subunit in the hippocampal region (Rampon et al., 2000).

In one study, object recognition memory was not impaired after partial damage to the hippocampus, even though spatial memory was impaired (Duva et al., 1997). These results can be understood in terms of lesion size. Partial lesions involving as much as 50% of total hippocampal volume did not impair recognition memory (Broadbent, Clark, and Squire, 2003). However, as the size of the hippocampal lesion increased from 50% to 100% of total hippocampal volume, a deficit gradually appeared and was severe after a complete lesion.

The distinction between recollection and familiarity is difficult if not impossible to apply to experimental animals, in part because methods are not available to reveal whether nonverbal animals have the capacity for episodic recollection (Tulving, 2002). In any case, it does seem more likely that rats and mice base their recognition performance on a capacity to detect familiarity than that they can reexperience the events of the learning episode itself. To the extent that rats and mice do base their recognition performance on the ability to discriminate between familiarity and novelty, the rodent data provide direct evidence for the importance of the hippocampus in detecting familiarity.

Formation of conjunctions and associations

Another view about the division of labor between the hippocampus and the adjacent medial temporal cortex, which is related to the recollection-familiarity distinction, is that the hippocampus might play an especially important role in forming associations between items that are to be learned and that the hippocampus itself is less important for the learning of single items (Henke et al., 1997, 1999; Kroll et al., 1996). Although it is true that neuroimaging studies of associative remembering sometimes reveal more activation within medial temporal lobe structures than tasks of single-item remembering, the typical finding is that the hippocampus and the parahippocampal gyrus behave similarly in this regard (Henke et al., 1997, 1999; Yonelinas et al., 2001; but see Davachi, Mitchell, and Wagner, 2003). A more direct test is to ask whether selective damage to the hippocampal region impairs associative remembering disproportionately and leaves single-item remembering relatively spared. In one study (Stark, Bayley, and Squire, 2002), recognition memory was tested for either pictures of houses or faces, on the one hand, or for house-face pairs, on the other hand. For both patients and controls, remembering the pairs was more difficult than remembering single items. However, remembering the pairs was not disproportionately difficult for the patients.

In a second study (Stark and Squire, 2003), which was based on earlier work by others (Kroll et al., 1996; Reinitz, Verfaellie, and Milberg, 1996), participants took a continuous recognition test involving two-part stimuli (e.g., JAMBARK). The test stimuli could be entirely novel (BARNDIRT), novel but with one previously encountered

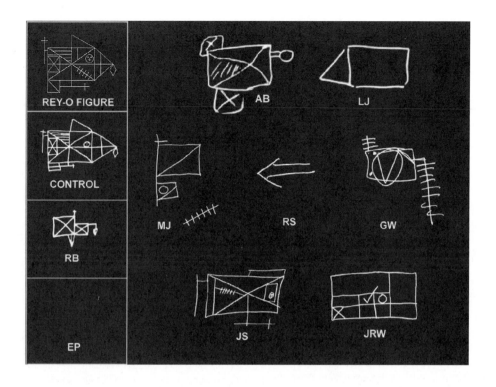

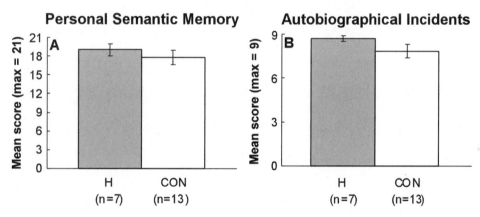

Personal Semantic Memory

Autobiographical Incidents

FIGURE 50.3 The upper panel shows performance on a test of nonverbal memory (the Rey–Osterrieth figure). Participants were asked to copy the figure illustrated in the small box in the upper left panel and, 10–15 minutes later, without forewarning, to reproduce it from memory. The reproduction by a representative healthy control is shown below the target figure. The left panel also shows the reproduction by amnesic patient R.B., who had histologically identified lesions involving the CA1 field of the hippocampus (Zola-Morgan, Squire, and Amaral, 1986). Patient E.P., who has large medial temporal lobe lesions, did not recall copying a figure and

declined to attempt a reproduction (lower left panel). The right panel shows reproductions by seven other amnesic patients who have bilateral damage limited primarily to the hippocampal region. The lower two panels (*A* and *B*) show the performance of the same seven patients (H) and 13 control subjects on the autobiographical memory interview, childhood portion (Kopelman, Wilson, and Baddeley, 1989). These data suggest that patients who fail to reproduce any of the complex figure (like E.P.) or who are deficient at producing remote memories will prove to have damage beyond the hippocampal region.

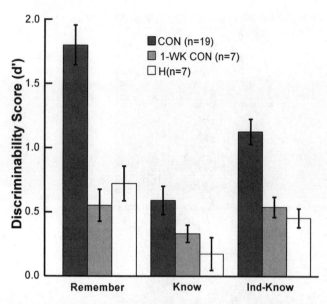

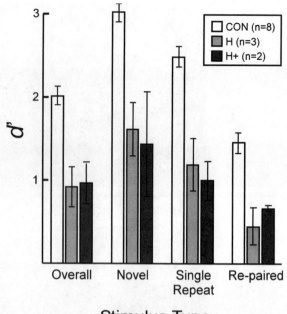

FIGURE 50.4 Recognition memory performance, expressed as discriminability scores (d′), for patients with damage limited primarily to the hippocampal region and controls. Patients were impaired both for items given remember judgments (Remember), for items given know judgments (Know), and for items given know judgments analyzed by an alternative method that assumes that remembering and knowing are independent processes (Ind-Know). A second control group (1-WK CON) was tested after a week. H, patients with damage limited primarily to the hippocampal region; CON, controls. Brackets show SEM. (From Manns et al., 2003.)

FIGURE 50.6 Combined performance on five tests of continuous recognition memory designed to assess associative and nonassociative components of memory. Overall discriminability (d′) scores (Overall) were calculated from the hit rate (probability of responding yes to true repetitions) and the overall false alarm rate (probability of responding yes to all other items). In addition, d′ scores were calculated using the hit rate and each of the three possible false alarm conditions: entirely novel stimuli (Novel), novel stimuli in which one component had been previously presented (Single Repeat), and novel stimuli in which both components had been previously presented but not together (Re-paired). H, patients with damage limited primarily to the hippocampal region; H+, patients with damage to both the hippocampal region and the parahippocampal gyrus; CON, controls. Brackets show SEM. (From Stark and Squire, 2003.)

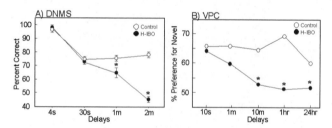

FIGURE 50.5 Delay-dependent memory impairment in rats with large ibotenic acid lesions of the hippocampus (H-IBO) on two different tests of recognition memory. (A) Performance on the delayed nonmatching-to-sample (DNMS). Both groups performed similarly on 4-s probe trials and on trials with a 30-s delay. The lesion group (n = 5) performed more poorly than the control group (n = 5) on the longer delays of 1 min and 2 min and failed to perform above chance on the 2-min delay trial. (B) Performance on the visual paired-comparison (VPC) task. The two groups performed similarly at the shorter delays (10 s, 1 min), but at the longer delays the lesion group (n = 8) performed more poorly than the control group (n = 16). Asterisks indicate impaired performance relative to the control group (P < 0.05). (From Clark, Zola, and Squire, 2000; Clark et al., 2001.)

component (JAMWOOD), novel but with both components recombined from other previously presented items (JAMDIRT), or true repetitions (JAMBARK). Participants were asked to endorse the true repetitions but to reject the other item types. An impairment that especially affected the ability to form conjunctions should reveal itself as a special difficulty in rejecting the recombined items. In this case, elements of the item would be familiar, but the elements would not be arranged in a previously encountered conjunction. In five different experiments involving different materials, patients with hippocampal damage exhibited impaired recognition memory. The impairment extended across all trial types, with no evidence that hippocampal damage selectively (or disproportionately) impaired the associative or conjunctive component of memory (figure 50.6). Accordingly, the hippocampal region appears to be important both for single-item remembering and for remembering associations between items. (For a suggestion that amnesic patients do worse at remembering associations than at remembering single items, irrespective of the nature and extent of damage, see Giovanello, Verfaellie, and Keane, 2003.)

This conclusion is not an argument against the existence of functional specialization with the medial temporal lobe. Indeed, the physiological data are consistent with the idea that the hippocampus carries out a more abstract, less stimulus-specific operation than the adjacent cortex that projects to it (Suzuki and Eichenbaum, 2000). We suggest that all these operations (both stimulus-specific and abstract) make essential contributions to single-item memory and associative memory, and that neither form of memory will be intact unless all the components of the medial temporal lobe memory system are functioning.

Retrograde memory: Animal studies

Impaired formation of long-term memory is the hallmark of the amnesic syndrome in humans and is the most prominent impairment in animal models of human amnesia. A second prominent feature of memory dysfunction is retrograde amnesia, which refers to a loss of memories that were acquired *before* the onset of amnesia. Retrograde memory loss is often temporally graded. That is, information learned long before the onset of memory impairment is often spared relative to information learned recently. It has long been recognized that the study of retrograde amnesia can reveal an enormous amount about the organization of normal memory.

Figure 50.7 illustrates the results of 19 studies published through 2002 in which animals were given equivalent amounts of training at two or more different times before damage to the hippocampal formation or the fornix. Of these 19 studies, the majority found temporally graded retrograde amnesia. That is, material learned shortly before surgery was impaired, but material learned remote from the time of surgery was spared. The typical extent of the retrograde amnesia was about 30 days. This pattern of findings suggests that the hippocampus (and related structures) is necessary for memory storage for only a limited time after learning. One account of the phenomenon suggests that memory is stored in the same neocortical structures that were involved in processing the relevant information during learning. Initially, the hippocampus serves to bind these cortical regions and to allow memory to be reactivated for retrieval. Over time and through a process of reorganization, the connections among the cortical regions are progressively strengthened until the cortical memory can be reactivated and retrieved independent of the hippocampus (Squire and Alvarez, 1995; also see McClelland, McNaughton, and O'Reilly, 1995). That is, memory that was initially hippocampus-dependent becomes hippocampus-independent.

The findings summarized in figure 50.7 count against an alternative suggestion that memories that are initially hippocampus-dependent remain permanently dependent on the hippocampus (Nadel and Moscovitch, 1997), insofar as this idea is meant to apply to the kind of memories typically studied in experimental animals. In this view, older memories are proposed to have a more redundant and spatially distributed representation within the hippocampus than recent memories. Temporally graded retrograde amnesia occurs because a partial lesion of the hippocampus is more likely to spare a distributed remote memory than a less distributed memory that was acquired recently. This idea predicts that temporally graded retrograde amnesia will not be observed when hippocampal lesions are complete (i.e., recent and remote memories will be similarly impaired). Yet the hippocampal lesions were complete in several of the studies summarized in figure 50.7 (e.g., panels 7, 15, and 19).

Retrograde memory: Spatial cognition

One influential view of hippocampal function, which grew out of the discovery of hippocampal place cells in the rodent, emphasizes its role in the acquisition and retrieval of spatial knowledge (O'Keefe and Nadel, 1978). By this view, the hippocampus constructs and stores spatial maps and is therefore essential for learning and remembering places, including places learned about long ago. This view has seemed at odds with the tradition of human neuropsychological research, which has long emphasized that patients with hippocampal damage have a broad impairment that includes spatial memory but also includes memory for words, faces, odors, and sounds.

In view of the finding that hippocampal damage typically produces temporally graded retrograde amnesia (see figure 50.7), the question naturally arises as to whether the phenomenon of temporally graded retrograde amnesia also extends to spatial memory. This question was addressed in a study of the severely amnesic patient E.P. (Teng and Squire, 1999). E.P. was asked to recall the spatial layout of the region where he grew up, and from which he moved away as a young adult more than 50 years earlier. E.P. performed as well as or better than age-matched controls who grew up in the same region and also moved away (figure 50.8). E.P. described how to travel from his home to other locations in his neighborhood, how to travel from one location to another, and he was able to construct alternative routes to travel between locations. He was also able to imagine himself in a particular orientation at a location and then to point toward a specific landmark. In contrast to his entirely normal performance on all these tests, E.P. demonstrated no knowledge of the neighborhood to which he moved after he became amnesic (see figure 50.8C).

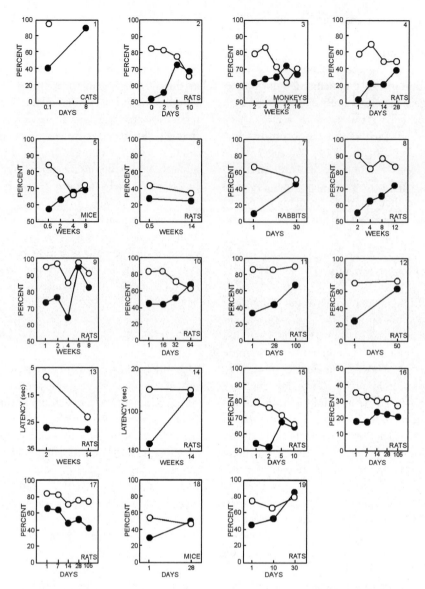

FIGURE 50.7 Summary of findings from 19 studies published through 2002 that examined retrograde amnesia prospectively. In each case, an equivalent amount of training was given at each of two or more times before damage to the hippocampal formation or fornix, and retention was assessed shortly after surgery. The data show the performance of control (CON) and operated animals (H, hippocampus; EC, entorhinal cortex; FX, fornix) as a function of training–surgery interval. Open circles and filled circles show the performance of control and operated animals, respectively. The performance score is usually in percent (0–100), so that a high score reflects good retention. In panels 13 and 14, the performance score is the latency to find a hidden goal, and here a low score reflects good retention. Studies: **1**. Uretsky and McCleary, 1969; adapted from figure 2. **2**. Winocur, 1990; adapted from figure 2. **3**. Zola-Morgan and Squire, 1990; figure 2. **4**. Kim and Fanselow, 1992;

figure 2. **5**. Cho, Beracochea, and Jaffard, 1993; figure 3. **6**. Bolhuis, Stewart, and Forrest, 1994; figure 4A. **7**. Kim, Clark, and Thompson, 1995; adapted from figure 3, 1st retention day. **8**. Cho and Kesner, 1996; figure 4. **9**. Wiig, Cooper, and Bear, 1996; adapted from figure 4A. **10**. Ramos, 1998; adapted from figure 6A. **11**. Maren, Aharonov, and Fanselow, 1999; adapted from figure 4A. **12**. Anagnostaras, Maren, and Fanselow, 1999; figure 3C. **13**. Mumby et al., 1999; adapted from figure 5. **14**. Kubie, Sutherland, and Miller, 1999; adapted from figures 3 and 5. **15**. Winocur, McDonald, and Moscovitch, 2001; adapted from figure 2. **16**. Sutherland et al., 2001; adapted from figure 8. **17**. Sutherland et al., 2001; adapted from figure 6B. **18**. Takehara et al., 2002; adapted from figure 6. **19**. Clark et al., 2002; adapted from figure 5.

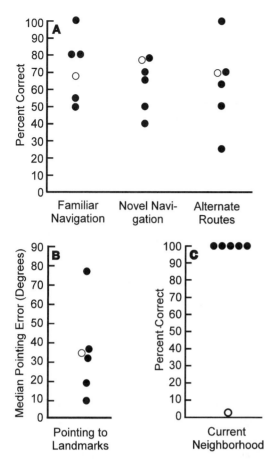

FIGURE 50.8 Performance of patient E.P. (open circles) and five controls (closed circles) on four tasks of topographical memory. (*A*) Score for three navigation tasks that asked about the neighborhood where participants grew up. The tasks required either recalling familiar routes, constructing novel routes, or describing alternative routes when the most direct route was blocked. (*B*) Median error in degrees when participants pointed to particular locations while imagining themselves oriented at other locations. For *A* and *B*, E.P. was tested twice; the score here is his average score. (*C*) Score on a navigation task within the neighborhood where participants currently reside. (Adapted from Teng and Squire, 1999.)

These findings show that the medial temporal lobe is not the permanent repository of spatial maps, and they support the view that the hippocampus and other structures in the medial temporal lobe are essential for the formation of long-term memories, both spatial and nonspatial, but not for the retrieval of very remote memories, either spatial or nonspatial.

In contrast to the findings for patient E.P., the few studies available from rodents have so far yielded mixed results. Two studies suggested that remote spatial memory might be spared after hippocampal lesions (Ramos, 1998; Kubie, Sutherland, and Miller, 1999). In contrast, in those studies involving the most widely used test of spatial memory for the rat (the Morris water maze), remote spatial memory was impaired after hippocampal lesions (see figure 50.7: panels

6, 13, 16, and 17). One study (Clark, Broadbent, and Squire, 2003) used three different tasks of spatial memory and introduced hippocampal lesions as long as 14 weeks after training. In all three tasks, rats with large hippocampal lesions exhibited impaired spatial memory. It is unclear why the findings for rodents and humans differ. One possibility is that tests of rodents' spatial memory may require some new learning, because the animal must update its location in space during the retention test (Knowlton and Fanselow, 1998). In contrast, human patients do not need to acquire new information in order to answer simple questions about their remote spatial memory.

Retrograde memory: Autobiographical recollection

Memories of autobiographical events are often complex, richly detailed narratives and have the defining characteristic of being unique to a particular time and place. One view has been that autobiographical memory, like other forms of declarative memory, gradually became independent of the medial temporal lobe through a process of consolidation or reorganization. A quite different view is that episodic memory is not subject to memory consolidation and remains dependent on the medial temporal lobe as long as a memory persists (Fujii, Moscovitch, and Nadel, 2000).

To choose between these views, we assessed remote autobiographical memory in eight well-characterized amnesic patients with damage limited primarily to the hippocampal region (n = 6) or with more extensive damage to the medial temporal lobe (n = 2; patients E.P. and G.P.; Bayley, Hopkins, and Squire, 2003). The patients and 25 age-matched control subjects were each asked to recollect memories from the first third of their lives, before the onset of amnesia (on average, from before age 16 years). Each participant was given 24 cue words one at a time (e.g., "river," "bottle," "nail") and asked to recollect a unique memory involving the cue word that was specific in time and place (Crovitz and Schiffman, 1974). Additional tests suggested that the narratives were recollections from memory rather than fabrications.

Figure 50.9 shows the results. Overall, the recollections of the patients and the recollections of the controls contained a similar number of details (±5%). Both groups also required a similar amount of time to begin their narrative, a similar amount of time to report their narrative, and received a similar number of prompts before beginning their narrative.

The results suggest that the hippocampal region and adjacent medial temporal lobe cortex are not essential for the recall of remote autobiographical events. It is noteworthy that some patients reported to have difficulty with autobiographical remembering have damage outside the medial temporal lobe (Moscovitch et al., 2000). For other single-case studies of patients with impaired autobiographical remembering (Hirano and Noguchi, 1998; Cipolotti et al., 2001), it

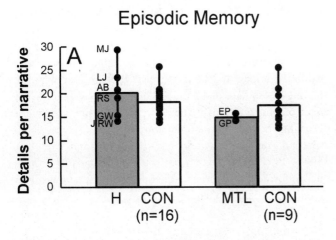

Episodic Memory

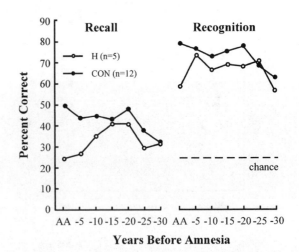

FIGURE 50.10 Recall and recognition performance on a test of news events that occurred from 1950 to 2002. The patients became amnesic in different years from 1976 to 2001, and the data for each patient (and for 2–3 controls matched to each patient) were aligned according to the year when the patient became amnesic. In this way an average score could be calculated for the period of amnesia (AA, anterograde amnesia) and for events that occurred during 5-year periods preceding the onset of amnesia. Standard errors ranged from 4% to 8% for recall and from 2% to 12% for recognition. H, patients with damage limited primarily to the hippocampal region; CON, controls. (From Manns, Hopkins, and Squire, 2003.)

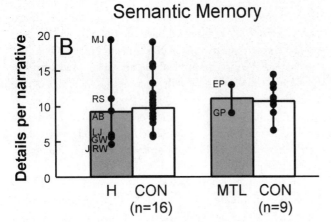

FIGURE 50.9 The number of details contained in narrative reports of remote autobiographical memories. Participants were given 24 cue words (e.g., "river," "bottle," "nail") and for each cue word were asked to recollect a specific event from the first third of their life that involved the word. (*A*) The mean number of details per narrative that described specific events (episodic memory). (*B*) The mean number of details per narrative that were recounted as part of an autobiographical memory but were not unique to a specific event (semantic memory). Each participant is represented by a solid circle, and patients are identified by their initials. H, patients with lesions limited primarily to the hippocampal region; MTL, postencephalitic patients with large medial temporal lobe lesions; CON, controls. (Adapted from Bayley, Hopkins, and Squire, 2003.)

will be important to evaluate carefully the possibility that damage has occurred beyond the medial temporal lobe. A number of considerations suggest that the neocortex supports the capacity for remote autobiographical remembering (particularly lateral temporal cortex, frontal cortex, and occipital cortex; for discussion, see Bayley, Hopkins, and Squire, 2003).

Retrograde memory: Semantic knowledge

An important question has been whether the hippocampal region is important for remembering facts (semantic memory) in the same way that it is important for remem-

bering spatial layouts and autobiographical events. One view is that the hippocampal region is uniquely important for remembering events and that adjacent cortical structures support memory for facts (Vargha-Khadem et al., 1997; Tulving and Markowitsch, 1998; for related views, see Brown and Aggleton, 2001; Yonelinas et al., 2002). Another view is that the hippocampal region is important for both event and fact memory (Squire and Zola, 1998; Manns and Squire, 2002).

Two studies of patients with limited hippocampal damage have addressed this issue. In the first study (Manns, Hopkins, and Squire, 2003), five amnesic patients took a free-recall test and a four-alternative multiple-choice test that asked about 251 news events from the years 1950–2002. The results were that the patients exhibited a significant impairment in learning about news events that occurred after they became amnesic (figure 50.10). In addition, the free-recall scores demonstrated temporally limited retrograde amnesia covering a period 1–10 years prior to the onset of amnesia. In contrast, patients had good access to knowledge about news events that occurred remote to the onset of amnesia (11–30 years earlier). Retrograde amnesia was not as evident in the recognition memory data. Nevertheless, the two patients for whom the most data were available (G.W. and R.S., figure 50.3) did exhibit an impairment that was evident in the fourth and sixth years prior to amnesia.

These findings support the notion that the human hippocampus is important for remembering facts as well as for remembering events (also see Rempel-Clower et al., 1996; Reed and Squire, 1998; Kapur and Brooks, 1999; see Zola-Morgan, Squire, and Amaral, 1986, for a report of patient R.B., in whom no retrograde amnesia was detected, but the tests of retrograde amnesia were not sufficiently sensitive to detect an impairment covering less than 10 years). It should be noted that the pattern of findings is the same in humans as in experimental animals, but in animals the retrograde amnesia ranges over weeks or months rather than years.

Tulving (1991) pointed out an important reason why it has been difficult to decide the question whether the hippocampal region is important for semantic memory. In tests of factual knowledge that are designed to assess semantic memory, normal individuals could be advantaged by being able to remember episodic details about the time and place in which they acquired the factual information. If so, impaired performance by patients on tests about facts could reflect poor episodic memory rather than poor semantic memory.

A second study considered this issue (Manns, Hopkins, and Squire, 2003). Six patients and 14 control subjects were asked whether famous persons were still living. The 126 famous persons had become known before 1970, and half of them had died between 1990 and 2001. Patients performed similarly to controls in discriminating famous names from fictitious names, presumably because these judgments depended on very remote memory (figure 50.11*a*). In contrast, the patients were significantly worse than controls when asked to decide whether the persons they had correctly judged to be famous were still living (figure 50.11*b*).

For three patients who became amnesic well after 1990 (G.W., R.S., and J.S., figure 50.3), a measure of retrograde amnesia could be obtained by considering test items (mean = 40) about persons who had died before the onset of their amnesia. Across the three patients, these events occurred from 1 year to 11 years before amnesia. Figure 50.11*c* shows that these three patients performed significantly worse than control subjects for the retrograde time period. Thus, the patients not only had difficulty acquiring factual knowledge after they became amnesic, they also had difficulty recollecting factual knowledge about events that occurred during the few years before they became amnesic.

To consider the possible impact of episodic memory on test performance, 13 of the 14 control subjects were asked to recollect any circumstances in which they had heard that an individual had died (either at the time of death or any time afterward). When those famous names were removed from the analysis, the patients still exhibited significant anterograde amnesia (figure 50.11*d*). Further, for the three patients in whom retrograde memory could be assessed, there was a trend (*P* = 0.10) toward an impairment when

the famous names associated with episodic memory were removed from this analysis (figure 50.11*e*).

Both these studies indicate that the hippocampal region is important for semantic memory and not just for episodic memory, just as it is important for both recollection and familiarity, and for both conjunction memory and single-item memory (for further discussion, see Suzuki, 2003). It should not be surprising that semantic memory can be deficient in memory-impaired patients but that it will nevertheless appear to be superior to episodic memory (Verfaellie, Koseff, and Alexander, 2000; Van der Linden et al., 2001). Semantic memory is usually based on multiple learning events (that is, it is subject to repetition), and therefore typically reflects stronger memory than episodic memory, which by definition is unique to a single event. We propose two conclusions: (1) semantic memory, like episodic memory, is dependent on the integrity of the hippocampal region, and (2) the impairment in semantic memory is proportional to the impairment in episodic memory, that is, the relationship in patients between semantic and episodic memory is the same as it is in healthy individuals.

We note that the suggestion that episodic and semantic memory do not describe specific functions of different components of the medial temporal lobe memory system does not count against the view that the anatomical components of the medial temporal lobe make distinct contributions to memory function (for further discussion, see Suzuki and Eichenbaum, 2000; Zola and Squire, 2000; Norman and O'Reilly, 2003).

Classical conditioning

Classical conditioning is a simple form of associative learning that has been studied extensively in vertebrate and invertebrate animals (Rescorla and Wagner, 1972; Carew and Sahley, 1986; Squire and Kandel, 1999). Perhaps the best understood example of classical conditioning in vertebrates is conditioning of the eyeblink response (Gormezano, 1962; Kim and Thompson, 1997), whereby a neutral conditioned stimulus (CS), such as a tone, is presented just prior to an unconditioned stimulus (US), such as a mild puff of air to the eye. After repeated pairings of the CS and the US, the CS elicits a learned or conditioned eyeblink response (CR) in advance of the US. In delay conditioning, the CS is presented and then remains on until the US is presented. The two stimuli then overlap and coterminate. In trace conditioning, an empty (i.e., trace) interval separates the CS offset and the US onset (figure 50.12).

Work with rabbits first demonstrated a clear distinction between these two forms of conditioning. The acquisition and retention of delay eyeblink conditioning require the cerebellum and associated brainstem structures (Christian and Thompson, 2003). No forebrain structures, including

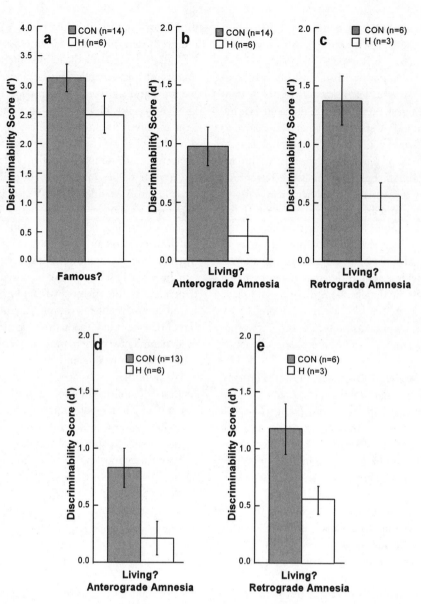

FIGURE 50.11 Performance on a test that asked whether famous persons were still living. The famous persons had become known before 1970, and half of them died between 1990 and 2001. (*a*) Patients performed similarly to controls in discriminating famous names from fictitious names but (*b*) were impaired at deciding which of the correctly identified famous persons had died during the period of anterograde amnesia. (*c*) For three of the patients, many of the deaths (mean = 40) had occurred prior to the onset of their amnesia, and these patients were impaired at making judgments about these names as well (retrograde amnesia). For a few names (13% of the test items) that control subjects had correctly identified as the names of persons who had died, control subjects were able to recollect episodic details about the circumstances in which they had learned of the deaths. When these test items were excluded (*d*), control subjects still performed better than the patients at deciding which of the correctly identified famous persons had died during the period of anterograde amnesia. (*e*) For three patients in whom retrograde amnesia could be assessed, there was a trend toward retrograde amnesia when the famous names associated with episodic memories were removed. H, patients with damage limited primarily to the hippocampal region; CON, controls. Brackets show SEM. (From Manns, Hopkins, and Squire, 2003.)

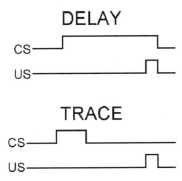

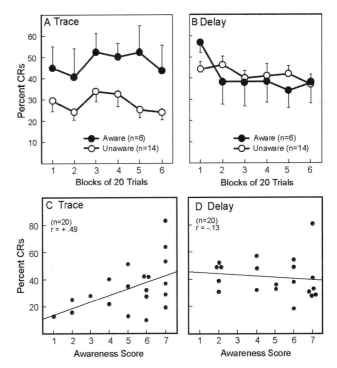

FIGURE 50.12 Schematic representation of delay classical conditioning (top) and trace classical conditioning (bottom). In delay conditioning, the conditioned stimulus (CS), for example a tone, is presented and remains on (upward deflection) until the unconditioned stimulus (US), for example a puff of air to the eye, is presented. The two stimuli then overlap and coterminate. In trace conditioning the CS is presented and then terminated. A silent or trace interval then follows before the presentation of the US. Single-cue conditioning involves a single CS, as illustrated here. Differential conditioning involves a CS$^+$ that precedes the US and a CS$^-$ that occurs in the absence of the US.

the hippocampus, are required (Mauk and Thompson, 1987). Because delay conditioning is independent of the forebrain and is intact in amnesia, it appears to be a quintessential example of nondeclarative memory. Successful trace eyeblink conditioning, like delay conditioning, requires the cerebellum (Woodruff-Pak, Lavond, and Thompson, 1985). However, trace conditioning differs from delay conditioning in that it additionally requires the hippocampus and neocortex. Thus, acquisition and retention of trace conditioning were severely disrupted in rabbits and rats when the hippocampus was damaged (Solomon et al., 1986; Moyer, Deyo, and Disterhoft, 1990; Kim, Clark, and Thompson, 1995; Weiss et al., 1999). In addition, trace conditioning in rabbits was disrupted by damage to medial prefrontal cortex (Kronforst-Collins and Disterhoft, 1998; Weible, McEchron, and Disterhoft, 2000). Findings in humans are consistent with the animal work (for review, see Clark, Manns, and Squire, 2002).

The difference between delay and trace eyeblink conditioning has recently come into sharper focus in studies that have explored the importance of awareness. In one study, older participants (51–75 years) were given single-cue *trace* conditioning (a single-tone CS, 1000-ms trace interval) while watching a silent movie. They also took a seven-item post-conditioning questionnaire after the first 10 conditioning trials that assessed awareness of the CS-US contingency (i.e., the CS predicts the US). Other participants (aged 50–76 years) watched the silent movie during single-cue *delay* conditioning and also took the questionnaire after the first 10 conditioning trials. In the case of trace conditioning, those who became aware of the CS-US relationship early in the session conditioned to a greater extent than those who were

FIGURE 50.13 Percent conditioned responses (CRs) across six blocks of 20 trials by participants who were classified as aware or unaware on the basis of their answers to seven true-or-false questions given after the first 10 trials. (*A*) Trace conditioning. (*B*) Delay conditioning. Brackets show SEM. (*C* and *D*) Relationship between the awareness score obtained after the first 10 trials and the strength of conditioning (percent CRs) across all 120 conditioning trials. (*C*) Performance of participants who received trace conditioning ($r = 0.49$, $P < 0.05$). (*D*) Performance of participants who received delay conditioning ($r = -0.13$, $P > 0.1$). (From Manns, Clark, and Squire, 2001.)

unaware of the CS-US relationship (figure 50.13*a*). Further, performance on the questionnaire after the first 10 conditioning trials predicted the magnitude of single-cue trace conditioning over the entire 120-trial conditioning session (figure 50.13*c*) (Manns, Clark, and Squire, 2001). Thus, single-cue trace conditioning appears to be importantly related to awareness. In contrast to the findings for single-cue trace conditioning, awareness was found to be unrelated to single-cue delay conditioning (figure 50.13*b*), and there was no relationship between awareness scores obtained early in conditioning and the magnitude of conditioning across the 120-trial conditioning session (figure 50.13*d*) (Manns, Clark, and Squire, 2001).

In delay and trace differential conditioning, the CS$^+$ (e.g., a tone) is followed by the US, and the CS$^-$ (e.g., a static noise) is presented alone. Successful differential conditioning occurs when more CRs are elicited by the CS$^+$ than by the CS$^-$. In differential conditioning, the participant can in principle learn a number of different facts about the stimulus contingencies (for example, the CS$^+$ predicts the US, the CS$^-$ does not predict the US, and the CS$^+$ and CS$^-$ are unrelated), and knowledge (awareness) of all these facts can be assessed.

When older individuals (59–78 years) were given a 17-item, true-or-false test after differential conditioning, awareness was found to be important for successful trace conditioning but not for successful delay conditioning (Clark and Squire, 1998). Further, four amnesic patients who had damage that included the hippocampus bilaterally failed to become aware, and also failed to acquire differential trace conditioning. By contrast, in the case of differential delay conditioning, awareness of the stimulus contingencies had no relationship to acquisition of the differential conditioned response.

In related studies, also with older participants, awareness was manipulated directly by fully explaining the stimulus contingencies prior to conditioning (Clark and Squire, 1999). The explanation facilitated trace conditioning and also improved postconditioning awareness scores. Other participants were asked to engage in a secondary (distraction) task during the conditioning session. These individuals failed to develop awareness and also failed to exhibit differential trace conditioning. By contrast, participants given this same distraction task during differential delay conditioning performed as well as participants who were not distracted.

In the case of successful differential trace eyeblink conditioning, the question arises whether awareness of the stimulus contingencies precedes, follows, or parallels the acquisition of differential trace conditioning. This question was addressed using a trial-by-trial ("online") measure of awareness during the course of differential trace conditioning. Successful differential trace eyeblink conditioning and awareness of the stimulus contingencies emerged approximately in parallel (Manns, Clark, and Squire, 2000). These studies indicate that awareness of the stimulus contingencies is important for successful differential trace conditioning but is unnecessary for differential delay conditioning. Nevertheless, some work has suggested a role for awareness in differential delay conditioning (Ross and Nelson, 1973; Knuttinen et al., 2001). As discussed elsewhere (Clark, Manns, and Squire, 2002; Manns, Clark, and Squire, 2002), these findings may be related to the poor discriminability of the two CSs or to scoring criteria that may inadvertently have included voluntary responses along with true conditioned responses.

Individuals who develop awareness of the stimulus contingencies may be successful at trace conditioning because they have acquired a representation that allows them to expect the US when the CS is presented. A method for evaluating the relationship of expectancy to conditioning performance was developed by Perruchet (1985). A sequence of trials is presented such that the US follows the CS only 50% of the time. Strings of one to four CS-alone trials are inter-

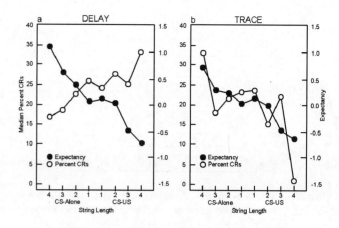

FIGURE 50.14   The relationship between expectancy of the US and conditioning performance for delay (a) and trace conditioning (b). Black circles indicate each group's expectancy of the US (on a scale of −3 to +3) as a function of the recent history of CS-alone and CS-US trials. String length refers to the number of consecutive trials, immediately prior to the trial on which a prediction was made, in which the CS had been presented alone or both the CS and the US had been presented. For both delay and trace conditioning, the subjective expectation of the US was highest following four CS-alone trials and lowest following four CS-US trials. White circles indicate the median percentage of CRs as a function of the recent history of CS-alone or CS-US trials. The performance of the group given delay conditioning (n = 20) was inversely related to expectation of the US. Thus, the probability of a CR was related to the associative strength of the CS and US (highest following a string of paired CS-US trials and lowest following a string of CS-alone trials). The results for trace conditioning (n = 18) were opposite. That is, conditioning performance mirrored the expectation of the US. CR probability was highest when expectation of the US was highest and lowest when expectation of the US was lowest. (Adapted from Clark, Manns, and Squire, 2001.)

mixed with strings of one to four CS-US trials. Before each trial, participants rate how much they expect the US on that trial. Figure 50.14 shows the percentage of conditioned responses (CRs) as a function of the recent history of CS-alone and CS-US trials (Clark, Manns, and Squire, 2001). The findings for delay conditioning (figure 50.14a) fully confirmed the findings reported previously (Perruchet, 1985). That is, the probability of a CR was related not to expectancy but to the associative strength of the CS and US. CRs became more likely as the number of consecutive CS-US trials increased, despite the fact that US expectancy decreased. The results for trace conditioning were opposite (figure 50.14b). The probability of a CR was positively related to expectancy of the air puff US. That is, CR probability was high when expectancy of the US was high and low when expectancy of the US was low. These findings show that expectation of the US has a different role in trace conditioning than it does in delay conditioning and support the idea that trace conditioning and delay conditioning are fundamentally different in their dependence on higher-order cognitive processes, such as awareness.

The studies outlined in this section can be understood in terms of the declarative and nondeclarative memory systems that support eyeblink classical conditioning. In both delay and trace conditioning paradigms, individuals sometimes develop declarative (conscious) knowledge about the stimulus contingencies and sometimes do not. For the most commonly studied forms of delay conditioning, declarative knowledge is superfluous to the acquisition of the CR, and conditioned performance can be supported by cerebellar and brainstem circuits (Christian and Thompson, 2003). Trace conditioning is fundamentally different. Trace conditioning resembles delay conditioning in that it also depends on the cerebellum (Woodruff-Pak, Lavond, and Thompson, 1985), but trace conditioning is additionally dependent on the hippocampus (Solomon et al., 1986; Moyer, Deyo, and Disterhoft, 1990; McGlinchey-Berroth et al., 1997; Weiss et al., 1999) and neocortex (Kronforst-Collins and Disterhoft, 1998; Weible, McEchron, and Disterhoft, 2000). Further, unlike delay conditioning, trace conditioning is strongly related to the acquisition of declarative knowledge (awareness) of the CS-US contingencies and to the degree to which the US is expected.

We suggest that for both trace and delay conditioning, the cerebellum is responsible for the acquisition, storage, and generation of the CR. Trace conditioning may additionally require declarative knowledge, because the trace interval makes it difficult for the cerebellum to process the CS and the US and form a motor memory. Indeed, electrophysiological studies have not detected activity in the cerebellum for longer than 100 ms after the termination of a single input pulse (Eccles, Ito, and Szentagothai, 1967). If, however, the hippocampus and neocortex have represented the stimulus contingencies, then it is possible that processed information about the CS can be transmitted to the cerebellum at a time during each trial that is optimal for cerebellar plasticity (immediately before and during the US). By this view, awareness of the contingencies, while not directly driving the acquisition of the conditioned response by the cerebellum, serves as an indicator that the hippocampus and related structures are effectively engaged by the task and working with the cerebellum so that the trace CR can be acquired.

The work reviewed in this chapter describes some of what has been learned recently about the function of the medial temporal lobe. Important matters for future study include identifying the separate contributions to memory that might be made by the separate anatomical components of the medial temporal lobe system and discovering the mechanism by which memories become independent of medial temporal lobe structures as time passes after learning. These and other questions will benefit from work that combines the study of humans with the study of experimental animals, and from work that explores the same tasks with both lesion analysis and neuroimaging.

REFERENCES

ANAGNOSTARAS, S. G., S. MAREN, and M. S. FANSELOW, 1999. Temporally graded retrograde amnesia of contextual fear after hippocampal damage in rats: Within-subjects examination. *J. Neurosci.* 19:1106–1114.

BADDELEY, A., F. VARGHA-KHADEM, and M. MISHKIN, 2001. Preserved recognition in a case of developmental amnesia: Implications for the acquisition of semantic memory? *J. Cogn. Neurosci.* 13:357–369.

BAKER, K. B., and J. J. KIM, 2002. Effects of stress and hippocampal NMDA receptor antagonism on recognition memory in rats. *Learn. Mem.* 9:58–65.

BAYLEY, P. J., R. O. HOPKINS, and L. R. SQUIRE, 2003. Successful recollection of remote autobiographical memories by amnesic patients with medial temporal lobe lesions. *Neuron* 38:135–144.

BAYLEY, P. J., and L. R. SQUIRE, 2002. Medial temporal lobe amnesia: Gradual acquisition of factual information by nondeclarative memory. *J. Neurosci.* 22:5741–5748.

BOLHUIS, J., C. A. STEWART, and E. M. FORREST, 1994. Retrograde amnesia and memory reactivation in rats with ibotenate lesions to the hippocampus or subiculum. *Q. J. Exp. Psychol.* 47:129–150.

BROADBENT, N. J., R. E. CLARK, and L. R. SQUIRE, 2003. Small dorsal hippocampal lesions impair spatial memory whereas large hippocampal lesions are required to impair novel object recognition. *Soc. Neurosci. Abstr.* 938.1.

BROWN, M. W., and J. P. AGGLETON, 2001. Recognition memory: What are the roles of the perirhinal cortex and hippocampus? *Nat. Rev. Neurosci.* 2:51–61.

CAREW, T. J., and C. L. SAHLEY, 1986. Invertebrate learning and memory: From behavior to molecules. *Annu. Rev. Neurosci.* 9:435–487.

CHO, Y. H., D. BERACOCHEA, and R. JAFFARD, 1993. Extended temporal gradient for the retrograde and anterograde amnesia produced by ibotenate entorhinal cortex lesions in mice. *J. Neurosci.* 13:1759–1766.

CHO, Y. H., and R. P. KESNER, 1996. Involvement of entorhinal cortex or parietal cortex in long-term spatial discrimination memory in rats: Retrograde amnesia. *Behav. Neurosci.* 110:436–442.

CHRISTIAN, K. M., and R. F. THOMPSON, 2003. Neural substrates of eyeblink conditioning: Acquisition and retention. *Learn. Mem.* 11:427–455.

CHUN, M. M., and E. A. PHELPS, 1999. Memory deficits for implicit contextual information in amnesic subjects with hippocampal damage. *Nat. Neurosci.* 2:844–847.

CIPOLOTTI, L., T. SHALLICE, D. CHAN, N. FOX, R. SCAHILL, G. HARRISON, J. STEVENS, and P. RUDGE, 2001. Long-term retrograde amnesia . . . the crucial role of the hippocampus. *Neuropsychologia* 39:151–172.

CLARK, R. E., N. J. BROADBENT, S. M. ZOLA-MORGAN, and L. R. SQUIRE, 2002. Anterograde amnesia and temporally-graded amnesia for a nonspatial memory task following lesions of hippocampus and subiculum. *J. Neurosci.* 22:4663–4669.

CLARK, R. E., N. J. BROADBENT, and L. R. SQUIRE, 2003. An examination of remote spatial memory with three spatial tasks following complete hippocampal lesions in rats. *Soc. Neurosci. Abstr* 938.2.

CLARK, R. E., J. R. MANNS, and L. R. SQUIRE, 2001. Trace and delay eyeblink conditioning: Contrasting phenomena of declarative and nondeclarative memory. *Psychol. Sci.* 12:304–308.

CLARK, R. E., J. R. MANNS, and L. R. SQUIRE, 2002. Classical conditioning, awareness, and brain systems. *Trends Cogn. Sci.* 6:524–531.

CLARK, R. E., and L. R. SQUIRE, 1998. Classical conditioning and brain systems: A key role for awareness. *Science* 280:77–81.

CLARK, R. E., and L. R. SQUIRE, 1999. Human eyeblink classical conditioning: Effects of manipulating awareness of the stimulus contingencies. *Psychol. Sci.* 10:14–18.

CLARK, R. E., A. N. WEST, S. M. ZOLA, and L. R. SQUIRE, 2001. Rats with lesions of the hippocampus are impaired on the delayed nonmatching-to-sample task. *Hippocampus* 11:176–186.

CLARK, R. E., S. M. ZOLA, and L. R. SQUIRE, 2000. Impaired recognition memory in rats after damage to the hippocampus. *J. Neurosci.* 20:8853–8860.

CROVITZ, H. F., and H. SCHIFFMAN, 1974. Frequency of episodic memories as a function of their age. *Bull. Psychonomi. Soc.* 4: 517–518.

DAVACHI, L., J. P. MITCHELL, and A. D. WAGNER, 2003. Multiple routes to memory: Distinct medial temporal lobe processes build item and source memories. *Proc. Natl. Acad. Sci. U.S.A.* 100: 2157–2162.

DAVIDSON, P. S., and E. L. GLISKY, 2002. Neuropsychological correlates of recollection and familiarity in normal aging. *Cogn. Affect. Behav. Neurosci.* 2:174–186.

DUVA, C. A., S. B. FLORESCO, G. R. WUNDERLICH, T. L. LAO, J. P. J. PINEL, and A. G. PHILLIPS, 1997. Disruption of spatial but not object-recognition memory by neurotoxic lesions of the dorsal hippocampus in rats. *Behav. Neurosci.* 111:1184–1196.

ECCLES, J. C., M. ITO, and J. SZENTAGOTHAI, 1967. *The Cerebellum as a Neuronal Machine.* New York: Springer-Verlag.

EICHENBAUM, H., and N. J. COHEN, 2001. *From Conditioning to Conscious Recollection: Memory Systems of the Brain.* New York: Oxford University Press.

ELDRIDGE, L. L., B. J. KNOWLTON, C. S. FURMANSKI, S. Y. BOOKHEIMER, and S. A. ENGEL, 2000. Remembering episodes: A selective role for the hippocampus during retrieval. *Nat. Neurosci.* 3:1068–1069.

FUJII, T., M. MOSCOVITCH, and L. NADEL, 2000. Memory consolidation, retrograde amnesia, and the temporal lobe. In *Handbook of Neuropsychology*, vol. 2, F. Boller, J. Grafman, and L. Cermak, eds. Amsterdam: Elsevier, pp. 223–250.

GIOVANELLO, K. S., M. VERFAELLIE, and M. M. KEANE, 2003. Disproportionate deficit in associative recognition in global amnesia. *Cogn. Affect. Behav. Neurosci.* 3:186–194.

GORMEZANO, I., 1962. Nicitating membrane: Classical conditioning and extinction in the albino rabbit. *Science* 138:33–34.

GREENE, A. J., B. A. SPELLMAN, J. A. DUSEK, H. B. EICHENBAUM, and W. B. LEVY, 2001. Relational learning with and without awareness: Transitive inference using nonverbal stimuli in humans. *Mem. Cognit.* 29:893–902.

HAMANN, S. B., and L. R. SQUIRE, 1995. On the acquisition of new declarative knowledge in amnesia. *Behav. Neurosci.* 109:1027–1044.

HENKE, K., A. BUCK, B. WEBER, and H. G. WIESER, 1997. Human hippocampus establishes associations in memory. *Hippocampus* 7:249–256.

HENKE, K., B. WEBER, L. KNEIFEL, H. G. WIESER, and A. BUCK, 1999. Human hippocampus associates information in memory. *Proc. Natl. Acad. Sci. U.S.A.* 96:5884–5889.

HIRANO, M., and K. NOGUCHI, 1998. Dissociation between specific personal episodes and other aspects of remote memory in a patient with hippocampal amnesia. *Percept. Motor Skills* 87: 99–107.

HOLDSTOCK, J. S., A. R. MAYES, N. ROBERTS, E. CEZAYIRLI, C. L. ISAAC, R. C. O'REILLY, and K. A. NORMAN, 2002. Under what condition is recognition spared relative to recall after selective hippocampal damage in humans? *Hippocampus* 12:341–351.

KAPUR, N., and D. J. BROOKS, 1999. Temporally-specific retrograde amnesia in two cases of discrete bilateral hippocampal pathology. *Hippocampus* 9:247–254.

KIM, J. J., R. E. CLARK, and R. F. THOMPSON, 1995. Hippocampectomy impairs the memory of recently, but not remotely, acquired trace eyeblink conditioned responses. *Behav. Neurosci.* 109:195–203.

KIM, J. J., and M. S. FANSELOW, 1992. Modality-specific retrograde amnesia of fear. *Science* 256:675–677.

KIM, J. J., and R. F. THOMPSON, 1997. Cerebellar circuits and synaptic mechanisms involved in classical eyeblink conditioning. *Trends Neurosci.* 20:177–181.

KNOWLTON, B. J., and M. S. FANSELOW, 1998. The hippocampus, consolidation, and on-line memory. *Curr. Opin. Neurobiol.* 8: 293–296.

KNUTTINEN, M. G., J. M. POUER, A. R. PRESTON, and J. F. DISTERHOFT, 2001. Awareness in classical differential eyeblink conditioning in young and aging humans. *Behav. Neurosci.* 115: 747–757.

KOPELMAN, M. D., B. A. WILSON, and A. D. BADDELEY, 1989. The autobiographical memory interview: A new assessment of autobiographical and personal semantic memory in amnesic patients. *J. Clin. Exp. Neuropsychol.* 11:724–744.

KROLL, N. E. A., R. T. KNIGHT, J. METCALFE, E. S. WOLF, and E. TULVING, 1996. Cohesion failure as a source of memory illusions. *J. Mem. Lang.* 35:176–196.

KRONFORST-COLLINS, M. A., and J. F. DISTERHOFT, 1998. Lesions of the caudal area of the rabbit medial prefrontal cortex impair trace eyeblink conditioning. *Neurobiol. Learn. Mem.* 2:147–162.

KUBIE, J. L., R. J. SUTHERLAND, and R. U. MILLER, 1999. Hippocampal lesions produce a temporally graded retrograde amnesia on a dry version of the Morris swimming task. *Psychobiology* 27:313–330.

MANNS, J. R., R. E. CLARK, and L. R. SQUIRE, 2000. Parallel acquisition of awareness and trace eyeblink classical conditioning. *Learn. Mem.* 7:267–272.

MANNS, J. R., R. E. CLARK, and L. R. SQUIRE, 2001. Single-cue delay eyeblink conditioning is unrelated to awareness. *Cogn. Affect. Behav. Neurosci.* 1:192–198.

MANNS, J. R., R. E. CLARK, and L. R. SQUIRE, 2002. Standard delay eyeblink classical conditioning is independent of awareness. *J. Exp. Psychol. Anim. Behav. Process* 28:32–37.

MANNS, J. R., R. O. HOPKINS, J. M. REED, E. G. KITCHENER, and L. R. SQUIRE, 2003. Recognition memory and the human hippocampus. *Neuron* 37:171–180.

MANNS, J. R., R. O. HOPKINS, and L. R. SQUIRE, 2003. Semantic memory and the human hippocampus. *Neuron* 38:127–133.

MANNS, J. R., and L. R. SQUIRE, 2001. Perceptual learning, awareness and the hippocampus. *Hippocampus* 11:776–782.

MANNS, J. R., and L. R. SQUIRE, 2002. The medial temporal lobe and memory for facts and events. In *Handbook of Memory Disorders*, A. Baddeley, M. D. Kopelman, and B. A. Wilson, eds. New York: Wiley, pp. 81–99.

MAREN, S., G. AHARONOV, and M. S. FANSELOW, 1999. Neurotoxic lesions of the dorsal hippocampus and Pavlovian fear conditioning in rats. *Behav. Brain Res.* 110:436–442.

MAUK, M. D., and R. F. THOMPSON, 1987. Retention of classically conditioned eyelid responses following acute decerebration. *Brain Res.* 403:89–95.

MCCLELLAND, J. L., B. L. MCNAUGHTON, and R. C. O'REILLY, 1995. Why there are complementary learning systems in the hippocampus and neocortex: Insights from the successes and failures of connectionist models of learning and memory. *Psychol. Rev.* 102:419–457.

McGLINCHEY-BERROTH, R., M. C. CARRILLO, J. D. E. GABRIELI, C. M. BRAWN, and J. F. DISTERHOFT, 1997. Impaired trace eyeblink conditioning in bilateral, medial-temporal lobe amnesia. *Behav. Neurosci.* 111:873–882.

MISHKIN, M., 1978. Memory in monkeys severely impaired by combined but not by separate removal of amygdala and hippocampus. *Nature* 273:297–298.

MOSCOVITCH, M., T. YASCHYSHYN, M. ZIEGLER, and L. NADEL, 2000. Remote episodic memory and retrograde amnesia: Was Endel Tulving right all along? In *Memory, Consciousness and the Brain: The Tallinn Conference*, E. Tulving, ed. Philadelphia: Psychology Press/Taylor and Francis, pp. 331–345.

MOYER, J. R., R. A. DEYO, and J. F. DISTERHOFT, 1990. Hippocampectomy disrupts trace eye-blink conditioning in rabbits. *Behav. Neurosci.* 104:243–252.

MUMBY, D. G., R. S. ASTURM, M. P. WEISAND, and R. J. SUTHERLAND, 1999. Retrograde amnesia and selective damage to the hippocampal formation: Memory for places and object discriminations. *Behav. Brain Res.* 106:97–107.

NADEL, L., and M. MOSCOVITCH, 1997. Memory consolidation, retrograde amnesia and the hippocampal complex. *Curr. Opin. Neurobiol.* 7:217–227.

NORMAN, K. A., and R. C. O'RIELLY, 2003. Modeling hippocampal and neocortical contributions to recognition memory: A complementary-learning-systems approach. *Psychol. Rev.* 110:611–646.

O'KANE, G., E. A. KENSINGER, and S. CORKIN, 2004. Evidence for semantic learning in profound amnesia: An investigation with patient H.M. *Hippocampus.* 14:417–425.

O'KEEFE, J., and L. NADEL, 1978. *The Hippocampus as a Cognitive Map*. London: Oxford University Press.

PERRUCHET, P., 1985. A pitfall for the expectancy theory of human eyelid conditioning. *J. Biol. Sci.* 20:163–170.

RAMOS, J. M., 1998. Retrograde amnesia for spatial information: A dissociation between intra- and extramaze cues following hippocampus lesions in rats. *Eur. J. Neurosci.* 10:3295–3301.

RAMPON, C., Y. P. TANG, J. GOODHOUSE, E. SHIMIZU, M. KYIN, and J. Z. TSIEN, 2000. Enrichment induces structural changes and recovery from nonspatial memory deficits in CA1 NMDAR1-knockout mice. *Nat. Neurosci.* 3:238–244.

REED, J. M., S. B. HAMANN, L. STEFANACCI, and L. R. SQUIRE, 1997. When amnesic patients perform well on recognition memory tests. *Behav. Neurosci.* 111:1163–1170.

REED, J. M., and L. R. SQUIRE, 1997. Impaired recognition memory in patients with lesions limited to the hippocampal formation. *Behav. Neurosci.* 111:667–675.

REED, J. M., and L. R. SQUIRE, 1998. Retrograde amnesia for facts and events: Findings from four new cases. *J. Neurosci.* 18:3943–3954.

REINITZ, M. T., M. VERFAELLIE, and W. P. MILBERG, 1996. Memory conjunction errors in normal and amnesic subjects. *J. Mem. Lang.* 35:286–299.

REMPEL-CLOWER, N., S. M. ZOLA, L. R. SQUIRE, and D. G. AMARAL, 1996. Three cases of enduring memory impairment following bilateral damage limited to the hippocampal formation. *J. Neurosci.* 16:5233–5255.

RESCORLA, R. A., and A. R. WAGNER, 1972. A theory of Pavlovian conditioning: Variations in the effectiveness of reinforcement and nonreinforcement. In *Classical Conditioning II: Current Theory and Research*, A. H. Black and W. F. Prokasy, eds. New York: Appleton-Century-Crofts, pp. 64–99.

ROSS, L. E., and M. N. NELSON, 1973. The role of awareness in differential conditioning. *Psychophysiology* 10:91–94.

SCHACTER, D. L., and E. TULVING, 1994. *Memory Systems 1994*. Cambridge, Mass.: MIT Press.

SCOVILLE, W. B., and B. MILNER, 1957. Loss of recent memory after bilateral hippocampal lesions. *J. Neurol. Neurosurg. Psychiatry* 20:11–21.

SHIMAMURA, A. P., and L. R. SQUIRE, 1987. A neuropsychological study of fact memory and source amnesia. *J. Exp. Psychol. Learn. Mem. Cognit.* 13:464–473.

SHIMAMURA, A. P., and L. R. SQUIRE, 1988. Long-term memory in amnesia: Cued recall, recognition memory, and confidence ratings. *J. Exp. Psychol. Learn. Mem. Cognit.* 14:763–770.

SOLOMON, P. R., E. R. VANDER SCHAAF, R. F. THOMPSON, and D. J. WEISZ, 1986. Hippocampus and trace conditioning of the rabbit's classically conditioned nictitating membrane response. *Behav. Neurosci.* 100:729–744.

SQUIRE, L. R., 1992. Memory and the hippocampus: A synthesis from findings with rats, monkeys, and humans. *Psychol. Rev.* 99:195–231.

SQUIRE, L. R. (in press). Memory systems of the brain: A brief history and current perspective. *Neurobiol. Learn. Mem.*

SQUIRE, L. R., and P. ALVAREZ, 1995. Retrograde amnesia and memory consolidation: A neurobiological perspective. *Curr. Opin. Neurobiol.* 5:169–177.

SQUIRE, L. R., and E. R. KANDEL, 1999. *Memory: From Mind to Molecules*. New York: W. H. Freeman.

SQUIRE, L. R., and B. J. KNOWLTON, 2000. The medial temporal lobe, the hippocampus, and the memory systems of the brain. In *The New Cognitive Neurosciences*, 2nd ed., M. S. Gazzaniga, ed. Cambridge, Mass.: MIT Press.

SQUIRE, L. R., and S. M. ZOLA, 1998. Episodic memory, semantic memory, and amnesia. *Hippocampus* 8:205–211.

SQUIRE, L. R., and S. ZOLA-MORGAN, 1983. The neurology of memory: The case for correspondence between the findings for human and nonhuman primate. In *The Physiological Basis of Memory*, J. A. Deutsch, ed. New York: Academic Press, pp. 199–268.

SQUIRE, L. R., and S. ZOLA-MORGAN, 1991. The medial temporal lobe memory system. *Science* 253:1380–1386.

STARK, C. E., P. J. BAYLEY, and L. R. SQUIRE, 2002. Recognition memory for single items and for associations is similarly impaired following damage to the hippocampal region. *Learn. Mem.* 9:238–242.

STARK, C. E. L., and L. R. SQUIRE, 2003. Hippocampal damage equally impairs memory for single items and memory for conjunctions. *Hippocampus* 13:281–292.

STEFANACCI, L., E. A. BUFFALO, H. SCHMOLCK, and L. R. SQUIRE, 2000. Profound amnesia following damage to the medial temporal lobe: A neuroanatomical and neuropsychological profile of patient E.P. *J. Neurosci.* 20:7024–7036.

SUTHERLAND, R. J., M. P. M. D. WEISEND, R. S. ASTUR, F. M. HANLON, A. KOERNER, M. J. THOMAS, Y. WU, S. N. MOSES, C. COLE, D. A. HAMILTON, and J. M. HOESING, 2001. Retrograde amnesia after hippocampal damage: Recent vs. remote memories in three tasks. *Hippocampus* 11:27–42.

SUZUKI, W. A., 2003. Declarative versus episodic: Two theories put to the test. *Neuron* 38:5–7.

SUZUKI, W. A., and H. EICHENBAUM, 2000. The neurophysiology of memory. *Ann. N. Y. Acad. Sci.* 911:175–191.

TAKEHARA, K., S. KAWAHARA, K. TAKATSUKI, and Y. KIRINO, 2002. Time-limited role of the hippocampus in the memory for trace eyeblink conditioning in mice. *Brain Res.* 951:183–190.

TENG, E., and L. R. SQUIRE, 1999. Memory for places learned long ago is intact after hippocampal damage. *Nature* 400:675–677.

THOMPSON, R. F., and D. J. KRUPA, 1994. Organization of memory traces in the mammalian brain. *Annu. Rev. Neurosci.* 17:519–550.

TULVING, E., 1985. Memory and consciousness. *Can. Psychologist* 26:1–12.

TULVING, E., 1991. Concepts in human memory. In *Memory: Organization and Locus of Change*, L. R. Squire, N. M. Weinberger, G. Lynch, and J. L. McGaugh, eds. New York: Oxford University Press, pp. 3–32.

TULVING, E., 2002. Episodic memory: From mind to brain. *Annu. Rev. Psychol.* 53:1–25.

TULVING, E., C. A. G. HAYMAN, and C. A. MACDONALD, 1991. Long-lasting perceptual priming and semantic learning in amnesia: A case experiment. *J. Exp. Psychol. Learn. Mem. Cognit.* 17:595–617.

TULVING, E., and H. J. MARKOWITSCH, 1998. Episodic and declarative memory: Role of the hippocampus. *Hippocampus* 8:198–204.

URETSKY, E., and R. A. MCCLEARY, 1969. Effect of hippocampal isolation on retention. *J. Comp. Physiol. Psychol.* 68:1–8.

VAN DER LINDEN, M., V. CORNIL, T. MEULEMANS, A. IVANOIU, E. SALMON, and F. COYETTE, 2001. Acquisition of a novel vocabulary in an amnesic patient. *Neurocase* 7:283–293.

VARGHA-KHADEM, F., D. GAFFAN, K. E. WATKINS, A. CONNELLY, W. VAN PAESSCHEN, and M. MISHKIN, 1997. Differential effects of early hippocampal pathology on episodic and semantic memory. *Science* 277:376–380.

VERFAELLIE, M., P. KOSEFF, and M. P. ALEXANDER, 2000. Acquisition of novel semantic information in amnesia: Effects of lesion location. *Neuropsychologia* 38:484–492.

WEIBLE, A. P., M. D. MCECHRON, and J. F. DISTERHOFT, 2000. Cortical involvement in acquisition and extinction of trace eyeblink conditioning. *Behav. Neurosci.* 114:1058–1067.

WEISS, C., H. BOUWMEESTER, J. M. POWER, and J. F. DISTERHOFT, 1999. Hippocampal lesions prevent trace eyeblink conditioning in the freely moving rat. *Behav. Brain Res.* 99:123–132.

WESTMACOTT, R., and M. MOSCOVITCH, 2001. Names and words without meaning: Incidental postmorbid semantic learning in a person with extensive bilateral medial temporal lobe damage. *Neuropsychology* 15:586–596.

WIIG, K. A., L. N. COOPER, and M. F. BEAR, 1996. Temporally graded retrograde amnesia following separate and combined lesions of the perirhinal cortex and fornix in the rat. *Learn. Mem.* 3:313–325.

WINOCUR, G., 1990. Anterograde and retrograde amnesia in rats with dorsal hippocampal or dorsomedial thalamic lesions. *Behav. Brain Res.* 38:145–154.

WINOCUR, G., R. M. MCDONALD, and M. MOSCOVITCH, 2001. Anterograde and retrograde amnesia in rats with large hippocampal lesions. *Hippocampus* 11:18–26.

WIXTED, J. T., and L. R. SQUIRE, 2004. Recall and recognition are equally impaired in patients with selective hippocampal damage. *Cogn. Affect. Behav. Neurosci.*

WOODRUFF-PAK, S. D., D. G. LAVOND, and R. F. THOMPSON, 1985. Trace conditioning: Abolished by cerebellar nuclear lesions but not lateral cerebellar cortex aspirations. *Brain Res.* 348:249–260.

YONELINAS, A. P., J. B. HOPFINGER, M. H. BUONOCORE, N. E. ROLL, and K. BAYNES, 2001. Hippocampal, parahippocampal and occipital-temporal contributions to associative and item recognition memory: An fMRI study. *Neuroreport* 12:359–363.

YONELINAS, A. P., N. E. KROLL, J. R. QUAMME, M. M. LAZZARA, M. J. SAUVE, K. F. WIDAMAN, and R. T. KNIGHT, 2002. Effects of extensive temporal lobe damage or mild hypoxia on recollection and familiarity. *Nat. Neurosci.* 5:1236–1241.

ZOLA, S., and L. R. SQUIRE, 2000. The medial temporal lobe and the hippocampus. In *The Oxford Handbook of Memory*, E. Tulving and F. I. M. Craik, eds. New York: Oxford University Press, pp. 485–500.

ZOLA-MORGAN, S., and L. R. SQUIRE, 1990. The primate hippocampal formation: Evidence for a time-limited role in memory storage. *Science* 250:288–290.

ZOLA-MORGAN, S., L. R. SQUIRE, and D. G. AMARAL, 1986. Human amnesia and the medial temporal region: Enduring memory impairment following a bilateral lesion limited to field CA1 of the hippocampus. *J. Neurosci.* 6:2950–2967.

ZOLA-MORGAN, S., L. R. SQUIRE, and S. J. RAMUS, 1994. Severity of memory impairment in monkeys as a function of locus and extent of damage within the medial temporal lobe memory system. *Hippocampus* 4:483–495.

51 Cognitive Control, Semantic Memory, and Priming: Contributions from Prefrontal Cortex

ANTHONY D. WAGNER, SILVIA A. BUNGE, AND DAVID BADRE

ABSTRACT *Cognitive control* refers to an ensemble of mechanisms that constrain our thoughts and responses in accordance with our goals. Functional brain imaging studies have provided important insights regarding the functional and neuroanatomical bases of cognitive control and have illustrated that cognitive control has an influence on and is influenced by long-term memory. This chapter provides an overview of elemental forms of cognitive control, their relation to working memory, and their dependence on prefrontal cortex (PFC). The interaction between cognitive control and memory is then considered within the context of retrieving goal-relevant knowledge from semantic memory, with a focus on understanding how PFC guides controlled retrieval. Finally, the nature of priming—a form of nondeclarative (or implicit) memory that is reflected as nonconscious effects of previous experience on future behavior—is described en route to illustrating how reductions in cognitive control demands can follow experience-based changes in nondeclarative memory.

Cognitive control refers to mechanisms that permit an individual to access and work with internal representations in a goal-directed manner. In so doing, cognitive control supports context-relevant stimulus processing, the retrieval and online maintenance of knowledge, and the transformation of representations to satisfy our goals. Prefrontal cortex (PFC) is a central component of the neural circuitry underlying cognitive control, including the control of memory; flexible behavior often depends on PFC mechanisms that support access to long-term knowledge. Accordingly, the specification of cognitive control processes, their dependence on PFC, and their interactions with long-term memory is of fundamental importance (Stuss and Benson, 1984;

Goldman-Rakic, 1987; Schacter, 1987b; Shallice, 1988; Petrides, 1994; Shimamura, 1995; Fuster, 1997; Miller and Cohen, 2001; Wagner, 2002).

In this chapter, we consider neuroimaging evidence regarding PFC contributions to cognitive control, and the interactions between control mechanisms and memory. We first delineate the elemental processes that constitute working memory and cognitive control, and their organization within PFC. We then provide an in-depth discussion of one control mechanism to illustrate how cognitive control can interact with long-term memory. This discussion considers how cognitive control supports retrieval from declarative (or explicit) memory, as revealed through PFC contributions to the controlled retrieval of task-relevant semantic knowledge. We conclude by exploring the relation between this PFC control mechanism and priming, a nondeclarative (or implicit) form of memory, to illustrate how reductions in cognitive control demands can follow experience-based changes in long-term memory.

Working memory and cognitive control

Language comprehension, problem solving, goal satisfaction, and other high-level cognitive functions depend on working memory, which refers to our ability to maintain and manipulate active representations (Miller, Galanter, and Pribram, 1960; Fuster and Alexander, 1971; Goldman-Rakic, 1987). Working memory is a multifaceted rather than unitary faculty. A prominent model of human working memory proposes that this ability depends on at least three components: a buffer for the short-term maintenance of verbal information, a buffer for the maintenance of visuospatial information, and a "central executive" that gates and manipulates representations held in these buffers (Baddeley and Hitch, 1974; Baddeley, 1986). This influential perspective has proved to be an effective framework for examining the architecture of working memory, although, as

ANTHONY D. WAGNER Department of Psychology and Neurosciences Program, Stanford University, Stanford, Calif.
SILVIA A. BUNGE Department of Psychology and Center for Mind and Brain, University of California at Davis, Davis, Calif.
DAVID BADRE Department of Brain and Cognitive Sciences, Massachusetts Institute of Technology, Cambridge, Mass.

we will see, working memory can also be conceptualized as an integrated set of cognitive control processes.

VERBAL WORKING MEMORY Verbal working memory constitutes the maintenance of speech-based (phonological) representations, as when we subvocally rehearse a phone number while preparing to dial it. Verbal working memory depends on a system termed the phonological loop, which consists of two components: a phonological store, which represents active phonological information, and an articulatory control process, which rehearses the contents of the store and reactivates long-term phonological knowledge (Baddeley and Hitch, 1974). Support for this architecture comes from behavioral and neuropsychological observations that the two components of the phonological loop are dissociable (Baddeley, 1986; Smith and Jonides, 1995).

Neuroimaging studies of verbal working memory consistently implicate frontal, parietal, and cerebellar regions that work together to support the phonological loop (Smith and Jonides, 1999; figure 51.1). Demands on the articulatory control process elicit activation in structures important for speech production, including left ventrolateral PFC (approximately Brodmann's area [BA] 44; Broca's area) and left premotor and supplementary motor cortices (BA 6) (Paulesu, Frith, and Frackowiak, 1993; Awh et al., 1996; Fiez et al., 1996). These frontal regions are thought to maintain active phonological representations stored in left or bilateral inferior parietal cortices (Awh et al., 1996; Jonides, Schumacher, et al., 1998; Bunge et al., 2001; but see Chein and Fiez, 2001). Cerebellar subregions may integrate inputs from ventrolateral PFC and parietal regions, providing a corrective signal that refines the rehearsal process (Desmond et al., 1997).

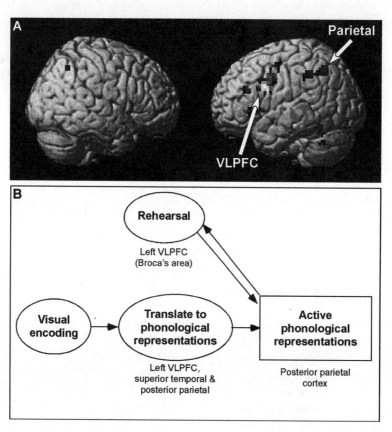

FIGURE 51.1 Neural correlates and component processes of phonological working memory. (*A*) Left ventrolateral prefrontal cortex (VLPFC) and posterior parietal cortex demonstrate greater activation during the encoding and maintenance of visually presented words. (Data from D. Badre and A. D. Wagner, 2004. Selection and conflict monitoring in prefrontal cortex: Assessing the specificity of cognitive control. *Neuron* 41:473–487. Used with permission.) (*B*) Component processes supporting phonological working memory and their neural substrates. Visually presented information is translated into phonological representations, which are actively represented (stored) in posterior parietal cortex. These representations passively decay over the course of seconds in the absence of subvocal rehearsal, which is mediated by left VLPFC (Broca's area). Recurrent loops between left VLPFC and posterior parietal cortex allow information to be actively maintained for a prolonged period. (Adapted with permission from E. E. Smith and J. Jonnides, 1998. Neuroimaging analyses of human working memory. *Proc. Natl. Acad. Sci. U.S.A.* 95:12061–12068. Copyright 1998, National Academy of Sciences, U.S.A.)

The contributions of specific PFC subregions to verbal working memory partially depend on the amount of information that must be maintained. Whereas control processes mediated by left ventrolateral PFC appear sufficient to maintain low working memory loads, when the amount of information to be maintained begins to approach an individual's working memory capacity limit, activation also emerges in bilateral dorsolateral PFC (BA 9/46) (Rypma et al., 1999). Dorsolateral PFC activation may reflect a shift to reliance on additional cognitive control processes, such as those supporting the "chunking" of information (but see Veltman, Rombouts, and Dolan, 2003). This interpretation is consistent with the idea that central executive mechanisms are engaged when working memory maintenance demands approach or exceed capacity limits (Baddeley and Hitch, 1974), and further suggests that, in humans, dorsolateral PFC supports nonmaintenance cognitive control processes, a hypothesis to which we will return.

SPATIAL AND OBJECT WORKING MEMORY Visuospatial working memory allows us to maintain visual representations of objects and knowledge of the position of objects in space. As with verbal working memory, this ability depends on PFC–posterior neocortical interactions (Chafee and Goldman-Rakic, 2000; Miller and Cohen, 2001). However, whereas verbal working memory is associated with left PFC, visuospatial working memory in humans is differentially associated with right-lateralized or bilateral PFC (D'Esposito et al., 1998; Smith and Jonides, 1999; Prabhakaran et al., 2000). Visuospatial working memory also engages occipitotemporal and parietal cortices that support object and spatial representations; PFC is thought to control the maintenance of spatial and object codes through reciprocal interactions with these posterior representations. One hypothesis regarding rehearsal in spatial working memory is that spatial information is maintained through shifts of spatial selective attention to location-specific representations (Awh and Jonides, 1998).

In contrast to the traditional two-store model of working memory, according to which object and spatial representations are maintained by a single buffer, termed the visuospatial sketchpad (Baddeley, 1986), recent evidence suggests that object and spatial working memory may be separable (e.g., Farah, 1988; Baddeley, 1994; Carlesimo et al., 2001). Behaviorally, spatial distraction impairs spatial working memory more than visual working memory, whereas visuo-object distraction has the reverse effect (e.g., Tresch, Sinnamon, and Seamon, 1993). At the neural level, single-cell recordings in infrahuman primates indicate that some PFC neurons maintain spatial representations, others maintain object representations, and yet others maintain an integration of spatial and object information (Rao, Rainer, and Miller, 1997; Rainer, Asaad, and Miller, 1998). Thus, segre-

gation and interaction characterize working memory for space and objects.

Object working memory and spatial working memory are not strictly topographically segregated in PFC. In infrahuman primates, object, spatial, and integrative neurons are present in ventrolateral and dorsolateral PFC (Rainer, Asaad, and Miller, 1998; figure 51.2), with there being a moderate bias for a greater proportion of object working memory neurons in ventrolateral PFC and spatial working memory neurons in dorsolateral PFC (Wilson, Ó Scalaidhe, and Goldman-Rakic, 1993). In humans, many neuroimaging studies have failed to observe a marked segregation between spatial and object working memory within PFC, with both forms of maintenance often eliciting activation in ventrolateral and dorsolateral PFC (e.g., McCarthy et al., 1996; D'Esposito et al., 1998; Nystrom et al., 2000). By contrast, other studies suggest that spatial working memory and object working memory are at least partially separable, with a subregion of the superior frontal sulcus being differentially associated with spatial working memory (Courtney et al., 1998; Haxby et al., 2000; Sala, Rama, and Courtney, 2003; see also Alain et al., 2001).

Although the degree of topographic segregation between spatial and object working memory in PFC remains uncertain, the collective data indicate that a comprehensive model of human working memory requires separable systems for object, spatial, and phonological information, and an understanding of how these different types of information are integrated. Neuropsychological, behavioral, and neuroimaging data also suggest that a fourth system may subserve working memory for semantic knowledge (e.g., Martin, Shelton, and Yaffee, 1994; Demb et al., 1995; Shivde and Anderson, 2001).

COGNITIVE CONTROL The central executive, as originally proposed, is a limited-capacity attentional system that coordinates working memory maintenance buffers and manipulates their contents (Baddeley, 1986). The executive also is thought to mediate selective attention and the inhibition of task-irrelevant representations. Although it was once conceptualized as a monolithic component of working memory, there is little behavioral evidence for a single executive processor (e.g., Towse and Houston-Price, 2001). Rather, executive functions, which may include both working memory manipulation *and* maintenance processes, likely emerge from a set of elemental cognitive control mechanisms.

Cognitive control refers to processes that constrain our thoughts and responses in accordance with our goals. Putative control functions include dual-task coordination and task switching (*task management*); retrieval of goal-relevant information from long-term memory (*controlled retrieval*); selection of appropriate responses (*response selection*) and

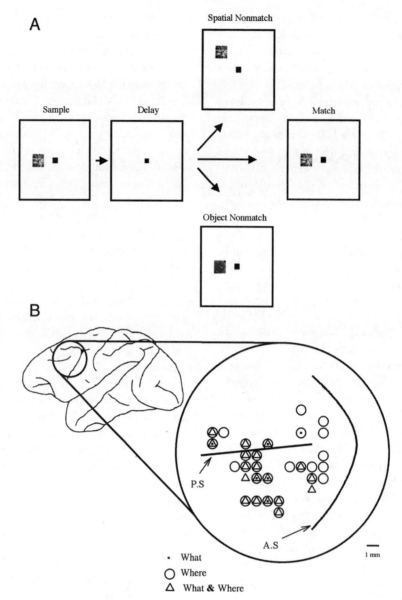

FIGURE 51.2   PFC neurons maintain object and spatial information, and the integration of object and space. (*A*) Delayed match-to-sample task. An initial sample is presented and must be maintained over a delay until a matching test stimulus appears. In this variant, the monkey must remember the sample stimulus ("what") and the location of the stimulus in space ("where"), and respond by releasing a lever only to stimuli that match on both dimensions. (*B*) Recording sites where neurons with what, where, or what-and-where delay activity were found. The arcuate sulcus (A.S.) and principal sulcus (P.S.) are delineated. (Reprinted with permission from G. Rainer, W. F. Asaad, and E. K. Miller, 1998. Memory fields of neurons in the primate prefrontal cortex. *Proc. Natl. Acad. Sci. U.S.A.* 95:15008–15013. Copyright 1998, National Academy of Sciences, U.S.A.)

inhibition of inappropriate responses (*response inhibition*); resolution of distraction from competing representations (*interference resolution*); transformation, reordering, or updating of information maintained in working memory (*manipulation*); and evaluation of whether information in working memory meets the criteria associated with one's goal (*monitoring*).

Biased competition theory   According to the biased competition framework (Desimone and Duncan, 1995), a similar neural mechanism may underlie each of the control functions just hypothesized (Miller and Cohen, 2001). Biased competition theory asserts that, in the absence of cognitive control, the representation most strongly activated by response cues in an automatic, bottom-up fashion will serve as the basis for behavior, irrespective of whether the representation is task relevant. However, cognitive control, in the form of top-down excitatory signals deriving from PFC, can bias information processing in favor of weaker but task-relevant representations, enhancing these representations and indirectly suppressing task-irrelevant competitors through lateral inhibitory interconnections between representations (Cohen,

Dunbar, and McClelland, 1990). This top-down bias signal is argued to constitute the fundamental basis of cognitive control, enabling the selection of appropriate goal representations, the retrieval of target knowledge from working memory and long-term memory (LTM), and the execution of context-appropriate responses (see also Shimamura, 1995).

Intimately related to the biased competition framework is the hypothesis that the anterior cingulate cortex (ACC) and PFC play distinct roles in cognitive control (Cohen, Braver, and O'Reilly, 1996; MacDonald et al., 2000; figure 51.3). From this perspective, the rostral zone of ACC serves to detect the presence of conflict (i.e., the simultaneous activation of multiple competing representations) and signals PFC to resolve the conflict by up-regulating control (i.e., increasing the top-down biasing of task-appropriate representations). Computational models and some neuroimaging data suggest that ACC may selectively detect conflict between competing responses (Botvinick et al., 2001; Milham et al., 2001; van Veen et al., 2001). However, other evidence points to a more general function, with ACC detecting conflict at multiple processing stages (see van Veen and Carter, 2002; Badre and Wagner, 2004).

Dissociable mechanisms in dorsolateral and ventrolateral PFC A complementary perspective on cognitive control is the hypothesis that "maintenance" and "manipulation" constitute interacting but dissociable control mechanisms that differentially depend on distinct PFC subregions. From this perspective, the rehearsal processes that support maintenance in verbal, object, and spatial working memory are themselves forms of cognitive control. Accordingly, ventrolateral PFC regions are argued to control the retrieval of task-relevant representations and their active maintenance. By contrast, dorsolateral PFC functions monitor the contents of working memory and/or manipulate active representations in the service of completing the current goal (Petrides, 1994; Owen, Evans, and Petrides, 1996; D'Esposito et al., 1998; but see Raye et al., 2002; Veltman, Rombouts, and Dolan, 2003).

Neuroimaging data provide empirical support for the differential roles of ventrolateral and dorsolateral PFC subregions in cognitive control. As already discussed, neuroimaging studies indicate that dorsolateral PFC is recruited at higher verbal working memory loads, suggesting that it is not involved in maintenance per se but instead may play a role in reorganizing or manipulating representations to facilitate maintenance (Rypma et al., 1999). Dorsolateral regions are also differentially engaged when we reorder (D'Esposito, Postle, Ballard, et al., 1999; Postle, Berger, and D'Esposito, 1999; Wagner, Maril, Bjork, et al., 2001) or update (Salmon et al., 1996; Garavan et al., 2000) representations in working memory (figure 51.4). Thus, dorsolateral PFC mechanisms

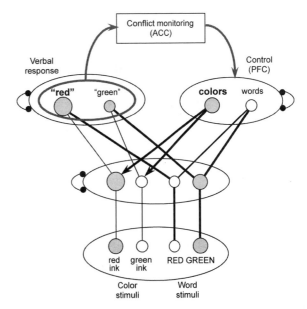

FIGURE 51.3 Model of PFC and ACC involvement during performance of the Stroop task. Circles represent processing units, which correspond to a population of neurons assumed to code a given piece of information. Lines represent connections between units, with heavier lines indicating stronger connections. Looped connections with black circles indicate mutual inhibition among units within that layer. Subjects must name the color that a word is printed in, rather than read the word. During presentation of a conflict stimulus (the word *green* displayed in red ink), the "colors" context unit is activated in PFC (indicated by gray fill), representing the current intent to name the color. This passes activation to the intermediate units in the color-naming pathway (indicated by arrows), which increases the activation of those units (indicated by larger size) and biases processing in favor of activity flowing along this pathway. This biasing effect favors activation of the response unit corresponding to the color input, even though the connection weights in this pathway are weaker than in the word pathway. Importantly, the need for this top-down bias from PFC is initially detected by ACC, which computes the level of conflict (or the presence of simultaneously active representations in the response layer). (Adapted with permission from M. M. Botvinick, T. S. Braver, D. M. Barch, C. S. Carter, and J. D. Cohen, 2001. Conflict monitoring and cognitive control. *Psychol. Rev.* 108:624–652; and from E. K. Miller and J. D. Cohen, 2001. An integrative theory of prefrontal cortex function. *Ann. Rev. Neurosci.* 24:167–202. With permission from the Annual Review of Neuroscience, Volume 24. © 2001 by Annual Reviews, www.annualreviews.org.)

may operate on and transform the contents of working memory.

In addition to its role in active maintenance, ventrolateral PFC supports the control of thought and action in ways that are just beginning to be understood. Subregions of ventrolateral PFC are implicated in the controlled retrieval and selection of task-relevant long-term knowledge (Petrides, 1994; Thompson-Schill et al., 1997; Badre and Wagner, 2002), a point to which we return in the next section. Other subregions of left ventrolateral PFC appear to resolve interference in verbal working memory (Jonides, Smith,

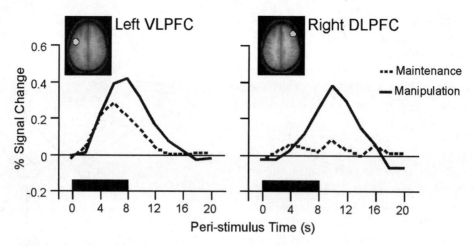

Figure 51.4 Hemodynamic responses in left VLPFC and right DLPFC during working memory maintenance alone or maintenance with manipulation. During each 8-s trial (indicated by black box), subjects either rehearsed a triplet of nouns (maintenance task) or maintained the triplet and reordered the words along a semantic dimension (manipulation task). The manipulation task recruited both VLPFC and DLPFC, whereas the maintenance task primarily recruited VLPFC. (Adapted from A. D. Wagner, A. Maril, R. A. Bjork, and D. L. Schacter, 2001. Prefrontal contributions to executive control: fMRI evidence for functional distinctions within lateral prefrontal cortex. *NeuroImage* 14:1337–1347. Copyright 2001, with permission from Elsevier.)

et al., 1998; D'Esposito, Postle, Jonides, et al., 1999; Bunge et al., 2001), with homologous right ventrolateral regions supporting interference resolution between nonverbal representations (Hazeltine et al., 2003). Right ventrolateral PFC regions are also active when we shift between alternate response criteria, as in the Wisconsin Card-Sorting Task (Konishi, Nakajima, Uchida, Kameyama, et al., 1998), and when we halt the execution of an inappropriate response (Konishi, Nakajima, Uchida, Sekihara, et al., 1998; Garavan, Ross, and Stein, 1999; Bunge et al., 2002; see also Aron et al., 2003).

Frontopolar control processes Extant data also implicate frontopolar cortex (FPC) as central to cognitive control. However, perhaps owing to a paucity of comparative data, FPC remains poorly understood at the functional level, even though neuroimaging studies consistently observe FPC activation during episodic retrieval, complex working memory, and higher-level cognitive tasks (Fletcher and Henson, 2001; Ramnani and Owen, 2004). Findings from the task management literature suggest that FPC is active when subjects must maintain a primary task goal or task-relevant information while simultaneously attending to a secondary goal or task (Koechlin et al., 1999; Braver and Bongiolatti, 2002; Badre and Wagner, 2004). An emerging literature on analogical reasoning further suggests that FPC is important for integrating disparate representations or relations (Christoff et al., 2001; Kroger et al., 2002). Given these findings, FPC involvement in episodic retrieval may reflect processes that integrate retrieved information with response criteria or context information held in working memory, thus permitting decisions about whether the retrieved information satisfies the mnemonic goal (e.g., Rugg and Wilding, 2000).

As suggested by this formulation of frontopolar function, one intriguing development over the past decade has been the emerging conceptualization of cognitive control as an ensemble of processes that intimately interact with mnemonic and cognitive systems. Accordingly, efforts to delineate cognitive control may benefit from approaches that examine the role of control processes in a variety of memory domains. With this in mind, we now turn to consider evidence regarding the interaction between cognitive control and LTM, with an in-depth discussion of a particular form of control (controlled retrieval). In the next section, we delineate how controlled retrieval serves to activate declarative knowledge structures through a top-down biasing of semantic memory. The chapter concludes with a consideration of how nondeclarative memory influences controlled retrieval demands.

Cognitive control and semantic memory

Recovering context-relevant meaning about the world allows us to flexibly use long-term knowledge to generate goal-consistent responses. Let us say that we need to pound in a nail and the only objects available are standard office supplies, such as a stapler, computer, and the like. Although information strongly associated with each concept (e.g., that staplers are used to bind documents) is of little assistance in this context, we are capable of accessing other weakly associated, but context-relevant, knowledge about the objects. Thus, we recall that staplers are heavy and fairly wieldy objects, whereas computers tend to be fragile. Such knowledge may ultimately support the inference that the stapler is a suitable substitute for a hammer. Importantly, our ability to retrieve this information requires processes that guide access to, or control the retrieval of, relevant knowledge when strongly associated semantic information is insufficient to meet task demands.

This example illustrates how some situations require control processes that guide retrieval from *semantic memory*, which is a declarative (or explicit) form of LTM that represents our general knowledge about the world, including facts, concepts, and vocabulary (Tulving, 1972). In this section, we consider when and how cognitive control mediates semantic retrieval. We begin by briefly introducing basic concepts regarding the organization of semantic knowledge, and then consider how semantic information can be retrieved through automatic or controlled processes. The consequences of left PFC lesions for semantic retrieval are subsequently discussed as a foundation for understanding neuroimaging data regarding the role of PFC in controlled semantic retrieval.

STRUCTURE OF SEMANTIC KNOWLEDGE   Our aim is to consider the contributions of PFC to cognitive control and to specify how control processes interact with LTM; as such, a full discussion of the structure of semantic knowledge is beyond the scope of this chapter (see Smith and Medin, 1981; Martin and Chao, 2001). However, a few characteristics of semantic memory are relevant for understanding the processes that retrieve semantic knowledge. First, semantic information is stored in a distributed, associative network that links conceptual representations and components of representations. Second, the associations between representations vary in strength, depending on the frequency of their prior co-occurrence, their overlap in features, and their categorical relations. Finally, multiple representations can compete for processing and retrieval through mutually inhibitory interactions.

At the neural level, semantic knowledge is distributed throughout posterior neocortex, including lateral and ventral regions of the temporal lobes (for review, see Martin and Chao, 2001). Patients suffering from the temporal variant of semantic dementia demonstrate a marked loss of semantic knowledge due to degeneration of temporal cortices, and more focal temporal lesions can result in category-specific dementia—the loss of knowledge associated with certain taxonomic categories. These latter deficits suggest that different semantic primitives correlate more strongly with certain categories, with their representation being differentially dependent on particular posterior cortical regions (Farah and McClelland, 1991; Martin and Chao, 2001; Thompson-Schill, 2003; but see Caramazza and Shelton, 1998). In line with this interpretation, neuroimaging studies demonstrate a systematic relation between activation in temporal cortical subregions and the processing of specific semantic categories or features (Martin and Chao, 2001). For example, subregions within inferotemporal cortex are dif-

ferentially active during the processing of living versus non-living concepts (figure 51.5), perhaps revealing markers of stored primitives related to visual versus functional semantics (e.g., Martin et al., 1996; Chao, Haxby, and Martin, 1999; Thompson-Schill et al., 1999; but see Pilgrim et al., 2002). Other putative primitives, such as knowledge about color versus action, result in functional dissociations in lateral temporal cortex (e.g., Martin et al., 1995; see also Kourtzi and Kanwisher, 2000; Kellenbach, Brett, and Patterson, 2003). Collectively, these data indicate that semantic knowledge is stored in a distributed (Haxby et al., 2001) but systematic manner in posterior neocortex.

Complementary data indicate that long-term semantic knowledge is not stored in PFC, although PFC mechanisms appear to affect our ability to work with semantic information. For example, multidimensional scaling reveals that the structure of semantic memory is similar in patients with PFC damage and in healthy control subjects (see figure 51.5), although such patients sometimes demonstrate difficulties in retrieving stored knowledge (Sylvester and Shimamura, 2002). These latter deficits beg the question, when and how does cognitive control interact with semantic memory to support knowledge retrieval?

MULTIPLE ROUTES TO MEMORY   Semantic retrieval constitutes the recovery of conceptual representations, and accordingly depends on processes that activate stored knowledge, essentially bringing long-term information into working memory. Behavioral evidence indicates that the retrieval of task-relevant semantic knowledge can occur in a relatively automatic (or bottom-up) fashion or in a more controlled (or top-down) manner, with these two retrieval routes representing the ends of a continuum (for review, see Neely, 1991).

Automatic retrieval occurs when the association between a retrieval cue and relevant knowledge is sufficiently strong that presentation of the cue serves to automatically activate, or make accessible, the target knowledge (figure 51.6). Automatic retrieval is thought to derive from an associative mechanism whereby bottom-up activation of the cue's representation serves to activate other, strongly associated representations. Automatic retrieval (1) occurs rapidly, (2) is obligatory, and (3) is context independent, resulting in recovery of strongly associated knowledge regardless of whether the knowledge is task relevant.

By contrast, *controlled retrieval* mechanisms are recruited when automatically retrieved knowledge is insufficient to meet task demands or when an individual comes to expect that the strategic retrieval of certain conceptual representations will aid performance. Controlled retrieval is thought to depend on a top-down bias mechanism whereby task or context representations facilitate activation of weakly associated, task-relevant knowledge (see figure 51.6).

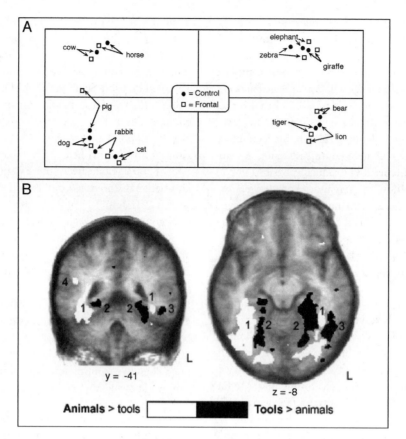

FIGURE 51.5 Multidimensional representation of semantic space and functional neuroanatomical dissociations in occipitotemporal cortices. (*A*) Two-dimensional semantic space for controls and patients with frontal lesions as revealed by multidimensional scaling. The close correspondence between patients and controls provides strong evidence that frontal cortex does not support storage of semantic knowledge. (Reprinted with permission from C. Y. Sylvester and A. P. Shimamura, 2002. Evidence for intact semantic representations in patients with frontal lobe lesions. *Neuropsychology* 16:197–207.) (*B*) Group-averaged statistical maps show differential activation across semantic domains in distinct occipitotemporal cortices. Lateral fusiform (1) and right superior temporal (4) cortices show greater activation during the processing of animals versus tools (white), whereas medial fusiform (2) and left middle to inferior temporal (3) cortices show preference for tools over animals (black). (Reprinted from A. Martin and L. L. Chao, 2001. Semantic memory and the brain: Structure and processes. *Curr. Opin. Neurobiol.* 11:194–201. Copyright 2001, with permission from Elsevier.)

Relative to automatic retrieval, controlled retrieval (1) is slower and more effortful, (2) can bias retrieval of task-relevant information even in the presence of more strongly associated but task-irrelevant information, and (3) can either directly or indirectly inhibit the retrieval of prepotent, task-irrelevant information.

SEMANTIC RETRIEVAL AND PREFRONTAL CORTEX   Left ventrolateral PFC lesions result in impairments on semantic tasks that require some form of cognitive control during semantic or lexical retrieval (e.g., Swick and Knight, 1996; Thompson-Schill et al., 1998; Metzler, 2001). For instance, although patients with Broca's aphasia, a language disorder that follows left PFC damage, show intact semantic priming effects that are due to automatic retrieval processes (Blumstein, Milberg, and Shrier, 1982; Hagoort, 1997), they fail to show normal levels of semantic priming when the cue–target associative strength is weak or ambiguous

(Milberg, Blumstein, and Dworetzky, 1987; Metzler, 2001) or when the context requires strategic assessment of the utility of primes in cuing upcoming targets (Milberg et al., 1995). Left PFC lesions also result in difficulty retrieving a weak associate of a cue when faced with competition from other associated knowledge (Thompson-Schill et al., 1998). Thus, deficits occur in situations in which healthy individuals likely use cognitive control to effectively access relevant semantic knowledge. Consistent with this interpretation, even temporary disruption of anterior left ventrolateral PFC with transcranial magnetic stimulation results in a performance deficit when controlled access to semantic knowledge is required, but not when stimuli are processed in a nonsemantic manner (Devlin, Matthews, and Rushworth, 2003).

Neuroimaging studies provide complementary high spatial resolution evidence that more precisely maps semantic processing functions to ventrolateral PFC. Extensive

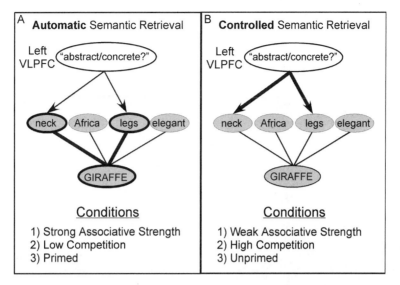

FIGURE 51.6 Two routes to the retrieval of semantic knowledge. (A) Schematic representation of *automatic retrieval* processes that support classification of a stimulus along a semantic dimension (here, abstract/concrete). Features are connected by associative links of varying strengths. The presentation of a retrieval cue (e.g., *giraffe*) results in bottom-up activation of strongly associated representations (denoted by thick lines). When the intrinsic connections are sufficient to retrieve relevant representations—owing to a strong cue–target association, low competition from irrelevant representations, or priming due to prior retrieval—limited demands are placed on top-down (controlled) retrieval processes. (B) Schematic representation of *controlled retrieval*. Owing to weak pre-existing associative links between the cue and relevant knowledge, competition from irrelevant information, or the absence of priming, knowledge necessary to meet task demands may not be successfully retrieved through automatic processes. In this case, a top-down bias mechanism, depending on left PFC regions that represent the conceptual context, facilitates retrieval of task-relevant information.

imaging data indicate that anterior left ventrolateral PFC (BA 47/45), which falls rostral and inferior to the left PFC region associated with phonological working memory, is engaged when access to semantic knowledge is required (Buckner, Raichle, and Petersen, 1995; Fiez, 1997; Poldrack et al., 1999; Wagner, 1999). For example, greater left PFC activation is observed during the retrieval of semantic knowledge associated with a word than during word reading (e.g., Petersen et al., 1988), and when making semantic relative to nonsemantic decisions about stimuli (e.g., Kapur et al., 1994; Gabrieli et al., 1996). This is the case even when task difficulty is greater during nonsemantic processing, indicating that left PFC activation is modulated by semantic retrieval demands rather than by demands on global attentional resources (Demb et al., 1995). Thus, extant data implicate anterior left ventrolateral PFC in some form of cognitive control that facilitates access to task-relevant semantic knowledge.[1]

COGNITIVE CONTROL AND RECOVERING MEANING The precise nature of this left ventrolateral PFC control process and its role in semantic retrieval remain controversial (e.g., Thompson-Schill et al., 1997; Gabrieli, Poldrack, and Desmond, 1998; Badre and Wagner, 2002; Gold and Buckner, 2002). From one perspective, left ventrolateral PFC supports controlled semantic retrieval, wherein PFC represents the conceptual context and biases retrieval of context-relevant information when that information is not recovered through automatic retrieval processes. By contrast, a selection hypothesis posits that left ventrolateral PFC does not support semantic retrieval (Thompson-Schill et al., 1997). Rather, retrieval is argued to emerge entirely within posterior neocortex, where knowledge associated with a given cue is retrieved upon cue presentation through bottom-up processes. Once representations are retrieved, left PFC selects those that are task relevant from among competing, irrelevant representations.

A critical prediction of the controlled retrieval hypothesis, but not the selection account, is that increased left PFC activity should occur when the associative strength between a retrieval cue and target knowledge is weak relative to when it is strong, and that this should be the case even when using a semantic processing task that requires minimal selection. A recent fMRI study (Wagner, Paré-Blagoev, et al., 2001) tested this prediction, varying controlled retrieval demands by (1) manipulating the preexperimental associative strength between the cue and the correct target and (2) further manipulating retrieval demands by varying the number of targets to be considered (figure 51.7) (cf. Thompson-Schill et al., 1997). fMRI results revealed that, even when selection demands are held constant and to a minimum, activation in anterior left ventrolateral PFC increases with the number of targets to be considered, and, critically, is greater when the cue–target associative strength is weak rather than

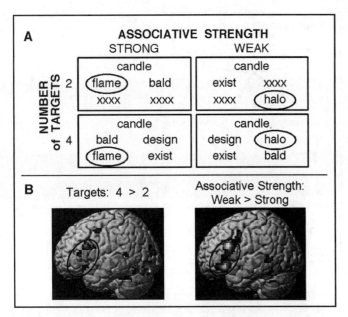

A **ASSOCIATIVE STRENGTH**

STRONG   WEAK

NUMBER of TARGETS

2

candle
(flame) bald
xxxx   xxxx

candle
exist   xxxx
xxxx   (halo)

4

candle
bald   design
(flame) exist

candle
design (halo)
exist   bald

B

Targets: 4 > 2

Associative Strength:
Weak > Strong

FIGURE 51.7   Left ventrolateral PFC is differentially engaged when controlled semantic retrieval demands are high. (*A*) Semantic decision task designed to manipulate controlled retrieval demands. On each trial, a cue (top word) was presented above either two or four target words. Participants determined which of the targets was most globally related to the cue word, with the correct response (circled) being either a strong or a weak associate of the cue. The factors of cue–target associative strength and number of targets were crossed. (*B*) fMRI revealed greater activation in left ventrolateral PFC (circled) as controlled retrieval demands increased, due either to having to retrieve information about four versus two possible targets or to a weak versus strong preexisting associative relation between the cue and the correct target. (Data from A. D. Wagner, E. J. Paré-Blagoev, J. Clark, and R. A. Poldrack, 2001. Recovering meaning: Left prefrontal cortex guides controlled semantic retrieval. *Neuron* 31:329–338. Copyright 2001, with permission from Elsevier.)

strong. Conceptually similar effects of associative strength on left PFC activation are also seen when subjects make categorical decisions about less prototypical exemplars (e.g., *bird-ostrich*) than about more prototypical exemplars (e.g., *bird-robin*) (Roskies et al., 2001), and when subjects make analogical reasoning decisions about weakly associated relative to strongly associated word pairs. Such findings indicate that left ventrolateral PFC is engaged when target semantic knowledge must be retrieved in a controlled manner.

It should be emphasized that controlled retrieval and selection demands are likely to be highly correlated, suggesting a possible reconciliation of the two perspectives (Badre and Wagner, 2002). Specifically, controlled retrieval is necessary when task-relevant information does not come to mind through automatic, bottom-up processes. This can occur either because task-relevant information is weakly associated with a presented retrieval cue, resulting in insufficient bottom-up activation, or because more strongly associated information competes with recovery of the target

knowledge, resulting in high selection demands. In both cases, a top-down bias signal may be required to effectively retrieve the relevant representation (see figure 51.6). Accordingly, controlled retrieval demands typically increase as selection demands increase, but also increase because of other factors that make automatic access to relevant information insufficient or ineffective, such as weak cue–target associative connections.

Cognitive control and priming: On the road to automaticity

The evidence discussed in the preceding section indicates that a controlled retrieval process interacts with declarative memory to support knowledge recovery, thus guiding flexible, goal-directed behavior. Because controlled retrieval is one end of a processing continuum, it is important to understand how knowledge recovery shifts from depending on more controlled to more automatic retrieval mechanisms. As we discuss in this final section, neuroimaging studies of repetition priming indicate that reductions in controlled retrieval demands follow experience-based modifications of semantic memory.

Repetition priming is a nondeclarative (or implicit) form of LTM that is expressed as an experience-based change in behavior, is not necessarily accompanied by conscious recollection, and is preserved following medial temporal lobe damage (Schacter, 1987a; Squire, 1992; Gabrieli, 1998). At the behavioral level, priming refers to instances in which an earlier encounter with a stimulus alters later responding to that same stimulus or to a related stimulus. Behavioral changes include an increased speed of responding, increased response accuracy, or biased responding.

Although there are multiple forms of priming, most instances fall into one of two broad categories, perceptual and conceptual (Roediger and McDermott, 1993). *Perceptual priming* refers to an enhanced ability to identify a stimulus due to previous exposure to the stimulus, whereas *conceptual priming* refers to facilitated processing of the meaning of a stimulus or enhanced access to a concept due to prior processing of the stimulus's meaning or retrieval of the concept. In this section, we discuss perceptual and conceptual priming, and describe neuroimaging correlates of these forms of nondeclarative memory. We then focus on the relation between conceptual priming and controlled retrieval, emphasizing how priming-related changes in PFC activation mark a shift from controlled to automatic retrieval.

PERCEPTUAL PRIMING   Perceptual priming is often revealed as either an increased likelihood of completing a perceptual fragment, such as a word stem (e.g., *sta___*), with a previously encountered stimulus (e.g., *stamp*), or a faster and more accurate identification of degraded stimuli as a result of prior exposure to those stimuli. Perceptual priming is sensitive to the degree of perceptual overlap between the initial and repeated encounter with a stimulus. For example, this form of priming is modality-specific, being greater when the initial and repeated encounters occur in the same modality as opposed to different modalities (Jacoby and Dallas, 1981). By contrast, perceptual priming is comparable irrespective of whether attention at study is focused on the meaning of the stimulus or on its structural form (Jacoby and Dallas, 1981).

Perceptual priming is thought to reflect learning in perceptual representation systems (Tulving and Schacter, 1990). Perceptual representation systems encode and retain pre-semantic perceptual information (in the form of perceptual records) about encountered words and objects, and are thought to depend on modality-specific sensory cortices. Perceptual representation systems include a word form system that can be further differentiated into visual and auditory systems that represent seen and spoken words, respectively, and a structural representation system that represents the visual form of objects.

Neuroimaging studies of perceptual priming typically demonstrate decreased activation in modality-sensitive cortical regions that were engaged during initial stimulus processing (Schacter and Buckner, 1998; Wagner and Koutstaal, 2002; figure 51.8), although increases are sometimes observed on repetition of unfamiliar stimuli (Schacter et al., 1995; Henson, Shallice, and Dolan, 2000). Priming-related activation decreases persist across delays of multiple days, indicating that such experience-based reductions in activation depend on a form of LTM (van Turennout, Ellmore, and Martin, 2000).

Neural priming effects in human sensory cortex resemble the phenomenon of repetition suppression in infrahuman primates, wherein repeated exposure to a stimulus leads to a reduction in the firing rate of neurons in higher-order

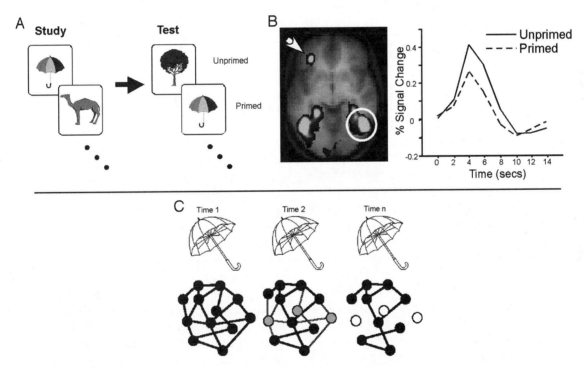

FIGURE 51.8 Repetition priming paradigm, neural priming effects, and a hypothesized neural "sharpening" mechanism. (A) On priming tasks, subjects initially study a set of stimuli; in this instance, making a semantic decision (size judgment) about visually presented objects. Subsequently, during the critical test, semantic decisions are made about previously studied (primed) and novel (unprimed) stimuli. (B) fMRI scanning during the critical test revealed priming-related activation reductions in fusiform cortex (circled) and left ventrolateral PFC (arrow); the former reflect neural correlates of perceptual priming and the latter reflect correlates of conceptual priming. (Data from W. Koutstaal, A. D. Wagner, M. Rotte, A. Maril, R. L. Buckner, and D. L. Schacter, 2001. Perceptual specificity in visual object priming: Functional magnetic resonance imaging evidence for a laterality difference in fusiform cortex. *Neuropsychologia* 39:184–199. Copyright 2001, with permission from Elsevier.) (C) Hypothesized experience-based changes in a neural network representing visual object features. Initially, neurons coding for relevant and irrelevant features respond during object processing, but each encounter serves to prune or sharpen the representation such that only neurons coding relevant features subsequently fire. Such a change may result in more efficient perception (i.e., behavioral priming) and an overall reduction in the mean firing rate of a population of neurons (i.e., repetition suppression or neural priming). (Reprinted from C. L. Wiggs and A. Martin, 1998. Properties and mechanisms of perceptual priming. *Curr. Opin. Neurobiol.* 8:227–233. Copyright 1998, with permission from Elsevier.)

visual regions (Desimone, 1996). Given this parallel, one hypothesis is that priming-related activation reductions in neuroimaging studies reflect a "sharpening" or "tuning" of perceptual representation systems (Wiggs and Martin, 1998). From this perceptive, multiple neurons are engaged during initial perception of a stimulus, with some coding less relevant features than others. In the course of this initial processing, the perceptual representation system is sharpened such that neurons that code unnecessary features of the stimulus are pruned, resulting in reduced responding by those neurons on reencounter with the stimulus (see figure 51.8). This sharpening of the representation may result in efficient stimulus reprocessing, thus giving rise to facilitated behavior. Although an intriguing possibility, priming-related activation reductions could also reflect a reduction in the duration of neural processing due to (1) experience-based strengthening of synaptic connections (see figure 51.6), thus resulting in more rapid network settling (Henson and Rugg, 2003), or (2) rapid stimulus-response learning and a shift to a response retrieval strategy of stimulus processing on reencounter (Dobbins et al., 2004).

CONCEPTUAL PRIMING   Conceptual priming refers to the increased likelihood of generating a concept in response to a test cue due to previous processing of the concept during an unrelated study phase. For example, when participants are presented with a category cue (e.g., "fruit") and are asked to generate the first few exemplars that come to mind, the probability of spontaneously generating a given exemplar (e.g., "cherry") is higher if the exemplar had appeared on a prior study list. Conceptual priming is also revealed on semantic classification tasks, wherein prior processing of a stimulus's meaning results in faster classification of the stimulus along a particular semantic dimension.

In contrast to perceptual priming, conceptual priming is modality-independent. For example, cross-modality priming (auditory study, visual test) is comparable to within-modality priming (visual study, visual test) on semantic classification tasks (Vaidya et al., 1997). Moreover, whereas perceptual priming is insensitive to the level of semantic elaboration during initial processing, conceptual priming is greater when semantic features of a stimulus are attended during study than when perceptual features are attended. Finally, conceptual priming is intact following focal lesions to modality-specific sensory cortices, whereas such lesions impair perceptual priming (e.g., Gabrieli et al., 1995). By contrast, conceptual priming is impaired in patients with Alzheimer's disease, who suffer pathological changes in amodal association areas of frontal, temporal, and parietal cortex, as well as in the medial temporal lobe (Heindel et al., 1989). This pattern suggests that temporal association cortices that represent semantic knowledge, and perhaps frontal cortices that permit controlled access to this knowledge, may

be important for conceptual priming (Swick and Knight, 1996).

In a pattern that parallels that seen during comparisons of automatic versus controlled retrieval conditions, neuroimaging investigations of conceptual priming reveal that the anterior and posterior extents of left ventrolateral PFC show reduced activation during repeated (primed) relative to initial (unprimed) semantic processing of stimuli (e.g., Raichle et al., 1994; Gabrieli et al., 1996; Wagner et al., 1997; Schacter and Buckner, 1998). For example, activation is weaker when making semantic classification decisions about primed relative to unprimed objects or words (see figure 51.8), and this is the case even following study–test retention intervals of more than 24 hours (Wagner, Maril, and Schacter, 2000). Reductions in left ventrolateral PFC activation are observed in patients with global amnesia, suggesting that these changes reflect computational benefits deriving from the nondeclarative memory processes that support conceptual priming at the behavioral level (Buckner and Koutstaal, 1998; Gabrieli, Poldrack, and Desmond, 1998). In addition to changes in PFC activation, conceptual priming is correlated with activation reductions in posterior cortical regions that may represent long-term conceptual knowledge, including ventral and lateral temporal cortices (e.g., Raichle et al., 1994; Blaxton et al., 1996). These outcomes indicate that conceptual priming stems from experience-based "tuning" of semantic memory, mirroring at the conceptual level the sort of processes hypothesized to underlie perceptual priming (cf. Dobbins et al., 2004).

The changes in semantic memory that support conceptual priming could emerge in a number of ways. For example, the tuning of semantic memory may constitute a sharpening of conceptual representations, perhaps through retrieval-induced suppression, whereby the initial retrieval of relevant stimulus features serves to suppress or inhibit less relevant features (Anderson, Bjork, and Bjork, 1994). Suppression of irrelevant features would reduce the degree to which these features compete for retrieval, thus facilitating the subsequent recovery of recently retrieved knowledge. In addition, modifications in semantic memory are likely to emerge at least partially from a strengthening of the connections or associations between a response cue and the initially retrieved relevant features associated with the cue/concept. This strengthening of cue–target associations facilitates subsequent retrieval of these target representations by increasing the effects of bottom-up inputs on knowledge recovery.

CONTROLLED RETRIEVAL AND CONCEPTUAL PRIMING   The consistent observation that reductions in left PFC activation accompany conceptual priming suggests that cognitive control demands can decline following experience-based changes in semantic memory (see figure 51.6). That is, PFC priming effects may mark the beginnings of a transition from reliance on more controlled to more automatic retrieval mechanisms (Raichle et al., 1994; Demb et al., 1995; Fletcher, Shallice, and Dolan, 2000). From this perspective, controlled semantic retrieval tunes semantic memory, strengthening the representations of initially recovered knowledge and perhaps weakening those of competing knowledge. Critically, this increased accessibility of recently relevant knowledge reduces the computational demands on controlled retrieval when this knowledge must be retrieved in the future. Such reductions in controlled retrieval demands reflect both an increased automaticity of target knowledge retrieval due to strengthened cue–target associations (Raichle et al., 1994) and a reduction of competition from task-irrelevant representations (Thompson-Schill, D'Esposito, and Kan, 1999). Thus, these neural priming effects illustrate the point that interactions between cognitive control and LTM are bidirectional: cognitive control affects retrieval from LTM, with the resulting changes in LTM affecting subsequent demands on cognitive control.

Conclusions

Memory systems can produce outputs based on bottom-up mechanisms that unfold automatically in response to inputs, although in many situations these outputs are insufficient to support flexible cognition. In such instances, cognitive control processes must be recruited to retrieve, maintain, and manipulate relevant knowledge and to select against or resolve interference from competing representations. The past decade of cognitive neuroscience research has highlighted that an understanding of cognitive control processes requires consideration of their intimate relation with memory. Future investigations undoubtedly will continue to delineate the elemental forms of control and their dependence on prefrontal cortex. In so doing, these efforts promise to provide important insights into the workings of memory, revealing how memory can be brought to bear, in a controlled manner, to support flexible behavior.

NOTE

1. Other evidence indicates that functional distinctions exist within left PFC. One putative distinction is that between anterior and posterior left ventrolateral PFC, based on semantic and phonological processing demands (for discussion, see Bookheimer, 2002; Buckner et al., 1995; Fiez, 1997; Gabrieli et al., 1998; Gold and Buckner, 2002; Poldrack et al., 1999; Wagner, Koutstaal et al., 2000).

REFERENCES

ALAIN, C., S. R. ARNOTT, S. HEVENOR, S. GRAHAM, and C. L. GRADY, 2001. "What" and "where" in the human auditory system. *Proc. Natl. Acad. Sci. U.S.A.* 98:12301–12306.

ANDERSON, M. C., R. A. BJORK, and E. L. BJORK, 1994. Remembering can cause forgetting: Retrieval dynamics in long-term memory. *J. Exp. Psychol. Learn. Mem. Cognit.* 20:1063–1087.

ARON, A. R., P. C. FLETCHER, E. T. BULLMORE, B. J. SAHAKIAN, and T. W. ROBBINS, 2003. Stop-signal inhibition disrupted by damage to right inferior frontal gyrus in humans. *Nat. Neurosci.* 6:115–116.

AWH, E., and J. JONIDES, 1998. Spatial working memory and spatial selective attention. In *The Attentive Brain*, R. Parasuraman, ed. Cambridge, Mass.: MIT Press, pp. 353–380.

AWH, E., J. JONIDES, E. E. SMITH, E. H. SCHUMACHER, R. A. KOEPPE, and S. KATZ, 1996. Dissociation of storage and rehearsal in verbal working memory: Evidence from PET. *Psychol. Sci.* 7:25–31.

BADDELEY, A. D., 1986. *Working Memory.* Oxford, England: Oxford University Press.

BADDELEY, A. D., 1994. Working memory: The interface between memory and cognition. In *Memory Systems 1994*, D. L. Schacter and E. Tulving, eds. Cambridge, Mass.: MIT Press, pp. 351–367.

BADDELEY, A. D., and G. J. HITCH, 1974. Working memory. In *The Psychology of Learning and Motivation: Advances in Research and Theory*, vol 8, G. H. Bower, ed. New York: Academic Press, pp. 47–89.

BADRE, D., and A. D. WAGNER, 2002. Semantic retrieval, mnemonic control, and prefrontal cortex. *Behav. Cogn. Neurosci. Rev.* 1:206–218.

BADRE, D., and A. D. WAGNER, 2004. Selection and conflict monitoring in prefrontal cortex: Assessing the specificity of cognitive control. *Neuron* 41:473–487.

BLAXTON, T. A., S. Y. BOOKHEIMER, T. A. ZEFFIRO, C. M. FIGLOZZI, W. D. GAILLARD, and W. H. THEODORE, 1996. Functional mapping of human memory using PET: Comparisons of conceptual and perceptual tasks. *Can. J. Exp. Psychol.* 50:42–56.

BLUMSTEIN, S. E., W. MILBERG, and R. SHRIER, 1982. Semantic processing in aphasia: Evidence from an auditory lexical decision task. *Brain Lang.* 17:301–315.

BOOKHEIMER, A., 2002. Functional MRI of language: New approaches to understanding the cortical organization of semantic processing. *Annu. Rev. Neurosci.* 25:151–188.

BOTVINICK, M. M., T. S. BRAVER, D. M. BARCH, C. S. CARTER, and J. D. COHEN, 2001. Conflict monitoring and cognitive control. *Psychol. Rev.* 108:624–652.

BRAVER, T. S., and S. R. BONGIOLATTI, 2002. The role of frontopolar cortex in subgoal processing during working memory. *NeuroImage* 15:523–536.

BUCKNER, R. L., and W. KOUTSTAAL, 1998. Functional neuroimaging studies of encoding, priming, and explicit memory retrieval. *Proc. Natl. Acad. Sci. U.S.A.* 95:891–898.

BUCKNER, R. L., M. E. RAICHLE, and S. E. PETERSEN, 1995. Dissociation of human prefrontal cortical areas across different speech production tasks and gender groups. *J. Neurophysiol.* 74:2163–2173.

BUNGE, S. A., E. HAZELTINE, M. D. SCANLON, A. C. ROSEN, and J. D. GABRIELI, 2002. Dissociable contributions of prefrontal and parietal cortices to response selection. *NeuroImage* 17:1562–1571.

BUNGE, S. A., K. N. OCHSNER, J. E. DESMOND, G. H. GLOVER, and J. D. GABRIELI, 2001. Prefrontal regions involved in keeping information in and out of mind. *Brain* 124:2074–2086.

CARAMAZZA, A., and J. R. SHELTON, 1998. Domain-specific knowledge systems in the brain: The animate-inanimate distinction. *J. Cogn. Neurosci.* 10:1–34.

CARLESIMO, G. A., R. PERRI, P. TURRIZIANI, F. TOMAIUOLO, and C. CALTAGIRONE, 2001. Remembering what but not where: Independence of spatial and visual working memory in the human brain. *Cortex* 37:519–534.

CHAFEE, M. V., and P. S. GOLDMAN-RAKIC, 2000. Inactivation of parietal and prefrontal cortex reveals interdependence of neural activity during memory-guided saccades. *J. Neurophysiol.* 83:1550–1566.

CHAO, L. L., J. V. HAXBY, and A. MARTIN, 1999. Attribute-based neural substrates in temporal cortex for perceiving and knowing about objects. *Nat. Neurosci.* 2:913–919.

CHEIN, J. M., and J. A. FIEZ, 2001. Dissociation of verbal working memory system components using a delayed serial recall task. *Cereb. Cortex* 11:1003–1014.

CHRISTOFF, K., V. PRABHAKARAN, J. DORFMAN, Z. ZHAO, J. K. KROGER, K. J. HOLYOAK, et al., 2001. Rostrolateral prefrontal cortex involvement in relational integration during reasoning. *NeuroImage* 14:1136–1149.

COHEN J. D., T. S. BRAVER, and R. C. O'REILLY, 1996. A computational approach to prefrontal cortex, cognitive control and schizophrenia: Recent developments and current challenges. *Philos. Trans. R. Soc. Lond. B Biol. Sci.* 351:1515–1527.

COHEN, J. D., K. DUNBAR, and J. L. McCLELLAND, 1990. On the control of automatic processes: A parallel distributed processing account of the Stroop effect. *Psychol. Rev.* 97:332–361.

COURTNEY, S. M., L. PETIT, J. M. MAISOG, L. G. UNGERLEIDER, and J. V. HAXBY, 1998. An area specialized for spatial working memory in human frontal cortex. *Science* 279:1347–1351.

DEMB, J. B., J. E. DESMOND, A. D. WAGNER, C. J. VAIDYA, G. H. GLOVER, and J. D. GABRIELI, 1995. Semantic encoding and retrieval in the left inferior prefrontal cortex: A functional MRI study of task difficulty and process specificity. *J. Neurosci.* 15:5870–5878.

DESIMONE, R., 1996. Neural mechanisms for visual memory and their role in attention. *Proc. Natl. Acad. Sci. U.S.A.* 93:13494–13499.

DESIMONE, R., and J. DUNCAN, 1995. Neural mechanisms of selective visual attention. *Annu. Rev. Neurosci.* 18:193–222.

DESMOND, J. E., J. D. GABRIELI, A. D. WAGNER, B. L. GINIER, and G. H. GLOVER, 1997. Lobular patterns of cerebellar activation in verbal working-memory and finger-tapping tasks as revealed by functional MRI. *J. Neurosci.* 17:9675–9685.

D'ESPOSITO, M., G. K. AGUIRRE, E. ZARAHN, D. BALLARD, R. K. SHIN, and J. LEASE, 1998. Functional MRI studies of spatial and nonspatial working memory. *Cogn. Brain Res.* 7:1–13.

D'ESPOSITO, M., B. R. POSTLE, D. BALLARD, and J. LEASE, 1999. Maintenance versus manipulation of information held in working memory: An event-related fMRI study. *Brain Cognit.* 41:66–86.

D'ESPOSITO, M., B. R. POSTLE, J. JONIDES, and E. E. SMITH, 1999. The neural substrate and temporal dynamics of interference effects in working memory as revealed by event-related functional MRI. *Proc. Natl. Acad. Sci. U.S.A.* 96:7514–7519.

DEVLIN, J. T., P. M. MATTHEWS, and M. F. RUSHWORTH, 2003. Semantic processing in the left inferior prefrontal cortex: A combined functional magnetic resonance imaging and transcranial magnetic stimulation study. *J. Cogn. Neurosci.* 15:71–84.

DOBBINS, I. G., D. M. SCHNYER, M. VERFAELLIE, and D. L. SCHACTER, 2004. Cortical activity reductions during repetition priming can result from rapid response learning. *Nature* 428:316–319.

FARAH, M. J., 1988. Is visual memory really visual? Overlooked evidence from neuropsychology. *Psychol. Rev.* 95:307–317.

FARAH, M. J., and J. L. McCLELLAND, 1991. A computational model of semantic memory impairment: Modality specificity and emergent category specificity. *J. Exp. Psychol. Gen.* 120:339–357.

FIEZ, J. A., 1997. Phonology, semantics, and the role of the left inferior prefrontal cortex. *Hum. Brain Mapp.* 5:79–83.

FIEZ, J. A., E. A. RAIFE, D. A. BALOTA, J. P. SCHWARZ, M. E. RAICHLE, and S. E. PETERSEN, 1996. A positron emission tomography study of the short-term maintenance of verbal information. *J. Neurosci.* 16:808–822.

FLETCHER, P. C., and R. N. HENSON, 2001. Frontal lobes and human memory: Insights from functional neuroimaging. *Brain* 124:849–881.

FLETCHER, P. C., T. SHALLICE, and R. J. DOLAN, 2000. "Sculpting the response space": An account of left prefrontal activation at encoding. *NeuroImage* 12:404–417.

FUSTER, J. M., 1997. *The Prefrontal Cortex: Anatomy, Physiology, and Neuropsychology of the Frontal Lobe.* Philadelphia: Lippincott-Raven.

FUSTER, J. M., and G. E. ALEXANDER, 1971. Neuron activity related to short-term memory. *Science* 173:652–654.

GABRIELI, J. D., 1998. Cognitive neuroscience of human memory. *Annu. Rev. Psychol.* 49:87–115.

GABRIELI, J. D., J. E. DESMOND, J. B. DEMB, A. D. WAGNER, M. V. STONE, C. J. VAIDYA, et al., 1996. Functional magnetic resonance imaging of semantic memory processes in the frontal lobes. *Psychol. Sci.* 7:278–283.

GABRIELI, J. D., D. A. FLEISCHMAN, M. A. KEANE, S. L. REMINGER, and F. MORRELL, 1995. Double dissociation between memory systems underlying explicit and implicit memory in the human brain. *Psychol. Sci.* 6:76–82.

GABRIELI, J. D., R. A. POLDRACK, and J. E. DESMOND, 1998. The role of left prefrontal cortex in language and memory. *Proc. Natl. Acad. Sci. U.S.A.* 95:906–913.

GARAVAN, H., T. J. ROSS, S. J. LI, and E. A. STEIN, 2000. A parametric manipulation of central executive functioning. *Cereb. Cortex* 10:585–592.

GARAVAN, H., T. J. ROSS, and E. A. STEIN, 1999. Right hemispheric dominance of inhibitory control: An event-related functional MRI study. *Proc. Natl. Acad. Sci. U.S.A.* 96:8301–8306.

GOLD, B. T., and R. L. BUCKNER, 2002. Common prefrontal regions coactivate with dissociable posterior regions during controlled semantic and phonological tasks. *Neuron* 35:803–812.

GOLDMAN-RAKIC, P. S., 1987. Circuitry of primate prefrontal cortex and regulation of behavior by representational memory. In *Handbook of Physiology*, Sect. 1, *The Nervous System*, vol. V, *Higher Functions of the Brain*, Part 1, F. Plum and V. Mountcastle, eds. Bethesda, Md.: American Physiological Society, pp. 373–417.

HAGOORT, P., 1997. Semantic priming in Broca's aphasics at short SOA: No support for an automatic semantic access deficit. *Brain Lang.* 56:287–300.

HAXBY, J. V., M. IDA GOBBINI, M. L. FUREY, A. ISHAI, J. L. SCHOUTEN, and P. PIETRINI, 2001. Distributed and overlapping representations of faces and objects in ventral temporal cortex. *Science* 293:2425–2430.

HAXBY, J. V., L. PETIT, L. G. UNGERLEIDER, and S. M. COURTNEY, 2000. Distinguishing the functional roles of multiple regions in distributed neural systems for visual working memory. *NeuroImage* 11:380–391.

HAZELTINE, E., S. A. BUNGE, M. D. SCANLON, A. C. ROSEN, and J. D. GABRIELI, 2003. Material-dependent and material-independent selection processes in the frontal and parietal lobes: An event-related fMRI investigation of response competition. *Neuropsychologia* 41:1208–1217.

HEINDEL, W. C., D. P. SALMON, C. W. SHULTS, P. A. WALLICKE, and N. BUTTERS, 1989. Neuropsychological evidence for multiple implicit memory systems: A comparison of Alzheimer's, Huntington's and Parkinson's disease patients. *J. Neurosci.* 9:582–587.

HENSON, R., and M. D. RUGG, 2003. Neural response suppression, haemodynamic repetition effects, and behavioral priming. *Neuropsychologia* 41:263–270.

HENSON, R., T. SHALLICE, and R. DOLAN, 2000. Neuroimaging evidence for dissociable forms of repetition priming. *Science* 287:1269–1272.

JACOBY, L. L., and M. DALLAS, 1981. On the relationship between autobiographical memory and perceptual learning. *J. Exp. Psychol. Gen.* 110:306–340.

JONIDES, J., E. H. SCHUMACHER, E. E. SMITH, R. A. KOEPPE, E. AWH, P. A. REUTER-LORENZ, et al., 1998. The role of parietal cortex in verbal working memory. *J. Neurosci.* 18:5026–5034.

JONIDES, J., E. E. SMITH, C. MARSHUETZ, and R. A. KOEPPE, 1998. Inhibition in verbal working memory revealed by brain activation. *Proc. Natl. Acad. Sci. U.S.A.* 95:8410–8413.

KAPUR, S., R. ROSE, P. F. LIDDLE, R. B. ZIPURSKY, G. M. BROWN, D. STUSS, et al., 1994. The role of the left prefrontal cortex in verbal processing: Semantic processing or willed action? *Neuroreport* 5:2193–2196.

KELLENBACH, M. L., M. BRETT, and K. PATTERSON, 2003. Actions speak louder than functions: The importance of manipulability and action in tool representation. *J. Cogn. Neurosci.* 15:30–46.

KOECHLIN, E., G. BASSO, P. PIETRINI, S. PANZER, and J. GRAFMAN, 1999. The role of the anterior prefrontal cortex in human cognition. *Nature* 399:148–151.

KONISHI, S., K. NAKAJIMA, I. UCHIDA, M. KAMEYAMA, K. NAKAHARA, K. SEKIHARA, et al., 1998. Transient activation of inferior prefrontal cortex during cognitive set shifting. *Nat. Neurosci.* 1:80–84.

KONISHI, S., K. NAKAJIMA, I. UCHIDA, K. SEKIHARA, and Y. MIYASHITA, 1998. No-go dominant brain activity in human inferior prefrontal cortex revealed by functional magnetic resonance imaging. *Eur. J. Neurosci.* 10:1209–1213.

KOURTZI, Z., and N. KANWISHER, 2000. Activation in human MT/MST by static images with implied motion. *J. Cogn. Neurosci.* 12:48–55.

KOUTSTAAL, W., A. D. WAGNER, M. ROTTE, A. MARIL, R. L. BUCKNER, and D. L. SCHACTER, 2001. Perceptual specificity in visual object priming: Functional magnetic resonance imaging evidence for a laterality difference in fusiform cortex. *Neuropsychologia* 39:184–199.

KROGER, J. K., F. W. SABB, C. L. FALES, S. Y. BOOKHEIMER, M. S. COHEN, and K. J. HOLYOAK, 2002. Recruitment of anterior dorsolateral prefrontal cortex in human reasoning: A parametric study of relational complexity. *Cereb. Cortex* 12:477–485.

MACDONALD, A. W., III, J. D. COHEN, V. A. STENGER, and C. S. CARTER, 2000. Dissociating the role of the dorsolateral prefrontal and anterior cingulate cortex in cognitive control. *Science* 288:1835–1838.

MARTIN, A., and L. L. CHAO, 2001. Semantic memory and the brain: Structure and processes. *Curr. Opin. Neurobiol.* 11:194–201.

MARTIN, A., J. V. HAXBY, F. M. LALONDE, C. L. WIGGS, and L. G. UNGERLEIDER, 1995. Discrete cortical regions associated with knowledge of color and knowledge of action. *Science* 270: 102–105.

MARTIN, A., C. L. WIGGS, L. G. UNGERLEIDER, and J. V. HAXBY, 1996. Neural correlates of category-specific knowledge. *Nature* 379:649–652.

MARTIN, R. C., J. R. SHELTON, and L. S. YAFFEE, 1994. Language processing and working memory: Neuropsychological evidence for separate phonological and semantic capacities. *J. Mem. Lang.* 33:83–111.

MCCARTHY, G., A. PUCE, R. T. CONSTABLE, J. H. KRYSTAL, J. C. GORE, and P. GOLDMAN-RAKIC, 1996. Activation of human prefrontal cortex during spatial and nonspatial working memory tasks measured by functional MRI. *Cereb. Cortex* 6:600–611.

METZLER C., 2001. Effects of left frontal lesions on the selection of context-appropriate meanings. *Neuropsychology* 15:315–328.

MILBERG, W., S. E. BLUMSTEIN, and B. DWORETZKY, 1987. Processing of lexical ambiguities in aphasia. *Brain Lang.* 31:138–150.

MILBERG, W.P., S. E. BLUMSTEIN, D. KATZ, F. GERSHBERG, and T. BROWN, 1995. Semantic facilitation in aphasia: Effects of time and expectancy. *J. Cogn. Neurosci.* 7:33–50.

MILHAM, M. P., M. T. BANICH, A. WEBB, V. BARAD, N. J. COHEN, T. WSZALEK, et al., 2001. The relative involvement of anterior cingulate and prefrontal cortex in attentional control depends on nature of conflict. *Cogn. Brain Res.* 12:467–473.

MILLER, E. K., and J. D. COHEN, 2001. An integrative theory of prefrontal cortex function. *Annu. Rev. Neurosci.* 24:167–202.

MILLER, G. A., E. GALANTER, and K. H. PRIBRAM, 1960. *Plans and the Structure of Behavior.* New York: Holt, Rinehart and Winston.

NEELY, J. H., 1991. Semantic priming effects in visual word recognition: A selective review of current findings and theories. In *Basic Processing in Reading: Visual Word Recognition*, D. Besner and G. W. Humphreys, eds. Hillsdale, N.J.: Erlbaum, pp. 264–336.

NYSTROM, L. E., T. S. BRAVER, F. W. SABB, M. R. DELGADO, D. C. NOLL, and J. D. COHEN, 2000. Working memory for letters, shapes, and locations: fMRI evidence against stimulus-based regional organization in human prefrontal cortex. *NeuroImage* 11:424–446.

OWEN, A. M., A. C. EVANS, and M. PETRIDES, 1996. Evidence for a two-stage model of spatial working memory processing within the lateral frontal cortex: A positron emission tomography study. *Cereb. Cortex* 6:31–38.

PAULESU, E., C. D. FRITH, and R. S. FRACKOWIAK, 1993. The neural correlates of the verbal component of working memory. *Nature* 362:342–345.

PETERSEN, S. E., P. T. FOX, M. I. POSNER, M. MINTUN, and M. E. RAICHLE, 1988. Positron emission tomographic studies of the cortical anatomy of single-word processing. *Nature* 331:585–589.

PETRIDES, M., 1994. Frontal lobes and behaviour. *Curr. Opin. Neurobiol.* 4:207–211.

PILGRIM, L. K., J. FADILI, P. FLETCHER, and L. K. TYLER, 2002. Overcoming confounds of stimulus blocking: An event-related fMRI design of semantic processing. *NeuroImage* 16:713–723.

POLDRACK, R. A., A. D. WAGNER, M. W. PRULL, J. E. DESMOND, G. H. GLOVER, and J. D. E. GABRIELI, 1999. Functional specialization for semantic and phonological processing in the left inferior frontal cortex. *NeuroImage* 10:15–35.

POSTLE, B. R., J. S. BERGER, and M. D'ESPOSITO, 1999. Functional neuroanatomical double dissociation of mnemonic and executive control processes contributing to working memory performance. *Proc. Natl. Acad. Sci. U.S.A.* 96:12959–12964.

PRABHAKARAN, V., K. NARAYANAN, Z. ZHAO, and J. D. GABRIELI, 2000. Integration of diverse information in working memory within the frontal lobe. *Nat. Neurosci.* 3:85–90.

RAICHLE, M. E., J. A. FIEZ, T. O. VIDEEN, A. M. K. MACLEOD, J. V. PARDO, P. T. FOX, et al., 1994. Practice-related changes in human brain functional anatomy during nonmotor learning. *Cereb. Cortex* 4:8–26.

RAINER, G., W. F. ASAAD, and E. K. MILLER, 1998. Memory fields of neurons in the primate prefrontal cortex. *Proc. Natl. Acad. Sci. U.S.A.* 95:15008–15013.

RAMNANI, N., and A. M. OWEN, 2004. Anterior prefrontal cortex: Insights into function from anatomy and neuroimaging. *Natl. Rev. Neurosci.* 5:184–194.

RAO, S. C., G. RAINER, and E. K. MILLER, 1997. Integration of what and where in the primate prefrontal cortex. *Science* 276: 821–824.

RAYE, C. L., M. K. JOHNSON, K. J. MITCHELL, J. A. REEDER, and E. J. GREENE, 2002. Neuroimaging a single thought: Dorsolateral PFC activity associated with refreshing just-activated information. *NeuroImage* 15:447–453.

ROEDIGER, H. L., and K. MCDERMOTT, 1993. Implicit memory in normal human subjects. In *Handbook of Neuropsychology*, vol. 8, F. Boller and J. Grafman, eds. New York: Elsevier, pp. 63–131.

ROSKIES, A. L., J. A. FIEZ, D. A. BALOTA, M. E. RAICHLE, and S. E. PETERSEN, 2001. Task-dependent modulation of regions in the left inferior frontal cortex during semantic processing. *J. Cogn. Neurosci.* 13:829–843.

RUGG, M. D., and E. L. WILDING, 2000. Retrieval processing and episodic memory. *Trends Cogn. Sci.* 4:108–115.

RYPMA, B., V. PRABHAKARAN, J. E. DESMOND, G. H. GLOVER, and J. D. GABRIELI, 1999. Load-dependent roles of frontal brain regions in the maintenance of working memory. *NeuroImage* 9:16–26.

SALA, J. B., P. RAMA, and S. M. COURTNEY, 2003. Functional topography of a distributed neural system for spatial and nonspatial information maintenance in working memory. *Neuropsychologia* 41:341–356.

SALMON, E., M. VAN DER LINDEN, F. COLLETTE, G. DELFIORE, P. MAQUET, C. DEGUELDRE, et al., 1996. Regional brain activity during working memory tasks. *Brain* 119:1617–1625.

SCHACTER, D. L. 1987a. Implicit memory: History and current status. *J. Exp. Psychol. Learn. Mem. Cognit.* 13:501–518.

SCHACTER, D. L., 1987b. Memory, amnesia, and frontal lobe dysfunction. *Psychobiology* 15:21–36.

SCHACTER, D. L., and R. L. BUCKNER, 1998. Priming and the brain. *Neuron* 20:185–195.

SCHACTER, D. L., E. REIMAN, A. VECKER, M. A. POLSTER, L. S. YUN, and L. A. COOPER, 1995. Brain regions associated with retrieval of structurally coherent visual information. *Nature* 376:587–590.

SHALLICE, T., 1988. *From Neuropsychology to Mental Structure*. New York: Cambridge University Press.

SHIVDE, G., and M. C. ANDERSON, 2001. Maintaining meaning: Evidence for semantic working memory. *Abstr. Psychonom. Soc.* 6.

SHIMAMURA, A. P., 1995. Memory and frontal lobe function. In *The Cognitive Neurosciences*, M. S. Gazzaniga, ed. Cambridge, Mass.: MIT Press, pp. 803–813.

SMITH, E. E., and J. JONIDES, 1995. Working memory in humans: Neuropsychological evidence. In *The Cognitive Neurosciences*, M. S. Gazzaniga, ed. Cambridge, Mass.: MIT Press, pp. 1009–1020.

SMITH, E. E., and J. JONIDES, 1998. Neuroimaging analyses of human working memory. *Proc. Natl. Acad. Sci. U.S.A.* 95: 12061–12068.

SMITH, E. E., and J. JONIDES, 1999. Storage and executive processes in the frontal lobes. *Science* 283:1657–1661.

SMITH, E. E., and D. L. MEDIN, 1981. *Concepts and Categories*. Cambridge, Mass.: Harvard University Press.

SQUIRE, L. R., 1992. Memory and the hippocampus: A synthesis from findings with rats, monkeys, and humans. *Psychol. Rev.* 99: 195–231.

STUSS, D. T., and D. F. BENSON, 1984. Neuropsychological studies of the frontal lobes. *Psychol. Bull.* 95:3–28.

SWICK, D., and R. T. KNIGHT, 1996. Is prefrontal cortex involved in cued recall? A neuropsychological test of PET findings. *Neuropsychologia* 34:1019–1028.

SYLVESTER, C. Y., and A. P. SHIMAMURA, 2002. Evidence for intact semantic representations in patients with frontal lobe lesions. *Neuropsychology* 16:197–207.

THOMPSON-SCHILL, S. L., 2003. Neuroimaging studies of semantic memory: Inferring "how" from "where." *Neuropsychologia* 41: 280–292.

THOMPSON-SCHILL, S. L., G. K. AGUIRRE, M. D'ESPOSITO, and M. J. FARAH, 1999. A neural basis for category and modality specificity of semantic knowledge. *Neuropsychologia* 37:671–676.

THOMPSON-SCHILL, S. L., M. D'ESPOSITO, G. K. AGUIRRE, and M. J. FARAH, 1997. Role of left inferior prefrontal cortex in retrieval of semantic knowledge: A reevaluation. *Proc. Natl. Acad. Sci. U.S.A.* 94:14792–14797.

THOMPSON-SCHILL, S. L., M. D'ESPOSITO, and I. P. KAN, 1999. Effects of repetition and competition on activity in left prefrontal cortex during word generation. *Neuron* 23:513–522.

THOMPSON-SCHILL, S. L., D. SWICK, M. J. FARAH, M. D'ESPOSITO, I. P. KAN, and R. T. KNIGHT, 1998. Verb generation in patients with focal frontal lesions: A neuropsychological test of neuroimaging findings. *Proc. Natl. Acad. Sci. U.S.A.* 95:15855–15860.

TOWSE, J. N., and C. M. T. HOUSTON-PRICE, 2001. Reflections on the concept of working memory. In *Working Memory in Perspective*, J. Andrade, ed. Hove, England: Psychology Press, pp. 240–260.

TRESCH, M. C., H. M. SINNAMON, and J. G. SEAMON, 1993. Double dissociation of spatial and object visual memory: Evidence from selective interference in intact human subjects. *Neuropsychologia* 31:211–219.

TULVING, E., 1972. Episodic and semantic memory. In *Organization of Memory*, E. Tulving and W. Donaldson, eds. New York: Academic Press, pp. 382–403.

TULVING, E., and D. L. SCHACTER, 1990. Priming and human memory systems. *Science* 247:301–306.

VAIDYA, C. J., J. D. GABRIELI, M. M. KEANE, L. A. MONTI, H. GUTIERREZ-RIVAS, and M. M. ZARELLA, 1997. Evidence for multiple mechanisms of conceptual priming on implicit memory tests. *J. Exp. Psychol. Learn. Mem. Cognit.* 23:1324–1343.

VAN TURENNOUT, M., T. ELLMORE, and A. MARTIN, 2000. Long-lasting cortical plasticity in the object naming system. *Nat. Neurosci.* 3:1329–1334.

VAN VEEN, V., and C. S. CARTER, 2002. The anterior cingulate as a conflict monitor: fMRI and ERP studies. *Physiol. Behav.* 77:477–482.

VAN VEEN, V., J. D. COHEN, M. M. BOTVINICK, V. A. STENGER, and C. S. CARTER, 2001. Anterior cingulate cortex, conflict monitoring, and levels of processing. *NeuroImage* 14:1302–1308.

VELTMAN, D. J., S. A. ROMBOUTS, and R. J. DOLAN, 2003. Maintenance versus manipulation in verbal working memory revisited: An fMRI study. *NeuroImage* 18:247–256.

WAGNER, A. D., 1999. Working memory contributions to human learning and remembering. *Neuron* 22:19–22.

WAGNER, A. D., 2002. Cognitive control and episodic memory: Contributions from prefrontal cortex. In *Neuropsychology of Memory*, L. R. Squire and D. L. Schacter, eds. New York: Guilford Press, pp. 174–192.

WAGNER, A. D., J. E. DESMOND, J. B. DEMB, G. H. GLOVER, and J. D. E. GABRIELI, 1997. Semantic repetition priming for verbal and pictorial knowledge: A functional MRI study of left inferior prefrontal cortex. *J. Cogn. Neurosci.* 9:714–726.

WAGNER, A. D., and W. KOUTSTAAL, 2002. Priming. In *Encyclopedia of the Human Brain*, vol. 4, V. S. Ramachandran, ed. San Diego, Calif.: Academic Press, pp. 27–46.

WAGNER, A. D., W. KOUTSTAAL, A. MARIL, D. L. SCHACTER, and R. L. BUCKNER, 2000. Task-specific repetition priming in left inferior prefrontal cortex. *Cereb. Cortex* 10:1176–1184.

WAGNER, A. D., A. MARIL, R. A. BJORK, and D. L. SCHACTER, 2001. Prefrontal contributions to executive control: fMRI evidence for functional distinctions within lateral prefrontal cortex. *NeuroImage* 14:1337–1347.

WAGNER, A. D., A. MARIL, and D. L. SCHACTER, 2000. Interactions between forms of memory: When priming hinders new learning. *J. Cogn. Neurosci.* 12:S2:52–60.

WAGNER, A. D., E. J. PARÉ-BLAGOEV, J. CLARK, and R. A. POLDRACK, 2001. Recovering meaning: Left prefrontal cortex guides controlled semantic retrieval. *Neuron* 31: 329–338.

WIGGS, C. L., and A. MARTIN, 1998. Properties and mechanisms of perceptual priming. *Curr. Opin. Neurobiol.* 8:227–233.

WILSON, F. A. W., S. P. Ó SCALAIDHE, and P. S. GOLDMAN-RAKIC, 1993. Dissociation of object and spatial processing domains in primate prefrontal cortex. *Science* 260:1955–1958.

52 Retrieval Processing in Human Memory: Electrophysiological and fMRI Evidence

MICHAEL D. RUGG

ABSTRACT Retrieval of an episodic memory requires coordination of a number of distinct cognitive processes. Preretrieval processes operate on retrieval cues to generate cue representations that optimize the match between the cue and the targeted memory representation, ecphoric processes support the recovery and representation of stored information, and postretrieval processes support monitoring and evaluation of the outcome of a retrieval attempt. The present chapter reviews recent evidence from event-related potential (ERP) and functional magnetic resonance (fMRI) studies of episodic retrieval. The evidence from these studies indicates that these three components of retrieval processing have distinct neural correlates and that pre- and postretrieval processing are both highly sensitive to variation in retrieval goals and retrieval strategy.

This chapter is concerned with mechanisms underlying the retrieval of episodic memories, defined here as information about unique events and their contexts (see Baddeley, Conway, and Aggleton, 2001, for a recent review). The chapter takes up two themes relating to the neural correlates of retrieval success and the evaluation of retrieved information that were addressed in previous editions of this book (Rugg, 1995; Rugg and Allan, 2000). In addition, a new theme is introduced, the processing of retrieval cues, research on which began only recently. Throughout, the focus is on retrieval in direct memory tests, when there is an intention to retrieve, rather than on the involuntary or unintentional episodic retrieval that can be elicited on indirect tests (Richardson-Klavehn, Gardiner, and Java, 1996).

The studies reviewed here all employed one of two different noninvasive measures of brain activity to investigate the neural correlates of retrieval processing (see Rugg, 1999, for further discussion). The event-related potential (ERP) method is a direct, online measure of item-related brain activity that permits the neural correlates of different retrieval processes to be described in terms of their timing, sensitivity to experimental manipulations, and characteristic patterns of activity over the scalp. Functional magnetic resonance (fMRI) employs an indirect hemodynamic measure of neural activity (blood oxygenation) and permits task- and stimulus-related differences in activity to be localized with a spatial resolution of less than 1 cm. The fMRI studies to which most attention is devoted employed event-related designs, analogous to those employed with ERPs. Such designs are of particular value because they make it possible to investigate differences in item-related brain activity associated with different experimental conditions or differential memory performance (e.g., hits vs. misses on a recognition memory task). Whereas fMRI has far better spatial resolution than the ERP method, the sluggishness of the BOLD response means that the temporal resolution of event-related fMRI signals is typically of the order of hundreds of milliseconds. This compares unfavorably with the millisecond-level resolution that can be attained with ERPs. Thus, the two methods provide complementary perspectives on event-related brain activity.

Theoretical framework

The theoretical perspective framing the studies reviewed in this chapter borrows ideas from a number of previous proposals about retrieval processing (e.g., Tulving, 1983; Johnson, Hashtroudi, and Lindsay, 1993; Burgess and Shallice, 1996; Koriat and Goldsmith, 1996; Schacter, Norman, and Koutstaal, 1998; Rugg and Wilding, 2000). As outlined in figure 52.1, a distinction is drawn between processes that operate on a retrieval cue in the course of an attempt to retrieve information from memory (preretrieval processes), processes that support the successful recovery and representation of information (ecphoric processes), and processes that operate on the outcome of a retrieval attempt (postretrieval processes). Pre- and postretrieval processes are considered to be under voluntary control. In the following sections, these processes are discussed in the context of relevant ERP and fMRI findings.

MICHAEL D. RUGG Center for the Neurobiology of Learning and Memory and Department of Neurobiology and Behavior, University of California, Irvine, Calif.

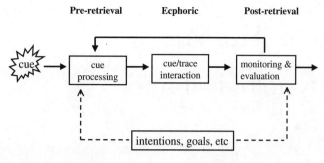

Pre-retrieval   Ecphoric   Post-retrieval

FIGURE 52.1   Stages in episodic retrieval processing.

An aspect of retrieval processing missing from figure 52.1 is retrieval mode. Retrieval mode refers to a hypothesized cognitive state or set that biases subjects to process stimulus events as retrieval cues, and to experience successful episodic retrieval autonoetically (Tulving, 1983; Wheeler, Stuss, and Tulving, 1997). Investigation of the neural correlates of retrieval mode requires contrasts between activity elicited during tasks with and tasks without an episodic retrieval component (Rugg and Wilding, 2000). In all of the studies reviewed here, contrasts are between different conditions of one or more retrieval tasks, and therefore do not speak to this issue.

Preretrieval processes

The retrieval of an episodic memory requires an appropriate interaction between a retrieval cue and an encoded memory representation (Tulving, 1983). The importance of retrieval cues and their processing is emphasized in the principles of transfer-appropriate processing (Morris, Bransford, and Franks, 1977) and encoding specificity (Tulving and Thomson, 1973). Broadly speaking, these principles hold that memory performance depends on the degree to which the processing engaged during encoding is recapitulated during retrieval. Implicit in these principles is the notion that people can vary how they process retrieval cues so as to optimize compatibility with targeted memory representations, and hence optimize the chances of successful retrieval.

According to Rugg and Wilding (2000), the ability to vary how a retrieval cue is processed requires the adoption of different "retrieval orientations," cognitive states or sets that bias cue processing in the service of the demands of a particular retrieval goal. Rugg and Wilding proposed that the neural correlates of the adoption of different retrieval orientations can be investigated by contrasting the activity elicited by physically identical retrieval cues when these are used to probe memory for different kinds of information. Rugg and Wilding further proposed that such contrasts should be restricted to retrieval cues bearing no relation to studied items (e.g., new items in a recognition memory test), so as to avoid confounding preretrieval processes with those

associated with retrieval success. They argued that whereas cues corresponding to unstudied items would fully engage preretrieval processes, they would engage ecphoric and postretrieval processes only to a limited degree.

Findings from a number of ERP studies suggest that the neural activity elicited by physically identical cues does indeed vary according to the nature of the information being sought. Johnson, Kounios, and Nolde (1997) employed an encoding manipulation (how difficult the object denoted by a word or a picture would be to draw versus the number of functions it might have) and reported that the ERPs elicited by both new and old test words in a subsequent source memory test (was the item studied as a word or a picture?) differed markedly according to study task. In Ranganath and Paller (1999), ERPs to new items over the left frontal scalp were more positive-going when the test required retrieval of specific as opposed to general information (classifying as old those test pictures with an exact versus an approximate correspondence to studied items).

Wilding (1999) compared ERPs elicited by new items on a source memory task according to the nature of the source judgment that was required (speaker voice versus type of study task) and reported that ERPs over the frontal scalp varied according to this manipulation. These findings were interpreted as evidence that the requirement to retrieve different kinds of source information influenced subjects' retrieval orientation. Consistent with the idea that retrieval orientation takes the form of a tonically maintained set or state, Wilding and Nobre (2001) found that task-dependent ERP effects were present only when the two source retrieval tasks were blocked, with no effects evident when the tasks were interleaved within a single test phase.

The findings from the foregoing studies suggest that retrieval cues receive differential processing according to task demands. All of the studies, however, employed at least one retrieval condition that required explicit recovery of contextual detail about the study episode. Rugg, Allan, and Birch (2000) employed a yes/no recognition task and investigated ERP correlates of cue processing according to whether old words had been studied in a deep or a shallow encoding task. ERPs to new items were more positive-going when they were intermixed with shallowly studied items than when they were intermixed with deeply studied items. Rugg and colleagues (2000) interpreted their findings as reflecting, in part, differences in cue processing brought about by the requirement to search for semantically versus nonsemantically encoded words. Interpretation of these findings is difficult, however, because of a confound between the encoding manipulation and test difficulty: new item accuracy was lower and response times were longer in the shallow condition, raising the possibility that the ERP effects merely reflected the greater retrieval effort required in this condition.

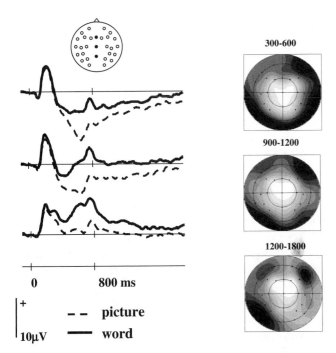

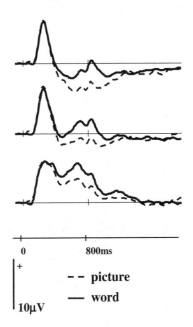

FIGURE 52.2 *Left:* Grand average ERP waveforms from Robb and Rugg (2002), recorded from the scalp sites indicated by the solid circles. The waveforms were elicited by words corresponding to unstudied items and are overlaid according to whether words or pictures were the sought-for material. Waveforms have been collapsed over the difficulty manipulation. *Right:* Scalp distribution (lighter shade indicates more positive-going) of the differences in amplitude between the two conditions, word versus picture, in three latency regions.

To remove this confound, Robb and Rugg (2002) crossed an encoding manipulation with two levels of task difficulty. In separate study-test cycles, subjects studied lists of pictures or words, and then undertook a yes/no recognition memory test with words as the test items. Test difficulty was manipulated by varying the length of the study list and the study–test delay. Regardless of difficulty, ERPs elicited by new test words differed markedly according to whether the study materials were words or pictures. The onset of this effect occurred around 250 ms after stimulus presentation and took the form of a topographically widespread, temporally sustained negativity in the waveforms elicited during the picture condition relative to the word condition (figure 52.2). The findings suggest that retrieval cues in tests of recognition memory are indeed processed differentially according to the form of the sought-for information.

These findings were extended by Herron and Rugg (2003a). Pictures and words were randomly interleaved within a common study block. In separate test phases, participants were instructed to respond positively to test words corresponding either to studied pictures or to studied words. Of importance, each test phase contained words corresponding to both classes of studied item. As shown in figure 52.3, the effect of the instructions was to induce differences

FIGURE 52.3 Grand average ERPs, from the same electrode sites as in figure 52.1, elicited by unstudied test words in Herron and Rugg (2003a) and overlaid according to whether words or pictures were the sought-for material.

in new-item ERPs that closely resembled those described by Robb and Rugg (2002; figure 52.2). Thus, ERP retrieval orientation effects can be obtained not only when relevant and irrelevant items have been encoded in a common list context, but also when the test list contains retrieval cues that correspond to both classes of item.

The findings of Robb and Rugg (2002) and Herron and Rugg (2003a), along with those described earlier, give credence to the idea that individuals vary their processing of retrieval cues according to the demands of the retrieval task. Thus, the findings suggest that the concept of retrieval orientation has utility. The findings also raise a number of important questions. One question relates to the time course of these putative ERP correlates of retrieval orientation. Although retrieval orientation is held to bias preretrieval processing, it is evident that there is considerable temporal overlap between the effects illustrated in figure 52.3 and the retrieval success (old vs. new) effects for the same experiment (see figure 52.6). One might argue that the time course of retrieval success effects offers little guide to how long a retrieval cue is employed to probe memory in the absence of success (Robb and Rugg, 2002). Nevertheless, the extent of the overlap raises the possibility that, in addition to differential preretrieval processes, the new-item ERP effects illustrated in figures 52.2 and 52.3 reflect other processes of later onset that are more properly considered postretrieval processes (e.g., monitoring of the outcome of a retrieval attempt).

Another question is whether the new-item ERP effects observed in Robb and Rugg (2002) and Herron and Rugg

(2003a) depended on the employment of a "copy cue" condition. In both studies, the critical comparison was between a condition in which study and test items were in the same physical format and a condition in which study and test formats differed. It will be of interest to determine whether similar ERP retrieval orientation effects can be obtained when the degree of physical overlap between different classes of study item and their retrieval cues is held constant.

A third issue concerns the conditions necessary for the development and subsequent maintenance of retrieval orientation effects. As already noted, there is evidence that individuals cannot easily switch between different retrieval orientations on a trial-by-trial basis (Wilding and Nobre, 2001). A related issue is whether a given retrieval orientation can be established and maintained solely on the basis of an instructional set, or whether it must be in some sense reinforced by successful retrieval of the sought-for information.

Finally, there is the important question of the loci of the neural activity reflected in the aforementioned ERP effects. This question cannot be answered at present: the diffuse scalp distribution of the effects offers no hints to their likely intracerebral origins and, at the time of writing, there are no directly relevant fMRI findings. One clue comes from an fMRI study reported by Ranganath, Johnson, and D'Esposito (2000), which employed a task manipulation similar to that employed in the ERP study of Ranganath and Paller (1999). In keeping with the distribution over the left frontal scalp of the new-item ERP differences reported for the general-versus-specific task manipulation in that study, Ranganath, Johnson, and D'Esposito (2000) reported that new test items elicited greater activity in left anterior prefrontal cortex during the specific than the general condition. This finding, perhaps not unexpectedly (Burgess and Shallice, 1996; Fletcher and Henson, 2001; Ranganath and Knight, 2002), implicates the prefrontal cortex in one example of differential cue processing. A role for prefrontal cortex in differential cue processing is also suggested by the findings of Dobbins and colleagues (2002, 2003). When word pairs or triplets were presented in a forced-choice task, activity differed in a variety of prefrontal regions (in most cases regardless of response accuracy), depending on whether discrimination required a source versus a yes/no recognition judgment (Dobbins et al., 2002, Experiment 1) or a source versus a recency judgment (Dobbins et al., 2002, Experiment 2; Dobbins et al., 2003).

Retrieval success

When an appropriately processed retrieval cue interacts with episodic memory representations that share some of the cue's attributes, information about a prior episode is retrieved from memory and accompanied by the phenome-nal experience of remembering. As attested to by a large body of evidence (e.g., Schacter and Dodson, 2001), this process is fallible. The discussion that follows, however, is concerned solely with veridical memory. It focuses on two areas where recent progress has been made: characterization of the neural correlates of episodic retrieval, and its strategic control.

NEURAL CORRELATES OF SUCCESSFUL EPISODIC RETRIEVAL Most recent ERP and fMRI studies of episodic retrieval have employed tests of recognition memory, often operationalizing the neural correlates of retrieval success as the contrast between the activity elicited by correctly classified old versus new items. As has been noted previously (e.g., Rugg and Henson, 2002), this contrast is problematic for several reasons, not least because it confounds recognition based on retrieval of episodic information ("recollection," in the terminology of "dual-process" models of recognition; Yonelinas, 2002) with that based on a different form of information about prior occurrence, an acontextual, strength-like index termed "familiarity." Thus, the contrast between old and new recognition test items will not yield a pure correlate of episodic retrieval.

In part motivated by this problem, from the early 1990s onward a number of ERP studies employed designs in which test items could be segregated according to whether recognition was primarily familiarity-driven or was also associated with recollection (for reviews, see Rugg, 1995; Friedman and Johnson, 2000; Rugg and Allan, 2000). The findings from these studies converge to suggest that ERPs elicited by recollected test items are characterized by a posteriorly distributed positivity, which, in recognition of its characteristic left-sided scalp distribution (figure 52.4), has been termed the left parietal old/new effect. The effect has been reported to be sensitive to several of the variables that have been held to selectively index or influence recollection on the basis of evidence from experimental psychology (e.g., Yonelinas,

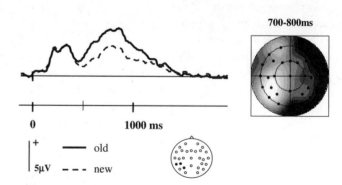

FIGURE 52.4 *Left:* ERP waveforms illustrating the left parietal old/new effect. Data were averaged over the three electrode sites indicated by the solid circles. *Right:* Scalp distribution of the effect (old − new). (Data from Tsivilis, Otten, and Rugg, 2001.)

2002). These variables include "remember" versus "know" judgments (e.g., Smith, 1993; Düzel et al., 1997), accurate versus inaccurate source memory judgments (Wilding and Rugg, 1996; Trott et al., 1997), associative versus item recognition (e.g., Donaldson and Rugg, 1998), "deep" versus "shallow" study tasks (e.g., Rugg et al., 1998), and recognition hits versus false alarms (e.g., Curran, 2000). In addition, the left parietal effect has been reported to be absent in memory-impaired patients in whom recognition memory is presumed to rely largely on familiarity (e.g., Smith and Halgren, 1989; Tendolkar et al., 1999; Düzel et al., 2001).

The foregoing evidence suggests strongly that the left parietal old/new effect is a correlate of recognition associated with recollection, but says little about its neural origins or functional significance. These issues have been informed by recent fMRI findings.

fMRI studies of recollection Since 1998, contrasts between neural activity elicited by old and new items have been reported in more than a dozen event-related fMRI studies of recognition memory (for review, see Rugg and Henson, 2002). Whereas the findings from these studies have proven remarkably consistent, only a few have employed experimental designs that permit recognized items to be segregated on the basis of level of recollection. Thus, whereas several regions (e.g., lateral and medial parietal cortex, anterior, dorsal and ventral prefrontal cortex, and, less consistently, medial temporal lobe) have been reported to show "retrieval success effects" in the form of greater activity for correctly classified old items, the functional significance of these fMRI old/new effects for the most part remains unclear. In the following discussion we focus on studies in which a direct contrast was performed between activity elicited by items according to their level of recollection.

Two of these studies contrasted activity for recognized test words accorded remember versus know judgments (Henson, Rugg, et al., 1999; Eldridge et al., 2000). In both studies, the contrast revealed relatively greater activity for remembered items in lateral parietal cortex (Brodmann area BA39/40; left only in the case of Henson, Rugg, et al., 1999), as well as left dorsal and anterior prefrontal cortex, and the posterior cingulate. In the study of Eldridge and colleagues (2000) but not that of Henson, Rugg, and colleagues (1999), greater activity was also reported for remembered items in the left hippocampal formation and adjacent medial temporal cortex.

In two other studies, activity was contrasted according to accuracy in a source memory task. In the study of Cansino and colleagues (2002), subjects studied pictures presented in one of four locations. The test requirement was to classify items as new or, if old, to indicate the location where they had been presented during study. Recollection was operationalized as the contrast between activity elicited by items

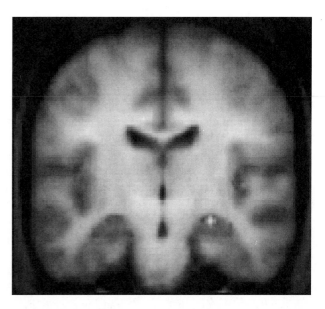

FIGURE 52.5 Right hippocampal region in a study by Cansino and colleagues (2002), where recognized items accorded a correct source judgment elicited greater activity than items accorded an incorrect judgment.

correctly judged old and accorded correct versus incorrect location judgments. The contrast revealed greater activity for "recollected" items in a variety of regions, some of which corresponded to those identified in one or both of the aforementioned remember/know studies. Among these regions were the hippocampal formation (figure 52.5) and lateral parietal cortex (BA 40) (in contrast to the previous studies, these effects were right lateralized, perhaps reflecting the employment of pictorial rather than verbal stimuli). Dobbins and colleagues (2003) had subjects study words in one of two encoding tasks. The test task involved the presentation of two old words, with the requirement to judge which had been encoded in a given task. Correct judgments were associated with greater activity than incorrect judgments in a variety of regions, including the left hippocampus and adjacent cortex, and left superior parietal cortex (BA 7/5), although not the more lateral parietal region (BA 40/39) identified in the preceding three studies.

Taken together, the findings from these four studies cannot be accounted for by such factors as the differential novelty of test items or whether an item is merely perceived to be old or new (cf. Wheeler and Buckner, 2003). Rather, the data demonstrate differences between activity elicited by items that were all correctly judged as old but that differed with respect to amount of recovered episodic information. Although the fMRI findings reported in these various studies differ in numerous respects, they converge to suggest that activity in both parietal cortex and the hippocampus is associated with recognition accompanied by recollection. Whereas the results for the hippocampus are unsurprising, given the wealth of lesion evidence supporting a role for this structure in the retrieval of recently acquired episodic information, the findings for the parietal cortex currently have no neuropsychological counterpart.

Relationship between ERP and fMRI correlates of recollection Inferences about the location of the generators of an ERP effect on the basis of the effect's scalp distribution are problematic. That said, it is evident that the scalp distribution of the left parietal old/new effect (figure 52.4) fits well with the hypothesis that it is generated in immediately underlying cortex. The fMRI findings of recollection-related activity in lateral parietal cortex add weight to this hypothesis. Indeed, it is tempting to assume that the effects observed with the two methods are neuroanatomically and functionally equivalent.

As indexed by ERPs, parietal old/new effects appear to onset sufficiently early (ca. 400–500 ms poststimulus) to reflect neural activity that could contribute causally to recollection-based memory judgments, but beyond that their functional significance is obscure. One early suggestion was that the left parietal old/new effect reflected hippocampally mediated, cortical reinstatement of retrieved information (Wilding and Rugg, 1996). This suggestion is consistent with the aforementioned findings that both left parietal and hippocampal activity are sensitive to recollection, although a functional relationship between recollection-related activity in the two regions remains to demonstrated. An alternative possibility, arguably more compatible with the role posited for parietal cortex in attention (Kastner and Ungerleider, 2000), is that the ERP and fMRI parietal effects reflect some kind of attentional shift or orienting triggered by successful episodic retrieval.

Finally, it should be noted that neither the ERP nor the fMRI data reviewed in the preceding discussion provide sufficient grounds to argue that the distinction between recollection and familiarity is honored at the neuroanatomical level (as has been proposed, for example, by Brown and Aggleton, 2001). The data are equally compatible with the view that the distinction between these two forms of memory is quantitative rather than qualitative, such that left parietal and hippocampal activity reflect the amount rather than the nature of the information retrieved. Evidence against this view, and in favor of the proposal that recognition based on recollection and familiarity does indeed have a distinct neural signature, is reviewed elsewhere (Rugg and Yonelinas, 2003).

CONTROL OF RETRIEVAL   In an earlier section, evidence was put forward suggesting that subjects can control their processing of retrieval cues by adopting specific retrieval orientations. It was proposed that this allows overlap between cues and a class of sought-for memory representations to be optimized, improving the likelihood of successful retrieval.

Another benefit of adopting a specific retrieval orientation might be to preclude the retrieval of unwanted information. That is, by constraining the way retrieval cues are processed, it may be possible to prevent irrelevant or potentially interfering memories from being retrieved. Thus, retrieval orientation might be better viewed as a mechanism for optimizing the selectivity rather than the amount of information retrieved from memory (see also Anderson and Bjork, 1994, and their discussion of cue bias).

Support for this proposal comes from the results of the ERP study of Herron and Rugg (2003a) that was described previously. The task employed in this study is an example of an exclusion task (Jacoby, 1991), in that subjects were required to endorse as old test words corresponding to one class of studied item (targets) but to reject test items belonging to the alternative class (the nontargets). One way in which this requirement could be met is by retrieving study information unselectively and discriminating between target and nontarget items on the basis of what was recollected. An alternative strategy would be to bias the processing of the test items so that they act as selective retrieval cues, and thus to bias retrieval in favor of target information. As can be seen from figure 52.6, in Herron and Rugg (2003a), both strategies appear to have been employed. When pictures were the target material, ERP old/new effects were observed for both correctly classified targets and nontargets. By contrast, when words were the targets, test items corresponding to nontargets elicited ERPs indistinguishable from those to new items. These findings suggest an asymmetry in the selectivity with which test items were employed to probe memory in the two conditions. When words were targets, subjects presumably were able to adopt a retrieval orientation that prevented test items corresponding to studied pictures from eliciting retrieval. When pictures were targets, however, selective cue processing was not possible, and subjects were

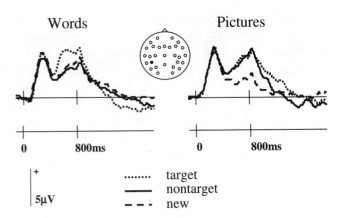

FIGURE 52.6 Grand average ERPs from a study by Rugg and Herron (2003a). An old/new effect is present for targets but not for nontargets when words are the sought-for material, but this effect is elicited by both classes of items when memory is probed for pictures. Electrode site is indicated in the insert.

forced to rely on postretrieval monitoring (see next section) to determine whether test items corresponded to a target or a nontarget.

The findings from a second study (Herron and Rugg, 2003b) add further weight to the idea that subjects can control the specificity with which retrieval cues are employed to probe memory. Subjects encoded words in two separate study lists and were subsequently required to endorse as old items from the second study list (targets) while rejecting both new items and items belonging to the first list (nontargets). The crucial manipulation was the memorability of target items; in one condition these were encoded in an elaborative study task that led to good subsequent memory, whereas in another condition the study task was more superficial and led to much poorer memory. Nontargets were encoded in identical tasks in the two conditions. Herron and Rugg (2003b) hypothesized that when target memory was good, subjects would base their judgments primarily on whether a test item elicited episodic information diagnostic of the target source, rejecting any item that failed to elicit such information. Thus, subjects would adopt a retrieval orientation directed toward recovery of information about target episodes. This strategy would be suboptimal when target memory is poor, however, because the failure to retrieve target information can no longer serve as a reliable basis for classifying an item as a nontarget. Hence, both target and nontarget source information should be retrieved. As shown in figure 52.7, these predictions were fulfilled: target items elicited a robust left parietal old/new effect in both conditions, but the effect was elicited by nontargets only when target memory was poor.

Findings similar to those of Herron and Rugg (2003b) had been reported previously by Dywan and colleagues (Dywan, Segalowitz, and Webster 1998; Dywan et al., 2001; Dywan, Segalowitz, and Arsenault, 2002). In the test phase of these experiments, previously studied words were presented along with new items, some of which repeated after

a lag of only a few trials, when they still required a no response. Whereas a parietal old/new effect was observed for studied items, no effect was detected (in young subjects) for the repeated nontargets. This finding converges with those described earlier to indicate that there are circumstances in which people can bias their processing of retrieval cues to prevent the recollection of potentially interfering memories.

Postretrieval processing

Postretrieval processes are engaged when the outcome of a retrieval attempt must be monitored or evaluated, for example, to allow a response to be chosen on the basis of the content of the retrieved information, or to evaluate the relevance of retrieved information in relation to a current behavioral goal. It is unlikely that such a diverse set of processes is neuroanatomically homogeneous. There is, however, evidence that right dorsolateral prefrontal cortex (BA9/46) plays a role in at least some forms of postretrieval processing.

One source of evidence pointing to a right frontal role in postretrieval processing comes from ERP studies describing the "right frontal" old/new effect. This effect, first described in a study of source memory (Wilding and Rugg, 1996), takes the form of a sustained positivity with a right frontal scalp maximum (figure 52.8). On the basis of its scalp distribution, time course, and apparent sensitivity to level of recollection, Wilding and Rugg (1996) proposed that the right frontal effect reflected the engagement of processes, supported by the right prefrontal cortex, that subjected retrieved episodic information to further processing in the service of task goals. This proposal received support from neuroimaging findings suggesting that right prefrontal activity covaries with the probability of successful retrieval (e.g., Rugg et al., 1996). It has subsequently become clear, however, that the right frontal ERP effect is not simply a correlate of successful episodic retrieval (e.g., Senkfor and Van Petten, 1998).

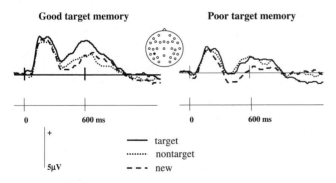

FIGURE 52.7   Grand average ERPs from a study by Herron and Rugg (2003b) illustrating a left parietal old/new effect for target but not for nontarget items when target memory is good, but for both classes of item when target memory is poor.

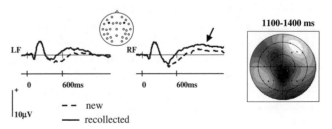

FIGURE 52.8   The right frontal ERP old/new effect. *Left:* Waveforms elicited by recognized old words accorded "remember" or correct source judgments (data collapsed to form a "recollected" category), overlain by waveforms elicited by correctly classified new items. Recording sites are indicated by solid circles. *Right:* Scalp distribution of the effect (recollected-new) for the period 1100–1400 ms poststimulus. (Data from Mark and Rugg, 1998.)

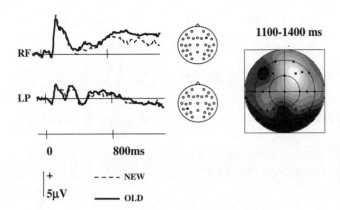

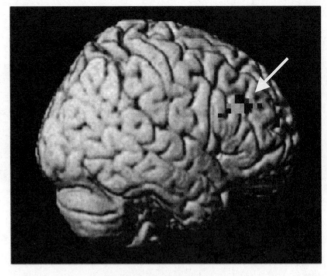

1100-1400 ms

FIGURE 52.9 *Left:* ERPs from right frontal and left parietal electrodes elicited by new items and correctly classified, "shallowly" studied old items. A right frontal old/new effect is evident in the absence of a left parietal effect, suggesting that recognition was accompanied by little or no recollection. *Right:* Scalp distribution of old/new effects in the latency range 1100–1400 ms, illustrating their right frontal maximum. (Data from Rugg et al., 2000.)

Indeed, recollection appears to be neither a necessary nor a sufficient condition for the generation of the effect. For example, Rugg and colleagues (2000) found that it could be elicited by items that, by virtue of their shallow encoding, were likely recognized on the basis of familiarity alone (figure 52.9).

In two recent event-related fMRI studies, the idea was explored that retrieval-related activity in one prefrontal region, the right dorsolateral prefrontal cortex, reflects the extent to which the outcome of a retrieval attempt is subjected to postretrieval monitoring. The starting point for these studies was the observation that recognized items attracting a know response elicited greater activity in this region than items endorsed as remembered (figure 52.10). To account for these findings, Henson, Rugg, and colleagues (1999) proposed that when information supporting a recognition judgment was relatively impoverished, as might often occur in the absence of recollection, monitoring operations would be engaged to a greater extent than when information was less equivocal (see also Fletcher and Henson, 2001). Henson and colleagues (2000) tested this proposal in a study in which recognition judgments were accompanied by confidence ratings. They predicted that judgments (whether old or new) made with low confidence would be associated with greater right dorsolateral activity than confident responses, which, they assumed, would reflect judgments based on information more strongly diagnostic of study status. This prediction was upheld.

In Rugg, Henson, and Robb (2003), two different retrieval tasks were employed. The study phases (in which words were presented in one of two different study contexts) and the structure of the test lists were held constant across the tasks. In the recognition task, studied items were classified as old regardless of the context in which they had been encoded.

FIGURE 52.10 Right dorsolateral prefrontal region (arrowed) where activity was greater for recognized test items endorsed as known rather than remembered, in the study of Henson and colleagues (1999). (See color plate 24.)

In the exclusion task, "old" responses were required to items studied in one of the two contexts, while words studied in the alternative context were to be given the same response as new items. Rugg and colleagues (2003) argued that the high levels of item memory engendered by the study tasks meant that postretrieval monitoring demands in the recognition task would be low. This would not be the case in the exclusion task, however, where a correct response to a studied item depended not merely on information that an item was old, but also on identification of the source of that information. (This prediction assumes that subjects do not adopt a retrieval orientation that is sufficiently selective to preclude retrieval of the nontargets.) The postretrieval operations necessitated by this latter requirement were expected to engage the right dorsolateral prefrontal cortex (see also Henson, Shallice, and Dolan, 1999). In contrast, as in the recognition task, a correct "new" judgment could be based on the mere detection of novelty, allowing responses to these items to be made on the basis of minimal monitoring and, therefore, with little dorsolateral prefrontal involvement. In keeping with these expectations, right dorsolateral activity failed to distinguish between old and new items in the recognition task but was elevated for both classes of old item in the exclusion condition (figure 52.11).

These findings, together with those of Henson and colleagues (1999, 2000) and the previous ERP results, demonstrate the variety of circumstances under which right dorsolateral prefrontal activity can be engaged during memory tests. The proposal here is that what these circumstances have in common is the need to monitor and evaluate the outcome of a retrieval attempt before selecting a response. Thus, although the cognitive operations supported

Target > New

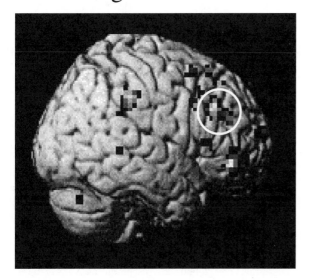

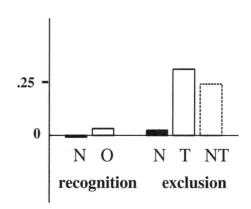

FIGURE 52.11   *Left:* Right dorsolateral region (circled) identified by the contrast between activity elicited by correctly classified target and new items in Rugg and colleagues (2003). *Right:* Activity (arbitrary units) elicited in this region by new (N) and old (O) items in the recognition task, and by new (N), target (T), and nontarget (NT) items in the exclusion task. (See color plate 25.)

by right dorsolateral prefrontal cortex are not engaged invariably when episodic retrieval is successful, they are nonetheless integral to the effective employment of episodic information in the control of behavior. This is illustrated by the memory deficits that can follow lesions of the prefrontal cortex, including dorsolateral regions, which appear to be attributable in part to impairment of postretrieval monitoring and evaluation (Ranganath and Knight, 2002). An interesting question for the future is the relationship between these operations and other functions that have been attributed to dorsolateral prefrontal cortex (for review, see Wood and Grafman, 2003).

ACKNOWLEDGMENTS   This work was supported by the Wellcome Trust and the U.K. Medical Research Council.

REFERENCES

ANDERSON, M. C., and R. A. BJORK, 1994. Mechanisms of inhibition in long term memory. In *Inhibitory Processes in Attention, Memory, and Language,* D. Dagenbach and T. H. Carr, eds. San Diego, Calif.: Academic Press, pp. 265–325.

BADDELEY, A., M. CONWAY, and J. AGGLETON, eds., 2001. *Episodic Memory* [special issue]. *Philos. Trans. R. Soc. Lond. B* 356.

BROWN, M. W., and J. P. AGGLETON, 2001. Recognition memory: What are the roles of the perirhinal cortex and hippocampus? *Nat. Rev. Neurosci.* 2:51–61.

BURGESS, P. W., and T. SHALLICE, 1996. Confabulation and the control of recollection. *Memory* 4:359–411.

CANSINO, S., P. MAQUET, R. J. DOLAN, and M. D. RUGG, 2002. Brain activity underlying encoding and retrieval of source memory. *Cereb. Cortex* 12:1048–1056.

CURRAN, T., 2000. Brain potentials of recollection and familiarity. *Mem. Cogn.* 28:923–938.

DOBBINS, I. G., H. FOLEY, D. L. SCHACTER, and A. D. WAGNER, 2002. Executive control during episodic retrieval: Multiple prefrontal processes subserve source memory. *Neuron* 35:989–996.

DOBBINS, I. G., H. J. RICE, A. D. WAGNER, and D. L. SCHACTER, 2003. Memory orientation and success: separable neurocognitive components underlying episodic recognition. *Neuropsychologia* 41:318–333.

DONALDSON, D. I., and M. D. RUGG, 1998. Recognition memory for new associations: Electrophysiological evidence for the role of recollection. *Neuropsychologia* 36:377–395.

DÜZEL, E., F. VARGHA-KHADEM, H. J. HEINZE, and M. MISHKIN, 2001. Brain activity evidence for recognition without recollection after early hippocampal damage. *Proc. Natl. Acad. Sci. U.S.A.* 98:8101–8106.

DÜZEL, E., A. P. YONELINAS, G. R. MANGUN, H. J. HEINZE, and E. TULVING, 1997. Event-related brain potential correlates of two states of conscious awareness in memory. *Proc. Natl. Acad. Sci. U.S.A.* 94:5973–5978.

DYWAN, J., S. J. SEGALOWITZ, and A. ARSENAULT, 2002. Electrophysiological response during source memory decisions in older and younger adults. *Brain Cogn.* 49:322–340.

DYWAN, J., S. J. SEGALOWITZ, and L. WEBSTER, 1998. Source monitoring: ERP evidence for greater reactivity to nontarget information in older adults. *Brain Cogn.* 36:390–430.

DYWAN, J., S. J. SEGALOWITZ, L. WEBSTER, K. HENDRY, and J. HARDING, 2001. Event-related-potential evidence for age-related differences in attentional allocation during a source monitoring task. *Dev. Neuropsychol.* 19:99–120.

ELDRIDGE, L. L., B. J. KNOWLTON, C. S. FURMANSKI, S. Y. BOOKHEIMER, and S. A. ENGEL, 2000. Remembering episodes: A selective role for the hippocampus during retrieval. *Nat. Neurosci.* 3:1149–1152.

FLETCHER, P. C., and R. N. HENSON, 2001. Frontal lobes and human memory: Insights from functional neuroimaging. *Brain* 124: 849–881.

FRIEDMAN, D., and J. R. JOHNSON, 2000. Event-related potential (ERP) studies of memory encoding and retrieval: A selective review. *Microsc. Res. Tech.* 5:6–28.

HENSON, R. N., M. D. RUGG, T. SHALLICE, and R. J. DOLAN, 2000. Confidence in recognition memory for words: Dissociating right prefrontal roles in episodic retrieval. *J. Cogn. Neurosci.* 12:913–923.

HENSON, R. N. A., M. D. RUGG, T. SHALLICE, O. JOSEPHS, and R. DOLAN, 1999. Recollection and familiarity in recognition memory: An event-related fMRI study. *J. Neurosci.* 19:3962–3972.

HENSON, R. N., T. SHALLICE, and R. J. DOLAN, 1999. Right prefrontal cortex and episodic memory retrieval: A functional MRI test of the monitoring hypothesis. *Brain* 122:1367–1381.

HERRON, J. E., and M. D. RUGG, 2003a. Retrieval orientation and the control of recollection. *J. Cogn. Neurosci.* 15:843–854.

HERRON, J. E., and M. D. RUGG, 2003b. Strategic influences on recollection in the exclusion task: Electrophysiological evidence. *Psychonom. Bull. Rev.* 10:703–710.

JACOBY, L. L., 1991. A process dissociation framework: Separating automatic from intentional uses of memory. *J. Mem. Lang.* 30: 513–541.

JOHNSON, M. K., S. HASHTROUDI, and D. S. LINDSAY, 1993. Source monitoring. *Psychol. Bull.* 114:3–28.

JOHNSON, M. K., J. KOUNIOS, and S. F. NOLDE, 1997. Electrophysiological brain activity and memory source monitoring. *Neuroreport* 8:1317–1320.

KASTNER, S., and L. G. UNGERLEIDER, 2000. Mechanisms of visual attention in the human cortex. *Annu. Rev. Neurosci.* 23:315–341.

KORIAT, A., and M. GOLDSMITH, 1996. Monitoring and control processes in the strategic regulation of memory accuracy. *Psychol. Rev.* 103:490–517.

MARK, R. E., and M. D. RUGG, 1998. Age effects on brain activity associated with episodic memory retrieval: An electrophysiological study. *Brain* 121:861–873.

MORRIS, C. D., J. D. BRANSFORD, and J. J. FRANKS, 1977. Levels of processing versus transfer appropriate processing. *J. Verb. Learn. Verb. Behav.* 16:519–533.

RANGANATH, C., M. K. JOHNSON, and M. D'ESPOSITO, 2000. Left anterior prefrontal activation increases with demands to recall specific perceptual information. *J. Neurosci.* 20:RC108.

RANGANATH, C., and R. T. KNIGHT, 2002. Prefrontal cortex and episodic memory: Integrating findings from neuropsychology and functional brain imaging. In *The Cognitive Neuroscience of Memory: Encoding and Retrieval*, A. Parker, E. L. Wilding, and T. J. Bussey, eds. Hove, England: Psychology Press, pp. 83–99.

RANGANATH, C., and K. A. PALLER, 1999. Frontal brain potentials during recognition are modulated by requirements to retrieve perceptual detail. *Neuron* 22:605–613.

RICHARDSON-KLAVEHN, A., J. M. GARDINER, and R. I. JAVA, 1996. Memory: Task dissociations, process dissociations, and dissociations of consciousness. In *Implicit Cognition*, G. Underwood, ed. New York: Oxford University Press, pp. 85–157.

ROBB, W. G. K., and M. D. RUGG, 2002. Electrophysiological dissociation of retrieval orientation and retrieval effort. *Psychol. Bull. Rev.* 9:583–589.

RUGG, M. D., 1995. ERP studies of memory. In *Electrophysiology of Mind*, M. D. Rugg and M. G. H. Coles, eds. New York: Oxford University Press, pp. 132–170.

RUGG, M. D., 1999. Functional neuroimaging in cognitive neuroscience. In *Neurocognition of Language*, P. Hagoort and C. Brown, eds. Oxford, England: Oxford University Press, pp. 15–36.

RUGG, M. D., and K. ALLAN, 2000. Memory retrieval: An electrophysiological perspective. In *The New Cognitive Neurosciences*, M. S. Gazzaniga, ed. Cambridge, Mass.: MIT Press, pp. 805–816.

RUGG, M. D., K. ALLAN, and C. S. BIRCH, 2000. Electrophysiological evidence for the modulation of retrieval orientation by depth of study processing. *J. Cogn. Neurosci.* 12:664–678.

RUGG, M. D., P. C. FLETCHER, C. D. FRITH, R. S. J. FRACKOWIAK, and R. J. DOLAN, 1996. Differential activation of the prefrontal cortex in successful and unsuccessful memory retrieval. *Brain* 119:2073–2083.

RUGG, M. D., and R. N. A. HENSON, 2002. Episodic memory retrieval: An (event-related) functional neuroimaging perspective. In *The Cognitive Neuroscience of Memory Encoding and Retrieval*, A. E. Parker, E. L. Wilding and T. Bussey, eds. New York: Psychology Press, pp. 3–37.

RUGG, M. D., R. N. HENSON, and W. G. ROBB, 2003. Neural correlates of retrieval processing in the prefrontal cortex during recognition and exclusion tasks. *Neuropsychologia* 41: 40–52.

RUGG, M. D., R. E. MARK, P. WALLA, A. M. SCHLOERSCHEIDT, C. S. BIRCH, and K. ALLAN, 1998. Dissociation of the neural correlates of implicit and explicit memory. *Nature* 392:595–598.

RUGG, M. D., and E. L. WILDING, 2000. Retrieval processing and episodic memory. *Trends. Cogn. Sci.* 4:108–115.

RUGG, M. D., and A. P. YONELINAS, 2003. Human recognition memory: A cognitive neuroscience perspective. *Trends Cogn. Sci.* 7:313–319.

SENKFOR, A. J., and C. VAN PETTEN, 1998. Who said what? An event-related potential investigation of source and item memory. *J. Exp. Psychol. Learn. Mem. Cogn.* 24:1005–1025.

SCHACTER, D. L., and C. S. DODSON, 2001. Misattribution, false recognition and the sins of memory. *Trans. R. Soc. Lond. B Biol. Sci.* 356:1385–1393.

SCHACTER, D. L., K. A. NORMAN, and W. KOUTSTAAL, 1998. The cognitive neuroscience of constructive memory. *Annu. Rev. Psychol.* 49:289–318.

SMITH, M. E., 1993. Neurophysiological manifestations of recollective experience during recognition memory judgments. *J. Cogn. Neurosci.* 5:1–13.

SMITH, M. E., and E. HALGREN, 1989. Dissociation of recognition memory components following temporal lobe lesions. *J. Exp. Psychol. Learn. Mem. Cogn.* 15:50–60.

TENDOLKAR, I., A. SCHOENFELD, G. GOLZ, G. FERNANDEZ, K. P. KUHL, R. FERSZT, and H. J. HEINZE, 1999. Neural correlates of recognition memory with and without recollection in patients with Alzheimer's disease and healthy controls. *Neurosci. Lett.* 263: 45–48.

TROTT, C. T., D. FRIEDMAN, W. RITTER, and M. FABIANI, 1997. Item and source memory: Differential age effects revealed by event-related potentials. *Neuroreport* 8:373–378.

TSIVILIS, D., L. J. OTTEN, and M. D. RUGG, 2001. Context effects on the neural correlates of recognition memory: An electrophysiological study. *Neuron* 31:497–505.

TULVING, E., 1983. *Elements of Episodic Memory*. Oxford, England: Oxford University Press.

TULVING, E., and D. M. THOMSON, 1973. Encoding specificity and retrieval processes in episodic memory. *Psychol. Rev.* 80:353–373.

WHEELER, M. E., and R. L. BUCKNER, 2003. Functional dissociation among components of remembering: Control, perceived oldness, and content. *J. Neurosci.* 23:3869–3880.

WHEELER, M. A., D. T. STUSS, and E. TULVING, 1997. Toward a theory of episodic memory: The frontal lobes and autonoetic consciousness. *Psychol. Bull.* 121:331–354.

WILDING, E. L., 1999. Separating retrieval strategies from retrieval success: An event-related potential study of source memory. *Neuropsychologia* 37:441–454.

WILDING, E. L., and A. C. NOBRE, 2001. Related Articles, task-switching and memory retrieval processing: Electrophysiological evidence. *Neuroreport* 12:3613–3617.

WILDING, E. L., and M. D. RUGG, 1996. An event-related potential study of recognition memory with and without retrieval of source. *Brain* 119:889–905.

WOOD, J. N., and J. GRAFMAN. Human prefrontal cortex: Processing and representational perspectives. *Nat. Rev. Neurosci.* 4:139–147.

YONELINAS, A. P., 2002. The nature of recollection and familiarity: A review of 30 years of research. *J. Mem. Lang.* 46:441–517.

53 Neural Correlates of Memory's Successes and Sins

RANDY L. BUCKNER AND DANIEL L. SCHACTER

ABSTRACT This chapter discusses memory as a constructive process that calls on strategic, controlled processes intermixed with more automatic processes to build a perception that is experienced as an incident from the past. Specific results suggest that frontal regions contribute to control processes that interact with posterior regions supplying retrieved content. Most often, memories are constructed accurately. Under certain conditions, however, memory errors that reveal the nature and fragility of memory processes arise. We discuss how properties of these brain networks enable retrieval goals to be achieved, yet sometimes give rise to inaccurate memories.

The intuitive view that memory retrieval represents an accurate revival of past experience has been challenged by a growing number of empirical observations. Foremost among them is the finding that individuals can hold strong beliefs about past events that never happened, often referred to as false memories (Roediger and McDermott, 1995). These observations suggest that memories are not products of a unitary and always accurate retrieval mechanism but instead rely on a collection of cobbled-together processes that aid memory decisions. Memory is a constructive process that depends on strategic, controlled processes intermixed with more automatic processes to build a perception that is experienced as an incident from the past (Bartlett, 1932; Jacoby, 1991; Schacter, Norman, and Koutstaal, 1998). The mechanisms are efficient yet not infallible, and probably exist because they work well most of the time. In this chapter, we explore the separate contributions of brain regions that participate in accessing past information and those that aid in detecting familiarity and representing the contents of memories. We discuss how properties of brain networks enable retrieval goals to be achieved, yet sometimes give rise to "memory sins" (Schacter, 1999, 2001), such as those that result in inaccurate memories.

RANDY L. BUCKNER Department of Psychology, Howard Hughes Medical Institute at Washington University, St. Louis, Mo.
DANIEL L. SCHACTER Department of Psychology, Harvard University, Cambridge, Mass.

Specific frontal regions contribute to control processes during remembering

A central point of this chapter is that multiple, interdependent processes support retrieval through interacting brain networks. Medial temporal/diencephalic structures, discussed thoroughly by Squire, Clark, and Bayley (this volume), are perhaps the best-understood contributors to memory. Areas within the medial temporal lobe appear to support memory processes that bind and/or associate new information that is required for retrieval for a period of time following learning (Eichenbaum and Cohen, 2001; see also Squire, Clark, and Bayley, this volume). An additional broad class of processes that contribute to retrieval is required when sought-after information cannot be automatically accessed, and strategic processes must be engaged. We refer to these as controlled processes because they involve attention-demanding operations that are sequential in nature, are sensitive to capacity limitations, and are influenced by retrieval context. Not all retrieval tasks require strategic processes. In some situations, retrieval cues can automatically result in a perception that information is from the past, suggesting certain retrieval processes can occur spontaneously and are not dependent on strategic operations. Models of performance on recognition tasks have, in particular, long proposed distinctions that capture these separate retrieval processes (Mandler, 1980; Jacoby, 1991).

Patients with frontal lobe lesions show impairments when retrieval requires controlled access to past information. Difficulties are greatest when retrieval cues are minimal (e.g., during free recall) or when weakly associated information must be retrieved (e.g., during source retrieval). Patients tend not to show organized retrieval groupings typical of healthy young adults (Gershberg and Shimamura, 1995), and sometimes can exhibit excessively high false alarm rates (Schacter, Curran, et al., 1996) or even confabulation (Moscovitch, 1989). For these reasons, interpretation of frontal deficits has focused on implementing strategies and monitoring the products of retrieval (e.g., Shallice and Burgess, 1991), in contrast to the pervasive memory deficits that result from lesions to medial temporal regions (Corkin, 1984; Squire, 1992; Eichenbaum and Cohen, 2001).

Complementing patient studies, imaging results in young, healthy adults have consistently shown frontal activation during performance of a wide range of retrieval tasks (for reviews, see Desgranges, Baron, and Eustasche, 1998; Cabeza and Nyberg, 2000; Fletcher and Henson, 2001; Buckner, 2003). Frontal activation during retrieval has generalized across different retrieval task formats (recall and recognition) and material types (words, pictures, and faces). Important to this discussion, three principles have emerged from imaging studies that help us to understand the role of frontal cortex in memory retrieval. Each principle is discussed separately.

1. *Frontal contributions to retrieval involve anatomically specific regions within frontal cortex that exhibit a roughly posterior to anterior organization.* For purposes of the present discussion, we will refer to subdivisions of the frontal cortex by their approximate Brodmann area (BA) numbers (Talairach and Tournoux, 1988; Petrides and Pandya, 1994). Posterior frontal regions, near BA 44 and 6, participate in many forms of controlled retrieval. It is important to note that these posterior regions modulate differentially, depending on the domain of information that is accessed, with greater left-lateralized recruitment during verbal retrieval tasks and greater right-lateralized recruitment during nonverbal tasks (Wagner et al., 1998; McDermott et al., 1999).

More anterior regions, near BA 45 and 47, show properties that reflect the degree of controlled processing demands. For example, when people are remembering recent episodes, recalling the details of an earlier event elicits strong activation in anterior prefrontal regions, whereas simply recognizing whether a presented cue item is old or new shows less activation (Nolde, Johnson, and D'Esposito, 1998; Dobbins et al., 2002; see also Cabeza, Locantore, and Anderson, 2003). Konishi and colleagues (2002), building on earlier neuropsychological paradigms (Milner, Corsi, and Leonard, 1991), recently noted enhanced activation in similar prefrontal regions when the difficulty in recalling the temporal details of an earlier episode was increased. Within the perceptual domain, Ranganath, Johnson, and D'Esposito (2000) observed increased activation of the left anterior prefrontal cortex as the level of perceptual detail required at the time of retrieval was manipulated. Wheeler and Buckner (2003; see also Velanova et al., 2003) similarly noted that, within the context of retrieving perceptual source details, a region near BA 45/47 was more active when the to-be-retrieved information was studied minimally, requiring the subject to devote more extensive controlled processing during retrieval, than when the information was repeatedly studied. It should also be noted that these regions are not exclusively devoted to tasks that involve remembering (see, e.g., Petersen et al., 1988; Demb et al., 1995; Gold and Buckner, 2002). They appear to participate as general processing resources

that are deployed during remembering and other forms of controlled processing (Buckner, 2003).

A final set of regions, in the right frontal cortex, at or near BA 9 (in what is often defined as dorsolateral prefrontal cortex, or DLPC), and also in frontopolar cortex (FPC) near BA 10, are commonly active during remembering. As we discuss later under point 3, regions within FPC can show a fundamentally distinct temporal profile that suggests a role in supporting an ongoing attention set, or retrieval mode, during remembering.

2. *Frontal contributions to control processes modulate based on retrieval demands and do not depend on mnemonic outcome at an individual event level; they are deployed during events that result in recognition failures as well as during events that elicit strong recollective experiences.* An important property of frontal contributions to remembering is that participation appears aligned with guiding or monitoring the act of retrieval and is not specific to successful acts of retrieval. That is, although modulation is prominent for the type of retrieval demand, similar levels of activation often occur for retrieval events in which information is successfully remembered (hits) and also for events in which information is correctly rejected as being new (Wheeler and Buckner, 2003; Velanova et al., 2003; Figure 53.1). The prevailing interpretation of these results is that frontal regions at or near BA 45/47 participate when a novel or weakly associated representation of the target information must be momentarily constructed to solve a task goal, with the exclusion of other possible but context-inappropriate representations (Thompson-Schill et al., 1997; Fletcher, Shallice, and Dolan, 2000; Gold and Buckner, 2002; see also Goldman-Rakic, 1987; Miller, 2000; Duncan, 2001; Mesulam, 2002; Wagner, Bunge, and Badre, this volume). Situations in which past experience or invariant rules allow a cue to directly specify the needed representation appear to minimize prefrontal involvement. Through poorly understood mechanisms, anterior prefrontal regions contribute to the dynamic selection of representations during long-term memory retrieval when remembering requires access to detailed, or weakly associated, information.

3. *Frontal-polar regions contribute to control processes that can be sustained across individual retrieval attempts, thereby suggesting a role in establishing an attentional set or retrieval mode.* Perhaps the most novel and perplexing finding to emerge from neuroimaging research on memory retrieval is that FPC regions, often right lateralized, are differentially activated when people are engaged in remembering episodes (for reviews, see Buckner, 1996; Tulving et al., 1994). Other forms of retrieval show considerably less activation in this region. For example, FPC regions activate minimally when a subject retrieves *any* word beginning with a certain stem cue (e.g., generating *street* in response to *str__*). But if the task requires using the stem cue to remember a word from a specific earlier study list of

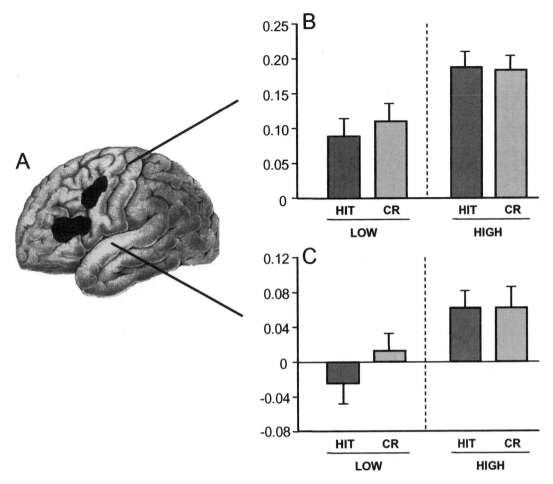

FIGURE 53.1 Specific frontal regions contribute to controlled processing during memory retrieval. (*A*) Approximate locations of two prefrontal regions that transiently modulate based on retrieval demands. The upper region is located at or near BA 44; the lower region is located at or near BA 45/47. (*B, C*) The magnitude (in percent MR signal change) for retrieval trials is plotted for each of the regions. Data from two conditions are displayed: LOW indicates low-control condition following extensive study; HIGH indicates high-control condition following minimal study. Items are separated based on hits (HIT, correctly recognized old items) and correct rejections (CR). Note that the prefrontal regions modulate based on the level of control required and not based on whether the item is a HIT or CR. (Adapted from Velanova et al., 2003.)

words, robust activation is observed (Squire et al., 1992). FPC regions also dissociate from other frontal regions because they do not modulate across verbal/nonverbal domain lines; they are right lateralized for retrieval of both word and faces (McDermott et al., 1999). Despite these observations, it has been surprisingly difficult to specify the nature of frontopolar contributions to remembering.

One puzzle is that the ability to detect FPC activation in brain imaging studies is influenced by the temporal structure of the memory paradigm and the exact time frame over which activity is recorded. Early paradigms, because of their methodological limitations, averaged activity over extended time periods during which many retrieval events were performed in rapid succession (e.g., Squire et al., 1992; Tulving et al., 1994; Fletcher et al., 1995; Buckner et al., 1995; Schacter, Alpert, et al., 1996; Rugg et al., 1996). Right frontal-polar activity was almost always observed during

remembering in these studies (Buckner, 1996). By contrast, more recent "event-related" paradigms that explore activity aligned to individual retrieval events less often note right FPC activity (but exceptions do exist), or note activity patterns that are temporally extended (e.g., Schacter, Buckner, et al., 1997; Henson et al., 2000).

A possible interpretation of these data is that FPC contributes to form an attentional set, or retrieval mode, that extends over multiple individual retrieval events (Düzel et al., 1999; Nyberg et al., 1995; figure 53.2). Preliminary evidence, based on a paradigm that can separate temporally extended activity correlates from those aligned with individual events (Donaldson, Petersen, Ollinger, et al., 2001; Donaldson and Buckner, 2002), suggests that right FPC contributions to memory retrieval can be associated with sustained, mode-related processes (Velanova et al., 2003). Further exploration will be required to explore this

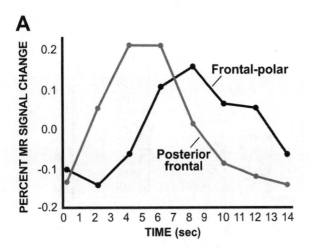

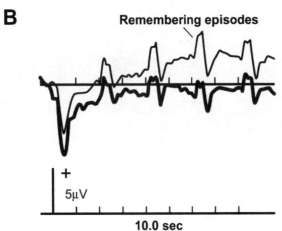

FIGURE 53.2 Frontal-polar regions contribute to sustained control processes associated with retrieval mode. (*A*) The time course of event-related fMRI responses (in percent MR signal change) is displayed for posterior frontal regions (near those displayed in figure 53.1) and frontopolar regions. Note the temporally delayed and extended responses between regions. (Adapted from Schacter, Buckner et al., 1997.) (*B*) The ERP waveform recorded from anterior scalp sites during remembering (episodic retrieval) in contrast to semantic retrieval. Note the slowly evolving, temporally extended waveform, suggestive of a sustained control process. (Adapted from Düzel et al., 1999.)

possibility. Many kinds of systems require context-dependent gating such that information is handled differently, depending on task context. FPC may maintain cognitive (attentional) sets during remembering, and other forms of cognitive task, that select one mode of processing over another across extended periods of time.

Parietal and frontal networks correlate with the perception that information is old

A hallmark feature of remembering is the ability to reconstruct a perception that is experienced as being from one's own past, including many content details of the original episode, such as visual and auditory impressions, and even the thoughts and emotions that were originally experienced. Component processes involved in remembering must therefore also represent the episode-specific contents of the memory, in addition to those that act to strategically access and evaluate that content.

A number of studies have recently converged to suggest that specific parietal and frontal regions contribute to processes associated with successful retrieval. Such results were anticipated by a meta-analysis of positron emission tomography (PET) data by Habib and Lepage (1999). In their analysis, they explored five blocked-task studies in which subjects recognized familiar items in contrast to new items. A network of regions, including medial parietal (near the precuneus), left lateral parietal cortex, and left anterior prefrontal cortex near BA 10, was more active for familiar items. Event-related functional magnetic resonance imaging (fMRI) studies have extended these findings. Konishi and colleagues (2000), using a procedure that could separate correctly identified old items (hits) from correct rejections, observed activation in almost the identical network of parietal and frontal regions (see also Henson et al., 2000). Henson and colleagues (1999) explored recognition using a variant of the remember-know paradigm (Tulving, 1985; Gardiner and Richardson-Klavehn, 2000) and also noted similar results. Wheeler and Buckner (2003) noted that activity in these regions tracked performance, being greater for hits than for misses and greater for false alarms than for correct rejections. Among the regions correlating with successful retrieval of past information, left lateral parietal cortex near BA 39/40 has been most consistent, paralleling a similar phenomenon that has been observed in studies using event-related potentials (ERP) (Smith and Guster, 1993; Wilding and Rugg, 1996; for review, see Rugg and Allen, 2000; figure 53.3).

Several additional observations suggest that a region in left posterior parietal cortex participates in both controlled and automatic forms of retrieval, so long as information is recognized as familiar. First, the region responds strongly to hits following study conditions that encourage familiarity-based as well as recollection-based recognition (Vellanova et al., 2003). In addition, the region is similarly responsive to fast and slow recognition decisions if they are sorted post hoc by response time (Donaldson, Petersen, and Buckner, 2001) and can occur spontaneously in situations where explicit retrieval decisions are not required by the task (Koutstaal et al., 2001; Donaldson, Petersen, and Buckner, 2001). McDermott and colleagues (2000) also noted that new combinations of familiar item components elicit activation (in contrast to new items), even when task instructions make recombined items nontargets. Finally, and perhaps most telling, increased activation is observed to

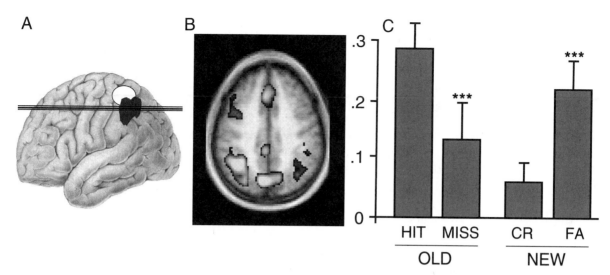

FIGURE 53.3 Left lateral parietal regions correlate with the perception that information is old during recognition. (A) Approximate location of a lateral parietal region that transiently modulates based on successful retrieval. (B) An event-related fMRI activation map of hits versus correction rejections shows a network of modulated regions, including medial and lateral parietal cortex. (Adapted from Konishi et al., 2000.) (C) The magnitude (in percent MR signal change) for retrieval trials, sorted by the history of the item (OLD versus NEW) and by the subject's response (HIT, MISS, CR, and FA). The response is greatest for OLD items reported as old (HIT) and least for NEW items reported as new (CR: correct rejections). Of interest, the response also correlates with memory errors being greater for HIT as compared with MISS responses, and also greater for FA (false alarms) as compared with CR. (Adapted from Wheeler and Buckner, 2003.) (See color plate 26.)

both remember and know decisions (Henson et al., 1999; Wheeler and Buckner, 2004).

Taken collectively, these results suggest a network of regions including left parietal cortex that, in some manner, correlates with the perception or decision that information is old. These regions presumably act in concert with frontal regions that deploy controlled processing resources, depending on the difficulty of the retrieval task. Several open questions persist with regard to neural correlates of retrieval success.

Foremost among these open questions is the relation between the results of imaging studies and findings in patients with damage to left parietal cortex and monkey single-unit physiology which emphasize spatial attention and motor intention. Historically, parietal cortex has not been discussed in terms of contributions to long-term retrieval. The imaging results suggest that contributions of parietal cortex should be reconsidered in the context of potential contributions to the perception that information is old and perhaps to a broader class of decision tasks, of which retrieval decisions are one form. Studies of patients with brain lesions in these regions during retrieval tasks, or other forms of detection task, will likely provide important new information, as will single-unit studies in monkeys that record from parietal cortex during old/new recognition decisions.

Additional open questions concern the generality of the findings and their boundary conditions. One unresolved issue has to do with whether correlates of successful recognition interact with the task context. Although the data provided earlier suggest a role for certain parietal regions in both controlled and automatic forms of retrieval, additional evidence suggests that other parietal regions modulate according to the form of the retrieval task. For example, Dobbins and colleagues (2003) compared a source judgment task with a recency judgment task and found a region in left parietal cortex that modulated by task, independent of whether the judgments were accurate. Source judgments require subjects to make decisions about the specific context encoded with an item, whereas recency judgments merely require subjects to note whether the item is old. Thus, these results suggest participation in processes that are differentially modulated, depending on task. Henson and colleagues (1999; see also Wheeler and Buckner, 2004) noted left lateral parietal regions that responded more to remember than to know decisions; these regions were just adjacent to the parietal region, discussed earlier, that responded strongly to both forms of retrieval decision. These results raise the possibility that either (1) multiple functionally heterogenous regions exist within posterior parietal cortex, with only a subset responding differentially to old information, or (2) interactions between processes associated with retrieval success and the task context contribute.

Domain-specific regions associated with content during remembering

The description of correlates of retrieval success raises the separate question of how the brain represents the episode-specific contents of a memory. There is considerable evidence from a variety of experimental approaches that certain regions of the brain that process incoming (bottom-up) perceptual information are also involved in representing that information during remembering (Farah, 1985; Kosslyn, 1994; Fallgatter, Mueller, and Strick, 1997, among others; see Buckner and Wheeler, 2001; for a recent review). Such an idea is quite old (James, 1890; Hebb, 1968) and shares similarities with the cognitive framework of transfer-appropriate processing, which postulates that memory performance is influenced by the overlap between the specific processes engaged during memory formation and retrieval (Morris, Bransford, and Franks, 1977; Blaxton, 1989; Roediger, Weldon, and Shallice, 1989).

Imaging studies based on both PET and fMRI suggest domain-specific reactivation during the retrieval of content-specific aspects of memories. Several studies in which subjects retrieved visual information showed activity increases in occipital and temporal cortex (e.g., Buckner et al., 1996; D'Esposito et al., 1997; Chen et al., 1998; Goebel et al., 1998; Ishai, Ungerleider, and Haxby, 2000; O'Craven and Kanwisher, 2000), whereas retrieval of auditory information resulted in increased activity in superior and middle temporal cortex (e.g., Halpern and Zatorre, 1999; Nyberg et al., 2000). Recently, Wheeler, Petersen, and Buckner (2000;

replicated in Wheeler and Buckner, 2003) had subjects study a set of picture and sound items extensively over several days, then tested them on a source memory task in which the subjects were asked to vividly recall the items and indicate whether they had been studied as pictures or as sounds. A subset of cortical regions activated during perception of pictures and sounds was reactivated during retrieval of those same forms of information (figure 53.4). A left-lateralized region along the fusiform gyrus was associated with both perception and retrieval of picture information; bilateral superior temporal regions were associated with both perception and retrieval of sounds. This observation generalized to visual objects studied during a single episodic exposure (Wheeler and Buckner, 2003).

An interesting further observation from these studies is that retrieval may selectively recruit high-level sensory regions in an efficient manner. That is, rather than modulating all regions in the sensory hierarchy (e.g., from early striate cortex to inferior temporal regions), reactivation during retrieval appears, under certain circumstances, to selectively modulate high-level sensory areas, depending on the content of the memory. For example, in the studies conducted by Wheeler and colleagues (2000, 2003), subjects retrieved visual objects in the service of a source retrieval task. Early visual areas near striate cortex did not modulate activity, while late visual

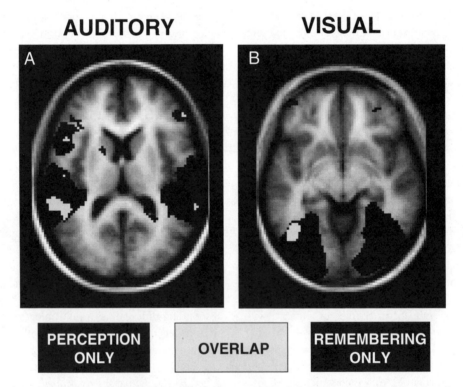

FIGURE 53.4   Late sensory regions reactivate during retrieval of sensory-specific information. (*A, B*) Regions active during the *perception* of auditory (*A*) and visual (*B*) information, superimposed on regions active during the *retrieval* of auditory and visual information. Bilateral temporal cortex is active during the perception of auditory information, with a subset of auditory regions reactivating during retrieval. Similar reactivation occurs in visual regions, again in late as opposed to early areas. (Adapted from Wheeler, Petersen, and Buckner, 2000.) (See color plate 27.)

regions showed robust modulation. The modulated visual regions were likely homologous to inferotemporal areas in monkeys that respond to object-level attributes and also to paired-associate learning (Sakai and Miyashita, 1991; Messinger et al., 2001). Thus, reactivation during remembering may rely on a top-down cascade of neural activity that includes sensory areas that process relatively high-level perceptual attributes while sparing early areas that process primitive attributes. Such a retrieval process is both elegant and efficient (see Hebb, 1968; Roland and Gulyas, 1994; Buckner and Wheeler, 2001, for similar discussion).

False memories reveal the constructive nature of remembering

We have examined some of the brain networks that allow people to retrieve prior experiences and thereby revisit and relive their personal pasts. Despite these impressive abilities, memory retrieval is far from perfect: people often forget and distort the past. Schacter (1999, 2001) has proposed that memory's imperfections can be divided into seven basic categories or "sins." Three of the seven sins involve different forms of forgetting (transience, absent-mindedness, and blocking), and one involves intrusive memories of traumatic events (persistence). Most pertinent to the present concerns, three of the sins concern distortions of past experiences, or "false memories": misattribution, suggestibility, and bias. *Misattribution* occurs when retrieved information is assigned to the wrong source (e.g., mistaking a previously imagined event for a real one). *Suggestibility* refers to the tendency to incorporate inaccurate information from external sources, such as misleading questions, into personal recollections. *Bias* involves the distorting influences of present knowledge, beliefs, and feelings on recollection of previous experience. All three of these memory sins provide potentially useful insights into the constructive nature of episodic retrieval processes because they reveal the various ways in which we piece together bits of information to form a coherent narrative about the past. Cognitive evidence concerning all three sins of commission is abundant and has been reviewed elsewhere (Schacter, 1999, 2001). Cognitive neuroscience evidence is so far largely restricted to the sin of misattribution. Here we focus on the misattribution error known as *false recognition*, which occurs when subjects are shown novel items (e.g., words or pictures) and incorrectly claim to have encountered them earlier in the experiment. False recognition is typically inferred from "old" responses to novel items that are in some way related to previously studied items, that is, false alarms above and beyond the "baseline" level of false alarms to unrelated novel items (cf. Underwood, 1965; Roediger and McDermott, 1995).

Roediger and McDermott (1995) provide an especially striking and influential demonstration of robust false recognition. They modified and extended a procedure developed initially by Deese (1959) in which subjects hear lists of associated words (e.g., *candy, sour, sugar, bitter, good, taste, tooth,* etc.) that all converge on a nonpresented "theme word" or false target (e.g., *sweet*). Roediger and McDermott reported exceptionally high levels of false recognition (e.g., 80%) to the theme words. The level of false recognition responses was indistinguishable from the hit rate to studied items, and false recognitions were accompanied by high confidence and a sense of detailed recollection. Numerous subsequent studies using the DRM (Deese, Roediger, McDermott) paradigm have delineated a variety of behavioral and cognitive properties of this powerful false recognition effect (e.g., Mather, Henkel, and Johnson, 1997; Norman and Schacter, 1997; Robinson and Roediger, 1997; Schacter, Israel, and Racine, 1999; Blair, Lenton, and Hastie, 2001; Gallo, Roediger, and McDermott, 2001; Brainerd et al., 2003; Neuschatz, Benoit, and Payne, 2003). Other behavioral studies have revealed potent false recognition effects using perceptually related nonverbal materials (e.g., Koutstaal et al., 1999; cf. Posner and Keele, 1968), and experimental paradigms where the source of repeated items must be recollected in order to respond accurately (e.g., Jennings and Jacoby, 1997; Schnider and Ptak, 1999; Dodson & Schacter, 2002).

Cognitive neuroscience evidence concerning such potent forms of false recognition comes from neuropsychological studies of brain-damaged patients and from brain imaging studies using fMRI, PET, and ERP methods. Of interest, the sources of misattribution align well with observations discussed in the earlier sections on veridical memory retrieval.

Amnesia and dementia influence false recognition. Neuropsychological evidence concerning the basis of robust false recognition has been provided by studies of amnesic patients as well as patients with dementia of the Alzheimer's type (DAT). Using the DRM semantic associates procedure, Schacter, Verfaellie, and Pradere (1996) found that amnesic patients with damage to either medial temporal (i.e., anoxia, encephalitis) or diencephalic (i.e., patients with Korsakoff's syndrome) regions produced fewer hits to studied items and more false alarms to unrelated lure words than did control subjects. Despite making more false alarms in response to the presentation of unrelated lures, amnesic patients produced significantly fewer false alarms in response to semantically related lure words; that is, they showed a smaller false recognition effect than did controls (see also Schacter et al., 1998; Melo, Winocur, and Moscovitch, 1999).

These findings extend to the domain of perceptual false recognition: after studying lists of perceptually related words (e.g., *lake, fake, sake*), amnesic patients committed fewer false recognition errors in response to the presentation of perceptually related lure words (e.g., *rake*) than did controls (Schacter, Verfaellie, and Anes, 1997). Koutstaal and colleagues (1999) examined false recognition of abstract visual patterns in amnesic patients, using a prototype recognition procedure that is similar in some respects to the paradigms used in the category learning experiments described earlier. Koutstaal and colleagues found robust false recognition of prototypes in control subjects and significantly reduced false recognition of prototypes in amnesic patients. Parallel results have been obtained in studies of patients with DAT, in whom severe episodic memory impairment is primarily attributable, at least in the early stages of DAT, to medial temporal lobe dysfunction, with results revealing reduced levels of robust false recognition—conceptual and perceptual—in DAT patients compared with nondemented older adults (Balota et al., 1999; Budson et al., 2000, 2001, 2003).

The overall pattern of results from the foregoing studies indicates that the medial temporal/diencephalic regions that are damaged in amnesic patients, and that have long been linked to veridical recognition, are also involved in false recognition. Specifically, it has been proposed (Schacter, Verfaellie, and Pradere, 1996; Schacter, Verfaellie, et al., 1998) that medial temporal areas are involved in the encoding and/or retrieval of semantic and perceptual gist (Brainerd, Reyna, and Kneer, 1995) or global similarity (Hintzman and Curran, 1994) information that supports robust false recognition. Amnesia and DAT typically reduce false recognition by impairing this proposed mechanism. However, the false recognition rate of amnesic and DAT patients can exceed that of control subjects when repeating study list items increases control subjects' episodic memory for previously studied words, thus allowing them, but not the patients, to suppress false recognition responses (Schacter et al., 1998; Budson et al., 2000).

Over the past several years, Schnider and colleagues have developed a different approach to studying false recognition in amnesic patients. In their continuous recognition paradigm, participants view a series of pictures, some of which are repeated, and are instructed to respond no to new pictures and yes to repeated ones. After the initial run, the same pictures are presented again in a separate run. Subjects are instructed to disregard whether a picture appeared in an earlier run and to respond yes only to picture recurrences within the same run. Schnider and colleagues (Schnider and Ptak, 1999; Schnider, 2001) focused on differences between amnesic patients who produced spontaneous confabulations (i.e., detailed false recollections) and those who did not. The two patients groups showed similar deficits on the first run and responded equally often to old pictures on the second run. However, on the second run, confabulating amnesics showed elevated false recognition of new pictures that had appeared previously in the first run. Elevated false recognition was associated with damage to the anterior limbic structures, including medial orbiotfrontal cortex, basal forebrain,

and related structures, which are often associated with confabulation (Schnider, 2001). In the Schnider paradigm, false recognition reflects a failure of source memory (cf. Schacter, Harbluk, and McLachlan, 1984; Shimamura and Squire, 1987) rather than a tendency to respond on the basis of semantic or perceptual gist information.

False recognition is increased in patients with frontal damage. Several case studies have shown dramatic increases of false recognition in patients with lesions of various regions within the frontal lobes. For instance, Parkin and colleagues (1996) reported elevated false recognition in a patient who had sustained a ruptured anterior communicating artery aneurysm that produced left frontal lobe atrophy. False recognition of nonpresented materials was accompanied by high confidence but was nearly eliminated when lure items were perceptually dissimilar to studied items. Subsequent research with this same patient (Parkin et al., 1999) suggested that J.B.'s problems resulted from a poorly focused retrieval description to guide memory search (Burgess and Shallice, 1996; Schacter, Norman, and Koutstaal, 1998). The poorly focused retrieval description, in turn, was attributed to encoding deficits that resulted in generic representations of target items that lack specific details.

In a case study similar to the foregoing reports, Schacter and Curran and their colleagues found extremely high levels of false recognition of words, nonsense syllables, pictures, and sounds in a patient (B.G.) who had suffered an infarction of the right frontal lobe (Schacter, Curran, et al., 1996; Curran et al., 1997; figure 53.5). As with J.B., however, false recognition in B.G. was reduced when lure items did not share the general features of studied items. Thus, for example, after studying pictures of animate objects from various categories, B.G. produced frequent false alarms to novel pictures from studied categories, but virtually never produced false alarms to pictures of animals (Schacter, Curran, et al., 1996). Subsequent experiments showed that false recognition in B.G. could also be reduced by requiring him to make encoding judgments that resulted in detailed recollections of studied items (Curran et al., 1997). The overall pattern of results suggests that when making recognition judgments, B.G. (like J.B.) relied excessively on general similarities between study and test items, probably reflecting retrieval monitoring deficits combined with some encoding problems.

Rapcsak and colleagues (1999) provided evidence for strategic retrieval deficits in studies that examined false recognition of faces in patients with frontal lobe damage. Previous studies by Rapcsak's group had demonstrated that patients with various types of frontal lobe lesions are prone to high levels of false recognition of unfamiliar faces (e.g., Rapcsak et al., 1996). The experiments by Rapcsak and colleagues (1999) indicated that frontal patients do not engage

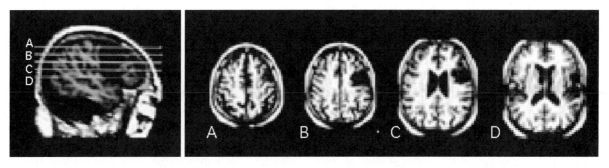

FIGURE 53.5 Lesion localization for patient B.G. in parasagittal and axial (horizontal) planes as revealed by MRI. The entire precentral gyrus is affected, as seen in the parasagittal view. The superior-inferior and lateral-medial extents of this lesion can be appreciated in a series of axial sections that proceed from superior to inferior (levels A–D). These images are derived from a T1-weighted structural image. Right is on the right. (See color plate 28.)

in strategic or effortful retrieval monitoring operations that are needed to check or oppose recognition decisions based on a general sense of familiarity with a face, which are sometimes triggered by the automatic activation of structural information that matches that of previously encountered faces. When patients were specifically instructed to use stricter decision criteria that produced more careful retrieval monitoring, false recognition of faces was greatly reduced, and no longer differed from that of control subjects. Ward and collaborators have documented a similar type of false facial familiarity in a detailed case study of a patient, M.R., whose recognition problems were associated with damage to the left frontal lobe (Ward et al., 1999; Ward and Jones, 2003). These results suggest that controlled processing resources supported by frontal cortex, when absent, lead to retrieval misattributions and errors.

Imaging studies suggest similarities and differences between true and false recognition. A number of studies have examined different types of false recognition with neuroimaging techniques. Several studies have examined the DRM semantic associates paradigm. Early studies using PET (Schacter, Reiman, et al., 1996), fMRI (Schacter et al., 1997), and ERP (Düzel et al., 1997; Johnson et al., 1997) support the general conclusion that the same or similar patterns of brain activity are observed during true and false recognition, with small differences occurring under restricted experimental conditions. More specifically, differences between true and false recognition were initially reported when true and false target were tested in separate blocks, with PET data indicating greater activation in the left superior temporal gyrus during true than during false recognition and trends toward more anterior prefrontal regions during false than during true recognition (Schacter, Reiman, et al., 1996), fMRI data suggesting greater right anterior frontal activity during false than during true recognition (Schacter, Buckner, et al., 1997), and ERP data indicating differences between true and false recognition in frontal and left temporoparietal electrode sites (Johnson et al., 1997). However, when true and false targets

were randomly intermixed during recognition testing, as can be done with ERPs and event-related fMRI, it was difficult to detect differences in brain activity underlying true and false recognition (Düzel et al., 1997; Johnson et al., 1997; Schacter et al., 1997). A preliminary interpretation is that, under typical conditions, the neural events that support veridical memory are largely similar and potentially causal in eliciting false memories. Blocked-task paradigms may allow distinct retrieval modes to be adopted. Conclusions from these early studies, however, have been added to by more recent work that suggests retrieved content can differ between true and veridical memories.

Cabeza and colleagues (2001), for example, noted that differences between true and false recognition can be increased when perceptual processing of target materials is increased during encoding (e.g., Schacter, Israel, and Racine, 1999). To promote perceptual encoding, Cabeza and colleagues instructed subjects (prior to scanning) to try to remember lists of semantic associates, and also to try to remember the source (a man or a woman) who presented the word lists; half the lists were presented (on videotape) by a man and half were presented by a woman. The general idea was that, during subsequent retrieval, previously studied words, but not semantically associated false targets, would activate regions initially involved in encoding perceptual (i.e., source) information, whereas regions involved in the encoding and retrieval of semantic information would show comparable activation during the two forms of recognition. The major finding of the study was a dissociation between two regions within the medial temporal lobe: parahippocampal gyrus, which showed greater activation during true than during false recognition, and hippocampus, which showed significant activation during both true and false recognition. The true > false parahippocampal activation (obtained under test conditions in which item types were randomly intermixed) suggests recovery of sensory-perceptual information, whereas the true = false hippocampal activation suggests recovery of semantic information (both findings are consistent with a number of other imaging findings discussed by

Cabeza and colleagues, 2001). Further, the finding of hippocampal activation during both true and false recognition of semantic associates converges with the previously mentioned findings of false recognition "deficits" in amnesic patients with medial temporal lobe damage.

Further neuroimaging evidence suggesting a role for recovery of sensory-perceptual information during true but not false recognition comes from a more recent event-related fMRI study by Slotnick and Schacter (in press). Subjects in this experiment studied abstract visual shapes that were all related to a nonpresented prototype and later made old/new recognition decisions about previously studied shapes, nonstudied prototypes, and new unrelated shapes. Behavioral data revealed significantly more "old" responses to studied shapes than nonstudied prototypes, which in turn were associated with more "old" responses than nonstudied unrelated shapes. Imaging analyses revealed greater activation for studied shapes than nonstudied prototypes in regions of extrastriate visual cortex, suggesting reactivation of encoded features of the studied visual shapes, paralleling the results suggested by the studies of veridical source retrieval discussed earlier (cf. Nyberg et al., 2000; Wheeler, Petersen, and Buckner, 2000; Wheeler and Buckner, 2003).

A number of studies have provided evidence for a possible role of frontally mediated control processes during true/false recognition decisions. Cabeza and colleagues (2001) reported greater activation in right ventromedial prefrontal cortex during false than true recognition, which they tentatively attributed to the engagement of verification or monitoring processes that are particularly demanding when subjects attempt to make old/new decisions about related lure items that elicit a powerful recollective experience but reduced recovery of sensory details (see also Schacter, Reiman, et al., 1996; Schacter et al., 1997). In a PET study, Treyer, Buck, and Schnider (2003) examined brain activation during the Schnider source discrimination paradigm discussed earlier, in which subjects must recollect whether test items appeared in the current run or a previous one, and found evidence for activation of a left orbitofrontal region under task conditions that required this difficult source discrimination to avoid false recognition (for related evidence, see Dobbins et al., 2002, 2003). Finally, in an ERP study of the DRM semantic associates procedure, Curran and colleagues (2001) performed a median split to compare high-performing subjects, who discriminated well between true and false items, with low-performing subjects, who did not. The high-performing subjects were characterized by more positive late right frontal ERPs than were low-performing subjects, perhaps reflecting retrieval monitoring operations that were more likely to be engaged by high- than low-performing subjects (see also Goldmann et al., in press).

Finally, although most imaging studies of false recognition have focused on retrieval processes, some studies have begun to explore the encoding origins of false recognition and related memory misattributions. For instance, Gonsalves and Paller (2000) recorded ERPs while subjects viewed pictures of common objects or generated images of objects. On a later source monitoring test, posterior ERPs at encoding were more positive when subjects falsely recognized pictures that they had only imagined, perhaps reflecting more vivid visual imagery at encoding for items later subject to misattribution. In an event-related fMRI study, Mitchell, Dodson, and Schacter (2003) examined a misattribution known as the illusion of truth, in which exposure to a statement increases subsequent confidence that the statement is true, even when people are cued that the statement is false. Subjects appear to misattribute familiarity with a previously exposed statement to increased truth value, but the illusion of truth can be reduced when subjects specifically recollect that a statement was cued false (Begg, Anas, and Farinacci, 1992). Mitchell and colleagues found that regions whose activation during encoding is associated with successful recollection—hippocampus and left inferior prefrontal gyrus—showed greater activation during encoding when subjects were able to later avoid the illusory truth effect than when they could not.

Conclusions

The present chapter summarizes results suggesting that the component processes involved in retrieval are cobbled together to allow information to be flexibly retrieved from the past. Studies of patients with frontal lesions have long supported a role for frontal cortex in strategic aspects of memory. Neuroimaging studies have recently provided insights into the anatomic specificity of frontal contributions to retrieval and have also suggested constraints on the nature of the contributions. Providing distinct contributions to retrieval, posterior regions, including (surprisingly) regions in left parietal cortex, appear to participate in some manner with the successful retrieval of information. Regions within sensory-processing hierarchies reactivate in support of content during remembering.

Reflecting the constructive nature of memory retrieval, these component processes do not always converge on a perfectly accurate representation during acts of remembering, resulting in misattributions, or false memories. Patients with damage to the medial temporal lobe and patients with frontal damage are particularly susceptible to such memory errors. Nonetheless, all of us are vulnerable to memory's sins, and benefit greatly from its successes.

ACKNOWLEDGMENTS This work was supported by the Howard Hughes Medical Institute (R.L.B), the James S. McDonnell Foundation (R.L.B.), and grants NIMH MH57506 (R.L.B.), NIA AG08441 (D.L.S.), and NIMH MH060951 (D.L.S.).

REFERENCES

BALOTA, D. A., M. J. CORTESE, J. M. DUCHEK, D. ADAMS, H. L. ROEDIGER III, K. B. MCDERMOTT, and B. E. YERYS, 1999. Veridical and false memory in healthy older adults and in dementia of the Alzheimer's type. *Cogn. Neuropsychol.* 16:361–384.

BARTLETT, F. C., 1932. *Remembering: A Study in Experimental and Social Psychology.* New York: Macmillan.

BEGG, I. M., A. ANAS, and S. FARINACCI, 1992. Dissociation of processes in belief: Source recollection, statement familiarity, and the illusion of truth. *J. Exp. Psychol. Gen.* 121:446–458.

BLAIR, I. V., A. P. LENTON, and R. HASTIE, 2002. The reliability of the DRM paradigm as a measure of individual differences in false memories. *Psychonom. Bull. Rev.* 9:590–596.

BLAXTON, T. A., 1989. Investigating dissociations among memory measures: Support for a transfer-appropriate processing framework. *J. Exp. Psychol. Learn. Mem. Cogn.* 15:657–668.

BRAINERD, C. J., D. G. PAYNE, R. WRIGHT, and V. F. REYNA, 2003. Phantom recall. *J. Mem. Lang.* 48:445–467.

BRAINERD, C. J., V. F. REYNA, and R. KNEER, 1995. False recognition reversal: When similarity is distinctive. *J. Mem. Lang.* 34:157–185.

BUCKNER, R. L., 1996. Beyond HERA: Contributions of specific prefrontal brain areas to long-term memory retrieval. *Psychonom. Bull. Rev.* 3:149–158.

BUCKNER, R. L., 2003. Functional-anatomic correlates of control processes in memory. *J. Neurosci.* 23:3999–4004.

BUCKNER, R. L., S. E. PETERSEN, J. G. OJEMANN, F. M. MEIZEN, L. R. SQUIRE, and M. E. RAICHLE, 1995. Functional anatomical studies of explicit and implicit memory retrieval tasks. *J. Neurosci.* 15:12–29.

BUCKNER, R. L., M. E. RAICHLE, F. M. MEIZEN, and S. E. PETERSEN, 1996. Functional anatomic studies of memory retrieval for auditory words and visual pictures. *J. Neurosci.* 16:6219–6235.

BUCKNER, R. L., and M. E. WHEELER, 2001. The cognitive neuroscience of remembering. *Nat. Rev. Neurosci.* 2:624–634.

BUDSON, A. E., K. R. DAFFNER, R. DESIKAN, and D. L. SCHACTER, 2000. When false recognition is unopposed by true recognition: Gist-based memory distortion in Alzheimer's disease. *Neuropsychology* 14:277–287.

BUDSON, A. E., R. DISIKAN, K. R. DAFFNER, and D. L. SCHACTER, 2001. Perceptual false recognition in Alzheimer's disease. *Neuropsychology* 15:230–243.

BUDSON, A. E., A. L. SULLIVAN, K. R. DAFFNER, and D. L. SCHACTER, 2003. Semantic versus phonological false recognition in aging and Alzheimer's disease. *Brain Cogn.* 51:251–261.

BURGESS, P. W., and T. SHALLICE, 1996. Confabulation and the control of recollection. *Memory* 4:359–411.

CABEZA, R., J. K. LOCANTORE, and N. D. ANDERSON, 2003. Lateralization of prefrontal activity during episodic memory retrieval: Evidence for the production-monitoring hypothesis. *J. Cogn. Neurosci.* 15:249–259.

CABEZA, R., and L. NYBERG, 2000. Imaging cognition. II: An empirical view of 2275 PET and fMRI studies. *J. Cogn. Neurosci.* 12:1–47.

CABEZA, R., S. M. RAO, A. D. WAGNER, A. R. MAYER, and D. L. SCHACTER, 2001. Can medial temporal lobe regions distinguish true from false? An event-related functional MRI study of vertical and illusory recognition memory. *Proc. Natl. Acad. Sci. U.S.A.* 98:4805–4810.

CHEN, W., T. KATO, X. H. ZHU, S. OGAWA, D. W. TANK, and K. UGURBIL, 1998. Human primary visual cortex and lateral geniculate nucleus activation during visual imagery. *Neuroreport* 9:3669–3674.

CORKIN, S., 1984. Lasting consequences of bilateral medial temporal lobectomy: Clinical course and experimental findings in H.M. *Semin. Neurol.* 4:249–259.

CURRAN, T., D. L. SCHACTER, M. K. JOHNSON, and R. SPINKS, 2001. Brain potentials reflect behavioral differences in true and false recognition. *J. Cogn. Neurosci.* 13:201–216.

CURRAN, T., D. L. SCHACTER, K. A. NORMAN, and L. GALLUCCIO, 1997. False recognition after a right frontal lobe infarction: Memory for general and specific information. *Neuropsychologia* 35:1035–1049.

DEESE, J., 1959. On the prediction of occurrence of particular verbal intrusions in immediate recall. *J. Exp. Psychol.* 58:17–22.

DEMB, J. B., J. E. DESMOND, A. D. WAGNER, C. J. VAIDYA, G. H. GLOVER, and J. D. E. GABRIELI, 1995. Semantic encoding and retrieval in the left inferior prefrontal cortex: A functional MRI study of task difficulty and process specificity. *J. Neurosci.* 15: 5870–5878.

DESGRANGES, B., J. C. BARON, and F. EUSTACHE, 1998. The functional neuroanatomy of episodic memory: The role of the frontal lobes, the hippocampal formation, and other areas. *Neuroimage* 8:198–213.

D'ESPOSITO, M., J. A. DETRE, G. K. AGUIRRE, M. STALLCUP, D. C. ALSOP, L. J. TIPPET, and M. J. FARAH, 1997. A functional MRI study of mental image generation. *Neuropsychologia* 35:725–730.

DOBBINS, I. G., H. FOLEY, D. L. SCHACTER, and A. D. WAGNER, 2002. Executive control during episodic retrieval: Multiple prefrontal processes subserve source memory. *Neuron* 35:989–996.

DOBBINS, I. G., H. J. RICE, A. D. WAGNER, and D. L. SCHACTER, 2003. Memory orientation and success: Separable neurocognitive components underlying episodic recognition. *Neuropsychologia* 41:318–333.

DODSON, C. S., and D. L. SCHACTER, 2002. Aging and strategic retrieval processes: Reducing false memories with a distinctiveness heuristic. *Psychol. Aging* 17:405–415.

DONALDSON, D. I., and R. L. BUCKNER, 2002. Effective paradigm design. In *Functional MRI: An Introduction to Methods*, P. Jezzard, P. M. Matthews, and S. M. Smith, eds. London: Oxford University Press, pp. 177–195.

DONALDSON, D. I., S. E. PETERSEN, and R. L. BUCKNER, 2001. Dissociating memory retrieval processes using fMRI: Evidence that priming does not support recognition memory. *Neuron* 31:1047–1059.

DONALDSON, D. I., S. E. PETERSEN, J. M. OLLINGER, and R. L. BUCKNER, 2001. Dissociating state and item components of recognition memory using fMRI. *NeuroImage* 13:129–142.

DUNCAN, J., 2001. An adaptive coding model of neural function in prefrontal cortex. *Nat. Rev. Neurosci.* 2:820–829.

DÜZEL, E., R. CABEZA, T. W. PICTON, A. P. YONELINAS, H. SCHEICH, H. J. HEINZE, and E. TULVING, 1999. Task-related and item-related brain processes of memory retrieval. *Proc. Natl. Acad. Sci. U.S.A.* 96:1794–1799.

DÜZEL, E., A. P. YONELINAS, G. R. MANGUN, H. J. HEINZE, and E. TULVING, 1997. Event-related brain potential correlates of two states of conscious awareness in memory. *Proc. Natl. Acad. Sci. U.S.A.* 94:5973–5978.

EICHENBAUM, H., and N. COHEN, 2001. *From Conditioning to Conscious Recollection: Memory Systems of the Brain.* New York: Oxford University Press.

FALLGATTER, A. J., T. J. MUELLER, and W. K. STRICK, 1997. Neurophysiological correlates of mental imagery in different sensory modalities. *Int. J. Psychophysiol.* 25:145–153.

FARAH, M. J., 1985. Psychophysical evidence for a shared representational medium for mental images and percepts. *J. Exp. Psychol. Gen.* 114:91–103.

FLETCHER, P. C., C. D. FRITH, P. M. GRASBY, T. SHALLICE, R. S. FRACKOWIAK, and R. J. DOLAN, 1995. Brain systems for encoding and retrieval of auditory-verbal memory: An in vivo study in humans. *Brain* 118:401–416.

FLETCHER, P. C., and R. N. HENSON, 2001. Frontal lobes and human memory: Insights from functional neuroimaging. *Brain* 124:849–881.

FLETCHER, P. C., T. SHALLICE, and R. J. DOLAN, 2000. "Sculpting the response space": An account of left prefrontal activation at encoding. *NeuroImage* 12:404–417.

GALLO, D. A., H. L. ROEDIGER III, and K. B. MCDERMOTT, 2001. Associative false recognition occurs without strategic criterion shifts. *Psychonom. Bull. Rev.* 8:579–586.

GARDINER, J. M., and A. RICHARDSON-KLAVEHN, 2000. Remembering and knowing. In *The Oxford Handbook of Memory*, E. Tulving and F. I. M. Craik, eds. New York: Oxford University Press, pp. 229–224.

GERSHBERG, F. B., and A. P. SHIMAMURA, 1995. Impaired use of organizational strategies in free recall following frontal lobe damage. *Neuropsychologia* 33:1305–1333.

GOEBEL, R., D. KHORRAM-SEFAT, L. MUCKLI, H. HACKER, and W. SINGER, 1998. The constructive nature of vision: Direct evidence from functional magnetic resonance imaging studies of apparent motion and motion imagery. *Eur. J. Neurosci.* 10:1563–1573.

GOLD, B., and R. L. BUCKNER, 2002. Common prefrontal regions coactivate with dissociable posterior regions during controlled semantic and phonological tasks. *Neuron* 35:803–812.

GOLDMANN, R. E., A. L. SULLIVAN, D. J. DROLLER, M. D. RUGG, T. CURRAN, T., P. J. HOLCOMB, D. L. SCHACTER, K. R. DAFFNER, and A. E. BUDSON, 2003. Late frontal brain potentials distinguish true and false recognition. *Neuroreport.*

GOLDMAN-RAKIC, P. S., 1987. Circuitry of primate prefrontal cortex and regulation of behavior by representational memory. In *The Handbook of Physiology:* Sect. 1, *The Nervous System*, vol. V, *Higher Functions of the Brain*, F. Plum and V. Mountcastle, eds. Bethesda, Md.: American Physiological Society, pp. 373–417.

GONSALVES, B., and K. PALLER, 2000. Neural events that underlie remembering something that never happened. *Nat. Neurosci.* 3:1316–1321.

HABIB, R., and M. LEPAGE, 1999. Novelty assessment in the brain. In *Memory, Consciousness, and the Brain*, E. Tulving, ed. Philadelphia: Psychology Press, pp. 265–277.

HALPERN, A. R., and R. J. ZATORRE, 1999. When that tune runs through your head: A PET investigation of auditory imagery for familiar melodies. *Cereb. Cortex* 9:697–704.

HEBB, D. O., 1968. Concerning imagery. *Pyschol. Rev.* 75:466–477.

HENSON, R. N., M. D. RUGG, T. SHALLICE, O. JOSEPHS, and R. J. DOLAN, 1999. Recollection and familiarity in recognition memory: An event-related functional magnetic resonance imaging study. *J. Neurosci.* 19:3962–3972.

HENSON, R. N., M. D. RUGG, T. SHALLICE, and R. J. DOLAN, 2000. Confidence in recognition memory for words: Dissociating right prefrontal roles in episodic retrieval. *J. Cogn. Neurosci.* 12:913–923.

HINTZMAN, D. L., and T. CURRAN, 1994. Retrieval dynamics of recognition and frequency judgments: Evidence for separate processes of familiarity and recall. *J. Mem. Lang.* 33:1–18.

ISHAI, A., L. G. UNGERLEIDER, and J. V. HAXBY, 2000. Distributed neural systems for the generation of visual images. *Neuron* 28:979–990.

JACOBY, L. L., 1991. A process dissociation framework: Separating automatic from intentional uses of memory. *J. Mem. Lang.* 30:513–541.

JAMES, W., 1890. *The Principles of Psychology.* New York: Henry Holt.

JENNINGS, J. M., and L. L. JACOBY, 1997. An opposition procedure for detecting age-related deficits in recollection: Telling effects of repetition. *Psychol. Aging* 12:352–361.

JOHNSON, M. K., S. F. NOLDE, M. MATHER, J. KOUNIOS, D. L. SCHACTER, and T. CURRAN, 1997. Test format can affect the similarity of brain activity associated with true and false recognition memory. *Psychol. Sci.* 8:250–257.

KONISHI, S., I. UCHIDA, T. OKUAKI, T. MACHIDA, I. SHIROUZU, and Y. MIYASHITA, 2002. Neural correlates of recency judgement. *J. Neurosci.* 22:9549–9555.

KONISHI, S., M. E. WHEELER, D. I. DONALDSON, and R. L. BUCKNER, 2000. Neural correlates of episodic retrieval success. *NeuroImage* 12:276–286.

KOSSLYN, S. M., 1994. *Image and Brain: The Resolution of the Imagery Debate*, Cambridge, Mass.: MIT Press.

KOUTSTAAL, W., D. L. SCHACTER, M. VERFAELLIE, C. J. BRENNER, and E. M. JACKSON, 1999. Perceptually based false recognition of novel objects in amnesics: Effects of category size and similarity to category prototypes. *Cogn. Neuropsychol.* 16:317–342.

KOUTSTAAL, W., A. D. WAGNER, M. ROTTE, A. MARIL, R. L. BUCKNER, and D. L. SCHACTER, 2001. Perceptual specificity in visual object priming: Functional magnetic resonance imaging evidence for a laterality difference in fusiform cortex. *Neuropsychologia* 39:184–199.

MANDLER, G., 1980. Recognizing: The judgment of previous occurrence. *Psychol. Rev.* 87:252–271.

MATHER, M., L. A. HENKEL, and M. K. JOHNSON, 1997. Evaluating characteristics of false memories: Remember/know judgments and memory characteristics questionnaire compared. *Mem. Cogn.* 25:826–837.

MCDERMOTT, K. B., 1997. Priming on perceptual implicit memory test can be achieved through presentation of associates. *Psychonom. Bull. Rev.* 4:582–586.

MCDERMOTT, K. B., R. L. BUCKNER, S. E. PETERSEN, W. M. KELLEY, and A. L. SANDERS, 1999. Set- and code-specific activation in the frontal cortex: An fMRI study of encoding and retrieval of faces and words. *J. Cogn. Neurosci.* 11:631–640.

MCDERMOTT, K. B., T. C. JONES, S. E. PETERSEN, S. K. LAGEMAN, and H. L. ROEDIGER III, 2000. Retrieval success is accompanied by enhanced activation in anterior prefrontal cortex during recognition memory: An event-related fMRI study. *J. Cogn. Neurosci.* 12:965–976.

MELO, B., G. WINOCUR, and M. MOSCOVITCH, 1999. False recall and false recognition: An examination of the effects of selective and combined lesions to the medial temporal lobe/diencephalon and frontal lobe structures. *Cogn. Neupsychol.* 16:343–359.

MESSINGER, A., L. R. SQUIRE, S. M. ZOLA, and T. D. ALBRIGHT, 2001. Neuronal representations of stimulus associations develop in the temporal lobe during learning. *Proc. Natl. Acad. Sci. U.S.A.* 98:12239–12244.

MESULAM, M.-M., 2002. The human frontal lobes: Transcending the default mode through contingent encoding. In *Principles of Frontal Lobe Function*, D. T. Stuss and R. T. Knight, eds. New York: Oxford University Press, pp. 8–31.

MILLER, E. K., 2000. The prefrontal cortex and cognitive control. *Nat. Rev. Neurosci.* 1:59–65.

MILNER, B., P. CORSI, and G. LEONARD, 1991. Frontal-lobe contribution to recency judgements. *Neuropsychologica.* 29:601–618.

MITCHELL, J. P., C. S. DODSON, and D. L. SCHACTER, 2003. Counteracting misattribution: An event-related fMRI study of illusory truth.

MORRIS, C. D., J. P. BRANSFORD, and J. J. FRANKS, 1977. Levels of processing versus transfer appropriate processing. *J. Verb. Learn. Verb. Behav.* 16:519–533.

MOSCOVITCH, M., 1989. Confabulation and the frontal systems: Strategic versus associated retrieval in neuropsychological theories of memory. In *Varieties of Memory and Consciousness: Essays in Honour of Endel Tulving*, H. L. Roediger III and F. I. M. Craik, eds. Hillsdale, N.J.: Erlbaum, pp. 133–155.

NEUSCHATZ, J. S., G. E. BENOIT, and D. G. PAYNE, 2003. Effective warnings in the Deese-Roediger-McDermott false-memory paradigm: The role of identifiability. *J. Exp. Psychol. Learn. Mem. Cogn.* 29:35–41.

NOLDE, S. F., M. K. JOHNSON, and M. D'ESPOSITO, 1998. Left prefrontal activation during episodic remembering: An event-related fMRI study. *Neuroreport* 15:3509–3514.

NORMAN, K. A., and D. L. SCHACTER, 1997. False recognition in young and older adults: Exploring the characteristics of illusory memories. *Mem. Cogn.* 25:838–848.

NYBERG, L., R. HABIB, A. R. MCINTOSH, and E. TULVING, 2000. Reactivation of encoding-related brain activity during memory retrieval. *Proc. Natl. Acad. Sci. U.S.A.* 26:11120–11124.

NYBERG, L., E. TULVING, R. HABIB, L. G. NILSSON, S. KAPUR, S. HOULE, R. CABEZA, and A. R. MCINTOSH, 1995. Functional brain maps of retrieval mode and recovery of episodic information. *Neuroreport* 7:249–252.

O'CRAVEN, K. M., and N. KANWISHER, 2000. Mental imagery of faces and places activates corresponding stumulus-specific brain regions. *J. Cogn. Neurosci.* 12:1013–1023.

PARKIN, A. J., C. BINDSCHAEDLER, L. HARSENT, and C. METZLER, 1996. Pathological false alarm rates following damage to the left frontal cortex. *Brain Cogn.* 32:14–27.

PARKIN, A. J., J. WARD, C. BINDSCHAEDLER, E. J. SQUIRES, and G. POWELL, 1999. False recognition following frontal lobe damage: The role of encoding factors. *Cogn. Neuropsychol.* 16:243–265.

PETERSEN, S. E., P. T. FOX, M. I. POSNER, M. MINTUN, and M. E. RAICHLE, 1988. Positron emission tomographic studies of the cortical anatomy of single-word processing. *Nature* 331:585–589.

PETRIDES, M., and D. N. PANDYA, 1994. Comparative architectonic analysis of the human and the macaque frontal cortex. In *Handbook of Neuropsychology*, vol. 9, F. Boller and J. Grafman, eds. Amsterdam: Elsevier, pp. 17–58.

POSNER, M. I., and S. W. KEELE, 1968. On the genesis of abstract ideas. *J. Exp. Psychol.* 77:353–363.

PAYNE, D. G., C. J. ELIE, J. M. BLACKWELL, and J. S. NEUSCHATZ, 1996. Memory illusions: Recalling, recognizing, and recollecting events that never occurred. *J. Mem. Lang.* 35:261–285.

RANGANATH, C., M. K. JOHNSON, and M. D'ESPOSITO, 2000. Left anterior prefrontal activation increases with demands to recall specific perceptual information. *J. Neurosci.* 20:RC108.

RAPCSAK, S. Z., M. R. POLSTER, M. L. GLISKY, and J. F. COMER, 1996. False recognition of unfamiliar faces following right hemisphere damage: Neuropsychological and anatomical observations. *Cortex* 32:593–611.

RAPCSAK, S. Z., S. L. REMINGER, E. L. GLISKY, A. W. KASZNIAK, and J. F. COMER, 1999. Neuropsychological mechanisms of false facial recognition following frontal lobe damage. *Cogn. Neuropsychol.* 16:267–292.

ROBINSON, K. J., and H. L. ROEDIGER III, 1997. Associative processes in false recall and false recognition. *Psychol. Sci.* 8:231–237.

ROEDIGER, H. L., III, and K. B. MCDERMOTT, 1995. Creating false memories: Remembering words not presented in lists. *J. Exp. Psychol. Learn. Mem. Cogn.* 21:803–814.

ROEDIGER, H. L., III, J. M. WATSON, K. B. MCDERMOTT, and D. A. GALLO, 2001. Factors that determine false recall: A multiple regression analysis. *Psychonom. Bull. Rev.* 8:385–407.

ROEDIGER, H. L., III, M. S. WELDON, and B. H. CHALLIS, 1989. Explaining dissociations between implicit and explicit measures of retention: A processing account. In *Varieties of Memory and Consciousness: Essays in Honore of Endel Tulving*, H. L. Roediger III and F. I. M. Craik, eds. Hillsdale, N.J.: Erlbaum, pp. 3–42.

ROLAND, P. E., and B. GULYAS, 1994. Visual imagery and visual representation. *Trends Neurosci.* 17:281–287.

RUGG, M. D., and K. ALLEN, 2000. Event-related potential study of memory. In *The Oxford Handbook of Memory*, E. Tulving and F. I. M. Craik, eds. New York: Oxford University Press, pp. 521–537.

RUGG, M. D., P. C. FLETCHER, C. D. FRITH, R. S. FRACKOWIAK, and R. J. DOLAN, 1996. Differential activation of the prefrontal cortex in successful and unsuccessful memory retrieval. *Brain* 119:2073–2083.

SAKAI, K., and Y. MIYASHITA, 1991. Neural organization for the long-term memory of paired associates. *Nature* 354:152–155.

SCHACTER, D. L., 1999. The seven sins of memory: Insights from psychology and cognitive neuroscience. *Am. Psychol.* 54:182–203.

SCHACTER, D. L., 2001. *The Seven Sins of Memory: How the Mind Forgets and Remembers.* Boston: Houghton Mifflin.

SCHACTER, D. L., N. M. ALPERT, C. R. SAVAGE, S. L. RAUCH, and M. S. ALBERT, 1996. Conscious recollection and the human hippocampal formation: Evidence from positron emission tomography. *Proc. Natl. Acad. Sci. U.S.A.* 93:321–325.

SCHACTER, D. L., R. L. BUCKNER, W. KOUTSTAAL, A. M. DALE, and B. R. ROSEN, 1997. Late onset of anterior prefrontal activity during retrieval of veridical and illusory memories: A single trial fMRI study. *NeuroImage* 6:259–269.

SCHACTER, D. L., T. CURRAN, L. GALLUCCIO, W. MILBERG, and J. BATES, 1996. False recognition and the right frontal lobe: A case study. *Neuropsychologia* 34:793–808.

SCHACTER, D. L., J. L. HARBLUK, and D. R. MCLACHLAN, 1984. Retrieval without recollection: An Experimental analysis of source amnesia. *J. Verb. Learn. Verb. Behav.* 23:593–611.

SCHACTER, D. L., L. ISRAEL, and C. RACINE, 1999. Suppressing false recognition in younger and older adults: The distinctiveness heuristic. *J. Mem. Lang.* 40:1–24.

SCHACTER, D. L., K. A. NORMAN, and W. KOUTSTAAL, 1998. The cognitive neuroscience of constructive memory. *Annu. Rev. Psychol.* 49:289–318.

SCHACTER, D. L., E. REIMAN, T. CURRAN, L. S. YUN, D. BANDY, K. B. MCDERMOTT, and H. L. ROEDIGER III, 1996. Neuroanatomical correlates of veridical and illusory recognition memory: Evidence from positron emission tomography. *Neuron* 17:267–274.

SCHACTER, D. L., M. VERFAELLIE, and M. D. ANES, 1997. Illusory memories in amnesic patients: Conceptual and perceptual false recognition. *Neuropsychology* 11:331–342.

SCHACTER, D. L., M. VERFAELLIE, M. D. ANES, and C. A. RACINE, 1998. When true recognition suppresses false recognition: Evidence from amnesic patients. *J. Cogn. Neurosci.* 10:668–679.

SCHACTER, D. L., M. VERFAELLIE, and D. PRADERE, 1996. The neuropsychology of memory illusions: False recall and recognition in amnesic patients. *J. Mem. Lang.* 35:319–334.

SCHNIDER, A., 2001. Spontaneous confabulation, reality monitoring, and the limbic system: A review. *Brain Res. Rev.* 36:150–160.

SCHNIDER, A., and R. PTAK, 1999. Spontaneous confabulations fail to suppress currently irrelevant memory traces. *Nat. Neurosci.* 2:677–681.

SHALLICE, T., and P. W. BURGESS, 1991. Deficits in strategy application following frontal lobe damage in man. *Brain* 114:727–741.

SHIMAMURA, A. P., and L. R. SQUIRE, 1987. A neuropsychological study of fact memory and source amnesia. *J. Exp. Psychol. Learn. Mem. Cogn.* 13:464–473.

SLOTNICK, S., and D. L. SCHACTER, 2004. A sensory signature that distinguishes true from false memories. *Nat. Neurosci.* 7:664–672.

SMITH, M. E., and K. GUSTER, 1993. Decomposition of recognition memory event-related potentials yields target, repetition, and retrieval effects. *Clin. Neurophysiol.* 86:335–343.

SQUIRE, L. R., 1992. Memory and the hippocampus: A synthesis from findings with rats, monkeys, and humans. *Psychol. Rev.* 99:195–231.

SQUIRE, L. R., J. G. OJEMANN, F. M. MIEZIN, S. E. PETERSEN, T. O. VIDEEN, and M. E. RAICHLE, 1992. Activation of the hippocampus in normal humans: A functional anatomical study of memory. *Proc. Natl. Acad. Sci. U.S.A.* 89:1837–1841.

TALAIRACH, J., and P. TOURNOUX, 1988. *Co-planar Stereotaxic Atlas of the Human Brain.* Stuttgart: Thieme.

THOMPSON-SCHILL, S. L., M. D'ESPOSITO, G. K. AGUIRRE, and M. J. FARAH, 1997. Role of left inferior prefrontal cortex in retrieval of semantic knowledge: A reevaluation. *Proc. Natl. Acad. Sci. U.S.A.* 94:14792–14797.

TREYER, V., A. BUCK, and A. SCHNIDER, 2003. Subcortical loop activation during selection of currently relevant memories. *J. Cogn. Neurosci.* 15:610–618.

TULVING, E., 1985. Memory and consciousness. *Can. Psychol.* 26:1–12.

TULVING, E., S. KAPUR, F. I. CRAIK, M. MOSCOVITCH, and S. HOULE, 1994. Hemispheric encoding/retrieval asymmetry in episodic memory: Positron emission tomography findings. *Proc. Natl. Acad. Sci. U.S.A.* 91:2012–2015.

UNDERWOOD, B. J., 1965. False recognition produced by implicit verbal responses. *J. Exp. Psychol.* 70:122–129.

VELANOVA, K., L. L. JACOBY, M. E. WHEELER, M. P. McAVOY, S. E. PETERSEN, and R. L. BUCKNER, 2003. Functional-anatomic correlates of sustained and transient processing components engaged during controlled retrieval. *J. Neurosci.* 23:8460–8470.

WAGNER, A. D., R. A. POLDRACK, L. L. ELDRIDGE, J. E. DESMOND, G. H. GLOVER, and J. D. E. GABRIELI, 1998. Material-specific lateralization of prefrontal activation during episodic encoding and retrieval. *Neuroreport* 9:3711–3717.

WARD, J., and A. JONES, 2003. Inappropriate association of semantics and context to novel stimuli can give rise to the false recognition of unfamiliar people. *Neuropsychologia* 41:538–549.

WARD, J., A. J. PARKIN, G. POWELL, E. J. SQUIRES, J. TOWNSHEND, and V. BRADLEY, 1999. False recognition of unfamiliar people: "Seeing film stars everywhere." *Cogn. Neuropsychol.* 16:293–315.

WHEELER, M. E., and R. L. BUCKNER, 2003. Functional dissociation among components of remembering: Control, perceived oldness, and content. *J. Neurosci.* 23:3869–3880.

WHEELER, M. E., and R. L. BUCKNER, 2004. *Functional-anatomic correlates of remembering and knowing. NeuroImage* 21:1337–1349.

WHEELER, M. E., S. E. PETERSEN, and R. L. BUCKNER, 2000. Memory's echo: Vivid remembering reactivates sensory-specific cortex. *Proc. Natl. Acad. Sci. U.S.A.* 97:11125–11129.

WILDING, E. L., and M. D. RUGG, 1996. An event-related potential study of recognition memory with and without retrieval of source. *Brain* 119:889–905.

VII LANGUAGE

Introduction

ALFONSO CARAMAZZA

COMPREHENDING or producing even the simplest sentence entails the coordinated functioning of various mechanisms, some dedicated specifically to linguistic processes, others shared by various cognitive tasks. We can consider as an example the production of a simple sentence, such as "He takes the candy from the jar." Even a superficial analysis of the task reveals the complexity of the process and the many mechanisms that must be engaged for its normal functioning. The major components of the process include the following. First, the speaker must formulate the semantic content or intention she wants to communicate. We know very little about this process, but it must be quite complex and must involve cognitive mechanisms distributed across large areas of the left and right hemispheres. Then the formulated intention must be realized in a specific linguistic form for communication. This entails the speaker's computing a sentence structure, selecting lexical items and their grammatical properties (e.g., noun), and establishing their order and specific forms (e.g., number agreement—take versus takes, say). Finally, the phonological representation of the utterance must guide the formulation of articulatory plans for producing speech. These processes all implicate other cognitive mechanisms, such as working memory. For example, if we assume that the selection of words is a serial process, it is clear that the content of the intended meaning the speaker is trying to communicate must be kept active while the speaker is selecting and structuring the lexical items that will convey the intended meaning. Thus, an exploration of language processing necessarily involves the analysis of complex, closely intertwined linguistic and cognitive operations. Because of this, our expectation should be that even the simplest language task, such as word production or comprehension, recruits large areas of the left and right hemispheres.

This prefatory comment is by way of illustrating the daunting task researchers face in trying to uncover the neural basis of language processing, and of asking whether the tools at our disposal are up to the task. The methods available to us include the classic lesion-deficit analysis of aphasic disorders and various neuroimaging techniques that vary in spatial and temporal resolution. Each approach has merits and limitations. But the more general issue is whether these instruments are too blunt to permit the fine-grained analysis that is needed to separate the contribution of the various mechanisms that are recruited even in simple tasks. For example, is it possible to identify the neural correlates of the various stages of processing in lexical access, that is, to distinguish among the retrieval of the semantic, grammatical, morphological, and phonological properties of words? Or are we limited to claims that are no more specific than the broad distinction between meaning and form? To put this point differently, is it possible to have as fine-grained a cognitive neuroscience theory of language as is being developed in the purely cognitive/linguistic domain? This is the challenge facing the cognitive neuroscientist of language.

This issue can be illustrated with an example from the lesion-deficit method (the study of aphasia). Language deficits are almost invariably complex disorders. This is not surprising since chronic language deficits are associated with large left hemisphere lesions, and it is unlikely that such lesions would affect only one processing mechanism. The more likely outcome is that the lesion affects several processing components. This conjecture is supported by the detailed analyses of patients' performance, which invariably reveal the contribution of multiple mechanisms. Furthermore, lesions can vary from patient to patient fairly radically even when their clinical symptoms seem to be quite similar.

Given this clinical reality, it is rather difficult to isolate the functional components implicated in a deficit, and nearly impossible to locate the laboriously identified mechanisms in distinct parts of the brain areas that are damaged. This is not to say that the study of aphasia does not allow meaningful inferences about the nature of language processes. To the contrary, investigations of individual patients can produce deep insights into the structure of linguistic representations and processes (see, e.g., Caramazza and Miceli, 1990). But this requires carrying out very extensive investigations and analyzing performance with many tasks to identify which of the various component processes involved in a language task are causally related to specific features of the observed deficit. Although such studies play an important role in constraining cognitive theories, they reveal little about the brain areas that are crucial for specific aspects of a cognitive process.

The studies that have attempted to locate component processes of language to specific brain regions have not carried out detailed investigations of individual patients but have instead relied on the performance on a single task administered to many patients (see Tranel et al., 2001, for a particularly elegant example of this approach). Although such studies may succeed in establishing correlations between levels of performance on a task and areas of brain damage, they reveal little about the cognitive mechanisms that are causally related to the impaired performance and, in turn, to the identified brain areas.

These limitations of the lesion-deficit method are not specific to this approach but apply also to neuroimaging methods. For example, functional magnetic resonance imaging (fMRI) studies typically report the performance of a group of subjects on a single task. Performance on a language task (say, sentence comprehension) involves many component processes, from the perception of the input to lexical access, to syntactic and semantic analysis, to working memory and other cognitive operations. This makes it difficult if not impossible to relate the individual components implicated in a given process with the patterns of neural activation.

Fortunately, the problems I have discussed here are not theoretical limitations but practical ones that can be overcome as we refine our methods of investigation and develop detailed theories of language processing. There are increasing indications that significant progress is being made in this direction; the chapters in this volume attest to this development.

Two chapters in this section address the processing of lexical forms. Indefrey and Cutler report a meta-analysis of fMRI studies in an attempt to identify common areas of activation that might correspond to auditory language recognition, and more specifically the phonological, lexical, and sentence-level components. They compared their results with electrophysiological, magnetoencelographic, and clinical findings and found that phonological, lexical, and sentence-level components are more clearly differentiated in the left than the right temporal lobe. Hillis and Rapp focus instead on the shared mechanisms involved in reading and writing. Their investigation relied primarily on evidence from the analysis of alexia and agraphia. They found that reading and writing probably share a common orthographic lexicon (our knowledge of the spelling of words). Hillis and Rapp also discuss evidence for the representation of sublexical processes and the graphemic buffer. Ramus also focuses on reading, but from the perspective of reading acquisition and developmental dyslexia. He identifies the primary cause of developmental dyslexia as a phonological deficit that results in impaired phonological awareness. Ramus links this deficit to a dysfunction of temporoparietal brain areas.

The grammatical component of language processing includes two parts: the syntactic operations involved in sentence parsing for comprehension and production, and the grammatical features of words. Friederici reviews PET, fMRI, and ERP studies of sentence comprehension. She argues that the results show a distinction between two types of syntactic processes: local phrase-structure building and syntactic integration. Friederici locates these processes in a neural network consisting of the frontal operculum and BA 44/45, the anterior portion of the STG and the basal ganglia, and the posterior portion of the STG. Shapiro and I investigated the neural representation of the grammatical properties of words. We considered evidence from neuropsychology, electrophysiology, fMRI, and transcranial magnetic stimulation (TMS) and concluded that the left frontal cortex is crucial for the representation of the grammatical and morphological properties of nouns and verbs.

The debate over whether language is acquired through a set of mechanisms dedicated specifically to that task or through a set of general-purpose cognitive mechanisms continues unabated. Mehler, Sebastián-Gallés, and Nespor discuss the biological basis of language and present evidence that the left perisylvian area is sensitive to language well before an infant has had any significant linguistic experience.

They also found that speech contains specific cues that could trigger specialized processing of the input. The evolutionary counterpart of language-as-a-special-faculty is discussed by Fitch. He presents comparative evidence for a species-specific biological component of human language. Fitch identifies three core components of the language faculty, imitation, reference, and recursion, and argues that only recursion is exclusively available to humans.

Although progress in developing a richly articulated cognitive neuroscience theory of language has been slow, we now seem poised to ask more detailed questions, which should lead to more rapid developments. The chapters in this section strongly encourage this optimism.

REFERENCES

MICELI, G., and A. CARAMAZZA, 1990. The structure of graphemic representations. *Cognition.* 37:243–297.

TRANEL, D., R. ADOLPHS, H. DAMASIO, and A. R. DAMASIO, 2001. A neural basis for the retrieval of words for action. *Cogn. Neuropsychol.* 18:655–674.

54 Prelexical and Lexical Processing in Listening

PETER INDEFREY AND ANNE CUTLER

ABSTRACT   This chapter presents a meta-analysis of hemodynamic studies on passive auditory language processing. We assess the overlap of hemodynamic activation areas and activation maxima reported in experiments involving the presentation of sentences, words, pseudowords, or sublexical or nonlinguistic auditory stimuli. Areas that have been reliably replicated are identified. The results of the meta-analysis are compared with electrophysiological, magnetoencephalographic, and clinical findings. We conclude that auditory language input is processed in a left posterior frontal and bilateral temporal cortical network. Within this network, no processing level is related to a single cortical area. The temporal lobes seem to differ with respect to their involvement in postlexical processing, in that the left temporal lobe has greater involvement than the right, and also in the degree of anatomical specialization for phonological, lexical, and sentence-level processing, with greater overlap on the right contrasting with a higher degree of differentiation on the left.

The listener's task in understanding spoken language is to extract meaning from an almost continuous stream of sound. The meaning—the message that speakers wish to convey—is expressed via a sequence of words and the relationships between those words (which can in turn be encoded, depending on the language, in the order in which the words occur, or in inflectional markings of various kinds applied to them). Whole utterance meanings are rarely stored in memory; the beauty of language is the possibility of expressing new meanings via combinations of known words. The words are, however, stored as known units, in some form (again, the form may be language dependent). Understanding spoken language thus requires recognition of the individual words that the speaker has uttered.

Laboratory tasks used to investigate this type of processing over the past four decades fall into two main groups: tasks that require attention to sublexical units and tasks that require attention to words. The first category includes the detection of target phonemes or fragments (e.g., "Press the button when you hear a word containing /b/" or ". . . containing *bot-*"), or the categorization of phonemes ("Does this syllable begin with /d/ or /t/?"). The second category

includes lexical decision ("Is this a real word or not?"), word spotting ("Press the button when you hear any real word in this input"), word reconstruction, mispronunciation detection and phoneme restoration (all tasks that require finding the word that most closely matches a slightly distorted input), and various adaptations or combinations of these (e.g., priming tasks, in which, for instance, a lexical decision on a second word may be affected by a preceding first word), as well as decisions about semantic properties of words ("abstract or concrete?"). All these tasks can involve measurement of response time; further, accuracy rates may also be informative, and in phoneme categorization the nature of the decision is crucial. (For an overview of the tasks, see Grosjean and Frauenfelder, 1997.)

Such research methods have yielded an enormous amount of knowledge that can guide neuroimaging approaches to prelexical and lexical processing in listening. Briefly, research on spoken-word recognition has produced no agreement on the nature of the prelexical representations (if any) involved in listening, but almost unanimous agreement on the following premises: (1) speech information is continuously mapped to the lexicon; (2) speech input can activate multiple candidate words simultaneously, including partial activation of words with partial support from the input; and (3) concurrently active word candidates compete with one another for recognition. Continuity is supported by evidence that coarticulatory information for upcoming phonemes can constrain lexical activation (e.g., Streeter and Nigro, 1979; Whalen, 1991; Marslen-Wilson and Warren, 1994; McQueen, Norris, and Cutler, 1999); multiple activation is supported by evidence that word fragments activate multiple possible completions (e.g., Zwitserlood, 1989; Connine, Blasko, and Wang, 1994; Zwitserlood and Schriefers, 1995; Soto-Faraco, Sebastián-Gallés, and Cutler, 2001) and by evidence of activation of words only spuriously present in the speech input, such as *lips* in *tulips* (Gow and Gordon, 1995; Tabossi, Burani, and Scott, 1995; Vroomen and de Gelder, 1997; Luce and Lyons, 1999); and competition is supported by evidence that the more words are potentially compatible with the input, the more difficult recognition of any one of them becomes (McQueen, Norris, and Cutler, 1994; Norris, McQueen, and Cutler, 1995;

PETER INDEFREY and ANNE CUTLER   Max-Planck Institute for Psycholinguistics, Nijmegen, The Netherlands.

759

Vroomen and de Gelder, 1995; Soto-Faraco, Sebastián-Gallés, and Cutler, 2001). A recent review of the evidence is presented by McQueen, Dahan, and Cutler (2003).

Agreement on the nature of prelexical representations is lacking because there is evidence compatible (1) with a continuous cascade of information through intervening levels at which, for instance, discrete phonemic representations play a role, (2) with alternative abstract representations such as syllables or featural bundles, or (3) with a model involving no intervening representations, where lexical mapping is achieved via computation of similarity to previously encountered acoustic forms.

Of course, behavioral tasks do not tap directly into the necessary processing steps involved in speech recognition; they all involve some decision component, so that observed effects could arise at the decision level rather than at levels normally involved in recognition. Thus, lexical effects in phoneme-level tasks need not imply that the prelexical evaluation of speech signals is directly influenced by lexical knowledge; it could be that explicit decisions about phonemic identity are informed by lexical information (see Norris, McQueen, and Cutler, 2000, for further discussion). It is for this reason necessary, and indeed standard, in behavioral research to seek converging evidence from a wide variety of tasks with differing behavioral profiles, and thanks to this strategy, these tasks have provided a wealth of evidence concerning lexical processing.

Neurophysiological and neuroimaging techniques attempt to achieve an unmediated reflection of processing. In this respect, reliance on the behavioral tasks normally used in spoken-word recognition research introduces potentially serious complications. In a contribution to the second edition of this book, Norris and Wise (2000) pointed out that the problem-solving and decision aspects of the most widely used tasks in this area of cognitive neuroscience, such as phoneme detection, lexical decision, or semantic categorization, may recruit many cognitive subsystems beyond those involved in speech processing, and that observed contrasts may reflect differences in secondary tasks rather than in relevant underlying processes. Giraud and Price (2001) made similar cautionary remarks.

In the present review, therefore, we endeavor to summarize what can be learned about prelexical and lexical processing from neuropsychological, neurophysiological, and neuroimaging studies in the absence of task confounds. To this purpose we assembled all available evidence uncontaminated by potential artifacts due to secondary tasks, as described in a subsequent section. We extended the scope of this evidence beyond studies involving just sublexical and lexical stimuli by including tone stimuli (to assess the involvement of simple auditory processing) and sentence stimuli (to assess the linguistic processing of which prelexical and lexical processing form a part).

Cerebral regions involved in language perception: A meta-analysis

PROCEDURES

Data set We queried the ISI Current Contents and Medline publication databases using the following combination of search terms: (PET *OR* Positron Emission Tomography *OR* fMRI *OR* functional Magnetic Resonance Imaging *OR* MEG *OR* Magnetencephalography *OR* magnetencephalographic) *AND* (auditory *OR* voice *OR* language *OR* sound *OR* speech). This query resulted in a set of 1058 neuroimaging studies using linguistic and nonlinguistic auditory stimuli (December 19, 2002). Based on the abstracts, 463 potentially relevant publications were selected. Among these, 36 publications (marked by an asterisk in the reference list) representing 55 experiments met the following criteria: (1) there was no task other than listening to the auditory stimuli, and (2) the activations were reported in Talairach coordinates or an equivalent coordinate system. In more than half of these experiments (table 54.1), auditory stimuli were compared with a condition in which no acoustic stimuli other than the inevitable background noise of the PET or fMRI scanning procedure were presented (henceforth called the silent control condition). Given this constant control condition, we assumed that activations from similar stimuli should similarly reflect acoustic and linguistic properties of the stimuli. Using a reliability estimate, we assessed the degree of anatomical overlap of activation areas in four experiments presenting sentences, 10 experiments presenting words, four experiments presenting pseudowords or meaningless syllables (monosyllabic pseudowords), and 10 experiments presenting nonlinguistic tone stimuli. It should be noted that a silent rest baseline is not without problems, because some brain regions seem to be activated during such a baseline. Binder and colleagues (1999) examined hemodynamic activations of silent rest compared with a simple perceptual task (listening to tones) and found significant blood flow increases in the left posterior frontal lobe, the left angular gyrus, and the bilateral cingulate gyri. This means that activations of auditory stimuli in these areas may be at least in part obscured when compared with silent rest. Binder and colleagues (1999) report that silent rest does not seem to activate the temporal lobes more strongly than tone stimuli do. Shulman and colleagues (1997) found greater temporal activation in left BA 20 for a silent fixation condition compared with passive viewing of nonlinguistic visual stimuli, but not compared with passive viewing of linguistic stimuli. Thus, although there may be some temporal lobe activation during silent rest, it is too weak to obscure hemodynamic responses during passive listening.

The remaining studies (table 54.2) investigated the neural substrate of specific aspects of the auditory stimuli presented in the active condition in comparison to various auditory

Table 54.1

Passive listening experiments with silent control conditions

Study	Stimulus	No. in Figure 54.2
Belin et al., 1998	200-ms frequency transition, 60/min	1
Belin et al., 1998	40-ms frequency transition, 60/min	2
Belin et al., 1999	Synthetic diphthong, 6/min	3
Binder et al., 2000	Tones, different frequencies, 90/min	4
Bookheimer et al., 1998	Pseudowords, 9/min	5
Celsis et al., 1999	Syllables, 180/min	6
Celsis et al., 1999	Tones, 500 and 700 Hz, 180/min	7
di Salle et al., 2001	Tones, 1000 Hz, 6/min	8
Engelien et al., 1995	Environmental sounds, 10/min	9
Fiez et al., 1996	Pseudowords, 60/min	10
Fiez et al., 1996	Words, 60/min	11
Giraud et al., 2000	Vowels vs. expecting vowels, 120/min	12
Holcomb et al., 1998	Tones, 1500 Hz and lower tones, 30/min	13
Jäncke et al., 1999	Tones, 1000 Hz, 60/min	14
Lockwood et al., 1999	Tones, 500 and 4000 Hz, 60/min	15
Mellet et al., 1996	Words, 30/min	16
Mirz et al., 1999	Music	17
Mirz et al., 1999	Sentences	18
Mirz et al., 1999	Tones, 1000 Hz	19
Mirz et al., 1999	Tones, 1000 and 4000 Hz	20
Mirz et al., 1999	Words	21
Müller et al., 1997	Sentences, 12/min	22
Petersen et al., 1988	Words, 60/min	23
Price et al., 1996	Words, 40/min	24
Price et al., 1996	Words, different rates	25
Suzuki, Kitano, et al., 2002	Words, 60/min	26
Suzuki, Kouzaki, et al., 2002	Tones, 1000 Hz, 60/min	27
Thivard et al., 2000	Tones with spectral maxima, 60/min	28
Warburton et al., 1996	Words, 4/min	29
Wise et al., 1991	Pseudowords, 40 or 60/min	30
Wong et al., 1999	Reversed sentences, 30/min	31
Wong et al., 1999	Sentences, 30/min	32
Wong et al., 1999	Words, 30/min	33
Wong et al., 2002	Reversed words, 15/min	34
Wong et al., 2002	Sentences, 12/min	35
Wong et al., 2002	Words, 15/min	36

Note: Studies listed in the table contributed to the meta-analyses (table 54.3 and figure 54.1) and the localization synopsis in figure 54.2. All experiments except numbers 3, 9, 12, 17, 31, and 34 were entered into the reliability analyses. Data from Experiments 1 and 2 as well as from Experiments 19 and 20 were collapsed in the reliability analyses, since the experiments were not independent.

TABLE 54.2

Passive listening experiments with heterogeneous auditory control conditions

Study	Stimulus vs. Control Stimulus	No. in Figure 54.3
Benson et al., 2001	CVC > CV > V	1
Binder et al., 1996	Words vs. tones	2
Binder et al., 2000	Pseudo words vs. tones	3
Binder et al., 2000	Reversed words vs. tones	4
Binder et al., 2000	Words vs. tones	5
Giraud et al., 2000	Amplitude modulated noise vs. noise	6
Giraud et al., 2000	Sentences vs. vowels	7
Giraud et al., 2000	Words vs. vowels	8
Hall et al., 2002	Frequency modulated vs. static tone	9
Hall et al., 2002	Harmonic vs. single tone	10
Jäncke et al., 2002	Syllables vs. 350-ms white noise bursts	11
Jäncke et al., 2002	Syllables vs. steady-state portion of vowel	12
Jäncke et al., 2002	Syllables vs. tones	13
Müller et al., 2002	90% 1000 Hz + 10% 500 Hz vs. 1000 Hz	14
Mummery et al., 1999	Words vs. signal-correlated noise	15
Price et al., 1996	Words vs. reversed words	16
Schlosser et al., 1998	Sentences vs. unknown language	17
Scott et al., 2000	Sentences vs. rotated sentences	18
Thivard et al., 2000	Frequency transition vs. stationary tone	19

Note: This table lists experiments that contributed to the localization synopsis in figure 54.3.

control stimuli. Because no two studies in this subset used the same combination of active and control stimuli, we refrained from testing anatomical overlap between experiments, and present the activation foci reported in these studies descriptively.

Anatomical coding The reported activation foci were coded in two ways to account for global activation patterns on a whole-brain level as well as for finer-grained anatomical differences within the temporal lobe. At the whole-brain level, the reported foci were entered in an anatomical reference system of 92 cortical regions, based on the parcellation of the cerebral cortex described by Rademacher and colleagues (1992), plus 16 subcortical and cerebellar regions. At the fine-grained level, the foci were entered in a coordinate system with millimeter resolution covering the temporal lobes. Activation foci reported in MNI coordinates were converted to the Talairach and Tournoux (1988) space using the nonlinear algorithm of Brett (1999, available at *www.mrc-cbu.cam.ac.uk/Imaging/mnispace.html*).

Reliability estimate Reliability estimates were calculated using the procedure of Indefrey and Levelt (2000, 2004). For any subset of experiments to be compared at the whole-brain level, we divided the average number of activated regions per experiment by the number of regions to obtain the chance probability for any particular region to be reported in one experiment. Assuming this probability, the chance level for a region to be reported as activated in a number of experiments is given by a binomial distribution. If this level was below 5%, we rejected the possibility that the agreement of reports about a given region was due to chance. It should be noted that the studies were not assigned weights reflecting design or number of subjects, so that activation overlaps that are reliable according to our criterion cannot necessarily be interpreted as statistically significant.

At the fine-grained level, we applied a similar reliability criterion to the reported locations of temporal lobe activation maxima on the lateral temporal planes. Assuming a two-dimensional cortical layer, we ignored location differences in the medial-lateral dimension, except for the most medial (absolute value of the x-coordinate <40) activation foci located on the superior temporal plane, which were analyzed separately. Owing to anatomical variability between subjects, the location of activation maxima may shift by several millimeters to over a centimeter between studies even if identical or highly similar experimental paradigms are used (Stromswold et al., 1996; Caplan, Alpert, and Waters, 1998; Caplan et al., 2000; Indefrey et al., 2004). To account for this variability, all reported activation foci were converted to focal activation areas extending ±5 mm from the original coordinates in the dorsal-ventral and the rostral-caudal

TABLE 54.3

Brain regions activated in passive listening versus a silent control condition

Lobe	Side	Region	Sentences	Words	Pseudowords	Tones
Frontal lobes	Right	Inferior frontal gyrus, pars triangularis	0 (4)	0 (10)	0 (4)	2 (10)
		Inferior frontal gyrus, pars opercularis	0 (4)	0 (10)	0 (4)	3 (10)
	Left	Inferior frontal gyrus, pars triangularis	0 (4)	2 (10)	0 (4)	0 (10)
		Inferior frontal gyrus, pars opercularis	0 (4)	0 (10)	0 (4)	2 (10)
		Inferior frontal gyrus, frontoorbital	3 (4)	0 (10)	0 (3)	0 (7)
Temporal lobes	Right	Anterior superior temporal gyrus	2 (4)	5 (10)	2 (4)	3 (10)
		Posterior superior temporal gyrus	3 (4)	8 (10)	4 (4)	9 (10)
		Anterior middle temporal gyrus	3 (4)	5 (10)	0 (4)	0 (10)
		Posterior middle temporal gyrus	3 (4)	5 (10)	2 (4)	2 (10)
	Left	Anterior superior temporal gyrus	4 (4)	4 (10)	2 (4)	2 (10)
		Posterior superior temporal gyrus	4 (4)	8 (10)	4 (4)	10 (10)
		Anterior middle temporal gyrus	4 (4)	3 (10)	1 (4)	1 (10)
		Posterior middle temporal gyrus	4 (4)	6 (10)	1 (4)	1 (10)

Note: Table lists brain regions found activated in more than one out of 28 experiments comparing passive listening with a silent control condition. Cells show the number of experiments reporting a given region in relation to the number of experiments covering it (in parentheses). Reliable activations are shaded in gray. Following Rademacher and colleagues (1992), the border between anterior and posterior temporal regions was located at the rostrolateral end of the first transverse sulcus, corresponding approximately to $y = -12$ in the coordinate system of Talairach and Tournous (1988).

dimensions. Dividing the mean focal activation area per experiment by the approximate total area of the lateral temporal plane, $3500\,mm^2$, we obtained an estimate for the chance probability of every $1\,mm^2$ pixel to be activated in a single experiment. For smaller sets of experiments the statistical power decreases, such that a relatively larger number of positive reports is required for an above-chance decision. The procedure controlled for the fact that the average number of activation foci may differ across stimuli, influencing the chances of coincidental agreements of findings between studies.

The reliability criterion we applied does not mean that atypical findings of activations in any single study are necessarily due to chance. The number of experiments *not* reporting activations was insufficient to consider a region as inactive at the chosen error probability level. Isolated observations, therefore, do not exclude the possibility that a region is active. They may, for example, reflect smaller activations detectable only with refined techniques or better scanning devices. Furthermore, the nature of the data does not allow interpretation in terms of relative strengths of activations of certain areas. Parameters such as item duration and frequency strongly influence activation patterns (Price et al., 1994, Price, Moore, and Frackowiak, 1996).

RESULTS AT THE WHOLE–BRAIN LEVEL   Overall, the brain activations observed during the presentation of auditory stimuli involve primarily the temporal and posterior inferior frontal lobes. Taking into account the complete data set from

all 55 experiments, only 13 (5 frontal, 8 temporal) of 108 regions were found to be activated in more than one study. Table 54.3 summarizes for these 13 regions the findings of the 28 experiments using sentences, words, pseudowords, or tone stimuli compared with silent control conditions. The table lists the number of experiments reporting a certain region as activated in relation to the number of experiments in which this region could have been found, given that it was covered by the field of view. Regions that by our criterion have been reliably replicated are shaded in gray in the table. For auditorily presented sentences and words, these regions include the bilateral anterior and posterior superior temporal gyri and the bilateral anterior and posterior middle temporal gyri. Sentences and words seem to differ, however, with respect to involvement of the left inferior frontal cortex. Whereas for sentence presentation, activation of the left fronto-orbital cortex (BA 47) was reliably replicated, activation of this region was not reported for auditorily presented words. Conversely, activation of the pars triangularis (BA 45) of the left inferior frontal gyrus was found in two of 10 experiments on word listening. Based on experiments with silent baseline conditions alone, this proportion is not reliable; however, BA 45 was also found to be activated in two (Binder et al., 1996; Price et al., 1996) of five experiments that used acoustically more complex control conditions. For passive listening to sentences, activation of the pars triangularis was reported only by Schlosser and colleagues (1998), in which the control condition was listening to an unknown language. Activation of frontal regions was not reliably replicated in experiments in which subjects listened to pseudowords or meaningless syllables. Only one study (Binder et al., 2000, comparing pseudowords to tones) found bilateral activation of the pars opercularis (BA 44). Temporal regions reliably found to be activated for pseudoword and syllable presentation are the bilateral anterior and posterior superior temporal gyri and the right posterior middle temporal gyrus. In contrast to linguistic stimuli, tone stimuli of varying spectral complexity seem to reliably activate the superior temporal gyri bilaterally, but not the middle temporal gyri. The reports of frontal activations elicited by tone stimuli agree to a reliable extent on the pars opercularis (BA 44) of the right inferior frontal gyrus.

FINE-GRAINED ANALYSIS OF THE TEMPORAL LOBES   In a finer-grained analysis of the patterns of reported activation foci in the temporal lobes, we first present the areas that, to date, can be considered reliable focal activation areas (figure 54.1) for different kinds of stimuli. This reliability estimate is based on overlap of reported activation maxima from experiments with silent baseline conditions (table 54.1, figure 54.2). We then describe the patterns of reported activation maxima obtained in experiments using acoustically or linguistically more complex control conditions (table 54.2, figure 54.3).

Sentences: Silent control   Both temporal lobes exhibit an anterior and a posterior region of reliable overlap of activation maxima (red areas in figure 54.1). In the *z*-dimension (ventral-dorsal), these areas are approximately centered on the superior temporal sulcus. The posterior regions reach dorsally into the primary auditory cortex but extend for the greater part more ventrally. In the right temporal lobe, the posterior activation maxima (figure 54.2, black squares) cluster less tightly than in the left.

Sentences: Acoustic or linguistic control   The control conditions used in three studies on passive sentence listening (Schlosser et al., 1998: unknown language; Giraud et al., 2000: vowels; Scott et al., 2000: spectrally rotated sentences) shared the acoustic and phonological properties of sentences to different extents, but did not involve semantic or syntactic processing. The resulting patterns of activation foci (figure 54.3, black squares) differ in hemisphere-specific ways from those found with a silent baseline (figure 54.2, black squares). In the right temporal lobe, no anterior temporal activation maxima are reported, and the maxima tend to cluster around the primary auditory cortex; in the left temporal lobe, roughly the opposite pattern is observed. Two studies (Schlosser et al., 1998; Giraud et al., 2000) report more posterior activation foci along the superior temporal sulcus than found in studies using a silent baseline.

Words: Silent control   As with sentences, passive listening to words seems to reliably elicit activation foci in two areas of both temporal lobes (figure 54.1, yellow). On the left, these two areas are posteriorly adjacent to the sentence areas. On the right, the posterior area largely overlaps with the sentence area and, in addition, includes the primary auditory cortex. Although some word foci (figure 54.2, light gray triangles) have been reported as far anterior as sentence foci (figure 54.2, black squares), the area of reliable overlap reaches less rostrally than the sentence area.

Words: Acoustic or linguistic control   Activation foci (figure 54.3, light gray triangles) shift toward the superior temporal sulcus in both hemispheres. It is mainly on the left that even more ventral activation foci in the middle and inferior temporal gyri are reported (Binder et al., 1996; Price et al., 1996). Similar to the pattern observed for sentences, anterior temporal activations are reported with acoustically complex control conditions on the left (Price et al., 1996) but not on the right.

Pseudowords/meaningless syllables: Silent control   The reported activation foci overlap reliably in the posterior primary auditory cortex and the adjacent superior temporal gyri in both temporal lobes (figures 54.1, green, and 54.2, dark gray triangles). These overlap areas are similar to those observed for words. On the left, a second more anterior area of overlap is caudally adjacent to that found for words. More anterior temporal activation of the right superior temporal lobe has been found in one study (Bookheimer et al., 1998) but to date is not reliable.

Pseudowords/meaningless syllables: Acoustic or linguistic control   The use of control conditions such as tones (Binder et al., 2000; Jäncke et al., 2002), noise bursts (Jäncke et al., 2002), or vowels (Benson et al., 2001; Jäncke et al., 2002) leads to a shift of activation maxima (figure 54.3, dark gray triangles) away from the auditory cortex. Activation foci are more frequently found in the posterior superior temporal planes than in studies of word or sentence listening. In contrast to word listening maxima, activation maxima for pseudowords are observed more ventrally than the superior temporal sulcus only on the right, not on the left (Benson et al., 2001; Jäncke et al., 2002).

Tones: Silent control   Activation maxima cover both auditory cortices and the posteriorly adjacent superior temporal cortices (figures 54.1, blue, and 54.2, hexagons). This also holds for medial superior temporal lobe activation maxima, which were analyzed separately (not shown in figure 54.1).

Tones: Acoustic control   Comparing frequency- or amplitude-modulated tones to stationary stimuli strongly reduces the number of activation foci (figure 54.3, hexagons) found near

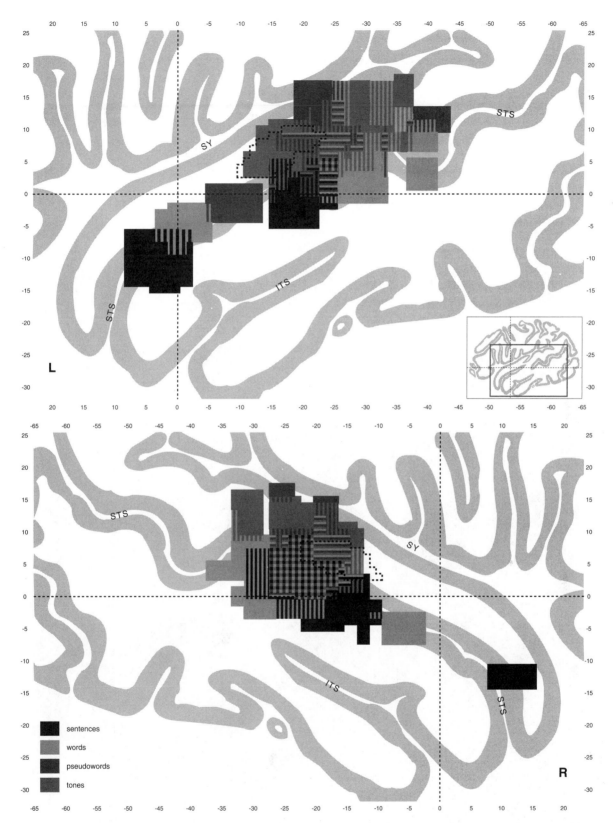

FIGURE 54.1 Meta-analysis results for passive listening experiments with silent control conditions. Colors indicate the areas of reliable overlap of activation foci for the different stimuli. Results are projected onto sagittal slices of the temporal lobe at Talairach *x*-coordinates −51 (upper panel) and +51 (lower panel). To facilitate orientation, the approximate contours of the 50%–75% probability volumes of the primary auditory cortices (Penhune et al., 1996) at *x* = −51 and *x* = +51 are indicated by a black line. Abbreviations: SY, sylvian fissure; STS, superior temporal sulcus; ITS, inferior temporal sulcus. (See color plate 29.)

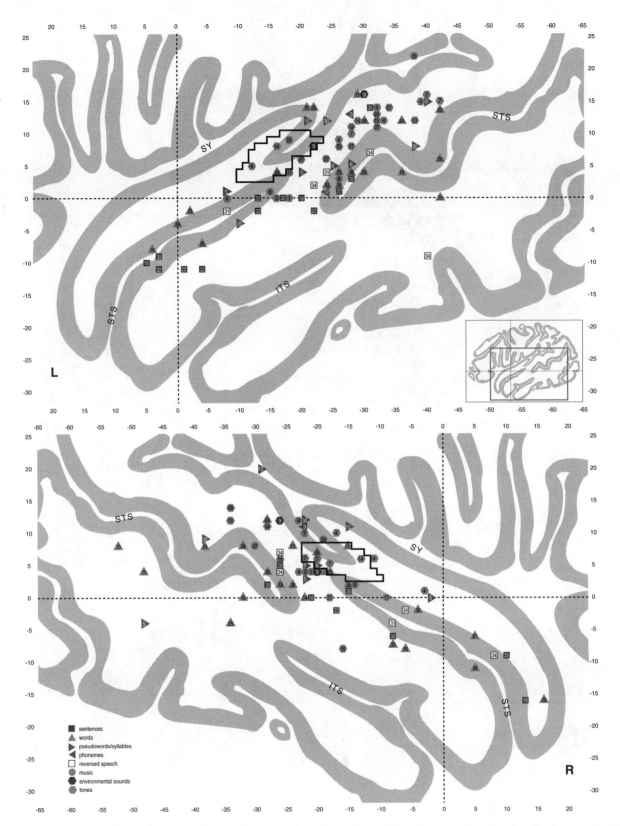

FIGURE 54.2 Synopsis of hemodynamic activation foci reported for passive listening experiments with silent control conditions. Numbers refer to the experiments listed in table 54.1. To facilitate orientation, the approximate contours of the 50%–75% probabil-ity volumes of the primary auditory cortices (Penhune et al., 1996) at $x = -51$ and $x = +51$ are indicated by a black line. Abbreviations: SY, sylvian fissure; STS, superior temporal sulcus; ITS, inferior temporal sulcus.

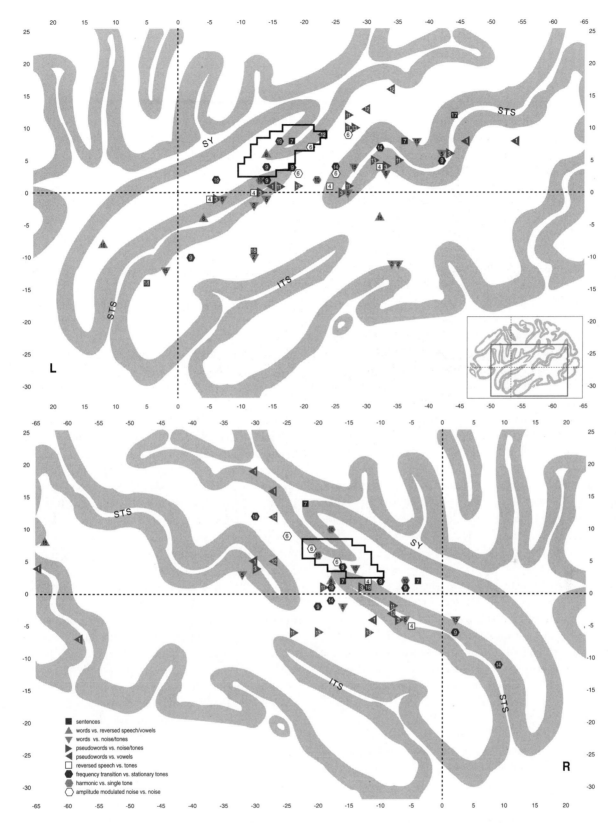

FIGURE 54.3 Synopsis of hemodynamic activation foci reported for passive listening experiments with heterogeneous auditory control conditions. Numbers refer to the experiments listed in table 54.2. To facilitate orientation, the approximate contours of the 50%–75% probability volumes of the primary auditory cortices (Penhune et al., 1996) at $x = -51$ and $x = +51$ are indicated by a black line. Abbreviations: SY, sylvian fissure; STS, superior temporal sulcus; ITS, inferior temporal sulcus.

the posterior superior temporal planes, suggesting that this part of the superior temporal gyrus does not specifically respond to such modulations. Similar to the linguistic stimuli, activation maxima for nonlinguistic auditory stimuli tend to be observed nearer to the superior temporal sulcus when compared to tone stimuli than when compared to silence. However, their reported location tends to be less ventral than that of linguistic stimuli, and also tends to respect the superior temporal sulcus as a ventral border in both hemispheres.

Structure-function relationships

GENERAL OBSERVATIONS Our synopsis suggests that no brain areas other than the posterior inferior frontal and the temporal cortex are reliably activated during passive listening to speech. As has been previously observed (Mazoyer et al., 1993; Binder et al., 1996), the temporal cortex activation areas for different kinds of auditory stimuli seem to show roughly the subset-superset relationships one might expect from the hierarchical organization of the acoustic, phonological, lexical semantic, and syntactic stimulus properties (see table 54.3). All auditory stimuli reliably activate the central and posterior parts of the superior temporal gyri. With increasing linguistic complexity, more ventral and anterior parts of the temporal lobes are recruited. This hierarchical relationship is not as clearly observed in the frontal lobes. For example, the right posterior inferior frontal gyrus, which is reliably activated by tone stimuli, is typically not activated by pseudoword, word, and sentence stimuli, although the latter kinds of stimuli have, besides their additional linguistic properties, many properties in common with the simpler acoustic stimuli.

Our meta-analysis of the overlap of activation maxima (as opposed to total activation areas) shows that there is also a systematic deviation from this expected subset-superset relationship in the temporal lobes. Rather than showing ever larger areas of reliable focal activation as one proceeds from nonlinguistic stimuli to stimuli with increasingly linguistic properties, the hemodynamic activation maxima observed for different kinds of auditory stimuli are clustered in a stimulus-dependent way on the lateral temporal plane of both hemispheres. This is most clearly seen in the anterior left temporal lobe, where the activation maxima for sentences, words, pseudowords, and tones are ordered along an anterior-to-central dimension. In the posterior left temporal lobe, activation maxima for pseudowords and syllables but not for words are reported in the superior temporal plane. Activation maxima for words but not for sentences are reported in the posterior middle/inferior temporal gyri. Considering that words share all the acoustic and linguistic properties of pseudowords, and sentences all the acoustic and linguistic properties of words, these patterns of reported

activation maxima do not seem to follow a "subtraction logic" according to which foci observed for listening to sentences compared to a silent baseline should reflect acoustic or phonological processing as well as semantic or syntactic processing. These findings suggest that the brain response to a particular auditory stimulus property is not uniform but actively adapted to the other properties of the stimulus. They can only be accounted for by assuming that those neuronal populations of the temporal cortex that are sensitive to the "highest" linguistic property of an auditory stimulus show the strongest and most consistent hemodynamic response, thus determining the location of the statistical activation maxima. According to this reasoning, the stimulus-specific patterns of reported activation maxima in passive listening experiments with a silent baseline condition provide information on the stimulus properties that particular cortical areas are sensitive to. In the following sections, we will attempt to draw some tentative conclusions about the temporal cortex regions subserving different levels of linguistic processing. To this end, we will also take into account the spatial distribution of activation foci found in comparisons with control conditions other than silence, as well as electrophysiological, MEG, and clinical data.

ACOUSTIC PROCESSING In both hemispheres, activation maxima for nonlinguistic acoustic stimuli compared to silence are reported in the primary auditory cortex and the posterior superior temporal plane, suggesting a role of these regions in acoustic processing. Activation of these areas starts 20–80 ms after the onset of pure-tone stimuli (Yvert et al., 2001). The precise location of activation maxima within these regions depends on acoustic properties such as sound pressure (Bilecen et al., 2002) and frequency (Lauter et al., 1985; Wessinger et al., 1997; Bilecen et al., 1998; Talavage et al., 2000; Le, Patel, and Roberts, 2001; Engelien et al., 2002; Schönwiesner, von Cramon, and Rübsamen, 2002). Activation of these regions is rarely observed for words or sentences compared to tones, so that these regions do not seem to be related to word-level processing (Binder et al., 1996). When spectrally or temporally more complex acoustic stimuli are compared with simpler ones, more ventral activation foci near the central (on the left also posterior) superior temporal sulcus are observed, so that a role of this part of the superior temporal sulci in acoustic processing is probable.

PHONETIC/PHONOLOGICAL PROCESSING At present, neuroimaging data do not allow for a distinction between phonetic and phonological processing. Throughout this chapter, we use the term phonological processing in the loose sense of a processing level operating on discrete categories. Although it is as yet unclear whether and how lexical access indeed involves discrete intermediate representations, there is clear evidence for categorical perception of speech sounds and for language-specific phonological constraints in speech processing (see Phillips, 2001, for a discussion of acoustic, phonetic, and phonological processing levels).

Pseudowords have all the properties of real words except for meaning. One might therefore assume phonological processing to be involved in activation observed with pseudoword presentation. At the same time, though, pseudowords are also acoustically more complex than most control stimuli that have been used (see Scott and Wise, 2004, for a detailed discussion of different control stimuli), so that stronger activation of a neural population for pseudowords compared with nonlinguistic stimuli is a necessary but not a sufficient condition for a role of this population in phonological processing. For this reason, we will have to consider additional evidence to achieve a tentative conclusion as to the neural structures involved in phonological processes.

In both hemispheres, activation maxima for pseudowords are reported in the central to posterior dorsal aspect of the superior temporal gyri (Wernicke's area), when compared to silent rest. Activation of the bilateral posterior superior temporal plane and the right central middle temporal gyrus by monosyllabic pseudowords does not seem to be cancelled out by tone, noise, or phonologically simpler control stimuli (Benson et al., 2001; Jäncke et al., 2002), suggesting a function in the processing of complex acoustic properties underlying linguistic stimuli or a phonological processing function. Furthermore, it is possible that the right and left temporal lobes differ in the kind of processing they support. Left-hemispheric dominance for phonemes as opposed to nonlinguistic acoustic stimuli has been observed in a number of mismatch negativity (MMN), mismatch field (MMF), and dipole modeling studies (e.g., Näätänen et al., 1997; Alho et al., 1998; Gootjes et al., 1999; Rinne et al., 1999; Szymanski, Rowley, and Roberts, 1999; Szymanski et al., 2001; also see Shtyrov et al., 1999, for converging evidence). While these findings suggest some specialization for language stimuli in the left temporal lobe, they do not prove phonological processing in the left superior temporal lobe or exclude phonological processing in the right temporal lobe (see Phillips, 2001, for detailed discussion of electrophysiological findings).

To distinguish between acoustic and phonological processing, Phillips and colleagues (2000) exploited phonemic category perception effects in an elegantly designed MEG study. Using stimuli from a /tæ-dæ/ voice onset time (VOT) continuum, they elicited an MMF response to infrequent /t/ phonemes with long VOTs when frequent stimuli with shorter VOTs varied acoustically within the phonemic category /d/, but not when the same amount of acoustic variation occurred across the phonemic /d-t/ boundary, preventing the perception of a standard phoneme. The MMF response occurred in a time window of 150–200 ms

after stimulus onset. The response had its source in the left auditory cortex (the right temporal lobe was not measured). In a near-infrared spectroscopy (NIRS) experiment, Minagawa-Kawai and colleagues (2002) demonstrated hemodynamic activation of the left auditory cortex and the adjacent planum temporale for between-category compared to equidistant within-category vowel length contrasts. The effect was bilateral in some subjects but was never right lateralized. Although it is debatable whether the observed category effects reflect phonological rather than phonetic categories, the effects clearly show that the processing of linguistic stimuli in the left auditory cortex, possibly also the adjacent posterior temporal plane and right homologue areas, goes beyond acoustic representations. Further electrophysiological evidence for phonological processing comes from a study by Dehaene-Lambertz, Dupoux, and Gout (2000), who showed that MMN responses can be sensitive to language-specific phonotactic constraints.

Note that the set of phonetic features studied so far is limited and does not allow the conclusion that all phonetically relevant distinctions are processed in the temporal lobes. In a recent fMRI study, Mathiak and colleagues (2002) compared the hemodynamic responses to two categorical perception tasks in which the identity of a word-medial consonant was signaled either by VOT or by the length of the preceding word-medial pause (closure time, CLT). In direct comparisons, they found stronger activation of the left supratemporal plane in the VOT condition and stronger frontal and cerebellar activation in the CLT condition. The latter finding confirmed clinical findings in patients with cerebellar atrophy, who did not show categorical perception for the CLT contrast (Ackermann et al., 1997). Clinical observations also suggest an involvement of the posterior superior temporal lobes in phonological processing. Bilateral lesions of the posterior superior temporal lobes (in some cases also left unilateral lesions; see Griffiths, Rees, and Green, 1999) may result in word deafness, an impairment of language perception with relatively spared processing of nonlinguistic auditory stimuli (Buchman et al., 1986; Griffiths, Rees, and Green, 1999; Poeppel, 2001). Unilateral lesions of the dominant posterior superior temporal gyrus, as in Wernicke's aphasia, may cause more subtle phonological processing deficits, such as problems with the discrimination of phonological contrasts, in particular place of articulation (Blumstein, 1995).

In sum, there is good evidence for a role of the central to posterior superior temporal gyri in phonetic or phonological processing. The left posterior superior temporal gyrus seems to be dominant. In contrast to the robust findings from studies using phoneme discrimination or monitoring tasks (Demonet et al., 1992, 1996) there is, to date, little evidence for involvement of the left posterior frontal cortex in phonological processing during passive listening.

LEXICAL PROCESSING Words and pseudowords activate wholly or partially matching candidate words; nonlinguistic stimuli do not. Activation of a word form can also make available conceptual information, so that syntactic and semantic properties of multiple lexical candidates may also be simultaneously active. Brain areas that are activated by pseudowords may thus to some extent reflect conceptual processing. Nonetheless, words differ from pseudowords in that there is a winner of the lexical competition process, and the successful retrieval of a lexical entry is necessary for word recognition to occur. It may therefore be assumed that brain areas that are activated more strongly for words than for pseudowords reflect additional syntactic and semantic processes involved in or subsequent to lexical recognition.

Activation foci for all linguistic stimuli but not for nonlinguistic stimuli are mainly reported for anterior and posterior parts of the left superior temporal sulcus (see also Giraud and Price, 2001), compared to both silent rest and acoustic control conditions. These areas may therefore be considered candidates for involvement in lexical access and competition processes. There is evidence that lexical access may be affected in patients with fluent aphasia, many of whom have lesions of the posterior part of the left superior temporal sulcus. In such patients, Milberg, Blumstein, and Dworetzky (1988) observed enhanced semantic facilitation by phonologically distorted primes (not only *cat*, but also the pseudoword *wat* primed "dog"). Since these patients can indeed discriminate *cat* from *wat*, Blumstein and Milberg (2000) locate the effect at the lexical level, assuming a lower threshold for the activation of lexical entries, or a general "overactivation" of lexical entries.

Regions in which activation maxima are found for words but not for pseudowords are the most likely candidates for a role in the retrieval of lexically stored information after resolution of the competition process. Compared to silent rest, reliable word activation maxima are found more ventrally and anteriorly than pseudoword maxima in both hemispheres. Due to a broader distribution of pseudoword foci, these location differences disappear with acoustic control conditions in the right hemisphere but not in the left. Here word activation foci are found more anteriorly (Price, Wise, et al., 1996; Mummery et al., 1999) and posteroventrally (Binder et al., 1996; Price, Wise, et al., 1996) than pseudoword foci. A possible relation of these areas to semantic processing has been suggested by a number of authors (for an overview, see Price, Indefrey, and van Turennout, 1999). More recently, Scott and colleagues (2000) assigned a particular role for the processing of "intelligible" speech to a left anterior superior temporal pathway, whereas Hickok and Poeppel (2000) suggested that the auditory-conceptual interface involves a posterior pathway to the left temporoparietal-occipital junction. Rather than supporting an exclusive role

of anterior or posterior temporal structures in semantic processing, the data reviewed here suggest that different parts of the left middle and inferior temporal gyri may be involved in lexical semantic (but possibly also lexical syntactic) processing during passive listening. In addition, Broca's area, in particular BA 45, seems to be involved in the retrieval of lexical information (Binder et al., 1996; Price, Wise, et al., 1996). This rather broad distribution of brain areas associated with lexical processing is also reflected in the heterogeneity of clinical findings. Auditory language comprehension deficits in Wernicke's aphasia do not seem to be strongly related to phonological deficits (Blumstein, 1995; Hickok and Poeppel, 2000). In patients with impaired comprehension, the lesions are typically not confined to the left superior temporal gyrus but extend ventrally and caudally into the middle temporal gyrus and the inferior parietal lobe (Damasio, 1992). Impairments of language comprehension with a relatively preserved ability to repeat heard words, suggesting intact word form representations, are found in transcortical sensory aphasia (TCSA) and semantic dementia. TCSA may result from lesions of the left temporoparietal or anterior temporal/inferior frontal cortex (Damasio, 1991; Berthier, 1999). Semantic dementia is a neurodegenerative disease affecting the left anterior and inferior medial temporal cortex. Although the observed impairments suggest that the left anterior temporal lobe is necessary for language comprehension, Scott and Wise (2004) point out that surgical removal of this region in epileptic patients does not seem to result in a semantic processing deficit (see also Hagoort et al., 1999). Although the neural substrate of language functions may of course have been altered in epileptic patients, the observation suggests that the TCSA and dementia data should be interpreted with caution.

In sum, the available evidence suggests that lexical processing involves anterior and posterior parts of the left superior temporal sulcus. Based on the differences observed between word and pseudoword activation patterns, it can be assumed that there are additional lexical retrieval processes for items that are recognized (win the lexical competition). These processes seem to recruit the left posterior inferior frontal gyrus as well as more anterior and posteroventral temporal areas reaching into the middle and inferior temporal gyri. It should be noted that this picture is almost certainly incomplete, considering the available data on category-specific semantic representations that were not targeted by the experiments analyzed here (see Shapiro and Caramazza, this volume).

SENTENCE-LEVEL PROCESSING Reliable focal activation areas for sentences but not words compared to silent rest are the temporal poles and the central regions of the middle temporal gyri, as well as the left posterior inferior frontal gyrus. With acoustic or phonological control conditions, left temporal pole activation has been confirmed by Scott and colleagues (2000), whereas the other regions either are no longer found or are found for other stimuli as well. These findings suggest the left temporal pole as the best candidate area for sentence-level processing in the temporal lobes. They do not allow a decision as to whether syntax, sentence-level meaning, or prosody is processed. Mazoyer and colleagues (1993), who were the first to observe bilateral temporal pole activations for sentences, found similar activations for meaningless pseudoword and syntactic prose sentences. Friederici, Meyer, and von Cramon (2000) also reported bilateral anterior temporal lobe activation, although more dorsally, for normal and pseudoword sentences. These findings suggest a syntactic rather than semantic function, a view that is also advocated by Dronkers and colleagues (1994) on the basis of clinical data. For aphasic patients with syntactic processing impairments (agrammatism), they found a common lesion area in the anterior temporal lobe that was spared in aphasic patients, who were not agrammatic. By contrast, Hagoort and colleagues (1999) did not find any syntactic deficit in epileptic patients who underwent anterior temporal lobe surgery. Such conflicting findings again point to the necessity of interpreting structure-function relations in clinical populations with caution, given that neural reorganization may have occurred to an unknown extent. If the left anterior temporal pole indeed has a syntactic function, one would expect this area to be more strongly activated for sentences than for words. Wong and colleagues (1999), however, did not find temporal pole activation but posterior inferior frontal (BA 47) activation in a direct comparison of sentences and words. The latter area was also found to be reliably activated in our comparison of sentences to silent rest, so it probably subserves a syntactic or semantic sentence-level processing function. BA 47 is ventrally adjacent to Broca's area (BA 44/45), which is typically found to be active in experiments using syntactic violation or judgment tasks (see Kaan and Swaab, 2002; see also Friederici, this volume, for an overview of frontal and temporal activations observed with such paradigms). Insofar as persisting syntactic processing deficits seem to require frontal lesions that go beyond BA 44 and 45 (Mohr et al., 1978), BA 47 may well play a role in syntactic processing. Further, because syntactic processing deficits can also occur after posterior superior temporal lesions (Caplan, Hildebrandt, and Makris, 1996), neither the left anterior temporal lobe nor the left inferior frontal lobe seems sufficient for syntactic natural language processing.

In sum, there is evidence suggesting involvement of the left temporal pole and the left posterior inferior frontal gyrus in sentence-level processing. To date, however, the exact role of these two areas is unclear.

Conclusions

Auditory language input is processed in a left posterior frontal and bilateral temporal cortical network. Within this network, no processing level is related to a single cortical area. Although auditory language processing activates both temporal lobes, they are not equipotential. In the right temporal lobe, activation foci for different auditory stimuli are found in largely overlapping areas, and there is to date no clear evidence for hemodynamic activation related to postlexical linguistic processing. In the left temporal lobe, the reported activation foci for different kinds of auditory stimuli show clearly distinguishable patterns, and areas that seem to be specialized for phonological (posterior superior temporal gyrus), lexical (anterior and posterior superior temporal sulcus/middle temporal gyrus, posterior inferior frontal gyrus), and sentence-level (temporal pole, posterior inferior frontal gyrus) processing can be identified with some confidence on the basis of the available evidence.

ACKNOWLEDGMENTS We thank Frauke Hellwig for creating the illustrations and Peter Hagoort and James McQueen for helpful comments on the text.

REFERENCES

ACKERMANN, H., S. GRABER, I. HERTRICH, and I. DAUM, 1997. Categorical speech perception in cerebellar disorders. *Brain Lang.* 60:323–331.

ALHO, K., J. F. CONNOLLY, M. CHEOUR, A. LEHTOKOSKI, M. HUOTILAINEN, J. VIRTANEN, R. AULANKO, and R. J. ILMONIEMI, 1998. Hemispheric lateralization in preattentive processing of speech sounds. *Neurosci. Lett.* 258:9–12.

BELIN, P., R. J. ZATORRE, R. HOGE, A. C. EVANS, and B. PIKE, 1999. Event-related fMRI of the auditory cortex. *NeuroImage* 10:417–429.*

BELIN, P., M. ZILBOVICIUS, S. CROZIER, L. THIVARD, and A. FONTAINE, 1998. Lateralization of speech and auditory temporal processing. *J. Cogn. Neurosci.* 10:536–540.*

BENSON, R. R., D. H. WHALEN, M. RICHARDSON, B. SWAINSON, V. P. CLARK, S. LAI, and A. M. LIBERMAN, 2001. Parametrically dissociating speech and nonspeech perception in the brain using fMRI. *Brain Lang.* 78:364–396.*

BERTHIER, M. 1999. *Transcortical Aphasias.* Hove, England: Psychology Press.

BILECEN, D., K. SCHEFFLER, N. SCHMID, K. TSCHOPP, and J. SEELIG, 1998. Tonotopic organization of the human auditory cortex as detected by BOLD-FMRI. *Hear. Res.* 126:19–27.

BILECEN, D., E. SEIFRITZ, K. SCHEFFLER, J. HENNING, and A. C. SCHULTE, 2002. Amplitopicity of the human auditory cortex: An fMRI study. *NeuroImage* 17:710–718.

BINDER, J. R., J. A. FROST, T. A. HAMMEKE, P. S. F. BELLGOWAN, S. M. RAO, and R. W. COX, 1999. Conceptual processing during the conscious resting state: A functional MRI study. *J. Cogn. Neurosci.* 11:80–93.

BINDER, J. R., J. A. FROST, T. A. HAMMEKE, P. S. F. BELLGOWAN, J. A. SPRINGER, J. N. KAUFMAN, and E. T. POSSING, 2000. Human temporal lobe activation by speech and nonspeech sounds. *Cereb. Cortex* 10:512–528.*

BINDER, J. R., J. A. FROST, T. A. HAMMEKE, S. M. RAO, and R. W. COX, 1996. Function of the left planum temporale in auditory and linguistic processing. *Brain* 119:1239–1247.*

BLUMSTEIN, S. E., 1995. The neurobiology of the sound structure of language. In *The Cognitive Neurosciences*, M. S. Gazzaniga, ed. Cambridge, Mass.: MIT Press, pp. 915–930.

BLUMSTEIN, S. E., and W. P. MILBERG, 2000. Language deficits in Broca's and Wernicke's aphasia: A singular impairment. In *Language and the Brain*, Y. Grodzinsky, L. P. Shapiro, and D. Swinney, eds. San Diego, Callif.: Academic Press, pp. 167–183.

BOOKHEIMER, S. Y., T. A. ZEFFIRO, T. A. BLAXTON, W. D. GAILLARD, B. MALOW, and W. H. THEODORE, 1998. Regional cerebral blood flow during auditory responsive naming: Evidence for cross-modality neural activation. *Neuroreport* 9:2409–2413.*

BUCHMAN, A. S., D. C. GARRON, J. E. TROSTCARDAMONE, M. D. WICHTER, and M. SCHWARTZ, 1986. Word deafness: 100 years later. *J. Neurol. Neurosurg. Psychiatry* 49:489–499.

CAPLAN, D., N. ALPERT, and G. WATERS, 1998. Effects of syntactic structure and propositional number on patterns of regional cerebral blood flow. *J. Cogn. Neurosci.* 10:541–552.

CAPLAN, D., N. ALPERT, G. WATERS, and A. OLIVIERI, 2000. Activation of Broca's area by syntactic processing under conditions of concurrent articulation. *Hum. Brain Mapp.* 9:65–71.

CAPLAN, D., N. HILDEBRANDT, and N. MAKRIS, 1996. Location of lesions in stroke patients with deficits in syntactic processing in sentence comprehension. *Brain* 119:933–949.

CELSIS, P., K. BOULANOUAR, B. DOYON, J. P. RANJEVA, I. BERRY, J. L. NESPOULOUS, and F. CHOLLET, 1999. Differential fMRI responses in the left posterior superior temporal gyrus and left supramarginal gyrus to habituation and change detection in syllables and tones. *NeuroImage* 9:135–144.*

CONNINE, C. M., D. G. BLASKO, and J. WANG, 1994. Vertical similarity in spoken word recognition: Multiple lexical activation, individual differences, and the role of sentence context. *Percept. Psychophys.* 56:624–636.

DAMASIO, A. R., 1992. Aphasia. *N. Engl. J. Med.* 326:531–539.

DAMASIO, H., 1991. Neuroanatomical correlates of the aphasias. In *Acquired Aphasia*, M. Taylor Sarno, ed. New York: Academic Press, pp. 45–71.

DEHAENE-LAMBERTZ, G., E. DUPOUX, and A. GOUT, 2000. Electrophysiological correlates of phonological processing: A cross-linguistic study. *J. Cogn. Neurosci.* 12:635–647.

DÉMONET, J. F., F. CHOLLET, S. RAMSAY, D. CARDEBAT, J. L. NESPOULOUS, R. WISE, A. RASCOL, and R. FRACKOWIAK, 1992. The anatomy of phonological and semantic processing in normal subjects. *Brain* 115:1753–1768.

DÉMONET, J. F., J. A. FIEZ, E. PAULESU, S. E. PETERSEN, and R. J. ZATORRE, 1996. Pet studies of phonological processing: A critical reply to Poeppel. *Brain Lang.* 55:352–379.

DI SALLE, F., E. FORMISANO, E. SEIFRITZ, D. E. J. LINDEN, K. SCHEFFLER, C. SAULINO, G. TEDESCHI, F. E. ZANELLA, A. PEPINO, R. GOEBEL, and E. MARCIANO, 2001. Functional fields in human auditory cortex revealed by time-resolved fMRI without interference of EPI noise. *NeuroImage* 13:328–338.*

DRONKERS, N. F., D. P. WILKINS, R. D. VANVALIN, B. B. REDFERN, and J. J. JAEGER, 1994. A reconsideration of the brain-areas involved in the disruption of morphosyntactic comprehension. *Brain Lang.* 47:461–463.

ENGELIEN, A., Y. H. YANG, W. ENGELIEN, J. ZONANA, E. STERN, and D. A. SILBERSWEIG, 2002. Physiological mapping of human auditory cortices with a silent event-related fMRI technique. *NeuroImage* 16:944–953.*

FIEZ, J. A., M. E. RAICHLE, D. A. BALOTA, P. TALLAL, and S. E. PETERSEN, 1996. PET activation of posterior temporal regions during auditory word presentation and verb generation. *Cereb. Cortex* 6:1–10.*

FRIEDERICI, A. D., M. MEYER, and D. Y. VON CRAMON, 2000. Auditory language comprehension: An event-related fMRI study on the processing of syntactic and lexical information. *Brain Lang.* 74:289–300.

GIRAUD, A. L., and C. J. PRICE, 2001. The constraints functional neuroimaging places on classical models of auditory word processing. *J. Cogn. Neurosci.* 13:754–765.

GIRAUD, A. L., E. TRUY, R. S. J. FRACKOWIAK, M. C. GREGOIRE, J. F. PUJOL, and L. COLLET, 2000. Differential recruitment of the speech processing system in healthy subjects and rehabilitated cochlear implant patients. *Brain* 123:1391–1402.*

GOOTJES, L., T. RAIJI, R. SALMELIN, and R. HARI, 1999. Left-hemisphere dominance for processing of vowels: A whole-scalp neuromagnetic study. *Neuroreport* 10:2987–2991.

GOW, D. W., and P. C. GORDON, 1995. Lexical and prelexical influences on word segmentation: Evidence from priming. *J. Exp. Psychol. Hum. Percept. Perform.* 21:344–359.

GRIFFITHS, T. D., A. REES, and G. G. R. GREEN, 1999. Disorders of human complex sound processing. *Neurocase* 5:365–378.

GROSJEAN, F., and U. H. FRAUENFELDER, eds., 1997. *A Guide to Spoken Word Recognition Paradigms*. Hove, England: Psychology Press.

HAGOORT, P., N. RAMSEY, G. J. RUTTEN, and P. VAN RIJEN, 1999. The role of the left anterior temporal cortex in language processing. *Brain Lang.* 69:322–325.

HALL, D. A., I. S. JOHNSRUDE, M. P. HAGGARD, A. R. PALMER, M. A. AKEROYD, and A. Q. SUMMERFIELD, 2002. Spectral and temporal processing in human auditory cortex. *Cereb. Cortex* 12:140–149.*

HICKOK, G., and D. POEPPEL, 2000. Towards a functional neuroanatomy of speech perception. *Trends Cogn. Sci.* 4:131–138.

HOLCOMB, H. H., D. R. MEDOFF, P. J. CAUDILL, Z. ZHAO, A. C. LAHTI, R. F. DANNALS, and C. A. TAMMINGA, 1998. Cerebral blood flow relationships associated with a difficult tone recognition task in trained normal volunteers. *Cereb. Cortex* 8:534–542.*

INDEFREY, P., F. M. HELLWIG, H. HERZOG, R. SEITZ, and P. HAGOORT, 2004. Neural responses to the production and comprehension of syntax in identical utterances. *Brain Lang.* 89:312–319.

INDEFREY, P., and W. J. M. LEVELT, 2000. The neural correlates of language production. In *The New Cognitive Neurosciences*, M. S. Gazzaniga, ed. Cambridge, Mass.: MIT Press, pp. 845–865.

INDEFREY, P., and W. J. M. LEVELT, 2004. The spatial and temporal signatures of word production components. *Cognition.* 92:101–144.

JÄNCKE, L., S. MIRZAZADE, and N. J. SHAH, 1999. Attention modulates activity in the primary and the secondary auditory cortex: A functional magnetic resonance imaging study in human subjects. *Neurosci. Lett.* 266:125–128.*

JÄNCKE, L., T. WÜSTENBERG, H. SCHEICH, and H. J. HEINZE, 2002. Phonetic perception and the temporal cortex. *NeuroImage* 15:733–746.*

KAAN, E., and T. Y. SWAAB, 2002. The brain circuitry of syntactic comprehension. *Trends Cogn. Sci.* 6:350–356.

LAUTER, J. L., P. HERSCOVITCH, C. FORMBY, and M. E. RAICHLE, 1985. Tonotopic organization in human auditory cortex revealed by positron emission tomography. *Hear. Res.* 20:199–205.

Le, T. H., S. Patel, and T. P. L. Roberts, 2001. Functional MRI of human auditory cortex using block and event-related designs. *Magn. Reson. Med.* 45:254–260.

Lockwood, A. H., R. J. Salvi, M. L. Coad, S. A. Arnold, D. S. Wack, B. W. Murphy, and R. F. Burkard, 1999. The functional anatomy of the normal human auditory system: Responses to 0.5 and 4.0 kHz tones at varied intensities. *Cereb. Cortex* 9:65–76.*

Luce, P. A., and E. A. Lyons, 1999. Processing lexically embedded spoken words. *J. Exp. Psychol. Hum. Percept. Perform.* 25:174–183.

Marslen-Wilson, W., and P. Warren, 1994. Levels of perceptual representation and process in lexical access: Words, phonemes, and features. *Psychol. Rev.* 101:653–675.

Mathiak, K., I. Hertrich, W. Grodd, and H. Ackermann, 2002. Cerebellum and speech perception: A functional magnetic resonance imaging study. *J. Cogn. Neurosci.* 14:902–912.

Mazoyer, B. M., N. Tzourio, V. Frak, A. Syrota, N. Murayama, O. Levrier, G. Salamon, S. Dehaene, L. Cohen, and J. Mehler, 1993. The cortical representation of speech. *J. Cogn. Neurosci.* 5:467–479.

McGuire, P. K., D. A. Silbersweig, and C. D. Frith, 1996. Functional neuroanatomy of verbal self-monitoring. *Brain* 119: 907–917.

McQueen, J. M., D. Dahan, and A. Cutler, 2003. Continuity and gradedness in speech processing. In *Phonetics and Phonology in Language Comprehension and Production: Differences and Similarities*, N. O. Schiller and A. S. Meyer, eds. Berlin, New York: Mouton de Gruyter, pp. 37–76.

McQueen, J. M., D. Norris, and A. Cutler, 1994. Competition in spoken word recognition: Spotting words in other words. *J. Exp. Psychol. Learn. Mem. Cogn.* 20:621–638.

McQueen, J. M., D. Norris, and A. Cutler, 1999. Lexical influence in phonetic decision making: Evidence from subcatgorical mismatches. *J. Exp. Psychol. Hum. Percept. Perform.* 25: 1363–1389.

Mellet, E., N. Tzourio, F. Crivello, M. Joliot, M. Denis, and B. Mazoyer, 1996. Functional anatomy of spatial mental imagery generated from verbal instructions. *J. Neurosci.* 16: 6504–6512.*

Milberg, W., S. Blumstein, and B. Dworetzky, 1988. Phonological processing and lexical access in aphasia. *Brain Lang.* 34:279–293.

Minagawa-Kawai, Y., K. Mori, I. Furuya, R. Hayashi, and Y. Sato, 2002. Assessing cerebral representations of short and long vowel categories by NIRS. *Neuroreport* 13:581–584.

Mirz, F., T. Ovesen, K. Ishizu, P. Johannsen, S. Madsen, A. Gjedde, and C. B. Pedersen, 1999. Stimulus-dependent central processing of auditory stimuli: A PET study. *Scand. Audiol.* 28: 161–169.*

Mohr, J. P., M. S. Pessin, S. Finkelstein, H. H. Funkenstein, G. W. Duncan, and K. R. Davis, 1978. Broca aphasia: Pathologic and clinical. *Neurology* 28:311–324.

Müller, B. W., M. Jüptner, W. Jentzen, and S. P. Müller, 2002. Cortical activation to auditory mismatch elicited by frequency deviant and complex novel sounds: A PET study. *NeuroImage* 17:231–239.*

Müller, R. A., R. D. Rothermel, M. E. Behen, O. Muzik, T. J. Mangner, and H. T. Chugani, 1997. Receptive and expressive language activations for sentences: A PET study. *Neuroreport* 8:3767–3770.*

Mummery, C. J., J. Ashburner, S. K. Scott, and R. J. S. Wise, 1999. Functional neuroimaging of speech perception in six normal and two aphasic subjects. *J. Acoust. Soc. Am.* 106:449–457.*

Näätänen, R., A. Lehtokoski, M. Lennes, M. Cheour, M. Huotilainen, A. Iivonen, M. Vainio, P. Alku, R. J. Ilmoniemi, A. Luuk, J. Allik, J. Sinkkonen, and K. Alho, 1997. Language-specific phoneme representations revealed by electric and magnetic brain responses. *Nature* 385:432–434.

Norris, D., J. M. McQueen, and A. Cutler, 1995. Competition and segmentation in spoken word recognition. *J. Exp. Psychol. Learn. Mem. Cogn.* 21:1209–1228.

Norris, D., J. M. McQueen, and A. Cutler, 2000. Merging information in speech recognition: Feedback is never necessary. *Behav. Brain Sci.* 23:299–325.

Norris, D., and R. Wise, 2000. The study of prelexical and lexical processes in comprehension: Psycholinguistics and functional neuroimaging. In *The New Cognitive Neurosciences*, M. S. Gazzaniga, ed. Cambridge, Mass.: MIT Press, pp. 867–880.

Penhune, V. B., R. J. Zatorre, J. D. MacDonald, and A. C. Evans, 1996. Interhemispheric anatomical differences in human primary auditory cortex: Probabilistic mapping and volume measurement from magnetic resonance scans. *Cereb. Cortex* 6:661–672.

Petersen, S. E., P. T. Fox, M. I. Posner, M. Mintun, and M. E. Raichle, 1988. Positron emission tomographic studies of the cortical anatomy of single-word processing. *Nature* 331:585–589.*

Phillips, C., 2001. Levels of representation in the electrophysiology of speech perception. *Cogn. Sci.* 25:711–731.

Phillips, C., T. Pellathy, A. Marantz, E. Yellin, K. Wexler, D. Poeppel, M. McGinnis, and T. Roberts, 2000. Auditory cortex accesses phonological categories: An MEG mismatch study. *J. Cogn. Neurosci.* 12:1038–1055.

Poeppel, D., 2001. Pure word deafness and the bilateral processing of the speech code. *Cogn. Sci.* 25:679–693.

Price, C., P. Indefrey, and M. van Turennout, 1999. The neural architecture underlying the processing of written and spoken word forms. In *The Neurocognition of Language*, C. M. Brown and P. Hagoort, eds. Oxford, England: Oxford University Press, pp. 211–240.

Price, C. J., C. J. Moore, and R. S. J. Frackowiak, 1996. The effect of varying stimulus rate and duration on brain activity during reading. *NeuroImage* 3:40–52.

Price, C. J., R. J. S. Wise, E. A. Warburton, C. J. Moore, D. Howard, K. Patterson, R. S. J. Frackowiak, and K. J. Friston, 1996. Hearing and saying: The functional neuro-anatomy of auditory word processing. *Brain* 119:919–931.*

Price, C. J., R. J. S. Wise, J. D. G. Watson, K. Patterson, D. Howard, and R. S. J. Frackowiak, 1994. Brain activity during reading: The effects of exposure duration and task. *Brain* 117:1255–1269.

Rademacher, J., A. M. Galaburda, D. N. Kennedy, P. A. Filipek, and V. S. Caviness, 1992. Human cerebral cortex: Localization, parcellation, and morphometry with magnetic-resonance-imaging. *J. Cogn. Neurosci.* 4:352–374.

Rinne, T., K. Alho, P. Alku, M. Holi, J. Sinkkonen, J. Virtanen, O. Bertrand, and R. Näätänen, 1999. Analysis of speech sounds is left-hemisphere predominant at 100–150 ms after sound onset. *Neuroreport* 10:1113–1117.

Schlosser, M. J., N. Aoyagi, R. K. Fulbright, J. C. Gore, and G. McCarthy, 1998. Functional MRI studies of auditory comprehension. *Hum. Brain Mapp.* 6:1–13.*

Schönwiesner, M., D. Y. von Cramon, and R. Rübsamen, 2002. Is it tonotopy after all? *NeuroImage* 17:1144–1161.

Scott, S. K., C. C. Blank, S. Rosen, and R. J. Wise, 2000. Identification of a pathway for intelligible speech in the left temporal lobe. *Brain* 12:2400–2406.*

SCOTT, S., and R. WISE, 2004. *The functional neuroanatomy of prelexical processing in speech perception. Cognition.* 92:13–45.

SHTYROV, Y., T. KUJALA, R. J. ILMONIEMI, and R. NÄÄTÄNEN, 1999. Noise affects speech-signal processing differently in the cerebral hemispheres. *Neuroreport* 10:2189–2192.

SHULMAN, G., M. CORBETTA, R. BUCKNER, J. FIEZ, F. MIEZIN, M. RAICHLE, and S. PETERSEN, 1997. Common blood flow changes across visual tasks. II. Decreases in cerebral cortex. *J. Cogn. Neurosci.* 9:648–663.

SOTO-FARACO, S., N. SEBASTIÁN-GALLÉS, and A. CUTLER, 2001. Segmental and suprasegmental mismatch in lexical access. *J. Mem. Lang.* 45:412–432.

STREETER, L. A., and G. N. NIGRO, 1979. The role of medial consonant transitions in word perception. *J. Acoust. Soc. Am.* 65:1533–1541.

STROMSWOLD, K., D. CAPLAN, N. ALPERT, and S. RAUCH, 1996. Localization of syntactic comprehension by positron emission tomography. *Brain Lang.* 52:452–473.

SUZUKI, M., H. KITANO, T. KITANISHI, R. ITOU, A. SHIINO, Y. NISHIDA, Y. YAZAWA, F. OGAWA, and K. KITAJIMA, 2002. Cortical and subcortical activation with monaural monosyllabic stimulation by functional MRI. *Hear. Res.* 163:37–45.*

SUZUKI, M., H. KOUZAKI, R. ITO, A. SHIINO, Y. NISHIDA, and H. KITANO, 2002. Cortical activation patterns in functional magnetic resonance images following monaural pure tone stimulation. *Neurosci. Res. Commun.* 30:197–206.*

SZYMANSKI, M. D., D. W. PERRY, N. M. GAGE, H. A. ROWLEY, J. WALKER, M. S. BERGER, and T. P. L. ROBERTS, 2001. Magnetic source imaging of late evoked field responses to vowels: Toward an assessment of hemispheric dominance for language. *J. Neurosurg.* 94:445–453.

SZYMANSKI, M. D., H. A. ROWLEY, and T. P. L. ROBERTS, 1999. A hemispherically asymmetrical MEG response to vowels. *Neuroreport* 10:2481–2486.

TABOSSI, P., C. BURANI, and D. SCOTT, 1995. Word identification in fluent speech. *J. Mem. Lang.* 34:440–467.

TALAIRACH, J., and P. TOURNOUX, 1988. *Co-planar Stereotaxic Atlas of the Human Brain. 3. Dimensional Proportional System: An Approach to Cerebral Imaging.* Stuttgart: Thieme.

TALAVAGE, T. M., P. J. LEDDEN, R. R. BENSON, B. R. ROSEN, and J. R. MELCHER, 2000. Frequency-dependent responses exhibited by multiple regions in human auditory cortex. *Hear. Res.* 150:225–244.

THIVARD, L., P. BELIN, M. ZILBOVICIUS, J. B. POLINE, and Y. SAMSON, 2000. A cortical region sensitive to auditory spectral motion. *Neuroreport* 11:2969–2972.*

VROOMEN, J., and B. DE GELDER, 1997. Activation of embedded words in spoken word recognition. *J. Exp. Psychol. Hum. Percept. Perform.* 23:710–720.

VROOMEN, J., and B. DE GELDER, 1995. Metrical segmentation and lexical inhibition in spoken word recognition. *J. Exp. Psychol. Hum. Percept. Perform.* 21:98–108.

WARBURTON, E., R. J. S. WISE, C. J. PRICE, C. WEILLER, U. HADAR, S. RAMSAY, and R. S. J. FRACKOWIAK, 1996. Noun and verb retrieval by normal subjects studies with PET. *Brain* 119:159–179.*

WESSINGER, C. M., M. H. BUONOCORE, C. L. KUSSMAUL, and G. R. MANGUN, 1997. Tonotopy in human auditory cortex examined with functional magnetic resonance imaging. *Hum. Brain Mapp.* 5:18–25.

WHALEN, D. H., 1991. Subcategorical phonetic mismatches and lexical access. *Percept. Psychophys.* 50:351–360.

WISE, R., F. CHOLLET, U. HADAR, K. FRISTON, E. HOFFNER, and R. FRACKOWIAK, 1991. Distribution of cortical neural networks involved in word comprehension and word retrieval. *Brain* 114:1803–1817.*

WONG, D., R. T. MIYAMOTO, D. B. PISONI, M. SEHGAL, and G. D. HUTCHINS, 1999. PET imaging of cochlear-implant and normal-hearing subjects listening to speech and nonspeech. *Hear. Res.* 132:34–42.*

WONG, D., D. B. PISONI, J. LEARN, J. T. GANDOUR, R. T. MIYAMOTO, and G. D. HUTCHINS, 2002. PET imaging of differential cortical activation by monaural speech and nonspeech stimuli. *Hear. Res.* 166:9–23.*

YVERT, B., A. CROUZEIX, O. BERTRAND, A. SEITHER-PREISLER, and C. PANTEV, 2001. Multiple supratemporal sources of magnetic and electric auditory evoked middle latency components in humans. *Cereb. Cortex* 11:411–423.

ZWITSERLOOD, P., 1989. The locus of the effects of sentential-semantic context in spoken-word processing. *Cognition* 32:25–64.

ZWITSERLOOD, P., and H. SCHRIEFERS, 1995. Effects of sensory information and processing time in spoken-word recognition. *Lang. Cogn. Processes* 10:121–136.

55 Cognitive and Neural Substrates of Written Language: Comprehension and Production

ARGYE E. HILLIS AND BRENDA C. RAPP

ABSTRACT   Written language is an important domain of investigation in cognitive neuroscience because reading and spelling are uniquely human cognitive tasks that are increasingly important in society. Furthermore, examining the extent to which reading and writing depend on the same cognitive processes and representations allows exploration of the relationship between comprehension and production or, more generally perception and action. Two sources of evidence regarding shared versus independent cognitive mechanisms in reading and spelling are reviewed: neurologically impaired subjects performance on various written language tasks and neuroanatomical substrates of reading and spelling revealed by lesion studies and functional imaging. This review leads to the conclusion that reading and spelling have in common at least some underlying cognitive processes and representations, involving specific left frontal, temporal, and parietal regions.

One reason for interest in understanding the cognitive and neural bases of written language processing is that literacy involves both comprehension (reading) and production (spelling). Accordingly, written language processing constitutes a domain within which to investigate longstanding questions concerning the relationship between recognition and production, perception, and action. These questions have been widely debated in other domains, such as spoken language, where it has been proposed that speech perception makes use of motor representations (Liberman and Mattingly, 1985). Similarly, in vision the possibility that perception and action may make use of the same neural substrates has received considerable attention (e.g., Rizzolatti et al., 1996; Decety and Grezes, 1999; Meltzoff, 1999). Thus, the domain of written language processing is particularly promising for investigating whether a set of representations and processes is shared by recognition and production, as the components and representational content of the processing architecture are understood in some detail.

ARGYE E. HILLIS   Department of Neurology, Johns Hopkins University School of Medicine, and Department of Cognitive Science, Johns Hopkins University, Baltimore, Md.

BRENDA C. RAPP   Department of Cognitive Science, Johns Hopkins University, Baltimore, Md.

In this chapter, we review current understanding of the cognitive and neural substrates of written language processing, focusing on the question, to what extent do reading and spelling share cognitive and neural substrates? A review of the relevant evidence will also serve to address more fundamental questions regarding the degree to which human cortex may become specialized for specific cognitive functions. The first section of the chapter reviews the cognitive processes involved in word reading, summarizing the rationale and evidence for proposing each of the cognitive components. In this section we consider the degree to which spelling entails the same or different representations and processes. In the second section, we evaluate the evidence from lesion studies and functional neuroimaging that specific neural regions are shared by reading and spelling.

Cognitive processes of reading

Figure 55.1 is a schematic representation of cognitive components that have been hypothesized to be required for reading a word (see Coltheart, Patterson, and Marshall, 1980, for a generally similar architecture, and Seidenberg and McClelland, 1988, and Plaut and Shallice, 1993, for connectionist architectures of reading incorporating distributed representations). Each component has been proposed on the basis of the computational requirements of reading and evidence from neurologically impaired subjects. For heuristic purposes, we describe these components as functionally independent, although there is strong evidence for at least some degree of interaction between processes in both reading and spelling (Hillis and Caramazza, 1991; Patterson and Lambon-Ralph, 1999; Rapp, Epstein and Tainturier, 2002). It should also be noted that processing may not be strictly serial, as shown in the figures; there may be activation of two or more components simultaneously.

FROM LETTER SHAPE TO GRAPHEMIC REPRESENTATION Reading a printed word begins with an adequate visual analysis. Various impairments in visual processing that are not specific to reading (or language) can interfere with

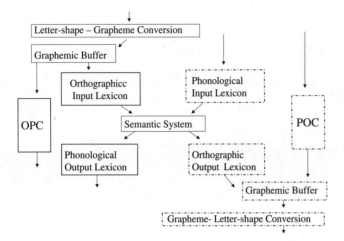

FIGURE 55.1 The independent-components account of the cognitive processes underlying reading and spelling. Reading (or shared) components are outlined with solid lines; spelling components are outlined with broken lines.

reading. For example, impaired processing of visual stimuli on the side of the viewer contralateral to the lesion (a type of hemispatial neglect) and other visual attentional deficits can affect reading in a variety of ways (Riddoch, 1991; Zihl, 1995). A review of these deficits is beyond the scope of this chapter.

Visual processes allow perception of letter shapes, which in turn are represented as *graphemes*—abstract letter identities that lack shape, font, or case. This transformation of letter shapes to graphemes allows the reader to appreciate that CHAIR and *chair* or *phaip* and PHAIP are identical. Evidence for such a process comes from cases of selective impairment in transforming visual to graphemic representations after brain damage, manifested by impaired matching of letters or letter strings presented in different font and case, and impaired recognition of written words despite recognition of the same words when they are spelled aloud (e.g., Reuter-Lorenz and Brunn, 1990).

ACCESSING LEXICAL ORTHOGRAPHIC REPRESENTATIONS The graphemic representation of a stimulus serves as the basis for activating stored word representations (lexical ortho-graphic representations) in the long-term memory store of familiar orthographic forms, referred to as the *orthographic lexicon*. Activation of a lexical orthographic representation allows, for example, recognition that the word *chair* is a familiar word, and failure to access such a representation indicates that *chare* is not. However, access to the lexical orthographic representation does not ensure understanding of the word; understanding requires access to its semantic representation (meaning). Evidence that lexical orthographic and semantic representations are relatively independent comes from individuals with focal brain damage who have impaired access to lexical orthographic representations in

reading, as evidenced by impaired oral reading and comprehension of familiar written words in the face of intact comprehension of the same spoken words (Patterson, Coltheart, and Marshall, 1985).

ACCESSING SEMANTIC REPRESENTATIONS The activated lexical orthographic representation serves to access the word's meaning, or semantic representation. The semantic system is shared by lexical processes, regardless of the modality of input or output, and therefore, individuals with impairment at the level of the semantic system show poor comprehension and production of both spoken and written words. They also show essentially equal error rates and types of errors (e.g., matching the word *toothbrush* to a picture of a comb) with spoken and written word input (Howard and Orchard-Lisle, 1984; Dickerson and Johnson, in press).

ACCESSING LEXICAL PHONOLOGICAL REPRESENTATIONS The activated semantic representation normally serves to activate a corresponding lexical phonological representation (pronunciation) of the word stored in the long-term memory repository of spoken word forms—the *phonological lexicon*. One hypothesis regarding access to the phonological lexicon is that each of the semantic features that together define the word activates all of the lexical phonological representations that share that feature. Thus, for toothbrush, the semantic feature <grooming tool> would activate lexical phonological representations of "toothbrush," "comb," "brush," "razor," and so on, and the feature <dental> would activate lexical phonological representations of "toothbrush," "toothpaste," "dentist," "braces," "fillings," "drills," and so on. In normal readers, only the target representation "toothbrush" receives activation from all of the semantic features of the stimulus, and so it will be selected for output. However, other semantically related words (e.g., in this example, "comb," "dentist," etc.) will also be somewhat activated. Therefore, if the target lexical phonological representation is not available because of damage, one of the other partially activated words will be selected. Thus, patient R.G.B., described by Caramazza and Hillis (1990), understood printed words well, as shown by his accurate definitions of printed words. Nevertheless, during oral reading of these words, he made semantically related errors. For example, he read the word *gray* as "blue" but defined it as "the color of hair when you get old." Unlike individuals with impaired lexical semantic processing, however, R.G.B. had spared word comprehension and relatively spared written naming of the same items that elicited semantic errors in oral production tasks (see also Bub and Kertesz, 1982; Rapp, Benzing, and Caramazza, 1997). Therefore, his semantic errors in oral reading were most likely due to impaired access to lexical phonological representations for output, with partial activation of the more accessible representations.

Other brain-injured individuals with impairments similarly affecting lexical phonological representations do not make semantic errors in oral reading. Instead, they may bypass the phonological lexicon and use sublexical orthography-to-phonology conversion mechanisms to sound out words and produce phonologically plausible responses (ONE → "own"). However, it should be noted that many connectionist models do not invoke separate lexical and sublexical mechanisms but demonstrate that many of the reported patterns of performance by brain-damaged subjects can be simulated by "damage" to a computational model with a single mechanism responsible for conversion of orthography to phonology, for both words and pseudowords (e.g., Seidenberg and McClelland, 1989; Plaut and Shallice, 1993).

SUBLEXICAL ORTHOGRAPHY-TO-PHONOLOGY CONVERSION Unfamiliar words or pseudowords do not access representations in the orthographic lexicon but instead are read using the sublexical orthography-to-phonology conversion system. This mechanism makes use of knowledge regarding the systematic relationships between sublexical units such as letters (or letter groups) and their corresponding sounds in order to reliably read stimuli such as *famp* as [fæmp] (rhyming with stamp).

Individuals who have impaired access to lexical orthographic representations may rely on sublexical orthography-to-phonology conversion mechanisms to read words aloud, as evidenced by "regularization" of irregular words (e.g., ONE read as "own"). However, reliance on sublexical mechanisms to read previously familiar words (sometimes referred to as surface dyslexia) does not reveal the locus of impairment within the lexical system (Patterson, Coltheart, and Marshall, 1985). Use of orthography-to-phonology conversion mechanisms can reflect impairment in accessing lexical orthographic representations, lexical semantic representations, or lexical phonological representations.

The relative independence of sublexical and lexical reading mechanisms is supported by the performance of neurologically impaired individuals who rely on sublexical orthography-to-phonology conversion mechanisms, as well as the performance of others who are selectively unable to use these sublexical processes. For example, Marshall and Newcombe (1973) described brain-damaged individuals who were unable to use orthography-to-phonology conversion mechanisms to sound out pseudowords but were able to correctly read many familiar words (see also Beauvois and Derousne, 1979; Funnell, 1983). Individuals with the complementary pattern of intact pseudoword reading accompanied by impaired reading of familiar words have also been described. For example, K.T., described by McCarthy and Warrington (1986), had preserved nonword reading (96% correct) but severely impaired reading of irregular words (26% correct) (see also Beauvois and Derouesne, 1981; Bub,

Cancelliere, and Kertesz, 1985; Shallice, 1988; and cases in Patterson, Coltheart and Marshall, 1985).

SUMMARY Evidence for each of the components of the reading system shown in figure 55.1 has been provided by studies of brain-damaged individuals whose patterns of performance across language tasks can be explained by assuming selective deficits for specific processing components. Thus, with regard to the question of the neural instantiation of the cognitive components of reading, these selective deficits constitute prima facie evidence that the cognitive operations of reading are instantiated in neural tissue with sufficient discreteness and independence that they can be selectively affected by brain lesions.

Cognitive mechanisms of spelling: Are they shared with reading?

One possibility is that spelling to dictation is simply the reverse of oral reading. According to such a hypothesis, spelling an auditorily presented word entails access to the lexical phonological representation of the word, followed by access to its semantic representation, and then to its orthographic representation. Similarly, when spelling an unfamiliar word or pseudoword (or when reading a word, if access to any of the lexical components has been disrupted), sublexical phonology-to-orthography conversion processes, consisting of the reverse operation of the orthography-to-phonology mechanism, are employed to yield a phonologically plausible spelling ("one" → W-U-N). On this account, the representations activated for written language production in spelling are just those activated during written language comprehension in reading (Allport and Funnell, 1981; Coltheart and Funnell, 1987; Behrmann and Bub, 1992) (figure 55.2). This organization has the appeal of parsimony. An alternative, however, is that reading and spelling share

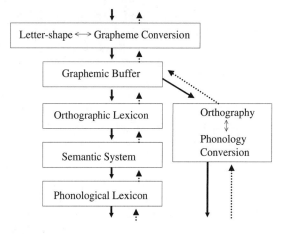

FIGURE 55.2 The shared-components account of the cognitive processes underlying reading and writing. Black arrows show access for reading; broken arrows show access for spelling.

only a common, amodal semantic system (see figure 55.1), and that all of the other processes are specific to reading or spelling.

It would seem to be a straightforward matter to adjudicate between these accounts: the association of deficits of reading and spelling would favor the shared-components account, while the dissociation of reading and spelling deficits would favor the independent-components account. However, associations can be interpreted under an independent-components account as arising from coincidental damage to components instantiated in neighboring neural substrates, so that brain damage would generally affect both regions or neither region. Furthermore, dissociations can be interpreted under a shared-components account as arising from deficits in the procedures involved in *accessing* the relevant components rather than from deficits affecting the components themselves (Allport and Funnell, 1981). The latter hypothesis is illustrated in figure 55.2, where the different arrow types indicate that reading and spelling may involve distinct procedures for accessing the same components. In that case, if access to a component is affected for reading, it may be intact for spelling, or vice versa. Therefore, evidence stronger than the mere association or dissociation of impairments is critical. More fine-grained similarities or differences regarding specific errors types, rates, and distributions would constitute more compelling evidence of shared or independent components. In the next section we review the relevant evidence, highlighting instances where this sort of more detailed information is available.

A SHARED SEMANTIC SYSTEM? Evidence that a single semantic system is shared by reading and writing comes from studies of patients who have impaired sublexical mechanisms for reading or spelling and who make essentially identical semantic errors across oral and written naming, oral reading, spelling to dictation, and comprehension (Hillis et al., 1990; Dickerson and Johnson, in press). Because there is strong evidence for a single semantic system shared across written/spoken and input/output modalities of language (Riddoch et al., 1988), we will not discuss this issue further.[1]

---

[1] Lexical-semantic impairments have been attributed to lesions or dysfunction of left posterior, superior temporal lobe in a variety of chronic lesion studies (Hart and Gordon, 1990; see Goodglass and Wingfield, 1997, for review), acute stroke studies (Hillis, Wityk et al., 2001), and temporary lesion studies (Lesser et al., 1986), whether lexical-semantic functions are studied with oral or written input or output. Functional imaging studies also show activation of this region during a variety of word comprehension tasks (Chertkow et al., 2000; Wise et al., 1991, 2001). These results are, therefore, also consistent with the hypothesis that lexical-semantic representations are shared by reading and writing.

A SHARED ORTHOGRAPHIC LEXICON? One piece of evidence indicating that a single set of lexical orthographic representations is used in both reading and spelling comes from reports of individuals who exhibit a high degree of consistency in the specific words that give rise to errors in both reading and spelling (Coltheart and Funnell, 1987; Behrmann and Bub, 1992; Friedman and Hadley, 1992). However, this high degree of consistency might be explained by an independent-components account if it is assumed that the factors that determine the likelihood of lexical access are the same for reading and spelling. For example, both input and output orthographic lexicons might well be sensitive to similar factors such as word frequency. Under conditions of damage, this would result in difficulty with low-frequency words in reading and spelling. Problematic to this interpretation, however, are studies reporting item-specific consistency even when factors such as word length and frequency have been partialed out (Coltheart and Funnell, 1987; Berhrmann and Bub, 1992).

Another source of evidence favoring shared orthographic representations comes from the treatment of acquired reading and spelling impairments. To illustrate, patient P.S.'s performance on reading and spelling tasks could be accounted for by assuming impairment affecting lexical orthographic representations used in both reading and spelling (Hillis, 1993). He could read aloud and spell pseudowords (e.g., filt) normally but made "regularization" errors in reading and spelling real, irregular words (e.g., *bread* read as "breed" and "bread" spelled as *bred*). In addition, he made homophone confusions in both reading and spelling. For example, he read *stake* correctly but understood it as meat from a cow. When trained to match written homophones to their definitions, he improved not only in reading comprehension but also in spelling the trained words; however, he showed no change in reading comprehension or spelling of untrained homophones. These results cannot be explained if the reading and spelling difficulties resulted simply from coincidental damage to nearby brain regions subserving independent components of reading and spelling.

A shared-components account must, however, also be able to account for reports of dissociations involving orthographic representations in reading but not spelling, and vice versa. In fact, these can fairly readily be understood as arising from difficulties in accessing lexical orthographic representations either from vision (in reading) or from semantics (in spelling), rather than from damage to a single lexicon.

For example, the dissociation of reading and spelling, often referred to as "alexia without agraphia" or "letter-by-letter reading" can be explained by assuming impaired access to orthographic representations from visual input. For instance, patient M.J., described by Chialant and Caramazza (1998), had excellent spelling abilities despite very impaired single-word reading. Although he could not understand written words, he could understand the same words if the letters were spelled aloud to him. His vision was intact in the left hemifield, but he typically could recognize words (with some errors) only after slowly reading the individual letters of the word. Most patients described with this pattern of performance have had lesions in the left occipital lobe, and the splenium of the corpus callosum. As a result, all visual information is initially processed in the right occipital lobe, and their performance can be explained by impaired transfer of visual representations in the right occipital lobe to the left hemisphere for oral production (for similar interpretations, see Dejerine, 1892; Geschwind, 1965; Damasio and Damasio, 1986; Chialant and Caramazza, 1998). Other, less anatomically based accounts similarly propose that this performance can be accounted for by impaired coupling of visual information and more abstract graphemic representations (Montant, Nazir, and Poncet, 1998).

A shared-components account must also be able to explain cases of impaired access to orthographic representations for spelling but not reading. These cases have been interpreted by positing impaired access to lexical orthographic representations specifically from semantics; such a deficit creates difficulties in spelling but leaves oral reading intact (Hillis, Rapp, and Caramazza, 1999).

In sum, for the orthographic lexicon, the finding of item consistency and remediation generalization across reading and spelling constitutes fairly strong positive evidence that lexical orthographic knowledge is shared in reading and spelling. Additionally, the reported dissociations between reading and spelling can also be readily accommodated within a shared-components framework.

SHARED SUBLEXICAL MECHANISMS? The case for shared sublexical mechanisms is considerably weaker. First, there are potentially problematic computational considerations. Namely, for many languages (e.g., English and French), orthography-phonology and phonology-orthography mappings are not symmetrical. In these languages there is far greater unpredictability (greater incidence of one-to-many mappings) in the conversion of sounds to letters (spelling) than in the mapping of letters to sounds (reading). For example, in English F is read as /f/ with 0.99 probability, while /f/ is spelled as F with only 0.78 probability. For this reason, simple bidirectional links weighted with the probabilities of the phoneme-grapheme mapping cannot be assumed. These facts create difficulties for the proposal that the phonology-to-orthography conversion process is simply the orthography-to-phonology conversion process operating in reverse.

With regard to the neuropsychological evidence, individuals who are unable to read pseudowords are generally unable to spell pseudowords. The French-speaking patient M.L.B. (Tainturier, 1996; Tainturier and Rapp, 2001) not only had associated difficulties in reading and spelling nonwords, she produced a very unusual error type on both tasks, and the distribution of error types across tasks was virtually identical. Nonetheless, a number of striking dissociations have been reported. For example, patient R.G. (Beauvois and Derousne, 1981) could spell pseudowords with 99% accuracy but was very poor in reading pseudowords despite relatively preserved reading of words. In contrast, patient M.H. (Bub and Kertesz, 1982) read three-letter pseudowords with 90% accuracy but was unable to spell any pseudowords. In order to account for these dissociations under a shared-components account, the selective inability to use sublexical mechanisms in one modality must be attributable to deficits arising before or after sublexical conversion systems and must not affect the processing of word stimuli. For example, a problem in phonological segmentation or in "holding" the phonological representation in a phonological buffer could be responsible for failures in spelling pseudowords but not actual words only if spelling words places fewer demands on such a buffer. Similarly, difficulties in "blending" sounds could account for selective impairment in orally reading pseudowords, if blending is more demanding for pseudowords than for words.

Despite the intriguing associations that have been reported, the computational issues and the absence of specific evidence supporting access accounts of the observed dissociations weaken the case for a shared phonology-to-orthography conversion process.

A SHARED GRAPHEMIC BUFFER? In addition to the central components of reading and spelling depicted in figures 55.1 and 55.2, there are additional, more peripheral components. One of these is the graphemic buffer, discussed fairly extensively in the context of spelling. In spelling (see figure 55.1), the grapheme string retrieved from the orthographic lexicon, or assembled via phonology-to-orthography conversion processes, must be held in short-term memory by the graphemic buffer while individual graphemes are converted to specific letter shapes for written spelling or to letter names for oral spelling. Evidence for a graphemic buffer comes from individuals who make similar errors in spelling across input and output modalities (oral and written spelling to dictation, written naming, and even delayed copying of words) and across stimulus types (words and pseudowords, irregular and regular words, low- and high-frequency words; Caramazza et al., 1987; Posteraro, Zinelli, and Mazzocchi, 1988; Caramazza and Miceli, 1990). Errors take the form of letter deletions, insertions, substitutions, and transposition, and, importantly, increase as a function of the length of the word. A length effect is expected, because longer stimuli place greater demands on a limited buffer.

The graphemic buffer might also be used in reading (see figure 55.2), where it would serve to maintain the activation of graphemes while they await identification in the orthographic lexicon or await sublexical processing (Tainturier and Rapp, 2003). It has been hypothesized that the demands on the graphemic buffer are greater for pseudoword reading than for word reading on the assumption that pseudoword reading requires greater serial processing of the buffered graphemic representations. In support of the shared buffer proposal, Tainturier and Rapp (2003) reported the case of M.C., who exhibited the classic symptoms of a graphemic buffer impairment in spelling, and also showed a strikingly similar pattern of performance in reading pseudowords. His spelling and reading exhibited length effects that were statistically indistinguishable across tasks. He also produced identical error rates and extremely similar distributions of error types across tasks.

In summary, although there is some rather striking evidence in its favor, the proposal of a shared buffer for reading and spelling is a relatively recent one. It is possible that clear and problematic dissociations have yet to be reported (see Posteraro, Zinelli, and Mazzucchi, 1998).

SHARED REPRESENTATIONS OF LETTER SHAPES? Disrupted selection of letter shapes for written spelling is manifested by letter substitutions in written spelling, such as "lamb" spelled as *lamd* and "tree" spelled as *tbee*, with relatively spared oral spelling (Zangwill, 1954; Kinsbourne and Rosenfield, 1974; Rothi and Heilman, 1981; Black et al., 1989; Rapp and Caramazza, 1997). In the reported cases there was no generalized motor problem or apraxia to explain these errors, and letters were well formed. These deficits have been ascribed to disrupted translation of abstract graphemes to letter shapes or to the letter-shape representations themselves. If these processes or representations used in spelling are shared by reading, then individuals with these spelling deficits should have similar difficulties in translating letter shapes to graphemes in reading. Rapp and Caramazza (1997) examined the abilities of two subjects with letter-shape selection deficits in spelling to perform input tasks such as matching letters across font (a/a) and case (a/A). One subject performed this task normally (100%), while the other one performed it poorly (78% correct). In addition, of three other patients described in the literature with apparently similar deficits in written spelling, two had spared letter recognition (Black et al., 1989; Lambert et al., 1994), and one was impaired (Rapp and Caramazza, 1989). Insofar as the literature reveals both associated and dissociated abilities in processing letter shapes in reading and spelling, more detailed evidence than simple accuracy rates would be useful. In one case of associated deficits (Rapp and Caramazza, 1997), the distribution of error types in letter recognition and in letter production were clearly distinct, thus weakening the case for shared letter-shape representations or shape-to-grapheme conversion processes.

SUMMARY Although the arguments are not unassailable, a reasonably strong case can be made for a shared orthographic lexicon (as well as a shared semantic system) in reading and spelling. However, with regard to the other components of written language comprehension and production, reliable dissociations and an absence of the necessary detailed counterevidence suggest that we should assume at least some differences in the component processes or representations.

Neural substrates of reading and spelling

Given the important difficulties of interpretation discussed in the previous section, evidence regarding the neural substrates that support the specific processing components of reading and spelling may provide additional relevant evidence regarding the overlap of components. Under a shared-components account, if there are particular brain regions that are essential for both reading and spelling, then damage to those regions should result in impairments in both reading and spelling. Similarly, those regions should be activated in reading and spelling, as documented by functional imaging.

Unfortunately, there are few if any lesion or functional imaging studies that directly provide the necessary evidence, because these studies investigate the neural regions involved in either one task or the other, but not both. However, by comparing studies that provide evidence of the neural substrates of particular components of each task, we can examine commonalities and differences. Even this goal is limited, because few studies have clearly identified the neural basis of individual components of either reading or writing, and there are conflicting results reported across studies.

One problem concerns the limitations of each of the current methodologies for identifying structure-function relationships. The most commonly used method is the chronic deficit-lesion correlation approach. The rationale of this approach is straightforward: If months or years after a stroke, a person can do all aspects of a language task except component X, the region of the brain affected by the stroke must be responsible for component X. The weaknesses are that (1) most patients with chronic deficits have large strokes covering numerous brain regions, and (2) there may be extensive reorganization of structure-function relationships after brain damage, such that other brain areas take over functions of the part that was damaged. Thus, if a patient recovers all but component X, it is difficult to determine which part of the large lesion was actually responsible for component X. These limitations can be lessened by studying patients immediately after onset of stroke, which permits the study of patients with small strokes before reorganization or recovery. A second problem is that computed tomography or conventional magnetic resonance imaging (MRI) does not always reveal the entire area of dysfunctional tissue that may contribute to the deficits (Hillis, Wityk, et al., 2002; Love et al., 2002).

Functional neuroimaging techniques (e.g., positron emission tomography, functional MRI [fMRI], event-related potentials, magnetoencephalography) can also play an important role in identifying areas of the brain activated during a particular task. One interpretative difficulty is that areas of activation are not necessarily brain areas that are essential to a given cognitive operation. Therefore, activation studies are complementary to lesion studies.

Converging evidence from various imaging methods relating a specific region to a particular cognitive component would be ideal. However, localization of function is limited by our understanding of the cognitive operations themselves. Thus, some of the components we have discussed may actually entail a number of discrete underlying subprocesses that take place in different brain regions. If so, disparate brain regions would be associated with what was assumed to be a single processing component. For example, what we have termed letter-shape selection may involve activating a particular abstract letter shape, and then activating a motor plan to execute the movements required to write the letter shape. The fact that only the former would plausibly be shared by reading could account for the observed associations and dissociations between letter-shape selection in reading versus spelling. It could also account for reports of impaired letter-shape selection after lesions to quite different locations, including very small lesions in premotor cortex (Brodmann's area 6, or BA 6; Anderson, Damasio, and Damasio, 1990; Hillis, Kane, et al., 2002), and other lesions involving the left angular gyrus or occipital gyrus (Rapp and Caramazza, 1997; Rapcsak and Beeson, 2002; figure 55.3). Furthermore, one fMRI study comparing writing minus oral naming and writing minus tapping (which require letter-shape selection

and other spelling processes) showed activation in premotor cortex (BA 6), as well as in other areas (Katanoda, Yoshikawa, and Sugashita, 2001). The precise role of each of these areas in what are likely to be different subcomponents of the letter-shape selection process is unclear.

Given the paucity of studies that isolate specific components of the reading or spelling process in exploring the neural substrates of these tasks, we will focus our review on studies investigating the neural basis of the one component that has been most thoroughly investigated, the orthographic lexicon. However, although we discuss the orthographic lexicon as a unitary entity, it should be noted that different types of lexical orthographic representations may depend on separate or additional neural mechanisms. For example, there is evidence that the posterior frontal cortex may be more important for accessing the lexical orthographic (and phonological) representations of verbs than nouns in word production (see Hillis et al., 2003, for evidence from spelling). In addition, damage to this region results in greater difficulty reading verbs than nouns (Nadeau, Gonzalez Rothi, and Crosson, 2000). It is possible that this region may be necessary for selecting a particular morphological form of a verb (e.g., *walk* versus *walking*), whereas other regions may be essential for accessing the orthographic representation of the stem for both nouns and verbs. This example underscores the possibility that each of the components just described may have dissociable subcomponents that depend on different neural regions.

Evidence for neural substrates of the orthographic lexicon

Evidence from Lesion Studies Most chronic lesion studies of reading have reported that lesions in the left temporoparieto-occipital junction, particularly the angular

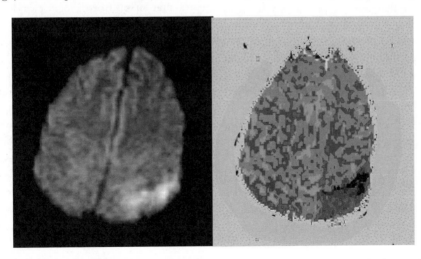

Figure 55.3 Diffusion-weighted (left) and perfusion-weighted (right) MR images taken 10 hours after the onset of stroke in a patient with selectively impaired access to the orthographic lexicon for reading and writing. The bright area on the diffusion-weighted image shows an acute infarct in the angular gyrus. The dark area on the perfusion-weighted image shows low blood flow in the angular gyrus. (See color plate 30.)

gyrus (BA 39), cause impairments in processing orthographic representations (Benson, 1979; Black and Behrmann, 1994). Similarly, in one study of acute stroke patients, infarct or low blood flow in the left angular gyrus was associated with impaired access to orthographic representations for reading (Hillis, Kane, Barker, et al., 2001). A description of a chronic stroke patient also demonstrated the association between low blood flow in the angular gyrus and impaired reading (Love et al., 2002).

With regard to spelling, lesions in the left angular gyrus (BA 39) have also been reported to be associated with impairments in processing orthographic representations for output in chronic stroke (Dejerine, 1892; Beauvois and Derouesne, 1981; Hatfield and Patterson, 1983; Roeltgen and Heilman, 1984; Vanier and Caplan, 1985; Goodman and Caramazza, 1986; Rapcsak and Beeson, 2002), as well as in acute stroke (Hillis, Kane, Jacobs, et al., 2001). Furthermore, in patients with Alzheimer's disease, impaired access to the orthographic lexicon in spelling (as manifested by impaired spelling of irregular but not regular words) has been associated with reduced metabolism in left angular gyrus (Peniello et al., 1995).

Taken together, these studies indicate that lesions of the left angular gyrus should consistently disrupt lexical orthographic representations in *both* reading and spelling. However, some patients with left angular gyrus lesions exhibit deficits in only one of these tasks. One possible explanation is that, in most reported cases, the individuals have been studied a long time after stroke, when they may have recovered function in either reading or writing (and other brain areas may have taken over the function, perhaps particularly in a trained task), creating an apparent dissociation between reading and spelling.[2] In support of this hypothesis, acute lesions of the angular gyrus generally disrupt both reading and spelling. To illustrate, the patient whose scans are shown in figure 55.3 had impaired access to orthographic representations in both reading and writing on day 1 of his stroke, when perfusion imaging showed low blood flow in left angular gyrus. At that time, although reading and spelling were impaired, auditory comprehension, oral naming, and spontaneous speech were not affected.

Lesions of other areas have also been shown to disrupt access to orthographic representations in reading. In particular, abnormalities in posteroinferior/middle temporal gyrus (lateral BA 37) have also been associated with impaired access to orthographic representations in reading in studies of acute stroke (Hillis, Kane, Barker, et al., 2001). Furthermore, Samuelsson (2000) reported a case in which an early

lesion in this area resulted in developmental dyslexia with impaired access to the orthographic lexicon but spared sublexical reading.

Similarly, in spelling, abnormalities of the left posteroinferior/middle temporal gyrus (lateral BA 37) are associated with impaired access to lexical orthographic representations for output (Patterson and Kay, 1982; Rapcsak, Rubens, and Laguna, 1990; Hillis, Kane, et al., 2002). Lesions to this area have also been implicated in certain cases of selective difficulty in spelling kanji (equivalent to lexical orthographic word forms) versus kana (Kawahata, Nagata, and Shishido, 1988; Soma et al., 1989; Sakurai et al., 1994).

In summary, studies of patients with both acute and chronic lesions have implicated the left angular gyrus (BA 39) and the posteroinferior/middle temporal areas (part of BA 37) in the processing of orthographic representations for both reading and spelling (figure 55.4). However, it is not yet understood in what ways these areas contribute differentially to written language processing.

EVIDENCE FROM FUNCTIONAL NEUROIMAGING INVESTIGATIONS There have been numerous functional neuroimaging studies of reading, and these have identified a large number of neural areas that are activated during reading (Petersen et al., 1988; Fiez and Petersen, 1998; Turkeltaub et al., 2002). However, studies that have attempted to isolate the regions most significant for orthographic representations have generally identified posteroinferior temporal-occipital regions that are largely coincident with those areas identified with orthographic representation in the lesion studies described in the previous section. Most studies have converged in identifying an area in the midportion of the left fusiform gyrus (part of BA 37, medial to the posteroinferior/middle temporal gyri) as especially activated in response to the visual presentation of words, legal pseudowords, and consonant strings, relative to nonalphabetic visual stimuli (Price et al., 1996; Puce et al., 1996; but see Howard et al., 1992). The area is active regardless of the spatial location of the stimuli (right or left visual field), is insensitive to typographic case, and displays quite reliable localization across subjects (e.g., Cohen et al., 2000, 2002; Dehaene et al., 2001, 2002). Furthermore, the area has been shown to be more sensitive to letters than digits (Polk et al., 2002) and selective for letters versus geometric shapes (Gros et al., 2001). Based on these characteristics it has been referred to as the visual word form area (VWFA).[3] Furthermore, this area has shown selective activation during visual presentation of kanji characters versus scrambled kanji (Uchida et al., 1999).

---

[2] Another explanation for this observation is that spelling and reading make use of distinct subareas within the angular gyrus.

[3] It may also be the basis for early latency (150–200 ms) electrical and magnetic signals recorded when subjects view written words (Nobre et al., 1995; Salmelin et al., 1996; Tarkiainen et al., 1999).

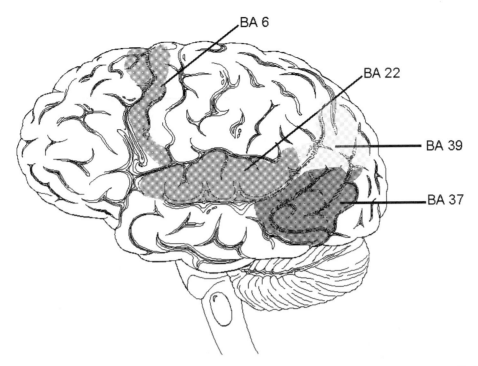

FIGURE 55.4 Schematic representation of the brain with the approximate locations of Brodmann's areas that are likely to be engaged in reading and spelling. (See color plate 31.)

Despite the converging evidence of activation of in this region, the specific functions of the VWFA are far from clear. Some functional neuroimaging studies have reported activation in this area when words are presented auditorily (Démonet et al., 1992, 1994; Chee et al., 1999; Buckner et al., 2000; Wise et al., 2000; Giraud and Price, 2001), in the tactile modality with blind subjects (Buchel, Price, and Friston, 1998), or with sign language in the deaf (Corina et al., in press). Others have found it to respond to visually but not auditorily presented words (Dehaene et al., 2002). The fact that the area is also responsive to Braille stimuli in the blind and to sign language in the deaf may indicate that either this area is available for representations in different modalities, depending on the specific circumstances of the individual (visually literate, blind, deaf), or that it serves to represent highly structured spatial representations that abstract away from modality.

A second important question concerns the content of the orthographic information represented in the VWFA. The fact that the area is strongly activated by both words and pseudowords and, at least in some studies, more so than by consonant strings (Price et al., 1996; Rees et al.,1999; Dehaene et al., 2002) has led to the suggestion that the VWFA is responsible for prelexical processing. Alternatively, the area could indeed represent the orthographic lexicon, which, at some point in the course of processing prior to lexical identification, may be equally activated by words and pseudowords.

In regard to spelling, functional neuroimaging studies involving alphabetic languages have also reported activation in part of BA 37 during tasks that require access to orthographic representations (Petrides, Alivisatos, and Evans, 1995; Rapp and Hsieh, 2001; Beeson et al., 2003). Beeson and colleagues specifically reported an activation focus that falls within the range of locations reported for reading by Cohen and colleagues (2002). However, the tasks used also involve other components of spelling, so it is not clear whether this activation is specific to accessing orthographic representations.

One puzzling finding is the relative absence of consistent angular gyrus (BA 39) activation during lexical orthographic processing in functional imaging studies, even though this site has been consistently identified as crucial for orthographic processing in lesion-deficit correlation studies of both spelling and reading. In an fMRI study of reading, Horowitz, Rusey, and Donohue (1998) did find evidence of correlated activity between angular gyrus and extrastriate occipital and temporal lobe regions during word reading, but such evidence is not common. In spelling, both Beeson and colleagues (2003) and Rapp and Hsieh (2001) reported that the majority, but not all, individual subjects show significant spelling-specific activation in the left angular gyrus. Thus, the left angular gyrus is inconsistently activated in reading and spelling tasks. Why this variability occurs is an intriguing question for future research.

SUMMARY The constraints on the shared components versus independent-components hypotheses provided by evidence of the neural substrates of the cognitive components of reading and spelling are very limited, although generally consistent with a shared-components account. With regard to chronic lesion studies, the limitations are due to the typically large size of lesions and the possibility of neural reorganization of function. Although acute lesion-deficit correlation studies can avoid these problems, few such studies have been reported. With regard to functional neuroimaging, there is a general paucity of studies designed to isolate specific components of reading and spelling processes. Only when such studies have been carried out will functional imaging contribute more significantly to determining whether reading and spelling share common neural and cognitive substrates.

Conclusions

To date, the bulk of the evidence regarding the relationship between written language comprehension and production has come from detailed case studies of brain-damaged individuals. This evidence, supported by the somewhat more limited observations regarding the neural substrates of written language processing, indicates that the most central and abstract aspects of our written language knowledge— semantic and lexical orthographic representations—are most likely shared for the purposes of written language comprehension and production. It is also apparent that conclusions regarding the shared or independent status of other representations and processes must await further evidence. Researchers' ability to develop this evidence awaits both more sophisticated techniques for investigating brain structure and activity and a better understanding of the cognitive operations required for written language processing.

Framing these results with the larger question of the relationship between perception and action, or between comprehension and production, leads to the question of whether findings in written language processing reflect general principles of cognition/brain organization, or whether literacy represents a special case. Unlike spoken language, vision, or navigation, literacy is generally considered to be an evolutionarily recent skill. For this reason, written language processing, like driving, playing chess, or playing the piano, is unlikely to have a specific genetic blueprint for its neural instantiation. Nevertheless, an understanding of the principles of neural instantiation of older as well as more recent additions to the human repertoire is important not only in its own right, but also because of its contribution to our understanding of the limitations and possibilities of the modifiable and plastic aspects of human cortex.

ACKNOWLEDGMENTS This work was supported in part by NIH grant RO1 DC05375 (A.H.)

REFERENCES

ALLPORT, D. A., and E. FUNNELL, 1981. Components of the mental lexicon. *Philos. Trans. R. Soc. Lond. B* 295:397–410.

ANDERSON, S. W., A. R. DAMASIO, and H. DAMASIO, 1990. Troubled letters but not numbers: Domain specific cognitive impairments following focal damage in frontal cortex. *Brain* 113:749–766.

BEAUVOIS, M. F., and J. DEROUESNE, 1979. Phonological alexia: Three dissociations. *J. Neurol. Neurosurg. Psychiatry* 42:115–1124.

BEAUVOIS, M. F., and J. DEROUSNE, 1981. Lexical or orthographic agraphia. *Brain* 104:21–49.

BEESON, P. M., S. Z. RAPCSAK, E. PLANTE, J. CHARGUALAF, A. CHUNG, S. C. JOHNSON, and T. P. TROUARD, 2003. The neural substrates of writing: A functional magnetic resonance imaging study. *Aphasiology* 17:647–665.

BEHRMANN, M., and D. BUB, 1992. Surface dyslexia and dysgraphia: Dual routes, single lexicon. *Cogn. Neuropsychol.* 9:209–251.

BENSON, D. F., 1979. *Aphasia, Alexia, and Agraphia.* New York: Churchill Livingstone.

BLACK, S., and M. BEHRMANN, 1994. Localization in alexia. In *Localization and Neuroimaging in Neuropsychology,* A. Kertesz, ed. San Diego, Calif.: Academic Press.

BLACK, S. E., M. BEHRMANN, K. BASS, and P. HACKER, 1989. Selective writing impairment: Beyond the allographic code. *Aphasiology* 3:265–277.

BUB, D., A. CANCELLIERE, and A. KERTESZ, 1985. Whole-word and analytic translation of spelling to sound in a non-semantic reader. In *Surface Dyslexia,* K. E. Patterson, J. C. Marshall, and M. Coltheart, eds. London: Erlbaum.

BUB, D., and A. KERTESZ, 1982. Evidence for lexico-graphic processing in a patient with preserved written over oral single word naming. *Brain* 105:697–717.

BUCHEL, C., C. PRICE, and K. FRISTON, 1998. A multimodal language region in the ventral visual pathway. *Nature* 394:274–277.

BUCKNER, R. L., W. KOUTSTAL, D. L. SCHACTER, and B. R. ROSEN, 2000. Functional MRI evidence for a role of frontal and inferior temporal cortex in amodal components of priming. *Brain* 123:620–640.

CARAMAZZA, A., and A. E. HILLIS, 1990. Where do semantic errors come from? *Cortex* 26:95–122.

CARAMAZZA, A., and G. MICELI, 1990. The structure of orthographic representations. *Cognition* 37:243–297.

CARAMAZZA, A., G. MICELI, G. VILLA, and C. ROMANI, 1987. The role of the graphemic buffer in spelling: Evidence from a case of acquired dysgraphia. *Cognition* 26:59–85.

CHEE, M. W. L., K. M. O'CRAVEN, R. BERGIDA, B. R. ROSEN, and R. L. SAVOY, 1999. Auditory and visual word processing studied with fMRI. *Hum. Brain Mapp.* 7:15–28.

CHERTKOW, H., C. WHATMOUGH, S. MURTHA, D. BUB, D. FUNG, and D. GOLD, 2000. PET activation during picture naming in Alzheimer's disease. *Brain Lang.* 74:345–347.

CHIALANT, D., and A. CARAMAZZA, 1998. Perceptual and lexical factors in a case of letter-by-letter reading. *Cogn. Neuropsychol.* 15:167–201.

COHEN, L., S. DEHAENE, L. NACCACHE, S. LEHERICY, G. DEHAENE-LAMBERTZ, M. A. HENAFF, et al., 2000. The visual word form area: Spatial and temporal characterization of an initial stage of reading in normal subjects and posterior split-brain patients. *Brain* 123:291–307.

COHEN, L., S. LEHERICY, F. CHOCHON, C. LEMER, S. RIVAUD, and S. DEHAENE, 2002. Language-specific tuning of visual cortex? Functional properties of the visual word form area. *Brain* 125:1054–1069.

COLTHEART, M., and E. FUNNELL, 1987. Reading and writing: One lexicon or two? In *Language Perception and Production: Shared Mechanisms in Listening, Reading, and Writing.* D. A. Allport, D. G. Mackay, W. Prinz, and E. Scheerer, eds. London: Academic Press.

COLTHEART, M., K. PATTERSON, and J. C. MARSHALL, 1980. *Deep Dyslexia.* London: Routledge and Kegan Paul.

CORINA, D. P., L. SAN JOSE-ROBERTSON, A. GUILLEMIN, J. HIGH, and A. R. BRAUN (in press). Language lateralization in a bimanual language. *J. Cogn. Neurosci.*

DAMASIO, A. R., and H. DAMASIO, 1986. Hemianopia, hemiachromatopsia and the mechanisms of alexia. *Cortex* 22:161–169.

DECETY, J., and J. GREZES, 1999. Neural mechanisms subserving the perception of human actions. *Trends Cogn. Sci.* 3:172–178.

DEHAENE, S., G. LECLEC'H, J. B. POLINE, D. LEBIHA, and L. COHEN, 2002. The visual word form area: A prelexical representation of visual words in the fusiform gyrus. *Neuroreport* 13:321–325.

DEHAENE, S., L. NACCACHE, L. COHEN, D. L. BIHAN, J. F. MANGIN, J. B. POLINE, and D. RIVIERE, 2001. Cerebral mechanisms of word masking and unconscious repetition priming. *Nat. Neurosci.* 4:752–758.

DEJERINE, J., 1892. Contribution à l'étude anatomo-pathologique et clinique des différentes variétés de cécité verbale. *Mem. Soc. Biol.* 4:61–90.

DÉMONET, J.-F., F. CHOLLET, S. RAMSAY, D. CARDEBAT, J.-L. NESPOULOUS, R. WISE, et al. 1992. The anatomy of phonological and semantic processing in normal subjects. *Brain* 115:1753–1768.

DÉMONET, J.-F., C. PRICE, R. WISE, and R. S. FRACKOWIAK, 1994. A PET study of cognitive strategies in normal subjects during language tasks: Influence of phonetic ambiguity and sequence processing on phoneme monitoring. *Brain* 117:671–682.

DICKERSON, J., and H. JOHNSON (in press). Sub-types of deep dyslexia: A case study of central deep dyslexia. *Neurocase.*

FIEZ, J. A., and S. E. PETERSEN, 1998. Neuroimaging studies of word reading. *Proc. Natl. Acad. Sci. U.S.A.* 95:914–921.

FRIEDMAN, R. B., and J. A. HADLEY, 1992. Letter-by-letter surface alexia. *Cogn. Neuropsychol.* 9:185–208.

FUNNELL, E., 1983. Phonological processes in reading: New evidence from acquired dyslexia. *Br. J. Psychol.* 74:159–180.

GESCHWIND, N., 1965. Disconnection syndromes in animals and man. *Brain* 88:237–294, 585–644.

GIRAUD, A. L., and C. J. PRICE, 2001. The constraints functional neuroimaging palces on classical models of auditory word processing. *J. Cogn. Neurosci.* 13:754–765.

GOODGLASS, H., and A. WINGFIELD, 1997. Word-finding deficits in aphasia: Brain-behavior relations and symptomatology. In *Anomia,* H. Goodglass, ed. London: Academic Press.

GOODMAN, R. A., and A. CARAMAZZA, 1986. Phonologically plausible errors: Implications for a model of the phoneme-grapheme conversion mechanism in the spelling process. In *Proceedings of the International Colloquium on Graphemics and Orthography,* G. Augst, ed., pp. 300–325.

GROS, H., K. BOULANOUAR, G. VIALLARD, E. CASSOL, and P. CELSIS, 2001. Event-related functional magnetic resonance imaging study of the extrastriate cortex response to a categorically ambiguous stimulus primed by letters and familiar geometric figures. *J. Cereb. Blood Flow Metab.* 21:1330–1341.

HART, J., and B. GORDON, 1990. Delineation of single-word semantic comprehension deficits in aphasia, with anatomical correlation. *Ann. Neurol.* 27:226–231.

HATFIELD, F. M., and K. PATTERSON, 1983. Phonological spelling. *Q. J. Exp. Psychol.* 35a:451–468.

HILLIS, A. E., 1993. The role of models of language processing in rehabilitation of language impairments. *Aphasiology* 7:5–26.

HILLIS, A. E., and A. CARAMAZZA, 1991. Mechanisms for accessing lexical representations for output: Evidence from a category-specific semantic deficit. *Brain Lang.* 40:106–144.

HILLIS, A. E., and A. CARAMAZZA, 1995. The compositionality of lexical-semantic representations: Clues from semantic errors in object naming. *Memory* 3:333–358.

HILLIS, A. E., A. KANE, P. BARKER, N. BEAUCHAMP, and R. WITYK, 2001. Neural substrates of the cognitive processes underlying reading: Evidence from magnetic resonance perfusion imaging in hyperacute stroke. *Aphasiology* 15:919–931.

HILLIS, A. E., A. KANE, M. JACOBS, P. BARKER, N. BEAUCHAMP, R. WITYK, and B. GORDON, 2001. Neural substrates of the cognitive processes underlying writing: Evidence from MR perfusion and diffusion imaging in hyperacute stroke. *Neurology* 56(Suppl 3):A158–A159.

HILLIS, A. E., A. KANE, E. TUFFIASH, N. BEAUCHAMP, P. B. BARKER, M. A. JACOBS, and R. WITYK, 2002. Neural substrates of the cognitive processes underlying spelling: Evidence from MR diffusion and perfusion imaging. *Aphasiology* 16:425–438.

HILLIS, A. E., B. C. RAPP, and A. CARAMAZZA, 1999. When a rose is a rose in speaking but a tulip in writing. *Cortex* 35:337–356.

HILLIS, A. E., B. C. RAPP, C. ROMANI, and A. CARAMAZZA, 1990. Selective impairment of semantics in lexical processing. *Cogn. Neuropsychol.* 7:191–244.

HILLIS, A. E., R. J. WITYK, P. B. BARKER, N. J. BEAUCHAMP, P. GAILLOUD, K. MURPHY, O. COOPER, and E. J. METTER, 2002. Subcortical aphasia and neglect in acute stroke: The role of cortical hypoperfusion. *Brain* 125:1094–1104.

HILLIS, A. E., R. WITYK, P. B. BARKER, and A. CARAMAZZA, 2003. Neural regions essential for writing verbs. *Nat. Neurosci.* 6:19–20.

HILLIS, A. E., R. J. WITYK, E. TUFFIASH, N. J. BEAUCHAMP, M. A. JACOBS, P. B. BARKER, and O. A. SELNES, 2001. Hypoperfusion of Wernicke's area predicts severity of semantic deficit in acute stroke. *Ann. Neurol.* 50:561–566.

HOROWITZ, B., J. M. RUSEY, and B. C. DONOHUE, 1998. Functional connectivity of the angular gyrus in normal reading and dyslexia. *Proc. Nat. Acad. Sci. U.S.A.* 95:8939–8944.

HOWARD, D., and V. ORCHARD-LISLE, 1984. On the origin of semantic errors in naming: Evidence from a case of a global aphasic. *Cogn. Neuropsychol.* 1:163–190.

HOWARD, D., K. PATTERSON, R. WISE, W. D. BROWN, K. FRISTON, C. WEILLER, and R. FRACKOWIAK, 1992. The cortical localization of the lexicons. *Brain* 115:1769–1782.

KATANODA, K., K. YOSHIKAWA, and M. SUGASHITA, 2001. A functional MRI study on the neural substrates for writing. *Hum. Brain Mapp.* 13:34–42.

KAWAHATA, N., K. NAGATA, and F. SHISHIDO, 1988. Alexia with agraphia due to the left posterior inferior temporal lobe lesion: Neuropsychological analysis and its pathogenetic mechanisms. *Brain Lang.* 33:296–310.

KINSBOURNE, M., and D. B. ROSENFIELD, 1974. Agraphia selective for written spelling. *Brain Lang.* 1:215–225.

LAMBERT, J., F. VIADER, F. EUSTACHE, and P. MORIN, 1994. Contribution to peripheral agraphia: A case of post-allographic impairment? *Cogn. Neuropsychol.* 11:35–55.

LESSER, R., M. LUDERS, N. DINNER, D. S. DINNER, G. KLEM, J. HAHN, and M. HARRISON, 1986. Electrical stimulation of Wernicke's area interferes with comprehension. *Neurology* 36:658–663.

LIBERMAN, A. M., and I. G. MATTINGLY, 1985. The motor theory of speech perception revisited. *Cognition* 21:1–36.

Love, T., D. Swinney, E. Wong, and R. Buxton, 2002. Perfusion imaging and stroke: A more sensitive measure of the brain bases of cognitive deficits. *Aphasiology* 16:873–883.

Marshall, J. C., and F. Newcombe, 1973. Patterns of paralexia: A psycholinguistic approach. *J. Psycholinguist. Res.* 2:175–199.

McCarthy, R. A., and E. K. Warrington, 1986. Phonological reading: Phenomena and paradoxes. *Cortex* 22:359–380.

Meltzoff, A. N. 1999. Origins of theory of mind, cognition and communication. *J. Commun. Disord.* 32:251–269.

Montant, M., T. A. Nazir, and M. Poncet, 1998. Pure alexia and the viewing position effect in printed words. *Cogn. Neuropsychol.* 15(1/2):93–140.

Nadeau, S. E., L. J. Gonzalez Rothi, and B. Crosson, 2000. *Aphasia and Language: Theory to Practice.* New York: Guilford Press.

Nobre, A. C., T. Allison, and G. McCarthy, 1994. Word recognition in the human inferior temporal lobe, *Nature* 372:260–263.

Patterson, K. E., and M. A. Lambon-Ralph, 1999. Selective disorders of reading? *Curr. Opin. Neurobiol.* 9:235–239.

Patterson, K. E., and J. Kay, 1982. Letter-by-letter reading: Psychological descriptions of a neurological syndrome. *Q. J. Exp. Psychol.* 34A:411–441.

Patterson, K. E., M. Coltheart, and J. C. Marshall, 1985. *Surface Dyslexia.* London: LEA.

Peniello, M.-J., J. Lambert, F. Eustache, M. C. Petit-Taboué, L. Barré, F. Viader, P. Morin, B. Lechevalier, and J.-C. Baron, 1995. A PET study of the functional neuroanatomy of writing impairment in Alzheimer's disease: The role of the left supramarginal and angular gyri. *Brain* 118:697–707.

Petersen, S. E., P. T. Fox, M. I. Posner, M. Mintun, and M. E. Raichle, 1988. Positron emission tomography studies of the cortical anatomy of single word processing. *Nature* 331:585–589.

Petrides, M., B. Alivisatos, and A. C. Evans, 1995. Functional activation of the human ventrolateral frontal cortex during mnemonic retrieval of verbal information. *Proc. Natl. Acad. Sci. U.S.A.* 92:5803–5807.

Plaut, D., and T. Shallice, 1993. Deep dyslexia: A case study in connectionist neuropsychology. *Cogn. Neuropsychol.* 10:377–500.

Polk, T. A., M. Stallcup, G. K. Aguirre, D. C. Aslop, M. D'Esposito, J. A. Detre, and M. J. Farah, 2002. Neural specialization for letter recognition. *J. Cogn. Neurosci.* 14:145–159.

Posteraro, L., P. Zinelli, and A. Mazzucchi, 1988. Selective impairment of the graphemic buffer in acquired dysgraphia: A case study. *Brain Lang.* 35:274–286.

Price, C. J., R. J. Wise, E. A. Warburton, C. J. Moore, D. Howard, K. Patterson, et al. 1996. Hearing and saying: The functional neuro-anatomy of auditory word processing. *Brain* 119:919–931.

Puce, A., T. Allison, M. Asgari, J. C. Gore, and G. McCarthy, 1996. Differential sensitivity of human visual cortex to faces, letterstrings, and textures: A functional magnetic resonance imaging study. *J. Neurosci.* 16:5205–5215.

Rapcsak, S. Z., and P. M. Beeson, 2002. Neuroanatomical correlates of spelling and writing. In *Handbook of Adult Language Disorders: Integrating Cognitive Neuropsychology, Neurology, and Rehabilitation,* A. E. Hillis, ed. Philadelphia: Psychology Press, pp. 71–99.

Rapcsak, S. Z., A. B. Rubens, and J. F. Laguna, 1990. From letters to words: Procedures for word recognition in letter-by-letter reading. *Brain Lang.* 38:504–514.

Rapp, B. C., L. Benzing, and A. Caramazza, 1997. The autonomy of lexical orthographic representations. *Cogn. Neuropsychol.* 14:71–104.

Rapp, B., and A. Caramazza, 1989. Letter processing in reading and spelling: Some dissociations. *Read. Writ. Interdiscip. J.* 1:13–33.

Rapp, B. C., and A. Caramazza, 1997. From graphemes to abstract letter shapes: Levels of representation in written spelling. *J. Exp. Psychol. Hum. Percept. Perform.* 23:1130–1152.

Rapp, B., C. Epstein, and M. J. Tainturier, 2002. The integration of information across lexical and sublexical processes in spelling. *Cogn. Neuropsychol.* 19:1–29.

Rapp, B., and L. Hsieh, 2001. *Functional magnetic resonance imaging of the cognitive components of the spelling process.* Presented at the Cognitive Neuroscience Society Meeting, San Francisco, Calif.

Rees, G., C. Russell, C. D. Frith, and J. Driver, 1999. Inattentional blindness versus inattentional amnesia for fixated but ignored words. *Science* 286:2504–2507.

Reuter-Lorenz, P. A., and J. L. Brunn, 1990. A prelexical basis for letter-by-letter reading: A case study. *Cogn. Neuropsychol.* 7: 1–20.

Riddoch, M. J., 1991. *Neglect and the Peripheral Dyslexias.* London: Erlbaum.

Riddoch, M. J., G. W. Humphreys, M. Coltheart, and E. Funnell, 1988. Semantic systems or system? Neuropsychological evidence re-examined. *Cogn. Neuropsychol.* 5:3–25.

Rizzolatti, G., L. Fadiga, V. Gallese, and L. Goassi, 1996. Premotor cortex and the recognition of motor actions. *Cogn. Brain Res.* 3:131–141.

Roeltgen, D. P., and K. M. Heilman, 1984. Lexical agraphia: Further support for the two strategy hypothesis of linguistic agraphia. *Brain* 107:811–827.

Rothi, L. J., and K. M. Heilman, 1981. Alexia and agraphia with spared spelling and letter recognition abilities. *Brain Lang.* 12:1–13.

Saffran, E. M., and H. B. Coslett, 1998. Implicit vs. letter-by-letter reading in pure alexia: A tale of two systems. *Cogn. Neuropsychol.* 15(1/2):141–165.

Sakurai, Y., K. Sakai, M. Sakuta, and M. Iwata, 1994. Naming difficulties in alexia with agraphia for kanji after a left posterior inferior temporal lesion. *J. Neurol. Neurosurg. Psychiatry* 57: 609–613.

Salmelin, R., E. Service, P. Kiesila, K. Uutela, and O. Salonen, 1996. Impaired visual word processing in dyslexia revealed with magnetoencephalography. *Ann. Neurol.* 40:157–162.

Samuelsson, S., 2000. Converging evidence for the role of occipital regions in orthographic processing? A case of developmental surface dyslexia. *Neuropsychologia* 38:351–362.

Seidenberg, M., and J. L. McClelland, 1989. A distributed, developmental model of visual word recognition and naming. *Psychol. Rev.* 96:523–568.

Shallice, T., 1988. *From Neuropsychology to Mental Structure.* Cambridge, England: Cambridge University Press.

Soma, Y., M. Sugishita, K. Kitamura, S. Maruyama, and H. Imanaga, 1989. Lexical agraphia in the Japanese language: Pure agraphia for Kanji due to left posteroinferior temporal lesions. *Brain* 112:1549–1561.

Sugishita, M., Y. Takayama, T. Shiono, K. Yoshikawa, and Y. Takahashi, 1996. Functional magnetic resonance imaging (fMRI) during mental writing with phonograms. *Neuroreport* 7:1917–1921.

Tainturier, M. J., 1996. Phonologically-based errors and their implications in the specification of phonology to orthography conversion processes. *Brain Cogn.* 32:148–151.

Tainturier, M. J., and B. Rapp, 2001. Spelling words. In *What Deficits Reveal about the Human Mind/Brain: A Handbook of Cognitive Neuropsychology,* B. Rapp, ed. Philadelphia: Psychology Press.

Tainturier, M. J., and B. Rapp, 2003. Is a single graphemic buffer used in reading and spelling? *Aphasiology* 17:537–562.

TARKIAINEN, A., P. HELENIUS, P. C. HANSEN, P. L. CORNELISSEN, and R. SALMELIN, 1999. Dynamics of letter string perception in the human occipitotemporal cortex. *Brain* 122:2119–2132.

TURKELTAUB, P. E., G. F. EDEN, K. M. JONES, and T. A. ZEFFIRO, 2002. Meta-analysis of the functional neuroanatomy of single-word reading: Method and validation. *NeuroImage* 16:765–780.

UCHIDA, I., H. KIKYO, K. NAKAJIMA, S. KONISHI, K. SEKIHARA, and Y. MIYASHITA, 1999. Activation of lateral extrastriate areas during orthographic processing of Japanese characters studied with fMRI. *NeuroImage* 9:208–215.

WISE, R. J. S., F. CHOLLET, U. HADAR, K. FRISTON, E. HOFFNER, and R. FRACKOWIAK, 1991. Distribution of cortical neural networks involved in word comprehension and word retrieval. *Brain* 114:1803–1817.

WISE, R. J. S., S. K. SCOTT, C. BLANK, C. J. MUMMERY, K. MURPHY, and E. A. WARBUTON, 2001. Separate neural subsystems within "Wernicke's area." *Brain* 124:83–95.

VANIER, M., and D. CAPLAN, 1985. CT correlates of surface dyslexia. In *Surface Dyslexia: Neuropsychological and Cognitive Studies of Phonological Reading*, K. E. Patterson, J. C. Marshall, and M. Coltheart, eds. London: Erlbaum.

ZANGWILL, O. L., 1954. Agraphia due to a left parietal glioima in a left-handed man. *Brain* 77:510–520.

ZIHL, J., 1995. Eye movement patterns in hemianopic dyslexia. *Brain* 118:891–912.

56 The Neural Basis of Syntactic Processes

ANGELA D. FRIEDERICI

ABSTRACT Due to a growing body of neuroscientific data, our knowledge concerning the neural basis of syntactic processes has advanced considerably. Findings from brain imaging studies suggest that syntactic processes are supported by a fronto-temporal network consisting of the frontal operculum, the posterior portion of Broca's area, and the superior temporal gyrus (STG). Evidence from electroencephalographic and magnetoencephalographic studies with healthy adults and patients, together with results from functional brain imaging, allow a functional specification of the different areas within the network. The frontal operculum and the anterior portion of the STG subserve processes of local structure building, whereas the posterior portion of the STG seems to be involved in the integration of syntactic and semantic information. Broca's area, in particular its posterior portion, comes into play when long-distance dependencies in complex syntactic structures are to be processed.

The ability to process language, and more specifically the capability of comprehending sentence structures, has been claimed to be uniquely human (Hauser, Chomsky, and Fitch, 2002; Sakai, Homai, and Hashimoto, 2003). Language comprehension depends not only on understanding the meaning of words but also, and crucially, on understanding the relations between different words (e.g., nouns and verbs) in a sentence. These relations are most relevant because they signal who is doing what to whom in the sentence. They are indicated by syntactic structures whose basic architecture is considered to be hierarchical. Online sentence comprehension must therefore be viewed as a process that extracts these structural hierarchies from sequential input. The underlying structure of a simple sentence such as example 1 is shown in figure 56.1. The sentence (S) is made up of a noun phrase (NP), which is the subject, and a verb phrase (VP), consisting of the verb (V) and a noun phrase that is the object.

(1) *The man greets the boy.*

The processing system can rely on a number of different information types that specify the hierarchical structure. These vary from language to language. Some languages, such as English, have a relatively fixed word order signaling the grammatical relations, such as subject (*man*) and object

(*boy*) in sentence 1. Other languages, such as German, have a relatively free word order and signal subjecthood and objecthood either by case marking in the article, for example nominative (NOM) and accusative (ACC), respectively, in sentence 2, or by subject-verb agreement in the case of ambiguous case marking (i.e., feminine noun phrase), such as singular (SING) and plural (PLUR) in sentences 3a and 3b.

(2a) *Der Mann* (NOM) *gruesst den* (ACC) *Jungen.*
      The (NOM) *man greets the* (ACC) *boy.*

(2b) *Den* (ACC) *Jungen grüßt der* (NOM) *Mann.*
      The (ACC) *boy greets the* (NOM) *man.*
      (The man greets the boy.)

(3a) *Die Professorinnen* (PLUR) *gruessen* (PLUR) *die Frau* (SING).
      The professors (PLUR) *greet* (PLUR) *the woman* (SING).

(3b) *Die Frau* (SING) *gruessen* (PLUR) *die Professorinnen* (PLUR).
      The woman (SING) *greet* (PLUR) *the professors* (PLUR).
      (The professors greet the woman.)

Since the subject has to agree in number with the verb, it is clear that in examples 3a and 3b, *die Professorinnen/the professors* is the subject of the sentence. Thus, different languages have different means to express information about syntactic structure. The human language processing system deals with these different languages quite easily.

The cognitive architecture of the language processing system, however, is still a matter of debate (see Frauenfelder and Tyler, 1987; Altmann, 1990; Pickering, Clifton, and Crocker, 2000). Although some researchers assume syntactic processes to be modular and to precede semantic processes in time (e.g., Frazier, 1978, 1987a,b; De Vincenzi, 1991; Gorrell, 1995), others view comprehension as a highly interactive, online process (e.g., Marslen-Wilson and Tyler, 1980; McClelland, John, and Taraban, 1989; MacDonald, Pearlmutter, and Seidenberg, 1994a,b; Trueswell and Tanenhaus, 1994). The crucial difference between the two views concerns the time course in which syntactic and semantic information interact: The so-called serial or

ANGELA D. FRIEDERICI Max Planck Institute for Human Cognitive and Brain Sciences, Leipzig, Germany.

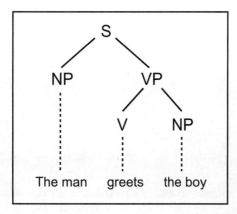

FIGURE 56.1 Hierarchical structure of a simple subject-verb-object sentence. Abbreviations: S, sentence; NP, noun phrase; VP, verb phrase.

syntax-first approach does not allow interaction during the initial stage of phrase structure building, but only during a later stage of processing, whereas the interactive approach holds that interaction takes place during all processing stages. Each of these views can call on ample empirical evidence from behavioral studies conducted on healthy participants. Therefore it is difficult to describe the cognitive architecture of the language processing system on the basis of these data alone.

Data from cognitive neuroscience serve as an additional source of empirical information, helping to outline the structure of the language comprehension system. There are at least four methods that provide relevant findings. Two methods allow the time course of neural activity to be traced, electroencephalography (EEG) and magnetoencephalography (MEG). Two other methods allow neural activity to be localized, functional magnetic resonance imaging (fMRI) and positron emission tomography (PET). Although the value of event-related potential (ERP) and field (ERF) data for modeling the time structure of language comprehension processes seems obvious, imaging data contribute to the debate on the cognitive architecture of the processing system in more indirect ways. Using imaging data to draw conclusions about cognitive architectures presupposes that functionally distinct processes are subserved by distinct brain systems. Under this presupposition, distinct brain activity patterns may be viewed as support for domain specificity. However, this presupposition has to be specified even further: here it is assumed that domain specificity can only be claimed if the activation pattern as a whole—that is, the entire neural network, and not selective parts of it—is specifically activated in response to a given task. Single brain areas within such a pattern may well be activated by other cognitive tasks as part of a different neural network and thus cannot be considered to be domain-specific in isolation. For example, Broca's area, which is activated together with other areas in syntactic tasks (Kaan and Swaab,

2002), is also activated during the processing of sequential information in nonlanguage domains (for a review see Schbotz and von Cramon, 2002), although in a network comprising different areas than those reported for language. Thus it appears that this area receives its specificity in distinct neural networks. Another approach to specifying language-brain relationships correlates particular brain lesions either with specific behavior or with specific brain activity patterns as measured by the different technologies.

In this chapter, I review data from the different methodological approaches, focusing on first, the description of the neural network responsible for syntactic processes, and second, the time course of syntactic processes.

The neural network for syntactic processes

The number of functional neuroimaging studies investigating sentence processing with a focus on syntactic processes has increased over the last several years. Early studies compared brain activation during the comprehension of sentences or short passages with resting baseline conditions or nonlanguage control conditions (e.g., Lechevalier et al., 1989; Mazoyer et al., 1993; Bottini et al., 1994; Bavelier et al., 1997; Müller et al., 1997). These studies found activation in a broadly distributed network of areas in the perisylvian region. One of these studies, however, investigated sentence processing and the processing of random word lists (including function words and content words). In this study, the left inferior frontal gyrus (IFG) and the left superior temporal gyrus (STG) were found to be active in the word list condition, and the left temporal pole and the left STG were found to be active in the sentence condition (Mazoyer et al., 1993). More recent studies have focused more directly on syntactic processes.

The various studies reported in the literature will be discussed with respect to three different aspects of syntactic processing: (1) the processing of syntactic violations, (2) the processing of syntactic structure as compared with word lists, and (3) the interaction of syntactic complexity with syntactic memory (i.e., the memory necessary to process long-distance syntactic dependencies). Only studies that deal with these issues at the sentence level are considered. The main areas of activation for these different studies are shown in figure 56.2.

SYNTACTIC VIOLATIONS Syntactic violations have been investigated in a number of fMRI experiments. Ni and colleagues (2000) investigated syntactic and semantic violations during visual sentence processing and observed a number of brain areas similarly active in both conditions. These areas included bilaterally, the IFG (BA 44, 45, and 47), the middle frontal gyri (BA 46/49), and the STG and MTG. However, no region specific for the processing of syntactic violations

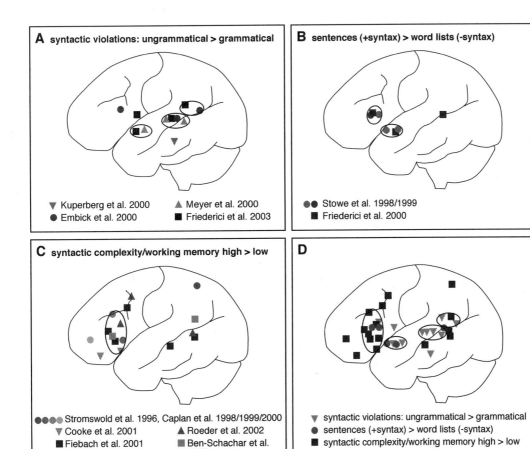

FIGURE 56.2   Main activations of the different sentence-level syntactic processing studies discussed in the text. (*A*) Activation foci for the processing of syntactic violations. (*B*) Activation for sentences versus word lists. (*C*) Activation foci for sentences of high syntactically complex and high syntactic memory demand. (*D*) Activation foci for all studies. (See color plate 32.)

could be identified. Kuperberg and colleagues (2000), comparing syntactic, semantic, and pragmatic violations, also found no area specifically activated by syntactic violations. More recently, Moro and colleagues (2001) reported a PET study on the processing of syntactic violations during visual sentence comprehension. In this study, however, pseudoword sentences were used. Activation of the anterior portion of the left insula and the right homolog of Broca's area (BA 44/45) was reported to be selectively increased for the violation conditions (i.e., word order violation and subject-verb agreement violation) compared with activation during presentation of the correct condition.

Meyer, Friederici, and von Cramon (2000) used syntactically correct and syntactically incorrect auditorily presented sentences. They observed stronger activation for incorrect than for correct sentences, mainly in the left temporal regions (i.e., planum polare, Heschl's gyrus, and planum temporale); a much weaker effect was observed in the frontal operculum. A recent study used an auditory event-related fMRI design (Friederici, Rüschemeyer, et al., 2003) to investigate the processing of syntactic and semantic violations. Both violation types caused increased activation in the pos-

terior portion of the left STG. Syntactic phrase structure violations revealed specific involvement of the anterior portion of the left STG and the left operculum adjacent to BA 44, as well as the putamen in the basal ganglia.

In a PET study, Indefrey and colleagues (2001) investigated the processing of syntactic errors in meaningless sentences using different syntactic and nonsyntactic tasks. Stimuli were presented visually in a whole-sentence format. They found that an area of the left dorsolateral prefrontal cortex, adjacent to Broca's area, is specifically involved in the detection of syntactic errors.

Embick and colleagues (2000) used an error detection paradigm in which subjects had to detect misspelled words or syntactic errors in sentences. They reported larger activation for the grammatical task in Broca's area as compared to Wernicke's area or the angular and supramarginal gyri. They interpreted this result as suggesting selective involvement of Broca's area in syntactic processing.

The definition of Broca's area normally does include BA 44 and 45 (Aboitiz and Garcia, 1997; Amunts et al., 1999). However, the cytoarchitectonic data from Amunts and colleagues (1999) suggest a possible functional distinction between the two Brodmann areas. Amunts and colleagues (1999) analyzed the laminar distributions of cell densities vertical to the cortical surface and found a systematic left-over-right asymmetry of all densities for BA 44, but not for BA 45 in the ten brains that were investigated. They suggest that the observed morphological asymmetry of BA 44 might provide a putative correlate for language function. More recently, they reported (Amunts et al., 2003) a differential developmental pattern for the two brain areas, with BA 45 reaching a left-over-right asymmetry at the age of 5 years and BA 44 reaching a left-over-right asymmetry only at the age of 11 years.

With the goal of specifying different subregions of Broca's area, namely, the pars opercularis (BA 44) and the pars triangularis (BA 45), Newman and colleagues (2003) conducted an fMRI study using different violation types. They compared violations of subject-verb agreement with violations due to an extra verb in the sentence (e.g., *The coach watched the poet and told the visitor took in the evening*). Increased activation in the pars opercularis was found for subject-verb agreement violation, whereas increased activation in the pars triangularis was observed for sentences with the extra verb. It is assumed that in the latter condition, thematic processing is hampered owing to the extra verb, whereas in the former condition, syntactic processing is tapped.

SYNTAX VERSUS WORD LISTS Friederici, Meyer, and von Cramon (2000) investigated syntactic processes in an auditory fMRI study by systematically varying the presence of semantic and syntactic information in the input. Participants had to judge whether the stimulus contained a syntactic structure and/or content words. Normal sentences and syntactically structured nonsense sentences (Jabberwocky), that is, the two conditions in which syntax was present, activated the anterior portion of the STG (planum polare) selectively, compared with the processing of word lists. Moreover, activation of the deep frontal operculum adjacent to BA 44, which was maximal in the left hemisphere, was observed only in the Jabberwocky condition, the condition in which only syntactic information was available.

Stowe and colleagues (1998, 1999) conducted a PET study in which word lists were directly compared with sentences of different complexity and found that activation of the anterior portion of the STG increased with sentences of increasing complexity. This result suggests that this part of the STG plays a major role in syntactic processing.

From the studies discussed so far, it appears that syntactic violations in a sentence do not automatically give rise to a specific activation pattern in Broca's area. Rather, it appears that the online processing of local syntactic violations elicits activity in the left frontal operculum or left insula rather than in Broca's area itself, whereas a syntactic error detec-

tion task can activate Broca's area. The anterior portion of the STG, in contrast, seems to be activated more generally as a function of syntactic online processing. This conclusion is in agreement with a recent fMRI study by Humphries and colleagues (2001) that compared sentence processing with processing of a sequence of environmental sounds conveying meaning similar to that expressable in a sentence (e.g., a gunshot followed by the sound of someone running away) and found increased activation in the anterior STG for the sentences.

SYNTACTIC COMPLEXITY/SYNTACTIC MEMORY A number of PET and fMRI studies have attempted to specify those brain areas in which activation varies systematically as a function of syntactic complexity. By comparing syntactically complex with syntactically less complex sentences and keeping the lexical elements identical, researchers have sought to subtract lexical-semantic processes and to look at pure syntactic processes. The majority of these studies have been carried out in English, a language in which variation in syntactic complexity is often directly confounded by working memory demands. Caplan and collaborators (Stromswold et al., 1996; Caplan, Alpert, and Waters, 1998, 1999; Caplan et al., 2000), for example, compared the processing of visually presented subject relative clauses (4a) and object relative clauses (4b). Sentence 4b presents a sentence structure in which the object of the sentence, according to some well-established linguistic theories (e.g., Chomsky, 1981; 2000), is moved from its original position indexed by "____" and leaves a trace behind (original sentence form: *The child spilled the juice*). The subscript i indicates the relation between the trace and the moved element (*that*). It should be noted that there are linguistic theories that do not make this specific assumption of movement when describing relative clause constructions (for a recent review, see Goldberg, 2003). But within the framework chosen by Caplan and colleagues, the difference between a subject relative clause and an object relative clause is described as a difference in the dependency between an element's position in the original structure and in the actual structure, as indicated in sentences 4a and 4b.

(4a) *The child spilled the juice$_i$ that ____$_i$ stained the rug.* (subject first)

(4b) *The juice$_i$ that the child spilled ____$_i$ stained the rug.* (object first)

In a PET study, the authors reported focal activation in the left pars opercularis (BA 44) for object relative clauses compared with subject relative clauses (Stromswold et al., 1996; Caplan, Alpert, and Waters, 1998). In later studies using different sentence material (cleft object versus cleft subject sentences) or different tasks (concurrent articulation),

BA 45 was also reported to show increased activation for object-first sentences compared with subject-first structures (Caplan, Alpert, and Waters, 1999; Caplan et al., 2000).

Just and colleagues (1996) conducted an fMRI study in English using three types of sentences with different syntactic complexity: sentences in which two simple clauses were conjoined by *and*, sentences with center-embedded subject relative clauses, and sentences with center-embedded object relative clauses. They reported increased activation as a function of syntactic complexity in left Broca's area and left Wernicke's area, and to a lesser degree in their right hemisphere homologs. The authors attributed the increased activation to the amount of cognitive resources necessary to perform the task, which may also include aspects of working memory. Similar conclusions were reached in an fMRI investigation of the processing of simple and center-embedded sentences in Japanese (Inui et al., 1998), in which left inferior frontal regions (BA 44 and 45) as well as the premotor area were found to be active. For these two studies, unfortunately, no coordinates of the activation foci are available.

Fiebach, Schlesewsky, and Friederici (2001) reported a study of native German speakers in which two factors confounded in early studies on syntactic complexity were varied systematically. These two factors are syntactic complexity (subject-initial vs. object-initial structures) and the distance between the moved element (filler) and its trace (long vs. short). Applying an event-related fMRI technique, Fiebach and colleagues found that activation in the IFG, or BA 44 extending to BA 45, increased as a function of the filler–trace distance and not as a function of complexity. They concluded that this brain area appears to be correlated with syntactic working memory involved in processing long-distance dependencies rather than with parsing of syntactic complexity.

A very similar finding was reported for English sentences in which the relevant factors, namely, working memory and syntactic complexity, were varied independently (Cooke et al., 2001). This study compared filler–trace dependencies of different length (long vs. short, tapping the factor working memory) in constructions of different complexity (subject vs. object relative clauses, tapping the factor syntactic complexity). Significant activation in BA 44/45 was observed only when the distance of the filler and its trace was long (seven words), and not when it was short (three words). This result was taken to indicate an involvement of this brain area in processing long-distance syntactic dependencies.

The combined findings from German and English studies suggest that BA 44/45 supports processes involved in the comprehension of noncanonical sentence structures whose demands on syntactic working memory are higher than those of sentences with a canonical word order. This interpretation is based on the assumption that once the filler is identified, it is maintained in memory until the parser reaches the element's original position. In English, in sentences like 4a and 4b, the filler can be identified as soon as the element *that* is encountered. In German, case marking can signal whether a particular element is in its canonical position (an accusative marked NP in the sentence beginning is clearly not canonical, as the accusative marks the direct object). A recent electrophysiological study using case-marked NPs in sentences similar to those in the study by Fiebach, Schlewesky, and Friederici (2002) provides support for this interpretation, as the observed brain activation started when the filler was identified and ended when the original position was reached.

Syntactic Complexity and Other Linguistic Factors
Three additional studies should be discussed in the present context. These varied the factor syntactic complexity systematically, crossing it either with the factor meaningfulness (Roeder et al., 2002), with the factor verb complexity (Ben-Shachar et al., 2003), or directly comparing the processing of syntactic complexity with processing of syntactic violations (Fiebach et al., in press).

Roeder and colleagues (2002) compared the processing of simple German sentences with more complex sentences in which elements were moved from their original position in the sentence. The syntactically easy and difficult conditions were realized in sentences containing real words and in sentences in which content words were replaced by pseudowords. Syntactic difficulty had its strongest effect (i.e., increased activation) in the left IFG and the left STG and MTG. This effect was more pronounced in meaningful as compared with pseudoword sentences.

Using Hebrew, Ben-Shachar and colleagues (2003) investigated syntactic transformations, that is, the processing of embedded object relative clauses compared with the processing of embedded sentential complements. The factor syntactic transformation was crossed with the factor verb complexity. Syntactic transformations were found to be correlated with activation in the left IFG (Broca's region) and in the posterior superior temporal sulcus bilaterally. The left posterior temporal sulcus was affected specifically by verb complexity.

A recent fMRI study by Fiebach and colleagues (in press) in German compared the processing of sentences containing syntactic violations with the processing of syntactically complex sentences. Syntactic complexity was modulated by moving increasingly more words from their canonical position in the sentence to a less common but nevertheless acceptable position. The authors reported greater activation in the left operculum for syntactic violations and greater activation of BA 44/45 for syntactic complexity.

Summary The findings reviewed here suggest that the left IFG as well as the left STG is involved in syntactic processes

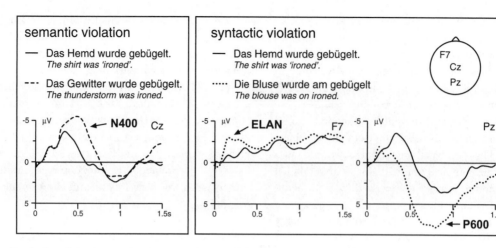

FIGURE 56.3 Examples of the three major language-related ERP components: N400, reflecting semantic processes, and ELAN and P600, reflecting syntactic processes.

(see figure 56.1). The left anterior portion of the STG appears to support online structure-building processes (figure 56.2*A*, *B*), with the anterior position possibly reflecting processes involved in accessing word category information (figure 56.2*B*). The posterior portion of the STG/STS seems to come into play during syntactic integration processes (figure 56.2*A*). The left IFG becomes active only under increased syntactic processing demands (figure 56.2*B*, *C*). Within the left IFG, two brain areas may be functionally separable: The left operculum appears to subserve local syntactic structure building (figure 56.2*B*), and the more superior and anterior portion of the IFG, namely BA 44/45, seems to support syntactic working memory (figure 56.2*C*) (which is presumably required to bridge the filler–trace distance).

The time course of syntactic processes

The time course of the neural activity related to syntactic processes can be measured by EEG, which registers the total postsynaptic electrical activity, and MEG, which registers its magnetic field. Event-related activity (ERP, ERF) is the brain's reaction to a particular stimulus type. In the language domain, different stimulus types have been shown to elicit ERP waveforms that are distinct with respect to their latency, amplitude, and topography.

One of these ERP components is known to reflect semantic processes. This component is a broadly distributed negativity in the waveform that peaks around 400 ms after the critical event. Because of its amplitude and latency, this component is designated N400. As this chapter is concerned with syntactic processes, I will not discuss this component in detail (for reviews, see Kutas and Van Petten, 1994; Kutas and Federmeier, 2000). It is important to keep in mind that the N400 has been interpreted functionally to reflect processes of semantic integration (Chwilla, Brown, and Hagoort, 1995).

With respect to syntactic processes, several different ERP effects have been reported: two transient ERP components and one sustained ERP effect. The two local components are (1) a left anterior negativity, which is present about 200–500 ms after a syntactically anomalous element, and (2) a bilaterally distributed positivity, which is present around 600 ms after the critical element (labeled P600, or sometimes the syntactic positive shift). An additional ERP effect observed in the context of syntactic processes is a sustained frontal negativity, maximal over the left hemisphere, that accumulates across the span of sentences whose comprehension demands syntactic memory. Examples of the N400, ELAN, and P600 are shown in figure 56.3. I will discuss each of the ERP components in turn.

LEFT ANTERIOR NEGATIVITY A number of studies have observed a left anterior negativity (LAN) as a function of syntactic processes.

The LAN as a marker of local phrase structure building Left anterior negativities have been found in the context of violations of local phrase structure, violations of subject-verb agreement, and violations of the verb argument structure. Some studies have found an early LAN, or ELAN (Friederici, 1995), between 150 and 200 ms, when the word category of the incoming element does not match the expectations based on the rules of the grammar (Neville et al., 1991; Friederici, Pfeifer, and Hahne, 1993; Hahne and Friederici, 1999; Hahne, 2001; Hahne and Jescheniak, 2001). Other studies investigating word category violation have reported an LAN that peaks somewhat later (Münte et al., 1993; Friederici, Hahne, and Mecklinger, 1996). The latency difference for this type of violation appears to be a function of when the relevant word category information is available to the parser. When this information is available early, owing to the fact that the word category information can be accessed rapidly, either in short function words as in example 5 (Neville et al., 1991) or in a prefix as in example 6 (Hahne and Friederici, 1999), the LAN occurs early, that is, with a short latency after word onset. Note that sentence 6 is incorrect, because the preposition obligatorily requires a noun (in the garden) to follow, but not a verb (in the greeted).

(5) *Max's of proof the theorem.

(6) *Der Präsident wurde im gegrüßt.
     The president was in the   greeted.

When the relevant information becomes available late in the critical word, for example, in the suffix of the main verb, as in 7a/7b (Friederici, Hahne, and Mecklinger, 1996) or only after accessing the entire lexical entry, as in 8a/8b (Münte et al., 1993), the latency of the word category-related LAN occurs 300 ms after word onset.

(7a) *Das Metall wurde zur veredelt.
      The metal was by the refined.

(7b) Veredelung
      refinement

(8a) *your write

(8b) your letter

More recently, a similar violation type was also investigated in Dutch (Hagoort, Wassenaar, and Brown, 2003). Word category violations were realized by presenting a verb in a noun position. Similar to previous studies, word category was marked in the suffix (schroef/propeller vs. schroeft/propelled). In this study, an anterior negativity between 300 and 500 ms with a bilateral instead of a left-lateralized distribution was observed.

Thus, the combined data suggest that the latency of the syntactic negativity elicited by a word category violation depends on the word category decision point.

It should be noted, however, that some studies have not found an LAN effect for presumed word category violations. In these studies, stimulus materials were created such that the crucial target word did not actually violate local syntactic word category-related rules; rather, it constituted a nonpreferred reading (Hagoort, Brown, and Groothusen, 1993; Ainsworth-Darnell, Shulman, and Boland, 1998). Therefore, it may not be surprising that no LAN was found.

LAN as a marker of morphosyntactic processes. The LAN between 300 and 500 ms after stimulus onset has been found in response to agreement violations in a number of different languages: for subject-verb agreement violations in

English (Kutas and Hillyard, 1983; Osterhout and Mobley, 1995), Dutch (Gunter, Stowe, and Mulder, 1997), German (Penke et al., 1997) and Italian (Angrilli et al., 2002); for article-noun gender agreement in German (Gunter et al., 2000); and for noun-verb gender agreement in Hebrew (Deutsch and Bentin, 2001).

Although a large number of studies across different languages consistently elicit an LAN in response to subject-verb agreement violations, two studies did not (Münte et al., 1997; Osterhout and Nicol, 1999). Münte and colleagues attributed the lack of an LAN effect to the "unobtrusive nature of the number mismatch." However, their material was ambiguous with respect to number marking of the target, and thus it is not clear that there was a local number mismatch. Osterhout and Nicol (1999) did report a "more negative-going" wave for the syntactic anomaly (tense violation) "over lateral sites, maximal over left anterior sites" in one experiment. In a follow-up experiment, ERPs were averaged over tense violation and reflexive-antecedent agreement violation. The averaged ERP did not reveal a reliable effect in the relevant time window (300–500 ms). Unfortunately, no separate ERPs for the different violation types were given. Thus, we cannot evaluate to what extent the ERP pattern was obscured by averaging two different violation types, namely, tense violation and reflexive-antecedent agreement violation, the latter of which is marked in pronominal elements. This, however, would be important, as the two violation types differ, in that the latter may be directly involved in thematic role assignment whereas the former is not. It is not unlikely that the two violation types elicit different ERP effects.

Verb argument processing. Violations of verb argument structure elicit an LAN under some conditions and an N400 under others. This may not be surprising, insofar as the argument structure of a verb specifies different aspects, namely, the number of arguments as well as the type of arguments a verb can take. However, only a few ERP studies have focused on this issue.

An LAN was observed in English for a noun phrase whose case marking indicated an argument position (i.e., subject) that was already occupied (Coulson, King, and Coutas, 1998), as in sentence 9.

(9) *The plane took we to paradise.

A study in German focused on two different aspects of verb argument structure information using the fact that, in German subordinate clauses, the verb is in clause-final position and thus occurs after all its arguments (Friederici and Frisch, 2000). An LAN was also found for the verb in sentence-final position when the preceding NPs did not match the argument structure required by the verb. For example, an LAN was elicited when the verb required a dative (DAT) marked NP (10b), and the preceding object NP was incorrectly marked accusative (ACC) instead (10a).

(10a) *Anna weiß, dass der Kommissar den₍ACC₎ Banker beistand.
       Anna knows, that the inspector the ₍ACC₎ banker helped.

(10b) Anna weiß, dass der Kommissar dem₍DAT₎ Banker beistand.
       Anna knows, that the inspector the₍DAT₎ banker helped.

However, an N400 was observed for the sentence-final verb when thematic role assignment was implausible, as in sentence 11, due to an incorrect number of arguments. In this example two arguments, *inspector* and *banker*, are presented instead of one, *inspector* (Friederici and Frisch, 2000). In such a sentence the second NP (*the banker*) cannot be assigned a thematic role, because the verb does not provide a free slot in its argument structure.

(11) *Anna weiß, dass der Kommissar₍NOM₎ denBanker₍ACC₎ abreiste.
      Anna knows that the inspector₍NOM₎ the banker₍ACC₎ left town.

The two violation types tap different aspects of verb argument structure information. Although the verb in sentence 10a is a two-place argument verb preceded by an incorrect morphosyntactically marked NP, the verb in sentence 11 is a one-place argument verb preceded by two arguments, both requiring thematic implementation—which, however, cannot be fulfilled. These two different aspects—morphosyntactic in one case and thematic in the other—appear to be reflected in two ERP component, the LAN and the N400, respectively.

In more recent studies, an N400 component was observed systematically in German sentences with case marking errors that signaled impossible thematic role assignment (Frisch and Schlesewsky, 2001). In languages with case marking, thematic roles and thereby semantic roles can be derived directly from the case itself. Bornkessel (2002) proposes that in heavily case-marked languages such as German, the parser must implement two parallel processing routes, one route that considers case whenever unambiguous and maps thematic roles directly on the basis of case information and another route that is used when noun phrases are marked ambiguously. The latter route considers other types of syntactic information, such as word order or subject-verb agreement, to achieve thematic role assignment. Thus, whereas the two routes may be active in case-marked languages, only the latter will be active in languages without overt case marking.

Late Centroparietal Positivity   A late centroparietal positivity labeled P600 has been observed as a function of (1) ambiguous syntactic structures, (2) syntactic violations, and (3) syntactic complexity.

Ambiguous sentence structures   The P600 was first shown in response to the disambiguating element in a structurally ambiguous sentence (Osterhout and Holcomb, 1992, 1993; Osterhout et al., 1994; Mecklinger et al., 1995). Friederici and Mecklinger (1996) formulated the assumption that the latency of the positivity varies as a function of the difficulty of structural reanalysis. The motivation for this proposal was their finding of a very early positivity (P345) for nonpreferred object relatives compared to subject relatives in German, but a later positivity (P600) for difficult-to-revise object-first complement sentences compared to subject-first complement sentences. These studies demonstrated that the P600 was elicited by an element signaling a necessary reanalysis of an initially preferred sentence interpretation. The P600 was thus considered to reflect structural processing.

Syntactic violations   A P600 effect has also been reported in a number of studies in various languages for outright syntactic violations, namely, phrase structure violations (Neville et al., 1991; Friederici, Hahne, and Mecklinger, 1996), subjacency violations (Neville et al., 1991; McKinnon and Osterhout, 1996), and agreement violations (Friederici, Pfeifer, and Hahne, 1993; Hagoort, Brown, and Groothusen, 1993; Gunter, Stowe, and Mulder, 1997; Coulson, King, and Coutas, 1998; Deutsch and Bentin, 2001). In most of these cases the P600 was preceded by an LAN component as part of a biphasic pattern. It has been proposed that this pattern reflects two stages of syntactic processing, with the (E)LAN marking the processing of syntactic anomaly and the P600 signaling syntactic repair (Friederici, 1995, 2002).

Syntactic complexity   A few studies have investigated whether the P600 is tied to processing syntactic anomalies, be they syntactic violations or preference violations, or whether this component reacts more generally to syntactic difficulty. Kaan and colleagues (2000) found that the P600 varied as a function of syntactic difficulty of integration and argued that the P600 should be viewed as a marker of syntactic integration difficulty. Friederici, Hahne, and Saddy (2002) compared the late positivity in response to syntactic violations and in response to syntactic complexity and observed a difference in the distribution of the two effects: the P600 was distributed centroparietally for the violation condition and more frontally for the complexity condition. In sum, it appears that the P600 most generally marks difficulty of syntactic integration processes, but that different aspects of integration processes find different brain signatures within the late positivity.

SUSTAINED LEFT FRONTAL NEGATIVITY   An additional ERP effect observed in relation to syntactic variation is a sustained frontal negativity that is not elicited by a syntactic violation but is assumed to reflect processes of syntactic working memory that are presumably necessary for the processing of sentences in noncanonical word order.

King and Kutas (1995) observed a sustained frontal negativity across the sentence for object-relative compared to subject-relative sentences. Structurally, the object-relative sentence (12a) differs from the subject-relative sentence (12b) in that the first NP in the relative clause (*the senator*) is the object.

(12a)   *The reporter who the senator attacked admitted the error.*

(12b)   *The reporter who attacked the senator admitted the error.*

The processing of sentence 12a requires additional memory resources, because the first NP has to be kept in memory until its "original" position in the sentence (after the verb) is reached.

A similar sustained frontal negativity was found for German sentences in which the two factors syntactic complexity (subject-first versus object-first) and syntactic working memory (distance between filler and its trace) were varied independently (Fiebach et al., 2002). A sustained left frontal negativity was observed for object-first sentences in which the distance between the object-NP and its original position was long. This sustained negativity was present across the sentence, that is, for each word between object-NP (filler) and its trace.

The interpretation that the sustained left frontal negativity observed in these two studies is a function of syntactic memory necessary to process a moved element is supported by the finding that this negativity is modulated by individual differences in working memory capacities. In both studies, two subject groups were defined on the basis of the Reading Span Test by Daneman and Carpenter (1980). The amplitude of the sustained negativity was larger for subjects with a low memory span than for those with a high memory span (King and Kutas, 1995; Fiebach, Schlesewsky, and Friederici, 2002).

SUMMARY   There are two transient components and one sustained ERP component correlated with syntactic processes. The sustained left frontal negativity has been shown to be related to processes involving syntactic memory, which are necessary to cope with long-distance dependencies. The two transient ERP effects, (E)LAN and P600, have been attributed to different stages of online syntactic processes during comprehension. ELAN and LAN are seen as a function of local phrase-structure building and interphrasal assignment (agreement and verb argument assignment),

respectively, and P600 is taken to reflect late processes of syntactic integration.

Bridging space and time of neural activity

Given the low temporal resolution of fMRI different aspects of syntactic processing—early and late processes—are not easily pulled apart. An obvious question is how those data specifying the neural network underlying syntactic processes in the fMRI can be brought together with data indicating different stages of online syntactic processing as measured by ERPs. In principle, there are two ways. The first method is to use dipole modeling to identify the location of the sources of a given ERP component. This modeling approach, however, relies on mathematical procedures and must therefore be considered an indirect way. An alternative approach is to investigate patients with circumscribed brain lesions in ERP experiments and to interpret the absence or modulation of particular ERP components as a function of the locus of the brain lesion. Here the caveat is that brain lesions are sometimes not circumscribed enough to allow precise localization, and, moreover, recovery processes may have affected the brain's original functional organization. With these precautionary thoughts in mind, I now turn to results from these two approaches.

DIPOLE MODELING APPROACH   The spatial parameters for the early syntactic processes as reflected in the ELAN component, for example, are hard to specify, because this component is usually part of a biphasic ERP pattern with a P600 as its second part. The interpretation of P600 as a component reflecting late processes of syntactic reanalysis and integration clearly separates it from the ELAN functionally. The particular question of which brain areas support the early phrase-structure-building processes reflected by the ELAN was been approached by using different dipole modeling techniques applied to MEG data for the early time window in which the ELAN usually occurs (Friederici et al., 2000; Gross et al., 1998; Knösche, Maess, and Friederici, 1999). When fMRI constraints were applied for the dipole location, two dipoles were found in the left hemisphere: a larger dipole in the left temporal brain region and a smaller one in the left inferior frontal brain region in the time window reflecting the ELAN (Friederici et al., 2000). This finding suggests involvement of the left temporal cortex as well as the inferior frontal cortex during early structure-building processes.

This interpretation is supported by a recent independent fMRI study that used the same stimulus material as the MEG study by Friederici and colleagues (2000). The fMRI data indicated activation in the frontal operculum adjacent to the inferior portion of BA 44, the anterior portion of STG, and the most posterior portion of STG and the basal ganglia (Friederici, Kotz, et al., 2003). Thus, it is likely that the former two brain areas support early phrase-structure building and that the latter two brain areas are involved in late integration processes. Unfortunately, so far no study has been able to successfully dipole model the late syntactic processes, and therefore our interpretation of the brain basis of this ERP component must remain indirect.

PATIENT APPROACH   ERP studies of patients who have sustained brain damage provide additional evidence. Using the same stimulus material as in the MEG and the fMRI studies (Friederici et al., 2000, 2003), researchers have shown that patients with left frontal cortical brain lesions do not exhibit an ELAN component in response to a phrase structure violation, but only a P600 (Friederici, Hahne, and von Cramon, 1998; Friederici, von Cramon, and Kotz, 1999). In contrast, patients with lesions in the left basal ganglia (Friederici, von Cramon, and Kotz, 1999) and with dysfunction of the basal ganglia due to Parkinson's disease do show an ELAN component, but a reduced P600 component (Friederici, von Cramon, and Kotz, 1999; Friederici et al., 2003). Thus, it appears that the P600 may partly depend on intact basal ganglia.

SUMMARY   The available literature suggests that the neural network supporting syntactic processes involves the IFG, the STG, and the basal ganglia. The anterior portion of the STG and the frontal operculum seem to subserve early syntactic processes, Broca's area (BA 44/45) appears to support the processing of memory-demanding complex sentences, and the most posterior portion of the STG and possibly the basal ganglia are involved in processes of syntactic integration.

Implications for psycholinguistic models

ERP and imaging studies provide rich evidence for a distinction between different types of syntactic processes such as local phrase-structure building and syntactic integration, on the one hand, and lexical-semantic processes on the other. This chapter has focused on syntactic processes whose neural network and ERP signatures are clearly distinct from those of lexical-semantic processes. The neural network for syntactic processes involves the frontal operculum and BA 44/45 in the IFG, and the anterior portion of the STG together with the basal ganglia and the posterior portion of the STG. The neural network for semantic processes consists of BA 45/47 in the IFG and the posterior portion of the MTG, together with the posterior portion of the STG (for an overview, see Friederici, 2002). The finding that the posterior portion of the STG is involved in syntactic as well as semantic processes suggests that this area is a candidate for processes of late integration during which syntactic and semantic processes interact (Friederici et al., 2003). Thus it appears that the combined data support views that assume

a separation of syntactic and semantic processes (different networks), but also partly those views that propose an interaction between syntax and semantics (posterior STG activation present in both).

But the issue that crucially distinguishes the different psycholinguistic models, namely, syntax-first versus interactive models, is, the time interaction between syntax and semantics takes place. Empirical neuroscientific evidence allowing a tentative answer to this issue comes from recent ERP studies in which the factors of syntactic violation and semantic anomaly were completely crossed (Gunter, Stowe, and Mulder, 1997; Gunter, Friederici, and Schriefers, 2000; Hahne and Friederici, 2002). These studies demonstrated that the (E)LAN was present independently of the semantic factor but the P600 can vary as a function of both.

These data do not support strong versions of interactive models that assume that all types of information interact at all times during sentence processing. These findings clearly indicate that syntactic and semantic processes are independent during early processing stages, and that interaction takes place during a stage of late integration. The results are thus compatible with those models that claim an early independence of syntactic processes from lexical-semantic aspects, and allow late interactions.

Conclusion

The description of the neural basis of language is a clear example of how cognitive modeling and neuroscience can stimulate each other. Neuroimaging needs input from cognitive models, in this case psycholinguistics, in order to be able to pose the right questions (and to construct the crucial material). Modeling psycholinguistic functions in turn can fruitfully use the input from neuroscience to constrain crucial aspects of the cognitive architecture of the language system.

REFERENCES

ABOITIZ, F., and R. GARCIA, 1997. The evolutionary origin of the language areas in the human brain: A neuroanatomical perspective. *Brain Res. Rev.* 25:381–396.

AINSWORTH-DARNELL, K., H. G. SHULMAN, and J. E. BOLAND, 1998. Dissociating brain responses to syntactic and semantic anomalies: Evidence from event-related brain potentials. *J. Mem. Lang.* 38:112–130.

ALTMANN, G. T. M., 1990. *Cognitive Models of Speech Processing: Psycholingutistic and Computational Perspectives.* Cambridge, Mass.: MIT Press.

AMUNTS, K., A. SCHLEICHER, U. BÜRGEL, H. MOHLBERG, H. B. M. UYLINGS, and K. ZILLES, 1999. Broca's region re-visited: Cytoarchitecture and intersubject variability. *J. Comp. Neurol.* 412:319–341.

AMUNTS, K., A. SCHLEICHER, A. DITTERICH, and K. ZILLES, 2003. Broca's region: Cytoarchitectonic asymmetry and developmental changes. *J. Comp. Neurol.* 465:72–89.

ANGRILLI, A., B. PENOLAZZI, F. VESPIGNANI, M. DE VINCENZI, R. JOB, L. CICCARELLI, D. PALOMBA, and L. STEGAGNO, 2002. Cortical brain responses to semantic incongruity and syntactic violation in Italian language: An event-related potential study. *Neurosci. Lett.* 322:5–8.

BAVELIER, D., D. CORINA, P. JEZZARD, S. PADMANABHAN, V. P. CLARK, A. KARNI, A. PRINSTER, A. BRAUN, A. LALWANI, J. P. RAUSCHECKER, R. TURNER, and H. NEVILLE, 1997. Sentence reading: A functional MRI study at 4 Tesla. *J. Cogn. Neurosci.* 9:664–686.

BEN-SHACHAR, M., T. HENDLER, I. KAHN, D. BEN-BASHAT, and Y. GRODZINSKY, 2003. The neural reality of syntactic transformations: Evidence from fMRI. *Psychol. Sci.* 14:433–440.

BORNKESSEL, I., 2002. *The argument dependency model: A neurocognitive approach to incremental interpretation.* Doctoral diss., University of Potsdam, MPI Series in Cognitive Neuroscience, no. 28.

BOTTINI, G., R. CORCORAN, R. STERZI, E. PAULESU, P. SCHENONE, P. SCARPA, R. FRACKOWIAK, and C. FRITH, 1994. The role of right hemisphere in interpretation of figurative aspects of language: A positron emission tomography activation study. *Brain* 117:1241–1253.

CAPLAN, D., N. ALPERT, and G. WATERS, 1998. Effects of syntactic structure and propositional number on patterns of regional cerebral blood flow. *J. Cogn. Neurosci.* 10:541–552.

CAPLAN, D., N. ALPERT, and G. WATERS, 1999. PET studies of syntactic processing with auditory sentence presentation. *NeuroImage* 9:348–351.

CAPLAN, D., N. ALPERT, G. WATERS, and A. OLIVIERI, 2000. Activation of Broca's area by syntactic processing under conditions of concurrent articulation. *Hum. Brain Mapp.* 9:65–71.

CHOMSKY, N., 1981. *Lectures on Government and Binding.* Dordrecht, The Netherlands: Foris.

CHOMSKY, N., 2000. *New Horizons in the Study of Language and Mind.* Cambridge, England: Cambridge University Press.

CHWILLA, D. J., C. BROWN, and P. HAGOORT, 1995. The N400 as a function of the level of processing. *Psychophysiology* 32:274–285.

COOKE, A., E. B. ZURIF, C. DEVITA, D. ALSOP, P. KOENIG, J. DETRE, J. GEE, M. PINANGO, J. BALOGH, and M. GROSSMAN, 2001. Neural basis for sentence comprehension: Grammatical and short-term memory components. *Hum. Brain Mapp.* 15:80–94.

COULSON, S., J. KING, and M. KUTAS, 1998. Expect the unexpected: Event-related brain responses of morpho-syntactic violations. *Lang. Cogn. Processes* 13:21–58.

DANEMAN, M., and P. A. CARPENTER, 1980. Individual differences in working memory and reading. *J. Verb. Learn. Verb. Behav.* 19: 77–103.

DE VINCENZI, M., 1991. *Syntactic parsing Strategies in Italian: The Minimal Chain Principle (Studies in Theoretical Psycholinguistics,* vol. 12). Dordrecht, The Netherlands: Kluwer Academic Publishers.

DEUTSCH, A., and S. BENTIN, 2001. Syntactic and semantic factors in processing gender agreement in Hebrew: Evidence from ERPs and eye movements. *J. Mem. Lang.* 45:200–224.

EMBICK, D., A. MARANTZ, Y. MIYASHITA, W. O'NEIL, and K. L. SAKAI, 2000. A syntactic specialization for Broca's area. *Pro. Nat. Acad. Sci. U.S.A.* 97:6150–6154.

FIEBACH, C. J., A. D. FRIEDERICI, K. MÜLLER, and D. Y. VON CRAMON, 2002. fMRI evidence for dual routes to the mental lexicon in visual word recognition. *J. Cogn. Neurosci.* 14:11–23.

FIEBACH, C. J., M. SCHLESEWSKY, and A. D. FRIEDERICI, 2002. Separating syntactic memory costs and syntactic integration costs during parsing: The processing of German WH-questions. *J. Mem. Lang.* 47:250–272.

FIEBACH, C. J., M. SCHLESEWSKY, I. D. BORNKESSEL, D. Y. VON CRAMON, and A. D. FRIEDERICI (in press). Distinct neural correlates of legal and illegal word order variations in German: How can fMRI inform cognitive models of sentence processing? In *The On-line Study of Sentence Comprehension,* M. Carreiras and C. Clifton, eds. Hove: Psychology Press, pp. 357–370.

FRAUENFELDER, U. H., and L. K. TYLER, 1987. The process of spoken word recognition: An introduction. *Cognition* 25:1–20.

FRAZIER, L., 1978. *On Comprehension Sentences: Syntactic Parsing Strategies.* Doctoral diss., University of Connecticut, Storrs.

FRAZIER, L., 1987a. Sentence processing: A tutorial review. In *Attention and Performance XII: The Psychology of Reading,* M. Coltheart, ed. London: Erlbaum.

FRAZIER, L., 1987b. Theories of sentence processing. In *Modularity in Knowledge Representation and Natural-Language Processing,* J. Garfield, ed. Cambridge, Mass.: MIT Press.

FRIEDERICI, A. D., 1995. The time course of syntactic activation during language processing: A model based on neuropsychological and neurophysiological data. *Brain Lang.* 50: 259–281.

FRIEDERICI, A. D., 2002. Towards a neural basis of auditory sentence processing. *Trends Cogn. Sci.* 6:78–84.

FRIEDERICI, A. D., and S. FRISCH, 2000. Verb-argument structure processing: The role of verb-specific and argument-specific information. *J. Mem. Lang.* 43:476–507.

FRIEDERICI, A. D., A. HAHNE, and A. MECKLINGER, 1996. The temporal structure of syntactic parsing: Early and late event-related brain potential effects elicited by syntactic anomalies. *J. Exp. Psychol. Learn. Mem. Cogn.* 22:1219–1248.

FRIEDERICI, A. D., A. HAHNE, and D. SADDY, 2002. Distinct neurophysiological patterns for aspects of syntactic complexity and syntactic repair. *J. Psycholinguist. Res.* 31:45–63.

FRIEDERICI, A. D., A. HAHNE, and D. Y. VON CRAMON, 1998. First-pass versus second-pass parsing processes in a Wernicke's and a Broca's aphasic: Electro-physiological evidence for a double dissociation. *Brain Lang.* 62:311–341.

FRIEDERICI, A. D., S. A. KOTZ, K. WERHEID, G. HEIN, and D. Y. VON CRAMON, 2003. Syntactic comprehension in Parkinson's disease: Investigating early automatic and late integrational processes using event-related brain potentials. *Neuropsychology* 17:133–142.

FRIEDERICI, A. D., and A. MECKLINGER, 1996. Syntactic parsing as revealed by brain responses: First-pass and second-pass parsing processes. *J. Psycholinguist. Res.* 25:157–176.

FRIEDERICI, A. D., M. MEYER, and D. Y. VON CRAMON, 2000. Auditory language comprehension: An event-related fMRI study on the processing of syntactic and lexical information. *Brain Lang.* 74:289–300.

FRIEDERICI, A. D., E. PFEIFER, and A. HAHNE, 1993. Event-related brain potentials during natural speech processing: Effects of semantic, morphological and syntactic violations. *Cogn. Brain Res.* 1:183–192.

FRIEDERICI, A. D., S.-A. RÜSCHEMEYER, A. HAHNE, and C. J. FIEBACH, 2003. The role of left inferior frontal and superior temporal cortex in sentence comprehension: Localizing syntactic and semantic processes. *Cereb. Cortex* 13:170–177.

FRIEDERICI, A. D., D. Y. VON CRAMON, and S. A. KOTZ, 1999. Language related brain potentials in patients with cortical and subcortical left hemisphere lesions. *Brain* 122:1033–1047.

FRIEDERICI, A. D., Y. WANG, C. S. HERRMANN, B. MAESS, and U. OERTEL, 2000. Localization of early syntactic processes in frontal and temporal cortical areas: A magnetoencephalographic study. *Hum. Brain Mapp.* 11:1–11.

FRISCH, S., and M. SCHLESEWSKY, 2001. The N400 reflects problems of thematic hierarchizing. *Neuroreport* 12:3391–3394.

GOLDBERG, A. E., 2003. Constructions: A new theoretical approach to language. *Trends Cogn. Sci.* 7:219–224.

GORRELL, P., 1995. *Syntax and Parsing*. Cambridge, England: Cambridge University Press.

GROSS, J., A. A. IOANNIDES, J. DAMMERS, B. MAESS, A. D. FRIEDERICI, and H.-W. MÜLLER-GÄRTNER, 1998. Magnetic field tomography analysis of continuous speech. *Brain Topogr.* 10:273–281.

GUNTER, T. C., A. D. FRIEDERICI, and H. SCHRIEFERS, 2000. Syntactic gender and semantic expectancy: ERPs reveal early autonomy and late interaction. *J. Cogn. Neurosci.* 12:556–568.

GUNTER, T. C., L. A. STOWE, and G. MULDER, 1997. When syntax meets semantics. *Psychophysiology* 34:660–676.

HAGOORT, P., C, BROWN, and J. GROOTHUSEN, 1993. The syntactic positive shift as an ERP measure of syntactic processing. *Lang. Cogn. Processes* 8:39–483.

HAGOORT, P., M. WASSENAAR, and C. M. BROWN, 2003. Syntax-related ERP-effects in Dutch. *Cogn. Brain Res.* 16:38–50.

HAHNE, A., and A. D. FRIEDERICI, 2002. Differential task effects on semantic and syntactic processes as revealed by ERPs. *Cogn. Brain Res.* 13:339–356.

HAHNE, A., and A. D. FRIEDERICI, 1999. Electrophysiological evidence for two steps in syntactic analysis: Early automatic and late controlled processes. *J. Cogn. Neurosci.* 11:194–205.

HAHNE, A., and J. D. JESCHENIAK, 2001. What's left if the Jabberwocky gets the semantics? An ERP investigation into semantic and syntactic processes during auditory sentence comprehension. *Cogn. Brain Res.* 11:199–212.

HAUSER, M. D., N. CHOMSKY, and T. W. FITCH, 2002. The faculty of language: What is it, who has it, and how did it evolve? *Science* 298:1569–1579.

HUMPHRIES, C., K. TOMLINSON, B. BUCHSBAUM, and G. HICKOK, 2001. Role of anterior temporal cortex in auditory sentence comprehension: An fMRI study. *Neuroreport* 12:1749–1752.

INDEFREY, P., P. HAGOORT, H. HERZOG, R. J. SEITZ, and C. M. BROWN, 2001. Syntactic processing in left prefrontal cortex is independent of lexical meaning. *NeuroImage* 14:546–555.

INUI, T., Y. OTSU, S. TANAKA, T. OKADA, S. NISHIZAWA, and J. KONISHI, 1998. A functional MRI analysis of comprehension processes of Japanese sentences. *Neuroreport* 9:3325–3328.

JUST, M. A., P. A. CARPENTER, T. A. KELLER, W. F. EDDY, and K. R. THULBORN, 1996. Brain activation modulated by sentence comprehension. *Science* 274:114–116.

KAAN, E., A. HARRIS, E. GIBSON, and P. HOLCOMB, 2000. The P600 as an index of syntactic integration difficulty. *Lang. Cogn. Processes* 15:159–201.

KAAN, E., and T. Y. SWAAB, 2002. The brain circuitry of syntactic comprehension. *Trends Cogn. Sci.* 6:350–356

KING, J. W., and M. KUTAS, 1995. Who did what and when: Using word- and clause-level ERPs to monitor working memory usage in reading. *J. Cogn. Neurosci.* 7:376–395.

KNÖSCHE, T., B. MAESS, and A. D. FRIEDERICI, 1999. Processing of syntactic information monitored by brain surface current density mapping based on MEG. *Brain Topogr.* 12:75–87.

KUPERBERG, G. R., P. K. MCGUIRE, E. T. BULLMORE, M. J. BRAMMER, S. RABE-HESKETH, I. C. WRIGHT, D. J. LYTHGOE, S. C. R. WILLIAMS, and A. S. DAVID, 2000. Common and distinct neural substrates for pragmatic, semantic, and syntactic processing of spoken sentences: An fMRI study. *J. Cogn. Neurosci.* 12:321–341.

KUTAS, M., and K. D. FEDERMEIER, 2000. Electrophysiology reveals semantic memory use in language comprehension. *Trends Cogn. Sci.* 4:463–470.

KUTAS, M., and S. A. HILLYARD, 1983. Event-related potentials to grammatical errors and semantic anomalies. *Mem. Cogn.* 11:539–550.

KUTAS, M., and C. VAN PETTEN, 1994. Psycholinguistics electrified: Event-related brain potential investigations. In *Handbook of Psycholinguistics*, M. A. Gernsbacher, ed. San Diego, Calif.: Academic Press, pp. 83–143.

LECHEVALIER, B., M. PETIT, F. EUSTACHE, J. LAMBERT, F. CHAPON, and F. VIADER, 1989. Regional cerebral blood flow during comprehension and speech (in cerebrally healthy subjects). *Brain Lang.* 37:1–11.

MACDONALD, M. C., N. J. PEARLMUTTER, and M. S. SEIDENBERG, 1994a. The lexical nature of syntactic ambiguity resolution. *Psychol. Rev.* 101:676–703.

MACDONALD, M. C., N. J. PEARLMUTTER, and M. S. SEIDENBERG, 1994b. Syntactic ambiguity resolution as lexical ambiguity resolution. In *Perspectives on Sentence Processing*, C. Clifton, Jr., L. Frazier, and K. Rayner, eds. Hillsdale, N.J.: Erlbaum, pp. 123–154.

MARSLEN-WILSON, W. D. and L. K. TYLER, 1980. The temporal structure of spoken language understanding. *Cognition* 8:1–71.

MAZOYER, B. M., N. TZOURIO, V. FRAK, A. SYROTA, N. MURAYAMA, O. LEVRIER, G. SALAMON, S. DEHAENE, L. COHEN, and J. MEHLER, 1993. The cortical representation of speech. *J. Cogn. Neurosci.* 5:467–479.

MCCLELLAND, J. L., M. ST. JOHN, and R. TARABAN, 1989. An interaction model of context effects in letter perception. Part I. An account of basic findings. *Lang. Cogn. Processes* 4:287–336.

MCKINNON, R., and L. OSTERHOUT, 1996. Constraints on movement phenomena in sentence processing: Evidence from event-related brain potentials. *Lang. Cogn. Processes* 11:495–523.

MECKLINGER, A., H. SCHRIEFERS, K. STEINHAUER, and A. D. FRIEDERICI, 1995. Processing relative clauses varying on syntactic and semantic dimensions: An analysis with event-related potentials. *Mem. Cogn.* 23:477–494.

MEYER, M., A. D. FRIEDERICI, and D. Y. VON CRAMON, 2000. Neurocognition of auditory sentence comprehension: Event-related fMRI reveals sensitivity to syntactic violations and task demands. *Cogn. Brain Res.* 9:19–33.

MORO, A., M. TETTAMANTI, D. PERANI, C. DONATI, S. F. CAPPA, and F. FAZIO, 2001. Syntax and the brain: Disentangling grammar by selective anomalies. *NeuroImage* 13:110–118.

MÜLLER, R.-A., R. D. ROTHERMEL, M. E. BEHEN, O. MUZIK, T. J. MANGNER, and H. T. CHUGANI, 1997. Receptive and expressive language activations for sentences: A PET study. *Neuroreport* 8:3767–3770.

MÜNTE, T. F., H. J. HEINZE, and G. R. MANGUN, 1993. Dissociation of brain activity related to syntactic and semantic aspects of language. *J. Cogn. Neurosci.* 5:335–344.

MÜNTE, T. F., A. SZENTKUI, B. M. WIERINGA, M. MATZKE, and S. JOHANNES, 1997. Human brain potentials to reading syntactic errors in sentences of different complexity. *Neurosci. Lett.* 235:105–108.

NEVILLE, H. J., J. NICOL, A. BARSS, K. I. FORSTER, and M. F. GARRETT, 1991. Syntactically based sentence processing classes: Evidence from event-related brain potentials. *J. Cogn. Neurosci.* 3:151–165.

NEWMAN, S. D., M. A. JUST, T. A. KELLER, J. ROTH, and P. A. CARPENTER, 2003. Differential effects of syntactic and semantic processing on the subregions of Broca's area. *Cogn. Brain Res.* 16:297–307.

NI, W., R. T. CONSTABLE, W. E. MENCL, K. R. PUGH, R. K. FULBRIGHT, S. E. SHAYWITZ, B. A. SHAYWITZ, J. C. GORE, and D. SHANKWEILER, 2000. An event-related neuroimaging study distinguishing form and content in sentence processing. *J. Cogn. Neurosci.* 12:120–133.

OSTERHOUT, L., and P. J. HOLCOMB, 1992. Event-related potentials and syntactic anomaly. *J. Mem. Lang.* 31:785–804.

OSTERHOUT, L., and P. J. HOLCOMB, 1993. Event-related potentials and syntactic anomaly: Evidence of anomaly detection during the perception of continuous speech. *Lang. Cogn. Processes* 8:413–437.

OSTERHOUT, L., P. J. HOLCOMB, and D. SWINNEY, 1994. Brain potentials elicited by garden-path sentences: Evidence of the application of verb information during parsing. *J. Exp. Psychol. Learn. Mem. Cogn.* 20:786–803.

OSTERHOUT, L., and L. A. MOBLEY, 1995. Event-related brain potentials elicited by failure to agree. *J. Mem. Lang.* 34:739–773.

OSTERHOUT, L., and J. NICOL, 1999. On the distinctiveness, independence, and time course of the brain responses to syntactic and semantic anomalies. *Lang. Cogn. Processes* 14:283–317.

PENKE, M., H. WEYERTS, M. GROSS, E. ZANDER, T. F. MUENTE, and H. CLAHSEN, 1997. How the brain processes complex words: An event-related potential study of German verb inflections. *Cogn. Brain Res.* 6:37–52.

PICKERING, M., C. CLIFTON, and M. CROCKER, 2000. *Architectures and Mechanisms of the Language Processing System.* Cambridge, England: Cambridge University Press.

ROEDER, B., O. STOCK, H. NEVILLE, S. BIEN, and F. ROESLER, 2002. Brain activation modulated by the comprehension of normal and pseudo-word sentences of different processing demands: A functional magnetic resonance imaging study. *NeuroImage* 15:1003–1014.

SAKAI, K. L., F. HOMAE, and R. HASHIMOTO, 2003. Sentence processing is uniquely human. *Neurosci. Res.* 46:273–279.

SCHUBOTZ, R. I., and D. Y. VON CRAMON, 2002. A blueprint for target motion: fMRI reveals perceived sequential complexity to modulate premotor cortex. *NeuroImage* 16:920–935.

STOWE, L. A., C. A. J. BROERE, A. M. J. PAANS, A. A. WIJERS, G. MULDER, W. VAALBURG, and F. ZWARTS, 1998. Localization components of a complex task: Sentence processing and working memory. *Neuroreport* 9:2995–2999.

STOWE, L. A., A. M. J. PAANS, A. A. WIJERS, F. ZWARTS, G. MULDER, and W. VAALBURG, 1999. Sentence comprehension and word repetition: A positron emission tomography investigation. *Psychophysiology* 36:786–801.

STROMSWOLD, K., D. CAPLAN, N. ALPERT, and S. RAUCH, 1996. Localization of syntactic comprehension by positron emission tomography. *Brain Lang.* 10:132–144.

TRUESWELL, J. C., and M. K. TANENHAUS, 1994. Toward a lexicalist framework of constraint-based syntactic ambiguity resolution. In *Perspectives on Sentence Processing*, C. Clifton, Jr., L. Frazier, and K. Rayner, eds. Hillsdale, N.J.: Erlbaum, pp. 155–180.

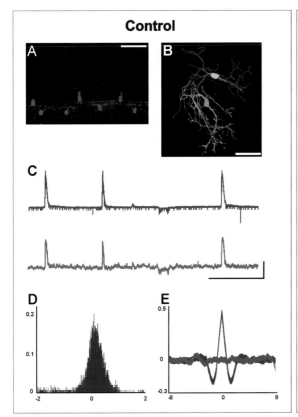

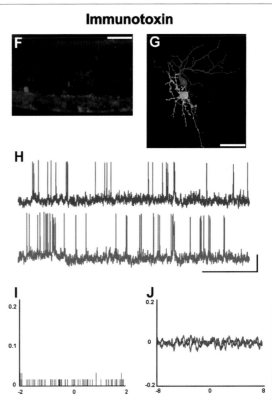

PLATE 1   (*A*) Photomicrograph of a P10 ferret retina injected with saline on P0. Regularly spaced starburst amacrine cells are shown in red after labeling by anti-choline acetyletransferase (ChAT) immunohistochemistry. Ganglion cell layer is to the bottom and photoreceptor layer is to the top of the photomicrograph. Scale bar = 100 μm.

(*B*) Two neighboring ganglion cells in a control retina. One was filled with a green dye and the other with a red dye, during the paired patch-clamp recording session. Scale bar = 25 μm.

(*C*) An example of current-clamp recordings from two neighboring ganglion cells in a control retina. Green trace shows the activity of one ganglion cell and red trace shows that of the neighboring cell. Highly correlated, periodic bursts of activity are clearly present. Horizontal scale = 1 minute, vertical scale = 20 mV.

(*D*) Cross-correlation of spiking activity for two neighboring control ganglion cells (shown in blue). There is a prominent peak near zero time lag. Red indicates the cross-correlation resulting from a random shuffle of the same spike data. This and all other ganglion cell pairs recorded in control P2–P10 retinas showed statistically significant correlations (n = 15 pairs).

(*E*) Cross-correlation of the membrane potential activity for two neighboring control ganglion cells (shown in blue). There is a prominent peak near zero time lag. Red indicates the cross-correlation of a random shuffle of the same membrane potential data. This and all other ganglion cell pairs recorded in control P2–P10 retinas showed statistically significant correlations in their activity patterns (n = 15 pairs).

(*F*) Photomicrograph of a P10 ferret retina that was injected with immunotoxin on P0. Most starburst amacrine cells are ablated.

However, a single starburst cell can be seen in red. Ganglion cell layer is to the bottom and photoreceptor layer is to the top. Scale bar = 100 μm.

(*G*) Two neighboring ganglion cells in an immunotoxin retina. One was filled with a green dye and the other with a red dye during the paired patch-clamp recording session. Scale bar = 25 μm.

(*H*) An example of current-clamp recordings from two neighboring ganglion cells in an immunotoxin-treated retina. Green trace shows the activity of one ganglion cell and red trace shows the activity of the neighboring cell. The spiking activity of these two cells does not appear correlated. Horizontal scale = 1 minute, vertical scale = 20 mV.

(*I*) Cross-correlation of spiking activity for two neighboring ganglion cells in an immunotoxin-treated retina (shown in blue). There is no peak in the correlation at any time lag, and the correlation resembles that of a random shuffle of the same spike data (shown in red). Neither this nor any other ganglion cell pair recorded from immunotoxin-treated P2–P10 retinas showed statistically significant correlations (n = 15 pairs).

(*J*) Cross-correlation of the membrane potential activity for two neighboring ganglion cells in an immunotoxin-treated retina (shown in blue). There is no peak in the correlation at any time lag and the correlation resembles that of a random shuffle of the same membrane potential data (shown in red). Neither this nor any other ganglion cell pair recorded from immunotoxin-treated P2–P10 retinas showed statistically significant correlations (n = 15 pairs). (All panels adapted from Huberman et al., 2003.)

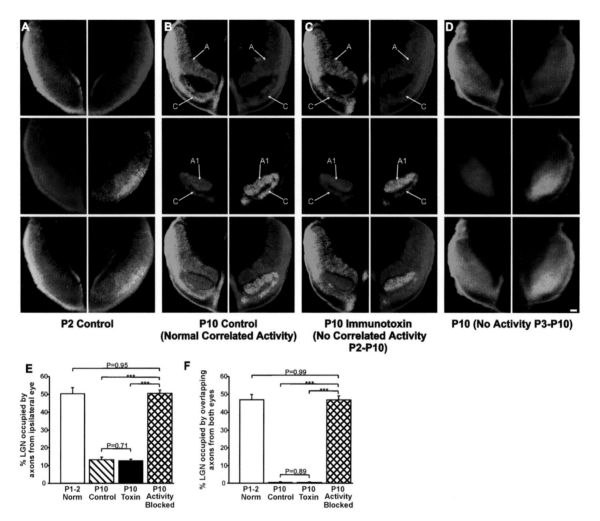

P2 Control

P10 Control (Normal Correlated Activity)

P10 Immunotoxin (No Correlated Activity P2-P10)

P10 (No Activity P3-P10)

PLATE 2 Development of eye-specific layers in the dLGN of (*A*) normal P2, (*B*) control P10, (*C*) P10 immunotoxin-treated, and (*D*) epibatidine-treated ferrets. (*A–D*) Axons from the right eye are shown in green and axons from the left eye are shown in red. Contralateral (top panels) and ipsilateral (middle panels) retinal inputs to the dLGN, and their merged representation (bottom panels) are shown. Tissue sections are in the horizontal plane: rostral is to the top and medial is to the center of each panel. Scale bar in A = 150 μm; scale bar in B–D = 100 μm. (All panels adapted from Huberman et al., 2003.)

(*A*) A normal P2 ferret. Inputs from the two eyes are still overlapped at this age; the contralateral eye projection is found throughout the nucleus, where it intermingles with axons from the ipsilateral eye.

(*B*) A control P10 ferret. Axons from the two eyes are completely segregated by this age. Arrows indicate the complementary "A" (contralateral eye) and A1 (ipsilateral eye) layers. C layers are also seen.

(*C*) A P10 ferret that received binocular intravitreal injections of immunotoxin on P0. Axons from the two eyes are segregated normally in these animals. Arrows indicate the complementary and "A" (contralateral eye) and A1 (ipsilateral eye) layers. Normal C layers are also evident.

(*D*) A P10 ferret that received binocular intravitreal injections of epibatidine (which blocks all retinal activity) every 48 hours from P3 to P10. Projections from the two eyes overlapped; there is no gap in the contralateral eye's projection, and the ipsilateral eye's projection is dramatically expanded.

(*E* and *F*) Quantification of the percent of dLGN area occupied by the ipsilateral eye projection (*E*) and overlapping axons from the two eyes (*F*) in the four treatment groups. Open bars: normal P1/2 ferrets (*n* = 8), hatched bars = control P10 ferrets (*n* = 12), black bars = P10 ferrets that received binocular injections of immunotoxin on P0 (*n* = 14), cross hatched bars = P10 ferrets that received binocular injections of epibatidine from P3 to P10 (*n* = 14). ***P < 0.0001; *t*-test; ±SEM.

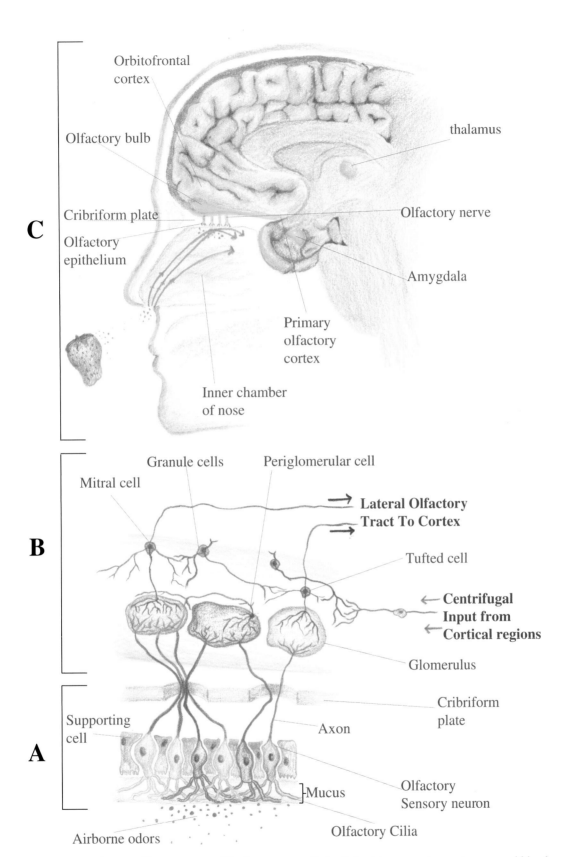

C

Orbitofrontal cortex

Olfactory bulb

thalamus

Cribriform plate

Olfactory epithelium

Olfactory nerve

Primary olfactory cortex

Amygdala

Inner chamber of nose

B

Granule cells

Periglomerular cell

Mitral cell

Lateral Olfactory Tract To Cortex

Tufted cell

Centrifugal Input from Cortical regions

Glomerulus

Cribriform plate

Supporting cell

Axon

A

Mucus

Olfactory Sensory neuron

Airborne odors

Olfactory Cilia

PLATE 3 Structure of the human olfactory system. The human olfactory system can be segregated into three primary compartments: epithelium, bulb, and cortex. (*A*) Olfactory epithelium. Each olfactory sensory neuron expresses one olfactory receptor gene. Like receptors project to one or a small number of glomeruli. (*B*) Organization of the olfactory bulb. Glomeruli receive input from olfactory sensory neurons and cortical olfactory regions. Mitral and tufted cell dendrites contact receptor axons within glomeruli. The axons of the mitral and tufted cells project widely to higher brain structures, as labeled in *C*. Lateral processing in the olfactory bulb occurs across two types of interneurons, periglomerular cells and granule cells. (*C*) Sagittal view of the human head. The olfactory bulb and epithelium are highlighted in yellow.

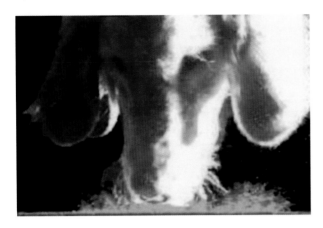

PLATE 4 Airflow visualization using Schlieren imaging, from the work of Gary Settles (Settles, 2001; Settles et al., 2003). These visualizations revealed that before sniffing inward, dogs may also sniff outward in a lateral trajectory in order to distribute particles so that they can be inhaled and smelled. As this image clearly depicts, sensation is an active process, and olfaction is a good case in point.

PLATE 5 fMRI results obtained in humans. Top row, from left to right: MR activity induced by natural sniffing, by trying to sniff with the nostrils occluded, by artificial airflows directed at the nostrils, and by sniffing with topical anesthesia in the nostrils. Middle row, from left to right: The implants used to restrict nasal flow and the effect of this on fMRI signal in piriform cortex. Bottom row: The corresponding activation patterns. Taken together, these results demonstrate that activity in primary olfactory cortex is strongly affected by the somatosensory stimulation of sniffing. (Reprinted from N. Sobel, V. Prabhakaran, J. E. Desmond, et al., 1998. Sniffing and smelling: Separate subsystems in the human olfactory cortex. *Nature* 392:282–286. Copyright 1998, with permission from the Nature Publishing Group.)

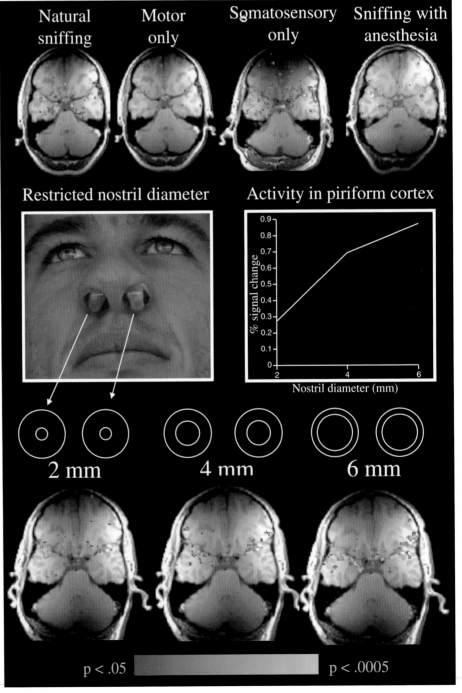

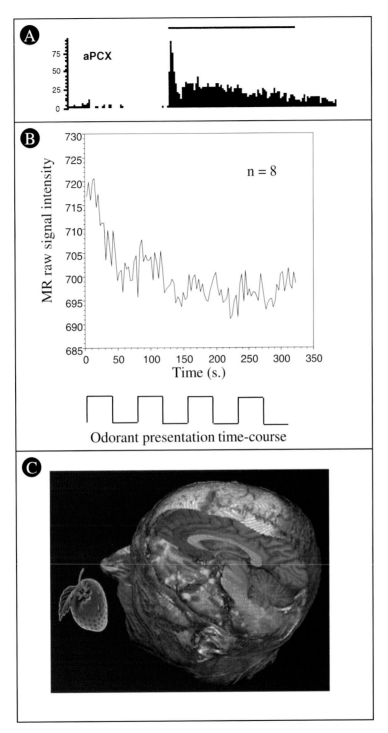

PLATE 6 Habituation in olfactory cortex. (*A*) Data from Wilson (1998) showing a multi-unit recording in piriform cortex of the rat in response to a 50 s continuous odor pulse (denoted by bar above data). (Reprinted with permission from D. A. Wilson, Habituation of odor responses in the rat anterior piriform cortex. *J. Neurophysiol.* 79:1425–1440. Copyright 1998 by the American Physiological Society.) (*B*) Mean time course of fMRI signal from the piriform cortex of eight human subjects. Note the striking similarity between the time course in *A* (from rat) and the first 50 s in *B* (from human). (*C*) Once this habituation was taken into consideration in models of the expected hemodynamic response, odorant-induced activity was readily measurable in human piriform cortex. Here data from eight subjects smelling vanillin are overlaid on the three-dimensional image.

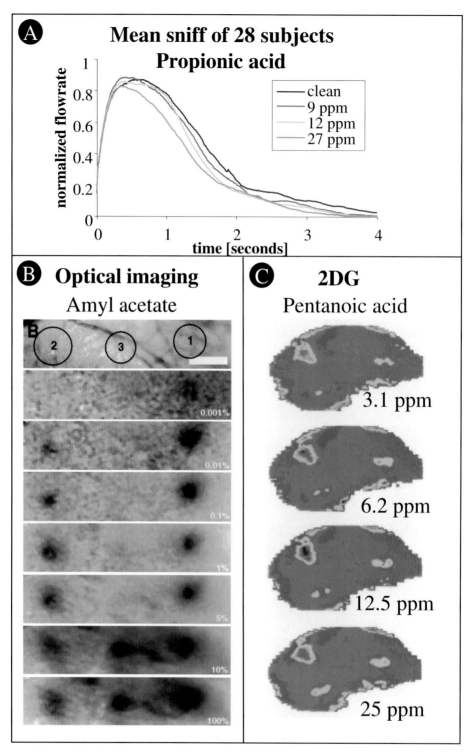

PLATE 7 Coding intensity. (*A*) The mean sniffs of 28 subjects in response to three concentrations of propionic acid and clean air. Higher concentrations of odor were sampled at lower airflow rates. Airflow rate was adjusted to meet odorant concentration within 160 ms. (Reprinted from B. N. Johnson, J. D. Mainland, N. Sobel, 2003. Rapid olfactory processing implicates subcortical control of an olfactomotor system. *J. Neurophysiol.* 90:1084–1094. Copyright 2003 the American Physiological Society. Used by permission.) (*B*) Effects of increasing odorant concentration on the optical image obtained in the anesthetized rodent. Increased concentration was reflected in increased spatial extent of glomerular response. (Reprinted from *Neuron*, vol. 23, B. D. Rubin and L. C. Katz, Optical imaging of odorant representations in the mammalian olfactory bulb, pp. 499–511, copyright 1999, with permission from Elsevier.) (*C*) Effects of increasing odorant concentration on the 2DG image obtained in the awake behaving rodent. Increased concentration had no impact on spatial patterns of glomerular response. As implicated in panel *A*, awake behaving animals would not sample high- and low-intensity odorants with equal vigor. Data obtained from the anesthetized animal will fail to reflect this essential olfactory mechanism. (Reprinted with permission from B. A. Johnson and M. Leon, Modular representations of odorants in the glomerular layer of the rat olfactory bulb and the effects of stimulus concentration. *J. Comp. Neural.* 422:496–509. Copyright 2000, used by permission of Wiley-Liss, Inc., a subsidiary of John Wiley & Sons, Inc.)

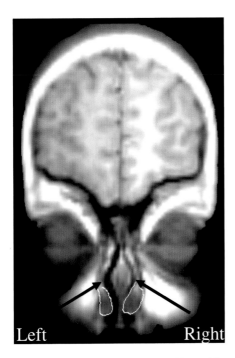

PLATE 8   A coronal image of the nasal passage. The turbinates are traced in white. In this subject the right turbinate is expanded, largely blocking the right nostril. Thus, this subject has an open left nostril with a high airflow rate (green) and an occluded right nostril with a low airflow rate (red).

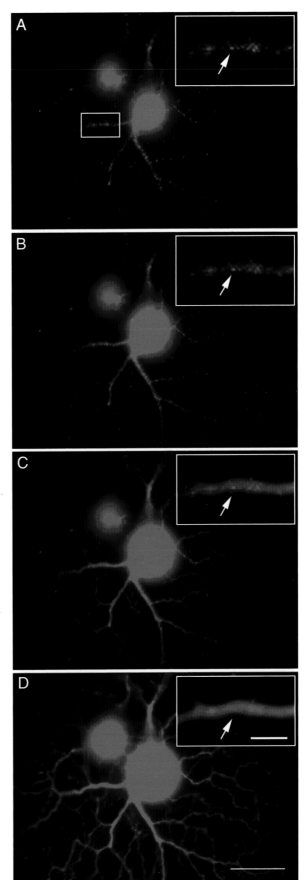

PLATE 9   In vitro photodynamic staining reveals the detailed dendritic morphology of ganglion cells after retrograde labeling from tracer injections into retinorecipient structures. (*A–D*) Sequence of photomicrographs showing the progress of photostaining in vitro that was initiated by a brief light exposure. Plane of focus is in the IPL on the dendritic tree of a parasol ganglion cell retrogradely labeled from injections of rhodamine-dextran into the LGN. (*A*) Tracer initially appears as small bright granules in the soma and dendrites. On exposure to light, the granules burst and release the fluorescent tracer, which diffuses throughout the cytoplasm. Here photostaining has already begun in the soma, which is brightly and uniformly labeled; tracer in the dendrites still appears as small bright granules. Area indicated by the box is enlarged in the inset, and a single granule is indicated by the arrow. (*B*) Photostaining has begun in the dendrites; some granules have burst, and tracer is beginning to diffuse through the dendrites. The tracer granule indicated by the arrow in the inset has not yet burst. (*C*) Photostaining continues as more granules burst and release tracer into the dendrites. (*D*) Photostaining is complete. Note that the granule indicated by the arrow in the insets has now burst. The entire dendritic tree is uniformly tracer labeled. Photostaining can be used to efficiently characterize the morphology of a large number of retrogradely labeled ganglion cells and also to selectively target individual morphological types in vitro for physiological analysis (Dacey, Peterson, et al., 2003). Scale bar = 50 μm; inset scale bar = 10 μm.

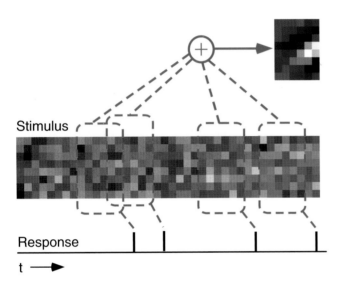

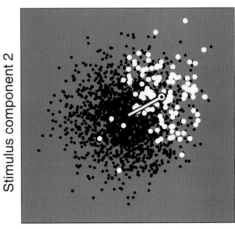

Stimulus component 2

Stimulus component 1

PLATE 10 Two alternative illustrations of the reverse correlation procedure. *Left:* Discretized stimulus sequence and observed neural response (spike train). On each time step, the stimulus consists of an array of randomly chosen values (eight, for this example), corresponding to the intensities of a set of individual pixels, bars, or any other fixed spatial patterns. The neural response at any particular moment in time is assumed to be completely determined by the stimulus segment that occurred during a prespecified interval in the past. In this figure, the segment covers six time steps, and lags three time steps behind the current time (to account for response latency). The spike-triggered ensemble consists of the set of segments associated with spikes. The spike-triggered average (STA) is constructed by averaging these stimulus segments (and subtracting off the average over the full set of stimulus segments).

Right: Geometric (vector space) interpretation of the STA. Each stimulus segment corresponds to a point in a *d*-dimensional space (in this example, $d = 48$) whose axes correspond to stimulus values (e.g., pixel intensities) during the interval. For illustration purposes, the scatter plot shows only two of the 48 axes. The spike-triggered stimulus segments (white points) constitute a subset of all stimulus segments presented (black points). The STA, indicated by the line in the diagram, corresponds to the difference between the mean (center of mass) of the spike-triggered ensemble and the mean of the raw stimulus ensemble. Note that the interpretation of this representation of the stimuli is only sensible under Poisson spike generation; the scatter plot depiction implies that the probability of spiking depends only on the position in the stimulus space.

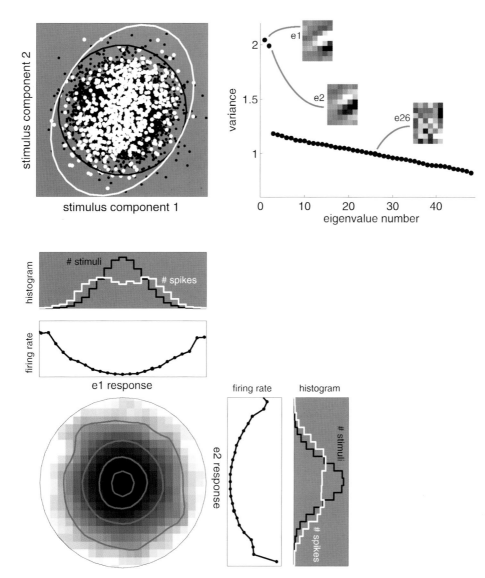

PLATE 11 Simulated characterization of a particular LNP model using spike-triggered covariance (STC). In this model, the Poisson spike generator is driven by the sum of the squares of two oriented linear filter responses. As in figure 23.1, filters are 6×8, and thus live in a 48-dimensional space. The simulation is based on a sequence of 50,000 raw stimuli, with a response containing 4500 spikes. *Top left:* Simulated raw and spike-triggered stimulus ensembles, viewed in a two-dimensional subspace that illustrates the model behavior. The covariance of these ensembles within this two-dimensional space is represented geometrically by an ellipse that is 3 SD from the origin in all directions. The raw stimulus ensemble has equal variance in all directions, as indicated by the black circle. The spike-triggered ensemble is elongated in one direction, as represented by the white ellipse. *Top right:* Eigenvalue analysis of the simulated data. The principal axes of the covariance ellipse correspond to the eigenvectors of the spike-triggered covariance matrix,

and the associated eigenvalues indicate the variance of the spike-triggered stimulus ensemble along each of these axes. The plot shows the full set of 48 eigenvalues, sorted in descending order. Two of these are substantially larger than the others and indicate the presences of two axes in the stimulus space along which the model responds. The others correspond to stimulus directions that the model ignores. Also shown are three example eigenvectors (6×8 linear filters). *Bottom, one-dimensional plots:* Spike-triggered and raw histograms of responses of the two high-variance linear filters, along with the nonlinear firing rate functions estimated from their quotient (see figure 23.3). *Bottom, two-dimensional plot:* The quotient of the two-dimensional spike-triggered and raw histograms provides an estimate of the two-dimensional nonlinear firing rate function. This is shown as a circular-cropped gray-scale image, where intensity is proportional to firing rate. Superimposed contours indicate four different response levels.

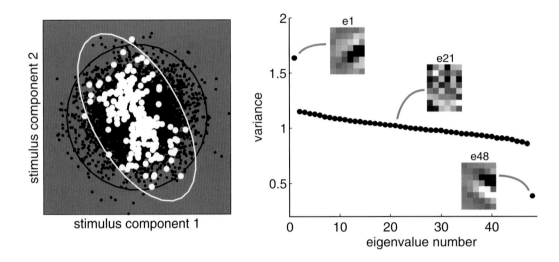

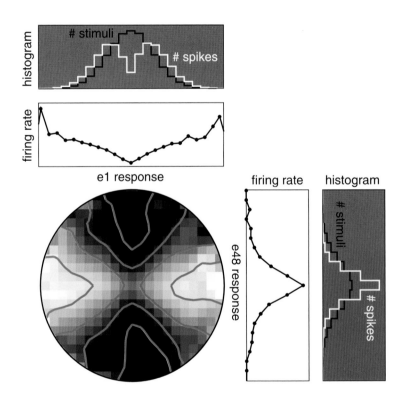

PLATE 12 Characterization of a simulated LNP model, constructed from the squared response of one linear filter divided by the sum of the squares of its own response and the response of another filter. The simulation is based on a sequence of 200,000 raw stimuli, with a response containing 8000 spikes. See text and caption of figure 23.4 for details.

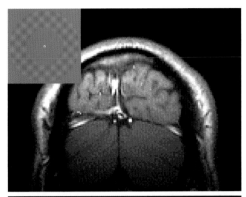

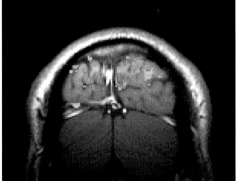

PLATE 13 Statistical parameter maps of cortical activity as a function of stimulus contrast. Gray scale image is an obliquely oriented anatomical slice passing through the posterior occipital lobe and cerebellum. Colors indicate regions that achieve a criterion statistical threshold.

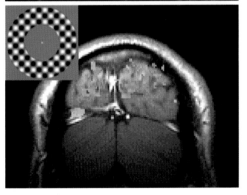

PLATE 14 Three time-varying synergies extracted from the entire kicking data set. The first three columns (W_1–W_3) represent the three extracted synergies as a color-coded activation time course of 13 muscles over 30 samples (300 ms total duration) normalized to the maximum sample. The three synergies capture different features of the kicking muscle patterns: W_1 and W_2 show a high level of activation, especially in extensors muscles (in particular the hip extensors RI and SM for the first synergy and the knee extensors VI and VE for the second). Mostly flexor muscles (IP, ST, TA, SA, BI) are recruited in W_3. The fourth column indicates the sign (flexion or extension) of the moment arms around hip, knee, and ankle joints of the 13 muscles included in each synergy. Abbreviations: HE, hip extension; HF, hip flexion; KE, knee extension; KF, knee flexion; AE, ankle extension; AF, ankle flexion.

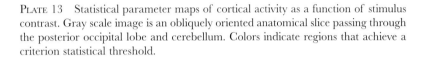

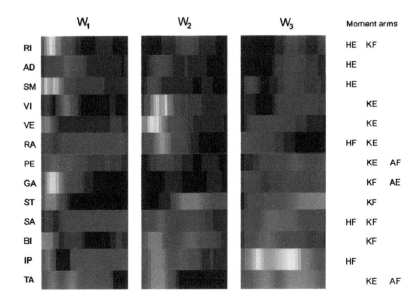

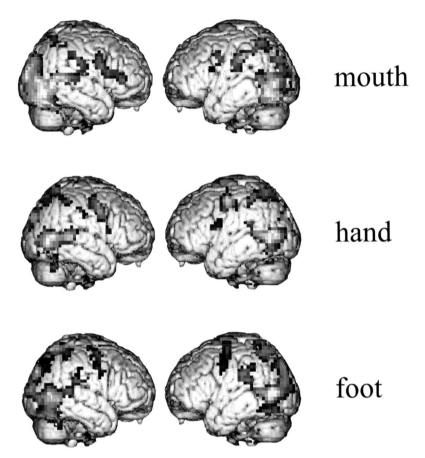

PLATE 15 Activations of frontal and parietal cortical areas during observation of mouth, hand and foot actions, rendered on a standard brain schema (Montreal Neurological Institute): mouth, biting an apple; hand, grasping a cup or a ball; foot, kicking a ball or pushing a brake. All actions were compared with the observation of a static face, hand, and foot, respectively.

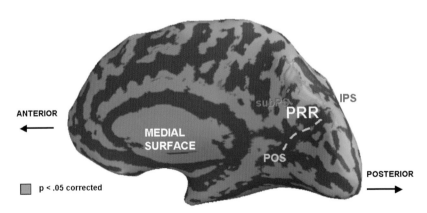

PLATE 16 Medial view of an inflated cerebral cortex, showing unfolded sulci and gyri and the location of the fMRI delay interval activation, as determined using multiple regression analysis (ten subjects, P < 0.05). GLM signal timecourses that were subjected to further ANOVA analysis were situated anterior to the parieto-occipital sulcus, posterior to the subparietal sulcus, medial to the intraparietal sulcus. (Reprinted with permission from J. D. Connolly et al., fMRI evidence for a "parietal reach region" in the human brain. *Exp. Brain Res.* 153:140–145. © 2003 by Springer-Verlag.)

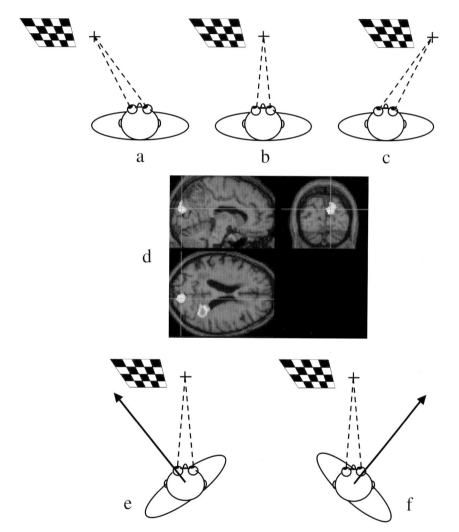

PLATE 17 Postural modulation of left visual neglect after right hemisphere damage. A left retinal stimulus that is neglected when gazing leftward (*a*) or straight ahead (*b*) may be detected or judged better when gazing rightward (*c*). Region in right occipital cortex (*d*) for a single case of left neglect after right parietal damage (lesion visible in transverse section) that showed higher activation specifically when patient was gazing rightward for left-minus-right retinal stimulation (see text for further details). Head-on-trunk posture can also modulate visual neglect (*e* and *f*). Performance for fixed retinotopic and craniotopic left visual stimulus can be improved with the trunk twisted leftward (*e*, arrow depicts straight-ahead direction from trunk) than with trunk straight or twisted rightward (*f*).

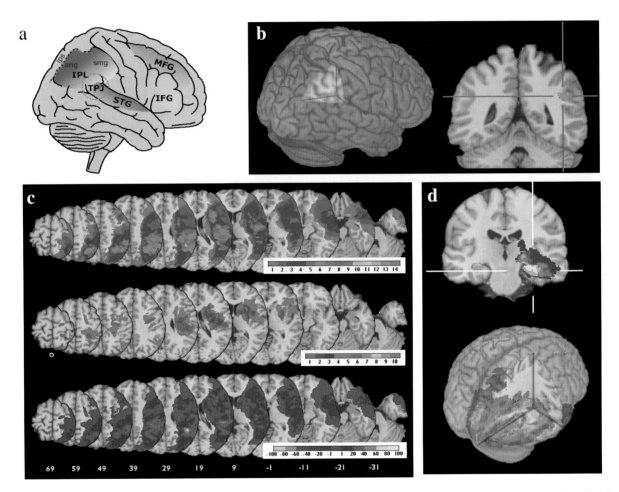

PLATE 18   Anatomy of neglect syndrome. (*a*) Regions associated with lesions in neglect patients include the right inferior parietal lobe (IPL), the temporoparietal junction (TPJ), the middle and inferior frontal gyri (MFG and IFG, respectively), and the superior temporal gyrus (STG). Subcortical lesions or white matter damage may also play a role (see text). Lesions in individual patients with neglect can often be large. (*b*) Region of maximum overlap for damage in neglect patients found in angular gyrus by Mort and colleagues (in press). Coronal section's shown at right of panel, with the location shown by the cutout at the left of the panel. (*c*) Detailed lesion anatomy from this study. Top row shows anatomy in neglect patients with right middle cerebral artery (CA) infarctions, middle row shows anatomy in right middle CA controls without neglect, and bottom row shows subtraction. Note the presence of an angular gyrus hotspot in *c*, plus other areas. (*d*) Coronal section and cutout showing lesion overlap for right posterior CA neglect patients minus nonneglect right posterior CA controls (from Mort and colleagues, 2003).

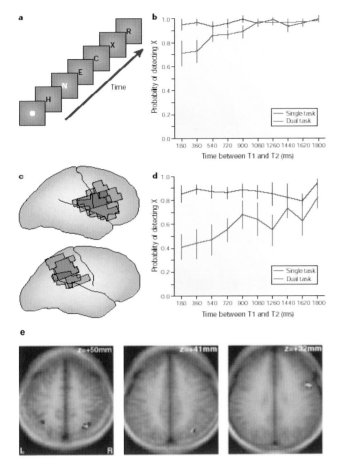

PLATE 19   (a–d) Prolonged "attentional blink" in neglect patients for rapid sequence of visual stimuli at central fixation (figure adapted with authors' permission from Husain and Rorden, 2003; data from Husain et al., 1997). (a) Schematic stimulus sequence. Observer must name the white letter (first target, T1) and detect whether or not an X (second target, T2) is presented afterward, on each trial. (b) Normal results show performance for T2 is impaired if presented shortly after T1, under dual-task conditions (i.e., when monitoring for both targets rather than for just T2). (c) In neglect patients with right parietal or frontal damage, this impairment is pathologically extended (d). (e) Activation of related brain areas is found in normals subjects (data from Marois et al., 2000) in similar attentional tasks on rapid visual streams at fixation (see also Wojciulik and Kanwisher, 1999).

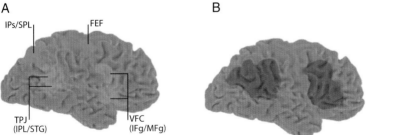

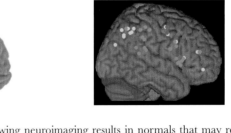

PLATE 20   (a) Distinct superior (blue) and inferior (yellow) attention-related networks (adapted with authors' permission from review by Corbetta and Shulman, 2002, on functional neuroimaging results in normals). They suggest the superior network is activated by preparatory attention, often bilaterally, while the inferior network is more strongly right lateralized, and associated with interruption of preexisting attentional states (as when a target suddenly appears on an unexpected side for invalidly cued trials; see main text). They argue that damage to this inferior right lateralized network may play a role in neglect, consistent with their view (see b) of brain areas commonly lesioned in neglect (see also figure 43.5).

When reviewing neuroimaging results in normals that may relate to neglect, Husain and Rorden (2003) emphasized similar inferior regions (see c, adapted with authors' permission from their review paper), arguing these do not solely play a role in interrupting existing attentional states but also in sustained attention (red circles here, coordinates of activation maxima from several studies), in nonspatial selective attention (yellow; c.f. figure 43.5e) in transaccadic spatial working memory (green), and salience detection (blue). Processes related to all these functions might thus be disrupted in many patients with neglect, in addition to their spatial bias toward the right side.

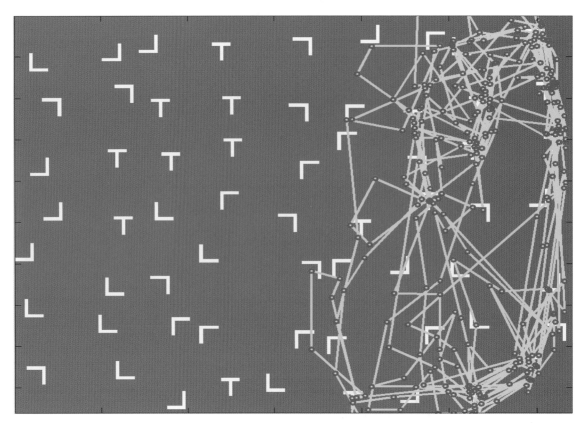

PLATE 21 Deficits in retaining the locations of targets already found, due to impaired spatial working memory, may contribute to pathological search in neglect. Shown are example eye movement data from a patient with neglect after right parietal damage searching for Ts among Ls, with the instruction to click on a response button only when a "new" T has been found (adapted with authors' permission from Husain et al., 2001). The patient revisits previously discovered targets many times and erroneously treats them as new discoveries, indicating a failure to retain the locations of targets already found across saccades. Such mistakes increase with the load on spatial working memory (e.g., for displays with more items, even though the probability of returning by chance should decrease for these).

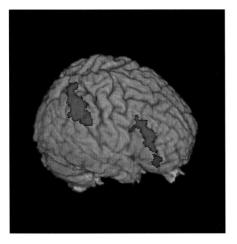

PLATE 22 Extensive dorsolateral and parietal activation (in red) is shown for event-related response inhibition. Activation (in blue) of the right inferior frontal gyrus was correlated with the CFQ score, suggesting a greater reliance on this right prefrontal area in subjects scoring highest on everyday absentmindedness (Garavan and Hester, 2004).

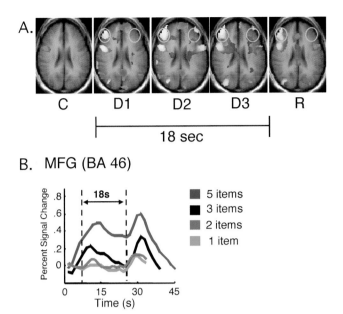

B. MFG (BA 46)

PLATE 23 Activation within middle frontal gyrus (area 46) during spatial working memory tasks increases with increasing load. (*A*) Statistical maps superimposed on anatomical axial section showing significant activations (in hot colors) during maintenance of five spatial locations, compared with a control condition. The same effect was not seen when activation during maintenance of three spatial locations was compared with a control condition. Middle frontal gyrus is delineated by blue circles (C = cue period, D1–D3 = three segments of delay period, 6 s each, R = response period). (*B*) Time course percent signal change in the middle frontal gyrus (area 46/9) during maintenance of one, two, three, and five locations. Dashed lines indicate beginning and end of delay period (18 s here). (Adapted from Leung, Gore, and Goldman-Rakic, 2002.)

PLATE 24 Right dorsolateral prefrontal region (arrowed) where activity was greater for recognized test items endorsed as known rather than remembered, in the study of Henson and colleagues (1999).

Target > New

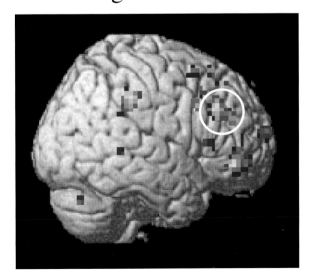

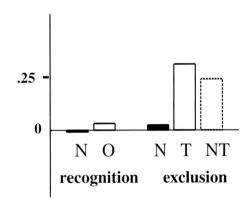

PLATE 25 *Left:* Right dorsolateral region (circled) identified by the contrast between activity elicited by correctly classified target and new items in Rugg and colleagues (2003). *Right:* Activity (arbitrary units) elicited in this region by new (N) and old (O) items in the recognition task, and by new (N), target (T), and nontarget (NT) items in the exclusion task.

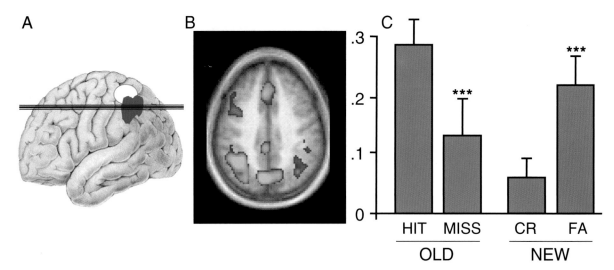

PLATE 26 Left lateral parietal regions correlate with the perception that information is old during recognition. (*A*) Approximate location of a lateral parietal region that transiently modulates based on successful retrieval. (*B*) An event-related fMRI activation map of hits versus correction rejections shows a network of modulated regions, including medial and lateral parietal cortex. (Adapted from Konishi et al., 2000.) (*C*) The magnitude (in percent MR signal change) for retrieval trials, sorted by the history of the item (OLD versus NEW) and by the subject's response (HIT, MISS, CR, and FA). The response is greatest for OLD items reported as old (HIT) and least for NEW items reported as new (CR: correct rejections). Of interest, the response also correlates with memory errors being greater for HIT as compared with MISS responses, and also greater for FA (false alarms) as compared with CR. (Adapted from Wheeler and Buckner, 2003.)

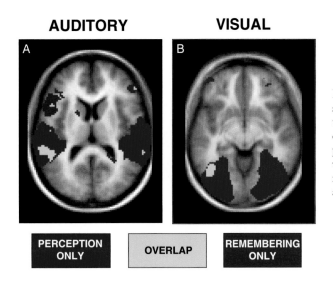

PLATE 27 Late sensory regions reactivate during retrieval of sensory-specific information. (*A, B*) Regions active during the *perception* of auditory (*A*) and visual (*B*) information, superimposed on regions active during the *retrieval* of auditory and visual information. Bilateral temporal cortex is active during the perception of auditory information, with a subset of auditory regions reactivating during retrieval. Similar reactivation occurs in visual regions, again in late as opposed to early areas. (Adapted from Wheeler, Petersen, and Buckner, 2000.)

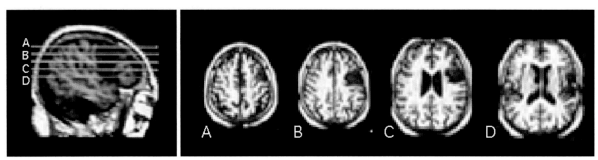

PLATE 28 Lesion localization for patient B.G. in parasagittal and axial (horizontal) planes as revealed by MRI. The entire precentral gyrus is affected, as seen in the parasagittal view. The superior-inferior and lateral-medial extents of this lesion can be appreciated in a series of axial sections that proceed from superior to inferior (levels A–D). These images are derived from a T1-weighted structural image. Right is on the right.

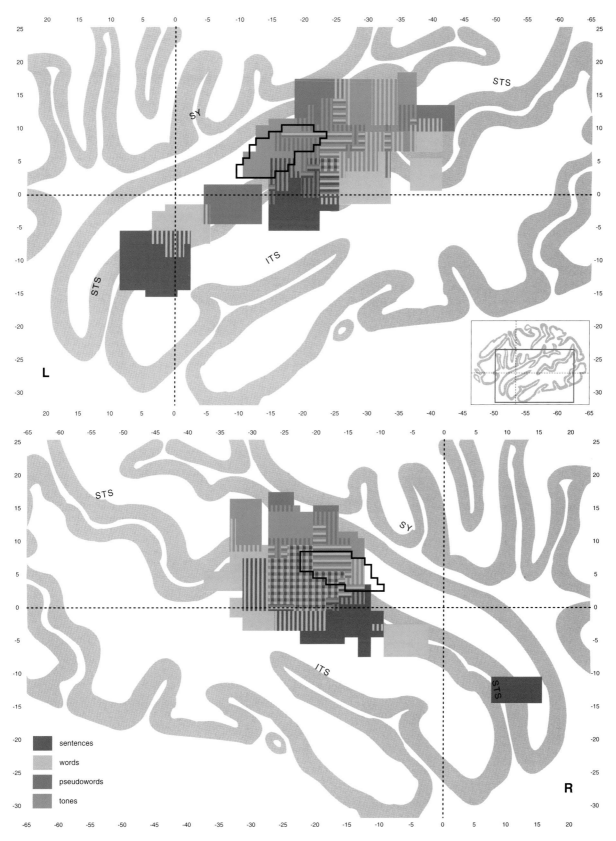

PLATE 29 Meta-analysis results for passive listening experiments with silent control conditions. Colors indicate the areas of reliable overlap of activation foci for the different stimuli. Results are projected onto sagittal slices of the temporal lobe at Talairach x-coordinates −51 (upper panel) and +51 (lower panel). To facilitate orientation, the approximate contours of the 50%–75% probability volumes of the primary auditory cortices (Penhune et al., 1996) at $x = -51$ and $x = +51$ are indicated by a black line. Abbreviations: SY, sylvian fissure; STS, superior temporal sulcus; ITS, inferior temporal sulcus.

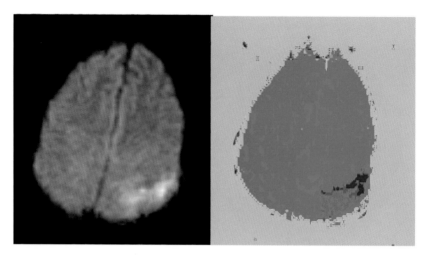

PLATE 30   Diffusion-weighted (left) and perfusion-weighted (right) MR images taken 10 hours after the onset of stroke in a patient with selectively impaired access to the orthographic lexicon for reading and writing. The bright area on the diffusion-weighted image shows an acute infarct in the angular gyrus. The dark area on the perfusion-weighted image shows low blood flow in the angular gyrus.

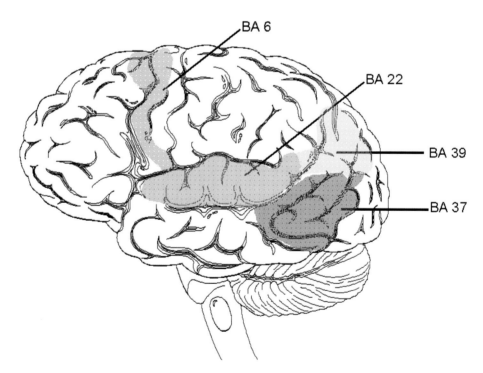

PLATE 31   Schematic representation of the brain with the approximate locations of Brodmann's areas that are likely to be engaged in reading and spelling.

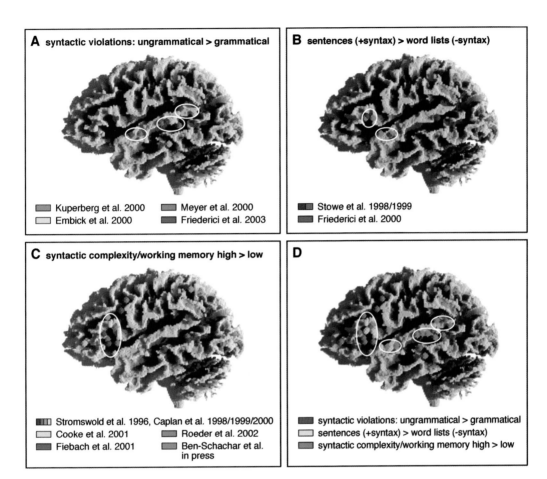

PLATE 32 Main activations of the different sentence-level syntactic processing studies discussed in the text. (*A*) Activation foci for the processing of syntactic violations. (*B*) Activation for sentences versus word lists. (*C*) Activation foci for sentences of high syntactically complex and high syntactic memory demand. (*D*) Activation foci for all studies.

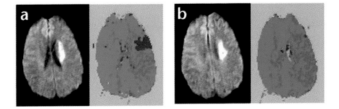

PLATE 33 Diffusion-weighted (left) and perfusion-weighted (right) imaging scans before and intervention to restore blood flow. (*a*) Scans obtained when written naming of verbs was impaired. (*b*) Scans obtained intervention, when written naming of verbs had recovered. (Reprinted with permission from Hillis et al., 2003.)

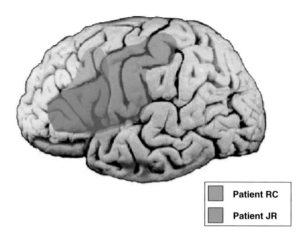

| | Patient RC |
| | Patient JR |

PLATE 34   Brain regions implicated in naming of nouns and verbs (Shapiro and Caramazza, 2003c). Patient R.C. (red) is relatively impaired at naming verbs, and presents with a lesion primarily affecting the left posterior frontal lobe and underlying structures. Patient J.R. (blue) is more impaired at noun production; he suffered a left middle cerebral artery infarction with damage extending from the frontal lobe posteriorly, including the sensory strip and the angular and supramarginal gyri. The left temporal lobe is largely spared, with the possible exception of the first temporal gyrus near the pole.

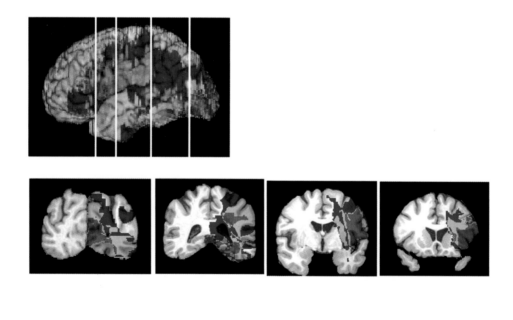

| 1 | 2 | 3 | 4 |

Number of Subjects in Overlap

PLATE 35   Areas of lesion overlap in 13 subjects with disproportionate impairments in action naming relative to naming of concrete entities. The figure shows three regions of maximal overlap: *1*, the left frontal operculum, underlying white matter, and anterior insula; *2*, the left mesial occipital cortex; and *3*, the paraventricular white matter underneath the supramarginal gyrus and posterior temporal region. Color bar indicates the number of subjects in the overlap. (Reprinted with permission from Tranel et al., 2001.)

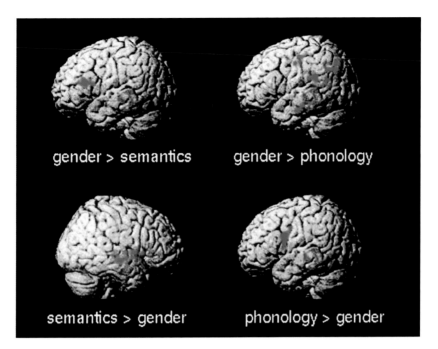

PLATE 36 Lateral see-through of activations observed with fMRI, contrasting conditions in which subjects viewed words and made decisions about their gender (masculine or feminine?), meaning (animal or artifact?), and phonology (does it contain a /tʃ/ or a /k/ sound?). (Reprinted with permission from Miceli et al., 2002.)

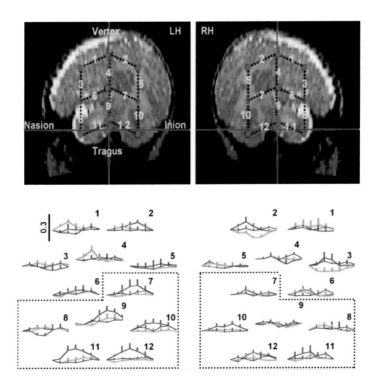

PLATE 37 OT study of a 2-month-old infant. Top panels show positioning of the fiber-optics on the infant's head. Numbers 1 to 12 in bottom panels refer to the left and the right channels depicted in the top panels. The vertical line to the left of channel 1 in the left hemisphere shows the value of the change in concentration of total hemoglobin. Red indicates the response to forward utterances, green the response to backward utterances, and blue, the response to the control condition (silence).

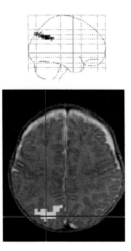

PLATE 38   Results from the study of Dehaene-Lambertz and colleagues (2002), showing that forward utterances produced more activation in the left hemisphere angular gyrus than did backward utterances.

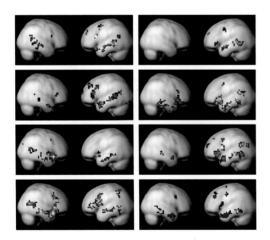

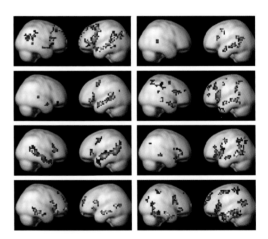

PLATE 39   The eight panels on the left depict cortical areas that showed significantly greater activation when native Koreans were processing French compared to Polish utterances. The eight panels on the right illustrate the cortical areas that showed significantly greater activation when native French speakers were processing French compared to Polish utterances. Although both populations had become equally fluent in French, a significantly greater area of the left hemisphere was activated in the native French speakers than in the native Korean speakers.

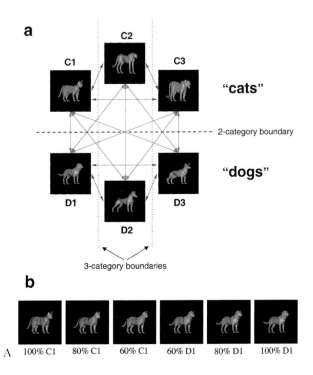

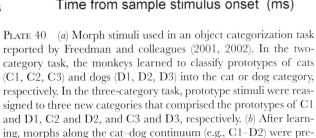

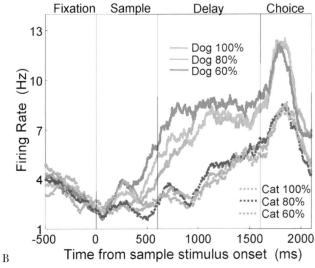

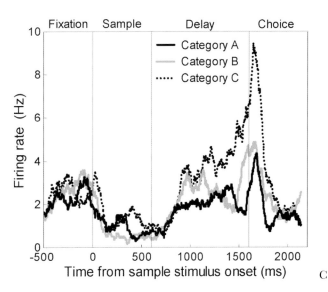

PLATE 40 (*a*) Morph stimuli used in an object categorization task reported by Freedman and colleagues (2001, 2002). In the two-category task, the monkeys learned to classify prototypes of cats (C1, C2, C3) and dogs (D1, D2, D3) into the cat or dog category, respectively. In the three-category task, prototype stimuli were reassigned to three new categories that comprised the prototypes of C1 and D1, C2 and D2, and C3 and D3, respectively. (*b*) After learning, morphs along the cat–dog continuum (e.g., C1–D2) were presented for classification. (*c*) Single-cell response of a dog-selective neuron to six levels of morph. During the delay and choice periods, the neuron demonstrated an increased response to stimuli containing a larger proportion of the dog prototype (i.e., Dog 100%, Dog 80%, Dog 60%) than the cat prototype. The response was categorical to the degree that the Dog 60% and Dog 80% stimuli elicited the same level of increased activity as the Dog 100% stimulus.

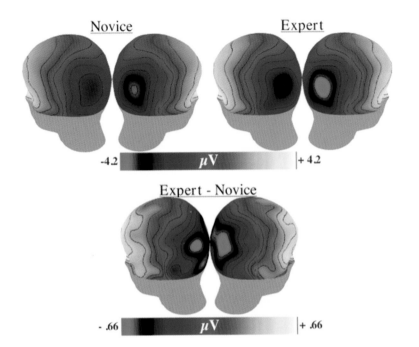

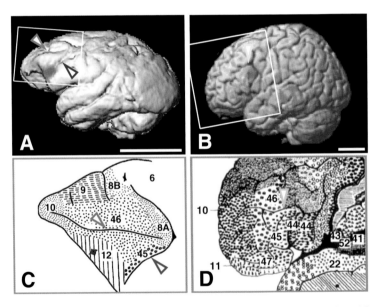

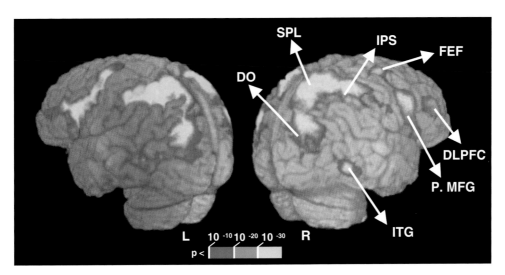

PLATE 43   Working memory network. The regions within this network were revealed by the contrast of working memory versus fixation control trials. The statistical group maps of functional activations are shown overlaid onto a three-dimensional rendering of the brain of a representative individual. The color bar indicates P values (uncorrected). Abbreviations: DLPFC, dorsolateral prefrontal cortex; DO, dorsal occipital; FEF, frontal eye field; IPS, intraparietal sulcus; ITG, inferior temporal gyrus; P. MFG, posterior middle frontal gyrus; SPL, superior parietal lobule. (Reprinted with permission from Cell Press.)

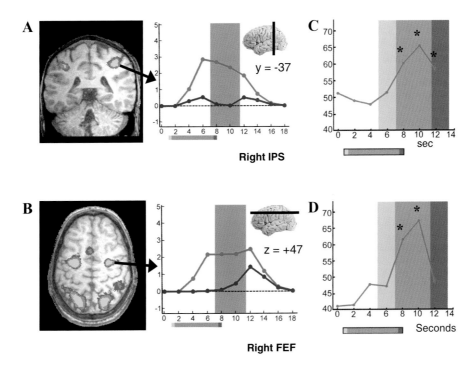

PLATE 44   (A, B) Performance-related activity in the intraparietal sulcus (IPS, A) and the frontal eye field (FEF, B) during the three phases of the working memory task: encoding, delay, and test. Performance-related activity was obtained by comparing activity for correct and incorrect trials at each task phase. Functional group maps are shown overlaid on structural scans from a representative individual. Arrow indicates the region from which the fitted hemodynamic responses were obtained. The level of the coronal section is indicated on the small whole-brain inset. The bar below the x-axis 24 codes the periods when the sample stimulus (light gray), the delay (intermediate gray), and the test stimulus (dark gray) occurred during the task. The vertical gray bar indicates the delay interval. (C, D) The contingency between signal amplitude and the subjects' performance was assessed with a logistic regression analysis for every time point within working memory trials. Activity at 8 and 10 s for the FEF and at 8, 10, and 12 s for the IPS significantly predicted performance ($P < 0.05$), such that for a 1% increase in fMRI signal, the probability of being correct for that trial increased from chance to close to 70% (y-axis).

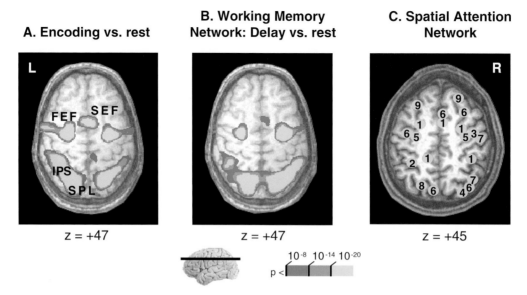

A. Encoding vs. rest

L

FEF SEF

IPS

SPL

z = +47

**B. Working Memory
Network: Delay vs. rest**

z = +47

**C. Spatial Attention
Network**

R

9   9
  6   6
  1   1
6   1 5 3 7
5   2 1   1
      8 6   7
              4 6

z = +45

p < 10^{-8} 10^{-14} 10^{-20}

PLATE 45   Regions involved in visual spatial attention and visual working memory. (*A*) Encoding versus rest on the working memory task. (*B*) Working memory network revealed by the contrast of working memory delay versus rest. (*C*) Regions in the spatial attention network as determined by a meta-analysis of imaging data. The statistical group map is shown overlaid on a structural scan of a representative individual. The level of the axial section is indicated on the small whole-brain inset. Numbers correspond to the following studies: *1*, Corbetta et al., 1993; *2*, Fink et al., 1997; *3*, Nobre et al., 1997; *4*, Vandenbergh et al., 1997; *5*, Corbetta et al., 1998; *6*, Kastner et al., 1999; *7*, Rosen et al., 1999; *8*, Corbetta et al., 2000; *9*, Hopfinger et al., 2000.

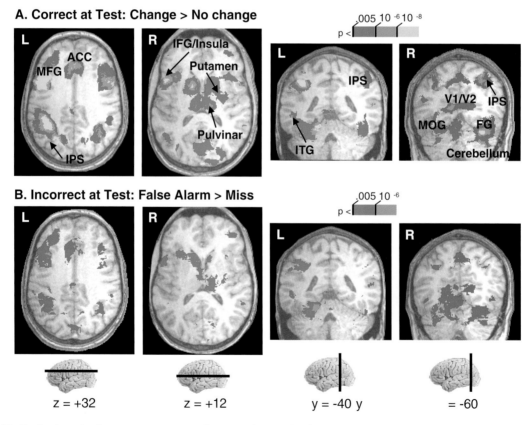

A. Correct at Test: Change > No change

L   R

ACC   IFG/Insula
MFG   Putamen

      Pulvinar
IPS

p < .005 10^{-6} 10^{-8}

L   R

IPS
      V1/V2   IPS
      MOG   FG
ITG   Cerebellum

B. Incorrect at Test: False Alarm > Miss

L   R

p < .005 10^{-6}

L   R

z = +32   z = +12   y = -40 y   = -60

PLATE 46   Similar brain activations occur on correct change and false alarm trials. (*A*) Functional group maps showing regions activated at test on correct change (nonmatch) compared to no-change (match) trials. (*B*) Functional group maps showing regions activated at test on incorrect no-change (false alarms) compared to incorrect change (miss) trials, at the same slice levels. Although the number of high-confidence, incorrect trials was small and the associated activations were weaker, comparing the two patterns of activation revealed a great deal of overlap. Statistical group maps are shown overlaid on structural scans from a representative individual. The level of the axial and coronal sections is indicated on the small whole-brain insets. The color bar indicates *P* values (uncorrected). (Reprinted with permission by Oxford University Press.)

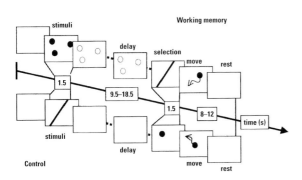

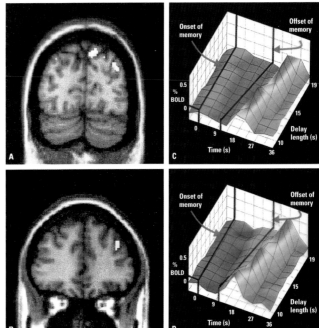

PLATE 47   In a study reported by Rowe and colleagues (2000), subjects had to hold in working memory the position of three dots for a variable length of time. At the end of the delay interval, a line that went through only one of the dots came on. The subjects had to point to where on the line there had been a dot. Area 9/46 acti-vation was associated with the offset operation (*B*) and not with the maintenance of information over the delay (*A*). *C* illustrates when during the time-course at the trial (*x*-axis) activation (*z*-axis) occured for trial of different length (*y*-axis).

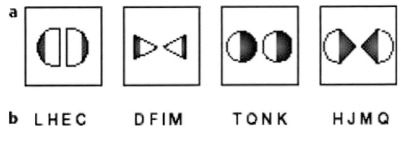

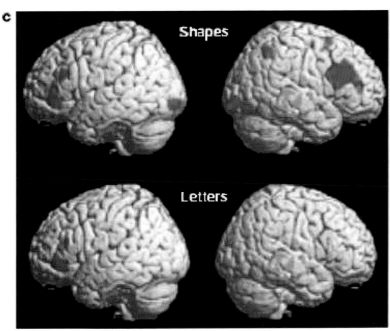

PLATE 48   Demonstration by Duncan and colleagues (2000) of an association of DLPFC activation with general intelligence (*g*) processes. (*a–c*) The activation differences between carrying out the IQ tasks, compared with performing cognitively undemanding control tasks using similar stimuli. The three tasks involved shapes, letters, and spatial relations.

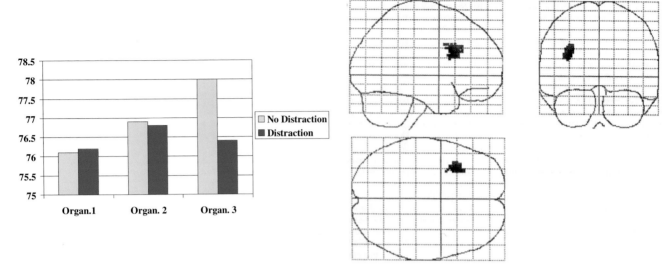

PLATE 49   Activations of a region of left DLPFC during the three different conditions of the memory organization study reported by Fletcher, Shallice, and Dolan (1998).

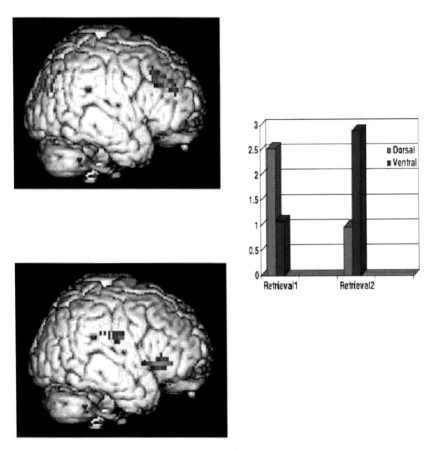

PLATE 50   Activations of the right DLPFC and the right insula/ VLPFC during the two critical conditions of the study reported by Fletcher, Shallice, Frith, and colleagues (1998), namely, organized list recall (retrieval 1) and paired associate recall (retrieval 2). Each was compared with its own control task, which involved only repetition.

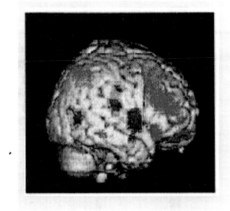

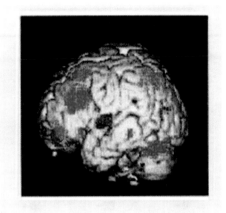

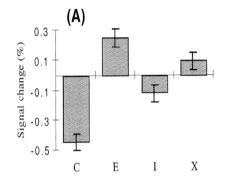

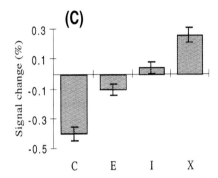

PLATE 51   Activations in the exclusion condition of the source memory study reported by Henson, Shallice, and Dolan (1999) (top) and of a left and right DLPFC voxel in each of the four conditions of the study. Abbreviations: E, encoding; X, exclusion retrieval; I, inclusion retrieval; C, control.

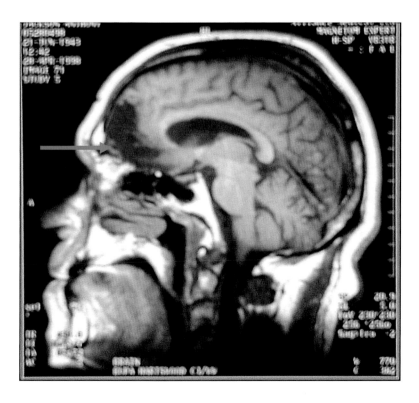

PLATE 52   The lesion of patient A.P. of Shallice and Burgess (1991) with a severe impairment of "intention marker" realization. The lesion affects BA 10 and 11 bilaterally.

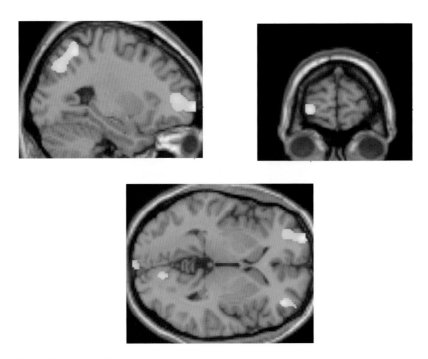

PLATE 53   Activation sites.

LGN and Visual Cortex Activation in Monkey B97

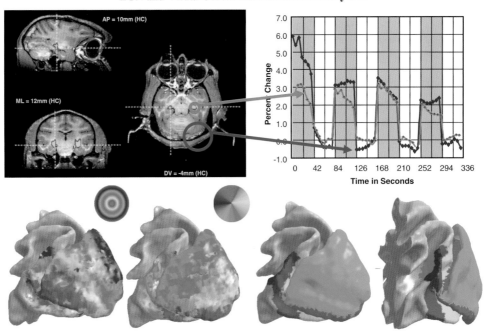

PLATE 54   Upper left panel shows activation of the lateral geniculate nucleus (LGN) and visual cortex. Yellow dotted lines indicate the LGN position. AP, anteroposterior; ML, mediolateral; DV, dorsoventral. Upper right panel shows the time course of the signal for the activated regions in LGN (red) and visual cortex (blue). The two lower left images show the retinotopic organization of the posterior visual areas as revealed with fMRI. Based on this organization, the boundaries of the areas can be defined as shown in the lower right two images: cyan: V1; magenta: V2; yellow: V3; red: V4; blue: V4t; green: MT(V5).

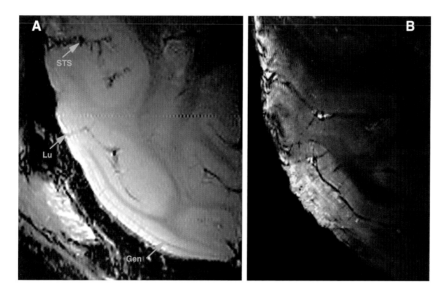

PLATE 55 Anatomical and functional scans acquired with an implanted surface coil. (*A*) T2*-weighted echo-planar image obtained with an actual resolution of $125 \times 125\,\mu\mathrm{m}^2$ and a section thickness of $720\,\mu\mathrm{m}$. (*B*) Similar image from another animal with slightly different acquisition parameters. The resolution is sufficient to visualize the susceptibility effects produced by small cortical vessels with an average diameter of $120\,\mu\mathrm{m}$. In color are the fMRI correlation coefficient maps.

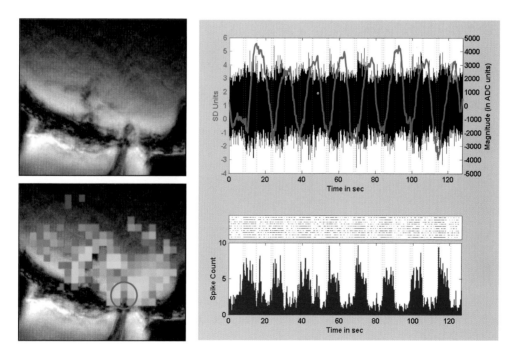

PLATE 56 Combined neurophysiology-fMRI experiments in alert, active monkeys. In the upper left panel an anatomical scan shows the position of the electrode tip. In the lower left panel the activation elicited by a rotating checkerboard is superimposed on the anatomical scan. Top right panel shows the time course of the comprehensive signal (LFPs and spiking activity), together with the BOLD (red thick line), response. Bottom right panel illustrates the raster plots and peristimulus histograms of spiking activity. Each dot is an action potential, and each bin shows the number of action potentials in 250 ms.

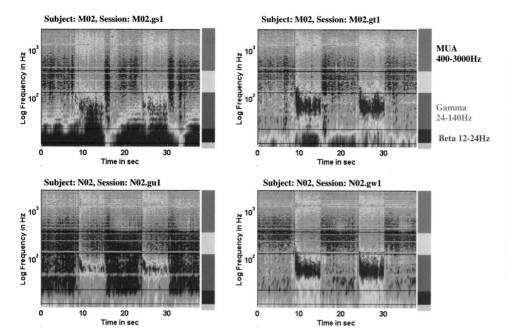

PLATE 57 Time-dependent frequency analysis of the neural signals. Two sessions from two animals are shown (see labels). The spectrograms were computed for windows of 250 ms. Frequency is plotted on the *y*-axis and time on the *x*-axis. At the right of each plot the MUA and LFP ranges are indicated. The red (gamma band) and blue (beta band) sections indicate two of the usual EEG bands. Changes in the power of the signal in the gamma band was best correlated with the hemodynamic response.

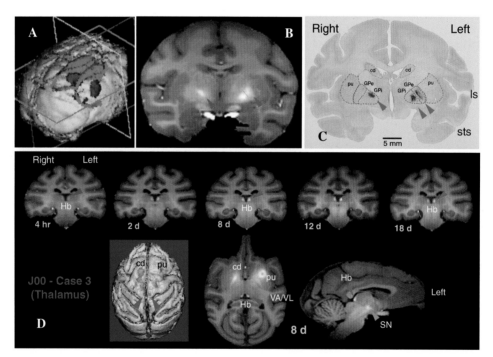

PLATE 58   (*A*) Dorsal view of the rendered brain showing the location and extent of the basal ganglia. (*B*) Manganese transfer to the globus pallidus 24.5 hours after injection into the caudate and putamen. Coronal MRI illustrates the specificity of distribution of Mn^{2+} signal in globus pallidum externum (GPe) and internum (GPi, arrowheads). Note the different spatial distributions of the MR-detectable tracer in the globus pallidus, precisely as expected given the known connectivity of the striatopallidal system: tracer is found in the dorsomedial portion of the GPe and GPi after caudate injection (right hemisphere), and in the ventrolateral or midportion of the GPe and GPi after putamen injection (left hemisphere). At this rostrocaudal level of the globus pallidus, a strong signal was observed only in the GPi on the caudate injection side. (*C*) Coronal

histology section showing the WGA-HRP labeling in the GPe and GPi (arrowheads) 24.5 hours after right caudate and left putamen injections. Note the similar distribution of Mn^{2+} signal and WGA-HRP labeling in the MRI and the histological section, respectively. (*D*) Transneuronal transfer of Mn^{2+} shown by signal changes in the thalamic nuclei over long time periods (4 hours–18 days) after MnCl$_2$ injection into the right caudate and left putamen. The upper row shows coronal MRIs from five different scans (4 hours, 2 days, 8 days, 12 days, and 18 days) illustrating the Mn^{2+} signal in the habenular thalamic nuclei (Hb, bright discrete regions; arrowheads). The lower row indicates the signal increases in the thalamic nuclei (VA/VL and Hb).

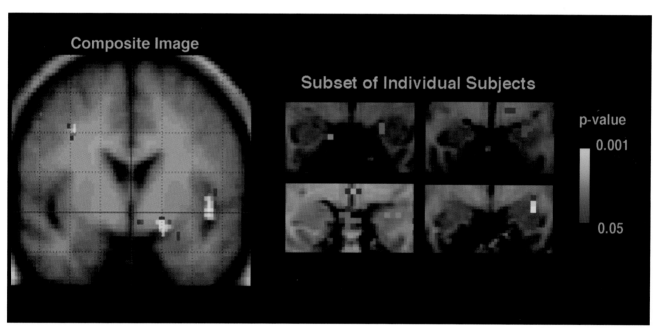

PLATE 59   Activation of the left amygdala in response to instructed fear. Shown are composite activation response to threat versus safe stimuli (left) and selected individual subjects' responses (right). (Adapted with permission from E. A. Phelps et al., Activation of the left amygdala to a cognitive representation of fear. *Nat. Neurosci.* 4:437–441. © 2001 by the Nature Publishing Group.)

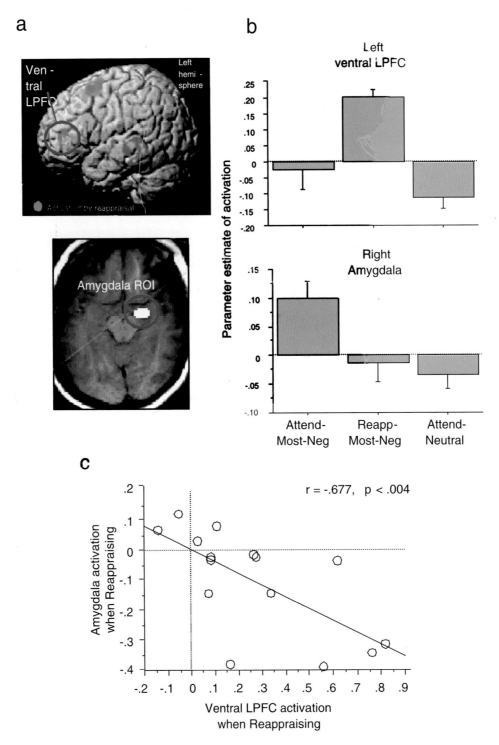

PLATE 60 (a) Activation of the left, ventral LPFC during reappraisal versus attended trials (top) and right amygdala activation
during attended versus reappraisal trials (bottom). (b) Parameter
estimates of activation to the right amygdala and left, ventral
LPFC. (c) Scatterplot depicting the correlation activation of the
amygdala and ventral LPFC for reappraisal versus attended trials.
(Adapted with permission from K. N. Ochsner et al., Rethinking
feelings: An fMRI study of the cognitive regulation of emotion.
J. Cogn. Neurosci. 14:1215–1229. © 2002 by the Society for
Neuroscience.)

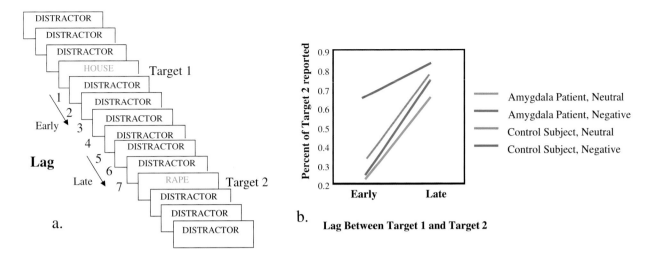

a.

b.

Lag Between Target 1 and Target 2

Amygdala Patient, Neutral
Amygdala Patient, Negative
Control Subject, Neutral
Control Subject, Negative

PLATE 61   (*a*) Schematic illustration of the attentional blink paradigm with an emotion word in the second target position. (*b*) Percent correct identification of target 2 reported in the early and late lag periods for negative and neutral words. Results are for normal control subjects and a patient with bilateral amygdala damage. (Adapted with permission from A. K. Anderson and E. A. Phelps, The human amygdala supports affective modulatory influences on visual awareness. *Nature* 411:305–309. © 2001 by the Nature Publishing Group.)

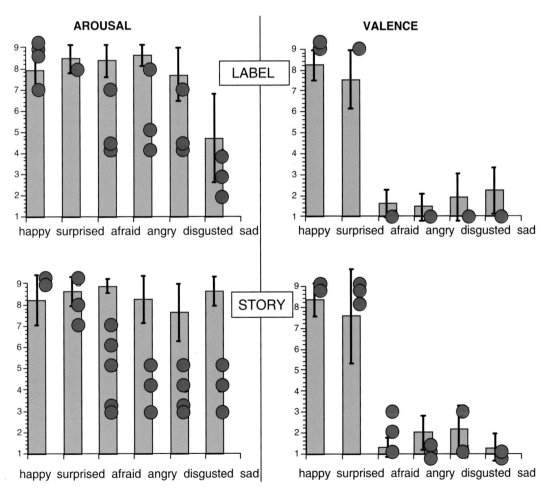

PLATE 62   Developmental damage to the amygdala impairs knowledge of the arousal of unpleasant emotions. Patient S.M.046 was impaired in her knowledge that negatively valenced emotions, especially fear and anger, are also highly arousing. The impairment was evident both for facial expressions of emotions (not shown) and for lexical stimuli such as the words for the emotions and stories depicting emotions. Bars indicate means ± SD of responses by normal controls; circles indicate responses from S.M.046.

Frequency

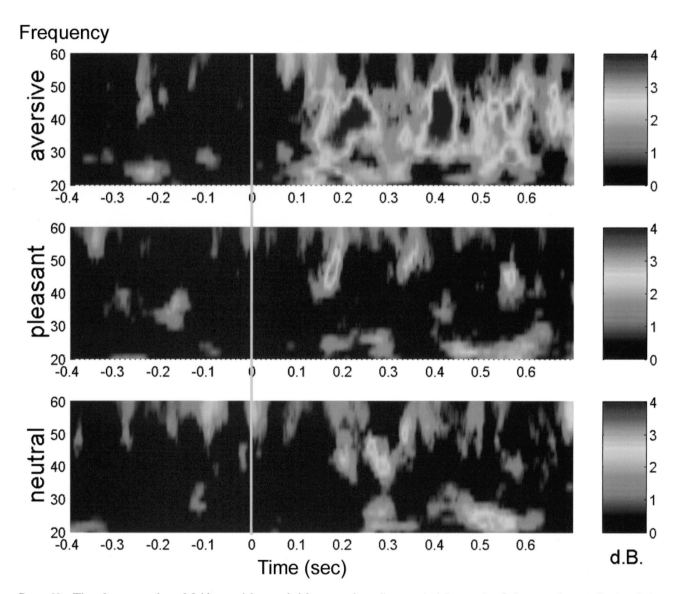

Time (sec)

PLATE 63   Time-frequency plots of field potentials recorded from the amygdala in response to visual stimuli. Time is shown on the x-axis (seconds) and the frequency of the recorded response (20–60 Hz) is shown on the y-axis. Stimulus onset is indicated by the yellow vertical bar at 0s. Color encodes amplitude of the response in dB. Stimuli were sorted into three emotion categories as shown; there were significantly larger responses to aversive stimuli than to pleasant or neutral stimuli.

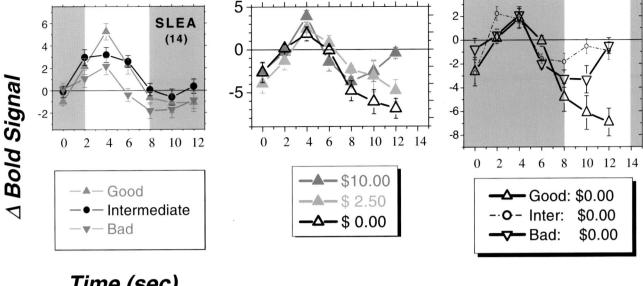

Time (sec)

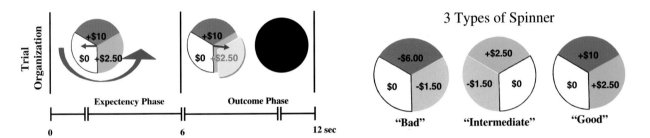

3 Types of Spinner

PLATE 64 These data illustrate an example of brain mapping efforts to temporally dissect subprocesses shown in figure 75.2, using an experimental design that applied principles of prospect theory and decision affect theory (Breiter et al., 2001). This study employed a single-trial-like design, shown at the bottom with three spinners. The trial sequence started with presentation of one of these spinners and continued with an arrow rotating on it. This rotating arrow would abruptly stop after 6s, at which time the sector on which it had landed would flash for 5.5s, indicating the subject had won or lost that amount of money. Given three spinners, each with three outcomes, this experiment sought to determine which putative reward/aversion regions in the brain would display differential expectancy and/or outcome effects. With one outcome ($0) shared across spinners, it could explicitly also evaluate counterfactual comparison effects (Mellers et al., 1997; Mellers, 2000). The evaluation of counterfactual comparison effects is necessary to determine that the experiment did produce expectancy effects, and the incorporation of expectancy effects is necessary to be able to interpret any outcome effects. The graphs at top display differential expectancy effects (left), differential outcome effects (middle), and counterfactual comparisons (right). The y-axes display normalized fMRI signal, while the x-axes display time in seconds. All time courses come from a region of signal change in the sublenticular extended amygdala (SLEA).

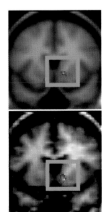

Monetary Expectancy

Cocaine Expectancy

PLATE 65 Expectancy of a monetary gain in the upper panel from a study involving a game of chance in healthy controls (Breiter et al., 2001), and expectancy of a cocaine infusion in the lower panel from a study of double-blind, randomized, cocaine versus saline infusions in cocaine-dependent subjects (Breiter et al., 1997; Breiter and Rosen, 1999). Results are shown in the radiological orientation as pseudocolor statistical maps juxtaposed on coronal group structural images in gray tone. Note the close anatomical proximity for NAc signal changes during positive expectancy in the context of uncertainty for both experiments.

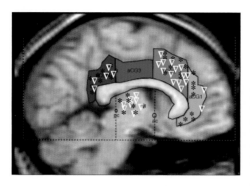

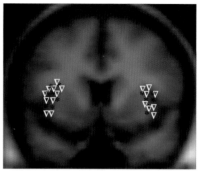

* Reward Effects
▽ Pain Effects

PLATE 66 The gray-tone structural images on the left in the sagittal orientation, and on the right in the coronal orientation (+6 mm anterior of the anterior commissure), juxtapose published neuroimaging data in humans from painful stimuli (Talbot et al., 1991; Coghill et al., 1994; Craig et al., 1996; Rainville et al., 1997; Davis, Kiss, et al., 1998; Davis, Kwan, et al., 1998; Becerra et al., 1999, 2001; Ploghaus et al., 1999; Sawamoto et al., 2000; Rainville, Bushnell, and Duncan, 2001) and from rewarding stimuli (Ketter et al., 1996, 2001; Berns, Cohen, and Mintun, 1997; Berns et al., 2001; Breiter et al., 1997, 2001; Thut et al., 1997; Blood et al., 1999; Bartels and Zeki, 2000; Elliott, Friston, and Dolan, 2000; Liu et al., 2000; Blood and Zatorre, 2001; Knutson, Adams, et al.,

2001; Knutson, Fong, et al., 2001; O'Doherty et al., 2001, 2002; Small et al., 2001; Bush et al., 2002; Elliott et al., 2003) in three brain regions traditionally reported as "classic" pain regions (Becerra et al., 2001). These regions include the thalamus (Thal in left image, between ac and pc), the cingulate cortex, and the anterior insula (INS in right image). The cingulate cortex is segmented into four units following the standardized methods of the Massachusetts General Hospital Center for Morphometric Analysis (Makris et al., 1999; Meyer et al., 1999); the aCG includes aCG1 and aCG2, while the posterior cingulate is the darkest segmentation unit. Note the close approximation of reported activation from stimuli of opposite valance.

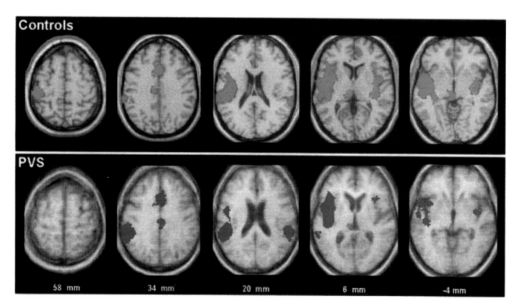

PLATE 67 Brain regions that activated during somatosensory stimulation in normal subjects (top panel) and 15 PVS subjects (bottom panel) are shown in lighter color on mean MRI templates for each group. Darker-colored regions in PVS images correspond to regions that activated significantly less in the patients than in the controls. (Reprinted with permission from S. Laureys et al., Cortical processing of noxious somatosensory stimuli in the persistent vegetative state. *NeuroImage* 17:732–741. © 2002 by Elsevier.)

Multi-focal brain injury

A   B   C

Anoxia

D   E

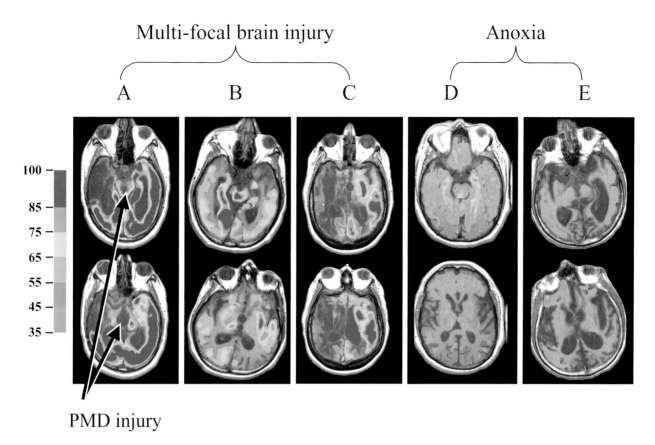

100 —
85 —
75 —
65 —
55 —
45 —
35 —

PMD injury

PLATE 68   Resting brain metabolism in five PVS patients (see text for details). (Reprinted with permission from N. Schiff et al., Residual cerebral activity and behavioral fragments in the persistent vegetative state. *Brain* 125:1210–1234. © 2002 by *Brain*.)

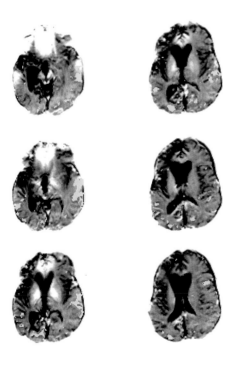

PLATE 69   fMRI responses to passive language stimuli (see text for details).

| | FORWARD | | BACKWARD | | OVERLAP |

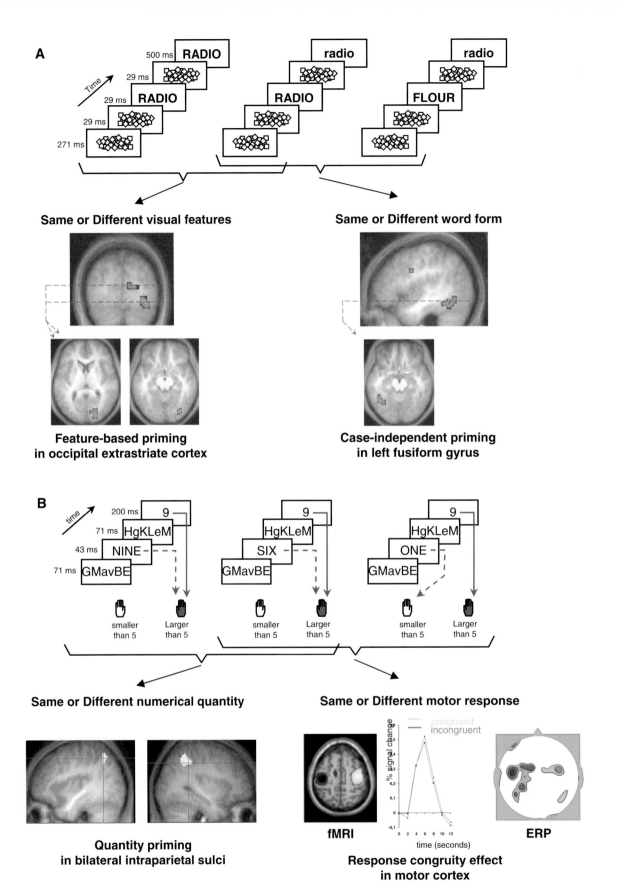

PLATE 70   Main paradigms used in neuroimaging studies of sub-liminal priming. (*A*) Word repetition paradigm, in which a word prime is flashed for 29 ms, hidden by forward and backward masking shapes (Dehaene et al., 2001, 2004). Repetition of the same physical stimulus as prime and target leads to feature-based priming in occipital cortex, while cross-case word repetition leads to case-independent priming in the left fusiform visual word form area. (*B*) Number comparison paradigm, in which a numerical prime is flashed for 43 ms, hidden by forward and backward letter strings (Dehaene, Naccache et al., 1998; Naccache and Dehaene, 2001a, 2001b; Naccache, Blandin, and Dehaene, 2002). Repeating the same quantity as prime and target leads to quantity-based priming in the left and right intraparietal sulci; repeating the same motor response leads to response priming in the left and right motor cortex. Together, these results indicate that a subliminal prime can proceed through an entire series of visual, semantic, and motor stages without entering consciousness.

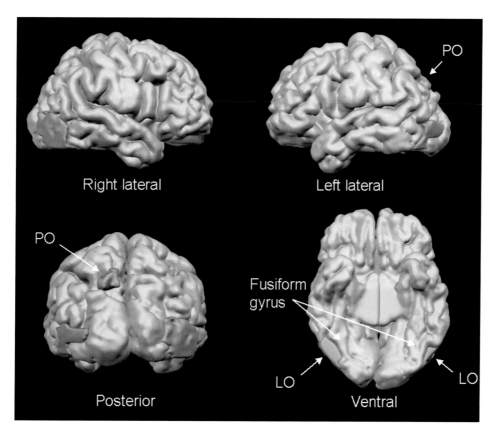

PLATE 71   Four views of D.F.'s brain, mathematically rendered to show pial surface. The lesions were reconstructed from high-resolution MRI sections and were then rendered on the pial surface in pale blue. Abbreviations: LO, lateral occipital area; PO, parieto-occipital area. (Adapted with permission from James et al., 2003.)

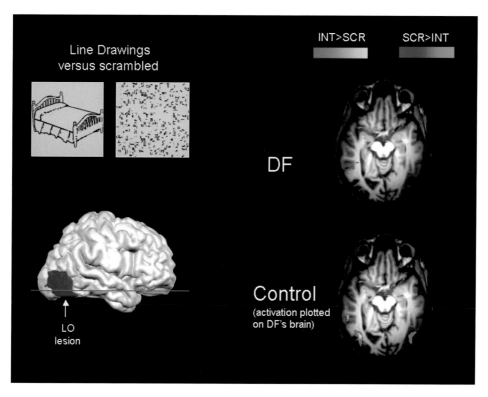

PLATE 72   An fMRI study of activation in D.F. on presentation of line drawings versus scrambled line drawings. D.F. shows essentially no differential activation with line drawings, whereas a control subject shows robust activation. The activation in the control subject has been stereotactically morphed to fit onto D.F.'s brain. Activation to the line drawings falls neatly into the LO lesions. (Adapted with permission from James et al., 2003.)

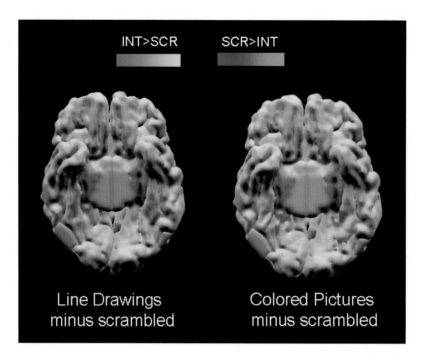

PLATE 73 Activation maps drawn on the ventral surface of D.F.'s brain that represent the comparison of intact line drawing with scrambled line drawing (left) and intact colored pictures with scrambled colored pictures (right). D.F. shows no fMRI activation for the line drawings but robust activation in the fusiform gyrus for the colored pictures. (Adapted with permission from James et al., 2003.)

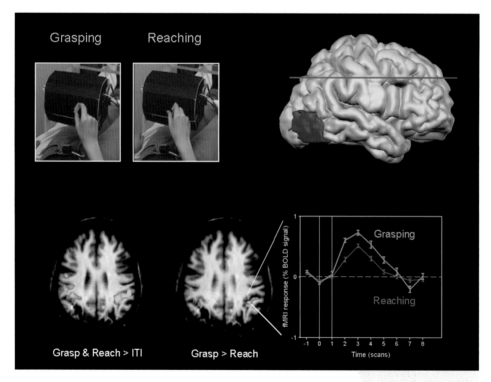

PLATE 74 The "grasparatus" devised by Culham and colleagues (2003) is shown in the upper left. The subject lies in the dark inside the MRI magnet. The solid shapes appear in front of the subject as the cylinder is made to rotate stepwise by a pneumatic motor. The target shape is presented by turning on a superbright LED behind the shape. The task is either to grasp the target shape or, in a control condition, to simply touch it with the knuckles. A section imaged through D.F.'s parietal lobe reveals selective activation in an anterior part of the IPS (area AIP) when she grasps the target object. This activation is similar to that seen in control subjects. (Adapted with permission from James et al., 2003.)

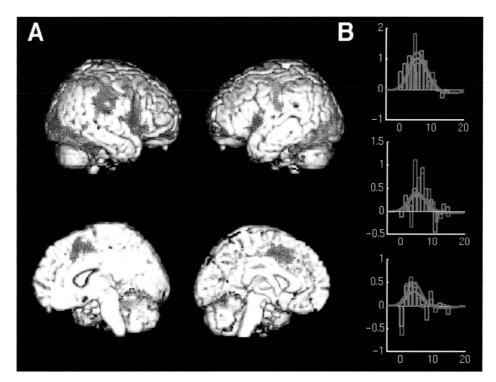

PLATE 75 Event-related activity associated with binocular rivalry perceptual switches. (*A*) Four views of the medial and lateral surfaces of a rendering of an anatomical template image in Talairach space, on which are superimposed areas where evoked activity was specifically related to perceptual transitions in either binocular rivalry (red) or physical stimulus alternation (green). Areas modulated by perception during both rivalrous and physical stimulus alternation, and the bilateral symmetry of the evoked activity are apparent. (*B*) Illustrative postevent histograms of the modulation of activity produced by transition events in rivalry (red) and physical stimulus alternation (green) conditions from three different subjects. The evoked activity (percent change in BOLD contrast) is shown as a function of postevent time (in seconds) for each subject, with the fitted models of hemodynamic response function superimposed in solid lines. The modulation of activity shown here is taken from a voxel in right anterior fusiform gyrus. (Reprinted with permission from E. D. Lumer et al., Neural correlates of perceptual rivalry in the human brain. *Science* 280:1930–1934. © 1998 by the American Association for the Advancement of Science.)

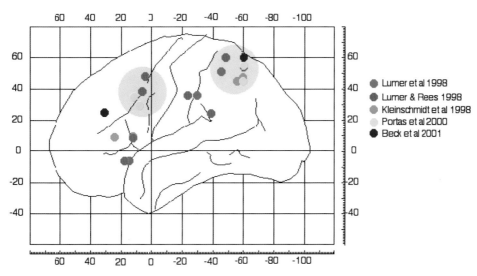

PLATE 76 Neural correlates of conscious vision in parietal and prefrontal cortex. Areas of parietal and prefrontal cortex that show activation correlated with changes in visual awareness in a number of selected studies (Lumer et al., 1998; Lumer and Rees, 1999; Kleinschmidt et al., 1998; Portas et al., 2000; Beck et al., 2001) are plotted on a standardized brain in Talairach space (Talairach and Tournoux, 1988). Each circle is placed at the center of a cluster of activation, with different shades representing different studies; overlapping loci from the same study are omitted for clarity. There is prominent clustering of activations in superior parietal and dorsolateral prefrontal cortex, highlighted by large, light circles.

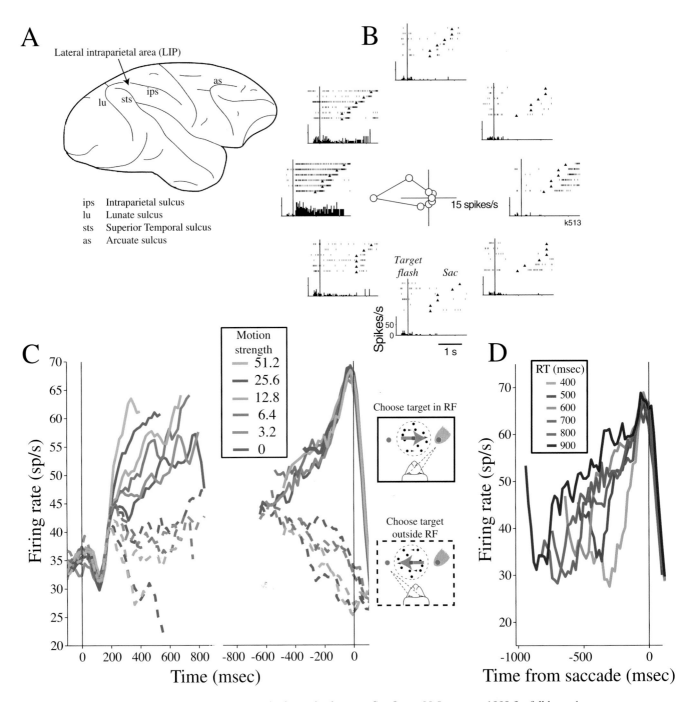

PLATE 77   A neural correlate of a decision process in the parietal cortex. See figure 88.5 on page 1235 for full legend.

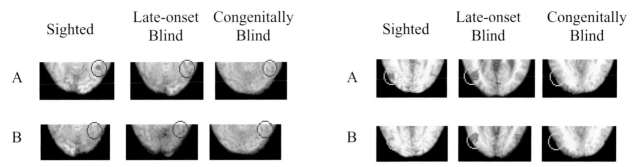

	Sighted	Late-onset Blind	Congenitally Blind			Sighted	Late-onset Blind	Congenitally Blind
A					A			
B					B			

PLATE 78   (*A*) Horizontal MRI images of the posterior part of the hemisphere at the level of the fusiform gyrus (right side on the right). Shown is the effect of visual imagery of a face for 10 s, compared with the effect of imagining a static, nonface pattern. In both sighted individuals and those with late-onset blindness (even though they had been blind for decades), there was clear and specific activation (red voxels) in the right FFA. (*B*) Effect of touching a doll's face on activity in FFA in the sighted (but blindfolded) late and congenitally blind, compared with the effect of touching a "scrambled" doll's face.

PLATE 79   (*A*) The effect of imagining, for 10 s, the visual impression of curtains opening and closing, compared with the effect of imagining the same curtains closed and stationary. The level of this section is through the visual motion area, V5 or MT, and this is clearly activated, at least on the left side, by this motion imagery in both sighted and late-blind individuals. (*B*) The effect of touching the surface of the palm with an unidentifiable moving object, compared with the effect of static placement of the same object on the hand. The visual motion area, MT/V5, is strongly activated only in the late blind.

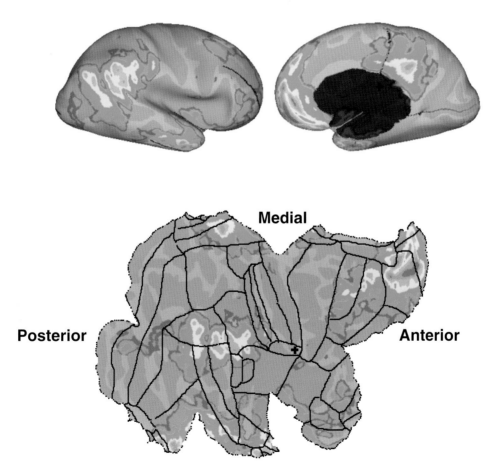

PLATE 80   Areas of the brain observed to decrease their activity during a wide variety of goal-directed behaviors and referred to in the text as task-independent decreases (TIDS). Here these data, representing nine different PET imaging experiments and 134 subjects (G. L. Shulman, Fiez, et al., 1997), are mapped to surface reconstructions of the right cerebral hemisphere from the *Human.colin* atlas (Holmes et al., 1998; Van Essen, 2002). The PET data are mapped to fiducial (3D) surface reconstructions registered to Talairach space (Talairach and Tournoux, 1988) and are displayed on inflated surfaces (top) and on a flat map (bottom). The fiducial markers on the flat map reflect Brodmann areas. Those of particular interest here are designated by their appropriate number. (For further details concerning these mapping strategies, see Van Essen, 2002.)

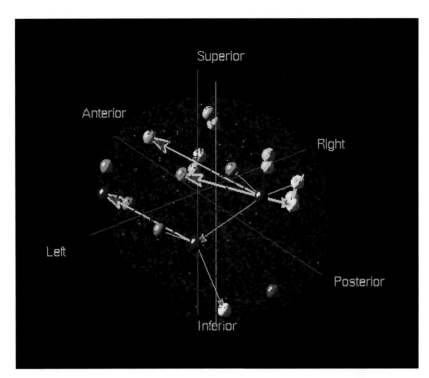

PLATE 81   In a connected network it is often useful to identify the optimal route by which to propagate a message through the system. Analytical techniques permit the assessment of the minimum-cost path (the path in which information loss is minimal or propagation delay is smallest) between a node in a connected network to other surrounding nodes. In this figure, the brain regions identified in a study of face processing by McIntosh (1998) are shown as spheroids in the standardized Talairach space. In the McIntosh study, path weights were determined through decomposition of the covariance matrix between brain regions. To examine the minimum-cost path from the region of the fusiform gyrus to its neighbors, the reported path weights may be subjected to Djikstra's Minimum-cost path analysis. The resulting paths shown here indicate both direct and indirect paths connecting the fusiform area to other regions distributed throughout the brain. This suggests the existence of both functional and effective connectivity in the processing of faces, in particular connectivity between FFA and regions of the frontal lobe putatively involved in executive functions. The strength of the connection is indicated by line thickness, and no connectivity is evident where two brain regions are not connected by a path.

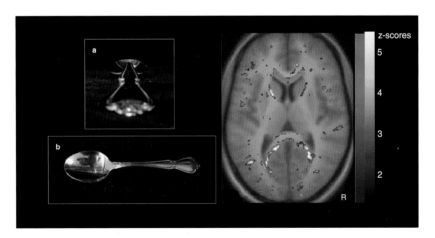

PLATE 82   Example object, a spoon, used in the study of Baird and colleagues. The spoon is shown in both unusual and usual perspectives. At right is a z-score statistical parametric map illustrating the results of a multiple regression analysis using DTI anisotropy and BOLD activation, in which the splenium of the corpus callosum is predictive of relatively faster reaction times and decreased BOLD response. Conversely, the genu of the corpus callosum was significantly predictive of longer reaction times and increased BOLD response in cortical regions of interest on a task that required individuals to name objects presented from unusual perspectives. (Images courtesy of Abigail Baird, Dartmouth College, Hanover, N.H.)

57 The Organization of Lexical Knowledge in the Brain: The Grammatical Dimension

KEVIN SHAPIRO AND ALFONSO CARAMAZZA

ABSTRACT Retrieving a word from the mental lexicon entails access to three types of knowledge: the word's meaning, its sound structure, and its grammatical properties. In this chapter, we outline what is currently known about how grammatical properties of words are represented in the brain, with an emphasis on neural structures that distinguish between words of different syntactic categories. Evidence from neuropsychology, neuroimaging, electrophysiology, and transcranial magnetic stimulation indicates that the left frontal cortex is a crucial component of circuits that process grammatical knowledge about words. Anatomically distinct subregions within this part of the brain may be engaged in various computations that govern the relations between words in speech.

In his *Cours de linguistique générale*, the foundational canon of the modern sciences of language, Saussure defined a linguistic sign as a psychological entity consisting of two elements, a concept and a sound pattern, that are connected in the brain by an associative link (de Saussure, 1916/1972). Such signs, or words, are taken to be the basic units of language, out of which more complex speech structures such as phrases and sentences can be built.

Accordingly, a great deal of work on the cognitive neuroscience of language has been devoted to illuminating the nature of the link between sounds and concepts, and the specific brain regions this lexical circuit encompasses. Some researchers have even been inspired to translate Saussure's formulation, albeit roughly, into neuroanatomical terms. A recent meta-analysis of 58 neuroimaging studies of lexical access (Indefrey and Levelt, 2000) parceled the left perisylvian cortex into areas engaged in the selection of words from concepts (viz., the left middle temporal lobe) and phonological code retrieval (left posterior temporal and inferior parietal lobe), as well as various postlexical phonological and articulatory processes (left posterior frontal lobe and superior temporal gyrus).

Although this model is interesting as far as it goes, it almost certainly presents an incomplete view of how knowledge about words is represented in the brain. Missing from the picture are the brain areas and cognitive mechanisms involved in processing grammatical information that governs the combination of words in speech, and the parsing of strings of words in comprehension. This includes information such as a word's syntactic category (noun, verb, and so forth), which defines the phrasal structure in which it is embedded and the various grammatical forms in which it can appear. In short, grammatical features are the glue that binds words into well-formed and coherent sentences. It would be remarkable if the neural circuitry subserving language use did not provide for their representation.

The representation of nouns and verbs in the brain

There is agreement among linguists that all natural languages incorporate distinctions between words of at least two syntactic categories, such as nouns and verbs (O'Grady, 1997). Such distinctions play a crucial rôle in the ordering of words in phrases and sentences and in the selection of functional elements, such as determiners (*a*, *the*), auxiliaries (*did*, *have*), and inflections (*-s*, *-ing*). Moreover, it has long been observed that access to words of different syntactic categories can be selectively impaired or spared in the aftermath of brain damage (Goodglass et al., 1966; Luria and Tsvetkova, 1967; Miceli et al., 1984). Knowledge of syntactic categories might therefore seem an ideal object of study for a researcher interested in the grammatical organization of the mental lexicon.

This impression should dissipate quickly on considering that a word's syntactic category is correlated with a raft of other variables, many of which are difficult to control in an experimental setting. For instance, verbs, compared to nouns, are typically less imageable, more abstract, more polysemous, acquired later, and associated with a greater number of inflectional variants (Gentner, 1981)—all factors that could (and probably do) contribute to neural and

KEVIN SHAPIRO and ALFONSO CARAMAZZA Cognitive Neuropsychology Laboratory and Department of Psychology, Harvard University, Cambridge, Mass.

behavioral differences observed in processing nouns and verbs. Nevertheless, a rapidly growing corpus of evidence from neuropsychology and neuroimaging suggests that syntactic category knowledge is represented independently of these variables, and that access to words of different syntactic categories can be spared or impaired selectively as a consequence of brain damage.

NOUN AND VERB DEFICITS IN NEUROPSYCHOLOGY Typically, patients with impairments in verb production have lesions in the left frontal lobe, while patients with noun production deficits have lesions in the left temporal lobe (Goodglass et al., 1966; Luria and Tsvetkova, 1967; Miceli et al., 1984; Damasio and Tranel, 1993; Daniele et al., 1994). Although this lesion-deficit pattern is reasonably clear (despite several exceptions, which we mention later), its explanation is not. Accounts of the double dissociation between noun and verb production can be grouped roughly into three clusters, roughly along the lines proposed by Bates and colleagues (1991): the semantic or semantic-conceptual hypothesis, the lexical-grammatical hypothesis, and the morphological hypothesis.

The *semantic hypothesis* holds that apparent noun-verb dissociations reflect differences in the cortical organization of semantic knowledge associated with the two categories. According to one variant, noun or verb deficits result from damage to brain systems involved in representing knowledge about objects and actions, respectively (Damasio and Tranel, 1993; Pulvermueller, Lutzenberger, and Preissl, 1999; Druks and Shallice, 2000). The object system is thought to involve posterior and inferior parts of the left temporal lobe, areas that represent visual form, whereas the action system is distributed more anteriorly in the motor planning areas of the left posterior frontal lobe. Another variant of the semantic hypothesis explains selective noun or verb impairments as reflecting the differential imageability of words of the two classes (Allport and Funnell, 1981; Bird, Howard, and Franklin, 2000).

The *lexical-grammatical hypothesis* states that the lexical system is organized in the brain along lines of grammatical category. In other words, information about a word's noun or verb status is stored at the form level (Miceli et al., 1984; Caramazza and Hillis, 1991). Unlike the semantic-conceptual hypothesis, this position does not appeal to (or rely on) any putative facts about the organization of the cerebral cortex. On the other hand, it is congenial to claims made in developmental psycholinguistics that the noun/verb distinction is either innately specified (Pinker, 1984) or else a product of the universal tendency of the language system to assign different grammatical roles to words associated with fundamentally different conceptual cores (O'Grady, 1997).

Finally, the *morphological hypothesis* argues that noun/verb distinctions are not represented explicitly in the lexicon but emerge in language use, when grammatical category is assigned to words retrieved in the course of comprehension or production. Some grammatical information is reflected overtly in the form of inflectional morphemes, which are specific to one or another syntactic category: for example, the English plural marker –s (which applies to nouns) and the past tense marker –ed (which applies to verbs).[1] Insofar as morphological processing is thought to depend on left frontal structures, including Broca's area, this hypothesis suggests that distinctions between words of different grammatical categories might be instantiated by frontal neural systems (Shapiro and Caramazza, 2003a).

Although these three hypotheses need not be construed as mutually exclusive, they make different predictions about the nature of grammatical category-specific deficits. The question most relevant to this chapter is whether noun and verb deficits are *not* always reducible to more general impairments in conceptual knowledge—in other words, whether there is empirical support for the lexical-grammatical or morphological hypothesis in at least some cases. Such cases would shed light on the cortical organization of grammatical knowledge.

One method of demonstrating that brain damage can affect access to words of a particular grammatical category independently of various semantic factors is simply to show that these factors cannot account for a patient's performance in producing nouns or verbs. For example, Berndt and colleagues (Berndt et al., 2002) constructed a sentence completion task in which the target words varied parametrically by syntactic category (noun or verb) and imageability (high or low). Some of the patients they tested using this task only showed effects of imageability. Others, however, only showed syntactic category effects, while a third group of patients showed an interaction between syntactic category and imageability, demonstrating that the two effects are independent, contrary to claims that imageability differences can account wholly for selective verb deficits in aphasia (Bird, Howard, and Franklin, 2000).

Results like these suggest that even if semantic-conceptual hypotheses can account for many cases of purported noun and verb deficits, there remain many cases in which the loss of grammatical knowledge is a central feature of a category-specific deficit. Nevertheless, a limitation of this approach is that it is virtually impossible to control for *all* of the semantic variables that might be confounded with a word's grammatical category. Providing a satisfactory demonstration of the neuropsychological independence of knowledge about grammatical categories will therefore require us to adopt a different tack. Namely, we must identify cases for which a semantic explanation is improbable a fortiori. At least two types of patients seem to fit the bill: those with impairments in the production of nouns or verbs limited to one output modality, and those whose impairments manifest in contexts that apparently require no access to semantic knowledge.

MODALITY-SPECIFIC DEFICITS   Among the more compelling reasons to believe that the organization of the brain reflects categorical distinctions between nouns and verbs is the observation that some neurological patients present with problems producing words of one category in only one modality of output (speech or writing). Such deficits may occur as a result of stroke (Caramazza and Hillis, 1991; Rapp and Caramazza, 1997, 2002) or in neurodegenerative disorders (Hillis, Tuffiash, and Caramazza, 2002). Syntactic category-specific deficits of this type cannot logically arise at the level of word meaning, at least on the assumption that a single semantic system supports lexical production and comprehension across modalities.

The majority of reported patients with modality-specific grammatical category impairments have more difficulty with verbs than nouns (Caramazza and Hillis, 1991; Rapp and Caramazza, 1998; Hillis, Tuffiash, and Caramazza, 2002) (though some patients do have modality-specific problems with nouns (Hillis and Caramazza, 1995; Rapp and Caramazza, 2002), suggesting that such deficits do not arise simply because verbs are more susceptible to impairment). Perhaps the clearest anatomical conclusion that can be drawn from these cases is that the written production of verbs depends on structures in the left posterior frontal and anterior parietal cortices, brain regions that were damaged in patient S.J.D (Badecker and Caramazza, 1991; Caramazza and Hillis, 1991) and patient P.W. (Rapp and Caramazza, 1998), both of whom suffered ischemic strokes.

Converging evidence for the importance of left posterior frontal cortex especially comes from a striking study by Hillis and colleagues (2003), who showed that in two patients, impaired written production of verbs (compared with spoken production of verbs, and written and spoken production of nouns) was linked to hypoperfusion of left posterior inferior frontal gyrus and precentral gyrus. When blood flow was restored to these regions, performance in writing verbs improved to ceiling for both patients (figure 57.1).

Curiously, the same brain regions—left parietal and posterior frontal cortices—seem to be implicated in verb production deficits irrespective of output modality. We have already mentioned the classic association between left frontal lesions and problems in verb production (Miceli et al., 1984). There is also evidence linking left parietal damage to poor verb production in patients with no frontal damage (Silveri and di Betta, 1997).

Why, then, does damaging these parts of the brain sometimes, but not always, result in problems restricted to either speaking or writing? One possibility is that the spoken and written representations of verbs have separate but adjacent neural substrates, and that lesion data are not sufficiently

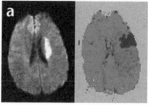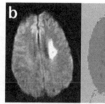

FIGURE 57.1   Diffusion-weighted (left) and perfusion-weighted (right) imaging scans before and intervention to restore blood flow. (*a*) Scans obtained when written naming of verbs was impaired. (*b*) Scans obtained intervention, when written naming of verbs had recovered. (Reprinted with permission from Hillis et al., 2003.) (See color plate 33.)

fine-grained to disentangle them. This possibility is consistent with the lexical-grammatical hypothesis of noun and verb deficits, which holds that grammatical category is represented at the level of lexical form.

On the other hand, it is also possible that reports of so-called modality-specific verb (or noun) deficits in fact conflate two independent deficits: a deficit in producing verbs (or nouns), which might be semantic in nature, and a deficit in producing spoken or written words. This account requires that both deficits be so mild as to yield little evidence of difficulty with the spared category in the impaired modality, and vice versa. Although it is difficult to imagine how such a constellation of deficits could produce patterns of performance where output in the spared category or modality is virtually at ceiling (Caramazza and Hillis, 1991), the "two-hit" story cannot be excluded on purely logical grounds.

Empirically, however, the story is challenged by the case of patient K.S.R., who presented with a remarkable modality-specific double dissociation, being worse with nouns in speech but worse with verbs in writing (Rapp and Caramazza, 2002; figure 57.2). Unfortunately from a neurolinguistic standpoint, K.S.R.'s lesion is very large, affecting the entire area of the left middle cerebral artery distribution (including the caudate, Broca's area, Wernicke's area, and the supramarginal gyrus). All the same, the deficits observed in K.S.R. and in patients with similar impairments suggest that syntactic category may be an organizational principle of the mental lexicon, that is, that word forms marked as nouns and verbs are represented or retrieved in different parts of the brain.[2]

MORPHOSYNTACTIC DEFICITS   A second in-principle argument against the sufficiency of the semantic-conceptual hypothesis comes from the study of patients whose problems with nouns or verbs seem to be bound up with problems in the use of grammatical inflections appropriate to words of the impaired category, such as the plural marker *–s* for nouns and the past tense marker *–ed* for verbs.

The category-specific omission or misuse of inflections does not appear to be determined by damage to a store

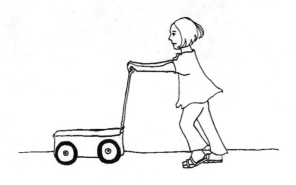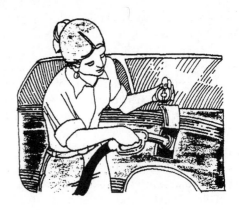

Speaking: "the girl is holding the [baig]"   "the man is putting gas in the car"
Writing: THE GIRL IS ACTIONS A WAGON   THE WOMAN IS HOLD GAS THE CAR

FIGURE 57.2   Examples of K.S.R.'s production of nouns and verbs in oral and written naming (Rapp and Caramazza, 2002).

of semantic knowledge, especially insofar as it can be demonstrated that patients with this kind of disorder have exactly the same problems with real nouns and verbs, on the one hand, and with meaningless nonce words used as nouns and verbs, on the other.

For example, patient J.R. correctly produced verb phrases such as *he judges* and *he wugs*, but not noun phrases such as *the judges* and *the wugs* (Shapiro, Shelton, and Caramazza, 2000). Patient R.C. exhibited a mirror deficit with verbs (Shapiro and Caramazza, 2003a), suggesting that category-specific morphosyntactic deficits do not arise because inflection is somehow more difficult or complex for one category than another. Nor does it seem to be the case that such deficits are evident only in languages that, like English, have relatively weak morphological marking: a Greek-speaking patient, S.K., had more trouble with verbal than with nominal morphology, even though both nouns and verbs are richly inflected in Greek (Tsapkini et al., 2002). A similar pattern obtained for the Italian-speaking patient M.R. (Laiacona and Caramazza, in press).

Problems with inflectional morphology do not seem to be inevitable corollaries of deficits in retrieving word forms or meanings. For example, patients H.G. (Shapiro and Caramazza, 2003b) and E.A. (Laiacona and Caramazza, in press) presented with profound impairments in verb and noun production, respectively, but performed at ceiling on various morphological tasks with words and nonce words of both categories. The occurrence of cases like J.R. and R.C., on the one hand, and H.G. and E.A. on the other underscores our argument that problems in naming nouns and verbs (or actions and objects) may be symptomatic of disorders at any of several different levels in the language production system—semantic-conceptual, lexical, and morphological.

Extension of this logic suggests that the knowledge relevant to noun and verb production at each level should have unique neural substrates. In other words, information about the meaning of nouns might be stored in one brain area, while word forms with the grammatical category label Noun might be represented in another region, and the rules for computing nominal inflections (such as the plural -*s*) might be processed in still a different part of the brain. Obviously, the lexical access system would have to include mechanisms for retrieving and integrating information from all three sources in the process of producing a noun or a verb.

If this model were correct, it would easily accommodate "exceptions" to the canonical observation that noun and verb deficits result from temporal and frontal damage, respectively. J.R.'s lesion, for example, encompasses the left posterior inferior frontal cortex and parts of the left inferior parietal cortex, including the angular and supramarginal gyri. This distribution differs from what has been described in most cases of patients with noun deficits, in which the lesions generally affect parts of the left middle and inferior temporal lobe.

One possible implication is that knowledge about the morphological properties of nouns is represented in the left frontal lobe but lexical knowledge about nouns, or semantic knowledge about concrete objects, relies primarily on temporal regions. Support for such a division of labor can be drawn with caution from the observation that some patients with predominantly temporal dementias (Robinson, Rossor, and Cipolotti, 1999) and with optic aphasia (Campbell and Manning, 1996; Druks and Shallice, 2000) exhibit problems with noun naming that appear to derive either from an impairment of semantic knowledge about objects or from an inability to activate lexical representations of object names on the basis of picture input.

Likewise, analysis of the lesions in patients R.C. and M.R. suggests that the brain regions critical for representing grammatical knowledge about verbs include parts of the left

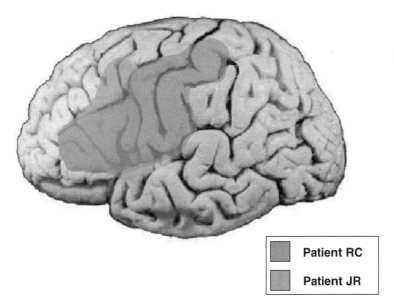

FIGURE 57.3 Brain regions implicated in naming of nouns and verbs (Shapiro and Caramazza, 2003c). Patient R.C. (red) is relatively impaired at naming verbs, and presents with a lesion primarily affecting the left posterior frontal lobe and underlying structures. Patient J.R. (blue) is more impaired at noun production;

he suffered a left middle cerebral artery infarction with damage extending from the frontal lobe posteriorly, including the sensory strip and the angular and supramarginal gyri. The left temporal lobe is largely spared, with the possible exception of the first temporal gyrus near the pole. (See color plate 34.)

frontal cortex superior and anterior to Broca's area (figure 57.3).[3] In fact, suppression of approximately this area using transcranial magnetic stimulation (TMS) in neurologically intact subjects interferes with the production of verbs and nonce words used as verbs in a task very similar to the one performed by R.C. (Shapiro et al., 2001).

Other prefrontal/premotor areas, along with more posterior cortical areas, are likely to be important for the semantic specification of verbs or action words. Poor retrieval of action words, rather than verbs as such, has been linked to damage affecting a number of other brain regions, including the anterior insula, left mesial occipital cortex, and paraventricular white matter underlying the supramarginal gyrus and posterior temporal region (Tranel et al., 2001; figure 57.4). Posterior parietal areas found to have been damaged in some patients with verb retrieval deficits could also be involved in representing semantic features of actions (Silveri and di Betta, 1997).

EVIDENCE FROM ELECTROPHYSIOLOGY   Although most neuropsychological studies on the representation of grammatical category knowledge have probed patients' written or spoken production, experiments using event-related potential recording ERP in neurologically intact subjects have naturally focused on input-driven processes, such as auditory and visual word recognition. Such studies have almost universally found that nouns and verbs elicit distinct event-related responses, especially when these words are presented in the context of phrases or sentences (Teyler et al., 1973; Federmeier et al., 2000).

The spatial distribution of ERPs elicited by nouns and verbs in various studies have been found to correspond to topographically or functionally distinct neural generators (Koenig and Lehmann, 1996; Federmeier et al., 2000; Kellenbach et al., 2002). However, there is considerable variability in the brain regions that have been linked to noun and verb recognition in different tasks. For example, Dehaene (1995) reported that classifying verbs produced left temporoparietal negativity around 260 ms, while Federmeier and colleagues (2000) found that reading unambiguous verbs in the context of sentences produced a left-lateralized anterior positivity not found for nouns. It is possible that such differences reflect access to different properties of verbs, with the more "semantic" task engaging posterior regions and the more "grammatical" task engaging frontal regions.

As is the case in neuropsychology, the interpretation of categorical differences in electrophysiological measures is not clear-cut. Pulvermueller and colleagues have argued that observed ERP differences between nouns and verbs reflect the differential dependence of nouns and verbs on cortical structures that encode, respectively, the visual features of objects and motor schemata relating to actions (Pulvermueller, 1999, 2001; Pulvermueller, Lutzenberger, and Preissl, 1999). Again, however, careful studies indicate that while the semantic-conceptual hypothesis may explain *some* observed differences in brain responses to nouns and verbs, it is not likely to provide an exhaustive account. For example, a study by Kellenbach and colleagues (2002) found that visual-perceptual/motor attributes and grammatical category exerted independent effects on the spatiotemporal

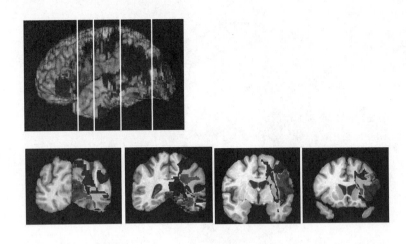

Number of Subjects in Overlap

FIGURE 57.4 Areas of lesion overlap in 13 subjects with disproportionate impairments in action naming relative to naming of concrete entities. The figure shows three regions of maximal overlap: *1*, the left frontal operculum, underlying white matter, and anterior insula; *2*, the left mesial occipital cortex; and *3*, the paraventricular white matter underneath the supramarginal gyrus and posterior temporal region. Color bar indicates the number of subjects in the overlap. (Reprinted with permission from Tranel et al., 2001.) (See color plate 35.)

distribution of ERPs in word reading and recognition (figure 57.5).

EVIDENCE FROM NEUROIMAGING Curiously, functional imaging studies have not revealed clear-cut dissociations between nouns and verbs. In experimental tasks ranging from word generation (Warburton et al., 1996) to word stem completion (Buckner et al., 2000) and semantic categorization (Tyler et al., 2001), nouns and verbs both activate a patchwork of areas in the left hemisphere, including temporal, parietal, and prefrontal regions, with no differences across grammatical category. One study using a lexical decision paradigm showed that some areas in the left hemisphere, including dorsolateral prefrontal cortex and parts of the parietal and temporal lobes, were activated more robustly for verbs than for nouns, but the experimenters did not find any areas in which nouns elicited greater activity (Perani et al., 1999).

One reason for this puzzling negative finding might be that the tasks used in neuroimaging studies to date have engaged processing mechanisms that do not distinguish between nouns and verbs. Not all of the components of the lexical production system need to be sensitive to the grammatical category of a word being produced, and it is possible that tasks like lexical decision (Perani et al., 1999; Tyler et al., 2001) and semantic categorization (Tyler et al., 2001), even in carefully designed studies, are not appropriate to reveal categorical differences between nouns and verbs.

None of these studies employed tasks that specifically tapped subjects' grammatical knowledge about words.

SUMMARY Notwithstanding the lack of converging data from neuroimaging, the evidence from neuropsychological and ERP studies seems to corroborate our contention that grammatical information about nouns and verbs is represented in the brain separately from word meaning. Whether this information is stored in the lexicon and retrieved during word production (the lexical-grammatical hypothesis) or assigned "on the fly" during the course of syntactic computations (the morphological hypothesis), or some combination of the two, is for the moment a matter of speculation. In either case, semantic information may still be important in determining how a word is used grammatically; for example, if the morphological hypothesis is correct, a word's meaning may pick out the inflectional wringer for which it is destined.

Anatomically speaking, there is considerable support for the idea that the processing of verbs depends heavily on left anterior brain regions, while noun processing depends on posterior regions. However, it is possible that this gross distinction reflects the organization of semantic features that correlate with the categories of nouns and verbs, with knowledge about the properties of objects localized in inferior temporal areas (the so-called ventral, or "what," pathway) while knowledge about actions is distributed in prefrontal areas implicated in the representation of motor schemata and/or in parietal areas important for the representation

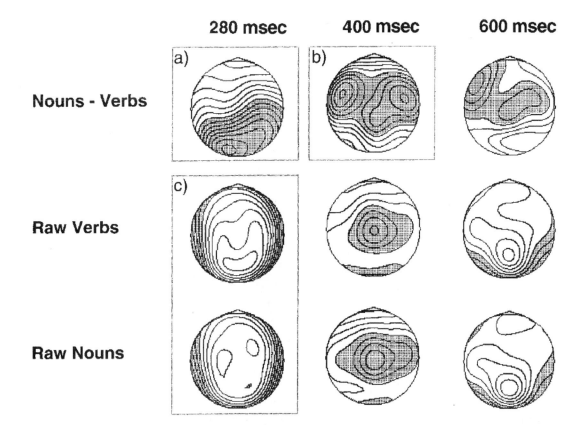

280 msec **400 msec** **600 msec**

Nouns - Verbs

Raw Verbs

Raw Nouns

FIGURE 57.5 Topographies of differences between grand mean ERPs to nouns and verbs (contour line spacing = 0.1 mV) and raw ERP distribution for nouns and verbs (contour line spacing = 0.4 mV). Shading indicates relatively more negativity. (Reprinted with permission from Kellenbach et al., 2002.)

of spatial relations between objects (the dorsal "where" pathway). Already, we should note, this is a departure from the Indefrey and Levelt (2000) model, which confines semantic processing to the middle temporal lobe.

When we consider the representation of knowledge about syntactic categories as such, the picture changes. The cognitive machinery that treats nouns and verbs as grammatical objects seems to rely on neural structures within the left prefrontal cortex, including and adjacent to Broca's area. At first glance, the data on this point are much stronger for verbs than for nouns; there is abundant evidence from neuropsychology and TMS that syntactic information about verbs is processed in the left prefrontal region, while the evidence for nouns derives largely from observation of patient J.R. However, when we look closely at the kinds of grammatical operations associated with noun production in various languages, especially the retrieval of grammatical gender, the case for involvement of the left frontal lobe in representing nouns is strengthened.

Grammatical features and function words

Languages vary in the repertoire of grammatical features they associate with lexical items. For example, in Italian and in many other languages, nouns have the property of grammatical gender, which is reflected in the phonological forms of local determiners and adjectives, as well as in pronominal referents. Thus, one can say of *la luce* (the light [feminine]) that *essa è chiara* (it is clear), or one can demand that someone should *spegnerla* (turn it off), but when referring to a source of light as *il lume* (masculine) one must say *esso è chiaro* and *spegnerlo*.

The assignment of feminine gender to *luce* and masculine gender to *lume* cannot be predicted on the basis of these words' semantic or phonological properties, and clearly has nothing to do with natural or biological gender. (As Mark Twain famously observed, the German word for turnip, *die Rübe*, is grammatically feminine, while the word for maiden, *das Mädchen*, is neuter.) Gender is, rather, an arbitrary association that must be learned by speakers of Italian, German, and numerous other languages (Corbett, 1991). Moreover, some patients with damage to posterior parts of the left hemisphere seem to be able to report the gender of words whose forms they cannot produce (Henaff Gonon, Bruckert, and Michel, 1989; Badecker, Miozzo, and Zanuttini, 1995). This suggests that knowledge of a noun's gender is retrieved by computations that are neurally distinct from those involved in accessing word form.

NEURAL CORRELATES OF GRAMMATICAL GENDER Several recent experiments have offered a glimpse of what the neural substrate of gender knowledge might look like. Miceli and colleagues (2002), using functional magnetic resonance imaging (fMRI), found that retrieving the grammatical gender of an Italian word activates a cortical network distinct from that engaged in processing the word's phonological and semantic features, comprising portions of the left middle and inferior frontal gyri and the left middle and inferior temporal gyri. Another fMRI study found that producing a German noun's definite determiner—a task that requires access to gender—produces activation in the anterior part of Broca's area (Heim, Opitz, and Friederici, 2002; figure 57.6). These results are complemented by an ERP study of sentence reading in German which showed that gender agreement violations elicit a left anterior negativity that is independent of semantic expectancy effects (Gunter, Friederici, and Schriefers, 2000).

Together, the findings from electrophysiology and neuroimaging suggest that a left frontal-temporal circuit is involved in retrieving the gender of nouns for speakers of several languages. If we assume that the posterior portion of this circuit is involved in lexical access to nouns (along with their associated gender), we may tentatively conclude that the grammatical processing of gender is primarily a function of the left frontal cortex, and specifically of cortical regions adjacent to or contained within Broca's area.

IS GENDER A MODEL GRAMMATICAL PROPERTY? Gender is an unusually clear-cut example of grammatical knowledge, in that gender features are associated arbitrarily with nouns in the mental lexicon and in many languages cannot logically be specified by phonological or semantic information (although correlations between gender and certain phonological or semantic properties may play a supporting role in access to gender information; Vigliocco and Franck, 2001). Studying how a word's gender is retrieved therefore makes for an excellent model of the representation of grammatical knowledge in the brain (see, e.g., van Turennout, Hagoort, and Brown, 1998, for an experiment that uses gender decision as a proxy for syntactic processing in general).

This approach has obvious shortcomings: not all languages have gender, and it is unclear how well observations about gender processing generalize to other kinds of grammatical features in various languages. On the other hand, the most interesting characteristic of grammatical gender systems is not that they partition the lexicon into arbitrary categories but that they control the selection of other grammatical material, such as determiners and agreement markers. For this reason it makes sense to view findings on the cortical substrates of gender knowledge not as a curiosity of functional anatomy (like the vermiform appendix) but as a window on the brain mechanisms engaged in the coordination of grammatical elements in speech.

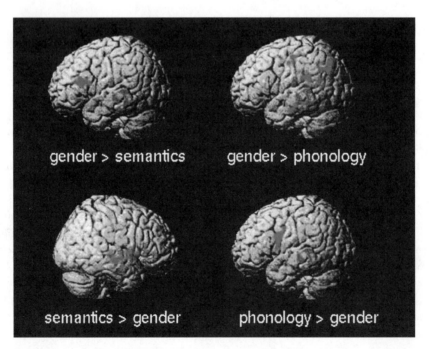

FIGURE 57.6 Lateral see-through of activations observed with fMRI, contrasting conditions in which subjects viewed words and made decisions about their gender (masculine or feminine?), meaning (animal or artifact?), and phonology (does it contain a /tʃ/ or a /k/ sound?). (Reprinted with permission from Miceli et al., 2002.) (See color plate 36.)

In fact, there is much reason to believe that the selection of grammatical or "function" words depends on structures in the left frontal lobe. We begin with the well-known fact that aphasic patients with frontal lesions often present with "agrammatic" speech, in which content words are mostly preserved but function words are largely omitted. This has been interpreted as evidence that such patients have difficulties processing the grammatical content of functional elements (Jakobson, 1956; Luria, 1970; Berndt and Caramazza, 1980).[4] By contrast, patients with more posterior lesions in the left hemisphere have few difficulties with function words but may be impaired in the production and comprehension of "content" words, such as nouns and verbs.

Electrophysiological measures have also been used to support the notion that function words are processed in frontal cortical areas. Neville and colleagues (Neville, Mills, and Lawson, 1992) reported differences in ERPs to function words and content words in sentence reading. Function words elicited a negative ERP component (N280) that was largest over anterior regions of the left hemisphere, while content words elicited a larger posteriorly distributed negativity (N400). Together with the neuropsychological data, these findings suggest that the production and intepretation of grammatical information is handled largely by neural structures in the left frontal lobe, while knowledge pertinent to a word's meaning may depend more on the temporal and parietal lobes.

Why the left frontal lobe?

LANGUAGE AND THE FRONTAL LOBE In the foregoing sections we have tried to make the case that grammatical knowledge is represented in the brain independently of knowledge about a word's meaning, or its phonological or orthographic form. Furthermore, we have described evidence that the representation of grammatical knowledge depends crucially on neural structures housed in the left frontal lobe.

It has been known at least since the seminal observations of Broca (1861) and Dax (1836/1865) that parts of the left frontal lobe are crucial for the production of speech. Even now, however, the functional role of this part of the brain in language use, and the nature of language deficits following frontal lobe damage, remain controversial.

On one side of the theoretical divide are those who have claimed that structures in the frontal lobe are critical for retrieving and utilizing abstract syntactic knowledge (Jakobson, 1956; Luria, 1970; Berndt and Caramazza, 1980; Zurif, 1980; Caplan, 2001). In the opposing camp are researchers who have argued that the left frontal lobe is primarily responsible for the motor output of speech (Lenneberg, 1973) or higher-level phonological processes (Indefrey and Levelt, 2000), and that apparent deficits in

grammatical processing can be reduced to problems with articulatory and phonological planning (Kean, 1978).

We might take the findings we have described in this chapter to bolster the position that the left frontal lobe specializes in representing the grammatical component of language (which is not to say, of course, that some frontal structures are not crucial for phonological and articulatory processes; in fact, it is clearly true that they are). The various fractionations in grammatical knowledge that can arise in the aftermath of frontal damage may reflect the greater dependence of certain operations on certain portions of a frontal circuit broadly engaged in grammatical processing.

THE LEFT FRONTAL CORTEX IN COGNITIVE NEUROSCIENCE What, then, are we to make of findings in other branches of cognitive neuroscience, for example, memory research, that implicate frontal brain structures in what appear to be very different sorts of cognitive tasks? We might adopt the position that such findings need not concern us: a given population of neurons in the frontal cortex could constitute a part of several circuits with distinct cognitive functions, just as a single stretch of DNA can encode multiple genes with different products. The present state of neurobiological knowledge does not seem to warrant much greater specificity (or generality) in assigning functions to particular patches of tissue within frontal cortex.

Certainly some of the functions that have been assigned to the left prefrontal region do not seem fully equipped to handle the phenomena we have described. It may be true, for instance, that some portions of the left prefrontal cortex are engaged in some kind of semantic processing (Petersen et al., 1989; Démonet et al., 1992; Mueller, Kleinhans, and Courchesne, 2003). But even were this so, it remains the case (as we have argued) that the retrieval of grammatical knowledge cannot be reduced to semantic processes, implying that this part of the brain would have to be capable of carrying out more than one kind of operation.

Other hypotheses about the role of the left prefrontal cortex are more directly compatible with the account we have presented. For example, a number of extraordinary studies of neuronal activation in primate frontal cortex have motivated the view that prefrontal neurons are specially adapted for categorization, that is, they classify input received from other parts of the brain into one or more discrete categories relevant to a task (Miller et al., 2003). In a representative experiment, monkeys were trained to respond differentially to exemplars of two categories (e.g., dogs or cats). Subsequently it was possible to identify neurons in prefrontal regions that fired whenever the subject was presented with an exemplar of one category, even when the features of the exemplar were intermediate between prototypes of the two categories (Freedman et al., 2001).

Language, as we have seen, relies heavily on mechanisms of categorization. A word that takes the plural ending -s must be categorized as a noun, even if its semantic properties bear more similarity to verbs (*departure*) or adjectives (*length*) than to prototypical nouns. Similarly, a meaningless nonce word like *wug* may instantly be assigned to one or another grammatical category based on its context (*wug* is a verb in *he wugs*). If the frontal lobes, and especially the left frontal lobe, are necessary for this kind of classification, it stands to reason that much of what we call grammatical knowledge should be rooted here.[5]

At the same time, access to grammatical knowledge entails retrieving not only the category to which a word belongs, but also the set of operations that apply to words of that category: for example, identifying a noun as the subject of a sentence, or forming the past tense of a verb in English by affixing the inflectional morpheme -*ed*. Computations of this sort are often described as syntactic algorithms, procedures, or rules, and are also thought to be the special province of frontal tissues (Jakobson, 1956; Luria, 1970; Caramazza and Zurif, 1976; Ullman, 2001), as we might naturally expect, given that rules are formulated over categories and that categories are useful only insofar as they are manipulated by rules.

Finally, we note that grammatical processes require a sort of cognitive workspace in which information about objects (including linguistic objects) assigned to abstract categories can be maintained and manipulated. Identifying grammatical knowledge with this aspect of language processing dovetails neatly with the view that the left lateral frontal cortex is engaged in working memory. Such a view is now widely held among memory researchers, despite a lack of consensus regarding the nature of the operations and the format of the representations handled by this part of the brain. At least some investigators have argued that the left prefrontal cortex specializes in the maintenance of verbal information in memory (Caplan and Waters, 1999; Smith and Jonides, 1999), a hypothesis that is clearly compatible with our account.

AN EVOLUTIONARY PERSPECTIVE   Cognitive processes that involve the implementation of rules, the maintenance of information in working memory, and the representation of categories all depend on a single remarkable skill: the ability to encode multiple bits of information quickly and efficiently in an abstract, propositional format. It is precisely this ability that enables the amazing combinatorial productivity of human language, making it more than a set of arbitrary associative pairings of the kind that can be learned by most animals. It is this ability, in other words, that allows for the brain to represent what we have called grammatical knowledge.

It may not be coincidental, then, that the phylogenesis of language coincided in evolutionary time with a ballooning in the size of the frontal lobe, such that human prefrontal cortex is more than twice the size predicted for a "typical" primate brain (Brodmann, 1912; Blinkov and Glezer, 1968). This is not an original observation on our part, to be sure (cf. Deacon, 1997), but it underscores the natural plausibility of locating in the frontal lobe the processing systems that govern the intricacies of fluent and grammatical speech.

ACKNOWLEDGMENTS   This work was supported in part by grant DC04542 (A.C.) from the National Institutes of Health and by a grant from the Sackler Scholars Program in Psychobiology (K.S.).

NOTES

1. Indeed, some researchers have speculated that grammatical categories are acquired in ontogeny by a statistical mechanism that observes patterns co-occurrence of grammatical morphemes, like verbal -*ed*, -*ing*, and -*s* (Maratsos and Chalkley, 1981; Cartwright and Brent, 1997).

2. For alternative explanations, see Rapp and Caramazza (2002) and Shapiro and Caramazza (2003c).

3. Similar regions were implicated in much earlier studies of "dynamic" aphasia by Luria and colleagues, one of the characteristics of which was impoverished performance in generating names of actions (verbs) relative to names of objects. Luria and Tsvetkova (1967) attributed this discrepancy to a disturbance in the "predicative function of speech."

4. A number of investigators have pointed out that clinical agrammatism does not imply a uniform deficit in function word production; rather, the types of function words that are spared or impaired varies from case to case (Goodglass and Menn, 1985; Miceli et al., 1989). For example, the production of freestanding functional elements (like prepositions) may dissociate from the production of inflectional morphemes (like -*s* and -*ed*; Thompson, Fix, and Gitelman, 2002), and inflectional morphemes may dissociate from derivational morphemes (like -*ize* and -*ness*). Further fractionations of this sort may suggest not only that the prefrontal lobe is specialized for processing grammatical knowledge, but that different classes of grammatical elements are handled by dissociable circuits within left frontal cortex.

5. Taking the view that frontal tissue is the neural soil in which representational categories sprout, we should not necessarily expect regularity across individuals in the subregions of frontal cortex devoted to particular kinds of categories, such as nouns or verbs. Indeed, it remains to be seen whether such regularity obtains. If it does, however, the organization of grammatical knowledge may owe much to the peculiarities of how information from other parts of the brain reaches the frontal lobe. For instance, it may be the case that grammatical knowledge about verbs is stored in prefrontal areas adjacent to areas involved in representing the motor schemata of prototypical actions, while operations relevant to nouns is stored in areas that receive input from visual or other sensory processing areas (Caramazza, 1994). Semantic input might then constitute a kernel for the eventual representation of grammatical knowledge.

REFERENCES

ALLPORT, D. A., and E. FUNNELL, 1981. Components of the mental lexicon. *Philos. Trans. R. Soc. Lond.* 295:397–410.

BADECKER, W., and A. CARAMAZZA, 1991. Morphological composition in the lexical output system. *Cogn. Neuropsychol.* 8:335–367.

BADECKER, W., M. MIOZZO, and R. ZANUTTINI, 1995. The two-stage model of lexical retrieval: Evidence from a case of anomia with selective preservation of grammatical gender. *Cognition* 57:193–216.

BATES, E., S. CHEN, O. J. TZENG, P. LI, et al., 1991. The noun-verb problem in Chinese aphasia. *Brain Lang.* 41:203–233.

BERNDT, R. S., and A. CARAMAZZA, 1980. A redefinition of the syndrome of Broca's aphasia: Implications for a neuropsychological model of language. *Appl. Psycholinguist.* 1:225–278.

BERNDT, R. S., A. N. HAENDIGES, M. W. BURTON, and C. C. MITCHUM, 2002. Grammatical class and imageability in aphasic word production: Their effects are independent. *J. Neurolinguist.* 15:353–371.

BIRD, H., D. HOWARD, and S. FRANKLIN, 2000. Why is a verb like an inanimate object? Grammatical category and semantic category deficits. *Brain Lang.* 72:246–309.

BLINKOV, S., and I. GLEZER, 1968. *The Human Brain in Figures and Tables.* New York: Plenum Press.

BROCA, P. P., 1861. Perte de la parole, ramollissement chronique et destruction partielle du lobe antérieur gauche du cerveau. *Bull. Soc. Anthropol.* 2:235–238.

BRODMANN, K., 1912. Neue Ergebnisse über die vergleichende histologische Localisation mit besonderer Berücksichtigung des Stinhirns. *Anat. Anzeig. Suppl.* 41:157–216.

BUCKNER, R. L., W. KOUTSTAAL, D. L. SCHACTER, and B. R. ROSEN, 2000. Functional MRI evidence for a role of frontal and inferior temporal cortex in amodal components of priming. *Brain* 123 (Pt. 3):620–640.

CAMPBELL, R., and L. MANNING, 1996. Optic aphasia: A case with spared action naming and associated disorders. *Brain Lang.* 53:183–221.

CAPLAN, D., 2001. Functional neuroimaging studies of syntactic processing. *J. Psycholinguist. Res.* 30:297–320.

CAPLAN, D., and G. S. WATERS, 1999. Verbal working memory and sentence comprehension. *Behav. Brain Sci.* 22:77–126.

CARAMAZZA, A., 1994. Parallels and divergences in the acquisition and dissolution of language. *Philos. Trans. R. Soc. Lond. B* 346:121–127.

CARAMAZZA, A., and A. E. HILLIS, 1991. Lexical organization of nouns and verbs in the brain. *Nature* 349:788–790.

CARAMAZZA, A., and E. ZURIF, 1976. Dissociation of algorithmic and heuristic processes in language comprehension: Evidence from aphasia. *Brain Lang.* 3:572–582.

CARTWRIGHT, T. A., and M. R. BRENT, 1997. Syntactic categorization in early language acquisition: Formalizing the role of distributional analysis. *Cognition* 63:121–170.

CORBETT, G. G., 1991. *Gender.* Cambridge, England: Cambridge University Press.

DAMASIO, A. R., and D. TRANEL, 1993. Nouns and verbs are retrieved with differently distributed neural systems. *Proc. Nat. Acad. Sci. U.S.A.* 90:4957–4960.

DANIELE, A., L. GIUSTOLISI, M. C. SILVERI, C. COLOSIMO, et al., 1994. Evidence for a possible neuroanatomical basis for lexical processing of nouns and verbs. *Neuropsychologia* 32:1325–1341.

DAX, M., 1836/1865. Observations tendant à prouver la coincidence constante des dérangements de la parole avec une lésion de l'hémisphère gauche du cerveau. *Compt. Rend. Hebdom. Séances Acad. Sci.* 61:534.

DE SAUSSURE, F., 1916/1972. *Cours de linguistique générale.* Paris: Editions Payot.

DEACON, T. W., 1997. *The Symbolic Species.* New York: Norton.

DEHAENE, S., 1995. Electrophysiological evidence for category-specific word processing in the normal human brain. *Neuroreport* 6:2153–2157.

DÉMONET, J. F., F. CHOLLET, S. RAMSAY, D. CARDEBAT, J. L. NESPOULOUS, R. J. S. WISE, et al., 1992. The anatomy of phonological and semantic processing in normal subjects. *Brain* 115:1753–1768.

DRUKS, J., and T. SHALLICE, 2000. Selective preservation of naming from description and the "restricted preverbal message." *Brain Lang.* 72:100–128.

FEDERMEIER, K. D., J. B. SEGAL, T. LOMBROZO, and M. KUTAS, 2000. Brain responses to nouns, verbs and class-ambiguous words in context. *Brain* 123:2552–2566.

FREEDMAN, D. J., M. RIESENHUBER, T. POGGIO, and E. K. MILLER, 2001. Categorical representation of visual stimuli in the primate prefrontal cortex. *Science* 291:312–316.

GENTNER, D., 1981. Some interesting differences between verbs and nouns. *Cogn. Brain Theory* 4:161–178.

GOODGLASS, H., B. KLEIN, P. CAREY, and K. JONES, 1966. Specific semantic word categories in aphasia. *Cortex* 2:74–89.

GOODGLASS, H., and L. MENN, 1985. Is agrammatism a unitary phenomenon? In *Agrammatism*, M.-L. Kean, ed. Orlando, Fla.: Academic Press, pp. 1–25.

GUNTER, T. C., A. D. FRIEDERICI, and H. SCHRIEFERS, 2000. Syntactic gender and semantic expectancy: ERPs reveal early autonomy and late interaction. *J. Cogn. Neurosci.* 12:556–568.

HEIM, S., B. OPITZ, and A. D. FRIEDERICI, 2002. Broca's area in the human brain is involved in the selection of grammatical gender for language production: Evidence from event-related functional magnetic resonance imaging. *Neurosci. Lett.* 328:101–104.

HENAFF GONON, M. A., R. BRUCKERT, and F. MICHEL, 1989. Lexicalization in an anomic patient. *Neuropsychologia* 27:391–407.

HILLIS, A. E., and A. CARAMAZZA 1995. Representation of grammatical categories of words in the brain. *J. Cogn. Neurosci.* 7:396–407.

HILLIS, A. E., E. TUFFIASH, and A. CARAMAZZA, 2002. Modality-specific deterioration in naming verbs in nonfluent primary progressive aphasia. *J. Cogn. Neurosci.* 14:1099–1108.

HILLIS, A. E., R. J. WITYK, P. B. BARKER, and A. CARAMAZZA, 2003. Neural regions essential for writing verbs. *Nat. Neurosci.* 6:19–20.

INDEFREY, P., and W. J. M. LEVELT, 2000. The neural correlates of language production. In *The New Cognitive Neurosciences*, M. S. Gazzaniga, ed. Cambridge, Mass.: MIT Press, pp. 845–865.

JAKOBSON, R., 1956. Two aspects of language in two types of aphasic disturbances. In *Fundamentals of Language*, R. Jakobson and M. Halle, eds. The Hague: Mouton.

KEAN, M.-L., 1978. The linguistic interpretation of aphasic syndromes: Agrammatism in Broca's aphasia, an example. *Cognition* 5:9–46.

KELLENBACH, M. L., A. A. WIJERS, M. HOVIUS, J. MULDER, and G. MULTER, 2002. Neural differentiation of lexico-syntactic categories or semantic features? Event-related potential evidence for both. *J. Cogn. Neurosci.* 14:561–577.

KOENIG, T., and D. LEHMANN, 1996. Microstates in language-related brain potential maps show noun-verb differences. *Brain Lang.* 53:169–182.

LAIACONA, M., and A. CARAMAZZA, in press. The noun/verb dissociation in language production: varieties of causes. *Cogn. Neuropsychol.*

LENNEBERG, E. H., 1973. The neurology of language. *Daedalus* 102:115–133.

LURIA, A. R., 1970. *Traumatic Aphasia*. The Hague: Mouton.

LURIA, A. R., and L. S. TSVETKOVA, 1967. Towards the mechanisms of "dynamic aphasia." *Acta Neurol. Psychiatr. Belg.* 67:1045–1057.

MARATSOS, M., and M. A. CHALKLEY, 1981. The internal language of children's syntax: The ontogenesis and representation of syntactic categories. In *Children's Language*, vol. 2, K. Nelson, ed. New York: Gardner Press, pp. 127–214.

MICELI, G., M. C. SILVERI, C. ROMANI, and A. CARAMAZZA, 1989. Variation in the pattern of omissions and substitutions of grammatical morphemes in the spontaneous speech of so-called agrammatic patients. *Brain Lang.* 36:447–492.

MICELI, G., M. C. SILVERI, G. VILLA, and A. CARAMAZZA, 1984. On the basis for the agrammatic's difficulty in producing main verbs. *Cortex* 20:207–220.

MICELI, G., P. TURRIZIANI, C. CALTAGIRONE, R. CAPASSO, F. TOMAIUOLU, and A. CARAMAZZA, 2002. The neural correlates of grammatical gender: An fMRI investigation. *J. Cogn. Neurosci.* 14:618–628.

MILLER, E. K., A. NIEDER, D. J. FREEDMAN, and J. D. WALLIS, 2003. Neural correlates of categories and concepts. *Curr. Opin. Neurobiol.* 13:198–203.

MUELLER, R.-A., N. KLEINHANS, and E. COURCHESNE, 2003. Linguistic theory and neuroimaging evidence: An fMRI study of Broca's area in lexical semantics. *Neuropsychologia* 41:1199–1207.

NEVILLE, H. J., D. L. MILLS, and D. S. LAWSON, 1992. Fractionating language: Different neural subsystems with different sensitive periods. *Cereb. Cortex* 2:244–258.

O'GRADY, W., 1997. *Syntactic Development*. Chicago: University of Chicago Press.

PERANI, D., S. F. CAPPA, T. SCHNUR, M. TETTAMANTI, S. COLLINA, M. M. ROSA, and F. FAZIO, 1999. The neural correlates of verb and noun processing: A PET study. *Brain* 122(Pt. 12):2337–2344.

PETERSEN, S. E., P. T. FOX, M. I. POSNER, M. MINTUM, and M. E. RAICHLE, 1989. Positron emission tomographic studies of the processing of single words. *J. Cogn. Neurosc.* 1:153–170.

PINKER, S., 1984. *Language Learnability and Language Development*. Cambridge, Mass.: Harvard University Press.

PULVERMUELLER, F., 1999. Words in the brain's language. *Behav. Brain Sci.* 22:253–336.

PULVERMUELLER, F., 2001. Brain reflections of words and their meaning. *Trends Cogn. Sci.* 5:517–524.

PULVERMUELLER, F., W. LUTZENBERGER, and H. PREISSL, 1999. Nouns and verbs in the intact brain: Evidence from event-related potentials and high-frequency cortical responses. *Cereb. Cortex* 9:497–506.

RAPP, B., and A. CARAMAZZA, 1997. The modality-specific organization of grammatical categories: Evidence from impaired spoken and written sentence production. *Brain Lang.* 56:248–286.

RAPP, B., and A. CARAMAZZA, 1998. A case of selective difficulty in writing verbs. *Neurocase* 4:127–139.

RAPP, B., and A. CARAMAZZA, 2002. Selective difficulties with spoken nouns and written verbs: A single case study. *J. Neurolinguist.* 15:373–402.

ROBINSON, G., M. ROSSOR, and L. CIPOLOTTI, 1999. Selective sparing of verb naming in a case of severe Alzheimer's disease. *Cortex* 35:443–450.

SHAPIRO, K., and A. CARAMAZZA, 2003a. Grammatical processing of nouns and verbs in left frontal cortex? *Neuropsychologia* 41:1189–1198.

SHAPIRO, K., and A. CARAMAZZA, 2003b. Looming a loom: Evidence for independent access to grammatical and phonological properties in verb retrieval. *J. Neurolinguist.* 16:85–111.

SHAPIRO, K., and A. CARAMAZZA, 2003c. The representation of grammatical categories in the brain. *Trends Cogn. Sci.* 7:201–206.

SHAPIRO, K., J. SHELTON, and A. CARAMAZZA, 2000. Grammatical class in lexical production and morphological processing: Evidence from a case of fluent aphasia. *Cogn. Neuropsychol.* 17:665–682.

SHAPIRO, K. A., A. PASCUAL-LEONE, F. M. MOTTAGHY, M. GANGITANO, and A. CARAMAZZA, 2001. Grammatical distinctions in the left frontal cortex. *J. Cogn. Neurosci.* 13:713–720.

SILVERI, M. C., and A. DI BETTA, 1997. Noun-verb dissociations in brain-damaged patients: Further evidence. *Neurocase* 3:477–488.

SMITH, E. E., and J. JONIDES, 1999. Storage and executive processes in the frontal lobes. *Science* 283:1657–1661.

TEYLER, T. J., R. A. ROEMER, T. F. HARRISON, and R. F. THOMPSON, 1973. Human scalp-recorded evoked-potential correlates of linguistic stimuli. *Bull. Psychonom. Soc.* 1.

THOMPSON, C. K., S. FIX, and D. GITELMAN, 2002. Selective impairment of morphosyntactic production in a neurological patient. *J. Neurolinguist.* 15:189–207.

TRANEL, D., R. ADOLPHS, H. DAMASIO, and A. R. DAMASIO, 2001. A neural basis for the retrieval of words for actions. *Cogn. Neuropsychol.* 18:655–674.

TSAPKINI, K., G. JAREMA, and E. KEHAYIA, 2000. A morphological processing deficit in verbs but not in nouns: A case study in a highly inflected language. *J. Neurolinguist.* 15:265–288.

TYLER, L. K., R. RUSSELL, J. FADILI, and H. E. MOSS, 2001. The neural representation of nouns and verbs: PET studies. *Brain* 124(Pt. 8):1619–1634.

ULLMAN, M. T., 2001. A neurocognitive perspective on language: The declarative/procedural model. *Nat. Rev. Neurosci.* 2:717–726.

VAN TURENNOUT, M., P. HAGOORT, and C. M. BROWN, 1998. Brain activity during speaking: From syntax to phonology in 40 milliseconds. *Science* 280:572–574.

VIGLIOCCO, G., and J. FRANCK, 2001. When sex affects syntax: Contextual influences in sentence production. *J. Mem. Lang.* 45:368–390.

WARBURTON, E., R. J. WISE, C. J. PRICE, C. WEILLER, U. HADAR, S. RAMSAY, and R. S. FRACKOWIAK, 1996. Noun and verb retrieval by normal subjects: Studies with PET. *Brain* 119 (Pt. 1):159–179.

ZURIF, E. B., 1980. Language mechanisms: A neuropsychological perspective. *Am. Scientist* 68:305–311.

58 The Neural Basis of Reading Acquisition

FRANCK RAMUS

ABSTRACT Learning to read is a recently invented cognitive challenge imposed to our hunter-gatherer's brain. Nevertheless, in societies where reading is taught systematically, it is acquired early on by most children, who ultimately achieve a high degree of mastery. Understanding reading acquisition therefore requires answers to the following questions: What cognitive resources does the child bring to the task? What is the nature of the input necessary for learning to occur? And how, starting with these cognitive resources, and under the influence of this input, does the brain partly reshape itself into a proficient reading machine? Attempting to answer these questions will take us from developmental and psycholinguistic models to teaching methods and to functional brain imaging studies of reading acquisition, while at the same time considering disruptions due to sensory deprivation or developmental dyslexia.

Unlike language, reading is not one of those "natural" human skills that may have evolved under the pressure of natural selection. Rather, like tennis or chess, it is a recent cultural invention (about 5000 years old), and one that places considerable demands on the cognitive system. Nevertheless, in societies where reading is taught systematically, it is acquired early on by most children, who go on to master it to a high degree of skill. Those who fail to do so (e.g., dyslexics) pose major issues of social integration.

As the study of adult reading shows, reading skill is achieved by a whole network of brain areas, some of which seem exquisitely specific and dedicated to the sole task of reading (see Hillis and Rapp, this volume). Understanding reading acquisition therefore requires answers to the following questions: What cognitive resources does the child bring to the task? What is the nature of the input necessary for learning to occur? And how, starting with these cognitive resources and under the influence of this input, does the brain partly reshape itself into a proficient reading machine?

Cognitive modeling of reading acquisition

Formally, the bare essentials of reading are a set of external symbols that represent words of the language, which, in

order to be understood and verbalized, need to be mentally represented and connected to the corresponding items of the mental lexicon. Every schoolchild starts with two mental lexicons, one storing the meanings of words, or the *semantic lexicon*, and one storing the forms of words, or the *phonological lexicon*, where phonology is an abstract representation of speech (except in deaf signers). Figure 58.1 shows a minimal information-processing model of this initial state with respect to the task of reading acquisition. In this and other models, the components are usually justified by psycholinguistic and neuropsychological data, as reported by Hillis and Rapp in chapter 55 (see also Morton, 1969, 1980; Caramazza, 1997b; Levelt, Roelofs, and Meyer, 1999; Coltheart et al., 2001; Ramus, 2001). One important aspect of this model is the distinction between the phonological lexicon and sublexical phonological representations, the latter being a temporary store for anything that can be represented in a phonological format and articulated, including words, phrases, and nonsense sequences of phonological units (e.g., nonwords).

Internally representing the set of written symbols means creating an *orthographic lexicon*, and those new representations need to be connected with the corresponding items in the semantic and phonological lexicons. Moreover, phonological representations are combinatorial: they are made of smaller units that include phonemes. Alphabetic writing systems exploit this natural combinatoriality: in those systems, written symbols are themselves combinations of smaller units (letters), which correspond more or less well to phonemes. Then, any string of letters can be mentally represented, which again justifies the existence of a sublexical (alphabetic) representation for letter strings. And there are obvious connections between representations of letter strings and the corresponding sublexical phonological representations. The mature reading system therefore has to resemble the one presented in figure 58.2 (see papers in Caramazza, 1997a).

Proficient readers typically access written words' meanings automatically and almost instantly; such high proficiency is commonly illustrated by the Stroop effect in most adult readers: people are slower to name the ink color (e.g., red) of a printed word if the word is a conflicting color name

---

FRANCK RAMUS Laboratoire de Sciences Cognitives et Psycholinguistique (EHESS/ENS/CNRS), Paris, France.

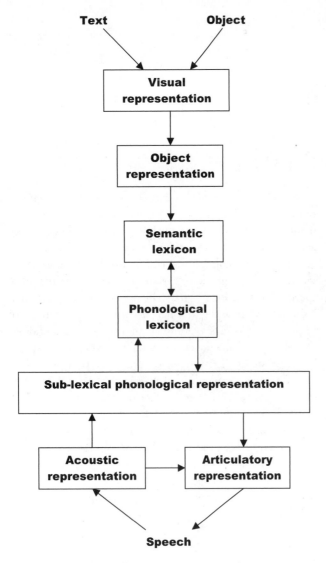

FIGURE 58.1   The initial state: logographic reading stage.

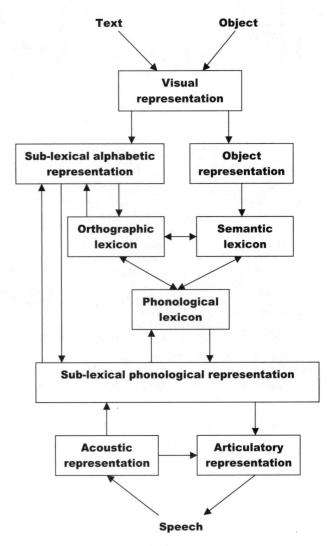

FIGURE 58.2   The final state: orthographic reading stage.

(green) (Stroop, 1935). This effect demonstrates how difficult it is to inhibit reading whenever a word is being looked at. For the child, getting there is a long and arduous way that involves specific teaching and massive exposure to print. Several models describe this process. There is little hope that one single specific model will be able to account for all cases of reading acquisition, if only because each developmental path depends on the child's own experience with print, his or her own cognitive style or capacities, and the instruction received (or the absence thereof). Nevertheless, keeping in mind this caveat, it seems possible to make general observations on how reading acquisition unfolds, at least within one particular writing system.

The standard model of reading acquisition in alphabetic systems has been proposed by Frith (1985, 1986; see Morton, 1989, for an information-processing account). It postulates that the child goes through three main stages, respectively called logographic, alphabetic, and orthographic. Between two stages, new representations are set up and new connections are established between representations.

In the *logographic* stage (figure 58.1), the child processes words just as if they were any other visual object or symbol. Word meanings are associated with global visual shapes and features, which means that word recognition is highly inaccurate, overly reliant on fonts, patterns, colors, and so on, and partly insensitive to precise letter order.

From there, it is assumed that alphabetic and phonics teaching are necessary to progress; that is, it is necessary to acquire an explicit knowledge of phonemes, their correspondences with letters, and how to merge those sounds into words. In this *alphabetic* stage, the child needs to visually represent words in a different format from other objects or symbols: he or she needs to represent ordered sequences of letters (in fact, abstract representations of letters, independent of font, size and color). Furthermore, these representations of letters must connect with their corresponding sounds in the child's sublexical phonological representation.

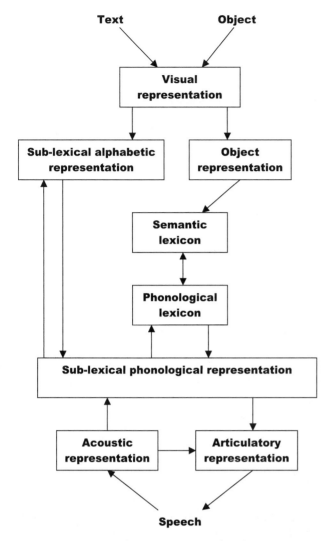

Text   **Object**

Visual representation

Sub-lexical alphabetic representation

Object representation

Semantic lexicon

Phonological lexicon

Sub-lexical phonological representation

Acoustic representation

Articulatory representation

Speech

FIGURE 58.3   An intermediate state: alphabetic reading stage.

This has a cognitive prerequisite, the ability to pay attention to units of this sublexical phonological level, and in particular to phonemes; this is called phoneme awareness, and is assumed to arise naturally in children at age 5 or 6. With this architecture in place (figure 58.3), the child can read by sounding out a sequence of letters and merging those sounds into a word. Word recognition occurs through the phonological lexicon. Of course, this way of reading is tedious and relatively inefficient, as it requires letter-by-letter processing, and in certain spelling systems, like that of English, the letter-sound correspondence is not reliable enough to ensure total accuracy. A further refinement of the alphabetic stage is to associate phonemes not just with single letters but with *graphemes*—letters or sequences of letters that have a more reliable correspondence with phonemes (for instance, in English, it is better to associate the grapheme "oa" with the phoneme [o] than try to sound out "o" and "a" separately).[1]

Finally, repeated exposure to the same words leads the child to store whole-word grapheme sequences, that is, to

create an orthographic lexicon. With this new component in the system (see figure 58.2), word recognition may occur through direct connections from the orthographic to the semantic lexicon. And reading aloud can proceed directly through the phonological lexicon (lexicalized phonological recoding; Share, 1995) without going through grapheme-phoneme conversion. There is good evidence that morphological units play an important role in the orthographic lexicon, as they may provide reliable, conveniently sized units that can be quickly assembled to recognize complex words. Through the accumulation of orthographic lexical items and their connections with phonological lexical items, new sublexical letter-sound regularities may implicitly be acquired (induced sublexical relations; Thompson, Cottrell, and Fletcher-Flinn, 1996). For instance, the child may implicitly learn that pronunciation of the sequence *eal* can be deduced systematically from the surrounding context (e.g., depending on whether it is followed by *s, t, e, i,* etc.)—something that is usually not explicitly taught. Therefore, in the mature reading system (see figure 58.2), the connections between sublexical alphabetic and phonological representations are in part explicitly learned grapheme-phoneme rules and in part implicitly acquired, more complex sublexical relations.

Many people are suspicious of models requiring discrete developmental stages. But this only happens if one takes the model too literally. It is not assumed that those developmental stages are disjoint periods demarcated by abrupt cognitive changes. Rather, they reflect three types of reading strategies that progressively take precedence over each other. The beginnings of the alphabetic stage may well see remnants of logographic reading. Furthermore, alphabetic reading is never entirely abandoned, since it is often necessary to read unknown words; rather, the more the orthographic lexicon grows, the less alphabetic reading is employed.

Perhaps the most valid criticism of Frith's (1985) model is that it assumes a particular class of teaching methods, based on explicit phonics instruction. Although there is a huge controversy as to whether phonics is an essential component of good teaching, it is a fact that other teaching methods exist, and that some children manage to become fluent readers without ever receiving explicit phonics instruction. For those children, the scenario certainly needs to be revised to a certain extent. Beyond the logographic stage, it seems that instead of going through an alphabetic stage, they start building directly an orthographic lexicon connected to the other two lexicons (albeit painstakingly, perhaps in the same way that Chinese children learn their language's characters) (figure 58.4). From there they acquire implicit sublexical relations (including standard grapheme-phoneme correspondences), so that their mature reading system closely resembles that of phonics-taught children (see figure 58.2),

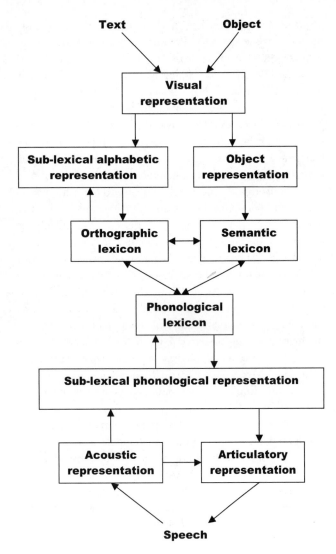

Text   **Object**

Visual representation

Sub-lexical alphabetic representation

Object representation

Orthographic lexicon

Semantic lexicon

Phonological lexicon

Sub-lexical phonological representation

Acoustic representation

Articulatory representation

Speech

FIGURE 58.4 An alternative intermediate stage without explicit phonic teaching.

except that the sublexical letter-sound connections are all implicit. This revised scenario seems to apply not only to students taught by "whole language" methods but also to precocious readers who learn to read by themselves without any reading instruction (Fletcher-Flinn and Thompson, 2000, 2004).

The present scenario of reading acquisition presupposes certain answers to the first two questions that we have raised: the necessary cognitive resources brought by the child to the task of learning to read would seem to include fully functional phonological (and therefore auditory), lexical, and visual systems. The input necessary for learning to occur includes massive exposure to written words, presented together with their phonological forms (at least at the beginning). Explicit instruction in letter sounds and grapheme-phoneme correspondences would seem to be a facilitating factor for most children, in that it does allow bootstrapping the formation of the orthographic lexicon; without it, the

child has to rely for a very long time on the simultaneous presentation of written and verbal forms to acquire new words, but with it, it is possible to read aloud, understand, and therefore learn new words by applying grapheme-phoneme correspondences. Nevertheless, this facilitating factor is not entirely necessary, and many children can do without it.

In the next section, these answers are refined by taking into consideration possible disorders of these systems and their impact on reading acquisition.

Insights from developmental disorders

FIFTY WAYS TO FAIL READING ACQUISITION Just as in a car, the failure of many different parts can prevent the car from functioning, there are many different ways in which reading acquisition can go wrong. The most obvious ones are cases of major sensory deprivation. Blindness, severe ophthalmologic impairments, or simply uncorrected hyperopia (farsightedness), preventing the formation of alphabetic representations, are major obstacles to the acquisition of reading. Similarly, deafness prevents the formation of phonological representations related to speech, and the units of sign language phonological representations have little to do with phonemes or letters, which makes the alphabetic principle meaningless to profoundly deaf people and leaves them only the possibility of logographic reading.

Another obvious cause of reading disability is mental retardation. More generally, it is well known that reading ability is correlated with intelligence quotient (IQ) (Snowling, 2000), so difficulties in learning to read are straightforwardly predicted at the bottom end of the IQ scale.

Language itself is of course a prerequisite of reading. At the very least, the child's vocabulary (i.e., semantic and phonological lexicons) sets an upper limit on the development of the orthographic lexicon, and reading comprehension can never be better than language comprehension. It is therefore not surprising that children with language impairments generally have problems acquiring reading.

Finally, there can also be more extrinsic factors: one can imagine a variety of emotional, social, or educational contexts in which the acquisition of reading can be difficult.

DEVELOPMENTAL DYSLEXIA It is quite remarkable that, even after the more obvious causes of failure are excluded, about 5% of schoolchildren still have great difficulty learning to read. Such a specific reading disability without apparent endogenous or exogenous cause is generally called developmental dyslexia. Even within this more limited diagnostic category, there appear to be a variety of causes. Traditionally, two distinct causes have been envisioned, visual and phonological.

Insofar as major ophthalmologic problems are already excluded from the definition of dyslexia, any remaining visual cause must be relatively subtle, that is, they have little impact on everyday life outside reading. This is reflected in the term "congenital word blindness," which was used to describe one of the very first cases of dyslexia ever reported (Morgan, 1896). Again, there are several possibilities: poor vergence, which would affect the capacity to focus at short distance, instability of binocular fixations, leading to unstable visual images, and poor saccade planning, which would affect fluent text reading, have been argued to be major causes of reading disability (Stein and Walsh, 1997). Another relevant disorder is visual stress, which is manifested in migraines, visual distortions, and apparent movements when the viewer is confronted with a high-contrast black-and-white page of text (Wilkins, 1995). Research into visual causes of dyslexia remains controversial and subject to intense debate (Skottun, 1997; Stein, Talcott, and Walsh, 2000). It is fair to say that there is evidence that both binocular control dysfunction and visual stress can be factors in reading disability and that visually based treatments can help in those cases (Bouldoukian, Wilkins, and Evans, 2002; Stein, Richardson, and Fowler, 2000), but most practitioners and scientists find that these visual disorders concern only a small fraction of dyslexic persons.

The other major and now most widely accepted explanation of developmental dyslexia has to do with the phonological system. The hypothesis is quite simply that a deficit in phonological representations and processing impairs the ability to access representations of phonemes and to associate them with graphemes (Shankweiler and Liberman, 1972; Vellutino, 1979; Stanovich, 1988; Snowling, 2000). This hypothesis is supported by widespread evidence that most dyslexic individuals have difficulty with at least three types of tasks involving phonological representations and processing (Morris et al., 1998): phoneme awareness tasks (such as swapping phonemes between two words to make spoonerisms), verbal short-term memory, and speeded naming of objects (or digits, letters, or colors). Among the different manifestations of the phonological deficit, it appears that poor phoneme awareness is the most proximal cause of reading difficulties. Phoneme awareness is the awareness that speech is combinatorial, made up of a limited number of sounds that are combined to make words. This is obviously crucial to mastering the alphabetic principle; the hypothesis is that dyslexic children have insufficient phoneme awareness and therefore have difficulty reaching the alphabetic stage of reading. The importance of the alphabetic stage in bootstrapping reading acquisition implies that the phonological deficit will have further developmental consequences, disrupting the whole acquisition of the reading system, notably the acquisition of the orthographic lexicon.

It is not entirely clear what the three different manifestations of the phonological deficit have in common so that they could be reduced to some common substrate. It can be argued that phoneme awareness requires a good verbal short-term memory to simultaneously pay attention to phonemes and to their combinations, so that a deficit in the latter would entail one in the former (Baddeley, 1979). It has also been argued that the rapid naming deficit is in fact independent from poor phoneme awareness, although often associated with it (Wolf and Bowers, 1999). However, discussions of the phonological deficit have seldom been framed within an information-processing model such as figure 58.2. Within such a framework, the exact locus of the phonological deficit remains uncertain. Some theorists would situate it at the lexical level, and rather in output processes (Elbro, 1996; Snowling, 2000), while others argue for a sublexical locus, either abstract (Ramus, 2001) or specific to input processes (Mody, Studdert-Kennedy, and Brady, 1997; Serniclaes et al., 2001). Unfortunately, it seems that investigations into the phonological deficit have not yet reached the degree of sophistication necessary to tease apart these hypotheses (Ramus, 2001).

Although most researchers agree that a phonological deficit is the most likely proximal cause of dyslexia, there is another debate regarding whether the deficit is specific to the phonological system or whether it is secondary to a more basic auditory impairment. There is some evidence that on average, dyslexic persons perform more poorly than controls on a range of auditory tasks (Tallal, 1980; Farmer and Klein, 1995; McAnally and Stein, 1996; Witton et al., 2002). It is perfectly plausible that a mild auditory disorder would have an impact on the development of the phonological system, deafness being only an extreme case in point. The question is whether the auditory disorders observed in dyslexic persons are of the nature and severity to cause the type of phonological disruption that leads to dyslexia. In fact, it seems that they are mostly unrelated to speech perception and phonological processing (Mody, Studdert-Kennedy, and Brady, 1997; Rosen and Manganari, 2001; Ramus et al., 2003). It also appears that auditory disorders are restricted to a subset of dyslexics (McArthur and Bishop, 2001; Amitay, Ahissar, and Nelken, 2002) and that they are not necessary for a phonological deficit to arise (Ramus et al., 2003; White et al., 2004). Overall, there is overwhelming evidence that for the vast majority of children with dyslexia, a specific deficit of the phonological system is the main culprit (see reviews in Ramus, 2003; Rosen, 2003).

Cognitive prerequisites of reading acquisition

Returning to the question of cognitive prerequisites, of course, every component of the reading system is important, whether it is visual, auditory, or more specifically linguistic; the total disruption of any one of them can prevent normal reading acquisition. Nevertheless, it is quite remarkable that even in the case of blindness, the visual medium can easily be replaced with a tactile one (Braille). This shows that the brain does not expect orthographic representations to come in a particular modality (indeed, it does not expect orthographic representations at all, as this is a cultural invention). Rather, it has the potential to create an orthographic lexicon in the relevant modality, whether visual or tactile. And when the new representations are combinatorial and their units are in a reliable correspondence to phonological units, then appropriate sublexical representations are also created and connected to sublexical phonology (Braille is also an alphabet).

The case of profound deafness is more complicated, because letters cannot connect to relevant phonological units. But even in this extreme case, partial information about relevant phonological units can be obtained by representing the speaker's articulatory gestures (lipreading), which provides certain phonetic features (e.g., rounding of the lips, labial articulation place) but not others (voicing). The missing phonetic features can even be complemented by a specific system of manual cues that the speaker can produce as he speaks (cued speech, Cornett, 1967). In this case, both speech comprehension and reading acquisition become accessible to deaf people. Furthermore, any residual hearing can also provide disambiguating cues and complement the representation of phonological units. So, it seems that when standard sublexical phonological representations are absent or insufficient, the brain can make appropriate ones with any combination of auditory and visual cues so as to properly connect them to alphabetic representations.

Different reading systems can provide more insights. When the units that make up the written symbols do not correspond to phonological units but to whole words or morphemes, as in Chinese characters, then no sublexical relations can be formed, and reading acquisition has to proceed through rote learning of all the arbitrary pairs of orthographic and phonological lexical items.[2] Nevertheless, most Chinese children are able to learn the few thousand characters that are most useful for everyday life. Other writing systems can also be based on different phonological units than phonemes: this is the case of the Japanese *hiragana*, where each character represents a syllable.[3] Because there are few different syllables in Japanese (unlike in English), this system is as easy to learn as an alphabet. Sublexical relations are then established between *hiragana* representations and the corresponding sublexical phonological units—that is, syllables.

The diversity of writing systems and the alternative reading strategies that are set up when one modality is not available show that there is little fixed or necessary in the architecture of the reading system; rather, when presented with a new set of lexical symbols, the brain has the capacity to create a new lexicon to represent them, and when their combinatorial structure bears any relationship with phonological or other related representations, it establishes the corresponding sublexical connections which significantly increase the efficiency of the acquisition process.

With such flexibility of reading acquisition, it can be expected to be relatively resistant to more moderate disruptions of any single component. Developmental dyslexia itself is seldom a total incapacity to learn to read: it makes the process significantly harder to the extent that the trouble can only partially be overcome, generally through alternative reading strategies requiring inordinate intellectual effort or prowess. Most ophthalmologic disorders do not prevent reading but rather disrupt its fluency to various degrees (Legge et al., 1985). Mild to moderate hearing loss, while disrupting the formation of accurate phonological representations and often disturbing speech perception and production, does not necessary lead to difficulties to learn to read (Briscoe, Bishop, and Norbury, 2001).

This leads us to a paradox. On the one hand, hearing loss that significantly disturbs phonological representations can still allow for normal reading acquisition; on the other, a rather mild phonological deficit (mild in the sense that it leaves speech production and comprehension intact) can impair reading acquisition very consistently in a large proportion of the population. This suggests that there is something special to normally developed phonology that dramatically facilitates reading acquisition and is disrupted in dyslexia, but not necessarily by moderate hearing loss. Phoneme awareness seems the most likely candidate, which justifiably makes it the single most important cognitive prerequisite to reading acquisition.

Reading acquisition in the brain

Putting together the rough sketch of reading acquisition outlined here and what we know of the correspondence between functional modules and brain areas (see Hillis and Rapp, this volume; Cutler and Indefrey, this volume), it becomes possible to make specific predictions concerning the specialization of the child's brain for reading. In particular, brain imaging studies performed on children at different stages of reading acquisition would be expected to reflect the emergence of new representations for alphabetic strings and orthographic lexical items. The results of such imaging studies could therefore be used to confirm or infirm theories of reading acquisition.

Unfortunately, the current state of the art can only give us a very preliminary picture. Functional brain imaging studies of children are scarce, and the tasks used and subtractions reported, together with the limited anatomical resolution, do not allow for a clear identification of the components of the lexical system. Nevertheless, it is possible to provide a rough overview.

The clearest brain/function mapping demonstrated in the reading system lies in alphabetic/orthographic processing; this has been reliably associated with the occipitotemporal region of the left hemisphere (see reviews in Pugh et al., 2001; McCandliss, Cohen, and Dehaene, 2003; and Hillis and Rapp, this volume). According to the analysis by Cohen and colleagues (2002), there seems to be a whole hierarchy of representations in this region (more than are sketched in figure 58.2), with the more posterior areas (in the occipital lobe) being specifically visual and perhaps related to processing of low-level visual features and letter shapes, while they seem to get progressively more abstract as they get more anterior in the ventral temporal lobe: the midportion of the left fusiform gyrus would support representations of abstract letter strings of both words and nonwords, while the more anterior portion might be more specific to words (however, in many studies this distinction is not explicitly made). Furthermore these reading-related areas are embedded within a larger ventral object recognition system with similar perceptual gradients (Lerner et al., 2001), so that one can see the development of this orthographic system as reflecting the specialization, under the pressure of the input, of object recognition areas that happen to be tuned to certain visual properties that are particularly suitable for representing letter strings (Cohen et al., 2002). From the fusiform gyrus, the hierarchy of more and more abstract orthographic representations seems to progress over the posterior portions of the inferior and medial temporal gyri, the latter being a possible locus for the orthographic lexicon (Simos, Breier, et al., 2002).

Developmentally, across a large group of children ages 7–17, B. A. Shaywitz and colleagues have shown that activation in those occipital-temporal areas during reading increases with reading skill[4] (B. A. Shaywitz et al., 2002; see also Booth et al., 2001; Schlaggar et al., 2002; Turkeltaub et al., 2003), which is consistent with the idea of the progressive formation of alphabetic and orthographic representations. From studies of developmental dyslexia, there is reliable evidence that these same areas are hypoactivated in both child and adult dyslexic subjects during reading tasks (e.g., S. E. Shaywitz et al., 1998; Brunswick et al., 1999; B. A. Shaywitz et al., 2002). This does not mean that a dysfunction in these areas is the cause of dyslexia; rather, it is compatible with the prediction that orthographic representations develop abnormally as a result of the phonological deficit.

The other major component in the reading system is the temporoparietal junction, including the posterior superior temporal gyrus (STGp), the angular gyrus, and the supramarginal gyrus, predominantly in the left hemisphere. A clear decomposition of this large region into functional areas has not been achieved yet, but it is assumed to be generally involved in the lexicon (with the angular gyrus another con-

tender for the seat of the orthographic lexicon; see Hillis and Rapp, this volume), in sublexical phonology (STGp and anterior supramarginal gyrus; Jacquemot et al., 2003) and in computing grapheme-phoneme correspondences (particularly the STGp; Simos, Breier, et al., 2002). Activation of the temporoparietal junction in reading occurs after activation of the occipitotemporal areas (Simos, Breier, et al., 2000; Simos, Breier, et al., 2002), consistent with the view that visual/alphabetic processing precedes phonological processing and lexical access. Interestingly, the left STGp seems to be activated more in children than in adults during tasks requiring word reading (Booth et al., 2001). This observation is again consistent with the idea that children rely more on alphabetic and less on orthographic strategies. Furthermore, activation in the neighboring left posterior superior temporal sulcus was found to be correlated with a measure of phonological awareness in children (Turkeltaub et al., 2003). In contrast, this area—indeed, the whole temporoparietal junction—has consistently been found to be activated less in dyslexic children and adults than in controls (Paulesu et al., 2001; Temple et al., 2001; Simos, Fletcher, Bergman, et al., 2002; Simos, Fletcher, Foorman, et al., 2002; see review by Temple, 2002), an observation consistent with the idea that dyslexic individuals have a phonological deficit and difficulties with grapheme-phoneme processing. Interestingly, dyslexic persons seem to compensate by hyperactivating the symmetrical right hemisphere areas compared with controls (S. E. Shaywitz et al., 1998; Simos, Fletcher, Bergman, et al., 2002; Simos, Fletcher, Foorman, et al., 2002). A remediation study further showed that, following a phonological awareness training program, dyslexic children not only improved behaviorally but also were able to involve their left STGp during nonword reading tasks significantly more than before the treatment (Simos, Fletcher, Bergman, et al., 2002).

Another way in which dyslexic individuals may compensate for their orthographic-phonological processing difficulties on tasks such as nonword reading is through increased involvement of the inferior frontal gyrus (Broca's area) bilaterally, another area that, in the left hemisphere, is often involved in reading (S. E. Shaywitz et al., 1998; Pugh et al., 2000; Temple et al., 2001). One possible explanation is that slow and effortful grapheme-phoneme processing may increase the load on verbal working memory, as the subject needs to keep in store the beginning of the word while processing the end, perhaps engaging in covert articulation or rehearsal. Moreover, this hyperactivation seems to increase with age in dyslexic persons (B. A. Shaywitz et al., 2002).

It is quite tempting to ascribe dyslexic subjects' difficulties to a congenital dysfunction of the left temporoparietal junction (Temple, 2002), resulting in disrupted sublexical phonological representations and difficulties in learning alphabetic reading, with further consequences for the acquisition of the orthographic lexicon. This hypothesis is compatible with some anatomical data indicating structural and metabolic anomalies in these areas of the brain in dyslexia (Galaburda et al., 1985; Rae et al., 1998; Brown et al., 2001). However, it bears emphasis that many areas of the brain in dyslexic persons have been found to be "different" (Habib, 2000), but no functional significance of these differences has been established.

Perhaps the currently most promising hypothesis is that of a partial disconnection of left temporoparietal areas from the temporo-occipital language areas (but see Paulesu et al., 1996, for another disconnection hypothesis). This hypothesis is supported by diffusion tensor imaging showing disruption in the underlying white matter (Klingberg et al., 2000) and becomes interesting in light of evidence that, unlike in controls, functional activations in the angular gyrus of dyslexic subjects fails to correlate with activations in the ventral orthographic system (Horwitz, Rumsey, and Donohue, 1998; Pugh et al., 2000; Simos et al., 2000).

Other hypotheses exist concerning the neurological origin of dyslexia, in particular related to alternative cognitive theories (auditory, visual). The most notable of those, the magnocellular theory (Stein, 2001), hypothesizes that magnocells in all sensory pathways are deficient, leading both to visual disorders causing reading difficulties and to auditory disorders causing the phonological deficit. Beyond the criticism already mentioned concerning the prevalence and the causal role of those sensory deficits, the magnocellular theory also faces more specific challenges. In particular, it predicts that dyslexics' sensory deficits will be observed for stimuli in a certain range of spatial and temporal frequencies characteristic of the response domain of magnocells. In the auditory domain, this translates into the hypothesis of a rapid auditory processing deficit proposed by Tallal (1980). The empirical evidence is highly contradictory, split between findings consistent and inconsistent with the theory (see reviews in Skottun, 2000; Ramus, 2003; Rosen, 2003). Overall, the magnocellular theory in its present state does not seem to be able to adequately characterize the sensory deficits of even the fraction of dyslexics that are so impaired.

Conclusion

The human brain has not evolved to learn to read, but it has the potential to acquire an additional lexicon in a new modality (usually visual). Representations for visual forms of words progressively settle in the occipitotemporal cortex, recruiting for their own purpose a subset of a functionally appropriate object recognition region. These new functional areas have to connect with the existing lexicon in the temporoparietal junction. In alphabetic writing systems, the acquisition of orthographic lexical items and their connection with phonological and semantic ones is greatly facili-

tated by the acquisition of sublexical relations between graphemes and phonemes. Such orthographic-phonological conversion is likely performed by the STGp. In developmental dyslexia, reading acquisition difficulties seem to stem from a specific phonological deficit consisting of an impaired phonological awareness, leading to poor ability to learn grapheme-phoneme correspondences. At the neural level, this may result from a dysfunction of the temporoparietal brain areas or of their underlying connections with orthographic representations.

ACKNOWLEDGMENTS   This work was supported by a grant from the Fyssen Foundation. I thank Uta Frith and Alfonso Caramazza for comments on a previous version of this chapter.

NOTES

1. This definition of the word grapheme is the one used in the reading literature and is different from the one used in neuropsychology, where it usually refers to abstract letter representations (e.g., Hillis and Rapp, this volume).

2. In fact, even in Chinese characters there are implicit sublexical relations that make it possible to guess the pronunciation of a new character slightly better than chance.

3. Actually each character represents a mora, where the mora is a phonological unit slightly smaller than the syllable. In Japanese, with a few exceptions, moras are almost always syllables, so it is a reasonable approximation to talk about a syllabic writing.

4. These authors found a correlation between activation in the occipitotemporal areas (as well as other areas) and *nonword reading*. However, nonword reading was the only reading measure reported, and it is usually highly correlated with reading skill of all types of words, so that the correlation should be expected to hold with reading skill more generally. In fact, considering the function attributed to those areas, one would predict the highest correlation with performance on a more specifically orthographic task.

REFERENCES

AMITAY, S., M. AHISSAR, and I. NELKEN, 2002. Auditory processing deficits in reading disabled adults. *J. Assoc. Res. Otolaryngol.* 3: 302–320.

BADDELEY, A. D., 1979. Working memory and reading. In *Processing of Visible Language*, vol. 1, P. A. Kolers, M. E. Wrolstadt, and H. Bouma, eds. New York: Plenum Press.

BOOTH, J. R., D. D. BURMAN, F. W. VAN SANTEN, Y. HARASAKI, D. R. GITELMAN, T. B. PARRISH, et al., 2001. The development of specialized brain systems in reading and oral language. *Neuropsychol. Dev. Cogn. Sect. C Child Neuropsychol.* 7:119–141.

BOULDOUKIAN, J., A. J. WILKINS, and B. J. EVANS, 2002. Randomised controlled trial of the effect of coloured overlays on the rate of reading of people with specific learning difficulties. *Ophthalmic Physiol. Opt.* 22:55–60.

BRISCOE, J., D. V. BISHOP, and C. F. NORBURY, 2001. Phonological processing, language, and literacy: A comparison of children with mild-to-moderate sensorineural hearing loss and those with specific language impairment. *J. Child. Psychol. Psychiatry* 42: 329–340.

BROWN, W. E., S. ELIEZ, V. MENON, J. M. RUMSEY, C. D. WHITE, and A. L. REISS, 2001. Preliminary evidence of widespread morphological variations of the brain in dyslexia. *Neurology* 56: 781–783.

BRUNSWICK, N., E. McCRORY, C. J. PRICE, C. D. FRITH, and U. FRITH, 1999. Explicit and implicit processing of words and pseudowords by adult developmental dyslexics: A search for Wernicke's Wortschatz? *Brain* 122(Pt. 10):1901–1917.

CARAMAZZA, A., 1997a. *Access of Phonological and Orthographic Lexical Forms: Evidence from Dissociations in Reading and Spelling. Journal of Cognitive Neuropsychology* [special issue]. New York: Psychology Press.

CARAMAZZA, A., 1997b. How many levels of processing are there in lexical access? *Cogn. Neuropsychol.* 14:177–208.

COHEN, L., S. LEHERICY, F. CHOCHON, C. LEMER, S. RIVAUD, and S. DEHAENE, 2002. Language-specific tuning of visual cortex? Functional properties of the Visual Word Form Area. *Brain* 125(Pt. 5):1054–1069.

COLTHEART, M., K. RASTLE, C. PERRY, R. LANGDON, and J. ZIEGLER, 2001. DRC: A dual route cascaded model of visual word recognition and reading aloud. *Psychol. Rev.* 108:204–256.

CORNETT, R. O., 1967. Cued speech. *Am. Ann. Deaf* 112:3–13.

ELBRO, C., 1996. Early linguistic abilities and reading development: A review and a hypothesis. *Read. Writ. Interdiscip. J.* 8:453–485.

FARMER, M. E., and R. M. KLEIN, 1995. The evidence for a temporal processing deficit linked to dyslexia: A review. *Psychon. Bull. Rev.* 2:460–493.

FLETCHER-FLINN, C. M., and G. B. THOMPSON, 2000. Learning to read with underdeveloped phonemic awareness but lexicalized phonological recoding: A case study of a 3-year-old. *Cognition* 74:177–208.

FLETCHER-FLINN, C. M., and G. B. THOMPSON, 2004. A mechanism of implicit lexicalized phonological recoding used concurrently with underdeveloped explicit letter-sound skills in both precocious and normal reading development. *Cognition* 90:303–335.

FRITH, U., 1985. Beneath the surface of developmental dyslexia. In *Surface Dyslexia*, K. E. Patterson, J. C. Marshall, and M. Coltheart, eds. London: Erlbaum, pp. 301–330.

FRITH, U., 1986. A developmental framework for developmental dyslexia. *Ann. Dyslexia* 36:69–81.

GALABURDA, A. M., G. F. SHERMAN, G. D. ROSEN, F. ABOITIZ, and N. GESCHWIND, 1985. Developmental dyslexia: Four consecutive patients with cortical anomalies. *Ann. Neurol.* 18:222–233.

HABIB, M., 2000. The neurological basis of developmental dyslexia: An overview and working hypothesis. *Brain* 123:2373–2399.

HORWITZ, B., J. M. RUMSEY, and B. C. DONOHUE, 1998. Functional connectivity of the angular gyrus in normal reading and dyslexia. *Proc. Natl. Acad. Sci. U.S.A.* 95:8939–8944.

JACQUEMOT, C., C. PALLIER, D. LE BIHAN, S. DEHAENE, and E. DUPOUX, 2003. Phonological grammar shapes the auditory cortex: A functional magnetic resonance imaging study. *J. Neurosci.* 23:9541–9546.

KLINGBERG, T., M. HEDEHUS, E. TEMPLE, T. SALZ, J. D. GABRIELI, M. E. MOSELEY, et al., 2000. Microstructure of temporo-parietal white matter as a basis for reading ability: Evidence from diffusion tensor magnetic resonance imaging. *Neuron* 25:493–500.

LEGGE, G. E., G. S. RUBIN, D. G. PELLI, and M. M. SCHLESKE, 1985. Psychophysics of reading: II. Low vision. *Vision Res.* 25:253–265.

LERNER, Y., T. HENDLER, D. BEN-BASHAT, M. HAREL, and R. MALACH, 2001. A hierarchical axis of object processing stages in the human visual cortex. *Cereb. Cortex* 11:287–297.

LEVELT, W. J., A. ROELOFS, and A. S. MEYER, 1999. A theory of lexical access in speech production. *Behav. Brain Sci.* 22:1–38.

McANALLY, K. I., and J. F. STEIN, 1996. Auditory temporal coding in dyslexia. *Proc. Nat. Acad. Sci.* 263:961–965.

McARTHUR, G. M., and D. V. M. BISHOP, 2001. Auditory perceptual processing in people with reading and oral language impairments: Current issues and recommendations. *Dyslexia* 7: 150–170.

McCANDLISS, B. D., L. COHEN, and S. DEHAENE, 2003. The visual word form area: Expertise for reading in the fusiform gyrus. *Trends Cogn. Sci.* 7:293–299.

MODY, M., M. STUDDERT-KENNEDY, and S. BRADY, 1997. Speech perception deficits in poor readers: Auditory processing or phonological coding? *J. Exp. Child Psychol.* 64:199–231.

MORGAN, W. P., 1896. A case of congenital word blindness. *B.M.J.* 2:1378.

MORRIS, R. D., K. K. STUEBING, J. M. FLETCHER, S. E. SHAYWITZ, G. R. LYON, D. P. SHANKWEILER, et al., 1998. Subtypes of reading disability: Variability around a phonological core. *J. Educ. Psychol.* 90:347–373.

MORTON, J., 1969. The interaction of information in word recognition. *Psychol. Rev.* 76:165–178.

MORTON, J., 1980. The logogen model and orthographic structure. In *Cognitive Processes in Spelling*, U. Frith ed. London: Academic Press, pp. 117–133.

MORTON, J., 1989. An information-processing account of reading acquisition. In *From Reading to Neurons*, A. M. Galaburda, ed. pp. 43–66. Cambridge, Mass.: MIT Press.

PAULESU, E., J.-F. DÉMONET, F. FAZIO, E. McCRORY, V. CHANOINE, N. BRUNSWICK, et al., 2001. Dyslexia: Cultural diversity and biological unity. *Science* 291:2165–2167.

PAULESU, E., U. FRITH, M. SNOWLING, A. GALLAGHER, J. MORTON, R. S. J. FRACKOWIAK, et al., 1996. Is developmental dyslexia a disconnection syndrome? Evidence from PET scanning. *Brain* 119:143–157.

PUGH, K. R., W. E. MENCL, A. R. JENNER, L. KATZ, S. J. FROST, J. R. LEE, et al., 2001. Neurobiological studies of reading and reading disability. *J. Commun. Disord.* 34:479–492.

PUGH, K. R., W. E. MENCL, B. A. SHAYWITZ, S. E. SHAYWITZ, R. K. FULBRIGHT, R. T. CONSTABLE, et al., 2000. The angular gyrus in developmental dyslexia: Task-specific differences in functional connectivity within posterior cortex. *Psychol. Sci.* 11:51–56.

RAE, C., M. A. LEE, R. M. DIXON, A. M. BLAMIRE, C. H. THOMPSON, P. STYLES, et al., 1998. Metabolic abnormalities in developmental dyslexia detected by ^{1}H magnetic resonance spectroscopy. *Lancet* 351:1849–1852.

RAMUS, F., 2001. Outstanding questions about phonological processing in dyslexia. *Dyslexia* 7:197–216.

RAMUS, F., 2003. Developmental dyslexia: Specific phonological deficit or general sensorimotor dysfunction? *Curr. Opin. Neurobiol.* 13:212–218.

RAMUS, F., S. ROSEN, S. C. DAKIN, B. L. DAY, J. M. CASTELLOTE, S. White, et al., 2003. Theories of developmental dyslexia: Insights from a multiple case study of dyslexic adults. *Brain* 126:841–865.

ROSEN, S., 2003. Auditory processing in dyslexia and specific language impairment: Is there a deficit? What is its nature? Does it explain anything? *J. Phonet.* 31:509–527.

ROSEN, S., and E. MANGANARI, 2001. Is there a relationship between speech and nonspeech auditory processing in children with dyslexia? *J. Speech Lang. Hear. Res.* 44:720–736.

SCHLAGGAR, B. L., T. T. BROWN, H. M. LUGAR, K. M. VISSCHER, F. M. MIEZIN, and S. E. PETERSEN, 2002. Functional neuroanatomical differences between adults and school-age children in the processing of single words. *Science* 296:1476–1479.

SERNICLAES, W., L. SPRENGER-CHAROLLES, R. CARRÉ, and J.-F. DÉMONET, 2001. Perceptual discrimination of speech sounds in developmental dyslexia. *J. Speech Lang. Hear. Res.* 44:384–399.

SHANKWEILER, D. P., and I. Y. LIBERMAN, 1972. Misreading: A search for causes. In *Language by Ear and by Eye: The Relationships Between Speech and Reading*, J. F. Kavanagh and I. G. Mattingly, eds. Cambridge, Mass.: MIT Press, pp. 293–317.

SHARE, D. L., 1995. Phonological recoding and self-teaching: Sine qua non of reading acquisition. *Cognition* 55:151–218.

SHAYWITZ, B. A., S. E. SHAYWITZ, K. R. PUGH, W. E. MENCL, R. K. FULBRIGHT, P. SKUDLARSKI, et al., 2002. Disruption of posterior brain systems for reading in children with developmental dyslexia. *Biol. Psychiatry* 52:101–110.

SHAYWITZ, S. E., B. A. SHAYWITZ, K. R. PUGH, R. K. FULBRIGHT, R. T. Constable, W. E. Mencl, et al., 1998. Functional disruption in the organization of the brain for reading in dyslexia. *Proc. Natl. Acad. Sci. U.S.A* 95:2636–2641.

SIMOS, P. G., J. I. BREIER, J. M. FLETCHER, E. BERGMAN, and A. C. PAPANICOLAOU, 2000. Cerebral mechanisms involved in word reading in dyslexic children: A magnetic source imaging approach. *Cereb. Cortex* 10:809–816.

SIMOS, P. G., J. I. BREIER, J. M. FLETCHER, B. R. FOORMAN, E. M. Castillo, and A. C. PAPANICOLAOU, 2002. Brain mechanisms for reading words and pseudowords: An integrated approach. *Cereb. Cortex* 12:297–305.

SIMOS, P. G., J. M. FLETCHER, E. BERGMAN, J. I. BREIER, B. R. FOORMAN, E. M. CASTILLO, et al., 2002. Dyslexia-specific brain activation profile becomes normal following successful remedial training. *Neurology* 58:1203–1213.

SIMOS, P. G., J. M. FLETCHER, B. R. FOORMAN, D. J. FRANCIS, E. M. CASTILLO, R. N. DAVIS, et al., 2002. Brain activation profiles during the early stages of reading acquisition. *J. Child Neurol.* 17:159–163.

SKOTTUN, B. C., 1997. The magnocellular deficit theory of dyslexia. *Trends Neurosci.* 20:397–398.

SKOTTUN, B. C., 2000. The magnocellular deficit theory of dyslexia: The evidence from contrast sensitivity. *Vision Res.* 40:111–127.

SNOWLING, M. J., 2000. *Dyslexia*, 2nd ed. Oxford: Blackwell.

STANOVICH, K. E., 1988. Explaining the differences between the dyslexic and the garden-variety poor reader: The phonological-core variable-difference model. *J. Learn. Disabil.* 21:590–604.

STEIN, J. F., 2001. The magnocellular theory of developmental dyslexia. *Dyslexia* 7:12–36.

STEIN, J. F., A. J. RICHARDSON, and M. S. FOWLER, 2000. Monocular occlusion can improve binocular control and reading in dyslexics. *Brain* 123(Pt. 1):164–170.

STEIN, J. F., J. TALCOTT, and V. WALSH, 2000. Controversy about the visual magnocellular deficit in developmental dyslexics. *Trends Cogn. Sci.* 4:209–211.

STEIN, J. F., and V. Walsh, 1997. To see but not to read: The magnocellular theory of dyslexia. *Trends Neurosci.* 20:147–152.

STROOP, J. R., 1935. Studies of interference in serial verbal reactions. *J. Exp. Psychol.* 12:643–662.

TALLAL, P., 1980. Auditory temporal perception, phonics, and reading disabilities in children. *Brain Lang.* 9:182–198.

TEMPLE, E., 2002. Brain mechanisms in normal and dyslexic readers. *Curr. Opin. Neurobiol.* 12:178–183.

TEMPLE, E., R. A. POLDRACK, J. SALIDIS, G. K. DEUTSCH, P. TALLAL, M. M. MERZENICH, et al., 2001. Disrupted neural responses to phonological and orthographic processing in dyslexic children: An fMRI study. *Neuroreport* 12:299–307.

THOMPSON, G. B., D. S. COTTRELL, and C. M. FLETCHER-FLINN, 1996. Sublexical orthographic-phonological relations early in the acquisition of reading: The knowledge sources account. *J. Exp. Child Psychol.* 62:190–222.

TURKELTAUB, P. E., L. GAREAU, D. L. FLOWERS, T. A. ZEFFIRO, and G. F. EDEN, 2003. Development of neural mechanisms for reading. *Nat. Neurosci.* 6:767–773.

VELLUTINO, F. R., 1979. *Dyslexia: Research and Theory*. Cambridge, Mass.: MIT Press.

WHITE, S., E. MILNE, S. ROSEN, P. C. HANSEN, J. SWETTENHAM, U. FRITH, et al., 2004. *The role of sensorimotor processing in dyslexia: A multiple case study of dyslexic children*. Unpublished manuscript.

WILKINS, A. J., 1995. *Visual Stress*. Oxford, England: Oxford University Press.

WITTON, C., J. F. STEIN, C. J. STOODLEY, B. S. ROSNER, and J. B. TALCOTT, 2002. Separate influences of acoustic AM and FM sensitivity on the phonological decoding skills of impaired and normal readers. *J. Cogn. Neurosci.* 14:866–874.

WOLF, M., and P. BOWERS, 1999. The "double-deficit hypothesis" for the developmental dyslexias. *J. Educ. Psychol.* 91:1–24.

59 Biological Foundations of Language Acquisition: Evidence from Bilingualism

JACQUES MEHLER, NÚRIA SEBASTIÁN-GALLÉS, AND MARINA NESPOR

ABSTRACT This chapter presents a comprehensive view of language acquisition based on the notion that humans have mechanisms that respond specifically to speech signals. Some speech signals trigger statistical computations while others trigger rule-like processes. We present evidence that human brains are tuned to speech signals at birth. Next, we show that infants extract statistical information from speech signals, but also that they extract structural regularities that cannot be solely due to the statistical information contained in the signal.

We present results from a large typological study that includes data from many different languages. The outcome supports the view that languages can be sorted into classes. Properties of those classes may bias children toward the postulation of some linguistic structures rather than other possible structures that go with languages in other classes.

Arguing in favor of the study of language acquisition using realistic scenarios, we review data from infants acquiring two languages at once. We base our presentation on a large-scale project comparing the acquisition of two related languages, Spanish and Catalan, and two distant languages, Spanish and Basque. We conclude with a review of studies of adults who ought to have been bilingual but have forgotten their first language. These adults are undistinguishable from native speakers of their language of adoption.

This chapter attempts to establish how the brain of humans is endowed with specialized processes that respond to properties of signals with specialized computation and biases that are essential to the progress of language acquisition.

Humans acquire the grammatical systems underlying language in a smooth and effortless fashion if neurological disorders do not intervene to upset the language learning processes. Chomsky (1967) used this straightforward evidence as a cornerstone of his linguistic theory, and a number of psycholinguists have included it in their proposals about the psychology of language (see Mehler, 1994; Pinker, 1994).

JACQUES MEHLER Cognitive Neuroscience Sector, International School for Advanced Studies, Trieste, Italy and CNRS, Paris, France.

NÚRIA SEBASTIÁN-GALLÉS Department of Psychology, Universitat de Barcelona, Barcelona, Spain.

MARINA NESPOR Department of Linguistics, Ferrara University, Ferrara, Italy.

(It should be noted that others do not; see Tomasello, 2000.) In this chapter, we attempt to explore the notion that speech, the usual source for learning a language, contains specific cues that trigger biases and special kinds of computations.

There is evidence that even in the initial state, speech activates specialized brain regions homologous to those that mediate language in adulthood. We take those observations as an indication of the existence of specific mechanisms for acquiring language. Just after birth, infants start learning the language they are exposed to out of the thousands of languages currently spoken in the world. How does such learning happen? We claim that cues in the speech signal trigger specific computations. In particular, we present evidence that humans are excellent statistical machines and excellent at deriving rule-like generalizations, and that the computation in which they engage depends on the cues delivered by the stimulus configuration. Next we show that despite the variability of natural languages, there is a reliable correlation between some abstract grammatical properties and the acoustical properties of the utterances of a language. This evidence supports the best-developed conjecture as to how grammar might be learned, namely, parameter-setting theory (see Chomsky, 1988). However, such an approach must also be considered in a far from exceptional language learning setting: one in which more than one language is present. Although most theoreticians tacitly assume that languages are learned in a monolingual environment, bilingualism is widespread. How does the brain/mind respond to such a situation? We present data from studies in very young infants who are exposed to two languages while still in the crib. We also review how bilingualism affects the neural representation of the first- and second-acquired languages. In particular, we present data from individuals who lost their first-acquired language in favor of a second language acquired relatively late. We conclude that despite the large number of languages and structures, the cultural specificities of bilingual acquisition, and the personal histories of the language learner, the mind's robust language acquisition device maintains its capacity to master the native language.

Theoretical perspectives on language acquisition

To understand the biological foundations of language, it is necessary to focus both on the species-specific disposition to acquire grammar and on the different types of mechanisms that guide acquisition despite the huge surface diversity of natural languages. Indeed, there are a number of suggestions that language acquisition and language use rely on more than one single kind of computation (see Marcus et al., 1999; Pinker, 1994; Peña et al., 2002).

EVIDENCE FOR SIGNAL-DRIVEN COMPUTATIONS Different investigators have shown that at least two mechanisms play an active role in language acquisition, namely, the extraction of statistical regularities in the input and the ability of the learner to hypothesize rules to characterize structural regularities. Saffran, Aslin, and Newport (1996) have stressed that statistical information is essential for lexical segmentation, and Marcus and colleagues (1999) have argued that infants use algebraic-like computations to discover structures in speech. Saffran, Aslin, and Newport (1996) have shown that 8-month-olds parse a continuous, monotonous speech stream into constituent "words" on the basis of conditional probabilities. That is, infants perceive dips in transition probability (TP) between syllables as signaling "word" boundaries. However, 7-month-olds also use algebraic-like rules to establish the structural regularities of the utterances generated by a very simple grammar (see Marcus et al., 1999). The stimuli Saffran and colleagues used are monotonous, continuous streams of syllables of equal length and intensity. In contrast, Marcus and colleagues used lists of three-syllable items separated by silence.

Peña and colleagues (2002) proposed that specific signals received during language acquisition trigger special kinds of computations that may affect syntactic acquisition even in prelexical infants. They suggested that statistical and rule-like computations play an important role in language acquisition. They went further to explore the conditions that might cause the mind to rely mainly on statistical computations or to project rule-like conjectures. They familiarized some participants to continuous, meaningless, monotonous streams of syllables and other participants to the same stream after subliminal silent gaps were added after each "word." The syllables in the stream formed three trisyllabic words; the first syllable of each word predicted the third syllable. The stream can be described as having three AxC families, where x is a variable syllable used to generate three words per family. Words had a transition probability dip after the last syllable. Participants heard the continuous stream for 14 minutes and were tested afterwards. Although they could recognize the "words" they heard during familiarization, they did not accept rule-based words or Ax*C items, where x* denotes a syllable that occurred during familiarization but

never between A and C. Thus, the authors concluded that participants had only computed transitional probabilities. However, when participants were familiarized with the stream containing silent subthreshold gaps, they accepted the rule-based words as familiar, suggesting that they had generalized to a rule-like conjecture, such as "if A then C, with a syllable between them." The inclusion of a minimal signal is thus sufficient to toggle the nature of participants' computations from statistical to rule-based. Trebling the duration of familiarization to the continuous stream to 30 minutes was insufficient for participants to extract the structural regularities present in the stream. However, reducing exposure to the stream with gaps to only 2 minutes was enough for participants to judge rule-like words as being familiar. Peña and colleagues hypothesized that when signals are unsegmented, statistics guides learning, whereas conjectures are automatically projected when minimal cues to segmentation are present.

To what extent are the human computational abilities during language acquisition signal-driven? This is a basic question whose answer might well clarify what the infant acquires during the first weeks of exposure to language. It is well known that infants pay attention to ambient language, and learn a great deal about speech from passive exposure to the signals in their surroundings. We know much less about how the gains made during the first few weeks may bias or guide the acquisition of the abstract properties of the surrounding language. We propose that just as gaps can drive computations in adults, so can some of the prosodic properties of speech drive computations in the infant.

SEPARATING LANGUAGES: THE DISCOVERY OF THE EXISTENCE OF DIFFERENT SOUND SYSTEMS As we stated in our opening comments, humans deploy their species-specific linguistic endowment to learn the properties of the surrounding language out of the thousands of existing languages to which they could be exposed. Psychologists often conjecture that associative learning underlies this acquisition. However, as argued in Chomsky's seminal writings, it seems unlikely that such a mechanism alone could account for language acquisition. We propose that the specific properties of the signal might guide the learning of (1) grammar, by giving cues to abstract properties, or (2) lexical properties, by computing statistical dependencies. This proposal is an extension of the prosodic bootstrapping hypothesis originally proposed by Morgan, Meier, and Newport (1987).

A prerequisite to language acquisition is the ability to distinguish linguistic from nonlinguistic signals (Colombo and Bundy, 1983) and to establish whether the input data represent one or more languages. If infants were unable to distinguish two languages to which they are exposed, they would be highly confused. Given that there is no evidence that early bilingual exposure causes a delay in language acquisition, we infer that bilingual infants must have ways to adjust their computations to each one of the input languages. How long does the bilingual infant take to acquire separate files for the languages in the surrounding environment? Some investigations of language production propose that infants do not differentiate the two languages present in the environment before their third year of life (Volterra and Taeschner, 1978; Redlinger and Park, 1980; Vihman, 1985; Genesee, 1989). However, neonates display behaviors that suggest that they begin to respond differently to some language pairs as early as they have been tested. Thus, procedures are needed to evaluate the linguistic representations of infants much earlier than their first word productions.

One way to explore this issue is to present infants with two languages, one for habituation and the other as a test. A large number of experiments have established that newborns discriminate some language pairs but fail to discriminate others. For instance, they distinguish Spanish versus English and English versus Japanese, but fail to distinguish Dutch versus English and Spanish versus Italian. In brief, as Mehler and colleagues (1988), Nazzi, Bertoncini, and Mehler (1998), and Ramus, Nespor, and Mehler (1999) have claimed, neonates and very young infants (less than 2 months old) discriminate languages if and only if the languages belong to different rhythmic classes, regardless of whether one of the languages is the one in their surroundings (see Christophe, 1998).

Phonologists such as Pike (1945), Abercrombie (1967), and Ladefoged (1975) were among the first to claim that lan-

guages differ in rhythm. Recently, Ramus, Nespor, and Mehler (1999) proposed that language rhythms can be described in terms of the patterns of alternation of vocalic and consonantal space (see Mehler and Christophe, 2000). This method of capturing language rhythms is also implicit in the work of some psycholinguists that explores cross-linguistic speech segmentation phenomena (Mehler et al., 1981; Cutler et al., 1983; Sebastián-Gallés et al., 1992; Otake et al., 1993).

According to the measures of Ramus, Nespor, and Mehler (1999), languages such as English, Dutch, or Polish, all supposedly stress-timed, cluster together. Spanish, Italian, and French, all supposedly syllable-timed, also cluster together. Japanese, a so-called mora-timed language, stands by itself, possibly because of the scarcity of languages included in the original measures.[1] The ability of newborns to discriminate among languages appears to depend on the ability to distinguish between languages belonging to these different rhythmic groups.

Subsequent work has added several unrelated languages to those plotted in the work of Ramus and colleagues (figure 59.1). It now appears that the languages that cluster with Japanese in the right part of figure 59.1, besides being mora-timed, tend to be complement-head (C-H) and/or agglutinative languages[2] or languages that have a relatively free word order. Indeed, the diagonal line in figure 59.1 divides languages into two groups, those that are head-complement (H-C), that is, English, Dutch, Polish, French, Spanish, Catalan, and Italian, and those that are mostly complement-

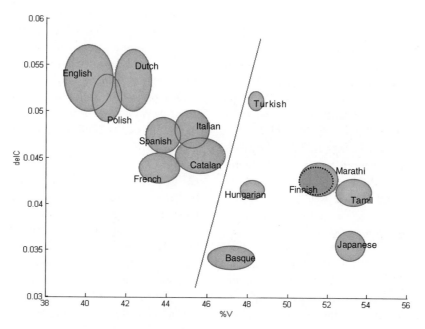

FIGURE 59.1   Fourteen languages plotted in the %V versus delC space first proposed by Ramus (1999, p. 150). All Romance languages and all Germanic languages (as well as Polish) tend to have low %V. We also present a selection of languages having higher values of %V. The diagonal line separates the languages into two groups. On the left are head-complement languages; the ones on the right tend to be complement-head languages.

head, that is, Basque, Hungarian, Turkish, Finnish, Japanese, Tamil, and Marathi. (It should be noted that Dutch and Hungarian are in fact "mixed" languages, because some phrases have a C-H order while others have H-C. However, Dutch is predominantly H-C, while Hungarian is mostly C-H.

A number of scientists have argued that prosodic bootstrapping is essential for the acquisition of abstract properties of grammars. Nespor, Guasti, and Christophe (1996), Christophe and Dupoux (1996), and Aslin and colleagues (1996) give specific examples to illustrate how prosodic bootstrapping might actually work. Nespor and colleagues (1996) argue that the correlation between the prominence of the phonological phrase (PP),[3] that is, its main stress and the value of the H-C parameter (Nespor and Vogel, 1986), might be used to set the head-direction parameter at a prelexical stage. In a recent study, Christophe and colleagues (2003) provided empirical support for this view. It is likely that both rightmost prominence in the PP and low values of %V will bias infants toward an H-C organization of syntax, as well as toward a cluster of morphological and phonological properties. Leftmost PP prominence and a high %V would bias them toward a C-H syntax and possibly also toward a cluster of properties such as agglutinative morphology, simple syllabic structure, and relatively free word order. Developmental psycholinguists may consider acoustic cues that correlate with syntactic parameters a solution to the paradox that Mazuka (1996) pointed out. Indeed, without robust cues in the signal, parameter setting would fail to explain how the infant goes from the input to syntax without lexical information. However, if the child had already acquired lexical items, setting parameters would become unnecessary. If infants could rely on prosodic cues, they would be able to set at least some parameters without knowledge of the lexicon (Mehler and Christophe, 2000). Rhythm may also provide the infant with information to bias lexical segmentation toward shorter or longer words: languages in the stress group, such as English and Dutch, would tend to have shorter words (given that they have over 16 different syllabic types), while languages in the mora group (e.g., Japanese) would tend to have longer words (since they have about three syllabic types; see Mehler and Nespor, 2003).

The infant brain's response to natural speech

Since Broca's original publication (Broca, 1861), investigators have realized that there is a privileged relationship between language and the left hemisphere. For some, language acquisition is responsible for the emergence of left hemisphere superiority (Lenneberg et al., 1964; Mills, Coffey-Corina, and Neville, 1993, 1997), whereas others believe structural biases present at birth cause greater left-hemispheric activation when infants hear speech stimuli

(Segalowitz and Chapman, 1980; Mehler and Christophe, 2000), mediating future aspects of language acquisition. After a flurry of studies in pursuit of answers to these questions, the availability of excellent imaging methods has allowed researchers to make progress. Two recent studies have shown that speech stimuli result in greater left-hemispheric activation in very young infants. One of these studies used optical topography to study neonates; the other study used fMRI to study 3-month-olds.

OPTICAL TOPOGRAPHY Peña and colleagues (in press) explored left hemisphere activity in 1-week-old neonates using a 24-channel optical topographical (OT) system. They assessed the change of total hemoglobin in response to auditory stimulation in 12 areas of the right hemisphere and 12 areas of the left hemisphere. Peña and colleagues stimulated the infants with normal speech (forward speech), with the same utterances played backward, and with silence. They found that acoustic stimulation resulted in greater activation in the left hemisphere than in the right (figure 59.2). Moreover, as the figure shows, temporal areas in the left hemisphere were significantly more activated by forward utterances than by backward utterances. No area of the right hemisphere was more activated by forward than by backward speech. This result is compelling, because backward speech (derived from forward utterances) is an optimal control for natural forward speech, since the two utterances are matched in pitch, intensity, and duration. Yet humans cannot produce either reverse prosody or some segments that appear in backward utterances, such as those that correspond to time-reversed stop and affricate consonants.

Peña and colleagues have thus demonstrated that the neonate's brain is particularly sensitive to language-like stimuli, or at least to stimuli that the human vocal tract can produce. These results attest to the early tuning of the human brain to the speech signals made by conspecifics. It is hardly necessary for the neonate to have gained experience from such stimuli in order for the brain to show the specificity of the response.

fMRI STUDIES In a study comparable to the one reported by Peña and colleagues, Dehaene-Lambertz, Dehaene, and Hertz-Pannier (2002) used fMRI in 3-month-old infants and found that auditory stimuli (forward and backward speech) gave rise to greater activity in the left hemisphere superior temporal lobe than did silence. Larger activations for forward than for backward utterances were found in the posterior areas of the left hemisphere (angular gyrus and the mesial parietal cortex; figure 59.3).

Both the OT and the fMRI studies found a left hemispheric superiority in processing sound stimuli. OT technology makes it possible to test neonates in a silent environment. Peña and colleagues found greater activation for forward

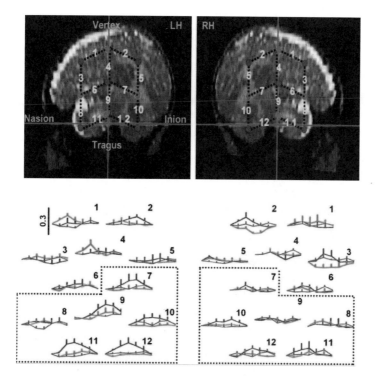

FIGURE 59.2   OT study of a 2-month-old infant. Top panels show positioning of the fiber-optics on the infant's head. Numbers 1 to 12 in bottom panels refer to the left and the right channels depicted in the top panels. The vertical line to the left of channel 1 in the left hemisphere shows the value of the change in concentration of total hemoglobin. Red indicates the response to forward utterances, green the response to backward utterances, and blue, the response to the control condition (silence). (See color plate 37.)

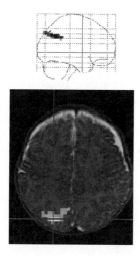

FIGURE 59.3   Results from the study of Dehaene-Lambertz and colleagues (2002), showing that forward utterances produced more activation in the left hemisphere angular gyrus than did backward utterances. (See color plate 38.)

than for backward utterances in the temporal areas of the left hemisphere, while Dehaene-Lambertz and colleagues found greater activation for forward than for backward utterances in the left angular gyrus and in left mesial parietal cortex in 3-month-olds. Despite the similarities of these two studies, the different results for backward versus forward utterances may reflect the fact that OT records total hemoglobin changes up to 2.5–3.0 cm from the infant's scalp, whereas fMRI can also record activations from deeper areas, such as the mesial parietal cortex. Age may also be partly responsible for the observed differences. However, it should also be noted that the older infants were tested in a magnet, that is, in a rather noisy environment, while the neonates were tested in silence.

In short, it appears from these two studies that the human brain is organized to respond to speech utterances in a specific fashion, displaying greater left hemispheric activation in perisylvian areas.

THE BRAIN-LANGUAGE LINK   These imaging results mesh well with the results of behavioral studies (e.g., Best, 1988; Segalowitz and Chapman, 1980; Bertoncini et al., 1989). If the initial left hemisphere advantage in processing speech indicates a language "organ," how is it possible that a patient who had failed to acquire language at 8 years could begin learning it after the damaged left hemisphere was surgically removed (Vargha-Khadem et al., 1997)? This situation indicates that the left hemisphere was blocking the ability of the right hemisphere to acquire language. Thus, it appears that the initial dominance of the left hemisphere for speech is just dominance: both hemispheres may have the potential to sustain language, but the specific cues used to signal speech are processed better by the left hemisphere. Recent work related to the cortical representation of speech and nonspeech sounds in very young infants (Holowka and Petitto, 2002) suggests that a similar left hemisphere dominance is also present for language production, and not only for language perception.

We have reviewed some of the evidence that suggests that the human brain is predisposed to language acquisition, a disposition that starts coming into play very shortly after birth. How well does this disposition adapt to different sociolinguistic conditions that the infant may encounter during language acquisition?

Bilinguals in the crib

Many studies that have investigated how grammatical knowledge is acquired have tacitly assumed that infants receive input from only one language. However, surveys show that more than half of the world's infants are confronted with input from more than one language, often from birth.

BILINGUAL LANGUAGE ACQUISITION   Discerning parents are amazed to notice how easily infants acquire the maternal language, or L1. Words, syntactic rules, and phonological knowledge grow ceaselessly. In less than 1 year, infants are able to identify some words, and they seem capable of extracting some of the fundamental properties of grammar (see Aslin et al., 1996; Nespor, Guasti, and Christophe, 1996; Jusczyk, 1997; Christophe et al., 2003). This is a striking achievement, yet it is even more striking to learn that very young infants have little if any difficulty learning two or more languages simultaneously. When one compares the achievement of infants with that of adults who are trying to learn a new language, let alone two, it becomes evident how powerful infants' language acquisition device is. Learning a new language is not as easy for adults as it is for infants. It is highly exceptional for individuals to attain a level of competence in a second language (L2) acquired after puberty comparable to that which is normally attained in L1 (see Johnson and Newport, 1989; Mayberry, 1993).

THE VOWEL SPACE   Infants raised with two rhythmically similar languages, Catalan and Spanish, were tested when they were $4^1/_2$ months old. The results showed that they were able to discriminate the two languages (Bosch and Sebastián-Gallés, 2001a). Therefore, the ability to sort languages that are in the same rhythmic class is attained much before the infant acquires lexical items, and before the monolingual infant identifies the phonemes in its maternal language (see Kuhl et al., 1992; Werker and Lalonde, 1988).

Because Spanish-Catalan bilingual infants cannot use rhythm to separate their languages, what other cues might they use to achieve separation? Several experiments may help answer this question. In one experiment, infants from monolingual Spanish families and monolingual Catalan families were tested to evaluate whether they were able to discriminate between Catalan and Spanish, as well as Italian (a Romance language) and English (a Germanic language), at $4^1/_2$ months of age (Bosch and Sebastián-Gallés, 2000a). Previous experiments with neonates and 2-month-olds had established that they fail to discriminate languages that belong to the same rhythmic class (see Mehler et al., 1988). In contrast to the procedure used to test neonates and 2-months-olds, Bosch and Sebastián-Gallés (2000a) used natural utterances in their experiments. Spanish has five vocalic phonemes, Italian has seven, and the five vowels common to the two languages have similar frequencies of occurrence. In contrast, Catalan has eight vowels, and its most frequent vowel is absent from both Italian and Spanish.[4] If infants are paying attention to vowel frequencies, they might be able to segregate Catalan utterances from both Spanish and Italian but would fail to discriminate Spanish from Italian.[5]

The results established that monolingual infants distinguish Catalan from both Spanish (as do Spanish-Catalan bilinguals) and Italian; however, they fail to distinguish Spanish from Italian. These results suggest that segmental distribution may provide information to individuate utterances as belonging to one or the other language that are in the same rhythmic category. Although by $4^1/_2$ months of age such distributional properties are used, we do not know whether younger infants perform similar computations.

Recent studies testing $4^1/_2$-month-old and 6-month-old bilingual Spanish-Catalan infants compared a native language (the one spoken by the mother) with a nonfamiliar language. These bilingual infants discriminated between their maternal language and a foreign language, regardless of whether it was in the same or a different rhythmic class (English and Italian were used) (figure 59.4).

The bilingual infants' pattern of results contrasts with that of the monolingual infants (Bosch and Sebastián-Gallés, 1997; 2001b). As shown in figure 59.4, bilingual infants orient faster to English and Italian than to Spanish or Catalan. Hence, 4-month-old bilingual infants may be aware that two languages are used in their environment. These results indicate that cognitive mechanisms (e.g., executive functions) may differ in matched monolingual and bilingual infants.

Taken together, the results indicate that bilingual infants attain the ability to differentiate languages of the same

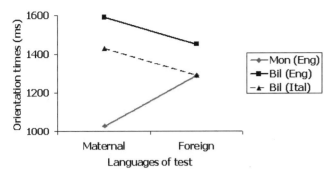

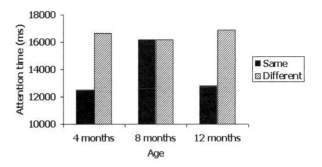

FIGURE 59.4 Figure shows mean orientation latencies of 4½-month-old infants from monolingual environments (either Catalan or Spanish) to maternal and English sentences (in gray; Mon (Eng)), and mean orientation latencies of infants from bilingual Spanish-Catalan environments to maternal and English sentences (solid black; Bil (Eng)) and maternal and Italian sentences (dashed black; Bil (Ital)). Monolingual infants oriented faster to the familiar (maternal) than to the unfamiliar (English) language. Bilingual infants showed the opposite pattern, they oriented slower to the familiar (language of the mother) than to the unfamiliar language. This pattern of results is observed both for an unfamiliar language within the same rhythmic category as the language of the mother (Italian) and for a language from a different rhythmic group (English). (Adapted from Bosch and Sebastián-Gallés, 1997.)

FIGURE 59.5 Time course of bilingual infants' discrimination capacities (as shown by the differences in mean attention times to same and different trials) to a Catalan-specific contrast (/e/-/ɛ/) during the first year of life. (Adapted from Bosch and Sebastián-Gallés, in press.)

rhythmic class earlier than monolingual infants. Future research may uncover whether this bilingual advantage arises when infants are asked to judge the familiar language against an unfamiliar language in the same rhythmic class. Whatever the outcome of those experiments, the refined discrimination ability of bilingual infants highlights the importance of perceptual learning.

At 6 months, monolingual infants respond preferentially to the vocalic contrasts used in their native language, and they appear to be attuned to vocalic contrasts earlier than to consonantal contrasts (Werker and Lalonde, 1988; Kuhl et al., 1992). Bilingual infants have a different developmental pattern than monolingual infants (Bosch and Sebastián-Gallés, in press). Four-month-old and 8-month-old infants from monolingual (Spanish or Catalan) and bilingual (Spanish-Catalan) households were tested on a vowel contrast present in Catalan but not in Spanish: /e/-/ɛ/ (/de'di/ versus /dɛ'di/). As expected, younger infants were able to perceive this contrast independently of the language of exposure, presumably on the basis of acoustic differences. By 8 months, infants from Catalan monolingual environments distinguished this contrast, but bilingual infants and Spanish monolingual infants did not. The behavior of the Spanish monolingual infants conformed to the previously attested decline in discrimination of contrasts that are absent from the linguistic input. The bilingual infants' behavior was unexpected, since they had received sufficient exposure to the /e/-/ɛ/ contrast. The bilingual infants receive exposure both to the /e/-/ɛ/ vowels and to the Spanish /E/ that falls

between the two Catalan vowels. Possibly, the vowel space in the pertinent region becomes so crowded that the infants represent a continuous distribution that gives rise to the infants' difficulty in discriminating the Catalan contrast (see Maye, Werker, and Gerken, 2002). Bilinguals infants, however, are also less frequently exposed to the Catalan /e/-/ɛ/ contrast than the Catalan monolinguals. To evaluate these conjectures, bilingual infants were tested with a vowel contrast existing both in Catalan and Spanish: /o/-/u/. At 8 months, bilingual infants failed to discriminate the two vowels, suggesting that mere exposure may not be sufficient to preserve the capacity to perceive a contrast. Furthermore, these results suggest that the phonetic representations of bilingual infants are not identical to those of monolingual infants until a few months later. Indeed, at 12 months, Spanish-Catalan bilingual children have no difficulty distinguishing /e/ from /ɛ/ or /o/ from /u/ (figure 59.5).

At this time, it is difficult to construct an accurate model of how bilinguals cope with the vowel space or with consonantal categories. What is clear, however, is that there are systematic behavioral differences between bilingual and monolingual infants that disappear by the time the infants begin to acquire the lexicon.

Phonotactics and the lexicon

At 6 months, infants start learning phonotactic regularities, that is, how segments co-occur (for a review, see Jusczyk, 1997). Phonotactic information is language-specific. For example, in English, words with an initial [s] can have another consonant to the right of [s]—*sphere, strategy*—whereas the corresponding Spanish words are *esfera* and *estrategia* because of the illegality of word-initial s+consonant clusters. To learn the phonotactics of their languages, bilingual users must segment speech into words and acquire separate lexicons for each language. Thus, it is possible that learning phonotactics may pose a problem for bilingual infants, particularly when they are raised with rhythmically similar languages in which prosodic cues do not mediate the segregation of utterances into language files.

Bilingual infants might first concentrate on one of their two languages, filtering out or ignoring the other language, or they might try to work on both languages in parallel. Presumably the second scenario is more likely when the languages that have to be mastered belong to two separate rhythmic classes; however, when the languages belong to the same class, such as Spanish and Catalan, the most likely prediction is that the infant will either be confused or will separate the languages on the basis of nonrhythmical cues.

If bilingual infants neglected one language, they should behave in their dominant language as monolingual infants do. If they do not, they might be acquiring the phonotactics of both languages simultaneously. However, bilingual infants receive half as much exposure in either one of the languages as monolingual infants, which might lead us to predict that bilingual infants will not behave exactly as monolingual infants in either case. Thus, bilingual infants may either have a similar performance in both languages that is inferior to that of monolingual infants or a performance that is better in one of the two languages but still not as good as that of monolingual controls for the dominant language.

Nine-month-old monolingual infants prefer to listen to lists of stimuli that conform to the phonotactics of their maternal language (Jusczyk, Luce, and Charles-Luce, 1994). Sebastián-Gallés and Bosch (2002) tested 10-month-old monolingual and bilingual Catalan-Spanish infants. They evaluated the infants' responses to items with Catalan phonotactic patterns that are absent in Spanish. Unlike Catalan, Spanish does not allow complex consonant clusters in word-final position. Therefore, a word ending in two or more consonants does not exist in Spanish. Although Catalan accepts word-final complex consonant clusters, not all consonant clusters are possible. (For instance, *pirn* could be a possible word in Catalan, but not *pikf*.) According to Jusczyk, Luce, and Charles-Luce (1994), monolingual Catalan infants should show a preference for the legal words when presented with lists containing legal or illegal word-final consonant clusters in Catalan. In contrast, Spanish monolingual infants ought to show no preference, since both types of stimuli are illegal in Spanish.

Sebastián-Gallés and Bosch (2002) confirmed these predictions (figure 59.6). The bilingual infants who had been mostly exposed to Catalan behaved as the monolingual Catalan infants, while the infants who had been mostly exposed to Spanish behaved as Spanish monolingual infants, showing no preference for one or the other type of stimulus. These results are more consistent with the hypothesis that, when acquiring phonotactic knowledge, bilingual infants focus on one language first rather than acquiring both systems in parallel or a single common system for both languages.

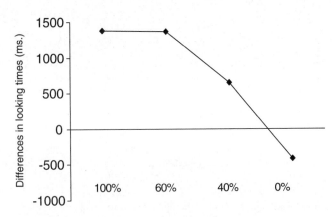

FIGURE 59.6 Sensitivity to Catalan-specific phonotactic constraints (mean differences in looking times for legal versus illegal Catalan codas) as a function of Catalan exposure (100% Catalan-monolingual infants, 0% Spanish-monolingual infants). (Adapted from Sebastián-Gallés and Bosch, 2002.)

Bilingual infants show language discrimination capacities that challenge the view that they are confused during early language acquisition. Moreover, the results presented suggest that bilingual infants display acquisition patterns that differ from those of monolingual infants. The neural substrate and the mechanisms responsible for these differences remain to be unveiled.

Unusual acquisition scenarios

The way in which the brain represents language has mostly been studied in adult monolingual university students or in patients. Here we present studies of special bilingual populations that are important because they inform us about the reliability of the language acquisition device and how it manifests itself under different conditions.

NEURAL REPRESENTATIONS OF L1 AND L2 IN BILINGUAL INDIVIDUALS Studies of highly proficient English-Italian and Catalan-Spanish bilingual individuals show that when participants listen to either of the languages, mostly very similar perisylvian areas of the left hemisphere are activated (see Perani et al., 1998). Likewise, Kim and colleagues (1997) studied a group of bilingual participants who had to implicitly produce short stories. The authors reported that the activations of L1 and L2 were indistinguishable from one another in participants who had acquired L2 early in life. Neville and colleagues (1998) studied English and American Sign Language (ASL) bilingual individuals and found that the left hemisphere perisylvian areas were activated similarly by English and ASL. This study included a group of participants who had acquired ASL and English during infancy. In these participants, oral and sign languages also activated overlapping areas of the left hemisphere. Moreover, a greater right hemisphere involvement was observed for ASL

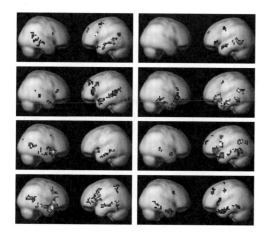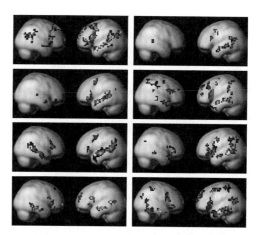

FIGURE 59.7   The eight panels on the left depict cortical areas that showed significantly greater activation when native Koreans were processing French compared to Polish utterances. The eight panels on the right illustrate the cortical areas that showed significantly greater activation when native French speakers were processing French compared to Polish utterances. Although both populations had become equally fluent in French, a significantly greater area of the left hemisphere was activated in the native French speakers than in the native Korean speakers. (See color plate 39.)

than for English (Paulesu and Mehler, 1998). A subsequent study (Newman et al., 2002) confirmed the involvement of both the right hemisphere and the left hemisphere in native ASL users and in highly proficient bilingual participants processing ASL. It is difficult to specify the role of the right hemisphere in ASL speakers. Aphasias in native users of ASL mostly arise after left hemisphere lesions, in contrast to what brain activation studies might suggest. Some researchers attribute the right hemisphere involvement in ASL processing to the spatial nature of signs and to the superiority of the right hemisphere in processing biological motion. But as Newman and colleagues point out, "The exact role of the RH in ASL processing has yet to be determined" (2002, p. 78).

Thus, a comparison of activation studies of oral-oral and oral-sign bilinguals suggests the following: (1) the oral-oral pairs show activation in overlapping areas of the left hemisphere in participants who have attained a high degree of proficiency in both languages, and (2) highly proficient oral-sign bilingual individuals have similar left hemisphere representations, but only native signers recruit larger areas of their right hemisphere. Thus, it appears that the modalities of the bilingual individuals' languages may affect the extent to which the neural representations overlap.

LOSING L1   Imaging has also been used to investigate whether a normally acquired, then forgotten L1 affects the way in which a later-acquired language is represented and processed. Pallier and colleagues (2003) studied eight Korean children who had been adopted by French families when they were more than 3 but less than 8 years old. These participants' French was indistinguishable from that of French monolingual participants on a number of behavioral tasks. After adoption, the participants' contact with Korean speakers was nil. Participants were given a number of behavioral tests and also took part in an event-related fMRI study.[6] Like the native speakers of French, in a classification of Korean and Japanese sentences, the Korean participants failed to identify the Korean utterances. In word recognition the Koreans and the control group were at chance levels. In figure 59.7 we display, for each one of the eight participants, the results of the imaging study in a French-Polish comparison. Polish may be considered the baseline condition because it was equally alien to Korean and native French participants.

The network activated by French in Korean participants is similar to the network described in previous studies on native French volunteers (see Mazoyer et al., 1993; Perani et al., 1995; Dehaene et al., 1997). Indeed, the network includes perisylvian areas in the left hemisphere, the pars triangularis, the left inferior frontal gyrus, and, to a much lesser extent, some contralateral temporal areas. The individual results for the French-Polish comparison uncover an interesting difference—the Korean group showed less extensive activation than the native French group. Interestingly, in the French-Korean comparison, a comparison that is critical to understanding whether some latent Korean is still present in the adoptees, the two groups were statistically alike. The study by Pallier and colleagues (2003) shows that the maternal language can be entirely reduced in participants who learned L1 for 3 or more years before switching exclusively to L2. Neither behavioral nor imaging data show differences between adopted participants and native French participants with respect to the Korean sentences.

Retraining experiments are helpful to assess whether despite these observations, some latent "knowledge" of L1 remains present. Ventureyra and colleagues (in press) reported results of behavioral tests on two groups of adopted

Koreans. One group had never been reexposed to Korean after learning French, while the other group had been reexposed to Korean after French had become their "native" language. The authors tested whether these groups could perform better on the discrimination of Korean contrasts than the native French speakers who have great difficulty discriminating the selected contrasts. The authors report that both groups of Koreans performed similarly to native French users. Thus, reexposure does not have an effect, since the two adopted Korean groups did not differ from one another.

The authors suggest that the usual problems encountered when learning an L2 after puberty may be due to the interference of L1 rather than to the crystallization of L1. However, we still can ask why interference is critical only if L2 is acquired after puberty. Indeed, children under the age of 10 tend to have little difficulty acquiring a second language when fully immersed in a different culture.

Conclusions

Recent studies of language acquisition have explored specific conditions that inform us about the robustness of the "language instinct." Imaging studies have strengthened our belief that the perisylvian areas of the left hemisphere are attuned to language long before the infant gains much experience about his or her surroundings. Furthermore, studies of the rhythmic properties of a fairly large number of languages have uncovered a correlation of syntactic and morphological properties with rhythm. This raises the possibility that such low-level cues might bias infants toward setting a parameter in one of its possible values. A number of future investigations will no doubt explore this conjecture in greater detail.

In this chapter, we have stressed the importance of studying the acquisition of language in realistic contexts. It is still unknown how the acquisition of language in bilingual societies affects language acquisition. We have presented a review of some investigations of Catalan-Spanish bilingual infants that will be complemented by a parallel study of infants raised with Basque and Spanish, the aim being to determine how the distance between the languages of the bilingual infant might affect the acquisition processes.

We ended with a review of some rather unique language acquisition situations that might clarify our views about standard circumstances. We have seen how differences in the modalities of the languages of the bilingual person might affect the neural representations of the two languages. We also reviewed a study of adults who had been adopted after having acquired, then forgotten, their maternal language. The study shows that such individuals are indistinguishable from native speakers of the adopted language. Imaging and behavioral studies failed to detect evidence of a residual knowledge of L1. Some hypotheses about how these studies

may help understand the more habitual bilingual learning situation were considered.

Throughout this chapter, we have tried to illustrate how pervasive the nature of the stimulating environment may be in triggering different processes. In our view, the evidence presented suggests that humans are attuned to specialized signals that trigger specific computations and biases.

ACKNOWLDGMENTS   This work was supported by grants from the Human Frontier Science Program (RGP 68/2002), the James McDonnell Foundation (Bridging Brain, Mind, and Behaviour Program), the Regione FVG (L.R. 3/98), and MIUR.

NOTES

1. Stress timing assumes that there is the same duration going from any one stress to the next. Syllable timing assumes that all syllable have roughly the same duration. Mora timing assumes that subsyllabic units (roughly CVs, syllabic Vs, geminates, and nasal segments in coda position) are equal in duration.

2. We are grateful to Dan Slobin for having suggested this as an additional property of languages that have a high %V.

3. Informally, a phonological phrase includes a syntactic head and all the elements that precede it in H-C languages or that follow it in C-H languages.

4. Specifically, whereas about 25% of Spanish and Italian vowels are mid-back ones (Spanish and Italian vowel /o/ and Italian vowel /ɔ/), in Catalan only 8% are mid-back vowels. In fact, in Catalan, central vowels /a/ and schwa count for more than half of the total number of vowels in fluent speech, whereas central vowels represent less than 25% of the vowels in either Spanish or Italian that have only [a].

5. In all the studies mentioned in this section, bilingual infants were exposed to both languages in a range varying from 50%/50%, that is, equal exposure to both languages, up to 35%/65% in the most unbalanced situation (in some studies the most unbalanced situation was 40%/60%).

6. Subjects had to listen to sentences in Korean, Japanese, Polish, Swedish, and Wolof and rate whether sentences were Korean or not, using a seven-point scale. Participants also read a series of French words; each visual word was followed by two spoken Korean words, and they had to guess which of the two was the corresponding translation. Participants also took part in an event-related fMRI procedure while listening to sentences in French, Korean, Japanese, and Polish. Three native speakers of each language had recorded the sentences used in this part of the experiment. While they were being scanned, participants had to judge whether a fragment belonged to the previously heard sentence or not. The aim of this task was to equalize the attention that the participants were paying to the utterances.

REFERENCES

ASLIN, R. N., J. Z. WOODWARD, N. P. LAMENDOLA, and T. G. BEVER, 1996. Models of word segmentation in fluent maternal speech to infants. In *Signal to Syntax: Bootstrapping from Speech to Grammar in Early Acquisition*, J. L. Morgan and K. Demuth, eds. Mahwah, N.J.: Erlbaum, pp. 117–134.

ABERCROMBIE, D., 1967. *Elements of General Phonetics*. Edinburgh: Edinburgh University Press.

BERTONCINI, J., J. MORAIS, R. BIJELJAC-BABIC, S. MACADAMS, I. PERETZ, and J. MEHLER, 1989. Dichotic perception and laterality in neonates. *Brain Cogn.* 37:591–605.

BEST, C. T., 1988. The emergence of cerebral asymmetries in early human development: A literature review and a neuroembryological model. In *Brain Lateralization in Children: Developmental Implications*, D. L. Molfese and S. J. Segalowitz, eds. New York: The Guilford Press, pp. 5–34.

BOSCH, L., and N. SEBASTIÁN-GALLÉS, 1997. Native-language recognition abilities in four-month-old infants from monolingual and bilingual environments. *Cognition* 65:33–69.

BOSCH, L., and N. SEBASTIÁN-GALLÉS, 2001a. Evidence of early language discrimination abilities in infants from bilingual environments. *Infancy* 2:29–49.

BOSCH, L., and N. SEBASTIÁN-GALLÉS, 2001b. Early language differentiation in bilingual infants. In *Trends in Bilingual Acquisition*, J. Cenoz and F. Genesee, eds. Amsterdam: John Benjamins, pp. 71–93.

BOSCH, L., and N. SEBASTIÁN-GALLÉS (in press). Simultaneous bilingualism and the perception of a language specific vowel contrast in the first year of life. *Lang. Speech.*

BROCA, P., 1861. Remarques sur le siège de la faculté du langage articulé, suivies d'une observation d'aphémie (perte de la parole). *Bull. Soc. Anat.* 6:330–357.

CHOMSKY, N., 1967. Recent contributions to the theory of innate knowledge. *Synthese* 17:2–11.

CHOMSKY, N., 1988. *Language and Problems of Knowledge.* Cambridge, Mass.: MIT Press.

CHRISTOPHE, A., and E. DUPOUX, 1996. Bootstrapping lexical acquisition: The role of prosodic structure. *Linguist Rev.* 13: 383–412.

CHRISTOPHE, A., and J. MORTON, 1998. Is Dutch native English? Linguistic analysis by 2-month-olds. *Dev. Sci.* 1:215–219.

CHRISTOPHE, A., M. NESPOR, M. T. GUASTI, and B. VAN OOYEN, 2003. Prosodic structure and syntactic acquisition: The case of the head-direction parameter. *Dev. Sci.* 6:213–222.

COLOMBO, J., and R. S. BUNDY, 1983. Infant response to auditory familiarity and novelty. *Infant Behav. Dev.* 6:305–311.

CUTLER, A., J. MEHLER, D. NORRIS, and J. SEGUI, 1983. A language-specific comprehension strategy. *Nature* 304:159–160.

DEHAENE, S., E. DUPOUX, J. MEHLER, L. COHEN, E. PAULESU, D. PERANI, P. F. VAN DE MOORTELE, S. LEHIRICY, and D. LE BIHAN, 1997. Anatomical variability in the cortical representation of first and second languages. *Neuroreport* 8:3809–3815.

DEHAENE-LAMBERTZ, G., S. DEHAENE, and L. HERTZ-PANNIER, 2002. Functional neuroimaging of speech perception in infants. *Science* 298:2013–2015.

GENESEE, F., 1989. Early bilingual development: One language or two? *J. Child Lang.* 16:161–179.

HOLOWKA, S., and L. A. PETITTO, 2002. Left hemisphere cerebral specialization for babies while babbling. *Science* 297:1515.

JOHNSON, J. S., and E. L. NEWPORT, 1989. Critical period effects in second language learning: The influence of maturational state on the acquisition of English as a second language. *Cogn. Psychol.* 21:60–99.

JUSCZYK, P. W., 1997. *The Discovery of Spoken Language Recognition.* Cambridge, Mass.: MIT Press.

JUSCZYK, P. W., P. A. LUCE, and J. CHARLES-LUCE, 1994. Infants' sensitivity to phonotactic patterns in the native language. *J. Mem. Lang.* 33:630–645.

KIM, K. H. S., N. R. RELKIN, L. KYOUNG-MIN, and J. HIRSCH, 1997. Distinct cortical areas associated with native and second languages. *Nature* 388:171–174.

KUHL, P. K., K. A. WILLIAMS, F. LACERDA, K. N. STEVENS, and B. LINDBLOM, 1992. Linguistic experiences alter phonetic perception in infants by 6 months of age. *Science* 255:606–608.

LADEFOGED, P., 1975. *A Course on Phonetics.* New York: Harcourt Brace Jovanovich.

LENNEBERG, E. H., I. A. NICHOLS, and E. F. ROSENBERGER, 1964. *Primitive Stages of Language Development in Mongolism.* Baltimore: Williams and Wilkins.

MARCUS, G. F., S. VIJAYAN, S. BANDI RAO, and P. M. VISHTON, 1999. Rule-learning in seven-month-old infants. *Science* 283:77–80.

MAYBERRY, R. I., 1993. First-language acquisition after childhood differs from second-language acquisition: The case of American Sign Language. *J. Speech Hear. Res.* 36:1258–1270.

MAYE, J., J. F. WERKER, and L. A. GERKEN, 2002. Infant sensitivity to distributional information can affect phonetic discrimination. *Cognition* 82:B101–B111.

MAZOYER, B., N. TZOURIO, J.-B. POLINE, L. PETIT, O. LEVRIER, and M. JOLIOT, 1993. Anatomical regions of interest versus stereotactic space: A comparison of two approaches for brain activation map analysis. In *Quantification of Brain Function*, K. Uemura, N. A. Lassen, Jones, and T. I. Kanno, eds. Amsterdam: Elsevier Science Publishers, pp. 511–518.

MAZUKA, R., 1996. How can a grammatical parameter be set before the first word? In *Signal to Syntax: Bootstrapping from Speech to Grammar in Early Acquisition*, J. L. Morgan and K. Demuth, eds. Mahwah, N.J.: Erlbaum, pp. 313–330.

MEHLER, J., 1994. Editorial. *Cognition* 50:1–6.

MEHLER, J., and A. CHRISTOPHE, 2000. Acquisition of languages: Infant and adult data. In *The New Cognitive Neurosciences*, 2nd ed., M. S. Gazzaniga, ed. Cambridge, Mass: MIT Press, pp. 897–908.

MEHLER, J., J. Y. DOMMERGUES, U. FRAUENFELDER, and J. SEGUI, 1981. The syllable's role in speech segmentation. *J. Verbal Learn. Verbal Behav.* 20:298–305.

MEHLER, J., and E. DUPOUX, 1994. *What Infants Know.* Cambridge, Mass.: Blackwell.

MEHLER, J., P. JUSCZYK, G. LAMBERTZ, N. HALSTED, J. BERTONCINI, and C. AMIEL-TISON, 1988. A precursor of language acquisition in young infants. *Cognition* 29:143–178.

MEHLER, J., and M. NESPOR, 2003. Linguistic rhythm and the acquisition of language. In *Structures and Beyond*, A. Belletti, ed. Oxford, England: Oxford University Press.

MILLS, D. L., S. A. COFFEY-CORINA, and H. J. NEVILLE, 1993. Language acquisition and cerebral specialization in 20-month-old infants. *J. Cogn. Neurosci.* 5:317–334.

MILLS, D. L., S. A. COFFEY-CORINA, and H. J. NEVILLE, 1997. Language comprehension and cerebral specialization from 13 to 20 months. *Dev. Neuropsychol.* 13:397–445.

MORGAN, J. L., R. P. MEIER, and E. L. NEWPORT, 1987. Structural packaging in the input to language learning: Contributions of prosodic and morphological marking of phrases to the acquisition of language. *Cogn. Psychol.* 19:498–550.

NAZZI, T., J. BERTONCINI, and J. MEHLER, 1998. Language discrimination by newborns: Towards an understanding of the role of rhythm. *J. Exp. Psychol. Hum. Percept Perform.* 24:756–766.

NESPOR, M., M. T. GUASTI, and A. CHRISTOPHE, 1996. Selecting word order: The rhythmic activation principle. In *Interfaces in Phonology*, U. Kleinhenz, ed. Berlin: Akademie Verlag, pp. 1–26.

NESPOR, M., and I. VOGEL, 1986. *Prosodic Phonology.* Dordrecht, The Netherlands: Foris.

NEVILLE, H. J., D. BAVELIER, D. CORINA, J. RAUSCHECKER, A. KARNI, A. LALWANI, A. BRAUN, V. CLARK, P. JEZZARD, and R.

Turner, 1998. Cerebral organization for language in deaf and hearing subjects: Biological constraints and effects of experience. *Proc. Natl. Acad. Sci.* 95:922–929.

Newman, A. J., D. Bavelier, D. Corina, P. Jezzard, and H. J. Neville, 2002. A critical period for right hemisphere recruitment in American Sign Language processing. *Nat. Neurosci.* 5:76–80.

Otake, T., G. Hatano, A. Cutler, and J. Mehler, 1993. Mora or syllable? Speech segmentation in Japanese. *J. Mem. Lang.* 32:258–278.

Pallier, C., S. Dehaene, J.-B. Poline, D. Lebihan, A.-M. Argenti, E. Dupoux, and J. Mehler, 2003. Brain imaging of language plasticity in adopted adults: Can a second language replace the first? *Cereb. Cortex* 13:155–161.

Paulesu, E., and J. Mehler, 1998. Right on in sign language. *Nature* 392:233–234.

Peña, M., L. Bonatti, M. Nespor, and J. Mehler, 2002. Signal-driven computations in speech processing. *Science* 298:604–607.

Peña, M., A. Maki, D. Kovacic, G. Dehaene-Lambertz, H. Koizumi, F. Bouquet, and J. Mehler (in press). Sounds and silence: An optical topography study of language recognition at birth. *Proc. Natl. Acad. Sci. U.S.A.*

Perani, D., S. F. Cappa, V. Bettinardi, S. Bressi, M. Gorno-Tempini, M. Matarrese, and F. Fazio, 1995. Different neural systems for the recognition of animals and man-made tools. *Neuroreport* 6:1637–1641.

Perani, D., E. Paulesu, N. Sebastián-Gallés, E. Dupoux, S. Dehaene, V. Bettinardi, S. Cappa, F. Fazio, and J. Mehler, 1998. The bilingual brain: Proficiency and age of acquisition of the second language. *Brain* 121:1841–1852.

Pike, K. L., 1945. *The Intonation of American English.* Ann Arbor: University of Michigan Press.

Pinker, S., 1994. *The Language Instinct.* London: Penguin Books.

Ramus, F., M. Nespor, and J. Mehler, 1999. Correlates of the linguistic rhythm in the speech signal. *Cognition* 73:265–292.

Redlinger, W., and T. Z. Park, 1980. Language mixing in young bilingual children. *J. Child Lang.* 7:337–352.

Saffran, J. R., R. N. Aslin, and E. L. Newport, 1996. Statistical Learning by 8-month-old Infants. *Science* 274:1926–1928.

Sebastián-Gallés, N., and L. Bosch, 2002. The building of phonotactic knowledge in bilinguals: The role of early exposure. *J. Exp. Psychol. Hum. Percept. Perform.* 28:974–989.

Sebastián-Gallés, N., E. Dupoux, J. Segui, and J. Mehler, 1992. Contrasting syllabic effects in Catalan and Spanish. *J. Mem. Lang.* 31:18–32.

Segalowitz, S. J., and J. S. Chapman, 1980. Cerebral asymmetry for speech in neonates: A behavioral measure. *Brain Lang.* 9:281–288.

Tomasello, M., 2000. Do young children have adult syntactic competence? *Cognition* 74:209–253.

Vargha-Khadem, F., L. J. Carr, E. Isaacs, E. Brett, C. Adams, and M. Mishkin, 1997. Onset of speech after left hemispherectomy in a nine-year-old boy. *Brain* 120:159–182.

Ventureyra, V. A. G., C. Pallier, and H.-Y. Yoo (in press). The loss of the first language phonetic perception in adopted Koreans. *J. Neurolinguist.*

Vihman, M. M., 1985. Language differentiation by the bilingual infant. *J. Child Lang.* 12:297–324.

Volterra, V., and T. Taeschner, 1978. The acquisition and development of language by bilingual children. *J. Child Lang.* 5:311–326.

Werker, J. F., and C. E. Lalonde, 1988. Cross-language speech perception: Initial capabilities and developmental change. *Dev. Psychol.* 24:672–683.

60 The Evolution of Language

W. TECUMSEH FITCH

ABSTRACT   Progress in understanding the evolution of language requires a highly interdisciplinary integration of a vast amount of data from many fields. I present a framework for integrating such data from a comparative biological perspective, based on Tinbergen's four "why questions": mechanism, ontogeny, phylogeny, and function. I discuss three human capacities widely agreed to be necessary for language, but not present in chimpanzees: vocal imitation (speech), semantic reference, and recursive syntax. Although the combination of these abilities appears to be unique to humans, comparative data provide insights into each of them considered separately. Converging data from neuroscience, molecular genetics, linguistics, evolutionary theory and ethology are placing ever-tighter constraints on phylogenetic and functional hypotheses about language evolution. I argue that integration of these data is both possible and necessary and that a deeper understanding of language evolution is within our grasp.

Any attempt to take language evolution seriously entails an integration of neo-Darwinian evolutionary theory, speech science, and modern theoretical linguistics. In this review, I present an integrative empirical framework that emphasizes nascent areas of agreement without neglecting unresolved controversies. I will adopt the pluralistic approach to biological questions developed by Tinbergen (1963) in ethology and widely accepted by contemporary evolutionary biologists. Tinbergen pointed out that there are several equally valid, complementary approaches to answering biological questions, which can be placed into four categories: mechanistic, ontogenetic, phylogenetic, and functional. *Mechanistic* questions address the physiological or neural mechanisms that underlie individual behavior, and *ontogenetic* questions concern the developmental processes by which these individual mechanisms are constructed. *Functional* questions address the selective value of the mechanisms: Why did (or do) ancestral organisms possessing certain mechanisms outreproduce conspecifics lacking them? *Phylogenetic* questions concern the evolutionary history of a mechanism or species. The answers to each of these four questions influence and constrain the others, and a full understanding of any biological trait demands rich and mutually consistent answers to all of them. This is as true of biolinguistics (the biological study of language and its evolution (Lenneberg, 1967; Lieberman, 1984; Jenkins, 1999)) as of any other biological enterprise. Thus, although any individual researcher will

W. TECUMSEH FITCH   School of Psychology, University of St. Andrews, St. Andrews, Fife, Scotland.

typically focus on one or two questions, the field as a whole must encourage, and attempt to integrate, research on all of them.

Biolinguistics: A comparative evolutionary approach

The comparative method—the use of comparisons among species to derive inferences about phylogenesis and function—is a pillar of evolutionary biology. Evolution occurs slowly, with the demoralizing consequence that laboratory experiments on evolution are at best tediously slow and more typically impossible. Fortunately, Darwin recognized that each living species represents an "experiment of nature," and by judiciously comparing extant species we often find that answers to important questions were provided long ago by evolution. The incorporation of comparative data by molecular biologists has led to stunning insights into the nature of genetic systems and the evolution of life (Carroll, Grenier, and Weatherbee, 2001), and comparative neuroscience has vastly enriched our understanding of neural mechanisms and their evolution (Allman, 1999). Although application of the comparative method to biolinguistics is just beginning, early results look promising (Hauser, Chomsky, and Fitch, 2002), and I will adopt this comparative approach here whenever possible.

A major conceptual hurdle in adopting the comparative approach to biolinguistics is the lack of language in extant nonhuman species: language is so different from the communication systems known in other animals that the very comparison may seem forced. Thus, we need to construct a model of language evolution that explains the undeniable differences between language and other communication systems in a manner that neither neglects the similarities nor trivializes the differences. Ultimately, a mature biolinguistics should be able to single out a set of crucial genetic changes, explain their effects in terms of brain development and neural function, relate these physiological mechanisms to the cognitive and computational principles of language, and understand why these particular changes were adaptive during our species's evolution. Although the answers to such questions seemed hopelessly distant a few decades ago, tantalizing findings in molecular genetics and the rapid progress that has been made in neurolinguistics and neural development offer grounds for cautious optimism, and substantial progress can be expected in the coming decades.

Defining the target: The faculty of language

Following Saussure (1916) and many others, I will refer to the system that underlies the human language capacity as the *faculty of language*, or FL. Thanks to FL, any normal human child given adequate exposure to a heterogeneous set of linguistic utterances will develop a linguistic ability that not only encompasses these past utterances but also provides a limitless capacity to generate and understand novel utterances in the same style, providing a remarkable capacity to share novel concepts between individual brains. The fact that each of us went through this acquisition process, with little fanfare or conscious effort, should not blind us to its complex nature. The language faculty is responsible for the enormous cognitive and cultural power of our species, for good or ill. An infant chimpanzee raised under the same circumstances and exposed to the same corpus of utterances will not develop this capacity. This logically entails the recognition of a species-specific biological component of human language, which I will denote "FL in the narrow sense" (FLN), making no assumptions about its particular nature. It should be noted that the existence of an FLN distinguishing humans from chimpanzees is a truism and by no means licenses disregarding the data on what a chimpanzee *does* acquire in this situation. Indeed, such data provide one of the richest sources of comparative evidence about what is and is not uniquely human (Savage-Rumbaugh et al., 1993). Such comparative data paint an increasingly rich picture of what humans share with other apes, other mammals, and other vertebrates, and of the important role the shared components play in human language abilities. Thus FL, in the broad and inclusive sense (FLB), includes a wide variety of subsystems that play a crucial role in language but are shared with other animals, and a small subset of systems, capacities, or propensities that are unique to our species (FLN). A core desideratum of biolinguistics is to identify the nature and status of all of these subsystems (Hauser, Chomsky, and Fitch, 2002).

The shared components of FLB include, uncontroversially, most aspects of the biological and neural functioning of the human organism: FLB rests on a broad, shared foundation of basic capabilities that we inherited from our prelinguistic ancestors. These components of FLB can be studied in other species to gain insight into their functions in humans. Comparative studies also provide the only grounds, logically speaking, for claims that some system or capacity is uniquely human.

Current data justify provisionally singling out at least three potential candidates for uniquely human components of FLN: imitation, semantic reference, and recursion. None of these capacities is definitional of FLN. They are simply hypotheses, open to debate and empirical test, about what might constitute the uniquely human component of the language capacity. For example, Alvin Liberman and his colleagues suggested that categorical perception of speech sounds was a component of FLN, but this hypothesis was rejected when categorical perception was discovered in chinchillas and monkeys (Morse and Snowdon, 1975; Kuhl and Miller, 1978). However, other aspects of speech perception and production might still be uniquely human but have not yet been studied in nonhuman animals. A topic of intense current interest concerns various aspects of social intelligence that comprise "theory of mind," and it seems possible that some of these are uniquely human components of FLN. Thus, the provisional list below is probably incomplete. It is intended simply as a starting point for discussion and empirical investigation.

IMITATION   Imitation is a fundamental human characteristic that underlies all aspects of human culture, including ritual, dance, visual art, games, music, and technological development. There is a large literature on imitation that makes many important distinctions among different types (e.g., mimicry vs. role-reversal imitation; Tomasello, 1999). Here I use the term in its simplest form: imitation is the ability to reproduce a novel signal or gesture produced by another individual. Vocal imitation in particular is a critical component of spoken language, without which a flexible but shared vocabulary could never develop. Although extremely sophisticated forms of imitation may be uniquely human, imitation in general is not. Indeed, a wide variety of species possess imitative abilities in the vocal domain, including birds, seals, and cetaceans (dolphins and whales). However, a clear and surprising conclusion of modern ethological studies is that our nearest relatives, the nonhuman primates, have very poor imitative capacities in any domain, and virtually no ability for vocal imitation. Apes do not "ape," and "monkey see, monkey do" is a highly misleading myth. Thus, imitation provides a nice example of the value of the comparative approach: we can both identify a phylogenetic lacuna between humans and apes that was spanned during our recent evolution, and we can study more distant relatives, such as birds and dolphins, to gain insights into the ontogeny, phylogeny, function, and mechanisms underlying vocal imitation (Fitch, 2000).

SEMANTIC REFERENCE   Semantic reference, which gives language meaning, is roughly the process by which streams of sound (or gestures, in signed language) are systematically associated with conceptual structures in a consistent, intentional, and socially shared manner (see Jackendoff, 2002, for further discussion). "*Intentional*" is used here in a technical sense (Dennett, 1983); in this context it simply means "designed for use in meaningful exchanges" and does not necessarily connote any conscious awareness or "intent." Bee dances are intentional (designed by evolution for communicating flower locations) but most likely are unconscious on the signaling bee's part. Reference and meaning are sine qua non for language, and distinguish music (another universal human behavior) from language. Reference presupposes several subcapabilities, including some very basic ones, such as the ability to associate sounds and events, that are broadly shared with other vertebrates. An interpretive component, an ability to interpret conspecific vocalizations, gestures, or body postures as indicating certain cognitive or emotional states in the signaler, is another widely shared subcapability underlying many animal communication systems. In some cases, as in alarm calling, the state indicated may be associated with an external event, such as the appearance of predators of various types (Cheney and Seyfarth, 1990), and such systems are often termed "functionally" referential to distinguish them from true reference. At least in birds and mammals, studies of "audience effects" further indicate the capability on the part of signalers to modify or inhibit their behavior, depending on the presence or type of conspecific (Evans and Marler, 1994). Finally, the honeybee dance language, while limited to locational information, seems to represent a simple form of reference (including displacement of the referent and interchangeability between signaler and receiver; see Hockett, 1960). Such similarities to reference in language have led some authors to posit, or even implicitly assume, that reference is a widely shared capacity, long predating language. This conclusion is unjustified, for two reasons.

First, in the animal communication systems just mentioned, the signalers emit vocalizations from a limited, species-specific, and genetically canalized repertoire, and thus the number of messages expressible is strictly, genetically, limited. This is not true of linguistic utterances, which occur in limitless variety. Second, linguistic reference entails a symmetry between signaler and receiver, such that both parties attribute nearly the same meaning to the same utterance. This does not appear to be the case in primate communication: although a vervet's cry of fear versus surprise may enable a listener to infer the presence of a leopard versus a snake, current data do not support the further supposition that the caller is intentionally (either consciously or unconsciously) referring to snakes or leopards (Seyfarth and Cheney, 2003). But it is precisely this design for communicating specific referents, pragmatically taking the listener's knowledge into account, and the propensity to interpret utterances as intentional in this way that give language its limitless extent and great power (Tomasello, 1999). Thus, despite the great value of comparative data on "functionally referential" animal communication systems, rich referentiality appears, on current knowledge, to be a unique capability of human language. Note that this is not true by definitional fiat, or tautologically. If we discovered tomorrow that the learned and indefinitely extensible songs of mock-

ingbirds are consistently associated with conceptual states and are used intentionally to inform other mockingbirds of these states, we would conclude, by the definition above, that mockingbirds have reference.

RECURSION Recursion is the capability that lends to language its limitless extensibility, especially in the realm of syntax and semantics. In computer science, recursive functions are those that "call themselves," taking their own past outputs as future inputs. Recursive functions are differentiated from the much broader category of iterative or "feedback" functions, whose past output simply influences their future behavior. Iterative functions are ubiquitous in both biology (e.g., in motor control) and engineering (e.g., thermostats or antilock brakes), whereas the computational apparatus underlying recursion seems to be considerably rarer in nature. Recursion allows relatively simple embedding operations to build indefinitely complex structures. In linguistic recursion the types of data that serve as input and output are complex and structured (usually depicted as treelike phrase structures), and the entire structure can be operated on repeatedly without being flattened out, blended, or averaged, or otherwise lost, as in the following:

Mary is rather witty.
John thinks (Mary is rather witty).
Susan said (John thinks (Mary is rather witty)).
I'm shocked that (Susan said (John thinks (Mary is rather witty)).

Such embedding of phrases within phrases is the hallmark of linguistic recursion.

Second, despite the continuously variable nature of the output medium (whether sound or gesture), linguistic structures such as words or sentences are discrete. Combined with the capacity of all recursive functions to generate an infinity of output, this discretization of the sensory signal provides the "discrete infinity" capacity that is central to linguistic recursion. This allows us to generate a limitless variety of utterances that vary in arbitrary but perceptible ways from one another. This capacity is central to the limitless expressivity characteristic of human language, as in other unlimited systems, such as chemistry or genetics (Studdert-Kennedy, 1998). Although some ability to iteratively construct hierarchical structures appears (like imitation) to be shared with birds and whales, although without any known semantic content, there is no evidence for such abilities in nonhuman primates.

Summarizing, I argue that at least three key characteristics of language, imitation, reference, and recursion, combine in our species to create the FLN. Although each component invites further study of similar capacities in other animals, the combination appears to be unique to our species. With three important mechanisms underlying FLN now identified, I will analyze language evolution from the fourfold Tinbergian perspective, starting with function.

Function

What selective advantages did our hominid ancestors obtain from the precursor mechanisms ancestral to those underlying the modern FL? Because this question is unabashedly adaptationist, and because some thinkers on language evolution have questioned the concept that language is an adaptation, it is important first to clarify this question. A founding insight of modern evolutionary theory is that adaptation is "an onerous concept" (Williams, 1966), to be invoked carefully and interrogated rigorously in each particular case. A wide variety of constraints prevent organisms from being perfectly adapted (the perfect organism would live forever and produce infinite offspring), and any organism possesses nonadaptive features. Of course, the fastest empirical way to discover subtle nonadaptive features is to provisionally assume adaptiveness, construct plausible adaptive hypotheses, and then reject them one by one. This methodological imperative to assign adaptation to the role of null hypothesis may account for the persistence of Panglossian caricatures of adaptationists but in no way indicates a neo-Darwinian conviction that all features are adaptations. Chomsky's view on the subject, that language as a whole is adaptive, was made clear in 1975: "There is an obvious selective advantage in the ability to discover the language of one's speech community" (Chomsky, 1975, p. 252). Misunderstanding appears to derive mainly from Chomsky's use of the term *language* in a technical sense to refer to certain core aspects of syntax (e.g., recursion/discrete infinity). That language as a whole is adaptive is hardly questioned by scholars today (Pinker and Bloom, 1990; Hauser, Chomsky, and Fitch, 2002; Jackendoff, 2002). Of course, both the particular aspects of FL that are, or are not, adaptations, and the nature of the specific functional benefits they confer, are open empirical questions.

The selective context(s) in which language, and particularly semantic reference, derived its advantage is a topic that has received inadequate attention. There is a widespread assumption that sexual selection and increased mating success played a critical role in the conferring of a selective advantage on individual language users. For example, ("females would surely have preferred mates whose communicative capacities so strikingly outclassed those of other available partners"—Bickerton, 1998, p. 353) and "that tribal chiefs are often both gifted orators and highly polygynous is a splendid prod to any imagination that cannot conceive of how linguistic skills could make a Darwinian difference" (Pinker and Bloom, 1990, p. 725). Mating success has also been invoked in the opposite context: "Subjacency has many virtues, but I am sure that it could not have

increased the chances of having fruitful sex" (Lightfoot, 1991, p. 69). Despite its apparent appeal among academics, I know of no data supporting the notion that "better language leads to more sex," either in modern or in traditional societies. Nonetheless, the sexual selection hypothesis for language evolution appears to be the default assumption by many if not most scholars (Miller, 2001).

An alternative, the "mother tongues" hypothesis, is that the adaptive value of language lies primarily in enhancing communication among kin, particularly between parents and offspring (Fitch, in press). According to this argument, kin selection provides a viable evolutionary route to the capacity to honestly communicate arbitrary information. Young primates have a long childhood during which they are cared for by, and learn from, their mother and other related individuals, and any communicative efficiencies that enhance this learning process would offer a selective advantage in terms of offspring survival. This period of dependence is particularly long in humans and chimpanzees, and thus by inference in our prelinguistic ancestors, making offspring survival of paramount importance in human and ape reproductive success. Two facts support kin selection rather than sexual selection as the driving force behind language evolution. First and most obvious is the remarkable precocity of language development. Sexually selected traits typically develop at puberty, but a 1-year-old child is already far along in the process of language acquisition, and language is fully functional in humans many years prior to sexual maturity. Second is the lack of strong sexual dimorphism in language abilities: sexually selected traits are typically more highly developed in males, but language is sexually egalitarian. What small differences exist are in favor of females, who have larger vocabularies, earlier linguistic maturation, excel at tongue-twisters, and are less likely than males to suffer congenital language disturbances (Henton, 1992). Both factors are compatible with the mother tongues hypothesis, which would select for early linguistic competence and female bias and argue against sexual selection for semantic reference. This topic deserves further investigation.

A second functional issue concerns internal versus external uses of language. Is (or was) the primary functional advantage of early language capabilities for private thought within an individual or for interindividual communication? Clearly, both uses provide benefits in modern humans. The former hypothesis has been favored by some authors (e.g., Bierwisch, 2001), largely because it neatly solves a logical problem: with whom would an individual with some new advantageous mutation speak? However, this problem disappears if the primary beneficiaries of communicative acts are one's own offspring, who are likely to share the mutation. Two further considerations blunt the internalist hypothesis further. First, while the ability to manipulate semantic conceptual structures internally is clearly of substantial value, it is unclear why such manipulation should occur in terms of externalizable words and phrases. The medium of "silent speech" is not a pure language of thought but manifests itself in the phonological forms of our speech community, complete with rhyme, alliteration, and other semantically superfluous traits. The phonological component is entailed by communication, but seems without value from the internalist perspective. Second, the value of internal language use derives in large part from its association with externally derived knowledge. It is precisely the value of this shared cultural knowledge that makes our internal dialogue so meaningful and useful (Tomasello, 1999). True, an ability to internally and idiosyncratically name objects and events for personal reference might have some mnemonic value. But the value of this is dwarfed by the vastly increased power of linguistic thought enabled by communication between individuals, and the cultural accretion of knowledge that results. Thus, although the internalist hypothesis might provide a phylogenetic starting point for certain aspects of FL, such as recursion, it cannot explain FL as a whole, and particularly not the phonological component that renders language so well-suited to communication between individuals and to the cultural transmission of knowledge.

Ontogeny

The vast field of language acquisition contributes to linguistics in general and to biolinguistics in particular. The speed and robustness of language acquisition in childhood are among the chief reasons that many linguists adopt a nativist viewpoint. A child exposed to a hodgepodge of primary linguistic data, some of it incomplete or erroneous, will nonetheless reliably arrive at an abstract rule system that overlaps almost completely with that of other individuals in its community. The richness of the rule system, compared with the messiness and incompleteness of the input (the so-called "poverty of the stimulus"), has led many thinkers to conclude that at least some aspects of this rule system must be innate. This is a complex and extremely controversial topic that I will mostly avoid here (see Crain, 1991, and commentary for further discussion). However, from the biolinguistic perspective advocated here, two points are worth making. First, the questions of "learnability" that traditionally dominate discussions of this topic should not be considered in a vacuum but must be balanced against issues of implementability that take the nature of neural and genetic mechanisms into account, and against issues of evolvability that take the phylogenetic and functional history of our species into account. Second, irrespective of the possible existence of innate rules, there is a vast amount of linguistic structure that varies completely between languages and thus must be learned, namely, the contents of the lexicon. Despite the underspecified nature of the lexical input (a child typically has simply an utterance, unparsed into words, and some context, unparsed into meaning, to work with), children do indubitably acquire a vast lexicon, very close to that of their community, without the aid of any innate lexical items. Lexical acquisition is thus an ability to which innate constraints on learning, rather than innate knowledge, must apply.

Research in lexical acquisition has highlighted the remarkable speed and accuracy with which children acquire word meanings and has uncovered a number of basic principles that children appear to use to constrain their inferences about meaning, such as the *mutual exclusivity assumption* (that each object receives a single label) or the *whole object assumption* (that words label entire objects) (Markman, 1990). This raises the possibility of innate constraints on lexical inference, which would be potential candidates for inclusion in the FLN. However, recent data (Markson and Bloom, 1997) suggest that these same principles apply equally to the learning of nonlinguistic facts. Thus, lexical acquisition may be a case in which innate cognitive constraints on social cognition and learning, independent of language and presumably with a longer evolutionary history, play a crucial role in language acquisition. If true, this is good news for biolinguists, for two reasons. First, it means we can use comparative data from nonhuman cognition to help understand this critical component of the language faculty, and second, it lightens the load that evolutionary explanations must bear by extending the origin of innate constraints much farther back into primate evolutionary history. The existence and importance of innate constraints on animal learning have been appreciated for many years (Garcia and Koelling, 1966), and to the extent that such shared constraints aid language acquisition, we have one less thing to explain in the recent evolution of our species. Lexical acquisition thus provides a nice example of how results of studies on ontogenetic, mechanistic, and evolutionary mechanisms can be both mutually informative and mutually constraining.

Phylogeny

Human ancestors diverged from chimpanzees 5–6 million years ago, a short time in evolutionary history (for instance, vertebrates diverged from other animals more than 500 million years ago, and mammals from birds more than 200 million years ago). During that time a suite of changes occurred, some of which left a fossil record. Fossils provide clear evidence of at least three "grades" of human evolution, namely, australopithecines, *Homo erectus*, and *Homo sapiens*. These phases are distinguished by their brain and body size, tools, and geographic distribution. The earliest change was bipedalism, which long preceded the brain expansion and increasingly sophisticated tool use that typify later stages of human evolution. Unfortunately, language leaves no fossils, and even peripheral aspects such as vocal tract anatomy are inadequately preserved in fossils for any consensus to have emerged about their timing (Fitch, 2000). Based on inferences from archaeological data, many experts estimate that full language emerged relatively recently (e.g., in the last 100,000 years or later; Mellars, 1998), but we have very little hard evidence to date this or previous stages, and all we know for certain is that all of the various capacities underlying human language evolved sometime during the last 6 million years, since our divergence from chimpanzees. Thus, models of language phylogeny are relatively unconstrained by fossil data, and a consequent indulgence in phylogenetic storytelling has given this component of the biolinguistic enterprise a poor reputation. However, nonfossil comparative data, though often neglected, can also constrain phylogenetic hypotheses, and can provide opportunities for testing them.

To give an example, it has frequently been suggested that the descent of the human larynx (Lieberman, 1984) resulted directly from bipedalism, gravity inevitably lowering the larynx in an upright organism (Wind, 1983), and this idea is sometimes treated as a fact (e.g., Boë et al., 2002). If true, the descent of the larynx would have occurred early, in *Australopithecus*. But an examination of the comparative data serves to reject this hypothesis. All birds are bipedal, spending their lives upright, but no species has a descended larynx. Among mammals, kangaroos have a hopping bipedal locomotory system that exerts considerable gravitational force on their internal organs. Although kangaroos share with humans antigravity specializations that are not seen in nonbipedal mammals, such as a closed inguinal canal (Coveney et al., 2002), their larynx lies in the normal, undescended mammalian position. This is one case out of many where comparative data can reject superficially plausible phylogenetic hypotheses that have been repeated for decades.

Another source of constraints on phylogenetic hypotheses is logical. If one explicitly anatomizes language into subcomponents, as I've done here, the simple requirement that the acquisition of each subcomponent had to serve some purpose (not necessarily identical to its current usage) puts rather stringent restrictions on the construction of plausible phylogenetic hypotheses. Although partial phylogenetic hypotheses are simple to generate (e.g., assuming that reference and imitation are already in place, and then discussing only recursion), constructing a plausible and complete chain of events stretching from our common ancestor with chimps to the present FL, consistent with all the available evidence, is much more challenging. By way of example, I will sketch a framework for language phylogenesis consistent with the data reviewed thus far.

Many theorists posit a distinct intermediate stage of language evolution in which the signaling medium, complexity, and selective advantage of the protolanguage differed from modern language. A popular dual-stage theory is the ges-

tural origins theory, dating back to at least Condillac (Hewes, 1973). Another detailed dual-stage model is that of Donald (1998), who posits a long intermediate "mimetic" stage of human culture in which humans had a rich imitative culture that included dance, social ritual, music, and tool making but lacked language. Putting some of these ideas together, I will offer a three-stage model that appears compatible with the currently available fossil and comparative data.

The first hypothetical stage, characterized by australopithecines, was prelinguistic. Upright posture led to increased tool use and exploitation of new resources (especially protein-rich carcasses), and led to larger brains, but communication remained chimplike. The second, or "protolinguistic" stage, associated with *Homo erectus*, was associated with prolonged selection for imitation, and corresponds to Donald's mimetic stage. Progressively greater imitative abilities enhanced social cohesion and cultural transmission, giving early *Homo* a huge advantage over other hominids. These were the first hominids to expand out of Africa, occupying most of the Old World. Although nonlinguistic, these mimetic hominids had a rich and extensible vocal repertoire (see also MacLarnon and Hewitt, 1999), based on imitation and surface-level recursion, comparable to that of mockingbirds or whales. However, these "songs" were only holistically or ritualistically related to meaning and were probably not referential or intentionally meaningful in a modern sense. Following Darwin's (1871) suggestion that early stages of language evolution were musical and used for courtship, a key role for such performances may have been mate choice, and thus driven by sexual selection. If so, these protolinguistic abilities would have been more highly developed in males. In the final, linguistic stage, in later *Homo*, the crucial transition to referential language was made, perhaps via an analytical "insight" that individual components of songlike utterances could be associated with individual components of concepts (e.g., objects vs. actions). In this last stage, kin communication played a crucial role, and the accurate communication of propositional information became the primary selective force driving further evolution to our current state (Fitch, in press). This hypothesis implies that we should seek "fossils" of protolanguage not in one-word utterances (Bickerton, 1998) but in complex music and song. Plausibly enough, music is a human universal, of uncertain selective value, precisely as we would expect of a holdover from an earlier evolutionary period. This music-as-protolanguage hypothesis highlights the value of comparing the formal structure and the neural basis of music and language (Lerdahl and Jackendoff, 1983; Zatorre, Belin, and Penhune, 2002).

Mechanism

The mechanisms underlying FL are a major focus of research in cognitive neuroscience. Earlier chapters in this section dealt with neural mechanisms underlying language, and the evolution of peripheral mechanisms involved in speech and phonology have been reviewed elsewhere in detail (MacNeilage, 1998; Fitch, 2000; Lieberman, 2000). An area of exciting recent progress is the isolation of a gene, FOXP2, that differs between humans and chimps and is linked to oromotor coordination. Increasing oromotor control in humans was a critical prerequisite for vocal imitation and thus speech, and these findings provide a new source of information on the nature and timing of the changes undergone in linguistic evolution. The importance of this gene was discovered in long-term studies (Vargha-Khadem et al., 1995) of a large family, KE, some members of which have inadequate oral motor control (incorrect early claims that their deficiency was exclusively linguistic [Gopnik, 1990] were based on incomplete data). By isolating first the chromosomal location and finally the gene underlying this problem, these researchers opened the door to a comparison of the gene in humans and great apes (Enard et al., 2002). This comparison revealed small but crucial differences in the gene (only two amino acids differ) for the FOXP2 protein, which regulates the expression of other genes. That small structural differences could have major phenotypic effects is exciting, because these are precisely the sorts of changes we must uncover to understand the substantial difference between humans and chimps in the context of nearly identical DNA. It is also intriguing that FOXP2 is a highly conserved protein that shows little functional variation among the other mammals examined. These very recent advances are a promising example of the power of a highly interdisciplinary biolinguistic approach, and we can await experiments in transgenic mice in which the precise effects of the human version of the gene on mammalian neural development and function can be examined.

An important open mechanistic topic is the medium of language output. Significant progress in the study of signed language (Klima and Bellugi, 1979; Bellugi, Poizner, and Klima, 1990) leaves little doubt that the visual/gestural mode for linguistic expression is perfectly capable of supporting the full richness of human linguistic communication. Further studies of Tadoma (a tactile method of linguistic interchange developed for deaf and blind children) suggest the same is true of tactile communication (Vivian, 1966). That alternative linguistic expressive modes are available and fully adequate reveals a fundamental fact about FL and its neural instantiation: human linguistic abilities transcend any particular sensorimotor channel. However, it is equally relevant that the audiovocal channel is adopted in all human societies with the requisite capacities (disregarding the recent cultural innovation of reading), making it possible that there has been specific selection on the human auditory system for increased speech efficiency, as posited by many speech

scientists (Lieberman, 1984; Liberman, 1996). An oft-stated advantage of speech is that it leaves the hands free, but signers communicate remarkably well while working with their hands, and in any case have a complementary advantage over speech during eating or drinking. Similarly, communication in total darkness and silently is possible with Tadoma. Such factors thus seem incomplete as explanations for the dominance of speech as the medium of modern language, suggesting that additional neural or cognitive factors are at work.

The communicative adequacy of sign has led many researchers, dating back to Condillac, to posit a gestural origin of language (Hewes, 1973): that in an earlier stage of evolution, humans communicated primarily via signed gestures and vocalization was ancillary. Gestural origin hypotheses derive some of their apparent, persistent appeal from the communicative adequacy of sign language and the putative similarity between chimp gestures and sign (though see Tomasello, 1999). Recently, the discovery of mirror neurons has reinvigorated interest in gestural origins (Rizzolatti and Arbib, 1998; Corballis, 2002) and in the origins of imitation. However, the well-documented ineptitude of monkeys for manual imitation blocks any facile equation of mirror neurons and imitation skills, though mirror neurons perhaps were a "preadaptation" for imitation and thus language. In any case, mirror neurons would support gestural origin hypotheses only if corresponding audiovocal mirror neurons, which respond similarly to a primate's own call and that of another primate, were absent (and this seems unlikely, Kohler et al., 2002). Finally, gestural origin theories do not explain the genesis of the speech mode or its ascent to total dominance among modern humans. Backward extrapolation from modern signing capabilities to a primitive protolanguage thus seems both overly literal and unnecessary, given current data.

Conclusion: Taking language evolution seriously

One of the central insights of modern linguistics is the startling complexity of natural language. The fact that thousands of hard-working and highly intelligent linguists and engineers have yet to implement a full grammar of any language, despite many decades of concerted effort, gives some insight into the magnitude of the problem, which is masked by the effortlessness with which children acquire language. A central question for biolinguistics, then, is where this complexity comes from. Early approaches suggested that much of it was innately specified, in terms of a large set of language-specific rules called Universal Grammar (Chomsky, 1965), as argued by many scholars (Pinker and Bloom, 1990; Pinker, 1994; Jackendoff, 2002). However, there is increasing interest within linguistics in an alternative conception, broadly labeled the Minimalist Program

(Chomsky, 1994). By this hypothesis, the syntactic component of language is simple but powerful, composed of two operators, Move and Merge, and the vast complexity and variability of natural languages are derived from the phonological output component and (in particular) the semantic or conceptual component. This conception is appealing from the biolinguistic perspective, for several reasons. It lightens the load for evolutionary explanations: that a complex, interconnected suite of genetically specified rules specific to language could evolve to fixation in all human populations, in the short time since our divergence with chimps, is far less likely than the evolution of a few specific but powerful new capabilities. Most of the complexity underlying Universal Grammar would then derive from cognitive constraints or innate conceptual primitives that we share with other animals. Processing constraints associated with the phonological interface, and computational constraints associated with bridging the phonological and semantic components, would drive additional complexities. All of these factors can be studied via the comparative method, employing the full suite of modern neuroscientific techniques along with computer models and traditional cognitive experimentation. There is also a methodological advantage to assuming FLN is simple but FLB complex and shared with other animals. Empirical evaluation of the traditional assumption of a complex, language-specific Universal Grammar awaits a future synthesis of genetics, neural development, neuroscience, and linguistics that seems dauntingly distant. In contrast, the minimalist perspective generates hypotheses that can be empirically tested today, and such hypotheses thus provide an effective empirical strategy for discovering what is, and what is not, part of FLN.

ACKNOWLEDGEMENTS   I thank Alfonso Caramazza, John Hyman, and David Raubenheimer for comments on the manuscript.

REFERENCES

ALLMAN, J. M., 1999. *Evolving Brains*. New York: Scientific American Library.

BELLUGI, U., H. POIZNER, and E. S. KLIMA, 1990. Mapping brain funcion for language: Evidence for sign language. In *Signal and Sense*, G. M. Edelman, W. E. Gall, and W. M. Cowan, eds. New York: Wiley, pp. 521–543.

BICKERTON, D., 1998. Catastrophic evolution: The case for a single step from protolanguage to full human language. In *Approaches to the Evolution of Language*, J. R. Hurford, M. Studdert-Kennedy, and C. Knight, eds. New York: Cambridge University Press, pp. 341–358.

BIERWISCH, M., 2001. The apparent paradox of language evolution: Can Universal Grammar be explained by adaptive selection? In *New Essays on the Origin of Language*, J. Traban and S. Ward, eds. Berlin: Mouton de Gruyter, pp. 55–81.

BOË, L.-J., J.-L. HEIM, K. HONDA, and S. Maeda, 2002. The potential Neandertal vowel space was as large as that of modern humans. *J. Phonet.* 30:465–484.

CARROLL, S. B., J. K. GRENIER, and S. D. WEATHERBEE, 2001. *From DNA to Diversity: Molecular Genetics and the Evolution of Animal Design*. Malden, Mass.: Blackwell Science.

CHENEY, D. L., and R. M. SEYFARTH, 1990. *How Monkeys See the World: Inside the Mind of Another Species*. Chicago: University of Chicago Press.

CHOMSKY, N., 1965. *Aspects of the Theory of Syntax*. Cambridge, Mass.: MIT Press.

CHOMSKY, N., 1975. *Reflections on Language*. New York: Pantheon.

CHOMSKY, N., 1994. *The Minimalist Program*. Cambridge, Mass.: MIT Press.

CORBALLIS, M. C., 2002. *From Hand to Mouth: The Origins of Language*. Princeton, N.J.: Princeton University Press.

COVENEY, D., G. SHAW, J. M. HUTSON, and M. B. RENFREE, 2002. The development of the gubernaculum and inguinal closure in the marsupial *Macropus eugenii*. *J. Anat. (Lond.)* 201:239–256.

CRAIN, S., 1991. Language acquisition in the absence of experience. *Behav. Brain Sci.* 14:597–650.

DARWIN, C., 1871. *The Descent of Man and Selection in Relation to Sex*. London: John Murray.

Dennett, D. C., 1983. Intentional systems in cognitive ethology: The "Panglossian paradigm" defended. *Behav. Brain Sci.* 6: 343–390.

DONALD, M., 1998. Mimesis and the Executive Suite: Missing links in language evolution. In *Approaches to the Evolution of Language*, J. R. Hurford, M. Studdert-Kennedy, and C. Knight, eds. New York: Cambridge University Press, pp. 44–67.

ENARD, W., M. PRZEWORSKI, S. E. FISHER, C. S. L. LAI, V. WIEBE, T. KITANO, A. P. MONACO, and S. PAÄBO, 2002. Molecular evolution of FOXP2, a gene involved in speech and language. *Nature* 418:869–872.

EVANS, C. S., and P. MARLER, 1994. Food-calling and audience effects in male chickens, *Gallus gallus*: Their relationships to food availability, courtship and social facilitation. *Anim. Behav.* 47:1159–1170.

FITCH, W. T., 2000. The evolution of speech: A comparative review. *Trends Cogn. Sci.* 4:258–267.

FITCH, W. T., 2004. Kin selection and "mother tongue": A neglected component in language evolution. In *The Evolution of Communication Systems: A Comparative Approach*, D. K. Oller and U. Griebel, eds. Cambridge, Mass.: MIT Press.

GARCIA, J., and R. A. KOELLING, 1966. Relation of cue to consequences in avoidance learning. *Psychonom. Sci.* 4:123–124.

GOPNIK, M., 1990. Feature-blind grammar and dysphasia. *Nature* 344:715.

HAUSER, M., N. CHOMSKY, and W. T. FITCH, 2002. The language faculty: What is it, who has it, and how did it evolve? *Science* 298:1569–1579.

HENTON, C., 1992. The abnormality of male speech. In *New Departures in Linguistics*, G. Wolf, ed. New York: Garland Publishing.

HEWES, G. W., 1973. Primate communication and the gestural origin of language. *Curr. Anthropol.* 14:5–24.

HOCKETT, C. F., 1960. Logical considerations in the study of animal communication. In *Animal Sounds and Communication*, W. E. Lanyon and W. N. Tavolga, eds. Washington, D.C.: American Institute of Biological Sciences.

JACKENDOFF, R., 2002. *Foundations of Language*. New York: Oxford University Press.

JENKINS, L. 1999. *Biolinguistics: Exploring the Biology of Language*. New York: Cambridge University Press.

KLIMA, E. S., and U. Bellugi, 1979. *The Signs of Language*. Cambridge, Mass.: Harvard University Press.

KOHLER, E., C. KEYSERS, M. A. UMILTÀ, L. FOGASSI, V. GALLESE, and G. RIZZOLATTI, 2002. Hearing sounds, understanding actions: Action representation in mirror neurons. *Science* 297:846–849.

KUHL, P., and J. D. MILLER, 1978. Speech perception by the chinchilla: Identification functions for synthetic VOT stimuli. *J. Acoust. Soc. Am.* 63:905–917.

LENNEBERG, E. H., 1967. *Biological Foundations of Language.* New York: Wiley.

LERDAHL, F., and R. JACKENDOFF, 1983. *A Generative Theory of Tonal Music.* Cambridge, Mass.: MIT Press.

LIBERMAN, A. M., 1996. *Speech: A Special Code.* Cambridge, Mass.: MIT Press.

LIEBERMAN, P., 1984. *The Biology and Evolution of Language.* Cambridge, Mass.: Harvard University Press.

LIEBERMAN, P., 2000. *Human Language and Our Reptilian Brain: The Subcortical Bases of Speech, Syntax and Thought.* Cambridge, Mass.: Harvard University Press.

LIGHTFOOT, D., 1991. Subjacency and sex. *Lang. Commun.* 11:67–69.

MacLARNON, A., and G. HEWITT, 1999. The evolution of human speech: The role of enhanced breathing control. *Am. J. Phys. Anthropol.* 109:341–363.

MacNEILAGE, P. F., 1998. The frame/content theory of evolution of speech production. *Behav. Brain Sci.* 21:499–546.

MARKMAN, E. M., 1990. Constraints children place on word meanings. *Cogn. Sci.* 14:57–77.

MARKSON, L., and P. BLOOM, 1997. Evidence against a dedicated system for word learning in children. *Nature* 385:813–815.

MELLARS, P., 1998. Neanderthals, modern humans and the archaeological evidence for language. In *The Origin and Diversification of Language,* N. G. Jablonski and L. C. Aiello, eds. San Francisco: Academy of Sciences.

MILLER, G. F., 2001. *The Mating Mind: How Sexual Choice Shaped the Evolution of Human Nature.* New York: Doubleday.

MORSE, P. A., and C. T. SNOWDON, 1975. An investigation of categorical speech discrimination by rhesus monkeys. *Percept. Psychophys.* 19:137–143.

PINKER, S., 1994. *The Language Instinct.* New York: William Morrow.

PINKER, S., and P. BLOOM, 1990. Natural language and natural selection. *Behav. Brain Sci.* 13:707–784.

RIZZOLATTI, G., and M. A. ARBIB, 1998. Language within our grasp. *Trends Neurosc.* 21:188–194.

SAUSSURE, F. D., 1916. *Course in General Linguistics.* New York: McGraw-Hill.

SAVAGE-RUMBAUGH, E. S., J. MURPHY, R. A. SEVCIK, K. E. BRAKKE, S. L. WILLIAMS, and D. M. RUMBAUGH, 1993. Language comprehension in ape and child. *Monogr. Soc. Res. Child Devel.* 58:1–221.

SEYFARTH, R. M., and D. L. CHENEY, 2003. Signalers and receivers in animal communication. *Ann. Rev. Psychol.* 54:145–173.

STUDDERT-KENNEDY, M., 1998. The particulate origins of language generativity: From syllable to gesture. In *Approaches to the Evolution of Language,* J. R. Hurford, M. Studdert-Kennedy, and C. Knight, eds. New York: Cambridge University Press, pp. 202–221.

TINBERGEN, N., 1963. On aims and methods of ethology. *Z. Tierpsychol.* 20:410–433.

TOMASELLO, M., 1999. *The Cultural Origins of Human Cognition.* Cambridge, Mass.: Harvard University Press.

VARGHA-KHADEM, F., K. WATKINS, K. ALCOCK, P. FLETCHER, and R. PASSINGHAM, 1995. Praxic and nonverbal cognitive deficits in a large family with a genetically-transmitted speech and language disorder. *Proc. Nat. Acad. Sci. U.S.A.* 92:930–933.

VIVIAN, R., 1966. The Tadoma method: A tactual approach to speech and speech reading. *Volta Rev.* 68:733–737.

WILLIAMS, G. C., 1966. *Adaptation and Natural Selection.* Princeton, N.J.: Princeton University Press.

WIND, J., 1983. Primate evolution and the emergence of speech. In *Glossogenetics: The Origin and Evolution of Language,* É. Grolier, ed. New York: Harwood Academic Publishers, pp. 15–35.

ZATORRE, R. J., P. BELIN, and V. B. PENHUNE, 2002. Structure and function of auditory cortex: Music and speech. *Trends Cogn. Sci.* 6:37–46.

VIII HIGHER COGNITIVE FUNCTIONS

Introduction

NIKOS K. LOGOTHETIS

DEPENDING ON WHO is speaking, the systematic investigation of the process of how we think is either the ultimate scientific inquiry or the biggest waste of time ever. The contributors to this section all subscribe to the first view, and examine those cognitive abilities that are often characterized as higher brain functions. Higher cognitive processes, also referred to occasionally as symbolic processes, typically include memory, attention, imagery, ideation, concept formation, generalization, abstraction, problem solving, thinking, reasoning, and planning. Their common characteristic is that they are usually inner activities of the organism as opposed a mere representation of immediate reactions to stimulation. Some of these processes elude direct observation by traditional behavioral testing. Evidence for their existence must be derived from verbal or other behaviors, since they are often descriptive of situations that have ceased to be.

With the establishment of noninvasive functional imaging methods such as positron emission tomography and functional magnetic resonance imaging, the behavioral study of higher cognitive functions is consistently combined with observations of the brain activations elicited by the subjects as they think or act, thereby offering a unique opportunity to investigate the organization of the neural systems underlying higher cognitive processing. Moreover, extensive research into animal cognition showed long ago that capacities such as concept formation, intelligence, and the building of knowledge have common foundations in humans and nonhuman primates, whose neural activity can be directly assessed with intracortical recordings.

This section is slightly biased toward higher cognitive capacities that can be studied in both humans and nonhuman primates. Hauser and Spelke focus on the foundations of human knowledge. They discuss evidence indicating that complex, culture-specific human behavior draws on a set of psychological and neural mechanisms that most likely evolved before humanity and as such are shared with other animals. They point out that such core knowledge systems and their behavioral expression emerge early in human development, are common to infants, children, and adults, and ultimately form the building blocks for the skills comprising human intelligence. Hauser and Spelke use on comparative evolutionary studies and studies of human development to demonstrate this fundamental principle in the evolution of the system for representing numbers of objects or events, and large approximate numerical magnitudes. Piazza and Dehaene take this theme further in a neuropsychological and physiological direction by reviewing relevant findings on the cognitive and system neuroscience of number sense. They show how functional imaging and neuropsychology clarify the cerebral substrates of numerical ability, and attempt to compare the human results with single-unit recordings that are considered by the authors to reveal the neural basis of numerical representation in monkeys.

The following three chapters shift the focus to the representation of objects. In his chapter, Tanaka discusses the processes of object categorization in humans and monkeys from the perspective of the cognitive and brain sciences. Emphasis is placed on the role that experience plays in the way objects are categorized and recognized in the world, and on the effects of categorization on the perceptual representation of object features. The next chapter examines the nature and spatial distribution of cortical object representations. Is the encoding of a complex stimulus instantiated in the spatial distribution of neuronal activity within an association area? Do distributions across areas reflect the multiplicity of stimulus attributes, such as stimulus appearance, movement, or the way it is acted upon? Are these distributions invariant over time, or do different phases of activation reflect different cognitive capacities (e.g., automatic vs. attention- and memory-guided behaviors)? Using neuroimaging evidence, Haxby, Gobbini, and Montgomery raise and address such questions, summarizing a number of elegant studies performed in normal human subjects. Object representations would be of little value if the neural associative network of the brain did not encode the relationships among objects as well as between objects and symbols to form a semantic memory system. Fujimichi, Naya, and Miyashita provide convincing evidence of possible neural mechanisms for such an associative network. They discuss how a memory engram is organized and introduce the neural representation of semantically linked symbols by using the paired-associate paradigm applied in experiments with monkeys.

The chapter contributed by Pessoa and Ungerleider deals with top-down mechanisms. The activation of parietal and frontal areas observed during the delay interval of working memory tasks is a reliable predictor of trial-by-trial performance; moreover, the same frontoparietal areas are engaged in directed attention. The authors point out the similarity between mechanisms affecting performance in both working memory and attention tasks and suggest that an overlapping yet partially segregated network of parietal and frontal areas may be associated with top-down and stimulus-driven attention. Historically, because of its pervasiveness in human mental life, mental imagery, in particular visual mental imagery, has often been assigned an important role in theories of the mind. Ganis, Thompson, Mast, and Kosslyn review evidence supporting the notion that visual imagery and visual perception share many common processes. They point out that two-thirds of the areas activated during visual imagery and perception are activated jointly. And, although many researchers have documented parallel deficits in imagery and perception following brain damage, other researchers have shown that one or the other ability can be disrupted independently, which would be expected only if certain brain areas are shared by the two functions. They also provide evidence, however, that different sets of processes can be used even when the same imagery task is being performed.

A plethora of evidence indicates that the prefrontal cortex is involved in higher cognitive functions. Early research suggested that prefrontal cortex is primarily concerned with the retention of information in working memory. Accumulating evidence, however, suggests that the functional role of this region may be more complicated, perhaps representing either general intelligence or our ability to select among our concurrent thoughts. More specifically, the content of working memory represented in the dorsolateral prefrontal cortex has been proposed to be much more abstract than what we would expect of buffers storing spatial location or object properties; correspondingly, the prefrontal neural assemblies underlying the retention of information have been conceived of as equipotential modules that can employed in a large diversity of tasks and that represent an individual's general intelligence. In his chapter, Shallice discusses such theories while detailing his approach, which views prefrontal cortex as containing a hierarchically organized supervisory system that modulates contention scheduling. The latter deals with the situation in which multiple productions have their conditions satisfied at the same time. According to this model, the role of anterior prefrontal cortex is that of a supervisory system that comes into play when the goal-controlling immediate behavior needs to be interrupted and replaced by a new set of goals, possibly prefigured by previously produced intentions.

The final chapter of this section deals with the physiological foundations of the imaging technology most frequently used in cognitive neuroscience and psychology, namely, functional magnetic resonance imaging. The potential of MRI for functional brain mapping in humans is well-established. The combination of this technique with electrophysiology has fully confirmed the long-standing assumption that the regional activations measured in MR neuroimaging do indeed reflect local increases in neural activity. In addition, it has been demonstrated that fMRI responses mostly reflect the input of a given cortical area and its local intracortical processing, including the activity of interneurons. In the final chapter of this section, I point out the usefulness of this technique in animal research and provide a number of examples showing the benefits of its application in experiments combining imaging with other invasive neuroscientific methodologies.

61 Evolutionary and Developmental Foundations of Human Knowledge: A Case Study of Mathematics

MARC D. HAUSER AND ELIZABETH SPELKE

ABSTRACT Studies of human infants and of adult nonhuman primates provide evidence for two systems of representation that serve as building blocks for the number concepts of educated, enculturated humans. One is a system for representing small, precise numbers of objects; the other is a system for representing large, approximate numerical magnitudes. Studies of the signature limits of these systems reveal striking homologies across human and nonhuman primates and across infants and adults, suggesting that the systems emerged before the human species and arise in human development before the acquisition of language or culture. Children take a major step beyond these systems when they come to understand verbal counting and the natural number concepts that counting both defines and supports. Nevertheless, even the most sophisticated number concepts of educated humans rely in part on the core knowledge systems with deep roots in our ontogenetic and phylogenetic past. In this respect, numerical cognition may serve as a prototype for understanding other distinctively human, culturally supported concepts and cognitive skills.

The core knowledge thesis

What are the brain and cognitive systems that allow humans to play baseball, compute square roots, cook soufflés, or navigate the Tokyo subways? It may seem that studies of human infants and of nonhuman animals will tell us little about these abilities, because only educated, enculturated human adults engage in organized games, formal mathematics, gourmet cooking, or map reading. In this chapter, we argue against this seemingly sensible conclusion. Instead, we suggest that when human adults exhibit complex, uniquely human, culture-specific skills, they draw on a set of psychological and neural mechanisms with two distinctive properties: they evolved before humanity and thus are shared with other animals, and they emerge early in human development and thus are common to infants, children, and adults.

MARC D. HAUSER and ELIZABETH SPELKE Department of Psychology, Harvard University, Cambridge, Mass.

These core knowledge systems form the building blocks for uniquely human skills. To understand what is special about human intelligence, therefore, we must study both the core knowledge systems on which it rests and the mechanisms by which these systems are orchestrated to permit new kinds of concepts and cognitive processes.

What is core knowledge? A wealth of research on nonhuman primates and on human infants suggests that a system of core knowledge is characterized by four properties (Hauser, 2000; Spelke, 2000). First, it is domain-specific: each system functions to represent particular kinds of entities such as conspecific agents, manipulable objects, places in the environmental layout, and numerosities. Second, it is task-specific: each system uses its representations to address specific questions about the world, such as "who is this?" (face recognition), "what does this do?" (categorization of artifacts), "where am I?" (spatial orientation), and "how many are here?" (enumeration). Third, it is relatively encapsulated: each core knowledge system uses only a subset of the information delivered by an animal's input systems and sends information only to a subset of the animal's output systems. Finally, its operation is relatively automatic and impervious to explicitly held beliefs and goals.[1] Each of these properties gives rise to a set of *signature limits* that cognitive and brain scientists can use to identify particular core systems and their products across development and evolution.

In this chapter, we use the domain of number to illustrate how core knowledge systems are assembled to permit uniquely human cognitive advances in mathematics. We first review the comparative literature on animals and developmental studies of infants. This research provides evidence for two core knowledge systems that serve as building blocks for the number concepts of educated humans: a system for representing exact, small numbers of objects or events and a system for representing large, approximate numerical magnitudes. We next show that as human children develop, they use these systems to construct the first uniquely human number concepts, the natural numbers. Finally, we explore how the core knowledge systems function in educated human adults, permitting us to embrace concepts and engage in cognitive processing that is unique in the living world.

Knowledge of number

Natural number concepts are so simple and clear to human intuition that one might suppose they are shared by many animals and rooted in early human development. Both suppositions, however, are wrong. *Homo sapiens sapiens* is the only extant species that ever fully comprehends natural number concepts, and this understanding emerges only at about 4 years of age. Even the most highly trained chimpanzees and the most nurtured and educated 2-year-old children fail to do so. What makes the natural number concepts so difficult for animals and young children to understand?

One way to see how difficult the natural number concepts are is to consider how children learn to express them through verbal counting. Although children in many cultures begin to engage in verbal counting as young as 2 years of age, most children do not understand either the meanings of number words or the workings of the counting routine until 2 years later. Children construct this understanding laboriously, well after they master the script of the counting routine. For example, a 2½-year-old child who can count six toy fishes reliably typically knows only the meaning of the first word in her counting routine; when asked for "one fish," she will pick one and show it; when asked for any other number, she will grab and show a handful—a number greater than one fish but otherwise unrelated to the correct cardinal value (Wynn, 1990). Furthermore, if a child at this age is told that the pile contains "four fishes" and then watches as two fishes are removed, she will maintain that the pile still contains "four fishes" (Condry, Gramzow, and Cayton, 2003). Although she uses the counting words correctly in the count routine, she evidently interprets each word above one as simply meaning "more than one." With months of counting experience, as well as other cognitive advances that are running in parallel, children progress from understanding the meaning of "one" to understanding "two," and then "three"; this progression is highly systematic, with no evidence of children learning other numbers in the integer count list first, nor learning the meaning of three before they learn the meaning of two (Wynn, 1990). After this slow, systematic, stepwise progression, children take a leap forward. They form the induction that each word in the counting routine gives the cardinal value of a set composed of a specific number of individuals, that each word denotes a set with one more individual than the previous word, and that

the succession of cardinal values picked out by the number words can be continued indefinitely, with no upper bound. By age 5, preschool children can apply this knowledge robustly, even to number words outside their counting range (Lipton, 2003).

A second way to see how difficult the natural number concepts are is to consider the performance of the chimpanzee named Ai (Matsuzawa, 1985, 1996; Biro and Matsuzawa, 1999; Kawai and Matsuzawa, 2000). For more than 20 years, Ai has been involved in hundreds of experiments probing not only her natural cognitive ability but her cognitive potential once trained. Some of the training has focused on production and comprehension of symbols for kinds of objects, properties, and numbers. She has learned remarkably well: presented with symbols for "two," "red," and "pencil," Ai reliably points to an image of two red pencils. Her pattern of learning number words, however, departs strikingly from that of children. At the start of her number word training, Ai was taught the arabic symbols for "one" and "two." Once she had learned these symbols and a new symbol for "three" was introduced, Ai applied the symbols for "two" and "three" indiscriminately to arrays of two or three objects. In the initial training, Ai evidently interpreted 1 as "one" and 2 as "more than one," as do young children. Ai eventually learned to apply 2 and 3 correctly, but the amount of training needed to make this incremental advance was no different than the amount of training needed for the first two integers. When the symbol 4 was introduced, Ai's performance fell to chance on 3; she evidently interpreted 3 as "more than two." This pattern of learning continued throughout Ai's number symbol training: she never developed a "learning set" for number and never came to interpret a new arabic numeral as symbolizing a new cardinal value. Although human children arrive at correct interpretations of all number words after learning the first three or four of them, Ai has not progressed beyond the symbol 9 after 20 years of training. This stagnation suggests that chimpanzees' understanding of the integers is based on a mechanism that is very different from that of human children. Chimpanzees such as Ai learn the integer list by brute association, mapping each symbol to a discrete quantity. Human children, in contrast, learn by making an induction from a limited body of evidence. Children induce that the integer list is created by a successor function, and this function generates an infinite list of numbers.

Because human infants and nonhuman animals lack natural number concepts, one might think that studies of these populations could not inform us about the nature of these concepts and the cognitive processes of children and adults who form and use them. We believe the opposite is the case. Children construct natural number concepts by drawing on two systems of core knowledge of numerosity: a system for representing the approximate cardinal values of large sets of objects or events, and a system for representing the exact number of object arrays or events with very small numbers of entities. These systems are spontaneously present and functional both in untrained nonhuman primates and in human infants. Moreover, human adults draw on the same two systems when they use natural number concepts. Comparative and developmental studies answer crucial questions about the nature of these core knowledge systems. We next review the main insights that they have yielded.

THE LARGE, APPROXIMATE NUMBER SYSTEM When human adults are presented with a large number of objects in a short period of time, they are unable to determine exactly how many dots are in the array without verbal counting. Under these conditions, however, adults do represent the approximate number of elements in the array. Evidence for this ability comes from three kinds of experiments. First, if adults are asked to estimate how many elements are in an array, their estimates are nonrandom: the mean estimated number rises linearly with increasing numerosity, and the variance of their estimate is proportional to numerosity (Whalen, Gallistel, and Gelman, 1999; Cordes, Gelman, and Gallistel, 2002). Second, if adults are asked to judge which of two dot arrays has more elements, their judgments are above chance, and accuracy varies with the ratio of the two numerosities; with better accuracy for larger ratio differences (Barth, Kanwisher, and Spelke, 2003). Findings from these experiments suggest that adults form representations of large, approximate numerosities and that their representations accord with Weber's law: the variability in a numerosity representation is proportional to the numerosity (Gallistel, 1990; Dehaene, 1997, 2003).

Further experiments shed light on the nature of adults' numerosity representations. First, adults can perform numerical estimations and numerical comparisons on arrays of various types, including sequences of actions (Whalen, Gallistel, and Gelman, 1999; Cordes, Gelman, and Gallistel, 2002), sequences of sounds and light flashes, and visuospatial arrays (Barth, 2001; Barth, Kanwisher, and Spelke, 2003). Second, adults can compare two numerosities as accurately when the elements in the two sets are presented in different modalities (auditory vs. visual) and formats (spatial vs. temporal) as when the elements in the two sets are the same in modality and format (Barth, 2001; Barth, Kanwisher, and Spelke, 2003). Third, adults can perform nonsymbolic arithmetic on approximate number representations of either two successive arrays of dots or one array of dots and one sequence of sounds; for example, they can mentally add the two numerosities and compare the sum with a third dot array or sound sequence. Nonsymbolic addition is almost as accurate as numerical comparison, and cross-modal addition is every bit as accurate as addition

within a single modality (Barth et al., 2004). These findings provide evidence that adults can form, and operate on, a remarkably abstract representation of approximate numerical magnitudes. What are the phylogenetic and ontogenetic origins of this capacity? Is there a parallel signature both within and across species?

The first insights into the large, approximate system of number representation came from studies of animal timing. One approach, involving operant conditioning with rats and pigeons, is called the peak procedure. On some proportion of trials, a key is illuminated, and if the subject contacts the key after some fixed period of time, a food reward is delivered. On the remaining proportion of unrewarded trials, the key is illuminated for a significantly longer and variable period of time. Contacting the key after the fixed latency period for reward serves no purpose, as no reward will be forthcoming. The relevant data come from these unrewarded trials. There is a peak in responding centered around the fixed latency period. For example, if the latency for reward is 20 s, subjects tend to contact the key for approximately 20 s, plus or minus a few seconds. Importantly, the variability in response is proportional to the length of the latency period. With shorter latencies, subjects respond with high accuracy and little error around the target latency; with longer latencies, the distribution around the target spreads out, revealing a higher error rate. This aspect of duration representations is called *scalar variability*. The interesting aspect of scalar variability with respect to the current discussion is that the same data emerge when the task involves number as opposed to time or latency. If the subject has to make contact with the key after some number of light flashes, or some other numbered event or action, the distribution of errors is proportional to numerosity. A classic example of such data is plotted in figure 61.1 (Platt and Johnson, 1971).

These results, plus many others that control for factors that might explain subjects' responses other than number (e.g., effort, motivation, non-numerical stimulus dimensions; Brannon and Terrace, 1998, 2000; Orlov et al., 2000; Roberts, Coughlin, and Roberts, 2000), provide evidence that trained rats, pigeons, rhesus macaques, and other animals are sensitive to the approximate number of relevant events in a sequence or objects in an array (Gallistel, 1990; Shettleworth, 1998; Hauser, 2000; Brannon and Terrace, 2001). Additional data reveal that subjects' discrimination is guided by Weber's law, such that the difficulty of any given numerical discrimination depends on the ratio of the two numerosities (e.g., 8 and 12 are just as discriminable as 16 and 24, and more discriminable than 8 and 10). Moreover, the same Weber ratio appears to characterize discrimination of the numerosities of different types of entities: objects, tones, light flashes, and self-generated actions. The Weber ratio limit is one important signature of this system of

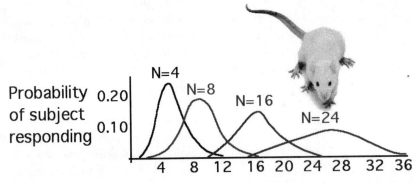

FIGURE 61.1 Plots of the probability of rats trying to access the feeding area as a function of the number of presses on a response lever and the number (N) required to load the feeding area with food. Data have been replotted from Platt and Johnson (1971).

representation. The lack of modality and format effects, which suggests that the system for representing numerosity is quite abstract, is a second signature property.

A different approach to assessing the large, approximate system in animals comes from training apes, like Ai, to represent and use symbols for cardinal values (Matsuzawa, 1985; Boysen and Bernston, 1989; Beran, 2001; Beran and Rumbaugh, 2001). Once Ai learned the nine arabic numerals, she was presented with a subset of the symbols in varying spatial positions on a monitor and was taught to touch the symbols in order of ascending numerosity. Results showed that she responded faster to symbols for lower numerosities than to symbols for higher ones, and when the ordinal distance between successive numbers was large than when it was small. These effects show the classic Weber signature of the large, approximate number system. In a different series of experiments, also focused on ordinality and serial position, Ai was presented with between three and five different numbers, with spatial position varying between trials. As soon as Ai pressed the first number in the ordinal sequence, white squares covered the remaining numbers, and Ai was required to recall not only the sequence of numbers but their location. Ai made more errors and responded more slowly when the two numbers were close together than when they were far apart. Thus, even though Ai was trained with arabic numerals, her performance and that of chimpanzees similarly tested (Boysen and Bernston, 1989; Boysen, 1997; Beran and Rumbaugh, 2001) show the Weber signature of the large number system.

In spite of the wealth of evidence for large, approximate number representations in nonhuman animals, the existence and nature of these representations has been little studied in human infants and children. For decades, studies of number representation in human infants focused only on exact discrimination of the smallest numerosities. Recently, however, investigators have begun to ask whether human infants are capable of forming the large, approximate numerical representations that are ubiquitous in nonhuman animals. The

answer is a clear yes, even though all of the animal studies cited earlier involved training, while none of the studies with human infants do.

In one series of studies (Xu and Spelke, 2000), 6-month-old infants were presented with visual arrays of 8 or 16 dots (figure 61.2). On a succession of habituation trials, the sizes and locations of dots varied, but the number was constant: 8 for half the infants and 16 for the others. After looking, time at the arrays had declined to half its initial level, infants were tested with new arrays presenting 8 or 16 dots in alternation. To ensure that any response to the test arrays was based on number as opposed to other continuous variables, the arrays with the two numerosities were equated in summed area and image size during habituation and were equated in item size and density at test; in a further study, the arrays were equated in contour length instead of summed area. Infants looked longer at the arrays presenting

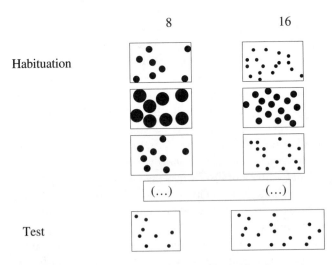

FIGURE 61.2 A sample of displays for the habituation and test phases of an experiment on human infant number discrimination (Xu and Spelke, 2000). These examples illustrate some of the variation between displays, designed to control for continuous covariates of number (e.g., continuous extent, density, etc.)

the change in numerosity, thereby providing evidence for numerosity discrimination (Xu and Spelke, 2000; Brannon, 2002).

Further studies tested whether infants' numerosity discrimination shows the Weber signature found in human adults and in nonhuman animals. At 6 months, infants successfully discriminated arrays in a 2:1 ratio (4 vs. 8, 8 vs. 16, and 16 vs. 32) and failed to discriminate arrays in a 3:2 ratio (4 vs. 6, 8 vs. 12, and 16 vs. 24) (Xu, Spelke, and Goddard, 2004; Xu, in press). At 9 months, infants successfully discriminated the latter arrays (Xu and Arriaga, 2004). These studies provide evidence that numerosity discrimination is characterized by the Weber signature at both ages, and that the critical discrimination ratio narrows with age.

Still further studies investigated infants' numerosity discrimination with sound sequences, using a head-turn preference procedure (Kemler Nelson et al., 1995). In one study (Lipton and Spelke, in press), 6-month-old infants were presented with sequences of 8 versus 16 natural sounds. On each familiarization trial, the quality and duration of the sounds varied but the number was constant. Then infants were tested with new sequences of 8 versus 16 sounds. To distinguish responses to number from responses to sequence duration, sound duration, sequence rate, or correlated variables such as the amount of sound, sequences were equated for sound duration and rate during familiarization and for sequence duration and total amount of sound during the test. Infants turned their heads for longer durations when the sequences with the novel numerosity were presented, again providing evidence of numerosity discrimination.

Tests for the set size ratio signature revealed three interesting findings. First, infants again showed this signature in their discrimination of sound sequences. Second, infants showed the same developmental change in sensitivity, with a decrease in the threshold ratio from 2.0 to 1.5 between 6 and 9 months. Third, infants showed exactly the same pattern of success and failure when tested with auditory temporal sequences as they had shown when tested with visual spatial arrays. The latter finding suggests that numerosity discrimination in infants shows a second signature of the system found in animals: it depends on an abstract process that is independent of sensory modality (visual or auditory) and stimulus mode (spatial vs. temporal).

As mentioned earlier, the studies of infants differ from those of animals in that infants represent number spontaneously, with no training. These findings raise the question of whether untrained animals also represent numerosity under the conditions used with infants, if such representations also show the Weber signature of the large, approximate number system, and if so, whether the ratio thresholds are the same or different. To address this issue, an experiment was designed (Hauser et al., 2003) with cotton-top tamarin monkeys using the same stimulus controls and same

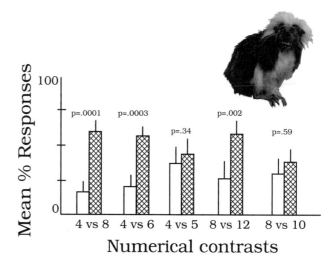

FIGURE 61.3   Results from familiarization-discrimination experiments on cotton-top tamarins (Hauser et al. 2003). The y-axis plots the mean proportion of responses (i.e., head orienting to a concealed speaker) to test items (speech syllables) with either the same (white bars) or different (cross-hatched bars) numbers as the familiarization sequence. P values are for Wilcoxon signed-ranks tests.

general methods as in the work with human infants (Lipton and Spelke, in press); the only significant methodological differences were in the use of speech syllables for the tamarins and in the implementation of a familiarization-discrimination procedure. As in previous work on tamarins with this method (Ramus et al., 2000; Hauser, Newport, and Aslin, 2001), we measured whether the subject turned in the direction of a concealed speaker when each test sequence was played. If subjects had extracted the common number of syllables from the familiarization phase of the session, then in the test phase they were expected to respond more to the tokens with a different number of syllables than to the tokens with the same number of syllables. Results provide clear evidence of the large, approximate number system, with successful discrimination at ratios of 2:1 and 3:2, but not 5:4 (figure 61.3).

Finally, very recent research has begun to ask what computations young children perform on large, approximate numerosities. From studies in young children (Barth et al., 2004), there is evidence that subjects can add two different numerosities. For example, children watch as one array of blue dots appears and then disappears behind an occluder; then a second array of blue dots appears and disappears behind the same occluder. Finally, children are presented with an array of red dots and are asked whether there are more blue or red dots. When tested with ratio differences of 1.75, 1.67, and 1.5 between the comparison dot array and the sum of the first two arrays, children performed well above chance, suggesting that this kind of representation can enter into computations of addition (Lamont, Barth, and Spelke, 2003; Barth et al., 2004). Recent studies of adult rhesus monkeys have begun to address similar issues of addition operations over large, approximate numerosities (Flombaum, 2002; Flombaum, Junge, and Hauser, 2004).

In summary, studies of trained animals, untrained animals, human infants, and preschool children all provide evidence for a core system of number representation. This system serves to represent the approximate cardinal values of large sets of objects or events with two well-established signatures, and evidence for a third underway. First, it is subject to a Weber limit on discrimination—discriminability depends on the set size ratio. Second, it is characterized by a common discrimination limit across modalities. The third signature concerns mathematical operations that take approximate mental magnitudes as input.

We now consider evidence for a second core system of number representation. The mechanisms underlying this system differ from the large, approximate system, and so do its limits.

THE SMALL, PRECISE NUMBER SYSTEM For more than a century, psychologists have recognized that there is something special about very small numbers. When human adults are asked to enumerate the exact number of elements in a visual array of dots, their response time rises linearly with increasing numerosity for all integers greater than 3. With the numbers 1–3, however, response times are fast and nearly flat. Although the nature and interpretation of this reaction time function has been much debated (Balakrishnan and Ashby, 1992), subjects' ability to identify small numbers rapidly, coupled with their introspections, suggests that a parallel process underlies enumeration of the smallest sets. Psychologists christened this preattentive, unconscious process *subitizing* (Mandler and Shebo, 1982; Butterworth, 1999).

Research over the past decade has revealed that this subitizing process has four signature properties. First, it is subject to a set size limit of three or four. Second, it operates when elements occupy distinct spatial positions, but not when they are superimposed on or embedded within one another (Trick and Pylyshyn, 1994). Third, it operates when distinct elements are separated by empty space, but not when they are joined by a grid of connecting lines (Trick and Pylyshyn, 1994; Scholl and Pylyshyn, 1999). Fourth, it operates when elements are stationary, when they move continuously while remaining in view, and when they move continuously with periods of brief occlusion; it fails to operate when elements appear and disappear discontinuously (Scholl and Pylyshyn, 1999) or when elements disperse and coalesce (Scholl, 2001; Mitroff, Scholl, and Wynn, 2004). Scholl and Pylyshyn have proposed that subitizing depends on mechanisms of object-directed attention, mechanisms that allow human adults to track three to four objects in parallel, provided that the objects are cohesive, bounded, and move continuously.

Over the past two decades, a wealth of experiments have provided evidence that this system of representation is shared by human infants. Wynn's (1992) celebrated study of "addition and subtraction" serves as an example. In one version of Wynn's experiment, 5-month-old infants viewed a puppet stage containing one object (a Mickey Mouse doll), and then the object was hidden behind a screen. Then a second, featurally identical object entered the scene and moved behind the same screen. To assess whether the infants had represented exactly two objects behind the screen, Wynn used the expectancy-violation method briefly mentioned in the last section: she raised the screen to reveal either the correct number of objects (two) or an incorrect number (one). Even though infants had seen only a single object on the stage at any given time, they looked longer at the one-object array. This looking pattern provides evidence that infants tracked each of the two objects over occlusion and formed a representation of both objects behind the screen. In subsequent versions of this study, infants were found to take correct account both of the addition and of the subtraction of an object, in arrays of as many as three objects. When shown larger numbers of objects, infants failed Wynn's task, looking equally long at possible and impossible outcomes.

Subsequent research reveals that Wynn's findings are highly robust, for they have been obtained from converging experiments using two other methods. In a box-search method (Feigenson and Carey, in press), 10- and 12-month-old infants watched as two objects were placed into a box, one at a time (1 + 1), and then one of the objects was surreptitiously removed. Then the infants were allowed to reach into the box and retrieve one object, and finally their subsequent reaching into the box was measured. In this condition, infants spent considerable time reaching back into the box. In contrast, they spent reliably less time reaching into the box if they initially saw only one object placed in the box, or if they were given the chance to remove two objects. This pattern of performance provides converging evidence that infants are capable of representing exactly two objects. In subsequent variations, infants were found to represent up to three objects. They failed this test, however, when larger numbers were presented, even larger numbers that differed by a large ratio.

The final method involves a two-box choice discrimination task (Feigenson, Carey, and Hauser, 2002). Here, an experimenter first presented infants with two widely separated boxes, placed different numbers of cookies into each box, walked away, and then allowed the infants to crawl to either of the boxes. Infants crawled reliably to the box with the greater number of cookies, provided that neither box contained more than three cookies. When larger numbers of cookies were placed in one or both boxes, in contrast, infants failed to show a preference in their approach patterns (figure 61.4).

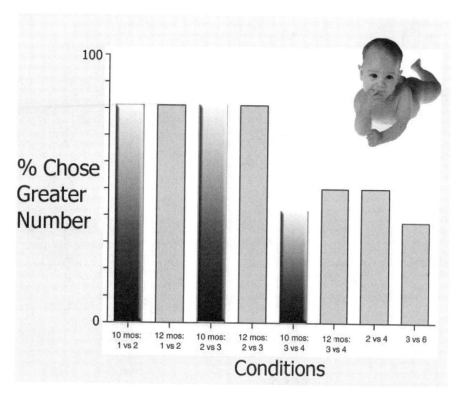

FIGURE 61.4 Responses of 10- and 12-month-old infants on a two-box choice test (Feigenson et al., 2002). The *y*-axis plots the proportion of subjects choosing the box with the greater number of cookies and the *x*-axis plots the conditions by age of subject.

These findings show that (1) infants' small number representations have the set size signature of adults' subitizing, and (2) infants' small number representations do not have the Weber signature of large number representations. Further studies of object representations in infants provide evidence for the other signatures of the adult object-tracking system as well (Scholl and Pylyshyn, 1999; Spelke, 2000; Scholl, 2001; Mitroff, Scholl, and Wynn, 2004). These findings suggest that a system for representing small numbers of objects is common to infants and adults and is distinct from the system for representing large numbers of objects.

Evidence for the small, exact number system in animals comes from the same methods used with human infants. The first experiment on animals to employ the looking time method involved a replication of Wynn's (1992) addition and subtraction experiments, focusing on a population of semi-free-ranging rhesus monkeys (Hauser, MacNeilage, and Ware, 1996). Monkeys were tested on Wynn's 1 + 1 = 2 versus 1 task and her 2 − 1 = 1 versus 2 task. There were four primary differences with Wynn's design. In contrast to Wynn, and most other studies with human infants, the rhesus experiments used (1) a between-subjects design, (2) no or minimal familiarization trials, (3) an experimenter in view, and (4) eggplants as test objects. In addition, since the rhesus monkeys lived on an island, subjects were free-ranging, with many potential distractions around the testing area. Despite these differences, analyses of both conditions revealed strik-

ing parallels, with subjects looking longer in both addition and subtraction conditions at the impossible event. In subsequent experiments, monkeys succeeded on the further tasks of 1 + 1 = 2 or 3, 1 small + 1 small = 1 big or 2 small, 2 + 1 = 2 or 3, and 2 + 1 = 3 or 4 (Hauser and Carey, 2004); they failed, however, when the outcome numbers exceeded three (e.g., 2 + 2 = 3 vs. 4 vs. 5) or when the number of times the representation required updating in short-term working memory was greater than two (figure 61.5). The 1 + 1 = 1 versus 2 versus 3 findings were replicated with captive cotton-top tamarins using a within-subject design (Uller, Hauser, and Carey, 2001), as well as with domesticated dogs (West and Young, 2002).

To further explore the limits on animals' spontaneous number capacity, Hauser and colleagues used the box search (Santos et al., 2002) and the two-box discrimination (Hauser, Carey, and Hauser, 2000) methods used with infants.[2] For both experiments, each subject was tested on only a single trial, thus eliminating any effects of experience or training. In the two-box discrimination task, an experimenter located a lone rhesus monkey and in the initial experiments, presented two empty boxes subsequently placed approximately 1 meter apart on the ground. Each box was then loaded up with different numbers of apple pieces, controlling for side and order of placement. The rhesus monkey selectively approached the box with the larger quantity for 2 versus 1, 3 versus 2, 4 versus 3, and 5 versus 3.

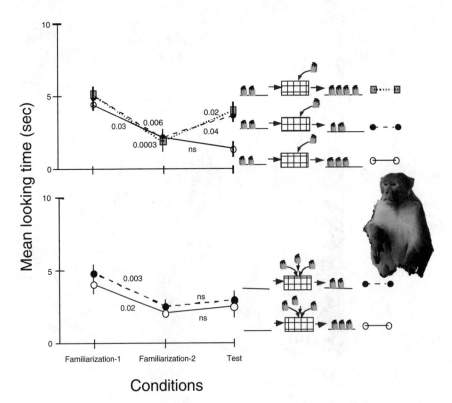

FIGURE 61.5   Looking time studies on rhesus monkeys, illustrating the updating and problem for 2 + 1 = 2 versus 3 versus 4 and 1 + 1 + 1 = 2 versus 3 (Hauser and Carey, 2004). The *y*-axis plots the mean amount of time (seconds) spent looking during the two familiarization trials and one test trial.

Rhesus monkeys might solve the two-box discrimination task by timing the events as opposed to counting the number of objects placed into each box. They might also solve this problem by quantifying volume as opposed to the number of pieces of apple. To address the time versus number confound, Hauser and colleagues reran all of the initial contrasts, but this time equated number of objects placed into each box by using a rock. In other words, when rhesus monkeys were presented with a comparison of two pieces of apple versus one piece of apple, the total number of objects was equated by placing a rock into the box with one piece of apple. Under these conditions, rhesus continued to pick the larger quantity in 2 versus 1, 3 versus 2, and 4 versus 3. To address the possibility that rhesus monkeys attend to volume over number, Hauser and colleagues placed three pieces of apple in one box and one piece of apple equal in volume to the three in the other box. Here again, subjects picked the box with three pieces of apple over the box with one piece.

A subsequent series of experiments involved the same general logic, but this time explored subtraction as opposed to addition (Sulkowski and Hauser, 2000). In the prototypical setup, subjects were shown two empty platforms, and then some number of objects were placed onto each, sequentially. An occluder was then placed in front of each platform, blocking the subject's view. The experimenter then reached down and removed some number of objects from one or both platforms. Independent of the particular setup or the number of objects removed, the rhesus monkey successfully picked the platform with more objects with all quantity pairs involving three or fewer objects. Thus, if one platform had three plums and the other had two plums and a rock, and the experimenter removed one plum from each, subjects approached the platform with two plums over the platform with one plum.

These two-box choice experiments suggest that rhesus monkeys can compute additions and subtractions over discrete objects, and for the addition experiments can discriminate the number of objects placed into each box when the ratio is 4:3. These conditions do not yet allow us to distinguish between the small and large systems. To distinguish between these systems, contrasts with larger numbers are needed. In subsequent conditions, Hauser and colleagues tested rhesus monkeys on 8 versus 4 and 8 versus 3, ratios that fall well within those discriminated for smaller numbers. Rhesus monkeys failed each of these conditions; their lack of discrimination cannot be accounted for by inattention, as only subjects who attended to the entire presentation were included in the final data set. These failures suggest that rhesus monkeys engage the small exact number system when tested in the two-box discrimination method. If the large approximate system had been available and engaged, they would have performed as well on 2 versus 1 as 8 versus 4.

In summary, the system used by human adults to apprehend small, exact numerosities is present and functional both in human infants and in two species of nonhuman primate. These findings suggest that this system is both ontogenetically and phylogenetically primitive. It is a second core system of numerical representation.

Putting the systems together

We have argued that human adults, adult nonhuman primates, and human infants share two capacities for numerical representation, one allowing approximate representations of large sets of entities and a second allowing exact representations of small numbers of objects. Because the performance of all these populations shows the same signature limits—especially the ratio limit of large number representations and the set size limit of small number representations—we suggest that these numerical representations depend on mechanisms that are homologous across monkeys, apes, and humans and are constant over human development. What, however, do these claims, and the evidence that they are based on, tell us about the uniquely human capacities for constructing the natural numbers? We hypothesize that humans depart from their closest living primate relatives by using these two systems in ontogeny to make sense of number words and the counting routine. Even after humans acquire the capacity to enumerate sets by counting, however, they retain the two core systems and use them during all quantitative reasoning tasks.

The two core systems found in infants and monkeys help to make sense of preschool children's otherwise puzzling interpretations of number words and the difficulty they experience in understanding verbal counting. When children first engage in the verbal counting routine, they know only that "one" picks out a single object, and that the other number words pick out larger sets of objects. At this stage, children may map "one" to their representations of objects, and they may map the other number words to their representations of large, approximate numerosities. When, over the next 1–2 years, children learn the meanings of the words *two* and *three*, they may map each of these terms to two representations at once: a representation of an array of objects (*two* refers to an array with an object and another object and no other objects) and a representation of an approximate numerosity (*two* refers to a very small set). Once children have learned these terms, they are in a position to notice that the progression from "two" to "three" in the counting routine corresponds both to the addition of one object to the set and to the increase in the cardinal value of the set. These inductions could form the basis for all the natural number concepts.

This account makes a set of predictions that can be tested with human adults, and, if confirmed, would explain both how children construct this system and why nonhuman animals will never do so, regardless of training. If children construct the natural number concepts by using natural language—number words and verbal counting—to link together core representations of small exact and large approximate numerosities, then the natural number concepts of adults may depend on three systems: the two core systems and natural language. Research has begun to test these predictions, with some success. In particular, adults given tasks that require representations of the natural numbers have been found to activate representations of large, approximate numerosities (Dehaene, 1997), and neurological patients with impaired abilities to form large, approximate number representations show impairments in natural number representations and mental arithmetic (Lemer et al., in press). These findings suggest that the core system for representing large, approximate numerosities partially underpins uniquely human natural number concepts. Moreover, adults who perform mental arithmetic on exact or approximate large numerosities show greater activation of language areas of the brain in the former case, and bilingual adults who learn new facts about large, exact numbers are better able to access that information in the language in which it was learned; in contrast, bilingual adults who learn new facts about large, approximate numbers or small, exact numbers are equally able to retrieve the facts in their two languages (Dehaene et al., 1999; Spelke and Tsivkin, 2001). These findings suggest that natural language is involved in the representation of uniquely human natural number concepts, but that language does not influence the approximate number representations that human adults share with infants and with nonhuman primates.

EvoDevo approaches to core knowledge

We have focused on number because it is one of the most comprehensively studied cognitive systems. The topic of numerical knowledge has been explored from both a phylogenetic and developmental perspective, using the tools of ethology, developmental psychology, cognitive science, neurobiology, linguistics and anthropology. Almost 50 years ago, in 1953, the Nobel laureate Nikolaas Tinbergen suggested that a comprehensive analysis of a particular behavior would require answers to four different questions: (1) What is its phylogenetic or historical background? (2) What is its original adaptive function? (3) What neurophysiological mechanisms are responsible for its expression? (4) How does it develop from its initial to the mature state? We have addressed each of these questions except the second. At present, we have little understanding of the adaptive pressures that led to either the shared core systems or the uniquely human system of the natural number concepts. Animals clearly benefit from quantifying small numbers precisely, as occurs when they form coalitions, when mothers track the number of offspring present, or when individuals engage in reciprocal exchanges (Gallistel, 1990; Hauser, 2000; Lyon, 2003). Animals also may benefit from the large, approximate system during foraging and intergroup aggression. But these are claims concerning current utility as opposed to original function. When it comes to our uniquely human capacities, such as verbal counting and natural number operations, our understanding of the relevant selective pressures is even less. Both our numerical and linguistic knowledge systems appear to rely on a generative mechanism to create a limitless range of meaningful expressions (Hauser, Chomsky, and Fitch, 2002), and it is not clear whether one mechanism evolved first for language and then for number or whether two distinct mechanisms evolved separately (Corballis, 1992, 1994; Bloom, 1994). Further phylogenetic and ontogenetic studies may help to shed light on these questions. For example, several small-scale societies such as the Hadza of Tanzania and the Piraha of Brazil have words for the first few integers and then use the equivalent of "many" for all other quantities (Dehaene, 1997; Butterworth, 1999; Gordon, 2004) These people have a fully expressive language that is based on the power of generativity, but they appear to lack a system of natural number concepts, relying exclusively on the small precise and large approximate systems (Gordon, 2004). Detailed anthropological studies of such cultures may help pinpoint some of the functional benefits of this system, as well as the social and ecological pressures that led to its emergence.

The framework outlined here, and applied specifically to numerical knowledge, has direct implications for cognitive neuroscientists interested in the cellular mechanisms that support the two core systems. As reviewed elsewhere (see Piazza and Dehaene, this volume), two recent studies with macaques provide exquisite evidence for a neural signature of the large, approximate system, with one study using a self-generated motor response (Sawamura, Shima, and Tanji, 2002) and the other using discrimination of static visual arrays (Nieder, Freedman, and Miller, 2002). Both studies entailed massive amounts of training prior to testing the subjects on their behavioral discrimination of different numerosities. If the trained macaques have an abstract representation of number, however, they should be capable of spontaneously transferring from one input modality to another and of performing numerical operations such as addition. To shed light on these numerical representations and operations, it would be highly desirable for neurophysiological studies to begin to employ the techniques currently being used by behaviorally oriented primatologists, reviewed above, to explore the spontaneously available resources for numerical discrimination.

Behind these specific suggestions is a more general one. When human adults form and use concepts that no other animal can attain, they do so by assembling a set of building blocks that are shared with other animals. These building blocks are part of core knowledge. Language may be a powerful device for assembling and coordinating the systems of core knowledge. Studies of nonlinguistic animals and prelinguistic infants, however, are uniquely placed to tell us what those systems are, how they evolved, and how they unfold over ontogeny.

NOTES

1. We assume here that even animals that lack belief-desire psychology (theory of mind) nonetheless have numerous actions that are volitional, planned, and goal-directed, and that the psychological mechanisms mediating these sorts of actions do not impinge on the output systems guiding the relationship between core knowledge and action.

2. Of historical interest, though most of the spontaneous methods used in animals were first implemented with human infants, the two-box discrimination task was first developed for rhesus monkeys and then used by Feigenson and colleagues (2002) with human infants.

REFERENCES

BALAKRISHNAN, J. D., and F. G. ASHBY, 1992. Subitizing: Magical numbers or mere superstition? *Psychol. Res.* 54:80–90.

BARTH, H. C., 2001. *Numerical Cognition in Adults: Representation and Manipulation of Nonsymbolic Quantities.* Doctoral diss., MIT, Cambridge, Mass.

BARTH, H. C., N. KANWISHER, and E. SPELKE, 2003. The construction of large number representation in adults. *Cognition* 86:201–221.

BARTH, H. C., K. LAMONT, J. S. LIPTON, S. DEHAENE, N. KANWISHER, and E. SPELKE, 2004. *Nonsymbolic arithmetic in adults and young children.* Unpublished manuscript.

BERAN, M. J., 2001. Summation and numerousness judgments of sequentially presented sets of items by chimpanzees (*Pan troglodytes*). *J. Comp. Psychol.* 115:181–191.

BERAN, M. J., and D. M. RUMBAUGH, 2001. "Constructive" enumeration by chimpanzees (*Pan troglodytes*) on a computerized task. *Anim. Cogn.* 4:81–89.

BIRO, D., and T. MATSUZAWA, 1999. Numerical ordering in a chimpanzee (*Pan troglodytes*): Planning, executing, and monitoring. *J. Comp. Psychol.* 113:178–195.

BLOOM, P., 1994. Generativity within language and other cognitive domains. *Cognition* 51:177–189.

BOYSEN, S. T., 1997. Representation of quantities by apes. *Adv. Study Behav.* 26:435–462.

BOYSEN, S. T., and G. G. BERNSTON, 1989. Numerical competence in a chimpanzee. *J. Comp. Psychol.* 103:23–31.

BRANNON, E. M., 2002. The development of ordinal numerical knowledge in infancy. *Cognition* 83:223–240.

BRANNON, E. M., and H. S. TERRACE, 1998. Ordering of the numerosities 1 to 9 by monkeys. *Science* 282:746–749.

BRANNON, E. M., and H. S. TERRACE, 2000. Representation of the numerosities 1–9 by rhesus macaques (*Macaca mulatta*). *J. Exp. Psychol. Anim. Behav. Processes* 26:31–49.

BRANNON, E. M., and H. S. TERRACE, 2001. The evolution and ontogeny of ordinal numerical ability. In *The Cognitive Animal*, M. Bekoff, C. Allen, and G. M. Burghardt, eds. Cambridge, Mass.: MIT Press.

BUTTERWORTH, B., 1999. *What Counts: How Every Brain Is Hardwired for Math.* New York: Free Press.

CONDRY, K., E. GRAMZOW, and G. CAYTON, 2003. *Toddler counting: Three-year-olds' inferences about addition and subtraction.* Presented at a meeting of the Society for Research in Child Development, Tampa, Fla.

CORBALLIS, M., 1992. On the evolution of language and generativity. *Cognition* 44:197–226.

CORBALLIS, M., 1994. The generation of generativity: A response to Bloom. *Cognition* 51:191–198.

CORDES, S., R. GELMAN, and C. R. GALLISTEL, 2002. Variability signatures distinguish verbal from nonverbal counting for both large and small numbers. *Psychol. Bull. Rev.* 8:698–707.

DEHAENE, S., 1997. *The Number Sense.* Oxford, England: Oxford University Press.

DEHAENE, S., 2003. The neural basis of the Weber-Fechner law: A logarithmic mental number line. *Trends Cogn. Sci.* 7:145–147.

DEHAENE, S., E. SPELKE, P. PINEL, R. STANESCU, and S. TSIVKIN, 1999. Sources of mathematical thinking: Behavioral and brain-imaging evidence. *Science* 284:970–974.

FEIGENSON, L., and S. CAREY (in press). Tracking individuals via object files: Evidence from infants' manual search. *Dev. Sci.*

FEIGENSON, L., S. CAREY, and M. D. HAUSER, 2002. The representations underlying infants' choice of more: Object files versus analog magnitudes. *Psychol. Sci.* 13:150–156.

FLOMBAUM, J., 2002. *The Evolution of Guesstimation.* Cambridge, Mass.: Harvard University Press.

FLOMBAUM, J., J. JUNGE, and M. D. HAUSER, 2004. *Monkeys spontaneously compute correct approximate sums following addition operations.* Unpublished manuscript.

GALLISTEL, C. R., 1990. *The Organization of Learning.* Cambridge, Mass.: MIT Press.

GORDON, P., 2004. *Numerical cognition without words: Evidence from Amazonia.* Unpublished manuscript.

HAUSER, M. D., 2000. *Wild Minds: What Animals Really Think.* New York: Henry Holt.

HAUSER, M. D., and S. CAREY, 2004. Spontaneous number representations of small numbers of objects by rhesus macaques: Examinations of content and format. *Cogn. Psychol.*

HAUSER, M. D., S. CAREY, and L. B. HAUSER, 2000. Spontaneous number representation in semi-free-ranging rhesus monkeys. *Proc. R. Soc. Lond.* 267:829–833.

HAUSER, M. D., N. CHOMSKY, and W. T. FITCH, 2002. The faculty of language: What is it, who has it, and how did it evolve? *Science* 298:1554–1555.

HAUSER, M. D., P. MACNEILAGE, and M. WARE, 1996. Numerical representations in primates. *Proc. Nat. Acad. Sci.* 93:1514–1517.

HAUSER, M. D., E. L. NEWPORT, and R. N. ASLIN, 2001. Segmenting a continuous acoustic speech stream: Serial learning in cotton-top tamarin monkeys. *Cognition* 78:B53–B64.

HAUSER, M. D., F. TSAO, P. GARCIA, and E. SPELKE, 2003. Evolutionary foundations of number: Spontaneous representation of numerical magnitudes by cotton-top tamarins. *Proc. R. Soc. Lond.* (online publication).

KAWAI, N., and T. MATSUZAWA, 2000. Numerical memory span in a chimpanzee. *Nature* 403:39–40.

KEMLER NELSON, D. G., P. W. JUSCZYK, D. R. MANDEL, J. MYES, A. TURK, and L. A. GERKEN, 1995. The headturn preference procedure for testing auditory perception. *Infant Behav. Dev.* 18:111–116.

LAMONT, K., H. C. BARTH, and E. SPELKE, 2003. *Can representations of large, approximate numerosities support addition in preschool children?* Paper presented at the 70th Biennial Meeting of the Society for Research in Child Development, Tampa, Fla.

LEMER, C., S. DEHAENE, E. SPELKE, and L. COHEN (in press). Approximate quantities and exact number words: Dissociable systems. *Neuropsychologia.*

LIPTON, J. S., 2003. *Preschool children's mapping of nonsymbolic numerosities.* Paper presented at the 70th Biennial Meeting of the Society for Research in Child Development, Tampa, Fla.

LIPTON, J. S., and E. S. SPELKE (in press). Origins of number sense: Large number discrimination in human infants. *Psychol. Sci.*

LYON, B. E., 2003. Egg recognition and counting reduce costs of avian conspecific brood parasitism. *Nature* 422:495–499.

MANDLER, G., and B. J. SHEBO, 1982. Subitizing: An analysis of its component processes. *J. Exp. Psychol. Gen.* 111:122.

MATSUZAWA, T., 1985. Use of numbers by a chimpanzee. *Nature* 315:57–59.

MATSUZAWA, T., 1996. Chimpanzee intelligence in nature and in captivity: Isomorphism of symbol use and tool use. In *Great Ape Societies*, W. C. McGrew, L. F. Marchant, and T. Nishida, eds. Cambridge, England: Cambridge University Press, pp. 196–209.

MITROFF, S. R., B. J. SCHOLL, and K. WYNN, 2004. *Divide and conquer: How object files adapt when a persisting object splits in two.* Unpublished manuscript.

NIEDER, A., D. J. FREEDMAN, and E. K. MILLER, 2002. Representation of the quanity of visual items in the primate prefrontal cortex. *Science* 297:1708–1711.

ORLOV, T., V. YAKOVLEV, S. HOCHSTEIN, and E. ZOHARY, 2000. Macaque monkeys categorize images by their ordinal number. *Nature* 404:77–80.

PLATT, J. R., and D. M. JOHNSON, 1971. Localization of position within a homogeneous behavior chain: Effects of error contingencies. *Learn. Motiv.* 2:386–414.

RAMUS, F., M. D. HAUSER, C. T. MILLER, D. MORRIS, and J. MEHLER, 2000. Language discrimination by human newborns and cotton-top tamarins. *Science* 288:349–351.

ROBERTS, W. A., R. COUGHLIN, and S. ROBERTS, 2000. Pigeons flexibly time or count on cue. *Psychol. Sci.* 11:218–222.

SANTOS, L. R., G. M. SULKOWSKI, G. M. SPAEPEN, and M. D. HAUSER, 2002. Object individuation using property/kind information in rhesus macaques (*Macaca mulatta*). *Cognition* 83:241–264.

SAWAMURA, H., K. SHIMA, and J. TANJI, 2002. Numerical representation for action in the parietal cortex of the monkey. *Nature* 415:918–922.

SCHOLL, B. J., 2001. Objects and attention: The state of the art. *Cognition* 80:1–46.

SCHOLL, B. J., and Z. W. PYLYSHYN, 1999. Tracking multiple items through occlusion: Clues to visual objecthood. *Cogn. Psychol.* 38:259–290.

SHETTLEWORTH, S., 1998. *Cognition, Evolution and Behavior.* New York: Oxford University Press.

SPELKE, E., 2000. Core knowledge. *Am. Psychol.* 55:1233–1243.

SPELKE, E., and S. TSIVKIN, 2001. Language and number: A bilingual training study. *Cognition* 78:45–88.

SULKOWSKI, G. M., and M. D. HAUSER, 2000. Can rhesus monkeys spontaneously subtract? *Cognition* 79:239–262.

TINBERGEN, N., 1963. On aims and methods in ethology. *Z. Tierpsychol.* 20:410–433.

TRICK, L., and Z. PYLYSHYN, 1994. Why are small and large numbers enumerated differently? A limited capacity preattentive stage in vision. *Psychol. Rev.* 101:80–102.

ULLER, C., M. D. HAUSER, and S. CAREY, 2001. Spontaneous representation of number in cotton-top tamarins (*Saguinus oedipus*). *J. Comp. Psychol.* 115:248–257.

WEST, R. E., and R. J. YOUNG, 2002. Do domestic dogs show any evidence of being able to count? *Anim. Cogn.* 5:183–186.

WHALEN, J., C. R. GALLISTEL, and R. GELMAN, 1999. Nonverbal counting in humans: The psychophysics of number representation. *Psychol. Sci.* 10:130–137.

WYNN, K., 1990. Children's understanding of counting. *Cognition* 36:155–193.

WYNN, K., 1992. Addition and subtraction by human infants. *Nature* 358:749–750.

XU, F. (in press). Numerosity discrimination in infants: Evidence for two systems of representations. *Cognition*.

XU, F., and R. ARRIAGA, 2004. *Large number discrimination in 10-month-old infants*. Unpublished manuscript.

XU, F., and E. S. SPELKE, 2000. Large number discrimination in 6-month old infants. *Cognition* 74:B1–B11.

XU, F., E. SPELKE, and S. GODDARD, 2004. *Number sense in human infants*. Unpublished manuscript.

62 From Number Neurons to Mental Arithmetic: The Cognitive Neuroscience of Number Sense

MANUELA PIAZZA AND STANISLAS DEHAENE

ABSTRACT Digits and number words are a very recent cultural invention in the evolution of the human species. Indeed, they arise from the specifically human and evolutionary recent ability to create and mentally manipulate complex symbols. However, the sense of numerosity is older. A sensitivity to numerical properties of the world is present in numerous nonhuman species as well as in babies. In this chapter we consider the most relevant findings on the cognitive neuroscience of number sense, showing how data from different domains, from cognitive psychology to electrophysiology, and in different species, from rats to humans, are providing us with complementary information on how the brain represents and manipulates numbers. In particular, we show how such sensitivity to numbers is rooted on a distinct neural circuitry, which has been reproducibly identified in different subjects and species with convergent methods. These observations lead to the hypothesis that an elementary number system is present very early in life in both humans and animals and constitutes the start-up tool for the development of symbolic numerical thinking that permeates so deeply our western technological societies.

Let us imagine a lioness with her pride on the Serengeti Plains, in Tanzania. One night, while alone, she hears a roar from an intruding lioness. Should she try to drive the intruder off? That would be an even match, thus ending in a possibly fatal fight. She decides not to act. The following night, when she is with four sisters, they hear the roars of three intruder lionesses. This time it is three versus five. The lionesses peer into each other's eyes, then launch the attack. But by the time they reach the expected location, they find no intruder. The roaring sounds they had heard came from loudspeakers set up by a researcher investigating the numerical capacity of animals. This research shows that generally, animals decide to attack back only when the number of defenders is superior to the number of intruders (McComb, Packer, and Pusey, 1994). The decision-making process of these animals seems to be based on a multimodal comparison between the number of defenders as perceived visually and the number of defenders as perceived auditorily. This suggests that the internal representation of number in animals can be quite abstract.

Numbers might be considered a very recent cultural invention in the evolution of the human species. Indeed, number words and digits arise from the specifically human and evolutionarily recent ability to create and mentally manipulate complex symbols. However, the sense of numbers is older. A sensitivity to numerical properties of the world is present in numerous nonhuman species, as well as in human babies, and its strong adaptive value is suggested by our lioness example. Such a sensitivity to numbers also seems to be rooted in a distinct neural circuitry that has been reproducibly identified in different subjects and species with convergent methods. These observations lead to the hypothesis that an elementary number system is present very early in life in both humans and animals, and constitutes the start-up tool for the development of the symbolic numerical thinking that permeates Western technological societies (Dehaene, 1997).

In this chapter, we consider the most relevant findings on the cognitive neuroscience of number sense, showing how data from different domains, from cognitive psychology to electrophysiology, provide complementary information on how the brain represents and manipulates numbers. We first consider how behavioral data have shed light on such a number sense in nonverbal organisms, either in animals or in human infants. Then we show how functional imaging and neuropsychology clarify the cerebral substrates of numerical ability. Finally, we explore the nature of the neural coding of numbers, as clarified by recent electrophysiological studies in monkeys.

Behavioral evidence for analogical representation of number

The ability to make numerical judgments has been tested in many different species of animals, including pigeons, rats, racoons, dolphins, and monkeys, in the wild and in more controlled experimental settings in laboratory, and using

MANUELA PIAZZA Service Hopitalier Frédéric Joliot and Department of Cognitive Neuroimaging, INSERM U562, Orsay Cedex, France.
STANISLAS DEHAENE Department of Cognitive Neuroimaging, INSERM U562, CEA, Orsay, France.

865

very different types of paradigms. Typically, animals are trained to respond differently to a variety of numerically defined stimuli, such as the number of visual stimuli, tones, motor responses, or reinforcements. However, because number usually covaries with some of the physical attributes of the stimuli, such as brightness, density, time, or hedonic value, reports of numerical abilities in animals are often met with skepticism. How can one be sure that animals are processing number rather than any other parameters of the stimulus? Two arguments have been used to demonstrate genuine numerical competence. First, animals can transfer numerosity between different modalities. For example, rats initially trained on distinct auditory and visual numerosity discrimination tasks could later generalize to novel sequences in which auditory and visual sequences were mixed (Church and Meck, 1984). This observation suggests that animals possess an abstract, amodal representation of number. Second, animals are able to generalize numerically relevant behavior to novel, nondifferentially rewarded stimuli (Meck and Church, 1983; Brannon and Terrace, 2000; Nieder, Freedman, and Miller, 2002; Sawamura, Shima, and Tanji, 2002). This finding indicates that they bring to the task more knowledge of numerical invariance than training alone could provide. For example, rats were trained to press one lever in response to a short two-tone sequence and another in response to a long eight-tone sequence. Although duration discrimination was sufficient for that initial performance, subsequently the rats generalized their behavior to novel, nondifferentially rewarded sequences in which duration was fixed and only number varied. This suggests that the animals were representing number during the initial training phase (Meck and Church, 1983).

An ability to discriminate sets on the basis of their number is also present in preverbal human infants. With the classic method of habituation and recovery of looking time, both newborns and preverbal infants have been shown to discriminate sets of visual objects, as well as tones or words that differ in the number of syllables, on the unique basis of their numerosity (e.g., Xu and Spelke, 2000). Again, there is suggestive evidence of cross-modal numerosity matching (Starkey, Spelke, and Gelman, 1983), as well as of processing of the numerosity of abstract entities such as collections, whose physical attributes can be well controlled (Wynn, Bloom, and Chiang, 2002). Such animal and infant data, taken together, suggest that the sensitivity to the numerical aspect of the world does not depend on an acquired ability to manipulate symbols but is based on a nonverbal amodal representation of numerosity.

This representation can also be adduced in human adults. When prevented from using language and counting procedures, adult humans can make approximate numerosity judgments similar to those of animals and infants. They too can transfer numerosity from different modalities (visual and auditory) and modes of stimulus presentation (sequential and simultaneous), and they do so without cost relative to a unimodal stimulus presentation (Barth, Kanwisher, and Spelke, 2003).

The parallels between human and animal behavior on number-related tasks are therefore numerous, but the most striking one is probably that they both seem to be governed by the very same metric (Gallistel and Gelman, 2000; figure 62.1). Number estimation performance in both humans and nonhuman animals is approximate, and becomes less and less accurate as the numbers increase. Furthermore, the variability in performance increases linearly with the size of the number involved, a property called scalar variability, or Weber's law, where the proportionality constant is called the Weber fraction. For example, rats instructed to press a lever a certain number of times will break off the sequence of lever presses with a probability that is roughly proportional to the percent deviation of the actual number of presses from the number of presses required to get the reward (Mechner, 1958; figure 62.1A). Likewise, monkeys instructed to judge whether successive visual displays have the same number of items make errors in direct proportion to the ratio of the two numbers. Thus, for larger numerical quantities, the two numerosities have to be numerically more distant for performance to reach the same level as the one obtained with smaller quantities (Nieder and Miller, 2003; figure 62.1B).

In humans, studies directly inspired by animal experiments show exactly the same type of metric. For example, Whalen, Gallistel, and Gelman (1999) presented numbers between 7 and 25 on a computer screen and asked subjects to press a button as fast as they could until they had felt they had made approximately the indicated number of button presses; verbal counting was prevented by asking subjects to recite words while performing the task. The results showed that both the mean estimate and its variability were proportional to target value, and that therefore the coefficient of variation (the ratio of the standard deviation to the mean) was constant across target size (figure 62.1C). Very similar results are found when humans were asked to estimate prices for different items; again, the standard deviation of price estimates was directly proportional to the mean price (Dehaene and Marques, 2002; figure 62.1D).

Moreover, Weber's law holds even when numerical judgments are not estimates but exact computations made over abstract numerical symbols, such as digits and number words. Such symbolic numerical judgments (e.g., choosing the larger number of 49 and 72) show magnitude effects exactly as nonsymbolic numerosity judgments do; they are influenced by the numerical difference between two values ("numerical distance effect") and by their absolute magnitude ("magnitude effect"), such that ultimately performance can be predicted by the ratio of the two numbers involved (Moyer and Landauer, 1967; Dehaene, 1992).

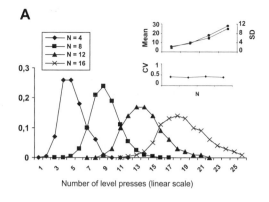

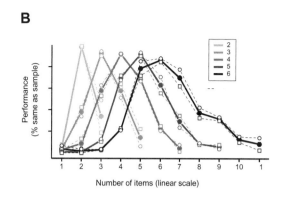

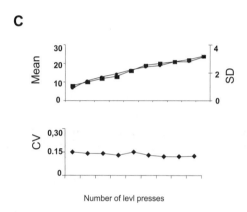

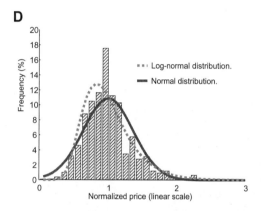

FIGURE 62.1 Evidence for Weber's law in animal and human numerical behavior. (A) The probability of rats breaking off a sequence of lever presses as a function of the number of presses in the sequence and the number required to get the reward. The inset shows the mean number of lever presses (circles) and standard deviation (squares). The coefficient of variation (CV), which is the ratio of the mean to the standard deviation, is constant, indicating Weber's law in estimation. (Redrawn from Mechner, 1958, and modified from Gallistel and Gelman, 2000.) (B) Behavioral performance of two monkeys on a same-different task where they judged whether a test stimulus contained the same or a different number of items as the sample display. Each curve represents the percent-

age of "same" response as a function of test numerosity, for a given sample numerosity. (Modified from Nieder and Miller, 2003.) (C) Behavioral performance of human adults who were asked to produce a given number of key presses. The mean number of presses (circles), standard deviation (squares), and the CV are striking similar to the rats' performance shown in A. (Redrawn from Gallistel and Gelman, 2000.) (D) Distribution of human adults' estimates of prices of items, after normalization by the mean price. The distribution is consistently skewed and is better fitted by a log-normal curve than by a normal curve. (From Dehaene and Marques, 2002.)

It has been a matter of debate whether Weber's law is better described by a linear continuum with increasing variability or by a nonlinear, perhaps logarithmic scale with constant variability. Some have argued that the linear model should be preferred, because it allows a simpler calculation of sums and differences (Gallistel and Gelman, 1992). Contrarily, others have proposed a logarithmic coding because this compressive scheme avoids an explosion in the size of the internal representation as the range of represented numerosities increases (Dehaene and Changeux, 1993). In fact, both assumptions accurately predict performance, and for a long time it was thought that the linear hypothesis and the logarithmic hypothesis could not be disentangled. Recently, however, detailed analyses of the exact shape of response distributions in both humans and animals have suggested that the internal scale is not linear but logarithmic. When plotted on a linear scale, performance curves are

asymmetric and are best fitted by a log-normal distribution (see figure 62.1D). However, they become symmetric when plotted on a logarithmic scale, and are then best fitted by a simple Gaussian with fixed variability (Dehaene et al., 2003; Nieder and Miller, 2003). Thus, the behavior of both humans and monkeys can be described in a more compact way by assuming a logarithmic scale than by assuming a linear internal scale for number.

Imaging number sense in humans

Given those behavioral observations, it has been proposed that animals and humans share a common and evolutionarily ancient mechanism for representing numerical quantities, and that this mechanism serves as a foundational core of numerical knowledge, providing humans with a start-up tool that permits the acquisition of numerical symbols (Dehaene,

1997; Butterworth, 1999; but see Simon, 1999, for an opposite view). The analogical representation of number would ground our intuition of what a given numerical size means, and of the proximity relations between numbers. It would be crucial in tasks that place strong emphasis on the quantitative aspects of numbers, such as the estimation of a price (Dehaene et al., 2003; figure 62.1*D*), the approximation of complex arithmetical problems (Dehaene et al., 1999; Spelke and Tsivkin, 2001), or the rough estimation of the number of elements in a set (Whalen, Gallistel, and Gelman, 1999). In support of this view, recent neuroimaging data show that an area of the brain is systematically activated whenever this putative core system for numerical quantities is called for—the horizontal segment of the intraparietal sulcus (IPS) in the parietal lobes.

The first investigation of the neural correlates of human numerical abilities showed increased metabolism in both parietal and frontal regions during complex calculation, using single-photon emission computed tomography (Roland and Friberg, 1985). This result was in agreement with earlier studies of patients with brain lesions, which had shown a crucial role for the parietal lobes in number processing. Since then, many studies using more refined functional imaging techniques such as PET and fMRI have yielded evidence for the recruitment of parietal regions on different number-related tasks. On the basis of a detailed review of the recent literature, and of a meta-analysis of some of the available activation images, we proposed that

parietal activation in number-related tasks can be segregated into three distinct sites, each associated with a distinct process (Dehaene et al., 2003): the posterior superior parietal lobule, associated with visuospatial processing; the angular gyrus of the left hemisphere, associated with verbal processing of numbers; and the horizontal segment of the IPS, the most plausible candidate for a domain-specific locus where numerical quantity is represented. In this chapter we focus mostly on the last site, the horizontal segment of the IPS, or HIPS (figure 62.2*A*). Several features of its responsiveness to experimental conditions suggest that this region encodes the analogical representation of numerical magnitude that grounds our intuition of what a given numerical size means, and of the proximity relations between numbers.

First, in calculation, the HIPS is more active when subjects estimate the approximate result of an addition problem than when they compute its exact solution, even when task difficulty is strictly controlled (Dehaene et al., 1999). This fits well with the approximate nature of the representation of numerical quantities. Within exact calculation, this region is also more active for operations that require a genuine manipulation of numerical quantities, such as subtraction, than for those that can be stored in rote verbal memory, such as multiplication (Lee, 2000). Moreover, its activation is modulated by semantic parameters such as the absolute magnitude of the numbers. It is larger and lasts longer during operations with large numbers than during operations with small numbers (Dehaene et al., 1999).

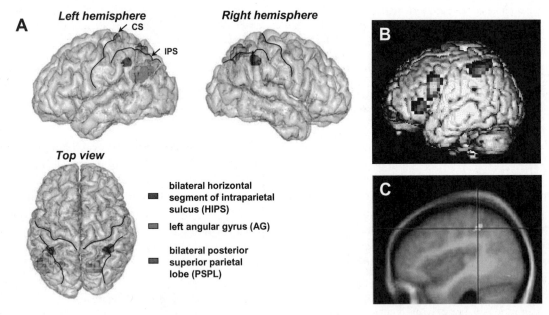

Figure 62.2 Brain imaging of number sense. (*A*) Three-dimensional representation of the three parietal sites of major activation in number processing individuated by a recent meta-analysis of fMRI studies of number processing. Abbreviations: CS, central sulcus; IPS, intraparietal sulcus. (From Dehaene et al., 2003.) (*B*) Regions whose activation increases with number size during calculation, including left HIPS, left premotor, and left inferior prefrontal areas. (From Stanescu et al., 2000.) (*C*) Region of reduced gray matter in a population of subjects with developmental dyscalculia. The location of impairment coincides with the left HIPS. (From Isaacs et al., 2001.)

Second, the HIPS is also active whenever a comparative operation that needs access to a numerical scale is called for. For instance, its activation is higher when subjects compare the magnitudes of two numbers than when subjects simply read them. Furthermore, its activation is modulated by the numerical distance separating the numbers (Pinel et al., 2001). The systematic contribution of this region to number comparison processes has also been replicated using scalp recordings of event-related potentials (Dehaene, 1996). The typical scalp signature of a numerical distance effect, moreover, has been observed in 5-year-old children, with a topography similar to that in adults for numbers presented either as arabic numerals or as sets of dots (Temple and Posner, 1998).

Third, the HIPS shows relatively robust category specificity for numbers when directly contrasted with different categories of objects or concepts. For example, in comparative judgments, it is more active when subjects are comparing numbers than when subjects are processing other categories of objects on non-numerical scales (such as the ferocity of animals, the relative positions of body parts, or the orientation of two visually presented characters; Pesenti et al., 2000; Thioux et al., 2002). Even on tasks that do not directly require a numerical judgment, such as simple detection tasks, the HIPS is the only region that shows higher activation when processing numbers than when processing letters of the alphabet or colors (Eger et al., 2003). Both control continua (letters and colors) were chosen because, like numbers, they show a distance effect (e.g., when detecting the letter M, it takes longer for a subject to reject the letter L than the letter C). Moreover, the alphabet also shares with numbers a strong serial component. However, both letters and colors lack quantitative meaning. Therefore, this experiment suggests that the HIPS activation for numbers relates to the processing of their quantitative meaning.

Fourth, the activation of the HIPS is independent of the particular modality of input used to present numbers. Arabic numerals, spelled-out number words, and even nonsymbolic stimuli like sets of dots or tones can activate this region if subjects attend to the corresponding number. In one study, subjects attended either to the numerosity or to the physical characteristics (color, pitch) of series of auditory and visual events. The right HIPS was active whenever subjects attended to number, regardless of the modality of the stimuli (Piazza, Mechelli, et al., 2003). In another study, activation of the bilateral HIPS was found to correlate directly with the numerical distance between two numbers in a comparison task, and this effect was observed whether the numbers were presented as words or as digits (Pinel et al., 2001). Finally, in a simple detection task, the HIPS was activated for numbers relative to letters and colors, irrespective of the visual or auditory modality of presentation (Eger et al., 2003). These results are consistent with the hypothesis that the HIPS encodes the abstract quantity meaning of numbers rather the numerical symbols themselves.

Fifth, quantity processing and HIPS activation were demonstrated even when subjects were not aware of having seen a numerical symbol (Naccache and Dehaene, 2001). In this experiment, subjects were asked to compare target numbers to a fixed reference of 5. Unbeknownst to them, just prior to presentation of the target, another number, the prime, was briefly present in a subliminal manner. fMRI revealed that the left and right intraparietal regions were sensitive to the unconscious repetition of the same number. When the prime and target corresponded to the same quantity (possibly in two different notations, such as ONE and 1), less parietal activation was observed than when the prime and target corresponded to two distinct quantities (e.g., FOUR and 1). This result suggests that this region comprises distinct neural assemblies for different numerical quantities, so that more activation can be observed when two such neural assemblies are activated than when only one is. It also indicates that this region can contribute to number processing in a subliminal fashion.

Finally, convincing evidence for the crucial role of the HIPS in numerical quantity representation comes from neuropsychological studies of impairments in number processing and calculation in adults, as well as in developmental cases. Several single-case studies indicate that numbers doubly dissociate from other categories of concepts at the semantic level. On the one hand, spared calculation and number comprehension abilities have been described in patients with grossly deteriorated semantic processing ("semantic dementia"; Remond-Besuchet et al., 1998; Butterworth, Cappelletti, and Kopelman, 2001). In both cases, the lesions broadly affected the left temporofrontal cortices while sparing the intraparietal regions. On the other hand, several cases demonstrate that the understanding of numbers and their relations can be specifically impaired in the context of otherwise preserved language and semantics (e.g., Delazer and Benke, 1997; Dehaene and Cohen, 1998). The majority of such cases result from lesions in the parietal regions, particularly in the left hemisphere.

Developmental studies confirm that impairments in arithmetic abilities correlate with abnormalities in the functional or anatomical organization of the HIPS. Levy, Reis, and Grafman (1999) reported the case of an adult with lifelong isolated dyscalculia but superior intelligence and reading ability, in whom the standard anatomical MRI appeared normal yet MR spectroscopy revealed a metabolic abnormality in the left inferior parietal area. Similarly, Isaacs and colleagues (2001) used voxel-based morphometry to compare gray matter density in adolescents born at equally severe grades of prematurity, half of whom suffered from dyscalculia. The only brain region that showed reduced gray matter associated with dyscalculia was the left IPS.

More recently, Molko and colleagues studied a population of females affected by Turner's syndrome, a syndrome characterized by a congenital abnormality of the X chromosome and often associated with defective development of number skills in the context of a normal general intelligence (Molko et al., 2003). They used voxel-based morphometry to compare the gray matter density of this dyscalculic Turner population with an age-, education-, and sex-matched group of controls. Results showed a region of reduced gray matter in the depth of the right HIPS. Morphometric analysis restricted to the cortical sulci showed that the length and depth of the right IPS were reduced in the patients with Turner's syndrome. Finally, the fMRI activation of this region differed significantly from activation in the control group for number-related tasks such as simple additions.

OTHER PARIETAL REGIONS INVOLVED IN NUMBER PROCESSING
Taken together, these data suggest that the HIPS is the most crucial cortical region for the correct development of numerical skills. Clearly, it is not the only system involved in number processing. Mental arithmetic relies on a highly composite set of processes, many of which are probably not specific to the number domain. For instance, studies of language interference in normal subjects suggest that language-based processes play an important role in exact but not approximate calculation (Spelke and Tsivkin, 2001). Likewise, concurrent performance of a spatial task interferes with subtraction but not multiplication, while concurrent performance of a language task interferes with multiplication but not subtraction (Lee and Kang, 2002). Such behavioral dissociations suggest that the neural bases of calculation must be heterogeneous.

A recent re-analysis of brain activation studies allowed us to individuate two satellite parietal systems that are often involved in numerical tasks, even if their primary function is not specific to numbers. We isolated a language-related region in the left angular gyrus associated with verbal processing of numbers and a visuospatial region in the posterior superior parietal lobe, presumably associated with spatial and nonspatial attention. On arithmetic tests, the left angular gyrus shows increasingly greater activation as the task puts greater requirement on verbal processing. For example, this region is more active in exact calculation than in approximation (Dehaene et al., 1999). This fits with behavioral data that indicate that exact arithmetic facts are stored in a language-specific format in bilinguals, while approximate knowledge is language independent (Spelke and Tsivkin, 2001). Moreover, within exact calculation, the left angular gyrus shows greater activation during operations that require access to a rote verbal memory of arithmetic facts, such as multiplication, than during operations that are not stored and require some form of quantity manipulation, such as subtraction.

The posterior superior parietal region is also frequently active, usually in synergy with the HIPS, for instance, in number processing during number comparison (Pesenti et al., 2000; Pinel et al., 2001), approximation (Dehaene et al., 1999), some subtraction tasks (Lee, 2000), and counting (Piazza et al., 2002; Piazza, Giacomini, et al., 2003). However, this region is clearly not specific to the number domain, because it plays a central role in attentional selection in space and time (Wojciulik and Kanwisher, 1999). Psychological experiments indicate that numbers have a strong serial and therefore spatial component, to the point that it has been metaphorically proposed that numbers are represented internally on a "number line," a quasi-spatial representation in which numbers are organized by their proximity (Moyer and Landaver, 1967; Dehaene, Bossini, and Giraux, 1993). It is therefore conceivable that the same process of covert attention that operates to select locations in space can also be engaged when attending to specific quantities on the number line.

According to the proposed tripartite organization of parietal activation during arithmetic suggested by our meta-analysis of existing neuroimaging studies, dissociations are expected between the types of arithmetic tasks that patients should or should not be able to perform according to the lesion site. For example, a lesion of the HIPS should affect all tasks requiring genuine manipulation of both symbolic and nonsymbolic numerical quantities, including approximation, subtraction, comparison, or estimation of numerosity. Lesions of the angular gyrus or other language-related regions of the left hemisphere should result in an impairment in retrieving arithmetic facts that are stored in verbal format, such as multiplication facts. Finally, lesions extending to the most posterior portion of the IPS or the superior parietal lobe should impair tasks that put strong emphasis on the visuospatial layout of number, such as bisection tasks (e.g., what number lies in the middle of 11 and 19?). Indeed, such dissociations have been reported in the literature. For example, some patients are much more impaired on subtraction than on multiplication (Dehaene and Cohen, 1997; Delazer and Benke, 1997; van Harskamp and Cipolotti, 2001). Such patients typically do not show language impairments but, in the rare case in which this has been investigated, may show difficulties in estimating the numerosity of arrays (Lemer et al., in press). Lesions are often reported around the left IPS. Other patients show the reverse dissociation, being more severely impaired on multiplication than on subtraction. They almost always have associated aphasia (Dehaene and Cohen, 1997; Cohen and Dehaene, 2000; Sandrini et al., 2003). Furthermore, the lesions in such patients often spare the intraparietal cortex and can affect multiple regions known to be engaged in language processing, such as the left perisylvian cortices, including the inferior angular gyrus, the left parietotemporal carrefour, or the left basal ganglia.

A recent study directly compared two acalculic patients, one with a focal lesion of the left parietal lobe and Gerstmann's syndrome and the other with semantic dementia with predominantly left temporal hypometabolism. As predicted by a numerical quantity deficit, the first patient was more impaired on subtraction than on multiplication, showed a severe slowness in approximation of calculation, and exhibited associated impairments in estimation and numerical comparison tasks, both with arabic numerals and with sets of dots. As predicted by a verbal deficit, the second patient was more impaired on multiplication than on subtraction, had intact approximation abilities, and showed preserved processing of nonsymbolic numerosities (Lemer et al., in press).

Support for the dissociation between quantity representation and the spatial scanning of the mental number line is provided by a study with unilateral neglect patients (Zorzi, Priftis, and Umiltà, 2002). It is a well-known, indeed, almost a defining feature of those patients that they perform poorly on spatial bisection tests. When asked to locate the middle of a line segment, neglect patients with right parietal lesions tend to indicate a location further to the right, consistent with their failure to attend to the left side of space. Zorzi and colleagues tested their performance on a numerical bisection task, where they were asked to find the middle of two numbers presented orally. Strikingly, the patients erred systematically, often selecting a number far larger than the correct answer (e.g., what number falls in the middle of 11 and 19? Patient's answer: 17). This suggests that spatial attention can be oriented on the left-to-right oriented number line, and that this attention-orienting process contributes to the resolution of simple arithmetic problems such as the bisection test. Interestingly, these patients were not acalculic and did not show deficits on other numerical tasks, such as simple arithmetic fact retrieval.

In summary, a review of neuropsychological dissociations between numerical operations indicates that most if not all cases so far described can be accommodated by the postulated dissociation between a quantity circuit (supporting subtraction and other quantity-manipulation operations), a verbal circuit (supporting multiplication and other rote memory-based operations), and a visuospatial circuit (supporting number bisection and other tasks on which the spatial sense of numbers is particularly relevant).

One intriguing discrepancy between the lesion and imaging studies relates to the lateralization of the core quantity circuit. In quantity-related dyscalculia, lesions are often restricted to the left hemisphere. However, imaging studies show bilateral parietal activation in quantity tasks. The exact role of the right hemisphere in number processing is therefore still unclear. Some neuropsychological studies have suggested a superiority of the right hemisphere, and in particular of the parietal region, in numerosity estimation tasks, such as estimating the number of dots in briefly presented arrays of elements (Warrington and James, 1967). Such a right hemisphere superiority in nonsymbolic numerical tasks was replicated in an imaging study of numerosity estimation, where parietal activation was indeed restricted to the right hemisphere (Piazza, Mechelli, et al., 2003). One possibility is that our core numerical system is initially bilateral and progressively becomes biased for symbolic manipulations of numbers in the left hemisphere and for nonsymbolic tasks in the right hemisphere. Such speculation, however, awaits confirmation.

The neural coding of numerosity

Recent electrophysiological studies have considerably improved our understanding of the neural bases of number sense. In 1993, Dehaene and Changeux presented a theoretical model of how numerical quantity could be represented at the single-neuron level. They proposed the existence of "numerosity detectors," neurons coarsely tuned to an approximate quantity. In 2002, two electrophysiological studies reported the first clear evidence of the existence of such neurons. The fine-grained analysis of those neurons' responses has proved extremely valuable for understanding the nature of the numerical representation underlying animal behavior.

The first pioneering study that investigated elementary numerosity discrimination abilities in animals at the neuronal level dates back to the work of Thompson and colleagues (1970). They recorded from cells in the posterior association cortex of the anesthetized cat (in an area that might be homologous to posterior parietal cortex in monkeys and humans) and found a handful of neurons that preferentially responded to a given numerosity, for instance, a sequence of three sounds or three light flashes. For many years, this finding stood alone. Very recently, however, two independent groups confirmed the existence of such "numerosity detectors" (Nieder, Freedman, and Miller, 2002; Sawamura et al., 2002). Sawamura and colleagues trained monkeys to push a lever five times in a row, then turn it five times, and so on. To prevent the monkeys from using time instead of number in deciding when to switch their actions, the time spent in a block of consecutive trials was varied between 20 and 46s and decorrelated from the number of movements performed. Neurons located in the superior parietal lobule, relatively superficially on the anterior bank of the IPS, responded selectively to numerical information. Although some of these cells responded specifically to a single number (which varied from one to five), for most cells the activity dropped off progressively with the numerical distance. Hence, a neuron coding preferentially for number three fired a little less for two and four, and even lesser for one or five.

This study represented an elegant effort to "read" the neural code supporting the representation of number in the monkey brain. However, some aspects of the task used made the interpretations of the results slightly problematic. First, the numerical information relevant to performing the task was related to the numerical position in a sequence (ordinal number) and not to the numerical quantity itself (cardinal number). Second, many of the neurons fired only for one of the two actions, thus showing both action and number tuning. It is not known whether these neurons would generalize to other numerical tasks.

A more recent study, however, reported neurons tuned to cardinal number, and performed fine-grained analysis of the neurons' tuning curves in parallel with a thorough analysis of the monkeys' behavior (Nieder et al., 2002; Nieder and Miller, 2003). Macaque monkeys were trained to perform a match-to-sample task on successively presented visual displays containing between one and five randomly arranged

items. During training, certain visual features inevitably covaried with numerosity. However, after training, the monkeys spontaneously generalized to novel displays in which all of the relevant non-numerical variables were controlled, suggesting that they were attending to number (figure 62.3).

Neurons were then recorded, initially only in the dorsolateral prefrontal cortex (Nieder, Freedman, and Miller, 2002). About one-third of the neurons there were tuned to a specific numerosity between one and five (the maximal numerosity that was tested). This finding was very similar to the findings of Sawamura, Shima, and Tanji (2002), but because the stimulation was visual it was possible to vary the stimulus extensively and verify to what extent neuronal response could be explained by other non-numerical parameters. The results indicated a remarkable degree of invariance to non-numerical parameters: a given neuron remained tuned to the same number across a broad variation of stimuli that controlled for object size, density, spacing, and spatial layout. Nevertheless, further tests will be necessary to assess

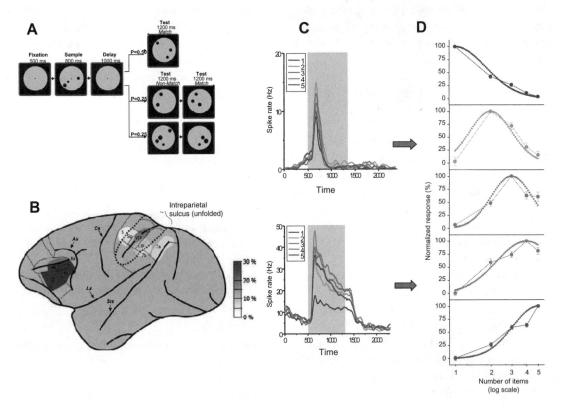

FIGURE 62.3   Evidence for Weber's law in neural coding. (Courtesy of Andreas Nieder and Earl Miller.) (*A*) Example of stimuli presented to monkeys instructed to perform a delayed match-to-sample number task on visual displays containing one to five items. (*B*) Recording sites in parietal and prefrontal cortex, with the percentage of numerosity-sensitive neurons observed in each subregion. (*C*) Responses (spike density functions) of two sample neurons, one preferentially responding to three and the other to four items. Each colored line shows the time course of activity for the five

tested numbers. Gray shading represents the sample period (800 ms). (*D*) Neural representation of number by a bank of visual numerosity detectors in the monkey prefrontal cortex. The different graphs represent the average activity of neurons tuned to different specific number (one to five from top to bottom). This population code for number coincides with the theoretical code proposed in Dehaene and Changeux's (1993) neuronal network model. (Modified from Nieder et al., 2002; Nieder and Miller, 2003; and Nieder and Miller, 2004.)

generalization to ordinal numerosity as well as to other modalities of auditory or motor stimulation.

One intriguing feature was the localization of such number-sensitive neurons in the prefrontal cortex. Intensive training may explain why many prefrontal neurons became sensitive to number in Nieder and Miller's (2003) study. However, human data suggested the intraparietal cortex, not the prefrontal cortex, as a crucial site for number processing. Although Sawamura and colleagues (2002) reported many number-tuned neurons in the superior parietal lobule, Nieder and colleagues (2002) reported finding only a small proportion of number neurons in area 7a of the inferior parietal lobule (about 7%). More recently, however, by recording in the depth of the IPS at a location that might correspond to area VIP, Nieder and Miller observed a much higher proportion of neurons tuned to numerosity (Nieder and Miller, 2004). Crucially, those neurons showed differential firing as a function of numerosity at a latency of about 80 ms, which is shorter than the value of 120 ms observed for prefrontal neurons. This is compatible with the hypothesis that numerosity is first extracted and represented in the IPS, and later transmitted to prefrontal circuits as needed for the requested task (Dehaene and Changeux, 1993). Furthermore, their localization in the depth of the IPS is a plausible monkey homologue to the site of activation observed in humans. Indeed, this localization was predicted by a human brain imaging study in which the activation during subtraction was found to be inserted within a network of visuomotor areas plausibly corresponding to areas AIP, MIP, V6A, and LIP in monkeys (Simon et al., 2002).

Several features of the response of those visual numerosity neurons illuminate the mechanisms of extraction and representation of number. First, their firing latency is independent of the number being represented. This result is not compatible with models that postulate a serial accumulator mechanism, which would therefore predict a linear increase in firing latency with numerosity (Gallistel and Gelman, 1992). It fits, however, with a parallel mechanism of numerosity abstraction as predicted by the Dehaene and Changeux (1993) model. A second important feature of number-coding neurons is that their tuning curves are broad, again suggesting approximate coding. Furthermore, this breadth is proportional to the neuron's preferred number. Thus, evidence for Weber's law can be observed at the single-neuron level, mirroring behavior. Finally, the neural tuning curves are asymmetrical on a linear scale but assume a Gaussian shape when plotted on a logarithmic scale (Nieder and Miller, 2003). Exactly like behavioral data, this suggests a compressive logarithmic neural encoding of numerical quantity.

Conclusion

The neurophysiological results reviewed in this chapter indicate that, down to a rather minute level of detail, the visual numerosity neurons observed by Nieder and Miller (2003) provide a plausible neuronal basis for the sense of number that is known to be present in animals and humans. Nevertheless, several experimental steps will be needed to confirm this hypothesis. More extensive studies in animals are needed to evaluate the abstractness and invariance of the neurons to multimodal stimuli. Investigating a greater range of numerosities, and examining the presence of those neurons in naive untrained animals, is crucial. Finally, reversible lesion or microstimulation studies are necessary to demonstrate that those neuronal representations play a causal role in the monkeys' numerical abilities. In parallel, experiments in humans with both nonsymbolic and symbolic numerical stimuli should attempt to demonstrate that a similar code for number is present in the human brain. This could be done with intracranial recordings, but it could also noninvasively using the "priming method" in fMRI (Naccache and Dehaene, 2001).

The number domain is one of the very few domains of cognitive neuroscience in which experimental studies can range from recordings of single neurons in the monkey to response-time studies of verbal symbols in humans. Such parallel studies in various species, performed using a range of experimental methods, are helping making sense of the human ability for mathematics through an integrated and progressively more coherent picture of the working brain.

REFERENCES

BARTH, H., N. KANWISHER, and E. SPELKE, 2003. The construction of large number representations in adults. *Cognition* 86:201–221.

BRANNON, E. M., and H. S. TERRACE, 2000. Representation of the numerosities 1–9 by rhesus macaques (*Macaca mulatta*). *J. Exp. Psychol. Anim. Behav. Processes* 26:31–49.

BUTTERWORTH, B., 1999. *The Mathematical Brain.* London: Macmillan.

BUTTERWORTH, B., M. CAPPELLETTI, and M. KOPELMAN, 2001. Category specificity in reading and writing: The case of number words. *Nat. Neurosci.* 4:784–786.

CHURCH, R. M., and W. H. MECK, 1984. The numerical attribute of stimuli. In *Animal Cognition*, H. L. Roilblat, T. G. Bever, and H. S. Terrace, eds. Hillsdale, N.J.: Erlbaum, pp. 445–464.

COHEN, L., and S. DEHAENE, 2000. Calculating without reading: Unsuspected residual abilities in pure alexia. *Cogn. Neuropsychol.* 17:563–583.

DEHAENE, S., 1992. Varieties of numerical abilities. *Cognition* 44:1–42.

DEHAENE, S., 1996. The organization of brain activations in number comparison: Event-related potentials and the additive-factors methods. *J. Cogn. Neurosci.* 8:47–68.

DEHAENE, S., 1997. *The Number Sense*. New York: Oxford University Press.

DEHAENE, S., S. BOSSINI, and P. GIRAUX, 1993. The mental representation of parity and numerical magnitude. *J. Exp. Psychol. Gen.* 122:371–396.

DEHAENE, S., and J.-P. CHANGEUX, 1993. Development of elementary numerical abilities: A neuronal model. *J. Cogn. Neurosci.* 5:390–407.

DEHAENE, S., and L. COHEN, 1997. Cerebral pathways for calculation: Double dissociation between rote verbal and quantitative knowledge of arithmetic. *Cortex* 33:219–250.

DEHAENE, S., and S. COHEN, 1998. Levels of representation in number processing. In *The Handbook of Neurolinguistics*, B. Stemmer and H. A. Whitaker, eds. New York: Academic Press, pp. 331–341.

DEHAENE, S., and J. F. MARQUES, 2002. Cognitive euroscience: Scalar variability in price estimation and the cognitive consequences of switching to the Euro. *Q. J. Exp. Psychol.* 55:705–731.

DEHAENE, S., M. PIAZZA, P. PINEL, and L. COHEN, 2003. Three parietal circuits for number processing. *Cogn. Neuropsychol.* 20:487–506.

DEHAENE, S., E. SPELKE, P. PINEL, R. STANESCU, and S. TSIVKIN, 1999. Sources of mathematical thinking: Behavioral and brain-imaging evidence. *Science* 284:970–974.

DELAZER, M., and T. BENKE, 1997. Arithmetic facts without meaning. *Cortex* 33:697–710.

EGER, E., P. STERZER, M. O. RUSS, A. L. GIRAUD, and A. KLEINSCHMIDT, 2003. A supramodal number representation in human intraparietal cortex. *Neuron* 37:719–725.

GALLISTEL, C. R., and I. GELMAN, 2000. Nonverbal numerical cognition: From reals to integers. *Trends Cogn. Sci.* 4:59–65.

GALLISTEL, C. R., and R. GELMAN, 1992. Preverbal and verbal counting and computation. *Cognition* 44:43–74.

ISAACS, E. B., C. J. EDMONDS, A. LUCAS, and D. G. GADIAN, 2001. Calculation difficulties in children of very low birthweight: A neural correlate. *Brain* 124:1701–1707.

LEE, K. M., 2000. Cortical areas differentially involved in multiplication and subtraction: A functional magnetic resonance imaging study and correlation with a case of selective acalculia. *Ann. Neurol.* 48:657–661.

LEE, K. M., and S. Y. KANG, 2002. Arithmetic operation and working memory: Differential suppression in dual tasks. *Cognition* 83:B63–B68.

LEMER, C., S. DEHAENE, E. SPELKE, and L. COHEN, (in press). Approximate quantities and exact number words: Dissociable systems. *Neuropsychologia*.

LEVY, L. M., I. L. REIS, and J. GRAFMAN, 1999. Metabolic abnormalities detected by H-MRS in dyscalculia and dysgraphia. *Neurology* 53:639–641.

MCCOMB, K., C. PACKER, and A. PUSEY, 1994. Roaring and numerical assessment in contests between groups of female lions. *Panthera leo. Anim. Behav.* 47:379–387.

MECK, W. H., and R. M. CHURCH, 1983. A mode control model of counting and timing processes. *J. Exp. Psychol. Anim. Behav. Processes* 9:320–334.

MECHNER, F., 1958. Probability relations within response sequences under ratio reinforcement. *J. Exp. Anal. Behav.* 1:109–121.

MOLKO, N., L. COHEN, J.-F. MANGIN, M. BRUANDET, D. LEBIHAN, and S. DEHAENE, 2003. Functional and structural alterations of the intraparietal sulcus in a developmental dyscalculia of genetic origin. *Neuron* 40:847–858.

MOYER, R. S., and T. K. LANDAUER, 1967. Time required for judgments of numerical inequality. *Nature* 215:1519–1520.

NACCACHE, L., and S. DEHAENE, 2001. The priming method: Imaging unconscious repetition priming reveals an abstract representation of number in the parietal lobes. *Cereb. Cortex* 11:966–974.

NIEDER, A., D. J. FREEDMAN, and E. K. MILLER, 2002. Representation of the quantity of visual items in the primate prefrontal cortex. *Science* 297:1708–1711.

NIEDER, A., and E. K. MILLER, 2003. Coding of cognitive magnitude: Compressed scaling of numerical information in the primate prefrontal cortex. *Neuron* 37:149–157.

NIEDER, A., and E. K. MILLER, 2004. A parieto-frontal network for visual numerical information in the monkey. *Proc. Natl. Acad. Sci. U.S.A.* 101(19):7457–7462.

PESENTI, M., M. THIOUX, X. SERON, and A. DEVOLDER, 2000. Neuroanatomical substrates of arabic number processing, numerical comparison, and simple addition: A PET Study. *J. Cogn. Neurosci.* 12:449–460.

PIAZZA, M., E. GIACOMINI, D. LE BIHAN, and S. DEHAENE, 2003. Single trial classification of parallel pre-attentive and serial attentive processes using fMRI. *Proc. R. Soc. Lond. B Biol. Sci.* 270:1237–1245.

PIAZZA, M., A. MECHELLI, B. BUTTERWORTH, and C. J. PRICE, 2002. Are subitizing and counting implemented as separate or functionally overlapping processes? *NeuroImage* 15:435–446.

PIAZZA, M., A. MECHELLI, C. PRICE, and B. BUTTERWORTH, 2003. *The quantifying brain: Functional neuroanatomy of numerosity estimation and counting*. Unpublished manuscript.

PINEL, P., S. DEHAENE, D. RIVIERE, and D. LE IHAN, 2001. Modulation of parietal activation by semantic distance in a number comparison task. *NeuroImage* 14:1013–1026.

REMOND-BESUCHET, C., M.-P. NOËL, X. SERON, M. THIOUX, M. BRUN, and X. ASPE, 1998. Selective preservation of exceptional arithmetical knowledge in a demented patient. *Math. Cognit.* 5:41–63.

ROLAND, P. E., and L. FRIBERG, 1985. Localization of cortical areas activated by thinking. *J. Neurophysiol.* 53:1219–1243.

SANDRINI, M., A. MIOZZO, M. COTELLI, and S. F. CAPPA, 2003. The residual calculation abilities of a patient with severe aphasia: Evidence for a selective deficit of subtraction procedures. *Cortex* 39:85–96.

SAWAMURA, H., K. SHIMA, and J. TANJI, 2002. Numerical representation for action in the parietal cortex of the monkey. *Nature* 415:918–922.

SIMON, O., J. F. MANGIN, L. COHEN, D. LE BIHAN, and S. DEHAENE, 2002. Topographical layout of hand, eye, calculation, and language-related areas in the human parietal lobe. *Neuron* 33:475–487.

SIMON, T. 1999. Finding the foundations of numerical thinking in a brain without numbers. *Trends Cogn. Sci.* 3:363–365.

SPELKE, E. S., and S. TSIVKIN, 2001. Language and number: A bilingual training study. *Cognition* 78:45–88.

STANESCU, R., P. PINEL, P.-F. VAN DE MOORTELE, D. LEBIHAN, L. COHEN, and S. DEHAENE, 2000. Cerebral bases of calculation processes: Impact of number size on the cerebral circuits for exact and approximative calculation. *Brain* 123:2240–2255.

STARKEY, P., E. S. SPELKE, and R. GELMAN, 1983. Detection of intermodal numerical correspondence by human infants. *Science* 222:179–181.

TEMPLE, E., and M. I. POSNER, 1998. Brain mechanisms of quantity are similar in 5-year-olds and adults. *Proc. Natl. Acad. Sci. U.S.A.* 95:7836–7841.

THIOUX, M., M. PESENTI, N. COSTES, A. DE VOLDER, and X. SERON, 2002. *Dissociating category-specific and task related cerebral activation during semantic processing.* Unpublished manuscript.

THOMPSON, R. F., K. S. MAYERS, R. T. ROBERTSON, and C. J. PATTERSON, 1970. Number coding in association cortex of the cat. *Science* 168:271–273.

VAN HARSKAMP, N. J., and L. CIPOLOTTI, 2001. Selective impairments for addition, subtraction and multiplication: Implications for the organisation of arithmetical facts. *Cortex* 37:363–388.

WARRINGTON, E. K., and M. JAMES, 1967. Tachistoscopic number estimation in patients with unilateral cerebral lesions. *J. Neurol.* 30:468–474.

WHALEN, J., C. R. GALLISTEL, and R. GELMAN, 1999. Non-verbal counting in humans: The psychophysics of number representation. *Psychol. Sci.* 10:130–137.

WOJCIULIK, E., and N. KANWISHER, 1999. The generality of parietal involvement in visual attention. *Neuron* 23:747–764.

WYNN, K., P. BLOOM, and W. C. CHIANG, 2002. Enumeration of collective entities by 5-month-old infants. *Cognition* 83:B55–B62.

XU, F., and E. S. SPELKE, 2000. Large number discrimination in 6-month-old infants. *Cognition* 74:B1–B11.

ZORZI, M., K. PRIFTIS, and, C. UMILTÀ, 2002. Brain damage: Neglect disrupts the mental number line. *Nature* 417:138–139.

63 Object Categorization, Expertise, and Neural Plasticity

JAMES W. TANAKA

ABSTRACT Drawing on results from neurophysiological and behavioral experiments with monkeys and humans, this chapter examines the role of categorization in object perception and object recognition. In perception, the process of categorization is critical for linking different retinal views of a stimulus to the same physical object. In recognition, a perceived object is categorized and identified as an exemplar of a particular object class (e.g., "animal," "dog," "beagle," "Spot"). The close tie between the processes of object categorization and object recognition argues that an object and its features cannot be defined independently of its category affiliation. This interdependency is illustrated in studies of expertise where experts recognize domain-specific objects at a level of finer perceptual detail than novices causing significant changes in neurophysiological function. This chapter views object recognition and categorization as a dynamic process that is continually changing according to the experience and task demands of the observer.

In cognitive neuroscience, object recognition lies at the boundary between visual perception and visual memory. Recognition occurs when a stimulus in the external environment activates a corresponding internal representation stored in visual memory. For example, outside my window I see something darting across the yard, and this image activates a visual memory for "cat," and on closer inspection activates the more specific memory for "my neighbor's cat." As decades of research have revealed, this seemingly effortlessness act of identification presents formidable computational challenges to scientists interested in studying the cognitive and neural basis of high level vision. The primary challenge in visual recognition concerns the issue of object invariance, that is, how are the infinite and multifaceted retinal images produced by stimuli in the world assigned to their appropriate representations in visual memory?

In this chapter, object invariance is posed as a problem of categorization. By definition, categorization is the operation by which dissimilar things are treated equivalently. At different levels of analysis, the recognition system is confronted with an array of images that vary in their visual appearance but must be categorized and regarded as similar. At a perceptual level in visual processing, different views of an object are classified and linked together in memory in order for the stimulus to be recognized from various perspectives. For example, although the front, side, and back views of my neighbor's cat are visually dissimilar, the cat is recognizable from multiple viewpoints because the different perspectives are categorized as instances of the same object.

Categorization also plays a critical role at higher cognitive levels of recognition. Typically, objects are recognized not as isolated, individual entities but as members of a broader category. For example, unless one is an expert, feline animals are recognized at the level of "cat" rather than at the level of a particular breed (e.g., Charteux, Siamese, Manx) or at the level of an individual animal (e.g., my neighbor's cat). In conventional object recognition, stimuli that are structurally dissimilar and that therefore vary in their visual appearance are nevertheless grouped together and recognized as examples of the same stimulus category. Thus, in vision, the processes of categorization operate at multiple scales of analysis, allowing the perceiver to generalize across different views of the same stimulus and to classify the stimulus as a representative of a general object class.

In this chapter, the interrelated processes of recognition and categorization are examined with respect to their cognitive and neural underpinnings. A recurrent theme in the chapter is the role that experience and learning play in shaping the categorization strategies of the perceiver and the neurophysiological properties that mediate these behaviors. In the first section, recognition invariance is described as a classification task in which previously acquired views of a stimulus are used to aid its recognition when seen from novel perspectives. The second section discusses how the cognitive demands of the categorization task determine which features of an object are encoded as most salient in memory. The effects of experience are directly addressed in the next section, where significant changes in cognitive and neurophysiological function are demonstrated as a result of perceptual expertise. In the final section, Riesenhuber and Poggio's model of object recognition provides a unifying framework for describing object categories that adapt to the task demands and experiences of the categorizer.

JAMES W. TANAKA Department of Psychology, University of Victoria, Victoria, British Columbia, Canada.

Categorization of object viewpoints

Because every change in the observer's viewpoint begets a new retinal image, a fundamental puzzle in vision concerns the activation of a singular object representation across changes in scale, translation, and orientation. For example, viewing a cat from a near or far distance or from the side or top yields a different retinal image, yet all of these images result in the recognition of a cat. Although in principle, the visual recognition system could generate a distinct memory corresponding to each object view, the amount of storage required to perform this operation is so large as to render this approach unworkable. As one solution, Marr and Nishihara (1978) proposed that the retinal image can be redescribed as a series of hierarchically arranged "sketches," beginning with simple local features and then organized at a higher level of shape contours, then complex surfaces, and finally as complete, three-dimensional (3D) objects. The computational advantage of the structural method is that the same object representation can be derived independent of the observer's viewpoint. According to the view-independent approach, object-centered representations are invariant not only across changes in the observer's viewpoint but also across the viewing experiences of the observer. Object-centered theories of recognition, such as Biederman's recogition-by-components (RBC) model (Biederman, 1987), claim that object representations are built from a limited set of geometric solids that are reliably accessed and retrieved regardless of the observer's viewpoint. The appeal of the object-centered explanation is that it solves the viewpoint problem through the use of a finite set of 3D visual primitives.

For all of its computational elegance, however, the object-centered approach fails to account for behavioral findings demonstrating the influence of perceptual experience on the recognition of novel objects. Specifically, behavioral studies have shown that participants are faster and more accurate in recognizing objects when those objects are displayed in a previously seen orientation than when they are shown in a novel orientation, even when the familiar and novel views are equated for informational content (Rock and DiVita, 1987; Tarr and Pinker, 1990; Edelman and Bülthoff, 1992). Moreover, the time to identify an object in a new orientation varies systematically as a function of its rotation from the nearest learned view, suggesting that multiple learned views of an object are stored in memory. These findings indicate that recognition is view-selective to the extent that recognition is affected by the previously learned viewpoints of the perceiver.

At the neurophysiological level, cells in the inferior temporal cortex (IT) are candidate neural structures for encoding the individual object views used in recognition. For example, single-cell recordings of IT neurons in monkeys selectively respond to familiar, complex stimuli, such as snowflake patterns (Tanaka et al., 1991) and faces (Gross, Rocha-Miranda, and Bender, 1972). In their study, Logothetis, Pauls, and Poggio (1995) trained monkeys to recognize 3D wire-shaped objects presented at multiple views of 0°, 60°, 120°, or 160° of rotation about the x-, y-, or z-axis. After training, a large proportion of IT cells responded selectively to a particular view of the target object. As the example in figure 63.1 shows, a view-selecitve cell responded maximally to the target object shown at one orientation and the cell's response decreased monotonically as the object was rotated away from this preferred view. This cell did not respond to other distracter objects containing similar visual features, such as the inverted V circled in figure 63.1, indicating a sensitivity to the orientation properties of the object rather than a local feature. View selectivity has also been shown in face perception, where IT neurons respond vigorously to faces presented in one orientation (e.g., frontal, three-quarters view, profile) and evince a corresponding drop-off in neural activity as the face rotates away from the preferred view (Perrett et al., 1991). At the neurophysiological level, the visual system registers information related not only to the identity of an object but also related to the viewing perspective from which it is encoded.

Computationally, recognition across viewpoints does not require the storage of every conceivable view of a familiar object. Instead, models of view-selective recognition (Poggio and Edelman, 1990; Ullman, 1998; Riesenhuber and Poggio, 2000) have shown that the novel views of familiar objects are recoverable from the storage of a finite number of 3D object views. According to these models, recognition of objects shown in novel views is achieved by combining the outputs of view-selective cells (Poggio and Edelman, 1990). This approach provides a viable solution to the problem of categorizing multiple views to the same object representation. The next section addresses the cognitive aspect of object recognition, namely, once a given object representation is activated, how is it assigned to a broader object category?

Object categories in humans and monkeys

OBJECT CATEGORIZATION AND ENTRY POINT RECOGNITION IN HUMANS   Although the same *chipping sparrow* object can be classified as an animal, a bird, a sparrow, or a chipping sparrow, it has been proposed that only one level of abstraction is dominant in object recognition. The critical point at which an object stimulus first makes contact with an object representation in memory has been referred to as the entry point in object recognition (Jolicoeur, Gluck, and Kosslyn, 1984). In human object recognition, the entry point in recognition is not arbitrary but the level at which category members share corresponding parts (Tversky and

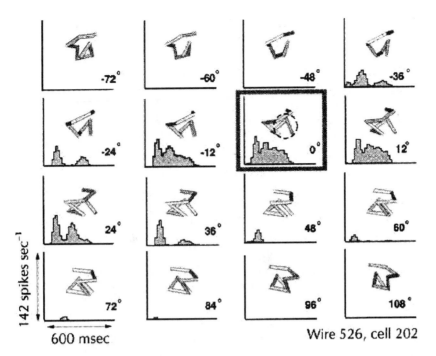

142 spikes sec⁻¹

600 msec

Wire 526, cell 202

FIGURE 63.1 Neuronal activity of a view-selective neuron in inferior temporal (IT) cortex. The cell's firing rate was maximal when the object was presented at a specific view (0°) and steadily declined as the object was rotated away from the preferred view. This cell did not demonstrate a selective response to distractor objects containing similar visual features, such as the circled inverted V feature in the illustration. This selectivity suggests that its response was based on the orientation properties of the object and not on a local feature.

Hemenway, 1984) and bear a perceptual resemblance to one another, the so-called basic level. Rosch and colleagues claimed that basic-level categories, such as "dog," "chair," or "bird," are derived from the perceptual and functional structure of object categories in the world. Therefore, basic levels and entry points in human object recognition can be defined independently of the experience of the perceiver. Supporting the primacy of the basic level in entry point recognition, it has been shown that familiar objects are most readily named and quickly identified at the basic level (Rosch et al., 1976), and this is the level at which new objects are most easily learned (Murphy and Smith, 1982). In contrast, categorizations that are superordinate to the basic level (e.g., "animal," "furniture") require additional processing time for semantic analysis, and categorizations that are subordinate to the basic level (e.g., "robin," "desk chair") require more time for perceptual processing (Jolicoeur, Gluck, and Kosslyn, 1984).

In humans, a diverse set of neural structures has been associated with basic-level categorization. For example, when participants are asked to judge whether two objects are members of the same basic-level category, posterior and anterior areas of fusiform gyrus as well as parietal cortex are activated relative to control conditions (Op de Beeck et al., 2000). Other studies have shown that the fusiform gyrus and right inferior frontal gyrus are activated during object decision tasks (Gerlack et al., 2000). In face processing, some researchers have argued that the fusiform gyrus responds to the general category of faces (Kanwisher, McDermott, and Chun, 1997), while others have hypothesized that generic face processing occurs in more occipital regions (Haxby et al., 1999). The absence of converging evidence from neuroimaging studies suggests that basic-level object processing does not occur in one specific area of the brain. Instead, a more plausible account is that basic-level recognition is distributed across many visual areas according to the properties of the object category (Martin et al., 1995).

OBJECT CATEGORIES IN MONKEYS The categories that qualify as basic to humans are also learnable by monkeys. After rheus monkeys were trained to make discriminations between trees and nontree objects, they were tested for their ability to categorize familiar and novel stimuli from the learned categories. Although novel stimuli were categorized more slowly (new: 306 ms, old: 283 ms) than the learned stimuli, they were categorized as accurately as old training stimuli (Vogels, 1999a). The transfer of category learning to new stimuli indicates that performance was not attributable to item-specific rote association but reflected encoding of a broader category structure.

Single-cell recordings in monkeys during category learning revealed that cells in IT showed differential activation to stimuli from the target category (trees) relative to nontarget stimuli (Vogels, 1999b). The nature of this activation was narrowly tuned to a few individual objects rather than broadly tuned to all of the items in the target category. The strong within-category selectivity suggests that category learning is not achieved by the activation of a group of "prototype" neurons responding to the characteristic features of the learned category. Instead, categorization behavior is supported by a population of individual, object-tuned neurons, each responding to the properties of a particular stimulus.

However, what is considered basic to humans is not necessarily basic to nonhuman primates. Monkeys demonstrate a surprising degree of flexibility in their ability to learn new object categories. For example, monkeys can learn superordinate level categories (animal versus nonanimal) quickly and can perform as accurately for novel stimuli as for familiar stimuli (Fabre-Thorpe, Richard, and Thorpe, 1998; Delorme, Richard, and Fabre-Thorpe, 2000). Furthermore, error analysis of the categorization responses revealed that decisions were not made on the basis of low-level visual features of color, texture, or form but on the kind of higher-order features, such as color *and* form, that have been identified by Kenji Tanaka and colleagues (1991).

CATEGORICAL OBJECT RECOGNITION   Rosch's structure-in-the-world position notwithstanding, object categories are not predetermined or immutable, but are adaptable and amendable to the goals and intentions of the categorizer (Barsalou, 1983). According to this adaptive view, categories emerge through interactions between the available information in the perceptual environment, the demands of the categorization task, and the experience of the categorizer (Schyns, 1998). The ability to quickly classify stimuli into meaningful categories while ignoring irrelevant perceptual differences has important ecological advantages. For a gazelle on the savanna, it would be more important to categorize a fast-approaching object as belonging to the general object class "lion" and significantly less important to distinguish this particular lion from other lions that it has encountered. The categories that are most immediate and relevant to the organism provide boundaries by which objects in the world are perceived and organized.

In this type of categorical perception, stimuli varying along a continuous dimension are differentiated relative to a category boundary. Stimuli lying on opposite sides of the category boundary are easily discriminated, whereas stimuli falling on the same side of the boundary are difficult to distinguish. The phenomenon of categorical perception has been well established in the speech perception literature, where sounds that vary according to the continuous dimension of voice onset are nevertheless perceived as members of one discrete phoneme category or another (Liberman et al., 1967). In vision, studies have shown that judgments about the expression (Calder et al., 1996), identity (Beale and Keil, 1995), and race (Levin and Beale, 2000) of a face are per-

formed categorically, as is the perception of common objects (Newell and Bulthoff, 2002).

Are there neurons in the visual object recognition system that code categorical relations in object stimuli? Cells in prefrontal cortex (PFC) share direct connections to neurons in IT and are involved in the acquisition of basic-level object categories (trees, fishes, faces) (Kobatake, Wang, and Tanaka, 1998). Using a match-to-sample task, Freedman and colleagues (2001, 2002) trained monkeys to categorize computer-generated stimuli as belonging to either the "cat" or "dog" category (figure 63.2*a*). The stimuli consisted of a continuum of images created by graphically morphing a prototypical dog image (dog:cat, 100:0) with a prototypical cat image (dog:cat, 0:100) to create four levels of dog and cat blends (dog:cat, 80:20, 60:40, 40:60, 20:80). Training continued until the monkeys classified prototypical stimuli and morph blends with 90% accuracy. After training, approximately 25% of the neurons in PFC were sensitive to the dog-cat category distinctions and responded with similar firing rates to stimuli from the same category and different firing rates to samples from the separate categories. Neuronal response, like behavioral response of the monkeys, was categorical in that the response to morph blends and category prototypes was equivalent. For example, the "dog" cell shown in figure 63.2*b* responded with same level of increased activity to 60:40 dog stimulus as the prototypical dog stimulus. Similarly, changing the relative contribution of the 60:40 dog stimulus to a 40:60 cat stimulus elicited the same baseline response as the prototypical cat stimulus. These findings indicate that PFC cells responded categorically to a range of inputs that varied along the graded continuum of morphs.

Given that the monkeys had no prior experience to the dogs and cats, it was likely that the selective response of the PFC neurons was a direct result of category learning. As a further test of the learning account, Freedman and colleagues retrained one of the monkeys to classify the morph stimuli into three new categories that were orthogonal to the previously learned dog-cat categories. After learning, it was found that PFC neurons exhibited differential responses to stimuli that were separated by these new category boundaries and did not distinguish stimuli that crossed the old category boundary between dogs and cats. These results indicate the flexibility of neurons in PFC to learn new task-relevant object categories and to unlearn old categories that are no longer meaningful to the animal.

OBJECT CATEGORIES AND OBJECT FEATURES   Categories constrain object perception by determining those features of an object that are diagnostic to the category and become perceptually salient to the categorizer. The link between categories and perception was demonstrated in a study by Schyns and Murphy (1994) in which they asked participants

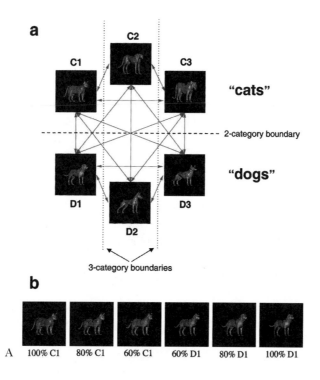

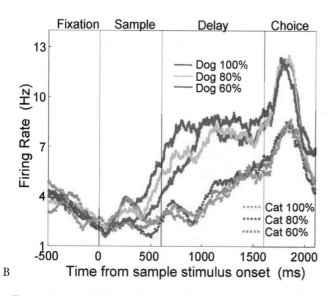

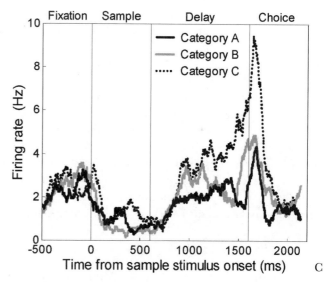

FIGURE 63.2 (*a*) Morph stimuli used in an object categorization task reported by Freedman and colleagues (2001, 2002). In the two-category task, the monkeys learned to classify prototypes of cats (C1, C2, C3) and dogs (D1, D2, D3) into the cat or dog category, respectively. In the three-category task, prototype stimuli were reassigned to three new categories that comprised the prototypes of C1 and D1, C2 and D2, and C3 and D3, respectively. (*b*) After learning, morphs along the cat–dog continuum (e.g., C1–D2) were pre-

sented for classification. (*c*) Single-cell response of a dog-selective neuron to six levels of morph. During the delay and choice periods, the neuron demonstrated an increased response to stimuli containing a larger proportion of the dog prototype (i.e., Dog 100%, Dog 80%, Dog 60%) than the cat prototype. The response was categorical to the degree that the Dog 60% and Dog 80% stimuli elicited the same level of increased activity as the Dog 100% stimulus. (See color plate 40.)

to categorize complex 3D shaded objects (Martian rocks) as Category A rocks or Category B rocks. Category A objects always included *part a*, whereas Category B objects always included *part b*. Before category learning, participants seldom identified part a or part b as a separate feature of the stimulus, but after category learning they always did so. When exposed to a novel group of rocks (Category C), all of which had parts a and b, the categorization groups delineated parts a and b as two distinct units, whereas naive subjects grouped parts a and b together as a single part. These results indicate a distinction between functional and perceptual parts of an object. Whereas perceptual parts correspond to points of the structural discontinuities in objects that allow them to be parsed into distinct subunits (Hoffman and Richards, 1985), functional parts are the perceptual features that are useful for categorization and cannot be defined independent of the categorization task or the learning history of categorizer.

At the neurophysiological level, neurons in IT become selectively tuned to the parts or features of an object that are diagnostic to a category. Sigala and Logothetis (2002) trained monkeys to categorize stimuli (faces or fish) into two categories. Each stimulus set contained four features, but only two of the features were diagnostic, that is, relevant to the categorization task. After categorization learning, 75% of the feature-selective neurons were more responsive to the diagnostic features than to the nondiagnostic features. These findings indicate that at the neuronal level, cells in IT become selectively tuned to the object features that are most diagnostic to the categorization task at hand and learn to ignore those features that are not.

The studies reviewed in this section demonstrate the interconnectivity between the observer's perceptions, categories, and goals in object processing. These studies show that the perceptual features of an object are constrained by the category in which it is placed, as determined by the goals and task demands of the observer. In the next section, the link between object categories and underlying brain activity is further examined in the context of perceptual expertise.

The plasticity of expertise

DOWNWARD SHIFTS IN ENTRY POINT RECOGNITION Although most people recognize objects at the basic level (e.g., "bird," "dog"), dog or bird experts recognize objects in their domain of expertise at more specific, subordinate levels of abstraction (Tanaka and Taylor, 1991; Johnson and Mervis, 1997). Behaviorally, object experts spontaneously name objects in their domain of expertise with subordinate labels (e.g., a bird expert identifies birds by their subordinate-level name, "sparrow" or "chipping sparrow"), list significantly more perceptual attributes at the subordinate level for expert objects, and are as fast to identify objects of expertise at the subordinate level as the basic level (Tanaka and Taylor,

1991). The downward shift in entry point recognition to subordinate-level categories is the hallmark of expertise (Gauthier and Tarr, 1997; Gauthier et al., 1998). These studies have shown that experts recognize objects in their domain at a fundamentally different level than novices.

Granted that relatively few individuals qualify as genuine object experts, it has been claimed that virtually everyone is an expert in the recognition of faces (Carey, 1992). As face experts, humans preferentially attend to faces in the environment and identify familiar faces at subordinate levels of abstraction. The level of categorization associated with normal face recognition constitutes a level that is even more subordinate than the level associated with other types of object expertise. For example, the relevant level of categorization for bird experts is the subspecies level (e.g., "chipping sparrow") and for car experts, it is the make, model, and year of an automobile (e.g., "2001 Honda Accord"). In comparison, the primary level of face recognition is at the level of the individual, in which there is only one person in the category, and so the individual can be identified by its proper name (e.g., "Elvis," "Tony Blair"). At the level of the individual face, faces share maximal perceptual similarity to other faces. Yet, as face experts, humans are as fast to identify familiar faces at the individual level (e.g., "Arnold Schwartzenegger") as they are to categorize faces at the basic level (e.g., "face") (Tanaka, 2001). Thus, similar to other types of expertise, face expertise results in a downward shift in entry point recognition. However, in contrast to other types of object expertise, face recognition represents expert object recognition in the extreme, where identification occurs at the level of the individual face.

Experts not only recognize familiar objects in their domain of expertise more quickly, specifically, and accurately than novices, they also seem to have an advantage in learning and discriminating novel, unfamiliar objects in their specialty area. After several days of practice, for example, greeble experts are able to learn new greebles from familiar greeble families faster than nongreeble experts (Gauthier et al., 1998). Similarly, participants trained to recognize birds at the species level (e.g., burrowing owl) demonstrated perceptual transfer in their ability to discriminate novel species of birds from the same family (e.g., screech owl). In contrast, participants trained to classify birds at the family level (e.g., owl) showed no evidence of perceptual transfer (Tanaka, Curran, and Sheinberg, in press). These findings suggest that subordinate-level categories play a crucial role in the transfer of perceptual abilities.

THE ELECTROPHYSIOLOGY OF FACE AND OBJECT EXPERTISE Behavioral changes produced by perceptual experience and expertise with faces and objects are mirrored by significant changes in brain function. Studies of event-related potentials (ERPs) have shown that face stimuli elicit an enhanced negative deflection in posterior recording sites approximately 170 ms post-stimulus onset relative to nonface objects (e.g., cars, flowers, furniture). The so-called face N170 is purported to reflect a specific set of neural operations that are specialized for the processing of face stimuli and are not recruited for the processing of other nonface stimuli (Bentin et al., 1996). An important question is whether the face N170 is specific to faces or whether it indicates a more global marker of perceptual expertise. To address this issue, Tanaka and Curran (2001) monitored the brain activity of dog and bird experts while they categorized pictures of common dogs and birds. The main finding was that experts showed an enhancement of the N170 component as a function of their expertise (figure 63.3). Specifically, whereas the brain activity of bird experts revealed an increased N170 to pictures of birds relative to pictures of dogs, dog experts showed a greater neurological response to dogs relative to birds. At a relatively early point in processing, the brain activity elicited by faces and expert objects is different from the brain activity produced by other objects.

Despite their similarities, it is controversial whether the face N170 and the expert N170 rely on common neural generators and whether they are indicative of similar cognitive operations (see discussion in Bentin and Carmel, 2002; Rossion, Curran, and Gauthier, 2002). In a recent study, Gauthier and colleagues (2003) reasoned that if the expert N170 and the face N170 reflected the holistic analysis associated with face and expert recognition, then the holistic processing of one type of expert object (e.g., cars) should interfere with the other type (e.g., faces). Consistent with this prediction, they found that concurrent holistic processing of faces and cars proved to be *more* disruptive to the face recognition performance of experts than novices. Critically, the difference in the N170 between faces and cars was also correlated with expertise, such that the car-face N170 difference was smaller for experts than for novices. Taken together, these results suggest that the N170 provides a metric by which holistic processes can be measured during face recognition and expert object recognition.

THE NEURAL SUBSTRATES OF FACE AND EXPERT OBJECT RECOGNITION   It is well established that ventral area of the temporal lobe of the right hemisphere, a region referred to as the fusiform face area (FAA), is selectively activated by the presentation of face stimuli relative to other stimuli (Sergent, Ohta, and MacDonald, 1992; Puce et al., 1995; Kanwisher, McDermott, and Chun, 1997). Neuropsychological studies have shown that damage to this area in humans can result in prosopagnosia, a condition in which patients experience a selective loss in their ability to recognize faces but not other objects. The specificity of this loss can be quite striking, as demonstrated by the case of the sheep farmer W.J., who lost his ability to recognize individual faces yet retained his ability to recognize individual sheep (McNeil and Warrington, 1993). These findings have led researchers to propose a domain-specific, face-processing module exclusively used for face recognition and not recruited for the recognition of nonface objects (Farah, 1995).

An alternative view is that face recognition taps into a general, expert recognition module that is activated by faces for most people and by objects of expertise for experts (Tarr and Gauthier, 2000). Support for the expert module account comes from neuroimaging studies in which the putative fusiform face area is similarly activated by objects of expertise. For example, studies of real-world experts showed that an overlapping pattern of FFA activity was found in response to faces in control participants, to car stimuli in car experts, and to bird stimuli in bird experts (Gauthier et al., 2000). A study of laboratory-trained experts revealed that as participants gained expertise in recognizing artificial greeble objects, there was a corresponding increase in FFA activity to greebles (Gauthier et al., 1999). The studies of real-world and laboratory-trained experts indicate that the fusiform gyrus is not reserved for the exclusive processing of faces. Instead, this brain area demonstrates a remarkable degree of plasticity as a consequence of perceptual experience and training.

Rather than specific to faces, it is argued that the fusiform gyrus carries out processes that are common to both expert object recognition and face recognition (Tarr and Gauthier, 2000). What are the computations that are common to face recognition and expert object recognition? Although faces are distinguished from other objects of expertise by their social importance and the age and frequency of exposure, expert object recognition shares important processing characteristics with face recognition. First, objects of expertise, like faces, are recognized at subordinate levels of abstraction, inducing a holistic rather than a parts-based recognition strategy. Second, object experts, like face experts, recognize objects in their domain quickly, accurately, and relatively automatically (Gauthier et al., 2000; Tanaka and Curran, 2001). According to the expertise approach, the FFA acts as a domain-general mechanism that responds flexibly to the task demands and experience of the perceiver (Tarr and Gauthier, 2000). In principle, other types of expert recognition with similar computational goals would be expected to recruit the resources of the FFA.

A perceptual and cognitive model of object categorization

This chapter has reviewed two fundamental problems in vision involving categorization. First, at a perceptual level, different views of the same object must be categorized and tagged as belonging to the same object stimulus. Second, at a conceptual level, different objects must be classified as belonging to the same object category. In Riesenhuber and

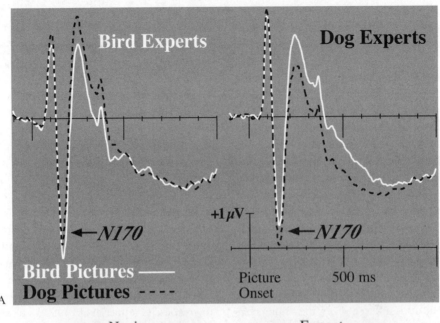

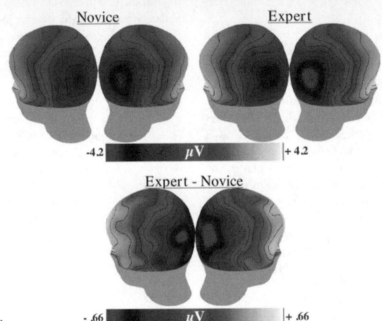

FIGURE 63.3 (*A*) Wave plots of the composite N170 channels for bird experts (left) and dog experts (right). For each group, event-related potentials are plotted separately for bird and dog stimuli. Bird experts showed an increased N170 response to pictures of birds, whereas dog experts showed an increased N170 response to pictures of dogs. (*B*) Topographic distribution of the expert N170. Top illustrations show the left and right views of the mean N170 voltages for novice and expert domains. Illustration at the bottom shows the mean differences between expert and novice domains. (See color plate 41.)

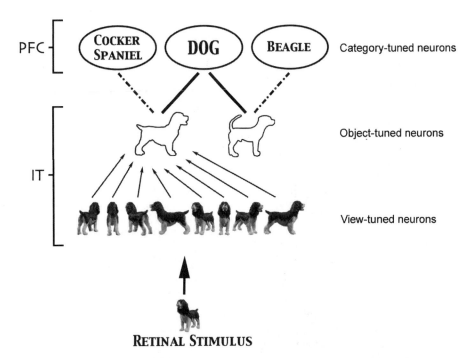

FIGURE 63.4 A perceptual and cognitive model of object categorization. At the perceptual level in Riesenhuber and Poggio's model, the retinal stimulus is encoded by view-tuned neurons in IT cortex and project their outputs to object-tuned neurons. Object-tuned neurons in turn achieve viewpoint independence by pooling signals across a subpopulation of view-tuned neurons. At the cognitive level, category-tuned neurons in PFC activate the task-relevant, object-tuned neurons. For basic-level categorization, the activation between the category-tuned neuron "dog" in PFC and the object-tuned neurons of cocker spaniel and beagle are strengthened (as indicated by the solid lines). In contrast, for subordinate-level categorization, only the connection between the category-tuned neuron "cocker spaniel" and its corresponding object-tuned neuron are activated (as indicated by dot-dashed line).

Poggio's model (2000), perceptual, view-based categorization and cognitive, object-based categorizations are handled by similar computations but carried out by distinct neural structures (figure 63.4).

During perceptual categorization, cells from primary visual and posterior infereotemporal regions encode specific views of an object. These view-selective or view-tuned neurons project their outputs to other object-tuned neurons in the anterior areas of the anterior inferior temporal (AIT) cortex. The inputs to the object-tuned neurons can activate representations of individual objects, such as a familiar face (e.g., "Joe Smith") or particular object (e.g., "my car"). By pooling together inputs from many view-tuned neurons, the corresponding object-tuned unit is activated in AIT.

At the cognitive level, top-down activation is provided by task-related or category-tuned neurons in PFC. This is the point at which a stimulus is categorized at either a basic (e.g., dog) or subordinate (e.g., cocker spaniel) level of abstraction. By projecting their outputs back to the object layer, the category-tuned neurons in PFC can modulate the activity of the object-tuned cells. According to this approach, PFC neurons act like the switch operator, strengthening incoming inputs according to the relevant object identification or categorization task at hand. Hence, a different constellation of object-based neurons in IT will be recruited by category-tuned neurons in PFC, depending on category level and task demands.

Downward shifts in expertise are triggered by strengthening the connections between the subordinate-level category-tuned neurons and object-based neurons. During the acquisition of expertise, subordinate-level category neurons in PFC are differentially activated over basic-level neurons. This subordinate-level bias is propagated back to the corresponding neurons in IT at the object level. In figure 63.4, activation of the category level of "cocker spaniel," for example, provides top-down feedback to a corresponding object-level unit that helps to differentiate this object-level unit from other subordinate level competitors, such as "beagle." The downward shift in recognition is produced by strengthening the connections between the category- and object-tuned neurons through extensive experience and feedback. When an object from the domain of expertise is represented as its input, the subordinate-level unit will be preferentially activated over the basic-level or superordinate-level representations.

The model proposed by Riesenhuber and Poggio is an extension of earlier exemplar-based theories of categorization in which a stimulus is classified according to its overall similarity to other category members (Nosofsky, 1991). For example, a stimulus would be classified as a dog if its similarity to other exemplars in the dog category is greater than its similarity to the exemplars from competing contrast categories, such as cats, birds, and horses. Exemplar-based theories have been successful in predicting the categorization behaviors of both monkeys (Sigala and Logothetis, 2002) and humans (Medin and Schaffer, 1978; Nosofsky, 1991). Prototype models, on the other hand, postulate that a stimulus is classified according to its similarity to a single, prototypical category representation (Posner and Keele, 1968; Reed and Freedman, 1973). Following this method, an object would be classified as a dog if its similarity to the prototypical representation for dogs were greater than its similarity to the prototypes from other contrast categories. Prototype accounts have been useful for explaining aftereffects (Leopold et al., 2001) and caricature effects (Rhodes, Brennan, and Carey, 1987) in face processing. Although there is less neurophysiological evidence to support the prototype position, it is still a hotly contested issue as to whether categorization is achieved by exemplars, prototypes, or a combination of the two representations.

Summary

Research in humans and monkeys on object categorization indicates that object categories are adaptive representations that are continually being created and modified in response to the perceptual experiences and demands of the observer. Whereas an object is imbued with physical properties of size, shape, color, and texture, the features of the object that are perceived, attended to, and ultimately encoded are dictated by the observer's category goals. At the neurophysiological level, object categories and strategies are reflected in the distinct firing patterns of individual neurons, the activation of specialized cell populations, and the recruitment of specific neural structures. Based on the converging behavioral and neurophysiological evidence presented in this chapter, a complete theory of object recognition will need to take into account the learning history and categorization goals of the organism.

ACKNOWLEDGMENTS   This work was supported by grants from the James S. McDonnell Foundation, National Institutes of Health, and National Sciences and Engineering Research Council of Canada. I would like to thank members of the Perceptual Expertise Network for their intellectual contributions to the chapter.

REFERENCES

BARSALOU, L. W., 1983. Ad hoc categories. *Mem. Cognit.* 11: 211–227.

BEALE, J. M., and F. C. KEIL, 1995. Categorical effects in the perception of faces. *Cognition* 57:217–239.

BENTIN, S., T. ALLISON, A. PUCE, E. PEREZ, and G. MCCARTHY, 1996. Electrophysiological studies of face perception in humans. *J. Cogn. Neurosci.* 8:551–565.

BENTIN, S., and D. CARMEL, 2002. Accounts for the N170 face-effect: A reply to Rossion, Curran & Gauthier. *Cognition* 85: 197–202.

BIEDERMAN, I., 1987. Recognition-by-Components: A theory of human image understanding. *Psychol. Rev.* 94:115–145.

CALDER, A. J., A. W. YOUNG, D. I. PERRETT, N. L. ETCOFF, and D. ROWLAND, 1996. Categorical perception of morphed facial expressions. *Vis. Cogn.* 3:81–117.

CAREY, S., 1992. Becoming a face expert. *Philos. Trans. R. Soc. Lond. B* 335:95–103.

DELORME, A., G. RICHARD, and M. FABRE-THORPE, 2000. Ultra-rapid categorisation of natural scenes does not reply on colour cues: A study in monkeys and humans. *Vision Res.* 40:2187–2200.

EDELMAN, S., and H. BÜLTHOFF, 1992. Orientation dependence in the recognition of familiar and novel views of three-dimensional objects. *Vision* 32:2385–2400.

FABRE-THORPE, M., G. RICHARD, and S. J. THORPE, 1998. Rapid categorization of natural images by rhesus monkeys. *Neuroreport* 9:303–308.

FARAH, M., 1995. Is face recognition "special"? Evidence from neuropsychology. *Behav. Brain Res.* 76:181–189.

FREEDMAN, D. J., M. RISENHUBER, T. POGGIO, and E. K. MILLER, 2001. Categorical representation of visual stimuli in the primate prefrontal cortex. *Science* 291:312–316.

FREEDMAN, D., M. RIESENHUBER, T. POGGIO, and E. K. MILLER, 2002. Visual categorization and primate prefrontal cortex: Neurophysiology and behavior. *J. Neurophysiol.* 88:929–941.

GAUTHIER, I., T. CURRAN, K. M. CURBY, and D. COLLINS, 2003. Perceptual interference supports a non-modular account of face processing. *Nat. Neurosci.* 6:428–432.

GAUTHIER, I., P. SKUDLARSKI, J. GORE, and A. ANDERSON, 2000. Expertise for cars and birds recruits brain areas involved in face recognition. *Nat. Neurosci.* 3:191–197.

GAUTHIER, I., and M. J. TARR, 1997. Becoming a "Greeble" expert: Exploring the face recognition mechanism. *Vision Res.* 37: 1673–1682.

GAUTHIER, I., M. J. TARR, A. W. ANDERSON, P. SKUDLARKSI, and J. C. GORE, 1999. Activation of the middle fusiform "face area" increases with expertise in recognizing novel objects. *Nat. Neurosci.* 2:568–573.

GAUTHIER, I., P. WILLIAMS, M. J. TARR, and J. W. TANAKA, 1998. Training "Greeble" experts: A framework for studying expert object recognition processes. *Vision Res.* 38:2401–2428.

GERLACK, C., I. LAW, A. GADE, and O. B. PAULSON, 2000. Categorization and category effects in normal object recognition: A PET study. *Neuropsychologia* 38:1693–1703.

GROSS, C. G., C. E. ROCHA-MIRANDA, and D. B. BENDER, 1972. Visual properties of neurons in inferotemporal cortex of the macaque. *J. Neurophysiol.* 35:96–111.

HAXBY, J. V., L. G. UNGERLEIDER, V. P. CLARK, J. L. SCHOUTEN, E. A. HOFFMAN, and A. MARTIN, 1999. The effect of face inversion on activity in human neural systems for face and object perception. *Neuron* 22:189–199.

HOFFMAN, D., and D. RICHARDS, 1985. Parts in recognition. *Cognition* 18:65–96.

JOHNSON, K., and C. MERVIS, 1997. Effects of varying levels of expertise on the basic level of categorization. *J. Exp. Psychol. Gen.* 126:248–277.

JOLICOEUR, P., M. A. GLUCK, and S. M. KOSSLYN, 1984. Pictures and names: Making the connection. *Cogn. Psychol.* 16:243–275.

KANWISHER, N., J. MCDERMOTT, and M. M. CHUN, 1997. The fusiform face area: A module in human extrastriate cortex specialized for face perception. *J. Neurosci.* 17:4302–4311.

KOBATAKE, E., G. WANG, and K. TANAKA, 1998. Effects of shape discrimination training on the selectivity of inferotemporal cells in adult monkeys. *J. Neurophysiol.* 80:324–330.

LEOPOLD, D. A., A. J. O'TOOLE, T. VETTER, and V. BLANZ, 2001. Prototype-referenced shape encoding revealed by high-level aftereffects. *Nat. Neurosci.* 4:89–94.

LEVIN, D. T., and J. M. BEALE, 2000. Categorical perception occurs in newly learned faces, other-race faces, and inverted faces. *Percept. Psychophys.* 62:386–401.

LIBERMAN, A. M., F. S. COOPER, D. P. SHANKWEILER, and M. STUDDERT-KENNEDY, 1967. Perception of the speech code. *Psychol. Rev.* 74:431–461.

LOGOTHETIS, N. K., J. PAULS, and T. POGGIO, 1995. Shape representation in the inferior temporal cortex of monkeys. *Curr. Biol.* 5:552–563.

MARR, D., and H. NISHIHARA, 1978. Representation and recognition of the spatial organization of three-dimensional shapes. *Proc. R. Soc. Lond. B* 200:269–294.

MARTIN, A., C. L. WIGGS, L. G. UNGERLEIDER, and J. V. HAXBY, 1995. Neural correlates of category-specific knowledge. *Nature* 379:649–652.

MCNEIL, J., and E. WARRINGTON, 1993. Prosopagnosia, a face-specific disorder. *Q. J. Exp. Psychol.* 46A:1–10.

MEDIN, D. L., and M. M. SCHAFFER, 1978. Context theory of classification learning. *Psychol. Rev.* 85:207–238.

MURPHY, G., and E. SMITH, 1982. Basic level superiority in picture categorization. *J. Verb. Learn. Verb. Behav.* 21:1–20.

NEWELL, F., and H. BULTHOFF, 2002. Categorical perception of familiar objects. *Cognition* 85:113–143.

NOSOFSKY, R. M., 1991. Tests of exemplar model for relating perceptual classification and recognition memory. *J. Exp. Psychol. Hum. Percept. Perform.* 17:3–27.

OP DE BEECK, H., E. BEATSE, J. WAGEMANS, S. SUNAERT, and P. VAN HECKE, 2000. The representation of shape in the context of visual object categorization tasks. *NeuroImage* 12:28–40.

PERRETT, D. I., M. W. ORAM, M. H. HARRIES, R. BEVAN, I. K. HIETANEN, P. J. BEASON, and S. THOMAS, 1991. Viewer-centered and object-centered coding of heads in the macaque temporal cortex. *Exp. Brain Res.* 86:150–175.

POGGIO, T., and S. EDELMAN, 1990. A network that learns to recognize three-dimensional objects. *Nature* 343:263–266.

POSNER, M. I., and S. W. KEELE, 1968. On the gensis of abstract ideas. *J. Exp. Psychol.* 77:353–363.

PUCE, A., T. ALLISON, J. C. GORE, and G. MCCARTHY, 1995. Face-sensitive regions in human extrastriate cortex studied by functional MRI. *J. Neurophysiol.* 74:1192–1199.

REED, S. K., and M. P. FREEDMAN, 1973. Perceptual vs. conceptual categorization. *Mem. Cognit.* 1:157–163.

RHODES, G., S. BRENNAN, and S. CAREY, 1987. Identification and ratings of caricatures: Implications for mental representations of faces. *Cogn. Psychol.* 19:473–497.

RIESENHUBER, M., and T. POGGIO, 2000. Models of object recognition. *Nat. Neurosci.* 3:1199–1204.

ROCK, I., and J. DIVITA, 1987. A case of viewer-centered object perception. *Cogn. Psychol.* 19:280–293.

ROSCH, E., C. MERVIS, W. GRAY, D. JOHNSON, and P. BOYES-BRAEM, 1976. Basic objects in natural categories. *Cogn. Psychol.* 8:382–439.

ROSSION, B., T. CURRAN, and I. GAUTHIER, 2002. A defense of subordinate-level expertise account for the N170 component. *Cognition* 85:189–196.

SCHYNS, P. G., 1998. Diagnostic recognition: Task constraints, object information, and their interactions. In *Object Recognition in Man, Monkey and Machine*, M. J. Tarr and H. H. Bulthoff, eds. Cambridge, Mass.: MIT Press.

SCHYNS, P. G., and G. L. MURPHY, 1994. The ontongeny of part representation in object concepts. In *The Psychology of Learning and Motivation*, vol. 31, D. Medin, ed. San Diego, Calif.: Academic Press, pp. 305–354.

SERGENT, J., S. OHTA, and B. MACDONALD, 1992. Functional neuroanatomy of face and object processing. *Brain* 115:15–36.

SIGALA, N., F. GABBIANI, and N. K. LOGOTHETIS, 2001. Visual categorization and object representation in monkeys and humans. *J. Cogn. Neurosci.* 14:1–12.

SIGALA, N., and N. K. LOGOTHETIS, 2002. Visual categorization shapes feature selectivity in the primate temporal cortex. *Nature* 415:318–320.

TANAKA, J. W., 2001. The entry point of face recognition: Evidence for face expertise. *J. Exp. Psychol. Gen.* 130:534–543.

TANAKA, J. W., and T. CURRAN, 2001. The neural basis of expert object recognition. *Psychol. Sci.* 12:43–47.

TANAKA, J. W., and M. TAYLOR, 1991. Object categories and expertise: Is the basic level in the eye of the beholder? *Cogn. Psychol.* 23:457–482.

TANAKA, J. W., T. CURRAN, and D. L. SHEINBERG (in press). The training of real world perceptual expertise. *Psychol. Sci.*

TANAKA, K., H. A. SAITO, Y. FUKADA, and M. MORIYA, 1991. Coding visual images of objects in the inferotemporal cortex of the macaque monkey. *J. Neurophysiol.* 66:170–189.

TARR, M. J., and I. GAUTHIER, 2000. FFA: A flexible fusiform area for subordinate-level visual processing automatized by expertise. *Nat. Neurosci.* 3:764–769.

TARR, M., and S. PINKER, 1990. When does human object recognition use a viewer-centered reference frame? *Psychol. Sci.* 19:253–256.

TVERSKY, B., and K. HEMENWAY, 1984. Objects, parts, and categories. *J. Exp. Psychol. Gen.* 113:169–193.

ULLMAN, S., ed., 1998. *Three-Dimensional Object Recogniton Based on the Combination of Views.* Cambridge, Mass.: MIT Press.

VOGELS, R., 1999a. Categorization of complex visual images by rhesus monkeys. Part I. Behavioral study. *Eur. J. Neurosci.* 11:1223–1238.

VOGELS, R., 1999b. Categorization of complex visual images by rhesus monkeys: Part 2. Single-cell study. *Eur. J. Neurosci.* 11:1239–1255.

64 Spatial and Temporal Distribution of Face and Object Representations in the Human Brain

JAMES V. HAXBY, M. IDA GOBBINI, AND K. MONTGOMERY

ABSTRACT Functional brain imaging has revealed that the functional architecture of ventral object vision pathway has a macroscopic organization. This architecture is characterized most commonly in terms of regions that demonstrate category-related response preferences, most notably the fusiform face area, which responds maximally during face perception, and the parahippocampal place area, which responds maximally to scenes and buildings. The representation of faces and object categories, however, extends beyond the boundaries of these regions that are defined by the stimuli that elicit maximal responses. Faces and other object categories evoke distinct patterns of response across expanses of ventral temporal cortex that include cortex that responds submaximally to the category being viewed. Thus, representations of faces are distributed locally within ventral temporal cortex. The representation of faces and objects also is distributed across other cortical areas. A second, locally distributed representation of faces and objects exists in lateral temporal cortex. Whereas the representation in ventral temporal cortex appears to contain information about the appearance of object form, the representation in lateral temporal cortex appears to contain information about how faces, bodies, and objects move. Neural responses to faces are also distributed across time. The early and late parts of responses to faces and objects show different effects of memory and attention and may reflect a differentiation between early feedforward processing and later processing with stronger effects of interregional interactions. Thus, the neural representations of faces and objects appear to be distributed in time as well as in space.

Functional brain imaging has revealed a complex, macroscopic organization in the functional architecture of the ventral object vision pathway. Numerous studies have found regions of ventral temporal cortex that consistently demonstrate category-related response preferences (Puce et al., 1996, 1998; Kanwisher, McDermott, and Chun, 1997; McCarthy et al., 1997; Epstein and Kanwisher, 1998; Aguirre, Zarahn, and D'Esposito, 1998; Haxby et al., 1999; Ishai et al., 1999; Chao, Haxby, and Martin, 1999; Chao, Martin, and Haxby, 1999; Downing, Jiang, et al., 2001; Hasson et al., 2003), most notably a region that responds maximally during face perception, the fusiform face area (Kanwisher, McDermott, and Chun, 1997; McCarthy et al., 1997), and a region that responds maximally during perception of scenes, interior spaces, and buildings, the parahippocampal place area (Epstein and Kanwisher, 1998). Faces and numerous other object categories, however, also evoke distinct patterns of response across wider expanses of ventral temporal cortex, including distinct patterns of response in cortical regions that respond submaximally to the category being viewed, suggesting that the representations of these categories extend beyond the regions defined by category preference. Thus, representations of faces and objects are distributed locally within ventral temporal cortex. A second, locally distributed representation of objects may exist in lateral temporal cortex, including regions in the posterior superior temporal sulcus (STS) and middle temporal gyrus (Puce et al., 1998; Haxby et al., 1999; Martin, Ungerleider, and Haxby, 1999; Hoffman and Haxby, 2000; Haxby, Hoffman, and Gobbini, 2000; Beauchamp et al., 2002, 2003). Whereas the representation in ventral temporal cortex appears to contain information about the appearance of object form, the representation in lateral temporal cortex appears to contain information about how faces, bodies, and objects move and about aspects of form that imply movement or can change with movement.

Faces and other categories of objects also evoke neural responses in cortical areas outside of the ventral object vision pathway (Martin et al., 1995, 1996; Hoffman and Haxby, 2000; Haxby, Hoffman, and Gobbini, 2000; Chao and Martin, 2000). These responses indicate the spontaneous activation of other information associated with objects, such as the emotion associated with a facial expression, the direction of attention indicated by eye gaze, the

JAMES V. HAXBY, M. IDA GOBBINI, and K. MONTGOMERY   Department of Psychology, Princeton University, Princeton, N.J.

phonological content associated with speech-related mouth movements, or the hand motion associated with tool use. Thus, the representation of visually presented objects appears to be not only distributed locally within the ventral object vision pathway but also extended across other cortical areas.

Neural responses to faces and objects are also distributed across time. Responses can differ for different objects as early as about 100 ms after an object appears. The early and late parts of responses to faces and objects show different effects of memory and attention (Bentin et al., 1996; Bentin and Deouell, 2000; Eimer, 2000a,b; Paller et al., 2000, 2003; Furey et al., 2001; Henson et al., 2003), and may reflect different levels of object differentiation (Sugase et al., 1999). Thus, the neural representations of faces and objects appear to be distributed in time as well as in space.

In this chapter, we review the functional neuroanatomy of face and object recognition, with an emphasis on explicating how representations are distributed in space and time. We will argue that the three different ways in which neural representations are distributed—locally, within cortical areas, extended across cortical areas, and extended over time—play three distinct functional roles in face and object processing. Local distribution of category-related activity within a cortical area reflects population responses that represent entities within a multidimensional representational space. Extended distribution of category-related activity across cortical areas reflects the spontaneous activation of different types of information that are associated with faces and objects and can play an integral role in accurate recognition. Distribution of neural activity across time reflects the evolution of a representation from early, coarse categorizing activity to finer within-category discriminations that are elaborated by input from multiple cortical areas.

Functional architecture of the ventral object vision pathway

Early functional imaging studies identified the ventral object vision pathway in regions of the inferior occipital, fusiform, and lingual gyri that were activated during the perception of faces, color, and shape (Lueck et al., 1989; Corbetta et al., 1990, 1991; Zeki et al., 1991; Haxby et al., 1991, 1994; Sergent, Ohta, and MacDonald, 1992). In 1995, Malach and colleagues showed that a region in lateral inferior occipital cortex responded more to intact, meaningful objects than to nonsense images, which they called the lateral occipital (LO) area (Malach et al., 1995). Malach and colleagues have further demonstrated that LO represents objects, insofar as the response of this area is invariant over manipulations of size and shape (Grill-Spector et al., 1999) and responds best when large-scale, holistic object features are intact (Lerner et al., 2001).

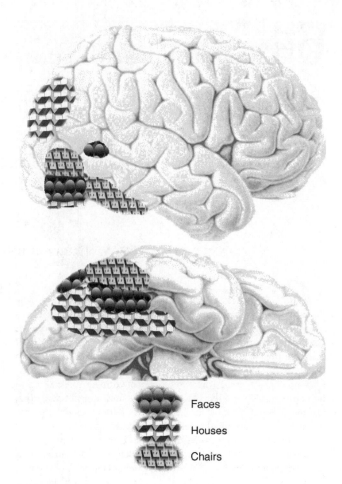

FIGURE 64.1 Locations of regions in occipitotemporal cortex that respond preferentially to faces, houses, and chairs. (Adapted from Ishai et al., 2000.)

The macroscopic functional architecture of the ventral object vision pathway was discovered by investigators searching for subregions that responded preferentially to some categories of faces or objects rather than others (Puce et al., 1996; Kanwisher, McDermott, and Chun, 1997; McCarthy et al., 1997; Aguirre, Zarahn, and D'Esposito, 1998; Epstein and Kanwisher, 1998; Chao, Haxby, and Martin, 1999; Chao, Martin, and Haxby, 1999; Haxby et al., 1999; Ishai et al., 1999; figures 64.1 and 64.2). Thus, most subsequent work has proceeded on the assumption that the identification of a region that responds maximally to a category indicates the location of neural activity that embodies the representation of that category or the perceptual processes that are recruited for that category.

CATEGORY-SPECIFIC MODULES A stricter version of this perspective holds that at least part of the object vision pathway is organized into "modules" for specific categories that have dedicated processors because of their biological significance (figure 64.2C). In 1997, Kanwisher, McDermott, and Chun (1997) and McCarthy and colleagues (1997) iden-

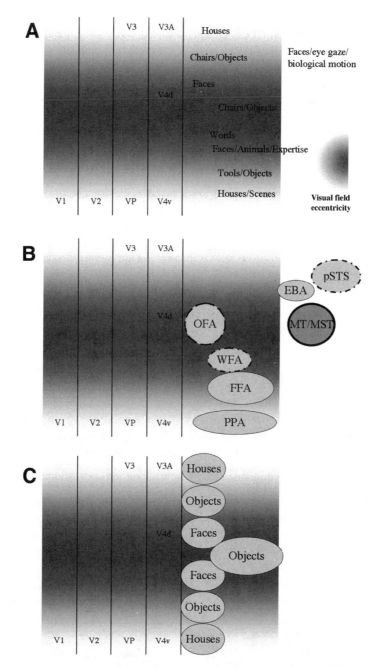

FIGURE 64.2 Schematic illustrations of different aspects of the functional organization of object-responsive extrastriate visual cortex. (*A*) The approximate locations of regions that respond preferentially to a variety of object categories are indicated by the category or process names. See text for complete references. The continuous eccentricity bias that spans from V1 to object-responsive cortex is illustrated with the gray-scale gradient. (*B*) The locations of regions that have been designated as category-selective modules (FFA, fusiform face area; PPA, parahippocampal place area; EBA, extrastriate body area), motion-selective (MT/MST), and other commonly referred-to regions (OFA, occipital face area; WFA, word form area; pSTS, posterior superior temporal sulcus). (*C*) A recent proposal for dividing object-responsive cortex into seven regions, defined by category selectivity, with a dorsal-ventral mirror organization. (Reprinted from U. Hasson et al., large-scale mirror-symmetry organization of human occipito-temporal object areas. *Neuron* 37:1027–1041. © 2003 by Elsevier.)

tified a region in the right fusiform gyrus that responded more to faces than to all other object categories. Kanwisher named this area the fusiform face area (FFA). Shortly thereafter, Epstein and Kanwisher (1998) found an area in the parahippocampal gyrus that responded preferentially to visual scenes depicting places, interior spaces, and buildings, which they named the parahippocampal place area (PPA). Other work has identified regions that respond preferentially to word forms, chairs, and tools, but none of these areas have a level of selectivity and a consistency across subjects to qualify as a module according to the strict criteria established by Kanwisher and colleagues. In 2001, the Kanwisher laboratory identified a third module, the extrastriate body parts area (EBA), in the lateral occipitotemporal cortex (Downing, Jiang et al., 2001), which they believed concluded the search for dedicated modules for specific object categories. They proposed that common objects are represented by a "general-purpose" recognition system, residing in cortex outside of these three modules (Downing, Jiang et al., 2001).

OTHER CATEGORY-RELATED REGIONS Aside from these special categories, numerous functional magnetic resonance imaging (fMRI) experiments found that other categories elicited different levels of activity in these and other regions of ventral occipitotemporal cortex and that faces and houses elicited strong responses in areas other than the FFA and PPA (figure 64.2B). Animal faces and whole animals with and without faces elicit strong responses in the FFA (Chao, Haxby, and Martin, 1999; Chao, Martin, and Haxby, 1999; Tong et al., 2000; but see Kanwisher, Stanley, and Harris, 1999). Face-responsive regions were also identified in the inferior occipital gyri (Halgren et al., 1999; Haxby et al., 1999) and the posterior STS (Puce et al., 1998; Chao, Haxby, and Martin, 1999; Chao, Martin, and Haxby, 1999; Haxby et al., 1999). Letter strings elicit a stronger response than other object categories in a region just lateral to the FFA (Puce et al., 1996; Fiez and Petersen, 1998; Hasson et al., 2002). Chairs elicit a stronger response than faces or houses in regions of the inferior temporal sulcus and middle occipital gyrus (Ishai et al., 1999, 2000). Tools elicit a stronger response than houses in a region just medial to the PPA and a stronger response in the posterior middle temporal gyrus (Chao, Haxby, and Martin, 1999). Chairs and tools both elicit a stronger response in the PPA than faces or animals. Houses, chairs, and tools all elicit a stronger response in the intraoccipital sulcus than faces or animals (Chao, Haxby, and Martin, 1999; Haxby et al., 1999; Ishai et al., 2000; Hasson et al., 2003).

Studies of category-related responding have clearly revealed that the ventral object vision pathway has a complex architecture, but it is not clear that its architecture is best described in terms of regions defined by their category selectivity. The functional architecture of the ventral object vision pathway is also characterized by other organizational dimensions, namely expertise (Gauthier et al., 1999; Gauthier, Tarr et al., 2000) and retinotopy (Levy et al., 2001; Malach, Levy, and Hasson, 2002; Hasson et al., 2002, 2003), which some believe may provide a more fundamental explanation for category-related responses.

VISUAL EXPERTISE AS AN ORGANIZING PRINCIPLE Gauthier and colleagues have argued that the FFA is not specialized for the category of faces but rather is specialized for perceptual processes that are associated with visual expertise. Visual expertise refers to the spontaneous recognition of exemplars from a category at a subordinate level rather than at the generic category level. They have shown that people who have acquired expertise in the visual recognition of specific categories of nonface objects—greebles, birds, cars—demonstrate stronger responses during viewing of these categories than are observed in people who are not experts (Gauthier et al., 1999; Gauthier, Skudlarski, et al., 2000).

RETINOTOPY IN OBJECT-RESPONSIVE CORTEX Malach and colleagues have shown that object-responsive cortex beyond the retinotopically defined visual areas (V1, V2, V3, VP, V3a, V4, V7, V8) also demonstrate a coarse retinotopy (figure 64.2A). The location of some object-selective regions may be related to eccentricity biases insofar as categories that require representation of finer details, such as faces and letters, are located in cortex with a more foveal bias, whereas buildings and landscapes are represented more in cortex with a peripheral bias. In a further refinement of this line of research, Hasson and colleagues (2003) have attempted to explain the functional architecture of object-responsive cortex in terms of seven regions (figure 64.2D)—two buildings regions, two face regions, and three objects regions, arranged with a dorsal to ventral mirror symmetry around the peripheral to foveal eccentricity maps—in an effort to account for the object-selectivity biases in terms of eccentricity biases. This work shows that retinotopy is one factor that may influence the topographic arrangement of category-related regions but is not in itself sufficient to explain smaller distinctions between object categories with equivalent eccentricity biases, such as faces versus letters or tools versus chairs versus shoes.

Locally distributed representations in occipitotemporal cortex

Describing the functional architecture of ventral temporal cortex in terms of regional category preferences provides a useful schema but has major shortcomings. First, it implies that the submaximal responses to a viewed object are discarded. If a response indicates the category being viewed based on response strength, low response levels indicate that the viewed object is simply something else and not the preferred object category. Second, an architecture based on regional category preferences has insufficient capacity to represent all conceivable categories of objects. The response to this shortcoming is the proposal that the number of regions dedicated to a specific category is limited to a small number of categories that have special biological significance, namely, faces, places, and body parts (Kanwisher, 2000; Downing, Jiang, et al., 2001). This proposal, however, highlights the third shortcoming of the regional model, namely, that such a model provides no account for how these special categories are represented, only where those representations reside in cortex, and is absolutely uninformative regarding how other categories may be represented, suggesting only that the remaining ventral temporal cortex may be somehow involved.

We have proposed that the representations of faces and other categories are distributed across ventral temporal cortex and that the representations of different categories overlap each other (Haxby, Ishai et al., 2000; Haxby et al., 2001). These representations can be studied with functional neuroimaging as patterns of response, in which the contrasts between strong and weak responses within those patterns, not just the peak activations, carry category-related information. Thus, our proposal explicitly posits that submaximal responses play a significant role in face and object representations. We would like to call the distribution of representations within one, well-defined, contiguous patch of cortex *local*, to distinguish this type of distribution from the distribution of representation across multiple, dispersed cortical areas, which we are calling *extended*. As we argue later, these two types of distribution play distinct roles in representing information associated with faces and objects.

We, like others, have consistently found regions of ventral temporal cortex that respond maximally to faces or houses or other categories of objects, such as tools and chairs (Chao, Haxby, and Martin, 1999; Chao, Martin, and Haxby, 1999; Haxby et al., 1999; Ishai et al., 1999, 2000). We also observed, however, that the responses to nonpreferred categories in these regions were significant and varied by category. We suspected that these nonmaximal responses to faces and objects may hold a key to solving a fundamental problem for representation in the ventral object vision pathway. The identification of category-selective regions cannot afford a comprehensive account of how faces and objects are represented in ventral temporal cortex. Perhaps certain categories of objects, such as faces and places, have specialized processors that have evolved because of their biological significance. The representation framework in the ventral pathway, however, must also distinguish between categories of uncertain biological significance, such as furniture versus clothing, and even among finer category distinctions, such as easy chairs versus desk chairs or dress shoes versus sport shoes. Clearly, there is not enough cortical real estate

in the ventral temporal lobe to provide a new, specialized region for every conceivable category. If, however, non-maximal responses also play a role in the representation of objects, meaning that different patterns of response in the same cortical space can represent different object categories, there are unlimited combinatorial possibilities that can accommodate an unlimited variety of categories.

We tested this hypothesis by measuring cortical patterns of response using fMRI while subjects viewed eight different categories of objects: faces, houses, cats, chairs, scissors, shoes, bottles, and phase-scrambled images (Haxby et al., 2001). We will summarize the design and results of this study here because of its importance for understanding how neural respresentations of faces and objects are locally distributed within a cortical area. If the full pattern of response codes the representation for a viewed object, not just activity in a region that responds maximally to that object's category, then all categories may be associated with distinct patterns of response. This implies that the pattern of non-maximal responses carries relevant information about the viewed object as well as the maximal responses. To test this aspect of our hypothesis more rigorously, we also analyzed whether distinct patterns of nonmaximal responses could be discerned for all categories.

In each individual subject we identified the cortical voxels that responded differentially to these categories in each of four anatomically defined volumes: ventral temporal cortex, lateral temporal cortex, inferior occipital cortex, and dorsal occipital cortex. The data for each subject were divided into statistically independent halves, namely, even-numbered and odd-numbered time series, and the patterns of response to each category were measured separately in each half of the data. We then analyzed whether the pattern of response to each category in one-half of the data could be classified correctly based on its similarity to the pattern of response to the same category in the other half of the data and its dissimilarity to the patterns of response to other categories. Overall accuracy was indexed by tabulating whether the within-category similarity was greater than the between-category similarity for each comparison between two categories. To gauge the contribution of nonmaximal responses to the information carried by the pattern of response, we tested whether the category being viewed could be identified based on the pattern of response in voxels that did not respond maximally either to the category being viewed or to the category to which it was being compared. For example, to test whether the pattern of nonmaximal responses to faces could be identified as compared to the pattern of nonmaximal responses to houses, all voxels that responded maximally to either faces or houses in either half of the data were excluded from the analysis.

The results showed that the category being viewed could be identified correctly, based on the full patterns of response in ventral temporal cortex, in 96% of pairwise comparisons. Illustrative examples of individual data and group results are shown in figure 64.3. When the analysis was restricted to cortex that responded submaximally to the two categories being compared, identification of the category being viewed was still 94% accurate. Clearly, the patterns of nonmaximal responses carry as much information about the category being viewed as do the maximal responses. The pattern of response that is distinctive for each category appears to subtend essentially the same expanse of ventral temporal cortex that can produce a different, distinctive pattern of response for each of the other categories.

REPLICATIONS IN HUMANS AND NONHUMAN PRIMATES The results of this study have been replicated and extended in a study by Spiridon and Kanwisher (2002), who showed further that these category-related patterns of response were not attributable to specific exemplars or to low-level features. They constructed their stimulus sets so that the patterns of response to one set of exemplars for each category could be compared to the patterns of response to a different set of exemplars, with minimal loss in the accuracy of identifying the category being viewed. They also tested the similarity of patterns of response to gray-scale photographs and patterns of response to line drawings, two visual depictions of the same object categories with markedly different low-level features, and showed again that the category being viewed could be identified with nearly as much accuracy as in the original experiment.

Category-related patterns of response in the ventral object vision pathway were first observed in humans using fMRI. Neurophysiological studies in monkeys, using single-unit recordings and optical imaging, had not revealed these patterns (Perrett et al., 1992). At best, clusters of face-selective cells had been identified, but these clusters were of uncertain size, and their location had not been associated with a consistent anatomical location. Moreover, within such a cluster, only 20% of neurons would demonstrate face selectivity (Rolls and Tovee, 1995; Rolls, 2000). Tanaka and colleagues have found evidence for small clusters of columns that respond to similar primitive object features or to different views of a face (Tanaka et al., 1991; Wang, Tanaka, and Tanifuji, 1996; Tsunoda et al., 2001; Tanaka, 2003) but have not reported any evidence for the sort of macroscopic structure that fMRI has demonstrated in humans.

To test whether these discrepant results in the ventral object vision pathways in the brains of humans and monkeys represent a lack of homology, Tsao and colleagues (in press) decided to study patterns of response to faces and objects in monkey cortex using fMRI and stimulus sets similar to those used in human studies. Surprisingly, they found that monkey cortex contains patches of inferior temporal (IT) cortex that respond preferentially to different object catgories, most notably faces and body parts. The location of the region that responded more strongly to faces than to other objects had been indicated in an earlier monkey fMRI study by a comparison between response to faces and scrambled images (Logothetis et al., 1999). Tsao and colleagues also examined patterns of response in object-responsive cortex using our methods and found distinctive patterns of response for all categories, and also that faces evoked a distinct pattern of response in cortex that responded maximally to other categories. These results indicate that the discrepancy between monkey and human results was due to differences between the neurophysiological methods used in monkeys and hemodynamic imaging.

PATTERNS OF RESPONSE: POPULATION ENCODING AS A VECTOR The patterns of response that we detected represent a fundamentally different type of information that can be extracted from a functional imaging data set compared with the information extracted by previous standard methods. Furthermore, these patterns suggest a different model for how information is represented by neural activity. Previous methods analyze how individual voxels respond differently to different stimulus or cognitive conditions. Whatever elicits the maximal response indicates the information that the cell populations in a given voxel are tuned to process. Patterns of response, by contrast, are vectors that reflect the activity in numerous voxels. Our analysis methods, based on correlations, were insensitive to the magnitude of responses and sensitive to the constellation of differences among the responses in different voxels. In other words, the critical information is the polar angle for the population vector, not its magnitude. Information about stimulus properties or cognitive state, therefore, is carried by differences between responses in different parts of a distributed cortical representation, not by the strength of the response in one piece of cortex. If we had analyzed a patch of cortex that responded uniformly more strongly to one category than to another, our method would have detected no difference.

OBJECT FORM TOPOGRAPHY Perhaps one of the most surprising implications of these results is that the relatively poor spatial resolution of fMRI could discern these category-related patterns of response. The voxel dimensions in the human imaging studies were 3 to 3.75mm (Haxby et al., 2001; Spiridon and Kanwisher, 2002). In the monkey study the voxel dimensions were 1.25mm (Tsao et al., in press). The maximally responsive regions, such as the FFA, the PPA, and the EBA, are low-spatial-frequency features that clearly fall within the spatial resolution of fMRI. The distinct, overlapping patterns of nonmaximal responses have spatial frequencies that are higher than those of category-selective regions but still low enough to be detected with functional imaging, meaning they must span numerous cortical

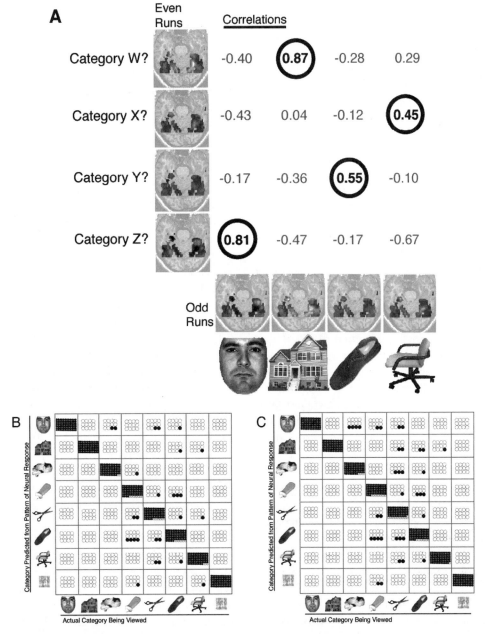

FIGURE 64.3 The category that a subject is viewing can be identified by the spatial pattern of response in ventral temporal cortex. (A) Within- and between-category correlations between patterns of response measured from even-numbered and odd-numbered time series in one subject. A correct identification is based on a higher within-category correlation than between-category correlation for a pairwise comparison between two categories. (C) Confusion matrix for identifying the category being viewed, based on all ventral temporal object-responsive cortex. Solid circles on the diagonal indicate correct identifications. Solid circles in the off-diagonal cells indicate misidentifications and show which category was incorrectly predicted. (D) Confusion matrix for identifying the category being viewed based only on ventral temporal object-responsive cortex that responded submaximally to the two categories in each pairwise comparison.

columns. If neurons or cortical columns were distributed randomly, in a salt-and-pepper fashion, with respect to their differential tuning to aspects of object appearance, functional neuroimaging would not be able to detect these category-related patterns of response. The fact that such patterns can be detected at the spatial resolution of functional neuroimaging indicates that the distributed representation of object information that is reflected by these patterns has a macroscopic structure that was previously unknown and remains unexplained. Understanding how the topographic arrangement of features or basis functions is organized at this macroscopic scale may be a key to deciphering the neural code that underlies face and object recognition. We have named this macroscopic organization *object form topography*.

DISTRIBUTED REPRESENTATIONS REFLECT POPULATION ENCODING   The distributed, category-related patterns of response within a ventral temporal cortex presumably reflect how information about face and object appearance is represented by a population encoding, expressed as a vector that is determined by the responses of numerous cell populations. A single unit in this population can carry information about different object categories (Riesenhuber and Poggio, 2002).

The principles of organization that underlie object form topography are unknown, but our results clearly show that the complete pattern of strong and weak responses carries information about face and object appearance. Whether the information carried by weak responses is used for object identification is unknown, but it seems unlikely that such information would be discarded. Moreover, a population code in which nonmaximal responses contribute information has a greater capacity to produce unique representations for an unlimited variety of faces and objects.

Representation of a simpler visual property, namely, color, illustrates how weak responses can play an integral role in representation by a population response. In color vision, the perceptual quality of a hue that evokes a maximal red response in red-green neurons is also dependent on small responses in yellow-blue neurons that determine whether that hue is perceived as being more orange or violet. Representation of even simpler visual properties, such as motion direction, also may rely on weak responses to make fine discriminations.

Representation of the individual identity of faces may rely on a population response in which strong and weak responses play integral roles (Young and Yamane, 1992; Rolls and Tovee, 1995; Rolls, 2000). Face-responsive cells in monkey anterior inferior temporal (AIT) cortex are broadly tuned to respond differentially to different individuals (Young and Yamane, 1992; Rolls and Tovee, 1995; Sugase et al., 1999). Each cell responds maximally to a few faces, responds with intermediate strength to most faces, and

responds weakly to a few faces (figure 64.4*A*). Thus, a single cell provides some information about face identity (about 0.33 bits, on average), but is not sufficient to identify any single face. The tuning functions for different cells, however, are quite independent, and the pattern of strong and weak responses in a population of 15–30 cells is sufficient to distinguish faces quite well (Young and Yamane, 1992; Rolls and Tovee, 1995).

Similarly, neurons in monkey IT cortex have complex tuning functions for objects other than faces (Sheinberg and Logothetis, 2001; figure 64.4*B*), and the population response of numerous cells presumably represents the appearance of a single object.

The basis functions that underlie the tuning functions for different face-responsive and object-responsive cell populations are unknown. Computational models of face and object perception suggest numerous possibilities (O'Toole, Vetter, and Blanz, 1999; Riesenhuber and Poggio, 1999; Ullman, Vidal-Naquet, and Sali, 2002), but neither single-unit recording studies nor functional neuroimaging studies have established any correspondences between the tuning functions of individual neurons or patches of cortex and a set of basis functions in a computational model of visual recognition. Single-unit studies have described such tuning functions empirically based on differential responses to diverse sets of objects and faces (Gross, Rocha-Miranda, and Bender, 1972; Desimone, 1991; Rolls and Tovee, 1995; Rolls, 2000; Sheinberg and Logothetis, 2001) or to simpler object primitive shapes derived subjectively based on experimenter intuitions (Tanaka, 1993, 1996). Imaging studies have described tuning functions based on object category (Kanwisher, McDermott, and Chun, 1997; Epstein and Kanwisher, 1998; Ishai et al., 1999; Tong et al., 2000; Downing, Jiang et al., 2001) or viewer expertise (Gauthier et al., 1999; Gauthier, Skudlarski et al., 2000). The discovery of category-related patterns of response, however, suggests that the basis functions that underlie the tuning functions of neurons in object-responsive cortex have an ordered structure that is reflected in their macroscopic spatial organization.

Extended distribution of representations across multiple areas

Face and object recognition elicits neural activity in numerous regions other than those in the ventral temporal cortex. Extrastriate visual cortices that demonstrate category-related response preferences also are found in inferior occipital, dorsal occipital, and lateral temporal cortices. In addition, numerous areas outside of extrastriate visual cortex appear to participate in face and object recognition. This extended distribution of activity across extrastriate visual and nonvisual cortices reflects the representation of a different kind of information than does the local distribution of activity

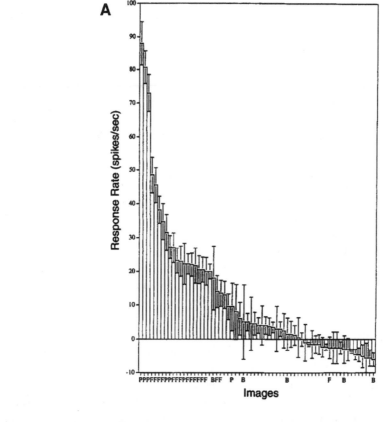

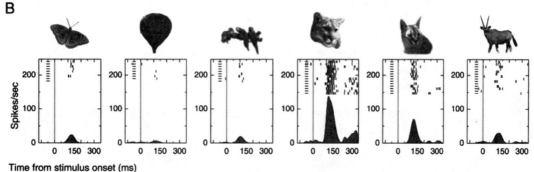

FIGURE 64.4 (*A*) Tuning function for one face-selective IT cell showing coarse coding for different face identities (F, full face; P, profile; B, body part; no letter, nonface natural scene). (Reprinted with permission from E. T. Rolls, functions of the primate temporal lobe cortical visual areas in invariant visual object 3147 and face recognition. *Neuron* 27:205–218. © 2000 by Elsevier.) (*B*) Tuning function for one object-selective IT cell showing complex tuning to disparate animate objects. (From Sheinberg and Logothetis, 2001.)

within a cortical area. Whereas distributed activity within ventral temporal cortex reflects a population response that represents the appearance of object form, activity in other areas represents other information associated with a face or object, such as how it can move, how it can be grasped, what sounds it might make, or what social message it might convey.

CATEGORY-RELATED ACTIVITY IN OTHER EXTRASTRIATE VISUAL AREAS   In visual cortices anterior to the retinotopically defined areas—V1, V2, VP, V3, V3A, V4, V7, and V8—category-related responses to faces and objects are seen in inferior occipital (including inferior and midoccipital gyri), dorsal occipital (in the dorsal occipital gyrus and intraoccipital sulcus), and lateral temporal (posterior STS and middle temporal gyrus) cortices. In our study (Haxby et al., 2001), the highest accuracy for identification of the category being viewed was found for patterns of response in ventral temporal cortex (96%), but high accuracies were also found for patterns of response in inferior occipital (92%) and lateral temporal (92%) cortices, with a lower but still significant level of accuracy for patterns of response in dorsal occipital cortices (87%).

A region in the posterior STS that responds more to faces than to other object categories appears to play a role in representing eye gaze direction, facial expression, and facial movement (Puce et al., 1998; Hoffman and Haxby, 2000). This area appears to play a more general role in interpretation of the intent of others and in social communication (Allison, Puce, and McCarthy, 2000). It also responds to whole-body movement (Bonda et al., 1996; Grossman et al., 2000; Beauchamp et al., 2002; Grossman and Blake, 2002), while judgments are being made about a person's character (Winston et al., 2002), and while the motion of simple geometric figures that implies intentional actions is being viewed (Castelli et al., 2000). Thus, activity in this region that is evoked by a face appears to play a role in interpreting the social meanings conveyed by that face, not the invariant structure that distinguishes the identity of that face (Haxby, Hoffman, and Gobbini, 2000). Activity that is evoked in this region by whole bodies and animals appears to be associated with the representation of how bodies move (Bonda et al., 1996; Grossman et al., 2000; Beauchamp et al., 2002; Grossman and Blake, 2002). The posterior STS region that responds to biological movement appears to abut a more inferior region in the middle temporal gyrus that responds more strongly to patterns of movement associated with inanimate artifacts, such as a broom, a saw, a hammer, or a pen (Beauchamp et al., 2002, in press). Thus, the lateral temporal cortex appears to contain a representation of patterns of movement that are associated with faces and objects (Martin, Ungerleider, and Haxby, 1999). Interestingly, these areas are immediately anterior and superior to human areas MT and MST, which are associated with the perception of simpler forms of motion. Martin has argued that information about typical patterns of movement is more important than information about object form for recognizing tools (Martin et al., 1996; Martin, Ungerleider, and Haxby, 1999). For example, saws come in radically different shapes but are members of the same category because of their function, cutting through a hard substance, which is achieved by a sawing motion. Presumably because of the central role played by function in the definition of tools, a category-specific agnosia for tools is typically associated with lesions in the middle temporal gyrus, not the ventral temporal cortex.

The roles played by the inferior and dorsal occipital areas in face and object representation remain unclear at this time. The face-responsive region in the inferior occipital gyri appears to abut both the face-responsive regions in the fusiform gyrus and the STS. We have suggested that it may provide input to both of these structures, implying that it plays a role in processing simpler features of facial structure (Haxby, Hoffman, and Gobbini, 2000).

DISTRIBUTED NEURAL SYSTEMS FOR FACE PERCEPTION   Face recognition also evokes activity in nonvisual areas associated with other types of information that is gleaned from faces. We have called the extrastriate visual areas that are associated with the representation of the invariant structure of a face (identity), changeable aspects of a face (eye gaze direction, expression), and face movement the *core system* for the visual analysis of faces. We have called the nonvisual areas that are recruited by face recognition the *extended system* (Haxby, Hoffman, and Gobbini, 2000; figure 64.5). The extended system is an open set of cortical and noncortical

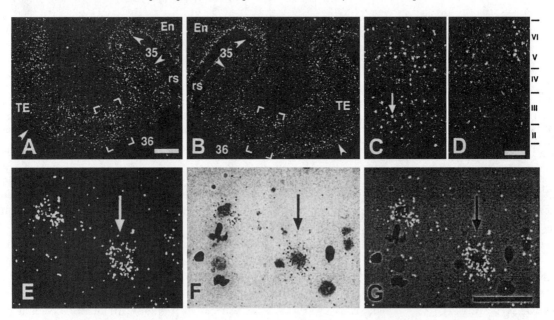

FIGURE 64.5   Model of the distributed human neural system for face perception. The extended system refers to nonvisual cortical areas that are recruited to glean information from faces related to person knowledge, emotion, spatial attention, and speech. (Adapted and elaborated from Haxby, Hoffman, and Gobbini, 2000.)

regions whose membership has expanded since we originally proposed our model.

A cortical area in the superior temporal gyrus that is activated by auditory speech is also activated by lip-reading with no auditory stimulus (Calvert et al., 1997; Calvert and Campbell, 2003). The amygdala and a cortical region in the anterior insula are associated with processing the emotional content of face expressions (Breiter et al., 1996; Morris et al., 1996; Phillips et al., 1997). An area in the intraparietal sulcus is activated by perception of averted eye gaze (Hoffman and Haxby, 2000), presumably because of the automatic shift of spatial attention that is elicited by such a stimulus (Friesen and Kingstone, 1998; Driver et al., 1999; Hietanen, 1999; Langton and Bruce, 1999).

Recognition of a familiar face is associated with an extensive constellation of neural responses in numerous brain areas, presumably reflecting the spontaneous activation of personal knowledge and emotions associated with that person. Activity elicited by familiar faces in the anterior middle temporal gyrus and the temporal poles has been associated with the spontaneous activation of biographical information (Gorno-Tempini et al., 1998; Leveroni et al., 2000; Nakamura et al., 2000). Activity in the anterior paracingulate cortex, the posterior STS, and the precuneus and posterior cingulate is associated with personal familiarity, suggesting that seeing a close relative or friend leads to the spontaneous activation of one's understanding of that person's intentions, personality traits, and other mental states (theory of mind) (Gobbini et al., 2004). The emotional response to a familiar person appears to be reflected in modulation of activity in the amygdala, with a reduced response for personally familiar faces, possibly reflecting how people feel less guarded around friends, but an increased response in mothers seeing their own child, perhaps related to maternal protectiveness.

DISTRIBUTED REPRESENTATION OF INFORMATION ABOUT TOOLS Martin has proposed a sensorimotor theory for the representation of knowledge about objects which holds that object representations reflect the sensory and motor attributes learned through experience with objects, and these attributes are represented in the cortical regions that process those sensory and motor attributes (Martin et al., 1996; Martin, Ungerleider, and Haxby, 1999; Martin and Chao, 2001). Accordingly, Martin and colleagues have shown that the perception of tools is associated with neural activity in the posterior middle temporal region associated with the perception of tool motion (Beauchamp et al., 2002) and in parietal and premotor regions associated with the representation of how objects can be grasped (Chao and Martin, 2002). These parietal and premotor areas are thought to be the human homologues of mirror neurons, which respond both during the performance of a hand movement and during the observation of someone else making the same movement (di Pellegrino et al., 1992; Gallese et al., 1996; Rizzolatti, Fogassi, and Gallese, 2001).

Temporal distribution of face and object processing

The neural response to a visual stimulus in the human brain begins about 80 ms after the stimulus appears, as measured with magnetoencephalography (MEG) or electroencephalography. Category-related responses are observed as early as 100–150 ms (Thorpe, Fize, and Marlot, 1996; Thorpe, 2002), suggesting a very fast, feedforward processing. Category-related responses continue for several hundreds of milliseconds thereafter, indicating that the neural activity that represents faces and objects is distributed over a substantial period of time. The early and late parts of this processing appear to play different roles in face and object processing.

The earliest category-related response to faces peaks around 170 ms after the appearance of a face, as measured with scalp electrodes or with MEG, called the N170 or M170, respectively (Bentin et al., 1996; Halgren et al., 2000; figure 64.6). Studies with intracranial electrodes in patients scheduled for epilepsy surgery show a similar response, but

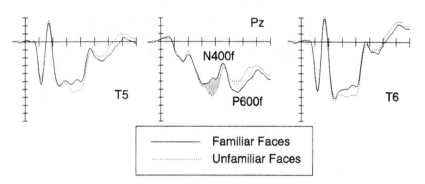

FIGURE 64.6 Evoked potential to familiar and unfamiliar faces illustrating the early, face-selective response (N170) at T5 and T6 that is not affected by familiarity and the late responses at Pz that are. (From Eimer, 2000a.)

at a slightly longer latency of approximately 200 ms (N200) (Allison et al., 1999). The onset of category-related differences leading to this peak, however, occurs at around 100 ms. Studies with intracranial electrodes and source localization of the evoked magnetic fields indicate that this early response is generated in the fusiform gyrus and in the STS (Allison et al., 1999; Halgren et al., 2000). The timing of this response suggests that it reflects a feedforward process, with little opportunity for modulation by feedback from other areas in the distributed network for face processing.

The N170 shows category-related properties, but it is not face-specific. Gauthier and colleagues have shown that this evoked potential is enhanced by expertise for object categories other than faces, such as cars and birds, suggesting that it reflects a process that can be adapted to nonface objects (Rossion et al., 2002).

Intracranial recordings have shown that neural activity in the fusiform cortex and in distant temporal, parietal, and frontal cortices demonstrates increased coherence around the time of the N170, with a phase lag of approximately 7 ms, suggesting that information processed by the N170 in fusiform cortex entrains neural activity in these other cortices, enabled by a one-synapse connection (Klopp et al., 2000). Intracranial recordings also have revealed later face-selective potentials, with latencies of approximately 350 ms (P350) and longer (N700) (Allison et al., 1999; McCarthy et al., 1999). The P350 appears to be more prominent over anterior ventral temporal cortex.

Whereas the early response appears to be driven primarily by feedforward connections, these later responses are susceptible to modulation by feedback connections from other regions that mediate attention and memory effects (see figure 64.6).

In a study of single-neuron responses in monkeys to faces and objects, Sugase and colleagues (1999) performed an information theory analysis to examine how much information was conveyed by early and late responses that contributed to discriminations between categories and to within-category discriminations between exemplars. They found that the tuning functions for early responses carried information that primarily was relevant for coarser between-category discriminations, whereas the tuning functions for later responses carried information that was relevant for finer within-category discriminations (figure 64.7). They proposed that the early responses could act like a header to direct further processing of a stimulus as an exemplar of an identified category. Bentin and Deouell (2000) similarly have argued that the N170 may initiate or stream further face processing.

Studies of memory effects suggest that late category-related responses, but not early category-related responses, in humans also carry information that is relevant for within-category discriminations. Repetition priming, long-term familiarity, and associated biographical knowledge have minimal or no effect on the N170 response to faces (Puce, Allison, and McCarthy, 1999; Bentin and Deouell, 2000;

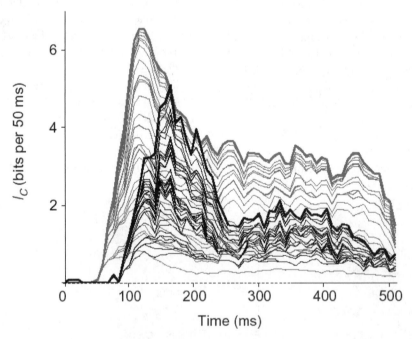

FIGURE 64.7 Information content for making between- and within-category discriminations (gray and black, respectively) from the responses of single IT neurons, plotted as a function of the time of activity after stimulus onset. Note that information content for between-category discriminations peaks earlier than the information content for within-category discriminations. (Reprinted with permission from Y. Sugase, S. Yamane, S. Veno, and K. Kawano, 1999. Global and fine information coded by single neurons in the temporal visual cortex. *Nature* 400:869–873. Copyright 1999 by Nature Publishing Group.)

Eimer, 2000a, 2000b; Henson et al., 2003; Paller et al., 2003). By contrast, familiarity and priming have consistent, large effects on later responses to faces (see figure 64.6). Trial-to-trial variation in the amplitude of the N170 is related to identity recognition performance (Liu, Harris, and Kanwisher, 2002), but this result suggests only that the information that is necessary for recognition is carried by the N170, but the act of recognition itself may occur later. The temporal locus for priming and familiarity effects differ slightly, with priming effects most evident from 250 to 400 ms and familiarity effects most evident later, from 400 to 600 ms. The distribution of these later responses that show memory effects also is different from the distribution of the N170. Whereas the N170 is most evident in electrodes placed over occipitotemporal cortex, memory effects are maximal in electrodes placed over parietal and frontal cortex.

In an MEG study (Furey et al., 2001), we found that only late responses to faces and houses, with latencies greater than 200 ms, were modulated by attention. Earlier responses were identical when subjects attended to faces or houses, but late responses were indistinguishable from category-related responses to single-exposure pictures of the attended category. A parallel fMRI study showed that the pattern of response in ventral temporal cortex reflected only the attended category. In other words, the face-related response in the fusiform cortex was eliminated by attention, but the early face-related evoked response was untouched. These results indicate that the pattern of hemodynamic responses in ventral temporal cortex reflects mostly later responses, which can be modulated by attention and memory.

Conclusions

The research summarized here shows that cortical representations of faces and objects are both spatially and temporally distributed. Category-related neural activity that is evoked by visually presented faces and other objects appears to begin in extrastriate regions in ventral and lateral occipitotemporal cortices. These early responses appear to reflect feedforward processes that are not strongly modulated by the effects of memory and attention. Because hemodynamic imaging is insensitive to these early category-related responses, their topography is not known in detail, and consequently it is unknown whether these early responses show the same local distribution of overlapping representations as do the later responses. In monkeys, early responses in IT cortex appear to carry more information about between-category distinctions than about finer within-category distinctions. The role of early responses in human face and object processing may similarly be related more to coarser between-category discriminations. These early between-category discriminations could initiate further processing that is relevant for the identified category. After the early

responses, further neural processing in extrastriate regions is in concert with neural activity in other brain areas. Thus, the extended distribution of face and object representations appears to be related to the later responses. The recruitment of the extended distribution can serve to elaborate the information contained in the representation, enable recognition of familiar faces and objects, and allow attention to modulate how the representation develops. The locally distributed representations within extrastriate visual cortical areas that are observed with neuroimaging reflect late neural responses in these areas that are modulated by the influence of the extended distribution. The relationship between the local distribution of early and late responses in extrastriate cortices is unknown, but single-unit studies in monkeys and recordings with intracranial electrodes indicate that they may be closely linked.

REFERENCES

AGUIRRE, G. K., E. ZARAHN, and M. D'ESPOSITO, 1998. An area within human ventral cortex sensitive to "building" stimuli: Evidence and implications. *Neuron* 21:373–383.

ALLISON, T., A. PUCE, and G. MCCARTHY, 2000. Social perception from visual cues: Role of the STS region. *Trends Cogn. Sci.* 4:267–278.

ALLISON, T., A. PUCE, D. D. SPENCER, and G. MCCARTHY, 1999. Electrophysiological studies of human face perception. I. Potentials generated in occipitotemporal cortex by face and non-face stimuli. *Cereb. Cortex* 9:415–430.

BEAUCHAMP, M. S., K. E. LEE, J. V. HAXBY, and A. MARTIN, 2002. Parallel visual motion processing streams for manipulable objects and human movements. *Neuron* 34:149–159.

BEAUCHAMP, M. S., K. E. LEE, J. V. HAXBY, and A. MARTIN, 2003. FMRI responses to video and point-light displays of moving humans and manipulable objects. *J. Cogn. Neurosci.* 15:991–1001.

BENTIN, S., T. ALLISON, A. PUCE, E. PEREZ, and G. MCCARTHY, 1996. Electrophysiological studies of face perception in humans. *J. Cogn. Neurosci.* 8:551–565.

BENTIN, S., and L. Y. DEOUELL, 2000. Structural encoding and identification in face processing: ERP evidence for separate mechanisms. *Cogn. Neuropsychol.* 17:35–54.

BONDA, E., M. PETRIDES, D. OSTRY, and A. EVANS, 1996. Specific involvement of human parietal systems and the amygdala in the perception of biological motion. *J. Neurosci.* 16:3737–3744.

BREITER, H. C., N. L. ETCOFF, P. J. WHALEN, W. A. KENNEDY, S. L. RAUCH, R. L. BUCKNER, M. M. STRAUSS, S. E. HYMAN, and B. R. ROSEN, 1996. Response and habituation of the human amygdala during visual processing of facial expression. *Neuron* 17:875–887.

CALVERT, G. A., E. T. BULMORE, M. J. BRAMMER, R. CAMPBELL, S. C. R. WILLIAMS, P. K. MCGUIRE, P. W. R. WOODRUFF, S. D. IVERSON, and A. S. DAVID, 1997. Activation of auditory cortex during silent lipreading. *Science* 276:593–596.

CALVERT, G. A., and R. CAMPBELL, 2003. Reading speech from still and moving faces: The neural substrates of visible speech. *J. Cogn. Neurosci.* 15:57–70.

CASTELLI, F., F. HAPPE, U. FRITH, and C. FRITH, 2000. Movement and mind: A functional imaging study of perception and interpretation of complex intentional movement patterns. *NeuroImage* 12:314–325.

Chao, L. L., J. V. Haxby, and A. Martin, 1999. Attribute-based neural substrates in temporal cortex for perceiving and knowing about objects. *Nat. Neurosci.* 2:913–919.

Chao, L. L., and A. Martin, 2000. Representation of manipulable man-made objects in the dorsal stream. *NeuroImage* 12:478–484.

Chao, L. L., A. Martin, and J. V. Haxby, 1999. Are face-responsive regions selective only for faces? *Neuroreport* 10:2945–2950.

Corbetta, M., F. M. Miezin, S. M. Dobmeyer, and S. E. Petersen, 1990. Attentional modulation of neural processing of shape, color, and velocity in humans. *Science* 248:1556–1559.

Corbetta, M., F. M. Miezin, S. M. Dobmeyer, G. L. Shulman, and S. E. Petersen, 1991. Selective and divided attention during visual discriminations of shape, color, and speed: Functional anatomy by positron emission tomography. *J. Neurosci.* 11:2383–2402.

Desimone, R., 1991. Face-selective cells in the temporal cortex of monkeys. *J. Cogn. Neurosci.* 3:1–8.

di Pellegrino, G., L. Fadiga, L. Fogassi, V. Gallese, and G. Rizzolatti, 1992. Understanding motor events: A neurophysiological study. *Exp. Brain Res.* 91:176–180.

Downing, P. E., Y. Jiang, M. Shuman, and N. Kanwisher, 2001. A cortical area selective for visual processing of the human body. *Science* 293:2470–2473.

Downing, P., J. Liu, and N. Kanwisher, 2001. Testing cognitive models of visual attention with fMRI and MEG. *Neuropsychologia* 39:1329–1342.

Driver, J., G. Davis, P. Ricciardelli, P. Kidd, E. Maxwell, and S. Baron-Cohen, 1999. Gaze perception triggers reflexive visuospatial orienting. *Vis. Cogn.* 6:509–540.

Eimer, M., 2000a. Event-related brain potentials distinguish processing stages involved in face perception and recognition. *Clin. Neurophysiol.* 111:694–705.

Eimer, M., 2000b. The face-specific N170 component reflects late stages in the structural encoding of faces. *Neuroreport* 11:2319–2324.

Epstein, R., and N. Kanwisher, 1998. A cortical representation of the local visual environment. *Nature* 392:598–601.

Fiez, J. A., and S. E. Petersen, 1998. Neuroimaging studies of word reading. *Proc. Natl. Acad. Sci. U.S.A.* 3:914–921.

Friesen, C., and A. Kingstone, 1998. The eyes have it! Reflexive orienting is triggered by nonpredictive gaze. *Psychonom. Bull. Rev.* 5:490–495.

Furey, M. L., T. Tanskanen, M. B. Beauchamp, S. Avikainen, J. V. Haxby, and R. Hari, 2001. Temporal characteristics of selective attention to faces and houses: A MEG study. *NeuroImage* 13(Suppl.):S316.

Gallese, V., L. Fadiga, L. Fogassi, and G. Rizzolatti, 1996. Action recognition in the premotor cortex. *Brain* 119:593–609.

Gauthier, I., P. Skudlarski, J. C. Gore, and A. W. Anderson, 2000. Expertise for cars and birds recruits brain areas involved in face recognition. *Nat. Neurosci.* 3:191–197.

Gauthier, I., M. J. Tarr, A. W. Anderson, P. Skudlarski, and J. C. Gore, 1999. Activation of the middle fusiform "face area" increases with expertise in recognizing novel objects. *Nat. Neurosci.* 2:568–573.

Gauthier, I., M. J. Tarr, J. Moylan, P. Skudlarski, J. C. Gore, and A. W. Anderson, 2000. The fusiform "face area" is part of a network that processes faces at the individual level. *J. Cogn. Neurosci.* 12:495–504.

Gobbini, I., E. Leibenluft, N. J. Santiago, and J. V. Haxby, 2004. Social and emotional attachment in the neural representation of faces. *NeuroImage* 22:1628–1635.

Gorno-Tempini, M. L., C. J. Price, O. Josephs, R. Vandenberghe, S. F. Cappa, N. Kapur, R. S. Frackowiak, and M. L. Tempini, 1998. The neural systems sustaining face and proper-name processing. *Brain* 121:2103–2118.

Grill-Spector, K., T. Kushnir, S. Edelman, G. Avidan, Y. Itzchak, and R. Malach, 1999. Differential processing of objects under various viewing conditions in the human lateral occipital complex. *Neuron* 24:187–203.

Gross, C. G., C. E. Rocha-Miranda, and D. B. Bender, 1972. Visual properties of neurons in inferotemporal cortex of the macaque. *J. Neurophysiol.* 35:96–111.

Grossman, E., M. Donnelly, R. Price, D. Pickens, V. Morgan, G. Neighbor, and R. Blake, 2000. Brain areas involved in perception of biological motion. *J. Cogn. Neurosci.* 12:711–720.

Grossman, E. D., and R. Blake, 2002. Brain areas active during visual perception of biological motion. *Neuron* 35:1167–1175.

Halgren, E., A. M. Dale, M. I. Sereno, R. B. Tootell, K. Marinkovic, and B. R. Rosen, 1999. Location of human face-selective cortex with respect to retinotopic areas. *Hum. Brain Mapp.* 7:29–37.

Halgren, E., T. Raij, K. Marinkovic, V. Jousmaki, and R. Hari, 2000. Cognitive response profile of the human fusiform face area as determined by MEG. *Cereb. Cortex* 10:69–81.

Hasson, U., M. Harel, I. Levy, and R. Malach, 2003. Large-scale mirror-symmetry organization of human occipito-temporal object areas. *Neuron* 37:1027–1041.

Hasson, U., I. Levy, M. Behrmann, T. Hendler, and R. Malach, 2002. Eccentricity bias as an organizing principle for human high-order object areas. *Neuron* 34:479–490.

Haxby, J. V., M. I. Gobbini, M. L. Furey, A. Ishai, J. L. Schouten, and P. Pietrini, 2001. Distributed and overlapping representations of faces and objects in ventral temporal cortex. *Science* 293:2425–2430.

Haxby, J. V., C. L. Grady, B. Horwitz, L. G. Ungerleider, M. Mishkin, R. E. Carson, P. Herscovitch, M. B. Schapiro, and S. I. Rapoport, 1991. Dissociation of spatial and object vision processing pathways in human extrastriate cortex. *Proc. Natl. Acad. Sci. U.S.A.* 88:1621–1625.

Haxby, J. V., E. A. Hoffman, and M. I. Gobbini, 2000. The distributed human neural system for face perception. *Trends Cogn. Sci.* 4:223–233.

Haxby, J. V., B. Horwitz, L. G. Ungerleider, J. M. Maisog, P. Pietrini, and C. L. Grady, 1994. The functional organization of human extrastriate cortex: A PET-rCBF study of selective attention to faces and locations. *J. Neurosci.* 14:6336–6353.

Haxby, J. V., A. Ishai, L. L. Chao, L. G. Ungerleider, and A. Martin, 2000. Object form topology in the ventral temporal lobe. *Trends Cogn. Sci.* 4:3–4.

Haxby, J. V., L. G. Ungerleider, V. P. Clark, J. L. Schouten, E. A. Hoffman, and A. Martin, 1999. The effect of face inversion on activity in human neural systems for face and object perception. *Neuron* 22:189–199.

Henson, R. N., Y. Goshen-Gottstein, T. Ganel, L. J. Otten, A. Quayle, and M. D. Rugg, 2003. Electrophysiological and haemodynamic correlates of face perception, recognition and priming. *Cereb. Cortex* 13:793–805.

Hietanen, J. K., 1999. Does your gaze direction and head orientation shift my visual attention? *Neuroreport* 10:3443–3447.

Hoffman, E. A., and J. V. Haxby, 2000. Distinct representations of eye gaze and identity in the distributed human neural system for face perception. *Nat. Neurosci.* 3:80–84.

ISHAI, A., L. G. UNGERLEIDER, A. MARTIN, and J. V. HAXBY, 2000. The representation of objects in the human occipital and temporal cortex. *J. Cogn. Neurosci.* 12:35–51.

ISHAI, A., L. G. UNGERLEIDER, A. MARTIN, J. L. SCHOUTEN, and J. V. HAXBY, 1999. Distributed representation of objects in the human ventral visual pathway. *Proc. Natl. Acad. Sci. U.S.A.* 96:9379–9384.

KANWISHER, N., 2000. Domain specificity in face perception. *Nat. Neurosci.* 3:759–763.

KANWISHER, N., J. MCDERMOTT, and M. M. CHUN, 1997. The fusiform face area: A module in human extrastriate cortex specialized for face perception. *J. Neurosci.* 17:4302–4311.

KANWISHER, N., D. STANLEY, and A. HARRIS, 1999. The fusiform face area is selective for faces not animals. *Neuroreport* 10:183–187.

KLOPP, J., K. MARINKOVIC, P. CHAUVEL, V. NENOV, and E. HALGREN, 2000. Early widespread cortical distribution of coherent fusiform face selective activity. *Hum. Brain Mapp.* 11:286–293.

LANGTON, S. R. H., and V. BRUCE, 1999. Reflexive visual orienting in response to the social attention of others. *Vis. Cogn.* 6:541–568.

LERNER, Y., T. HENDLER, D. BEN-BASHAT, M. HAREL, and R. MALACH, 2001. A hierarchical axis of object processing stages in the human visual cortex. *Cereb. Cortex* 11:287–297.

LEVERONI, C. L., M. SEIDENBERG, A. R. MAYER, L. A. MEAD, J. R. BINDER, and S. M. RAO, 2000. Neural systems underlying the recognition of familiar and newly learned faces. *J. Neurosci.* 20:878–886.

LEVY, I., U. HASSON, G. AVIDAN, T. HENDLER, and R. MALACH, 2001. Center-periphery organization of human object areas. *Nat. Neurosci.* 4:533–539.

LIU, J., A. HARRIS, and N. KANWISHER, 2002. Stages of processing in face perception: An MEG study. *Nat. Neurosci.* 5:910–916.

LOGOTHETIS, N. K., H. GUGGENBERGER, S. PELED, and J. PAULS, 1999. Functional imaging of the monkey brain. *Nat. Neurosci.* 2:555–562.

LUECK, C. J., S. ZEKI, K. J. FRISTON, M.-P. DEIBER, P. COPE, V. J. CUNNINGHAM, A. A. LAMMERTSMA, C. KENNARD, and R. S. J. FRACKOWIAK, 1989. The color centre in the cerebral cortex of man. *Nature* 340:386–389.

MALACH, R., I. LEVY, and U. HASSON, 2002. The topography of high-order human object areas. *Trends Cogn. Sci.* 6:176–184.

MALACH, R., J. B. REPPAS, R. R. BENSON, K. K. KWONG, H. JIANG, W. A. KENNEDY, P. J. LEDDEN, T. J. BRADY, B. R. ROSEN, and R. B. TOOTELL, 1995. Object-related activity revealed by functional magnetic resonance imaging in human occipital cortex. *Proc. Natl. Acad. Sci. U.S.A.* 92:8135–8139.

MARTIN, A., and L. L. CHAO, 2001. Semantic memory and the brain: Structure and processes. *Curr. Opin. Neurobiol.* 11:194–201.

MARTIN, A., J. V. HAXBY, F. M. LALONDE, C. L. WIGGS, and L. G. UNGERLEIDER, 1995. Discrete cortical regions associated with knowledge of color and knowledge of action. *Science* 270:102–105.

MARTIN, A., L. G. UNGERLEIDER, and J. V. HAXBY, 1999. Category specificity and the brain: The sensory/motor model of semantic representations of objects. In *The New Cognitive Neurosciences*, M. S. Gazzaniga, ed. Cambridge, Mass.: MIT Press, pp. 1023–1036.

MARTIN, A., C. L. WIGGS, L. G. UNGERLEIDER, and J. V. HAXBY, 1996. Neural correlates of category-specific knowledge. *Nature* 379:649–652.

MCCARTHY, G., A. PUCE, J. C. GORE, and T. ALLISON, 1997. Face-specific processing in the human fusiform gyrus. *J. Cogn. Neurosci.* 9:605–610.

MORRIS, J., C. D. FRITH, D. I. PERRETT, D. ROWLAND, A. W. YOUNG, A. J. CALDER, and R. J. DOLAN, 1996. A differential neural response in the human amygdala to fearful and happy facial expressions. *Nature* 383:812–815.

NAKAMURA, K., R. KAWASHIMA, N. SATO, A. NAKAMURA, M. SUGIURA, T. KATO, K. HATANO, K. ITO, H. FUKUDA, T. SCHORMANN, and K. ZILLES, 2000. Functional delineation of the human occipito-temporal areas related to face and scene processing. A PET study. *Brain* 123:1903–1912.

O'TOOLE, A. J., T. VETTER, and V. BLANZ, 1999. Three-dimensional shape and two-dimensional surface reflectance contributions to face recognition: An application of three-dimensional morphing. *Vision Res.* 39:3145–3155.

PALLER, K. A., B. GONSALVES, M. GRABOWECKY, V. S. BOZIC, and S. YAMADA, 2000. Electrophysiological correlates of recollecting faces of known and unknown individuals. *NeuroImage* 11:98–110.

PALLER, K. A., C. A. HUTSON, B. B. MILLER, and S. G. BOEHM, 2003. Neural manifestations of memory with and without awareness. *Neuron* 38:507–516.

PERRETT, D., J. K. HIETANEN, M. W. ORAM, and P. J. BENSON, 1992. Organization and functions of cells responsive to faces in the temporal cortex. *Philos. Trans. R. Soc. Lond. Series B Biol. Sci.* 335:25–30.

PHILLIPS, M. L., A. W. YOUNG, C. SENIOR, M. BRAMMER, C. ANDREW, A. J. CALDER, E. T. BULLMORE, D. I. PERRETT, D. ROWLAND, S. C. WILLIAMS, J. A. GRAY, and A. S. DAVID, 1997. A specific neural substrate for perceiving facial expressions of disgust. *Nature* 389:495–498.

PUCE, A., T. ALLISON, M. ASGARI, J. C. GORE, and G. MCCARTHY, 1996. Differential sensitivity of human visual cortex to faces, letterstrings, and textures: A functional magnetic resonance imaging study. *J. Neurosci.* 16:5205–5215.

PUCE, A., T. ALLISON, S. BENTIN, J. C. GORE, and G. MCCARTHY, 1998. Temporal cortex activation in humans viewing eye and mouth movements. *J. Neurosci.* 18:2188–2199.

PUCE, A., T. ALLISON, and G. MCCARTHY, 1999. Electrophysiological studies of human face perception. III. Effects of top-down processing on face-specific potentials. *Cereb. Cortex* 9: 445–458.

RIESENHUBER, M., and T. POGGIO, 1999. Hierarchical models of object recognition in cortex. *Nat. Neurosci.* 2:1019–1025.

RIESENHUBER, M., and T. POGGIO, 2002. Neural mechanisms of object recognition. *Curr. Opin. Neurobiol.* 12:162–168.

RIZZOLATTI, G., L. FOGASSI, and V. GALLESE, 2001. Neurophysiological mechanisms underlying the understanding and imitation of action. *Nat. Rev. Neurosci.* 2:661–670.

ROLLS, E. T., 2000. Functions of the primate temporal lobe cortical visual areas in invariant visual object and face recognition. *Neuron* 27:205–218.

ROLLS, E. T., and M. J. TOVEE, 1995. Sparseness of the neuronal representation of stimuli in the primate temporal visual cortex. *J. Neurophysiol.* 73:713–726.

ROSSION, B., I. GAUTHIER, V. GOFFAUX, M. J. TARR, and M. CROMMELINCK, 2002. Expertise training with novel objects leads to left-lateralized facelike electrophysiological responses. *Psychol. Sci.* 13:250–257.

SERGENT, J., S. OHTA, and B. MACDONALD, 1992. Functional neuroanatomy of face and object processing: A positron emission tomography study. *Brain* 115:15–36.

SHEINBERG, D. L., and N. K. LOGOTHETIS, 2001. Noticing familiar objects in real world scenes: The role of temporal cortical neurons in natural vision. *J. Neurosci.* 21:1340–1350.

SPIRIDON, M., and N. KANWISHER, 2002. How distributed is visual category information in human occipito-temporal cortex? An fMRI study. *Neuron* 35:1157–1165.

SUGASE, Y., S. YAMANE, S. UENO, and K. KAWANO, 1999. Global and fine information coded by single neurons in the temporal visual cortex. *Nature* 400:869–873.

TANAKA, K., 1993. Neuronal mechanisms of object recognition. *Science* 262:685–688.

TANAKA, K., 1996. Inferotemporal cortex and object vision. *Annu. Rev. Neurosci.* 19:109–139.

TANAKA, K., 2003. Columns for complex visual object features in the inferotemporal cortex: Clustering of cells with similar but slightly different stimulus selectivities. *Cereb. Cortex* 13:90–99.

TANAKA, K., H. SAITO, Y. FUKADA, and M. MORIYA, 1991. Coding visual images of objects in the inferotemporal cortex of the macaque monkey. *J. Neurophysiol.* 66:170–189.

THORPE, S., 2002. Ultra-rapid scene categorization with a wave of spikes. *Lecture Notes Comput. Sci.* 2525:1–15.

THORPE, S., D. FIZE, and C. MARLOT, 1996. Speed of processing in the human visual system. *Nature* 381:520–522.

TONG, F., K. NAKAYAMA, M. MOSCOVITCH, O. WEINRIB, and N. KANWISHER, 2000. Response properties of the human fusiform face area. *Cogn. Neuropsychol.* 17:257–279.

TSAO, D. Y., W. A. FREIWALD, T. A. KNUTSEN, J. B. MANDEVILLE, and R. B. H. TOOTELL (in press). Faces and objects in macaque cerebral cortex. *Nat. Neurosci.*

TSUNODA, K., Y. YAMANE, M. NISHIZAKI, and M. TANIFUJI, 2001. Complex objects are represented in macaque inferotemporal cortex by the combination of feature columns. *Nat. Neurosci.* 4:832–838.

ULLMAN, S., M. VIDAL-NAQUET, and E. SALI, 2002. Visual features of intermediate complexity and their use in classification. *Nat. Neurosci.* 5:682–687.

WANG, G., K. TANAKA, and M. TANIFUJI, 1996. Optical imaging of functional organization in the monkey inferotemporal cortex. *Science* 272:1665–1668.

WINSTON, J. S., B. A. STRANGE, J. O'DOHERTY, and R. J. DOLAN, 2002. Automatic and intentional brain responses during evaluation of trustworthiness of faces. *Nat. Neurosci.* 5:277–283.

YOUNG, M. P., and S. YAMANE, 1992. Sparse population coding of faces in the inferotemporal cortex. *Science* 256:1327–1331.

ZEKI, S., J. D. G. WATSON, C. J. LUECK, K. J. FRISTON, C. KENNARD, and R. S. J. FRACKOWIAK, 1991. A direct demonstration of functional specialization in human visual cortex. *J. Neurosci.* 11:641–649.

65 Associative Memory: Representation, Activation, and Cognitive Control

RYOKO FUJIMICHI, YUJI NAYA, AND YASUSHI MIYASHITA

ABSTRACT The investigation of the neural basis of semantic networks has been markedly facilitated by reducing complex associative networks to elementary associative links between two objects and then inquiring about the neural mechanisms underlying such elementary associative links in animal models. In this chapter, we examine associative memory in terms of its representation, activation, and cognitive control. Macaque monkeys were trained to memorize visual objects by association. First, we provide evidence that associations between semantically linked visual objects are formed in neural representations in the temporal neocortex and limbic cortex. We then discuss how such memory engrams are activated, highlighting two different retrieval processes: "active" and "automatic." The automatic memory retrieval signal flows backward from the limbic cortex, while during the active retrieval process, a top-down signal from the prefrontal cortex reaches the temporal cortex, as revealed in partial split-brain studies. The process of active retrieval could be involved where memory traces are explored through inferential strategies, either implicitly or explicitly, which then raises the question of how such inferential processes are cognitively controlled. To answer this, we used the Feeling-of-Knowing paradigm and identified brain areas associated with the metamemory system that supervises the retrieval process and exerts cognitive control.

Imagination is a wonderful gift that improves with use. We now attempt to stimulate your imagination to help you recall a whole portrait of this chapter in an image (figure 65.1).

A few days ago, I found a piece of paper with a strange scribble in my suitcase:

In the house, a place of work,
Teams of busy monkeys lurk,
Directed in their search for truth
By their leader, on the roof.

Up the hill, and through the door,
Worms come wriggling on the floor,
Advancing to their wormy doom—
A hen will eat them in that room.

The eggs she makes from such nutrition
Will come in one of two conditions—

Some will hatch, to our surprise,
Instead of chickens, butterflies.

Others yet, still smooth and round,
Are seized by monkeys on the ground
And sent, for better understanding,
To their friends upon the landing.

The clever simians there debate
Each egg, and what will be its fate.
It is the task of these macaques
To relay their instructions back.

Some they order broken wide,
Freeing the butterfly inside.
The house now shimmers with the sight
Of *Lepidoptera* in flight.

Hatched or broken, all will go
To the garden down below,
Where blooms of Cogitation grow,
And winds of Reason gently blow.

The image of the house on the hill in its various components helps organize and locate the issues discussed in this chapter. We can think of the monkey as an agent of "the Society of Mind" (Minsky, 1986), or as a neural assembly (Hebb, 1949). Each egg appears to have two possible destinies, to be broken or to be hatched. In either case, a butterfly representing the worm's associative component is born. By the end of the chapter, the structure of the memory systems and the somewhat complicated visual associative processes described herein should come into focus through the imagination's passing and recollection of the house on the hill.

Various forms of memory can be classified as declarative (explicit) or nondeclarative (implicit) on the basis of how information is stored and recalled (see Squire, Clark, and Bayley, this volume; Buckner and Schacter, this volume). Declarative memory underlies the learning of facts and personal experiences. Nondeclarative memory includes forms of perceptual and motor memory. Declarative memory can be further classified as episodic (a memory for events and personal experience) or semantic (Tulving, 1972). According to Tulving (1972), semantic memory is "a mental thesaurus,

RYOKO FUJIMICHI, YUJI NAYA, and YASUSHI MIYASHITA The University of Tokyo School of Medicine, Hongo, Tokyo, Japan.

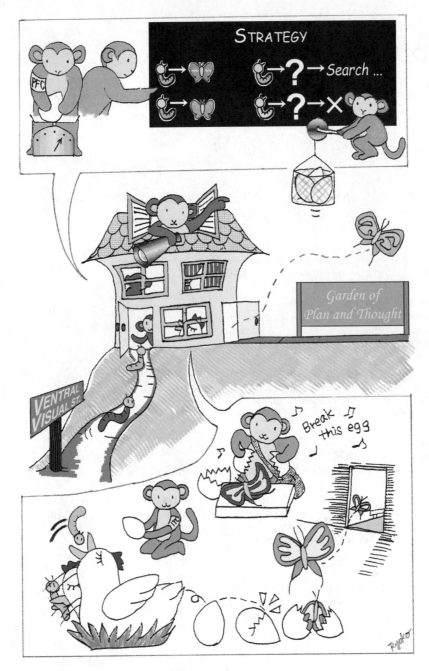

FIGURE 65.1 The house on the hill.

organized knowledge a person possesses about words and other verbal symbols, their meaning and referents, about relations among them, and about rules, formulas, and algorithms for the manipulation of these symbols, concepts, and relations. . . ." According to Lindsay and Norman (1977), such knowledge "contained within human memory forms an interrelated web of concepts and actions. Knowledge of one topic is related to knowledge of others. The human memory system makes possible the tracing of the relationships among the knowledge within the database." They also noted that "much of our knowledge is probably encoded in combina-tions of network representations, sensory images, and motor control images."

If we think of semantic memory in these terms, and as reflecting relationships among symbols, a prototypical semantic memory system in the brain would take the form of overlapped collections of each cell assembly for objects or their neuronal associative networks. In this chapter, we will provide evidence obtained by others and ourselves of possible neural mechanisms for such an associative network. We will first discuss how a memory engram is organized, and introduce the neural representation of semantically linked

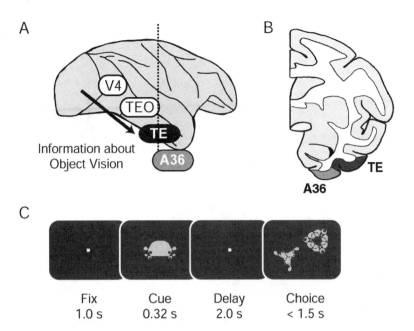

C

Fix	Cue	Delay	Choice
1.0 s	0.32 s	2.0 s	< 1.5 s

FIGURE 65.2 (*A*) Lateral view of a macaque brain. TE is located at the final processing stage of the ventral visual pathway. A36 is thought to be a part of the medial temporal lobe system. V4, visual area 4; TEO, area TEO. (*B*) Coronal cross-section indicated by the horizontal line on the ventral view in panel *A*. The black and gray areas indicate the locations of the recoding sites in TE and A36, respectively. (*C*) Sequence of events in one trial of the PA task. Fix-ation points and cue stimuli were presented at the center of a video monitor. Choice stimuli were presented randomly in two of four positions on the video monitor. (Modified with permission from Y. Naya, M. Yoshida, and Y. Miyashita, Backward spreading of memory-retrieval signal in the primate temporal cortex. *Science* 291:661–664. Copyright 2001 by the American Association for the Advancement of Science.)

symbols. We will then discuss how memory engrams are activated, highlighting two different retrieval processes, active and automatic. Finally, we will make further reference to a metamemory system that supervises the retrieval process and exerts cognitive control.

Representation of visual objects: Organizing a memory engram

Neuronal correlates of associative long-term memory were first reported in the monkey inferior temporal (IT) cortex by Miyashita (1988) and Sakai and Miyashita (1991). Their single-unit recordings identified two mnemonic properties of IT neurons: (1) IT neurons can acquire stimulus selectivity through learning in adulthood, and (2) their activity can link representations of temporally associated but geometrically unrelated stimuli. How these memory neurons function as basic elements of semantic networks, and how semantic networks are created through interaction among multiple representations in temporal cortical areas, is now firmly established (Miyashita and Chang, 1988; Miyashita and Hayashi, 2000). In that regard, investigation of the neural basis of semantic networks has been greatly facilitated by reducing complex associative networks to elementary associative links between two objects, and then asking what the neural mechanisms underlying such elementary associative links might be (Miyashita, 1993). The pair-association (PA)

memory task is the best-known neuropsychological test with which to tap the memory of such an elementary pair-wise associative relation (e.g., *Wechsler Memory Scale–Revised*; Wechsler, 1987). In the following section, we discuss how investigations using the PA task revealed the neuronal machinery of associative memory in the IT cortex.

FORWARD PROCESSING OF PAIR-ASSOCIATION MEMORY The IT cortex contains two cytoarchitectonically distinct but mutually interconnected areas: area TE (TE) and area 36 (A36) (Suzuki and Amaral, 1994; Saleem and Tanaka, 1996; figure 65.2*A*, *B*). TE is a unimodal neocortex located at the final stage of the ventral visual pathway, which processes object vision (Logothetis, Pauls, and Poggio, 1995; Tanaka, 1996; Sheinberg and Logothetis, 1997; Janssen, Vogels, and Orban, 2000). A36, on the other hand, is a limbic polymodal association area and a component of the medial temporal lobe memory system, which is involved in the formation of declarative memory (Zola-Morgan and Squire, 1990; Murray, Gaffan, and Mishkin, 1993; Higuchi and Miyashita, 1996; Yakovlev et al., 1998; Murray and Bussey, 1999; Liu and Richmond, 2000; Brown and Aggleton, 2001). Naya, Yoshida, and Miyashita (2003) found that association between the representations of different but semantically linked objects proceeds from TE to A36. To do this, they trained monkeys to perform the PA memory task in which meaningless computer-generated pictures were sorted

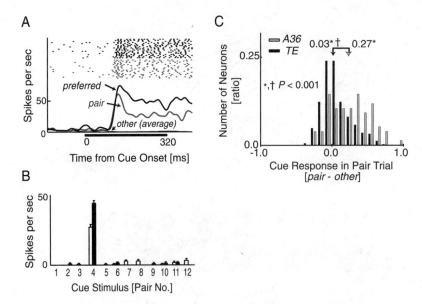

A

B

C

FIGURE 65.3 Stimulus-selective responses to both paired associates. *A* and *B* show data from a representative A36 neuron. (*A*) Raster displays and PSTHs in trials where the preferred stimulus (preferred, thick black line) or its paired associate (pair, thick gray line) served as a cue. PSTH and the trials were temporally aligned at the cue onset. The black lines indicate responses to the preferred cue stimulus (preferred, thick black line) or its paired associate (pair, thick gray line). The thin black line denotes the averaged responses in the other trials (other). The horizontal gray bar indicates the cue presentation period.

(*B*) Mean discharge rates during the cue period (60–320 ms from the cue onset) for each cue presentation. Twelve pairs of stimuli are labeled on the abscissa. The open and filled bars in pair 1, for example, refer to the responses to stimulus 1 and 1′, respectively. Error bars denote SEM.

(*C*) Distribution of response amplitudes in pair trials. The cue responses were quantified for each neuron as follows. The mean

firing rate during the cue period in the pair trials was calculated by subtracting that in the other trials from the raw value. The subtracted values were then normalized to the mean firing rates during the cue period in the preferred trials. The ordinate indicates the frequency of neurons in each bin normalized to the total number of the cue-selective neurons ($n = 76$ in A36, gray bar; $n = 347$ in TE, black bar). The distributions in both areas were shifted significantly toward more positive values (asterisk, $P < 0.001$, Wilcoxon's signed-rank test); moreover, the distribution of A36 neurons was shifted to significantly higher values than that of TE neurons (dagger, $P < 0.001$, Kolmogorov–Smirnov test). (Modified with permission from Y. Naya, M. Yoshida, and Y. Miyashita, Forward processing of long-term associative memory in monkey inferotemporal cortex. *J. Neurosci.* 23:2861–2871. © 2003 by the Society for Neuroscience.)

randomly into pairs. We refer to each member of a pair as a paired associate. The monkeys were trained to memorize combinations of paired associates, which could not be predicted otherwise. In each trial of the task, a cue stimulus was presented, and the monkey was rewarded when it chose the paired associate of the cue (figure 65.2*C*). After training, extracellular spike discharges were recorded from single neurons in TE and A36.

A total of 2368 neurons were recorded from A36 (510 neurons) and TE (1858 neurons) in the three monkeys performing the PA task. Of those, 475 neurons (85 neurons in A36 and 390 neurons in TE) showed responses to the cue presentation for at least one stimulus among the 24 learned stimuli (visually responsive cells). Out of them, 423 neurons (76 neurons in A36 and 347 neurons in TE) showed significant ($P < 0.01$, ANOVA) stimulus selectivity during the cue period (60–320 ms from cue onset) (cue-selective cells). The responses of a representative cue-selective neuron in A36 are shown in figure 65.3*A* and *B*. Note that one stimulus elicited the strongest response from this neuron during the cue

period (figure 65.3*A*, thick black line; *B*, solid bar in pair 4). This neuron was also activated when the paired associate of the preferred stimulus was presented (figure 65.3*A*, thick gray line; *B*, open bar in pair 4). In contrast to the robust responses to this stimulus pair, this neuron responded only negligibly when stimuli from any of the other pairs were presented as cue stimuli (figure 65.3*A*, thin black line, the averaged responses to the other 22 stimuli). This type of neuron, which is found in the IT cortex and is referred to as a *pair-coding neuron*, selectively responds to both paired associates (pair-coding response). This property indicates that memory storage is organized such that single neurons can code both paired associates in the PA task.

The pair-coding responses in A36 were compared with those in TE by examining the distributions of the response amplitude for the pair trials (figure 65.3*C*, A36, gray; TE, black). It was found that the distribution was significantly shifted toward positive values in both areas (A36, median = 0.27; TE, median = 0.03; $P < 0.001$ in both areas, Wilcoxon's signed-rank test), with the distribution of responses for the

A36 neurons shifted to significantly higher values than the distribution for the TE neurons ($P < 0.001$, Kolmogorov–Smirnov test). Thus, in addition to the preferred stimulus, neurons in both A36 and TE responded selectively to the paired associate of the preferred stimulus, and the response was more prominent in A36 than in TE. In addition, the percentage of pair-coding neurons among the cue-selective neurons was significantly higher in A36 (33%) than in TE (4.9%) ($P < 0.001$, χ^2 test) (Naya, Yoshida, and Miyashita, 2003). This means that although neurons in both areas acquire stimulus selectivity through associative learning, the effect is engraved more intensely on the neuronal representation in A36 than in TE. The dramatic increase in the percentage of pair-coding neurons observable in going from TE to A36 indicates that the association between representations of paired associates proceeds forward through this anatomical hierarchy of the IT cortex.

CIRCUIT REORGANIZATION DURING FORMATION OF THE PAIR-ASSOCIATION MEMORY It has long been hypothesized that memory engrams of declarative knowledge, as exemplified by the emergence of pair-coding neurons, develop with a structural and functional reorganization of neural circuits in the cerebral association cortices. (Squire and Zola-Morgan, 1991; Miyashita, 1993; Mishkin et al., 1997; Jones, 2000; Martin, Grimwood, and Morris, 2000). This reorganization of neural circuits would be accomplished through a cellular program of gene expression leading to increased protein synthesis and then to alteration of synaptic connections (Bailey and Kandel, 1993). To date, this hypothetical framework has been primarily investigated in invertebrates and lower mammals, in which it is difficult to examine the organization of semantic memory. Still, the hypothesis as applied to semantic memory has been tested in a series of molecular biological studies carried out in monkeys (Okuno and Miyashita, 1996; Tokuyama et al., 2000, 2002), showing that up-regulation of mRNA-encoding proteins thought to be involved in structural reorganization occurred during formation of the pair-association memory. In this series of studies, the RT-PCR mRNA quantitation was combined with three unique experimental strategies. The first strategy entailed the use of split-brain monkeys, which were prepared by transecting the anterior commissure and the entire extent of the corpus callosum (Hasegawa et al., 1998). The fact that there was no interhemispheric transfer of mnemonic engrams in this preparation (Gazzaniga, 1995; Hasegawa et al., 1998) enabled us to compare mRNA expression within individual monkeys (figure 65.4A), thereby eliminating genetic and cognitive variations between individuals. The second strategy entailed the use of a visual discrimination (VD) task rather than a no-task condition as the control (figure 65.4A). This enabled the motivational and attentional states in the two hemispheres, as well as the input of visual stimuli, to be appropriately balanced. The third strategy entailed training monkeys to first learn a rule or strategy component of the tasks using training stimulus sets, after which a test stimulus set was introduced for new learning of the declarative components of the task. Before the learning process with the test stimulus was complete, the animals were perfused, and expression of mRNA in the brains was evaluated. This enabled investigation of gene expression during formation of associative memory but not during formation of procedural memory.

Using the approach just described, it was found that expression of mRNA encoding brain-derived neurotrophic factor (BDNF) was significantly higher in A36 of the PA hemisphere than in the VD hemisphere ($P < 0.05$) (figure 65.4B). In the early visual cortex (e.g., V1 or V4), by contrast, expression of BDNF mRNA did not differ in the two hemispheres (V1, $P > 0.60$; V4, $P > 0.87$), indicating that the increased expression of BDNF mRNA level in A36 did not reflect a difference in the amount of visual input. The RT-PCR analysis also showed that expression of the mRNA encoding trkB, a specific receptor for BDNF (Bonhoeffer, 1996; McAllister, Katz, and Lo, 1999), was slightly increased in A36 of the PA hemisphere, though the increase did not reach statistical significance. The expression of the mRNA encoding the immediate-early gene zif268 was also selectively up-regulated in A36 during formation of PA memory (Tokuyama et al., 2002). On the other hand, expression of a housekeeping gene, β-actin, did not differ between the two hemispheres in any of the cortical areas examined.

The spatial distribution of the BDNF mRNA was visualized using in situ hybridization (figure 65.5). Notably, BDNF mRNA-positive cells accumulated as a "patchy" cluster in A36 of the PA hemisphere but not in the same area of the VD hemisphere, which suggests that up-regulation of BDNF expression is associated with neurons located within the patches in A36. These patches were most prominent in layers V/VI, but were also observed in layers II/III (figure 65.5C), extending for at least 0.4 mm along the anteroposterior axis. In contrast to the PA hemisphere, the VD hemisphere contained only scattered BDNF mRNA-positive cells in layers V/VI of A36 (figure 65.5B, D). And when the magnitude of the local increase of BDNF mRNA expression was estimated by grain-counting analysis (framed areas, figure 65.5A, B), it was found that significantly more neurons in the PA hemisphere expressed detectable levels of BDNF mRNA than in the VD hemisphere ($9.1\% \pm 0.7\%$ in the PA hemisphere vs. $3.7\% \pm 0.6\%$ in the VD hemisphere; $\chi^2 = 72.4$, $P < 0.001$). In area 35 of the PA hemisphere, expression of BDNF mRNA also seemed slightly stronger than in the VD hemisphere, but there were no differences in the patterns of BDNF mRNA expression in any other regions of the PA and VD hemispheres.

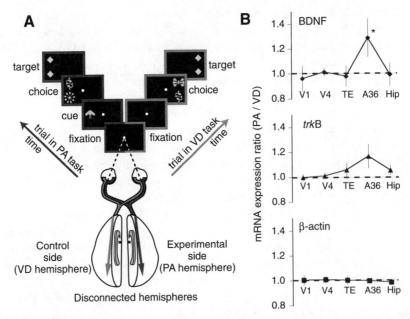

A

target · choice · cue · fixation

trial in PA task · time

trial in VD task · time

Control side (VD hemisphere)

Experimental side (PA hemisphere)

Disconnected hemispheres

B

BDNF

mRNA expression ratio (PA / VD)

V1 · V4 · TE · A36 · Hip

*trk*B

V1 · V4 · TE · A36 · Hip

β-actin

V1 · V4 · TE · A36 · Hip

FIGURE 65.4 (*A*) Visual memory tasks for split-brain monkeys. Stimulus configuration for two visual memory tasks in different visual hemifields. Each split-brain monkey was trained to perform both a pair-association (PA) task and a visual discrimination (VD) task. During visual fixation, visual stimuli for the PA task were presented to one visual hemifield, while visual stimuli for the VD task were presented in the other hemifield. Using this configuration, split-brain monkeys did the PA task with one hemisphere (PA hemisphere) and the VD task with the other hemisphere (VD hemisphere).

(*B*) Intra-animal comparison of levels of expression of BDNF, *trk*B, and β-actin mRNA in the PA and VD hemispheres. In each

cortical area of each monkey, the mRNA expression ratio was calculated by dividing the level of mRNA expression in the PA (experimental) hemisphere by that in the VD (control) hemisphere. The mRNA expression ratios were then averaged across animals and plotted for the indicated five cortical areas (mean ± SEM). Expression of BDNF mRNA was significantly higher in A36 of the PA hemisphere than A36 of the VD hemisphere. An asterisk indicates a significant difference between the PA and VD hemispheres ($P < 0.05$). (Modified with permission from W. Tokuyama et al., BDNF upregulation during declarative memory formation in monkey inferior temporal cortex. *Nat. Neurosci.* 3:1134–1142. © 2000 by the Nature Publishing Group.)

BDNF is thought to mediate activity-dependent synaptic plasticity, even in mature nervous systems (Thoenen, 1995; Bonhoeffer, 1996; McAllister, Katz, and Lo, 1999). Consistent with that idea, its expression is regulated by changes in neuronal activity. Moreover, since *zif*268 encodes a transcription factor, its expression could function as a trigger for a cascade of gene activation that leads to the cellular events underlying neuronal reorganization. Thus, analysis of the formation of PA memory has provided the first evidence supporting the hypothesis that BDNF contributes to the reorganization of neural networks, and that perhaps this reorganization is initiated by *zif*268, which triggers a cascade of gene activation.

The location of the focal patch expressing BDNF approximates the location of aggregates of pair-coding neurons detected by single-unit recording (referred to as a hotspot; Naya, Yoshida, and Miyashita, 2003; Yoshida, Naya, and Miyashita, 2003). A combined anatomical-physiological analysis recently showed that structural reorganization does indeed occur at hotspots and that the fiber terminals of picture-selective neurons in TE are retracted out of the hotspot in A36 but remain to project within the hotspot (Yoshida, Naya, and Miyashita, 2003). We therefore suggest

that BDNF expression may induce axonal and synaptic reorganization in the hotspot in A36, and that such reorganization of local networks is detected electrophysiologically as a change in neuronal stimulus selectivity, typically as the emergence of pair-coding neurons.

Activation of memory engrams: Active versus automatic retrieval

There appear to be two types of memory retrieval processes, automatic and active. Their differences are illustrated in the following example. Readers who loved adventure stories when they were young would strongly associate a beautiful fairy called Tinker Bell with the boy who would not grow up, Peter Pan. It would then be easy to recall Tinker Bell's name from Peter Pan's name; it would be automatic. On the other hand, if you were asked the name of the author who wrote *Peter Pan*, you would likely find it more difficult to recall the author's name—James M. Barrie.

Now, sometimes one needs no effort to recall, and at other times one must strive for a successful recall. We refer to the former as automatic retrieval and to the latter as active retrieval (Petrides, 2000; Fletcher and Henson, 2001). In the

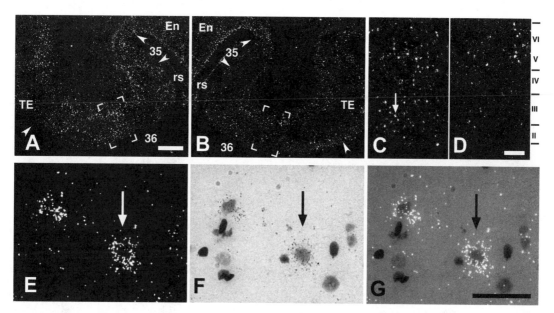

FIGURE 65.5   In situ hybridization of BDNF mRNA. (*A–D*) Distribution of BDNF mRNA in the IT gyrus of the PA (*A*) and VD (*B*) hemispheres. BDNF mRNA accumulated in a patch in A36 of the PA hemisphere (framed area), but not in A36 of the VD hemisphere. The framed areas in *A* and *B* are enlarged in *C* and *D*, respectively. BDNF mRNA-positive cells were observed in layers V/VI and in layers II/III of the PA hemisphere (*C*); the image of the cell marked by the arrow is defined in *E–G*. Abbreviations: En, entorhinal cortex; 35, area 35; 36, area 36; TE, area TE; rs, rhinal sulcus. Arrowheads mark the boundaries between different cortical areas.

(*E–G*) BDNF mRNA-positive cells in layers II/III of the PA hemisphere. The cell marked by an arrow in *C* is enlarged and shown in dark-field (*E*), bright-field (*F*), and bright-field with epi-illumination (*G*). Silver grains were concentrated around lightly Nissl-stained neuronal nuclei. Cortical layers of A36 are indicated along the margin of *D*. Scale bars = 1 mm (*A*, *B*), 250 μm (*C*, *D*), 50 μm (*E–G*). (Modified with permission from W. Tokuyama et al., BDNF upregulation during declarative memory formation in monkey inferior temporal cortex. *Nat. Neurosci.* 3:1134–1142. © 2000 by the Nature Publishing Group.)

previous section, we discussed visual associative memory stored in the IT cortex. It follows that such long-term memory could then be retrieved from the IT cortex by either of these two processes. In this section, we will suggest that whether retrieval is automatic or active depends on whether the retrieval signal is created within the network of the IT cortex or runs from the prefrontal (PF) cortex to the IT cortex. We begin by introducing a study that showed that the automatic memory retrieval signal flows backward through the IT cortex, from A36 to TE.

AUTOMATIC RETRIEVAL SIGNAL: BACKWARD SPREAD OF MEMORY RETRIEVAL SIGNAL IN THE INFERIOR TEMPORAL CORTEX   The theory of semantic network visualizes a retrieval of an item as activation of a corresponding node at the network. The neural correlate of such a node activation was first reported in the PA task by Sakai and Miyashita (1991). They found a group of IT neurons that showed an activation related to the retrieval of the paired associates from a cue stimulus. The response is referred to as pair-recall response. Using a modified PA task (PA with a color switch task), Naya, Sakai, and Miyashita (1996) showed that this pair-recall response indeed corresponded to the recall of the visual image in subject's mind, since IT

neurons started to fire just after a color switch that signaled the necessity and timing of memory retrieval during its delay period and the IT neurons also stopped to fire just after another color switch that signaled retrieval of other memorized items. Such change of neuronal discharge did not occur when a color switch signaled a simple maintenance of short-term memory. Therefore, this type of delay activity in the IT cortex represents the internal target that is retrieved from long-term memory. Recently, it was reported that this target-related activity is transmitted backward, from A36 to TE, as illustrated later (Naya, Yoshida, and Miyashita, 2001).

The responses of a representative A36 neuron showing the target-related activity specified by a cue stimulus (Sakai and Miyashita, 1991; Naya, Sakai, and Miyashita, 1996) are shown in figure 65.6*A* and *B*. One stimulus elicited the strongest response during the cue period, and the response continued into the delay period (upper panel). In the trial when the paired associate of this preferred stimulus was presented as a cue, the neurons in both A36 and TE exhibited the highest delay activity among the stimuli (lower panel). This type of activity is referred to as target-related. The onset of the target-related activity of the TE neuron was later than that of the A36 neuron (lower panel).

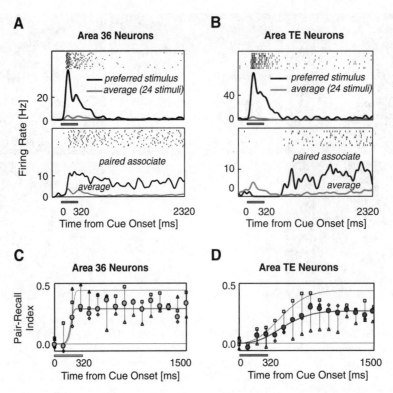

FIGURE 65.6   Neuronal activity related to memory retrieval, as shown by a single cell in A36 (*A*) and in TE (*B*). For the raster displays (*A* and *B*), PSTHs were temporally aligned at the cue onset in trials where the preferred stimulus (upper panel) or its paired associate (lower panel) served as a cue. Black lines indicate responses to the preferred cue stimulus (upper panel) or its paired associate (lower panel); gray lines indicate mean responses to all 24 stimuli. (*C, D*) Temporal dynamics of averaged PRI(*t*) for the population of stimulus-selective neurons (A36, n = 45; TE, n = 69). Mean values of PRI(*t*) were plotted every 100 ms for A36 (*C*) and TE (*D*) neurons (solid circle, total; open diamond, monkey 1; open square, monkey 2; open triangle, monkey 3). Thick lines (in *C* and *D*, respectively) indicate the best-fit Weibull functions for the population-averaged PRI(*t*) in the two areas (A36, TRT, 181 ms, TRD, 76 ms; TE, 493 ms, 602 ms). Thin lines indicate the same but for the neurons whose PRI(*t*) increased above the 5% significance level (A36, 197 ms, 69 ms; TE, 472 ms, 625 ms). (Modified with permission from Y. Naya, M. Yoshida, and Y. Miyashita, Backward spreading of memory-retrieval signal in the primate temporal cortex. *Science* 291:661–664. Copyright 2001 by the American Association for the Advancement of Science.)

The time course of the target-related delay activity of each neuron was examined by considering the responses to all cue stimuli. The partial correlation coefficients of instantaneous firing rates at time *t* for each cue stimulus were calculated with the visual responses to its paired associate (pair-recall index, PRI). The time courses of the average PRI(*t*) across the population of stimulus-selective neurons were found to differ significantly in A36 and TE (repeated-measures ANOVA, *P* < 0.0001) (figure 65.6*C, D*). The PRI(*t*) for the A36 neurons began to increase during the cue period and developed with a rapid time course. The PRI(*t*) for the TE neurons, by contrast, increased slowly and reached a plateau in the middle of the delay period. To summarize this section, memory-retrieval signals appeared first in A36, after which TE neurons were gradually recruited to represent the sought target. Thus, mnemonic information that was extracted from long-term storage spread backward, from A36 to TE.

TOP-DOWN SIGNALING APPEARS WHEN ACTIVE RETRIEVAL IS REQUIRED   A clinical case study helps us to highlight the

active retrieval in humans and provides a clue to an experimental model with which to investigate active retrieval (Sidtis et al., 1981). In that study, an epileptic patient who had undergone a posterior callosotomy was presented with a word in his left visual field. He could never read the word directly, although he claimed to "see" its image in his mind. He was nevertheless able to eventually identify the word using inferential strategies based on his mental image. His limited ability suggests that his right hemisphere was transmitting to his left hemisphere semantic information about the stimulus, but not the actual stimulus. After the callosum was completely sectioned, semantic information was no longer transferred from the right hemisphere to the left. Hasegawa and colleagues (1998) combined this posterior split-brain paradigm with the associative memory task in monkeys. In the posterior split-brain monkey, in which the posterior corpus callosum and the anterior commissure are sectioned, the cortex receives bottom-up visual information only from the contralateral visual field (figure 65.7*A*). With this paradigm, long-term memory acquired through stimulus-

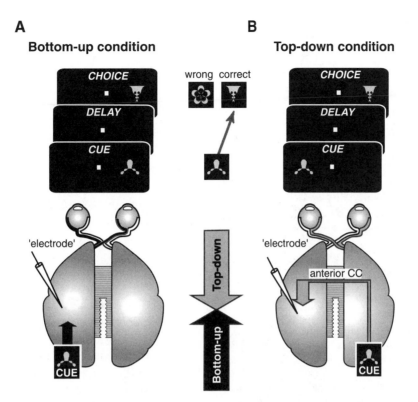

A **Bottom-up condition**

B **Top-down condition**

FIGURE 65.7 The posterior split-brain paradigm. (*A*) Bottom-up condition. Visual stimuli (cue and choice pictures) were presented in the hemifield contralateral to the recording site (electrode) in the IT cortex. The monkeys were trained to memorize visual stimulus-stimulus associations among 20 cue and 5 choice pictures. In each trial, while the monkey held a lever and maintained fixation, cue and choice pictures were sequentially presented parafoveally with a delay. If the choice picture was the correct one associated with the cue, the monkey had to release the lever. Bottom-up sensory signals (black arrow) would be detected in this condition.

(*B*) Top-down condition. The protocol was the same as in *A*, but the cue was presented in the hemifield ipsilateral to the recording site; the choice was presented contralaterally. In posterior split-brain monkeys, the sensory signal does not reach visual areas in the opposite hemisphere. In this condition, only top-down signals (gray arrow) could activate IT neurons through feedback connections from the prefrontal cortex. (Modified with permission from H. Tomita et al., Top-down signal from prefrontal cortex in executive control of memory retrieval. *Nature* 401:699–703. © 1999 by the Nature Publishing Group.)

stimulus association does not transfer interhemispherically via the anterior corpus callosum; nonetheless, when the visual cue was presented to one hemisphere, the anterior callosum could instruct the other hemisphere to retrieve the correct stimulus specified by the cue. Thus, although visual long-term memory is stored in the temporal cortex, memory retrieval is under the executive control of the PF cortex.

Direct proof of the existence of a top-down signal from the PF cortex to the temporal cortex and of its contribution to the active retrieval process was provided by single-unit recordings from the posterior split-brain preparation (Tomita et al., 1999). In this protocol, inferior temporal neurons in one hemisphere ("electrode" in figure 65.7*A*) are to be activated by bottom-up visual inputs when an object is presented in the visual hemifield contralateral to the recording site. When the object is presented in the ipsilateral hemifield, however, these neurons should not be able to receive bottom-up visual inputs. Any neural activation should therefore reflect top-down inputs from the PF cortex (figure 65.7*B*). It was found that a considerable number of IT

neurons did indeed receive top-down signals from the PF cortex; the activity of one such IT neuron is shown in figure 65.8. This neuron was not only activated by contralateral presentation of stimuli (figure 65.8, bottom-up response, black), but was also activated by ipsilateral presentation of stimuli (figure 65.8, top-down response, gray). In these neurons, which showed stimulus selectivity in both top-down and bottom-up responses, the latency was significantly longer in the top-down condition ($P < 0.001$). These top-down responses were abolished after transection of the remaining anterior corpus callosum. The partial split-brain studies in human and monkeys reveal the events occurring during the active retrieval process, which are indicative of purely top-down signaling.

Imaging studies carried out in humans have further confirmed that the PF cortex plays a key role in the active retrieval process. Activation of the PF cortex during memory retrieval is widely observed in functional neuroimaging studies employing a variety of psychological paradigms and test modalities, including recognition tests, word stem tasks,

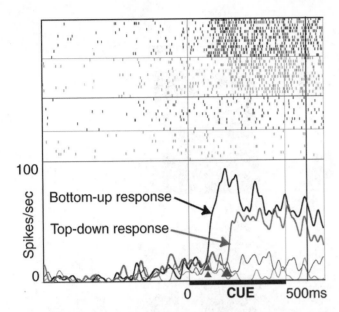

FIGURE 65.8 Activity of a single IT cell in the top-down condition (top-down, gray; bottom-up, black). Raster displays, PSTHs were temporally aligned at the cue onset. In the PSTH, thick lines show responses to the preferred cue, whereas thin lines show responses to a null cue. The onset of the top-down response (arrowhead) was later than that of the bottom-up response (double arrowhead). (Modified with permission from H. Tomita et al., Top-down signal from prefrontal cortex in executive control of memory retrieval. *Nature* 401:699–703. © 1999 by the Nature Publishing Group.)

word fragment tasks, paired associates tasks, free recall, and recency judgment (Squire et al., 1992; Shallice et al., 1994; Buckner, Raichle, and Petersen, 1995; Schacter, Buckner, and Koutstaal, 1998; Wagner et al., 1998; Konishi et al., 2002). Among these studies, Fletcher and colleagues (1998) found that the right dorsal PF cortex (BA 9/46) is strongly activated when monitoring demands were emphasized, while the right ventral PF cortex (BA 45) showed greater activation when external cuing was emphasized. Wagner and colleagues (1998) suggested that right PF activation reflected retrieval attempts, including initiation of retrieval search or evaluation of the products of retrieval. In addition, Cadoret, Pike, and Petrides (2001) attempted to identify more focal areas that were specifically related to active retrieval by matching the retrieval and control conditions in terms of depth of encoding, decision making, and postretrieval monitoring. They found activity related to active retrieval to be selectively increased within area 47/12 in the ventrolateral PF cortex. Earlier anatomical studies had shown that area 47/12 is strongly connected with the inferotemporal cortical region (Barbas, 1988; Ungerleider, Gaffan, and Pellack, 1989). Thus, we suggest that the source of the top-down signaling reported by Tomita and colleagues (1999) may be a homologue of BA 47/12. A process of active retrieval could be involved where memory traces are accessed through inferential strategies, either implicit or explicit, which then raises the question of how such inferential processes are cognitively controlled.

Metamemory: Cognitive control of memory system

As students, we probably experienced a situation in which we were unable to answer a question on a closed-format test but were sure we could have answered correctly if the question was in a multiple-choice format. In fact, we accessed related items in our semantic network, since there is a positive correlation between the objective score on the recognition test and the degree of subjective feeling of whether one knew the answer or not. Metamemory refers to knowledge about one's memory capabilities and knowledge about strategies that can aid memory (Shimamura, 1995). Metamemory requires execution of extensive retrieval process and, at the same time, supervises the retrieval process. Kikyo, Ohki, and Miyashita (2002) successfully identified brain areas related to a metamemory system in humans using a "feeling-of-knowing" paradigm, which is a well-established tool for assessing metamemory system (figure 65.9A). The feeling-of-knowing is a subjective sense of knowing a word before recalling it—a sense that "I know that I know it." Based on the recall-judgment-recognition paradigm (Hart, 1965), subjects in this experiment were asked to recall word answers for general information questions during fMRI scans. After the scans, the subjects wrote their answers to the recalled questions and were instructed to judge their degree of feeling-of-knowing to the non-recalled questions on a three-point scale, where 3 = "I definitely could recall the answer if given hints or more time"; 2 = "I probably would recognize the answer"; and 1 = "I definitely did not know." Event-related fMRI with a parametric analysis showed stronger activity in the bilateral inferior frontal gyri (BA 47), left medial frontal gyrus (BA 46/9, BA 10), and ACC/SMA (BA 32/24/6) when people have a greater feeling-of-knowing (figure 65.9B; see also Maril et al., 2003). These activation areas are referred to here as the feeling-of-knowing regions. Among these feeling-of-knowing regions, subregions in the bilateral inferior frontal gyri (BA 47) were not recruited for successful recall processes, suggesting a specific role for these regions in human metamemory system. One of the feeling-of-knowing regions was located in the anterior portion of the left medial frontal gyzus, BA 10. This area was regarded as part of the memory areas in the anterior PF cortex in some literatures and was related to retrieval strategy and/or "third level of executive control" (Fletcher and Henson, 2001).

Future perspective

The extensive investigations described in this chapter have been revealing a whole picture of the semantic memory

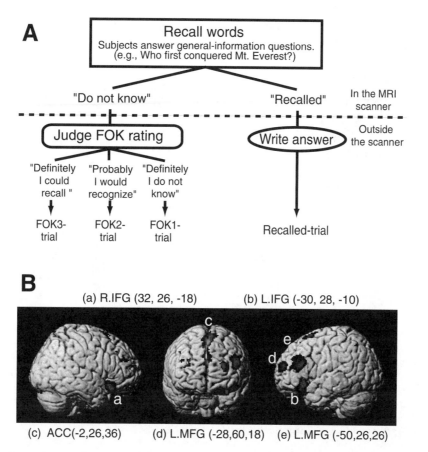

A

Recall words
Subjects answer general-information questions.
(e.g., Who first conquered Mt. Everest?)

"Do not know"   "Recalled"   In the MRI scanner

Judge FOK rating   Write answer   Outside the scanner

"Definitely I could recall "   "Probably I would recognize"   "Definitely I do not know"

FOK3-trial   FOK2-trial   FOK1-trial   Recalled-trial

B

(a) R.IFG (32, 26, -18)   (b) L.IFG (-30, 28, -10)

(c) ACC(-2,26,36)   (d) L.MFG (-28,60,18)   (e) L.MFG (-50,26,26)

FIGURE 65.9 (*A*) Experimental procedures in the feeling-of-knowing trials. Subjects were required to recall word answers to general-information questions during fMRI. By pressing buttons, they indicated whether or not they recalled the target words. Then, outside the scanner, they judged their degree of feeling-of-knowing to the nonrecalled questions on a scale of 1 to 3, or they wrote their answers to the recalled questions. Each trial was sorted into trial type (Recalled, FOK3, FOK2, FOK1) according to the participant's judgment and was subjected to event-related fMRI analysis.

(*B*) Regions involved in feeling-of-knowing and/or successful recall. A subset of the feeling-of-knowing regions was also activated in successful recall (c, d, and e). A subset of the feeling-of-knowing regions in the bilateral IFGs was not activated in successful recall (a and b). A small subset of the feeling-of-knowing region in the left IFG was also activated in successful recall, but its cluster size did not reach significance, given the correction for the whole-brain multiple comparisons. Identifications: c, bilateral caudate nuclei/thalami; d, left middle frontal gyrus; e, ACC/SMA; f, left superior parietal lobule/inferior parietal lobule; g, precuneus. (Modified with permission from H. Kikyo, K. Ohki, and Y. Miyashita, Neural correlates for feeling-of-knowing: An fMRI parametric analysis. *Neuron* 36:177–186. © 2002 by Elsevier.)

system. There are, however, still pieces missing that will be needed to make the picture complete. For example, in the metamemory system, how are the active retrieval subsystem and its cognitive control subsystem integrated? How does each component of the identified distributed metamemory network in the PF cortex differentially support those subsystems? Is there any specific molecular or cellular basis for those differential functional subsystems? It is anticipated that a number of missing pieces will be found when the gap between the information provided by invasive studies carried out in monkeys and that provided by noninvasive human imaging studies is filled (Logothetis et al., 1999; Miyashita and Hayashi, 2000). Most of the detailed knowledge of the anatomy, function, and cellular basis of the cortex has come from studies in monkeys (Felleman and Van Essen, 1991; Miyashita, 1993; Gaffan, 1994; Fuster, 1995; Goldman-

Rakic, 1995; Desimone, 1996; Miller, 2000; Logothetis, 2002). With that as background, using the same methods to study humans and monkeys would advance our understanding of the neural organization of higher-order cognitive function. For example, fMRI may bridge this gap by enabling direct comparison of the functional organization of the brains of monkeys and humans (Logothetis et al., 1999, 2001; Hayashi et al., 1999; Vanduffel et al., 2001; see also Logothetis, this volume). Using that approach, Nakahara and colleagues (2002) observed that, when subjects performed a high-level cognitive task, transient activation related to cognitive set shifting occurred in focal regions of PF cortex in both monkeys and humans (figure 65.10), and that these functional homologues were located in cytoarchitectonically equivalent regions in the posterior part of ventrolateral PF cortex. Such comparative imaging also has the

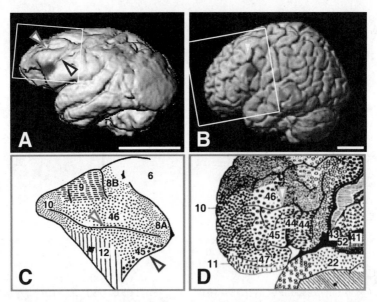

FIGURE 65.10 Comparison of shift-related activation in the PF cortex in monkeys and humans. Lateral views of 3D-rendered brain image in which the activation shown was superimposed (*A*, monkeys; *B*, humans). In the human data, a prominent activation focus in the posterior part of the inferior frontal sulcus is shown. Other activations in the precentral gyrus and in the anterior insula were also observed. For reference, cytoarchitectonic maps of macaque monkeys by Walker (1940, *C*) and that of humans by Brodmann (1910, *D*) are presented. These maps correspond approximately to areas in the white squares in *A* and *B*. Green arrowhead points to the principal sulcus, blue arrowhead to the inferior ramus of the arcuate sulcus, and yellow arrowhead to the inferior frontal sulcus. Scale bar = 30 mm. (Modified with permission from K. Nakahara, T. Hayashi, S. Konishi, and Y. Miyashita, Functional MRI of macaque monkeys performing a cognitive set-shifting task. *Science* 295:1532–1536. Copyright 2002 by the American Association for the Advancement of Science.) (See color plate 42.)

potential to provide significant new insights into the evolution of cognition in primates.

We began this chapter with an image of a house on a hill. Visual object information (a worm) reaches the final processing stage of the ventral visual pathway (climbing up the hill). There are cases in which the eggs hatch naturally (automatic retrieval). On the other hand, if the cell assemblies in the PF cortex (fairy monkeys on the second floor) and those in the IT cortex (monkeys on the first floor) interact, a top-down signal triggers active retrieval from long-term memory storage (eggs are broken by monkeys). In any case, butterflies (their paired associates) would flutter into the backyard. It would be interesting to know what a monkey in the garret would actually do. Our future goal is to put the missing pieces in their appropriate places, one by one, and in that way make the image of the house completely clear.

REFERENCES

BAILEY, C. H., and E. R. KANDEL, 1993. Structural changes accompanying memory storage. *Annu. Rev. Physiol.* 55:397–426.

BARBAS, H., 1988. Anatomic organization of basoventral and mediodorsal visual recipient prefrontal regions in the rhesus monkey. *J. Comp. Neurol.* 276:313–342.

BONHOEFFER, T., 1996. Neurotrophins and activity-dependent development of the neocortex. *Curr. Opin. Neurobiol.* 6:119–126.

BROWN, M. W., and J. P. AGGLETON, 2001. Recognition memory: What are the roles of the perirhinal cortex and hippocampus? *Nat. Rev. Neurosci.* 2:51–61.

BUCKNER, R. L., M. E. RAICHLE, and S. E. PETERSEN, 1995. Dissociation of human prefrontal cortical areas across different speech production tasks and gender groups. *J. Neurophysiol.* 74: 2163–2173.

CADORET, G., G. B. PIKE, and M. PETRIDES, 2001. Selective activation of the ventrolateral prefrontal cortex in the human brain during active retrieval processing. *Eur. J. Neurosci.* 14:1164–1170.

DESIMONE, R., 1996. Neural mechanisms for visual memory and their role in attention. *Proc. Natl. Acad. Sci. U.S.A.* 93:13494–13499.

FELLEMAN, D. J., and D. C. VAN ESSEN, 1991. Distributed hierarchical processing in the primate cerebral cortex. *Cereb. Cortex* 1: 1–47.

FLETCHER, P. C., and R. N. HENSON, 2001. Frontal lobes and human memory: Insights from functional neuroimaging. *Brain* 124: 849–881.

FLETCHER, P. C., T. SHALLICE, C. D. FRITH, R. S. FRACKOWIAK, and R. J. DOLAN, 1998. The functional roles of prefrontal cortex in episodic memory. II. Retrieval. *Brain* 121:1249–1256.

FUSTER, J. M., 1995. In *Memory in the Cerebral Cortex: An Empirical Approach to Neural Networks in the Human and Nonhuman Primate*. Cambridge, Mass.: MIT Press.

GAFFAN, D., 1994. Scene-specific memory for objects: A model of episodic memory impairment in monkeys with fornix transection. *J. Cogn. Neurosci.* 6:305–320

GAZZANIGA, M. S., 1995. Principles of human brain organization derived from split-brain studies. *Neuron* 14:217–228.

GOLDMAN-RAKIC, P. S., 1995. Cellular basis of working memory. *Neuron* 14:477–485.

HART, J. T., 1965. Memory and the feeling-of-knowing experience. *J. Educ. Psychol.* 56:208–216.

Hasegawa, I., T. Fukushima, T. Ihara, and Y. Miyashita, 1998. Callosal window between prefrontal cortices: Cognitive interaction to retrieve long-term memory. *Science* 281:814–818.

Hayashi, T., S. Konishi, I. Hasegawa, and Y. Miyashita, 1999. Mapping of somatosensory cortices with functional magnetic resonance imaging in anaesthetized macaque monkeys. *Eur. J. Neurosci.* 11:4451–4456.

Hebb, D. O., 1949. *The Organization of Behavior: A Neuropsychological Theory.* New York: Wiley.

Higuchi S., and Y. Miyashita, 1996. Formation of mnemonic neuronal responses to visual paired associates in inferotemporal cortex is impaired by perirhinal and entorhinal lesions. *Proc. Natl. Acad. Sci. U.S.A.* 93:739–743.

Janssen, P., R. Vogels, and G. A. Orban, 2000. Selectivity for 3D shape that reveals distinct areas within macaque inferior temporal cortex. *Science* 288:2054–2056.

Jones, E. G., 2000. Cortical and subcortical contributions to activity-dependent plasticity in primate somatosensory cortex. *Annu. Rev. Neurosci.* 23:1–37.

Kikyo, H., K. Ohki, and Y. Miyashita, 2002. Neural correlates for feeling-of-knowing: An fMRI parametric analysis. *Neuron* 36: 177–186.

Konishi, S., I. Uchida, T. Okuaki, T. Machida, I. Shirouzu, and Y. Miyashita, 2002. Neural correlates of recency judgment. *J. Neurosci.* 22:9549–9555.

Lindsay, P. H., and D. A. Norman, 1977. *Human Information Processing: An Introduction to Psychology.* Orlando, Fl.: Harcourt Brace Jovanovich.

Liu Z., and B. J. Richmond, 2000. Response differences in monkey TE and perirhinal cortex: Stimulus association related to reward schedules. *J. Neurophysiol.* 83:1677–1692.

Logothetis, N. K., 2002. The neural basis of the blood-oxygen-level-dependent functional magnetic resonance imaging signal. *Philos. Trans. R. Soc. Lond. B Biol. Sci.* 357:1003–1037.

Logothetis, N. K., H. Guggenberger, S. Peled, and J. Pauls, 1999. Functional imaging of the monkey brain. *Nat. Neurosci.* 2:555–562.

Logothetis, N. K., J. Pauls, M. Augath, T. Trinath, and A. Oeltermann, 2001. Neurophysiological investigation of the basis of the fMRI signal. *Nature* 412:150–157.

Logothetis, N. K., J. Pauls, and T. Poggio, 1995. Shape representation in the inferior temporal cortex of monkeys. *Curr. Biol.* 5:552–563.

Maril, A., J. S. Simons, J. P. Mitchell, B. L. Schwartz, and D. L. Schacter, 2003. Feeling-of-knowing in episodic memory: An event-related fMRI study. *NeuroImage* 18:827–836.

Martin, S. J., P. D. Grimwood, and R. G. Morris, 2000. Synaptic plasticity and memory: An evaluation of the hypothesis. *Annu. Rev. Neurosci.* 23:649–711.

McAllister, A. K., L. C. Katz, and D. C. Lo, 1999. Neurotrophins and synaptic plasticity. *Annu. Rev. Neurosci.* 22:295–318.

Miller, E. K., 2000. The prefrontal cortex and cognitive control. *Nat. Rev. Neurosci.* 1:59–65.

Minsky, M., 1986. *The Society of Mind.* New York: Simon and Schuster.

Mishkin, M., W. A. Suzuki, D. G. Gadian, and F. Vargha-Khadem, 1997. Hierarchical organization of cognitive memory. *Philos. Trans. R. Soc. Lond. B Biol. Sci.* 352:1461–1467.

Miyashita, Y., 1988. Neuronal correlate of visual associative long-term memory in the primate temporal cortex. *Nature* 335:817–820.

Miyashita, Y., 1993. Inferior temporal cortex: Where visual perception meets memory. *Annu. Rev. Neurosci.* 16:245–263.

Miyashita, Y., and H. S. Chang, 1988. Neuronal correlate of pictorial short-term memory in the primate temporal cortex. *Nature* 331:68–70.

Miyashita Y., and T. Hayashi, 2000. Neural representation of visual objects: Encoding and top-down activation. *Curr. Opin. Neurobiol.* 10:187–194.

Murray, E. A., and T. J. Bussey, 1999. Perceptual-mnemonic functions of the perirhinal cortex. *Trends Cogn. Sci.* 3:142–151.

Murray, E. A., D. Gaffan, and M. Mishkin, 1993. Neural substrates of visual stimulus-stimulus association in rhesus monkeys. *J. Neurosci.* 13:4549–4561.

Nakahara, K., T. Hayashi, S. Konishi, and Y. Miyashita, 2002. Functional MRI of macaque monkeys performing a cognitive set-shifting task. *Science* 295:1532–1536.

Naya, Y., K. Sakai, and Y. Miyashita, 1996. Activity of primate inferotemporal neurons related to a sought target in pair-association task. *Proc. Natl. Acad. Sci. U.S.A.* 93:2664–2669.

Naya, Y., M. Yoshida, and Y. Miyashita, 2001. Backward spreading of memory-retrieval signal in the primate temporal cortex. *Science* 291:661–664.

Naya, Y., M. Yoshida, and Y. Miyashita, 2003. Forward processing of long-term associative memory in monkey inferotemporal cortex. *J. Neurosci.* 23:2861–2871.

Okuno, H., and Y. Miyashita, 1996. Expression of the transcription factor Zif268 in the temporal cortex of monkeys during visual paired associate learning. *Eur. J. Neurosci.* 8:2118–2128.

Petrides, M., 2000. Frontal lobes and memory. In *Handbook of Neuropsychology*, F. Boller and J. Grafman, eds. Amsterdam: Elsevier, pp. 67–84.

Sakai, K., and Y. Miyashita, 1991. Neural organization for the long-term memory of paired associates. *Nature* 354:152–155.

Saleem, K. S., and K. Tanaka, 1996. Divergent projections from the anterior inferotemporal area TE to the perirhinal and entorhinal cortices in the macaque monkey. *J. Neurosci.* 16:4757–4775.

Schacter, D. L., R. L. Buckner, and W. Koutstaal, 1998. Memory, consciousness and neuroimaging. *Philos. Trans. R. Soc. Lond. B Biol. Sci.* 353:1861–1878.

Shallice T., P. Fletcher, C. D. Frith, P. Grasby, R. S. Frackowiak, and R. J. Dolan, 1994. Brain regions associated with acquisition and retrieval of verbal episodic memory. *Nature* 368:633–635.

Sheinberg, D. L., and N. K. Logothetis, 1997. The role of temporal cortical areas in perceptual organization. *Proc. Natl. Acad. Sci. U.S.A.* 94:3408–3413.

Shimamura, A. P., 1995. Memory and frontal lobe function. In *The Cognitive Neurosciences*, M. Gazzaniga, ed. Cambridge, Mass.: MIT Press.

Sidtis, J. J., B. T. Volpe, J. D. Holtzman, D. H. Wilson, and M. S. Gazzaniga, 1981. Cognitive interaction after staged callosal section: Evidence for transfer of semantic activation. *Science* 212:344–346.

Squire, L. R., J. G. Ojemann, F. M. Miezin, S. E. Petersen, T. O. Videen, and M. E. Raichle, 1992. Activation of the hippocampus in normal humans: A functional anatomical study of memory. *Proc. Natl. Acad. Sci. U.S.A.* 89:1837–1841.

Squire, L. R., and S. Zola-Morgan, 1991. The medial temporal lobe memory system. *Science* 253:1380–1386.

Suzuki, W. A., and D. G. Amaral, 1994. Perirhinal and parahippocampal cortices of the macaque monkey: Cortical afferents. *J. Comp. Neurol.* 350:497–533.

Tanaka, K., 1996. Inferotemporal cortex and object vision. *Annu. Rev. Neurosci.* 19:109–139.

THOENEN, H., 1995. Neurotrophins and neuronal plasticity. *Science* 270:593–598.

TOKUYAMA, W., T. HASHIMOTO, Y. X. LI, H. OKUNO, and Y. MIYASHITA, 1998. Highest trkB mRNA expression in the entorhinal cortex among hippocampal subregions in the adult rat: Contrasting pattern with BDNF mRNA expression. *Brain Res. Mol. Brain Res.* 62:206–215.

TOKUYAMA, W., H. OKUNO, T. HASHIMOTO, Y. X. LI, and Y. MIYASHITA, 2000. BDNF upregulation during declarative memory formation in monkey inferior temporal cortex. *Nat. Neurosci.* 3:1134–1142.

TOKUYAMA, W., H. OKUNO, T. HASHIMOTO, Y. X. LI, and Y. MIYASHITA, 2002. Selective zif268 mRNA induction in the perirhinal cortex of macaque monkeys during formation of visual pair-association memory. *J. Neurochem.* 81:60–70.

TOMITA, H., M. OHBAYASHI, K. NAKAHARA, I. HASEGAWA, and Y. MIYASHITA, 1999. Top-down signal from prefrontal cortex in executive control of memory retrieval. *Nature* 401:699–703.

TULVING, E., 1972. Episodic and semantic memory. In *Organization of Memory*, E. Tulving and W. Donaldson, eds. New York: Academic Press.

UNGERLEIDER, L. G., D. GAFFAN, and V. S. PELAK, 1989. Projections from inferior temporal cortex to prefrontal cortex via the uncinate fascicle in rhesus monkeys. *Exp. Brain Res.* 76:473–484.

VANDUFFEL, W., D. FIZE, J. B. MANDEVILLE, K. NELISSEN, P. VAN HECKE, B. R. ROSEN, R. B. TOOTELL, and G. A. ORBAN, 2001. Visual motion processing investigated using contrast agent-enhanced fMRI in awake behaving monkeys. *Neuron* 32:565–577.

WAGNER, A. D., J. E. DESMOND, G. H. GLOVER, and J. D. GABRIELI, 1998. Prefrontal cortex and recognition memory: Functional-MRI evidence for context-dependent retrieval processes. *Brain* 121:1985–2002.

WECHSLER, D., 1987. *Wechsler Memory Scale-Revised*. San Antonio, Tex.: Psychological Corporation, Harcourt Brace Jovanovich.

YAKOVLEV, V., S. FUSI, E. BERMAN, and E. ZOHARY, 1998. Inter-trial neuronal activity in inferior temporal cortex: A putative vehicle to generate long-term visual associations. *Nat. Neurosci.* 1:310–317.

YOSHIDA, M., Y. NAYA, and Y. MIYASHITA, 2003. Anatomical organization of forward fiber projections from area TE to perirhinal neurons representing visual long-term memory in monkeys. *Proc. Natl. Acad. Sci. U.S.A.* 100:4257–4262.

ZOLA-MORGAN, S. M., and L. R. SQUIRE, 1990. The primate hippocampal formation: Evidence for a time-limited role in memory storage. *Science* 250:288–290.

66 Top-Down Mechanisms for Working Memory and Attentional Processes

LUIZ PESSOA AND LESLIE G. UNGERLEIDER

ABSTRACT Maintaining information in working memory, such as when we rehearse the route to a restaurant, and directing attention, such as when we search for a familiar face in the crowd, are two fundamental cognitive capabilities of the primate brain. Both activities are considered top-down, because they depend on goal-directed processes that rely on previous knowledge, and not on incoming sensory stimulation. Top-down processes should be contrasted to bottom-up ones, such as the deployment of attention in reaction to a sudden movement in the periphery of the visual field, which is a sensory-driven, reflexive process. Understanding the neural bases of top-down control involved in working memory and visual attention is among the most challenging goals of cognitive neuroscience. In this chapter, we review neuroimaging studies that have investigated this question in the past decade or so. The picture that emerges from this line of research points to considerable overlap between the neural substrates that control working memory and those that control attention. At the same time, there is growing evidence that the control structures for attention differ according to the type of attentive process, in that goal-directed and reflexive attention appear to be mediated by separable networks of frontal and parietal regions.

The control of working memory

Working memory refers to the process of actively maintaining relevant information in mind for brief periods of time. In a typical working memory paradigm, on each trial a sample stimulus is presented, followed by a delay of several seconds, and then a test stimulus is shown. The subject's task is to indicate whether or not the test stimulus matches the sample. This type of working memory task requires primarily maintenance operations, in which the short-term memory store is emptied after each trial.

Working memory has been extensively investigated in monkeys, where the importance of prefrontal regions has been established. Lesions of the dorsolateral prefrontal

LUIZ PESSOA Department of Psychology, Brown University, Providence, R.I.

LESLIE G. UNGERLEIDER Laboratory of Brain and Cognition, National Institute of Mental Health, National Institutes of Health, Bethesda, Md.

cortex (DLPFC), especially within and surrounding the principal sulcus (Brodmann's area [BA] 46), greatly impair working memory performance (Goldman and Rosvold, 1970; Bauer and Fuster, 1976; Funahashi, Bruce, and Goldman-Rakic, 1993). At the same time, results from single-cell studies have demonstrated that prefrontal neurons show stimulus-specific sustained discharge during the delay period (Fuster and Alexander, 1971; Kubota and Niki, 1971; for reviews, see Goldman-Rakic, 1995; Fuster, 1997). This sustained activity has been interpreted to be the neural correlate of maintenance processes that take place during the delay, and thus has been taken to be the neural signature of working memory (Fuster, 2001). Sustained activity during the delay interval is not confined, however, to the prefrontal cortex. Depending on the type of stimulus, cells with sustained responses have been found in the inferior temporal (IT) cortex (for visual patterns or color stimuli; Fuster and Jervey, 1982; Chelazzi et al., 1998), the parietal cortex (for visuospatial stimuli; Chafee and Goldman-Rakic, 1998, 2000), and the premotor cortex (for particular motor responses; Bruce and Goldberg, 1985).

In tasks similar to those used in monkeys, functional brain imaging studies in humans have also provided evidence supporting the role of prefrontal regions in working memory by demonstrating sustained signals during delay intervals (Cohen et al., 1997; Courtney et al., 1997; for review, see D'Esposito, 2001). The prefrontal regions that show this activity include the middle frontal gyrus (MFG) (BA 9/46), thought to be the human homologue of the principal sulcul region of the DLPFC in monkeys, as well as more ventral regions in the inferior frontal gyrus (IFG) (BA 44, 45, 47). As in monkeys, several studies in humans have shown that regions outside of prefrontal cortex also exhibit sustained delay activity, including the IT cortex (Courtney et al., 1998), the parietal cortex (D'Esposito et al., 1998; Jonides et al., 1998; Rowe et al., 2000), and the premotor cortex (Courtney et al., 1998; Petit et al., 1998).

What determines successful performance on a working memory task? Results from single-cell studies help clarify

919

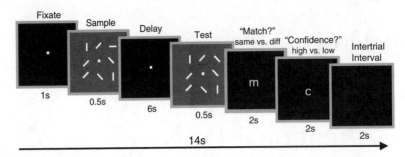

FIGURE 66.1   Experimental design. In working memory trials, subjects indicated whether the sample and test displays were the same or different (note that the bar orientation on the upper right changed in the present case). They also indicated the confidence of their response (high vs. low).

how neural activity may contribute to behavioral performance. It has been reported that, on trials in which monkeys make errors, activity during the delay interval fails to be sustained (Fuster, 1973; Rosenkilde, Bauer, and Fuster, 1981; Watanabe, 1986a,b; Funahashi, Bruce, and Goldman-Rakic, 1989), suggesting that activity during the delay bridges the gap between the sample and test stimuli to enable monkeys to correctly match them. However, interpreting the precise relationship between delay activity and performance as investigated in single-cell studies is often problematic. For example, the analysis of error trials has been typically assessed on a very limited number of such trials. Monkeys are generally trained to perform at very high levels of performance (90% correct or higher), such that only very few error trials are available for a given cell, largely precluding a quantitative assessment of the relationship between neuronal firing during working memory delays and behavioral performance. Additionally, in single-cell studies, it is possible that for incorrect trials the monkey never encoded the sample stimulus effectively, which in turn would lead to reduced neural activity during the delay.

In a recent functional magnetic resonance imaging (fMRI) study, we investigated how the moment-to-moment activity within cortical regions, as indexed by fMRI, contributes to success or failure on individual trials of a working memory task (Pessoa, Gutierrez, et al., 2002). Specifically, we examined how the entire network of regions engaged in visual working memory was differentially activated during trials that led to correct and incorrect outcomes. We hypothesized that different components of the task, namely, encoding, delay, and test, would engage different nodes of the working memory network to a greater extent on correct trials than on incorrect trials and provide the neural correlates of working memory performance. In particular, we hypothesized that fMRI activity during the delay interval would be stronger and more sustained on correct than on incorrect trials, and thus would predict task performance.

The task we employed to investigate this question is shown in figure 66.1. In working memory trials, after a 1-s fixation,

a sample visual display was presented for 0.5 s, followed by a 6-s fixation and a test display for 0.5 s. Subjects were then prompted by a display with the letter m (for memory) to indicate same or different by using two hand-held buttons. "Same" meant the test matched the sample, and "different" meant it did not match. Subjects also indicated the confidence level of their response by indicating high or low (via button presses) when c appeared on the display. Each of the two response periods lasted 2 s. Finally, a blank screen terminated the trial, which lasted 2 s (intertrial interval). Subjects were instructed to maintain fixation for those displays with a fixation spot. Subjects also performed control trials that did not have any maintenance demands, for which they were instructed to maintain fixation and press both buttons in both response periods.

To explore the neural substrates of working memory performance on a trial-by-trial basis, we first isolated the entire network of regions involved in working memory independent of performance by comparing fMRI signals for working memory and control trials. The main regions revealed by this contrast included dorsal occipital, inferior temporal, parietal, and premotor and prefrontal cortex, as illustrated on a surface rendering of the left and right hemispheres in figure 66.2. Having isolated the working memory network, we then probed how it was differentially activated according to task performance. This was accomplished by comparing correct and incorrect trials during each task phase—encoding, maintenance, and test. Our results demonstrated that different nodes were activated to a greater extent for correct compared to incorrect trials during the distinct components of the task. Additionally, as we anticipated, signals during the delay interval were both stronger and more sustained for correct compared to incorrect trials. For the purpose of this section, we will confine our discussion to the results pertaining only to the delay interval.

Regions exhibiting differential signals during the delay, namely, stronger activity during correct relative to incorrect trials, were almost exclusively in frontal and parietal cortex and included the DLPFC, frontal eye field (FEF), and sup-

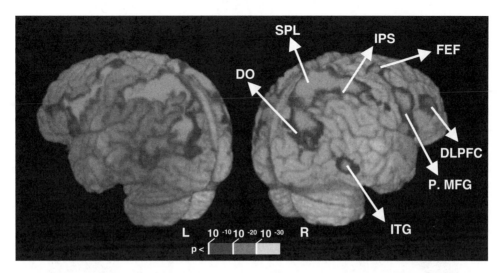

FIGURE 66.2 Working memory network. The regions within this network were revealed by the contrast of working memory versus fixation control trials. The statistical group maps of functional activations are shown overlaid onto a three-dimensional rendering of the brain of a representative individual. The color bar indicates P values (uncorrected). Abbreviations: DLPFC, dorsolateral prefrontal cortex; DO, dorsal occipital; FEF, frontal eye field; IPS, intraparietal sulcus; ITG, inferior temporal gyrus; P. MFG, posterior middle frontal gyrus; SPL, superior parietal lobule. (Reprinted with permission from Cell Press.) (See color plate 43.)

plementary eye field (SEF) in frontal cortex, and the superior parietal lobule (SPL) and intraparietal sulcus (IPS) in parietal cortex. As illustrated in figure 66.3A and B for the right IPS and right FEF, respectively, activity in these regions on correct trials rose during encoding, was sustained through the delay interval and at test, and declined thereafter. No such sustained activity during the delay was observed on incorrect trials. But could it be that stronger delay activity during correct trials relative to incorrect trials simply reflected ineffective encoding during incorrect trials? In other words, for incorrect trials, subjects might have failed to encode the stimulus, thereby preventing them from any attempt to maintain the encoded item. To address this possibility, we performed additional analyses confined to only those trials with stronger than average encoding-related activation. The results obtained in this manner were virtually identical to the ones shown in figure 66.3, arguing that strongly encoded items do not predict good performance in the absence of sustained signals in frontal and parietal cortex during the delay.

In order to quantify the relationship between fMRI signal amplitude and performance, we used a logistic regression analysis. This analysis revealed that the strength of the fMRI signal during the delay interval reliably predicted task performance. For example, a 1% increase in signal in the right IPS or right FEF increased the likelihood of success to close to 70% (figure 66.3C and D, respectively), and in the left DLPFC to close to 65%. A significant logistic regression fit was also obtained for the SPL, but not for the SEF. Our results thus provide direct evidence linking sustained activity during the delay interval with behavioral success on a trial-by-trial basis.

Both single-cell and lesion studies in monkeys have demonstrated that the DLPFC (BA 9/46) is centrally involved in working memory (Goldman-Rakic, 1995; Fuster, 1997), and in humans the corresponding region is commonly activated on working memory tasks (for reviews, see Cabeza and Nyberg, 2000; D'Esposito, 2001). Our study showed not only that the DLPFC is involved in working memory but also that its contribution to correct performance is significant (see also Sakai, Rowe, and Passingham, 2002).

Another region that showed a significant contribution of sustained delay signals for working memory performance included the FEF in the precentral sulcus extending forward into the superior frontal sulcus (BA 6/8). Several imaging studies have revealed working memory-related activity in the vicinity of the precentral sulcus and the superior frontal sulcus. Although such activity has often been attributed to hand or eye movements within premotor cortex, working memory studies that have explicitly controlled all motor responses have also observed activations in this region (Jonides et al., 1993; Smith et al., 1995; Courtney et al., 1996). Critically, sustained activity has been demonstrated in the superior frontal sulcus during the delay interval of working memory tasks (Courtney et al., 1998; Postle et al., 2000), and this activity appears to be greater for spatial than for object working memory (Courtney et al., 1998).

Within parietal cortex, bilateral SPL (BA 7) and IPS (BA 40) also exhibited differential delay signals. This finding is consistent with previous imaging work demonstrating SPL activation associated with both spatial and verbal working memory tasks, and IPS activation associated with object working memory tasks as well (for reviews, see Cabeza and Nyberg, 2000; D'Esposito, 2001). Recently, Rowe and col-

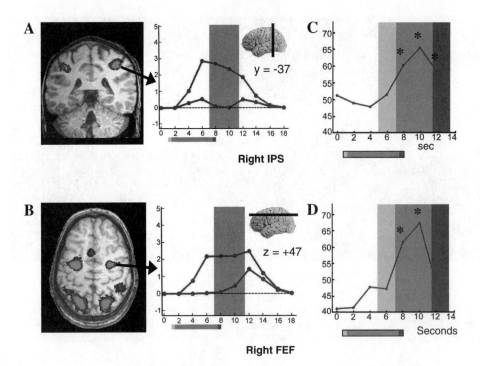

Right IPS

Right FEF

FIGURE 66.3 (*A, B*) Performance-related activity in the intraparietal sulcus (IPS, *A*) and the frontal eye field (FEF, *B*) during the three phases of the working memory task: encoding, delay, and test. Performance-related activity was obtained by comparing activity for correct and incorrect trials at each task phase. Functional group maps are shown overlaid on structural scans from a representative individual. Arrow indicates the region from which the fitted hemodynamic responses were obtained. The level of the coronal section is indicated on the small whole-brain inset. The bar below the *x*-axis 24 codes the periods when the sample stimulus (light gray),

the delay (intermediate gray), and the test stimulus (dark gray) occurred during the task. The vertical gray bar indicates the delay interval. (*C, D*) The contingency between signal amplitude and the subjects' performance was assessed with a logistic regression analysis for every time point within working memory trials. Activity at 8 and 10 s for the FEF and at 8, 10, and 12 s for the IPS significantly predicted performance (*P* < 0.05), such that for a 1% increase in fMRI signal, the probability of being correct for that trial increased from chance to close to 70% (*y*-axis). (See color plate 44.)

leagues (2000) have suggested that the posterior IPS may be especially important for maintenance processes, as it exhibited sustained activity over long working memory delays (close to 20 s).

Taken together, neuroimaging studies reveal a frontoparietal network of brain regions that is critical for working memory. This network includes the IPS and SPL in parietal cortex and the FEF and DLPFC in frontal cortex, which were shown in our study to reliably predict task performance on a trial-by-trial basis.

The control of attention

Attention and working memory are closely related cognitive processes, which has led to the idea that they may share common neural mechanisms (Desimone and Duncan, 1995; Kastner and Ungerleider, 2000; Awh and Jonides, 2001). For instance, when we attempt to find a famous painting in a museum gallery, presumably we maintain in mind some mental representation of the painting and attentively compare the paintings around the gallery to the one we are looking for. In this section, we will review the neural sub-

strates of the control of visuospatial attention, and compare them with those associated with working memory. As the close link between these two types of mechanisms suggests, their neural substrates show a large degree of overlap.

What we perceive depends critically on where we direct our attention. Attention to a location dramatically improves the accuracy and speed of detecting a target at that location. Attention has been shown not only to increase perceptual sensitivity for target discrimination but also to reduce the interference caused by nearby distracters. Moreover, attention is highly flexible and can be deployed in a manner that best serves the organism's momentary behavioral goals: either to locations, to visual features, or to objects. Also, attention can be based on internal goals (e.g., finding a familiar face in the crowd) or can depend on the external environment (as when a loud alarm sounds).

Visual attention has been studied extensively in single-cell recording experiments in monkeys and neuroimaging studies in humans. These experiments have shown that attention affects activity in areas of the brain that process stimulus features, such as color, motion, texture, and shape. The paradigmatic finding in monkeys is that when attention is directed to a single stimulus, there is an increase in the firing rate of neurons that respond to the attended stimulus (Motter, 1993, 1994). In similar fashion, increases in fMRI signals in humans have been reported for attended relative to unattended items. Such attentional effects have been observed in many visual cortical areas, including V1, V2, V4, TEO, and MT.

If attention modulates activity in visual processing areas, what is the source of these attentional effects? In humans, studies of patients suffering from attentional deficits due to brain damage (such as in the neglect syndrome; Mesulam, 1981; Rafal, 1998), as well as functional brain imaging studies of healthy individuals performing attentionally demanding tasks, have revealed a distributed network of higher-order areas in frontal and parietal cortex that appears to be involved in the generation and control of attentional top-down feedback signals. Further, there exists an anatomical substrate for such top-down influences, inasmuch as tract-tracing studies in monkeys have demonstrated direct feedback projections to extrastriate visual areas V4 and TEO from parietal cortex (in particular, area LIP) and to IT cortex (area TE) from prefrontal cortex, as well as indirect feedback projections to areas V4 and TEO from prefrontal cortex via parietal cortex (Cavada and Goldman-Rakic, 1989; Ungerleider, Gaffan, and Pelak, 1989; Webster, Bachevelier, and Ungerleider, 1994).

Our working memory study described earlier in this chapter (see figure 66.1) provided the opportunity to compare circuits involved in working memory with those involved in goal-directed attention. For this purpose, we investigated the activations revealed by the contrast of the encoding phase of the trial relative to a similar period during control trials in which subjects simply viewed a blank screen, and compared those activations with working memory-related ones. We reasoned that the contrast involving encoding would reveal regions involved in goal-directed attention because, behaviorally, a key component of successfully performing the task involved directing attention to the to-be-encoded stimulus array. The most robust activations revealed by this contrast involved a frontoparietal network of regions (figure 66.4A) consisting of the SPL (BA 7), the anterior IPS (BA 40), the FEF (BA 6), and the SEF (BA 6/32). Also consistently activated were the precuneus (BA 18/19), the precentral gyrus (BA 6), the dorsolateral portion of the MFG (DLPFC, BA 46), and the IFG/anterior insula (BA 44) (these latter regions are not shown in figure 66.4).

At the same time, as described earlier, working memory delay-related activations (revealed by the contrast of working memory and control trials during the delay period) were observed in several brain regions (figure 66.4B), including the SPL (BA 7), anterior IPS (BA 40), FEF (BA 6), SEF (BA 6), and DLPFC of the MFG (BA 9/46), with the strongest activations observed in the SPL, FEF, and SEF at a relatively dorsal plane (z = +47 in Talairach space). The remarkable overlap between the regions engaged by goal-directed attention and working memory maintenance (compare figure 66.4A and B) lends further credence to the idea that the two

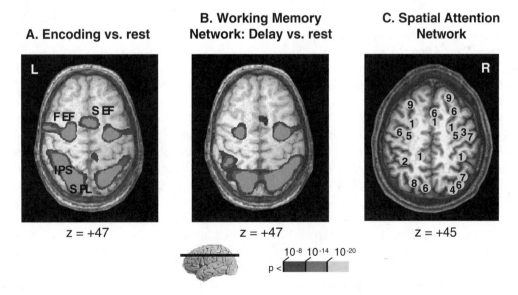

FIGURE 66.4 Regions involved in visual spatial attention and visual working memory. (A) Encoding versus rest on the working memory task. (B) Working memory network revealed by the contrast of working memory delay versus rest. (C) Regions in the spatial attention network as determined by a meta-analysis of imaging data. The statistical group map is shown overlaid on a structural scan of a representative individual. The level of the axial section is indicated on the small whole-brain inset. Numbers correspond to the following studies: 1, Corbetta et al., 1993; 2, Fink et al., 1997; 3, Nobre et al., 1997; 4, Vandenbergh et al., 1997; 5, Corbetta et al., 1998; 6, Kastner et al., 1999; 7, Rosen et al., 1999; 8, Corbetta et al., 2000; 9, Hopfinger et al., 2000. (See color plate 45.)

functions share key mechanisms and neural structures, consistent with several proposals (Mesulam, 1981, 1990; Desimone and Duncan, 1995; Awh and Jonides, 2001).

Recently, we performed a meta-analysis of foci of activation from 10 studies across several independent laboratories (Kastner and Ungerleider, 2000; Pessoa, Kastner, and Ungerleider, 2002). The results of this analysis, shown in figure 66.4C, reveal that a frontoparietal network of regions consisting of areas in the SPL, IPS, FEF, and SEF is consistently activated in a variety of tasks involving visuospatial attention (Corbetta et al., 1993, 1998; Fink et al., 1997; Nobre et al., 1997; Vandenberghe et al., 1997; Culham et al., 1998; Gitelman et al., 1999; Kim et al., 1999; Rosen et al., 1999). In addition, but less consistently, activations in the lateral prefrontal cortex in the region of the MFG and the anterior cingulate cortex (ACC) have also reported. A common feature among the visuospatial tasks in these experiments is that subjects were asked to maintain fixation at a central spot and to direct attention covertly to peripheral target locations in order to detect a stimulus (Corbetta et al., 1993, 1998; Nobre et al., 1997; Gitelman et al., 1999; Kim et al., 1999; Rosen et al., 1999), to discriminate it (Fink et al., 1997; Vandenberghe et al., 1997; Kastner et al., 1999), or to track its movement (Culham et al., 1998). Thus, there appears to be a general spatial attention network that operates independently of the specific requirements of the visuospatial task.

The results of the meta-analysis provide further support for the idea that the activation sites revealed by the contrast of the encoding phase of the working memory task relative to rest were indeed involved in goal-directed attention. As can be observed in figure 66.4, there was a large degree of concordance between encoding-related activations (figure 66.4A) and sites involved in spatial attention (figure 66.4C).

Although activations outside of visual cortex in attention tasks have been indicative of regions involved in attentional control, in many of these studies, it was not possible to separate signals associated with visual cues that prime the subject to expect potential subsequent visual targets from signals associated with the attended targets themselves. This was because cues and targets typically follow each other in rapid succession. More recent neuroimaging studies, however, have attempted to explicitly investigate top-down modulation in attentional paradigms by disentangling cue- and target-related activity by, for instance, introducing a longer interval between the two (e.g., Kastner et al., 1999; Hopfinger, Buonocore, and Mangun, 2000). In this way, the effects of attention in the presence and in the absence of visual stimulation can be assessed. The reasoning is that purely target-related activity should be observed in visual processing areas that respond to the specific stimulus (e.g., area MT to moving stimuli). By contrast, expectation- or cue-related activity that is uncontaminated by ensuing target-related activity should reflect mainly top-down signals and should be observed in regions of the brain that control attention.

Attention-related signals in the human visual cortex in the absence of visual stimulation were investigated by Kastner and colleagues (1999) by including an expectation period preceding the presentation of visual stimuli. The expectation period was initiated by a cue presented briefly next to the fixation point 11 s before the onset of the stimuli. At the appearance of the cue, subjects covertly shifted attention to the peripheral target location in anticipation of a target stimulus that would appear there. In this way, the effects of attention in the absence and in the presence of visual stimulation could be identified. Directed attention in the absence of visual stimulation activated the same distributed network of areas as directed attention in the presence of visual stimulation and included the FEF, the SEF, and the SPL. The increase in activity in these frontal and parietal areas during the expectation period (in the absence of visual input) was sustained throughout the expectation period and the attended visual presentations. These results suggest that the activity reflected the attentional operations of the task per se, and not the effects of attention on visual processing.

Converging evidence for a frontoparietal network of regions involved in attentional control comes from additional imaging studies. For example, by using a spatial attention Posner-type task, Corbetta and colleagues (2000) showed that the IPS was uniquely active when attention was directed toward and maintained at a relevant location (preceding target presentation), suggesting that the IPS is a top-down source of biasing signals observed in visual cortex. The same investigators (Shulman et al., 1999) found, when studying attention to motion, cue-related activity in FEF, as well as in several sites in the IPS. Finally, Hopfinger, Buonocore, and Mangun (2000) obtained evidence for a wider attentional control network, including the superior frontal gyrus, MFG, SPL, IPS, and superior temporal gyrus. This latter region has been identified in lesion studies as a key site responsible for neglect (Karnath, Ferber, and Himmelbach, 2001). Interestingly, a recent fMRI study indicates that the top-down control of attention to visual features draws on a network of areas that largely overlaps with the one revealed by spatial attention tasks (Giesbrecht and Mangun, in press; Giesbrecht et al., 2004). This raises the possibility that the control of attention may rely on a common network of brain regions, irrespective of the attribute attended (see also Vandenberghe et al., 2001).

Taken together, these studies provide evidence that a distributed frontoparietal attentional network may be the source of feedback that generates the top-down biasing signals modulating activity in visual cortex. This would explain the finding that functional brain imaging studies using different visuospatial attention tasks have described very similar attentional networks.

Top-down versus bottom-up attentional control

Thus far we have considered top-down mechanisms needed for the control of working memory and goal-directed attention. Further, we have shown how similar frontoparietal networks are likely engaged by both processes. Goal-directed attention is often referred to as *endogenous* attention. Goal-directed attention provides a fundamental mechanism by which behaviorally relevant information is favored relative to less important items. However, another type of attention, often referred to as *exogenous* attention, also plays an important role in guiding the allocation of processing resources and thereby in shaping behavior. For example, we can consider the case of a person trekking in the desert when a sudden movement is observed in the periphery of his or her visual field. In such a case, attention is involuntarily directed to that location, allowing the person to ascertain the nature of the moving object, for instance, whether it is just a squirrel or whether it is a threatening snake. Thus, endogenous attention is under top-down control, while exogenous attention is largely stimulus driven.

The distinction between endogenous and exogenous attention can be explored in the context of change detection. Detecting changes in an ever-changing environment is highly advantageous, and may be critical for survival. In the real world, changes are often accompanied by transients of some sort, such as motion signals that attract attention to their location (Yantis and Johnson, 1990; Remington, Johnston, and Yantis, 1992). In general, the attention-catching effect of a sudden or distinctive stimulus can be shown by flashing a light at a certain location in space and comparing the time it takes for subjects to react to a subsequent stimulus at that location to the time it takes to react when no initial flashing takes place (Posner and Cohen, 1984). Moreover, evidence indicates that when an item is seen to change (e.g., from a vertical to a horizontal bar), attention is drawn to the location of that item to facilitate visual processing. For example, Thornton and Fernandez-Duque (2000) showed that subjects are faster to discriminate a subsequent target at the location of a change than at a distant location (see also Smilek, Eastwood, and Meriklee, 2000; Rensink, 2002), indicating that a change can function as an orienting cue.

Interestingly, changes may occur in the absence of accompanying transients, such as those occurring during saccades, blinks, or flicker. Under these circumstances, changes can be quite difficult to detect, and even large changes may go unnoticed in the absence of focused attention (Rensink, O'Regan, and Clark, 1997; Rensink, 2002). In such situations, goaldirected attention (endogenous attention) appears necessarily to be focused on the region of space in which a change occurs at the time the change takes place. When this is not the case because of, say, saccades or flicker, "change blindness" will ensue (e.g., an engine repeatedly appearing and disappearing from the photograph of an airplane may go unnoticed). In most instances, however, changes in the environment are in fact accompanied by transients. Thus, change detection is associated with two related but distinct events, namely, a reflexive deployment of attention that can have an orienting function, akin to exogenous attention, and a goal-directed allocation of attention that may be instrumental in allowing changes to be perceived in demanding situations.

To investigate the neural correlates of attentional mechanisms involved in change detection that are more closely tied to exogenous attention, we compared activations on correct change versus correct no-change trials during the test phase of our working memory task (see figure 66.1). To minimize the contributions of varying attentional states that might have occurred during the long experimental fMRI session, we analyzed only high-confidence, correct trials. Contrasting detected versus undetected changes, as Beck and colleagues (2001) did in their study of change detection, would have involved correct (detected) and incorrect (undetected) trials, which likely would have included contributions due to variations in the subject's attentional state. Indeed, Ress, Backus, and Heeger (2000) attributed fluctuations in activity in V1 to trial-to-trial fluctuations in attention, which, they suggested, accounted for the variability in behavioral performance on a target detection task. We have also proposed that such fluctuations in attention have a similar role on behavioral performance in the context of our working memory task (Pessoa, Gutierrez, et al., 2002). Thus, we reasoned that by analyzing correct trials only, we would minimize the potentially large contributions of varying attentional states.

The contrast of correct change versus correct no-change trials during the test phase revealed activations in frontoparietal sites (figure 66.5A) that included the anterior IPS (BA 40), the precuneus (BA 19), the superior frontal gyrus (SFG; BA 6/8), the MFG (BA 9), the ACC (BA 32), and the IFG/anterior insula (BA 44). We also observed change-related responses to the stimulus array in cortical visual areas, most notably in the ITG. Subcortically, the right putamen, the cerebellum and pulvinar, both mainly on the right, showed greater activation on correct trials for the change compared to no-change contrast. Our interpretation of these results is that change detection activates frontal and parietal regions via bottom-up mechanisms, thereby triggering attentional mechanisms located in these regions, which then function via top-down feedback to deploy attention to the location of a change, enabling further, more elaborate processing of the stimulus. Moreover, subcortical sites, such as the pulvinar, may also participate in the deployment of

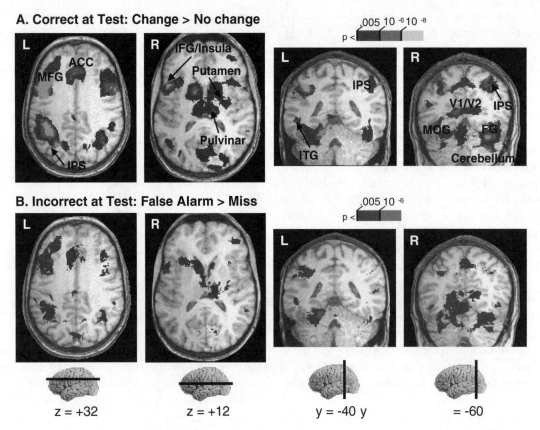

A. Correct at Test: Change > No change

B. Incorrect at Test: False Alarm > Miss

z = +32   z = +12   y = -40   y = -60

FIGURE 66.5 Similar brain activations occur on correct change and false alarm trials. (*A*) Functional group maps showing regions activated at test on correct change (nonmatch) compared to no-change (match) trials. (*B*) Functional group maps showing regions activated at test on incorrect no-change (false alarms) compared to incorrect change (miss) trials, at the same slice levels. Although the number of high-confidence, incorrect trials was small and the asso-ciated activations were weaker, comparing the two patterns of activation revealed a great deal of overlap. Statistical group maps are shown overlaid on structural scans from a representative individual. The level of the axial and coronal sections is indicated on the small whole-brain insets. The color bar indicates *P* values (uncorrected). (Reprinted with permission by Oxford University Press.) (See color plate 46.)

attention and thereby contribute to the processing of the stimulus.

In a task involving a decision, such as determining whether a change occurred or not, do brain activations follow the physical stimulus or the subject's report? To investigate this question, we asked whether the same areas activated by correctly detecting a change were also more active when the subjects reported a change but none had actually occurred? If this were true, then the pattern of activation for false alarms (on incorrect match trials) compared to misses (on incorrect nonmatch trials) should be similar to the one observed for rejects (on correct nonmatch trials) compared to hits (on correct match trials). On trials identified as false alarm trials, no physical change occurred, but subjects reported perceiving a change with high confidence; for miss trials, a physical change occurred, but subjects reported that no change occurred, again with high confidence. Although the number of high-confidence, incorrect trials was small and the associated activations were generally weaker, this contrast revealed a network of activations with a striking

degree of overlap with the network observed when subjects correctly detected a change (compare figure 66.5*A* and *B*). Thus, we suggest that reporting a change, whether or not it actually occurred, generates virtually the same pattern of activation.

A related dissociation between physical parameters and perceptual reports has been observed in the visual cortex of monkeys observing threshold or ambiguous stimuli. For example, Bradley, Chang, and Andersen (1998) showed that the responses of MT neurons to bistable, rotating cylinders defined by structure-from-motion cues were linked to the perception of which surface was perceived in front. This was also true for error trials in which the monkey's behavioral response reflected neuronal responses (the cell's preferred depth) rather than the physical cues of the stimulus. In another single-cell study, Thompson and Schall (1999, 2000) probed the neural substrates of target detection and showed that neural responses in the FEF to a target stimulus were greater when the target was detected than when it was missed. Moreover, neural responses were greater on false alarm trials than on trials in which the target was absent.

What is the relationship between change-related activations, on the one hand, and those associated with goal-directed attention, on the other hand? Although there was overlap between the locations of activations found during change detection at test and those for goal-directed attention, such as the anterior IPS, a notable feature of the comparison was the *lack* of overlap at more dorsal brain sites. In particular, the SPL, FEF, and SEF were strongly driven by goal-directed attention but not by the detection of a change. Conversely, regions strongly recruited during the detection of a change that were not recruited by goal-directed attention included the pulvinar and the cerebellum.

Thus, the most conspicuous feature of the networks activated by change detection and goal-directed attention was that they were largely nonoverlapping, with the notable exception of the anterior IPS, which was shared by both networks. Moreover, it appears that attentional processes associated with goal-directed attention recruit more dorsal cortical territories in both frontal and parietal cortex than those associated with change detection. Regions triggered by change detection were generally situated more ventrally (compare figures 66.4*A* and 66.5*A*) and included the MFG, the ACC, and the IFG/anterior insula. Importantly, processes engaged by working memory maintenance recruited the same dorsal frontoparietal regions associated with goal-directed attention (compare figure 66.4*A* and *C*).

Discussion

We reviewed evidence from fMRI studies that a frontoparietal network is critically involved in the top-down control of spatial attention. This is a similar network as the one proposed by Mesulam (1980), based on studies of patients with brain lesions. This frontoparietal network shows a remarkable degree of overlap with the one involved in maintaining information during the delay period of a working memory task. Both networks rely heavily on dorsal areas of the brain. Such congruence of activated sites agrees well with the idea that goal-directed attention and working memory share common mechanisms. Indeed, it has been proposed that they should not be viewed as separate processes, but instead as interdependent ones. For instance, Desimone (1998) proposed that attention is derived, at least in part, from the impact of short-term memory mechanisms (i.e., working memory) on cortical sensory representations.

We also reviewed evidence from our working memory study that change-detection activations involve a different network of regions that is situated more ventrally. We interpreted change-related activations as associated with a more reflexive deployment of attention toward the location of the change, akin to exogenous attention. Behavioral studies

demonstrate that endogenous and exogenous attention involve different mechanisms. For example, the facilitation due to a sensory cue in exogenous attention (e.g., a bright flash) appears more rapidly (~50 ms) than that observed in goal-directed attention. Moreover, unlike what is observed in endogenous attention, sensory cues produce a prolonged inhibition of processing (called inhibition of return) after the initial facilitation. Thus, it is generally believed that endogenous and exogenous attention comprise distinct systems (Jonides, 1981). Our findings of overlapping but separable dorsal and ventral neural systems subserving processes more closely tied to top-down and stimulus-driven attention, respectively, is thus consistent with the separation between these two types of attentional processes, as suggested by behavioral experiments.

Our proposal shares its key elements with the one advanced by Corbetta and Shulman (2002). Based on their own studies, as well as neuroimaging and patient reports, they postulated the existence of two anatomically segregated but interacting networks for spatial attention. According to their scheme, a dorsal frontoparietal system is involved in the generation of attentional sets associated with goal-directed stimulus-response selection (endogenous attention). Key nodes within this largely bilateral network would include the SPL, IPS, and FEF. A second, more ventral system that is strongly lateralized to the right hemisphere is proposed to detect behaviorally relevant stimuli and to work as an alerting mechanism for the first system when these stimuli are detected outside the focus of processing (exogenous attention). In our working memory study, we did not find evidence for a right lateralization of the ventral network engaged by change detection. One reason could be that change detection behaves slightly differently from more direct exogenous mechanisms recruited, for instance, by a loud sound or a flashing stimulus. Interestingly, in our study, the dorsal and ventral networks intersected at the anterior IPS, which may constitute a common processing node that links the two networks. In general, endogenous and exogenous attention strongly interact in the generation of behavior (see Corbetta and Shulman, 2002) and, in neural terms, such interactions may be mediated by anatomical connections known to exist between the dorsal and ventral networks (Distler et al., 1993; Webster, Bachevalier, and Ungerleider, 1993), as well as common anatomical regions, such as the IPS.

We also found evidence in our working memory study for the involvement of subcortical structures in exogenous attention, including the pulvinar and the cerebellum. Single-cell studies in monkeys reveal that the pulvinar nucleus of the thalamus has an important role in selective attention processes (Chalupa, 1977; Petersen, Robinson, and Keys, 1985). As summarized by Robinson and Petersen (1992), pulvinar cells generate signals related to the salience of visual objects and are involved in the selection of salient targets and the filtering of nonsalient distracters. In monkeys, pulvinar lesions lead to impairments in active visual scanning (Ungerleider and Christensen, 1979), and inactivation of the pulvinar produces a slowing down of attention shifts (Petersen, Robinson, and Morris, 1987). In humans, the right pulvinar is the principal site in the thalamus associated with spatial neglect (Karnath, Himmelbach, and Rorden, 2002). Imaging studies in humans also have obtained evidence of pulvinar involvement in attentional processes (LaBerge and Buchsbaum, 1990; Corbetta et al., 1991), although not consistently. In our working memory study, we found robust and consistent pulvinar activation, which we suggest was involved in the deployment of spatial attention to the location of the change.

Like the pulvinar, the cerebellar cortex was strongly activated when subjects detected a change. There is now evidence that the cerebellum has functions beyond those of motor processing (Middleton and Strick, 1994; Fiez et al., 1996; Schmahmann, 1996; Thach, 1996). In particular, based on studies of patients with cerebellar lesions, it has been proposed that the cerebellum mediates rapid shifts in attention (Akshoomoff and Courchesne, 1992, 1994). In an fMRI study to test cerebellar involvement in attentional processes, Le, Pardo, and Hu (1998) compared a condition of shifting attention to a condition of sustained attention, which revealed lateral cerebellar activation (see also Allen et al., 1997). Thus, our findings are consistent with the idea that the cerebellum is involved in attentional processes in general, and in the detection of change in particular.

Conclusion

In this chapter, we reviewed studies that show that frontal and parietal brain regions are centrally involved in the control of working memory and attention. Results from imaging studies, including our own, suggest that sites important for working memory are strongly involved in goal-directed (endogenous) attention and involve a dorsal frontoparietal network, including the SPL, IPS, FEF, and SEF. At the same time, reflexive (exogenous) attention relies on an overlapping but distinct network that also involves frontoparietal sites but is located more ventrally to encompass the MFG, ACC, and IFG. Moreover, this network includes subcortical sites such as the pulvinar and the cerebellum. A key site of overlap between the two networks is the anterior IPS. Distinguishing the precise functional contributions of the different nodes subserving the top-down control of attention and working memory, as well as those involved in reflexive attention, is a task for future investigations.

ACKNOWLEDGMENTS We thank David Sturman for assistance in preparation of the manuscript. This work was supported by the National Institute of Mental Health Intramural Research Program.

REFERENCES

AKSHOOMOFF, N. A., and E. COURCHESNE, 1992. A new role for the cerebellum in cognitive operations. *Behav. Neurosci.* 106:731–738.

AKSHOOMOFF, N. A., and E. COURCHESNE, 1994. ERP evidence for a shifting attention deficit in patients with damage to the cerebellum. *J. Cogn. Neurosci.* 6:388–399.

ALLEN, G., R. B. BUXTON, E. C. WONG, and E. COURCHESNE, 1997. Attentional activation of the cerebellum independent of motor movement. *Science* 275:1940–1943.

AWH, E., and J. JONIDES, 2001. Overlapping mechanisms of attention and spatial working memory. *Trends Cogn. Sci.* 5:119–126.

BAUER, R. H., and J. M. FUSTER, 1976. Delayed-matching and delayed-response deficit from cooling dorsolateral prefrontal cortex in monkeys. *J. Comp. Physiol. Psychol.* 90:293–302.

BECK, D. M., G. REES, C. D. FRITH, and N. LAVIE, 2001. Neural correlates of change detection and change blindness. *Nat. Neurosci.* 4:645–650.

BRADLEY, D. C., G. C. CHANG, and R. A. ANDERSEN, 1998. Encoding of three-dimensional structure-from-motion by primate area MT neurons. *Nature* 392:714–717.

BRUCE, C. J., and M. E. GOLDBERG, 1985. Primate frontal eye fields. I. Single neurons discharging before saccades. *J. Neurophysiol.* 53:603–635.

CABEZA, R., and L. NYBERG, 2000. Imaging cognition. II. An empirical review of 275 PET and fMRI studies. *J. Cogn. Neurosci.* 12:1–47.

CAVADA, C., and P. S. GOLDMAN-RAKIC, 1989. Posterior parietal cortex in rhesus monkey. II. Evidence for segregated cortico-cortical networks linking sensory and limbic areas with the frontal lobe. *J. Comp. Neurol.* 287:422–445.

CHAFEE, M. V., and P. S. GOLDMAN-RAKIC, 1998. Matching patterns of activity in primate prefrontal area 8a and parietal area 7ip neurons during a spatial working memory task. *J. Neurophysiol.* 79:2919–2940.

CHAFEE, M. V., and P. S. GOLDMAN-RAKIC, 2000. Inactivation of parietal and prefrontal cortex reveals interdependence of neural activity during memory-guided saccades. *J. Neurophysiol.* 83:1550–1566.

CHALUPA, L. M., 1977. A review of cat and monkey studies implicating the pulvinar in visual function. *Behav. Biol.* 20:149–167.

CHELAZZI, L., J. DUNCAN, E. K. MILLER, and R. DESIMONE, 1998. Responses of neurons in inferior temporal cortex during memory-guided visual search. *J. Neurophysiol.* 80:2918–2940.

COHEN, J. D., W. M. PERLSTEIN, T. S. BRAVER, L. E. NYSTROM, D. C. NOLL, J. JONIDES, and E. E. SMITH, 1997. Temporal dynamics of brain activation during a working memory task. *Nature* 386:604–608.

CORBETTA, M., E. AKBUDAK, T. E. CONTURO, A. Z. SNYDER, J. M. OLLINGER, H. A. DRURY, M. R. LINENWEBER, S. E. PETERSEN, M. E. RAICHLE, D. C. VAN ESSEN, and G. L. SHULMAN, 1998. A common network of functional areas for attention and eye movements. *Neuron* 21:761–773.

CORBETTA, M., J. M. KINCADE, J. M. OLLINGER, M. P. McAVOY, and G. L. SHULMAN, 2000. Voluntary orienting is dissociated from target detection in human posterior parietal cortex. *Nat. Neurosci.* 3:292–297.

CORBETTA, M., F. M. MIEZIN, S. DOBMEYER, G. L. SHULMAN, and S. E. PETERSEN, 1991. Selective and divided attention during visual discriminations of shape, color, and speed: Functional anatomy by positron emission tomography. *J. Neurosci.* 11:2382–2402.

CORBETTA, M., F. M. MIEZIN, G. L. SHULMAN, and S. E. PETERSEN, 1993. A PET study of visuospatial attention. *J. Neurosci.* 13:1202–1226.

CORBETTA, M., and G. L. SHULMAN, 2002. Control of goal-directed and stimulus-driven attention in the brain. *Nat. Rev. Neurosci.* 3:201–215.

COURTNEY, S. M., L. PETIT, J. M. MAISOG, L. G. UNGERLEIDER, and J. V. HAXBY, 1998. An area specialized for spatial working memory in human frontal cortex. *Science* 279:1347–1351.

COURTNEY, S. M., L. G. UNGERLEIDER, K. KEIL, and J. V. HAXBY, 1996. Object and spatial visual working memory activate separate neural systems in human cortex. *Cereb. Cortex* 6:39–49.

COURTNEY, S. M., L. G. UNGERLEIDER, K. KEIL, and J. V. HAXBY, 1997. Transient and sustained activity in a distributed neural system for human working memory. *Nature* 386:608–611.

CULHAM, J. C., S. A. BRANDT, P. CAVANAGH, N. G. KANWISHER, A. M. DALE, and R. B. TOOTELL, 1998. Cortical fMRI activation produced by attentive tracking of moving targets. *J. Neurophysiol.* 80:2657–2670.

DESIMONE, R., 1998. Visual attention mediated by biased competition in extrastriate visual cortex. *Philos. Trans. R. Soc. Lond.* 353:1245–1255.

DESIMONE, R., and J. DUNCAN, 1995. Neural mechanisms of selective attention. *Annu. Rev. Neurosci.* 18:193–222.

D'ESPOSITO, M., 2001. Functional neuroimaging of working memory. In *Handbook of Functional Neuroimaging of Cognition*, R. Cabeza and A. Kingstone, eds. Cambridge, Mass.: MIT Press, pp. 293–327.

D'ESPOSITO, M., G. K. AGUIRRE, E. ZARAHN, D. BALLARD, R. K. SHIN, and J. LEASE, 1998. Functional MRI studies of spatial and nonspatial working memory. *Cogn. Brain Res.* 7:1–13.

DISTLER, C., D. BOUSSAOUD, R. DESIMONE, and L. G. UNGERLEIDER, 1993. Cortical connections of inferior temporal area TEO in macaques. *J. Comp. Neurol.* 334:125–150.

FIEZ, J. A., E. A. RAIFE, D. A. BALOTA, J. P. SCHWARZ, M. E. RAICHLE, and S. E. PETERSEN, 1996. A positron emission tomography study of the short-term maintenance of verbal information. *J. Neurosci.* 16:808–822.

FINK, G. R., R. J. DOLAN, P. W. HALLIGAN, J. C. MARSHALL, and C. D. FRITH, 1997. Space-based and object-based visual attention: Shared and specific neural domains. *Brain* 120:2013–2028.

FUNAHASHI, S., S. J. BRUCE, and P. S. GOLDMAN-RAKIC, 1989. Mnemonic coding of visual space in the monkey's dorsolateral prefrontal cortex. *J. Neurophysiol.* 61:1–19.

FUNAHASHI, S., C. J. BRUCE, and P. S. GOLDMAN-RAKIC, 1993. Dorsolateral prefrontal lesions and oculomotor delayed response performance: Evidence for mnemonic "scotomas." *J. Neurosci.* 13:1479–1497.

FUSTER, J. M., 1973. Unit activity in prefrontal cortex during delayed-response performance: Neuronal correlates of transient memory. *J. Neurophysiol.* 36:61–78.

FUSTER, J. M., 1997. *The prefrontal cortex: Anatomy, Physiology, and Neuropsychology of the Frontal Lobes*. New York: Raven Press.

FUSTER, J. M., 2001. The prefrontal cortex: An update: Time is of the essence. *Neuron* 30:319–333.

FUSTER, J. M., and G. E. ALEXANDER, 1971. Neuron activity related to short-term memory. *Science* 173:652–654.

FUSTER, J. M., and J. P. JERVEY, 1982. Neuronal firing in the inferotemporal cortex of the monkey in a visual memory task. *J. Neurosci.* 2:361–375.

GIESBRECHT, B., and G. R. MANGUN, (in press) The neural mechanisms of top-down control. In *The Cognitive and Neural Bases of Spatial Neglect*, H. O. Karnath, D. Milner, and G. Vallar, eds. Oxford, England: Oxford University Press.

GIESBRECHT, B., M. G. WOLDORFF, A. W. SONG, and G. R. MANGUN, 2004. *Neural mechanisms of top-down control during spatial and feature attention*. Unpublished manuscript.

GITELMAN, D. R., A. C. NOBRE, T. B. PARRISH, K. S. LABAR, Y. H. KIM, J. R. MEYER, and M. MESULAM, 1999. A large-scale distributed network for covert spatial attention: Further anatomical delineation based on stringent behavioural and cognitive controls. *Brain* 122:1093–1106.

GOLDMAN, P. S., and H. E. ROSVOLD, 1970. Localization of function within the dorsolateral prefrontal cortex of the rhesus monkey. *Exp. Neurol.* 27:291–304.

GOLDMAN-RAKIC, P. S., 1995. Cellular basis of working memory. *Neuron* 14:477–485.

HOPFINGER, J. B., M. H. BUONOCORE, and G. R. MANGUN, 2000. The neural mechanisms of top-down attentional control. *Nat. Neurosci.* 3:284–291.

JONIDES, J., 1981. In *Attention and Performance XI*, M. I. Posner, and O. Marin, eds. Hillsdale, N.J.: Erlbaum, pp. 187–205.

JONIDES, J., E. H. SCHUMACHER, E. E. SMITH, R. A. KOEPPE, E. AWH, P. A. REUTER-LORENZ, C. MARSHUETZ, and C. R. WILLIS, 1998. The role of parietal cortex in verbal working memory. *J. Neurosci.* 18:5026–5034.

JONIDES, J., E. E. SMITH, R. A. KOEPPE, E. AWH, S. MINOSHIMA, and M. A. MINTUN, 1993. Spatial working memory in humans as revealed by PET. *Nature* 363:623–625.

KARNATH, H. O., S. FERBER, and M. HIMMELBACH, 2001. Spatial awareness is a function of the temporal not the posterior parietal lobe. *Nature* 411:950–953.

KARNATH, H. O., M. HIMMELBACH, and C. RORDEN, 2002. The subcortical anatomy of human spatial neglect: Putamen, caudate nucleus and pulvinar. *Brain* 125:350–360.

KASTNER, S., M. A. PINSK, P. DE WEERD, R. DESIMONE, and L. G. UNGERLEIDER, 1999. Increased activity in human visual cortex during directed attention in the absence of visual stimulation. *Neuron* 22:751–761.

KASTNER, S., and L. G. UNGERLEIDER, 2000. Mechanisms of visual attention in the human cortex. *Annu. Rev. Neurosci.* 23:315–341.

KIM, Y. H., D. R. GITELMAN, A. C. NOBRE, T. B. PARRISH, K. S. LABAR, and M. M. MESULAM, 1999. The large-scale neural network for spatial attention displays multifunctional overlap but differential asymmetry. *NeuroImage* 9:269–277.

KUBOTA, K., and H. NIKI, 1971. Prefrontal cortical unit activity and delayed alternation performance in monkeys. *J. Neurophysiol.* 34:337–347.

LABERGE, D., and M. S. BUCHSBAUM, 1990. Positron emission tomographic measurements of pulvinar activity during an attention task. *J. Neurosci.* 10:613–619.

LE, T. H., J. V. PARDO, and X. HU, 1998. 4 T-fMRI study of nonspatial shifting of selective attention: Cerebellar and parietal contributions. *J. Neurophysiol.* 79:1535–1548.

MESULAM, M. M., 1981. A cortical network for directed attention and unilateral neglect. *Ann. Neurol.* 10:309–325.

MESULAM, M. M., 1990. Large-scale neurocognitive networks and distributed processing for attention, language, and memory. *Ann. Neurol.* 28:597–613.

MIDDLETON, F. A., and P. L. STRICK, 1994. Anatomical evidence for cerebellar and basal ganglia involvement in higher cognitive function. *Science* 266:458–461.

MOTTER, B. C., 1993. Focal attention produces spatially selective processing in visual cortical areas V1, V2, and V4 in the presence of competing stimuli. *J. Neurophysiol.* 70:909–919.

MOTTER, B. C., 1994. Neuronal correlates of attentive selection for color or luminance in extrastriate area V4. *J. Neurosci.* 14:2178–2189.

NOBRE, A. C., G. N. SEBESTYEN, D. R. GITELMAN, M. M. MESULAM, R. S. J. FRACKOWIAK, and C. D. FRITH, 1997. Functional localization of the system for visuospatial attention using positron emission tomography. *Brain* 120:515–533.

PESSOA, L., and L. G. UNGERLEIDER, 2004. Neural correlates of change detection and change blindness in a working memory task. *Cereb. Cortex* 14:511–520.

PESSOA, L., E. GUTIERREZ, P. B. BANDETTINI, and L. G. UNGERLEIDER, 2002. Neural correlates of visual working memory: fMRI amplitude predicts task performance. *Neuron* 35:975–987.

PESSOA, L., S. KASTNER, and L. G. UNGERLEIDER, 2002. Attentional control of the processing of neural and emotional stimuli. *Cogn. Brain Res.* 15:31–45.

PETERSEN, S. E., D. L. ROBINSON, and J. D. MORRIS, 1987. Contributions of the pulvinar to visual spatial attention. *Neuropsychologia* 25:97–105.

PETERSEN, S. E., D. L. ROBINSON, and W. KEYS, 1985. Pulvinar nuclei of the behaving rhesus monkey: Visual responses and their modulation. *J. Neurophysiol.* 54:867–886.

PETIT, L., S. M. COURTNEY, L. G. UNGERLEIDER, and J. V. HAXBY, 1998. Sustained activity in the medial wall during working memory delays. *J. Neurosci.* 18:9429–9437.

POSNER, M. I., and Y. COHEN, 1984. Components of attention. In *Attention and Performance*, H. Bouman and D. Bowhuis, eds. Hillsdale, N.J.: Erlbaum, pp. 531–556.

POSTLE, B. R., J. S. BERGER, A. M. TAICH, and M. D'ESPOSITO, 2000. Activity in human frontal cortex associated with spatial working memory and saccadic behavior. *J. Cogn. Neurosci.* 12:2–14.

RAFAL, R., 1998. Neglect. In *The Attentive Brain*, R. Parasuraman, ed. Cambridge, Mass.: MIT Press, pp. 489–525.

REMINGTON, R. W., J. C. JOHNSTON, and S. YANTIS, 1992. Involuntary attentional capture by abrupt onset. *Percept. Psychophys.* 51:279–290.

RENSINK, R. A., 2002. Change detection. *Annu. Rev. Psychol.* 53:245–277.

RENSINK, R. A., J. K. O'REGAN, and J. J. CLARK, 1997. To see or not to see: The need for attention to perceive changes in scenes. *Psychol. Sci.* 8:368–373.

RESS, D., B. T. BACKUS, and D. J. HEEGER, 2000. Activity in primary visual cortex predicts performance in a visual detection task. *Nat. Neurosci.* 3:940–945.

ROBINSON, D. L., and S. E. PETERSEN, 1992. The pulvinar and visual salience. *Trends Neurosci.* 15:127–132.

ROSEN, A. C., S. M. RAO, P. CAFFARRA, A. SCAGLIONI, J. A. BOBHOLZ, S. J. WOODLEY, T. A. HAMMEKE, J. M. CUNNINGHAM, T. E. PRIETO, and J. R. BINDER, 1999. Neural basis of endogenous and exogenous spatial orienting: A functional MRI study. *J. Cogn. Neurosci.* 11:135–152.

ROSENKILDE, C. E., R. H. BAUER, and J. M. FUSTER, 1981. Single cell activity in ventral prefrontal cortex of behaving monkeys. *Brain Res.* 209:375–394.

ROWE, J. B., I. TONI, O. JOSEPHS, R. S. FRACKOWIAK, and R. E. PASSINGHAM, 2000. The prefrontal cortex: Response selection or maintenance within working memory? *Science* 288:1656–1660.

SAKAI, K., J. B. ROWE, and R. E. PASSINGHAM, 2002. Active maintenance in prefrontal area 46 creates distractor-resistant memory. *Nat. Neurosci.* 5:479–484.

SCHMAHMANN, J. D., 1996. From movement to thought: Anatomical substrates of the cerebellar contribution to cognitive processing. *Hum. Brain Mapp* 4:174–198.

SHULMAN, G. L., J. A. OLLINGER, E. AKBUDAK, T. E. CONTURO, A. Z. SNYDER, S. E. PETERSEN, and M. CORBETTA, 1999. Areas involved in encoding and applying directional expectations to moving objects. *J. Neurosci.* 21:9480–9496.

SMILEK, D., J. D. EASTWOOD, and P. M. MERIKLE, 2000. Does unattended information facilitate change detection? *J. Exp. Psychol. Hum. Percept. Perform.* 26:480–487.

SMITH, E. E., J. J. JONIDES, R. A. KOEPPE, E. AWH, E. H. SCHUMACHER, and S. MINOSHIMA, 1995. Spatial versus object working memory: PET investigations. *J. Cogn. Neurosci.* 7:337–356.

THACH, W. T., 1996. On the specific role of the cerebellum in motor learning and cognition: Clues from PET activation and lesion studies in man. *Behav. Brain Sci.* 19:411–431.

THOMPSON, K. G., and J. D. SCHALL, 1999. The detection of visual signals by macaque frontal eye field during masking. *Nat. Neurosci.* 2:283–288.

THOMPSON, K. G., and J. D. SCHALL. 2000. Antecedents and correlates of visual detection and awareness in macaque prefrontal cortex. *Vision Res.* 40:1523–1538.

THORNTON, I. M., and D. FERNANDEZ-DUQUE, 2000. An implicit measure of undetected change. *Spatial Vision* 14:21–44.

UNGERLEIDER, L. G., and C. A. CHRISTENSEN, 1979. Pulvinar lesions in monkeys produce abnormal scanning of a complex visual array. *Neuropsychologia* 17:493–501.

UNGERLEIDER, L. G., D. GAFFAN, and V. S. PELAK, 1989. Projections from inferior temporal cortex to prefrontal cortex via the uncinate fascicle in rhesus monkeys. *Exp. Brain Res.* 76:473–484.

VANDENBERGHE, R., J. DUNCAN, P. DUPONT, R. WARD, J. POLINE, G. BORMANS, J. MICHIELS, L. MORTELMANS, and G. A. ORBAN, 1997. Attention to one or two features in left or right visual field: A positron emission tomography study. *J. Neurosci.* 17:3739–3750.

VANDENBERGHE, R., D. R. GITELMAN, T. B. PARRISH, and M. MESULAM, 2001. Location- or feature-based targeting of peripheral attention. *NeuroImage* 14:37–47.

WATANABE, M., 1986a. Prefrontal unit activity during delayed conditional go/no-go discrimination in the monkey. I. Relation to the stimulus. *Brain Res.* 382:1–14.

WATANABE, M., 1986b. Prefrontal unit activity during delayed conditional go/no-go discrimination in the monkey. II. Relation to go and no-go responses. *Brain Res.* 382:15–27.

WEBSTER, M. J., J. BACHEVALIER, and L. G. UNGERLEIDER, 1993. Subcortical connections of inferior temporal areas TE and TEO in macaques. *J. Comp. Neurol.* 335:73–91.

WEBSTER, M. J., J. BACHEVELIER, and L. G. UNGERLEIDER, 1994. Connections of inferior temporal areas TEO and TE with parietal and frontal cortex in macaque monkeys. *Cere. Cortex* 4:470–483.

YANTIS, S., and D. N. JOHNSON, 1990. Mechanisms of attentional priority. *J. Exp. Psychol. Hum. Percept. Perform.* 16:812–825.

67 The Brain's Mind's Images: The Cognitive Neuroscience of Mental Imagery

GIORGIO GANIS, WILLIAM L. THOMPSON, FRED MAST, AND STEPHEN M. KOSSLYN

ABSTRACT Visual mental imagery is a fundamental aspect of human cognition. However, the scientific study of visual mental imagery has been difficult because it is intimately intertwined with an individual's inherently private phenomenology. Over the last two decades, powerful new methods have augmented the more traditional (behavioral and brain lesion) techniques for studying cognition in general and visual mental imagery in particular. In this chapter, we review convergent findings obtained by using multiple methods (studies of behavior, neuroimaging, transcranial magnetic stimulation, and deficits following brain damage) to investigate visual mental imagery. These findings support two general principles: (1) visual imagery shares many neural processes with visual perception, and (2) visual imagery is not a unitary process, but arises from the interaction of a host of subprocesses.

Unlike visual perception, visual mental imagery typically takes place in the absence of external visual stimuli. Indeed, visual mental images can be characterized as short-term memory representations of visual events that give rise to the experience of "seeing with the mind's eye." Such representations are based on stored visual long-term memories, but they are not necessarily restricted to visual memories of specific events that were actually experienced; visual images, although based on stored memories, can be transformed and combined in novel ways, resulting in images of events or objects that were never perceived. In fact, visual images typically can be transformed in multiple ways; for instance, we can imagine how an object would look if an external force were applied to it (shifting it, compressing it, or even crush-

ing it). Moreover, transformations can be carried out with different processes. For example, it is possible to imagine the results of an external force rotating an object versus an object being rotated by one's own actions, and different brain areas are active in the two cases (Wraga et al., 2003). Although the focus of this chapter is on visual mental imagery, we will also discuss motor imagery and illustrate some of the ways in which motor processes are intertwined with visual mental imagery. The latter is well illustrated by the close similarity of eye movement sequences during visual imagery and visual perception of the same visual pattern, and by the functional role that such eye movements may have in visual imagery (Laeng and Teodorescu, 2002).

Because of its pervasiveness in human mental life, mental imagery, and in particular visual mental imagery, historically has often been assigned an important role in theories of the mind. For instance, among the Greek philosophers, Plato used the metaphor of a mental artist painting pictures in the soul (*Philebus* 39c), and Aristotle, by saying that "The soul never thinks without a mental image" (*De Anima* 431a 15–20), attributed a key role in mental function to imagery. However, the private nature of visual mental imagery has complicated its scientific study. For over half a century, until about 1960, the behaviorist school questioned the scientific validity of mental imagery because it was not directly associated with observable behavior that could be measured objectively, which thereby violated the central tenet of their "black-box" approach. With the decline of behaviorism and the advent of the cognitive revolution in the 1960s and 1970s, researchers again began to study the nature of the internal representations used in visual mental imagery, and issues about such representations actually became the focus of an intense debate.

On one side, some theories (Pylyshyn, 1973, 2002) hypothesized that the depictive aspects of visual mental images of which we are conscious are epiphenomenal, that is, they play no role in information processing, just as the heat thrown off by a light bulb is epiphenomenal in the

GIORGIO GANIS Department of Psychology, Harvard University, Cambridge, Mass., and Department of Radiology, Massachusetts General Hospital, Boston, Mass.

WILLIAM L. THOMPSON Department of Psychology, Harvard University, Cambridge, Mass.

FRED MAST Department of Psychology, University of Zurich, Zurich, Switzerland.

STEPHEN M. KOSSLYN Department of Psychology, Harvard University, Cambridge, Mass., and Department of Neurology, Massachusetts General Hospital, Boston, Mass.

process of reading. These theories postulated that visual mental images rely on a language-like representational format. On the other side were theories proposing that mental images rely on representations in which the geometric properties of the representation itself correspond to those of the object being represented. In its original formulation, this theory was proposed in a computer graphics framework; that is, visual images were conceptualized as patterns of points within two-dimensional (2D) arrays akin to those in a computer video buffer (Kosslyn, 1980). Numerous behavioral studies attempted to resolve this issue but were ultimately unsuccessful in providing conclusive evidence. Indeed, Anderson (1978) argued that (1) such behavioral results are inherently ambiguous and could be explained equally well by theories positing either depictive or language-like representations, and (2) that only convergent, nonbehavioral evidence eventually could resolve this issue. Indeed, progress in neuroscience and cognitive neuroscience over the last three decades has yielded huge amounts of knowledge about the functioning of the primate visual system, and this knowledge in turn has been crucial in constraining and inspiring accounts of visual mental imagery (Kosslyn, 1994; Kosslyn et al., 2001). Relying on this type of evidence, the computational theory originally put forward by Kosslyn (1980) was translated into neurophysiological terms by proposing links with specific neural structures. For example, the 2D arrays that were posited to support depictive representations may correspond to patterns of neural activation in topographically organized visual areas (Kosslyn, 1994). This approach has led to numerous empirical predictions, many of which have born fruit. Because approaches such as the one proposed by Pylyshyn discard neurocognitive evidence as irrelevant for the understanding of visual mental imagery (Pylyshyn, 1973, 2002), they will not be discussed further in this context.

Cognitive neuroscience of visual mental imagery

A large amount of research in the field of visual mental imagery can be described as an effort toward articulating two principles. The first principle is that many processes are used in common during both visual imagery and visual perception (Farah, 1984; Kosslyn, 1994; Kosslyn, Ganis, and Thompson, 2001). The second principle, implicit in the first, is that imagery is the result of the operation of a host of subprocesses. The most convincing evidence in support of these principles comes from the convergence of multiple lines of research and methods.

Cognitive neuroscience approaches

Researchers have typically adopted three complementary approaches to investigate visual mental imagery and, more generally, visual cognition: (1) the neuropsychological approach, which entails observing patterns of impairment following brain damage, (2) the brain imaging approach, which entails recording patterns of neural activation using brain imaging technologies, and (3) the virtual lesion approach, which is akin to the neuropsychological approach but in which deficits are temporarily induced by transcranial magnetic stimulation (TMS) (a variant of the virtual lesion approach uses TMS to probe the excitability of cortical areas in various experimental situations).

Without question, the brain imaging approach is very powerful because it allows researchers to monitor the entire brain while it is engaged in a task of interest. Regardless of the specific spatial and temporal resolution characteristics of each neuroimaging method, one limitation of this approach is that, even with sophisticated parametric designs, it can only provide correlational information between cognitive processes and "brain activation" measures (which are more or less directly related to neural activity). In contrast, the neuropsychological approach in principle can provide evidence of causal links between neural structures and behavior; however, it has well-known limitations, including the following: (1) brain damage typically is diffuse and distributed, (2) it usually affects structures that are functionally unrelated, and (3) it is followed by substantial neural reorganization and compensation. The "virtual lesion" approach afforded by TMS provides a way to disrupt local neural activation and determine whether such activation has a causal role in carrying out a process of interest. Moreover, the effect of TMS is transient, can be targeted to structures that are involved in a specific function, and is not followed by neural reorganization. However, among other limitations, TMS has limited spatial resolution, and the method can be targeted toward only superficial parts of the brain.

Thus, because each approach has specific strengths and weaknesses, the combination of the three approaches has provided more powerful evidence about the neural bases of visual mental imagery than any of them could have provided in isolation.

Visual mental imagery and early visual areas

Most of the research in the field has been designed to discover whether visual imagery and visual perception share common processes. This research has typically focused specifically on the issue of whether early visual areas in the occipital lobe are involved in visual mental imagery. These areas (V1/V2 in the primate literature, also known as areas 17/18 in the human and cat literature) are the first cortical sites to receive visual information originating from the retina. Crucially, early visual areas are retinotopically organized, that is, the spatial distribution of activation in the retina is represented in a topographic manner on the cortical surface. Evidence that visual mental imagery engages retinotopically organized areas in spatially meaningful ways, as vision does, provides strong support for the view that visual mental imagery relies on depictive representations. Such findings cannot be easily explained by assuming propositional representations without invoking numerous post-hoc assumptions (Kosslyn, Thompson, and Ganis, 2002). The retinotopic organization of primate early visual cortex has been widely demonstrated, in nonhuman primates (Tootell et al., 1982), and in humans (e.g., Sereno et al., 1995; Engel, Glover, and Wandell, 1997). The fact that this organization has a functional role in human vision is demonstrated, for instance, by patients who sustained focal damage to early visual cortex and exhibit scotomas (blind spots) in the corresponding parts of the visual field (e.g., Rizzo and Robin, 1996).

EARLY VISUAL CORTEX AND MENTAL IMAGERY: EVIDENCE FROM NEUROIMAGING   The first coordinate of this retinotopic organization, visual eccentricity (i.e., the distance from the center of the visual field), is represented along the caudal/rostral axis in early visual cortex: the central parts of the visual field are represented in the most caudal parts of early visual cortex, while more peripheral parts are represented increasingly rostrally. Thus, a crucial test of whether this aspect of the topographic organization in early visual cortex is used by visual mental imagery is whether visual mental images of large objects activate more rostral locations in early visual cortex than those of small objects. Three studies tested this possibility. Kosslyn and colleagues (1993, Experiment 3) asked participants to visualize letters of the alphabet either at a very small size (as small as possible while still being distinguishable) or at a very large size (as large as possible without the letter seeming to overflow the "visual field") while their brains were scanned using position emission tomography (PET). The participants were asked to retain the image for 4s and then answer a question about the appearance of the letter (such as whether it had any curved lines). The PET data revealed that when participants visualized the letters at a small size, caudal V1 was activated; conversely, when the letters were imaged at the larger size, a more rostral part of V1 became active. Tootell and colleagues (1998) essentially replicated this study, using a single participant in a functional magnetic resonance imaging (fMRI) study. The most interesting aspect of this study was that the results were analyzed using a cortical unfolding algorithm, and thus the authors could establish convincingly that the size at which the imaged letters were formed altered the location of activation in area 17 per se. Finally, adopting the same line of reasoning, Kosslyn and colleagues (1995) asked participants to memorize the appearance of line drawings of common objects (such as a boat or a bell). The participants were later asked to form vivid visual images of the objects

(they were cued with the name of the object), to retain the image for 4s, and to make a judgment about the object's appearance (such as whether the right side was higher than the left). The objects were to be imaged at one of three sizes: small (0.25° of visual angle), medium (4°), or large (16°). The PET data revealed that activation in early visual cortex lined up according to image size, with small images activating the most caudal portions, medium-sized images activating somewhat more rostral parts, and large images activating the most rostral parts of V1 and V2, as would be expected if imagery relied on topographic representations.

The second coordinate of the retinotopic organization, polar angle (i.e., the angle formed with the vertical meridian), is represented on the cortex in a direction approximately orthogonal to that of visual eccentricity. A study by Klein and colleagues (2004) used fMRI to test the hypothesis that polar angle in visual mental imagery is represented in a way comparable to how polar angle is represented during visual perception. Participants were asked to perceive or visualize horizontal and vertical checkerboard wedges, like the ones used in visual retinotopy studies. For the majority of participants, both visual mental imagery and vision evoked patterns of activation that were consistent with the retinotopic organization of early visual cortex. Specifically, visualizing the vertically oriented wedges activated portions of V1/V2 around the vertical meridian, and visualizing the horizontally oriented wedges activated portions of V1/V2 around the horizontal meridian.

These findings extend previous results and provide strong support for the view that geometric spatial structure, both of perceived and of visualized objects, is directly related to detectable activation patterns in early topographically organized visual cortex (areas 17 and 18).

Despite evidence that early visual cortex is engaged during visual mental imagery, some brain imaging studies have failed to find signs of such engagement. A vigorous debate has emerged regarding the reasons for this inconsistency. A recent meta-analysis of neuroimaging studies of visual mental imagery by Kosslyn and Thompson (2003) addressed this issue by examining the factors that contribute to the activation (or nonactivation) of early visual cortex during imagery. They detailed three theories that might lead to such a prediction. The first is identified as perceptual anticipation theory, which essentially corresponds to the theory of imagery developed by Kosslyn (1994). The theory posits that during visual imagery, the expectation of seeing a particular object or part becomes so strong that the image is primed and activation is sent from the memory store in the temporal lobes backward to early visual cortex, where object shape is reconstructed topographically. The second theory Kosslyn and Thompson called propositional theory, according to which early visual areas should not be activated during imagery, and any findings of activation are false positives probably due to weaknesses in the methodology. Finally, methodological factors theory takes the opposite view from propositional theory, namely, that visual imagery should always activate early visual cortex. This theory predicts that failure to find such activation is a result of methodological limitations. Kosslyn and Thompson examined 59 studies of mental imagery and coded them on six variables (attributes of the studies) related to the theories. These variables were (1) the use of a task requiring visualization of high-resolution details; (2) the requirement to visualize shapes (not spatial relations, which may be processed in the parietal, not occipital, lobe); (3) the visualization of specific exemplars (not prototypic images); (4) the number of participants; (5) the power of the brain imaging technique used; and (6) the use of a resting baseline for task comparison, which is uncontrolled. The first three variables were associated with perceptual anticipation theory and the last three were associated with the other two theories, although with completely opposite predictions for each theory. The methodological factors theory would predict that early visual cortex would be activated when a study included larger numbers of participants, more powerful imaging techniques, and a controlled nonresting baseline, whereas the propositional theory would predict that artifactual activation might be found with the opposite valence on these variables. The results of a logistic regression analysis revealed that two variables associated with perceptual anticipation theory (visualization of high-resolution details and visualization of shapes, not spatial relations) and two variables associated with methodological factors theory (brain imaging technique and type of baseline task) predicted whether a study found activation in early visual cortex. Kosslyn and colleagues (1995) had previously shown that resting baselines may lead to hypermetabolism in early visual areas and thus may mask task activation that would otherwise be detected. Kosslyn and Thompson also performed a correlational analysis with 15 additional variables that differed among the studies (such as whether participants were tested in complete darkness, had their eyes open or closed, and had to make a judgment). Nine of the 21 total variables were found to be correlated with the presence or absence of early visual cortex activation in a study. These nine variables were then submitted to a forward stepwise logistic regression. The results of this regression analysis were similar to the first, theory-based analysis: the requirement to note high-resolution details and to visualize shapes predicted activation, as did the imaging technique used. Mazard and colleagues (in press) report converging findings when they performed a meta-analysis of data from their own laboratory. They found that early visual cortex was not activated when the task relied on spatial relations but was activated when shapes had to be visualized and evaluated. In short, the variability in results from different studies was not haphazard but rather reflected systematic ways in which the studies differed.

Another reason why some studies failed to detect activation in early visual areas during imagery hinges on the issue of "nonresponders" in neuroimaging studies. Kosslyn and Thompson (2003) report in their meta-analytic review that in about 24% of participants (in tasks where individual brain data are reported and early visual cortex was activated in the majority of participants during the task) early visual areas were not activated during imagery. The reasons for such nonactivation are controversial: participants may adopt a different task performance strategy, or detection of brain activation may be hindered by characteristics of individual brain anatomy or physiology. In any case, if about one-fourth of participants fit into the "nonresponder" category, there is a high probability that a large minority of participants will be nonresponders in any given study. For example, in a study with 12 participants, there is a 35% probability that one-third or more of the participants will be nonresponders. When data are averaged in a group analysis, effects can be masked by null responses from a minority of participants in the group, leading to many subthreshold results that go undetected. This is particularly true in studies that used single-photon emission computed tomography (SPECT) and PET, where almost all data are averaged. Consistent with this idea, most of the neuroimaging studies that failed to find activation of early visual cortex during imagery did in fact use PET or SPECT. In contrast, a substantial majority of fMRI studies of imagery have reported finding activation in topographic parts of visual cortex.

EARLY VISUAL CORTICAL LESIONS AND VISUAL MENTAL IMAGERY: EVIDENCE FROM NEUROPSYCHOLOGY AND TMS
Although the neuroimaging results appear to lend support to depictive theories of image representation, it is possible that the activation found in early visual cortex using fMRI or PET during imagery plays no functional role. It could be the case, for instance, that other brain regions actually represent visual images and that the activation found in early visual areas is merely epiphenomenal—a by-product of activation in other brain regions, playing no functional role in visual mental imagery, like the LED on the power button of an electric appliance.

Evidence suggesting that early visual cortex is necessary to perform at least some types of visual mental imagery comes from neuropsychological studies. Visual imagery impairments have been reported in patients with unilateral occipital infarcts that produce hemianopia. One study with detailed testing of visual imagery was reported by Butter and colleagues (1997). These researchers tested a group of eight hemianopic patients on a visual image scanning task that required participants to judge whether an arrow was pointing at one of a set of dots they had recently seen but were no longer visible. The patients made more errors when the arrow pointed to the side ipsilateral to their hemianopia than when the arrow pointed to the other side. However, because no neuroanatomical scanning was performed in three of the eight patients and only CT scans were obtained in the remaining five, it is impossible to tell whether the lesion involved only area 17.

In addition, Farah, Soso, and Dasheiff (1992) examined the spatial extent of images in a patient before and after removal of the occipital lobe in one hemisphere. Consistent with the findings of Butter and colleagues (1997), Farah and colleagues found that the horizontal "visual angle" subtended by visual mental images of objects was reduced by about half after the surgery. This finding suggests that half the horizontal extent of the "imagery field" was removed by the surgery. In contrast, the vertical extent of objects in images remained the same. Given that vertical extent is represented in both occipital lobes, this finding makes sense, and also provides a control against the possibility that the brain damage had simply made the task more difficult overall.

This picture is complicated by reports of patients who are cortically blind from bilateral damage to primary visual cortex but appear to have preserved visual imagery (Chatterjee and Southwood, 1995; Goldenberg, Mullbacher, and Nowak, 1995). These cases do not necessarily refute the hypothesis that early visual cortex is used in visual mental imagery because (1) it is possible that "islands" of intact cortex may support the spared imagery abilities; (2) some of the tasks used may have not been appropriate, for instance because the imagery questions could be answered without the use of high-resolution visual information (e.g., by using semantic information); and (3) although early visual cortex may typically be used during visual mental imagery, in some cases higher-level visual areas can compensate if these structures are damaged. For instance, many shape tasks can be converted to spatial relations tasks. In fact, one of us once examined a patient who had extensive damage to occipital cortex. When asked which uppercase letters have any curved lines, she literally "drew" each one in the air, and reflected on the movements her finger made; this patient apparently was using a spatial strategy, which was slow and cumbersome but allowed her to perform the task. The fact that spatial processes can be used in the service of visual mental imagery is shown by eye movements, which may help to arrange the component parts correctly when people generate images. Indeed, Laeng and Teodorescu (2002) have shown that people are less accurate when asked about visual details in images while they have to keep their gaze fixed. In general, area 17 may be engaged during visual imagery, if it is available, when a task requires high-resolution inspection of shapes (Kosslyn and Thompson, 2003). However, if area 17 is damaged, the processes that would take place there may take place in the next available visual area (area 18), perhaps

in a less efficient manner. This may lead one to predict, for instance, slower response times when cortically blind individuals perform imagery tasks; to our knowledge, this hypothesis has not been tested.

TMS, by creating transient virtual lesions in selected brain regions, in principle can address the issue of causality without many of the problems associated with neuropsychological studies. For example, Kosslyn and colleagues (1999) delivered repetitive TMS (rTMS) at 1 Hz to the medial occipital cortex of five participants before they performed an imagery task in which they were asked to visualize sets of stripes and make judgments about them; there was also a parallel perception task in which participants made the same judgments on the basis of actually viewing the sets of stripes. This type of stimulation is known to decrease cortical excitability (e.g., Boroojerdi et al., 2000) and presumably diminishes the efficiency of local processing. PET data (in a different set of participants) demonstrated that this task led to activation of early visual cortex. In both imagery and vision, the participants' performance was impaired when TMS was applied to early visual areas relative to a sham TMS condition in which the TMS coil was placed on the same location on the head but at such an orientation that TMS did not target the brain. This result supports the hypothesis that early visual areas play a critical role in performing imagery tasks, and thus the activation of these areas is not epiphenomenal.

VISUAL MENTAL IMAGERY AND HIGHER-LEVEL VISUAL AREAS: EVIDENCE FROM NEUROPSYCHOLOGY A major subdivision of function in the primate visual system is between the ventral and the dorsal streams (Ungerleider and Mishkin, 1982). The ventral stream, which includes portions of the occipital lobe and ventrolateral temporal regions, is generally involved in the analysis of shape and color, and damage to this stream can disrupt the ability to recognize and identify visual stimuli (visual agnosias). In contrast, the dorsal stream, which includes portions of the occipital lobe and posterior parietal regions, is involved in processing spatial and motion information; damage to this stream can disrupt the ability to locate stimuli (e.g., spatial disorientation). If visual mental imagery employs some of the same neural structures that support vision, one would expect this same distinction between the ventral and dorsal stream to hold in visual mental imagery. Indeed, some patients show precisely the corresponding pattern of impairment. For instance, one patient described by Levine, Warach, and Farah (1985) was impaired at color (achromatopsia) and face recognition (prosopagnosia) and showed a similar impairment when describing faces and the color of objects from memory. In contrast, this patient could make spatial judgments satisfactorily. However, another patient described in the same study exhibited spatial disorientation and was impaired at describing spatial relations from memory, but could recognize faces and colors well.

Focusing on the ventral stream, different visual areas are selectively engaged by different visual attributes and object classes. Some occipitotemporal areas are engaged preferentially by color, some by faces, and some by other objects, as reflected in the pattern of visual deficits observed in patients following brain damage. For instance, some patients are selectively unable to recognize colors, whereas others are unable to recognize faces. A number of patients have been reported to show remarkable similarities in the pattern of deficit between visual imagery and vision. For instance, achromatopic patients show color imagery deficits (Riddoch and Humphreys, 1987; Sacks and Wasserman, 1987; Ogden, 1993), whereas prosopagnosic patients show face imagery deficits (e.g., Shuttleworth, Syring, and Allen, 1982; Levine, Warach, and Farah, 1985). A patient described by Sartori and Job (1988) had specific problems in identifying pictures of animals, and also had a similar selective problem in visual imagery. A classic review by Farah (1984) summarized data from 28 cases of visual agnosia. Half of the patients had similar deficits in visual imagery. Of the remaining patients, six were not tested for visual imagery, and three had seemingly intact visual imagery but underwent no objective tests (e.g., drawing from memory). Overall, this pattern of similarity supports the idea that at least parts of these occipitotemporal areas are shared by visual imagery and vision.

However, a closer look at the literature does reveal some exceptions to the parallelism between visual imagery and vision as a result of damage to higher-level visual areas (e.g., Behrmann, Moscovitch, and Winocur, 1994; Servos and Goodale, 1995; Bartolomeo et al., 1998). In some cases it is possible to argue that the tasks employed did not necessarily rely on visual mental imagery. For instance, it has been argued that it is possible to draw from memory by relying on motor memories that bypass visual imagery (Kosslyn et al., 1985; Dijkerman and Milner, 1997): a patient might be impaired at visual mental imagery but still be able to draw a picture of an object from memory. Some of these studies, however, used tasks that almost certainly require visual mental imagery. For instance, Servos and Goodale (1995) used a reinterpretation task that requires visual mental images to be composed by transforming and combining images of elementary shapes (e.g., rotate the letter D counterclockwise by 90° and place it on top of a V; which object does it resemble? The answer: an ice cream cone). The patient studied by Servos and Goodale (1995) showed severe object agnosia but performed normally on such a visual mental imagery task. Cases of impaired vision and preserved visual imagery, such as the one just discussed, can be accommodated within a shared-systems framework by assuming that visual processes such as object recognition and identifi-

cation rely (in part) on low- and midlevel visual processes that are not required by visual imagery. This assumption is reasonable because much of low- and midlevel visual processes are involved in grouping, figure–ground segregation, and so on (Marr, 1982). When such preprocessing stages are compromised, visual object identification may be impaired, but visual imagery may be largely preserved. This interpretation is supported by cases such as those described by Behrmann, Moscovitch, and Winocur (1994) and Bartolomeo and colleagues (1998), in which patients with severe visual agnosia but normal visual imagery performed poorly on midlevel visual processes, such as those required to identify overlapping line drawings.

The opposite pattern of impairment, that is, impaired visual imagery with preserved perception, has been accommodated within a shared-systems framework by assuming that visual imagery is more complex and demanding than visual perception and therefore is more sensitive to brain damage (Farah, 1984; Goldenberg, 1993) or that the damage affects brain regions involved in activating stored information to generate images. Such processes might also be involved in top-down perception, but to our knowledge, researchers have not investigated whether impairments in imagery are accompanied by impairments in top-down perception.

VISUAL MENTAL IMAGERY AND HIGHER-LEVEL VISUAL AREAS: EVIDENCE FROM NEUROIMAGING AND TMS Neuroimaging studies have complemented the picture painted by neuropsychological studies. A general finding is that higher-level visual areas are often activated during visual mental imagery (Ishai, Ungerleider, and Haxby, 2000; O'Craven and Kanwisher, 2000; Ishai, Haxby, and Ungerleider, 2002), consistent with the neuropsychological findings. Furthermore, the specific pattern of activation during visual imagery is very similar to that found during vision. For instance, fMRI studies have found that portions of the same distinct ventral temporal regions that respond preferentially to pictures of faces and places show a similar pattern of selectivity during visual imagery of faces and places (O'Craven and Kanwisher, 2000). A similar pattern has been observed with pictures of faces, houses, and chairs (Ishai, Ungerleider, and Haxby, 2000). Usually, although many of the same brain regions are activated during visual imagery and during vision, the overlap is not complete (Kosslyn et al., 1997; Ishai, Ungerleider, and Haxby, 2000; O'Craven and Kanwisher, 2000; Ishai, Haxby, and Ungerleider, 2002) or the activation is not identical. For example, in the fMRI study reported by Ishai and collaborators (Ishai, Ungerleider, and Haxby, 2000), participants saw objects from different categories or visualized them. Activation in some ventral stream regions was clearly modulated by category type during vision. However, only small portions of these regions exhibited a similar pattern of activation during visual imagery, which suggests that the remaining portions were engaged during vision but not during visual imagery. As noted earlier, such findings are to be expected, given the pattern of dissociations between vision and visual imagery found in some brain-damaged patients: because the neural networks supporting vision and visual imagery are not completely overlapping, damage to the common areas will cause parallel deficits, whereas damage restricted to the nonoverlapping areas may produce independent deficits in visual imagery or visual perception.

Another general finding from neuroimaging experiments is that different visual imagery tasks engage different brain areas, often in a way that is consistent with the neuropsychological findings. Visuospatial tasks such as mental rotation (i.e., imagining how an object would look if it were rotated) tend to engage parietal regions in the "where" stream (Cohen et al., 1996; Richter et al., 1997; Kosslyn et al., 1998; Jordan et al., 2001; Ng et al., 2001), whereas tasks that require visualizing the shape of objects tend to engage early visual cortex and occipitotemporal regions in the "what" stream (Kosslyn et al., 1995; Ishai, Ungerleider, and Haxby, 2000; O'Craven and Kanwisher, 2000; Ishai, Haxby, and Ungerleider, 2002). It is also important to note the role of eye movements during mental imagery (e.g., Laeng and Teodorescu, 2002) when interpreting these neuroimaging findings. There is good evidence for frontal (e.g., the frontal eye fields) and superior parietal activation during voluntary saccades. However, only a few studies have examined saccade-related responses in early visual cortex, and the results are still controversial (Paus et al., 1995; Kimmig et al., 2001).

The regions that constitute the core of the ventral stream are too deep within the brain to be targeted by TMS; thus, no virtual lesions experiments using TMS have been carried out, for instance, to impair face recognition by stimulation of face-sensitive areas in the fusiform gyrus. However, a number of TMS studies have been performed to assess whether the dorsal stream is causally involved in spatial imagery. For instance, repetitive TMS to the right parietal cortex interferes with spatial imagery. For example, such TMS disrupts the mental clock task, in which participants hear one or more probes, such as "4:30," and visualize an analogue clock with the hands corresponding to the given time; next, they answer a spatial question about the specific hand configurations, such as whether the angle between them is smaller than 90°.

Motor imagery

Which specific brain regions are engaged during visual mental imagery depends crucially on the details of the task as well as on the details of what is visualized. In this section,

we briefly discuss the case of motor imagery, in part to illustrate the importance of the strategies employed during mental imagery.

When people imagine performing a particular movement (e.g., tying a shoe) and indicate when they would have finished the action, the estimated time for this movement is remarkably similar to the time it actually takes to execute the movement (Decety and Jeannerod, 1995; Papaxanthis et al., 2002). While performing these types of tasks, people report that they imagine themselves performing the movement in question. Numerous studies have demonstrated that this type of motor imagery can be dissociated from purely visual mental imagery. For example, several neuroimaging studies have shown that areas involved in motor execution also play a role in motor imagery, and these areas are not generally active during visual mental imagery. For example, Lafleur and colleagues (2002) demonstrated that repeated imagery of foot movements is accompanied by changes in brain activation over time similar to those that occur when the movements are actually executed. Moreover, behavioral studies have shown that mentally practicing a specific movement can improve the speed, accuracy, and strength of motor execution (Feltz and Landers, 1983; Yue and Cole, 1992; Yáguez et al., 1998). This finding suggests that motor imagery engages some of the same neural systems that are engaged during actual execution of the movements. In addition to their theoretical importance, such findings have remarkable applied potential, for example in brain rehabilitation or in competitive sports. But what do we know about the neural mechanisms underlying motor imagery?

Georgopoulos and colleagues (1989) showed that motor areas are involved in motor imagery. They recorded the activity from single cells in primary motor cortex in monkeys while the animals planned to move a handle along an arc. Neurons in the arm area (contralateral to the performing hand) are tuned for the orientation of the arm; the activation of these individual neurons can be combined into a summary measure, referred to as population vector, that encodes the direction of the arm. The temporal analysis of neural activity revealed a sequence starting with the population vector oriented toward the initial position of the handle and ending in the direction of the end position of the handle. It is noteworthy that this activity precedes the motor execution, which thus suggests a relation between motor imagery and motor planning. This systematic succession of activation shown for neuronal populations in motor cortex resembles the process of mental rotation. Thus, it is of interest that some neuroimaging studies implicate motor areas when humans perform mental rotation tasks. For example, Richter and colleagues (2000) used the multiarmed angular stimuli made out of blocks first described by Shepard and Metzler (1971). Participants were shown pairs of such stimuli, one of which could be rotated with respect to the other. The task was to decide whether the two examples shown in each pair were the same or mirror-reversed. The results showed bilateral activation of the superior parietal lobules, the premotor cortex, the supplementary motor cortex, and the left primary motor cortex. The PET study of Kosslyn and colleagues (1998), however, showed no activation in any frontal motor area when these types of objects had to be rotated mentally, whereas the fMRI study of Cohen and colleagues (1996) showed premotor activation in only half the subjects they tested.

STRATEGIES IN MOTOR IMAGERY AND MENTAL TRANSFORMATION OF IMAGES: EVIDENCE FROM NEUROIMAGING Why is it that motor areas are activated during mental rotation in only some people? One possibility is that participants may use different strategies when they solve mental rotation tasks. For example, one strategy is based on what one would see if an object were rotated by an external force, whereas another strategy is based on what one would see if an object were manipulated and rotated by hand. Kosslyn, Thompson, and colleagues (2001) tested this idea by asking participants to perform the same mental rotation task that differed only in the instructions. Participants saw a wooden model of the multiarmed angular Shepard–Metzler stimulus described above. Then, either they saw the stimulus being rotated by an electric motor, or they actually rotated the stimulus using their own hand. They were told to imagine the stimuli being rotated in exactly the same way with which they were familiarized during the instruction. Area M1 was activated during mental rotation only when participants were asked to physically manipulate the model prior to the task and later to imagine such rotation. This result demonstrates that people can voluntarily adopt a given strategy, which they can later use to perform mental rotation tasks. Therefore, whether motor areas are used during mental rotation depends more on the strategy used than on the nature of the stimulus that has to be rotated mentally.

Another form of mental transformation involves imagined rotations of one's own body, which are required for egocentric perspective transformations. Findings from neuropsychological studies suggest that perspective transformations rely in part on mechanisms that are not drawn on during mental rotation of objects. Lesions of the left hemisphere, near the parietal-temporal-occipital junction, can be associated with poor performance in egocentric perspective transformations (Ratcliff, 1979), whereas right-sided lesions can be associated with impaired performance on mental rotation of objects (Farah and Hammond, 1988; Corballis, 1997). A right-hemisphere advantage for mental rotation of objects has also been reported when the stimuli are selectively presented to the left or right visual field (Ditunno and Mann, 1990). However, a specialization of the right hemi-sphere for mental rotation is still controversial (Cohen et al., 1996; Alivisatos and Petrides, 1997).

Zacks and colleagues (1999) studied imagined body transformations. Using fMRI, they found a strongly lateralized left-sided activation at the parietal-temporal-occipital junction. During the task, participants evaluated schematic pictures of human figures that were holding a white ball in one hand and a black ball in the other; they decided whether the figure's right or left hand was holding the black ball. The lateralization in brain activation was reversed when the task was altered so that participants could perform it by using an object-based mental rotation strategy (they mentally rotated an inverted figure to the upright orientation). In addition, Zacks and colleagues (1999) found activation in and around the premotor cortex during imagined body transformations. Taken together, this line of research suggests the existence of two different processing systems, one responsible for egocentric perspective transformations and the other responsible for object-based transformations.

Activation within motor areas has also been documented in studies such as the one by Parsons and colleagues (1995), which required participants to make left-right judgments about visually presented hands. The hand stimuli appeared either in the left or right visual hemifield, and participants were not allowed to make any actual hand movements during the PET scans. This task activated the supplementary motor area of the left hemisphere, and also the prefrontal and insular motor areas in the hemisphere contralateral to the visual hemifield. Parsons and colleagues (1995) also found activation in other areas, including the superior and inferior premotor cortex, posterior and inferior parietal cortex, basal ganglia, cerebellum (all bilaterally activated), and primary visual areas (contralateral to the visual hemifield).

MOTOR IMAGERY: EVIDENCE FROM TMS The fact that motor areas are sometimes activated during mental transformation, however, does not answer the question of whether the activated areas are functionally involved in carrying out the task. We can ask whether the motor activation is purely incidental or whether it reflects processing mechanisms that are used to solve the cognitive task. Ganis and colleagues (2000) used TMS to investigate this issue. They administered TMS to the left primary motor cortex (approximately over the right-hand area) while subjects mentally rotated pictures of hands and feet that were presented in the right visual hemifield. These same pictures of hands had been shown to activate left primary motor cortex in a previous study (Kosslyn et al., 1998). Single magnetic pulses to the left motor cortex slowed down the participants' responses when the pulses were delivered with a 650 ms delay after the visual stimulus. The mental rotation of hands was impaired more than the rotation of feet, consistent with the fact that the site of TMS stimulation was right above the area controlling hand movements. Within the spatial resolution limits of TMS, these results indicate that TMS of primary motor cortex disrupted the processing mechanisms that were required to perform the task. However, this result does not necessarily imply that the computation itself takes place in motor cortex. Numerous areas are engaged when people perform mental rotation tasks, and it is possible that the motor cortex relays information that was computed elsewhere in the brain.

In short, there is converging evidence from neurophysiology and neuroimaging, as well as from behavioral studies, that mental imagery can engage the motor system. Such findings begin to illuminate the ways in which motor and visual processes are nested and intertwined. Future research should better elucidate the functional role of motor imagery with respect to various motor processes such as premotor planning, action selection, and motor execution.

Conclusions

Much research on mental imagery has focused on developing and supporting two general principles. The first is that visual imagery and visual perception share many common processes. As we have seen, there is ample evidence that this assumption is correct. However, we have also seen that imagery and perception do not draw on precisely the same systems; Kosslyn, Thompson, and Alpert (1997) and Ganis, Thompson, and Kosslyn (in press), for example, found substantial but not complete overlap between the areas activated during visual imagery and perception. And, although many researchers have documented parallel deficits in imagery and perception following brain damage, other researchers have shown that one or the other ability can be disrupted independently, as would be expected if only some brain areas were shared by the two functions. The second principle is that imagery arises from the operation of a host of distinct processes. We have seen that people can adopt different strategies for accomplishing the same image transformations, and that different brain areas are activated by the different strategies. Such findings indicate that different sets of processes can be used to perform the same task. We expect much future research on imagery to focus more tightly on this second principle, further articulating the specific processes that work together to give rise to imagery.

REFERENCES

ALIVISATOS, B., and M. PETRIDES, 1997. Functional activation of the human brain during mental rotation. *Neuropsychologia* 35:111–118.

ANDERSON, J. R., 1978. Arguments concerning representations for mental imagery. *Psychol. Rev.* 85:249–277.

BARTOLOMEO, P., A. C. BACHOUD-LEVI, B. DE GELDER, G. DENES, G. DALLA BARBA, P. BRUGIERES, et al., 1998. Multiple-domain dissociation between impaired visual perception and preserved mental imagery in a patient with bilateral extrastriate lesions. *Neuropsychologia* 36:239–249.

BEHRMANN, M., M. MOSCOVITCH, and G. WINOCUR, 1994. Intact visual imagery and impaired visual perception in a patient with visual agnosia. *J. Exp. Psychol. Hum. Percept. Perform.* 20:1068–1087.

BOROOJERDI, B., A. PRAGER, W. MUELLBACHER, and L. G. COHEN, 2000. Reduction of human visual cortex excitability using 1-Hz transcranial magnetic stimulation. *Neurology* 54:1529–1531.

BUTTER, C. M., S. M. KOSSLYN, D. MIJOVIC-PRELEC, and A. RIFFLE, 1997. Field-specific deficits in visual imagery following hemianopia due to unilateral occipiral infarcts. *Brain* 120:217–228.

CHATTERJEE, A., and M. H. SOUTHWOOD, 1995. Cortical blindness and visual imagery. *Neurology* 45:2189–2195.

COHEN, M. S., S. M. KOSSLYN, H. C. BREITER, G. J. DiGIROLAMO, W. L. THOMPSON, A. K. ANDERSON, et al., 1996. Changes in cortical activity during mental rotation: A mapping study using functional MRI. *Brain* 119(Pt. 1):89–100.

CORBALLIS, M. C., 1997. Mental rotation and the right hemisphere. *Brain Lang.* 57:100–121.

DECETY, J., and M. JEANNEROD, 1995. Fitt's law in mentally simulated movements. *Behav. Brain Res.* 72:127–134.

DIJKERMAN, H. C., and A. D. MILNER, 1997. Copying without perceiving: motor imagery in visual form agnosia. *Neuroreport* 8:729–732.

DITUNNO, P. L., and V. A. MANN, 1990. Right hemisphere specialization for mental rotation in normals and brain damaged subjects. *Cortex* 26:177–188.

ENGEL, S. A., G. H. GLOVER, and B. A. WANDELL, 1997. Retinotopic organization in human visual cortex and the spatial precision of functional MRI. *Cereb. Cortex* 7:181–192.

FARAH, M. J., 1984. The neurological basis of mental imagery: A componential analysis. *Cognition* 18:245–272.

FARAH, M. J., and K. M. HAMMOND, 1988. Mental rotation and orientation-invariant object recognition: Dissociable processes. *Cognition* 29:29–46.

FARAH, M. J., M. J. SOSO, and R. M. DASHEIFF, 1992. Visual angle of the mind's eye before and after unilateral occipital lobectomy. *J. Exp. Psychol. Hum. Percept. Perform.* 18:241–246.

FELTZ, D. L., and D. M. LANDERS, 1983. The effects of mental practice on motor skill learning and performance: A meta-analysis. *J. Sport Psychol.* 5:25–57.

GANIS, G., J. P. KEENAN, S. M. KOSSLYN, and A. PASCUAL-LEONE, 2000. Transcranial magnetic stimulation of primary motor cortex affects mental rotation. *Cereb. Cortex* 10:175–180.

GANIS, G., W. L. THOMPSON, and S. M. KOSSLYN, in press. Brain areas underlying visual imagery and visual perception: An fMRI study. *Cogn. Brain Res.*

GEORGOPOULOS, A. P., J. T. LURITO, M. PETRIDES, A. B. SCHARTZ, and J. T. MASSEY, 1989. Mental rotation of the neuronal population vector. *Science* 243:234–236.

GOLDENBERG, G., 1993. The neural basis of mental imagery. *Baillieres Clin. Neurol.* 2:265–286.

GOLDENBERG, G., W. MULLBACHER, and A. NOWAK, 1995. Imagery without perception: A case study of anosagnosia for cortical blindness. *Neuropsychologia* 33:1373–1382.

ISHAI, A., J. V. HAXBY, and L. G. UNGERLEIDER, 2002. Visual imagery of famous faces: Effects of memory and attention revealed by FMRI. *NeuroImage* 17:1729–1741.

ISHAI, A., L. G. UNGERLEIDER, and J. V. HAXBY, 2000. Distributed neural systems for the generation of visual images. *Neuron* 28:979–990.

JORDAN, K., H. J. HEINZE, K. LUTZ, M. KANOWSKI, and L. JANCKE, 2001. Cortical activations during the mental rotation of different visual objects. *NeuroImage* 13:143–152.

KIMMIG, H., M. W. GREENLEE, M. GONDAN, M. SCHIRA, J. KASSUBEK, and T. MERGNER, 2001. Relationship between saccadic eye movements and cortical activity as measured by fMRI: Quantitative and qualitative aspects. *Exp. Brain Res.* 141: 184–194.

KLEIN, I., J. DUBOIS, F. KHERIF, J. F. MANGIN, G. FLANDIN, J. B. POLINE, M. DENIS, S. M. KOSSLYN, and D. LE BIHAN, 2004. *Retinotopic organization of visual mental images as revealed by functional magnetic resonance imaging.* Unpublished manuscript.

KOSSLYN, S. M., 1980. *Image and Mind.* Cambridge, Mass.: Harvard University Press.

KOSSLYN, S. M., 1994. *Image and Brain.* Cambridge, Mass.: Harvard University Press.

KOSSLYN, S. M., N. M. ALPERT, W. L. THOMPSON, V. MALJKOVIC, S. B. WEISE, C. F. CHABRIS, S. E. HAMILTON, and F. S. BUONANNO, 1993. Visual mental imagery activates topographically organized visual cortex: PET investigations. *J. Cogn. Neurosci.* 5:263–287.

KOSSLYN, S. M., G. J. DIGIROLAMO, W. L. THOMPSON, and N. M. ALPERT, 1998. Mental rotation of objects versus hands: Neural mechanisms revealed by positron emission tomography. *Psychophysiology* 35:151–161.

KOSSLYN, S. M., G. GANIS, and W. L. THOMPSON, 2001. Neural foundations of imagery. *Nat. Rev. Neurosci.* 2:635–642.

KOSSLYN, S. M., J. D. HOLTZMAN, M. S. GAZZANIGA, and M. J. FARAH, 1985. A computational analysis of mental image generation: Evidence from functional dissociations in split-brain patients. *J. Exp. Psychol. Gen.* 114:311–341.

KOSSLYN, S. M., A. PASCUAL-LEONE, O. FELICIAN, S. CAMPOSANO, J. P. KEENAN, W. L. THOMPSON, G. GANIS, K. E. SUKEL, and N. M. ALPERT, 1999. The role of area 17 in visual imagery: Convergent evidence from PET and rTMS. *Science* 284:167–170.

KOSSLYN, S. M., and W. L. THOMPSON, 2003. When is early visual cortex activated during visual mental imagery? *Psychol. Bull.* 129:723–746.

KOSSLYN, S. M., W. L. THOMPSON, and N. M. ALPERT, 1997. Neural systems shared by visual imagery and visual perception: A positron emission tomography study. *NeuroImage* 6:320–334.

KOSSLYN, S. M., W. L. THOMPSON, and G. GANIS, 2002. Mental imagery doesn't work like that. *Behav. Brain Sci.* 25:198–200.

KOSSLYN, S. M., W. L. THOMPSON, I. J. KIM, and N. M. ALPERT, 1995. Topographical representations of mental images in primary visual cortex. *Nature* 378:496–498.

KOSSLYN, S. M., W. L. THOMPSON, M. WRAGA, and N. M. ALPERT, 2001. Imagining rotation by endogenous vs. exogenous forces: Distinct neural mechanisms. *Neuroreport* 12:2519–2525.

LAENG, B., and D. S. TEODORESCU, 2002. Eye scanpaths during visual imagery reenact those of perception of the same visual scene. *Cogn. Sci.* 26:207–231.

LAFLEUR, M. F., P. L. JACKSON, F. MALOUIN, C. L. RICHARDS, A. C. EVANS, and J. DOYON, 2002. Motor learning produces parallel dynamic functional changes during the execution and imagination of sequential foot movements. *NeuroImage* 16:142–157.

LEVINE, D. N., J. WARACH, and M. FARAH, 1985. Two visual systems in mental imagery: Dissociation of "what" and "where" in imagery disorders due to bilateral posterior cerebral lesions. *Neurology* 35:1010–1018.

MARR, D., 1982. *Vision: A Computational Investigation into the Human Representation and Processing of Visual Information.* San Francisco, Calif.: W.H. Freeman.

MAZARD, A., N. TZOURIO-MAZOYER, F. CRIVELLO, B. MAZOYER, and E. MELLET (in press). A PET meta-analysis of object and spatial mental imagery. *Eur. J. Cogn. Psychol.*

NG, V. W., E. T. BULLMORE, G. I. DE ZUBICARAY, A. COOPER, J. SUCKLING, and S. C. WILLIAMS, 2001. Identifying rate-limiting nodes in large-scale cortical networks for visuospatial processing: An illustration using fMRI. *J. Cogn. Neurosci.* 13:537–545.

O'CRAVEN, K. M., and N. KANWISHER, 2000. Mental imagery of faces and places activates corresponding stiimulus-specific brain regions. *J. Cogn. Neurosci.* 12:1013–1023.

OGDEN, J. A., 1993. Visual object agnosia, prosopagnosia, achromatopsia, loss of visual imagery, and autobiographical amnesia following recovery from cortical blindness: Case M.H. *Neuropsychologia* 31:571–589.

PAPAXANTHIS, C., M. SCHIEPPATI, R. GENTILI, and T. POZZO, 2002. Imagined and actual arm movements have similar durations when performed under different conditions of direction and mass. *Exp. Brain Res.* 143:447–452.

PARSONS, L. M., P. T. FOX, J. H. DOWNS, T. GLASS, T. B. HIRSCH, C. C. MARTIN, P. A. JERABEK, and J. L. LANCASTER, 1995. Use of implicit motor imagery for visual shape discrimination as revealed by PET. *Nature* 375:54–58.

PAUS, T., S. MARRETT, K. J. WORSLEY, and A. C. EVANS, 1995. Extraretinal modulation of cerebral blood flow in the human visual cortex: Implications for saccadic suppression. *J. Neurophysiol.* 74:2179–2183.

PYLYSHYN, Z., 1973. What the mind's eye tells the mind's brain: A critique of mental imagery. *Psychol. Bull.* 80:1–25.

PYLYSHYN, Z., 2002. Mental imagery: In search of a theory. *Behavi. Brain Sci.* 25:157–237.

RATCLIFF, G., 1979. Spatial thought, mental rotation, and the right cerebral hemisphere. *Neuropsychologia* 17:49–54.

RICHTER, W., R. SOMORJAI, R. SUMMERS, M. JARMASZ, R. S. MENON, J. S. GATI, A. P. GEORGOPOULOS, C. TEGELER, K. UGURBIL, and K. SEONG-GI, 2000. Motor area activity during mental rotation studied by time-resolved single-trial fMRI. *J. Cogn. Neurosci.* 12:310–320.

RICHTER, W., K. UGURBIL, A. GEORGOPOULOS, and S. G. KIM, 1997. Time-resolved fMRI of mental rotation. *Neuroreport* 8:3697–3702.

RIDDOCH, M. J., and G. W. HUMPHREYS, 1987. A case of integrative visual agnosia. *Brain* 110(Pt. 6):1431–1462.

RIZZO, M., and D. A. ROBIN, 1996. Bilateral effects of unilateral visual cortex lesions in human. *Brain* 119(Pt. 3):951–963.

SACKS, O., and R. WASSERMAN, 1987. The case of the color-blind painter. *New York Review of Books,* November 19, pp. 25–34.

SARTORI, G., and R. JOB, 1988. The oyster with four legs: A neuropsychological study on the interaction of visual and semantic information. *Cogn. Neuropsychol.* 5:105–132.

SERENO, M. I., A. DALE, J. B. REPPAS, K. K. KWONG, J. W. BELLIVEAU, T. J. BRADY, et al., 1995. Borders of multiple visual areas in humans revealed by functional magnetic resonance imaging. *Science* 268:889–893.

SERVOS, P., and M. A. GOODALE, 1995. Preserved visual imagery in visual form agnosia. *Neuropsychologia* 33:1383–1394.

SHEPARD, R. N., and J. METZLER, 1971. Mental rotation of three-dimensional objects. *Science* 171:701–703.

SHUTTLEWORTH, E. C., JR., V. SYRING, and N. ALLEN, 1982. Further observations on the nature of prosopagnosia. *Brain Cognit.* 1:307–322.

TOOTELL, R. B. H., N. K. HADJIKANI, J. D. MENDOLA, S. MARRETT, and A. M. DALE, 1998. From retinotopy to recognition: fMRI in human visual cortex. *Trends Cogn. Sci.* 2:174–183.

Tootell, R. B., M. S. Silverman, E. Switkes, and R. L. de Valois, 1982. Deoxyglucose analysis of retinotopic organization in primate striate cortex. *Science* 218:902–904.

Ungerleider, L. G., and M. Mishkin, 1982. Two cortical visual systems. In *The Analysis of Visual Behavior*, D. J. Ingle, M. A. Goodale, and R. J. W. Mansfield, eds. Cambridge, Mass.: MIT Press, pp. 549–586.

Wraga, M., W. L. Thompson, N. M. Alpert, and S. M. Kosslyn, 2003. Implicit transfer of motor strategies in mental rotation. *Brain Cogn.* 52:135–143.

Yáguëz, L., D. Nagel, H. Hoffman, A. G. M. Canavan, E. Wist, and V. Hömberg, 1998. A mental route to motor learning: Improving trajectorial kinematics through imagery training. *Behavi. Brain Res.* 90:95–106.

Yue, G., and K. J. Cole, 1992. Strength increases from the motor program: comparison of training with maximal voluntary and imagined muscle contractions. *J. Neurophysiol.* 67:1114–1423.

Zacks, J., B. Rypma, J. D. E. Gabrieli, B. Tversky, and G. H. Glover, 1999. Imagined transformations of bodies: An fMRI investigation. *Neuropsychologia* 37:1029–1040.

68 The Fractionation of Supervisory Control

TIM SHALLICE

ABSTRACT Three different frameworks for understanding the functions of different regions of prefrontal cortex—working memory, general intelligence, the Supervisory System approach—are compared. Three different lines of neuropsychological evidence are discussed with respect to the third of these frameworks. The contrasting functions of the human left and right dorsolateral prefrontal cortex are then considered. The left is held to be involved in top-down strategic modulation of lower-level systems while the right is considered to be more concerned with the control of checking that on-going behaviour accords with task goals. Finally, the functions of anterior prefrontal cortex are assessed; it is argued that they are concerned with changes in cognitive mode, particularly when that involves the realization of previously set-up intentions.

Approaches to prefrontal cortex

It is standard to view the prefrontal cortex as the seat of a high-level system (or systems) that receives input from more specific lower-level systems and that in turn modulates or controls the operation of the lower-level systems (e.g., Shallice, 1982; Goldman-Rakic, 1987). The prefrontal cortex is internally highly complex, with major functional differences between the lateral, orbital, and medial surfaces, along with increasing abstraction of function as one moves toward the frontal pole. Historically, however, the most deeply investigated region has been the dorsolateral region. The operation of these regions has been viewed within a number of different conceptual frameworks. This chapter considers these various frameworks.

THE WORKING MEMORY APPROACH The best-known framework is the working memory framework, which stemmed initially from Jacobsen's (1935) findings of a delayed response deficit in monkeys with frontal lobe lesions. The working memory framework became the dominant conceptual framework when it was shown with single-cell recordings that many units in dorsolateral prefrontal cortex (DLPFC) remained active during the delay (e.g., Fuster and Alexander, 1971). This approach was broadened by Goldman-Rakic (1987), who argued that a more dorsal area

around sulcus principalis is the seat of spatial working memory, but a more inferior area on the lateral surface holds working memories for the identity of stimuli.

Which operations related to working memory might be affected by prefrontal lesions? First, it should be noted that in the delayed response tasks, a deficit occurs with only one spatial position having to be held. Yet the capacity for spatial span—the ability to reproduce without delay a string of spatial positions by pointing—is about six positions in humans, and dramatic loss of capacity is typically found following right parietal lesions in humans (De Renzi and Nichelli, 1975). Indeed, patients with prefrontal lesions often are not impaired on spatial span tasks. Thus, patients with prefrontal lesions in a study reported by Owen and colleagues (1990) were impaired when spatial information had to be used in a more complex way, but they were unimpaired on spatial span per se. Therefore, damage to DLPFC lesions does not appear to impair the short-term spatial memory store. Possibly it affects the maintenance of spatial attention.

The situation is similar for verbal span. Rypma and D'Esposito (1999) found that on a verbal span task, activation of DLPFC became greater only when six items rather than two were being processed while the information was encoded, and load had no effect during the delay period. Instead, changes in memory load affected activation of parietal cortex during the delay. Moreover, patients with highly selective impairments of verbal span are typically found to have left parietotemporal lesions (Warrington and Shallice, 1969; Shallice and Vallar, 1990). Thus, the processing carried out in DLPFC would seem to be primarily concerned with activities other than the mere retention of information in working memory, which is the responsibility of parietotemporal cortex.

A dramatic demonstration that area 9/46 is involved in operations rather than storage per se can be found in the neuroimaging study reported by Rowe and colleagues (2000) (figure 68.1). In this study, maintenance of information in working memory was associated with bilateral activation of Brodmann's area (BA) 8 and of the parietal cortex. The critical mid-dorsolateral area (area 9/46) was activated only when the information being held in working memory was

TIM SHALLICE Institute of Cognitive Neuroscience, University College London, London, U.K.

943

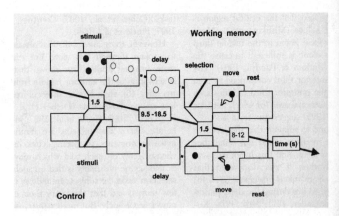

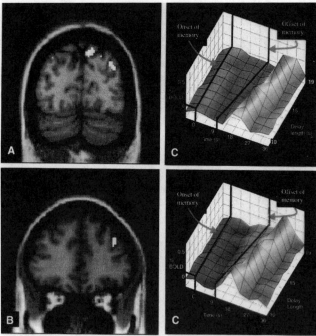

FIGURE 68.1 In a study reported by Rowe and colleagues (2000), subjects had to hold in working memory the position of three dots for a variable length of time. At the end of the delay interval, a line that went through only one of the dots came on. The subjects had to point to where on the line there had been a dot. Area 9/46 activation was associated with the offset operation (*B*) and not with the maintenance of information over the delay (*A*). *C* illustrates when during the time-course at the trial (*x*-axis) activation (*z*-axis) occured for trial of different length (*y*-axis). (See color plate 47.)

used to effect the response. Thus, DLPFC appears to be involved in cognitive operations rather than storage.

DORSOLATERAL PREFRONTAL CORTEX AS THE SEAT OF 'G'   A second conceptual framework holds that the critical function being effected by DLPFC is linked to working memory but also holds that it has a much more complex content than have the buffers being used to store spatial information. Duncan and colleagues (2000) have argued that the lateral prefrontal cortex contains highly adaptive cells that form the seat of general intelligence, designated *g*. They introduced three main lines of evidence. First, many of the cells in this region adapt their triggering features very flexibly to the specific task (Duncan and Miller, 2002). Second, Duncan and Owen (2000) performed a meta-analysis of functional imaging studies each of which examined a single variable related to the following factors: task novelty, response competition, working memory load, working memory delay, and perceptual difficulty. They compared activations for all pairs of conditions that differed on only one of the dimensions; for instance, a condition with response competition was contrasted to one without it but that was otherwise identical. They found that in regard to anterior structures, the maxima all lay in the anterior cingulate cortex and in a swathe down the two lateral prefrontal cortices. More specifically, this second set of maxima was thought to be clustered around the middle and posterior part of the inferior frontal sulcus

(IFS) and more ventrally along the frontal operculum. Critically, however, the five different types of contrast did not localize differentially within these regions. The areas of activation all overlapped. The third line of evidence came from a functional imaging experiment that contrasted three types of task that loaded heavily on *g* but otherwise had no apparent structural (i.e., lower-level processes) in common. All were odd-one-out tests. However, one was of shapes, the second was of relations between letters in a string, and the third involved spatial relations. When each of the three was compared with a structurally similar task that loaded much less on *g*, they all significantly activated the lateral prefrontal cortex (figure 68.2).

Duncan (2001) has drawn an analogy between the functional role of this region and the working memory of a production system model called SOAR (Newell, 1990). Production systems are artificial intelligence systems that have operations based on productions. These are condition-action pairs: when the conditions of a production are satisfied by perceptual representations or representations currently in working memory, then an action occurs, which can be an output or a new input to working memory. SOAR is one of the two symbolic models that have been most used to simulate in detail a wide range of cognitive processes. Its working memory contains elements that represent states of the environment, elements that correspond to its goals at various different levels, and elements that correspond to the

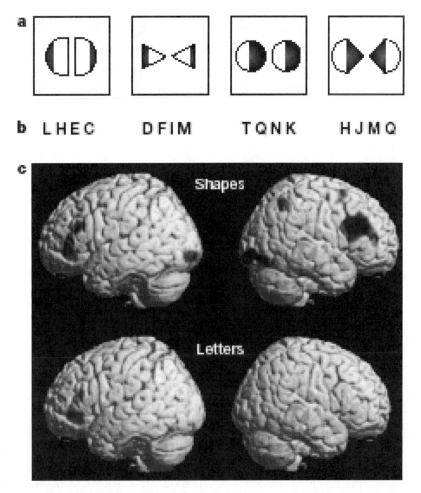

FIGURE 68.2   Demonstration by Duncan and colleagues (2000) of an association of DLPFC activation with general intelligence (*g*) processes. (*a–c*) The activation differences between carrying out the IQ tasks, compared with performing cognitively undemanding control tasks using similar stimuli. The three tasks involved shapes, letters, and spatial relations. (See color plate 48.)

working memory outputs of previously executed productions. Thus, this approach can be related to the previous one, but it greatly broadens the concept of what the contents of the active working memory contain.

Duncan's approach makes two strong challenges. First, in principle, it allows one to characterize how much individual tasks would require a higher-level system, in that one could specify how much demand they would make on SOAR's working memory. Second, and much more controversially, it views the lateral prefrontal cortex as having a unitary function, if a very broad and abstract one.

THE SUPERVISORY SYSTEM APPROACH   Although the SOAR analogy could in principle be used to assess how much individual tasks require a high-level control system, in practice SOAR has proved to be an inadequate model of human cognition (Cooper and Shallice, 1995). Computationally, the most interesting aspect of SOAR, and what made it superior to earlier symbolic models of cognition, is that it makes a basic division between situations in which appropriate

actions can be routinely carried out and those in which the system cannot initially "decide" what to do, where it confronts an impasse. The system then uses special procedures to deal with the impasse and produce a plausible approach.

The third approach to lateral prefrontal (and also frontal pole) function makes qualitatively the same distinction, but the model is tailored to the specific requirements of a biological processor that modulates a variety of lower-level systems. This model views the prefrontal cortex as containing a Supervisory System that modulates a lower-level system of action and thought selection—known as contention scheduling (Norman and Shallice, 1986; Shallice and Burgess, 1996; figure 68.3). The basic functional division between Supervisory and non-Supervisory Systems echoes that in SOAR: contention scheduling implements routine actions. However, the successful carrying out of nonroutine actions is held to require the additional use of the Supervisory System. As with the SOAR framework, contention scheduling was also proposed to operate analogously to a production system. Production systems are placed in a

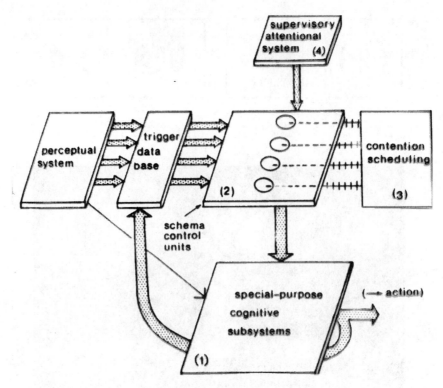

FIGURE 68.3   The original version of the Supervisory System model.

quandary when more than one production has its conditions satisfied at the same time. If all are executed, they may conflict with each other or remove each other's preconditions for selection. SOAR's impasse procedure is one way of dealing with the problem. In contention scheduling, a selection is made of which production (in our terminology, schema) will control the special-purpose processing systems it requires. This is based on McDermott and Forgy's (1978) approach to conflict resolution. Each schema has a salience measure, activation, and there is mutually inhibitory competition to determine which schema achieves an activation level that exceeds the selection threshold (see Cooper and Shallice, 2000, for an implemetation). This schema then operates by utilizing the processing subsystems it requires. This has similarities to the operation of the basal ganglia (see Gurney, Prescott, and Redgrave, 2001).

Evidence for the Supervisory System approach   Many different types of evidence support the idea that prefrontal cortex is involved in nonroutine as opposed to routine operations. These various lines of evidence include animal studies (e.g., Butter, 1964), neuropsychological studies (e.g., Shallice and Evans, 1978), electrophysiological studies (e.g., Knight, 1984), and functional imaging studies (e.g., Raichle et al., 1994; Jueptner et al., 1997).

More specifically, in the model, damage to the Supervisory System in prefrontal cortex leads to behavior controlled by contention scheduling. Behavior should then inevitably

be controlled by the schema that perceptual or working memory triggers, operating in an overlearned fashion, lead to be the strongest activated. Here we can consider three examples; the first two come from studies of neurological patients.

Della Malva and colleagues (1993) showed patients a series of cards that were either pictures (in one experiment) or words (in another). The cards told a story or made up a sentence, but were presented in a mixed-up order. Participants were asked to put the cards in order. There were two key conditions. In one, the original sequences contained a "capturing pair" of items in which two pictures (or words) appeared strongly associated but in fact represented very different stages of the story. Control subjects and patients with posterior lesions solved the two types of sequence equally well. By contrast, patients with anterior lesions were 15% worse if they had to overcome a capturing pair. The capturing pair triggers an overlearned thought schema in contention scheduling. It cannot be inhibited when the Supervisory System is damaged.

A more dramatic example was provided by Verin and colleagues (1993). Subjects were presented with two squares on a screen and had to guess which was correct. After the subject had guessed, the squares disappeared. At 15 s later, the squares reappeared, the subject guessed again, and so on. Which response was correct was dictated by a simple alternating sequence. Control subjects made an average of more than three errors before a sequence of ten correct responses. Patients with frontal lesions, however, made on average only 0.1 errors. They alternated spontaneously from trial 1. This can be explained if in contention scheduling the "move to nonrepeated target" is the dominant schema. This is plausible, as evinced by 6-year-old children showing the same behavior. It is unclear how a working memory or *g* account can explain this finding.

The third example used transanial magnetic stimulation (TMS). In a study reported by Jahanshahi and colleagues (1998), subjects attempted to generate a random string of single digits. As Baddeley (1986) showed, to produce a random string of numbers, subjects must inhibit the currently activated cognitive schema after each digit is produced. An unrelated schema must then be activated to produce the next digit. In the current framework, this process would require the inhibition of perceptual or memory triggers, and would therefore require a Supervisory System. Baddeley asked subjects to produce digits in time to the beat of a metronome. He showed that the degree of randomness declined as the rate of digit production increased. At the speed used by Jahanshahi and colleagues of one digit every 1.2 s, subjects frequently use the schemas of counting upward or downward in ones, the most routine procedure, or in twos, a somewhat less routine procedure. TMS over the left DLPFC increased the incidence of the most routine response, counting in ones, and decreased the rate of counting up or down in twos.

The internal organization of a Supervisory System

Three different lines of ideas support the view that higher-level modulating systems are not internally equipotential, as the *g* account claims. First, post-SOAR artificial intelligence systems that operate in nonroutine situations can require not just an all-purpose working memory in addition to productions, but a number of computationally quite distinct high-level processes (see Fox and Das, 2000).

Second, from the perspective of classical neurobiology, Petrides (1994) has argued that we need to distinguish between the functions of the ventrolateral prefrontal cortex (VLPFC) and DLPFC, but in a different way from Goldman-Rakic. VLPFC is held by Petrides to be involved in "active maintenance" operations, with the dorsolateral region being involved in "manipulation" operations. A series of experiments on spatial and verbal working memory using both PET and fMRI (see, e.g., Owen et al., 1999) have provided support for Petrides's position.

Third, functional imaging evidence now suggests that there is a set of distinct regions with putatively different cognitive functions in the lateral and anterior parts of prefrontal cortex. The evidence comes from a somewhat surprising source. Since the mid-1990s, some of the most frequently used functional imaging paradigms that give rise to pre-

frontal activations have been those involving episodic memory. It has been found that many different regions are activated in a large variety of different combinations according to the specific paradigm. Thus, Henson, Shallice, and Dolan (1999) and Rugg, Henson, and Robb (2003) consider the following regions to have different functional roles, or at least to be differently activated in a fairly consistent pattern across different type of episodic memory paradigm: left anterior, right anterior, and, in particular, left and right dorsolateral and left and right frontal operculum—both of which pairs appear to have different functions in the two hemispheres (see also Lepage et al., 2000; Fletcher and Henson, 2001).

Amnesic deficits do not occur following lesions to the frontal lobe, except most typically in the context of aneurysms of the anterior communicating artery on their posterior inferior medial surface, and most plausibly when the lesion involves the basal forebrain, which is a key structure for the cholinergic input to the hippocampus (Damasio et al., 1985). Lesions of the lateral surface do not generally give rise to problems of core memory processing. However, many episodic memory experiments require the subject to carry out, in addition to core memory operations, a series of other cognitive processes that tend to be similar for each test stimulus in a given condition. For instance, in a "source memory" experiment in which the subject must attempt to decide whether a test recognition stimulus that occurred earlier did so in the same or a somewhat different setting, complex cognitive operations as well as memory operations occur. Thus, it is plausible that most of the prefrontal regions activated realize different cognitive operations rather than specifically memory operations.

A first attempt to specify what the internal organization of a Supervisory System might be was made by Shallice and Burgess (1996; figure 68.4). A basic assumption of the model is that a key process in coping with a nonroutine situation is to develop and apply what would be termed phenomenologically an appropriate strategy. In terms of the model, a strategy corresponds to the operation of a schema (or set of schemas) in contention scheduling, which is activated above threshold only as a result of top-down output from the Supervisory System.

Lateralized dorsolateral functions

STRATEGY PRODUCTION AND EXECUTION The basic set of ideas can be applied to the cognitive processes involved in episodic memory experiments. Thus, it has been known for many years that the optimum strategy for retaining a list containing related items is to produce an abstract structure that ties the items into a structured whole (Mandler, 1967). Participants standardly reorder the input items for rehearsal into subcategories when a list that contains them is presented in

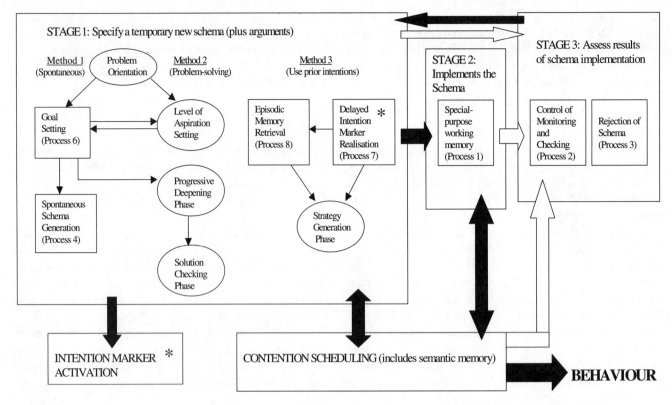

STAGE 1: Specify a temporary new schema (plus arguments)

Method 1 (Spontaneous)   Problem Orientation   Method 2 (Problem-solving)

Method 3 (Use prior intentions)

STAGE 2: Implements the Schema

STAGE 3: Assess results of schema implementation

Goal Setting (Process 6)

Level of Aspiration Setting

Episodic Memory Retrieval (Process 8)

Delayed Intention Marker Realisation (Process 7) *

Special-purpose working memory (Process 1)

Control of Monitoring and Checking (Process 2)

Rejection of Schema (Process 3)

Spontaneous Schema Generation (Process 4)

Progressive Deepening Phase

Strategy Generation Phase

Solution Checking Phase

INTENTION MARKER * ACTIVATION

CONTENTION SCHEDULING (includes semantic memory)

BEHAVIOUR

FIGURE 68.4   The Supervisory System component of the Mark II Supervisory System model of Shallice and Burgess (1996).

random order. Our group (Fletcher, Shallice, and Dolan, 1998) presented subjects auditorily with sets of 16 words each for 32 s. In each list, four words were drawn from each of four subcategories of the same broad semantic domain (e.g., for the domain food, there were four different meats, four kinds of fish, four breads, and four fruits). Subjects were given the sets of words in three different ways. The presentation order of the words could either be with each subcategory occurring in a block (procedure 1) or in one of two forms of random sequence, either with prior knowledge of what the subcategories are (procedure 2) or with no knowledge of it (procedure 3). In addition, we followed the argument of Moscovitch (1994) that a demanding secondary task would impair frontal executive processes, which was directly supported in an earlier study (Shallice et al., 1994). Thus, at the same time as listening to the lists, participants had to carry out a sensorimotor task involving moving a joystick to an indicated position. This involved otherwise identical input and output processes unrelated to those used in the memory encoding task. Two forms of this task differed in how easy it was for subjects to anticipate the next stimulus. In one case the sensorimotor task was completely predictable and in the other case it was random. The two sensorimotor task conditions were combined factorially with the three methods of list presentation to give six conditions in all.

Subjects underwent positron emission tomography (PET) as they encoded the lists. Later they were tested on how well

they remembered them. The lists were equally well remembered in all conditions but one, in which the list structure was random and subjects were given no prior information as to the subcategories (procedure 3) *and* subjects had the demanding rather than the easy secondary task. In this condition, subjects recalled significantly less. Moreover, their recall was less well organized into categories. Subjects were not able to effectively use the strategy of organizing the words in the list into the four subcategories.

In only one region did the level of activation show a critical interaction of the secondary task with the list presentation procedure. This was a left dorsolateral area just above the IFS. There was a large effect of difficulty of distraction on the degree of activation in this region for procedure 3 but not for the other two procedures, mirroring its effect on the ability to produce a satisfactory organization for the list (figure 68.5). Thus, the creation and/or use of an appropriate strategy in the situation appeared to depend on a specific region of the left lateral prefrontal cortex. It might be objected that what was impaired in the critical condition was the ability to abstract, and not the ability to produce a strategy. But producing a strategy typically requires a participant to abstract over aspects of the situations where action has previously not been sufficiently successful. I will assume the two processes involve the same structures.

Reverting to a nonmemory domain, this result is analogous to the very different study of Jahanshahi and col-

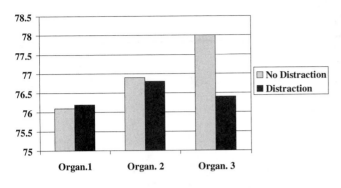
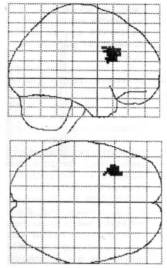
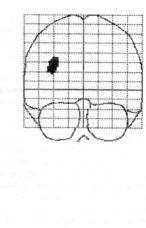

FIGURE 68.5 Activations of a region of left DLPFC during the three different conditions of the memory organization study reported by Fletcher, Shallice, and Dolan (1998). (See color plate 49.)

leagues, in which it was only TMS of the left DLPFC that led to a greater relapse into routine behavior, and therefore left DLPFC could be presumed to be the region required in top-down activation of other schemas (for related ideas, see Frith, 2000; Braver, Cohen, and Barch, 2002). TMS of the right DLPFC did not produce an equivalent effect. fMRI findings led to a similar conclusion, namely, that the left dorsolateral region was the most critical area (Jahanshahi et al., 2000).

CHECKING STRATEGY EXECUTION IN NONROUTINE SITUATIONS An obvious objection to the claim that there is a degree of lateralization in the top-down modulation functions of prefrontal cortex is that in these experiments, lateralization occurs simply because of the material used. However, the right DLPFC has been selectively activated using the same material in other memory situations. For instance, one such study (Fletcher, Shallice, Frith, et al., 1998) was a complement to the encoding study just discussed. This study involved retrieving organized lists of words. Five minutes before scanning in the experimental, so-called internally cued condition, subjects were presented with an organized list, which, as in the previous study, contained four items each from four related subcategories. During PET, subjects received the stimulus "next" every 4 s and had to attempt to recall another word from the list. In the control, externally cued condition, there were 16 much more specific categories in each list, each with a different cue (e.g., for *nan*, the cue was *Indian bread*). A different cue was presented every 4 s at retrieval. In addition, two word repetition tasks acted as control tasks, one for each of the types of retrieval cue used in the two retrieval conditions. When results were compared with results on the corresponding repetition control condi-

tions, both retrieval tasks gave rise to significantly greater activation in a large region of the right frontal cortex. In complete contrast to the organization-at-encoding task, there were no effects in *left* prefrontal cortex.

This left-right contrast reflects the Hemisphere Encoding and Retrieval Asymmetry generalization of Tulving, Kapur, and Craik (1994) (see Cabeza and Nyberg, 2000; Lepage et al., 2000; Fletcher and Henson, 2001). However, in addition, there was an unexpected double dissociation in the activation produced within the right prefrontal cortex. In right DLPFC, internally cued recall gave rise to significantly greater activation than externally cued recall. By contrast, in the posterior ventral prefrontal cortex there was significantly greater activation in the externally cued condition, which involved paired associate recall (figure 68.6).

Neuropsychological evidence exists concerning the failure of the relevant process. Stuss and colleagues (1994) gave subjects lists of the same length as in our study—16 words—to remember. Indeed, some lists contained four subcategories, as in our procedure. The task was free recall. A group of patients with right prefrontal lesions and a second group of patients with left frontal lesions were compared with normal control subjects. Patients with left frontal lesions performed worse than the others on free recall. However, it was the result in the patients with right frontal lesions that was particularly relevant. This group, but not patients with left lesions, produced a significantly larger number of repeated items on the free recall protocols, more than double the rate of controls.

Why might these effects be associated with the right DLPFC? When dealing with novel situations, it is necessary to continuously check the appropriateness of the behavior to be produced. We therefore proposed that the process

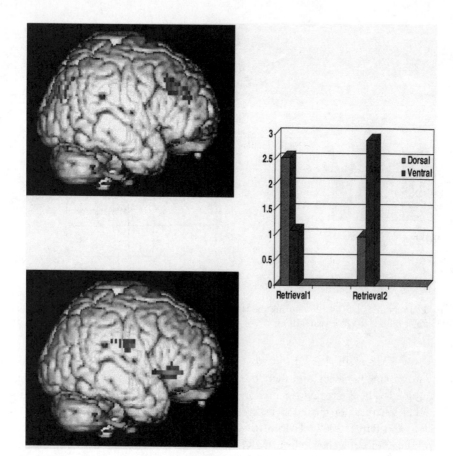

FIGURE 68.6 Activations of the right DLPFC and the right insula/VLPFC during the two critical conditions of the study reported by Fletcher, Shallice, Frith, and colleagues (1998), namely, organized list recall (retrieval 1) and paired associate recall (retrieval 2). Each was compared with its own control task, which involved only repetition. (See color plate 50.)

damaged in the patients with right frontal lesions studied by Stuss and colleagues (1994) comes into play when checking or monitoring operations are required. Such processes are much more necessary when retrieving a structured list than when retrieving single words. This is especially the case because the single words cannot be potentially confused with any other words being recalled, as they are known to be members of the specific category indicated by the cue words and the category is not repeated across the experiment.

Since then our group has completed a number of memory experiments involving contrasts between conditions in which different degrees of checking would be expected. In some cases, as in the study reported by Fletcher and colleagues, the right but not the left DLPFC was activated in the critical contrast where more checking was required. This occurred in a study of Henson, Rugg, and colleagues (1999) in which subjects had to rate for each word they remembered in a word recognition task whether they could clearly "recollect" the word being presented earlier or just "knew" it had occurred but had no specific memory. The latter condition is slower and would typically require a further check that fails. A similar result also occurred when the correct response had to be distinguished from competing similar

alternatives (Henson et al., 2002). In these cases, only the right DLPFC was activated in the critical contrast.

However, in other studies (e.g., Henson, Shallice, and Dolan, 1999: Henson et al., 2000) the left DLPFC was also significantly activated relative to a control baseline. Typical of these studies was the study of Henson, Shallice, and Dolan (1999), which used a so-called source memory paradigm derived from Jacoby (1996). Participants had to determine whether a previously presented item was in exactly the same setting as when it had occurred before. No responses had to be given to items that had occurred but in a slightly different setting; they were excluded. This condition was contrasted with one in which subjects had only to decide whether or not each item had occurred before—an inclusion decision. The former condition obviously requires more checking. The study used a blocked analysis procedure, standard in early functional imaging experiments. However, the results have been essentially replicated by Rugg, Henson, and Robb (2003), in a study that used an event-related design.

In the study by Henson and colleagues, both DLPFCs were activated in the exclusion retrieval condition. However, the right DLPFC region activated was much larger than the

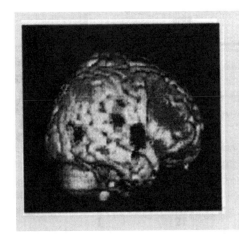

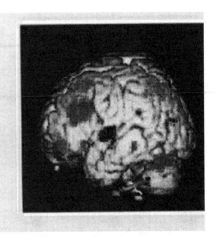

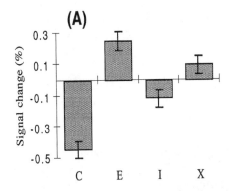

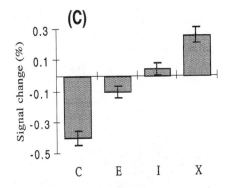

FIGURE 68.7   Activations in the exclusion condition of the source memory study reported by Henson, Shallice, and Dolan (1999) (top) and of a left and right DLPFC voxel in each of the four con-ditions of the study. Abbreviations: E, encoding; X, exclusion retrieval; I, inclusion retrieval; C, control. (See color plate 51.)

left. Moreover, the pattern of activation across conditions for the two DLPFCs was subtly different (figure 68.7). The right DLPFC was much more activated by retrieval processes requiring checking (exclusion) than by encoding. A very different pattern was found in left DLPFC. Thus the balance between the top-down process required at encoding and the checking process required at retrieval is quite different between the two regions. Even when both dorsolateral regions are activated by processes requiring checking, the right region tends to be activated more.

In a memory experiment, alternative explanations are difficult to reject because we do not have a componential analysis of all the subprocesses involved. For instance, could activation of the right DLPFC merely indicate the degree of effort being made at retrieval? Early EEG studies by Wilding and Rugg (1996) showed that there is a right frontal wave at retrieval that occurs very late; it does not begin until at least 1400 ms after stimulus, which clearly favors a checking account.

More conclusive, however, is that right DLPFC effects occur in paradigms with no relation to memory. For example, Posner and Petersen (1990) argued that right

DLPFC was involved in vigilance operations. Another example, from the language domain, is provided by the study of Sharp, Scott, and Wise (2003). Participants in that study had to make semantic or syllabic decisions about words presented either normally or phonologically degraded. The use of phonologically degraded stimuli led to decreased accuracy, especially for the semantic task, which would lead to greater checking. Increased activation of right DLPFC regions occurred even though the stimuli were verbal.

NEUROPSYCHOLOGICAL EVIDENCE   Easier to analyze than functional imaging experiments are neuropsychological ones. If a set of isolable subsystems is involved, then a full componential analysis of the tasks employed is less necessary than for functional imaging, particularly for the processes not affected by the lesion. Moreover, experimenters can be helped by the nature of the errors made. Thus, Reverberi and colleagues (2002) looked at what effects frontal lesions might have on acquisition of a rule. The patients saw a series of cards, each containing 10 circles in a 2 × 5 array. One circle was blue, and it moved from card to card in a prede-termined fashion according to a rule that changed every five to nine cards. Patients had to guess where on the next card the blue circle would be. Burgess and Shallice (1996) had already shown that patients with frontal lesions were impaired on this task. However to contrast rule attainment with a situation involving checking, an analogous set of cards, each with a red rather than blue circle, was introduced into each rule near the end of the sequence. The red circles moved according to a different rule. Subjects were told they only had to touch the red circle on each card, but as soon as the blue cards returned they were to resume obeying the "blue card rule."

Patients with left lateral lesions were very poor at acquiring the rule. By contrast, those with right lateral lesions were completely normal at acquiring the blue card rules. However, their rate of "capture errors" on returning to the blue cards was three times that of normal controls. They continued obeying the red card rule when the blue card rule should have been followed. They failed to check that the rule most activated implicitly was the correct one.

This section has reviewed in some detail studies identifying activation in DLPFC regions to show that as with parietal regions, there may be strong lateralization effects on functions, such as strategy production and checking/ monitoring, that are not related to language per se. However, earlier it was argued that there are at least five different prefrontal regions with different cognitive functions involved in episodic memory paradigm. The next section therefore briefly considers the more anterior regions.

Anterior prefrontal systems

Classically, in single-cell recording studies, much more attention has been paid to dorsolateral and ventrolateral regions of prefrontal cortex than to the frontal polar regions. With functional imaging, however, activations have been increasingly recorded in the frontopolar region, or BA 10. In a recent meta-analysis, Christoff and Gabrieli (2000) found that during reasoning tasks frontopolar activation occurred at least as frequently as dorsolateral activation. However, activation of this area also occurred on a variety of other tasks, such as ones requiring subjects to create an order over a set of items, with each being selected just once, on certain working memory tasks, on tasks requiring information about the self, on episodic memory retrieval, and on a few others.

A general characteristic of these tasks is their complexity, and consequently it is very rare to have an adequate componential analysis of the task. When we lack a componential analysis of tasks, then neuropsychological findings, particularly strong dissociations, provide a much easier basis for initial analysis. However, few neuropsychological studies compare the effect of lesions of frontal polar regions with the effect of lesions of other areas of prefrontal cortex.

There is, however, an exception. Eslinger and Damasio (1985) described patient E.V.R. who had intact performance on cognitive tests of prefrontal function but was incapable of organizing himself over time in everyday life situations. E.V.R. became the starting point for Damasio's (1996) "somatic marker" theory, which he linked to the orbital prefrontal damage incurred by the patient. However, Shallice and Burgess (1991) produced an alternative account. They described three patients with frontal lobe damage who exhibited a similar dissociation between intact performance on standard cognitive tasks sensitive to frontal lobe damage and disordered performance on everyday life tasks. These three patients, however, all failed at one particular type of cognitive task: a task that involved the carrying out of multiple subtasks during which the patient had to follow a small set of simple rules. The subtasks had no relation to each other, and no cue was available as to when a participant had to switch from one subtask to another. The three patients tended to fixate on one of the tasks. It appeared that the need to carry out other tasks did not lead to interruption of ongoing behavior, as in normal subjects. Shallice and Burgess (1991) argued that their patients had lost the ability to set up or realize "intentional markers" that affect the need to alter behavior at some stage in the future according to one-off current requirements.

The best localized of the lesions in the three patients was bilateral and affected the frontopolar regions, BA 10 and 11 (figure 68.8). A later group study used a task working on similar principles with three unrelated subtasks. Patients with left anterior prefrontal lesions had no difficulty learning the task rules, remembering them, developing an appropriate strategy, or remembering what they had done when asked. However, such patients scored very poorly on the test as a whole. They did not switch sufficiently and broke task rules, both of which require setting up specifications for control of behavior at some time later. In an attempt to isolate the "intentional marker" component more formally in an imaging situation, Burgess, Quayle, and Frith (2001) asked subjects to carry out tasks of two types. One type was an "ongoing task," which subjects had to carry out for roughly 30 stimuli. In one condition this was the only type of task subjects had to perform. However, in two conditions subjects were instructed they had another task, an "intention" task, to carry out. In one condition, intention maintenance, the intention task was never realized. In another condition, intention realization, it became relevant about once every six stimuli.

The study utilized four different ongoing and intention tasks involving different lower-level cognitive domains (figure 68.9). The results were based on conjunction analyses over the four basic sets of tasks. Realization of an intention by comparison with its maintenance activated the right thalamus and right DLPFC, possibly suggesting successful moni-

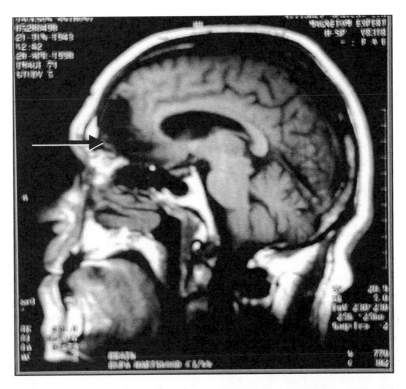

FIGURE 68.8   The lesion of patient A.P. of Shallice and Burgess (1991) with a severe impairment of "intention marker" realization. The lesion affects BA 10 and 11 bilaterally. (See color plate 52.)

toring. Maintenance of an intention by comparison with carrying out the ongoing task by itself also activated the right dorsolateral prefrontal region, but also, critically, the left and right frontal pole.

The region activated in this comparison, especially the left prefrontal region (−30, 62, −6), was in a virtually identical position to that found in another study of Koechlin and colleagues (1999; −36, 57, 9) and was similar to ones in related studies of Okuda and colleagues (1998) and Burgess, Scott, and Frith (2003). In the critical condition in the study reported by Koechlin and colleagues, subjects also had to do two tasks. Presented with a study of letters such as *A, B, L, t, e, a*, they had to decide whether successively presented letters were also in immediate succession in the word *tablet*. However, they, too, had a second task, which applied only when there was a change from uppercase to lowercase letters. Then subjects had to decide whether the letter was a *t*.

Koechin and colleagues called their critical condition "branching," emphasizing a need to return to a main task after carrying out a subroutine. Burgess and colleagues preferred the more general notion of anticipatory processing of McCarthy and Warrington (1990) and linked it to the old *Gestalt* views of Lewin and Zeigarnick regarding "goal tension," which would be the processing basis of holding and realizing an intention. In the model presented earlier (see figure 68.4), these views would correspond to the delayed intention realization process.

Conclusions

In the perspective presented in this chapter, control of nonroutine behavior involves a variety of different types of subsystem, each with abstract specifications. At the lowest supervisory level, Petrides's understanding of ventrolateral cortex as concerned with maintenance of ongoing operations can be developed. It has been suggested to hold the process of posing specific top-down requirements for particular lower-level systems such as language processing, short-term memory, or episodic memory (see, e.g., Henson, Shallice, and Dolan, 1999). Damage would lead to specific impairments, such as dynamic aphasia or rare forms of amnesia. These impairments have not been considered in this chapter.

At the next higher level would be dorsolateral structures. For these, the subject's task and immediate goals are well-defined and are the dominant motivational influences on cognition in the immediately preceding few-second period. What is required is a strategy to implement the task, and to check that the behavior that follows satisfies the task goals. It has been argued that in the human brain, the systems responsible for these processes are relatively lateralized to the left and right, respectively, at least for verbal and symbolic processing.

At the next higher level are situations where the cognitive mode needs to change or where the task and its goals, while abstractly active, have not been controlling behavior in the preceding few seconds. The goal structure currently con-

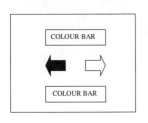

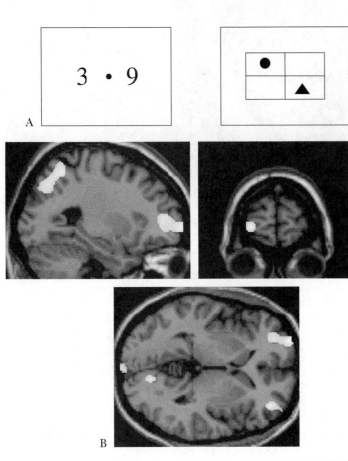

FIGURE 68.9 (*A*) Stimuli used by Burgess, Quayle, and Frith (2001) in their study of maintenance and realization of intentions for convolution of the critical maintenance of intention condition compared with the ongoing task, across the four different types of ongoing task. (*B*) Activation sites. (See color plate 53.)

trolling immediate behavior needs to be interrupted, and a new set of goals, possibly prefigured by previously produced intentions, needs to be brought into play. This, it is suggested, is the role of the anterior prefrontal cortex. The different subprocesses, however, are not independent processes. Collectively they form a supervisory system for coping with nonroutine situations by top-down modulation of systems implementing the routine.

REFERENCES

BADDELEY, A. D., 1986. *Working Memory*. Oxford, England: Oxford University Press.

BRAVER, T. S., J. D. COHEN, and D. M. BARCH, 2002. The role of prefrontal cortex in normal and disordered cognitive control: A cognitive neuroscience perspective. In *Frontal Lobe Function*, D. Stuss and R. T. Knight, eds. Oxford, England: Oxford University Press, pp. 428–447.

BURGESS, P., A. QUAYLE, and C. D. FRITH, 2001. Brain regions involved in prospective memory as determined by positron emission tomography. *Neuropsychologia* 39:545–555.

BURGESS, P. W., S. K. SCOTT, and C. D. FRITH, 2003. The role of rostral frontal cortex (area 10) in prospective memory: A lateral versus medial dissociation. *Neuropsychologia* 41:906–916.

BURGESS, P., and T. SHALLICE, 1996. Bizarre responses, rule detection and frontal lobe lesions. *Cortex* 32:241–260.

BUTTER, C. M., 1964. Habituation to novel stimuli in monkeys with selective frontal lesions. *Science* 144:313–315.

CABEZA, R., and L. NYBERG, 2000. Imaging cognition. II. An empirical review of 275 PET and fMRI studies. *J. Cogn. Neurosci.* 12:1–47.

CHRISTOFF, K., and J. D. E. GABRIELI, 2000. The frontopolar cortex and human cognition: Evidence from a rostrocaudal hierarchical organisation within the human prefrontal cortex. *Psychobiology* 28:168–186.

COOPER, R., and T. SHALLICE, 1995. SOAR and the case for unified theories of cognition. *Cognition* 55:115–149.

COOPER, R., and T. SHALLICE, 2000. Contention scheduling and the control of routine activities. *Cogn. Neuropsychol.* 17:297–338.

DAMASIO, A. R., 1996. The somatic marker hypothesis and the possible functions of the prefrontal cortex. *Philos. Trans. R. Soc. Series B* 351:1413–1420.

DAMASIO, A. R., N. R. GRAFF-RADFORD, P. J. ESLINGER, H. DAMASIO, and R. KAWASHIMA, 1985. Amnesia following basal forebrain lesions. *Arch. Neurol.* 42:263–271.

DE RENZI, E., and P. NICHELLI, 1975. Verbal and non-verbal short-term memory impairment following hemispheric damage. *Cortex* 11:341–354.

DELLA MALVA, C. L., D. T. STUSS, J. D'ALTON, and J. WILLMER, 1993. Capture errors and sequencing after frontal brain lesions. *Neuropsychologia* 31:363–372.

D'ESPOSITO, M., G. K. AGUIRRE, E. ZARAHN, and D. BALLARD, 1998. Functional MRI studies of spatial and non-spatial working memory. *Cogn. Brain Res.* 7:1–13.

DUNCAN, J., 2001. An adaptive coding model of neural function in prefrontal cortex. *Nat. Rev. Neurosci.* 2:820–829.

DUNCAN, J., and E. K. MILLER, 2002. Cognitive focus through adaptive neural coding in the primate prefrontal cortex. In *Principles of Frontal Lobe Function*, J. Duncan and E. K. Miller, eds. New York: Oxford University Press, pp. 278–291.

DUNCAN, J., and A. M. OWEN, 2000. Common regions of the human frontal lobe recruited by diverse cognitive demands. *Trends Neurosci.* 23:475–483.

DUNCAN, J., R. J. SEITZ, J. KOLODNY, D. BOR, H. HERZOG, A. AHMED, F. N. NEWELL, and H. EMSLIE, 2000. A neural basis for general intelligence. *Science* 289:457–460.

ESLINGER, P. J., and A. R. DAMASIO, 1985. Severe disturbance of higher cognition after bilateral frontal lobe ablation: Patient EVR. *Neurology* 35:1731–1741.

FLETCHER, P., and R. N. A. HENSON, 2001. Frontal lobes and human memory: Insights from functional imaging. *Brain* 124:849–881.

FLETCHER, P. C., T. SHALLICE, and R. J. DOLAN, 1998. The functional roles of prefrontal cortex in episodic memory. I. Encoding. *Brain* 121:1239–1248.

FLETCHER, P. C., T. SHALLICE, C. D. FRITH, R. S. J. FRACKOWIAK, and R. J. DOLAN, 1998. The functional roles of prefrontal cortex in episodic memory. II. Retrieval. *Brain* 121:1249–1256.

FOX, J., and S. K. DAS, 2000. *Safe and Sound: Artificial Intelligence in Hazardous Applications.* Menlo Park, Calif.: AAAI Press.

FRITH, C. D., 2000. The role of dorsolateral prefrontal cortex in the selection of action as revealed by functional imaging. In *Control of Cognitive Processes: Attention and Performance*, S. Monsell and J. Driver, eds. Cambridge, Mass.: MIT Press, pp. 549–565.

FUSTER, J. M., and G. E. ALEXANDER, 1971. Neuron activity related to short-term memory. *Science* 173:652–654.

GOLDMAN-RAKIC, P., 1987. Circuitry of primate prefrontal cortex and regulation of behaviour. In *Handbook of Physiology: The Nervous System*, F. Plum, ed. Bethesda, Md.: American Psychological Society, pp. 373–417.

GURNEY, K., T. J. PRESCOTT, and P. REDGRAVE, 2001. A computational model of action selection in the basal ganglia. I. A new functional anatomy. *Biol. Cybernet.* 84:401–410.

HENSON, R. N. A., M. D. RUGG, T. SHALLICE, and R. J. DOLAN, 2000. Confidence in word recognition: dissociating right prefrontal roles in episodic retrieval. *J. Cogn. Neurosci.* 12:913–923.

HENSON, R. N. A., M. D. RUGG, T. SHALLICE, O. JOSEPHS, and R. J. DOLAN, 1999. Recollection and familiarity in recognition memory: An event-related fMRI study. *J. Neurosci.* 19:3962–3972.

HENSON, R. N. A., T. SHALLICE, and R. J. DOLAN, 1999. The role of right prefrontal cortex in episodic retrieval: An fMRI test of the monitoring hypothesis. *Brain* 122:1367–1381.

HENSON, R. N. A., T. SHALLICE, O. JOSEPHS, and R. J. DOLAN, 2002. Functional magnetic resonance imaging of proactive interference during spoken recall. *NeuroImage* 17:543–558.

JACOBSEN, C. F., 1935. Functions of frontal association cortex in primates. *Arch. Neurol. Psychiatry* 33:558–560.

JACOBY, L. L., 1996. Associating automatic and consciously controlled effects of study-test compatibility. *J. Mem. Lang.* 35:32–52.

JAHANSHAHI, M., G. DIRNBERGER, R. FULLER, and C. D. FRITH, 2000. The role of the dorsolateral prefrontal cortex in random number generation: A study with positron emission tomography. *NeuroImage* 12:713–725.

JAHANSHAHI, M., P. PROFICE, R. G. BROWN, M. C. RIDDING, G. DIRNBERGER, and J. C. ROTHWELL, 1998. The effects of transcranial magnetic stimulation over the dorsolateral prefrontal cortex on suppression of habitual counting during random number generation. *Brain* 121:1533–1544.

JUEPTNER, M., K. M. STEPHAN, C. D. FRITH, D. J. BROOKS, R. S. J. FRACKOWIAK, and R. E. PASSINGHAM, 1997. Anatomy of motor learning. I. Frontal cortex and attention to action. *J. Neurophysiol.* 77:1313–1324.

KNIGHT, R. T., 1984. Decreased response to novel stimuli after prefrontal lesions in man. *Electroencephalogr. Clin. Neurophysiol.* 59:9–20.

KOECHLIN, E., G. BASSO, P. PIETRINI, S. PANZER, and J. GRAFMAN, 1999. The role of prefrontal cortex in cognition. *Nature* 399:148–151.

LEPAGE, M., O. GHAFFAR, E. NYBERG, and E. TULVING, 2000. Prefrontal cortex and episodic memory retrieval mode. *Proc. Natl. Acad. Sci. U.S.A.* 97:506–511.

MANDLER, G., 1967. Organizational memory. In *The Psychology of Learning and Motivation*, K. Spence and J. T. Spence eds. New York: Academic Press, pp. 327–372.

McCARTHY, R. A., and E. K. WARRINGTON, 1990. *Cognitive Neuropsychology.* London: Academic Press.

McDERMOTT, J., and C. FORGY, 1978. Production system conflict resolution strategies. In *Pattern-Directed Inference Systems*, D. A. Waterman and F. Hayes-Roth, eds. New York: Academic Press.

MOSCOVITCH, M., 1994. Cognitive resources and dual-task interference effects in normal people: The role of the frontal lobes and medial temporal cortex. *Neuropsychology* 8:524–533.

NEWELL, A., 1990. *Unified Theories of Cognition.* Cambridge, Mass.: Harvard University Press.

NORMAN, D. A., and T. SHALLICE, 1986. Attention to action: Willed and automatic control of behaviour. In *Consciousness and Self Regulation: Advances in Research*, vol. IV, R. J. Davidson, G. E. Schwartz, and D. Shapiro, eds. New York: Plenum Press, pp. 1–18.

OKUDA, J., T. FUJII, A. YAMADORI, R. KAWASHIMA, T. TSUKIURA, and R. FUKATSU, 1998. Participation of the prefrontal cortex in prospective memory: Evidence from a PET study in humans. *Neurosci. Lett.* 253:127–130.

OWEN, A. M., J. D. DOWNES, B. J. SAHAKIAN, C. E. POLKEY, and T. W. ROBBINS, 1990. Planning and spatial working memory following frontal lobe lesions in man. *Neuropsychologia* 28:1021–1034.

OWEN, A. M., N. J. HERROD, D. K. MENON, J. C. CLARK, S. P. DOWNEY, T. A. CARPENTER, P. S. MINHAS, F. E. TURKHEIMER, E. J. WILLIAMS, T. W. ROBBINS, B. J. SAHAKIAN, M. PETRIDES, and J. D. PICKARD, 1999. Redefining the functional organisation of spatial and non-spatial working memory processes within human lateral prefrontal cortex. *Eur. J. Neurosci.* 11:567–574.

PETRIDES, M., 1994. Frontal lobes and working memory: Evidence from investigations of the effects of cortical excisions in non-human primates. In *Handbook of Neuropsychology*, F. Boller and J. Grafman, eds. Amsterdam: Elsevier, pp. 59–84.

POSNER, M. I., and S. E. PETERSEN, 1990. The attention system of the human brain. *Annu. Rev. Neurosci.* 13:25–42.

RAICHLE, M. E., J. A. FIEZ, T. O. VIDEEN, A.-M. K. MacLEOD, J. V. PARDO, P. T. FOX, and S. E. PETERSEN, 1994. Practice related changes in human brain functional anatomy during nonmotor learning. *Cereb. Cortex* 4:8–26.

REVERBERI, C., A. LAVARONI, G. L. GIGLI, M. SKRAP, and T. SHALLICE, 2002. Inductive inferences and frontal cortex. *Cortex* 38:899–902.

ROWE, J., I. TONI, O. JOSEPHS, R. S. J. FRACKOWIAK, and R. E. PASSINGHAM, 2000. Separate fronto-parietal systems for selection versus maintenance in working memory. *Science* 288:1656–1660.

RUGG, M. D., R. N. A. HENSON, and W. G. K. ROBB, 2003. Neural correlates of retrieval processing in the prefrontal cortex during recognition and exclusion tasks. *Neuropsychologia* 41:40–52.

RYPMA, B., and M. D'ESPOSITO, 1999. The roles of prefrontal brain regions in components of working memory: Effects of memory load and individual differences. *Proc. Nati. Acad. Sci. U.S.A.* 96:6558–6563.

SHALLICE, T., 1982. Specific impairments of planning. *Philos. Trans. R. Soc. Lond. B* 298:199–209.

SHALLICE, T., and P. BURGESS, 1991. Deficits in strategy application following frontal lobe damage in man. *Brain* 114:727–741.

SHALLICE, T., and P. W. BURGESS, 1996. Domains of supervisory control and the temporal organisation of behaviour. *Philos. Trans. R. Soc. Lond. B* 351:1405–1412.

SHALLICE, T., and M. E. EVANS, 1978. The involvement of the frontal lobes in cognitive estimation. *Cortex* 14:294–303.

SHALLICE, T., P. C. FLETCHER, C. D. FRITH, P. GRASBY, R. S. J. FRACKOWIAK, and R. J. DOLAN, 1994. Brain regions associated with the acquisition and retrieval of verbal episodic memory. *Nature* 386:633–635.

SHALLICE, T., and G. VALLAR, 1990. The impairment of auditory-verbal short-term storage. In *Neuropsychological Impairments of Short-Term Storage*, G. Vallar and T. Shallice eds. Cambridge, England: Cambridge University Press.

SHARP, D. J., S. K. SCOTT, and R. J. S. WISE, (in press). Monitoring and the controlled processing of meaning: Distinct prefrontal systems. *NeuroImage*.

STUSS, D., M. P. ALEXANDER, C. PALUMBO, L. BUCKLE, L. SAYER, and J. POGUE, 1994. Organisational strategies of patients with unilateral or bilateral frontal lobe injury in word list learning tasks. *Neuropsychology* 8:355–373.

TULVING, E., S. KAPUR, and F. I. M. CRAIK, 1994. Hemispheric encoding/retrieval asymmetry in episodic memory: Positron emission tomography findings. *Proc. Natl. Acad. Sci. U.S.A.* 91: 2012–2015.

VERIN, M., A. PARTIOT, B. PILLON, C. MALAPANI, Y. AGID, and B. DUBOIS, 1993. Delayed response tasks and prefrontal lesions in man: Evidence for self-generated patterns of behaviour with poor environmental modulation. *Neuropsychologia* 31:1379–1396.

WARRINGTON, E. K., and T. SHALLICE, 1969. The selective impairment of auditory verbal short-term memory. *Brain* 92:885–896.

WILDING, E. L., and M. D. RUGG, 1996. An event-related potential study of recognition memory with and without retrieval of source. *Brain* 119:889–906.

69 Functional MRI in Monkeys: A Bridge Between Human and Animal Brain Research

NIKOS K. LOGOTHETIS

ABSTRACT Understanding the distributed, synergistic activity of large neural populations requires more than single microelectrode-based measurements of neuron spiking, as the latter provide very little information on spatiotemporal cooperativity and global, associational operations in a given brain structure. Single-cell recordings, large electrode or tetrode-array recordings, monitoring of action potentials and slow waves, and certainly neuroimaging must all be used to obtain the information required for studying the brains capacity to generate various behaviors. Instrumental in bringing about the integration of such information has been the continuous development and improvement of anatomic, physiologic, and neuroimaging techniques. The most commonly applied neuroimaging technique is magnetic resonance imaging (MRI), with its functional variants (fMRI) that can be employed to measure different aspects of hemodynamic responses. The combination of this technique with electrophysiology has fully confirmed the long-standing assumption that the regional activations measured in MR neuroimaging do indeed reflect local increases in neural activity. In addition, it has been demonstrated that fMRI responses mostly reflect the input of a given cortical area and its local intracortical processing, including the activity of excitatory and inhibitory interneurons. Also, studies in the nonhuman primate show that MRI visible tracers and microstimulation serve as ideal tools for the study of dynamic connectivity in the living animal. This chapter describes some recent developments that permit the combination of fMRI with a number of other invasive neuroscientific techniques. It discusses the structural and functional neurovascular coupling and presents data showing the power of MRI in revealing anatomical connectivity and eventually functional organization of the large networks underlying cognition.

Understanding brain function requires not only a comprehension of the physiological workings of individual neurons and glia cells but also a detailed map of the brain's functional architecture and a description of the connections between populations of neurons, the networks that ultimately underlie perception and cognition. In vivo neuroimaging, especially the spatiotemporally resolved magnetic resonance imaging (MRI), together with its functional variant, fMRI, is therefore of obvious importance and is cur-

rently the best tool available to link cognition and action with their neural substrates in humans. Equally interesting and important, however, is the employment of this technique in animals. Its application in the nonhuman primate, the most frequently used laboratory animal for studying the neural basis of cognition, enables us to investigate levels of neural organization that cannot be studied by microelectrodes alone. The local processing captured by microelectrodes can best be understood by simultaneously studying different loci in different brain areas. The latter can be optimally assessed if the dynamic distributed activity patterns related to any sensorimotor event can be reliably tracked in individual animals.

This review deals with spatiotemporally resolved fMRI in monkeys and its combination with other invasive neuroscientific techniques. The emphasis is on simultaneous imaging and electrophysiology experiments aimed at elucidating the neural basis of the blood-oxygen-level-dependent (BOLD) signal. A brief description of the principles of energy metabolism and neurovascular coupling then follows. Finally, a few approaches that permit the study of anatomical and functional architecture of the brain in the live animal are introduced.

The BOLD contrast mechanism

The BOLD contrast mechanism was first described in rat studies (Ogawa, Lee, Kay, et al., 1990; Ogawa, Lee, Nayak, et al., 1990). BOLD contrast is basically produced by field inhomogeneities induced by deoxyhemoglobin (dHb), which is confined to the intracellular space of the red blood cells, which in turn are restricted to the blood vessels. Magnetic susceptibility differences between the dHb-containing compartments and the surrounding space generate magnetic field gradients across and near the compartment boundaries. Pulse sequences designed to be sensitive to such susceptibility differences generate signal alterations whenever the concentration of dHb changes. On neural activation, any increases in dHb would be expected to enhance

NIKOS K. LOGOTHETIS Max Planck Institute for Biological Cybernetics, Tübingen, Germany.

957

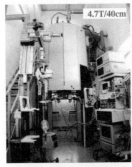
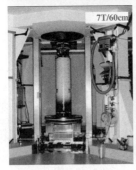
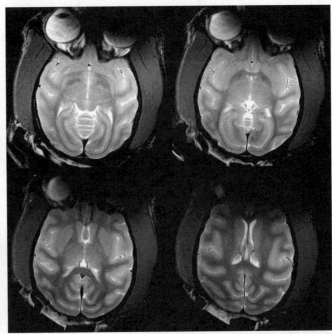

FIGURE 69.1   Left panel shows the BOLD fMRI scanning devices. Two vertical 4.7T, 40-cm-diameter and 7T, 60-cm-diameter bores (Bruker Medical Inc., Germany) were used to image monkey brains. The magnets have local passive shielding to permit the use of neurophysiology and anesthesia equipment. Primate chairs and special transport systems were designed and built for positioning the monkey within the magnets. Right panel shows a typical anatomical scan (multisection multi-echo, spin-density image).

the field inhomogeneities and reduce the BOLD signal. Yet a few seconds after the onset of stimulation, the BOLD signal actually increases. This enhancement reflects an increase in cerebral blood flow (CBF) that overcompensates for the increase in oxygen and ultimately delivers an oversupply of oxygenated blood (Fox and Raichle, 1986; Fox et al., 1988).

Ogawa's seminal studies excited great interest in applying BOLD fMRI to humans. In 1992, three groups simultaneously and independently obtained results in humans with BOLD imaging (Bandettini et al., 1992; Kwong et al., 1992; Ogawa et al., 1992), initiating the flood of fMRI publications that have been appearing in scientific journals ever since.

Research over the last decade has established that BOLD contrast depends not only on blood oxygenation but also on CBF and cerebral blood volume (CBV), a complex response controlled by several parameters. Despite this complexity, much progress has been made toward quantitatively elucidating various aspects of the BOLD signal and the way it relates to the hemodynamic and metabolic changes that occur in response to elevated neuronal activity (for detailed reading and references, see Kim and Ugurbil, 1997; Moonen, Bandettini, and Baert, 1999; Buxton, 2002; Jezzard, Matthews, and Smith, 2002). BOLD fMRI has been performed successfully in anesthetized and conscious animals, including rodents, rabbits, cats, bats, and recently monkeys (for reviews, see Logothetis, 2002, 2003).

BOLD MRI in monkeys

Figure 69.1 (left panel) shows the systems used to image the monkey brain. Two vertical scanners (4.7T and 7T, with 40- and 60-cm diameters), resonators, primate chairs, and special transport systems were designed and built to position the anesthetized or alert monkey inside the magnet (e.g., Logothetis et al., 1999). Figure 69.1 (right) shows a typical high-resolution anatomical scan (voxel size $0.375 \times 0.375 \times 2\,mm^3$) obtained in an alert, trained monkey with the 4.7T system. Figure 69.2 shows the functional results obtained in an anesthetized animal (Logothetis et al., 1999). Thresholded z-score maps showing brain activation are color-coded and superimposed on anatomical scans. The activation was elicited by a polar-transformed checkerboard pattern rotating in alternating directions. Robust BOLD signals in the lateral geniculate nuclei (LGN) and the striate cortex were routinely obtained.

One way to examine the specificity of the BOLD signal is to exploit the well-established retinotopic organization of the visual system (e.g., figure 69.2). In humans, retinotopy can be reliably demonstrated in fMRI by using slowly moving, phase-encoded retinotopic stimuli (Engel et al., 1994). The same approach can be used to study the retinotopical organization of the monkey visual areas (Brewer et al., 2002). The maps obtained in this manner are in excellent agreement with those obtained in monkeys using anatomical and physiological techniques. In contrast to the

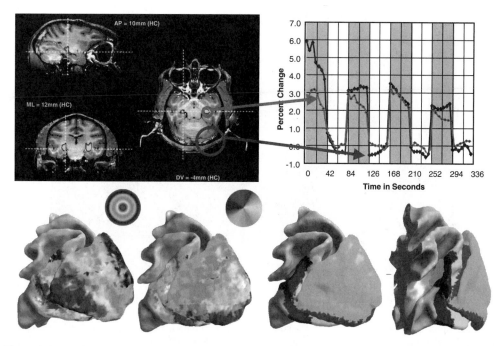

FIGURE 69.2 Upper left panel shows activation of the lateral geniculate nucleus (LGN) and visual cortex. Yellow dotted lines indicate the LGN position. AP, anteroposterior; ML, mediolateral; DV, dorsoventral. Upper right panel shows the time course of the signal for the activated regions in LGN (red) and visual cortex (blue). The two lower left images show the retinotopic organization of the posterior visual areas as revealed with fMRI. Based on this organization, the boundaries of the areas can be defined as shown in the lower right two images: cyan: V1; magenta: V2; yellow: V3; red: V4; blue: V4t; green: MT(V5). (See color plate 54.)

latter techniques, however, noninvasive mapping of the retinotopic areas of individual monkeys may prove to be a valuable tool for a number of longitudinal investigations, including studies of learning, plasticity, and reorganization (see, e.g., Kaas et al., 1990; Darian-Smith and Gilbert, 1995).

In animal experiments, very high-resolution structural and functional imaging can be performed with small, tissue-compatible, intraosteally implantable radiofrequency coils (Logothetis et al., 2002). Tiny voxel sizes can be obtained with good signal-to-noise and contrast-to-noise ratios, revealing both structural and functional cortical architecture in great detail. Figure 69.3A shows an example of a T$_2$*-weighted echo-planar image (EPI) obtained with an actual resolution of $125 \times 125\,\mu m^2$ and a section thickness of $720\,\mu m$. The contrast sensitivity of the image is sufficient to reveal the characteristic striation of the primary visual cortex. The dark line shown by the white arrow (Gen) is the well-known, approximately 200-μm-thick Gennari line formed by the axons of pyramidal and spiny stellate cells contained in the middle cortical layer (lamina IVB). Figure 69.3B shows fMRI correlation coefficient maps (in color) superimposed on the actual EPI (T$_2$*-weighted) images of a monkey during visual block design stimulation. The sections are around the lunate sulcus, and activation extends into the primary and secondary visual cortices (V1 and V2). Both robust activation and good anatomical detail can be discerned.

Neural correlates of the BOLD fMRI signal

Functional MRI cannot directly measure neural responses. Instead, it capitalizes on the interconnections among CBF, energy demand, and neural activity. The successful application of the method in cognitive neuroscience ultimately depends on a comprehensive understanding of the relationship between the fMRI signal and the underlying neuronal activity. A number of studies in humans and animals have already combined fMRI with electroencephalography (EEG; e.g., Menon et al., 1997; Krakow et al., 1999) or optical imaging recordings of intrinsic signals (Hess et al., 2000). But optical imaging also measures hemodynamic responses (Bonhoeffer and Grinvald, 1996) and thus can offer very little direct evidence of the underlying neural activity, while EEG studies typically suffer from poor spatial resolution and relatively imprecise localization of the electromagnetic field patterns associated with neural current flow. Recently, combined intracortical recordings and BOLD fMRI were successfully obtained in both anesthetized and conscious monkeys. The BOLD response was found to directly reflect an increase in neural activity, correlating in particular with those electrical signals that are thought to represent synaptic inputs and local intracortical processing. Before I discuss these findings, I will briefly review the kind of activities that can be monitored using intracortical electrodes (for a more detailed review, see Logothetis, 2002, 2003).

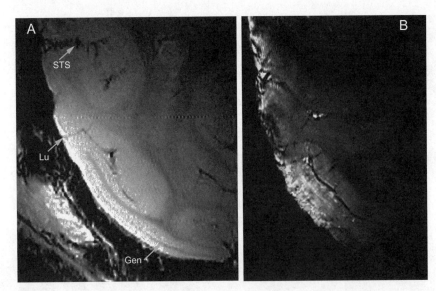

Figure 69.3   Anatomical and functional scans acquired with an implanted surface coil. (*A*) T2*-weighted echo-planar image obtained with an actual resolution of $125 \times 125\,\mu m^2$ and a section thickness of $720\,\mu m$. (*B*) Similar image from another animal with slightly different acquisition parameters. The resolution is sufficient to visualize the susceptibility effects produced by small cortical vessels with an average diameter of $120\,\mu m$. In color are the fMRI correlation coefficient maps. (See color plate 55.)

SPIKES AND SUBTHRESHOLD ACTIVITY   The signal measured by a microelectrode at any given neural site represents the mean extracellular field potential (mEFP) resulting from the weighted sum of all sinks (negativities caused by Na^+ or Ca^{2+} moving from the extracellular to the intracellular space) and sources (positivities) along multiple cells. If a microelectrode with a small tip is placed close to the soma or axon of a neuron, then the measured mEFP directly reports the spike traffic of that neuron and frequently that of its immediate neighbors as well. Recent studies in rats, for instance, show that tetrodes placed close (within $50\,\mu m$) to pyramidal neurons in the hippocampus provide accurate information on a number of their parameters, such as latency, amplitude, and shape of action potentials, the accuracy being monitored with simultaneous intracellular recordings (Harris et al., 2000; Henze et al., 2000).

The firing rate of such well-isolated neurons has been the critical measure for comparing neural activity to sensory processing or behavior ever since the early development of microelectrodes. A great deal has been learned since then, and the single-electrode, single-unit recording technique still remains the method of choice in many behavioral experiments with conscious animals. However, it has the drawback of providing information mainly on single receptive fields, providing no access to subthreshold integrative processes or the associational operations taking place at a given site. Moreover, it suffers from an element of bias toward certain cell types (for references, see Logothetis, 2002, 2003). Spikes generated by large neurons remain above the noise level over a greater distance from the cell than spikes from small neurons, so microelectrodes sample their somas or axons preferentially, a prediction supported by experimental work.

It follows that the measured spikes may actually represent only very small populations of neurons, which in the cortex are by and large the principal cells (e.g., pyramidal cells in cerebral cortex and Purkinje neurons in cerebellar cortex).

If the impedance of the microelectrode is sufficiently low and its exposed tip is slightly further away from the spike-generating sources, so that action potentials do not predominate in the neural signal, then the electrode can monitor the totality of the potentials in that region. The EFPs recorded under these conditions are related both to integrative processes (dendritic events) and to spikes generated by several hundreds of neurons. The two different signal types can be segregated by frequency band separation. A high-pass filter cutoff of approximately 300–400 Hz is used in most recordings to obtain multiple-unit spiking activity (MUA), and a low-pass filter cutoff of about 300 Hz is used to obtain the so-called local field potentials (LFPs).

A large number of experiments have presented data indicating that such a band separation does indeed reflect the activity of different neural processes. Depending on the recording site and the electrode properties, the MUAs are a weighted sum of the extracellular action potentials of all neurons within a sphere of approximately 140–300 μm radius, with the electrode at its center (Grover and Buchwald, 1970; Legatt, Arezzo, and Vaughan, 1980; Henze et al., 2000). Spikes produced by the synchronous firings of many cells can, in principle, be enhanced by summation and thus detected over larger distances (e.g., Arezzo, Legatt, and Vaughan, 1979).

The low-frequency range of the mEFP signal, the LFPs, primarily represent slow events reflecting cooperative activity in neural populations. Until recently these signals were thought to represent exclusively synaptic events. Evidence for this came from combined EEG and intracortical recordings showing that the slow-wave activity in the EEG is largely independent of neuronal spiking (Fromm and Bond, 1964; Ajmone-Marsan, 1965; Buchwald, Hala, and Schramm, 1965). These studies showed that, unlike the multiunit activity, the magnitude of the slow field fluctuations is not correlated with cell size but instead reflects the extent and geometry of dendrites in each recording site. Cells in the so-called open field geometrical arrangement, in which dendrites face in one direction and somata in another, produce strong dendrite-to-soma dipoles when they are activated by synchronous synaptic input. Other cortical neurons are oriented horizontally, and contribute less efficiently or not at all to the sum of potentials. The pyramidal cells, with their apical dendrites running parallel to each other and perpendicular to the pial surface, form an ideal open field arrangement and contribute maximally to both the macroscopically measured EEG and the LFPs.

Thus, LFPs reflect primarily a weighted average of synchronized dendrosomatic components of the synaptic signals of a neural population, most likely from within 0.5–3 mm of the electrode tip (Mitzdorf, 1987; Juergens, Guettler, and Eckhorn, 1999). Yet it has also been shown that LFPs may be partly due to the existence of other types of slow activity unrelated to synaptic events, including voltage-dependent membrane oscillations (e.g., Kamondi et al., 1998) and spike afterpotentials. To be more specific, the soma-dendritic spikes in the neurons of the central nervous system are generally followed by afterpotentials, a brief delayed depolarization, the *afterdepolarization*, and a longer-lasting *afterhyperpolarization*, which are thought to play an important role in the control of excitation-to-frequency transduction (e.g., Granit, Kernell, and Smith, 1963; Harada and Takahashi, 1983; Gustafsson, 1984). Afterpotentials, which were shown to be generated by calcium-activated potassium currents (e.g., Harada and Takahashi, 1983; Walton and Fulton, 1986; Higashi et al., 1993; Chandler et al., 1994; Kobayashi et al., 1997) have a duration on the order of tens of milliseconds and most likely contribute to the generation of the LFP signals (Buzsaki, 1931; Buzsaki et al., 1988).

In summary, MUA mostly represents the spiking of neurons, with single-unit recordings mainly reporting on the activity of the projection neurons that form the exclusive output of a cortical area. LFPs, on the other hand, represent slow waveforms, including synaptic potentials, afterpotentials of somatodendritic spikes, and voltage-gated membrane oscillations, that reflect the input of a given cortical area as well as its local intracortical processing.

LFPs, MUA, AND THE BOLD RESPONSE   One way to determine which cellular events contribute to the generation of the hemodynamic response measured in neuroimaging is to examine the correlation of LFPs, MUA, and single-neuron activity with the hemodynamic response in combined imaging-physiology experiments (Logothetis, Pauls, Augath, et al., 2001; figure 69.4). At first sight, all these signals seemed to be correlated with the BOLD signal. However, in all experiments, increases in the LFP range were greater in both spectral power and reliability. Furthermore, correlation analysis showed that LFPs are better predictors of the BOLD response than multiunit spiking. In fact, it was demonstrated that spike rate is nothing but a "fortuitous" predictor of the BOLD signal, simply because the firing of neurons itself usually happens to correlate with the LFPs. In cases in which there is a dissociation between these signals, BOLD is only predicted by the LFPs. In sites exhibiting strong multiunit response adaptation, for example, MUA returned to the baseline approximately 2.5 s after stimulus onset, while the activity underlying the LFPs remained elevated for the entire duration of the visual stimulus, being the only neural signal to be associated with the BOLD response. Similarly, results from ongoing research in our laboratory involving the injection of various neurotransmitters show that selective blocking of MUA has minimal effects on the BOLD responses averaged over regions coextensive with the spread of the injected substance. Finally, a dissociation between spikes and CBF has been also demonstrated in microstimulation studies in the cerebellar cortex (Mathiesen et al., 1998).

BOLD REFLECTS THE INPUT AND LOCAL PROCESSING OF AN AREA   Taken together, these results suggest that changes in the LFPs are more closely related to the evolution of the BOLD signal than are changes in the spiking activity of single or multiple neurons. In other words, the BOLD signal mainly reflects the incoming specific or association inputs into an area and the processing of this input information by the local cortical circuitry (including excitatory and inhibitory interneurons). Of course, the incoming subcortical or cortical input to an area will often generate the kind of output activity typically measured in intracortical recordings. In this case, the spike rate will indeed be correlated with the measured BOLD signal. If the activity of large projection neurons, however, is shunted by concurrent modulatory input, the incoming afferent signals and the ongoing intracortical activity will still elicit strong hemodynamic responses (figure 69.5). In such cases, spiking activity measured with microelectrodes will be a poor predictor of the BOLD response. A number of experiments demonstrate the plausibility of this explanation.

In a recent study, Tolias and colleagues (2001) used an adaptation technique (Grill-Spector et al., 1999) to study the brain areas processing motion information. They repeatedly imaged a monkey's brain while the animal viewed continuous motion in a single, unchanging direction. Under these

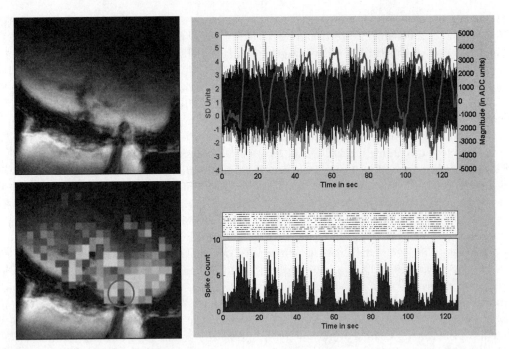

FIGURE 69.4   Combined neurophysiology-fMRI experiments in alert, active monkeys. In the upper left panel an anatomical scan shows the position of the electrode tip. In the lower left panel the activation elicited by a rotating checkerboard is superimposed on the anatomical scan. Top right panel shows the time course of the comprehensive signal (LFPs and spiking activity), together with the BOLD (red thick line), response. Bottom right panel illustrates the raster plots and peristimulus histograms of spiking activity. Each dot is an action potential, and each bin shows the number of action potentials in 250 ms. (See color plate 56.)

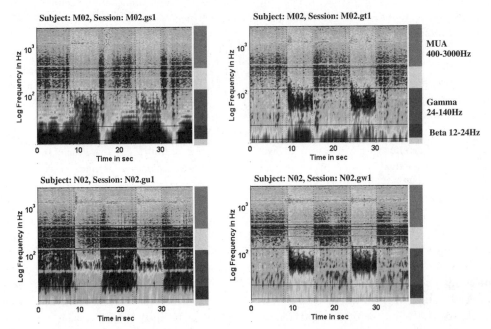

FIGURE 69.5   Time-dependent frequency analysis of the neural signals. Two sessions from two animals are shown (see labels). The spectrograms were computed for windows of 250 ms. Frequency is plotted on the *y*-axis and time on the *x*-axis. At the right of each plot the MUA and LFP ranges are indicated. The red (gamma band) and blue (beta band) sections indicate two of the usual EEG bands. Changes in the power of the signal in the gamma band was best correlated with the hemodynamic response. (See color plate 57.)

conditions, the BOLD response adapts. When the direction of motion reverses abruptly, the measured activity immediately shows a partial recovery, or rebound. The extent of this rebound was considered to be an index of the average directional selectivity of neurons in any given activated area. The results confirmed previous electrophysiological studies revealing a distributed network of visual areas (V1, V2, V3, V5/MT) in the monkey that process information about the direction of visual motion.

Surprisingly, however, strong activation was also observed in area V4, which is only weakly involved in motion processing (e.g., Desimone and Schein, 1987). Such a discrepancy can be explained on the basis of the arguments developed earlier. Areas V4 and MT are interconnected (Felleman and Van Essen, 1983; Ungerleider and Desimone, 1986). Although they process separate stimulus properties, each area may influence the sensitivity of the others by providing some kind of "modulatory" input, which in and of itself is insufficient to drive the pyramidal cells recorded in a typical electrophysiology experiment. In such cases, BOLD fMRI will reveal significant activation and will appear to provide results that do not match those of neurophysiology.

Similarly, attentional effects on the neurons of the striate cortex have been very difficult to measure in monkey electrophysiology experiments (Luck et al., 1997; McAdams and Maunsell, 1999). Yet for similar tasks, strong attentional effects are readily measurable with fMRI in human V1 (Tong and Engel, 1910; Gandhi, Heeger, and Boynton, 1999; Kastner and Ungerleider, 2000).

How does neural activity control BOLD?

BASICS OF BRAIN ENERGY METABOLISM The brain's demand for substrate requires adequate delivery of oxygen and glucose via elaborate mechanisms regulating CBF. Not surprisingly, these mechanisms are closely coupled with regional neural activity. Experimental evidence for such coupling was provided over 100 years ago in laboratory animals (Roy and Sherrington, 1890). Sherrington's seminal study was followed by the systematic investigations of Kety and Schmidt (1948), who introduced the nitrous oxide technique, a global flow measurement method that initially seemed to disprove the notion of a local coupling of CBF and neural activity (Sokoloff, 1960). However, the regional coupling of metabolic rate and neural activity was soon verified with methods allowing local CBF measurements. Although such methods had been used in conscious laboratory animals since the early 1960s (Sokoloff, 1981), a precise quantitative assessment of the relationship between neural activity and regional blood flow was possible only after the introduction of the deoxyglucose autoradiographic technique that enabled spatially resolved measurements of glucose metabolism in laboratory animals (Sokoloff et al., 1977). The

results of a large number of experiments with the [^{14}C]deoxyglucose method have in fact revealed a clear relationship between local cerebral activation and glucose consumption (Sokoloff, 1977).

The first quantitative measurements of regional brain blood flow and oxygen consumption in humans were performed using the radiotracer techniques, followed by the introduction of position emission tomography (PET) (for a historical review, see Raichle, 2000). With PET, it could be shown that maps of activated brain regions can be produced by detecting the indirect effects of neural activity on variables such as CBF (Fox et al., 1986), CBV (Fox and Raichle, 1986), and blood oxygenation (Fox and Raichle, 1986; Fox et al., 1988; Frostig et al., 1990). At the same time, optical imaging of intrinsic signals demonstrated the precision of neurovascular coupling by constructing detailed maps of cortical microarchitecture in both the anesthetized and the alert animal (Bonhoeffer and Grinvald, 1996).

STRUCTURAL NEUROVASCULAR COUPLING It has been demonstrated that the density of the vascular network largely correlates with the average activity of any given region. The spatial correlations reported by a large number of investigators have been mainly between vascular density and the number of synapses rather than the number of neurons. For instance, Duvernoy and colleagues (Duvernoy, Delon, and Vannson, 1981) demonstrated that based on its density, the human cortical vascular network can be subdivided into four layers parallel to the surface. These layers systematically overlap with certain portions of the cytoarchitectonically defined Brodmann laminae. Notably, the first Duvernoy layer, consisting of vessels oriented approximately parallel to neural fibers, is entirely within the lower part of the molecular layer (Layer I), which in the rodent has the lowest concentration of cell bodies and highest density of synapses (Schuz and Palm, 1989). Similarly, in the primate, this layer has the lowest concentration of neurons, the highest concentration of astrocytes, and a high density of synapses (O'Kusky and Colonnier, 1982).

Similar vascularization patterns to those reported by Duvernoy were also found in animal studies (Zheng, LaMantia, and Purves, 1991). Lamina I had the lowest and IVc the highest vascularization, with a IVc/I ratio of 3.3 : 1 (averaged across animals). Interestingly, the IVc/I ratio of synaptic density in the striate cortex of macaque is 2.43 : 1, that of astrocytes is 1.2 : 1, and that of neurons is 78.8 : 1. Assuming some similarity in the distribution of neurons, synapses, and astrocytes between squirrel monkeys and macaques, the recent data would also support the notion that vascular density is correlated with the density of perisynaptic elements rather than neuronal somata. Similar results were obtained in different cortical areas of rodents. For instance, endovascular casts revealed capillary densities resembling the whisker barrel pattern characterizing the somatosensory cortex of rats (Cox, Woolsey, and Rovainen, 1993) and the spatial patterns of stimulus-induced activation in the auditory cortex of chinchillas (Harrison et al., 2002). It seems that an anatomical neurovascular association does indeed exist, setting the basis and the limitations of the regional coupling between neural activity and metabolism. Furthermore, this anatomical neurovascular coupling also suggests that blood supply is better correlated with the density of axonal terminals and dendrites than with the number of neurons and ultimately their action potentials.

FUNCTIONAL NEUROVASCULAR COUPLING The cerebral metabolic rate (CMR) is commonly expressed in terms of oxygen consumption ($CMRO_2$) because glucose metabolism is about 90% aerobic and therefore parallels oxygen consumption (Siesjo, 1978; Ames, 2000). The $CMRO_2$ is likely to vary with neuronal firing properties, shape, and size, whereby large projection neurons, which maintain energy-consuming processes such as ion pumping over a large membrane surface, may have larger energy requirements (for detailed references, see Volterra, Magistretti, and Haydon, 2002). Moreover, neurons are not the only elements contributing to the energy metabolism of the brain; glia and vascular endothelial cells do so as well. In fact, research suggests a tightly regulated glucose metabolism in all brain cell types. An interesting case is the glia cell known as the astrocyte. The structural and functional characteristics of astrocytes makes them ideal bridges between the neuropil and the intraparenchymal capillaries. They are indeed massively connected with both neurons and the brain's vasculature and express receptors and uptake sites with which the neurotransmitters released during synaptic activity can interact.

It has been suggested that for each synaptically released glutamate molecule taken up with two to three Na^+ ions by an astrocyte, one glucose molecule enters the same astrocyte, two ATP molecules are produced through glycolysis, and two lactate molecules are released and consumed by neurons, to yield 18 ATPs through oxidative phosphorylation. Neuronal signals of some sort can therefore trigger receptor-mediated glycogenolysis in astrocytes in a manner similar to peripheral hormones in their target cells. Such signals can be ions or molecules that transiently accumulate in the extracellular space after neuronal activity and/or fast neurotransmitters eliciting both hemodynamic and metabolic responses in anticipation of or at least in parallel with the regional activation.

Recent studies were able to establish a quantitative relationship between imaging signals and the cycling of certain cerebral neurotransmitters (Magistretti et al., 1999; Rothman et al., 1999), as synaptic activity is tightly coupled to glucose uptake (Pellerin and Magistretti, 1994; Takahashi

et al., 1995). More specifically, stoichiometric studies using NMR spectroscopy suggest that the utilization of glutamate (Glu), the dominant excitatory neurotransmitter of the brain (about 90% of the synapses in gray matter are excitatory; Braitenberg and Schuez, 1998), is equal to the rate at which this molecule is converted to glutamine (Gln) in the brain (Sibson et al., 1998). The Glu to Gln conversion occurs in the astrocytes and the required energy is provided by glycolysis. Astrocytes are in fact enriched in glucose transporters. The transporters are driven by the electrochemical gradient of Na^+; for this reason there is a tight coupling between Glu and Na^+ uptake. Both Glu to Gln conversion and Na^+ restoration require ATP. Gln is subsequently released by astrocytes and taken up by the neuronal terminals to be reconverted to Glu (for a review, see Magistretti and Pellerin, 1999). Calculations based on these findings suggest that the energy demands of glutamatergic neurons account for 80%–90% of total cortical glucose usage in rats (Sibson et al., 1998) and humans (Pan et al., 2000).

These findings are in agreement with microstimulation experiments in which the increase in glucose utilization is assessed during orthodromic and antidromic stimulation, the former activating both pre- and postsynaptic terminals and the latter activating only postsynaptic terminals. Increases were observed only during orthodromic stimulation (Kadekaro, Crane, and Sokoloff, 1985; Kadekaro et al., 1987; Nudo and Masterton, 1986; for a review, see Jueptner and Weiller, 1995). Taken together, these results seem to suggest that brain energy consumption is due to presynaptic activity (restoration of gradients) and neurotransmitter cycling.

Others, however, have challenged the notion that presynaptic activity is the major energy consumer in the brain (Attwell and Laughlin, 2001). Based on computations of the number of vesicles released per action potential, the number of postsynaptic receptors activated per vesicle released, the metabolic consequences of activating a single receptor and changing ion fluxes, and neurotransmitter recycling, these investigators concluded that the greater part of energy expenditure is attributable to the postsynaptic effects of glutamate (about 34% of the energy in rodents and 74% in humans is attributable to excitatory postsynaptic currents).

Finally, an interesting alternative was recently proposed, namely, that the hemodynamic responses are probably driven by neurotransmitter-related signaling rather than by direct local energy needs of the brain (Attwell and Iadecola, 2002). There is indeed evidence that blood flow in a number of brain structures, including neocortex, cerebellum, and hippocampus, may be controlled directly by glutamate and GABA. In the cerebellar cortex, for example, the activation of parallel fibers releases glutamate and leads to the depolarization of Purkinje cells and interneurons. These cells in turn release GABA. Notably, the increased blood flow that typically follows the activation of parallel fibers is blocked by inhibitors of non-NMDA glutamate receptors, nitric oxide synthase, and adenosine receptors (Li and Iadecola, 1994), while microinjections of glutamate have vascular effects similar to those observed during stimulation of the parallel fibers (Yang and Iadecola, 1996). In neocortex and hippocampus, microinjection of neurotransmitters dilates pial arterioles and/or precapillary microvessels, an effect attenuated by inhibitors of nitric oxide synthase (NOS) (Faraci and Breese, 1993; Fergus and Lee, 1997). According to these latter findings, CBF may be driven by neurotransmitter-related signaling, being correlated with but not triggered by the utilization of energy.

The study of networks with MRI

CONNECTIVITY STUDIES WITH PARAMAGNETIC TRACERS Neuroanatomical corticocortical and corticosubcortical connections have been examined mainly by means of degeneration methods (Jones and Powell, 1970; Seltzer and Pandya, 1978) and anterograde and retrograde tracer techniques (Saint-Cyr, Ungerleider, and Desimone, 1990; Felleman and Van Essen, 1991; Saleem et al., 2000). Although such studies have demonstrated the value of the information gained from the investigation of the topographic connections between different brain areas, they do require fixed, processed tissue for data analysis and therefore cannot be applied to an animal participating in longitudinal studies, where consecutive studies examining an entire circuit could be carried out in the same subjects.

MRI-visible tracers that are infused into a specific brain region and are transported anterogradely or retrogradely along the axon may therefore enable us to study connectivity in the living animal. Such paramagnetic tracer studies may also be used to validate and further develop noninvasive fiber tracking techniques such as diffusion tensor MRI (see, e.g., Le et al., 2001) that permit the study of connectivity even in the human brain.

Manganese (Mn^{2+}) is an interesting example of an MRI-visible contrast agent. The axonal transport of its radioactive isotope ($^{54}Mn^{2+}$) was first studied using histological methods (Sloot and Gramsbergen, 1994; Tjalve et al., 1996; Takeda et al., 1998). Although these studies were carried out with the goal of understanding the regional specificity of Mn^{2+} distribution, they indicated the usefulness of Mn^{2+} as an anterograde neuronal tract tracer. Mn^{2+} distribution and transport has been also studied with MRI in rats and mice (London et al., 1989; Pautler, Silva, and Koretsky, 1998; Lin et al., 2001; Watanabe, Michaelis, and Frahm, 2001). Injection of $MnCl_2$ into the naris or eye yields a clear signal enhancement in the olfactory and visual pathways (Pautler, Silva, and Koretsky, 1998; Watanabe, Michaelis, and Frahm, 2001). Furthermore, the possibility that the transport of

manganese may pass across synapses was suggested by a number of studies (Pautler, Silva, and Koretsky, 1998; Takeda et al., 1998; Henriksson, Tallkvist, and Tjalve, 1999). Pautler and colleagues (Pautler, Silva, and Koretsky, 1998) indicated that Mn^{2+} must have traversed a synapse to explain the enhancements detected in the olfactory cortex of the mouse following the injection of its olfactory bulb. In contrast, Watanabe and colleagues (Watanabe, Michaelis, and Frahm, 2001) reported that the signal enhancement they observed in their rat study was confined to regions known to receive direct projections from the retina, and concluded that it did not constitute evidence for transsynaptic crossing of Mn^{2+}.

A recent study using manganese provided a detailed account of both the specificity and the transsynaptic transfer of this substance (see figure 69.6 for details). Injections were made into the striatum (Saleem et al., 2002). Its projections were confirmed histologically in the same animals by injecting WGA-HRP at the same sites where $MnCl_2$ had been injected. The size and location of the projection foci in the striatal targets were comparable with those found in both the MRI and histology images. By injecting WGA-HRP at the same sites as $MnCl_2$, we also confirmed for each animal the absence of a direct connection from the injection sites to various brain structures (e.g., thalamic nuclei). In this study, manganese was actually found in a number of structures receiving no direct projections from the injected sites.

MRI AND ELECTRICAL MICROSTIMULATION Our knowledge of connectivity and functional organization could profit a great deal from the combination of MRI with electrical microstimulation. The latter is established as an important neurobiological tool for the study of areal representation and the functional properties of CNS output structures. A new method was recently developed that combines this technique with fMRI for the detailed study of neural connectivity in the live animal. Specially constructed microelectrodes were used to directly stimulate a selected subcortical or cortical area while simultaneously measuring changes in brain activity, which was indexed by the BOLD signal (Logothetis, Pauls, Oeltermann, et al., 2001). The exact location of the stimulation site was determined by means of anatomical scans as well as by studying the physiological properties of neurons. Electrical stimulation was delivered using a biphasic pulse generator attached to a constant-current stimulus isolation unit. The compensation circuit, designed to minimize interference generated by the switching gradients during recording, was always active, minimizing the gradient-induced currents in the range of the stimulation current. Local microstimulation of striate cortex yielded both local BOLD signals and activation of areas V2, V3, and MT. Microstimulation of dLGN resulted in the activation of

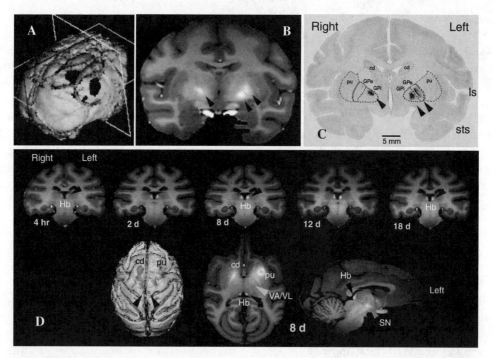

FIGURE 69.6 (*A*) Dorsal view of the rendered brain showing the location and extent of the basal ganglia. (*B*) Manganese transfer to the globus pallidus 24.5 hours after injection into the caudate and putamen. Coronal MRI illustrates the specificity of distribution of Mn²⁺ signal in globus pallidum externum (GPe) and internum (GPi, arrowheads). Note the different spatial distributions of the MR-detectable tracer in the globus pallidus, precisely as expected given the known connectivity of the striatopallidal system: tracer is found in the dorsomedial portion of the GPe and GPi after caudate injection (right hemisphere), and in the ventrolateral or midportion of the GPe and GPi after putamen injection (left hemisphere). At this rostrocaudal level of the globus pallidus, a strong signal was observed only in the GPi on the caudate injection side. (*C*) Coronal

histology section showing the WGA-HRP labeling in the GPe and GPi (arrowheads) 24.5 hours after right caudate and left putamen injections. Note the similar distribution of Mn²⁺ signal and WGA-HRP labeling in the MRI and the histological section, respectively. (*D*) Transneuronal transfer of Mn²⁺ shown by signal changes in the thalamic nuclei over long time periods (4 hours–18 days) after MnCl₂ injection into the right caudate and left putamen. The upper row shows coronal MRIs from five different scans (4 hours, 2 days, 8 days, 12 days, and 18 days) illustrating the Mn²⁺ signal in the habenular thalamic nuclei (Hb, bright discrete regions; arrowheads). The lower row indicates the signal increases in the thalamic nuclei (VA/VL and Hb). (See color plate 58.)

striate cortex as well as areas V2, V3, and MT. The findings show that microstimulation combined with fMRI can be an exquisite tool for finding and studying target areas of electrophysiological interest.

Conclusions

The suitability of MRI for functional brain mapping is firmly established. BOLD fMRI has been successfully implemented in conscious human subjects as well as in animals such as rats, cats, and monkeys. The use of high magnetic fields improves both signal specificity and spatial resolution. MRI studies, in which voxels may contain as few as 600–800 cortical neurons, can help us understand how neural networks are organized, and how small cell assemblies contribute to the activation patterns revealed in fMRI. The combination of this technique with electrophysiology has fully confirmed the long-standing assumption that the regional activations measured in MR neuroimaging do indeed reflect local increases in neural activity. In addition,

it has been demonstrated that fMRI responses mostly reflect the input of a given cortical area and its local intracortical processing, including the activity of excitatory and inhibitory interneurons. Finally, MRI-visible tracers and microstimulation appear to be ideal for the study of connectivity in the living animal.

ACKNOWLEDGMENTS This work was supported by the Max Planck Society.

REFERENCES

AJMONE-MARSAN, C., 1965. Electrical activity of the brain: Slow waves and neuronal activity. *Isr. J. Med. Sci.* 1:104–117.

AMES, A., 2000. CNS energy metabolism as related to function. *Brain Res. Brain Res. Rev.* 34:42–68.

AREZZO, J., A. D. LEGATT, and H. G. J. VAUGHAN, 1979. Topography and intracranial sources of somatosensory evoked potentials in the monkey. I. Early components. *Electroencephalogr. Clin. Neurophysiol.* 46:155–172.

ATTWELL, D., and C. IADECOLA, 2002. The neural basis of functional brain imaging signals. *Trends Neurosci.* 25:621–625.

ATTWELL, D., and S. B. LAUGHLIN, 2001. An energy budget for signaling in the grey matter of the brain. *J. Cereb. Blood Flow Metab.* 21:1133–1145.

BANDETTINI, P. A., E. C. WONG, R. S. HINKS, R. S. TIKOFSKY, and J. S. HYDE, 1992. Time course EPI of human brain function during task activation. *Magn. Reson. Med.* 25:390–397.

BONHOEFFER, T., and A. GRINVALD, 1996. Optical imaging based on intrinsic signals. In *Brain Mapping: The Methods*, A. W. Toga and J. C. Mazziotta, eds. New York: Academic Press, pp. 55–97.

BRAITENBERG, V., and A. SCHUEZ, 1998. *Cortex: Statistics and Geometry of Neuronal Connectivity*. Berlin: Springer-Verlag.

BREWER, A. A., W. PRESS, N. K. LOGOTHETIS, and B. WANDELL, 2002. Visual areas in macaque cortex measured using functional MRI. *J. Neurosci.* 22:10416–10426.

BUCHWALD, J. S., E. S. HALA, and S. SCHRAMM, 1965. A comparison of multi-unit activity and EEG activity recorded from the same brain site in chronic cats during behavioral conditioning. *Nature* 205:1012–1014.

BUXTON, R., 2002. *An Introduction to Functional Magnetic Resonance Imaging: Principles and Techniques*. New York: Cambridge University Press.

BUZSAKI, G., 1931. Theta oscillations in the hippocampus. *Neuron* 33:325–340.

BUZSAKI, G., R. G. BICKFORD, G. PONOMAREFF, L. J. THAL, R. MANDEL, and F. H. GAGE, 1988. Nucleus basalis and thalamic control of neocortical activity in the freely moving rat. *J. Neurosci.* 8:4007–4026.

CHANDLER, S. H., C. F. HSAIO, T. INOUE, and L. J. GOLDBERG, 1994. Electrophysiological properties of guinea pig trigeminal motoneurons recorded in vitro. *J. Neurophysiol.* 71:129–145.

COX, S. B., T. A. WOOLSEY, and C. M. ROVAINEN, 1993. Localized dynamic changes in cortical blood flow with whisker stimulation corresponds to matched vascular and neuronal architecture of rat barrels. *J. Cereb. Blood Flow Metab.* 13:899–913.

DARIAN-SMITH, C., and C. D. GILBERT, 1995. Topographic reorganization in the striate cortex of the adult cat and monkey is cortically mediated. *J. Neurosci.* 15:1631–1647.

DESIMONE, R., and S. J. SCHEIN, 1987. Visual properties of neurons in area V4 of the macaque: Sensitivity to stimulus form. *J. Neurophysiol.* 57:835–868.

DUVERNOY, H. M., S. DELON, and J. L. VANNSON, 1981. Cortical blood vessels of the human brain. *Brain Res. Bull.* 7:519–579.

ENGEL, S. A., D. E. RUMELHART, B. A. WANDELL, A. T. LEE, G. H. GLOVER, E.-J. CHICHILNISKY, and M. N. SHADLEN, 1994. fMRI of human visual cortex. *Nature* 369:525.

FARACI, F. M., and K. R. BREESE, 1993. Nitric oxide mediates vasodilatation in response to activation of N-methyl-D-aspartate receptors in brain. *Circ. Res.* 72:476–480.

FELLEMAN, D. J., and D. C. VAN ESSEN, 1983. The connections of area V4 of macaque extrastriate cortex. *Soc. Neurosci. Abstr.* 9:153.

FELLEMAN, D. J., and D. C. VAN ESSEN, 1991. Distributed hierarchical processing in the primate cerebral cortex. *Cereb. Cortex* 1: 1–47.

FERGUS, A., and K. S. LEE, 1997. Regulation of cerebral microvessels by glutamatergic mechanisms. *Brain Res.* 754:35–45.

FOX, P. T., M. A. MINTUN, M. E. RAICHLE, F. M. MIEZIN, J. M. ALLMAN, and D. C. VAN ESSEN, 1986. Mapping human visual cortex with positron emission tomography. *Nature* 323:806–809.

FOX, P. T., and M. E. RAICHLE, 1986. Focal physiological uncoupling of cerebral blood flow and oxidative metabolism during somatosensory stimulation in human subjects. *Proc. Natl. Acad. Sci. U.S.A.* 83:1140–1144.

FOX, P. T., M. E. RAICHLE, M. A. MINTUN, and C. DENCE, 1988. Nonoxidative glucose consumption during focal physiologic neural activity. *Science* 241:462–464.

FROMM, G. H., and H. W. BOND, 1964. Slow changes in the electrocorticogram and the activity of cortical neurons. *Electroencephalogr. Clin. Neurophysiol.* 17:520–523.

FROSTIG, R. D., E. E. LIEKE, D. Y. TS'O, and A. GRINVALD, 1990. Cortical functional architecture and local coupling between neuronal activity and the microcirculation revealed by in vivo high-resolution optical imaging of intrinsic signals. *Proc. Natl. Acad. Sci. U.S.A.* 87:6082–6086.

GANDHI, S. P., D. J. HEEGER, and G. M. BOYNTON, 1999. Spatial attention affects brain activity in human primary visual cortex. *Proc. Natl. Acad. Sci. U.S.A.* 96:3314–3319.

GRANIT, R., D. KERNELL, and R. S. SMITH, 1963. Delayed depolarization and the repetitive response to intracellular stimulation of mammalian motoneurones. *J. Physiol. (Lond.)* 168:890–910.

GRILL-SPECTOR, K., T. KUSHNIR, S. EDELMAN, G. AVIDAN, Y. ITZCHAK, and R. ITZCHAK, 1999. Differential processing of objects under various viewing conditions in the human lateral occipital complex. *Neuron* 24:187–203.

GROVER, F. S., and J. S. BUCHWALD, 1970. Correlation of cell size with amplitude of background fast activity in specific brain nuclei. *J. Neurophysiol.* 33:160–171.

GUSTAFSSON, B., 1984. Afterpotentials and transduction properties in different types of central neurones. *Arch. Ital. Biol.* 122:17–30.

HARADA, Y., and T. TAKAHASHI, 1983. The calcium component of the action potential in spinal motoneurones of the rat. *J. Physiol.* 335:89–100.

HARRIS, K. D., D. A. HENZE, J. CSICSVARI, H. HIRASE, and G. BUZSAKI, 2000. Accuracy of tetrode spike separation as determined by simultaneous intracellular and extracellular measurements. *J. Neurophysiol.* 84:401–414.

HARRISON, R. V., N. HAREL, J. PANESAR, and R. J. MOUNT, 2002. Blood capillary distribution correlates with hemodynamic-based functional imaging in cerebral cortex. *Cereb. Cortex* 12:225–233.

HENRIKSSON, J., J. TALLKVIST, and H. TJALVE, 1999. Transport of manganese via the olfactory pathway in rats: Dosage dependency of the uptake and subcellular distribution of the metal in the olfactory epithelium and the brain. *Toxicol. Appl. Pharmacol.* 156:119–128.

HENZE, D. A., Z. BORHEGYI, J. CSICSVARI, A. MAMIYA, K. D. HARRIS, and G. BUZSAKI, 2000. Intracellular features predicted by extracellular recordings in the hippocampus in vivo. *J. Neurophysiol.* 84:390–400.

HESS, A., D. STILLER, T. KAULISCH, P. HEIL, and H. SCHEICH, 2000. New insights into the hemodynamic blood oxygenation level-dependent response through combination of functional magnetic resonance imaging and optical recording in gerbil barrel cortex. *J. Neurosci.* 20:3328–3338.

HIGASHI, H., E. TANAKA, H. INOKUCHI, and S. NISHI, 1993. Ionic mechanisms underlying the depolarizing and hyperpolarizing afterpotentials of single spike in guinea-pig cingulate cortical neurons. *Neuroscience* 55:129–138.

JEZZARD, P., P. M. MATTHEWS, and S. M. SMITH, 2002. *Functional Magnetic Resonance Imaging: An Introduction to Methods*. Oxford, England: Oxford University Press.

JONES, E. G., and T. P. S. POWELL, 1970. An anatomical study of converging sensory pathways within the cerebral cortex of the monkey. *Brain* 93:793–820.

JUEPTNER, M., and C. WEILLER, 1995. Does measurement of regional cerebral blood flow reflect synaptic activity? Implications for PET and fMRI. *NeuroImage* 2:148–156.

JUERGENS, E., A. GUETTLER, and R. ECKHORN, 1999. Visual stimulation elicits locked and induced gamma oscillations in monkey intracortical- and EEG-potentials, but not in human EEG. *Exp. Brain Res.* 129:247–259.

KAAS, J. H., L. A. KRUBITZER, Y. M. CHINO, A. L. LANGSTON, E. H. POLLEY, and N. BLAIR, 1990. Reorganization of retinotopic cortical maps in adult mammals after lesions of the retina. *Science* 248:229.

KADEKARO, M., A. M. CRANE, and L. SOKOLOFF, 1985. Differential effects of electrical stimulation of sciatic nerve on metabolic activity in spinal cord and dorsal root ganglion in the rat. *Proc. Natl. Acad. Sci. U.S.A.* 82:6010–6013.

KADEKARO, M., W. H. VANCE, M. L. TERRELL, H. J. GARY, H. M. EISENBERG, and L. SOKOLOFF, 1987. Effects of antidromic stimulation of the ventral root on glucose utilization in the ventral horn of the spinal cord in the rat. *Proc. Natl. Acad. Sci. U.S.A.* 84:5492–5495.

KAMONDI, A., L. ACSADY, X. J. WANG, and G. BUZSAKI, 1998. Theta oscillations in somata and dendrites of hippocampal pyramidal cells in vivo: Activity-dependent phase-precession of action potentials. *Hippocampus* 8:244–261.

KASTNER, S., and L. G. UNGERLEIDER, 2000. Mechanisms of visual attention in the human cortex. *Annu. Rev. Neurosci.* 23:315–341.

KETY, S. S., and C. F. SCHMIDT, 1948. Nitrous oxide method for the quantitative determination of cerebral blood flow in man: Theory, procedure, and normal values. *J. Clin. Invest.* 27:475–483.

KIM, S. G., and K. UGURBIL, 1997. Comparison of blood oxygenation and cerebral blood flow effects in fMRI: Estimation of relative oxygen consumption change. *Magn. Reson. Med.* 38:59–65.

KOBAYASHI, M., T. INOUE, R. MATSUO, Y. MASUDA, O. HIDAKA, Y. KANG, and T. MORIMOTO, 1997. Role of calcium conductances on spike afterpotentials in rat trigeminal motoneurons. *J. Neurophysiol.* 77:3273–3283.

KRAKOW, K., F. G. WOERMANN, M. R. SYMMS, P. J. ALLEN, L. LEMIEUX, G. J. BARKER, J. S. DUNCAN, and D. R. FISH, 1999. EEG-triggered functional MRI of interictal epileptiform activity in patients with partial seizures. *Brain* 122:1679–1688.

KWONG, K. K., J. W. BELLIVEAU, D. A. CHESLER, I. E. GOLDBERG, R. M. WEISSKOFF, B. P. PONCELET, D. N. KENNEDY, B. E. HOPPEL, M. S. COHEN, and R. TURNER, 1992. Dynamic magnetic resonance imaging of human brain activity during primary sensory stimulation. *Proc. Natl. Acad. Sci. U.S.A.* 89:5675–5679.

LE, B., J. F. MANGIN, C. POUPON, C. A. CLARK, S. PAPPATA, N. MOLKO, and H. CHABRIAT, 2001. Diffusion tensor imaging: Concepts and applications. *J. Magn. Reson. Imaging* 13:534–546.

LEGATT, A. D., J. AREZZO, and H. G. J. VAUGHAN, 1980. Averaged multiple unit activity as an estimate of phasic changes in local neuronal activity: Effects of volume-conducted potentials. *J. Neurosci. Methods* 2:203–217.

LI, J., and C. IADECOLA, 1994. Nitric oxide and adenosine mediate vasodilation during functional activation in cerebellar cortex. *Neuropharmacology* 33:1453–1461.

LIN, C. P., W. Y. I., TSENG, H. C. CHENG, and J. H. CHEN, 2001. Validation of diffusion tensor magnetic resonance axonal fiber imaging with registered manganese-enhanced optic tracts. *NeuroImage* 14:1035–1047.

LOGOTHETIS, N. K., 2002. On the neural basis of the BOLD fMRI signal. *Philos. Trans. R. Soc. Lond. (Biol.)* 357:1003–1037.

LOGOTHETIS, N. K., 2003. The underpinnings of the BOLD functional magnetic resonance imaging signal. *J. Neurosci.* 23:3963–3971.

LOGOTHETIS, N. K., H. GUGGENBERGER, S. PELED, and J. PAULS, 1999. Functional imaging of the monkey brain. *Nat. Neurosci.* 2:555–562.

LOGOTHETIS, N. K., H. MERKLE, M. AUGATH, T. TRINATH, and K. UGURBIL, 2002. Ultra-high resolution fMRI in Monkeys with implanted RF coils. *Neuron* 35:227–242.

LOGOTHETIS, N. K., J. PAULS, M. AUGATH, T. TRINATH, and A. OELTERMANN, 2001. Neurophysiological investigation of the basis of the fMRI signal. *Nature* 412:150–157.

LOGOTHETIS, N. K., J. PAULS, A. OELTERMANN, M. AUGATH, and T. TRINATH, 2001. Studying connectivity with electrical microstimulation and fMRI. *Soc. Neurosci. Abstr.* 27:821.

LONDON, R. E., G. TONEY, S. A. GABEL, and A. FUNK, 1989. Magnetic resonance imaging studies of the brains of anesthetized rats treated with manganese chloride. *Brain Res. Bull.* 23:229–235.

LUCK, S. J., L. CHELAZZI, S. A. HILLYARD, and R. DESIMONE, 1997. Neural mechanisms of spatial selective attention in areas V1, V2, and V4 of macaque visual cortex. *J. Neurophysiol.* 77:24–42.

MAGISTRETTI, P. J., and L. PELLERIN, 1999. Cellular mechanisms of brain energy metabolism and their relevance to functional brain imaging. *Philos. Trans. R. Soc. Lond. Ser. B Biol. Sci.* 354:1155–1163.

MAGISTRETTI, P. J., L. PELLERIN, D. L. ROTHMAN, and R. G. SHULMAN, 1999. Neuroscience: Energy on demand. *Science* 283:496–497.

MATHIESEN, C., K., CAESAR, N. AKGOREN, and M. LAURITZEN, 1998. Modification of activity-dependent increases of cerebral blood flow by excitatory synaptic activity and spikes in rat cerebellar cortex. *J. Physiol.* 512:555–566.

MCADAMS, C. J., and J. H. MAUNSELL, 1999. Effects of attention on orientation-tuning functions of single neurons in macaque cortical area V4. *J. Neurosci.* 19:431–441.

MENON, V., J. M. FORD, K. O. LIM, G. H. GLOVER, and A. PFEFFERBAUM, 1997. Combined event-related fMRI and EEG evidence for temporal-parietal cortex activation during target detection. *Neuroreport* 8:3029–3037.

MITZDORF, U., 1987. Properties of the evoked potential generators: Current source-density analysis of visually evoked potentials in the cat cortex. *Int. J. Neurosci.* 33:33–59.

MOONEN, C. T., P. A. BANDETTINI, and A. L. BAERT, 1999. *Functional MRI.* Berlin: Springer-Verlag.

NUDO, R. J., and R. B. MASTERTON, 1986. Stimulation-induced [14]C2-deoxyglucose labeling of synaptic activity in the central auditory system. *J. Comp. Neurol.* 245:553–565.

O'KUSKY, J., and M. COLONNIER, 1982. A laminar analysis of the number of neurons, glia, and synapses in the adult cortex (area 17) of adult macaque monkeys. *J. Comp. Neurol.* 210:278–290.

OGAWA, S., T. M. LEE, A. R. KAY, and D. W. TANK, 1990. Brain magnetic resonance imaging with contrast dependent on blood oxygenation. *Proc. Natl. Acad. Sci. U.S.A.* 87:9868–9872.

OGAWA, S., T. M. LEE, A. S. NAYAK, and P. GLYNN, 1990. Oxygenation-sensitive contrast in magnetic resonance image of rodent brain at high magnetic fields. *Magn. Reson. Med.* 14:68–78.

OGAWA, S., D. W. TANK, R. MENON, J. M. ELLERMANN, S. G. KIM, H. MERKLE, and K. UGURBIL, 1992. Intrinsic signal changes accompanying sensory stimulation: Functional brain mapping with magnetic resonance imaging. *Proc. Natl. Acad. Sci. U.S.A.* 89:5951–5955.

PAN, J. W., D. T. STEIN, F. TELANG, J. H. LEE, J. SHEN, P. BROWN, G. CLINE, G. F. MASON, G. I. SHULMAN, D. L. ROTHMAN, and H. P. HETHERINGTON, 2000. Spectroscopic imaging of glutamate C4 turnover in human brain. *Magn. Reson. Med.* 44:673–679.

PAUTLER, R. G., A. C. SILVA, and A. P. KORETSKY, 1998. In vivo neuronal tract tracing using manganese-enhanced magnetic resonance imaging. *Magn. Reson. Med.* 40:740–8.

PELLERIN, L., and P. J. MAGISTRETTI, 1994. Glutamate uptake into astrocytes stimulates aerobic glycolysis: A mechanism coupling neuronal activity to glucose utilization. *Proc. Natl. Acad. Sci. U.S.A.* 91:10625–10629.

RAICHLE, M. E., 2000. A brief history of human functional brain mapping. In *The Systems*, A. W. Toga and J. C. Mazziotta, eds. San Diego, Calif.: Academic Press, pp. 33–75.

ROTHMAN, D. L., N. R. SIBSON, F. HYDER, J. SHEN, K. L. BEHAR, and R. G. SHULMAN, 1999. In vivo nuclear magnetic resonance spectroscopy studies of the relationship between the glutamate-glutamine neurotransmitter cycle and functional neuroenergetics. *Philos. Trans. R. Soci. Lond. Ser. B Biol. Sci.* 354:1165–1177.

ROY, C. S., and C. S. SHERRINGTON, 1890. On the regulation of the blood supply of the brain. *J. physiol. (Lond.)* 11:85–108.

SAINT-CYR, J. A., L. G. UNGERLEIDER, and R. DESIMONE, 1990. Organization of visual cortical inputs to the striatum and subsequent outputs to the pallido-nigral complex in the monkey. *J. Comp. Neurol.* 298:129–156.

SALEEM, K. S., J. PAULS, M. AUGATH, T. TRINATH, B. A. PRAUSE, and N. K. LOGOTHETIS, 2002. Magnetic resonance imaging of neuronal connections in the macaque monkey. *Neuron* 34: 685–700.

SALEEM, K. S., W. SUZUKI, K. TANAKA, and T. HASHIKAWA, 2000. Connections between anterior inferotemporal cortex and superior temporal sulcus regions in the macaque monkey. *J. Neurosci.* 20:5083–5101.

SCHUZ, A., and G. PALM, 1989. Density of neurons and synapses in the cerebral cortex of the mouse. *J. Comp. Neurol.* 286:442–455.

SELTZER, B., and D. N. PANDYA, 1978. Afferent cortical connections and architectonics of the superior temporal sulcus and surrounding cortex in the rhesus monkey. *Brain Res.* 149:1–24.

SIBSON, N. R., A. DHANKHAR, G. F. MASON, D. L. ROTHMAN, K. L. BEHAR, and R. G. SHULMAN, 1998. Stoichiometric coupling of brain glucose metabolism and glutamatergic neuronal activity. *Proc. Natl. Acad. Sci. U.S.A.* 95:316–321.

SIESJO, BO. K., 1978. *Brain Energy Metabolism.* New York: John Wiley & Sons.

SLOOT, W. N., and J. B. GRAMSBERGEN, 1994. Axonal transport of manganese and its relevance to selective neurotoxicity in the rat basal ganglia. *Brain Res.* 19:124–132.

SOKOLOFF, L., 1960. The metabolism of the central nervous system in vivo. In *Handbook of Physiology-Neurophysiology*, J. Field, H. W. Magoun, and V. E. Hall, eds. Washington, D.C.: American Physiological Society, pp. 1843–1864.

SOKOLOFF, L., 1977. Relation between physiological function and energy metabolism in the central nervous system. *J. Neurochem.* 29:13–26.

SOKOLOFF, L., 1981. Relationships among local functional activity, energy metabolism, and blood flow in the central nervous system. *Fed. Proc.* 40:2311–2316.

SOKOLOFF, L., M. REIVICH, C. KENNEDY, M. H. DESROSIERS, C. S. PATLAK, K. D. PETTIGREW, O. SAKURADA, and M. SHINOHARA, 1977. The [C14]deoxyglucose method for the measurement of local cerebral glucose utilization: Theory, procedure and normal values in the conscious and anesthetized albino rat. *J. Neurochem.* 28:897–916.

TAKAHASHI, S., B. F. DRISCOLL, M. J. LAW, and L. SOKOLOFF, 1995. Role of sodium and potassium ions in regulation of glucose metabolism in cultured astroglia. *Proc. Natl. Acad. Sci. U.S.A.* 92: 4616–4620.

TAKEDA, A., Y. KODAMA, S. ISHIWATARI, and S. OKADA, 1998. Manganese transport in the neural circuit of rat CNS. *Brain Res. Bull.* 45:149–152.

TJALVE, H., J. HENRIKSSON, J. TALLKVIST, B. S. LARSSON, and N. G. LINDQUIST, 1996. Uptake of manganese and cadmium from the nasal mucosa into the central nervous system via olfactory pathways in rats. *Pharmacol. Toxicol.* 79:347–356.

TOLIAS, A. S., S. M. SMIRNAKIS, M. A. AUGATH, T. TRINATH, and N. K. LOGOTHETIS, 2001. Motion processing in the macaque: Revisited with functional magnetic resonance imaging. *J. Neurosci.* 21:8594–8601.

TONG, F., and S. A. ENGEL, 1910. Interocular rivalry revealed in the human cortical blind-spot representation. *Nature* 411:195–199.

UNGERLEIDER, L. G., and R. DESIMONE, 1986. Cortical connections of visual area MT in the macaque. *J. Comp. Neurol.* 248:190–222.

VOLTERRA, A., P. J. MAGISTRETTI, and P. G. HAYDON, 2002. *The Tripartite Synapse: Glia in Synaptic Transmission.* Oxford, England: Oxford University Press.

WALTON, K., and B. P. FULTON, 1986. Ionic mechanisms underlying the firing properties of rat neonatal motoneurons studied in vitro. *Neuroscience* 19:669–683.

WATANABE, T., T. MICHAELIS, and J. FRAHM, 2001. Mapping of retinal projections in the living rat using high-resolution 3D gradient-echo MRI with Mn^{2+}-induced contrast. *Magn. Reson. Med.* 46:424–429.

YANG, G., and C. IADECOLA, 1996. Glutamate microinjections in cerebellar cortex reproduce cerebrovascular effects of parallel fiber stimulation. *Am. J. Physiol.* 271:R1568–R1575.

ZHENG, D., A.-S. LAMANTIA, and D. PURVES, 1991. Specialized vascularization of the primate visual cortex. *J. Neurosci.* 11: 2622–2629.

IX EMOTION AND SOCIAL NEUROSCIENCE

Introduction

TODD F. HEATHERTON, ELIZABETH A. PHELPS,
AND JOSEPH E. LEDOUX

IN THE PREVIOUS edition of this book, Joseph LeDoux (2000) noted that the study of emotion, though long neglected, had become one of the major growth areas in cognitive neuroscience. Indeed, as demonstrated by the six superb chapters on emotion in the 2nd edition, the rediscovery of the "hot" aspects of cognition, along with the corresponding demonstration that animal models of emotion applied well to the human brain, placed research examining the neural basis of emotions at the absolute forefront of cognitive neuroscience. The neuroscientific study of emotion has continued to flourish, and in doing so it has led scientists to recognize that other hot aspects of cognition are equally due for attention, namely, the social aspects of cognition. In additional to foundational chapters on emotion, this section expands in this new edition to include the social brain.

The interdisciplinary field of cognitive neuroscience has provided ample evidence of the benefits of examining psychological constructs across multiple levels of analysis, from the molecular to the cultural. The nine chapters in this section cross many levels, from the role of gene expression in learning and memory to brain regions that subserve sensitivity to societal norms and embarrassment. Cacioppo and Berntson detail many of the advantages of multilevel analyses and trace the history of these efforts in social and affective neuroscience. Of course, a multilevel approach works only if people consider interactions across levels, such as how basic affective processes influence cognition and how cognitive processes modulate affect. This approach is evident at least in some degree in each chapter in this section, even as the primary focus tends to be at adjoining levels of analysis. What is clear is that research using multiple approaches is moving the field toward the ultimate goal of developing

973

coherent models of how the brain makes emotion and performs its social function.

One overriding theme in the previous edition was the role of the amygdala in emotional processes. There was a remarkable convergence of evidence highlighting the important role of the amygdala across animal species and paradigms. The importance of the amygdala continues to hold center stage in the neuroscience of emotion, as is evident in many of the present chapters. Schafe and LeDoux review the importance of the amygdala in fear. Rapid advances in neuroscience methods over the past 5 years have provided researchers with the opportunity to study the biochemical and molecular mechanisms that underlie learning and memory. For instance, research has demonstrated an important role of gene expression in long-term potentiation, which is perhaps the most likely candidate for the physiological basis of fear conditioning. Schafe and LeDoux also review research on the fascinating phenomenon of reconsolidation, in which recalled fear memories can be disrupted by processes similar to those active during consolidation of new memories. In the next chapter, Phelps describes imaging and patient studies demonstrating the crucial role of the amygdala in human emotion and cognition. Her research investigates the role of the amygdala in affective learning and attention/perception. She also describes recent research on the cognitive and social basis of fear learning, such as learning through instruction and observation. The chapter by Adolphs reviews research showing that damage to the amygdala can impair the processing of social cues of emotion.

Of course, the amygdala is not the only brain structure that is important for emotion. The hippocampus plays an important role both in contextual fear conditioning and in the memory of emotional events. Sapolsky addresses how stress affects memory processes as a function of the type of stress and type of memory. Although some degree of stress facilitates emotional memories, chronic and severe stress can have devastating consequences, especially for hippoccampal-dependent memory and cognition. At the same time, severe stress can lead to enhanced consolidation of amygdala-dependent memories. Understanding how specific forms of stress can have an impact on different brain structures and cognitive processes is important for understanding the effects of traumatic experiences on psychological processes. In their chapter, Breiter and Gasic propose an information backbone consisting of many brain regions, especially in the mesolimbic dopamine pathway, that is responsible for processing reward and aversive input. The existence of this integrated system is supported by recent imaging and neurophysiological studies. This system might have important implications for understanding and classifying various psychiatric disorders based on deficits in processing reward and aversive inputs.

Three of the chapters focus on the role of the prefrontal cortex in social cognition and social emotions. Since the last edition an entirely new field has emerged, which some have called the social brain sciences. This new field encompasses research using the approaches of evolutionary psychology, social cognition, and especially neuroscience (e.g., patient studies, brain imaging) to study social behavior. As previously noted by Adolphs (2003), the social brain sciences represent a sometimes uneasy alliance between evolutionary psychology and social cognition. The successful marriage of these two areas is due to their adopting the methods of neuroscience and largely restricting the domain of empirical study to emotional aspects of cognition. Thinking about other people entails emotional responses that thinking about vegetables, say, does not. The social and emotional aspects of the brain are inexorably linked, with the adaptive significance of emotions being closely linked to their social value, and nearly all social interaction produces affective responses.

Of course, interest in understanding the neural basis of social behavior is not new. Since the time of Phineas Gage, it has been known that damage to certain brain regions (e.g., the medial prefrontal cortex) interferes with social and emotional competence while not affecting cognitive competence in other domains. Indeed, Cacioppo and Berntson's chapter traces much of this history. More recently there has been growing interest among social psychologists and cognitive neuroscientists in using brain imaging to study social cognition. This research has identified a number of brain regions that appear to subserve highly specialized social capacities, such as recognition of faces and emotional expressions, theory of mind, social emotions such as empathy, judging trustworthiness and attractiveness, cooperation, and so forth. The gist of these studies is that "people" are given privileged status by the brain as it processes objects in the environment (see Mitchell, Heatherton, and Macrae, 2002).

The social brain sciences approach is providing new insights into long-standing questions regarding social behavior. For example, Macrae, Heatherton, and Kelley describe research demonstrating how brain imaging was able to resolve a long-standing debate in social psychology regarding the processes responsible for the self-referentially enhancement effect in memory. The special role of self is also evident in Klein's chapter, in which he examines how people store information about themselves. He concludes that there is a subsystem of semantic memory that is dedicated to storing personality trait information in summary form, and that this system is not dependent on intact episodic memory (as revealed by studies of amnesic patients.). As Klein notes, the advent of cognitive neuroscience has allowed researchers to examine vexing questions about the self that were first raised, but not answered, by William James.

It is clear from recent research that many aspects of social behavior rely on specialized regions of the prefrontal cortex. For instance, Macrae, Heatherton, and Kelley discuss the importance of the medial prefrontal cortex for many aspects of social cognition, such as theory of mind. In their chapter, Beer, Shimamura, and Knight review various executive functions of prefrontal cortex, such as how dorsolateral regions are involved in control over attention. They also discuss the important role of the prefrontal cortex, especially orbitofrontal cortex, in the integration of emotion and cognition. Their studies of patients with prefrontal brain injury document impairments in the social domain, such as understanding how other people interpret their behavior, a capacity that requires theory of mind. The social brain sciences are in their infancy, with scholars from widely diverse areas (e.g., social psychology, neuroscience, philosophy, anthropology) working together and across levels of analysis to understand fundamental questions about human social nature. At the same time, there has been rapid progress in identifying the neural basis of many social behaviors. Many of the chapters in this section reflect this new field and describe some of the exciting new discoveries about human social behavior.

The chapters in this section make it clear that the study of emotion continues to be a strong growth area in cognitive neuroscience. Moreover, it has expanded to include the closely connected social brain. As an organ that has evolved to solve adaptive problems, the brain relies on emotional processes to solve challenges to successful adaptation. For humans, many of the most pernicious adaptive problems involve other humans, such as selecting mates, cooperating in hunting and gathering, forming alliances, competing over scarce resources, and even warring with neighboring groups. Interacting with other humans produces emotion, and these emotions serve as guidelines for successful group living. For example, behaviors such as lying, cheating, or stealing are discouraged by social norms in all societies because they decrease survival and reproduction for other group members. They also elicit vigorous emotional responses, knowing whether to trust somebody requires intact emotional processing systems, as is made clear by Adolphs's chapter. Hence, any true understanding of human nature will require a full consideration of both the emotional and the social brain. We expect that research on this topic will continue to be on the cutting edge of cognitive neuroscience in the next decade.

REFERENCES

ADOLPHS, R., 2003. Cognitive neuroscience of human social behavior. *Nat. Rev. Neurosci.* 4:165–178.

LEDOUX, J. E., 2000. Introduction. In *The New Cognitive Neurosciences*, M. S. Gazzaniga, ed. Cambridge, Mass.: MIT Press, pp. 1065–1066.

MITCHELL, J. P., T. F. HEATHERTON, and C. N. MACRAE, 2002. Distinct neural systems subserve person and object knowledge. *Proc. Natl. Acad. Sci. U.S.A.* 99:15238–15243.

70 Social Neuroscience

JOHN T. CACIOPPO AND GARY G. BERNTSON

ABSTRACT   The past decade has seen the emergence of the interdisciplinary field of social neuroscience, which involves collaborations between cognitive scientists, social psychologists, neuroscientists, anthropologists, geneticists, biologists, neurologists, endocrinologists, and many others in related disciplines. Social neuroscience employs multiple methods of investigation with humans and other animals to address questions concerning interactions between mind, brain, and the social world.

A few well-publicized clinical cases in the nineteenth century provided early signs of the role of the brain, particularly the frontal and temporal lobes, in social cognition, interpersonal processes, and behavior. The most famous is the case of Phineas Gage, a young American railroad construction supervisor who, in 1848, accidentally detonated a dynamite blast, sending a tamping rod rocketing through his eye and skull and decimating portions of the orbitofrontal and ventromedial cortex (Damasio et al., 1994). Gage was knocked over but may not have lost consciousness, and could speak and walk following the accident (Haas, 2001). He was taken to a local physician, John Harlow, who treated his wound, blood loss, and subsequent infection (Harlow, 1868). Gage soon recovered from the life-threatening nature of his accident, but he did not recover his former self. Prior to the accident, Gage was characterized as energetic, friendly, and reliable. Within a few months after the accident, he began acting in a fitful, irreverent, grossly profane manner, showing little deference to other workers. Described as impatient and obstinate yet capricious and vacillating, Gage was unable to proceed with any plans (Haas, 2001). He became incapable of holding a job or planning his future, and his friends complained that Gage was no longer the person they had known. He died penniless on May 21, 1860, 13 years after the accident, more an abomination than a shadow of his former self.

The twentieth century saw remarkable advances in the neurosciences, cognitive sciences, and social sciences, although scientific ventures and advances across these broad domains were quite limited until cognitive scientists and neuroscientists began to collaborate to unravel puzzles of the brain and mind (e.g., Gazzaniga, 1999; Kandel and Squire,

JOHN T. CACIOPPO   Department of Psychology, University of Chicago, Chicago, Ill.

GARY G. BERNTSON   Departments of Psychology and Psychiatry, Ohio State University, Columbus, Oh.

2000). The case of Phineas Gage, as well as those of Paul Broca's patient, Leborgne, who was known as "Tan," because this was the only word he was left able to speak (Schiller, 1979), and Angelo Mosso's patient, Bertino, who suffered a head injury that left him with part of his frontal lobes exposed to observation (Mosso, 1881), contributed to two foundational principles in cognitive neuroscience: (1) a lesion of circumscribed areas of the brain could cause the loss of very specific mental or nervous functions in humans (Haas, 2001), and (2) activity in circumscribed areas of the brain could reflect very specific mental or nervous functions in humans (Raichle, 2000). The greatest specificity of neurofunction mapping is found within the motor and sensory systems, and the extent of neurological differentiation for some integrative functions continues to be debated. Nevertheless, contemporary research continues to reveal anatomical differentiation even among higher-level psychological processes, and this differentiation is increasingly apparent as neural and psychological conceptions are refined in the light of interdisciplinary research. Although there is likely a limit to neurofunctional specificity, and although distributed processing clearly exists within neural circuits, appreciation of the boundaries of neural specificity and differentiation will be vitally important in the ultimate understanding of brain–behavior relations.

Throughout most of the twentieth century, the neurosciences emphasized cellular processes and neural substrates and production mechanisms for behavior, largely rejecting or ignoring mentalist and functionalist theories, whereas the social sciences emphasized multivariate systems, situational influences, and applications. These differences resulted in very different subject samples, research traditions, and technical demands, leaving what some regard as an unbridgeable abyss between social and biological approaches (Scott, 1991). The notion that billions of neurons can give rise to the human mind also inclined many neuroscientists to regard the social aspects of the mind as unimportant in the search for basic principles or as too complicated to sustain scientific progress (Wilson, 1998). As a result, some of the most distinguishing human traits, ranging from notions of the self and morality to social identity to culture, were left unstudied. This oversight is interesting in light of the intimation from the cases of Gage, Leborgne, and Bertino that the brain is not simply an information processing organ but also organizes information in a form that distinguishes self from others, biases information processing in ways that protects the self from actual and symbolic threats to support reproductive success, and promotes social identity, cooperation, and civil-social discourse.

As the twenty-first century dawns, evidence is accumulating showing that social factors have profound implications for basic development, structure, or processes of the brain or mind, and that comprehensive theories of the human mind and behavior may require the integrative study of behavior across multiple levels of organization, ranging from the biological to the social (e.g., Cacioppo and Berntson, 1992; Cacioppo, Berntson et al., 2000). This is less surprising when one considers that genes not only underlie cellular processes and behavior but are sculpted by an organism's adaptation to the environment (Lewontin, 2000). For humans, this is a social environment. For infants to survive, they must instantly engage their parents in protective behavior, and parents must care enough about their offspring to nurture and protect them (Bowlby, 1969). Although food is essential for survival, positive tactile contact has been found to be a stronger determinant of mother-infant attachment than feeding (Harlow and Harlow, 1973). Across history, cultures, and the life span, solitary confinement and ostracism are universal in their aversive and deleterious effects on humans (Felthous, 1997; Williams, 1997), and social isolation is as large a risk factor for broad-based morbidity and mortality as cigarette smoking (House, Landis, and Umberson, 1988).

The capacity for symbolic group identity, which appears to be unique to humans, extends the rewards of cooperative exchange beyond a dyad to groups, alliances, institutions, and societies (Brewer and Miller, 1996). Accordingly, functional magnetic resonance imaging (fMRI) research indicates that cooperation among humans activates the same neural systems as do appetitive stimuli and symbolic rewards (Rilling et al., 2002). Communication and coordination among humans is served by a language system, and its development unfolds even in the rare instances in which language is not modeled, heard, or taught (e.g., Goldin-Meadow and Mylander, 1984). Even when humans are grown, they are not particularly formidable physical specimens. Human survival depends not on individual might but on collective abilities, and the human brain has evolved accordingly.

Although multilevel research may be a challenging enterprise, the payoff can be substantial. Especially challenging are efforts to integrate information across levels of analyses, but this is precisely what is necessary for the ultimate interdisciplinary convergence on mind–body issues. The ultimate goal of multilevel analysis is to mutually calibrate concepts, relate measures, and integrate information across levels so as to inform processes and constrain theories at multiple levels of analysis (Berntson and Cacioppo, in press). This process represents reductionism, not in the sense of substitutionism,

but in the sense of better science based on the value of data derived from distinct levels of analysis to constrain and inspire the interpretation of data derived from others (Berntson and Cacioppo, in press; Cacioppo and Berntson, 1992). This chapter reviews a perspective that developed from this work, namely, social neuroscience (cf. Cacioppo et al., 2002).

The social brain: Information processing with a twist

Among the major evolutionary advantages in humans is the striking development of the human cerebral cortex, especially the frontal and temporal regions. The cerebral cortex is a mantle of approximately 30 billion neurons interconnected by about 100,000 km of axons. The frontal and temporal lobes constitute 32% and 23% of the cerebral cortex, respectively, reducing the somatosensory cortices that dominate lower mammalian brains to minority status in the human brain. The expansion of the frontal regions in the human brain is largely responsible for the human capacity for reasoning, planning, and performing mental simulations, and, as illustrated in the cases of Phineas Gage and Bertino, an intact frontal region contributes to the human ability to reason, remember, and work together (e.g., Adolphs, 1999, 2003; Frith and Frith, 2001). The temporal regions, in turn, play essential roles in social perception and communication (e.g., Brothers, 1990; Allison, Puce, and McCarthy, 2000).

Human information processing capacities remain woefully insufficient even with the expansion of the cortices, however. The sensory load from the physical environment is minor in comparison with the quantity and complexity of the information that comes from other individuals, groups, alliances, and cultures—as well as the potential for treachery from each. It is perhaps understandable why social cognition is not a rational information process but instead is rife with the operation of self-interest, self-enhancement, and self-protective processes. These emergent properties from the operation of the human brain, sculpted by adaptive and reproductive successes and failures, provide a view on cognitive neuroscience that otherwise may not be readily apparent.

In the twentieth century, the nuances of social cognition and social processes, including unconscious processes, were plumbed primarily through the clever experimental designs and measures of verbal reports, judgments, and reaction time. These methods were limited in what they could reveal about the processes and mechanisms underlying social behavior, though. Social cognition and behavior are often affect-laden or habitual, and nuances deriving from these features proved difficult to capture fully using subjective measures and response latencies to semantic (e.g., lexical decision) tasks (Zajonc, 1980). As important as these developments are, the same scientific forces that fueled the emergence of cognitive neuroscience are fueling the development of social neuroscience: theory and methods in the neurosciences constrain and inspire hypotheses in the behavioral and social sciences, foster experimental tests of otherwise indistinguishable theoretical explanations, and increase the comprehensiveness and relevance of social and behavioral theories (Cacioppo and Berntson, 1992; Cacioppo et al., 2002; Ochsner and Lieberman, 2001).

Specifically, studies of the neurophysiological structures and functions associated with psychological events were limited in the nineteenth century and much of the twentieth century to animal models, postmortem examinations, and observations of the occasional unfortunate individual who suffered trauma to or disorders of the brain. Although these studies indicated a connection between brain regions and social processes (Klein and Kihlstrom, 1998; see Adolphs, this volume), sustained progress in the field of social neuroscience awaited developments in electrophysiological recording, brain imaging, neurochemical studies, and gene mapping techniques within the neurosciences. Contemporary studies of racial prejudice, for instance, have utilized facial electromyography (Vanman, 2001), event-related brain potentials (ERPs; Ito and Cacioppo, 1999), and fMRI (Phelps et al., 2000) to investigate specific representations and processing stages. And advances in ambulatory recording and its combination with experience sampling methods have removed the tether of the laboratory to permit in vivo investigations of biology and social behavior (Shiffman and Stone, 1998; Hawkley et al., 2003).

Social processes and behavior: Multipurpose or specialized neural mechanisms?

One of the fundamental questions in the field is whether specific social constructs, processes, and representations have a single neural locus. The neural and hormonal substrates for sexual and reproductive responses notwithstanding, is social information processed by specialized neural circuitry? There are two complementary strategies for addressing this question: one can examine the function or functions associated with a particular neural locus or region to determine if it exclusively serves social information processing, or one can place the focus on a specific social process or function to examine the different neural mechanisms through which this function is achieved.

In a seminal thesis based primarily on neurophysiological recordings in nonhuman primates, Brothers (1990) proposed that the superior temporal sulcus (STS) is involved in integrative processing of conspecifics' behavior, and the amygdala and orbitofrontal cortex are subsequently involved in specifying the socioemotional relevance of social information. Kanwisher (e.g., Kanwisher, McDermott, and Chun,

1997; Kanwisher, 2000), using fMRI data, emphasized the role of the fusiform gyrus in face processing, and Damasio and colleagues (e.g., Damasio, 1994), focusing primarily on data from humans with brain lesions, have emphasized the role of the frontal (ventromedial prefrontal, orbitofrontal) cortex, amygdala, and somatosensory cortex (insula, S1, S2) in social perception, cognition, and decision making. More specifically, the thalamus, amygdala, ventral striatum, basal forebrain, hypothalamus, and periacqueductal gray area have been suggested to be components of a circuit involved in rapid, automatic social behaviors, the insular cortex and somatosensory cortices may play a role in feelings and social emotions (e.g., sympathy, empathy, guilt), and the ventromedial cortex and basal forebrain in conjunction with associative areas appear involved in more elaborative processing of social stimuli and contexts (Damasio, 1999). Drawing primarily from data from brain lesion studies, Adolphs (1999, 2001, 2003) has suggested that social cognition draws on neural mechanisms for perceiving, recognizing, and evaluating stimuli, and these and subsequent mechanisms are then used to construct complex central representations of the social environment. These central processes involve the fusiform gyrus and the STS in the temporal region, as well as the amygdala, orbitofrontal cortex, anterior and posterior cingulate cortices, and right somatosensory-related cortices. Like nonsocial information processing, the central processes of social cognition modulate effector systems, including the motor and premotor cortices, basal ganglia, hypothalamus, and periacqueductal gray (see Adolphs, this volume; Phelps, this volume). Thus, the neural mechanisms underlying social behavior are only beginning to be explored, with current evidence cautioning that multiple processing pathways may be involved.

Disputes have emerged regarding whether certain nuclei (e.g., fusiform gyrus) function to process social information (e.g., faces; Kanwisher, 2000) or more generic forms of information (e.g., objects about which there is expertise; Farah et al., 1998; Gauthier et al., 2000, 2003) and about the specific contribution to social cognition made by various nuclei. These disputes depend in part on the conceptualization of localization and in part on the conceptualization of what is localized. Rather than nuclei serving a single social process, for instance, the extant data suggest that a small set of cortical areas may be active in a wide range of psychological functions from action to perception to theory of mind, but across those functions the networks in which they participate may be quite different.

Ideas about the anatomical basis of functional localization in the cortex were debated for hundreds of years, until research on primary sensory cortices (e.g., Munk, 1881; Tunturi, 1952) and on somatosensory regions (e.g., Schaltenbrand and Woolsey, 1964) refuted the hypothesis that the brain was a homogeneous tissue that depended on total mass to carry out functions. The more recent discovery of mirror neurons in monkeys also cautions against a premature assignment of function to structures and at the same time illustrates the potential brain localization of social information processing. Mirror neurons are a class of neurons in the ventral premotor cortex of monkeys in area F5 that become active when the monkey makes a particular action or when it observes another individual making a similar action (Rizzolatti, Fogassi, and Gallese, 2001). The same neurons also respond when the monkey perceives an object that affords specific kinds of motor behaviors (Rizzolatti and Fadiga, 1998; Grezes and Decety, 2002), but they do not otherwise tend to respond to the presentation of an object of an action, or to the mimicking of an action in the absence of the object. Kohler and colleagues (2002) recorded from individual neurons in the F5 area of monkeys homologous to Broca's area in humans. They found that individual neurons responded when the monkey performed specific motor behaviors, when the monkey observed other individuals performing the same behavior, and when the monkeys heard but could not see the same behavior being performed by another. These results indicate that visual and audiovisual mirror neurons code not the visual analysis of the action per se but the goal and meaning of the actions of both oneself and others, as well as the perspective one takes on those actions (Ruby and Decety, 2001).

More generally, well-defined localization of sensory and motor functions poses as a hypothesis but does not prove that more complex integrative processing by the brain is similarly compartmentalized. Brothers (1990), for instance, suggested that the amygdala was an essential component of a set of nuclei involved in social cognition. Kluver and Bucy first demonstrated notable emotional and social effects of lesions to the anterior temporal lobes and the amygdalae, including affective blunting and hypersexuality, effects that have also been observed in humans (see Nahm, 1997). Monkeys with amygdalectomies have also been reported to be socially ostracized by their troop (Dicks, Myers, and Kling, 1969). This led to the view, subsequently challenged (Amaral et al., 2003), that the amygdala was essential for the normal perception and production of expressive displays and behaviors and that damage to the amygdala undermined an animal's capacity for effective social interactions.

The amygdala has been implicated in surprisingly fundamental aspects of human social cognition. One such demonstration was based on the social inferences elicited by Heider and Simmel's (1946) short film of three geometric shapes in motion. The relative distances among these three shapes, and their positions in and about a large rectangle, varied during the film. Heider and Simmel reported that everyone who watched the film attributed individual identities, social categories, and interpersonal relationships, motives, and emotions to the geometric shapes. However, Adolphs (1999,

Box 2) reported that when S.M., an individual with selective bilateral cystic lesions of the amygdala attributable to Urbach-Wiethe syndrome, viewed this film, she did not spontaneously make social attributions or draw social inferences but instead simply described the movement of geometric shapes. S.M.'s description was exceptional not because it was inaccurate (indeed, it was entirely accurate, in contrast to the story told by normal viewers) but because she saw no social meaning beyond the movement of the geometric shapes (Adolphs, 1999).

S.M.'s intelligence is not impaired, and she is capable of normal social encounters, although she is less likely to recognize fear or untrustworthy facial expressions as fearful or potentially dangerous. When S.M. was told how others viewed Heider and Simmel's film and was asked if she could see the social story that was unfolding, she was able to do so (Adolphs, 2000, personal communication). Together, the interesting study of S.M. suggests she was capable of ascribing social meaning to the movement of the shapes, but in the absence of the input from the amygdala she failed to do so automatically (Adolphs, 1999).

The amygdala, perhaps because of its role in affective processing (see LeDoux, this volume; Phelps, this volume), has also been implicated in evaluative aspects of social information processing. Phelps and colleagues (2000) tested Caucasian participants in an fMRI study and found that activation of the amygdala to black versus white faces correlated with the participants' racial evaluation as measured by the Implicit Association Test (IAT), an implicit measure of race bias (Greenwald, McGhee, and Schwartz, 1998). This result was interpreted as indicating that the amygdala was involved in indirect or nonconscious responses to racial groups, and hence in performance on the IAT (e.g., Phelps, Cannistraci, and Cunningham, 2000). Of course, the correlation between the IAT and amygdala activity may reflect the operation of a broader neural circuit rather than the function of the amygdala per se. To examine this possibility, Phelps, Cannistraci, and Cunningham (2003) conducted a follow-up study in which they compared the responses to the IAT of two groups of participants: a group of patients with bilateral amygdala damage and a matched control group. Phelps and colleagues (2003) replicated prior research on the IAT (and related measures) in the control group. They further demonstrated, however, that the patient group did not differ from the control group on any of their measures. That is, they showed comparably negative evaluation toward blacks on the IAT, suggesting that the amygdala is not critical for the indirect or nonconscious responses to racial groups.

In Adolph's (1999) report of S.M. and in Phelps's studies of racial prejudice, the amygdala appears to be involved in, but not necessary for, social cognition. Using macaque monkeys, Amaral and colleagues (Prather et al., 2001;

Amaral et al., 2003) examined the role of the amygdala in social cognition using a more circumscribed lesion of the amygdala and quantitative measures of dyadic social interactions.

Amaral and colleagues (2003) observed the social behavior of monkeys with ibotenic acid lesions of the amygdala and controls matched for age, sex, and dominance. Results revealed that the lesion of the amygdala appears to reduce social inhibitions. For instance, the lesioned monkeys did not go through the normal period of evaluation of an unfamiliar monkey before engaging in social interactions. As a result, the lesioned monkeys initiated more affiliative social behavior than the control monkeys. More interestingly, the lesioned monkeys were not shunned because of their early and non-normative forwardness toward the control monkeys, but instead the control monkeys were more likely to reciprocate, generating more affiliative social behaviors toward the lesioned than the control monkeys. Amaral and colleagues (2003) concluded, "The inevitable conclusion from this study is that in dyadic social interactions, monkeys with extensive bilateral lesions of the amygdala can interpret and generate social gestures and initiate and receive more affiliative social interactions than controls" (p. 238). Amaral and colleagues suggested that the amygdala functions to suppress the engagement of objects and conspecifics while an evaluation of the potential threat is conducted. In the absence of a functioning amygdala, conspecifics are not regarded as potentially dangerous or the social context is regarded as safe, and therefore social interactions are engaged. The very different picture painted of the role of the amygdala in prior work, Amaral and colleagues have suggested, may be due to lesions that went beyond the amygdala and to differences in the treatment and housing of the lesioned and control animals.

Importantly, the amygdala appears to play a role in threat appraisals generally, not only in the evaluation of potential dyadic partners (Amaral et al., 2003). The latency to retrieve a food reward from in front of a stimulus object is slowed in normal animals when the stimulus has fear-provoking qualities (e.g., a rubber snake), but the latency of lesioned monkeys is not altered in this test environment.

Prather and colleagues (2001) evaluated whether the amygdala was essential not for the emission of social behaviors but for the learning of social behaviors. Young monkeys underwent the same bilateral lesion of the amygdala at 2 weeks of age. Steps were taken to ensure opportunities for normal social development and to avoid the behavioral differences associated with nursery rearing. Results reveal interactions with the mother that are similar for lesioned and control animals. The lesioned animals also showed little fear of normally fear-provoking objects (e.g., a rubber snake), although they did show less social interaction and more fear grimaces and screams in novel dyadic social interactions.

Most social behaviors, however, were indistinguishable between lesioned and control animals.

In sum, the research on the essential role of the amygdala in social cognition suggests two principles: (1) even though the dramatic expansion of the human brain may have been fueled by the complexities of social interactions and communication, the central processes that evolved to accommodate this complexity are not necessarily limited to social information processing; and (2) the study of the social functions of brain mechanisms can advance our understanding of the specific nature of brain function. The amygdala does not operate in isolation, of course, and cortical as well as subcortical areas may be active in a wide range of behavioral functions. When thinking about the assignment of a function to a specific region (e.g., amygdala), it is important to consider the possibility that a given region may participate in very different networks. Indeed, Passingham, Stephan, and Kötter (2002) reviewed evidence that cortical region have unique patterns of corticocortical connections, and it is these more distributed subsystems of brain regions that produce the observed (more localized) differences in neural activity during different tasks.

Heterarchical organization of the central nervous system

In the preceding section, we reviewed representative work on a neural region, the amygdala, that is putatively essential for social cognition. In this section, we examine an essential function underlying adaptive behavior, evaluative processes, that is responsible for an organism's ability to differentiate hostile from hospitable stimuli. As one might expect, there is overlap in these two approaches. The evidence just reviewed on the amygdala indicates that in the absence of a functioning amygdala, primates appear not to have the capacity to differentiate hostile from hospitable conspecifics. However, the central nervous system (CNS) builds in redundant systems for achieving a variety of intraorganismic (e.g., regulatory) and behavioral functions (e.g., Berntson et al., 1993; Berntson, Cacioppo, and Sarter, 2003). We recall that patient S.M. did not spontaneously view Heider and Simmel's film of geometric objects as having a social connotation, but she was able to do so when prompted.

Differentiating hostile from hospitable others and events is such a critical capacity that all animals have rudimentary reflexes for categorizing and approaching or withdrawing from certain classes of stimuli, and for providing metabolic support for these actions. Evaluative discriminations are performed in simple organisms by hard-wired stimulus-response connections or fixed-action patterns, and human infants are also endowed with a finite set of hard-wired evaluative discriminations, including a startle response to sudden, intense noises and retreat from nociceptive stimuli (Berntson et al., 1993; Berntson, Cacioppo, and Sarter, 2003). The defensive withdrawal reflex is organized at the level of the spinal cord, and it can be classically conditioned for protection from nociceptive stimulation. A remarkable feature of humans is the extent to which the evaluative discrimination of stimuli is shaped by learning, cognition, modeling, and culture.

The nineteenth-century neurologist John Hughlings Jackson emphasized the hierarchical structure of the brain, and the re-representation of functions at multiple levels within this neural hierarchy (Jackson, 1884/1958). Primitive protective responses to aversive stimuli are organized at the level of the spinal cord, as is apparent in flexor (pain) withdrawal reflexes, which can be seen even after spinal transection. These primitive protective reactions are expanded and embellished at higher levels of the nervous system. The evolutionary development of higher neural systems, such as the limbic system, endowed organisms with an expanded behavioral repertoire, including escape reactions, aggressive responses, and even the ability to anticipate and avoid aversive encounters (Berntson et al., 1993). Evolution not only endowed humans with primitive, lower-level adaptive reactions, it also sculpted the remarkable information processing capacities of the highest levels of the brain. Thus, the neurobehavioral mechanisms underlying evaluative processes are not localized to a single level of organization within the brain but rather are represented at multiple levels of the nervous system. At progressively higher (more rostral) levels of organization (spinal, brainstem, limbic, cortical regions) there is a general expansion in the range and relational complexity of contextual controls and in the breadth and flexibility of discriminative and adaptive responses (Berntson et al., 1993).

Adaptive flexibility of higher-level systems has costs, given the finite information processing capacity of neural circuits (Berntson, Cacioppo, and Sarter, 2003). Greater flexibility implies a less rigid relationship between inputs and outputs, a greater range of information that must be processed, and a slower, serial-like mode of processing. Consequently, the evolutionary layering of higher processing levels onto lower substrates has adaptive advantage in that lower and more efficient processing levels may continue to be utilized, and may be sufficient in some circumstances (Berntson, Sarter, and Cacioppo, 1998; Berntson, Cacioppo, and Sarter, 2003). Higher neurobehavioral processes, however, can come to suppress or bypass pain withdrawal reflexes. If an individual unknowingly touches a hot flame, the individual reflexively withdraws his or her hand from the painful fire. If, however, the person hears a child on the other side of a wall of flames, he or she can override this defensive reflex and push through the flames. This is neither the only nor the most likely action that such an individual would take: he or she would likely show a more flexible, contextually appropriate response such as looking for a doorway or passage to the child that was not engulfed by flames, or donning fire-retardant covering (e.g., wet blanket) before challenging the flames to retrieve the child.

Although we might have the impression that we are the captains of our course, primitive evaluative dispositions can exert powerful influences on behavior. Boysen and colleagues (1996) illustrated this principle in a study of chimpanzees who had been trained extensively in simple arithmetic operations (counting, addition, subtraction) using arabic numerals. The animal could see two reinforcement pans, each of which was baited with different quantities of candies on each trial. A reversed reinforcement contingency was implemented such that the animal received the candies from the pan to which it did not point. Thus, it was in the chimpanzee's best interest to select the smaller of the two candy arrays in order to obtain the remaining, larger quantity. Even after hundreds of training trials across dozens of sessions, performance was significantly below chance. Moreover, this performance worsened at higher reward ratios, where the animals stood to benefit the most. This was true for all chimps in the study.

We posited that the inherent evaluative disposition based on the perceptual features of the candy arrays interfered with optimal performance based on the underlying rule structure of the task (Boysen et al., 1996). To test this hypothesis, the chimps performed the same task, but rather than candy arrays being used as stimuli, placards with corresponding arabic numerals were substituted. Thus, the animal received the number of candies that corresponded to the nonselected numeral. This change led to an immediate above-chance performance. When the candies were again used as experimental stimuli, performance fell immediately to below-chance levels, and when the arabic numerals were used, performance rose immediately to above chance. These results suggested that the chimps had acquired the rules of the task, but this knowledge, or at least its effect on behavior, was obscured by a potent competing disposition arising from the intrinsic incentive properties of the candy arrays. Lower-level evaluative processing is generally adaptive, but there are situations in which it is not. It is therefore interesting to note that these data further suggest that humans evolved the capacity to work with symbolic representations of the world because symbols helped minimize the powerful and sometimes maladaptive dictates of lower evaluative dispositions.

The anatomical systems underlying such judgments and behavior remain to be clarified, although the amygdala, nucleus accumbens, and the prefrontal cortex likely play important roles. This circuit is sufficient for simple or foreground conditioning but not for contextual (or background) conditioning, which is dependent on cortical circuits (Phillips and LeDoux, 1992, 1994). These data are consistent with the thesis that the acquisition and representation of affective (evaluative) dispositions can operate at multiple, interrelated levels of the neuraxis and suggest that the rapid responses by the chimps that failed to take into consideration the contextual contingency information were served by neural structures in the limbic region, whereas the chimps' responses to the symbols that reflected a consideration of the reverse contingency information may have been served by the prefrontal regions. In the latter regard, it is interesting to note that the ventromedial and lateral portions of the orbitofrontal cortex have been associated with the abstract representation of reward (O'Doherty et al., 2001). Identifying the specific nature, timing, and integration of the neural processes operating across multiple levels of the neuraxis, the antecedents and moderators of these processes, and the unique consequences resulting from effectors governed by these different processes remains an important scientific challenge.

An important neural modulator of the level of processing appears to be the basal forebrain cortical cholinergic system. This system is the primary source of cholinergic innervation of the cerebral cortex, which sets the functional tone of cortical processing (see, e.g., Berntson, Shafi, and Sarter, 2002; Bentson, Shafi et al., 2003). It is degeneration within this system that leads to the global dementia of Alzheimer's disease, and activation of this system promotes attentional processing of threat-related stimuli (Berntson, Sarter, and Cacioppo, 1998). Projections of this system to the medial prefrontal cortex may be particularly important in mediating anxiety-like reactions to contextual stimuli (Hart, Sarter, and Berntson, 1999) but would likely be less critical for simple fear conditioning. Because the basal forebrain cholinergic system acts as a gain control switch over cortical processing, it would likely be an important contributor to the level of processing. Thus, pharmacological blunting of this system by anxiolytic benzodiazepine agonists such as chlordiazepoxide (Librium) attenuates cortical/cognitive processing and results in a relative downward shift in processing levels (see Berntson, Sarter, and Cacioppo, 1998). What remains unclear is how psychological states and processes might affect activity within this level-switching system. This is an important topic for future research.

An implication of the rapid operation of lower evaluative mechanism is that their ascending input might mildly predispose an individual's thoughts, feelings, or preferences for a stimulus. Consistent with this notion, individuals become more positive toward initially neutral and unfamiliar Chinese ideographs when they are first exposed to the stimuli with their arms in a state associated with approach reactions (flexing the arm, as if pulling something toward them) than when they are first exposed to the stimuli with their arms in a state associated with avoidance reactions (extending the arm, as if pushing something away), even though participants are unaware of any link between their arm positions and motivational or affective responses (Cacioppo, Priester, and Berntson, 1993). The presence of

prior knowledge or feelings about the stimuli should diminish these subtle ascending influences, a prediction supported by Priester, Cacioppo, and Petty (1996): the effects of arm flexion and extension on subsequent preferences for stimuli were evident for neutral, pronounceable and novel nonwords (e.g., *balet*), but not for neutral, familiar words (e.g., *table*).

It is also clear that visceral feedback can impact cortical and cognitive processing and may serve as a bottom-up regulator of the level of functional processing. Systemic epinephrine, for example, potentiates the cerebral auditory-evoked response and enhances memory processes—effects that are dependent in part on the basal forebrain cholinergic system (Berntson, Cacioppo, and Sarter, 2003; Power, Thal, and McGaugh, 2002). Thus, it is clear that lower-level states can bias high-level processes, and higher-level processes are known to reciprocally impact lower-level functions. This neurobehavioral heterarchy parallels the levels of psychological function in attitude formation, as considered earlier. An important research direction will be to elucidate the links and relations between the neurobiological and psychological domains. Knowledge of the underlying neurobiology may guide the development of psychological theories (and vice versa) and may suggest specific hypotheses. For example, in view of the attenuating effects of benzodiazepine agonists on the basal forebrain cholinergic system, these pharmacological agents would be predicted to have effects on attitude formation that parallel the effects of limited information, or attentional distraction.

In sum, the localization hypothesis has considerable intuitive appeal and undeniable empirical support. As processes become more complex, localization becomes more distributed, if for no other reason than that more processes are involved. Moreover, because of levels of organization in the CNS, even simple processes such as motor acts have multiple representations (e.g., pyramidal, extrapyramidal). Social processes, too, may be re-represented across levels of the neuraxis and distributed broadly in the cortices. The refined feelings of social acceptance or rejection, approval or disapproval, and admiration or condemnation may serve as powerful motivational forces guiding thought and behavior, but these feelings represent the product of a host of resident processes that have evolved over millennia. There is no singular central process underlying all evaluations, attitudes, or preferences, nor are all evaluative processes automatic. Instead, there are multiple neurobehavioral mechanisms across the neuraxis that serve evaluative processes and behavior. Relative to caudal mechanisms, rostral mechanisms are slower, more serial-like, characterized by greater response flexibility, and subject to greater contextual control and, thus, more culturally appropriate behavior—reflective of qualities that are more distinctively those of the human social animal. Hence, although the features that most define what it means to be human depend on rostral neurobehavioral mechanisms, a comprehensive understanding of social processes and behavior requires an understanding not only of these rostral mechanisms but also of their integration with the full range of neural and humoral mechanisms that contribute to the social brain.

Conclusion

As neuroscientific approaches are applied to more complex questions, what were thought to be basic principles are being revisited. This is the case for principles in the neurosciences as well as the social sciences. Social neuroscience is premised on the notion that biological, cognitive, and social levels of analysis, and a dialogue and integrative collaborations among scientists working at these levels of analyses, will contribute to more comprehensive explanations of the human mind and behavior.

ACKNOWLEDGMENTS This work was supported by National Institute of Aging grant No. PO1 AG18911, National Science Foundation grant No. BCS-0086314, and National Institute of Mental Health grant No. P50MH52384-01A1.

REFERENCES

ADOLPHS, R., 1999. Social cognition and the human brain. *Trends Cogn. Sci.* 3:469–479.

ADOLPHS, R., 2001. The neurobiology of social cognition. *Curr. Opin. Neurobiol.* 11:231–239.

ADOLPHS, R., 2003. Cognitive neuroscience of human social behaviour. *Neurosci. Rev.* 4:165–178.

ALLISON, T., A. PUCE, and G. McCARTHY, 2000. Social perception from visual cues: Role of the STS region. *Trends Cogn. Sci.* 4:267–278.

AMARAL, D. G., J. P. CAPITANIO, M. JOURDAIN, W. A. MASON, S. P. MENDOZA, and M. PRATHER, 2003. The amygdala: Is it an essential component of the neural network for social cognition? *Neuropsychologica* 41:235–240.

BERNTSON, G. G., S. T. BOYSEN, and J. T. CACIOPPO, 1993. Neurobehavioral organization and the cardinal principle of evaluative bivalence. *Ann. N.Y. Acad. Sci.* 702:75–102.

BERNTSON, G. G., and J. T. CACIOPPO, in press. Multilevel analyses and reductionism: Why social psychologists should care about neuroscience and vice versa. In *Essays in Social Neuroscience*, J. T. Cacioppo and G. G. Berntson, eds. Cambridge, Mass.: MIT Press, p. 11.

BERNTSON, G. G., J. T. CACIOPPO, and M. SARTER, 2003. Bottom-up: Implications for neurobehavioral models of anxiety and autonomic regulation. In *Handbook of Affective Sciences*, R. J. Davidson, K. R. Sherer, and H. H. Goldsmith, eds. New York: Oxford University Press, pp. 1105–1116.

BERNTSON, G. G., M. SARTER, and J. T. CACIOPPO, 1998. Anxiety and cardiovascular reactivity: The basal forebrain cholinergic link. *Behav. Brain Res.* 94:225–248.

BERNTSON, G. G., R. SHAFI, D. KNOX, and M. SARTER, 2003. Blockade of epinephrine priming of the cerebral auditory evoked response by cortical cholinergic deafferentation. *Neuroscience* 116:179–186.

BERNTSON, G. G., R. SHAFI, and M. SARTER, 2002. Specific contributions of the basal forebrain corticopetal cholinergic system to electroencephalographic activity and sleep/waking behavior. *Eur. J. Neurosci.* 16:2453–2461.

BOWLBY, J., 1969. *Attachment and Loss.* Vol. 1, *Attachment.* New York: Basic Books.

BOYSEN, S. T., G. G. BERNTSON, M. B. HANNAN, and J. T. CACIOPPO, 1996. Quantity-based choices: Interference and symbolic representations in chimpanzees (*Pan troglodytes*). *J. Exp. Psychol. Anim. Behav. Processes* 22:76–86.

BREWER, M. B., and N. MILLER, 1996. *Intergroup Relations.* Berkshire, U.K.: Open University Press (Brooks/Cole).

BROTHERS, L., 1990. The social brain: A project for integrating primate behavior and neurophysiology in a new domain. *Concepts Neurosci.* 1:27–51.

CACIOPPO, J. T., and G. G. BERNTSON, 1992. Social psychological contributions to the decade of the brain: The doctrine of multilevel analysis. *Am. Psychol.* 47:1019–1028.

CACIOPPO, J. T., G. G. BERNTSON, R. ADOLPHS, C. S. CARTER, R. J. DAVIDSON, M. K. McCLINTOCK, B. S. McEWEN, M. J. MEANEY, D. L. SCHACTER, E. M. STERNBERG, S. S. SUOMI, and S. E. TAYLOR, 2002. *Foundations in Social Neuroscience.* Cambridge, Mass.: MIT Press.

CACIOPPO, J. T., G. G. BERNTSON, J. F. SHERIDAN, and M. K. McCLINTOCK, 2000. Multi-level integrative analyses of human behavior: Social neuroscience and the complementing nature of social and biological approaches. *Psychol. Bull.* 126:829–843.

CACIOPPO, J. T., J. R. PRIESTER, and G. G. BERNTSON, 1993. Rudimentary determinants of attitudes. II. Arm flexion and extension have differential effects on attitudes. *J. Pers. Soc. Psychol.* 65:5–17.

DAMASIO, A. R., 1994. *Descartes' Error: Emotion, Reason, and the Human Brain.* New York: Grosset/Putnam.

DAMASIO, A. R., 1999. *The Feeling of What Happens: Body and Emotion in the Making of Consciousness.* New York: Harcourt.

DAMASIO, H., T. GRABOWSKI, R. FRANK, A. M. GALABURDA, and A. R. DAMASIO, 1994. The return of Phineas Gage: Clues about the brain from the skull of a famous patient. *Science* 264:1102–1105.

DICKS, D., R. E. MYERS, and A. KLING, 1969. Uncus and amygdala lesions: Effects on social behavior in the free ranging rhesus monkey. *Science* 165:69–71.

FARAH, M. J., K. D. WILSON, M. DRAIN, and J. N. TANAKA, 1998. What is "special" about face perception? *Psychol. Rev.* 105:482–498.

FELTHOUS, A. R., 1997. Does "isolation" cause jail suicides? *J. Am. Acad. Psychiatry Law* 25:285–294.

FRITH, U., and C. FRITH, 2001. The biological basis of social interaction. *Curr. Direct. Psychol. Sci.* 10:151–155.

GAUTHIER, I., T. CURRAN, K. M. CURBY, and D. COLLINS, 2003. Perceptual interference supports a non-modular account of face processing. *Nat. Neurosci.* 6:428–432.

GAUTHIER, I., P. SKUDLARSKI, J. C. GORE, and A. W. ANDERSON, 2000. Expertise for cars and birds recruits brain areas involved in face recognition. *Nat. Neurosci.* 3:191–197.

GAZZANIGA, M. S., ed., 1999. *The New Cognitive Neurosciences*, 2nd ed. Cambridge, Mass.: MIT Press.

GAZZANIGA, M. S., and J. E. LEDOUX, 1978. *The Integrated Mind.* New York: Plenum Press.

GOLDIN-MEADOW, S., and C. MYLANDER, 1984. Gestural communication in deaf children: The effects and noneffects of parental input on early language development. *Monogr. Soc. Res. Child Dev.* 49:1–121.

GREENWALD, A. G., D. E. MCGHEE, and J. L. K. SCHWARTZ, 1998. Measuring individual differences in implicit cognition: The Implicit Association Test. *J. Pers. Soc. Psychol.* 74:1464–1480.

GREZES, J., and J. DECETY, 2002. Does visual perception of the object afford action? Evidence from a neuroimaging study. *Neuropsychologia* 40:212–222.

HAAS, L. F., 2001. Phineas Gage and the science of brain localization. *Neurol. Neurosurg. Psychiatry* 71:761.

HARLOW, H. F., and M. K. HARLOW, 1973. Social deprivation in monkeys. In *Readings from the Scientific American: The Nature and Nurture of Behavior*, San Francisco: W. H. Freeman, pp. 108–116.

HARLOW, J. M., 1868. Recovery from the passage of an iron rod through the head. *Publications Mass. Med. Soc.* 2:327–347.

HART, S., M. SARTER, and G. G. BERNTSON, 1999. Cholinergic inputs to the rat medial prefrontal cortex mediate potentiation of the cardiovascular defensive response by the anxiogenic benzodiazepine receptor partial inverse agonist FG7142. *Neuroscience* 94:1029–1038.

HAWKLEY, L. C., M. H. BURLESON, G. G. BERNTSON, and J. T. CACIOPPO, 2003. Loneliness in everyday life: Cardiovascular activity, psychosocial context, and health behaviors. *J. Personality Soc. Psychol.* 85:105–120.

HEIDER, F., and M. SIMMEL, 1944. An experimental study of apparent behaviour. *Am. J. Psychol.* 57:243–259.

HOUSE, J. S., K. R. LANDIS, and D. UMBERSON, 1988. Social relationships and health. *Science* 241:540–545.

ITO, T. A., and J. T. CACIOPPO, 1999. Measuring racial prejudice with event-related potentials. *Psychophysiology* 36:S62.

JACKSON, J. H., 1884/1958. Evolution and dissolution of the nervous system (Croonian Lectures). In *Selected writings of John Hughlings Jackson*, J. Taylor, ed. New York: Basic Books.

KANDEL, E. R., and L. R. SQUIRE, 2000. Neuroscience: Breaking down scientific barriers to the study of brain and mind. *Science* 290:1113–1120.

KANWISHER, N., 2000. Domain specificity in face perception. *Nat. Neurosci.* 3:759–763.

KANWISHER, N., J. MCDERMOTT, and M. CHUN, 1997. The fusiform face area: A module in human extrastriate cortex specialized for face perception. *J. Neurosci.*

KLEIN, S. B., and J. F. KIHLSTROM, 1998. On bridging the gap between social-personality psychology and neuropsychology. *Pers. Soc. Psychol. Rev.* 2:228–242.

KOHLER, E., C. KEYSERS, M. A. UMILTÀ, L. FOGASSI, V. GALLESE, and G. RIZZOLATTI, 2002. Hearing sounds, understanding actions: Action representation in mirror neurons. *Science* 297:846–848.

LEWONTIN, R., 2000. *The Triple Helix.* Cambridge, Mass.: Harvard University Press.

MOSSO, A., 1881. *Ueber den Kreislauf des Blutes im menschlichen Gehirn.* Leipzig: Verlag von Veit & Co.

MUNK, H., 1881. *Uber die Funktionen der Grosshirnrinde.* Berlin: Hirschwald.

NAHM, F. K., 1997. Heinrich Klüver and the temporal lobe syndrome. *J. Hist. Neurosci.* 6:193–208.

O'DOHERTY, J., M. L. KRINGELBACH, E. T. ROLLS, J. HORNAK, and C. ANDREWS, 2001. Abstract reward and punishment representations in the human orbitofrontal cortex. *Nat. Neurosci.* 4:95–102.

OCHSNER, K. N., and M. D. LIEBERMAN, 2001. The emergence of social cognitive neuroscience. *Am. Psychol.* 56:717–734.

PASSINGHAM, R. E., K. E. STEPHAN, and R. KÖTTER, 2002. The anatomical basis of functional localization in the cortex. *Nat. Rev. Neurosci.* 3:1–11.

PHELPS, E. A., C. J. CANNISTRACI, and W. A. CUNNINGHAM, 2003. Intact performance on an indirect measure of race bias following amygdala damage. *Neuropsychologia* 41:203–208.

PHELPS, E. A., K. J. O'CONNER, W. A. CUNNINGHAM, E. S. FUNAYAMA, J. C. GATENBY, J. C. GORE, and M. R. BANAJI, 2000. Performance in indirect measure of race evaluation predicts amygdala activation. *J. Cogn. Neurosci.* 12:729–738.

PHILLIPS, R, G., and J. E. LEDOUX, 1992. Differential contribution of amygdala and hippocampus to cued and contextual fear conditioning. *Behav. Neurosci.* 106:274–285.

PHILLIPS, R. G., and J. E. LEDOUX, 1994. Lesions of the dorsal hippocampal formation interfere with background but not foreground contextual fear conditioning. *Learn. Mem.* 1:34–44.

POWER, A. E., L. J. THAL, and J. L. MCGAUGH, 2002. Lesions of the nucleus basalis magnocellularis induced by 192 IgG-saporin block memory enhancement with posttraining norepinephrine in the basolateral amygdala. *Proc. Nat. Acad. Sci.* 99:2315–2319.

PRATHER, M. D., P. LAVANEX, M. L. MAULDIN-JOURDAIN, W. A. MASON, J. P. CAPITANIO, S. P. MENDOZA, et al., 2001. Increased social fear and decreased fear of objects in monkeys with neonatal amygdala lesions. *Neuroscience* 106:653–658.

PRIESTER, J. R., J. T. CACIOPPO, and R. E. PETTY, 1996. The influence of motor processes on attitudes toward novel versus familiar semantic stimuli. *Personality Soc. Psychol. Bull.* 22:442–447.

RAICHLE, M. E., 2000. A brief history of human functional brain mapping. In *Brain Mapping: The Systems*, A. W. Toga and J. C. Mazziotta, eds. San Diego, Calif.: Academic Press, pp. 33–77.

RILLING, J. K., D. A. GUTMAN, T. R. ZEH, G. PAGNONI, G. S. BERNS, and C. D. KILTS, 2002. A neural basis for social cooperation. *Neuron* 35:395–405.

RIZZOLATTI, G., and L. FADIGA, 1998. Grasping objects and grasping action meanings: The dual role of monkey rostroventral premotor cortex (area F5). *Novartis Found. Symp.* 218:81–95.

RIZZOLATTI, G., L. FOGASSI, and V. GALLESE, 2001. Neurophysiological mechanisms underlying the understanding and imitation of action. *Nat. Rev. Neurosci.* 2:661–670.

RUBY, P., and J. DECETY, 2001. Effect of subjective perspective taking during simulation of action: A PET investigation of agency. *Nat. Neurosci.* 4:546–550.

SCHALTENBRAND, G., and C. N. WOOLSEY, 1964. Cerebral *Localization and Organization: Proceedings of a Symposium Sponsored by the World Federation of Neurology, Held at Lisbon, Portugal, October, 1960.* Madison: University of Wisconsin Press.

SCHILLER, F., 1979. *Paul Broca.* Berkeley, Calif.: University of California Press.

SCOTT, T. R., 1991. A personal view of the future of psychology departments. *Am. Psychol.* 46:975–976.

SHIFFMAN, S., and A. A. STONE, 1998. Introduction to the special section: Ecological momentary assessment in health psychology. *Health Psychol.* 17:3–5.

TUNTURI, A. R., 1952. A difference in the representation of auditory signals for the left and right ears in the isofrequency contours of right ectosylvian auditory cortex of the dog. *J. Comp. Physiol. Psychol.* 168:712–727.

VANMAN, E. J., 2001. Saying one thing and doing another: Predicting behavior using psychophysiologic markers of attitudes (Abstract). *Psychophysiology* 38(Suppl. 1):S14.

WILLIAMS, K. D., 1997. Social ostracism. In *Aversive Interpersonal Behaviors*, R. M. Kowalski, ed. New York: Plenum Press, pp. 133–170.

WILSON, E. O., 1998. *Consilience.* New York: Alfred P. Knopf.

ZAJONC, R. B., 1980. Feeling and thinking: Preferences need no inferences. *Am. Psychol.* 35:157–193.

71 The Neural Basis of Fear

GLENN E. SCHAFE AND JOSEPH E. LeDOUX

ABSTRACT   The fear memory system of the brain has received extensive experimental attention. In this chapter we first review what is known about simple fear conditioning at the behavioral, neural systems, and cellular levels. We then discuss certain higher-level processes in the fear memory system, including contextual fear conditioning, reconsolidation of fear, fear extinction, instrumental fear learning, and declarative memory modulation by emotionally relevant stimuli.

Emotion research in the neurosciences has waxed and waned over the last century. Early attempts to define the "emotional brain" were largely overshadowed by the ensuing cognitive revolution in psychology, which left little room for the study of emotional processing by the brain or the role of emotion in guiding ongoing behavior (LeDoux, 1996). In recent years, however, great progress has been made in understanding the brain pathways and structures underlying one especially important emotion, fear. In particular, much has been learned about how the brain *learns* to fear an object or situation, how learned fears can guide the acquisition of behaviors that are instrumental in avoiding danger, and how fear can augment the strength of memory formation of significant life events. In this chapter, we describe what is known about the neurobiological basis of each of these types of fear memory.

Pavlovian fear conditioning as a model system

Much of what we have learned about the neural basis of fear has come from studies of Pavlovian fear conditioning, particularly in laboratory rats. In this paradigm, the animal is typically placed in an experimental chamber and presented with an innocuous stimulus, such as a tone (the conditioned stimulus, CS), that is copresented or paired with an aversive stimulus, such as a brief electric shock to the feet (the unconditioned stimulus, US). Before conditioning, the CS does not elicit defensive behavior. After as little as one CS-US pairing, however, the animal begins to exhibit a range of conditioned responses (CRs), both to the tone CS and to the context (i.e., the conditioning chamber) in which conditioning occurs. In

GLENN E. SCHAFE   Department of Psychology, Yale University, New Haven, Conn.

JOSEPH E. LeDOUX   W.M. Keck Foundation Laboratory of Neurobiology, Center for Neural Science, New York University, New York, N.Y.

rats, these responses include "freezing" or immobility (the rats' species-typical behavioral response to a threatening stimulus), autonomic and endocrine responses (such as changes in heart rate and blood pressure, defecation, and increased levels of circulating stress hormones), and other changes, among them the potentiation of reflexes such as the acoustic startle response (Blanchard and Blanchard, 1969; Kapp et al., 1979; Smith et al., 1980; LeDoux et al., 1988; Roozendaal, Koolhaas, and Bohus, 1991; Davis, Walker, and Lee, 1997). Thus, as the result of simple associative pairing, the CS comes to elicit many of the same defensive responses that are elicited by naturally aversive or threatening stimuli (figure 71.1).

Basic circuits of the fear conditioning memory system

INPUT PATHWAYS   The neural circuitry underlying Pavlovian fear conditioning, particularly auditory fear conditioning, has been well characterized (figure 71.2). Anatomical and lesion studies have suggested that auditory fear conditioning involves the transmission of CS information about the tone from cortical and subcortical areas of the auditory system to the lateral nucleus of the amygdala (LA), an area that is critical for fear conditioning. Cells in the LA receive projections from areas of the auditory thalamus, including the medial division of the thalamic medial geniculate body (MGm) and the posterior intralaminar nucleus (PIN), and also from the auditory cortex (area TE3) (LeDoux, Ruggiero, and Reis, 1985; LeDoux, Farb, and Romanski, 1991; Bordi and LeDoux, 1992; Romanski and LeDoux, 1993; McDonald, 1998; Doron and LeDoux, 1999). Each of these pathways contains the excitatory neurotransmitter glutamate (LeDoux and Farb, 1991; Farb et al., 1992). Electrophysiological studies have shown that the inputs from MGm/PIN and TE3 converge onto single cells in the LA (Li, Stutzman, and LeDoux, 1996), and that these same cells are also responsive to the foot shock US (Romanski et al., 1993). Thus, individual cells in the LA are well-suited to integrate information about the tone and shock during fear conditioning, suggesting that the LA is a critical locus of the cellular events underlying fear acquisition. Consistent with this notion, behavioral studies have demonstrated that acquisition of auditory fear conditioning is disrupted both by conventional electrolytic or neurotoxic lesions of the LA and by reversible functional inactivation targeted to the LA

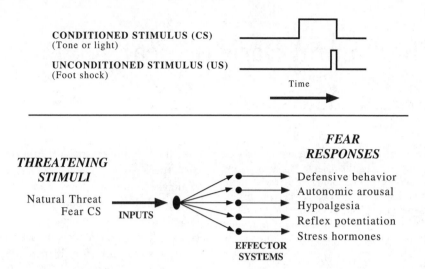

FIGURE 71.1   Pavlovian fear conditioning. *Top*, Fear conditioning involves the presentation of an initially innocuous stimulus, such as a tone (conditioned stimulus, CS), that is paired or associated with a noxious stimulus, such as a brief electric shock to the feet (uncon-ditioned stimulus, US). *Bottom*, Before conditioning, the CS elicits little response from the animal. After conditioning, the CS elicits a wide range of behavioral and physiological responses that are char-acteristically elicited by naturally aversive or threatening stimuli.

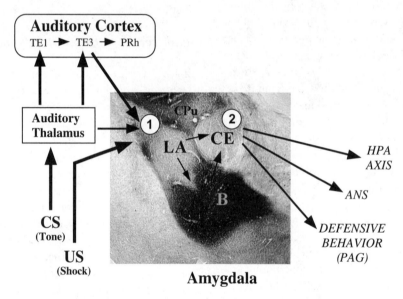

FIGURE 71.2   Anatomy of the fear system. *1*. Auditory fear con-ditioning involves the transmission of CS sensory information from areas of the auditory thalamus and cortex to the lateral amygdala (LA), where it can converge with incoming somatosensory infor-mation from the foot shock US. It is in the LA that alterations in synaptic transmission are thought to encode key aspects of the learning. *2*. During fear expression, the LA engages the central nucleus of the amygdala (CE), which projects widely to many areas of the forebrain and brainstem that control the expression of fear CRs, including freezing, HPA axis activation, and alterations in car-diovascular activity.

(LeDoux et al., 1990; Kim, Rison, and Fanselow, 1993; Campeau and Davis, 1995; Muller et al., 1997; Wilensky, Schafe, and LeDoux, 2000).

Pretraining lesions of the MGm/PIN have also been shown to impair auditory fear conditioning (LeDoux et al., 1986), but pretraining lesions of the auditory cortex do not (LeDoux, Sakaguchi, and Reis, 1984; Romanski and LeDoux, 1992). Thus, the thalamic pathway between the MGm/PIN and the LA appears to be particularly important for auditory fear conditioning. This is not to say, however, that cortical input to the LA is not essential. Indeed, the electrophysiological responses of cells in the auditory cortex are modified during fear conditioning (Edeline, Pham, and Weinberger, 1993). Further, when conditioning depends on the ability of the animal to make fine discriminations between different auditory CSs, the auditory cortex appears to be required (Jarrell et al., 1987).

OUTPUT PATHWAYS The LA is important for fear acquisition; its connections with other amygdaloid nuclei, including the basal nucleus (B) and the central nucleus of the amygdala (CE), are essential for fear expression (Paré, Smith, and Paré, 1995; Pitkänen, Savander, and LeDoux, 1997). However, damage confined to the LA and CE disrupts auditory fear conditioning (Amorapanth, LeDoux, and Nader, 2000; Nader et al., 2001), suggesting that a direct connection from LA to CE is sufficient to mediate fear conditioning. Projections from the LA to the basal nucleus are also important but appear to be involved exclusively in more instrumental aspects of fear learning (Amorapanth, LeDoux, and Nader, 2000). We will return to this topic in a later section.

The CE is well connected to areas of the forebrain, hypothalamus, and brainstem that control hard-wired behavioral, endocrine, and autonomic responses associated with fear conditioning. Projections from the CE to the periaqueductal gray, for example, have been shown to be important for mediating behavioral and endocrine responses such as freezing and hypoalgesia (Helmstetter and Landeira-Fernandez, 1990; Helmstetter and Tershner, 1994; De Oca et al., 1998), while projections to the lateral hypothalamus have been implicated in the control of conditioned cardiovascular responses (Iwata, LeDoux, and Reis, 1986). Of note, while lesions of these individual areas can selectively impair the expression of individual CRs, damage to the CE interferes with the expression of all fear CRs (LeDoux, 2000). Thus, the CE is typically thought of as the principal output nucleus of the fear system that acts to orchestrate the collection of hard-wired, and typically species-specific, responses that underlie defensive behavior.

SYNAPTIC PLASTICITY AND FEAR CONDITIONING The LA is not only the principal site of sensory input to the amygdala,

it also appears to be an essential locus of plasticity during fear conditioning. For example, individual cells in the LA alter their response properties when CS and US are paired during fear conditioning. Specifically, LA cells that are initially weakly responsive to auditory input respond vigorously to the same input after fear conditioning (Quirk, Repa, and LeDoux, 1995; Quirk, Armony, and LeDoux, 1997; Quirk, Armony, Repa, et al., 1997; Maren, 2000.) Thus, a change occurs in the function of LA cells as a result of training, a finding that has contributed to the view that neural plasticity in the LA encodes key aspects of fear learning and memory storage (Quirk, Armony, Repa, et al., 1997; Fanselow and LeDoux, 1999; Maren, 1999; Blair et al., 2001).

Interestingly, recent single-unit studies have suggested that there are two populations of cells in the LA that undergo plastic changes during fear conditioning, and in unique ways (Repa et al., 2001). The first is a more dorsal population (near the border of the striatum) that shows enhanced firing to the CS in the initial stages of training and testing and is sensitive to fear extinction (figure 71.3). These so-called transiently plastic cells exhibit short-latency changes (within 10–15 ms after tone onset) that are consistent with the involvement of rapid, monosynaptic thalamic input. The second population of cells occupies a more ventral position in the LA. In contrast to the transiently plastic cells, these more ventral cells exhibit enhanced firing to the CS throughout training and testing, and do not appear to be sensitive to extinction. Further, these long-term plastic cells exhibit longer latencies (within 30–40 ms after tone onset), indicative of a polysynaptic pathway. Thus, it has been hypothesized that a network of neurons within the LA is responsible for triggering and storing fear memories, respectively (Repa et al., 2001; Medina, Repa, and LeDoux, 2002).

ROLE OF LONG-TERM POTENTIATION IN FEAR CONDITIONING What mechanism might mediate the change that occurs in the LA as a result of conditioning? One of the leading candidates is long-term potentiation (LTP), an activity-dependent form of plasticity that was initially discovered in the hippocampus (Bliss and Lomø, 1973). LTP has also been demonstrated, both in vivo and in vitro, in each of the major auditory input pathways to the LA, including the thalamic and cortical auditory pathways (Clugnet and LeDoux, 1989; Chapman et al., 1990; Rogan and LeDoux, 1995; Huang and Kandel, 1998; Weisskopf, Bauer, and LeDoux, 1999). This includes tetanus-induced LTP, which appears to be NMDA receptor dependent (Huang and Kandel, 1998; Bauer, Schafe, and LeDoux, 2002), and also "associative" LTP, which is induced following pairing of subthreshold presynaptic auditory inputs with postsynaptic depolarizations of LA cells (Huang and Kandel, 1998; Weisskopf, Bauer, and LeDoux, 1999; Bauer, Schafe, and LeDoux,

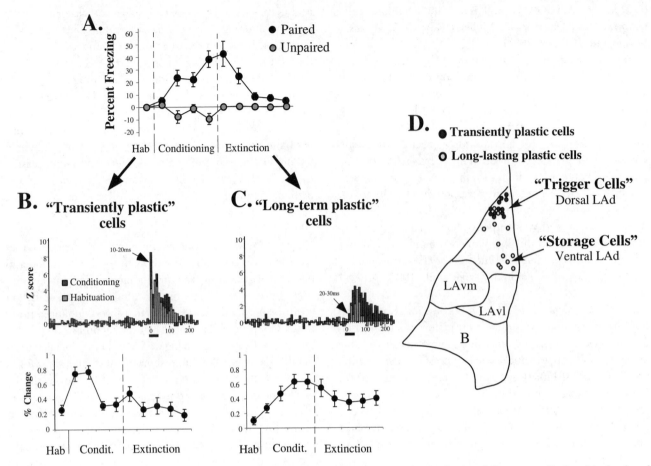

FIGURE 71.3   Plasticity in the LA during fear conditioning. Pairing of CS and US during fear conditioning leads to changes in fear behavior (*A*) and also to changes in the responsiveness of single LA cells to auditory stimuli. During fear conditioning, there are two populations of cells that undergo plastic change. (*B*) "Transiently plastic cells" are generally short latency and show enhanced firing shortly after training and during the initial phases of extinction, but not at other times. (*C*) "Long-term plastic cells" are generally longer latency and show enhanced firing throughout training and extinc-tion. (*D*) "Transiently plastic cells" are generally found in the dorsal tip of the LAd, where they may serve to trigger the initial stages of memory formation. "Long-term plastic cells," on the other hand, are found in the ventral regions of the LAd and may be important for long-term, extinction-resistant memory storage. (Adapted with permission from J. C. Repa et al., Two different lateral amygdala cell populations contribute to the initiation and storage of memory. *Nat. Neurosci.* 4:724–731. © 2001 by the Native Publishing Group.)

2002). Unlike that induced by a tetanus, associative LTP in the LA is dependent on L-type voltage-gated calcium channels (VGCCs) (Weisskopf, Bauer, and LeDoux, 1999; Bauer, Schafe, and LeDoux, 2002).

A number of findings have converged to support the hypothesis that fear conditioning is mediated by an associa-tive LTP-like process in the LA (figure 71.4). First, LTP induction at thalamic inputs to the LA has been shown to enhance auditory processing, and thus natural information flow, in the LA (Rogan and LeDoux, 1995). Second, fear conditioning has been shown to lead to electrophysiological changes in the LA very similar to those observed following artificial LTP induction, and these changes persist over days (McKernan and Shinnick-Gallagher, 1997; Rogan, Staubli, and LeDoux, 1997). Third, associative LTP in the LA has been shown to be sensitive to the same contingencies as fear

conditioning. That is, when presynaptic trains precede the onset of postsynaptic depolarizations 100% of the time, LTP is strong. However, if noncontingent depolarizations of the postsynaptic LA cell are interleaved within the same number of contiguous pairings, LTP is much weaker (Bauer, LeDoux, and Nader, 2001). Thus, the change in synaptic efficacy within the LA induced by LTP depends on the con-tingency between pre- and postsynaptic activity rather than simply on temporal contiguity—and it is contingency rather than temporal pairing that is known to be critical for asso-ciative learning, including fear conditioning (Rescorla, 1968).

Finally, fear conditioning and LTP induction have been characterized by a common pharmacological substrate. Fear conditioning, for example, is impaired by pharmacological blockade of either NMDA receptors (Miserendino et al.,

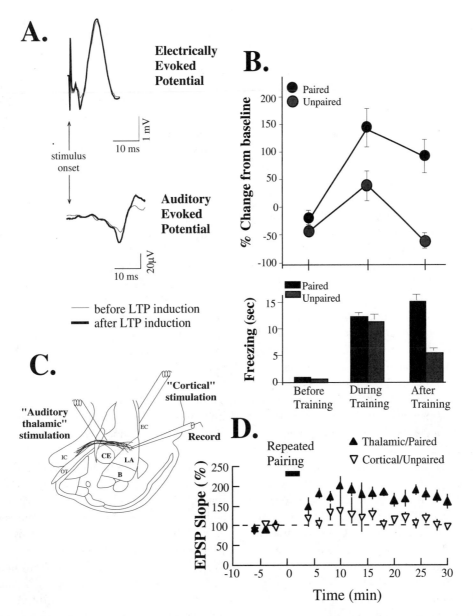

FIGURE 71.4   LTP in the LA. (*A*) Top graph shows LTP induced in the LA following high-frequency electrical stimulation of the MGm/PIN. The trace represents a stimulation-evoked field potential in the LA before and after LTP induction. Following artificial LTP induction, bottom trace shows that processing of naturalistic auditory stimuli is also enhanced in the LA. The trace represents an auditory-evoked field potential in the LA before and after LTP induction. (*B*). Top graph shows that fear conditioning leads to electrophysiological changes in the LA in a manner similar to LTP. The figure represents percent change in the slope of the auditory-evoked field potential in the LA before, during, and after conditioning in both paired and unpaired rats. Bottom graph shows freezing behavior across training and testing periods. Both paired and unpaired groups showed equivalent freezing behavior during training, but only the paired group showed an enhanced neural response. (*C*) Associative LTP is induced in the amygdala slice by pairing trains of presynaptic stimulation of fibers coming from the auditory thalamus with depolarization of LA cells. Stimulation of fibers coming from cortical areas serves as a control for input specificity. (*D*) LTP induced by pairing as measured by the change in the slope of the EPSP over time. In this case, the thalamic pathway received paired stimulation, whereas the cortical pathway received unpaired stimulation (i.e. trains and depolarizations, but in a non-contingent manner). The black bar represents the duration of the pairing.

1990; Kim et al., 1991; Rodrigues, Schafe, and LeDoux, 2001) or L-type VGCCs (Bauer, Schafe, and LeDoux, 2002) in the amygdala. Thus, Ca^{2+} entry through both NMDA and L-type VGCCs in the LA appears to set in motion a process that is essential for both synaptic plasticity and memory formation.

Biochemical and Molecular Mechanisms of Fear Conditioning In recent years, a great deal of research has focused on understanding the biochemical and molecular mechanisms that underlie learning and memory. This research has included fear conditioning, which, perhaps because of its simplicity, has been a particularly attractive model for this endeavor. Many of the recent studies have drawn on a larger literature that has focused on the biochemical events that underlie LTP, particularly in the hippocampus, to ask whether fear conditioning might be subserved by similar cellular mechanisms.

In the hippocampus, LTP is thought to involve the activation of a variety of protein kinase signaling pathways by increases in intracellular Ca^{2+} in the postsynaptic cell at the time of induction. Many protein kinase signaling pathways have been implicated in LTP, including the Ca^{2+}/calmodulin-dependent protein kinase (CaMK), protein kinase C (PKC), the cAMP-dependent protein kinase (PKA), and the extracellularly regulated kinase/mitogen-activated protein kinase (ERK/MAPK) (Silva et al., 1992; Huang, Li, and Kandel, 1994; Nguyen and Kandel, 1996; English and Sweatt, 1997). These kinases, when activated by elevations in intracellular Ca^{2+} at the time of LTP induction, are thought to have a variety of distinct actions. Both the alpha isoform of CaMKII (αCaMKII) and PKC, for example, are known to undergo rapid autophosphorylation, a state in which these enzymes can remain active in the absence of further Ca^{2+} entry (Soderling and Derkach, 2000). In this state, αCaMKII is thought to translocate to the postsynaptic density, where it can transiently influence the conductances of NMDA and AMPA receptors that are necessary for the induction and early, protein- and RNA synthesis-independent phase of LTP (Soderling and Derkach, 2000). PKA and ERK/MAPK, on the other hand, are thought to translocate to the cell nucleus, where they can engage activators of transcription, including the cAMP response element-binding protein (CREB) and cAMP response element (CRE)-mediated gene expression (Impey et al., 1996; Impey, Obrietan, et al., 1998). It is the activation of CREB- and CRE-mediated genes that ultimately leads to the protein- and RNA synthesis-dependent functional changes that are thought to underlie long-term synaptic plasticity and memory formation (Frank and Greenberg, 1994; Yin and Tully, 1996; Silva et al., 1998).

Of note, these same intracellular processes have been implicated in fear conditioning. Many of these studies have used molecular genetic methods in which the molecules of interest have been manipulated in knockout or transgenic mouse lines. For example, Silva and colleagues demonstrated early on that mice lacking two critical isoforms of CREB, α and δ, have impaired memory consolidation for auditory and contextual fear conditioning and hippocampal LTP (Bourtchuladze et al., 1994). The same laboratory has recently followed up on these findings and demonstrated that induced overexpression of a dominant negative isoform of CREB in the forebrain impairs fear memory formation (Kida et al., 2002). Other studies have shown that mice that overexpress R(AB), an inhibitory isoform of PKA in the forebrain, have impaired memory consolidation of fear conditioning, as well as impaired hippocampal LTP (Abel et al., 1997). Further, mice deficient in *Ras*, an upstream regulator of the ERK/MAPK signaling pathway, have impaired memory formation of auditory fear conditioning and amygdala LTP (Brambilla et al., 1997). Finally, deletion of the β isoform of PKC or overexpression of an active form of CaMKII specifically in the amygdala and striatum results in impaired fear conditioning (Mayford et al., 1996; Weeber et al., 2000).

More recent studies have used pharmacological or viral transfection methods to examine the involvement of these molecules in memory formation and LTP specifically in the amygdala. For example, recent studies have shown that LTP at thalamic and cortical inputs to the LA requires RNA and protein synthesis, PKA, and ERK/MAPK (Huang, Martin, and Kandel, 2000). Further, infusions of drugs into the LA that specifically block RNA or protein synthesis or PKA activity impair the formation of fear memories (Bailey et al., 1999; Schafe and LeDoux, 2000), and overexpression of the transcription factor CREB in the LA facilitates fear memory formation (Josselyn et al., 2001). Consistent with a role for each of these intracellular processes in long-term plasticity, it is long-term rather than short-term memory that is affected by these manipulations. Other recent studies have shown that ERK/MAPK is activated in the LA following fear conditioning, and pharmacological blockade of this activation following intra-LA infusions of ERK/MAPK inhibitors impairs long-term memory of fear conditioning (Schafe et al., 2000). Thus, many of same biochemical signaling pathways and molecular events that are involved in LTP also appear to be necessary for fear conditioning in the amygdala (figure 71.5).

Interestingly, the cells that express activated ERK/MAPK after fear conditioning occupy a more ventral position in the LA, in the same anatomical location as cells that exhibit long-term plasticity during and after fear conditioning (Repa et al., 2001). In fact, very little activated ERK is observed in the dorsal region of the LA, the site of the majority of CS-US convergence and of cells that exhibit rapid, and transient, plastic changes during fear conditioning (Romanski

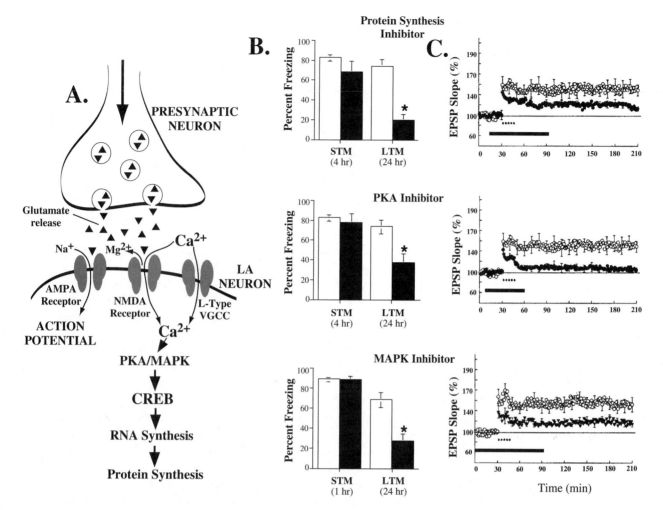

FIGURE 71.5 Molecular pathways underlying fear conditioning. (A) In many systems, LTP involves the release of glutamate and Ca²⁺ influx through either NMDA receptors or L-type VGCCs. The increase in intracellular Ca²⁺ leads to the activation of protein kinases, such as PKA and ERK/MAPK. Once activated, these kinases can translocate to the nucleus, where they activate transcription factors such as CREB. The activation of CREB by PKA and ERK/MAPK promotes CRE-mediated gene transcription and the synthesis of new proteins. (B) Fear memory formation in the amygdala has also recently been shown to require protein synthesis, PKA, and ERK/MAPK activation. In these studies, rats received intra-amygdala infusions of anisomycin (a protein synthesis inhibitor, top), Rp-cAMPS (a PKA inhibitor, middle), or U0126 (an MEK inhibitor, which is an upstream regulator of ERK/MAPK activation, bottom) at or around the time of training, and were assayed for both short-term memory (1–4 hours later) and long-term memory (24 hours later) of auditory fear conditioning. In each figure, vehicle-treated rats are represented by the white bars and drug-treated animals are represented by the black bars. *$P < 0.05$ relative to vehicle controls. (C) Amygdala LTP has recently been shown to be require the same biochemical processes. In these studies, reported by Huang and colleagues (2000), amygdala slices were treated with either anisomycin (top), KT5720 (a PKA inhibitor, middle), or PD098059 (an MEK inhibitor, bottom) before to and during tetanus of the thalamic pathway. In each experiment, field recordings were obtained from the LA and expressed across time as a percentage of baseline. (Adapted with permission from Y. Y. Huang et al., Both protein kinase A and mitogen-activated protein kinase are required in the amygdala for the macromolecular synthesis-dependent late phase of long-term potentiation. *J. Neurosci.* 20:6317–6325. © 2000 by the Society for Neuroscience.)

et al., 1993; Repa et al., 2001). This pattern of findings is consistent with the hypothesis that fear conditioning induces long-term plastic change and memory formation in a ventral population of cells in the LA via the ERK/MAPK signaling cascade. It remains unknown whether this involves a rapid "transfer" of plasticity between dorsal and ventral cells in the LA during fear conditioning or an independent, parallel process.

As noted earlier, most recent studies have focused on postsynaptic mechanisms and their role in amygdala LTP and memory formation (for a review, see Schafe et al., 2001). Growing evidence, however, suggests that synaptic plasticity and memory formation in the LA involves a presynaptic process. McKernan and Shinnick-Gallagher (1997), for example, showed that auditory fear conditioning occludes paired-pulse facilitation at cortical inputs to the LA, a type of short-term plasticity that is largely believed to be presynaptic. Similarly, Huang and Kandel (1998) observed that LTP at cortical inputs to the LA occludes paired-pulse facilitation in this pathway. Further, bath application, but not postsynaptic injection, of a PKA inhibitor impairs LTP in LA neurons (Huang and Kandel, 1998). Conversely, bath application of forskolin, a PKA activator, in the presence of antagonists of postsynaptic NMDAR and AMPAR receptors induces LTP and occludes PPF at cortical inputs (Huang and Kandel, 1998), suggesting that the presynaptic component of LTP in this pathway is PKA dependent. More recently, Tsvetkov and colleagues (2002) showed that auditory fear conditioning itself, in addition to LTP, occludes paired-pulse facilitation at cortical inputs to LA (Tsvetkov et al., 2002). Thus, although more work will be required, it is clear from the available evidence that a complete understanding of memory formation and synaptic plasticity in the LA will require attention to both sides of the synapse.

Beyond "simple" fear conditioning: Extended circuitry

CONTEXTUAL FEAR CONDITIONING In a typical auditory fear conditioning experiment, the animal learns to fear not only the tone that is paired with the foot shock but also the context in which conditioning occurs. Contextual fear may also be induced by the presentation of foot shocks alone within a novel environment. In the laboratory, fear of the context is measured by returning the rat to the conditioning chamber on the test day and measuring freezing behavior (Blanchard, Dielman, and Blanchard, 1968; Fanselow, 1980).

In comparison with auditory fear conditioning, much less is known about the neural system underlying contextual fear. Much of the work examining the neuroanatomical substrates of contextual fear has relied exclusively on lesion methods, and, as in auditory fear conditioning, the amygdala appears to play an essential role. For example, lesions

of the amygdala, including the LA and basal nucleus, have been shown to disrupt both acquisition and expression of contextual fear conditioning (Phillips and LeDoux, 1992; Kim, Rison, and Fanselow, 1993; Maren, 1998), as has reversible functional inactivation targeted to the LA (Muller et al., 1997). Contextual fear conditioning is also impaired by infusion of NMDA receptor antagonists, RNA and protein synthesis inhibitors, and inhibitors of PKA into the amygdala (Kim et al., 1991; Bailey et al., 1999; Goosens, Holt, and Maren, 2000; Rodrigues, Schafe, and LeDoux, 2001). Collectively, these findings suggest that essential aspects of the memory are encoded and stored in the amygdala. At this time, however, there is little data that allows us to distinguish between the involvement of different amygdala subnuclei in contextual fear, although recent lesion evidence suggests that the LA and anterior basal nuclei are critical, but not the posterior basal nucleus (Goosens and Maren, 2001). The CE is, of course, essential for the expression of contextual fear, as it is for auditory fear conditioning (Goosens and Maren, 2001).

The hippocampus has also been implicated in contextual fear conditioning, although its exact role has been difficult to define. A number of studies have shown that electrolytic and neurotoxic lesions of the hippocampus disrupt contextual but not auditory fear conditioning (Kim and Fanselow, 1992; Phillips and LeDoux, 1992; Kim, Rison, and Fanselow, 1993; Maren, Aharonov, and Fanselow, 1997). However, only lesions created shortly after training disrupt contextual fear conditioning (figure 71.6). If rats are subjected to hippocampal lesions 28 days after training, there is no memory impairment (Kim and Fanselow, 1992). This "retrograde gradient" of recall suggests that hippocampal-dependent memories are gradually stabilized over time in other regions of the brain for permanent storage, an idea that is consistent with the findings of hippocampal-dependent declarative memory research in humans (Milner, Squire, and Kandel, 1998).

What role does the hippocampus play in contextual fear? One prominent view is that it is necessary for forming a representation of the context in which conditioning occurs and for providing the amygdala with that information during training for CS-US integration (Phillips and LeDoux, 1992; Young, Bohenek, and Fanselow, 1994; Frankland et al., 1998). In support of this view, the hippocampal formation has been shown to project to the basal nucleus of the amygdala (Canteras and Swanson, 1992), which provides a potential neuroanatomical substrate through which contextual fear associations can be formed (Maren and Fanselow, 1995; but see Goosens and Maren, 2001). Further, it has recently been shown that intrahippocampal infusions of the protein synthesis inhibitor anisomycin impair the ability of the hippocampus to form a contextual representation, but not the ability of the animal to form a context-shock association

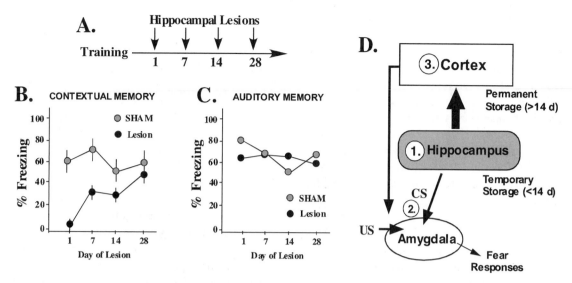

FIGURE 71.6 Hippocampal-dependent contextual fear. Contextual fear conditioning requires the dorsal hippocampus, but only for a limited time. (*A*) Experimental protocol from Kim and Fanselow (1992), in which rats were trained with tone-shock pairings and then given lesions of the dorsal hippocampus either 1, 7, 14, or 28 days later. (*B*) Contextual memory was impaired when lesions were given 1 day after training, but not if they were given 28 days after training. (*C*) Auditory fear conditioning was not affected by hippocampal lesions. In each panel, the lesioned rats are represented by the black circles. (*A–C* reprinted with permission from J. J. Kim and M. S. Fanselow, Modality-specific retrograde amnesia of fear. *Science* 256:675–677. © 1992 by the American Association for the Advancement of Science.) (*D*) A model of the neural system underlying contextual fear conditioning. The hippocampus (*1*) is necessary for forming an initial representation of the context and for providing that information as a CS to the amygdala (*2*) during fear conditioning. In the amygdala, the contextual CS can converge with the foot shock US, and it is here that the memory of contextual fear is thought to be formed. Over time, however, the "contextual memory" formed by the hippocampus is stabilized in the cortex (*3*) for permanent storage. At this point, the hippocampus is not necessary to retrieve the memory.

(Barrientos, O'Reilly, and Rudy, 2002). In these experiments, the immediate shock deficit paradigm was used to tease apart the contribution of the hippocampus to learning about a context and learning to fear one. Normally, immediate shock (i.e., a shock given soon after introduction to the conditioning chamber) is not sufficient to support contextual fear conditioning, presumably because it takes time for the hippocampus to form a representation of the context in which the animal finds itself. However, if the animal is *preexposed* to the conditioning chamber briefly on the day before training, it can subsequently acquire contextual fear following immediate shock, presumably because the animal now enters the training situation with a contextual representation already intact (Fanselow, 1980). In the study of Barrientos and colleagues (2002), rats were given an infusion of anisomycin or vehicle into the dorsal hippocampus immediately after exposure to a novel context on the day before they received immediate shock, or immediately after receiving immediate shock on the day after they received preexposure. The findings showed that intrahippocampal anisomycin resulted in impaired contextual learning only in the first group (Barrientos, O'Reilly, and Rudy, 2002). This important finding suggests that protein synthesis in the hippocampus is necessary for learning about contexts, but not for contextual fear conditioning.

It is clear, however, that the hippocampus undergoes plastic changes during fear conditioning, some of which may be necessary for memory formation of contextual fear. For example, intrahippocampal infusion of the NMDA receptor antagonist APV impairs contextual fear conditioning (Young, Bohenek, and Fanselow, 1994; Stiedl et al., 2000), and contextual but not auditory fear conditioning is impaired in mice that lack the NR1 subunit of the NMDA receptor exclusively in area CA1 of the hippocampus (Rampon et al., 2000). Further, fear conditioning leads to increases in the activation of αCaMKII, PKC, ERK/MAPK, and CRE-mediated gene expression in the hippocampus (Atkins et al., 1998; Hall, Thomas, and Everitt, 2000; Impey, Smith, et al., 1998). These findings add support to the notion that NMDA receptor-dependent plastic changes in the hippocampus, in addition to the amygdala, are required for contextual fear conditioning. However, it should be emphasized that the exact contribution of these plastic changes to contextual fear conditioning remains unclear. For example, most of these studies cannot distinguish between a role for NMDA receptor-mediated plasticity in the formation of contextual representations as opposed to a role in fear memory acquisition and storage. Further, regulation of intracellular signaling cascades in the hippocampus by fear conditioning, while potentially indicative of some type of memory storage, does not necessarily indicate that these changes are related to the acquisition *fear* memories. They may be related to declarative or explicit memories of the training experience that are acquired at the same time as fearful memories (LeDoux, 2000). Indeed, a number of studies have shown that hippocampal cells undergo plastic changes during and after fear conditioning (Doyère et al., 1995; Moita et al., 2003), including auditory fear conditioning, which is spared following hippocampal lesions (Kim and Fanselow, 1992). Clearly, more research is needed before a convincing picture of the role of the hippocampus in contextual fear conditioning emerges.

RETRIEVAL AND REACTIVATION OF FEAR MEMORIES What happens when a fear memory is remembered? The picture of fear conditioning that we have painted thus far is consistent with traditional thinking about memory formation, according to which memories are laid down by a process characterized by increasing stabilization. Newly acquired memories, for example, are thought to be inherently unstable, acquiring stability only over time as protein- and RNA synthesis-dependent processes kick in. Over the years, however, a number of studies have challenged this linear notion of memory formation. In these studies, amnesic manipulations at or around the time of memory retrieval, rather than at the time of initial learning, appeared to result in loss of the memory on subsequent recall tests (see Sara, 2000). These findings suggest that the retrieval process renders a memory susceptible to disruption in a manner very similar to a newly formed memory.

Recent studies using fear conditioning paradigms have rekindled interest in this phenomenon. For example, infusion of the protein synthesis inhibitor anisomycin into the amygdala immediately after retrieval of auditory fear conditioning has recently been shown to impair memory recall on subsequent tests (Nader, Schafe, and LeDoux, 2000). This effect was clearly dependent on retrieval of the memory; that is, no subsequent memory deficit was observed if exposure to the CS was omitted. Further, the effect was observed not only when the initial recall test and drug infusion were given shortly after training (i.e., 1 day), but also if they were given 14 days later, suggesting that the effect could not be attributable to disruption of late phases of protein synthesis necessary for the initial training episode. Thus, following active recall of a fear memory, that memory appears to undergo a second wave of consolidation (or so-called reconsolidation) that requires protein synthesis in the amygdala. Although little is currently known about the biochemical events that underlie this process, recent studies have shown that transient overexpression of a dominant negative isoform of CREB at the time of memory retrieval impairs reconsolidation of auditory and contextual fear conditioning (Kida et al., 2002), suggesting that a nuclear event is involved. Future

experiments will be required for a full appreciation of how reconsolidation differs at the cellular level from the initial process of memory encoding and storage.

Reconsolidation does not appear to be unique to the amygdala; hippocampal-dependent contextual memories also appear to be sensitive to manipulation at the time of retrieval. In a recent study, Debiec, LeDoux, and Nader (2002) gave rats intrahippocampal infusions of anisomycin following recall of contextual fear conditioning and found that memory retrieval was impaired on subsequent tests. Interestingly, reconsolidation of contextual fear was impaired even when memory reactivation and intrahippocampal anisomycin treatment were given 45 days after the initial training session, a time when lesion studies have shown that contextual memories should no longer depend on the hippocampus (Kim and Fanselow, 1992). The initial experiments by Kim and Fanselow, however, used only a single recall test after training and hippocampal lesions; the ability of the animal to recall contextual fear on subsequent tests was not examined. Surprisingly, when Debiec and colleagues reactivated the contextual memory prior to creating a lesion of the hippocampus, even as long as 45 days after training, subsequent recall was impaired (Debiec, LeDoux, and Nader, 2002). Thus, hippocampal-dependent contextual memories appear to undergo both a cellular and a systems-level reconsolidation following memory retrieval. That is, recall of an older, hippocampal-independent contextual memory must return to the hippocampus during retrieval and undergo a protein synthesis-dependent process of reconsolidation to be maintained. As in most hippocampal studies, however, it remains unclear what information is being reconsolidated, the memory of the context or the contextual fear memory.

EXTINCTION OF FEAR Extinction is a process whereby repeated presentations of the CS in the absence of the US leads to a weakening of the expression of conditioning responding. Although extinction of conditioned fear has been well documented in the behavioral literature, we known comparatively little about its neurobiological substrate. However, the medial prefrontal cortex (mPFC), and in particular the ventral mPFC, appears to play an important role. Early studies, for example, showed that selective lesions of the ventral mPFC retard the extinction of fear to an auditory CS while having no effect on initial fear acquisition (Morgan, Romanski, and LeDoux, 1993; Morgan and LeDoux, 1995; but see Gewirtz, Falls, and Davis, 1997). Further, neurons in the mPFC alter their response properties as a result of extinction (Garcia et al., 1999). Interestingly, a recent study suggests that the mPFC may not be necessary for fear extinction per se but rather in the long-term recall of extinguished fear (see figure 71.7). For example, rats with mPFC lesions are able to extinguish

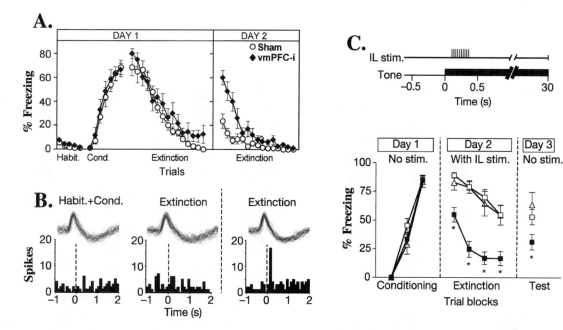

FIGURE 71.7 The role of the medial prefrontal cortex (mPFC) in long-term retention of fear extinction. (*A*) Rats with lesions of the mPFC can acquire and extinguish auditory fear conditioning normally (Day 1). However, they cannot retain their memory for extinction (Day 2; 24 hours later). In each panel, the lesioned animals are represented by the black circles. (Adapted with permission from G. J. Quirk et al., The role of ventromedial prefrontal cortex in the recovery of extinguished fear. *J. Neurosci.* 20:6225–6231. © 2000 by the Society for Neuroscience.) (*B*) Single cells in the mPFC are generally unresponsive to tones during training and within a session, but show impaired extinction between sessions (Quirk et al., 2000). Further, neurons in the mPFC fire strongly to a tone CS after behavioral extinction has occurred, and artificial stimulation of the mPFC that resembles responding in an extinguished rat is sufficient to inhibit behavioral expression of fear in nonextinguished rats (Milad and Quirk, 2002). Thus, it appears clear that the mPFC plays an essential role in long-term retention and/or expression of fear extinction. The question of whether the mPFC is a "site of storage" of extinction or simply a region that is necessary for the long-term expression of extinguished memories remains to be examined.

Interestingly, a number of studies have suggested that the amygdala may be an essential site of plasticity underlying fear extinction. Infusions of NMDA receptor antagonists or inhibitors of ERK/MAPK into the amygdala have been shown to impair fear extinction (Falls, Miserendino, and Davis, 1992; Lu, Walker, and Davis, 2001). Conversely, both systemic and intra-amygdala infusions of partial agonists of the NMDA receptor facilitate fear extinction (Walker et al., 2002; figure 71.8). These experiments suggest that some type of activity-dependent synaptic plasticity must take place in the amygdala during extinction learning, as it does during initial learning. After the memory of extinction is formed,

extinction (Day 1) but signal vigorously during long-term recall of extinction (Day 2; 24 hours later). (*C*) Direct stimulation of the mPFC during the early phases of extinction (Day 2) results in a dramatic reduction in fear, which is longlasting (Day 3; 24 hours later). In each figure, the stimulated animals are represented by the black squares. (*B* and *C* adapted with permission from M. R. Milad and G. J. Quirk, Neurons in medial prefrontal cortex signal memory for fear extinction. *Nature* 420:70–74. © 2002 by the Nature Publishing Group.)

the amygdala may then signal the mPFC to inhibit ongoing fear responses. Indeed, McDonald and colleagues have shown that the mPFC projects to GABAergic intercalated cells that are situated between the lateral and basal amygdala and the CE (McDonald, Mascagni, and Guo, 1996), and these cells may be important for regulating fear responses. Additional experiments will be necessary to define the exact contribution of connections between mPFC and the amygdala in extinction processes, as well as the detailed biochemical mechanisms responsible for promoting fear extinction.

INSTRUMENTAL FEAR LEARNING In addition to its role in the rapid, reflexive learning that characterizes Pavlovian fear conditioning, the amygdala contributes to other fear-related aspects of behavior. Pavlovian fear conditioning, for example, is useful for learning to detect a dangerous object or situation, but the animal must also be able to use this information to guide ongoing behavior that is instrumental in avoiding that danger. In some experimental situations, the animal must learn to make a response (e.g., move away, press a bar, turn a wheel) that will allow it to avoid presentation of a shock or danger signal, a form of learning known as active avoidance. In other situations, the animal must learn

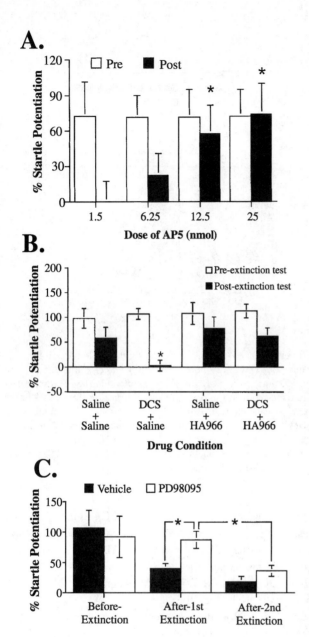

FIGURE 71.8 The amygdala and fear extinction. Extinction of fear-potentiated startle (FPS) can be impaired or facilitated by pharmacological manipulations of the amygdala. (*A*) Extinction of FPS is impaired in a dose-dependent manner following infusion of AP5, an NMDA receptor antagonist, into the amygdala. White bars represent preextinction startle baselines; black bars represent the amount of startle potentiation after an extinction session in each group. Note that with increasing doses there is less extinction. (Adapted with permission from W. A. Falls et al., Extinction of fear-potentiated startle: Blockade by infusion of an NMDA antagonist into the amygdala. *J. Neurosci.* 12:854–863. © 1992 by the Society for Neuroscience). (*B*) Extinction of FPS can be facilitated by infusion of a partial agonist of the NMDA receptor in the amygdala. Rats that were given intra-amygdala infusions of D-cycloserine (DCS; DCS/Saline), a partial agonist of the glycine recognition site of the NMDA receptor, had facilitated extinction relative to controls (Saline/Saline). This effect could be reversed by HA966 (DCS/HA966), an antagonist of the glycine recognition site that has no effect on extinction itself (Saline/HA966). In each group, white bars represent preextinction startle baselines; black bars represent the amount of startle potentiation after drug treatment and an extinction session. (Adapted with permission from D. L. Walker et al., Facilitation of conditioned fear extinction by systemic administration or intra-amygdala infusions of D-cycloserine as assessed with fear-potentiated startle in rats. *J. Neurosci.* 22:2343–2351. © 2002 by the Society for Neuroscience.) (*C*) Intra-amygdala infusion of on MAP kinase inhibitor (PD98095) blocks extinction of FPS. Rats were infused with PD98095 before the 1st extinction session. The 2nd extinction session was given drug-free. Note the absence of extinction on the 1st session. In each group, black bars represent preextinction startle baselines, while white bars represent the amount of startle potentiation after an extinction session. (Adapted with permission from K. T. Lu et al., Mitogen-activated protein kinase cascade is involved in extinction of fear-potentiated startle. *J. Neurosci.* 21:RC162. © 2001 by the Society for Neuroscience.)

not to respond, also known as passive avoidance. Both of these are examples of instrumental conditioning, and the amygdala plays a vital role in each.

Earlier we mentioned that only the LA and CE were critical for Pavlovian fear conditioning. However, we have recently begun to appreciate the significance of projections from the LA to the basal nucleus of the amygdala from studies that employ fear learning tasks that involve both classic and instrumental components (Killcross, Robbins, and Everitt, 1997; Amorapanth, LeDoux, and Nader, 2000). Amorapanth, LeDoux, and Nader (2000), for example, first trained rats to associate a tone with foot shock (the Pavlovian component). Next, rats learned to move from one side of a two-compartment box to the other to avoid presentation of the tone (the instrumental component), a so-called

escape-from-fear task. Findings showed that while lesions of the LA impaired both types of learning, lesions of the CE impaired only the Pavlovian component (i.e., the tone-shock association). Conversely, lesions of the basal nucleus impaired only the instrumental component (learning to move to the second compartment). Thus, different outputs of the LA appear to mediate Pavlovian and instrumental behaviors elicited by a fear-arousing stimulus (Amorapanth, LeDoux, and Nader, 2000; figure 71.9). It is important to note, however, that these findings do not indicate that the basal nucleus is a site of motor control or a locus of memory storage for instrumental learning. Rather, the basal amygdala likely guides fear-related behavior and reinforcement learning via its projections to nearby striatal regions that are known to be necessary for instrumental learning and reward processes (Robbins et al., 1989; Everitt, Cador, and Robbins, 1989; Everitt et al., 1999).

Pavlovian fear conditioning is an implicit form of learning and memory. However, during most emotional experiences, including fear conditioning, explicit or conscious memories are also formed. These occur through the opera-

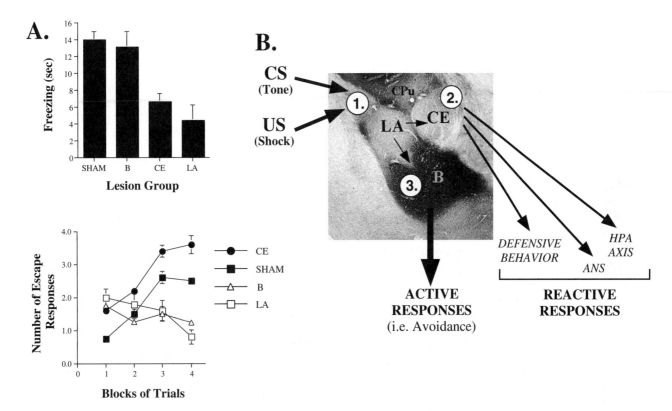

FIGURE 71.9   Active versus reactive fear. (A) Top graph shows percent freezing in rats given auditory fear conditioning after receiving selective amygdala lesions. Auditory fear conditioning is impaired by lesions of the CE and LA, but spared by lesions of the basal nucleus. Bottom graph shows number of escape responses across blocks of five trials during training in a one-way active avoidance task. Lesions of both LA and the basal nucleus impair this task; lesions of CE do not. (B) The data are consistent with a model in which projections between LA and CE are sufficient for Pavlovian fear conditioning (reactive responses), while projections between LA and the basal nucleus are necessary for instrumental avoidance learning (active responses). (Modified with permission from P. Amorapanth, J. E. LeDoux, and K. Nader, 2000. Different lateral amygdala outputs mediate reactions and actions elicited by a fear-arousing stimulus. *Nat. Neurosci.* 3:74–79. © 2000 by the Nature Publishing Group.)

tion of the medial temporal lobe memory system involving the hippocampus and related cortical areas (Milner, Squire, and Kandel, 1998; Eichenbaum, 2000). The role of the hippocampus in the explicit memory of an emotional experience is much the same as its role in other kinds of experiences, with one important exception. During a fearful or emotionally arousing experiences, the amygdala activates neuromodulatory systems in the brain and hormonal systems in the body via its projections to the hypothalamus, which can drive the hypothalamic-pituitary-adrenal (HPA) axis. Neurohormones released by these systems can in turn feed back to modulate the function of forebrain structures such as the hippocampus and serve to enhance the storage of the memory in these regions (McGaugh, 2000). The primary support for this model comes from studies of inhibitory avoidance learning, a type of passive avoidance learning in which the animal must learn not to enter a chamber in which it has previously received a shock. In this paradigm, various pharmacological manipulations of the amygdala that affect neurotransmitter or neurohormonal systems modulate the strength of the memory. For example,

immediate posttraining blockade of adrenergic or glucocorticoid receptors in the amygdala impairs memory retention of inhibitory avoidance, while facilitation of these systems in the amygdala enhances acquisition and memory storage (McGaugh et al., 1993; McGaugh, 2000). The exact subnuclei in the amygdala that are critical for memory modulation remain unknown, as are the areas of the brain where these amygdala projections influence memory storage. Candidate areas include the hippocampus and entorhinal and parietal cortices (Izquierdo et al., 1997). Indeed, it would be interesting to know whether the changes in unit activity or the activation of intracellular signaling cascades in the hippocampus during and after fear conditioning, as discussed earlier, might be related to the formation of such explicit memories, and how regulation of these signals depends on the integrity of the amygdala and its neuromodulators. A recent study has shown that stimulation of the basal nucleus of the amygdala can modulate the persistence of LTP in the hippocampus (Frey et al., 2001), which provides a potential mechanism whereby the amygdala can modulate hippocampal-dependent memories.

Summary

Basic research in emotion, especially that of fear and fear learning, has made a remarkable comeback in the neurosciences. In as little as 20 years, we have traced the neural circuits that underlie memory formation of fear conditioning, listened as cells in the amygdala alter their responsiveness to conditioned stimuli as animals acquire defensive behaviors, and looked into the cells of the amygdala in an effort to understand how these enduring changes are encoded at the biochemical or molecular level. Although much work remains to be done, a strong foundation has been laid for the further study of fear-related processes, including those related to reconsolidation, fear extinction, and memory modulation by emotional experiences. It is not yet known whether the findings of amygdala research might apply in a general way to other emotions. However, given the current enthusiasm for emotion research within the neurosciences, it would appear to be only a matter of time before the neural systems and mechanisms underlying other emotions are characterized.

ACKNOWLEDGMENTS   This work was supported in part by National Institutes of Health grants MH 46516, MH 00956, MH 39774, and MH 11902, and by a grant from the W.M. Keck Foundation to New York University.

REFERENCES

ABEL, T., P. V. NGUYEN, M. BARAD, T. A. DEUEL, E. R. KANDEL, and R. BOURTCHOULADZE, 1997. Genetic demonstration of a role for PKA in the late phase of LTP and in hippocampus-based long-term memory. *Cell* 88:615–626.

AMORAPANTH, P., J. E. LeDoux, and K. NADER, 2000. Different lateral amygdala outputs mediate reactions and actions elicited by a fear-arousing stimulus. *Nat. Neurosci.* 3:74–79.

ATKINS, C. M., J. C. SELCHER, J. J. PETRAITIS, J. M. TRZASKOS, and J. D. SWEATT, 1998. The MAPK cascade is required for mammalian associative learning. *Nat. Neurosci.* 1:602–609.

BAILEY, D. J., J. J. KIM, W. SUN, R. F. THOMPSON, and F. J. HELMSTETTER, 1999. Acquisition of fear conditioning in rats requires the synthesis of mRNA in the amygdala. *Behav. Neurosci.* 113:276–282.

BARRIENTOS, R. M., R. C. O'REILLY, and J. W. RUDY, 2002. Memory for context is impaired by injecting anisomycin into dorsal hippocampus following context exploration. *Behav. Brain Res.* 134:299–306.

BAUER, E. P., J. E. LeDoux, and K. NADER, 2001. Fear conditioning and LTP in the lateral amygdala are sensitive to the same stimulus contingencies. *Nat. Neurosci.* 4:687–688.

BAUER, E. P., G. E. SCHAFE, and J. E. LeDoux, 2002. NMDA receptors and L-type voltage-gated calcium channels contribute to long-term potentiation and different components of fear memory formation in the lateral amygdala. *J. Neurosci.* 22:5239–5249.

BLAIR, H. T., G. E. SCHAFE, E. P. BAUER, S. M. RODRIGUES, and J. E. LeDoux, 2001. Synaptic plasticity in the lateral amygdala: A cellular hypothesis of fear conditioning. *Learn. Mem.* 8:229–242.

BLANCHARD, R. J., and D. C. BLANCHARD, 1969. Crouching as an index of fear. *J. Comp. Physiol. Psychol.* 67:370–375.

BLANCHARD, R. J., T. E. DIELMAN, and D. C. BLANCHARD, 1968. Postshock crouching: Familiarity with the shock situation. *Psychonom. Sci.* 10:371–372.

BLISS, T. V. P., and T. LOMØ, 1973. Long-lasting potentiation of synaptic transmission in the dentate area of the anaesthetized rabbit following stimulation of the perforant path. *J. Physiol.* 232:331–356.

BORDI, F., and J. LeDoux, 1992. Sensory tuning beyond the sensory system: An initial analysis of auditory properties of neurons in the lateral amygdaloid nucleus and overlying areas of the striatum. *J. Neurosci.* 12:2493–2503.

BOURTCHOULADZE, R., B. FRENGUELLI, J. BLENDY, D. CIOFFI, G. SCHUTZ, and A. J. SILVA, 1994. Deficient long-term memory in mice with a targeted mutation of the cAMP-responsive element-binding protein. *Cell* 79:59–68.

BRAMBILLA, R., N. GNESUTTA, L. MINICHIELLO, G. WHITE, A. J. ROYLANCE, C. E. HERRON, M. RAMSEY, D. P. WOLFER, V. CESTARI, C. ROSSI-ARNAUD, S. G. GRANT, P. F. CHAPMAN, H. P. LIPP, E. STURANI, and R. KLEIN, 1997. A role for the Ras signalling pathway in synaptic transmission and long-term memory. *Nature* 390:281–286.

CAMPEAU, S., and M. DAVIS, 1995. Involvement of the central nucleus and basolateral complex of the amygdala in fear conditioning measured with fear-potentiated startle in rats trained concurrently with auditory and visual conditioned stimuli. *J. Neurosci.* 15:2301–2311.

CANTERAS, N. S., and L. W. SWANSON, 1992. Projections of the ventral subiculum to the amygdala, septum, and hypothalamus: A PHAL anterograde tract-tracing study in the rat. *J. Comp. Neurol.* 324:180–194.

CHAPMAN, P. F., E. W. KAIRISS, C. L. KEENAN, and T. H. BROWN, 1990. Long-term synaptic potentiation in the amygdala. *Synapse* 6:271–278.

CLUGNET, M. C., and J. E. LeDoux, 1989. Synaptic plasticity in fear conditioning circuits: Induction of LTP in the lateral nucleus of the amygdala by stimulation of the medial geniculate body. *J. Neurosci.* 10:2818–2824.

DAVIS, M., 1997. Neurobiology of fear responses: The role of the amygdala. *J. Neuropsychiatry Clin. Neurosci.* 9:382–402.

DAVIS, M., D. L. WALKER, and Y. LEE, 1997. Roles of the amygdala and bed nucleus of the stria terminalis in fear and anxiety measured with the acoustic startle reflex: Possible relevance to PTSD. *Ann. N.Y. Acad. Sci.* 821:305–331.

DE OCA, B. M., J. P. DeCOLA, S. MAREN, and M. S. FANSELOW, 1998. Distinct regions of the periaqueductal gray are involved in the acquisition and expression of defensive responses. *J. Neurosci.* 18:3426–3432.

DEBIEC, J., J. E. LeDoux, and K. NADER, 2002. Cellular and systems reconsolidation in the hippocampus. *Neuron* 36:527–538.

DORON, N. N., and J. E. LeDoux, 1999. Organization of projections to the lateral amygdala from auditory and visual areas of the thalamus in the rat. *J. Comp. Neurol.* 412:383–409.

DOYÈRE, V., C. REDINI-DEL NEGRO, G. DUTRIEUX, G. LE FLOCH, S. DAVIS, and S. LAROCHE, 1995. Potentiation or depression of synaptic efficacy in the dentate gyrus is determined by the relationship between the conditioned and unconditioned stimulus in a classical conditioning paradigm in rats. *Behav. Brain Res.* 70:15–29.

EDELINE, J.-M., P. PHAM, and N. M. WEINBERGER, 1993. Rapid development of learning-induced receptive field plasticity in the auditory cortex. *Behav. Neurosci.* 107:539–551.

EICHENBAUM, H., 2000. A cortical-hippocampal system for declarative memory. *Nat. Rev. Neurosci.* 1:41–50.

ENGLISH, J. D., and J. D. SWEATT, 1997. A requirement for the mitogen-activated protein kinase cascade in hippocampal long term potentiation. *J. Biol. Chem.* 272:19103–19106.

EVERITT, B. J., M. CADOR, and T. W. ROBBINS, 1989. Interactions between the amygdala and ventral striatum in stimulus-reward associations: Studies using a second-order schedule of sexual reinforcement. *Neuroscience* 30:63–75.

EVERITT, B. J., J. A. PARKINSON, M. C. OLMSTEAD, M. ARROYO, P. ROBLEDO, and T. W. ROBBINS, 1999. Associative processes in addiction and reward: The role of amygdala-ventral striatal subsystems. *Ann. N.Y. Acad. Sci.* 877:412–438.

FALLS, W. A., M. J. MISERENDINO, and M. DAVIS, 1992. Extinction of fear-potentiated startle: Blockade by infusion of an NMDA antagonist into the amygdala. *J. Neurosci.* 12:854–863.

FANSELOW, M. S., 1980. Conditional and unconditional components of postshock freezing. *Pavlovian J. Biol. Sci.* 15:177–182.

FANSELOW, M. S., and J. E. LEDOUX, 1999. Why we think plasticity underlying Pavlovian fear conditioning occurs in the basolateral amygdala. *Neuron* 23:229–232.

FARB, C. R., C. AOKI, T. MILNER, T. KANEKO, and J. LEDOUX, 1992. Glutamate immunoreactive terminals in the lateral amygdaloid nucleus: A possible substrate for emotional memory. *Brain Res.* 593:145–158.

FRANK, D. A., and M. E. GREENBERG, 1994. CREB: A mediator of long-term memory from mollusks to mammals. *Cell* 79: 5–8.

FRANKLAND, P. W., V. CESTARI, R. K. FILIPKOWSKI, R. J. MCDONALD, and A. J. SILVA, 1998. The dorsal hippocampus is essential for context discrimination but not for contextual conditioning. *Behav. Neurosci.* 112:863–874.

FREY, S., J. BERGADO-ROSADO, et al. 2001. Reinforcement of early long-term potentiation (early-LTP) in dentate gyrus by stimulation of the basolateral amygdala: Heterosynaptic induction mechanisms of late-LTP. *J. Neurosci.* 21(10):3697–3703.

GARCIA, R., R. M. VOUIMBA, M. BAUDRY, and R. F. THOMPSON, 1999. The amygdala modulates prefrontal cortex activity relative to conditioned fear. *Nature* 402:294–296.

GEWIRTZ, J. C., W. A. FALLS, and M. DAVIS, 1997. Normal conditioned inhibition and extinction of freezing and fear-potentiated startle following electrolytic lesions of medical prefrontal cortex in rats. *Behav. Neurosci.* 111:712–726.

GOOSENS, K. A., W. HOLT, and S. MAREN, 2000. A role for amygdaloid PKA and PKC in the acquisition of long-term conditional fear memories in rats. *Behav. Brain Res.* 114:145–152.

GOOSENS, K. A., and S. MAREN, 2001. Contextual and auditory fear conditioning are mediated by the lateral, basal, and central amygdaloid nuclei in rats. *Learn. Mem.* 8:148–155.

HALL, J., K. L. THOMAS, and B. J. EVERITT, 2000. Rapid and selective induction of BDNF expression in the hippocampus during contextual learning. *Nat. Neurosci.* 3:533–535.

HELMSTETTER, F. J., and J. LANDEIRA-FERNANDEZ, 1990. Conditional hypoalgesia is attenuated by naltrexone applied to the periaqueductal gray. *Brain Res.* 537:88–92.

HELMSTETTER, F. J., and S. A. TERSHNER, 1994. Lesions of the periaqueductal gray and rostral ventromedial medulla disrupt antinociceptive but not cardiovascular aversive conditional responses. *J. Neurosci.* 14:7099–7108.

HUANG, Y. Y., and E. R. KANDEL, 1998. Postsynaptic induction and PKA-dependent expression of LTP in the lateral amygdala. *Neuron* 21:169–178.

HUANG, Y. Y., X. C. LI, and E. R. KANDEL, 1994. cAMP contributes to mossy fiber LTP by initiating both a covalently mediated early phase and macromolecular synthesis-dependent late phase. *Cell* 79:69–79.

HUANG, Y. Y., K. C. MARTIN, and E. R. KANDEL, 2000. Both protein kinase A and mitogen-activated protein kinase are required in the amygdala for the macromolecular synthesis-dependent late phase of long-term potentiation. *J. Neurosci.* 20: 6317–6325.

IMPEY, S., M. MARK, E. C. VILLACRES, S. POSER, C. CHAVKIN, and D. R. STORM, 1996. Induction of CRE-mediated gene expression by stimuli that generate long-lasting LTP in area CA1 of the hippocampus. *Neuron* 16:973–982.

IMPEY, S., K. OBRIETAN, S. T. WONG, S. POSER, S. YANO, G. WAYMAN, J. C. DELOULME, G. CHAN, and D. R. STORM, 1998. Cross talk between ERK and PKA is required for Ca^{2+} stimulation of CREB-dependent transcription and ERK nuclear translocation. *Neuron* 21:869–883.

IMPEY, S., D. M. SMITH, K. OBRIETAN, R. DONAHUE, C. WADE, and D. R. STORM, 1998. Stimulation of cAMP response element (CRE)-mediated transcription during contextual learning. *Nat. Neurosci.* 1:595–601.

IWATA, J., J. E. LEDOUX, and D. J. REIS, 1986. Destruction of intrinsic neurons in the lateral hypothalamus disrupts the classical conditioning of autonomic but not behavioral emotional responses in the rat. *Brain Res.* 368:161–166.

IZQUIERDO, I., J. A. QUILLFELDT, M. S. ZANATTA, J. QUEVEDO, E. SCHAEFFER, P. K. SCHMITZ, and J. H. MEDINA, 1997. Sequential role of hippocampus and amygdala, entorhinal cortex and parietal cortex in formation and retrieval of memory for inhibitory avoidance in rats. *Eur. J. Neurosci.* 9:786–793.

JARRELL, T. W., C. G. GENTILE, L. M. ROMANSKI, P. M. MCCABE, and N. SCHNEIDERMAN, 1987. Involvement of cortical and thalamic auditory regions in retention of differential bradycardia conditioning to acoustic conditioned stimuli in rabbits. *Brain Res.* 412:285–294.

JOSSELYN, S. A., C. SHI, W. A. CARLEZON, JR., R. L. NEVE, E. J. NESTLER, and M. DAVIS, 2001. Long-term memory is facilitated by cAMP response element-binding protein overexpression in the amygdala. *J. Neurosci.* 21:2404–2412.

KAPP, B. S., R. C. FRYSINGER, M. GALLAGHER, and J. R. HASELTON, 1979. Amygdala central nucleus lesions: Effect on heart rate conditioning in the rabbit. *Physiol. Behav.* 23:1109–1117.

KIDA, S., S. A. JOSSELYN, S. P. DE ORTIZ, J. H. KOGAN, I. CHEVERE, S. MASUSHIGE, and A. J. SILVA, 2002. CREB required for the stability of new and reactivated fear memories. *Nat. Neurosci.* 5:348–355.

KILLCROSS, S., T. W. ROBBINS, and B. J. EVERITT, 1997. Different types of fear-conditioned behaviour mediated by separate nuclei within amygdala. *Nature* 388:377–380.

KIM, J. J., J. P. DECOLA, J. LANDEIRA-FERNANDEZ, and M. S. FANSELOW, 1991. N-Methyl-D-aspartate receptor antagonist APV blocks acquisition but not expression of fear conditioning. *Behav. Neurosci.* 105:126–133.

KIM, J. J., and M. S. FANSELOW, 1992. Modality-specific retrograde amnesia of fear. *Science* 256:675–677.

KIM, J. J., R. A. RISON, and M. S. FANSELOW, 1993. Effects of amygdala, hippocampus, and periaqueductal gray lesions on short- and long-term contextual fear. *Behav. Neurosci.* 107:1–6.

LEDOUX, J. E., 1996. *The Emotional Brain.* New York: Simon and Schuster.

LEDOUX, J. E., 2000. Emotion circuits in the brain. *Annu. Rev. Neurosic.* 23:155–184.

LeDoux, J. E., P. Cicchetti, A. Xagoraris, and L. M. Romanski, 1990. The lateral amygdaloid nucleus: Sensory interface of the amygdala in fear conditioning. *J. Neurosci.* 10:1062–1069.

LeDoux, J. E., and C. R. Farb, 1991. Neurons of the acoustic thalamus that project to the amygdala contain glutamate. *Neurosci. Lett.* 134:145–149.

LeDoux, J. E., C. R. Farb, and L. M. Romanski, 1991. Overlapping projections to the amygdala and striatum from auditory processing areas of the thalamus and cortex. *Neurosci. Lett.* 134:139–144.

LeDoux, J. E., J. Iwata, P. Cicchetti, and D. J. Reis, 1988. Different projections of the central amygdaloid nucleus mediate autonomic and behavioral correlates of conditioned fear. *J. Neurosci.* 8:2517–2529.

LeDoux, J. E., J. Iwata, D. Pearl, and D. J. Reis, 1986. Disruption of auditory but not visual learning by destruction of intrinsic neurons in the rat medial geniculate body. *Brain Res.* 371:395–399.

LeDoux, J. E., A. Sakaguchi, and D. J. Reis, 1984. Subcortical efferent projections of the medial geniculate nucleus mediate emotional responses conditioned by acoustic stimuli. *J. Neurosci.* 4:683–698.

LeDoux, J. E., D. A. Ruggierio, and D. J. Reis, 1985. Projections to the subcortical forebrain from anatomically defined regions of the medial geniculate body in the rat. *J. Comp. Neurol.* 242:182–213.

Li, X. F., G. E. Stutzmann, and J. E. LeDoux, 1996. Convergent but temporally separated inputs to lateral amygdala neurons from the auditory thalamus and auditory cortex use different postsynaptic receptors: In vivo intracellular and extracellular recordings in fear conditioning pathways. *Learn. Mem.* 3:229–242.

Lu, K. T., D. L. Walker, and M. Davis, 2001. Mitogen-activated protein kinase cascade in the basolateral nucleus of amygdala is involved in extinction of fear-potentiated startle. *J. Neurosci.* 21:RC162.

Maren, S., 1998. Overtraining does not mitigate contextual fear conditioning deficits produced by neurotoxic lesions of the basolateral amygdala. *J. Neurosci.* 18:3088–3097.

Maren, S., 1999. Long-term potentiation in the amygdala: A mechanism for emotional learning and memory. *Trends Neurosci.* 22:561–567.

Maren, S., 2000. Auditory fear conditioning increases CS-elicited spike firing in lateral amygdala neurons even after extensive overtraining. *Eur. J. Neurosci.* 12:4047–4054.

Maren, S., G. Aharonov, and M. S. Fanselow, 1997. Neurotoxic lesions of the dorsal hippocampus and Pavlovian fear conditioning in rats. *Behav. Brain Res.* 88:261–274.

Maren, S., and M. S. Fanselow, 1995. Synaptic plasticity in the basolateral amygdala induced by hippocampal formation stimulation in vivo. *J. Neurosci.* 15:7548–7564.

Mayford, M., M. E. Bach, Y. Y. Huang, L. Wang, R. D. Hawkins, and E. R. Kandel, 1996. Control of memory formation through regulated expression of a CaMKII transgene. *Science* 274:1678–1683.

McDonald, A. J., 1998. Cortical pathways to the mammalian amygdala. *Prog. Neurobiol.* 55:257–332.

McDonald, A. J., F. Mascagni, and L. Guo, 1996. Projections of the medial and lateral prefrontal cortices to the amygdala: A *Phaseolus vulgaris* leucoagglutinin study in the rat. *Neuroscience* 71:55–75.

McGaugh, J. L., 2000. Memory: A century of consolidation. *Science* 287:248–251.

McGaugh, J. L., I. B. Introini-Collison, L. F. Cahill, C. Castellano, C. Dalmaz, M. B. Parent, and C. L. Williams, 1993. Neuromodulatory systems and memory storage: Role of the amygdala. *Behav. Brain Res.* 58:81–90.

McKernan, M. G., and P. Shinnick-Gallagher, 1997. Fear conditioning induces a lasting potentiation of synaptic currents in vitro. *Nature* 390:607–611.

Medina, J. F., J. C. Repa, and J. E. LeDoux, 2002. Parallels between cerebellum- and amygdala-dependent conditioning. *Nat. Rev. Neurosci.* 3:122–131.

Milad, M. R., and G. J. Quirk, 2002. Neurons in medial prefrontal cortex signal memory for fear extinction. *Nature* 420:70–74.

Milner, B., L. R. Squire, and E. R. Kandel, 1998. Cognitive neuroscience and the study of memory. *Neuron* 20:445–468.

Miserendino, M. J. D., C. B. Sananes, K. R. Melia, and M. Davis, 1990. Blocking of acquisition but not expression of conditioned fear-potentiated startle by NMDA antagonists in the amygdala. *Nature* 345:716–718.

Moita, M. A., S. Rosis, Y. Zhou, J. E. LeDoux, and H. T. Blair, 2003. Hippocampal place cells acquire location-specific responses to the conditioned stimulus during auditory fear conditioning. *Neuron* 37:485–497.

Morgan, M. A., and J. E. LeDoux, 1995. Differential contribution of dorsal and ventral medial prefrontal cortex to the acquisition and extinction of conditioned fear in rats. *Behav. Neurosci.* 109:681–688.

Morgan, M. A., L. M. Romanski, and J. E. LeDoux, 1993. Extinction of emotional learning: Contribution of medial prefrontal cortex. *Neurosci. Lett.* 163:109–113.

Muller, J., K. P. Corodimas, Z. Fridel, and J. E. LeDoux, 1997. Functional inactivation of the lateral and basal nuclei of the amygdala by muscimol infusion prevents fear conditioning to an explicit conditioned stimulus and to contextual stimuli. *Behav. Neurosci.* 111:683–691.

Nader, K., P. Majidishad, P. Amorapanth, and J. E. LeDoux, 2001. Damage to the lateral and central, but not other, amygdaloid nuclei prevents the acquisition of auditory fear conditioning. *Learn. Mem.* 8:156–163.

Nader, K., G. E. Schafe, and J. E. LeDoux, 2000. Fear memories require protein synthesis in the amygdala for reconsolidation after retrieval. *Nature* 406:722–726.

Nguyen, P. V., and E. R. Kandel, 1996. A macromolecular synthesis-dependent late phase of long-term potentiation requiring cAMP in the medial perforant pathway of rat hippocampal slices. *J. Neurosci.* 16:3189–3198.

Paré, D., Y. Smith, and J. F. Paré, 1995. Intra-amygdaloid projections of the basolateral and basomedial nuclei in the cat: *Phaseolus vulgaris*-leucoagglutinin anterograde tracing at the light and electron microscopic level. *Neuroscience* 69:567–583.

Phillips, R. G., and J. E. LeDoux, 1992. Differential contribution of amygdala and hippocampus to cued and contextual fear conditioning. *Behav. Neurosci.* 106:274–285.

Pitkänen, A., V. Savander, and J. E. LeDoux, 1997. Organization of intra-amygdaloid circuitries in the rat: an emerging framework for understanding functions of the amygdala. *Trends Neurosci.* 20:517–523.

Quirk, G. J., J. L. Armony, and J. E. LeDoux, 1997. Fear conditioning enhances different temporal components of toned-evoked spike trains in auditory cortex and lateral amygdala. *Neuron* 19:613–624.

Quirk, G. J., J. L. Armony, J. C. Repa, X.-F. Li, and J. E. LeDoux, 1997. Emotional memory: A search for sites of plasticity. *Cold Spring Harbor Symp. Biol.* 61:247–257.

QUIRK, G. J., C. REPA, and J. E. LEDOUX, 1995. Fear conditioning enhances short-latency auditory responses of lateral amygdala neurons: Parallel recordings in the freely behaving rat. *Neuron* 15:1029–1039.

QUIRK, G. J., G. K. RUSSO, J. L. BARRON, and K. LEBRON, 2000. The role of ventromedial prefrontal cortex in the recovery of extinguished fear. *J. Neurosci.* 20:6225–6231.

RAMPON, C., Y. P. TANG, J. GOODHOUSE, E. SHIMIZU, M. KYIN, and J. Z. TSIEN, 2000. Enrichment induces structural changes and recovery from nonspatial memory deficits in CA1 NMDAR1-knockout mice. *Nat. Neurosci.* 3:238–244.

REPA, J. C., J. MULLER, J. APERGIS, T. M. DESROCHERS, Y. ZHOU, and J. E. LEDOUX, 2001. Two different lateral amygdala cell populations contribute to the initiation and storage of memory. *Nat. Neurosci.* 4:724–731.

RESCORLA, R. A., 1968. Probability of shock in the presence and absence of CS in fear conditioning. *J. Comp. Physiol. Psychol.* 66:1–5.

ROBBINS, T. W., M. CADOR, J. R. TAYLOR, and B. J. EVERITT, 1989. Limbic-striatal interactions in reward-related processes. *Neurosci. Biobehav. Rev.* 13:155–162.

RODRIGUES, S. M., G. E. SCHAFE, and J. E. LEDOUX, 2001. Intraamygdala blockade of the NR2B subunit of the NMDA receptor disrupts the acquisition but not the expression of fear conditioning. *J. Neurosci.* 21:6889–6896.

ROGAN, M. T., and J. E. LEDOUX, 1995. LTP is accompanied by commensurate enhancement of auditory-evoked responses in a fear conditioning circuit. *Neuron* 15:127–136.

ROGAN, M., U. STAUBLI, and J. LEDOUX, 1997. Fear conditioning induces associative long-term potentiation in the amygdala. *Nature* 390:604–607.

ROMANSKI, L. M., M. C. CLUGNET, F. BORDI, and J. E. LEDOUX, 1993. Somatosensory and auditory convergence in the lateral nucleus of the amygdala. *Behav. Neurosci.* 107:444–450.

ROMANSKI, L. M., and J. E. LEDOUX, 1992. Equipotentiality of thalamo-amygdala and thalamo-cortico-amygdala circuits in auditory fear conditioning. *J. Neurosci.* 12:4501–4509.

ROMANSKI, L. M., and J. E. LEDOUX, 1993. Information cascade from primary auditory cortex to the amygdala: Corticocortical and corticoamygdaloid projections of temporal cortex in the rat. *Cereb. Cortex* 3:515–532.

ROOZENDAAL, B., J. M. KOOLHAAS, and B. BOHUS, 1991. Attenuated cardiovascular, neuroendocrine, and behavioral responses after a single footshock in central amygdaloid lesioned male rats. *Physiol. Behav.* 50:771–775.

SARA, S. J., 2000. Retrieval and reconsolidation: Toward a neurobiology of remembering. *Learn. Mem.* 7:73–84.

SCHAFE, G. E., C. M. ATKINS, M. W. SWANK, E. P. BAUER, J. D. SWEATT, and J. E. LEDOUX, 2000. Activation of ERK/MAP kinase in the amygdala is required for memory consolidation of Pavlovian fear conditioning. *J. Neurosci.* 20:8177–8187.

SCHAFE, G. E., and J. E. LEDOUX, 2000. Memory consolidation of auditory pavlovian fear conditioning requires protein synthesis and protein kinase A in the amygdala. *J. Neurosci.* 20: RC96.

SCHAFE, G. E., K. NADER, H. T. BLAIR, and J. E. LEDOUX, 2001. Memory consolidation of Pavlovian fear conditioning: A cellular and molecular perspective. *Trends Neurosci.* 24:540–546.

SILVA, A. J., C. F. STEVENS, S. TONEGAWA, and Y. WANG, 1992. Deficient hippocampal long-term potentiation in alpha-calcium-calmodulin kinase II mutant mice. *Science* 257:201–206.

SILVA, A. J., J. H. KOGAN, P. W. FRANKLAND, and S. KIDA, 1998. CREB and memory. *Annu. Rev. Neurosci.* 21:127–148.

SMITH, O. A., C. A. ASTLEY, J. L. DEVITO, J. M. STEIN, and R. E. WALSH, 1980. Functional analysis of hypothalamic control of the cardiovascular responses accompanying emotional behavior. *Fed. Proc.* 39:2487–2494.

SODERLING, T. R., and V. A. DERKACH, 2000. Postsynaptic protein phosphorylation and LTP. *Trends Neurosci.* 23:75–80.

STIEDL, O., K. BIRKENFELD, M. PALVE, and J. SPIESS, 2000. Impairment of conditioned contextual fear of C57BL/6J mice by intracerebral injections of the NMDA receptor antagonist APV. *Behav. Brain Res.* 116:157–168.

TSVETKOV, E., W. A. CARLEZON, F. M. BENES, E. R. KANDEL, and V. Y. BOLSHAKOV, 2002. Fear conditioning occludes LTP-induced presynaptic enhancement of synaptic transmission in the cortical pathway to the lateral amygdala. *Neuron* 34:289–300.

WALKER, D. L., K. J. RESSLER, K.-T. LU, and M. DAVIS, 2002. Facilitation of conditioned fear extinction by systemic administration or intra-amygdala infusions of D-cycloserine as assessed with fear-potentiated startle in rats. *J. Neurosci.* 22:2343–2351.

WEEBER, E. J., C. M. ATKINS, J. C. SELCHER, A. W. VARGA, B. MIRNIKJOO, R. PAYLOR, M. LEITGES, and J. D. SWEATT, 2000. A role for the beta isoform of protein kinase C in fear conditioning. *J. Neurosci.* 20:5906–5914.

WEISSKOPF, M. G., E. P. BAUER, and J. E. LEDOUX, 1999. L-Type voltage-gated calcium channels mediate NMDA-independent associative long-term potentiation at thalamic input synapses to the amygdala. *J. Neurosci.* 19:10512–10519.

WILENSKY, A. E., G. E. SCHAFE, and J. E. LEDOUX, 2000. The amygdala modulates memory consolidation of fear-motivated inhibitory avoidance learning but not classical fear conditioning. *J. Neurosci.* 20:7059–7066.

YIN, J. C., and T. TULLY, 1996. CREB and the formation of long-term memory. *Curr. Opin. Neurobiol.* 6:264–268.

YOUNG, S. L., D. L. BOHENEK, and M. S. FANSELOW, 1994. NMDA processes mediate anterograde amnesia of contextual fear conditioning induced by hippocampal damage: Immunization against amnesia by context preexposure. *Behav. Neurosci.* 108: 19–29.

72 The Human Amygdala and Awareness: Interactions Between Emotion and Cognition

ELIZABETH A. PHELPS

ABSTRACT Traditional approaches to the study of human cognition considered emotion as a distinct process that could be studied independently. Initial investigations of the neuroscience of emotion supported this distinction by identifying brain structures, such as the amygdala, that appeared to be specialized for emotion. However, recent studies indicate that the amygdala interacts extensively with brain systems linked to cognition and awareness, suggesting a means for the interaction of emotion and cognition. Cognition and awareness can influence the amygdala through the verbal communication of emotion information or the cognitive control of emotional responses. The amygdala can influence cognition and awareness by altering the retention of memory with arousal and facilitating attention and perception. Evidence from cognitive neuroscience suggests that in order to understand the neural systems of cognition, a consideration of its interaction with emotion is necessary.

The relation between emotion and cognition has been a topic of debate since the days of the early philosophers. Aristotle suggested that emotion (the sensitive soul) and cognition (the rational soul) are different grades of the human soul, with only the rational soul (cognition) being unique to humans. The influence of this early philosophical work laid the groundwork for future discussions concerning cognition and its relation to emotion. In the 1980s, the psychologists Robert Zajonc and Richard Lazarus debated the appropriate role for emotion in our understanding of cognition. Zajonc (1980, 1984) argued that emotional responses can occur independently and prior to cognition and awareness, whereas Lazarus (1981, 1984) emphasized that emotional responses are dependent on cognitive interpretations.

Investigations of the neural systems of emotion are beginning to contribute to this debate. The amygdala, a small, almond-shaped structure in the medial temporal lobe, is a brain region that seems to be specialized for emotion (e.g., LeDoux, 1996, 2002). Animal models of the role of the amygdala in emotion processing have suggested it is a critical structure in the acquisition and expression of fear learn-

ing. Using a fear conditioning paradigm, researchers such as Joseph LeDoux (1996), Michael Davis (2000), and Bruce Kapp (e.g., Kapp et al., 1992) have traced the pathways for fear learning from stimulus input to response output (see Schafe and LeDoux, this volume). When these paradigms were extended to humans, the separation between emotion and cognition became apparent. Consistent with the animal models, patients with amygdala damage failed to demonstrate normal fear conditioning as assessed by physiological measures of autonomic nervous system arousal (Bechara et al., 1995; LaBar et al., 1995). However, these same patients indicated a cognitive awareness and understanding of the parameters of fear conditioning. The acquisition of the ability to remember and explicitly report the procedures of fear conditioning depended on a neighboring temporal lobe structure, the hippocampus (Bechara et al., 1995).

For example, patient S.P., who had sustained bilateral amygdala damage, and normal control subjects were presented with a blue square paired with a shock to the wrist. After several pairings, the normal control subjects began to show a physiological arousal response to the blue square presented alone, indicating acquisition of a conditioned fear response. S.P. failed to show an arousal response to the blue square. When S.P. was shown the data indicating that she did not demonstrate a normal conditioned fear response as assessed by autonomic arousal, she commented,

I knew that there was an anticipation that the blue square, at some particular point in time, would bring on one of the volt shocks. But even though I knew that, and I knew that from the very beginning, except for the very first one I was surprised. That was my response—I knew it was going to happen. I expected that it was going to happen. So I learned from the very beginning that it was going to happen: blue and shock. And it happened. I turned out to be right, it happened!

It is clear that S.P. was aware of the fear conditioning procedure, even though she failed to show a conditioned fear response (Phelps, 2002). Patients with hippocampal damage and an intact amygdala show the opposite pattern of results.

ELIZABETH A. PHELPS Department of Psychology, New York University, New York.

That is, they are unable to explicitly report the relation between the different stimuli, but they show normal conditioned responses (Bechara et al., 1995).

This dissociation between the neural systems of conditioned fear responses and explicit memory for the procedures of fear conditioning suggests that the amygdala can operate independently of awareness and cognitive interpretation. This independence, however, is limited. More recent research suggests that the relationship between the amygdala and cognitive awareness is more complex. In this chapter, I will outline how emotion and cognition interact through the amygdala. The relation between the amygdala and cognitive processes is bidirectional, with the amygdala influencing cognition and awareness, and vice versa.

Cognition to emotion: Cognition and awareness influence the amygdala

The amygdala is often described as a brain structure that is specialized for emotional processing (LeDoux, 2002). Most of the research examining amygdala function across species has highlighted its role in fear; however, more recent research has suggested it may also be involved in the processing of arousing, positive stimuli (e.g., Hamann et al., 1999; LaBar et al., 2001; Anderson, Christoff, Stappen, et al., 2003). There are two primary ways in which cognitive processes have been shown to influence the amygdala.

FEAR LEARNING THROUGH INSTRUCTION In the classic fear conditioning paradigm, a previously neutral stimulus acquires aversive properties by being paired with an aversive event. For instance, a person could be afraid of a neighborhood dog because the dog once bit that individual. This would be analogous to learning with fear conditioning. The previously neutral dog has acquired aversive properties by virtue of the individual's direct, personal experience of a painful bite. However, a person could also acquire a fear response to a neighborhood dog, not because it bit that person but because a neighbor told him or her that it was a mean dog that might bite. This type of symbolic communication is a common means of learning in human experience. In this case, the individual was verbally instructed about the aversive nature of the dog. This is an example of an *instructed fear* paradigm.

Animal models of the role of the amygdala in fear conditioning have suggested that the amygdala is critical in both the acquisition and expression of conditioned fear (LeDoux, 1996; but see also Cahill et al., 1999). In contrast, learning through verbal communication, or instruction, does not require the amygdala. During instructed fear, the subject is told that a particular stimulus, for example a blue square, predicts the possible occurrence of an aversive event, such as a shock to the wrist. This ability to understand and

remember the relationship between the blue square and shock depends on neural systems underlying language and episodic memory. Instructed fear results in the subject's acquiring an awareness of the aversive properties of the blue square without any direct, personal aversive experience. The question is, does the amygdala play any role in this cognitive means of fear learning?

In an effort to address this question, subjects participating in a functional magnetic resonance imaging (fMRI) study were instructed that they might receive a mild shock to the wrist when a blue square was presented (the threat stimulus). They were told that they would never receive a shock when a yellow square was presented (the safe stimulus). Although none of the subjects actually received a shock, all of the subjects reported that they believed a shock would be presented (Phelps et al., 2001). Consistent with this subjective report, subjects showed greater physiological arousal during presentations of the threat stimulus (blue squares) than during presentation of the safe stimulus (yellow squares). In addition, subjects showed an increase in blood-oxygen-level-dependent (BOLD) signal in the left amygdala during presentations of the threat relative to presentations of the safe stimulus, indicating amygdala involvement in the processing of instructed fear (figure 72.1).

In an effort to determine the specific role of the left amygdala in instructed fear, brain-injured patients with right, left, or bilateral amygdala damage participated in a similar study. Normal control subjects and patients with damage confined to the right amygdala demonstrated a greater or potentiated startle reflex response to the threat stimulus than to the safe stimulus, an indication of a fear response to verbal threat. Patients whose damage included the left amygdala failed to show a potentiated startle response to the threat stimulus (Funayama et al., 2001).

These results suggest that the left amygdala mediates the physiological expressions of fears that are learned through verbal communication. In such a situation, awareness of the emotional properties of the stimulus, independent of direct experience, results in amygdala involvement. In fear conditioning, awareness is not even necessary for the expression of a learned fear response. Öhman and colleagues (Öhman and Soares, 1993; Esteves, Dimberg, and Öhman, 1994) have shown that subliminal, masked presentations of a conditioned stimulus result in a conditioned response. This begs the question of whether awareness is necessary for the expression of instructed fear learning.

To investigate this question, Olsson and Phelps (in press) assessed physiological fear responses to both masked (subliminal) and unmasked (supraliminal) presentations of stimuli that had been linked to aversive, emotional consequences (i.e., a shock to the wrist). Some of the subjects learned this link through fear conditioning in which the stimulus was paired with the shock. Others learned through

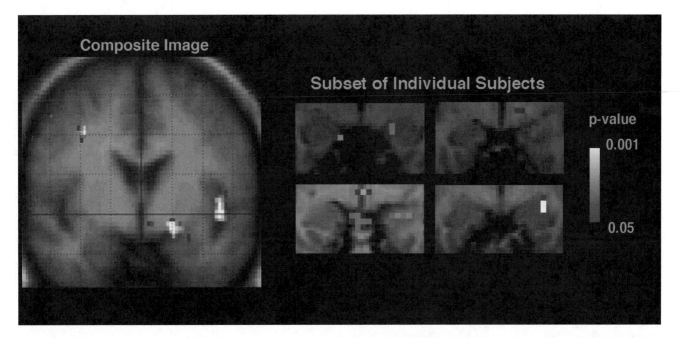

FIGURE 72.1 Activation of the left amygdala in response to instructed fear. Shown are composite activation response to threat versus safe stimuli (left) and selected individual subjects' responses (right). (Adapted with permission from E. A. Phelps et al., Activation of the left amygdala to a cognitive representation of fear. *Nat. Neurosci.* 4:437–441. © 2001 by the Nature Publishing Group.) (See color plate 59.)

instruction. They were told that a particular stimulus predicted a shock. A third group learned this link through observation. They watched a confederate who received a shock paired with a specific stimulus. None of the subjects in the instruction or observation learning conditions actually received a shock. During unmasked (supraliminal) presentations of the stimulus linked to shock, all subjects showed similar levels of physiological arousal (as measured by skin conductance), indicating that fear learning occurred in all conditions. When the stimulus linked with shock was presented briefly and masked (subliminal presentation) subjects who had undergone the fear conditioning procedure continued to show an arousal response, replicating earlier results (Öhman and Soares, 1993; Esteves, Dimberg, and Öhman, 1994). In contrast, subjects who had learned through instruction failed to show any response to the masked stimuli. This suggests that awareness is necessary for the expression of fear learning through instruction. Interestingly, the results from subjects in the observation condition were similar to those in the fear conditioning condition. Vicarious learning through observation resulted in expression of the learned fear response when the stimulus linked to shock was presented both subliminally and supraliminally. The results from the observation learning group are consistent with the idea that vicarious experience may more directly mirror the neural (Rizzolatti, Fogassi, and Gallese, 2002; Carr et al., 2003) and behavioral (e.g., Öhman and Mineka, 2001) effects of learning through personal experience.

Demonstrating the amygdala's involvement in instructed fear learning is important because in everyday human experience, symbolic and vicarious means of communication are a primary means of knowledge transfer. This indicates that animal models of neural systems of fear conditioning may be applicable to a wider range of human behavior. Unlike fear conditioning, learning through instruction requires only the left amygdala for expression, whereas damage to either the right or left amygdala leads to deficits of conditioned fear (LaBar et al., 1995). This laterality difference may be due to the fact that instructed fear depends on left-hemisphere-dominant functions, such as verbal communication and cognitive interpretation (e.g., Gazzaniga, 2000). When learning through instruction or observation, there is an awareness of the emotional properties of the stimulus that is acquired without any direct aversive experience. This suggests that the amygdala is important in the expression of cognitive fears that are imagined and anticipated but never actually experienced.

EMOTION REGULATION   Another means by which cognition and interpretation have been shown to influence the amygdala is emotion regulation. Emotion regulation refers to using a cognitive strategy or attentional focus to alter emotional reactions. It is not uncommon in everyday human experience to attempt to modulate a negative emotional state by focusing on nonemotional or positive aspects of a situation. The common phrase "the glass is half-full" (as opposed to half-empty) refers to a strategy of focusing on positive rather than negative possible interpretations or consequences of a situation. This is an example of the emotion regulation strategy of reappraisal.

Typical studies of reappraisal ask subjects to view scenes or film clips of emotional events (see Gross, 2002, for a review). Subjects are instructed either to simply attend to the stimuli or to reinterpret the events depicted in a way that makes them less negative. For example, if a scene shows a group of people crying outside of a church, a common interpretation is that the scene depicts a funeral. Another possible interpretation is that the scene depicts a wedding in which there are tears of joy. Subjects who are instructed to reappraise the scene are encouraged to focus on possible nonemotional or positive interpretations of the scenes. Subjects who successfully reappraise the emotional significance of an event report less distress and show decreases in physiological arousal responses to the negative emotional stimuli.

In an effort to assess whether cognitive reappraisal can alter amygdala function, Ochsner and colleagues (2002) presented subjects with pictures of emotional scenes and asked them either to attend to the pictures or to reappraise the situations depicted. Consistent with previous studies, subjects rated their subjective reaction to the emotional, negative scenes as less negative on the reappraisal trials relative to the attended trials. Using fMRI, Ochsner and colleagues found that the presentation of negative scenes on the attended trials resulted in more activation of the amygdala relative to the reappraisal trials (see Schaefer et al., 2002, for a similar finding). During the reappraisal trials there was relatively more activation of the left lateral prefrontal cortex (LPFC), a region that has also been implicated in the executive control of working memory (e.g., Smith and Jonides, 1999; Miller and Cohen, 2001). There was a negative correlation between these two brain areas. Subjects who showed greater left LPFC activation in response to viewing the negative scenes on the reappraisal (vs. attend) trials also showed less amygdala activation (figure 72.2). Our current understanding of the neuroanatomical connections between the amygdala and the prefrontal cortex suggests that the LPFC may not be altering amygdala function through direct projections (McDonald, 1991; Stefanacci and Amaral, 2002) but by a more indirect route. This research suggests that the ability to engage executive control processes during reappraisal can change the amygdala's response.

In addition, studies examining the influence of attentional demands on amygdala function have found that in limited circumstances, a distracting attentional task can also influence the amygdala response. Although most studies examining the effect of attention on the amygdala have reported that the allocation of attention has no effect on the strength of the amygdala response to an emotional stimulus (Vuillemier et al., 2001; Anderson, Christoff, and Panitz,

2003), there are exceptions. Pessoa, McKenna, and Gutierrez (2002) used a demanding attention task that required subjects to respond to stimuli presented in the peripheral region of perceptual space. This task was conducted while fearful faces and neutral faces were presented at the center of the screen. When attentional demands were minimal, there was greater amygdala activation in response to the fearful versus neutral faces. However, the amygdala response to fearful faces was diminished during the peripheral attention task (see also Anderson, Christoff, Panitz, et al., 2003). This highlights a situation where the focus of attention can influence amygdala processing. Along with the reappraisal study mentioned earlier, these studies indicate that the amygdala's reaction to an emotional situation can be altered by cognitive demands and interpretation.

SUMMARY: COGNITION TO EMOTION   Studies of fear conditioning in humans suggest that the amygdala plays a role in the acquisition and expression of learned fear, irrespective of awareness of the emotional properties of the stimulus and more cognitive means of learning. These results highlight the independence of the neural systems of emotion and cognition. However, this evidence from fear conditioning does not rule out a role for awareness and cognitive intrepretation in amygdala processing. Both symbolic means of emotional learning (i.e., language) and cognitive strategies can alter amygdala function. It appears that cognition may influence the amygdala and emotional reactions in a range of circumstances.

Emotion to cognition: The amygdala's influence on cognition and awareness

The demonstration that the amygdala's response can depend on cognition indicates the complex relationship between emotion and cognition. There is also evidence to suggest that cognition and awareness can depend on the amygdala. In many ways, the amygdala is well situated to influence cognition. There are direct projections between the amygdala and both mnemonic and sensory processing regions (e.g., Stefanacci and Amaral, 2000; Amaral, Behniea, and Kelly, 2003). Consistent with its neuroanatomical connectivity, it has been suggested the amygdala can influence cognition and awareness in two different ways: by modulating memory and by modulating attention or perception.

THE AMYGDALA AND EPISODIC MEMORY   The most important development in memory research that has emerged in the last 50 years is the recognition of many kinds of memory and corresponding memory systems. In humans, the most dominant type of memory is episodic memory (also called declarative or explicit memory), which allows us to be aware of past events. Episodic memory depends on the hippocampal complex for acquisition, and damage to this brain

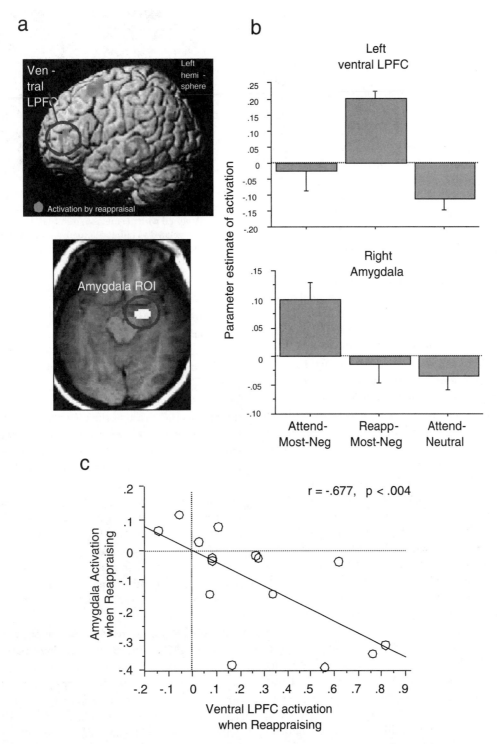

FIGURE 72.2 (a) Activation of the left, ventral LPFC during reappraisal versus attended trials (top) and right amygdala activation during attended versus reappraisal trials (bottom). (b) Parameter estimates of activation to the right amygdala and left, ventral LPFC. (c) Scatterplot depicting the correlation activation of the amygdala and ventral LPFC for reappraisal versus attended trials. (Adapted with permission from K. N. Ochsner et al., Rethinking feelings: An fMRI study of the cognitive regulation of emotion. *J. Cogn. Neurosci.* 14:1215–1229. © 2002 by the Society for Neuroscience.) (See color plate 60.)

region results in extreme difficulty in everyday functioning. One of the ways in which the amygdala can alter cognition and awareness is by modulating the hippocampal memory system. Research on emotion and memory has shown that discrete or mild arousal can enhance episodic memory performance (e.g., Christianson, 1992). Consistent with this behavioral data, McGaugh and colleagues (e.g., McGaugh, 2000) have identified a pathway by which the amygdala can influence hippocampal processing with arousal. In a series of studies, they have shown that the amygdala modulates the consolidation of hippocampal-dependent memories. Hippocampal consolidation is a slow process by which memories become more or less stable over time. By enhancing consolidation with arousal, the amygdala is altering the storage component of episodic memory formation (McGaugh et al., 1992).

To demonstrate that the amygdala modulates memory storage, McGaugh and colleagues disrupted or enhanced amygdala processing in rats *after* encoding, and examined the effect of arousal on memory. For example, Packard and Teather (1998) gave rats a maze-learning task that depended on the hippocampus. Immediately after learning, some of the rats received intra-amygdala injections of amphetamine and others received saline. Those rats whose amygdalas were pharmacologically excited after learning showed better retention for the maze. The mechanism by which the amygdala modulates consolidation is related to the neurohormonal changes that occur with arousal. Physiological arousal is linked to activation of the β-adrenergic system in the amygdala. Drugs that block the action of the β-adrenergic system also block the effect of arousal on episodic memory in both rats (e.g., McGaugh et al., 1992) and humans (e.g., Cahill et al., 1994). McGaugh (2002) and colleagues have suggested that one of the adaptive functions of having a long consolidation process for the storage of hippocampal-dependent memories is to allow time for the arousal response to enhance the retention of events linked to emotional consequences.

A number of studies have shown that the human amygdala plays a role in the long-term recollection of arousing events. Brain imaging studies have observed a correlation between the strength of the amygdala response to an emotional stimulus at encoding and the likelihood of successful recollection at a later time (e.g., Cahill et al., 1996; Hamann et al., 1999; Canli et al., 2000). Patients with damage to the amygdala fail to show arousal-enhanced memory (e.g., Cahill et al., 1995). If arousal, via the amygdala, is modulating the storage of episodic memory, there should be different forgetting curves for arousing and nonarousing stimuli. This has been demonstrated in a number of behavioral studies (see Christianson, 1992). In a classic study, Kleinsmith and Kaplan (1963) presented subjects with word-digit pairs. Half of the words were emotional and arousing

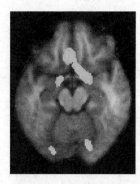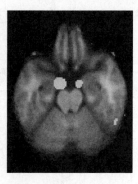

FIGURE 72.3 Amygdala activity during encoding correlated with subsequent memory for positive (left) and negative (right) picture stimuli. (Adapted with permission from S. B. Hamann et al., Amygdala activity related to enhanced memory for pleasant and aversive stimuli. *Nat. Neurosci.* 2:289–293. © 1999 by the Nature Publishing Group.)

and half were neutral. Subjects were given a cued recall task in which they were presented with the word and asked to recall the digit. Some of the subjects were given the memory task immediately after encoding and others were tested a day later. Comparing across the groups, there was forgetting over time for the neutral word-digit pairs, but memory for the arousing word-digit pairs did not diminish over time. Consistent with the idea that the amygdala enhances consolidation or storage processes, patients with amygdala damage, unlike normal controls, show similar patterns of forgetting for arousing and neutral words (LaBar and Phelps, 1998). In addition, using positron emission tomography (PET), Hamann and colleagues (1999) found that amygdala activity at encoding for positive and negative arousing scenes predicted recognition success 1 month later (figure 72.3). There was no relation between amygdala activation and memory performance on an immediate test of recollection. Thus, both research in patients and neuroimaging studies support a role for the human amygdala in the storage of episodic memories.

By influencing the retention of hippocampal-dependent memories, the amygdala alters the information that can be recollected over time. Long-term memory and awareness for events can be modulated by the amygdala. Although many other factors influence the retention of both emotional and nonemotional events (e.g, Phelps et al., 1998; Schacter, 2001), arousal, via the amygdala, is one of the mechanisms by which emotion can influence cognition and awareness.

EMOTIONAL MODULATION OF ATTENTION/PERCEPTION Research on the neural systems of memory and emotion suggest that the amygdala can modulate the storage component of episodic memory. It has also been suggested that emotion can affect the encoding stage of memory by altering attention or perceptual processing (e.g., Christianson and Loftus, 1991). Although there is no direct evidence that the

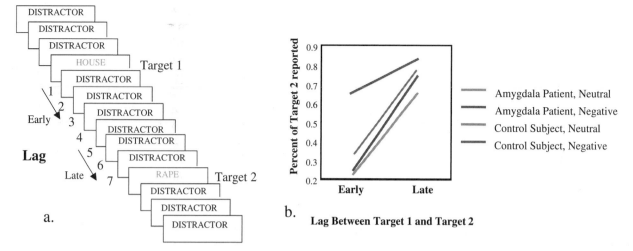

a.

b.

Lag Between Target 1 and Target 2

Figure 72.4   (a) Schematic illustration of the attentional blink paradigm with an emotion word in the second target position. (b) Percent correct identification of target 2 reported in the early and late lag periods for negative and neutral words. Results are for normal control subjects and a patient with bilateral amygdala damage. (Adapted with permission from A. K. Anderson and E. A. Phelps, The human amygdala supports affective modulatory influences on visual awareness. *Nature* 411:305–309. © 2001 by the Nature Publishing Group.) (See color plate 61.)

amygdala affects memory by enhancing encoding, there are data indicating that the amygdala may play a role in the modulation of attention or perception.

The claim that emotion can influence attention or perception has been documented in behavioral studies. Emotion has been shown both to capture attention (e.g., Fox et al., 2001) and to enhance attentional processing (e.g., Öhman, Flykt, and Esteves, 2001), depending on the task. At present, there is evidence that the human amygdala may play a role in the enhancement of attentional processing. This evidence comes from studies of the attentional blink. In this task, subjects are presented with stimuli very quickly. For instance, a series of 15 words may be presented at a rate of one every 10 ms. In this type of rapid serial visual presentation (RSVP) paradigm, the stimuli are presented too quickly for the subjects to encode each item, and subjects are unable to report the items that appeared. However, if the subjects are told that they can ignore most of the items, for instance those printed in black ink, and selectively focus on a few items, for instance those printed in green ink, then the subjects are usually able to attend selectively to the few target items and report them (figure 72.4a). The ability of the subjects to report more than one item in an RSVP paradigm depends on the timing of the presentation of the items. If a second target item appears soon after the first target item (i.e., during the early lag period), subjects have more difficulty reporting the item than if a second target item is presented later in the visual stream (during the late lag period). It is as if noticing and encoding the first target creates a short refractory period during which it is difficult to notice and encode the second target item. This brief refractory period is described metaphorically as an attentional blink.

Anderson and Phelps (2001) manipulated the emotional salience of the second target item. When the second target presented in the early lag period was an emotional, arousing word it was more likely to be reported than a neutral word. There was an attenuation of the attentional blink effect with emotion. In order to assess the role of the amygdala in the enhancement of attentional processing, patients with right, left, and bilateral amygdala damage performed the attentional blink paradigm with emotional and neutral items in the second target position. Unlike normal control subjects, patients with left amygdala damage showed similar decrements in reporting neutral and emotional items when those items appeared in the early lag period (figure 72.4b). These patients failed to exhibit the normal emotional attenuation of the attentional blink effect.

The attentional blink results indicate that in situations where attentional resources are limited, emotional stimuli are more likely to reach awareness. It has also been demonstrated that patients with attentional neglect are more likely to perceive emotional stimuli in the neglected field than neutral stimuli (Vuilleumier and Schwartz, 2001), consistent with the idea that perceiving emotional stimuli requires fewer attentional resources. The amygdala plays a role in this enhanced attentional processing. However, it is unclear exactly how the amygdala may affect performance.

One possibility is that the amygdala enhances attentional performance by altering perceptual encoding. Research with nonhuman animals has suggested two possible mechanisms by which the amygdala may influence perception. The first mechanism suggests that emotional learning, such as fear conditioning, can alter the cortical representation of stimuli linked to potential aversive consequences (Weinberger,

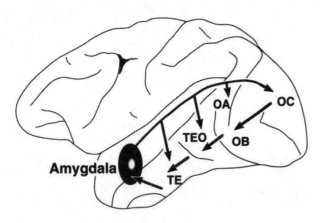

FIGURE 72.5 Schematic illustration of the relationship of the amygdala with visually related cortices in of the temporal and occipital lobes. (Adpated with permission from D. J. Amaral et al., Topographic organization of projections from the amygdala to the visual cortex in the macaque monkey. *Neuroscience* 118:1099–1120. © 1992 by the Society for Neuroscience.)

1995). For instance, if a tone of a specific frequency is repeatedly paired with a shock, eventually the cortical representation of that tone is changed in such a way that the rat is now especially sensitive to tones of that frequency. Through emotional learning, the amygdala is providing feedback allowing sensory cortical representations to be tuned for enhanced perception of emotional stimuli.

The second mechanism by which the amygdala can alter perceptual processing is more general. The amygdala has reciprocal connections with sensory cortical processing regions (figure 72.5). LeDoux and colleagues have shown that there are two pathways by which the amygdala can receive information about the emotional significance of a stimulus (see Schafe and LeDoux, this volume). The amygdala receives crude sensory input quickly via a subcortical route that bypasses cortical processing. It also receives more fully processed sensory information from cortical sensory regions. Because of the reciprocal connections with sensory cortex, the amygdala can provide feedback to perceptual systems in the presence of emotional stimuli. Through projections back to sensory cortical regions, the amygdala may enhance further perceptual processing in the presence of emotional or threatening stimuli, resulting in an overall heightened perceptual vigilance (Kapp, Supple, and Whalen, 1994; Whalen, 1998).

Although the evidence for a role of the human amygdala in the modulation in perception is not conclusive, several recent neuroimaging, patient, and behavioral studies are consistent with this idea. For instance, neuroimaging studies have demonstrated that the amygdala can respond to emotional stimuli presented subliminally, so quickly that subjects are unaware of their presentation (Morris, Öhman, and Dolan, 1998; Whalen et al., 1998). It has also been shown that there is enhanced activation of the visual cortex to visual emotional stimuli (e.g., Kosslyn et al., 1996). The magnitude of this enhanced visual cortex activation in response to emotional stimuli is correlated with the strength of amygdala activation in response to these same stimuli (Morris, Buchel, and Dolan, 2001). Together, these neuroimaging results are consistent with a mechanism by which the amygdala receives information about the emotional nature of a stimulus early in visual processing and then modulates further perceptual processing by influencing activity in the visual cortex (see figure 72.5).

Although subjects' lack of awareness does not necessarily indicate a subcortical pathway for perception, these neuroimaging results suggest that the amygdala detects emotion early in stimulus processing. Studies of patients with blindsight provide more direct support for the idea that the emotion can be perceived without complete perceptual processing. Damage to the striate cortex in the occipital lobe, an early visual region, can result in blindsight. Affected patients appear blind, but they are able to detect some simple visual stimuli through a pathway that bypasses the striate cortex. Recent studies have demonstrated that patients with blindsight can detect emotion in facial expressions (de Gelder, Vroomen, and Pourtois, 1999). They also show physiological evidence of fear conditioning to visually conditioned stimuli (Hamm et al., 2003). These results indicate that emotional information from visual stimuli that are not fully processed by the visual cortex can be perceived, consistent with the idea of a subcortical pathway for conveying emotional information to the amygdala.

Studies in patients with blindsight and neglect suggest that the amygdala may pick up on emotional information that has not been fully perceptually processed. But these studies do not specify how perception could be affected by these early signals. A few recent studies have started to explore the precise perceptual mechanisms that may be influenced by emotion or the amygdala. An fMRI study by Vuillemier and colleagues (2003) showed that the amygdala is particularly sensitive to low-spatial-frequency visual information in emotional stimuli. It is suggested that the subcortical pathway for conveying information about emotional, threatening stimuli to the amygdala may primarily code low-spatial-frequency information. In addition, Ling and colleagues (2004) recently demonstrated that emotion can enhance visual contrast sensitivity, particularly when cued by covert attention. These recent studies are starting to specify exactly how emotion and the amygdala can influence perceptual processing.

Our understanding of the role of the human amygdala in perception and attention is rapidly progressing, but the precise mechanisms are still not known. Studies on the role of the amygdala in attention provide support for the notion that the amygdala modulates enhanced awareness for emotional events in situations with limited attentional resources. Although there is not yet any evidence that the human amyg-

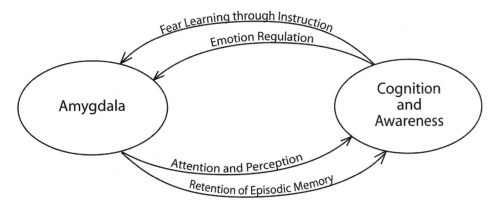

FIGURE 72.6   Schematic illustration of the current understanding of the complex interactions between the amygdala and cognition and awareness.

dala underlies any specific perceptual process, the bulk of evidence from a range of techniques strongly supports the hypothesis that the amygdala enhances perceptual processing when cued by emotional stimuli.

By modulating attention and perception with emotion, the amygdala gives priority to emotionally salient stimuli in cognitive processing. Emotion, via the amygdala, alters the ease with which stimuli are available to conscious awareness. How this enhanced awareness influences cognition broadly remains to be determined. Through its influence on attention and perception, the amygdala could potentially have a significant impact on a range of cognitive processes, including working memory, categorization, and episodic memory encoding.

SUMMARY: EMOTION TO COGNITION   Evolutionary arguments support the idea that emotion should influence cognitive processes. In order to survive in a changing environment, it is especially important that an organism remember those stimuli and events that are linked to emotional consequences. It is also important to be particularly vigilant and aware of emotional stimuli in the environment in order to allow for quick assessment and reaction. Research examining the role of the human amygdala suggests it may play a critical role in enhancing memory, attention, and perception with emotion.

Conclusions

Research on the cognitive neuroscience of emotion has provided a fresh perspective on the debate concerning the role of emotion in cognition. Traditionally, emotion has not been considered an important component in efforts to understand cognition (Neisser, 1976; Anderson, 1999). Because certain brain structures seem to be specialized for processing emotion, such as the amygdala, it could be argued that the traditional approach of studying emotion independently

from cognition is justified. However, as outlined in this chapter, there are complex interactions between neural systems that are more or less specialized for cognition and emotion (figure 72.6).

Learning through fear conditioning seems to depend on the amygdala, with little influence from cognition and awareness. However, cognition and awareness influence the amygdala in a number of ways. Fear learning through symbolic means (verbal communication) can alter amygdala function, and the expression of this learning depends on the amygdala. This relationship illustrates that the amygdala plays a role in the expression of fears that are generated through imagination. Cognitive and attentional strategies that regulate emotional reactions have also been shown to change the amygdala's response to a situation. This relationship demonstrates cognitive control over an amygdala response. The amygdala can also influence cognition and awareness. By modulating the retention of episodic memory with arousal, the amygdala helps determine which information in the environment will be accessible for later conscious recollection. The amygdala also influences online stimulus processing by altering the ease with which emotional information can reach awareness with limited attentional resources. The amygdala's influence on attention may be related to enhanced perceptual processing with emotion.

Researchers' efforts to understand the function of the human amygdala have led to the conclusion that understanding the neural systems of emotion requires a consideration of cognition and vice versa. A separation between emotion and cognition seems artificial when one is trying to understand everyday human function in a social environment. Although emotion may be considered a specific topic within the study of cognition, much as memory and attention are considered separate topics, research on the cognitive neuroscience of emotion highlights the fact that our efforts to understand the neural systems of cognition must include the study of emotion.

REFERENCES

AMARAL, D. G., H. BEHNIEA, and J. L. KELLY, 2003. Topographic organization of projections from the amygdala to the visual cortex in the macaque monkey. *Neuroscience* 118(4):1099–1120.

ANDERSON, A. K., K. CHRISTOFF, I. STAPPEN, D. PANITZ, D. G. GHAHREMANI, G. GLOVER, J. D. E. GABRIELLI, and N. SOBEL, 2003. Dissociated neural representations of intensity and valence in human olfaction. *Nat. Neurosci.* 6:196–202.

ANDERSON, A. K., K. CHRISTOFF, D. PANITZ, E. DEROSA, and J. D. GABRIELI, 2003. Neural correlates of the automatic processing of threat facial signals. *J. Neurosci.* 23(13):5627–5633.

ANDERSON, A. K., and E. A. PHELPS, 2001. The human amygdala supports affective modulatory influences on visual awareness. *Nature* 411:305–309.

ANDERSON, J. K., 1999. *Cognitive Psychology and Its Implications*, 5th ed. San Francisco: Freeman.

BECHARA, A., D. TRANEL, H. DAMASIO, R. ADOLPHS, C. ROCKLAND, and A. R. DAMASIO, 1995. Double dissociation of conditioning and declarative knowledge relative to the amygdala and hippocampus in human. *Science* 269:1115–1118.

CAHILL, L., R. BABINSKY, H. J. MARKOWITSCH, and J. L. MCGAUGH, 1995. The amygdala and emotional memory. *Science* 377:295–296.

CAHILL, L., R. J. HAIER, J. FALLON, M. T. ALKIRE, C. TANG, D. KEATOR, J. WU, and J. L. MCGAUGH, 1996. Amygdala activity at encoding correlated with long-term, free recall of emotional information. *Proc. Natl. Acad. Sci. U.S.A.* 93:8016–8021.

CAHILL, L., B. PRINS, M. WEBER, and J. L. MCGAUGH, 1994. β-Adrenergic activation and memory for emotional events. *Nature* 371:702–704.

CAHILL, L., N. M. WEINBERGER, B. ROOZENDAAL, and J. L. MCGAUGH, 1999. Is the amygdala a locus of "conditioned fear"? Some questions and caveats. *Neuron* 23:227–228.

CANLI, T., Z. ZHAO, J. BREWER, J. D. E. GABRIELI, and L. CAHILL, 2000. Event-related activation in the human amygdala associates with later memory for individual emotional experience. *J. Neurosci.* 20:RC99:1–5.

CARR, L., M. IACOBONI, M. C. DUBEAU, J. C. MAZZIOTTA, and G. L. LENZI, 2003. Neural mechanisms of empathy in humans: A relay from neural systems for imitation to limbic areas. *Proc. Natl. Acad. Sci. U.S.A.* 100(9):5497–5502.

CHRISTIANSON, S. A., 1992. *The Handbook of Emotion and Memory: Research and Theory.* N.J.: Lawrence Erlbaum Associates.

CHRISTIANSON, S. A., and E. F. LOFTUS, 1991. Remembering emotional events: The fate of detailed information. *Cogn. Emotion* 5:81–108.

DAVIS, M., 2000. The role of the amygdala in conditioned fear and anxiety. In *The Amygdala: A Functional Analysis*, 2nd ed., J. P. Aggleton, ed. New York: Oxford University Press, pp. 213–287.

DEGELDER, B., J. VROOMEN, G. POURTOIS, and L. WEISKRANTZ, 1999. Non-conscious recognition of affect in the absence of striate cortex. *Neuroreport* 10:3759–3763.

ESTEVES, F., U. DIMBERG, and A. ÖHMAN, 1994. Automatically elicited fear: Conditioned skin conductance responses to masked facial expressions. *Cogn. Emotion* 8:393–413.

FOX, E., R. RUSSO, R. BOWLES, and K. DUTTON, 2001. Do threatening stimuli draw or hold attention in visual attention in subclinical anxiety. *J. Exper. Psychol. Gen.* 130:681–700.

FUNAYAMA, E. S., C. G. GRILLON, M. DAVIS, and E. A. PHELPS, 2001. A double dissociation in the affective modulation of startle in humans: Effects of unilateral temporal lobectomy. *J. Cogn. Neurosci.* 13:721–729.

GAZZANIGA, M. S., 2000. Cerebral specialization and interhemispheric communication: Does the corpus callosum enable the human condition? *Brain* 123:1293–1326.

GROSS, J. J., 2002. Emotion regulation: Affective, cognitive, and social consequences. *Psychophysiology* 39:281–291.

HAMANN, S. B., T. D. ELY, S. T. GRAFTON, and C. D. KILTS, 1999. Amygdala activity related to enhanced memory for pleasant and aversive stimuli. *Nat. Neurosci.* 2(3):289–293.

HAMM, A. O., A. I. WEIKE, H. T. SCHUPP, T. TRIEG, A. DRESSEL, and C. KESSLER, 2003. Affective blindsight: Intact fear conditioning to a visual cue in a cortically blind patient. *Brain* 136:267–275.

KAPP, B. S., W. F. SUPPLE, and P. J. WHALEN, 1994. Stimulation of the amygdaloid central nucleus produces EEG arousal. *Behav. Neurosci.* 108:81–93.

KAPP, B. S., P. J. WHALEN, W. F. SUPPLE, and J. P. PASCOE, 1992. Amygdaloid contributions to conditioned arousal and sensory information processing. In *The Amygdala: Neurobiological Aspects of Emotion, Memory and Mental Dysfunction*, J. P. Aggleton, ed. pp. 229–254.

KLEINSMITH, L. J., and S. KAPLAN, 1963. Paired-associate learning as a function of arousal and interpolated interval. *J. Exper. Psychol.* 65(2):190–193.

KOSSLYN, S. M., L. M. SHIN, W. L. THOMPSON, P. J. MCNALLY, S. L. RAUCH, R. K. PITMAN, and N. M. ALPERT, 1996. Neural effects of visualizing and perceiving aversive stimuli: A PET investigation. *Neuroreport* 7:1569–1576.

LABAR, K. S., D. R. GITELMAN, T. B. PARRISH, Y. H. KIM, A. C. NOBRE, and M. M. MESULAM, 2001. Hunger selectively modulates corticolimbic activation to food stimuli in humans. *Behav. Neurosci.* 115:493–500.

LABAR, K. S., J. E. LEDOUX, D. D. SPENCER, and E. A. PHELPS, 1995. Impaired fear conditioning following unilateral temporal lobectomy in humans. *J. Neurosci.* 15:6846–6855.

LABAR, K. S., and E. A. PHELPS, 1998. Role of the human amygdala in arousal mediated memory consolidation. *Psychol. Sci.* 9:490–493.

LAZARUS, R. S., 1981. A cognitivist's reply to Zajonc on emotion and cognition. *Am. Psychol.* 36(2):222–223.

LAZARUS, R. S., 1984. On the primacy of cognition. *Am. Psychol.* 39(2):124–129.

LEDOUX, J. E., 1996. *The Emotional Brain: The Mysterious Underpinnings of Emotional Life.* New York: Simon & Schuster.

LEDOUX, J. E., 2002. *The Synaptic Self: How Our Brain Became Who We Are.* New York: Viking-Penguin.

LING, S., E. PHELPS, B. HOLMES, and M. CARRASCO, 2004. Emotion potentiates attentional effects in early vision [Abstract]. Vision Sciences Society, annual meeting, Sarasota, Florida.

MCDONALD, A. J., 1991. Organization of amygdala projections to the prefrontal cortex and associated striatum in the rat. *Neuroscience* 44:1–14.

MCGAUGH, J. L., 2000. Memory—a century of consolidation. *Science* 287:248–251.

MCGAUGH, J. L., I. B. INTROINI-COLLISION, L. CAHILL, K. MUNSO, and K. C. LIANG, 1992. Involvement of the amygdala in neuromodulatory influences on memory storage. In *The Amygdala: Neurobiological Aspects of Emotion, Memory, and Mental Dysfunction*, J. P. Aggleton, ed. New York, NY: Wiley-Liss, pp. 431–451.

MILLER, E. K., and J. D. COHEN, 2001. An integrative theory of prefrontal cortex function. *Annu. Rev. Neurosci.* 24:167–202.

MORRIS, J. S., C. BUCHEL, and R. J. DOLAN, 2001. Parallel neural responses in amygdala subregions and sensory cortex during implicit fear conditioning. *NeuroImage* 13:1044–1052.

Morris, J. S., A. Öhman, and R. J. Dolan, 1998. Conscious and unconscious emotional learning in the human amygdala. *Nature* 393:467–470.

Neisser, U., 1976. *Cognition and Reality: Principles and Implications of Cognitive Psychology*. San Francisco: Freeman

Öhman, A., A. Flykt, and F. Esteves, 2001. Fear, phobias, and preparedness: Toward an evolved model of fear and fear learning. *J. Exper. Psychol. Gen.* 130:466–478.

Öhman, A., and S. Mineka, 2001. Fears, phobias, and preparedness: Toward an evolved module of fear and fear learning. *Psychol. Rev.* 108(3):483–522.

Öhman, A., and J. J. F. Soares, 1993. On the automatic nature of phobic fear: Conditioned electrodermal responses to masked fear-relevant stimuli. *J. Abnormal Psychol.* 102:1221–1132.

Olsson, A., and E. A. Phelps (in press). Learned fear of "unseen" faces after Pavlovian, observational and instructed fear. *Psychol. Sci.*

Oschner, K. N., S. A. Bunge, J. J. Gross, and J. D. E. Gabrielli, 2002. Rethinking feelings: An fMRI study of the cognitive regulation of emotion. *J. Cogn. Neurosci.* 14:1215–1229.

Packard, M. G., and L. Teather, 1998. Amygdala modulation of hippocampal-dependent and caudate nucleus-dependent memory processes. *Proc. Natl. Acad. Sci. U.S.A.* 91:8477–8481.

Pessoa, L., M. McKenna, and L. G. Gutierrez, 2002. Neural processing of emotional faces requires attention. *Proc. Natl. Acad. Sci. U.S.A.* 99:11458–11463.

Phelps, E. A., 2002. Emotions. In *Cognitive Neuroscience: The Biology of Mind*, 2nd ed., M. S. Gazzaniga, R. B. Ivry, and G. R. Mangun, eds. New York: W.W. Norton & Company, pp. 537–576.

Phelps, E. A., D. S. LaBar, A. K. Anderson, K. J. O'Conner, R. K. Fulbright, and D. S. Spencer, 1998. Specifying the contributions of the human amygdala to emotional memory: A case study. *Neurocase* 4:527–540.

Phelps, E. A., K. J. O'Connor, J. C. Gatenby, C. Grillon, J. C. Gore, and M. Davis, 2001. Activation of the left amygdala to a cognitive representation of fear. *Nat. Neurosci.* 4:437–441.

Rizzolatti, G., L. Fogassi, and V. Gallese, 2002. Motor and cognitive functioins of the ventral premotor cortex. *Curr. Opin. Neurobiol.* 12:149–154.

Schacter, D. L., 2001. *The Seven Sins of Memory: How the Mind Forgets and Remembers*. Boston: Houghton Mifflin.

Schaefer, S. M., D. C. Jackson, R. J. Davidson, D. Y. Kimberg, and S. L. Thompson-Schill, 2002. Modulation of amygdalar activity by the conscious regulation of negative emotion. *J. Cogn. Neurosci.* 14:913–921.

Smith, E. E., and J. Jonides, 1999. Storage and executive processes in the frontal lobes. *Science* 283:1657–1661.

Stefanacci, L., and D. G. Amaral, 2000. Topographic organization of cortical inputs to the lateral nucleus of the macaque monkey amygdala: a retrograde tracing study. *J. Compar. Neurosci.* 421(1):52–79.

Stefanacci, L., and D. G. Amaral, 2002. Some observations on cortical inputs to the macaque monkey amygdala: an anterograde tracing study. *J. Compar. Neurosci.* 451(4):301–323.

Vuilleumier, P., J. L. Armony, J. Driver, and R. J. Dolan, 2001. Effects of attention and emotion on face processing in the human brain: An event-related fMRI study. *Neuron* 30:829–841.

Vuilleumier, P., J. L. Armony, J. Driver, and R. J. Dolan, 2003. Distal spatial frequency sensitivities for processing faces and emotional expressions. *Nat. Neurosci.* 6:624–631.

Vuilleumier, P., and S. Schwartz, 2001. Beware and be aware: Capture of spatial attention by fear-related stimuli in neglect. *Neuroreport* 12:1119–1122.

Weinberger, D. R., 1995. Retuning the brain by fear conditioning. In *The Cognitive Neurosciences*, M. S. Gazzaniga, ed. Cambridge, Mass.: MIT Press, pp. 1071–1090.

Whalen, P. J., 1998. Fear, vigilance, and ambiguity: Initial neuroimaging studies of the human amygdala. *Curr. Direct. Psychol. Sci.* 7(6):177–188.

Whalen, P. J., S. L. Rauch, N. L. Etcoff, S. C. McInerney, M. B. Lee, and M. A. Jenike, 1998. Masked presentations of emotional facial expressions modulate amygdala activity without explicit knowledge. *J. Neurosci.* 18(1):411–418.

Zajonc, R. B., 1980. Feeling and thinking: Preferences need no inferences. *Am. Psychol.* 35(2):151–175.

Zajonc, R. B., 1984. On the primacy of affect. *Am. Psychol.* 39(2):117–123.

73 Processing of Emotional and Social Information by the Human Amygdala

RALPH ADOLPHS

ABSTRACT Studies in animals have implicated the amygdala in social and emotional information processing. Within the past decade, the role of this structure has also been investigated in humans, using a variety of techniques. Perhaps best explored is its function in social judgments about facial expressions, the focus of this review. Lesion studies, electrophysiology, and functional imaging have all been brought to bear on this topic, and these approaches have begun to sketch the processes whereby the amygdala links perceptual representations of emotional sensory stimuli with the elicitation of behavioral and cognitive responses. These responses, in turn, both guide social behavior and generate social knowledge. The chapter closes with a preview of future directions that this line of research suggests.

A framework for the neurobiology of emotion and social cognition

In less than a decade, the study of emotion has morphed from a neglected topic to one of the hot frontiers of cognitive neuroscience. This reversal had several causes: the realization that emotion dysfunction is a hallmark of essentially all psychiatric diseases, as well as a highly salient component of healthy function; the development of new techniques, notably functional imaging, that permit an unprecedented examination of its neural substrates; and the development of theoretical frameworks within which new hypotheses can be tested and data can be interpreted. Most important, these frameworks have sought to integrate emotion into the architecture of cognition in general, rescuing the field from its prior isolation. A key contribution to the rapid expansion of the field have been data from lesion studies, because they allow researchers to assign causal roles to neural structures. Lesion studies have demonstrated dissociations between perception and emotion, recognition and emotion, emotion and feeling, and emotion and reason, and thus have outlined the neural systems that process emotionally salient stimuli,

link them to emotional responses, modulate cognition by emotion, and generate emotional feelings.

Despite the deluge of recent data, our understanding of emotion is confused. Different investigators use terms with different meanings, and researchers in different disciplines often find it difficult to understand one another. The reasons for this difficulty are some of the same reasons that make the study of cognition in general difficult, but they are more acute in the study of emotion. They arise from our pretheoretical beliefs about emotions and feelings. Everyone believes that people have emotions, just as they believe that people have thoughts. But when we start taking apart people and investigating the internal mechanisms required for such attributions, we necessarily lose the person we started with. Does it make sense to attribute emotions (or thoughts) to parts of our bodies, including our brains? It probably makes no more sense to attribute an emotion to my stomach, my adrenal glands, or my amygdala than it does to attribute a visual percept to my visual cortices. Processes occurring in these structures are constituents of what makes a whole person have an emotion or a visual percept, but they are not to be confused synecdochically with the organism of which they are a part. Let me reiterate this, as it should be an obvious point. Autonomic responses, neuronal activity in the amygdala or in any other isolated brain region, are never identical with emotions, because emotions depend on a complex, multidimensional pattern of concerted processes occurring in many places at various points in time. What is needed is an account of emotional and social information processing that describes the constituent internal processes and the roles that they play.

What, then, is a starting framework within which we can investigate emotions? It is useful to draw on three different theories of emotion here (there are others that are relevant, but these three serve as a starting point). One theory, in line both with an evolutionary approach to emotion and aspects of appraisal theory, concerns the domain of information that specifies emotion processing. In short, emotions concern, or derive from, information that is of direct

RALPH ADOLPHS Division of Humanities and Social Sciences, California Institute of Technology, Pasadena, Calif.

relevance to the homeostasis and survival of an organism (Darwin, 1872/1965; Frijda, 1986; Damasio, 1994), that is, the significance that the situation has for the organism, both in terms of its immediate impact and in terms of the organism's plans and goals in responding to the situation (Lazarus, 1991). Fear and disgust are obvious examples of such emotions. The notion of homeostasis and survival needs to be extended to the social world to account for social emotions, such as shame, guilt, or embarrassment, that regulate social behavior in groups. Emotions thus pertain to the value of a stimulus or of a behavior—value to the organism's own survival, or to the survival of one's offspring or relatives, or to a larger social group.

This first point, the domain specificity of emotional information, tells us what distinguishes emotion processing from information processing in general, but leaves open two further questions: How broadly should we construe this domain, and how is such specificity implemented? In regard to the first question, the domain includes social and basic emotions, but also states such as pain, hunger, and any other information that has a bearing on survival. Is this too broad? Philosophers worry about such distinctions, but for the present, we as neuroscientists can simply acknowledge that indeed, the processing of emotions should (and, as it turns out, does) share mechanisms in common with the processing of thirst, hunger, pain, sex, and any other category of information that motivates behavior (Panksepp, 1998; Rolls, 1999). In regard to the second question, the implementation of value-laden information, an answer will require information about the perceptual properties of a stimulus to be associated with information about the state of the organism perceiving that stimulus. Such information about the organism could be sensory (somatosensory in a broad sense, meaning information about the impact that the stimulus has on homeostasis) or motor (information about the action plans triggered by the stimulus). This brings us to the remaining two of the three emotion theories.

The first emotion theory, then, acknowledges that emotion processing is domain-specific and relates to the value that a stimulus has for an organism in a broad sense. The second emotion theory of relevance here concerns the cause-and-effect architecture of behavior, bodily states, and central states. Readers will be familiar with the theories of William James, Walter Cannon, and later thinkers that debated the primacy of bodily states (James, 1884; Cannon, 1927). Are we afraid first, and then we run away from the bear, or do we have an emotional bodily response to the bear first, whose perception in turn constitutes our feeling afraid? This debate has been very muddled, for at least two reasons: the failure to distinguish emotions from feelings, and the ubiquitous tendency for a single causal scheme.

It is useful to conceive of emotions as central states that are only dispositionally linked to certain physiological states of the body, or certain behaviors, or certain feelings of which we are aware. An emotion is thus a neural state (or, better, a collection of processes) that operates in a domain-specific manner on information. However, the mechanism behind assigning value to such information depends on an organism's reactive and proactive response to the stimulus. The proactive component prepares the organism for action, and the reactive component reflects the response to a stimulus. It is the coordinated web of action preparations, stimulus responses, and an organism's internal mapping of these that constitutes a central emotional state. Viewed this way, an emotion is neither cause nor consequence of a physiological response; it emerges in parallel with an organism's interaction with its environment, in parallel with physiological response, and in parallel with feeling. Behavior, physiological response, and feeling all causally affect one another, and none of them in isolation is co-extensive with the emotion, although we certainly use observations of them to infer an emotional state.

The third emotion theory to be considered here is the set of theories concerning appraisal. The issue under debate is the extent to which an emotion (or a social behavior) can ensue automatically and with only a coarse evaluation of a stimulus (Zajonc, 1980), or whether an emotion requires more elaborate cognitive appraisal of the significance that the stimulus has for an organism and of the behaviors appropriate to maximizing an adaptive response (Scherer, 1988; Lazarus, 1991). As with the James–Cannon debate, the answer here is, both. There is good evidence that some stimuli trigger emotional responses very rapidly and in the absence of conscious awareness, but also that elaborate cognitive processing and evaluation play key roles, for instance in emotion regulation. To some extent these components may occur on different temporal scales.

The findings from cognitive neuroscience corroborate the three points made earlier: emotional and social information processing is domain-specific, pertaining to maintenance of homeostasis in a changing and interactive environment; it unfolds in a complex, iterative way over time that involves perception, response, and feeling; and it draws on both relatively fast and coarse perceptual processing and more complex cognitive appraisals. Emotional and social information processing includes multiple perceptual routes, iterative feedback between emotion responses and their representation, and extensive regulation at several levels (Adolphs, 2002; figure 73.1). These multiple perceptual routes result in information processing that is temporally dispersed. The dispersion in time in turn drives emotional responses that also occur on multiple temporal scales: some are rapid and relatively automatic, others require extensive evaluation of the stimulus and are often volitionally modulated. Responses on different time scales interact, as shown clearly in some of the most popular paradigms for studying

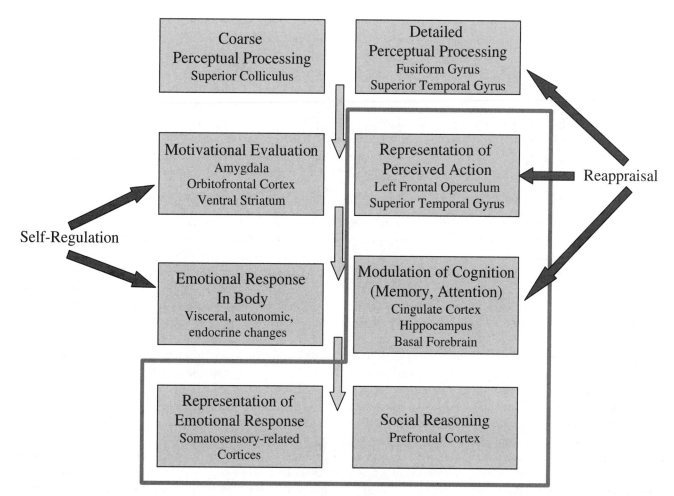

FIGURE 73.1   Processes that contribute to emotional and social information processing. Shown are some of the routes by which socially relevant information guides social behavior. Several features are important to note. There are multiple information processing streams that differ in the extent to which they recruit emotions, in the extent to which they are available for conscious awareness and control, and in their speed and elaboration. The causal relations among these processing components are complex and include extensive feedback (not shown). There are also notable metacognitive influences: adult humans stand out in the ability to regulate their social behavior based on awareness and effort (arrows indicating Self-Regulation and Reappraisal). This schematic summarizes an overall information processing architecture that includes many more structures than are discussed in the chapter. (Reproduced from Adolphs, 2003.)

emotions. For instance, emotional modulation of the startle reflex shows such an interaction: the startle reflex itself is extremely rapid and automatic, but it is modulated by the valence of visual stimuli via a pathway involving projections from the amygdala to the nucleus reticularis pars caudalis, as well as by cognitive evaluation of stimuli.

Emotional responses to stimuli in turn are represented centrally, and are themselves modulated continuously. The emotional information that is processed thus varies in time, as does the emotional response, and the feeling of the emotion. The subsequent sections of this chapter review what we know about the contribution made by a specific structure, the amygdala, to these processes, with an emphasis on findings gleaned from lesion studies. All of the points made in this introductory discussion will turn out to be relevant for understanding what the amygdala does as it participates in processing emotionally relevant information.

Early perception of socially relevant stimuli

Certain features of stimuli, such as certain facial configurations that signal emotions, can be processed rapidly, in part by subcortical mechanisms. For instance, processing of subliminally presented facial expressions of fear activates the amygdala (Whalen et al., 1998), possibly reflecting the operation of a circuit from the superior colliculus (SC) to the amygdala via the pulvinar thalamus. This interpretation is in line with functional imaging studies showing correlated activation of the SC, the pulvinar thalamus, and the amygdala in response to subliminally presented facial expressions that had been associated with an aversive stimulus (Morris,

Ohman, and Dolan, 1999), a pattern of activation that was recently replicated in a subject with blindsight when discriminating emotional facial expressions in the blind visual field (Morris et al., 2001).

Regions of nonprimary sensory cortices already appear to be relatively specialized to process certain socially relevant attributes of stimuli. The evidence is best in regard to faces, for which higher-order visual cortices can be regarded as an assembly of modules that process distinct attributes, as borne out by a variety of lesion studies, scalp and intracranial recordings, and a rapidly growing list of functional imaging studies. The data point to the fusiform gyrus in processing the structural, static properties of faces, which are reliable indicators of personal identity, and to regions more anterior and dorsal in the temporal lobe (such as the superior temporal gyrus and SC) in processing information about the changeable configurations of faces, such as facial expressions, eye movements, and mouth movements (McCarthy, 1999; Haxby, Hoffman, and Gobbini, 2000). Activation along the superior temporal sulcus (STS) and superior temporal gyrus (STG) has been found when subjects view stimuli depicting biological motion, such as eye gaze shifts, mouth movements, and point-light displays of whole-body biological motion, and more abstract movements of geometric shapes, likely reflecting the role of this region in processing biological motion information on the basis of which we make social attributions. Processing in this region may draw on both dorsal and ventral visual streams in integrating shape and motion information, and it may reflect a comparison of the observed action with the viewer's simulation of it. The fusiform gyrus, the STG, and other, less-well-specified regions of occipitotemporal cortex could thus be thought of as an interconnected system of regions that together construct a spatially distributed perceptual representation of different aspects of the face. There is good evidence that activation in all of these regions can be modulated by attention (Vuilleumier et al., 2001) and by the context in which the visual social signal appears (Pelphrey et al., 2003; Wicker et al., 2003).

An important recent lesion study showed that the amygdala is also critical to mediate visual attention. When words are flashed visually in a rapid serial stream, there is a well-known phenomenon called the *attentional blink*: when subjects are asked to identify a particular word that appears in the stream, their ability to detect a subsequent word within a short time window after the initially identified one is severely impaired. However, when the subsequent word to be detected is highly emotional, it can be detected even when it falls within the attentional blink window. Apparently, the initial allocation of attention to a target compromises subjects' ability to detect an immediately subsequent one, but emotional salience provides an independent boost that can override this blink—a boost that depends on the amygdala.

Lesions of the amygdala do not impair the attentional blink itself but the ability of emotion to override it (Anderson and Phelps, 2001). The finding is in line with the idea that the amygdala modulates the access of visual information to subsequent cognitive processing on the basis of the emotional value of the information.

The above anatomical investigations are complemented by data on the timing of face-processing components. Studies using event-related potentials (ERPs) and magnetoencephalography (MEG) show that some coarse categorization, such as sex and emotion categorization, can occur at latencies as short as 100 ms. Peak activity related to face-specific processing near the fusiform gyrus is seen around 170–200 ms (Allison et al., 1994). Although the construction of a detailed structural representation of the face thus seems to require about 170 ms, it appears that some rapid, coarse categorization can occur with substantially shorter latencies, presumably indicating coarse perceptual routes parallel to a full structural encoding of the stimulus. Perception of emotionally and socially relevant stimuli should be seen as an ongoing process extended in time, driven both by a collection of bottom-up processes and by top-down modulation.

The amygdala's role in processing emotional and social information

Although it is difficult to define exactly what constitutes higher-level processing, there are at least three domains that probably qualify: multistep processing that involves volition, thinking about other people's minds, and awareness of one's feelings. There is clear evidence that emotional and social information contributes to decision making, reasoning, and other processes that can be influenced volitionally. By definition, social information processing also includes abilities by which we attribute mental states (such as goals, intentions, and emotions) to other people, dubbed theory of mind. Regions in prefrontal cortex, including ventral and medial prefrontal and cingulate cortex, participate in these processes. Structures that function to construct components of a self model, such as visceral and somatic sensory cortices in parietal lobe and insula, participate in these processes as well and are critical for feeling an emotion (Adolphs, 2003a).

The amygdala's role in these higher processes is quite unclear. Although there have been reports of impaired decision making (Bechara et al., 1999) or theory-of-mind abilities (Stone et al., 2003) in subjects with bilateral amygdala damage, it is plausible to assign the impairments in those cases to a defect in more basic emotional information processing rather than specific to the higher function (Adolphs, 2003a). There is also evidence from functional imaging studies that volitional modulation of emotion modulates activation of the amygdala (Ochsner et al., 2002; Schaefer et al.,

2002), but again, this does not show that the amygdala subserves volitional emotional processing, merely that it can be influenced by such processing. Finally, there is no evidence to suggest that the amygdala itself is critical for feeling emotions (Adolphs, 1999; Anderson and Phelps, 2002).

The evidence thus far points to a role for the amygdala in processing information at a level somewhat "higher" than basic perception but "below" the level of explicit reasoning and thinking about social information. This picture is extremely vague, but it serves to roughly locate the contribution that the amygdala makes at the interface of bottom-up perceptual processing and a whole host of other cognitive processes. What the amygdala does is not like what a reflex does (although it modulates reflexes), nor is it like thinking (although it modulates our thoughts), but rather is something more ubiquitous that pervades the organization of thought and behavior at all levels.

RECOGNIZING EMOTION FROM FACES   The first definitive demonstration that the human amygdala plays a critical role in recognizing emotion came from two patients with bilateral damage to the amygdala (Adolphs et al., 1994; Young et al., 1995). Both patients had largely normal visuopercep-

tual function but were impaired at recognizing certain kinds of information from faces shown to them. In particular, both showed an inability to recognize normally emotions from facial expressions; that is, they had an emotion agnosia.

The patient my colleagues and I studied, S.M.046, had selective and complete bilateral amygdala damage due to Urbach-Wiethe disease (also known as lipoid proteinosis), a rare genetic disorder of epithelial tissue caused by a mutation in the extracellular matrix protein 1 gene (Hamada et al., 2002). Patients with this disease show medial temporal lobe calcifications and atrophy in about 50% of cases (Hofer, 1973). In S.M.046's case, the damage was confined to the amygdala and the very anterior portions of entorhinal cortex (Tranel and Hyman, 1990; figure 73.2). Her lesion and her neuropsychological profile have remained stable over more than a decade of study (Adolphs and Tranel, 2000). Despite her normal ability to recognize sex, identity, and other information from faces, S.M.046 is severely impaired in her ability to recognize certain emotions. The impairment is most notable for fear, but includes to some extent emotions that are conceptually close to fear, such as surprise and anger (Adolphs et al., 1994, 1995). Her dysfunction is clearly an agnosia, since S.M.046 is able to

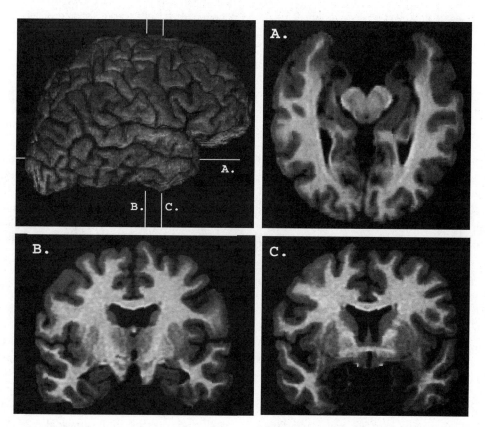

FIGURE 73.2   Neuroanatomy of S.M.046. Shown at top left is a three-dimensional reconstruction of S.M.'s brain from MR images, showing the planes of section of the other cuts. The symmetrical region of low signal in the anteromedial temporal lobe is due to calcification and atrophy of tissue within the entire amygdala as well as anterior entorhinal cortex. The damage resulted from a rare genetic disease, Urbach-Wiethe disease.

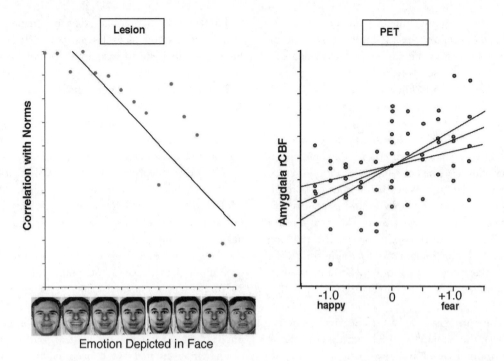

FIGURE 73.3 The amygdala's role in processing fearful facial expressions. *Left*, Impaired recognition of fear following bilateral amygdala damage. Shown are data from S.M.046 on rating the intensity of emotions shown in facial expressions. Subjects were shown morphs of prototypical facial expressions of emotions and asked to rate the intensity of each of the six basic emotions signaled by these stimuli. The *x*-axis shows the face stimuli and the *y*-axis shows the correlation of S.M.046's ratings with normal ratings; thus, values close to 1 reflect normal recognition, whereas values close to 0 reflect very impaired recognition. *Right*, Activation of the amygdala when normal subjects viewed facial expressions. When normal subjects with intact amygdalae were shown morphs between happy and fearful faces, regional cerebral blood flow within the amygdala correlated with the degree of fear shown in the face stimulus. (Data from Morris et al., 1996; © 1996 by MacMillan Press.)

discriminate normally even very faint morphs of the same emotions that she failed to recognize (Adolphs and Tranel, 2000). Moreover, she is able to use the word *fear* appropriately in conversation, and is able to generate considerable conceptual knowledge about that emotion. When asked to rate the intensity of emotion signaled by a facial expression, S.M.046 gave very abnormal (low) ratings to expressions of fear (figure 73.3). She also showed a converse impairment: when asked to draw facial expressions of emotions for which we supplied the name, she was able to draw all except fear (Adolphs et al., 1995). She thus showed a bidirectional disconnection between the concept of fear and the facial expressions that normally signal that emotion.

While S.M.046's impairment is strikingly specific to fear, at least on certain tasks, other patients with bilateral damage to the amygdala show impairments in facial emotion recognition that are not as specific but typically encompass several negative emotions, often including but not limited to fear. In a study of nine such patients, we found a pattern of impairments that extended across rating the intensity of multiple negative emotions, especially fear, anger, and disgust (Adolphs, Tranel, et al., 1999; figure 73.4). Other studies have pointed to disproportionate impairments in recogniz-

ing fear (Calder et al., 1996; Broks et al., 1998), more subtle impairments in various negative emotions that depend on the particular task and analysis (Schmolck and Squire, 2001), or impairments that might be attributable to difficulty of the task alone (Rapcsak et al., 2000; Adolphs, 2002).

Data from functional imaging studies have helped to narrow down these possibilities. Although there was an initial flurry of findings showing amygdala activation in response to fearful facial expressions (Breiter et al., 1996; Morris et al., 1996), some aspects of which are still supported by more recent studies (Whalen et al., 2001), those findings are now supplemented by others showing that the amygdala is activated by multiple emotional expressions (Blair et al., 1999; Yang et al., 2002), but differentially so. It does not look as if the amygdala is activated equally by expressions of all emotions or that its activation can be explained merely by the difficulty of the task required. On the other hand, it remains unclear exactly what emotion category it might be specialized to process.

We are thus faced with a key question: How domain-specific is processing in the amygdala? As in some regions of temporal extrastriate cortex, responses within the amygdala seem disproportionate for social visual information such as

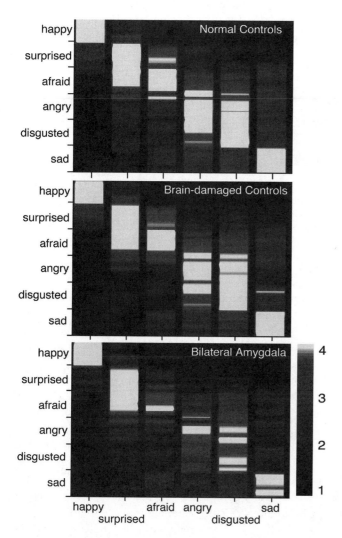

FIGURE 73.4 Impaired recognition of multiple negative emotions in nine subjects with bilateral amygdala damage. On the same task as in figure 73.3, a group of nine subjects with bilateral amygdala damage showed variable impairments across not only fear but also other negatively valenced emotions, compared to either brain-damaged or normal controls. Each of the three graphs shows data for normal controls, brain-damaged controls, and subjects with amygdala damage. The x- and y-axes represent the labels on which faces are rated and the face stimuli, respectively. The gray scale codes the intensity they assigned to the face on that emotion label.

faces, and the lesion studies certainly point to a role in recognizing only certain negatively valenced emotions, perhaps especially fear; but clearly its role is not restricted entirely to processing information about fear. There are at least three possibilities here: (1) the amygdala is specialized to process a particular basic emotion, fear; (2) the amygdala processes a region of two-dimensional affect space, namely, those emotions that are both negatively valenced and highly arousing; and (3) the amygdala processes a particular ecological category of emotions, for instance those related to threat and

danger (Adolphs, Tranel, et al., 1999; Adolphs, 2002), those requiring the resolution of ambiguity (Whalen, 1999), or perhaps those requiring a mapping of an observed emotional state onto a different emotion in the perceiver (e.g., anger elicits fear, not anger).

There are several further considerations in interpreting the data thus far. The lesion studies are complicated by the fact that different stimuli, different tasks, and different analyses have often been used. The patients present many differences also, both in terms of the details of their lesions and in terms of the cognitive background within which the amygdala damage results in impaired emotion processing. Most of the patients have damage also to extra-amygdalar structures that is often quite substantial. Even within the amygdala, the damage can vary, and studies have not attempted to distinguish between damage in different amygdala nuclei. These difficulties aside, it nonetheless seems possible to extract from the different studies a common pattern of disproportionately impaired recognition of only certain emotions, perhaps those that are both negatively valenced and of high arousal, such as fear. Is this because fearful facial expressions signal a particular type of information whose processing depends on the integrity of the amygdala? Or is processing of fear-related information distinguished in some other ways unrelated to emotion? These are tricky questions to which we as yet do not have definitive answers. There is, for instance, the possibility that certain tasks ask subjects to categorize fear at a level that is subordinate to the level of categorization required for happiness or sadness (which could be thought of as prototypes of the more superordinate categories "happy" and "unhappy"). It might be that fear is simply more confusable with certain emotions, like surprise and anger, than happiness is confusable with any emotion (Adolphs, 2002). In support of such a possibility, we described a patient with extensive bilateral temporal lobe damage, including damage to the amygdala, who essentially recognized only two superordinate emotion categories, happy and unhappy, and who misclassified fear into the happy category (Adolphs, Tranel, and Damasio, 2003). Future studies will need to be very careful in controlling for these factors.

A natural follow-up to the findings just presented is the specificity of the impairment for faces. We examined this issue by showing subjects social scenes under two conditions: in one condition the scenes contained emotional facial expressions, in the second the faces were erased in the scenes. Not surprisingly, normal and brain-damaged controls found it easier to recognize the emotion from scenes when they contained emotional expressions than when the expressions had been erased. By contrast, subjects with amygdala damage showed no such advantage. In fact, they were much worse at recognizing emotions from scenes when the scenes

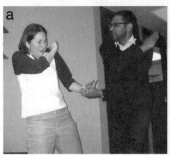 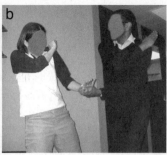 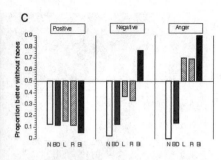

FIGURE 73.5   Recognition of emotion from social scenes is disproportionately severe when the scenes contain facial expressions. (*a*) Subjects with either unilateral or bilateral amygdala damage were more impaired in recognizing negatively valenced emotions from complex visual scenes only when those scenes contained facial expressions. (*b*) When faces in the scenes were erased, the subjects' performances became normal. (*c*) Accuracy in recognizing basic emotions from these stimuli: whereas normal controls (NC) and brain-damaged controls (BDC) always performed much better on the second set of stimuli, with the faces present, subjects with either

unilateral left (L), right (R), or bilateral (bi) amygdala damage showed the inverse pattern of performance specifically for negatively valenced emotions. What was even more surprising, some subjects with bilateral amygdala damage were severely impaired in recognizing scenes when the scenes contained facial expressions, but actually performed better than controls when faces had been erased, possibly suggesting that they learn to partly compensate for their impaired recognition of emotion from faces by developing greater sensitivity to social cues other than faces.

contained faces than when they did not (Adolphs and Tranel, 2003; figure 73.5)! Furthermore, there was even an indication that subjects with bilateral amygdala damage were better than normals in recognizing emotions from scenes when faces had been erased. Taken together, these findings emphasize the importance of the face in signaling emotional information, and the importance of the amygdala in processing precisely that information. Subjects with amygdala damage are sensitive to emotion signaled by the face but are unable to use it normally in order to recognize the emotion; when the face is removed, however, they are able to use information normally from context, body posture, or other cues in order to judge the emotion.

SOCIAL JUDGMENT FROM FACES   What is the significance of the emotion recognition impairment described in the previous section for real-life behavior? It is worth noting that we do not typically use information from faces solely to determine another person's emotional state, but rather to make social judgments regarding the other person's intentions and dispositions and to guide our own behavior toward them. We examined this issue by asking subjects to judge the approachability and trustworthiness of unfamiliar faces. These faces showed people in natural poses, not different strong emotional expressions (the expressions were neutral or smiling). We found a specific impairment in subjects with bilateral amygdala damage: whereas they judged approachable- and trustworthy-looking people normally, they failed to judge unapproachability and untrustworthiness (Adolphs, Tranel, and Damasio, 1998). The impairment consisted of two distinct components: first, subjects with bilateral amygdala damage exhibited an overall positive bias in judging everyone to look more trustworthy and approachable than

normally judged; second, they were able to rank-order very trustworthy- or approachable-looking people normally but failed to rank-order individuals who were normally judged to look untrustworthy or unapproachable (figure 73.6). This impairment extends the impaired recognition of basic emotions we have described to more complex social judgments. Possibly the two sets of impairments are related: recognition of facial expressions may be impaired disproportionately for those emotions that signal threat or danger in the environment in general, and social judgment may be impaired in regard to threat or danger in the social environment in particular. The impaired ability to judge untrustworthiness is also consistent with the real-life behavior of these subjects, which often features an overly trusting and friendly personality.

This finding from lesion studies has been corroborated by functional imaging studies. A recent study showed that activation within the amygdala correlated with the degree of judged untrustworthiness of the face that was shown to subjects (Winston et al., 2002). Moreover, this correlation held, even when other factors such as expression, sex, ethnicity, and eye gaze were controlled for. There is thus something about the physiognomy of the face on the basis of which we normally judge trustworthiness, and the amygdala is one structure mediating such judgments.

Just as difficult questions arose in regard to the amygdala's specificity for processing fear, there are analogous (broader) questions concerning its role in processing domain-specific social information. We followed up on the experiments described in the preceding section by investigating the preferences that subjects exhibit for nonsocial stimuli, such as pictures of landscapes. To our surprise, we found that subjects with bilateral amygdala damage showed the same

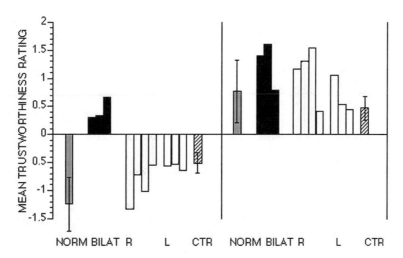

FIGURE 73.6   The amygdala in social judgments of trustworthiness. Bilateral damage to the amygdala (BILAT) selectively impairs the ability to judge untrustworthiness from faces, whereas unilateral damage (R, L), or brain damage elsewhere (BDC) does not. The two graphs plot mean ratings of untrustworthiness assigned by subjects to 50 faces that are normally rated the most untrustworthy looking (left, normative ratings, NORM) and to 50 faces normally rated the most trustworthy looking (right).

inability to judge aversive nonsocial stimuli: they judged pictures of landscapes, nonsense drawings, colored spheres, and colored Mondrians to be abnormally positive when asked how much they liked them (Adolphs and Tranel, 1999b). It thus appears as though bilateral damage to the amygdala impairs an ability to judge aversive, dangerous, or in some way undesirable stimuli in a manner that is not completely domain-specific. Similar observations have been made in nonhuman primates following experimentally introduced amygdala lesions (Emery et al., 2001).

RECOGNIZING EMOTION FROM AUDITORY STIMULI   By comparison to the amygdala's role in recognizing emotions from faces, its role in recognition of emotion from auditory stimuli is very unclear. This is surprising. Given the multimodal nature of sensory inputs to the amygdala, one would certainly expect impairments in emotion processing to be parallel across sensory modalities. A small number of functional imaging studies have reported activation of the amygdala to prosodic or other emotional auditory stimuli (Phillips et al., 1998), although some have reported deactivation of the amygdala instead (Morris, Scott, and Dolan, 1999). Some lesion studies have found impaired ability to recognize fear from auditory stimuli following bilateral amygdala damage (Scott et al., 1997), whereas others have not (Anderson and Phelps, 1998; Adolphs and Tranel, 1999a).

We investigated the role of the amygdala in recognizing emotion from prosody and found no significant impairment following bilateral amygdala damage (Adolphs and Tranel, 1999a). Curiously, however, we did find some evidence of variable impairment following temporal lobectomy (Adolphs, Tranel, and Damasio, 2001). A particularly unexpected finding was of a disproportionate impairment in recognizing emotions from faces or from prosody following left

or right amygdala damage, respectively (Adolphs, Tranel, and Damasio, 2002). Although this finding suggests different roles for the left and the right amygdala in processing emotional and social information from certain sensory modalities, it is important to keep in mind that the lesions of the patients in this study (patients with epilepsy who had undergone a temporal lobectomy) included not only unilateral amygdala lesions but also lesions in surrounding cortex and other structures in the anteromedial temporal lobe.

The evidence for the amygdala's role in recognizing emotion from nonprosodic auditory stimuli (e.g., screams, growls, sirens) is more encouraging. Some lesion studies, including unpublished findings with our patient S.M.046, have pointed to such a role (Scott et al., 1997).

RECOGNIZING EMOTION FROM LEXICAL INFORMATION   Although some functional imaging studies have found amygdala activation to lexical emotional stimuli (Isenberg et al., 1999; Phelps et al., 2001; Hamann and Mao, 2002), lesion studies have generally suggested that the amygdala is not essential for recognizing or judging emotional and social information from explicit, lexical stimuli such as stories. Our studies with S.M.046 are a good case in point: S.M.046 can label emotions from scenarios presented in stories, and she can retrieve considerable declarative knowledge about all emotions, including fear.

There is, however, an interesting wrinkle to this story. S.M.046 does not know that some unpleasant emotions are arousing! In order to probe the categories of emotions whose recognition is impaired, we asked subjects to rate emotional stimuli not in terms of their intensity on basic emotions, as done in the studies cited earlier, but in terms of their valence (pleasantness or unpleasantness) and arousal. Normal subjects judge emotions such as fear and anger to be both unpleasant and highly arousing. S.M.046, by contrast, judged them to be unpleasant but of low arousal (Adolphs, Russell, and Tranel, 1999). This impairment in recognizing arousal from unpleasant emotions held across labels for the emotions, stories depicting emotions, and facial expressions of emotions, thus reflecting impaired conceptual knowledge in general, irrespective of the nature of the stimulus. For instance, when told a story about someone driving a car down a steep mountain road who had lost the brakes, she correctly recognized that the situation would be very unpleasant, but also gave the highly abnormal judgment that it would make one feel sleepy and relaxed. The impairment was especially striking, since S.M.046 was able to judge arousal normally from positive emotions.

We found a similar impairment in two other subjects who, like S.M.046, had bilateral amygdala damage that was sustained relatively early in life. However, three subjects with complete bilateral amygdala damage due to encephalitis sustained in adulthood showed no such impairment (Adolphs et al., 1997; figure 73.7). How can we reconcile these findings? Our explanation is that normal acquisition of conceptual knowledge of certain emotions depends on the integrity of the amygdala during development. Bilateral amygdala damage would preclude normal emotional arousal responses to stimuli signaling fear or anger: the absence of such responses, as well as of cognitive modulation, explains the online impairment in recognizing fear from facial expressions in such patients. But they would still know, as a declarative fact, what fear is, and how arousing it should be, provided they have experienced such arousal in the past. Developmental damage to the amygdala would prevent such knowledge from arising normally, with the observed impaired knowledge that fear and anger are arousing emotions. This developmental consequence is probably analogous to the consequences of developmental frontal lobe damage: like patients with amygdala damage, they are impaired in their ability to trigger normal emotional responses to stimuli during development, and as in patients with developmental damage to the amygdala but not as in patients with adult-onset damage to either amygdala or prefrontal cortex, this translates into an impaired concept of some aspects of emotional or social knowledge.

ELECTROPHYSIOLOGICAL RESPONSES IN THE HUMAN AMYGDALA Single-unit recordings from the monkey amygdala have found neurons whose responses are modulated by the emotional significance of stimuli (Rolls, 1999). Of note, this modulation can be independent of the perceptual properties of the stimulus. For instance, the very same stimulus can evoke differential amygdala activity, depending on its prior association with reward or punishment (Nishijo, Ono, and Nishino, 1988). We have recorded field potentials and single-unit activity from the amygdala of neurosurgical patients who were undergoing epilepsy monitoring. As in the animal studies, we found neurons whose responses were selectively modulated by the emotion category of stimuli. In our case, these were complex visual stimuli, and we checked to be sure that responses could not be attributed to factors such as differences in luminance or color composition of the categories. The responses we found showed an increase in activity that was selective for aversive stimuli—pictures of mutilation, threat, and war (Oya et al., 2002; figure 73.8). An interesting additional finding was the suggestion of a differential electrophysiological signature (power at different frequency bands), depending on whether the images showed bodily injury to people or disgusting items (e.g., dirty toilets, cockroaches). These latter findings raise the intriguing possibility that different neurons within the amygdala, or possibly even the same neurons participating in a different network, can encode different aspects of emotional information. We have obtained similar findings also when patients were presented with olfactory stimuli: as for the visual stimuli, the neurons responded selectively by increasing their firing rates to unpleasant olfactory stimuli.

Summary

We can now tie some of these diverse strands together. The human amygdala appears to be important both for the acquisition and for the online processing of emotional stimuli. Its role is disproportionate for a particular category of emotional information, possibly that pertaining to evaluating potential threat in the environment. Its processing encompasses both the elicitation of emotional responses in the body and changes in other cognitive processes, such as attention and memory. When these effects occur online, as an emotional stimulus is processed, they also contribute to the acquisition of certain components of concepts of emotions, namely, those components of knowledge dependent on prior emotional responses. This is why damage to the amygdala early in life, as we saw in the case of S.M.046, compromises not only emotional responses and recognition of emotional stimuli, but also abstract knowledge of particular aspects of emotion concepts, specifically that unpleasant emotions can be arousing, an attribute that is particularly pertinent for the emotions fear and anger.

I have highlighted the amygdala as a structure that mediates between perceptual representations of stimuli and the modulation of cognition, but the amygdala should be thought of as only one component of a neural system. Other components with a related function include ventral and medial regions of the prefrontal cortex and the basal ganglia. In many studies these regions are coactivated, and

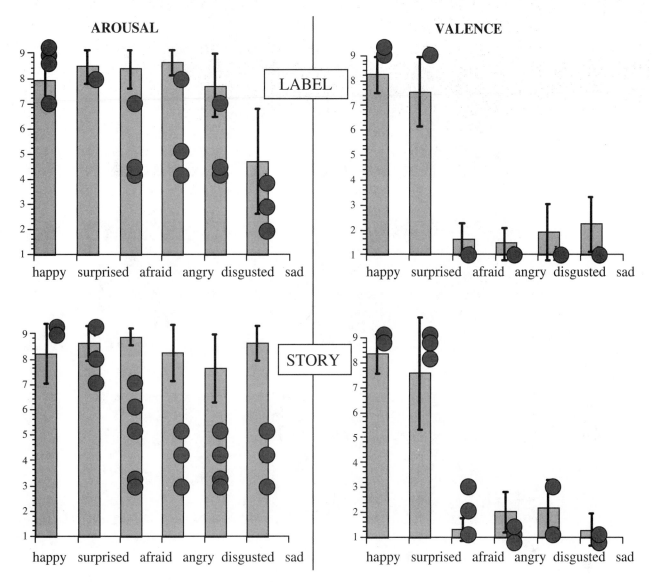

FIGURE 73.7 Developmental damage to the amygdala impairs knowledge of the arousal of unpleasant emotions. Patient S.M.046 was impaired in her knowledge that negatively valenced emotions, especially fear and anger, are also highly arousing. The impairment was evident both for facial expressions of emotions (not shown) and for lexical stimuli such as the words for the emotions and stories depicting emotions. Bars indicate means ± SD of responses by normal controls; circles indicate responses from S.M.046. (See color plate 62.)

in many ways their functions overlap. It remains an important question, therefore, to describe the ways in which they differ. One hypothesis is that the amygdala and the ventral striatum subserve relatively rapid, automatic, and coarse emotional processing driven largely by features of the stimulus, and that sectors of the prefrontal cortex modulate such processing by providing information about the context in which the stimulus occurred and by introducing volitional effects on information processing. This scheme is probably too simple, because it is likely that amygdala and ventral striatum also participate in these latter functions—indeed, there are data demonstrating that their activations can be modulated volitionally, perhaps via top-down influences

from prefrontal cortex. Another reason the scheme is likely to be simplistic is that it does not account for the different roles that different amygdala nuclei will play.

Future questions

The findings reviewed in this chapter leave us with some important open questions (Adolphs, 2003b). Several of these questions return to issues we identified at the beginning of the chapter. To what extent is social information processing domain-specific, and to what extent does it draw on more general motivational and emotional processing? Where in the causal relations between processes do feelings come in?

Frequency

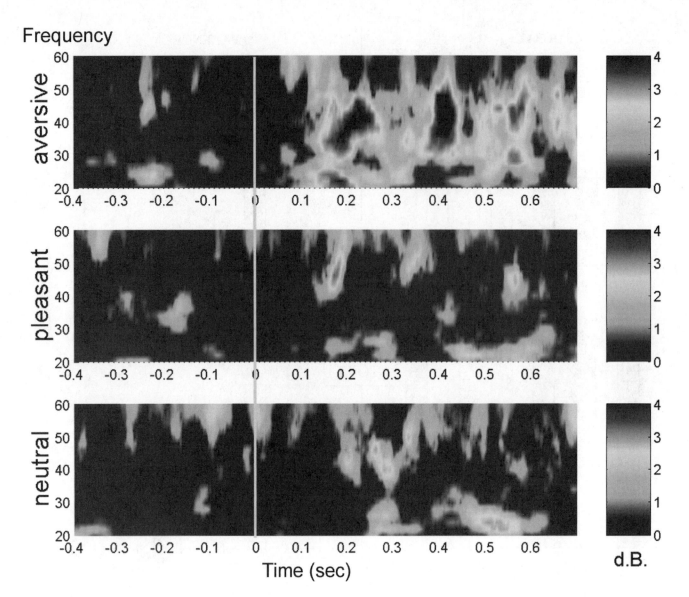

FIGURE 73.8 Time-frequency plots of field potentials recorded from the amygdala in response to visual stimuli. Time is shown on the x-axis (seconds) and the frequency of the recorded response (20–60 Hz) is shown on the y-axis. Stimulus onset is indicated by the white vertical bar at 0s. Grayscale encodes amplitude of the response in dB. Stimuli were sorted into three emotion categories as shown; there were significantly larger responses to aversive stimuli than to pleasant or neutral stimuli. (See color plate 63.)

What role does more extensive cognitive and volitional processing play in emotion and social information processing?

The evidence reviewed clearly points to some domain specificity in the processing of socially relevant information: there are brain mechanisms specialized to detect faces and process threat-related stimuli. But this observation still leaves open two possibilities: such specializations may reflect the operation of systems that are truly specialized to process social information, or they may reflect the fact that social stimuli make particular processing demands, which are, however, subserved by domain-general systems. The question of domain specificity thus concerns the factors that are driving this specificity: are they properties of the stimuli,

tasks, or behaviors or properties of the neural architecture that subserves the processing of such stimuli, tasks, or behaviors?

Although the amygdala does not appear directly essential for feeling emotions, it likely plays an indirect role by triggering components of emotional responses that can in turn be felt. Pilot data from our laboratory indicate that S.M.046 does not feel emotions normally when she views film clips or listens to music, but she can provide relatively normal ratings of feelings when given abstract information or when instructed to feel a certain way. These observations, together with the finding that patients with lesions of the amygdala endorse normal ratings on scales of dispositional affect, make it likely that the amygdala serves to link perceptual representations of external stimuli to the modulation of cognition and behavior, and therefore can indirectly have an influence on the feelings such stimuli elicit.

ACKNOWLEDGMENTS This work was supported by the National Institutes of Health, the Sloan Foundation, the E.J.L.B. Foundation, the Klingenstein Fund, and the James S. McDonnell Foundation.

REFERENCES

ADOLPHS, R., 1999. The human amygdala and emotion. *Neuroscientist* 5:125–137.

ADOLPHS, R., 2002. Recognizing emotion from facial expressions: Psychological and neurological mechanisms. *Behav. Cogn. Neurosci. Rev.* 1:21–61.

ADOLPHS, R., 2003a. Cognitive neuroscience of human social behavior. *Nat. Rev. Neurosci.* 4:165–178.

ADOLPHS, R., 2003b. Investigating the cognitive neuroscience of social behavior. *Neuropsychologia* 41:119–126.

ADOLPHS, R., G. P. LEE, D. TRANEL, and A. R. DAMASIO, 1997. Bilateral damage to the human amygdala early in life impairs knowledge of emotional arousal. *Soc. Neurosci. Abstr.* 23:1582.

ADOLPHS, R., J. A. RUSSELL, and D. TRANEL, 1999. A role for the human amygdala in recognizing emotional arousal from unpleasant stimuli. *Psychol. Sci.* 10:167–171.

ADOLPHS, R., and D. TRANEL, 1999a. Intact recognition of emotional prosody following amygdala damage. *Neuropsychologia* 37:1285–1292.

ADOLPHS, R., and D. TRANEL, 1999b. Preferences for visual stimuli following amygdala damage. *J. Cogn. Neurosci.* 11:610–616.

ADOLPHS, R., and D. TRANEL, 2000. Emotion recognition and the human amygdala. In *The Amygdala: A Functional Analysis*, J. P. Aggleton, ed. New York: Oxford University Press, pp. 587–630.

ADOLPHS, R., and D. TRANEL, 2003. Amygdala damage impairs recognition of emotion from scenes only when they contain facial expressions. *Neuropsychologia* 41:1281–1289.

ADOLPHS, R., D. TRANEL, and A. R. DAMASIO, 1998. The human amygdala in social judgment. *Nature* 393:470–474.

ADOLPHS, R., D. TRANEL, and A. DAMASIO, 2003. Dissociable neural systems for recognizing emotions. *Brain Cognit.* 52:61–69.

ADOLPHS, R., D. TRANEL, and H. DAMASIO, 2001. Emotion recognition from faces and prosody following temporal lobectomy. *Neuropsychology* 15:396–404.

ADOLPHS, R., D. TRANEL, and H. DAMASIO, 2002. Neural systems for recognizing emotion from prosody. *Emotion* 2:23–51.

ADOLPHS, R., D. TRANEL, H. DAMASIO, and A. DAMASIO, 1994. Impaired recognition of emotion in facial expressions following bilateral damage to the human amygdala. *Nature* 372:669–672.

ADOLPHS, R., D. TRANEL, H. DAMASIO, and A. R. DAMASIO, 1995. Fear and the human amygdala. *J. Neurosci.* 15:5879–5892.

ADOLPHS, R., D. TRANEL, S. HAMANN, A. YOUNG, A. CALDER, A. ANDERSON, E. PHELPS, G. P. LEE, and A. R. DAMASIO, 1999. Recognition of facial emotion in nine subjects with bilateral amygdala damage. *Neuropsychologia* 37:1111–1117.

ALLISON, T., H. GINTER, G. MCCARTHY, A. C. NOBRE, A. PUCE, M. LUBY, and D. D. SPENCER, 1994. Face recognition in human extrastriate cortex. *J. Neurophysiol.* 71:821–825.

ANDERSON, A. K., and E. A. PHELPS, 1998. Intact recognition of vocal expressions of fear following bilateral lesions of the human amygdala. *Neuroreport* 9:3607–3613.

ANDERSON, A. K., and E. A. PHELPS, 2001. Lesions of the human amygdala impair enhanced perception of emotionally salient events. *Nature* 411:305–309.

ANDERSON, A. K., and E. A. PHELPS, 2002. Is the human amygdala critical for the subjective experience of emotion? Evidence of intact dispositional affect in patients with amygdala lesions. *J. Cogn. Neurosci.* 14:709–720.

BECHARA, A., H. DAMASIO, A. R. DAMASIO, and G. P. LEE, 1999. Different contributions of the human amygdala and ventromedial prefrontal cortex to decision-making. *J. Neurosci.* 19:5473–5481.

BLAIR, R. J. R., J. S. MORRIS, C. D. FRITH, D. I. PERRETT, and R. J. DOLAN, 1999. Dissociable neural responses to facial expressions of sadness and anger. *Brain* 122:883–893.

BREITER, H. C., N. L. ETCOFF, P. J. WHALEN, W. A. KENNEDY, S. L. RAUCH, R. L. BUCKNER, M. M. STRAUSS, S. E. HYMAN, and B. R. ROSEN, 1996. Response and habituation of the human amygdala during visual processing of facial expression. *Neuron* 17:875–887.

BROKS, P., A. W. YOUNG, E. J. MARATOS, P. J. COFFEY, A. J. CALDER, C. ISAAC, A. R. MAYES, J. R. HODGES, D. MONTALDI, E. CEZAYIRLI, N. ROBERTS, and D. HADLEY, 1998. Face processing impairments after encephalitis: Amygdala damage and recognition of fear. *Neuropsychologia* 36:59–70.

CALDER, A. J., A. W. YOUNG, D. ROWLAND, D. I. PERRETT, J. R. HODGES, and N. L. ETCOFF, 1996. Facial emotion recognition after bilateral amygdala damage: Differentially severe impairment of fear. *Cogn. Neuropsychol.* 13:699–745.

CANNON, W. B., 1927. The James-Lange theory of emotions: A critical examination and an alternative theory. *Am. J. Psychol.* 39:106–124.

DAMASIO, A. R., 1994. *Descartes' Error: Emotion, Reason, and the Human Brain.* New York: Grosset/Putnam.

DARWIN, C., 1872/1965. *The Expression of the Emotions in Man and Animals.* Chicago: University of Chicago Press.

EMERY, N. J., J. P. CAPITANIO, W. A. MASON, C. J. MACHADO, S. P. MENDOZA, and D. G. AMARAL, 2001. The effects of bilateral lesions of the amygdala on dyadic social interactions in rhesus monkeys. *Behav. Neurosci.* 115:515–544.

FRIJDA, N. H., 1986. *The Emotions.* New York: Cambridge University Press.

HAMADA, T., et al., 2002. Lipoid proteinosis maps to 1q21 and is caused by mutations in the extracellular matrix protein 1 gene (ECM1). *Hum. Mol. Genet.* 11:833–840.

HAMANN, S., and H. MAO, 2002. Positive and negative emotional verbal stimuli elicit activity in the left amygdala. *Neuroreport* 13:15–19.

HAXBY, J. V., E. A. HOFFMAN, and M. I. GOBBINI, 2000. The distributed human neural system for face perception. *Trends Cogn. Sci.* 4:223–233.

HOFER, P.-A., 1973. Urbach-Wiethe disease: A review. *Acta Dermatol. Venerol.* 53:5–52.

ISENBERG, N., D. SILBERSWEIG, A. ENGELIEN, S. EMMERICH, K. MALAVADE, M. BEATTIE, A. C. LEON, and E. STERN, 1999. Linguistic threat activates the human amygdala. *Proc. Natl. Acad. Sci. U.S.A.* 96:10456–10459.

JAMES, W., 1884. What is an emotion? *Mind* 9:188–205.

LAZARUS, R. S., 1991. *Emotion and Adaptation.* New York: Oxford University Press.

MCCARTHY, G., 1999. Physiological studies of face processing in humans. In *The New Cognitive Neurosciences*, M. S. Gazzaniga, ed. Cambridge, Mass.: MIT Press, pp. 393–410.

MORRIS, J. S., B. DE GELDER, L. WEISKRANTZ, and R. J. DOLAN, 2001. Differential extrageniculostriate and amygdala responses to presentation of emotional faces in a cortically blind field. *Brain* 124:1241–1252.

MORRIS, J. S., C. D. FRITH, D. I. PERRETT, D. ROWLAND, A. W. YOUNG, A. J. CALDER, and R. J. DOLAN, 1996. A differential neural response in the human amygdala to fearful and happy facial expressions. *Nature* 383:812–815.

MORRIS, J. S., A. OHMAN, and R. J. DOLAN, 1999. A subcortical pathway to the right amygdala mediating "unseen" fear. *Proc. Natl. Acad. Sci. U.S.A.* 96:1680–1685.

MORRIS, J. S., S. K. SCOTT, and R. J. DOLAN, 1999. Saying it with feeling: Neural responses to emotional vocalizations. *Neuropsychologia* 37:1155–1163.

NISHIJO, H., T. ONO, and H. NISHINO, 1988. Single neuron responses in amygdala of alert monkey during complex sensory stimulation with affective significance. *J. Neurosci.* 8: 3570–3583.

OCHSNER, K., S. A. BUNGE, J. J. GROSS, and J. D. E. GABRIELI, 2002. Rethinking feelings: An fMRI study of the cognitive regulation of emotion. *J. Cogn. Neurosci.* 14:1215–1229.

OYA, H., H. KAWASAKI, M. A. HOWARD, and R. ADOLPHS, 2002. Electrophysiological responses in the human amygdala discriminate emotion categories of complex visual stimuli. *J. Neurosci.* 22:9502–9512.

PANKSEPP, J., 1998. *Affective Neuroscience*. New York: Oxford University Press.

PELPHREY, K. A., J. D. SINGERMAN, T. ALLISON, and G. MCCARTHY, 2003. Brain activation evoked by the perception of gaze shifts: The influence of timing and context. *Neuropsychologia* 41: 156–170.

PHELPS, E. A., K. J. O'CONNOR, J. C. GATENBY, J. C. GORE, C. GRILLON, and M. DAVIS, 2001. Activation of the left amygdala to a cognitive representation of fear. *Nat. Neurosci.* 4:437–441.

PHILLIPS, M. L., A. W. YOUNG, S. K. SCOTT, A. J. CALDER, C. ANDREW, V. GIAMPIETRO, S. C. R. WILLIAMS, E. T. BULLMORE, M. BRAMMER, and J. A. GRAY, 1998. Neural responses to facial and vocal expressions of fear and disgust. *Proc. R. Soc. Lond Ser. B* 265:1809–1817.

RAPCSAK, S. Z., S. R. GALPER, J. F. COMER, S. L. REMINGER, L. NIELSEN, A. W. KASZNIAK, M. VERFAELLIE, J. F. LAGUNA, D. M. LABINER, and R. A. COHEN, 2000. Fear recognition deficits after focal brain damage. *Neurology* 54:575–581.

ROLLS, E. T., 1999. *The Brain and Emotion*. New York: Oxford University Press.

SCHAEFER, S. M., D. C. JACKSON, R. J. DAVIDSON, G. K. AGUIRRE, D. Y. KIMBERG, and S. L. THOMPSON-SCHILL, 2002. Modulation of amygdalar activity by the conscious regulation of negative emotion. *J. Cogn. Neurosci.* 14:913–921.

SCHERER, K. R., 1988. Criteria for emotion-antecedent appraisal: A review. In *Cognitive Perspectives on Emotion and Motivation*, V. Hamilton, G. H. Bower, and N. H. Frijda, eds. Dordrecht, Holland: Martinus Nijhoff, pp. 89–126.

SCHMOLCK, H., and L. R. SQUIRE, 2001. Impaired perception of facial emotions following bilateral damage to the anterior temporal lobe. *Neuropsychology* 15:30–38.

SCOTT, S. K., A. W. YOUNG, A. J. CALDER, D. J. HELLAWELL, J. P. AGGLETON, and M. JOHNSON, 1997. Impaired auditory recognition of fear and anger following bilateral amygdala lesions. *Nature* 385:254–257.

STONE, V. E., S. BARON-COHEN, A. W. YOUNG, A. J. CALDER, and J. KEANE, 2003. Acquired theory of mind impairments in patients with bilateral amygdala lesions. *Neuropsychologia* 41:209–220.

TRANEL, D., and B. T. HYMAN, 1990. Neuropsychological correlates of bilateral amygdala damage. *Arch. Neurol.* 47:349–355.

VUILLEUMIER, P., J. L. ARMONY, J. DRIVER, and R. J. DOLAN, 2001. Effects of attention and emotion on face processing in the human brain: An event-related fMRI study. *Neuron* 30:829.

WHALEN, P. J., 1999. Fear, vigilance, and ambiguity: Initial neuroimaging studies of the human amygdala. *Curr. Direct. Psychol. Sci.* 7:177–187.

WHALEN, P. J., S. L. RAUCH, N. L. ETCOFF, S. C. MCINERNEY, M. B. LEE, and M. A. JENIKE, 1998. Masked presentations of emotional facial expressions modulate amygdala activity without explicit knowledge. *J. Neurosci.* 18:411–418.

WHALEN, P. J., L. M. SHIN, S. C. MCINERNEY, H. FISCHER, C. I. WRIGHT, and S. L. RAUCH, 2001. A functional MRI study of human amygdala responses to facial expressions of fear versus anger. *Emotion* 1:70–83.

WICKER, B., D. I. PERRETT, S. BARON-COHEN, and J. DECETY, 2003. Being the target of another's emotion: A PET study. *Neuropsychologia* 41:139–146.

WINSTON, J. S., B. A. STRANGE, J. O'DOHERTY, and R. J. DOLAN, 2002. Automatic and intentional brain responses during evaluation of trustworthiness of faces. *Nat. Neurosci.* 5:277–283.

YANG, T. T., V. MENON, S. ELIEZ, C. BLASEY, C. D. WHITE, A. J. REID, I. H. GOTLIB, and A. L. REISS, 2002. Amygdalar activation associated with positive and negative facial expressions. *Neuroreport* 13:1737–1741.

YOUNG, A. W., J. P. AGGLETON, D. J. HELLAWELL, M. JOHNSON, P. BROKS, and J. R. HANLEY, 1995. Face processing impairments after amygdalotomy. *Brain* 118:15–24.

ZAJONC, R. B., 1980. Feeling and thinking: Preferences need no inferences. *Am. Psychol.* 35:151–175.

74 Stress and Cognition

ROBERT M. SAPOLSKY

ABSTRACT Considerable experimental and clinical data demonstrate that stress (defined as a challenge to homeostasis) can alter cognition. This chapter reviews this subject, concentrating on three broad areas of findings. First, major and/or sustained stress can impair hippocampal-dependent declarative memory; this has been demonstrated in a number of species, including humans, and the neuroendocrine and cellular mechanisms underlying the phenomenon are relatively well understood. As a second point, milder and more transient stressors enhance hippocampal-dependent cognition, via mechanisms that are less well delineated. The enhancing and disruptive effects, when combined, form an "inverse-U"-shaped curve; this makes sense, in that we tend to define mild and transient stressors as being "stimulatory," a situation that we intuit as associated with enhanced cognition. Finally, stressors, over their full range of severities, enhance implicit learning associated with vigilance and fear-conditioning. Such enhancement is centered in the amygdala, and the mechanisms underlying it are of considerable relevance to the understanding of anxiety disorders and posttraumatic stress disorder.

Early in the twentieth century, Cannon described the fight-or-flight response to challenges to homeostasis (now termed stressors). Canon viewed the stress response, the body's effort to reestablish homeostasis, as beneficial. By the 1930s, Selye had described the other side of the stress response: its prolonged activation due to chronic stress can be pathogenic. This dichotomy between the adaptive and deleterious nature of the acute and chronic stress response, respectively, is the central concept of stress physiology.

The core of the stress response consists of activating the sympathetic nervous system and adrenocortical axis. The former occurs within seconds, triggering secretion by sympathetic nerve endings of epinephrine (adrenaline) and norepinephrine. The adrenocortical axis begins at the hypothalamus, where stress releases corticotropin-releasing hormone (CRH) and related hormones within seconds. They stimulate pituitary secretion of adrenocorticotropic hormone. This triggers the adrenal gland within minutes to release steroid hormones called glucocorticoids (GCs), cortisol in primates and corticosterone in most rodents.

The sympathetic nervous system and GCs mobilize energy from storage sites and increase cardiovascular tone to enhance energy delivery to exercising muscle. They also

ROBERT M. SAPOLSKY Department of Biological Sciences, Stanford University, and Department of Neurology and Neurological Sciences, Stanford University School of Medicine, Stanford, Calif.

inhibit growth, digestion, tissue repair, and reproduction until more auspicious times. The hormones also constrain immunity from overactivity during stress.

During chronic stress, however, excessive GCs and sympathetic nervous system activation become damaging, with increased risks of insulin-resistant diabetes, hypertension, immunosuppression, and reproductive impairments (Sapolsky, Romero, and Munck, 2000).

Severe or prolonged stress, or equivalent exposure to synthetic GCs (e.g., prednisone, dexamethasone, hydrocortisone), can also have adverse effects in the brain. These effects are centered in the hippocampus, a structure with ample receptors for and sensitivity to GCs, and the disruption involves impairment of hippocampal-dependent cognition. But, equally important, the effects of stress are not uniformly disruptive. Instead, two exceptions occur. First, whereas severe acute stressors impair hippocampal-dependent cognition, mild acute stressors enhance it. This forms an inverted U pattern, where optimal hippocampal-dependent cognition occurs with mild, acute stress (a circumstance often termed *stimulation*), with cognition less optimal in the absence of stimulation or during a more severe stressor. And second, whereas severe stress impairs hippocampal-dependent cognition, it enhances amygdala-dependent cognition. This plays a role in autonomic fear conditioning and is relevant to understanding anxiety and the cognitive consequences of trauma.

Stress and disruption of hippocampal-dependent memory

ANIMAL STUDIES Stress or GCs disrupt hippocampal-dependent spatial memory in rodents. As initial correlative evidence, basal GC levels rise (Sapolsky, 1992) and spatial memory declines with age in rodents (Gallagher and Burwell, 1989), and the greater the rise in GC levels, the greater is the cognitive impairment (Issa et al., 1990; Yau et al., 1995).

These findings are difficult to interpret. Potentially, elevated GC levels could impair hippocampal function. However, the hippocampus helps to mediate negative feedback regulation of GC secretion via inhibition of hypothalamic CRH release (Jacobson and Sapolsky, 1991); therefore, the causality could be reversed. Thus, hippocampal damage produces GC hypersecretion. Therefore, either elevated GC levels could be impairing hippocampal-dependent cognition in aged rodents, and/or hippocampal damage could be the cause of cognitive impairments and the GC hypersecretion.

As evidence for the first scenario, rats adrenalectomized in midage and maintained on minimal GCs thereafter are spared age-related declines in spatial memory (Landfield, Baskin, and Pitler, 1981). Conversely, excessive lifelong stress accelerates hippocampal senescence (Kerr et al., 1991).

In young rats, hippocampal-dependent memory is impaired by various stressors, including brief exposure to a predator smell, weeks of daily restraint, or months of rotating group membership (Altenor, Kay, and Richter, 1977; Bodnoff et al., 1995; Conrad et al., 1996; Diamond et al., 1999). Moreover, exposure to equivalent stress levels of GCs also disrupts spatial memory (Dachir et al., 1993; Luine, Spencer, and McEwen, 1993; Bardgett et al., 1994; Endo et al., 1999; Bisagno et al., 2000; Sousa et al., 2000). Impairments could reflect effects on acquisition, consolidation, or retrieval; of these, retrieval appears to be the most sensitive to the disruptive GC effects (De Quervain, Roozendaal, and McGaugh, 1998; Roozendaal et al., 2003).

Finally, not only does cumulative lifelong exposure to GCs influence hippocampal aging, but older rats are more vulnerable than young rats to the impairing effects of acute GC administration (Bodnoff et al., 1995). This increased susceptibility could reflect peripheral physiological effects. For example, if hepatic clearance of GCs declines with age, the amount of GCs reaching the brain would increase, artifactually enhancing the disruption of cognition. However, clearance is unchanged with age (Sapolsky, Krey, and McEwen, 1983).

Stress and GCs affect nonhuman primates similarly. Among male tree shrews, social subordinance elevates basal GCs and impairs hippocampal-dependent memory. Pharmacological GC exposure is similarly impairing, although more rapidly and transiently (Ohl et al., 2000).

Thus, in the rat and nonhuman primate, severe or sustained stressors, or equivalent exposure to exogenous GCs, impair hippocampal-dependent cognition. Aged rats are more vulnerable, and cumulative lifelong GC exposure contributes to the functional declines in the aged hippocampus.

HUMAN STUDIES Stress can disrupt declarative memory in humans (hippocampal-dependent memory in humans is generally considered to be declarative; whether rodents are capable of hippocampal-dependent, nonspatial declarative memory is controversial [Bunsey and Eichenbaum, 1996; Willingham, 1998]). Early evidence came from studies of Cushing's syndrome, in which various types of tumors cause GC hypersecretion. The syndrome was long noted to cause memory impairments, and formal testing has demonstrated selective deficits in declarative memory in patients that correlated with the severity of GC excess (Starkman et al., 1992).

Gerontology studies link elevated GC levels and impaired cognition. Human aging does not involve GC excess to the same extent as in rodents. Nonetheless, elevated basal GC levels occur in elderly humans who tend toward the most pronounced age-related declines in cognition, even after controlling for socioeconomic status, health, health-related behaviors, and psychosocial characteristics (Seeman et al., 1997). In impressive prospective studies, cognitive function and GC profiles were characterized in elderly individuals. At follow-up 1–6 years later, the subset with increases in basal GC levels over that time had declines in hippocampal-dependent cognition. Implicit memory was preserved, and no memory impairments occurred among other subjects (Lupien et al., 1995, 1998; Seeman et al., 1997). In one case, increased basal GC concentrations and declining cognition were accompanied by selective hippocampal volume loss (Lupien et al., 1998).

In a second gerontological approach, the response of the adrenocortical axis to an inhibitory negative feedback signal is characterized; elderly individuals most resistant to such suppression are most impaired in declarative memory (O'Brien, Schweitzer, and Ames, 1994). In a third approach, subjects are exposed to an acute stressor. Those with the strongest GC response have been shown to have the worst declarative memory (e.g., Meaney et al., 1995; Kelly, Hayslip, and Servaty, 1996; Lupien and McEwen, 1997).

Interpreting these correlative studies is complex. First, as in aged rodents, elevated GC concentrations in elderly humans could either cause or be caused by hippocampal dysfunction. Moreover, studies involving exposure of subjects to a stressor typically utilize a cognitive stressor. Therefore, poor performance may be elevating GC levels rather than elevated GC levels impairing performance.

As with rodent studies, the clearest demonstration that GCs can impair hippocampal-dependent cognition is to independently manipulate GC levels. This has been done in studies of patients administered exogenous GCs (to suppress overactive immune or inflammatory responses). Most GC treatment regimens are transient and nonsystemic (e.g., hydrocortisone cream for an inflamed rash, or hydrocortisone injection into a swollen joint). There is no evidence for cognitive consequences of such benign use. However, numerous individuals receive high-dose systemic GCs continuously or intermittently over long periods. Such exposure causes complex and idiosyncratic behavioral effects. Most commonly, high-dose systemic GCs initially are pleasurable and energizing, but with more prolonged exposure memory impairment and depression occur (cf. Varney, Alexander, and MacIndoe, 1984). This echoes the dichotomy concerning the response to stressors. Specifically, the acute stress response (as is typical of most mammalian stressors) is adaptive and mobilizes energy to, among other sites, the brain. Moreover, transient exposure to mildly elevated GC levels is reinforcing, releasing dopamine in the nucleus accumbens reward pathways (Piazza and Le Moal, 1997). It is only with prolonged stress that the deleterious consequences of the stress response emerge.

These clinical impressions have been formally tested. Such studies control for the cognitive consequences of the serious disease state that prompted the GC administration, requiring matching patients for disease (in addition to age, sex, or IQ), in which the patients were administered GCs or nonsteroidal alternatives. In one study, only the cohort treated with prednisone, 15 mg/day for more than a year, had deficits in hippocampal-dependent paragraph recall, with implicit memory unimpaired (Keenan et al., 1996). Moreover, as little as 3 months of treatment with higher doses (40–60 mg/day) produces similar deficits (Keenan et al., 1996).

There are also case reports of GC overdoses. In one, a woman was prescribed prednisone an order of magnitude higher than intended (producing 15 days of exposure to doses of 250–300 mg/day), impairing hippocampal and cortical function (Wolkowitz et al., 1997).

The adverse GC effects are particularly worrisome in pediatric medicine. For example, high- but not low-dose prednisone regimens cause memory deficits in asthmatic children (Bender, Lerner, and Poland, 1991); a confound is that higher doses are used for more severe cases of asthma which, because of its hypoxic potential, can alter brain status itself. In one well-controlled study, high-dose prednisone treatment in children with leukemia impaired hippocampal-dependent cognition, independent of the effects of radiation or of other drugs administered (Waber et al., 2000).

Despite the careful nature of these studies, it has been difficult to match not only for disease but also for disease severity. Thus, we must consider studies showing hippocampal impairment in healthy human volunteers administered GCs. Stated broadly, they show that exogenous GCs disrupt hippocampal-dependent cognition while sparing implicit memory. These studies have utilized dosages and time courses of GC exposure used clinically, ranging from a single dose (e.g., Wolkowitz, Reuss, and Weingartner, 1990; Kirschbaum et al., 1996; de Quervain et al., 2000) to 10 days of twice daily dosing (Young et al., 1999).

Given these findings, what facets of declarative memory are impaired? In many studies, GCs were administered prior to the learning and recall phases of a task, making it impossible to distinguish among effects on acquisition, consolidation, and retrieval. However, some allow these to be dissociated, reporting that GCs impair consolidation of new declarative information (Newcomer et al., 1994, 1999; Schmidt et al., 1999; Young et al., 1999). An elaboration on this approach combined the facts that declarative memory for a task is consolidated during sleep and that GCs decline during sleep. Infusion of GCs during slow-wave sleep dis-

rupts such consolidation (Born and Fehm, 1999). When GCs are administered some hours before both the task and sleep, they disrupt sleep consolidation without impairing presleep acquisition (Plihal, Pietrowsky, and Born, 1999).

Other studies show that GCs can disrupt recall (i.e., where GC treatment came after acquisition and consolidation) (Bender, Lerner, and Kollasch, 1988; Newcomer et al., 1994; Lupien and McEwen, 1997; Schmidt et al., 1999; Young et al., 1999; de Quervain et al., 2000; Wolf et al., 2001). Some report the recall deficit to involve omission errors (failure to recall items on a list) (Schmidt et al., 1999), and others report commission errors (supposed memory of items that were not on a list) (Wolkowitz, Reuss, and Weingartner, 1990; Wolkowitz et al., 1993).

These studies involve nonphysiological patterns of GC exposure (due to supraphysiological doses, or the use of synthetic GCs bound by only one of the two types of corticosteroid receptors). This raises the issue of whether stress, or physiological levels of endogenous GCs, also impairs declarative memory. This has been shown with a psychosocial stressor (the Trier Social Stress Test; Kirschbaum et al., 1996) and cortisol administration that elevated concentrations into the stress range (Newcomer et al., 1999).

Finally, GCs can also impair cognition involving the frontal cortex (reviewed in Arnsten, 2000), which is more of a GC target in primates than in rodents (based on density of corticosteroid receptors; Sanchez et al., 2000). As correlative evidence, among elderly human subjects with mild cognitive impairment, elevated basal GC levels predicted impaired performance on a frontal task, namely, immediate paragraph recall (Wolf et al., 2002). Moreover, GC administration in young adults impaired working memory and strategic organizing of declarative information (Kirschbaum et al., 1996; Lupien, Gillin, and Hauger, 1999; Young et al., 1999; Wolf et al., 2001), and impaired response inhibition in squirrel monkeys (Lyons et al., 2000).

How might these findings combine into a picture of the effects of stress on cognition? A frequent interpretation is that stress and GCs disrupt foreground-background distinctions. This can involve impaired filtering out of irrelevant stimuli (thereby causing commission errors; Wolkowitz et al., 1993), or decreased use of relevant cues (causing omission errors; Lupien and McEwen, 1997). There is disagreement as to whether GCs impair foreground-background contrast by altering specific cognitive realms (e.g., Newcomer et al., 1994) or whether this result occurs secondarily as a result of impaired attention (e.g., Wolkowitz et al., 1993). As evidence against impaired attention, stress and GCs should also disrupt implicit tasks, were attention being impaired, but this has been reported not to occur (Kirschbaum et al., 1996; Plihal, Pietrowsky, and Born, 1999; Young et al., 1999). Moreover, studies demonstrating impaired declarative memory report no change in levels of arousal or attention

(Bender et al., 1988; Lupien et al., 1994; Newcomer et al., 1994).

Although GCs can disrupt both consolidation and recall, the latter is more easily impaired (e.g., de Quervain et al., 2000). With moderate stress, recall of prior information is impaired, whereas consolidation of new information is not. This observation has prompted a thoughtful speculation: "It does not imply that memory is impaired, but rather that behaviour is *switched* to a more-opportune response that is adapted to the actual condition" (de Kloet et al., 1998; emphasis added). This appealing idea will be reprised.

Mechanisms underlying the adverse effects of stress and GCs

STRESS AND THE PLASTICITY OF SYNAPSES   GCs disrupt hippocampal function through various mechanisms. Beginning at the reversible level, GCs can impair synaptic plasticity. Rapid stimulation of a hippocampal neuron will "strengthen" its synaptic relationship with postsynaptic neurons, such that subsequent stimulation is more likely to evoke an action potential in postsynaptic neurons. Various forms of such plasticity exist, including long-term potentiation (LTP) and primed burst potentiation (PBP), and are thought to be models for, or perhaps even the underpinnings of, learning and memory.

Over the course of hours to days, stressors that disrupt cognition disrupt LTP and, even more readily, PBP in various hippocampal cell fields (Foy et al., 1987; Shors et al., 1989; Diamond et al., 1990; Diamond, Fleshner, and Rose, 1994; Shors and Dryver, 1994; Xu, Anwyl, and Rowan, 1997; Mesches et al., 1999; Diamond and Park, 2000). Moreover, both premortem stress and in vitro GCs disrupt LTP in hippocampal slices (Mesches et al., 1999; Zhou et al., 2000).

These effects are GC dependent, as stress levels of exogenous GCs are similarly disruptive (Diamond et al., 1989, 1992; Pavlides, Watanabe, and McEwen, 1993; Diamond, Fleshner, and Rose, 1994), and are receptor mediated. The hippocampus contains two receptors for GCs, with high-affinity mineralocorticoid receptors (MR) occupied heavily basally, and low-affinity glucocorticoid receptors (GR) occupied heavily only during major stressors. Commensurate with this, stress disrupts synaptic plasticity via GR (Pavlides, Watanabe, and McEwen, 1993; Pavlides et al., 1995; Xu, Anwyl, and Rowan, 1997). At the peak of an action potential, potassium channels open, allowing positively charged potassium to flow extracellularly. Such channels not only remain open long enough to repolarize the neuron back to the negative resting potential, they also transiently allow the potential to become even more negative. This phenomenon (termed afterhyperpolarization, or AHP) transiently reduces neuronal excitability, resulting in the refractory period, a brief period of quiescence. GCs, via GR, prolong AHP,

decreasing the likelihood that neurons will achieve the high firing rate needed for LTP or PBP. Moreover, norepinephrine inputs into the hippocampus can augment CA1 activity, and this augmentation can be blunted by glucocorticoids (Joels and de Kloet, 1992; Hesen and Joels, 1993; Kerr et al., 1989, 1992).

Long-term depression (LTD), which opposes LTP and PBP, involves synaptic alterations that decrease excitability, through mechanisms roughly the opposite of those involved in LTP. Initially, LTD appeared to be a model for forgetting. A priori, forgetting should arise from prolonged lack of synaptic stimulation. However, LTD is an active process and, importantly, is a subthreshold version of LTP. A high frequency of action potentials causes massive calcium mobilization in the postsynaptic neuron's dendritic spine, triggering LTP. In contrast, a lower frequency of action potentials, mobilizing calcium to a lesser degree, triggers LTD. Thus, in a synaptic network involved in an excitatory volley, LTP is induced in the most excited synapses and, rather than there merely being the absence of LTP in less excited neighboring synapses, the actively inhibited process of LTD occurs. This constitutes a mechanism for spatially sharpening signals.

Stress and GCs enhance LTD under conditions where they disrupt LTP (Pavlides et al., 1995; Kim, Foy, and Thompson, 1996; Xu, Anwyl, and Rowan, 1997). Given the spatial sharpening function of LTD, this could be a route for GCs' disrupting foreground-background contrasts.

STRESS AND NEURAL NETWORKS   The potential for the remodeling of neuronal processes is extraordinary. Neurons can regrow axons and can form new dendritic branches and synapses in response to injury, exercise, or environmental enrichment.

Stress can block such plasticity. For example, lesions of inputs into the hippocampus from the fimbria-fornix or the entorhinal cortex cause compensatory sprouting of surviving axons; such sprouting is inhibited by glucocorticoids (Scheff and DeKosky, 1983).

A more pertinent example occurs outside the context of brain injury. A few days to weeks of stress cause retraction of dendrites in the rodent and nonhuman primate hippocampus (Woolley, Gould, and McEwen, 1990; Watanabe, Gould, and McEwen, 1992; Magarinos et al., 1996; Sousa et al., 2000). Atrophy involves loss of apical dendritic branch points and decreased length of apical dendrites (Woolley, Gould, and McEwen, 1990; Watanabe et al., 1992; Sunanda et al., 1997; Bisagno et al., 2000; Conrad et al., 1999), and is GC dependent, being replicated by exposure to stress levels of GCs and blocked by GC synthesis inhibitors (Magarinos and McEwen, 1995). Potentially, dendritic retraction disconnects neural networks, with adverse functional consequences; commensurate with that, stressors that cause atrophy also impair cognition (Conrad et al., 1996; Bisagno et al., 2000). Finally, when stress or GC exposure abates, neurons slowly rebuild the atrophied processes (Conrad et al., 1999).

Dendritic atrophy involves the release of the excitatory neurotransmitter glutamate and its binding to NMDA glutamate receptors, as it is blocked by NMDA receptor antagonists (Watanabe, Gould, and McEwen, 1992) and by phenytoin (dilantin), which inhibits glutamate release (Watanabe et al., 1992; Magarinos and McEwen, 1995). Serotonin may also be involved, because the atypical anti-depressant tianeptine, which decreases serotonergic tone (the opposite effect of SSRIs such as Prozac), blocks stress-induced dendritic atrophy (Conrad et al., 1999; Czeh et al., 2001). Pharmacological interventions that block the atrophy also block the cognitive impairments, further linking the two (Luine et al., 1994).

Stress-induced atrophy may be clinically relevant. Brain imaging of patients with Cushing's syndrome reveals selective decreases in hippocampal volume (Starkman et al., 1992), with covariation among the severity of GC excess, the extent of volume loss, and the extent of cognitive impairment. The volume loss most likely arises from dendritic atrophy; this is because of the plausible mediating mechanisms, only the dendritic atrophy has been shown to be reversible, and with the correction of the cushingoid GC excess, hippocampal volume normalizes over subsequent months (Starkman et al., 1999).

STRESS AND THE BIRTH AND DEATH OF NEURONS A dogma of neuroscience is that because adult neurons do not divide, the maximal number of neurons occurs perinatally, declining thereafter. It is now accepted that neurogenesis occurs in the adult hippocampus in rodents and primates and is induced by injury, exercise, and environmental enrichment (Gould and Gross, 2002). New neurons form functional synapses (Van Praag et al., 2002), which may contribute to learning and memory (Shors, Chua, and Falduto, 2001). Moreover, some estimates of the rate of neurogenesis suggest that entire cell fields in the rodent hippocampus are replaced over the lifetime (Gould and Gross, 2002).

Over the course of days to weeks, stress and GCs can inhibit hippocampal neurogenesis in rodents and primates (Gould and Gross, 2002). The underlying mechanisms are unknown; also unknown is whether and how fast neurogenesis resumes when stress or GC exposure abates.

As a next mechanism by which stress impairs hippocampal function, GCs compromise the ability of neurons to survive insults, including seizure, hypoxia, and hypoglycemia. Although the mechanisms underlying such "endangerment" are understood (Sapolsky, 1999), the relevance to the present issue is minimal, because these GC actions will impair hippocampal-dependent cognition only in the context of a coincidental insult.

Finally, severe stress or GC exposure for months (in a rodent) to years (primates) can kill CA3 pyramidal neurons and damage surviving ones (Landfield, Baskin, and Pitler, 1981; Sapolsky, Krey, and McEwen, 1985; Uno et al., 1989; Sapolsky et al., 1990; Kerr et al., 1991). Whether stress of such severity ever occurs physiologically is unclear. Some authors have speculated that the stress-induced atrophy of dendrites, despite disrupting function, constitutes an early defense against glutamatergic excitotoxicity by disconnecting networks (McEwen, 1999).

These GC effects on the birth and survival of neurons may be relevant to two disorders (reviewed in Sapolsky, 2000). Major depression involves elevated GC concentrations in about half of subjects, and hippocampal-dependent cognitive impairments as well. Reports indicate selective loss of hippocampal volume in prolonged depression. Similarly, posttraumatic stress disorder (PTSD) involves either elevated GC concentrations or enhanced cellular sensitivity to GCs, along with cognitive impairments. Selective hippocampal volume loss occurs in PTSD arising from combat trauma or repeated childhood abuse. Volume loss (and some degree of cognitive impairment) persists after depression has resolved, or after the trauma has passed. This argues against the reversible atrophy of dendrites as causing the volume loss. Whether the cause is neuron death or attenuated neurogenesis, as both, is unknown.

Thus, excessive stress or GC exposure impairs hippocampal-dependent cognition, with various possible mediating mechanisms. Stress and GCs also impair frontocortical function. There are some insights into the mechanisms underlying this. Major stressors increase dopamine and norepinephrine turnover in the frontal cortex. The dopamine excess has been speculated to impair signaling in distal dendrites of frontal neurons (via D_1 receptor activation), while the norepinephrine excess hypothesized to increase background transsynaptic noise in proximal dendrites (via $NE\alpha_1$ receptor activation). The net result is impairment of signal-to-noise ratios, thereby disrupting frontal function (Arnsten, 2000). In addition, regimens of GC administration that decrease dendritic complexity in the hippocampus cause a reorganization within the prefrontal cortex, with atrophy of distal and elaboration of proximal parts of apical dendrites (Wellman, 2001). The functional significance of this reorganization is unclear.

The disruptive effects of stress on hippocampal function clearly represent stress having "bad" effects on neural plasticity. However, stress and GCs can have quite different effects on cognition.

Stress and its capacity to enhance cognition

The preceding section implies a monolithic stress-cognition relationship. That it to say, in the absence of stress (with minimal circulating levels of GCs or epinephrine), cognition is optimal, and every incremental exposure to stress (or the hormonal mediators of it) incrementally impairs cognition.

Intuitively, this explanation is dissatisfying: a world without stress or challenge leaves us in a torpor, anything but our most cognitively capable. This principle is relevant to every stage of life, influencing the toys for a newborn to the activities for the elderly. We learn best not in the absence of challenge but when optimally *stimulated*, which consists of a receiving challenge that is substantial but not insurmountable, and is not open-ended. Basically, stimulation is mild and transient stress.

As discussed, this relationship produces an inverted U. The transition from basal state to mild stress enhances cognition, while the transition from basal state to severe or prolonged stressors impairs cognition.

This inverted U is amply documented (Kim and Diamond, 2002). Mild stress (henceforth synonymous with stimulation) enhances conditioning of contextual cues of stressors (Oiztl and de Kloet, 1992; Cahill et al., 1994; LeDoux, 2000; Dolan, 2002). In a demonstration of this relationship, subjects were read one of two stories. The stories were identical in the beginning and end but differed in the affective content of the middle, with one story having a disturbing scene. Weeks later, recall of the arousing middle section was enhanced relative to recall of the middle section of the control story, while recall for the beginnings and endings was unchanged (Cahill et al., 1994).

Furthermore, severe stressors that disrupt hippocampal-dependent cognition enhance it when experienced in milder forms (Luine et al., 1994, 1996; Bodnoff et al., 1995; Conrad et al., 1996; Sandi, Loscertales, and Guanza, 1997; McLay, Freeman, and Zadina, 1998; Beck and Luine, 1999; Luine, 2002). Although administration of elevated levels of epinephrine or GCs disrupts cognition, lesser amounts stimulate (Conrad et al., 1999; Joels, 2001; Cahill and Alkire, 2003). Of importance, mild stress facilitates hippocampal-independent procedural memory, as well as hippocampal-dependent explicit memory. Moreover, whereas major stressors impair frontal cortical-dependent cognition, milder versions are enhancing (Arnsten, 2000).

Mechanisms underlying the enhancing effects of stress

ELECTROPHYSIOLOGICAL MEASURES Just as the disruptive effects of severe stress on cognition and synaptic plasticity occur in parallel, acute stressors have electrophysiological correlates as well. Although severe stressors disrupt LTP and PBP, milder versions are enhancing (Diamond et al., 1992; Hesen and Joels, 1993; Pavlides et al., 1994; Vaher et al., 1994; Beck and Luine, 1999).

NEUROENDOCRINE FACTORS GCs significantly mediate the inverted U. As discussed, GCs bind to both high-affinity

MR and the lower-affinity GR. Basally, neural MR are heavily occupied by GCs, and GR are only minimally occupied. Mild stress causes maximal MR occupancy, while GR are only heavily or maximally occupied during major stressors.

Commensurate with this, the enhancing effects of mild stress on cognition, LTP, and PBP are MR-mediated (Diamond et al., 1992; Pavlides et al., 1994, 1995; Vaher et al., 1994; Oitzl, Fluttert, and de Kloet, 1998). MR occupancy reduces 5HT-1a receptor-mediated potassium currents, thereby shortening AHP duration (Joels and de Kloet, 1992). Conversely, GR mediates the disruptive effects of major stressors on cognition and synaptic plasticity (Oitzl and de Kloet, 1992; Pavlides et al., 1995; Conrad et al., 1999). These results have been shown with the use of MR- and GR-specific agonists and antagonists.

As a complication, the enhancement/disruption dichotomy may reflect not merely an MR/GR dichotomy but also the contrast between heavy MR plus moderate GR occupancy versus heavy GR occupancy (de Kloet et al., 1988; Oitzl and de Kloet, 1992; Shors, Weiss, and Thompson, 1992; Korte et al., 1996; Roozendaal, Portillo-Marquez, and McGaugh, 1996; Conrad et al., 1999).

As noted, moderate epinephrine levels enhance cognition while high levels disrupt it, suggesting a mechanism similar to that seen with GCs. However, epinephrine receptors do not have similar traits to those for GCs (i.e., both receptors in the same cells, and with dramatic differences in receptor affinity). Other potential mechanisms could generate inverted Us with epinephrine effects, but they have not been demonstrated.

THE NEUROANATOMY OF ENHANCEMENT Where in the brain does stress enhance cognition? Although the hippocampus is central to declarative memory, procedural tasks are centered in extrapyramidal sites. Insofar as mild stress facilitates both types of cognition, this suggests the involvement of a third site with projections to hippocampus and extrapyramidal sites.

The amygdala serves this role. The amygdala is well known for its role in fear conditioning. But it also mediates the enhancing effects of mild stress on cognition. Electrical stimulation of the amygdala following a training task enhances consolidation (Goddard, 1964). In humans, an emotional event activates the amygdala, with the extent of activation predicting the extent of consolidation about the event (Cahill et al., 1996). Conversely, lesioning of the amygdala (or of its basolateral nucleus) blocks the enhancing effects of mild stress.

How mild stress activates the amygdala is understood (Roozendaal, 2000; McGaugh, 2003). Sympathetic epinephrine and norepinephrine stimulate the afferent branch of the vagus nerve, which stimulates the nucleus of the tractus solitarius (NTS), which then stimulates the amygdala (Williams, 2001). This pathway can be blocked by antagonizing noradrenergic receptors in the vagus with beta-blockers. Moreover, as shown with local microinfusions of GR antagonists, GCs act within the NTS, amygdala, and hippocampus to facilitate the effects of the sympathetic nervous system.

Interactions between the enhancing and the disruptive effects of stress

The preceding section laid out a clear dichotomy: acute, mild stress enhances cognition, while severe stressors disrupt cognition. In actuality, the two halves of the inverted U overlap. Under circumstances in which mild acute stress enhances posttraining consolidation in rats, imposition of a new stressor (of a similar duration and magnitude, as measured by the GC response) during the consolidation period disrupts consolidation (de Kloet, Oitzl, and Joels, 1999). Moreover, mild stress-induced enhancement of posttraining consolidation of new information disrupts retrieval of information about a previous task (de Quervain, Roozendaal, and McGaugh, 1998).

Initially, these findings suggest an unappealing conclusion that the same mild stressor can enhance some types of cognition while disrupting others. A more insightful interpretation is that stress shifts focus, as discussed earlier (de Kloet, Oitzl, and Joels, 1999). Thus, in the first instance, a new stressor makes consolidation of information about the prior stressor less pressing. In the second, consolidation of information about the ongoing stressor supercedes retrieving information about a prior experience. This reframing suggests that the amygdala and hippocampus help shift focus to proximal stressors. Of note, however, this model applies only to retrieval of information about a prior, *unrelated* stressor. Retrieving information about the prior experience of related stressors (i.e., how one successfully coped that previous time) can be adaptive.

Stress, trauma, and the amygdala

As reviewed, mild stress enhances implicit learning concerned with procedural memory of skills and habits. But the amygdala influences implicit memory that activates the autonomic nervous system. Consider an individual robbed at gunpoint. The event most likely activated the sympathetic nervous system, causing the individual to freeze with fear, breathe rapidly and shallowly, heart racing. Such activation depends on amygdaloid projections to hypothalamus and brainstem autonomic nuclei. Most probably, the next time the person is in the neighborhood of the robbery, the sympathetic nervous system will be activated; an autonomic response has been conditioned.

To accomplish this, the amygdala responds to information relayed from sensory cortices. Potentially, the conditioned response can be activated by thought (e.g., awareness of having to travel to that neighborhood), utilizing projections from frontal and other associational cortices to the amygdala. Or there can be autonomic activation without conscious awareness of the evoking stimulus (say, the brief glint of something resembling a gun). In experimental settings, such preconscious activation can be evoked subliminally. This engages projections from thalamic sensory nuclei directly to the amygdala, bypassing the cortex and delivering arousing information prior to conscious awareness.

In these scenarios, the trauma has sensitized the amygdala and its autonomic outflow to subsequent stimuli associated with that trauma; stress can potentiate autonomic conditioning. For example, stressors can enhance the frequency and magnitude of Pavlovian eyeblinks in response to a conditioned stimulus (Servatius and Shors, 1994; Korte, 2001; Shors, Chua, and Falduto, 2001), or can enhance conditioned freezing in the rat (Conrad et al., 1999; Korte, 2001). Stress-induced GC secretion is necessary but not sufficient for such enhancement.

Therefore, stressors can impair hippocampal-dependent cognition while facilitating amygdala-dependent cognition. Paralleling this, stressors that impair LTP and atrophy hippocampal dendrites facilitate amygdaloid LTP (LeDoux, 2000) and extend dendritic processes in the amygdala and its initial projection site, the bed nucleus of the striae terminalis (Vyas et al., 2002; Vyas, Bernal, and Chattarji, 2003). The mechanisms underlying these amygdaloid effects are unknown.

These opposing actions of stress in the hippocampus and amygdala prompted an important model relevant to anxiety (LeDoux, 1996). In the face of trauma, hippocampal-dependent consolidation of information about the event may be compromised, minimizing declarative memory of the event. Yet there is likely to be robust, amygdaloid-dependent autonomic conditioning. Therefore, the next time the individual is exposed to stimuli associated with the trauma, there may be a florid autonomic response without any conscious knowledge about its cause. This approximates free-floating anxiety.

Sex differences, stress, and cognition

Sex differences exist in the effects of stress on cognition. Initially, the most parsimonious summary of these differences is that females are less vulnerable to the disruptive effects of stress. For example, 21 days of intermittent restraint stress in rats impairs spatial memory in males but enhances it in females (Luine et al., 1994; Bowman, Zrull, and Luine, 2001). The stress paradigm increased levels of inhibitory GABA in the hippocampus of males, but not females, while enhancing serotonin and norepinephrine levels in females, but not males. The identical stressor also impairs Y maze performance more persistently in males (Conrad et al., 2003). In humans, under conditions where the Trier Social Stress Test did not significantly impair declarative memory in either sex, males showed an inverse relationship between GC concentrations and performance (Wolf et al., 2001).

These sex differences could reflect motivational differences. However, stress preferentially impairs male performance on tasks that do not involve reward (Luine, 2002). Alternatively, the sex differences could reflect different magnitudes of the stress response. However, the GC stress response does not differ by sex in these studies (Luine et al., 1994; Bowman, Zrull, and Luine, 2001; Wolf et al., 2001).

Estrogen appears relevant. The steroid enhances cognition and increases hippocampal sprouting, neurogenesis, and synaptogenesis (Garcia-Segura, Azcoitia, and DonCarlos, 2001). Moreover, in stressed rodents and humans, cognitive sparing in females is maximal under high estrogen conditions (i.e., during proestrus; Luine et al., 1994; Bowman, Zrull, and Luine, 2001; Wolf et al., 2001) and is lessened by ovariectomy (Luine et al., 1994; Bowman, Zrull, and Luine, 2001). That it is lessened rather than eliminated suggests the importance of perinatal estrogenic effects, or of nonestrogenic effects. Psychosocial stress impairs cognition more in elderly women than in men (Wolf et al., 2001), and high basal GC levels predict poor declarative and working memory in aged women but not men (Seeman et al., 1997; Carlson and Sherwin, 1999). However, this vulnerability is eliminated by estrogen replacement therapy (Carlson and Sherwin, 1999).

Despite these findings, females are not always less vulnerable than males to the effects of stress on hippocampal-dependent memory. Most exceptions concern implicit learning. For example, uncontrollable, intermittent tail shock enhances eyeblink conditioning and trace conditioning in male while disrupting it in female rats (Servatius and Shors, 1994; Wood and Shors, 1998; Wood, Beylin, and Shors, 2001). The effect in males depends on perinatal testosterone exposure (Shors and Miesegaes, 2002); disruption in females is maximal in proestrus (Shors et al., 1998) and is blunted by ovariectomy or estrogen receptor blockade (Wood and Shors, 1998).

Therefore, stress seemingly disrupts declarative memory in males while sparing or enhancing it in females, and blunts implicit conditioning in females while augmenting it in males. Sullying this dichotomy, acute stress enhances associative memory or trace conditioning in male rats (Shors, Weiss, and Thompson, 1992; Shors, Chua, and Falduto, 2001; Wood, Beylin, and Shors, 2001) while impairing it in females in an estrogen-dependent manner (Wood and Shors, 1998; Shors et al., 1998; Wood, Beylin, and Shors, 2001). It is controversial whether trace conditioning is a declarative

or an implicit task; regardless, it is hippocampus dependent. Thus, stress can augment a declarative or hippocampal-dependent task in males but not in females. Of relevance, a similar stressor increases dendritic spine density in the male hippocampus but decreases it in proestrous females (Shors, Chua, and Falduto, 2001).

Finally, some sex differences do not qualify as "better" or "worse," but merely different. Females tend to respond to local cues and males to global ones. When blockade of beta-receptors in the sympathetic nervous system impairs memory for an arousing event, women are more impaired in local memories and men are more impaired in global ones (Cahill and van Stegeren, 2003).

Conclusions

Memory is not monolithic but instead exists in multiple forms. Similarly, stress is not monolithic in its effects on memory. Instead, the effects depend on stressor type, intensity, and duration, and on the type of memory.

Throughout this review, events that weaken synaptic strength or cause dendritic retraction have been termed disruptive, while those strengthening synapses or elaborating dendrites have been termed facilitative or enhancing. By these definitions, stress has facilitative effects in the amygdala. Insofar as this can produce fear and anxiety, these locally facilitative effects are disruptive, potentially tragically so, at the organismal level.

This is not mere semantics. Anxiety disorders are extremely common and, at their extremes (e.g., PTSD), they are devastating. This point is particularly pressing given the conservative estimate of hundreds of thousands of New Yorkers who will succumb to PTSD related to the events of September 11 (Galea et al., 2002; Schlenger et al., 2002). Understanding the "good" and "bad" (in both the reductive and organismal sense) effects of stress on the brain is critical.

REFERENCES

ALTENOR, A., E. KAY, and M. RICHTER, 1977. The generality of learned helplessness in the rat. *Learn. Motiv.* 8:54–61.

ARNSTEN, A., 2000. Stress impairs prefrontal cortical function in rats and monkeys: Role of dopamine D1 and norepinephrine alpha-1 receptor mechanisms. *Prog. Brain Res.* 126:183–192.

BARDGETT, M., G. TAYLOR, J. CSERNANSKY, J. NEWCOMER, and B. NOCK, 1994. Chronic corticosterone treatment impairs spontaneous alternation behavior in rats. *Behav. Neural Biol.* 61:186–190.

BECK, K., and V. LUINE, 1999. Food deprivation modulates chronic stress effects on object recognition in male rats: Role of monoamines and amino acid. *Brain Res.* 830:56–71.

BENDER, B. G., J. A. LERNER, and E. KOLLASCH, 1988. Mood and memory changes in asthmatic children receiving corticosteroids. *J. Am. Acad. Child. Adolesc. Psychiatry* 27:720–725.

BENDER, B., J. LERNER, and J. POLAND, 1991. Association between corticosteroids and psychologic change in hospitalized asthmatic children. *Ann. Allergy* 66:414.

Bisagno, V., M. Ferrini, H. Rios, L. Zieher, and S. Wikinski, 2000. Chronic corticosterone impairs inhibitory avoidance in rats: Possible link with atrophy of hippocampal CA3 neurons. *Pharm. Biochem. Behav.* 66:235–240.

Bodnoff, S., A. Humphreys, J. Lehman, D. Diamond, G. Rose, and M. Meaney, 1995. Enduring effects of chronic corticosterone treatment on spatial learning, synaptic plasticity, and hippocampal neuropathology in young and mid-aged rats. *J. Neurosci.* 15:61–69.

Born, J., and H. Fehm, 1999. HPA activity during human sleep: A coordinating role for the limbic hippocampal system. *Exp. Clin. Endocrinol. Metab.* 106:153–162.

Bowman, R., M. Zrull, and V. Luine, 2001. Chronic restraint stress enhances radial arm maze performance in female rats. *Brain Res.* 904:279.

Bunsey, M., and H. Eichenbaum, 1996. Conservation of hippocampal memory function in rats and humans. *Nature* 379: 255–257.

Cahill, L., and M. T. Alkire, 2003. Epinephrine enhancement of human memory consolidation: Interaction with arousal at encoding. *Neurobiol. Learn. Mem.* 79:194–198.

Cahill, L., R. J. Haier, J. Fallon, M. T. Alkire, C. Tang, D. Keator, J. Wu, and J. L. McGaugh, 1996. Amygdala activity at encoding correlated with long-term, free recall of emotional information. *Proc. Natl. Acad. Sci. U.S.A.* 93:8016–8021.

Cahill, L., B. Prins, M. Weber, and J. McGaugh, 1994. Beta-adrenergic activation and memory for emotional events. *Nature* 371:702–704.

Cahill, L., and A. van Stegeren, 2003. Sex-related impairment of memory for emotional events with beta-adrenergic blockade. *Neurobiol. Learn. Mem.* 79:81–88.

Carlson, L., and B. Sherwin, 1999. Relationships among cortisol, DHEAS and memory in a longitudinal study of healthy elderly men and women. *Neurobiol. Aging* 20:315–324.

Conrad, C., L. Galea, Y. Kuroda, and B. McEwen, 1996. Chronic stress impairs rat spatial memory on the Y maze, and this effect is blocked by tianeptine pretreatment. *Behav. Neurosci.* 110:1321–1334.

Conrad, C., K. Grote, R. Hobbs, and A. Ferayorni, 2003. Sex differences in spatial and non-spatial Y-maze performance after chronic stress. *Neurobiol. Learn. Mem.* 79:32–40.

Conrad, C., J. LeDoux, A. Magarinos, and B. McEwen, 1999. Repeated restraint stress facilitates fear conditioning independently of causing hippocampal CA3 dendritic atrophy. *Behav. Neurosci.* 113:902–913.

Czeh, B., T. Michaelis, T. Watanabe, J. Frahm, G. de Biurrun, M. van Kampen, A. Bartolomucci, and E. Fuchs, 2001. Stress-kinduced changes in cerebral metabolites, hippocampal volume, and cell proliferation are prevented by antidepressant treatment with tianeptine. *Proc. Natl. Acad. Sci. U.S.A.* 98:12796–12801.

Dachir, S., T. Kadar, B. Robinzon, and A. Levy, 1993. Cognitive deficits induced in young rats by long-term corticosterone administration. *Behav. Neural Biol.* 60:103–109.

de Kloet, E., S. de Kock, V. Schild, and H. Veldhuis, 1988. Antiglucocorticoid RU 38486 attenuates retention of a behavior and disinhibits the hypothalamic-pituitary-adrenal axis at different sites. *Neuroendocrinology* 47:109–115.

de Kloet, E. R., M. S. Oitzl, and M. Joels, 1999. Stress and cognition: Are corticosteroids good or bad guys? *Trends Neurosci.* 22:422–426.

de Kloet, E. R., E. Vreugdenhil, M. S. Oitzl, and M. Joels, 1998. Brain corticosteroid receptor balance in health and disease. *Endocr. Rev.* 19:269–301.

de Quervain, D., B. Roozendaal, and J. McGaugh, 1998. Stress and glucocorticoids impair retrieval of long-term spatial memory. *Nature* 394:787–790.

de Quervain, D., B. Roozendaal, R. Nitsch, J. McGaugh, and C. Hock, 2000. Acute cortisone administration impairs retrieval of long-term declarative memory in humans. *Nat. Neurosci.* 3:313–317.

Diamond, D., M. Bennett, D. Engstrom, M. Fleshner, and G. Rose, 1989. Adrenalectomy reduces the threshold for hippocampal primed burst potentiation in the anesthetized rat. *Brain Res.* 492:356–360.

Diamond, D. M., M. C. Bennett, M. Fleshner, and G. M. Rose, 1992. Inverted-U relationship between the level of peripheral corticosterone and the magnitude of hippocampal primed burst potentiation. *Hippocampus* 2:421–430.

Diamond, D., M. Bennett, K. Stevens, R. Wilson, and G. Rose, 1990. Exposure to a novel environment interferes with the induction of hippocampal primed burst potentiation in the behaving rat. *Psychobiology* 18:273–281.

Diamond, D., M. Fleshner, and G. Rose, 1994. Psychological stress repeatedly blocks hippocampal primed burst potentiation in behaving rats. *Behav. Brain Res.* 62:1–9.

Diamond, D., and C. Park, 2000. Predator exposure produces retrograde amnesia and blocks synaptic plasticity: Progress toward understanding how the hippocampus is affected by stress. *Ann. N.Y. Acad. Sci.* 911:453–455.

Diamond, D., C. Park, K. Heman, and G. Rose, 1999. Exposing rats to a predator impairs spatial working memory in the radial arm water maze. *Hippocampus* 9:542–552.

Dolan, R., 2002. Emotion, cognition and behavior. *Science* 298: 1191–1197.

Endo, Y., J. Nishimura, S. Kogayashi, and F. Kimura, 1999. Chronic stress exposure influences local cerebral blood flow in the rat hippocampus. *Neuroscience* 93:551–563.

Foy, M., M. Stanton, S. Levine, and R. Thompson, 1987. Behavioral stress impairs long-term potentiation in rodent hippocampus. *Behav. Neural Biol.* 48:138–149.

Galea, S., H. Resnick, J. Ahern, J. Gold, M. Bucuvalas, D. Kilpatrick, J. Stuber, and D. Vlahov, 2002. PTSD in Manhattan, New York City, after the September 11th terrorist attacks. *J. Urban Health Bull. N.Y. Acad Med.* 79:340–353.

Gallagher, M., and R. Burwell, 1989. Relationship of age-related decline across several behavioral domains. *Neurobiol. Aging* 10:691–708.

Garcia-Segura, L., I. Azcoitia, and L. DonCarlos, 2001. Neuroprotection by estradiol. *Prog. Neurobiol.* 63:29–60.

Goddard, G., 1964. Amygdaloid stimulation and learning in the rat. *J. Comp. Physiol. Psych.* 58:23–30.

Gould, E., and C. Gross, 2002. Neurogenesis in adult mammals: Some progress and problems. *J. Neurosci.* 22:619–623.

Hesen, W., and M. Joels, 1993. Modulation of carbachol responsiveness in rat CA1 pyramidal neurons by corticosteroid hormones. *Brain Res.* 627:157–167.

Issa, A., W. Rowe, S. Gauthier, and M. Meaney, 1990. Hypothalamic-pituitary-adrenal activity in aged, cognitively impaired and cognitively unimpaired rats. *J. Neurosci.* 10:3247–3254.

Jacobson, L., and R. Sapolsky, 1991. The role of the hippocampus in feedback regulation of the hypothalamic-pituitary-adrenocortical axis. *Endocrine Rev.* 12:118–134.

Joels, M., 2001. Corticosteroid actions in the hippocampus. *J. Neuroendocrinol.* 13:657–669.

Joels, M., and E. R. de Kloet, 1992. Control of neuronal excitability by corticosteroid hormones. *Trends Neurosci.* 15:25–30.

KEENAN, P., M. JACOBSON, R. SOLEYMANI, M. MAYES, M. STRESS, and D. YALDOO, 1996. The effect on memory of chronic prednisone treatment in patients with systemic disease. *Neurology* 47:1396–1403.

KELLY, K., B. HAYSLIP, and H. SERVATY, 1996. Psychoneuroendocrinological indicators of stress and intellectual performance among older adults: An exploratory study. *Exp. Aging Res.* 22:393–398.

KERR, D., L. CAMPBELL, M. APPLEGATE, A. BRODISH, and P. LANDFIELD, 1991. Chronic stress-induced acceleration of electrophysiologic and morphometric biomarkers of hippocampal aging. *J. Neurosci.* 11:1316–1322.

KERR, D., L. CAMPBELL, S. HAO, and P. LANDFIELD, 1989. Corticosteroid modulation of hippocampal potentials: Increased effect with aging. *Science* 245:1505–1509.

KERR, D. S., L. W. CAMPBELL, O. THIBAULT, and P. W. LANDFIELD, 1992. Hippocampal glucocorticoid receptor activation enhances voltage-dependent Ca^{2+} conductances: relevance to brain aging. *Proc. Natl. Acad. Sci. U.S.A.* 89:8527–8531.

KIM, J., and D. DIAMOND, 2002. The stressed hippocampus, synaptic plasticity and lost memories. *Nat. Rev. Neurosci.* 3:453–462.

KIM, J., M. FOY, and R. THOMPSON, 1996. Behavioral stress modifies hippocampal plasticity through NMDA receptor activation. *Proc. Natl. Acad. Sci. U.S.A.* 93:4750–4753.

KIRSCHBAUM, C., O. T. WOLF, M. MAY, W. WIPPICH, and D. H. HELLHAMMER, 1996. Stress- and treatment-induced elevations of cortisol levels associated with impaired declarative memory in healthy adults. *Life Sci.* 58:1475–1483.

KORTE, S., 2001. Corticosteroids in relation to fear, anxiety and psychopathology. *Neurosci. Biobehav. Rev.* 25:117–131.

KORTE, S., E. DE KLOET, B. BUWALDA, S. BOPUMAN, and B. BOHUS, 1996. Antisense to the glucocorticoid receptor in hippocampal dentate gyrus reduces immobility in forced swim test. *Eur. J. Pharmacol.* 301:19–25.

LANDFIELD, P., R. BASKIN, and T. PITLER, 1981. Brain-aging correlates: Retardation by hormonal-pharmacological treatments. *Science* 214:581–584.

LEDOUX, J., 1996. *The Emotional Brain.* New York: Simon and Schuster.

LEDOUX, J., 2000. Emotion circuits in the brain. *Annu. Rev. Neurosci.* 23:155–184.

LUINE, V., 2002. Sex differences in chronic stress effects on memory in rats. *Stress* 5:205–216.

LUINE, V., C. MARTINEZ, M. VILLEGAS, A. MAGARINOS, and B. MCEWEN, 1996. Restraint stress reversibly enhances spatial memory performance. *Physiol. Behav.* 59:27–32.

LUINE, V., R. SPENCER, and B. MCEWEN, 1993. Effects of chronic corticosterone ingestion on spatial memory performance and hippocampal serotonergic function. *Brain Res.* 616:65–70.

LUINE, V., M. VILLEGAS, C. MARTINEZ, and B. MCEWEN, 1994. Repeated stress causes reversible impairments of spatial memory performance. *Brain Res.* 639:167–170.

LUPIEN, S., M. DE LEON, S. DE SANTI, A. CONVIT, C. TARSHISH, N. NAIR, M. THAKUR, B. MCEWEN, R. HAUGER, and M. MEANEY, 1998. Cortisol levels during human aging predict hippocampal atrophy and memory deficits. *Nat. Neurosci.* 1:69–73.

LUPIEN, S. J., C. J. GILLIN, and R. L. HAUGER, 1999. Working memory is more sensitive than declarative memory to the acute effects of corticosteroids: A dose-response study in humans. *Behav. Neurosci.* 113:420–430.

LUPIEN, S., A. LECOURS, I. LUSSIER, G. SCHWARTZ, N. NAIR, and M. MEANEY, 1994. Basal cortisol levels and cognitive deficits in human aging. *J. Neurosci.* 14:2893–2903.

LUPIEN, S., A. LECOURS, G. SCHWARTZ, S. SHARMA, R. HAUGER, M. MEANEY, and N. NAIR, 1995. Longitudinal study of basal cortisol levels in healthy elderly subjectds: Evidence for sub-groups. *Neurobiol. Aging* 17:95–105.

LUPIEN, S., and B. MCEWEN, 1997. The acute effects of corticosteroids on cognition: Integration of animal and human model studies. *Brain Res. Rev.* 24:1–27.

LYONS, D., J. LOPEZ, C. YANG, and A. SCHATZBERG, 2000. Stress-level cortisol treatment impairs inhibitory control of behavior in monkeys. *J. Neurosci.* 20:7816–7821.

MAGARINOS, A. and B. MCEWEN, 1995. Stress-induced atrophy of apical dendrites of hippocampal CA3c neurons: involvement of glucocorticoid secretion and excitatory amino acid receptors. *Neuroscience* 69:89–98.

MAGARINOS, A. and B. MCEWEN, 2000. Experimental diabetes in rats causes hippocampal dendritic and synaptic reorganization and increased glucocorticoid reactivity to stress. *Proc. Natl. Acad. Sci. U.S.A.* 97:11056–11061.

MAGARINOS, A., B. MCEWEN, G. FLUGGE, and E. FUCHS, 1996. Chronic psychosocial stress causes apical dendritic atrophy of hippocampal CA3 pyramidal neurons in subordinate tree shrews. *J. Neurosci.* 16:3534–3542.

MCEWEN, B., 1999. Stress and hippocampal plasticity. *Annu. Rev. Neurosci.* 22:105–122.

MCGAUGH, J., 2003. *Emotion and Memory.* New York: Weidenfeld and Nicolson.

MCGAUGH, J., L. CAHILL, R. HAIER, J. FALLON, M. ALKIRE, C. TANG, D. KEATOR, J. WU, and J. MCGAUGH, 1996. Amygdala activity an encoding correlated with long-term, free recall of emotional information. *Proc. Natl. Acad. Sci. U.S.A.* 93:8016–8021.

MCGAUGH, J., and G. GODDARD, 1964. Amygdaloid stimulation and learning in the rat. *J. Comp. Phys. Psych.* 58:23–30.

MCGAUGH, S., and C. WILLIAMS, 2001. Contribution of brain stem structures in modulating memory storage processes. In *Memory Consolidation: Essays in Honor of James L. McGaugh*, P. Gold and W. Greenough, eds. New York: American Psychological Association, pp. 141–163.

MCLAY, R., S. FREEMAN, and J. ZADINA, 1998. Chronic corticosterone impairs memory performance in the Barnes maze. *Physiol. Behav.* 63:933–937.

MEANEY, M., D. O'DONNELL, W. ROWE, B. TANNENBAUM, A. STEVERMAN, M. WALKER N. NAIR, and S. LUPIEN, 1995. Individual differences in HPA activity in later life and hippocampal aging. *Exp. Gerontol.* 30:229–251.

MESCHES, M., M. FLESHNER, K. HEMAN, G. ROSE, and D. DIAMOND, 1999. Exposing rats to a predator blocks primed burst potentiation in the hippocampus in vitro. *J. Neurosci.* 19:RC18.

NEWCOMER, J., S. CRAFT, T. HERSHEY, K. ASKINS, and M. BARDGETT, 1994. Glucocorticoid-induced impairment in declarative memory performance in adult human. *J. Neurosci.* 14:2047–2053.

NEWCOMER, J., G. SELKE, A. MELSON, T. HERSHEY, S. CRAFT, K. RICHARDS, and A. ALDERSON, 1999. Decreased memory performance in healthy humans induced by stress-level cortisol treatment. *Arch. Gen. Psychiatry* 56:527–533.

O'BRIEN, J., I. SCHWEITZER, and D. AMES, 1994. Cortisol suppression by dexamethasone in the healthy elderly: Effects of age, dexamethasone levels and cognitive function. *Biol. Psychiatry* 36:389–394.

OHL, F., T. MICHAELIS, G. VOLLMANN-HONSDORF, C. KIRSCHBAUM, and E. FUCHS, 2000. Effect of chronic psychosocial stress and long-term cortisol treatment on hippocampus-mediated memory and hippocampal volume: A pilot-study in tree shrews. *Psychoneuroendocrinology* 25:357–363.

OITZL, M., and E. DE KLOET, 1992. Selective corticosteroid antagonists modulate specific aspects of spatial orientation learning. *Behav. Neurosci.* 106:62–71.

OITZL, M., M. FLUTTERT, and E. DE KLOET, 1998. Acute blockade of hippocampal glucocorticoid receptors facilitates spatial learning in rats. *Brain Res.* 797:159–166.

PAVLIDES, C., A. KIMURA, A. MAGARINOS, and B. McEWEN, 1994. Type I adrenal steroid receptors prolong hippocampal long-term potentiation. *Neuroreport* 5:2673–2677.

PAVLIDES, C., Y. WATANABE, A. MARGARINOS, and B. McEWEN, 1995. Opposing roles of type I and type II adrenal steroid receptors in hippocampal long-term potentiation. *Neuroscience* 68: 387–394.

PAVLIDES, C., WATANABE, and B. McEWEN, 1993. Effects of glucocorticoids on hippocampal long-term potentiation. *Hippocampus* 3:183–192.

PIAZZA, P., and M. LE MOAL, 1997. Glucocorticoids as a biological substrate of reward: Physiological and pathophysiological implications. *Brain Res. Rev.* 25:359–378.

PLIHAL, W., R. PIETROWSKY, and J. BORN, 1999. Dexamethasone blocks sleep-induced improvement of declarative memory. *Psychoneuroendocrinology* 24:313–331.

ROOZENDAAL, B., 2000. Glucocorticoids and the regulation of memory consolidation. *Psychoneuroendocrinology* 25:213–238.

ROOZENDAAL, B., Q. GRIFFITH, J. BURANDAY, D. DE QUERVAIN, and J. McGAUGH, 2003. The hippocampus mediates glucocorticoid-induced impairment of spatial memory retrieval: Dependence upon the basolateral amygdala. *Proc. Natl. Acad. Sci. U.S.A.* 100: 1328–1330.

ROOZENDAAL, B., G. PORTILLO-MARQUEZ, and J. McGAUGH, 1996. Basolateral amygdala lesions block glucocorticoid-induced modulation of memory for spatial learning. *Behav. Neurosci.* 100: 1074–1083.

SANCHEZ, M., L. YOUNG, P. PLOTSKY, and T. INSEL, 2000. Distribution of corticosteroid receptors in the rhesus brain: Relative absence of GR in the hippocampal formation. *J. Neurosci.* 20: 4657–4668.

SANDI, C., M. LOSCERTALES, and C. GUANZA, 1997. Experience-dependent facilitating effect of corticosterone on spatial memory formation in the water maze. *Eur. J. Neurosci.* 9:637–642.

SAPOLSKY, R., 1992. Do glucocorticoid concentrations rise with age in the rat? *Neurobiol. Aging* 13:171–174.

SAPOLSKY, R., 1999. Stress, glucocorticoids and their adverse neurological effects: Relevance to aging. *Exp. Gerontol.* 34:721–735.

SAPOLSKY, R., 2000. Glucocorticoids and hippocampal atrophy in neuropsychiatric disorders. *Arch. Gen. Psychiatry* 57:925–935.

SAPOLSKY, R., L. KREY, and B. McEWEN, 1983. The adrenocortical stress-response in the aged male rat: Impairment of recovery from stress. *Exp. Gerontol.* 18:55–61.

SAPOLSKY, R., L. KREY, and B. McEWEN, 1985. Prolonged glucocorticoid exposure reduces hippocampal neuron number: Implications for aging. *J. Neurosci.* 5:1221–1227.

SAPOLSKY, R., M. ROMERO, and A. MUNCK, 2000. How do glucocorticoids influence the stress-response? Integrating permissive, suppressive, stimulatory, and preparative actions. *Endocrine Rev.* 21:55–71.

SAPOLSKY. R., H. UNO, C. REBERT, and C. FINCH, 1990. Hippocampal damage associated with prolonged glucocorticoid exposure in primates. *J. Neurosci.* 10:2897–2902.

SCHEFF, S., and S. DEKOSKY, 1983. Steroid suppression of axon sprouting in the hippocampal dentate gyrus of the adult rate: Dose-response relationship. *Exp. Neurol.* 82:183–191.

SCHLENGER, W., J. CADDELL, L. EBERT, B. JORDAN, K. ROURKE, D. WILSON, L. THALJI, J. DENNIS, J. FAIRBANK, and R. KULKA, 2002. Psychological reactions to terrorist attacks: Findings from the National Study of Americans' Reactions to September 11. *JAMA* 288:581–588.

SCHMIDT, L., N. FOX, M. GOLDBERG, C. SMITH, and J. SCHULKIN, 1999. Effects of acute prednisone administration on memory, attention and emotion in healthy human adults. *Psychoneuroendocrinology* 24:461–483.

SEEMAN, T., B. McEWEN, B. SINGER, M. ALBERT, and J. ROWE, 1997. Increase in urinary cortisol excretion and memory declines: MacArthur studies of successful aging. *J. Clin. Endocrinol. Metab.* 82:2458–2467.

SERVATIUS, R., and T. SHORS, 1994. Exposure to inescapable stress persistently facilitates associative and nonassociative learning in rats. *Behav. Neurosci.* 108:1101–1106.

SHORS, T., C. CHUA, and J. FALDUTO, 2001. Sex differences and opposite effects of stress on dendritic spine density in the male versus female hippocampus. *J. Neurosci.* 21:6292–6297.

SHORS, T., and E. DRYVER, 1994. Effect of stress and long-term potentiation (LTP) on subsequent LTP and the theta burst response in the dentate gyrus. *Brain Res.* 666:232–238.

SHORS, T. J., C. LEWCZYK, M. PACYNSKI, P. R. MATHEW, and J. PICKETT, 1998. Stages of estrous mediate the stress-induced impairment of associative learning in the female rat. *Neuroreport* 9:419–423.

SHORS, T., and G. MIESEGAES, 2002. Testosterone in utero and at birth dictates how stressful experience will affect learning in adulthood. *Proc. Natl. Acad. Sci. U.S.A.* 99:13955–13960.

SHORS, T., T. SEIB, S. LEVINE, and R. THOMPSON, 1989. Inescapable versus escapable shock modulates long-term potentiation in the rat hippocampus. *Science* 244:224–226.

SHORS, T., C. WEISS, and R. THOMPSON, 1992. Stress-induced facilitation of classical conditioning. *Science* 257:537–539.

SOUSA, N., N. V. LUKOYANOV, M. D. MADEIRA, O. F. ALMEIDA, and M. M. PAULA-BARBOSA, 2000. Reorganization of the morphology of hippocampal neurites and synapses after stress-induced damage correlates with behavioral improvement. *Neuroscience* 97:253–266.

STARKMAN, M., S. GEBARSKI, S. BERENT, and D. SCHTEINGART, 1992. Hippocampal formation volume, memory dysfunction, and cortisol levels in patients with Cushing's syndrome. *Biol. Psychiatry* 32:756–765.

STARKMAN, M. N., B. GIORDANI, S. S. GEBARSKI, S. BERENT, M. A. SCHORK, and D. E. SCHTEINGART, 1999. Decrease in cortisol reverses human hippocampal atrophy following treatment of Cushing's disease. *Biol Psychiatry* 46:1595–1602.

UNO, H., R. TARARA, J. ELSE, M. SULEMAN, and R. SAPOLSKY, 1989. Hippocampal damage associated with prolonged and fatal stress in primates. *J. Neurosci.* 9:1705–1711.

VAHER, P., V. LUINE, E. GOULD, and B. McEWEN, 1994. Effects of adrenalectomy on spatial memory performance and dentate gyrus morphology. *Brain Res.* 656:71–78.

VAN PRAAG, H., A. SCHINDER, B. CHRISTIE, N. TONI, T. PALMER, and F. GAGE, 2002. Functional neurogenssis in the adult hippocampus. *Nature* 415:1030–1034.

VARNEY, N., B. ALEXANDER, and J. MACINDOE, 1984. Reversible steroid dementia in patients without steroid psychosis. *Am. J. Psychiatry* 141:369–372.

VYAS, A., S. BERNAL, and S. CHATTARJI, 2003. Effects of chronic stress on dendritic arborization in the central and extended amygdala. *Brain Res.* 965:290–294.

VYAS, A., R. MITRA, R. B. SHANKARANARAYANA, and S. CHATTERJI, 2002. Chronic stress induces contrasting patterns of dendritic remodeling in hippocampal and amygdaloid neurons. *J. Neurosci.* 22:6810–6818.

WABER, D., S. CARPENTIERI, N. KLAR, L. SILVERMAN, M. SCHWENN, C. A. HURWITZ, P. MULLENIX, N. TARBELL, and S. SALLAN, 2000. Cognitive sequelae in children treated for acute lymphoblastic leukemia with dexamethasone or prednisone. *J. Pediatr. Hematol. Oncol.* 22:206–215.

WATANABE, Y., E. GOULD, H. A. CAMERON, D. C. DANIELS, and B. S., MCEWEN, 1992. Phenytoin prevents stress- and corticosterone-induced atrophy of CA3 pyramidal neurons. *Hippocampus.* 2:431–435.

WATANABE, Y., E. GOULD, and B. MCEWEN, 1992. Stress induces atrophy of apical dendrites of hippocampal CA3 pyramidal neurons. *Brain Res.* 588:341–348.

WELLMAN, C. L., 2001. Dendritic reorganization in pyramidal neurons in medial prefrontal cortex after chronic corticosterone administration. *J. Neurobiol.* 49:243–253

WILLIAMS, C., 2001. Contribution of brainstem structures in modulating memory storage processes. In P. Gold, W. Greenough, eds. *Memory consolidation: Essays in honor of James L. McGaugh.* Washington, D.C.: American Psychological Association, pp. 141–63.

WILLINGHAM, D., 1998. What differentiates declarative and procedural memories: Reply to Cohen, Poldrack, and Eichenbaum. *Memory* 6:689–699.

WOLF, O., A. CONVIT, E. THORN, and M. DE LEON, 2002. Salivary cortisol day profiles in elderly with mild cognitive impairment. *Psychoneuroendocrinology* 27:777–789.

WOLF, O., N. SCHOMMER, D. HELLHAMMER, B. MCEWEN, and C. KIRSCHBAUM, 2001. The relationship between stress-induced cortisol levels and memory differs between men and women. *Psychoneuroendocrinology* 26:711–720.

WOLKOWITZ, O., V. REUS, J. CANICK, B. LEVIN, and S. LUPIEN, 1997. Glucocorticoid medication, memory and steroid psychosis in medical illness. *Ann. N.Y. Acad. Sci.* 823:81–96.

WOLKOWITZ, O., V. REUSS, and H. WEINGARTNER, 1990. Cognitive effects of corticosteroids. *Am. J. Psychiatry* 147:1297–1310.

WOLKOWITZ, O., H. WEINGARTNER, D. RUBINOW, D. JIMERSON, M. KLING, W. BERRETINI, K. THOMPSON, A. BREIER, A. DORAN, V. REUS, and D. PICKAR, 1993. Steroid modulation of human memory: Biochemical correlates. *Biol. Psychiatry* 33:744–751.

WOOD, G., A. BEYLIN, and T. SHORS, 2001. The contribution of adrenal and reproductive hormones to the opposing effects of stress on trace conditioning in males versus females. *Behav. Neurosci.* 115:175–187.

WOOD, G., and T. SHORS, 1998. Stress facilitates classical conditioning in males, but inhibits classical conditioning in females through activational effects of ovarian hormones. *Proc. Natl. Acad. Sci. U.S.A.* 31:4066–4070.

WOOLLEY, C., E. GOULD, and B. MCEWEN, 1990. Exposure to excess glucocorticoids alters dendritic morphology of adult hippocampal pyramidal neurons. *Brain Res.* 531:225–232.

XU, L., R. ANWYL, and M. ROWAN, 1997. Behavioural stress facilitates the induction of long-term depression in the hippocampus. *Nature* 387:497–500.

YAU, J., T. OLSSON, R. MORRIS, M. MEANEY, and J. SECKL, 1995. Glucocorticoids, hippocampal corticosteroid receptor gene expression and antidepressant treatment: Relationship with spatial learning in young and aged rats. *Neuroscience* 66:571–871.

YOUNG, A., B. SAHAKIAN, T. ROBBINS, and P. COWEN, 1999. The effects of chronic administration of hydrocortisone on cognitive function in normal male volunteers. *Psychopharmacology* 145:260–266.

ZHOU, J., J. ZHENG, Y. ZHANG, and J. ZHOU, 2000. Corticosterone impairs cultured hippocampal neurons and facilitates Ca^{2+} influx through voltage-dependent Ca^{2+} channel. *Acta Pharmacol. Sinica* 21:156–163.

75 A General Circuitry Processing Reward/Aversion Information and Its Implications for Neuropsychiatric Illness

HANS C. BREITER AND GREGORY P. GASIC

ABSTRACT Neuroimaging experiments in humans have provided strong evidence for a generalized circuitry that processes reward/aversion information. Composed of an extended set of subcortical gray matter regions and the surrounding paralimbic cortical girdle, these neural systems form the core of an information backbone (iBM) for motivated behavior. Components of this iBM appear to be affected in several neuropsychiatric illnesses. Circuitry-based quantitative measures of these IBM components, as heritable and state indices, may provide better etiologic insights than the diagnostic categories based on statistical clusters of behaviors and symptoms used in current psychiatric diagnosis. Recent studies have alluded to parallels between the events at the molecular and brain circuitry levels during presentation of motivationally salient stimuli. This chapter will explore how integrative systems biology approaches can bridge the distributed neural circuits responsible for the processing of reward/aversion function and the networks of genes responsible for the development and maintenance of these neural circuits. These combined genetics and integrative neuroscience approaches have the potential to redefine our conceptualization of neuropsychiatric illnesses with the implementation of objective quantitative measures.

Motivation neuroscience and modern cosmology focus on a similar set of questions by looking in at the brain and looking out at the universe, respectively. In the case of modern cosmology, the question is, what is the nature of that which we perceive? Or, how does something come out of nothing? In the case of motivation neuroscience, the question is, how do we perceive, have any control over this perception, and exercise free will in general? Or, why is there directed action?

The concept of motivation relates to the question of how organisms make choices, direct behavior, or plan action across time. Directed action or motivated behavior can be defined as goal-directed behavior that optimizes the fitness of an individual organism (or social group) on the basis of input from a number of evaluative processes regarding potential goal objects in the environment, remembered consequences of previous behavior, internal homeostatic and socially acquired needs, and perceived needs in other organisms. The combined neural systems that produce this directed behavior on the basis of such internal evaluative processes are essential to what we call motivation (Watts and Swanson, 2002). Central to these neural systems are multiple modulatory subsystems that have evolved to allow the organism to assign a value to objects in the environment so as to work for "rewards" and avoid "punishments" (aversive outcomes). These subsystems include an extended set of subcortical gray matter regions (nucleus accumbens [Nac], caudate, putamen, sublenticular extended amygdala [SLEA], amygdala, hippocampus, hypothalamus, and thalamus) (Heimer et al., 1997) and domains of the paralimbic girdle (including the orbitofrontal cortex [GOb], insula, cingulate cortex, parahippocampus, and temporal pole) (Mesulam, 2000). Dopaminergic neurons in the substantia nigra, the retrotuberal field, and the ventral tegmental area (herein jointly referred to as the ventral tegmentum, VT) modulate a number of these regions (Schultz, 2002). Less is known about the roles of nondopaminergic neuromodulatory systems (noradrenergic, serotonergic, cholinergic, steroid hormones, and neuropeptides) that produce a balance between excitatory and inhibitory synaptic neurotransmission to guide motivated behavior. The role of these interconnected regions in relation to reward-focused behavior was first noted by Olds and Milner (1954) and expanded by a number of pioneering investigators over subsequent decades (Everitt, 1978; Gallistel, 1978; Wise, 1978; LeDoux et al., 1985). Within the past decade, neuroimaging studies

HANS C. BREITER Departments of Psychiatry and Radiology, Harvard Medical School, and Athinoula Martinos Center for Biomedical Imaging, Massachusetts General Hospital, Boston, Mass.

GREGORY P. GASIC Departments of Psychiatry and Radiology, Harvard Medical School, and Athinoula Martinos Center for Biomedical Imaging, Massachusetts General Hospital, Boston, Mass.

have further facilitated research into how an extensive set of deep gray matter and cortical brain regions process motivationally significant information.

A number of philosophers since the times of Aquinas, Spinoza, and Bentham have raised the question of how the experience of reward is perceived across categories of stimuli that reinforce behavior, and how these rewarding stimuli are experienced relative to aversive or painful events (Spinoza, 1883; Aquinas, 1993; Bentham, 1996). Employing multiple categories of rewarding and aversive stimuli, neuroimaging studies in humans have yielded evidence of a generalized circuitry (at the limits of their current resolution) processing rewarding and aversive stimuli. They demonstrate that motivationally salient features of monetary gains and losses, infusions of drugs of abuse, consumption of fruit juice, processing of beautiful faces or music, experiences of somatosensory pain, and harbingers of aversive events all activate a common distributed set of neural groups in evaluating painful and hedonic stimuli (Breiter, Etcoff, et al., 1996; Breiter et al., 1997, 2001; Aharon et al., 2001; Becerra et al., 2001; Berns et al., 2001; Blood and Zatorre, 2001; Knutson, Adams, et al., 2001; Phelps et al., 2001; O'Doherty et al., 2002; Elliott et al., 2003). Electrophysiological studies of rodents further suggest that distinguishable local circuits within these neural groups activate selectively to distinct categories of reward input (Carelli, Ijames, and Crumling, 2000; Carelli, 2002). Additional studies have begun to dissect the functions processing reward/aversion information into their subcomponent processes (Breiter and Rosen, 1999; Breiter et al., 2001). The convergence of results from these human studies with others in phylogenetically lower species (LeDoux, 2000; Kelley and Berridge, 2002; Robbins and Everitt, 2002) supports the existence of an informational backbone (iBM) that processes reward/aversion input.

Components of this iBM have been shown to be affected in several neuropsychiatric illnesses (Breiter, Rauch, et al., 1996; Volkow et al., 1997; Goldstein et al., 1999; Schneier et al., 2000; Crespo-Facorro et al., 2001; Hyman and Malenka, 2001; Manji, Drevets, and Charney, 2001; Saxena et al., 2001; Nestler et al., 2002). Neuroimaging research strongly suggests that these illnesses are characterized by distinct circuit-based alterations. If some of these alterations prove heritable, they may serve as endophenotypes for future genetic linkage studies. Endophenotypes are heritable quantitative traits that indicate an individual's risk of developing a disease but are not a hallmark of disease progression (Almasy and Blangero, 2001). Circuitry-based quantitative traits, along with state-sensitive alterations, may be better indications of the neural system's biology (O'Brien et al., 2000; Hill, 2001; Stoll et al., 2001) than the diagnostic categories, based on statistical associations of behavioral signs and symptoms, that are currently used for psychiatric diagnosis.

Emerging studies have alluded to a correspondence between events at the molecular and brain circuitry levels during the presentation of motivationally salient stimuli (Sutton and Breiter, 1994; Becerra et al., 2001; Barrot et al., 2002). This correspondence across scales of brain function suggests that we are observing similar molecular patterns in distributed neural networks responsible for an emerging systems behavior (Ben-Shahar et al., 2002). As a means to develop these interlinked concepts, this chapter will discuss (1) a general model of motivation with its implications for understanding the processing of reward/aversion information (i.e., via an iBM), (2) the brain circuitry associated with this iBM mediating reward/aversion function, (3) neuroimaging evidence implicating dysfunction in components of this reward/aversion circuitry in neuropsychiatric illness, and (4) how integrative neuroscience can bridge between the neural systems responsible for reward/aversion function and the networks of genes responsible for the development and maintenance of these neural circuits. These integrative neuroscience approaches to systems biology at multiple scales have the potential to redefine our conceptualization of neuropsychiatric illnesses through the use of objective quantitative measures.

Theoretical basis for motivation

In everyday life, organisms such as humans make choices to guide their behavior, integrating unconscious and conscious mental processes. These processes involve systematic evaluation of (1) goal objects in the environment, (2) memories of outcomes from previous behaviors focused on goal objects, (3) internal physiological and mental needs, and (4) the perceived social needs of other cooperative and competitive organisms. The confluence of these evaluative processes has classically been referred to as a *drive* or *motivational state* that acts as a postulate to explain the intensity and direction of behavior (Breiter and Rosen, 1999). In the context of evolutionary survival, or selection of fitness, motivational states seek to choose goal objects and activities that will maximize personal fitness over time.

Motivational states commonly require planning over time, or planning in parallel of alternative behaviors and choices. Not all drives that control behavior have a well-defined temporal relationship to environmental events (i.e., curiosity) (Breiter and Rosen, 1999; Kupferman, Kandel, and Iversen, 2000), yet all drives target outcomes characterized by variable arousal and satiation/relief. Motivational states represent an impetus for the evaluation of organism needs in time, linked to active (intentional, rather than stimulus-response based) detection of environmental opportunities to fulfill these needs. Multiple motivational states can be present concurrently (e.g., a person camping during winter becomes cold, tired, and hungry). Homeostatic and biological needs

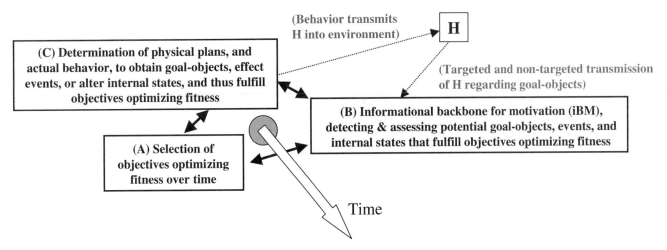

FIGURE 75.1 During communication, information (H), as defined by Shannon and Weaver (1949), is received and decoded by processes that allow incoming information to be linked to the set of communicable messages. Messages communicated from the organism are encoded and transmitted in the form of behavior. Self-organizing organisms always generate entropy as an outcome, which acts as a force behind the development of complexity in coding/decoding systems such as the brain, and their evolution toward greater complexity (Prigogine, 1985). Given the interdependence of these sets of brain processes on each other, they function as if they were all orthogonal to time.

related to glucose level, osmolality, oxygen saturation of hemoglobin, or thermoregulation may thus be arrayed with interorganism and social objectives related to issues such as defense, shelter, procreation, hierarchical ordering, or curiosity. The collective neuronal and physiological processes that mediate drives based on such needs and linked intentional activity can be collectively referred to as motivation.

Current thinking about motivational function is a direct challenge to the simple stimulus-response model of behaviorism. Behaviorism framed goal objects in the environment as having organizing effects on behavior in stimulus-response relationships. Goal objects or stimuli that produced repeated approach behaviors or response repetitions were called rewards. As an incentive for approach behavior, a rewarding stimulus could act either via a memory or via salient sensory properties (i.e., a food odor) of the stimulus. Rewarding stimuli that reinforced previous behavior, in contrast, would increase the probability that preceding behavioral responses would be repeated (i.e., drug self-administration). This behavioral perspective made it difficult to frame problems such as target detection by the brain, and its stimulus-response framework did not allow for symbolic manipulation as described by Chomskian linguistics. These types of issues led to a conceptual revolt manifested by cognitive neuroscience (Marr, 1982; Kosslyn and Shin, 1992; Hauser, Chomsky, and Fitch, 2002; Miller, 2003), neurocomputation (McClelland and Rumelhart, 1985; Churchland and Sejnowski, 1992), judgment and decision making (Mellers, Schwartz, and Cooke, 1998; Shizgal, 1999), emotion neuroscience (LeDoux, 1996; Davidson, Lewis, et al., 2002), evolutionary ecology (Krebs and Davies, 1997; Glimcher, 2003), and a more "pragma-

tist" perspective framed by nonlinear dynamics (Freeman and Barrie, 1994; Freeman, 2001).

A general schema for motivational function synthesizing these viewpoints, and consistent with recent neurocomputational evidence (Sutton and Barto, 1981; Freeman and Barrie, 1994; Dayan, Kakade, and Montague, 2000), is illustrated in figure 75.1. This schema ascribes to motivated behavior at least three fundamental operations (Breiter and Rosen, 1999). These operations include a number of processes: (1) evaluation of homeostatic and social needs, and selection of objectives to meet these needs; (2) sensory perception of potential goal objects that may meet these objectives, assessment of potential reward/aversion outcomes related to these goal objects, and comparison of these assessments against a memory of prior outcomes; and (3) assessment, planning, and execution of action to obtain or avoid these outcomes (Herrnstein, 1971; Herrnstein and Loveland, 1974; Mazur and Vaughan, 1987; Rachlin, Raineri, and Cross, 1991; Mazur, 1994; Shizgal, 1997, 1999; Breiter and Rosen, 1999). Because these operations rely on intricate feedback loops, they are not necessarily sequential but orthogonal to time. In humans, the third operation encompasses a number of potential actions: (1) modulation of attention-based filtering of perceptual input, (2) organization of motor output to obtain goal objects, and (3) the use of cognitive and logic systems (and their symbolic output in the form of language) to increase the range of goal objects that can be obtained or events that can be experienced (Breiter and Rosen, 1999).

The intentional behaviors that are the output of this model could be considered a form of communication (Shannon and Weaver, 1949) as well as a means for modulating sensory input to the brain that is distinct from top-down adaptation of this input once it is in modality-specific processing streams (Friston, 2002). The reference to communication theory is not accidental, since it helped fuel the revolt against behaviorism. In the 1940s, Claude Shannon and colleagues devised a schema for understanding communication in its broadest sense, namely, how one mind or mechanism affects another. These ideas were focused on the technical constraints on communication and never addressed the "semantic problem" or the "effectiveness problem" of communication. The integration of ideas from communication theory and empirical work in neural systems biology has occurred only recently in domains such as sensory representation (Churchland and Sejnowski, 1992), serial response learning and novelty assessment (Berns, Cohen, and Mintun, 1997), reward prediction (Schultz, Dayan, and Montague, 1997), conditional probability computation (Breiter and Rosen, 1999), and nonlinear dynamics underpinning decision making (Freeman and Barrie, 1994; Freeman, 2001). With this melding of communication theory and integrative systems biology, attempts have been made to address the semantic problem posed by interorganism communication, and what constitutes meaning for a biological system. Two viable hypotheses have been advanced, which could be considered two sides of the same coin. One hypothesis links meaning in biological systems to the intersection of intentional behaviors between organisms (Freeman, 2001). The alternative hypothesis frames meaning in the context of organism optimization of fitness over time and tissue metabolic needs (Breiter and Rosen, 1999). For the latter hypothesis, interorganism communication involves message sets defined by genomic and epigenomic control of the bioenergetics of metabolism.

A number of the general operations and processes illustrated in figure 75.1 have been the target of experimental dissection. For example, a set of hypothetical informational subprocesses appears to be active when an animal seeks and finds a stimulus with motivational salience (Pfaffmann et al., 1977; Kunst-Wilson and Zajonc, 1980; Haxby et al., 1991; Freeman and Barrie, 1994; Shizgal, 1997, 1999; Breiter and Rosen, 1999; Damasio, 1999b; Zeki, 2001; Beauchamp et al., 2002; Dayan and Balleine, 2002; Heckers et al., 2002; figure 75.2). These subprocesses include (1) receiving input from the environment or internal milieu across multiple channels, (2) representing it by transient neuronal activity, (3) evaluating it for sensory modality-specific characteristics such as color and motion, (4) combining it across modality at theoretical convergence zones as potential percepts, (5) encoding it into memory and contrasting it with other stimulus memories, and (6) evaluating it for features (rate, delay, intensity, amount, category) that are relevant to organizing behavior. Feature evaluation appears to include (1) categorical identification of putative rewards or aversive stimuli, (2)

evaluation of goal object intensity (i.e., strength) and amount in the context of potential hedonic deficit states, and (3) extraction of rate and delay information from the object of worth, to allow computation of a rate function to model temporal behavior (Gallistel, 1990) and of a probability function for possible outcomes (Kahneman and Tversky, 1979; Tversky and Kahneman, 1992) (see figure 75.2). How the output of these valuation and probability (i.e., expectation) subprocesses is combined remains an area of active discussion and inquiry (Shizgal, 1999).

For the model in figures 75.1 and 75.2, a reward is an operational concept for the positive value that an animal attributes to a goal object, a behavioral act, an internal physical state, or a cue associated with the same. Rewards with a direct temporal connection to homeostatic regulation depend heavily on the physiological state of the organism (Cabanac, 1971; Aharon et al., 2001), and an animal can assign a positive or aversive value to the stimulus, depending on its internal state and its previous experience with the stimulus. Although they are often referred to as deficit states vis-à-vis the physiological needs of the organism (e.g., hunger, thirst, body temperature), rewards are not trivial to define in the case of social rewards (e.g., personal or social aspirations). Social rewards do not always have a clear relationship to deficit states (Cabanac, 1971; Cabanac, Duclaux, and Spector, 1971; Aharon et al., 2001) and may provide insurance over time for satiating some motivational states or avoiding aversive outcomes (LeDoux, 1996; Adolphs, 2003) (figure 75.3). In contrast, aversive events can be directly defined as deficit states whose reduction could be considered rewarding. Rewarding and aversive outcomes are not just affected by these potential deficit states but depend on an assessment of the value and probabilities for alternative payoffs that do not occur (i.e., counterfactual comparisons dependent on memory). A simple example of the effects of counterfactual comparison might be the feeling that you were not very fortunate when you and a friend sauntered down a sidewalk and simultaneously found money, but she found a twenty-dollar bill and you found a one-dollar bill (Mellers, Schwartz, and Ritov, 1997) (see figure 75.2).

Objectives for optimizing fitness observed in figures 75.1 and 75.2 focus on meeting short-term homeostatic needs and projected long-term needs via the insurance provided by social interaction and planning (Adolphs, 2003). They are represented by multiple motivational states whose differing temporal demands produce a complex layering for competing behavioral incentives. This idea was first recognized by Darwin (1872), who hypothesized that motivational states form the basis for emotion. He theorized that the outward projection of emotion, such as by facial expression, represented communication between organisms of internal motivational states. Experimental evidence supporting the thesis of internal sources for emotion was suggested by the work

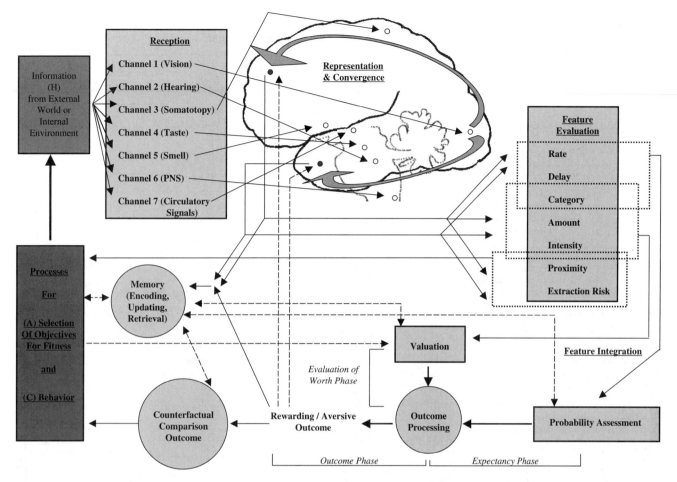

FIGURE 75.2   The theorized processes of the informational back-bone for sensory perception, memory, and reward/aversion assessment can be extensively dissected into subprocesses, reflecting one interpretation of research from evolutionary ecology (Shizgal, 1997; Glimcher, 2003) and behavioral finance (Kahneman and Tversky, 1979; Tversky and Kahneman, 1992; Shizgal, 1999). Dashed lines indicate subprocesses theorized to interact with feedback leading to nonlinear system function (Freeman and Barrie, 1994; Freeman, 2001), whereas solid lines connect subprocesses as steps in the algorithmic processing of information. The postulated early subprocesses are (1) information reception along discrete channels and representation (hollow points in cartoon of brain), (2) convergence of processed informational measures such as detected motion, color, and contrast for vision (thus the ventral and dorsal processing streams represented by arrows moving to solid points), and (3) convergence of represented information from distinct receptive channels for construction of a percept (Haxby et al., 1991; Damasio, 1999b; Zeki, 2001; Beauchamp et al., 2002; Dayan and Balleine, 2002). The postulated later subprocesses include the extraction of informational features necessary to match putative goal objects to internally determined objectives that optimize fitness over time (A). Such motivationally relevant features include rate, delay, category, amount, and intensity information, which are integrated during computation of probability functions and valuation functions, along with input regarding proximity and extraction risk (i.e., "cost" assessments) needed for general cost-benefit analyses (Breiter and Rosen, 1999; Shizgal, 1999). Dotted lines group features integrated in such computations (Gallistel, 1990) for the determination of rewarding and aversive outcomes. Memory encoding, updating, and retrieval functions are necessary for these subprocesses and for the evaluation of counterfactual comparisons (Mellers et al., 1997; Mellers, 2000).

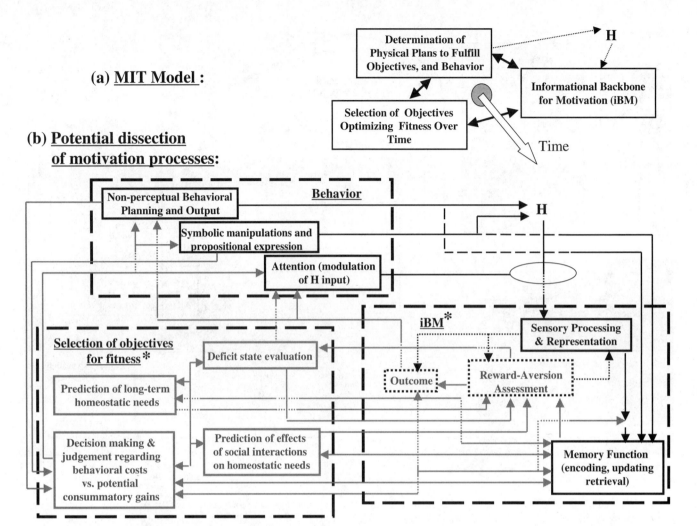

(a) MIT Model :

(b) Potential dissection of motivation processes:

FIGURE 75.3 The abbreviated schematic of the MIT model is shown in *a* to orient the description of its partial dissection into processes shown in *b*. Solid black compartment lines in *a* are dashed bold black lines in *b*. Compartments and connections in solid black represent processes and their interactions for which substantial, though not complete, neuroscience data have been accumulated. Compartments and interactions in light gray represent ones for which there is behavioral research, and beginning neuroscience data are available (Cabanac, 1971; Gallistel, 1990; Adolphs, 2003), but substantially less is known about them than for processes in solid black. Processes and interactions in small black dashes represent ones for which a significant body of neuroscience has begun to accumulate, although we remain far from the level of knowledge currently available for the processes in solid black. The informational backbone for motivation (iBM), and the operation for selection of objectives that optimize fitness over time, are starred to emphasize a synthetic view that their processes comprise those that together constitute the experience of emotion (Darwin, 1872; James, 1884; LeDoux, 1996; Damasio, 1999a).

of Cannon (Cannon and Britton, 1925) and others (LaBar et al., 1998; LeDoux, 2000; Davis and Whalen, 2001; Cain, Kapp, and Puryear, 2002), in contrast to another theory on emotion from James and Lange (James, 1884; Lange, 1985), which posited that sensory inputs regarding bodily function were central to emotional experience. Experimental data also supported the James–Lange thesis (Damasio, 1999a). Both of these perspectives on emotional function are represented by processes within the general schema for motivation (see figure 75.3). This suggests that emotion may be conceptualized within the schema of motivation, potentially allowing it to be readily linked to processes (see figure 75.3) that have been a strong focus of cognitive neuroscience

research, and synthesizing the original perspectives of Darwin and James.

In figure 75.3, the processes shown in solid black represent ones that are supported by behavioral and neuroscience data. These processes determining input and output to the organism appear to be more readily observed via experimentation than the processes shown with light gray lines and small black dashes. The processes shown in light gray are supported by emerging behavioral data, but much remains to be known regarding their systems biology. The processes in small black dashes (also see subprocesses at the bottom of figure 75.2), in contrast, have become associated with neural activity in a distributed set of deep brain regions, suggesting that they are part of an iBM for motivation. Intriguingly, they may represent a generalized circuitry for processing rewarding and aversive events.

Neural basis for a general reward/aversion system underlying motivated behavior

Animal studies aimed at understanding the neural systems that evaluate stimuli as aversive or rewarding have examined the role of the many projection fields of the VT dopamine neurons, such as the NAc, the SLEA of the basal forebrain, the amygdala, and the hypothalamus, and multiple fields in the paralimbic girdle (Lindvall and Bjorklund, 1974; Heimer et al., 1997; Mesulam, 2000; Watts and Swanson, 2002). In the past 5 years, human neuroimaging studies have implicated homologous systems for reward/aversion and have begun to dissect the contributions of individual brain regions.

Among the first human neuroimaging studies to observe activity in a subset of these regions during the processing of rewarding stimuli were three studies using monetary or drug infusion rewards (Berns, Cohen, and Mintun, 1997; Breiter et al., 1997; Thut et al., 1997). The drug infusion study (Breiter et al., 1997) involved double-blind cocaine versus saline infusions and specifically targeted multiple projection fields of the VT dopamine neurons. It was performed with chronic cocaine-dependent subjects, and thus its results, although linking subjective reports of euphoria and craving (i.e., a monofocused motivational state) to reward circuitry activity, could not be separated from neuro-adaptations to subject drug abuse. Follow-up studies in healthy controls using monetary reward, social reward in the form of beautiful faces, and thermal aversive stimuli confirmed the initial findings with cocaine and provided strong evidence for a generalized circuitry that processes stimuli with motivational salience (Breiter et al., 1997, 2001; Aharon et al., 2001; Becerra et al., 2001). The monetary reward study was modeled after a game of chance and temporally segregated expectancy effects from outcomes in reward regions (figure 75.4). It incorporated principles from Kahneman and Tversky's prospect theory, along with Mellor's decision affect theory (Kahneman and Tversky, 1979; Tversky and Kahneman, 1992; Mellers et al., 1997; Mellers, 2000), and observed rank ordering of signal responses in a set of reward regions that reflected the differential expectancy conditions. It further observed rank ordering of signal responses to differential monetary outcomes. For an outcome shared across expectancy conditions, strong effects of expectancy on subsequent outcomes, namely, "counterfactual comparisons" (Mellers et al., 1997; Mellers, 2000), were measured. At the high spatial resolution of that 3T functional magnetic resonance imaging (fMRI) study, a number of reward regions were activated by expectancy or outcome effects, whereas a few regions were activated by differential expectancies, outcomes, and counterfactual comparisons. Subsequent studies of monetary reward have expanded significantly both on the observation of differential expectancy responses in some reward regions (Knutson, Adams, et al., 2001) and on the observation of differential outcome effects (Elliott et al., 2003). Other strong experiments with different categorical rewards have shown segregation of expectancy and outcome effects, but not counterfactual comparison effects (Berns et al., 2001; O'Doherty et al., 2002). Given the degree of agreement across the results of several research groups and overlap across studies within the same research group (e.g., similar expectancy findings in the NAc) for a monetary stimulus (Breiter et al., 2001) and retrospectively for a cocaine infusion stimulus (Breiter and Rosen, 1999) (figure 75.5b), there is evidence that subsystems of reward function are conserved across stimulus category and are amenable to dissection (figures 75.5a).

In contrast to these monetary reward studies, presentation of social stimuli in the form of beautiful versus average faces addressed the issue of valuation (see figure 75.2). The study objectively quantified the reinforcement value of each stimulus by incorporating a key-press procedure, which determined the effort that experimental subjects wished to expend to increase or decrease their viewing time of each face. In addition, this study suggested that nonrewarding stimuli might produce a different regional signal profile to rewarding stimuli (Aharon et al., 2001), an observation that was further supported by a study using thermal pain (Becerra et al., 2001). Together, these studies in healthy controls noted that "classic" reward circuitry (including the NAc, SLEA, amygdala, VT, and GOb) processes both rewarding and aversive stimuli, with salient similarities and differences in the pattern of regional responses (see figure 75.5a).

In the context of these studies, the segregation of neural systems that process aversive stimuli from those that process rewarding stimuli could be considered artificial (Kelley and Berridge, 2002). The "classic reward system," comprised of subcortical gray structures, is activated by aversive stimuli such as thermal pain, expectancies of bad outcomes, and social stimuli that are not wanted (Aharon et al., 2001; Becerra et al., 2001; Breiter et al., 2001). In parallel, "classic pain circuitry," comprised of paralimbic cortical and thalamic structures, is activated by rewarding stimuli (for references, see the caption to figure 75.5c). This commonality in neuroimaging activation patterns in healthy humans across stimuli with positive and negative outcomes (see figure 75.5c) argues that an extended set of subcortical gray matter and paralimbic cortical regions should be considered a generalized system for the processing of reward/aversion information.

A general survey of studies presenting rewarding stimuli to humans indicates that this extended set of reward/

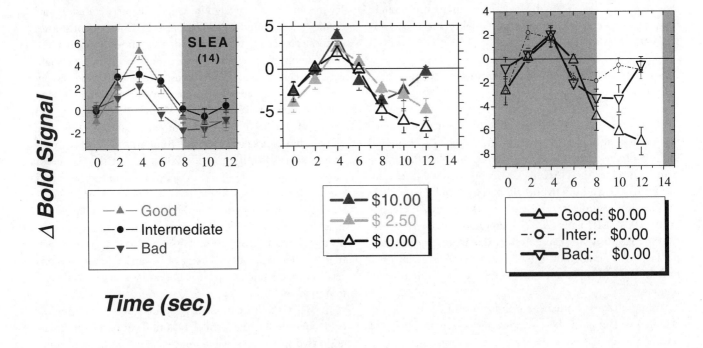

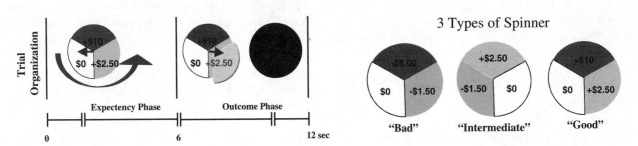

FIGURE 75.4 These data illustrate an example of brain mapping efforts to temporally dissect subprocesses shown in figure 75.2, using an experimental design that applied principles of prospect theory and decision affect theory (Breiter et al., 2001). This study employed a single-trial-like design, shown at the bottom with three spinners. The trial sequence started with presentation of one of these spinners and continued with an arrow rotating on it. This rotating arrow would abruptly stop after 6 s, at which time the sector on which it had landed would flash for 5.5 s, indicating the subject had won or lost that amount of money. Given three spinners, each with three outcomes, this experiment sought to determine which putative reward/aversion regions in the brain would display differential expectancy and/or outcome effects. With one outcome ($0) shared across spinners, it could explicitly also evaluate counterfactual comparison effects (Mellers et al., 1997; Mellers, 2000). The evaluation of counterfactual comparison effects is necessary to determine that the experiment did produce expectancy effects, and the incorporation of expectancy effects is necessary to be able to interpret any outcome effects. The graphs at top display differential expectancy effects (left), differential outcome effects (middle), and counterfactual comparisons (right). The y-axes display normalized fMRI signal, while the x-axes display time in seconds. All time courses come from a region of signal change in the sublenticular extended amygdala (SLEA). (See color plate 64.)

aversion regions responds across multiple categories of rewarding stimuli (for references, see the caption to figure 75.6) although individual subsets of neurons may respond to one type of rewarding stimulus but not another. As some studies in figure 75.6 focused only on select brain regions, such as the GOb, anterior cingulate cortex, or amygdala, or they did not have the spatial resolution to observe a subset of subcortical regions, the relative prevalence of activations noted for some of these regions is skewed. Rank ordering of the prevalence of activations across reward studies indicates that although the majority of studies involved a motor com-

ponent for the experimental task, the majority of activations reported did not involve regions associated with some aspect of motor control (i.e., dorsal caudate, putamen, globus pallidus, posterior cingulate gyrus, and thalamus). In addition, experiments using the passive presentation of social/aesthetic stimuli, appetitive stimuli, and drug stimuli produced activation patterns in subcortical gray matter and paralimbic cortex that overlapped those produced by tasks that included motor performance. Evidence summarized in figure 75.6 makes it difficult to argue that classic reward circuitry (i.e., NAc, SLEA, amygdala, VT, GOb) is uniquely

Expectancy			Outcome							
Region	**Cocaine**	**Monetary Reward**	**Region**	**Cocaine**		**Monetary Reward**	**Beauty**		**Pain**	
				(1)	**(2)**		**(+)**	**(-)**	**(+)**	**(-)**
GOb R			GOb R	↑¹	↑¹	↑³	(↑²)		↑²	
L	↑²	↑²	L	↑¹	↑¹	↑³				
NAc R	↑¹	↑¹	NAc R	↑¹	↑¹	↑¹	↑¹	(↓¹)		↓
L	↑¹	↑¹	L	↑¹				↓¹		↓
SLEA R		↑¹	SLEA R	(↑¹)	↑¹	↑¹	(↑¹)		↑¹	
L			L	↑¹				↑¹		
Amygdala R			Amygdala R	(↓¹)	↑¹	↑¹				
L		↑¹	L	↓¹		↑¹		(↑¹)		(↓¹)
VT R			VT R	↑¹	↑¹	↑¹			↑¹	
L			L	↑¹	↑¹		(↑¹)	↑¹	↑¹	

A

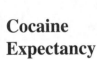

Monetary Expectancy

Cocaine Expectancy

B

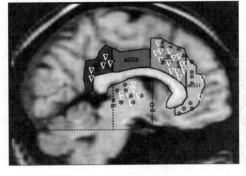

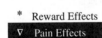

*   Reward Effects

▽   Pain Effects

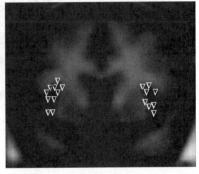

C

FIGURE 75.5 (a) Tabular results from studies at one laboratory (Aharon et al., 2001; Becerra et al., 2001; Breiter et al., 1997, 2001; Breiter and Rosen, 1999) regarding the analysis of expectancy, or of outcome, show common and divergent patterns of activation. Up arrows indicate positive signal changes, while down arrows stand for negative signal change. Raised numeric notation signifies more than one focus of signal change in that region, whereas brackets indicate the signal change was statistically subthreshold for that study. Two separate cocaine infusion studies are listed, as are positive and negative valuation results for the beautiful faces experiment and the thermal pain experiment. Bilateral NAc and left GOb are observed in both studies with expectancy conditions. The right GOb, right NAc, right SLEA, and potentially the left VT are observed during the outcome conditions for most of the experiments.

(b) Expectancy of a monetary gain in the upper panel from a study involving a game of chance in healthy controls (Breiter et al., 2001), and expectancy of a cocaine infusion in the lower panel from a study of double-blind, randomized, cocaine versus saline infusions in cocaine-dependent subjects (Breiter et al., 1997; Breiter and Rosen, 1999). Results are shown in the radiological orientation as pseudocolor statistical maps juxtaposed on coronal group structural images in gray tone. Note the close anatomical proximity for NAc signal changes during positive expectancy in the context of uncertainty for both experiments. (See color plate 65.)

(c) The gray-tone structural images on the left in the sagittal orientation, and on the right in the coronal orientation (+6 mm anterior of the anterior commissure), juxtapose published neuroimaging data in humans from painful stimuli (Talbot et al., 1991; Coghill et al., 1994; Craig et al., 1996; Rainville et al., 1997; Davis, Kiss, et al., 1998; Davis, Kwan, et al., 1998; Becerra et al., 1999, 2001; Ploghaus et al., 1999; Sawamoto et al., 2000; Rainville, Bushnell, and Duncan, 2001) and from rewarding stimuli (Ketter et al., 1996, 2001; Berns, Cohen, and Mintun, 1997; Berns et al., 2001; Breiter et al., 1997, 2001; Thut et al., 1997; Blood et al., 1999; Bartels and Zeki, 2000; Elliott, Friston, and Dolan, 2000; Liu et al., 2000; Blood and Zatorre, 2001; Knutson, Adams, et al., 2001; Knutson, Fong, et al., 2001; O'Doherty et al., 2001, 2002; Small et al., 2001; Bush et al., 2002; Elliott et al., 2003) in three brain regions traditionally reported as "classic" pain regions (Becerra et al., 2001). These regions include the thalamus (Thal in left image, between ac and pc), the cingulate cortex, and the anterior insula (INS in right image). The cingulate cortex is segmented into four units following the standardized methods of the Massachusetts General Hospital Center for Morphometric Analysis (Makris et al., 1999; Meyer et al., 1999); the aCG includes aCG1 and aCG2, while the posterior cingulate is the darkest segmentation unit. Note the close approximation of reported activation from stimuli of opposite valance. (See color plate 66.)

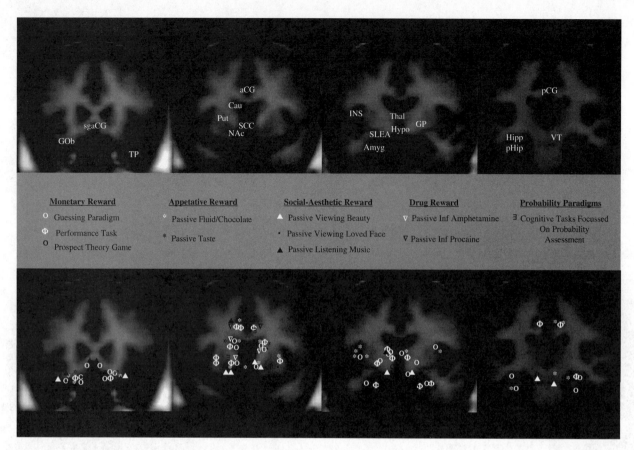

FIGURE 75.6   The top and bottom rows of images indicate, respectively, the anatomy of subcortical gray matter regions and paralimbic cortex, and reported localization in these regions of significant signal change for a number of distinct categories of rewarding stimuli. The gray-tone structural images are coronal slices taken (left to right) +18 mm, +6 mm, −6 mm, and −21 mm relative to the anterior commissure. Abbreviations for anatomy follow the schema adapted from the Massachusetts General Hospital Center for Morphometric Analysis (Breiter et al., 1997, 2001; Makris et al., 1999; Meyer et al., 1999). In this diagram, subcortical gray matter implicated in the processing of reward and aversion input includes the NAc (nucleus accumbens), Put (putamen), Cau (caudate), SCC (subcallosal cortex), Amyg (amygdala), SLEA (sublenticular extended amygdala), Hypo (hypothalamus), GP (globus pallidus), Thal (thalamus), Hipp (hippocampus), VT (ventral tegmentum). Components of the paralimbic girdle include: sgaCG (subgenual anterior cingulate gyrus), GOb (orbitofrontal cortex), aCG (anterior cingulate gyrus), pCG (posterior cingulate gyrus), INS (insula), pHip (parahippocampus), and TP (temporal

pole). The black, white, and gray-tone symbols on the lower row of brain slices show reported activation surveyed from 26 studies of reward function in healthy controls (Volkow et al., 1995, 1996, 1997; Ketter et al., 1996; Berns, Cohen, and Mintun, 1997; Elliott, Friston, and Dolan, 2000; Thut et al., 1997; Blood et al., 1999; Breiter and Rosen, 1999; Bartels and Zeki, 2000; Delgado et al., 2000; Liu et al., 2000; Aharon et al., 2001; Berns et al., 2001; Blood and Zatorre, 2001; Breiter et al., 2001, 2002; Drevets et al., 2001; Kampe et al., 2001; Knutson et al., 2001, 2003; O'Doherty et al., 2001, 2002; Small et al., 2001; Kahn et al., 2002; Elliott et al., 2003). These include ten studies with monetary reward (five with a guessing paradigm determining compensation, four with a performance task determining compensation, and one with a prospect theory-based game of chance). Four studies focused on appetitive reward with fruit juice, chocolate, or pleasant tastes, while five studies focused on some aspect of social reward (two with beautiful faces, one with passive viewing of a loved face, and two with music stimuli). Five studies involved amphetamine or procaine reward, and two studies focused on a probabilistic paradigm.

involved with reward functions, as a proportionate number of activation foci are also reported in the rest of the paralimbic girdle.

In evaluating this evidence in support of a generalized circuitry encompassing both subcortical gray matter and paralimbic cortices for the assessment of reward/aversion information, we need to consider some minor caveats to the studies surveyed. First, the majority of studies surveyed in figure 75.6 utilized monetary reward, which is theorized to be a ready substitute for most other categories of reward (Cabanac, 1992; Mellers, Schwartz, and Cooke, 1998). In the monetary reward studies, expectancy effects are known to be salient, but most of these reports did not take expectancy into account, and thus the results reflect a combination of expectancy and outcome effects (see figures 75.2 and 75.4). Second, all of the drugs infused into healthy controls have known global effects along with purported regional effects, making the association of regional activation to subjective reports of euphoria less certain. Finally, with the exception of a study using chocolate stimuli, none of these reward studies controlled for the presence of a deficit state, thus raising the question of how to gauge the relative reward value of these stimuli. Despite these general concerns, there now appears to be strong similarity between the conclusion drawn from animal and human studies on the neural basis for reward/aversion (Aharon et al., 2001; Becerra et al., 2001; Breiter et al., 2001; Kelley and Berridge, 2002).

The converging evidence for a general circuitry processing reward/aversion information, an important component of emotion function, has potential implications for characterizing the range of healthy emotion function and its malfunction. The systems biology of reward/aversion assessment, like the systems biology of all other subprocesses (e.g., attention, memory, symbolic discourse), represents an interface in the interactions of genome, epigenome, and environment. Across the interface of all motivation subprocesses, the interaction of genome, epigenome, and environment determines the set of all possible behavior. This interface can be sampled in a concentrated fashion to cover or characterize a particular behavioral function in an individual, resulting in a quantitative representation of the algorithmic steps, or set of algorithms, necessary for that behavioral function (e.g., valuation in the context of reward/aversion assessment of a goal object). If multiple samplings are obtained in each individual, covering particular subprocesses, the results can be overlaid and evaluated for correlations across the individuals studied. The correlations that are identified define a complex set of physiological and/or mechanistic interrelationships. These interrelationships can be grouped into functionally related clusters, or systems biology maps (e.g., in cardiovascular function, one can observe vascular, heart, renal, endocrine, and morphometric clusters). Within such clusters or systems biology maps, these

physiological and/or mechanistic relationships can also be defined as quantitative phenotypes, which can be clustered and assigned designations as normal and abnormal.

Implications of a generalized reward/aversion circuitry for psychiatric illness

Traditionally, major psychiatric disorders have been characterized on the basis of behaviors observed in patients and their subjective reports of symptoms. This phenomenological description of categorical outward signs, exophenotypes, produced the nosology of illness characterization that is the American Psychiatric Association's *Diagnostic and Statistical Manual* (*DSM*; 1994). Recently, it has been proposed that neuroscience approaches may replace current symptom-based characterizations of illness, or exophenotypes, by developing a unitary basis for psychiatric and neurological illnesses using a nosology based on genes, molecules, neuronal organelles, and specific neural systems (Cowan, Harter, and Kandel, 2000; Cowan, Kopnisky, and Hyman, 2002). Such a nosology, focused on descriptions of brain structure and function, would have to consider the impact of time, because many of these neuropsychiatric diseases appear to have a neurodevelopmental and/or neurodegenerative component (Breiter et al., 1994; Tager-Flusberg, 1999; Lewis and Levitt, 2002). At this point, we shall examine the current evidence for a neural systems approach, at least in the domain of reward/aversion function, for characterizing and distinguishing the major psychiatric illnesses (i.e., Axis I disorders in the *DSM*).

A growing body of neuroimaging work argues that neuropsychiatric illnesses can be distinguished by alterations in circuitry function observable with positron emission tomography, single-photon emission computed tomography, magnetoencephalography, magnetic resonance spectroscopy, or fMRI (David, Blamire, and Breiter, 1994; Buchbinder and Cosgrove, 1998). Furthermore, as morphometric MRI studies allude to the heritability of structural alterations (Thompson et al., 2001; Narr et al., 2002), a circuitry-based nosology would rely on the identification of endophenotypes for psychiatric disorders (Drevets, 1998; Almasy and Blangero, 2001; Gershon et al., 2001; Manji, Drevets, and Charney, 2001; Lenox, Gould, and Manji, 2002). The presence of these endophenotypes would have implications for characterizing the genetic, molecular, subcellular, and cellular mechanisms that produce them (Egan et al., 2001; Manji, Drevets, and Charney, 2001; Hariri et al., 2002; Hyman, 2002; Caspi et al., 2003). Circuitry-based phenotypes have been hypothesized for disorders such as depression, in that subtyping of depressed patients appears critical for reducing variability in the patterns of regional activity observed with functional imaging (Drevets, 1998, 2001). When structural and functional imaging studies of depression with large cohort sizes or replicated findings are grouped, at least three

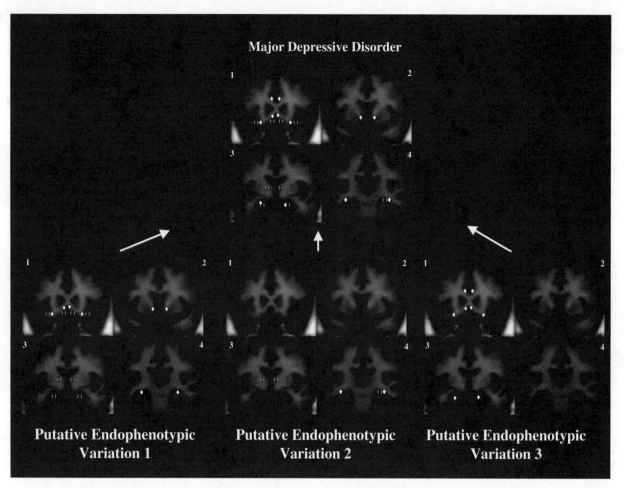

Major Depressive Disorder

Putative Endophenotypic Variation 1

Putative Endophenotypic Variation 2

Putative Endophenotypic Variation 3

FIGURE 75.7 (*a*) The same structural scans shown in figure 75.6 are displayed here, grouped two by two and numbered to correspond with the anterior-to-posterior orientation. The three groupings of brain sections at the bottom of the figure display changes in the structure, function, or morphology of subcortical gray matter and paralimbic cortices for the following three groupings of studies. Studies grouped as "putative endophenotype variation 1" were focused on recurrent depression with strong familiality (sometimes referred to as familial pure depressive disorder). Studies grouped as "putative endophenotype variation 2" were focused on primary depression with and without obsessive-compulsive features and without manifested familial connections. Studies grouped as "putative endophenotype variation 3" were focused on primary and sec-

ondary depression in older subjects who were studied postmortem (see text for references). Regions with differences in resting brain metabolism from healthy baselines are noted with an O symbol, while regions with differences in regional morphology or volume from healthy baselines are noted with a diamond. Most of these studies were not performed with a family segregation design, yet they do suggest the potential for circuitry-based endophenotypes for major depressive disorder. Aggregation of such data across studies, as done for the four sections shown at the top of the figure, point to a strong focus on the generalized reward/aversion system for circuitry-based alterations characterizing major depressive disorder. Such circuitry-based subtypes may aid treatment planning in the future.

putative phenotypes are observed. Distinct patterns of structural and functional alterations are observed for (1) recurrent depression with strong familial loading (i.e., familial pure depressive disorder), (2) primary depression with and without obsessive-compulsive disorder (OCD) and without manifested familial connections, and (3) primary and secondary depression in older subjects studied postmortem (Krishnan et al., 1991; Drevets, 1998, 2000, 2001; Ongur, Drevets, and Price, 1998; Drevets et al., 1999; Rajkowska et al., 1999; Bremner et al., 2000, 2002; Fava and Kendler, 2000; Manji, Drevets, and Charney, 2001; Rajkowska, Halaris, and Selemon, 2001; Sapolsky, 2001; Saxena et al., 2001; Botteron

et al., 2002; Nestler et al., 2002) (figure 75.7). A number of studies that used neuroimaging to compare individuals with neuropsychiatric disorders with unaffected controls have documented qualitative differences (presence or absence of a regional signal) and quantitative differences (numeric alterations in the mean or median signal) that allude to circuit-based phenotypes that may be heritable markers, or endophenotypes (Breiter, Rauch, et al., 1996; Fowler et al., 1996; Bush et al., 1999; Drevets, 2000; Heckers et al., 2000; Manoach et al., 2000, 2001; Schneier et al., 2000).

To date, no project has used a unitary set of experimental paradigms to classify the major categories of psychiatric

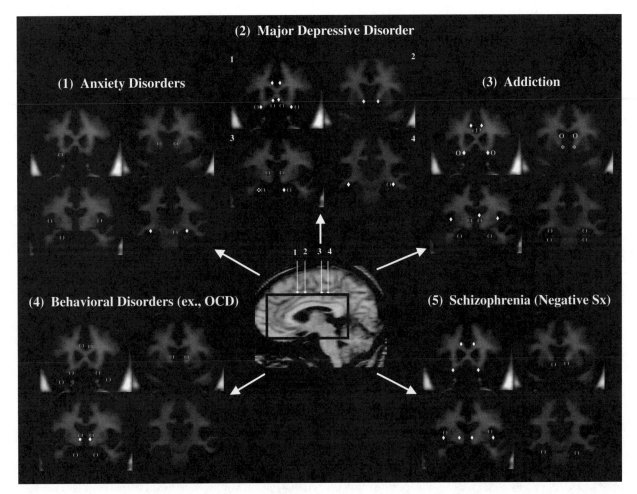

FIGURE 75.8   The groupings of structural images in gray tone are the same as in figure 75.7. Groupings 1 to 5 are placed like the spokes of a wheel around a central sagittal section showing the approximate location of each coronal section relative to a black rectangle around brain regions containing the subcortical gray matter and paralimbic cortices hypothesized to produce reward/aversion functions. Each grouping represents a partial consolidation of findings from the neuroimaging literature comparing patient groups with healthy controls on the basis of (1) resting metabolism, blood flow, or receptor binding, (2) blood flow or metabolic responses to normative stimuli (i.e., pictures of emotional faces that are rapidly masked in an effort to present them subconsciously to subjects with posttraumatic stress disorder), (3) structural differences, or (4) magnetic resonance spectroscopy measures (see text for references). As in figure 75.7, regions with functional differences (measures 1 and 2) between subjects and healthy controls are noted with an "O" symbol, while regions with differences in regional morphology, volume, or spectroscopy signal from healthy baselines (measures 3 and 4) are noted with a diamond. Regions with an asterisk are noted when a set of studies implicates a difference between patients and healthy controls for a large region, and a more recent study with significantly better spatial resolution in healthy controls notes an effect to the same experimental paradigm (i.e., amphetamine infusions) localized to a specific subregion (i.e., the NAc vs. the basal ganglia). The clinical groupings used for groupings 1 to 5 in the figure are listed above each set of sections and described in detail in the text. This schema supports the hypothesis that neuropsychiatric illness may lend itself to objective diagnosis by use of circuitry-based neuroimaging measures.

illness on the basis of their patterns of circuitry function or structural differences. However, by compiling studies that compare patients with unaffected controls for each of the major categories of neuropsychiatric illnesses on the basis of (1) patterns of resting brain metabolism, blood flow, or receptor binding, (2) functional differences in responses to normative stimuli (i.e., pictures of emotional faces that are rapidly masked in an effort to present them subconsciously), (3) volumes of brain structure, or (4) quantifiable chemical signatures of neuronal integrity, in brain systems that collectively process reward/aversion information, we can already observe patterns characteristic to each disorder (figure 75.8). In the consolidation of neuropsychiatric imaging results in figure 75.8, anxiety disorders (1), major depressive disorder (2), and addiction (3) were placed as a potential continuum along the top of the figure, with behavioral disorders (4) and schizophrenia (5) placed in the lower part of the figure to separate them. Anxiety disorder (1) involved a grouping of studies on posttraumatic stress disorder, social phobia, and simple phobia, and included one study aggregating data from symptom provocation studies that did not involve a healthy control group (Rauch et al., 1997, 2000; Schneier et al., 2000; Schuff et al., 2001). Major depression (2) involved the grouping of studies described for figure 75.7 (Krishnan et al., 1991; Drevets, 1998, 2000, 2001; Ongur, Drevets, and Price, 1998; Drevets et al., 1999; Rajkowska et al., 1999; Bremner et al., 2000, 2002; Fava and Kendler, 2000; Manji, Drevets, and Charney, 2001; Rajkowska, Halaris, and Selemon, 2001; Sapolsky, 2001; Saxena et al., 2001; Botteron et al., 2002; Nestler et al., 2002). Addiction (3) involved the grouping of multiple stimulant addictions (Volkow et al., 1991, 1997, 2000, 2001; Grant et al., 1996; Childress et al., 1999; Li et al., 1999; Garavan et al., 2000; Goldstein et al., 2001; Franklin et al., 2002). Behavioral disorders (4) were grouped following more recent suggestions to place OCD on a continuum with tics (Tourette's sydrome), attention-deficit/hyperactivity disorder, and other behavioral problems such as conduct disorder and oppositional behavior, and learning disabilities (Jankovic, 2001). For figure 75.8, studies of OCD were grouped (Baxter et al., 1987, 1988; Nordahl et al., 1989; Swedo et al., 1989; Sawle et al., 1991; Perani et al., 1995; Breiter, Rauch, et al., 1996; Fitzgerald et al., 2000; Graybiel and Rauch, 2000; Saxena et al., 2001). Lastly, schizophrenia (5) involved a grouping of studies that used subjects who were not actively psychotic. Also, given the focus on an iBM involving subcortical gray matter and paralimbic cortices, the schizophrenia grouping was focused on its possible relevance to negative symptoms, such as amotivation, avolition, and anhedonia (Andreasen et al., 1994; Goldstein et al., 1999; Heckers et al., 2000; Manoach et al., 2000, 2001; Crespo-Facorro et al., 2001).

In general, examination of circuitry-based phenotypes for the general categories of anxiety disorder, major depressive disorder, addiction, behavioral disorders, and schizophrenia reveals differences between patient and control groups primarily in subcortical gray matter and paralimbic cortices. These brain regions are implicated in mediating a number of subprocesses, such as reward/aversion assessment, that are fundamental to emotional function and the generation of motivated behavior (Berns, Cohen, and Mintun, 1997; Breiter and Rosen, 1999; Shizgal, 1999; LeDoux, 2000; Mesulam, 2000; Schultz, 2000; Breiter et al., 2001; Davis and Whalen, 2001; Anderson and Phelps, 2002; Robbins and Everitt, 2002; Watts and Swanson, 2002; Wise, 2002; Adolphs, 2003).

Such observations do not imply that a unitary nosology based on the circuitry of one or two motivation subprocesses would be complete. There already is strong evidence that disorders such as schizophrenia represent manifestations of abnormal circuitry function in many cortical regions and functional domains outside the circuitry implicated in the subprocess of reward/aversion assessment (Shenton et al.,

2001; Sawa and Snyder, 2002). The characterization and distinction of neuropsychiatric illnesses on the basis of abnormalities in circuitry for reward/aversion assessment represents perhaps one dimension of a multidimensional schema for circuitry-based (or systems-based) characterization of neuropsychiatric diseases. Other dimensions might include processes shown in figure 75.3 for attention and memory (Seidman et al., 1998; Wagner et al., 1998; Donaldson, Petersen, and Buckner, 2001), or processes involved with sensory perception (Bonhomme et al., 2001). At the interface between genome, epigenome, and environment, the systems biology of any number of brain subprocesses involved with motivated behavior may be dysfunctional in concert with that of reward/aversion assessment, producing neuropsychiatric signs and symptoms.

Future prospects: Implications of linking reward/aversion circuitry to gene function

If an organism is defined by the interaction of its genome-epigenome with the environment, then all disease states can be represented as a failure of the organism to adapt effectively to its environment. One view to building a new nosology of psychiatric disease is via common circuitry alterations, which represent adaptation failures on an immediate time scale (see figures 75.7 and 75.8). Other views are based on alterations in genetic, molecular, and neuronal function, which represent adaptation failures on a broader time scale. In any given individual, maladaptive changes can manifest at the genetic, molecular, and organelle level and are a by-product of the "capacitors" and "gain controls" responsible for species-wide adaptations to a changing environment over time (Kirschner and Gerhart, 1998; Rutherford and Lindquist, 1998; True and Lindquist, 2000; Vrana et al., 2000; Beaudet and Jiang, 2002; Queitsch, Sangster, and Lindquist, 2002). Given that circuitry and molecular genetic functions are interrelated, it is likely that neural systems-level descriptors (e.g., the reward/aversion systems described in the previous section) and molecular-genetic-level descriptors may both be necessary components for the characterization of all neuropsychiatric illness.

Arguments in favor of the future use of molecular-genetic-level descriptors to characterize psychiatric illness come from characterizations of less prevalent neuropsychiatric diseases with established neurodegenerative and neurodevelopmental causes (Breiter et al., 1994; Tager-Flusberg, 1999; Lewis and Levitt, 2002). For instance, prion diseases and many of the neurodegenerative diseases with patterns of mixed Mendelian and/or non-Mendelian inheritance (i.e., Alzheimer's disease, Parkinson's disease, frontotemporal dementias, Huntington's disease) have a strong component of their etiology from two processes. One process involves the dysfunction and/or cell death of a subset of brain neurons that express an aberrant gene product, while a second process involves the non-cell-autonomous consequences (e.g., altered homeostasis) of this neuronal vulnerability. These diseases result from an inability to maintain mutant proteins: (1) in a properly folded and/or functional state, (2) in their proper subcellular organelles, or (3) at appropriate steady-state levels to prevent their gain-of-function role (Gusella et al., 1983; Huntington's Disease Collaborative Research Group, 1993; Cummings and Zoghbi, 2000; Collinge, 2001; Heppner et al., 2001; Nicotera, 2001; Dunah et al., 2002; Okazawa et al., 2002; Shahbazian et al., 2002; Watase et al., 2002). Ultimately, the energy state of the cell and/or mitochondrial function may become impaired and normal transport processes may likewise be affected.

Protection against degenerative disease can be conferred by overexpression of some members of a family of heat-shock proteins that keep proteins in a folded state and are up-regulated during cellular stress conditions (Sherman and Goldberg, 2001; Li et al., 2002; Opal and Zoghbi, 2002). Aging causes these cellular defense proteins to decline, possibly heralding the onset of neurodegenerative disease whose prevalence increases with age (Sherman and Goldberg, 2001; Li et al., 2002; Opal and Zoghbi, 2002). Lindquist and colleagues have proposed that molecular systems that keep proteins in a folded state serve as "capacitors" for cellular evolution (Kirschner and Gerhart, 1998; Rutherford and Lindquist, 1998; True and Lindquist, 2000; Queitsch, Sangster, and Lindquist, 2002).

Another category of adaptation failure is proposed in the form of heritable alterations in gene expression that do not rely on alterations in DNA sequence (e.g., methylation of DNA bases) but on the parental origin of the DNA (epigenetic modifications such as imprinting). For example, Down syndrome, Turner's syndrome, and Praeder-Willi and Angelman syndromes are neuropsychiatric diseases that can be caused by alterations in gene dosage and/or imprinting rather than by mutations in the DNA itself (Tager-Flusberg, 1999; Nicholls and Knepper, 2001; Sapienza and Hall, 2001; Beaudet and Jiang, 2002). Such observations have led to a "rheostat" model for gene expression, which acts as a gain control to allow rapid and reversible attenuation of gene expression (over generations and during development). Alterations in such a gain-control mechanism may ultimately explain a spectrum of related neuropsychiatric diseases (Vrana et al., 2000; Beaudet and Jiang, 2002).

The molecules that serve as the putative gain control (i.e., rheostat) and capacitors for producing adaptive phenotypic variation function in a substantial and stepwise fashion rather than an incremental and progressive one. Variations in both systems may be present in neuropsychiatric diseases such as Rett syndrome (Amir et al., 1999; Zoghbi, 2001; Shahbazian et al., 2002; Watase et al., 2002). The molecular

genetic basis of such neuropsychiatric diseases may be the outcome of evolutionary events that strike a delicate balance between minimizing deleterious mutations while allowing phenotypic variations that are adaptive to a species in a changing environment (Kirschner and Gerhart, 1998; Rutherford and Lindquist, 1998; True and Lindquist, 2000; Vrana et al., 2000; Beaudet and Jiang, 2002; Queitsch, Sangster, and Lindquist, 2002; Shahbazian and Zoghbi, 2002).

These molecular genetic variations, which may be adaptive or maladaptive in a changing environment, produce changes observable at a number of spatiotemporal scales of brain function or levels of organization (figure 75.9). The parsimonious description of scales of brain function and their embedding remains a topic of active discussion (see Churchland and Sjenowski, 1992; Freeman, 2001). There is also an open question of whether the dynamic principles governing information processing at one level of organization are applicable to other levels of organization (i.e., neural scale invariance) (Sutton and Breiter, 1994). For at least one brain region, the NAc, a qualitative similarity is noted between reports of transcription factor cAMP response element-binding protein (CREB) activity in response to aversive and rewarding stimuli (Pliakas et al., 2001; Barrot et al., 2002) and the signal representing distributed group function observed with fMRI to similar aversive and rewarding stimuli (Breiter et al., 1997, 2001; Becerra et al., 2001). Reverse engineering how activity is linked across levels of brain organization will have implications for reductive understanding of health and disease. As a coarse example of an integrative neuroscience approach to brain disease, circuitry-based endophenotypes should be identifiable for any given psychiatric disease, allowing researchers to constrain future genetic association and linkage studies (figure 75.10). Such a top-down approach for integrative neuroscience was utilized to find an EEG-based endophenotype in individuals susceptible to alcohol dependence, forging an association with a locus that contains a subunit of the $GABA_A$ receptor (Reich et al., 1999; Williams et al., 1999; Porjesz et al., 2002).

The linkage of systems-level measures to molecular-genetic-level descriptors assumes that the probability of illness manifestation will be related to (1) the probability associated with having a specific allele(s) at a particular locus (loci), (2) the probability of having a particular endophenotype, and (3) the probability of having a particular set of epigenetic elements (e.g., this might be expressed as P(illness) ≈ P(allele, locus) × P(EndophenotypeN, t) × P(Epigenome, t)). Epigenetic elements appear to be species-specific (Vrana et al., 2000), and may explain significant differences in phenotypes between species that otherwise have 99% sequence similarity (Enard et al., 2002). Phylogenetically lower animal species may help to a limited degree in elucidating the abnormalities at discrete spatiotemporal scales of brain function characterizing human functional illness.

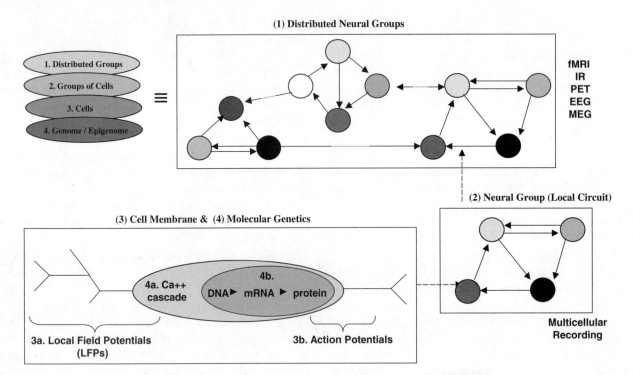

FIGURE 75.9 As a rough approximation, brain processes can be analogized to a set of nested scales of function. The genome/epigenome is nested in cells (neural and glial), which in turn are nested in neural groups as local circuits, which in turn are nested in sets of interconnected groups that are distributed across the brain and modulated by monoaminergic and hormonal systems. The scale of distributed neural groups can be sampled using a number of distinct technologies, including tomographic imaging modalities such as fMRI and PET. Local circuits or neural groups, comprised of excitatory and inhibitory synapses, axonal and dendrodendritic circuits, can be sampled by multicellular recording techniques. The individual cell, with its intracellular signaling and surface receptors, can also be characterized by measures of local field potential and sequences of action potentials. From the scale of molecular genetics to that of distributed neural groups, reductionistic explanation of empirical observation using linkage of measures across scale has to occur both from top down and bottom up to be self-sufficient. Given the nesting of scales, and the measurable relationship of information processing at one scale to another, dense sampling of one scale of brain function will reflect processes at the other scales (see figure 75.10).

Epigenetic issues may partly explain replication difficulties across gene linkage studies of psychiatric illness. Another salient challenge may be the use of coarse clinical measures and dichotomous behavioral distinctions rather than quantitative markers (endophenotypes) to cluster subjects for these studies. Activity in a variable number of distinct, distributed neural groups may yield multiple endophenotypes for an illness yet produce indistinguishable symptom/sign clusters. The scale of distributed cell groups controls behavior, and is biased by genetic/epigenetic function. Weinberger and colleagues have demonstrated with fMRI that genetic variations in COMT and 5-HT transporter are correlated with fMRI signal changes in human amygdala and prefrontal cortex, respectively (Egan et al., 2001; Hariri et al., 2002). These types of studies represent a bottom-up approach to complement findings from the top-down approach. In some diseases, such as Huntington's, a single major disease locus may be enough to produce the endophenotypes and exophenotypes that characterize the illness. In contrast, oligogenetic and polygenic diseases (Beaudet et al., 2001), such as Parkinson's disease and most neuropsychiatric illnesses, appear to involve more than one genetic locus. In such cases, future genome-wide linkage and association studies using circuit-based endophenotypes will have to demonstrate that variant alleles at multiple loci (when quantitative trait loci become quantitative trait nucleotides) are both necessary and sufficient to produce the alterations in the functional subprocesses and their mediating neurocircuitry.

ACKNOWLEDGMENTS   We would like to thank the following individuals for helpful comments on the manuscript: Arthur Beaudet, David Colman, Steven Hyman, Michael Moskowitz, Eric Nestler, Jerrold Rosenbaum, and Huda Zohgbi. We thank Frederick Sheahan for editorial assistance and commentary.

This work was supported by funding from the National Institute of Drug Abuse (grant nos. 14118 and 09467), the Office of National Drug Control Policy–Counterdrug Technology Assessment Center (ONDCP-CTAC), and the Massachusetts General Hospital Department of Radiology. This work was further supported in part by the National Center for Research Resources (P41RR14075), the Mental Illness and Neuroscience Discovery (MIND) Institute, and the Division on Addictions, Harvard Medical School.

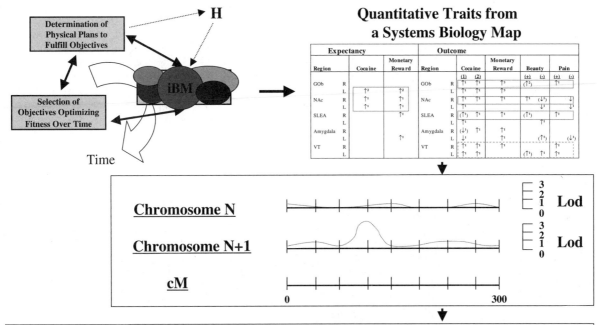

FIGURE 75.10 This schematic illustrates one potential top-down approach to integrative neuroscience, such as might be used for identifying the genes associated with a susceptibility or resistance to addiction. Overlapping sampling of circuitry processing reward/aversion input (cartoon at top left) from families with addiction could be used to produce a systems biology map (cartoon top right) that identifies quantitative traits with a demonstrated familiality and little alteration with disease progression. These endophenotypes could then be used in a multipoint genetic linkage analysis to chromosomal loci (schematic in center and bottom). This top-down approach would define disease susceptibility by continuous quantitative traits measured from systems biology (as via neuroimaging), and might perform a total genome scan and a multipoint linkage analysis using a variance component approach (for quantitative and potential qualitative traits). Analysis of microsatellite repeats and SNP markers could then drive gene identification.

REFERENCES

ADOLPHS, R., 2003. Cognitive neuroscience of human social behaviour. *Nat. Rev. Neurosci.* 4:165–178.

AHARON, I., N. ETCOFF, D. ARIELY, C. F. CHABRIS, E. O'CONNOR, and H. C. BREITER, 2001. Beautiful faces have variable reward value: fMRI and behavioral evidence. *Neuron* 32:537–551.

ALMASY, L., and J. BLANGERO, 2001. Endophenotypes as quantitative risk factors for psychiatric disease: Rationale and study design. *Am. J. Med. Genet.* 105:42–44.

American Psychological Association, 1994. *Diagnostic and Statistical Manual of Mental Disorder S–IV.* Bethesda, Md.: American Psychological Association.

AMIR, R. E., I. B. VAN DEN VEYVER, M. WAN, C. Q. TRAN, U. FRANCKE, and H. Y. ZOGHBI, 1999. Rett syndrome is caused by mutations in X-linked MECP2, encoding methyl-CpG-binding protein 2. *Nat. Genet.* 23:185–188.

ANDERSON, A. K., and E. A. PHELPS, 2002. Is the human amygdala critical for the subjective experience of emotion? Evidence of intact dispositional affect in patients with amygdala lesions. *J. Cogn. Neurosci.* 14:709–720.

ANDREASEN, N. C., S. ARNDT, V. SWAYZE, 2nd, T. CIZADLO, M. FLAUM, D. O'LEARY, J. C. EHRHARDT, and W. T. YUH, 1994. Thalamic abnormalities in schizophrenia visualized through magnetic resonance image averaging. *Science* 266:294–298.

AQUINAS, T., 1993. Summa Theologiae: Feelings. In *Aquinas: Selected Philosophical Writings.* T. McDermott, ed. New York: Oxford University Press, pp. 156–168.

BARROT, M., J. D. A. OLIVIER, L. I. PERROTTI, R. J. DiLEONE, O. BERTON, A. J. EISCH, S. IMPEY, D. R. STORM, R. L. NEVE, J. C. YIN, et al., 2002. CREB activity in the nucleus accumbens shell controls gating of behavioral responses to emotional stimuli. *Proc. Natl. Acad. Sci. U.S.A.* 99:11435–11440.

BARTELS, A., and S. ZEKI, 2000. The neural basis of romantic love. *Neuroreport* 11:3829–3834.

BAXTER, L. R., JR., M. E. PHELPS, J. C. MAZZIOTTA, B. H. GUZE, J. M. SCHWARTZ, and C. E. SELIN, 1987. Local cerebral glucose metabolic rates in obsessive-compulsive disorder: A comparison with rates in unipolar depression and in normal controls. *Arch. Gen. Psychiatry* 44:211–218.

BAXTER, L. R., JR., J. M. SCHWARTZ, J. C. MAZZIOTTA, M. E. PHELPS, J. J. PAHL, B. H. GUZE, and L. FAIRBANKS, 1988. Cerebral glucose metabolic rates in nondepressed patients with obsessive-compulsive disorder. *Am. J. Psychiatry* 145:1560–1563.

BEAUCHAMP, M. S., K. E. LEE, J. V. HAXBY, and A. MARTIN, 2002. Parallel visual motion processing streams for manipulable objects and human movements. *Neuron* 34:149–159.

BEAUDET, A. L., and Y. H. JIANG, 2002. A rheostat model for a rapid and reversible form of imprinting-dependent evolution. *Am. J. Hum. Genet.* 70:1389–1397.

BEAUDET, A. L., C. R. SCRIVER, W. S. SLY, and D. VALLE, 2001. Genetics, biochemistry, and molecular bases of variant human phenotypes. In *The Metabolic and Molecular Basis of Inherited Disease.* C. R. Scriver et al., eds. New York: McGraw-Hill, pp. 3–44.

BECERRA, L. R., H. C. BREITER, M. STOJANOVIC, S. FISHMAN, A. EDWARDS, A. R. COMITE, R. G. GONZALEZ, and D. BORSOOK, 1999. Human brain activation under controlled thermal stimulation and habituation to noxious heat: An fMRI study. *Magn. Reson. Med.* 41:1044–1057.

BECERRA, L., H. C. BREITER, R. WISE, R. G. GONZALEZ, and D. BORSOOK, 2001. Reward circuitry activation by noxious thermal stimuli. *Neuron* 32:927–946.

BEN-SHAHAR, Y., A. ROBICHON, M. B. SOKOLOWSKI, and G. E. ROBINSON, 2002. Influence of gene action across different time scales on behavior. *Science* 296:741–744.

BENTHAM, J., 1996. *An Introduction to the Principles of Morals and Legislation,* J. H. B. and H. L. A. Hart, eds. Oxford: Clarendon Press.

BERNS, G. S., J. D. COHEN, and M. A. MINTUN, 1997. Brain regions responsive to novelty in the absence of awareness. *Science* 276:1272–1275.

BERNS, G. S., S. M. MCCLURE, G. PAGNONI, and P. R. MONTAGUE, 2001. Predictability modulates human brain response to reward. *J. Neurosci.* 21:2793–2798.

BLAZQUEZ, P. M., N. FUJII, J. KOJIMA, and A. M. GRAYBIEL, 2002. A network representation of response probability in the striatum. *Neuron* 33:973–382.

BLOOD, A. J., R. J. ZATORRE, P. BERMUDEZ, and A. C. EVANS, 1999. Emotional responses to pleasant and unpleasant music correlate with activity in paralimbic brain regions. *Nat. Neurosci.* 2:382–387.

BLOOD, A. J., and R. J. ZATORRE, 2001. Intensely pleasurable responses to music correlate with activity in brain regions implicated in reward and emotion. *Proc. Natl. Acad. Sci. U.S.A.* 98:11818–11823.

BONHOMME, V., P. FISET, P. MEURET, S. BACKMAN, G. PLOURDE, T. PAUS, M. C. BUSHNELL, and A. C. EVANS, 2001. Propofol anesthesia and cerebral blood flow changes elicited by vibrotactile stimulation: A positron emission tomography study. *J. Neurophysiol.* 85:1299–1308.

BOTTERON, K. N., M. E. RAICHLE, W. C. DREVETS, A. C. HEATH, and R. D. TODD, 2002. Volumetric reduction in left subgenual prefrontal cortex in early onset depression. *Biol. Psychiatry* 51:342–344.

BREITER, H. C., I. AHARON, D. KAHNEMAN, A. DALE, and P. SHIZGAL, 2001. Functional imaging of neural responses to expectancy and experience of monetary gains and losses. *Neuron* 30:619–639.

BREITER, H. C., N. F. ETCOFF, P. J. WHALEN, W. A. KENNEDY, L. R. SCOTT, R. L. BUCKNER, M. M. STRAUSS, S. E. HYMAN, and B. R. ROSEN, 1996. Response and habituation of the human amygdala during visual processing of facial expression. *Neuron* 17:875–887.

BREITER, H. C., P. A. FILIPEK, D. N. KENNEDY, L. BAER, D. A. PITCHER, M. J. OLIVARES, P. F. RENSHAW, and V. S. CAVINESS, JR., 1994. Retrocallosal white matter abnormalities in patients with obsessive-compulsive disorder. *Arch. Gen. Psychiatry* 51:663–664.

BREITER, H. C., R. L. GOLLUB, R. M. WEISSKOFF, D. N. KENNEDY, N. MAKRIS, J. D. BERKE, J. M. GOODMAN, H. L. KANTOR, D. R. GASTFRIEND, J. P. RIORDEN, et al., 1997. Acute effects of cocaine on human brain activity and emotion. *Neuron* 19:591–611.

BREITER, H. C., S. L. RAUCH, K. K. KWONG, J. R. BAKER, R. M. WEISSKOFF, D. N. KENNEDY, A. D. KENDRICK, T. L. DAVIS, A. JIANG, M. S. COHEN, et al., 1996. Functional magnetic resonance imaging of symptom provocation in obsessive-compulsive disorder. *Arch. Gen. Psychiatry* 53:595–606.

BREITER, H. C., and B. R. ROSEN, 1999. Functional magnetic resonance imaging of brain reward circuitry in the human. *Ann. N.Y. Acad. Sci.* 877:523–547.

BREMNER, J. D., M. NARAYAN, E. R. ANDERSON, L. H. STAIB, H. L. MILLER, and D. S. CHARNEY, 2000. Hippocampal volume reduction in major depression. *Am. J. Psychiatry* 157:115–118.

BREMNER, J. D., M. VYTHILINGAM, E. VERMETTEN, A. NAZEER, J. ADIL, S. KHAN, L. H. STAIB, and D. S. CHARNEY, 2002. Reduced volume of orbitofrontal cortex in major depression. *Biol. Psychiatry* 51:273–279.

BUCHBINDER, B. R., and G. R. COSGROVE, 1998. Cortical activation MR studies in brain disorders. *Magn. Reson. Imaging Clin. North Am.* 6:67–93.

BUSH, G., J. A. FRAZIER, S. L. RAUCH, L. J. SEIDMAN, P. J. WHALEN, M. A. JENIKE, B. R. ROSEN, and J. BIEDERMAN, 1999. Anterior cingulate cortex dysfunction in attention-deficit/hyperactivity disorder revealed by fMRI and the Counting Stroop. *Biol. Psychiatry* 45:1542–1552.

BUSH, G., B. A. VOGT, J. HOLMES, A. M. DALE, D. GREVE, M. A. JENIKE, and B. R. ROSEN, 2002. Dorsal anterior cingulate cortex: A role in reward-based decision making. *Proc. Natl. Acad. Sci. U.S.A.* 99:523–528.

CABANAC, M., 1971. Physiological role of pleasure. *Science* 173:1103–1107.

CABANAC, M., 1992. Pleasure: The common currency. *J. Theor. Biol.* 155:173–200.

CABANAC, M., R. DUCLAUX, and N. H. SPECTOR, 1971. Sensory feedback in regulation of body weight: Is there a ponderostat? *Nature* 229:125–127.

CAIN, M. E., B. S. KAPP, and C. B. PURYEAR, 2002. The contribution of the amygdala to conditioned thalamic arousal. *J. Neurosci.* 22:11026–11034.

CANNON, W. D., and S. W. BRITTON, 1925. Pseudoaffective mediadrenal secretion. *Am. J. Physiol.* 72:283–294.

CARELLI, R. M., 2002. Nucleus accumbens cell firing during goal-directed behaviors for cocaine vs. "natural" reinforcement. *Physiol. Behav.* 76:379–387.

CARELLI, R. M., S. G. IJAMES, and A. J. CRUMLING, 2000. Evidence that separate neural circuits in the nucleus accumbens encode cocaine versus "natural" (water and food) reward. *J. Neurosci.* 20:4255–4266.

CASPI, A., K. SUGDEN, T. E. MOFFITT, A. TAYLOR, I. W. CRAIG, H. HARRINGTON, J. MCCLAY, J. MILL, J. MARTIN, A. BRAITHWAITE, et al., 2003. Influence of life stress on depression: Moderation by a polymorphism in the 5-HTT gene. *Science* 301:386–389.

CHILDRESS, A. R., P. D. MOZLEY, W. MCELGIN, J. FITZGERALD, M. REIVICH, and C. P. O'BRIEN, 1999. Limbic activation during cue-induced cocaine craving. *Am. J. Psychiatry* 156:11–18.

CHURCHLAND, P., and T. SEJNOWSKI, 1992. *The Computational Brain.* Cambridge, Mass.: MIT Press.

COGHILL, R. C., J. D. TALBOT, A. C. EVANS, E. MEYER, A. GJEDDE, M. C. BUSHNELL, and G. H. DUNCAN, 1994. Distributed processing of pain and vibration by the human brain. *J. Neurosci.* 14:4095–4108.

COLLINGE, J., 2001. Prion diseases of humans and animals: Their causes and molecular basis. *Annu. Rev. Neurosci.* 24:519–550.

COWAN, W. M., D. H. HARTER, and E. R. KANDEL, 2000. The emergence of modern neuroscience: Some implications for neurology and psychiatry. *Annu. Rev. Neurosci.* 23:343–391.

COWAN, W. M., K. L. KOPNISKY, and S. E. HYMAN, 2002. The human genome project and its impact on psychiatry. *Annu. Rev. Neurosci.* 25:1–50.

CRAIG, A. D., E. M. REIMAN, A. EVANS, and M. C. BUSHNELL, 1996. Functional imaging of an illusion of pain. *Nature* 384:258–260.

CRESPO-FACORRO, B., S. PARADISO, N. C. ANDREASEN, D. S. O'LEARY, G. L. WATKINS, L. L. PONTO, and R. D. HICHWA, 2001. Neural mechanisms of anhedonia in schizophrenia: A PET study of response to unpleasant and pleasant odors. *JAMA* 286:427–435.

CUMMINGS, C. J., and H. Y. ZOGHBI, 2000. Trinucleotide repeats: Mechanisms and pathophysiology. *Annu. Rev. Genomics. Hum. Genet.* 1:281–328.

DAMASIO, A., 1999a. *The Feeling of What Happens.* London: William Heinemann.

DAMASIO, A. R., 1999b. How the brain creates the mind. *Sci. Am.* 281:112–117.

DARWIN, C., 1872. *The Expression of the Emotions in Man and Animals.* London: John Murray.

DAVID, A., A. BLAMIRE, and H. BREITER, 1994. Functional magnetic resonance imaging: A new technique with implications for psychology and psychiatry. *Br. J. Psychiatry* 164:2–7.

DAVIDSON, R. J., D. A. LEWIS, L. B. ALLOY, D. G. AMARAL, G. BUSH, J. D. COHEN, W. C. DREVETS, M. J. FARAH, J. KAGAN, J. L. MCCLELLAND, et al., 2002. Neural and behavioral substrates of mood and mood regulation. *Biol. Psychiatry* 52:478–502.

DAVIDSON, R. J., D. PIZZAGALLI, J. B. NITSCHKE, and K. PUTNAM, 2002. Depression: Perspectives from affective neuroscience. *Annu. Rev. Psychol.* 53:545–574.

DAVIS, K. D., Z. H. KISS, L. LUO, R. R. TASKER, A. M. LOZANO, and J. O. DOSTROVSKY, 1998. Phantom sensations generated by thalamic microstimulation. *Nature* 391:385–387.

DAVIS, K. D., C. L. KWAN, A. P. CRAWLEY, and D. J. MIKULIS, 1998. Event-related fMRI of pain: Entering a new era in imaging pain. *Neuroreport* 9:3019–3023.

DAVIS, M., and P. J. WHALEN, 2001. The amygdala: Vigilance and emotion. *Mol. Psychiatry* 6:13–34.

DAYAN, P., and B. W. BALLEINE, 2002. Reward, motivation, and reinforcement learning. *Neuron* 36:285–298.

DAYAN, P., S. KAKADE, and P. R. MONTAGUE, 2000. Learning and selective attention. *Nat. Neurosci.* 3(Suppl):1218–1223.

DONALDSON, D. I., S. E. PETERSEN, and R. L. BUCKNER, 2001. Dissociating memory retrieval processes using fMRI: Evidence that priming does not support recognition memory. *Neuron* 31:1047–1059.

DREVETS, W. C., 1998. Functional neuroimaging studies of depression: The anatomy of melancholia. *Annu. Rev. Med.* 49:341–361.

DREVETS, W. C., 2000. Functional anatomical abnormalities in limbic and prefrontal cortical structures in major depression. *Prog. Brain Res.* 126:413–431.

DREVETS, W. C., 2001. Neuroimaging and neuropathological studies of depression: Implications for the cognitive-emotional features of mood disorders. *Curr. Opin. Neurobiol.* 11:240–249.

DREVETS, W. C., E. FRANK, J. C. PRICE, D. J. KUPFER, D. HOLT, P. J. GREER, Y. HUANG, C. GAUTIER, and C. MATHIS, 1999. PET imaging of serotonin 1A receptor binding in depression. *Biol. Psychiatry* 46:1375–1387.

DUNAH, A. W., H. JEONG, A. GRIFFIN, Y. M. KIM, D. G. STANDAERT, S. M. HERSCH, M. M. MOURADIAN, A. B. YOUNG, N. TANESE, and D. KRAINC, 2002. Sp1 and TAFII130 transcriptional activity disrupted in early Huntington's disease. *Science* 296:2238–2243.

EGAN, M. F., T. E. GOLDBERG, B. S. KOLACHANA, J. H. CALLICOTT, C. M. MAZZANTI, R. E. STRAUB, D. GOLDMAN, and D. R. WEINBERGER, 2001. Effect of COMT Val108/158 Met genotype on frontal lobe function and risk for schizophrenia. *Proc. Natl. Acad. Sci. U.S.A.* 98:6917–6922.

ELLIOTT, R., K. J. FRISTON, and R. J. DOLAN, 2000. Dissociable neural responses in human reward systems. *J. Neurosci.* 20:6159–6165.

ELLIOTT, R., J. L. NEWMAN, O. A. LONGE, and J. F. DEAKIN, 2003. Differential response patterns in the striatum and orbitofrontal cortex to financial reward in humans: A parametric functional magnetic resonance imaging study. *J. Neurosci.* 23:303–307.

ENARD, W., P. KHAITOVICH, J. KLOSE, S. ZOLLNER, F. HEISSIG, P. GIAVALISCO, K. NIESELT-STRUWE, E. MUCHMORE, A. VARKI, R. RAVID, et al., 2002. Intra- and interspecific variation in primate gene expression patterns. *Science* 296:340–343.

EVERITT, B. J., 1978. Monoamines and sexual behaviour in non-human primates. *Ciba Found. Symp.* 62:329–358.

FAVA, M., and K. S. KENDLER, 2000. Major depressive disorder. *Neuron* 28:335–341.

FITZGERALD, K. D., G. J. MOORE, L. A. PAULSON, C. M. STEWART, and D. R. ROSENBERG, 2000. Proton spectroscopic imaging of the thalamus in treatment-naive pediatric obsessive-compulsive disorder. *Biol. Psychiatry* 47:174–182.

FOWLER, J. S., N. D. VOLKOW, G. J. WANG, N. PAPPAS, J. LOGAN, R. MACGREGOR, D. ALEXOFF, C. SHEA, D. SCHLYER, A. P. WOLF, et al., 1996. Inhibition of monoamine oxidase B in the brains of smokers. *Nature* 379:733–736.

FRANKLIN, T. R., P. D. ACTON, J. A. MALDJIAN, J. D. GRAY, J. R. CROFT, C. A. DACKIS, C. P. O'BRIEN, and A. R. CHILDRESS, 2002. Decreased gray matter concentration in the insular, orbitofrontal, cingulate, and temporal cortices of cocaine patients. *Biol. Psychiatry* 51:134–142.

FREEMAN, W. J., 2001. *How Brains Make Up Their Minds.* New York: Columbia University Press.

FREEMAN, W. J., and J. M. BARRIE, 1994. Chaotic oscillations and the genesis of meaning in cerebral cortex. In *Temporal Coding in the Brain,* G. Buszaki et al., eds. Berlin: Springer-Verlag.

FRISTON, K., 2002. Beyond phrenology: What can neuroimaging tell us about distributed circuitry? *Annu. Rev. Neurosci.* 25:221–250.

GALLISTEL, C. R., 1978. Self-stimulation in the rat: Quantitative characteristics of the reward pathway. *J. Comp. Physiol. Psychol.* 92:977–998.

GALLISTEL, C. R., 1990. *The Organization of Learning.* Cambridge, Mass.: MIT Press.

GARAVAN, H., J. PANKIEWICZ, A. BLOOM, J. K. CHO, L. SPERRY, T. J. ROSS, B. J. SALMERON, R. RISINGER, D. KELLEY, and E. A. STEIN, 2000. Cue-induced cocaine craving: Neuroanatomical specificity for drug users and drug stimuli. *Am. J. Psychiatry* 157:1789–1798.

GERSHON, E. S., J. R. KELSOE, K. S. KENDLER, and J. D. WATSON, 2001. A scientific opportunity. *Science* 294:957.

GLIMCHER, P., 2003. *Decisions, Uncertainty, and the Brain: The Science of Neuroeconomics.* Cambridge, Mass.: MIT Press.

GOLDSTEIN, J. M., J. M. GOODMAN, L. J. SEIDMAN, D. N. KENNEDY, N. MAKRIS, H. LEE, J. TOURVILLE, V. S. CAVINESS, JR., S. V. FARAONE, and M. T. TSUANG, 1999. Cortical abnormalities in schizophrenia identified by structural magnetic resonance imaging. *Arch. Gen. Psychiatry* 56:537–547.

GOLDSTEIN, R. Z., N. D. VOLKOW, G. J. WANG, J. S. FOWLER, and S. RAJARAM, 2001. Addiction changes orbitofrontal gyrus function: Involvement in response inhibition. *Neuroreport* 12: 2595–2599.

GRANT, S., E. D. LONDON, D. B. NEWLIN, V. L. VILLEMAGNE, X. LIU, C. CONTOREGGI, R. L. PHILLIPS, A. S. KIMES, and A. MARGOLIN, 1996. Activation of memory circuits during cue-elicited cocaine craving. *Proc. Natl. Acad. Sci. U.S.A.* 93:12040–12045.

GRAYBIEL, A. M., and S. L. RAUCH, 2000. Toward a neurobiology of obsessive-compulsive disorder. *Neuron* 28:343–347.

GUSELLA, J. F., N. S. WEXLER, P. M. CONNEALLY, S. L. NAYLOR, M. A. ANDERSON, R. E. TANZI, P. C. WATKINS, K. OTTINA, M. R. WALLACE, A. Y. SAKAGUCHI, et al., 1983. A polymorphic DNA marker genetically linked to Huntington's disease. *Nature* 306:234–238.

HARIRI, A. R., V. S. MATTAY, A. TESSITORE, B. KOLACHANA, F. FERA, D. GOLDMAN, M. F. EGAN, and D. R. WEINBERGER, 2002. Serotonin transporter genetic variation and the response of the human amygdala. *Science* 297:400–403.

HAUSER, M. D., N. CHOMSKY, and W. T. FITCH, 2002. The faculty of language: What is it, who has it, and how did it evolve? *Science* 298:1569–1579.

HAXBY, J. V., C. L. GRADY, B. HORWITZ, L. G. UNGERLEIDER, M. MISHKIN, R. E. CARSON, P. HERSCOVITCH, M. B. SCHAPIRO, and S. I. RAPOPORT, 1991. Dissociation of object and spatial visual processing pathways in human extrastriate cortex. *Proc. Natl. Acad. Sci. U.S.A.* 88:1621–1625.

HECKERS, S., T. CURRAN, D. GOFF, S. L. RAUCH, A. J. FISCHMAN, N. M. ALPERT, and D. L. SCHACTER, 2000. Abnormalities in the thalamus and prefrontal cortex during episodic object recognition in schizophrenia. *Biol. Psychiatry* 48:651–657.

HECKERS, S., A. P. WEISS, N. M. ALPERT, and D. L. SCHACTER, 2002. Hippocampal and brain stem activation during word retrieval after repeated and semantic encoding. *Cereb. Cortex* 12:900–907.

HEIMER, L., R. E. HARLAN, G. F. ALHEID, M. M. GARCIA, and J. DE OLMOS, 1997. Substantia innominata: A notion which impedes clinical-anatomical correlations in neuropsychiatric disorders. *Neuroscience* 76:957–1006.

HEPPNER, F. L., C. MUSAHL, I. ARRIGHI, M. A. KLEIN, T. RULICKE, B. OESCH, R. M. ZINKERNAGEL, U. KALINKE, and A. AGUZZI, 2001. Prevention of scrapie pathogenesis by transgenic expression of anti-prion protein antibodies. *Science* 294:178–182.

HERRNSTEIN, R. J., 1971. Quantitative hedonism. *J. Psychiatr. Res.* 8:399–412.

HERRNSTEIN, R. J., and D. H. LOVELAND, 1974. Hunger and contrast in a multiple schedule. *J. Exp. Anal. Behav.* 21:511–517.

HILL, A. V., 2001. The genomics and genetics of human infectious disease susceptibility. *Annu. Rev. Genomics Hum. Genet.* 2:373–400.

The Huntington's Disease Collaborative Research Group, 1993. A novel gene containing a trinucleotide repeat that is expanded and unstable on Huntington's disease chromosomes. *Cell* 72:971–983.

HYMAN, S. E., 2002. Neuroscience, genetics, and the future of psychiatric diagnosis. *Psychopathology* 35:139–144.

HYMAN, S. E., and R. C. MALENKA, 2001. Addiction and the brain: The neurobiology of compulsion and its persistence. *Nat. Rev. Neurosci.* 2:695–703.

JAMES, W., 1884. What is an emotion? *Mind* 9:188–205.

JANKOVIC, J., 2001. Tourette's syndrome. *N. Engl. J. Med.* 345: 1184–1192.

KAHNEMAN, D., and A. TVERSKY, 1979. Prospect theory: An analysis of decision under risk. *Econometrica* 47:263–291.

KELLEY, A. E., and K. C. BERRIDGE, 2002. The neuroscience of natural rewards: Relevance to addictive drugs. *J. Neurosci.* 22:3306–3311.

KETTER, T. A., P. J. ANDREASON, M. S. GEORGE, C. LEE, D. S. GILL, P. I. PAREKH, M. W. WILLIS, P. HERSCOVITCH, and R. M. POST, 1996. Anterior paralimbic mediation of procaine-induced emotional and psychosensory experiences. *Arch. Gen. Psychiatry* 53:59–69.

KETTER, T. A., T. A. KIMBRELL, M. S. GEORGE, R. T. DUNN, A. M. SPEER, B. E. BENSON, M. W. WILLIS, A. DANIELSON, M. A. FRYE, P. HERSCOVITCH, et al., 2001. Effects of mood and subtype on cerebral glucose metabolism in treatment-resistant bipolar disorder. *Biol. Psychiatry* 49:97–109.

KIRSCHNER, M., and J. GERHART, 1998. Evolvability. *Proc. Natl. Acad. Sci. U.S.A.* 95:8420–8427.

KNUTSON, B., C. M. ADAMS, G. W. FONG, and D. HOMMER, 2001. Anticipation of increasing monetary reward selectively recruits nucleus accumbens. *J. Neurosci.* 21:RC159.

KNUTSON, B., G. W. FONG, C. M. ADAMS, J. L. VARNER, and D. HOMMER, 2001. Dissociation of reward anticipation and outcome with event-related fMRI. *Neuroreport* 12:3683–3687.

KOSSLYN, S. M., and L. M. SHIN, 1992. The status of cognitive neuroscience. *Curr. Opin. Neurobiol.* 2:146–149.

KREBS, J., and N. DAVIES, 1997. *Behavioural Ecology; An Evolutionary Perspective.* Oxford, England: Blackwell Science.

KRISHNAN, K. R., P. M. DORAISWAMY, G. S. FIGIEL, M. M. HUSAIN, S. A. SHAH, C. NA, O. B. BOYKO, W. M. MCDONALD, C. B. NEMEROFF, and E. H. ELLINWOOD, JR., 1991. Hippocampal abnormalities in depression. *J. Neuropsychiatry Clin. Neurosci.* 3:387–391.

KUNST-WILSON, W. R., and R. B. ZAJONC, 1980. Affective discrimination of stimuli that cannot be recognized. *Science* 207: 557–558.

KUPFERMAN, I., E. R. KANDEL, and S. IVERSEN, 2000. Motivational and addictive states. In *Principles of Neural Science*, T. Jessell, E. R. Kandel, and J. H. Schwartz, eds. New York: McGraw-Hill, pp. 998–1013.

LABAR, K. S., J. C. GATENBY, J. C. GORE, J. E. LEDOUX, and E. A. PHELPS, 1998. Human amygdala activation during conditioned fear acquisition and extinction: A mixed-trial fMRI study. *Neuron* 20:937–945.

LANGE, C. G., 1985. *Om Sindsbevaegelser et Psyko. Fysiolog. Studie.* Kromar, Copenhagen.

LEDOUX, J., 1996. *The Emotional Brain.* New York: Simon and Schuster.

LEDOUX, J. E., 2000. Emotion circuits in the brain. *Annu. Rev. Neurosci.* 23:155–184.

LEDOUX, J. E., A. SAKAGUCHI, J. IWATA, and D. J. REIS, 1985. Auditory emotional memories: Establishment by projections from the medial geniculate nucleus to the posterior neostriatum and/or dorsal amygdala. *Ann. N.Y. Acad. Sci.* 444:463–464.

LENOX, R. H., T. D. GOULD, and H. K. MANJI, 2002. Endophenotypes in bipolar disorder. *Am. J. Med. Genet.* 114:391–406.

LEWIS, D. A., and P. LEVITT, 2002. Schizophrenia as a disorder of neurodevelopment. *Annu. Rev. Neurosci.* 25:409–432.

Li, Y. J., W. K. Scott, D. J. Hedges, F. Zhang, P. C. Gaskell, M. A. Nance, R. L. Watts, J. P. Hubble, W. C. Koller, R. Pahwa, et al., 2002. Age at onset in two common neurodegenerative diseases is genetically controlled. *Am. J. Hum. Genet.* 70:985–993.

Li, S. J., Y. Wang, J. Pankiewicz, and E. A. Stein, 1999. Neurochemical adaptation to cocaine abuse: Reduction of *N*-acetyl aspartate in thalamus of human cocaine abusers. *Biol. Psychiatry* 45:1481–1487.

Lindvall, O., and A. Bjorklund, 1974. The organization of the ascending catecholamine neuron systems in the rat brain as revealed by the glyoxylic acid fluorescence method. *Acta Physiol. Scand. Suppl.* 412:1–48.

Liu, Y., J. H. Gao, H. L. Liu, and P. T. Fox, 2000. The temporal response of the brain after eating revealed by functional MRI. *Nature* 405:1058–1062.

Makris, N., J. W. Meyer, J. F. Bates, E. H. Yeterian, D. N. Kennedy, and V. S. Caviness, 1999. MRI-based topographic parcellation of human cerebral white matter and nuclei. II. Rationale and applications with systematics of cerebral connectivity. *NeuroImage* 9:18–45.

Manji, H. K., W. C. Drevets, and D. S. Charney, 2001. The cellular neurobiology of depression. *Nat. Med.* 7:541–547.

Manoach, D. S., R. L. Gollub, E. S. Benson, M. M. Searl, D. C. Goff, E. Halpern, C. B. Saper, and S. L. Rauch, 2000. Schizophrenic subjects show aberrant fMRI activation of dorsolateral prefrontal cortex and basal ganglia during working memory performance. *Biol. Psychiatry* 48:99–109.

Manoach, D. S., E. F. Halpern, T. S. Kramer, Y. Chang, D. C. Goff, S. L. Rauch, D. N. Kennedy, and R. L. Gollub, 2001. Test-retest reliability of a functional MRI working memory paradigm in normal and schizophrenic subjects. *Am. J. Psychiatry* 158:955–958.

Manoach, D. S., K. A. Lindgren, M. V. Cherkasova, D. C. Goff, E. F. Halpern, J. Intriligator, and J. J. Barton, 2002. Schizophrenic subjects show deficient inhibition but intact task switching on saccadic tasks. *Biol. Psychiatry* 51:816–826.

Marr, D., 1982. *A Computational Investigation Into the Human Representation and Processing of Visual Information.* San Francisco: Freeman.

Mazur, J. E., 1994. Effects of intertrial reinforcers on self-control choice. *J. Exp. Anal. Behav.* 61:83–96.

Mazur, J. E., and W. Vaughan, Jr., 1987. Molar optimization versus delayed reinforcement as explanations of choice between fixed-ratio and progressive-ratio schedules. *J. Exp. Anal. Behav.* 48:251–261.

McClelland, J. L., and D. E. Rumelhart, 1985. Distributed memory and the representation of general and specific information. *J. Exp. Psychol. Gen.* 114:159–197.

Mellers, B. A., 2000. Choice and the relative pleasure of consequences. *Psychol. Bull.* 126:910–924.

Mellers, B. A., A. Schwartz, and A. D. Cooke, 1998. Judgment and decision making. *Annu. Rev. Psychol.* 49:447–477.

Mellers, B. A., A. Schwartz, K. Ho, and I. Ritov, 1997. Decision affect theory: How we feel about risky options. *Psychol. Sci.* 8:423–429.

Mesulam, M., 2000. *Principles of Behavioral and Cognitive Neurology.* Oxford, England: Oxford University Press.

Meyer, J. W., N. Makris, J. F. Bates, V. S. Caviness, and D. N. Kennedy, 1999. MRI-based topographic parcellation of human cerebral white matter. *NeuroImage* 9:1–17.

Miller, G. A., 2003. The cognitive revolution: A historical perspective. *Trends Cogn. Sci.* 7:141–144.

Narr, K. L., T. D. Cannon, R. P. Woods, P. M. Thompson, S. Kim, D. Asunction, T. G. van Erp, V. P. Poutanen, M. Huttunen, J. Lonnqvist, et al., 2002. Genetic contributions to altered callosal morphology in schizophrenia. *J. Neurosci.* 22:3720–3729.

Nestler, E. J., M. Barrot, R. J. DiLeone, A. J. Eisch, S. J. Gold, and L. M. Monteggia, 2002. Neurobiology of depression. *Neuron* 34:13–25.

Nicholls, R. D., and J. L. Knepper, 2001. Genome organization, function, and imprinting in Prader-Willi and Angelman syndromes. *Annu. Rev. Genomics. Hum. Genet.* 2:153–175.

Nicotera, P., 2001. A route for prion neuroinvasion. *Neuron* 31:345–348.

Nordahl, T. E., C. Benkelfat, W. E. Semple, M. Gross, A. C. King, and R. M. Cohen, 1989. Cerebral glucose metabolic rates in obsessive compulsive disorder. *Neuropsychopharmacology* 2:23–28.

O'Brien, S. J., G. W. Nelson, C. A. Winkler, and M. W. Smith, 2000. Polygenic and multifactorial disease gene association in man: Lessons from AIDS. *Annu. Rev. Genet.* 34:563–591.

O'Doherty, J., M. L. Kringelbach, E. T. Rolls, J. Hornak, and C. Andrews, 2001. Abstract reward and punishment representations in the human orbitofrontal cortex. *Nat. Neurosci.* 4:95–102.

O'Doherty, J., E. T. Rolls, S. Francis, R. Bowtell, and F. McGlone, 2001. Representation of pleasant and aversive taste in the human brain. *J. Neurophysiol.* 85:1315–1321.

O'Doherty, J. P., R. Deichmann, H. D. Critchley, and R. J. Dolan, 2002. Neural responses during anticipation of a primary taste reward. *Neuron* 33:815–826.

Okazawa, H., T. Rich, A. Chang, X. Lin, M. Waragai, M. Kajikawa, Y. Enokido, A. Komuro, S. Kato, M. Shibata, et al., 2002. Interaction between mutant ataxin-1 and PQBP-1 affects transcription and cell death. *Neuron* 34:701–713.

Olds, J., and P. M. Milner, 1954. Positive reinforcement produced by electrical stimulation of the septal area and other regions of the rat brain. *J. Comp. Physiol. Psychol.* 47:419–427.

Ongur, D., W. C. Drevets, and J. L. Price, 1998. Glial reduction in the subgenual prefrontal cortex in mood disorders. *Proc. Natl. Acad. Sci. U.S.A.* 95:13290–13295.

Opal, P., and H. Y. Zoghbi, 2002. The role of chaperones in polyglutamine disease. *Trends Mol. Med.* 8:232–236.

Perani, D., C. Colombo, S. Bressi, A. Bonfanti, F. Grassi, S. Scarone, L. Bellodi, E. Smeraldi, and F. Fazio, 1995. [18F]FDG PET study in obsessive-compulsive disorder: A clinical/metabolic correlation study after treatment. *Br. J. Psychiatry* 166:244–250.

Phelps, E. A., K. J. O'Connor, J. C. Gatenby, J. C. Gore, C. Grillon, and M. Davis, 2001. Activation of the left amygdala to a cognitive representation of fear. *Nat. Neurosci.* 4:437–441.

Pliakas, A. M., R. R. Carlson, R. L. Neve, C. Konradi, E. J. Nestler, and W. A. Carlezon, Jr., 2001. Altered responsiveness to cocaine and increased immobility in the forced swim test associated with elevated cAMP response element-binding protein expression in nucleus accumbens. *J. Neurosci.* 21:7397–7403.

Ploghaus, A., I. Tracey, J. S. Gati, S. Clare, R. S. Menon, P. M. Matthews, and J. N. Rawlins, 1999. Dissociating pain from its anticipation in the human brain. *Science* 284:1979–1981.

Porjesz, B., L. Almasy, H. J. Edenberg, K. Wang, D. B. Chorlian, T. Foroud, A. Goate, J. P. Rice, S. J. O'Connor, J. Rohrbaugh, et al., 2002. Linkage disequilibrium between the beta frequency of the human EEG and a GABAA receptor gene locus. *Proc. Natl. Acad. Sci. U.S.A.* 99:3729–3733.

Prigogine, I., 1985. The rediscovery of time. In *Science and Complexity*, S. Nash, ed. Northwood, Middlesex, England: Science Reviews.

QUEITSCH, C., T. A. SANGSTER, and S. LINDQUIST, 2002. Hsp90 as a capacitor of phenotypic variation. *Nature* 417:618–624.

RACHLIN, H., A. RAINERI, and D. CROSS, 1991. Subjective probability and delay. *J. Exp. Anal. Behav.* 55:233–244.

RAINVILLE, P., M. C. BUSHNELL, and G. H. DUNCAN, 2001. Representation of acute and persistent pain in the human CNS: Potential implications for chemical intolerance. *Ann. N.Y. Acad. Sci.* 933:130–141.

RAINVILLE, P., G. H. DUNCAN, D. D. PRICE, B. CARRIER, and M. C. BUSHNELL, 1997. Pain affect encoded in human anterior cingulate but not somatosensory cortex. *Science* 277:968–971.

RAJKOWSKA, G., A. HALARIS, and L. D. SELEMON, 2001. Reductions in neuronal and glial density characterize the dorsolateral prefrontal cortex in bipolar disorder. *Biol. Psychiatry* 49:741–752.

RAJKOWSKA, G., J. J. MIGUEL-HIDALGO, J. WEI, G. DILLEY, S. D. PITTMAN, H. Y. MELTZER, J. C. OVERHOLSER, B. L. ROTH, and C. A. STOCKMEIER, 1999. Morphometric evidence for neuronal and glial prefrontal cell pathology in major depression. *Biol. Psychiatry* 45:1085–1098.

RAUCH, S. L., C. R. SAVAGE, N. M. ALPERT, A. J. FISCHMAN, and M. A. JENIKE, 1997. The functional neuroanatomy of anxiety: A study of three disorders using positron emission tomography and symptom provocation. *Biol. Psychiatry* 42:446–452.

RAUCH, S. L., P. J. WHALEN, L. M. SHIN, S. C. MCINERNEY, M. L. MACKLIN, N. B. LASKO, S. P. ORR, and R. K. PITMAN, 2000. Exaggerated amygdala response to masked facial stimuli in posttraumatic stress disorder: A functional MRI study. *Biol. Psychiatry* 47:769–776.

REICH, T., A. HINRICHS, R. CULVERHOUSE, and L. BIERUT, 1999. Genetic studies of alcoholism and substance dependence. *Am. J. Hum. Genet.* 65:599–605.

ROBBINS, T. W., and B. J. EVERITT, 2002. Limbic-striatal memory systems and drug addiction. *Neurobiol. Learn. Mem.* 78:625–636.

RUTHERFORD, S. L., and S. LINDQUIST, 1998. Hsp90 as a capacitor for morphological evolution. *Nature* 396:336–342.

SAPIENZA, C., and J. G. HALL, 2001. Genome imprinting in human disease. In *The Metabolic and Molecular Bases of Inherited Disease,* C. R. Scriver et al., eds. New York: McGraw-Hill.

SAPOLSKY, R. M., 2001. Depression, antidepressants, and the shrinking hippocampus. *Proc. Natl. Acad. Sci. U.S.A.* 98:12320–12322.

SAWA, A., and S. H. SNYDER, 2002. Schizophrenia: diverse approaches to a complex disease. *Science* 296:692–695.

SAWAMOTO, N., M. HONDA, T. OKADA, T. HANAKAWA, M. KANDA, H. FUKUYAMA, J. KONISHI, and H. SHIBASAKI, 2000. Expectation of pain enhances responses to nonpainful somatosensory stimulation in the anterior cingulate cortex and parietal operculum/posterior insula: An event-related functional magnetic resonance imaging study. *J. Neurosci.* 20:7438–7445.

SAWLE, G. V., N. F. HYMAS, A. J. LEES, and R. S. FRACKOWIAK, 1991. Obsessional slowness: Functional studies with positron emission tomography. *Brain* 114(Pt. 5):2191–2202.

SAXENA, S., A. L. BRODY, M. L. HO, S. ALBORZIAN, M. K. HO, K. M. MAIDMENT, S. C. HUANG, H. M. WU, S. C. AU, and L. R. BAXTER, JR., 2001. Cerebral metabolism in major depression and obsessive-compulsive disorder occurring separately and concurrently. *Biol. Psychiatry* 50:159–170.

SCHNEIER, F. R., M. R. LIEBOWITZ, A. ABI-DARGHAM, Y. ZEA-PONCE, S. H. LIN, and M. LARUELLE, 2000. Low dopamine D(2) receptor binding potential in social phobia. *Am. J. Psychiatry* 157:457–459.

SCHUFF, N., T. C. NEYLAN, M. A. LENOCI, A. T. DU, D. S. WEISS, C. R. MARMAR, and M. W. WEINER, 2001. Decreased hippocampal *N*-acetylaspartate in the absence of atrophy in posttraumatic stress disorder. *Biol. Psychiatry* 50:952–959.

SCHULTZ, W., 2000. Multiple reward signals in the brain. *Nat. Rev. Neurosci.* 1:199–207.

SCHULTZ, W., 2002. Getting formal with dopamine and reward. *Neuron* 36:241–263.

SCHULTZ, W., P. DAYAN, and P. R. MONTAGUE, 1997. A neural substrate of prediction and reward. *Science* 275:1593–1599.

SEIDMAN, L. J., H. C. BREITER, J. M. GOODMAN, J. M. GOLDSTEIN, P. W. WOODRUFF, K. O'CRAVEN, R. SAVOY, M. T. TSUANG, and B. R. ROSEN, 1998. A functional magnetic resonance imaging study of auditory vigilance with low and high information processing demands. *Neuropsychology* 12:505–518.

SHAHBAZIAN, M. D., B. ANTALFFY, D. L. ARMSTRONG, and H. Y. ZOGHBI, 2002. Insight into Rett syndrome: MeCP2 levels display tissue- and cell-specific differences and correlate with neuronal maturation. *Hum. Mol. Genet.* 11:115–124.

SHAHBAZIAN, M. D., and H. Y. ZOGHBI, 2002. Rett syndrome and MeCP2: Linking epigenetics and neuronal function. *Am. J. Hum. Genet.* 71:1259–1272.

SHANNON, C. E., and W. WEAVER, 1949. *The Mathematical Theory of Communication.* Urbana: University of Illinois Press.

SHENTON, M. E., C. C. DICKEY, M. FRUMIN, and R. W. MCCARLEY, 2001. A review of MRI findings in schizophrenia. *Schizophr. Res.* 49:1–52.

SHERMAN, M. Y., and A. L. GOLDBERG, 2001. Cellular defenses against unfolded proteins: A cell biologist thinks about neurodegenerative diseases. *Neuron* 29:15–32.

SHIZGAL, P., 1997. Neural basis of utility estimation. *Curr. Opin. Neurobiol.* 7:198–208.

SHIZGAL, P., 1999. On the neural computation of utility: Implications from studies of brain stimulation reward. In *Well-Being: The Foundations of Hedonic Psychology,* D. Kahneman, E. Diener, and N. Schwarz, eds. New York: Russell Sage Foundation, pp. 502–506.

SMALL, D. M., R. J. ZATORRE, A. DAGHER, A. C. EVANS, and M. JONES-GOTMAN, 2001. Changes in brain activity related to eating chocolate: From pleasure to aversion. *Brain* 124:1720–1733.

SPINOZA, B., 1883. On the origin and nature of emotions. In *The Ethics,* R. H. M. Elwes, ed. Princeton, N.J.: Princeton University Press, pp. 1–132.

STOLL, M., A. W. COWLEY, JR., P. J. TONELLATO, A. S. GREENE, M. L. KALDUNSKI, R. J. ROMAN, P. DUMAS, N. J. SCHORK, Z. WANG, and H. J. JACOB, 2001. A genomic-systems biology map for cardiovascular function. *Science* 294:1723–1726.

SUTTON, J., and H. C. BREITER, 1994. Neural scale invariance: An integrative model with implications for neuropathology. *World Congress Neural Netw.* 4:667–672.

SUTTON, R. S., and A. G. BARTO, 1981. Toward a modern theory of adaptive networks: Expectation and prediction. *Psychol. Rev.* 88:135–170.

SWEDO, S. E., M. B. SCHAPIRO, C. L. GRADY, D. L. CHESLOW, H. L. LEONARD, A. KUMAR, R. FRIEDLAND, S. I. RAPOPORT, and J. L. RAPOPORT, 1989. Cerebral glucose metabolism in childhood-onset obsessive-compulsive disorder. *Arch. Gen. Psychiatry* 46:518–523.

TAGER-FLUSBERG, H., 1999. *Neurodevelopmental Disorders.* Cambridge, Mass.: MIT Press.

TALBOT, J. D., S. MARRETT, A. C. EVANS, E. MEYER, M. C. BUSHNELL, and G. H. DUNCAN, 1991. Multiple representations of pain in human cerebral cortex. *Science* 251:1355–1358.

THOMPSON, P. M., T. D. CANNON, K. L. NARR, T. VAN ERP, V. P. POUTANEN, M. HUTTUNEN, J. LONNQVIST, C. G. STANDERTSKJOLD-NORDENSTAM, J. KAPRIO, M. KHALEDY, et al., 2001. Genetic influences on brain structure. *Nat. Neurosci.* 4:1253–1258.

THUT, G., W. SCHULTZ, U. ROELCKE, M. NIENHUSMEIER, J. MISSIMER, R. P. MAGUIRE, and K. L. LEENDERS, 1997. Activation of the human brain by monetary reward. *Neuroreport* 8:1225–1228.

TRUE, H. L., and S. L. LINDQUIST, 2000. A yeast prion provides a mechanism for genetic variation and phenotypic diversity. *Nature* 407:477–483.

TVERSKY, A., and D. KAHNEMAN, 1992. Advances in prospect theory: Cumulative representation of uncertainty. *J. Risk Uncertainty* 5:297–323.

VOLKOW, N. D., L. CHANG, G. J. WANG, J. S. FOWLER, Y. S. DING, M. SEDLER, J. LOGAN, D. FRANCESCHI, J. GATLEY, R. HITZEMANN, et al., 2001. Low level of brain dopamine D2 receptors in methamphetamine abusers: Association with metabolism in the orbitofrontal cortex. *Am. J. Psychiatry* 158:2015–2021.

VOLKOW, N. D., J. S. FOWLER, A. P. WOLF, R. HITZEMANN, S. DEWEY, B. BENDRIEM, R. ALPERT, and A. HOFF, 1991. Changes in brain glucose metabolism in cocaine dependence and withdrawal. *Am. J. Psychiatry* 148:621–626.

VOLKOW, N. D., Y. S. DING, J. S. FOWLER, G. J. WANG, J. LOGAN, J. S. GATLEY, S. DEWEY, C. ASHBY, J. LIEBERMANN, R. HITZEMANN, et al., 1995. Is methylphenidate like cocaine? Studies on their pharmacokinetics and distribution in the human brain. *Arch. Gen. Psychiatry* 52:456–463.

VOLKOW, N. D., G. J. WANG, J. S. FOWLER, S. J. GATLEY, Y. S. DING, J. LOGAN, S. L. DEWEY, R. HITZEMANN, and J. LIEBERMAN, 1996. Relationship between psychostimulant-induced "high" and dopamine transporter occupancy. *Proc. Natl. Acad. Sci. U.S.A.* 93:10388–10392.

VOLKOW, N. D., G. J. WANG, M. W. FISCHMAN, R. W. FOLTIN, J. S. FOWLER, N. N. ABUMRAD, S. VITKUN, J. LOGAN, S. J. GATLEY, N. PAPPAS, et al., 1997. Relationship between subjective effects of cocaine and dopamine transporter occupancy. *Nature* 386:827–830.

VOLKOW, N. D., G. J. WANG, J. S. FOWLER, D. FRANCESCHI, P. K. THANOS, C. WONG, S. J. GATLEY, Y. S. DING, P. MOLINA, D. SCHLYER, et al., 2000. Cocaine abusers show a blunted response to alcohol intoxication in limbic brain regions. *Life Sci.* 66:PL161–167.

VRANA, P. B., J. A. FOSSELLA, P. MATTESON, T. DEL RIO, M. J. O'NEILL, and S. M. TILGHMAN, 2000. Genetic and epigenetic incompatibilities underlie hybrid dysgenesis in Peromyscus. *Nat. Genet.* 25:120–124.

WAGNER, A. D., D. L. SCHACTER, M. ROTTE, W. KOUTSTAAL, A. MARIL, A. M. DALE, B. R. ROSEN, and R. L. BUCKNER, 1998. Building memories: Remembering and forgetting of verbal experiences as predicted by brain activity. *Science* 281:1188–1191.

WATASE, K., E. J. WEEBER, B. XU, B. ANTALFFY, L. YUVA-PAYLOR, K. HASHIMOTO, M. KANO, R. ATKINSON, Y. SUN, D. L. ARMSTRONG, et al., 2002. A long CAG repeat in the mouse Sca1 locus replicates SCA1 features and reveals the impact of protein solubility on selective neurodegeneration. *Neuron* 34:905–919.

WATTS, A. G., and L. W. SWANSON, 2002. Anatomy of motivation. In *Stevens' Handbook of Experimental Psychology: Learning, Motivation, and Emotion*, vol. 3., H. Pasher and C. R. Gallistel, eds. New York: Wiley.

WILLIAMS, J. T., H. BEGLEITER, B. PORJESZ, H. J. EDENBERG, T. FOROUD, T. REICH, A. GOATE, P. VAN EERDEWEGH, L. ALMASY, and J. BLANGERO, 1999. Joint multipoint linkage analysis of multivariate qualitative and quantitative traits. II. Alcoholism and event-related potentials. *Am. J. Hum. Genet.* 65:1148–1160.

WISE, R. A., 1978. Catecholamine theories of reward: A critical review. *Brain Res.* 152:215–247.

WISE, R. A., 2002. Brain reward circuitry: Insights from unsensed incentives. *Neuron* 36:229–240.

ZEKI, S., 2001. Localization and globalization in conscious vision. *Annu. Rev. Neurosci.* 24:57–86.

ZOGHBI, H. Y., 2001. Rett syndrome. In *The Metabolic and Molecular Bases of Inherited Disease*, C. R. Scriver, et al., eds. New York: McGraw-Hill.

76 A Self Less Ordinary: The Medial Prefrontal Cortex and You

C. NEIL MACRAE, TODD F. HEATHERTON, AND WILLIAM M. KELLEY

ABSTRACT Questions of self have perplexed thinkers for centuries. What is the nature of self-knowledge? How does one recognize oneself? Is self-referential processing supported by distinct neural operations? Reflecting contemporary interest in core aspects of social-cognitive functioning, discussion in this chapter centers on the issue of what it might mean to be a social agent in possession of a self. In pursuit of this objective, consideration is given to the role of medial prefrontal cortex (MPFC) in self-referential processing and in mentalizing (i.e., theory of mind), cognitive operations that are fundamental components of human social cognition.

Is there anything, apart from a really good chocolate cream pie and receiving a large unexpected check in the post, to beat finding yourself.

—Bill Bryson, *Neither Here Nor There*

As Bill Bryson observes, finding yourself can be a pretty big deal. A beguiling feature of the human condition is the constant quest for self-knowledge and personal understanding. Setting self apart from others, identifying one's true inner nature, and establishing one's unique place in the world are goals that motivate the behavior of most healthy individuals. Why else would people pierce their nipples, backpack across the globe, or lie on a bed of nails for apparent entertainment? In the search for personal enlightenment, the truth must surely be out there, if only one could find it. Regrettably, however, the truth (or at least some approximation thereof) is notoriously difficult to find.

Questions of self have perplexed thinkers for centuries, so much so that many have denied that the topic is even worthy of experimental scrutiny. For some, self is little more than a "ghost in the machine" (Ryle, 1949), a cognitive specter that has neither scientific status nor credibility. Yet this is patently not the self with which we are all familiar, the self that guides our daily actions in a purposive, meaningful manner. Whether we select cheesecake, apple pie, or chocolate ice cream, one thing is abundantly clear: we (or rather I) do the choosing. In the realm of everyday experience, ghost, ghoul, or bogeyman fall short of capturing the role of self in social

cognition. An arguably better metaphor is that of self as agent, if without the gadgets and bald adversary.

What unquestionably impeded scientific understanding of self for many years was that, as an agent, self was very much of the secret variety. Lurking in the cognitive shadows, self was difficult to detect, isolate, and measure. As a result, it had all the properties of a metaphysical entity, and thus was to be avoided. The advent of cognitive psychology, however, dramatically reshaped the experimental landscape. Armed with a host of new methods and measuring instruments, psychologists were able to explore the cognitive operations (and structures) that guide human behavior. Self (and self-function) was suddenly exposed. This public unveiling of self has since been taken a step further with the rise of cognitive neuroscience and the emergence of functional brain imaging (e.g., positron emission tomography [PET], functional magnetic resonance imaging [fMRI], magnetoencephalography [MEG]) as an exploratory tool. Suddenly, hitherto baffling questions have become empirically tractable and open to debate. What is the nature of self-knowledge? How does one recognize oneself? Is self-referential processing supported by distinct neural operations? Questions that were previously outside the purview of scientific investigation are now amenable to direct empirical inquiry. Reflecting this contemporary interest in core aspects of social-cognitive functioning, the discussion in this chapter centers on the issue of what it might mean to be a social agent in possession of a self. As is the case in any emerging area of inquiry, more questions will inevitably be raised than answers provided. Nevertheless, we hope to demonstrate the utility of applying a social brain sciences approach to an obdurate problem in social psychology—the nature and status of self-referential processing. In pursuit of this objective, we will consider the functional significance of medial prefrontal cortex (MPFC) in self-referential processing and in mentalizing (i.e., theory of mind), cognitive operations that are fundamental components of human social cognition.

The search for self

Although a common term in everyday parlance, formal definitions of the self have proved to be elusive. Kihlstrom and

C. NEIL MACRAE, TODD F. HEATHERTON, and WILLIAM M. KELLEY Department of Psychological and Brain Sciences, Dartmouth College, Hanover, N.H.

Klein (1997), however, have provided one useful conceptual framework. Emphasizing the role of self as a repository of personal knowledge, Kihlstrom and Klein suggested that this material may fall into four broad categories: (1) a fuzzy set of context-specific selves (e.g., self at work, self in relationships), (2) a narrative self that provides one with a sense of temporal continuity (e.g., historical me vs. current me), (3) an image-based representation of self (e.g., visual self-image), and (4) an associative network that contains material pertaining to one's personality, autobiographical memory, and behavioral record (e.g., self-knowledge). These distinct aspects of self suggest that any cortical representation of self-knowledge is likely to be distributed across a network of brain regions, much like other forms of semantic and episodic knowledge. But might this conception of self necessarily obscure potentially unique aspects of self-referential processing? Is self really just an ordinary cognitive structure?

An arguably unique human talent is the ability to reflect on one's immediate past ("Why did I kiss the secretary?") and to consider one's possible future ("Will her husband kill me?"). Indeed, it is this introspective ability that has prompted some leading thinkers to raise a number of vexing questions about the nature and status of the self (James, 1890). In the corridors of academia, this debate has centered on two fundamental questions. Is the self a unique cognitive structure? Does self-referential processing (i.e., considering information in the context of self) have some privileged status in the brain, or is it functionally equivalent to semantic processing about other classes of stimuli, such as speedboats, foodstuffs, and lingerie (Markus, 1977; Rogers, Kuiper, and Kirker, 1977; Bower and Gilligan, 1979; Maki and McCaul, 1985; Klein and Kihlstrom, 1986; Klein and Loftus, 1988)? Put simply, is self-referential processing special in any way?

Initial behavioral research suggested that self-referential processing may indeed possess some unique cognitive qualities (Rogers, Kuiper, and Kirker, 1977). The basis for this conclusion was the so-called self-reference effect in memory (see Symons and Johnson, 1997). Pioneering research by Rogers and colleagues showed that when trait adjectives (e.g., *happy*) were processed with reference to the self (e.g., "Does happy describe you?"), subsequent memory performance was better than when the items were processed only for their general meaning (e.g., "Does happy mean the same as optimistic?"). This classic levels-of-processing effect (Craik and Tulving, 1975) has since been replicated on many occasions, prompting researchers to consider the cognitive status of self-referential processing (Symons and Johnson, 1997). For the most part, controversy has centered on whether the self-reference effect in memory is indicative of the special functional role played by the self in human cognition.

Two putative explanations have been offered for the self-reference effect in memory. One account suggests that self is a unique cognitive structure that possesses special mnemonic abilities, hence the enhanced memorability of material processed in relation to self (Rogers, Kuiper, and Kirker, 1977; Maki and McCaul, 1985). An alternative viewpoint, however, argues that the self plays no special or unique role in cognition (i.e., no distinct structure or neural process is dedicated to self-referential processing). Rather, the memory enhancement that accompanies self-referential processing can be interpreted as a standard depth-of-processing effect (Klein and Kihlstrom, 1986; Greenwald and Banaji, 1989). The wealth of personal information that resides in memory encourages the elaborative encoding of material that is processed in relation to self (Klein and Loftus, 1988). In turn, this elaborative encoding enhances the memorability of self-relevant information. In other words, self is a powerful encoding device.

A frustrating feature of these competing accounts, however, is that they are difficult to evaluate using purely behavioral measures, because they make identical experimental predictions (i.e., enhanced memory for self-relevant material). For this reason, researchers have recently turned to neuroimaging techniques in an attempt to identify the basis of the self-reference effect in memory. As we shall discover, the message that emerges from this work is a provocative one. As a cognitive structure, self may be less ordinary than researchers have hitherto supposed (cf. Klein and Kihlstrom, 1986; Greenwald and Banaji, 1989).

Using PET, Craik and colleagues (1999) investigated the neural substrates of the self-reference effect in memory. The results of this study were intriguing, though frustratingly incomplete. During self-referential processing, distinct activations were observed in frontal regions, notably MPFC and areas of right prefrontal cortex. However, because these activations were not accompanied by a behavioral advantage for items processed in relation to self, it was not possible to conclude that the observed frontal activity was indicative of self-referential processing. Noting this limitation, Kelley and colleagues (2002) used event-related fMRI in an attempt to identify the neural signature of self-referential mental activity. In a standard self-reference paradigm, participants judged trait adjectives in one of three ways: *self* ("Does the trait describe you?), *other* ("Does the trait describe George Bush?"), and *case* ("Is the trait presented in uppercase letters?"). These judgments were expected to produce varying levels of subsequent memory performance (i.e., self > other > case). More important, they enabled Kelley and colleagues (2002) to test the competing explanations that have been offered for the self-reference effect in memory. Previous functional imaging studies have identified multiple regions within the left frontal cortex that are responsive to elaborate semantic encoding (Kapur et al., 1994; Demb et al., 1995; Gabrieli et al., 1996; Wagner et al., 1998; see also Buckner, Kelley, and Petersen, 1999). Thus, if the self-reference effect simply reflects the operation of such a process, then one would expect to observe elevated levels of activation in these left frontal areas when traits are judged in relation to self (figure 76.1*A*). If, however, the effect results from the properties of a unique cognitive self, then one might expect self-referential mental activity to engage brain regions that are distinct from those involved in general semantic processing (Craik et al., 1999).

Critically, Kelley and colleagues (2002) observed activity in areas of prefrontal cortex, notably MPFC (Brodmann's area [BA] 10), during self-referential processing (figure 76.1*B*). This result is noteworthy, as it suggests that MPFC may play a prominent role in the self memory system (Conway and Pleydell-Pearce, 2000). But what exactly is the nature of this role? Activity in MPFC accompanies self-referential processing, but does this activity contribute to the formation of memories in the brain? Reflecting the distributed nature of memory function, the neural correlates of memory formation appear to be related to the characteristics of the to-be-encoded material. Whereas the encoding of verbal information preferentially activates areas of left dorsal and inferior prefrontal cortex (Kapur et al., 1994; Demb et al., 1995; Dolan and Fletcher, 1997; Brewer et al., 1988; Kelley et al., 1998; Henson et al., 1999; Kirchhoff et al., 2000; Otten and Rugg, 2001; Otten, Henson, and Rugg, 2001), encoding of nonverbal, pictorial information is often associated with elevated levels of activity in homologous regions of right prefrontal cortex (Brewer et al., 1998; Kelley et al., 1998; Wagner et al., 1998). Emotional intensity is yet another factor that moderates the neural processes that support subsequent remembering, such that differential amygdala activation correlates with the memorability of emotional experiences (Cahill et al., 1996; Hamann et al., 1999; Canli et al., 2000; Hamann, 2001). These findings suggest that, depending on the characteristics of the to-be-encoded material, discrete brain regions support the memorability of prior experience.

In such a distributed system, it is probable that other cortical areas also contribute to memory formation, particularly if task demands encourage reliance on distinct processing operations. Thus, the MPFC activity that is indicative of self-referential processing may support the formation of self-relevant memories (Kelley et al., 2002). To investigate this possibility, Macrae and colleagues (in press) measured brain activity while participants judged the relevance of a series of personality characteristics. Afterward, memory for the items was tapped in a surprise recognition task. By contrasting brain activation elicited by items that were subsequently remembered with those that were forgotten (Brewer et al., 1998; Wagner et al., 1998), it was possible to identify brain regions that predict successful recognition. Importantly, Macrae and colleagues showed that subsequent memory was predicted by activity in MPFC during the encoding phase of

the task (i.e., the greater the MPFC activity, the more likely an item was to be remembered) (figure 76.2). Thus, not only does activity in MPFC track with self-referential processing, it also contributes to the formation of self-relevant memories. In this respect, MPFC would appear to be a critical component of the human memory system.

The observation that MPFC plays a critical role in self-referential processing is supported by evidence from a number of sources. Gusnard and colleagues (2001) used a block design fMRI paradigm to examine judgments about affectively normed pictures and observed MPFC activity that was preferentially associated with introspective judgments. Similarly, Johnson and colleagues (2002) found MPFC to be implicated in the mental operation of self-reflection. In their task, participants were required to respond to a series of questions that demanded access to either personal knowledge (e.g., "I have a quick temper") or general semantic knowledge (e.g., "10 seconds is more than a minute"). The results revealed that self-reflective thought was accompanied by activity in anterior regions of MPFC. The available neuropsychological evidence also confirms that MPFC plays a prominent role in self-referential processing (Stuss and Benson, 1986; Wheeler, Stuss, and Tulving, 1997). Impairments in the ability to self-reflect, introspect, and daydream have long been associated with damage to areas of prefrontal cortex. Indeed, Wheeler, Stuss, and Tulving (1997) have argued that persons with damage to specific areas of PFC may be unable to reflect on personal knowledge. It is possible that the self-reference effect in memory (Kelley et al., 2002) depends on an intact ability to be self-reflective, and that neural activity in MPFC reflects the operation of just such a process.

Thus, the message that emerges from research on the neural correlates of self-referential mental activity is quite unequivocal. When reflecting on aspects of self-knowledge—whether these be personality characteristics, autobiographical facts, or personal beliefs and opinions—MPFC plays a critical role in the execution of self-reflective thought. From this observation, one would therefore suspect that MPFC is a key component in the neural network that regulates core aspects of social-cognitive functioning (Baron-Cohen, 1995). As we shall discover, this intuition is bolstered when one considers other fundamental aspects of human social cognition. A central feature of social cognition is the ability to understand other minds, that is, to feel what other people feel and to know what other people know. Through the possession of what is termed a theory of mind, people are able to understand the goals and intentions that guide the behavior of others (Baron-Cohen, 1995; Frith and Frith, 1999). Interestingly, this core social-cognitive ability is also closely associated with activity in MPFC, thereby giving rise to an intriguing question: Could it be that the ability to understand others is related in some way to the process of

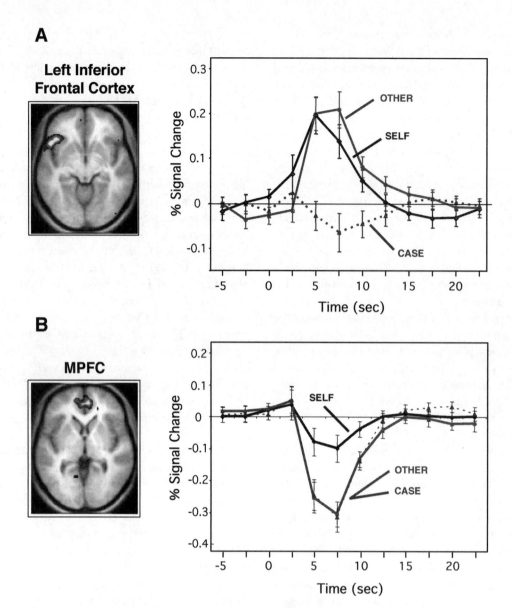

A

Left Inferior Frontal Cortex

B

MPFC

FIGURE 76.1 (*A*) LPFC activation, averaged across participants, demonstrates a greater response for semantic-based judgments than for surface-based judgments. The statistical image, comparing the two semantic tasks to the nonsemantic task, was created using a random effects model. Time courses are shown separately for each trial type. Time courses were generated in an unbiased manner using a region of interest (ROI) defined from an overall statistical image that compared all three tasks to baseline. Thus, each task contributed equally to the generation of the ROI. The ROI included all contiguous voxels within 10 mm of the peak that reached the significance level (*P* = 0.0001). (Reprinted with permission from W. M. Kelley et al., typist-repeat from part *B*, below.)

(*B*) Statistical activation maps directly comparing self and other trials demonstrate greater activity during self encoding trials in MPFC. Displayed at the bottom left is an axial section through the activation foci averaged across participants. Time courses are shown separately for each trial type. Time courses were computed for each condition within a three-dimensional region surrounding the peak voxel identified from an overall statistical image that compared all three tasks to baseline. Regions were defined using an automated algorithm that identified all contiguous voxels within 10 mm of the peak that reached the significance level (*P* < 0.0001). MPFC was the only brain region that was uniquely sensitive to self-encoding trials. (Reprinted with permission from W. M. Kelley et al., Finding the self: An event-related fMRI study. *J. Cogn. Neurosci.* 14:785–794. © 2002 by the Society for Neuroscience.)

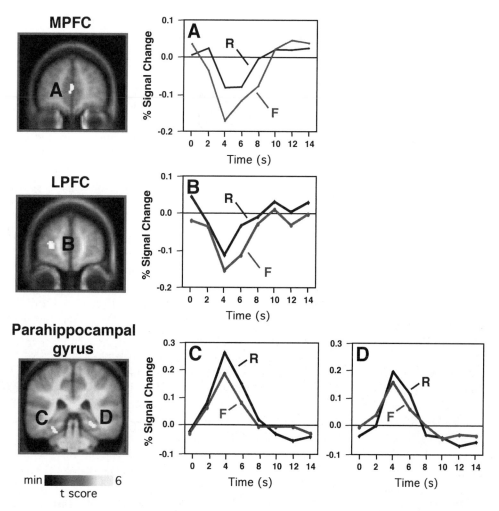

FIGURE 76.2 Statistical activation maps reveal brain regions that demonstrate greater activity during self-descriptive judgments of words later remembered relative to words later forgotten. Images are coronal sections averaged across participants. Greater activation was observed in medial prefrontal cortex (MPFC) (A: −1, 50, 5; BA 10), left anterior prefrontal cortex (LPFC) (B: −24, 58, 1; BA 10), and bilateral regions of the parahippocampal gyrus (C: −26, −31, −16, and D: 27, −33, −8). Time courses were computed for each condition in an unbiased manner by generating regions of interest from a combined statistical map compared to baseline. An automated algorithm identified all contiguous voxels within 10 mm of the peak that reached the significance level ($P < 0.0001$). The left side of the image corresponds to the left side of the brain. Regions were defined in an unbiased manner by comparing all self-reference trials to the baseline fixation task. (From Macrae et al., in press.)

self-understanding? We now turn to a consideration of this issue.

Understanding others

Humans are social animals. We live in groups and form and maintain important relationships with other people. Central to the ability to live harmoniously with others is the possession of a theory of mind, a capacity to understand the mental states—beliefs, desires, intentions—that give rise to human behavior. As Gallager and Frith (2003) observe, "one aspect of social cognition sets us apart from other primates. It underpins our ability to deceive, cooperate, and empathize, and to read others' body language. It also enables us to accurately anticipate other people's behavior, almost as if we had read their minds. This exceptional capacity is known as having a 'theory of mind,' or mentalizing" (p. 77). Given the pivotal role played by mentalizing in human social cognition, a rapidly emerging literature has attempted to identify the neural underpinnings of this ability (Baron-Cohen, 1995; Frith and Frith, 1999; Blakemore and Decety, 2001; Siegal and Varley, 2002; Gallagher and Frith, 2003). The emerging viewpoint is that theory of mind may be supported by a domain-specific, innate cognitive mechanism (Leslie, 1987; Fodor, 1992; Leslie and Thaiss, 1992). The emphasis in functional imaging investigations has been to try to identify the neural basis of this mechanism. Although distributed widely throughout the brain, the cortical implementation of the ability to mindread is known to involve a raft of frontal operations (Shallice, 2001). Of particular interest in the present context, MPFC is acknowledged to be a critical component of the neural system that supports mentalizing (Gallagher and Frith, 2003).

Notwithstanding the various methods that have been used to investigate the neural substrates of theory-of-mind reasoning, a highly consistent pattern of results has emerged. When behavioral tasks tap people's ability to understand the beliefs and desires of others, activity in medial areas of the frontal lobe is observed (Frith and Frith, 1999; Gallagher and Frith, 2003). In the first study of this kind, Fletcher and colleagues (1995) measured neural activity while participants performed a story comprehension task in which they had to understand the mental states of others. In one such story, for example, participants had to work out that an actor's behavior (giving himself up to the police) was based on his assumption about the policeman's beliefs (the policeman knew he had robbed a shop). As the policeman's beliefs were not made explicit in the story, mental state attribution (i.e., theory-of-mind reasoning) was required to perform the task. To isolate the neural operations involved in mental state attribution, Fletcher and colleagues (1995) compared stories of the sort just described with others that required only an understanding of physical events. The results were revealing. Mental state attribution was accompanied by activation in MPFC. Comparable effects have been observed using pictorial materials. Gallagher and associates (2000) presented participants with cartoons that either did or did not require mental state attribution to be understood. Again, when mental state attribution was required to comprehend the material, activity in MPFC was observed.

Reflecting the obligatory operation of mental state attribution in human social cognition, this process can also be triggered by low-level perceptual stimulus inputs. In a seminal study, Heider and Simmel (1944) demonstrated that even basic geometric shapes can elicit the attribution of complex internal states (e.g., beliefs, hopes), if their patterns of movement are appropriate. Would, then, such geometric shapes also trigger the MPFC activity that is indicative of theory-of-mind reasoning? To investigate this issue, Castelli and associates (2000) presented participants with cartoon animations, some of which were intended to trigger mental state attribution. In the theory-of-mind condition, participants observed an interaction between two shapes (a big and a small triangle) that was scripted in such a way as to imply the operation of a complex mental state (e.g., intention to deceive). This was contrasted with animations in which the contingency between the objects was purely physical or the pattern of motion was random. Despite the impoverished nature of the stimulus materials, when the pattern of motion implied the operation of complex mental states, activity in MPFC was observed. These findings are important, because they further demonstrate the inherently social nature of the human mind and the ease with which the machinery of

mental state attribution can be activated. Cortical areas that contribute to an agentic (i.e., higher-order) interpretation of human behavior (i.e., MPFC) can also be triggered by appropriate patterns of biological motion (Blakemore and Decety, 2001).

Of course, to understand how other people think or feel, one must engage in some tricky mental gymnastics. Psychologically speaking, one must put oneself in another person's shoes. This ability to take the perspective of others is also supported by activity in MPFC. In a clever study, Goel and associates (1995) required participants to reason about other people's thoughts regarding specific objects (e.g., "Would Christopher Columbus know what to do with a CD?"). Activity in MPFC was observed during this task, suggesting that this cortical area supports people's ability to mentalize. Subsequent research has corroborated this observation. Gallagher, Jack, and Frith (2002) measured neural activity while participants played a computerized version of the game rock, paper, scissors under different instructional conditions. Of critical interest were the conditions in which participants believed they were playing against either the experimenter (i.e., agentic perspective) or a computer (i.e., mechanistic perspective). When these conditions were compared, mentalizing (i.e., agentic perspective) was associated with neural activity in MPFC (see also McCabe et al., 2001). The emerging picture, then, is pretty clear. When the participant is observing action, adopting the perspective of another person, or inferring the mental state of an actor performing a social behavior, activity is observed in MPFC (Fletcher et al., 1995; Goel et al., 1995; Brunet et al., 2000; Castelli et al., 2000; Gallagher et al., 2000; Vogeley et al., 2001).

The observation that mentalizing and self-referential processing both yield activity in MPFC gives rise to an interesting question: What is the relationship between theory-of-mind reasoning and self-reflective processing (i.e., self-consciousness)? Are they one and the same thing? When performing theory-of-mind tasks, do participants use their own mental states to predict or explain the behavior of others (Gallese and Goldman, 1998)? Although the literature addressing this question is somewhat limited, the preliminary findings are intriguing. Although mentalizing and self-reflection are not functionally identical, they do share common neural operations, notably activity in MPFC (see Vogeley et al., 2001; Vogeley and Fink, 2003). What this suggests is that self-reflection may be a component of the neural system that enables people to understand and empathize with others. To chart a smooth passage through life's choppy waters, one must have a conceptualization of how self functions in different settings. Damasio (1999) refers to this relationship between subject and environment as the "core self," a structure that is reinstated from moment to moment. Of importance, this reactivation of the core self relies on medial cortical structures, including MPFC. Understanding how other people deal with the vagaries of daily life (e.g., environmental demands) may similarly rely on the medial cortical structures that give one's own existence a sense of coherence and agency. In this way, self may make up part of the lens through which the behavior of others is construed. One task for future research will be to investigate this possibility.

Medial prefrontal cortex and you

That MPFC consistently shows elevated levels of activity during self-referential processing and mental state attribution gives rise to an important question: What is the functional significance of MFPC activity during these tasks? In this respect, an interesting framework has been offered by Raichle and colleagues (Gusnard et al., 2001; Raichle et al., 2001) that relates MPFC function to default processing in the brain. The impetus for this viewpoint is the observation that responses in MPFC are almost always observed as decreases in activation relative to a resting baseline (Gusnard and Raichle, 2001). MPFC appears to be part of a network of brain regions that consistently exhibit task-related decreases in activity (Shulman et al., 1997). Decreases in these regions appear to be largely task independent, occurring across a wide variety of goal-directed activities. The consistency of this pattern of deactivations prompted Raichle and colleagues (2001, p. 676) to suggest the existence of "an organized, baseline default mode of brain function that is suspended during specific goal-directed behaviors."

This description fits nicely with the finding that baseline metabolic activity in MPFC is high at rest (Raichle et al., 2001) and provides a context in which to consider self-related effects in cognition. Self-referential mental activity may be the signature of stimulus-independent thought (Antrobus et al., 1970; Teasdale et al., 1995). That is, it is what people spontaneously do when they are not actively engaged in the processing of externally generated information. In this regard, self-relevant mental activity may be categorized not by its unique difference from resting brain activity but by its similarity to spontaneous neural activity. As Kjaer, Nowak, and Lou (2002, p. 1084) have argued, "the activity pattern of reflective self-awareness is indistinguishable from the metabolically highly active structures thought to constitute the baseline of conscious states."

But if MPFC function is tied to self-reflection, why does theory-of-mind reasoning also modulate activity in this area? One possibility is that self-reflection and mental state attribution share a common component process, specifically, metacognition. This may explain why theory-of-mind tasks report activity in MPFC. As we have already noted, these tasks typically require participants to mentalize about the beliefs, knowledge, and desires of others, hence to rely on metacognition for their successful execution (Fletcher et al.,

1995; Goel et al., 1995). If true, of course, then any other social-cognitive task with a metacognitive component might also be expected to recruit MPFC. As it turns out, this appears to be the case. A rapidly emerging literature is revealing that MPFC plays a prominent role in fundamental aspects of social-cognitive functioning, such as the simulation of other minds, the use and representation of social knowledge, moral reasoning, and self-referential mental activity (Anderson et al., 1999; Castelli et al., 2000; Adolphs, 2001; Milne and Grafman, 2001; Kelley et al., 2002; Mitchell, Heatherton, and Macrae, 2002). Although these studies have typically reported increased activity in MPFC, it is important to note that these increases have been observed relative to some other active task (Brunet et al., 2000; Castelli et al., 2000; Gallagher et al., 2000), thereby obscuring whether any changes occurred relative to a resting baseline (but see, Gusnard et al., 2001; Kelley et al., 2002; Mitchell, Heatherton, and Macrae, 2002). If compared to a resting baseline task (e.g., fixating a crosshair), these various manifestations of social-cognitive reasoning may all be associated with deactivations in MPFC.

With the emergence of social cognitive neuroscience as a distinct area of inquiry, researchers are shedding new light on some old problems in experimental social psychology. Here we considered one such thorny topic, the nature and status of self-referential mental processing. Although it is evident that MPFC plays a significant functional role in self-reflection, numerous questions remain. These largely center on the role of metacognition in social-cognitive functioning and the component cognitive operations that subserve social thought. What is beyond dispute, however, is that self-discovery far outweighs the benefits of a culinary delight or an unexpected financial windfall.

REFERENCES

ADOLPHS, R., 2001. The neurobiology of social cognition. *Curr. Opin. Neurobiol.* 11:231–239.

ANDERSON, S. W., A. BECHARA, H. DAMASIO, D. TRANEL, and A. R. DAMASIO, 1999. Impairment of social and moral behavior related to early damage in human prefrontal cortex. *Nat. Neurosci.* 2:1032–1037.

ANTROBUS, J. S., J. L. SINGER, S. GOLDSTEIN, and M. FORTGANG, 1970. Mindwandering and cognitive structure. *Trans. N.Y. Acad. Sci.* 32:242–252.

BARON-COHEN, S., 1995. *Mindblindness: An Essay on Autism and Theory of Mind.* Cambridge, Mass.: MIT Press.

BLAKEMORE, S. J., and J. DECETY, 2001. From the perception of action to the understanding of intention. *Nat. Rev. Neurosci.* 2:561–567.

BOWER, G. H., and S. G. GILLIGAN, 1979. Remembering information related to one's self. *J. Res. Pers.* 13:420–432.

BREWER, J. B., Z. ZHAO, J. E. DESMOND, G. H. GLOVER, and J. D. E. GABRIELI, 1998. Making memories: Activity that predicts how well visual experience will be remembered. *Science* 281:1185–1187.

Brunet, E., Y. Sarfati, M. C. Hardy-Bayle, and J. Decety, 2000. A PET investigation of the attribution of intentions with a non-verbal task. *NeuroImage* 11:157–166.

Bryson, B., 1993. *Neither Here Nor There*. London: Avon Books.

Buckner, R. L., W. M. Kelley, and S. E. Petersen, 1999. Frontal cortex contributes to human memory formation. *Nat. Neurosci.* 2:311–314.

Cahill, L., R. J. Haier, J. Fallon, M. T. Alkire, C. Tang, D. Keator, J. Wu, and J. L. McGaugh, 1996. Amygdala activity at encoding correlated with long-term, free recall of emotional information. *Proc. Natl. Acad. Sci. U.S.A.* 93:8016–8021.

Canli, T., Z. Zhao, J. Brewer, J. D. Gabrieli, and L. Cahill, 2000. Event-related activation in the human amygdala associates with later memory for individual emotional experience. *J. Neurosci.* 20:RC99.

Castelli, F., F. Happé, U. Frith, and C. Frith, 2000. Movement and mind: A functional imaging study of perception and interpretation of complex intentional movement patterns. *NeuroImage* 12:314–325.

Conway, M. A., and C. W. Pleydell-Pearce, 2000. The construction of autobiographical memories in the self memory system. *Psychol. Rev.* 107:261–288.

Craik, F. I. M., T. M. Moroz, M. Moscovitch, D. T. Stuss, G. Winocur, E. Tulving, and S. Kapur, 1999. In search of the self: A positron emission tomography study. *Psychol. Sci.* 10: 26–34.

Craik, F. I. M., and E. Tulving, 1975. Depth of processing and the retention of words in episodic memory. *J. Exp. Psychol. Gen.* 104:268–294.

Damasio, A. R., 1999. *The Feeling of What Happens: Body and Emotion in the Making of Consciousness*. New York: Harcourt Brace.

Demb, J. B., J. E. Desmond, A. D. Wagner, C. J. Vaidya, G. H. Glover, and J. D. E. Gabrieli, 1995. Semantic encoding and retrieval in the left inferior prefrontal cortex: A functional MRI study of task difficulty and process specificity. *J. Neurosci.* 15:5870–5878.

Dolan, R. J., and P. C. Fletcher, 1997. Dissociating prefrontal and hippocampal function in episodic memory encoding. *Nature* 388:582–585.

Fletcher, P. C., F. Happé, U. Frith, S. C. Baker, R. J. Dolan, R. S. J. Frackowiak, and C. D. Frith, 1995. Other minds in the brain: A functional imaging study of "theory of mind" in story comprehension. *Cognition* 57:109–128.

Fodor, J. A., 1992. A theory of the child's theory of mind. *Cognition* 44:283–296.

Frith, C. D., and U. Frith, 1999. Interacting minds: A biological basis. *Science* 286:1692–1695.

Gabrieli, J. D. E., J. E. Desmond, J. B. Demb, A. D. Wagner, M. V. Stone, C. J. Vaidya, and G. H. Glover, 1996. Functional magnetic resonance imaging of semantic memory processes in the frontal lobes. *Psychol. Sci.* 7:278–283.

Gallagher, H. L., and C. D. Frith, 2003. Functional imaging of "theory of mind." *Trends Cogn. Sci.* 7:77–83.

Gallagher, H. L., F. Happé, N. Brunswick, P. C. Fletcher, U. Frith, and C. D. Frith, 2000. Reading the mind in cartoons and stories: An fMRI study of "theory of mind" in verbal and nonverbal tasks. *Neuropsychologia* 38:11–21.

Gallagher, H. L., A. I. Jack, and C. D. Frith, 2002. Imaging the intentional stance. *NeuroImage* 16:814–821.

Gallese, V., and A. Goldman, 1998. Mirror neurons and the simulation theory of mind-reading. *Trends Cogn. Sci.* 2:493–501.

Goel, V., J. Grafman, N. Sadato, and M. Hallett, 1995. Modeling other minds. *Neuroreport* 6:1741–1746.

Greenwald, A. G., and M. R. Banaji, 1989. The self as a memory system: Powerful, but ordinary. *J. Pers. Soc. Psychol.* 57: 41–54.

Gusnard, D. A., E. Akbudak, G. L. Shulman, and M. E. Raichle, 2001. Medial prefrontal cortex and self-referential mental activity: Relation to a default mode of brain function. *Proc. Natl. Acad. Sci. U.S.A.* 98:4259–4264.

Gusnard, D. A., and M. E. Raichle, 2001. Searching for a baseline: Functional imaging and the resting human brain. *Nat. Rev. Neurosci.* 2:685–694.

Hamann, S., 2001. Cognitive and neural mechanisms of emotional memory. *Trends Cogn. Sci.* 5:394–400.

Hamann, S. B., T. D. Ely, S. T. Grafton, and C. D. Kilts, 1999. Amygdala activity related to enhanced memory for pleasant and aversive stimuli. *Nat. Neurosci.* 2:289–293.

Heider, F., and M. Simmel, 1944. An experimental study of apparent behavior. *Am. J. Psychol.* 57:243–259.

Henson, R. N., M. D. Rugg, T. Shallice, O. Josephs, and R. J. Dolan, 1999. Recollection and familiarity in recognition memory: An event-related functional magnetic resonance imaging study. *J. Neurosci.* 19:3962–3972.

James, W., 1890. *Principles of Psychology*, vol. 1. New York: Henry Holt.

Johnson, S. C., L. C. Baxter, L. S. Wilder, J. G. Pipe, J. E. Heiserman, and G. P. Prigatano, 2002. Neural correlates of self-reflection. *Brain* 125:1808–1814.

Kapur, S., F. I. M. Craik, E. Tulving, A. A. Wilson, S. Houle, and G. M. Brown, 1994. Neuroanatomical correlates of encoding in episodic memory: Levels of processing effects, *Proc. Natl. Acad. Sci. U.S.A.* 91:2008–2011.

Kelley, W. M., F. M. Miezin, K. B. McDermott, R. L. Buckner, M. E. Raichle, N. J. Cohen, J. M. Ollinger, E. Akbudak, T. E. Conturo, A. Z. Snyder, and P. E. Petersen, 1998. Hemispheric specialization in human dorsal frontal cortex and medial temporal lobe for verbal and nonverbal memory encoding. *Neuron* 20:927–936.

Kelley, W. M., C. N. Macrae, C. L. Wyland, S. Caglar, S. Inati, and T. F. Heatherton, 2002. Finding the self: An event-related fMRI study. *J. Cogn. Neurosci.* 14:785–794.

Kihlstrom, J. F., and S. B. Klein, 1997. Self-knowledge and self-awareness. In *The Self Across Psychology: Self Recognition, Self-awareness, and the Self Concept*, J. G. Snodgrass and R. L. Thompson, eds. *Ann. N.Y. Acad. Sci.* 818:4–17.

Kirchhoff, B. A., A. D. Wagner, A. Maril, and C. E. Stern, 2000. Prefrontal-temporal circuitry for episodic encoding and subsequent memory. *J. Neurosci.* 20:6173–6180.

Kjaer, T. W., M. Nowak, and H. C. Lou, 2002. Reflective self-awareness and conscious states: PET evidence for a common midline parietofrontal core. *NeuroImage* 17:1080–1086.

Klein, S. B., and J. F. Kihlstrom, 1986. Elaboration, organization, and the self-reference effect in memory. *J. Exp. Psychol. Gen.* 115:26–38.

Klein, S. B., and J. Loftus, 1988. The nature of self-referent encoding: The contributions of elaborative and organizational processes. *J. Pers. Soc. Psychol.* 55:5–11.

Leslie, A. M., 1987. Pretense and representation in infancy: The origins of "theory of mind." *Psychol. Rev.* 94:412–426.

Leslie, A. M., and L. Thaiss, 1992. Domain specificity in conceptual development: Neuropsychological evidence from autism. *Cognition* 43:225–251.

Macrae, C. N., J. M. Moran, T. F. Heatherton, J. F. Banfield, and W. M. Kelley, in press. *Medial prefrontal activity predicts memory for self*. Cerebral Cortex.

MAKI, R. H., and K. D. McCAUL, 1985. The effects of self-reference versus other reference on the recall of traits and nouns. *Bull. Psychon. Soc.* 23:169–172.

MARKUS, H., 1977. Self-schemata and processing information about the self. *J. Pers. Soc. Psychol.* 35:63–78.

McCABE, K., D. HOUSER, V. SMITH, and T. TROUARD, 2001. A functional imaging study of cooperation in two-person reciprocal exchange. *Proc. Natl. Acad. Sci. U.S.A.* 98:11832–11835.

MILNE, E., and J. GRAFMAN, 2001. Ventromedial prefrontal cortex lesions in humans eliminate implicit gender stereotyping. *J. Neurosci.* 21:RC150.

MITCHELL, J. P., T. F. HEATHERTON, and C. N. MACRAE, 2002. Distinct neural systems subserve person and object knowledge. *Proc. Natl. Acad. Sci. U.S.A.* 99:15238–15243.

OTTEN, L. J., R. N. HENSON, and M. D. RUGG, 2001. Depth of processing effects on neural correlates of memory encoding: Relationship between findings from across- and within-task comparisons. *Brain* 124:399–412.

OTTEN, L. J., and M. D. RUGG, 2001. Electrophysiological correlates of memory encoding are task-dependent. *Cogn. Brain Res.* 12:11–18.

RAICHLE, M. E., A. M. MACLEOD, A. Z. SNYDER, W. J. POWERS, D. A. GUSNARD, and G. L. SHULMAN, 2001. A default mode of brain function. *Proc. Natl. Acad. Sci. U.S.A.* 98:676–682.

ROGERS, T. B., N. A. KUIPER, and W. S. KIRKER, 1977. Self-reference and the encoding of personal information. *J. Pers. Soc. Psychol.* 35:677–688.

RYLE, G., 1949. *The Concept of Mind.* London: Hutchison.

SHALLICE, T., 2001. "Theory of mind" and the prefrontal cortex. *Brain* 124:247–248.

SHULMAN, G. L., J. A. FIEZ, M. CORBETTA, R. L. BUCKNER, F. M. MIEZIN, M. E. RAICHLE, and S. E. PETERSEN, 1997. Common blood flow changes across visual tasks. II. Decreases in cerebral cortex. *J. Cogn. Neurosci.* 9:648–663.

SIEGAL, M., and R. VARLEY, 2002. Neural systems involved in "theory of mind." *Nat. Rev. Neurosci.* 3:463–471.

STUSS, D. T., and D. F. BENSON, 1986. *The Frontal Lobes.* New York: Raven Press.

SYMONS, C. S., and B. T. JOHNSON, 1997. The self-reference effect in memory: A meta-analysis. *Psychol. Bull.* 121:371–394.

TEASDALE, J.-D., B.-H. DRITSCHEL, M.-J. TAYLOR, L. PROCTOR, C. A. LLOYD, I. NIMMO-SMITH, and A. D. BADDELEY, 1995. Stimulus-independent thought depends on central executive resources. *Mem. Cogn.* 23:551–559.

VOGELEY, K., P. BUSSFIELD, A. NEWEN, S. HERRMANN, F. HAPPE, P. FALKAI, W. MAIER, N. J. SHAH, G. R. FINK, and K. ZILLS, 2001. Mind reading: Neural mechanisms of theory of mind and self-perspective. *NeuroImage* 14:170–181.

VOGELEY, K., and G. R. FINK, 2003. Neural correlates of the first-person perspective. *Trends Cogn. Sci.* 7:38–42.

WAGNER, A. D., D. L. SCHACTER, M. ROTTE, W. KOUTSTAAL, A. MARIL, A. M. DALE, B. R. ROSEN, and R. L. BUCKNER, 1998. Building memories: Remembering and forgetting of verbal experiences as predicted by brain activity. *Science* 281:1188–1191.

WHEELER, M. A., D. T. STUSS, and E. TULVING, 1997. Toward a theory of episodic memory: The frontal lobes and autonoetic consciousness. *Psychol. Bull.* 121:331–354.

77 The Cognitive Neuroscience of Knowing One's Self

STANLEY B. KLEIN

ABSTRACT The unified self of everyday experience may actually be composed of several functionally and neurally isolable components. These include episodic memories of one's own life, representations of one's own personality traits, facts about one's personal history (semantic personal knowledge), the experience of personal agency and continuity through time, and the ability to reflect on one's own thoughts and experiences (Klein, 2001). One component of the self—knowledge of one's own personality traits—is surprisingly resilient in the face of brain damage and developmental disorders. Personality knowledge can be preserved and even updated without any retrievable episodic memory. More strikingly, a pattern of category-specific dissociations within semantic memory suggests that the human cognitive architecture may include a subsystem that is functionally specialized for the acquisition, storage, and retrieval of trait self-knowledge. The ability to retrieve accurate information about one's own personality traits can be preserved despite damage to the systems that retrieve information from other content-based categories of semantic knowledge, including knowledge of other people's personality traits, knowledge of one's own personal history, knowledge of cultural history, and knowledge of facts about animals, foods, and objects. Neuropsychological case studies reveal dissociations not only of storage and retrieval but also of acquisition; personality knowledge may be acquired via learning mechanisms that are functionally distinct from those that cause the acquisition of knowledge about other domains. Taken together, the cognitive and neuropsychological evidence suggests that personality self-knowledge is acquired through domain-specific learning mechanisms, stored in proprietary databases, and retrieved via functionally specialized search engines.

Who is the I that knows the bodily me, who has an image of myself and a sense of identity over time, who knows that I have propriate strivings? I know all these things, and what is more, I know that I know them. But who is it who has this perspectival grasp? . . . It is much easier to feel the self than to define the self.

—G. W. Allport, *Patterns and Growth in Personality*

What *is* the self? Philosophers and scientists pursuing an answer to this deep ontological question immediately find themselves immersed in a host of metaphysical questions about mind and body, subject and object, object and process, the homunculus, free will, self-awareness, and a variety of other puzzling matters (e.g., Williams, 1973; Cassam, 1994;

STANLEY B. KLEIN Department of Psychology, University of California, Santa Barbara, Santa Barbara, Calif.

Bermudez, 1998; Gallagher and Shear, 1999). The enduring nature of these problems has led some to question whether a conceptual understanding of the self is possible in practice (e.g., Olson, 1999; Uttal, 2000) or in principle (e.g., McGinn, 1991).

Although researchers are deeply interested in the complex questions and controversies raised by the problem of the ontology of self, that is not the focus of this chapter. Instead, the focus is on what can be thought of as *first-person epistemology:* how we come to know who and what we are (e.g., Crispin, Smith, and Macdonald, 1998). The cognitive architecture of an individual is able to learn about the individual it is situated in, and even experience itself as a knower. A cognitive account of the mechanisms, databases, and search engines that allow this information about the self to be acquired, stored, and retrieved should be possible, even if some of the more troubling ontological questions remain unanswered.

A brief history of social-cognitive explorations of self

In his book, *Consciousness Regained*, Nicholas Humphrey (1984) made a strong case for the proposition that our ability to reflect on the self—the capacity to experience ourselves as thinking, feeling, wanting, doing beings—is likely what gave rise to psychology in the first place. Indeed, no less an authority than William James (1890) proclaimed the self to be the fundamental unit of analysis for a science of mental life, the problem about which everything else revolves. Yet academic psychology, influenced by arguments from "black-box" behaviorism, largely ignored questions about the mental representation of self-knowledge until the late 1970s.

With the rise of the cognitive sciences, various components of the self began to be cashed out as computational systems and the databases they access. For example, research on theory of mind reframed Humphrey's "ability to reflect upon the self" as the ability to form metarepresentations: representations about other mental representations, whether one's own or others (e.g., Baron-Cohen, Leslie, and Frith, 1985; Leslie, 1987). In Leslie's (1987, 2000) account, these representations are data files with a particular format, including slots for an *agent* (e.g., "I," "you," "Lowell"), that agent's *attitude* toward a proposition (e.g., "believes," "doubts," "hopes"), and an embedded proposition (e.g., "It is raining," "I will become anxious at the zoo"). Because the agent can be the self and the embedded proposition can itself be a metarepresentation, this data format allows the formation of self-reflective representations, such as "I believe that I will become anxious at the zoo."

The computational machinery that produces metarepresentations appears to come online at about 18 months (e.g., Leslie, 1987; Baron-Cohen, 1995), and it can be selectively impaired. For example, individuals with autism understand that photographs—physical representations of the world—can misrepresent the facts, but have difficulty understanding that beliefs—mental representations about the world—can do the same (Leslie and Thaiss, 1992). Autism, it has been argued, disrupts the development of metarepresentational machinery (Baron-Cohen, 2000; Leslie, 2000); schizophrenia may be a late-onset breakdown of the same system (Frith, 1992; Frith and Frith, 1992; Gallagher, 2000). If true, then the ability to reflect on one's own mental states should be impaired in both disorders, and this appears to be the case (e.g., Frith, 1992; Baron-Cohen, 1995).

But where does the information about the self that a metarepresentation represents come from? How is it derived, where is it stored, and how is it retrieved? Metarepresentational machinery may permit a cognitive architecture to reflect on the thoughts, desires, reactions, personality, and other properties of the individual in which it is situated. But it can do so only if that information is represented somewhere in the architecture. Recognizing this, social and personality psychologists began to examine how knowledge about the self is stored in memory. It was known that we store vast amounts of information about our own personality traits and those of others (e.g., Wiggins, 1973). The question is, in what data formats and storage systems is that knowledge represented, and what are the mechanisms whereby it is retrieved?

Investigations in social psychology centered on whether the representation of knowledge about the self differed from representations of knowledge about other social and nonsocial entities (for reviews, see Greenwald, 1981; Kihlstrom and Klein, 1994; Linville and Carlston, 1994). Speculation about the uniqueness of self-knowledge was fueled by theoretical and experimental work on the role of self in information processing. Particularly influential in this regard was the demonstration by Rogers, Kuiper, and Kirker (1977) that asking someone whether a trait adjective, such as *kind*, is self-descriptive leads to better recall of that adjective than asking the person to make other judgments about it (e.g., "Does the word *kind* describe you?" versus "What does *kind* mean?"; see also Bower and Gilligan, 1979; Klein and Kihlstrom, 1986; Klein and Loftus, 1988; for review, see Symons and Johnson, 1997). Given the recall superiority found for self-referential

judgments, it seemed to a number of investigators that self-knowledge might have properties that distinguish it from other structures in memory (e.g., Rogers, 1981; Greenwald and Pratkanis, 1984). Explaining these properties soon became the dominant focus of research exploring how self-knowledge is represented in and retrieved from memory (for review, see Higgins and Bargh, 1987; Kihlstrom and Klein, 1994; Linville and Carlston, 1994).

THE SELF AND MEMORY   How does a person know that he or she possesses some traits but not others? How is this knowledge represented in and retrieved from memory? These questions have been asked within the context of debates about multiple memory systems (for recent reviews of the memory systems debate, see Schacter and Tulving, 1994; Foster and Jelicic, 1999).

Psychologists generally agree that memory stores two basic types of information, procedural and declarative (e.g., Tulving, 1983, 1995; Cohen and Eichenbaum, 1993; Parkin, 1993; Schacter and Tulving, 1994). Procedural memory makes possible the acquisition and retention of motor, perceptual, and cognitive skills (e.g., knowing how to ride a bike); it consists in the nonconscious expression of previously acquired behavioral skills and cognitive procedures (e.g., Tulving, 1985; Tulving and Schacter, 1990; Parkin, 1993). Declarative memory consists in facts and beliefs about the world (e.g., knowing that canaries are yellow; knowing that Eli pitched a shutout yesterday). Conceptually, the difference between procedural and declarative memory coincides with Ryle's (1949) classic distinction between *knowing how* (operating on the environment in ways difficult to verbalize) and *knowing that* (stating knowledge in the form of propositions).

Tulving (1983, 1985, 1993a) distinguishes two types of declarative memory: episodic and semantic (see also Cermak, 1984; Wood, Brown, and Felton, 1989; Parkin, 1993; Moscovitch et al., 2000). Semantic memory is relatively generic, context-free knowledge about the world, such as *apples are edible*, *2 + 2 = 4*, and *Sacramento is the capital of California*. Semantic memory usually lacks a source tag: it is experienced as knowledge without regard to where and when that knowledge was obtained (e.g., Tulving, 1983, 1993a, 1995; Perner and Ruffman, 1994; Gennaro, 1996; Wheeler, Stuss, and Tulving, 1997). Most semantic memory makes no reference to the self; it can, however, contain propositions expressing facts about the self (e.g., *Stan Klein was born in New York*), just as it can about other things in the world. But this information is known in the same way that one knows that apples are edible; it is not recalled or reexperienced.

In contrast to semantic memory, episodic memory records events as having been experienced by the self at a particular (and unique) point in space and time; when retrieved, these events are reexperienced in a quasi-perceptual way, with conscious awareness that "this happened to *me*" (e.g., Tulving, 1983, 1993a; Suddendorf and Corballis, 1997; Wheeler, Stuss, and Tulving, 1997). Every episodic memory by definition entails a mental representation of the self as the agent or recipient of some action, or as the stimulus or experiencer of some state (Kihlstrom, 1997). Examples of episodic memory are *I remember attending a concert yesterday evening* and *I recall having met with my graduate student last Monday.*

Not surprisingly it is the episodic component of declarative memory that traditionally has been the focus of interest for psychologists studying the relation between self and memory. This is because retrieval from episodic memory is assumed to have a self-referential quality thought to be largely absent from other types of memorial experience (i.e., semantic and procedural; for discussion, see Klein, 2001; Kihlstrom, Beer, and Klein, 2002; Klein, Cosmides, Tooby, and Chance, 2002). By contrast, semantic memory is not accompanied by awareness of reexperiencing one's personal past (e.g., Tulving, 1993a, 1995; Perner and Ruffman, 1994; Wheeler, Stuss, and Tulving, 1997). I may *know* where I was born, but I do not know this by virtue of having recalled or reexperienced my birth. That is why this bit of personal history would be considered semantic knowledge, despite its being about oneself.

KNOWING ONESELF: SOURCES OF FIRST-PERSON DATA IN MEMORY Episodic memories of a personal past are clearly one source of information about the self (and others). It would be strange, however, if these were the only source of data about oneself. Many decisions require quick and accurate judgments of one's own personality traits and those of others (e.g., Will standing up to him make me anxious?). But making these judgments would be a slow process indeed if the only database with pertinent information was the episodic store: each time a judgment was needed, episodic memories would have to be retrieved, and the behavioral events they represent would have to be analyzed for evidence of the trait in question.

Better to have answers precomputed and available for whenever they are needed. Trait generalizations are precomputed summaries of the dispositions one manifested in various behavioral episodes. Research over the past 10 years has provided evidence that the semantic memory system contains a subsystem that stores information about one's own personality traits in the form of trait generalizations (e.g., *Self: Usually stubborn*). These trait summaries form a fast-access database that provides quick answers to decision processes that require trait judgments.

In the next section I review converging evidence that this trait summary database exists, based on studies of individuals with normal cognitive function and individuals with varying degrees of cognitive impairment (e.g., amnesia,

autism, Alzheimer's dementia). From these studies, a tentative model is emerging of how representations from episodic and semantic memory interact to generate a conception of oneself (Klein, Cosmides, Tooby, and Chance, 2002). This model will be discussed after the evidence is reviewed.

Does the mind store trait summaries?

Two explanations have been offered for how personality trait judgments are made. The abstraction view proposes direct retrieval of precomputed trait summaries; the computational view eschews trait summaries and proposes instead that trait judgments are computed online, on the basis of retrieved episodes (for reviews, see Klein and Loftus, 1993a; Kihlstrom and Klein, 1994).

According to the computational view, there is a mechanism that makes trait judgments online by retrieving trait-relevant behaviors from episodic memory and computing their similarity to the trait being judged (e.g., Bower and Gilligan, 1979; Locksley and Lenauer, 1981; Smith and Zarate, 1992; Keenan, 1993). For example, if asked whether I am friendly, this mechanism would search the episodic memory store for trait-consistent episodes (in this case, records of events in which my behavior was friendly). The judgment would be computed from the episodes retrieved (based, e.g., on how diagnostic they were of friendliness or on how fast a given number could be retrieved).

According to the abstraction view, information about one's personality traits is abstracted from specific behaviors, either as they happen or on the basis of episodic memories of these behaviors. These abstractions are stored in the form of precomputed trait summaries (e.g., Buss and Craik, 1983; Klein, Loftus, Trafton, and Fuhrman, 1992; Klein and Loftus, 1993a; Lord, 1993). Trait judgments are made by direct retrieval from this store. When a trait summary is retrieved, trait-consistent episodes are not retrieved along with it (because the information they provide would be redundant). Trait-consistent episodes are consulted only when the search engine fails to retrieve a trait summary (e.g., when a summary does not exist yet for a particular trait).

Note that these two views carry very different predictions about the need to access episodic memories when making trait judgments. If the computational view is correct, then trait-consistent episodes must be retrieved to make a trait judgment. If the abstraction view is correct, then trait-consistent episodes will not be retrieved in making trait judgment, except under unusual circumstances (e.g., the absence of a summary). These predictions have been extensively tested through paradigms that take advantage of priming, encoding specificity, and encoding variability. Priming results are described in the next section (for converging results using the other methods, see Klein, Loftus, and Plog, 1992; Klein, Loftus, and Burton, 1989).

TESTING FOR TRAIT SUMMARIES IN COGNITIVELY NORMAL INDIVIDUALS The logic of tests using priming paradigms is straightforward. The computational view requires the retrieval of trait-consistent episodes; this means that being asked whether a trait describes you should activate trait-consistent behavioral episodes, allowing faster recall of them subsequently. No priming of trait-consistent episodes is predicted by the abstraction view (except in cases where summaries are absent).

Tests using priming paradigms support the abstraction view, not the computational view (Klein and Loftus, 1993a,b; Klein, Loftus, and Burton, 1989; Klein, Loftus, Trafton, and Fuhrman, 1992; Klein, Cosmides, Tooby, and Chance, 2002). Klein, Loftus, and colleagues presented each subject with many pairs of tasks; each pair involved a particular trait adjective (e.g., *stubborn*). Subjects were asked to retrieve a memory in which they displayed behavior relevant to the trait in question (e.g., "Recall a specific incident in which you behaved in a stubborn manner"). The dependent measure was the response latency for this recall task when it was the second task of the pair. The independent variable was the nature of the initial task, the prime.

The prime was either a describe task, a control task, or a filler task. The *describe* task asked subjects to judge whether the trait adjective was self-descriptive (e.g., "Does this describe you: *Stubborn?*"). The control task varied depending on the experiment; sometimes it was a *define* task (e.g., "Think of the definition of the word *stubborn*"), sometimes it was looking at a blank screen. Control tasks were ones that that do not elicit retrieval of trait-consistent behavioral episodes.

If the computational view is correct, then trait-consistent episodes will be activated and analyzed whenever one is asked to decide whether a trait describes oneself, that is, by performing the describe task. If trait-consistent episodic memories are activated by the describe task, then one should be able to retrieve those memories faster after performing a describe task than after performing a control task. This was not the case: when subjects were asked to recall a specific behavioral incident in which they manifested a particular trait (recall task), those who had first made a self-descriptiveness judgment were no faster than those who had not (e.g., Klein, Loftus, and Burton, 1989; Klein and Loftus, 1990, 1993a; Klein, Loftus, Trafton, and Fuhrman, 1992). Yet the procedure used is known to be sensitive enough to detect episodic priming when it occurs (e.g., Babey, Queller, and Klein, 1998; Klein, Loftus, Trafton, and Fuhrman, 1992; Sherman and Klein, 1994; Sherman et al., 1998). (For experiments showing that this result obtains regardless of how central a trait is to one's self-concept, see Klein, Cosmides, Tooby, and Chance, 2001; Klein, Loftus, Trafton, and Fuhrman, 1992.)

The fact that making a trait judgment did not prime episodic memories of trait-consistent behaviors is consistent with the abstraction view. That view holds that trait judgments can be made by directly retrieving trait summaries; no supporting evidence from episodic memory need be accessed. Klein and Loftus concluded from this series of results that people can answer questions about their own personality traits by accessing these trait summaries, without activating memories of episodes in which their behavior exemplified the trait.

Other research showed that the presence or absence of a trait summary is the variable that explains whether trait-consistent episodes are primed. When a trait summary is absent (as it is when trait-relevant behavioral experience is severely limited), trait-consistent episodes are indeed activated in the course of making trait judgments (e.g., Klein and Loftus, 1993a). The same holds when making judgments of others: trait-consistent episodes are not primed when summaries exist but are primed when they are absent (e.g., Babey, Queller, and Klein, 1998; Sherman and Klein, 1994).

Additional support for the independence of episodic and semantic trait self-knowledge in brain-intact people recently was presented by Craik and colleagues (1999). Using positron emission tomography, these investigators discovered that requiring participants to judge trait adjectives for self-descriptiveness produced activation of cortical areas associated with semantic memory retrieval (left frontal regions) but not those associated with episodic memory retrieval (right frontal regions).[1] Similar findings have been reported by investigators employing functional magnetic resonance imaging (fMRI) technology (e.g., Kircher et al., 2000; Kelley et al., 2002; Zhang et al., 2002; Zysset et al., 2002; but see Keenan et al., 2001). Morin (2002), in a recent review of the literature on self-referential encoding and neuroimaging, concludes that the evidence points toward a left hemisphere involvement.[2]

These studies, all performed on individuals with normal cognitive function, converge on the following conclusion regarding "first-person epistemology": we can know what we are like by retrieving trait summaries from semantic memory. We do not have to compute the answer online based on information retrieved from episodic memory (e.g., Klein, Loftus, Trafton, and Fuhrman, 1992; Klein and Loftus, 1993a; Klein, Loftus, and Sherman, 1993, 1996; Schell, Klein, and Babey, 1996; Klein, Babey, and Sherman, 1997).

EVIDENCE FROM INDIVIDUALS WITH IMPAIRED COGNITIVE FUNCTION Given the automatic and flawless way in which different systems of memory normally interact, it is difficult to disentangle their respective contributions to knowledge about the self. However, because neuropsychological disorders of memory can be selective (i.e., patients may exhibit normal or near normal performance in some domains and profound impairments in others; e.g., Parkin and Leng, 1993; Parkin, 1996; Mayes, 2000), they can provide a window into the operation of a component system in relative isolation, without the influence of other systems. By revealing differential patterns of impaired and preserved performance, the study of patients with neuropsychological impairments can illuminate aspects of a system's function and structure that are difficult to detect under normal operating conditions (e.g., Shallice, 1988; Tulving, 1983; Weiskrantz, 1997).

A SOCIAL NEUROPSYCHOLOGICAL APPROACH TO UNDERSTANDING THE SELF: FIVE CASE STUDIES   Klein and Loftus (1993a; see also Klein and Kihlstrom, 1998) proposed that the study of patients with amnesia—patients such as K.C., whose amnesia has been extensively studied by Tulving (1993b)—would prove to be a particularly effective method for examining the respective contributions of episodic and semantic memory to the creation of self-knowledge. This is because amnesic patients often experience highly selective memory loss, typically displaying intact semantic memory with impaired access to episodic memory (e.g., Tulving, 1983, 1995; Cermak, 1984; Parkin, 1987; Moscovitch et al., 2000). Amnesic patients therefore present a unique opportunity to test alternative models of self-knowledge: tests of trait knowledge can be conducted in amnesic patients with assurance that episodic memory for traits is not involved.

For example, if semantic memory contains a database of personality trait summaries, then an amnesic patient should be able to know what he or she is like despite being unable to recall the particular experiences from which that knowledge was derived. Neuropsychological data are now available from five patients. The dissociations found in these individuals speak strikingly to this and other issues involving how knowledge about oneself is acquired and represented in memory.

K.C. Patient K.C. permanently lost his entire fund of episodic memory following a motorcycle accident (see Tulving, 1993b). He also underwent a marked personality change after the accident. Nevertheless, K.C. was able to describe his postmorbid personality with considerable accuracy (his mother's ratings served as the criterion; Tulving, 1993b). The fact that K.C. could accurately report his own personality traits supports the view that knowing oneself does not require retrieval of episodic memories. It is consistent with the hypothesis that personality information is stored independently from episodic memory, in the form of trait summaries.

It should be noted that K.C.'s self-knowledge reflected his postmorbid personality, not his premorbid personality. This means that K.C. not only had access to semantic knowledge of his own personality traits, he was also able to acquire new knowledge about his personality. Yet this updating occurred without his being able to recall any information about the behavioral episodes on which this updating was based. (It is unclear how K.C.'s updating was achieved; one possibility is that it occurred "online," as each new behavioral episode was unfolding.)

W.J. W.J. suffered a concussive blow to the head shortly after completing her first quarter in college (Klein, Loftus, and Kihlstrom, 1996). Interviews conducted shortly after her accident revealed that W.J. had forgotten much of what had happened during the preceding 12 months, a period of time that included her first quarter at college. To document her deficit in episodic memory, Klein, Loftus, and Kihlstrom (1996) used the autobiographical memory cuing task originated by Galton (1879) and popularized by Crovitz (e.g., Crovitz and Schiffman, 1974) and Robinson (1976). W.J. was asked to try to recall specific personal events related to each of a list of cue words (e.g., *car*, *sing*, *brave*) and to provide for each recollection as precise a date as possible. On initial testing, she was unable to recollect personal events from recent years. Over the next month, however, her amnesia remitted completely, and when she was retested 4 weeks later, her performance had improved to the point that it was indistinguishable from that of neurologically healthy women who served as controls.

On two occasions, during her amnesia and after its resolution, W.J. was asked to provide personality ratings describing what she was like during her first quarter at college. While she was amnesic, W.J. was able to describe her personality; more important, the ratings she made during her amnesic period agreed with those she made afterward. Thus, while W.J. was amnesic she knew what she had been like in college, even though she could not episodically recollect any personal events or experiences from that time period.

Could W.J.'s judgments while amnesic be based on her continued access to episodic recollections of high school or earlier, periods not covered by her amnesia? Probably not. W.J., like many freshmen, manifested somewhat different personality traits in college than she did in high school. Yet her self-ratings during the amnesic period reflected her college personality (for data and analyses, see Klein, Loftus, and Kilstrom, 1996). This suggests that W.J.'s ratings were based on semantic knowledge of her personality during her time at college, not on recollections of episodes long past.

D.B. The case of D.B. (like that of K.C.) shows that one can have accurate knowledge of one's own personality traits even with a total loss of episodic memory (Klein, Rozendal, and Cosmides, 2002). Patient D.B. was a 79-year-old man who became profoundly amnesic as a result of anoxia following cardiac arrest. On both informal questioning and psychological testing, D.B. was unable to consciously recollect a single thing he had ever done or experienced from any period of his life. In addition to his dense retrograde episodic amnesia, he also sustained severe anterograde episodic memory impairment, rendering him incapable of recollecting events that had transpired only minutes earlier.

To test D.B.'s semantic self-knowledge, we asked him on two separate occasions to judge a list of personality traits for self-descriptiveness. We also asked D.B.'s daughter (with whom he lived) to rate D.B. on the same traits. Our findings revealed that D.B.'s ratings were both reliable ($r = 0.69$ across sessions) and consistent with the way he is perceived by others ($r = 0.64$ between D.B. and his daughter). (Age-matched controls showed $rs = 0.74$ and 0.57 across sessions and raters, respectively.) D.B. thus appeared to have accurate and detailed knowledge about his personality even though he had no conscious access to any specific actions or experiences on which that knowledge was based. (For related findings, see Cermak and O'Connor, 1983; Evan et al., 1993; Tulving, 1993b; Starkstein, Sabe, and Dorrego, 1997; Kircher et al., 2000; for review, see Klein, Cosmides, Tooby, and Chance, 2002.)

D.B. manifested a clear dissociation between episodic and semantic self-knowledge. But can semantic knowledge of one's own personality traits dissociate from other types of semantic knowledge? Further testing of D.B. suggested that it can.

D.B.'s semantic memory was also affected by his illness, although this impairment was far less severe than that affecting his episodic memory (Klein, Rozendal, and Cosmides, 2002). For example, although he knew a variety of general facts about his life, he showed a number of striking gaps in his life story: he knew the name of the high school he attended and where he was born, but could not recall the names of any friends from his childhood or the year of his birth. He also showed spotty knowledge of facts in the public domain. For example, although he was able to accurately recount a number of details about certain historical events (e.g., the Civil War), his knowledge of other historical facts was seriously compromised (e.g., he claimed that America was discovered by the British in 1812). Despite these impairments in D.B.'s more general semantic knowledge, his knowledge of his own personality was intact. This result suggests a dissociation *within* semantic memory: between general semantic knowledge and semantic knowledge of one's own personality traits.

Additional testing revealed a dissociation between D.B.'s knowledge of his own personality traits and the traits of others. D.B. could not retrieve accurate knowledge of his daughter's personality traits: the correlation between D.B.'s ratings of his daughter and her self-ratings was not reliable ($r = 0.23$), and was less than half that found between control parents' ratings of their child and the child's self-ratings ($r = 0.61$). Thus, although D.B.'s ability to retrieve accurate knowledge of his own personality was intact (no different from that of age-matched controls), he had lost the ability to retrieve accurate personality information about his adult daughter, with whom he lived.

In short, D.B.'s case goes well beyond the usual episodic/semantic distinction. It suggests category-specific dissociations within semantic memory. His ability to retrieve trait self-knowledge was intact; his ability to retrieve his daughter's traits was impaired; and his knowledge about the world at large (and specific facts about himself) was impaired. This pattern raises the possibility that the human cognitive architecture includes a subsystem of semantic memory that is functionally specialized for the storage and retrieval of trait self-knowledge. More data relevant to this claim come from the cases of R.J. and K.R.

R.J. Patients K.C., W.J., and D.B. lost access to episodic memory as a result of brain trauma. However, there also are cases of individuals in whom episodic memory failed to develop in the first place (e.g., Vargha-Khadem et al., 1997; Ahern, Wood, and McBrien, 1998). Such developmental dissociations are interesting because they permit inferences about the origins of self-knowledge that are not licensed by the discovery of dissociations caused by brain trauma in adults.

Consider, for example, the hypothesis that semantic self-knowledge, despite being functionally independent of episodic memory, initially is constructed from a database of episodic memories. This hypothesis cannot be ruled out by cases like D.B. and W.J.; their intact semantic self-knowledge could have been derived from episodic memories during the years prior to the brain trauma that caused their episodic loss as adults. But consider the implications of finding an individual who never developed the ability to access episodic memories, yet has intact semantic self-knowledge. This developmental dissociation would suggest that building a semantic database of trait self-knowledge does not require access to a database of episodic memories.

Autism is a developmental disorder that has been hypothesized to impair normal development of the cognitive machinery that supports metarepresentations (Baron-Cohen, Leslie, and Frith, 1985; Leslie, 1987; Baron-Cohen, 1995). It has been proposed that episodic memories are stored in and retrieved via metarepresentations (e.g., Perner, 1991; Cosmides and Tooby, 2000). If so, then autism should disrupt the normal development of episodic memory. To test this prediction, Klein, Chan, and Loftus (1999) assessed the episodic memory of R.J., a 21-year-old man with autism.

Compared with ability-matched controls, R.J. was found to be severely impaired on a variety of tests of recall, especially when memory for personally experienced events was tested (e.g., the Galton-Crovitz task). Although his impairment was developmental in origin, his episodic performance was similar to that found in classic amnesia caused by brain trauma (similar findings have been reported by Boucher and Warrington, 1976; Boucher, 1981; and Millward et al., 2000; but see Minshew and Goldstein, 1993).

Despite this deficit in episodic retrieval, R.J. demonstrated reliable and accurate knowledge of his personality traits. His test-retest correlations were high ($r = 0.86$; IQ-matched controls, $r = 0.78$). Moreover, the correlation between R.J.'s trait self-ratings and his mother's ratings of him was significant ($r = 0.56$) and did not differ reliably from that obtained from control mother-son pairs ($r = 0.50$). R.J.'s self-ratings also were compared with ratings of R.J. obtained from one of his teachers; the correlation again was reliable ($r = 0.49$) and comparable to those obtained between control mother-son pairs.

These findings suggest that R.J.'s knowledge of what he is like accurately reflects how he is perceived by people with whom he interacts. But how did he acquire this trait self-knowledge? His case suggests that conscious access to a database of episodic memories is unnecessary. R.J. cannot retrieve episodic memories now and, because his impairment is developmental in origin, he probably never developed this ability in the first place. All four cases—W.J., D.B., K.C., and R.J.—show that trait self-knowledge can exist independently of episodic access, but R.J.'s developmental dissociation suggests that the acquisition of trait self-knowledge does not require episodic access (as does K.C.'s ability to update).

As in the case of D.B., further tests of R.J. suggested content-specific dissociations within semantic memory. Klein, Cosmides, Costabile, and Mei (2002) asked R.J. to judge features of common objects (e.g., "Is a lemon sour?" "Is a balloon round?"). R.J.'s answers were reliable across sessions ($r = 0.77$). However, they did not correlate with those provided by others of the same mental age. There was high agreement among IQ-matched controls, with correlations among their answers ranging from 0.78 to 0.81. In contrast, correlations between R.J.'s answers and theirs ranged from 0.18 to 0.33.

R.J.'s atypical semantic knowledge is not due to a general inability to understand or answer questions; his ability to answer personality questions is fine. This pattern of consensually accurate personality knowledge coexisting with odd, nonconsensual knowledge of foods, animals, and objects is surprising. One would think the evidence of one's senses would allow the easy acquisition of knowledge about tastes, shapes, and colors. Indeed, words like *sweet*, *tall*, and *large* are more concrete and have more obvious referents than personality terms such as *kind*, *friendly*, and *ungrateful*. Nevertheless, an individual with autism was able to learn his own personality traits but was unable to acquire consensually held knowledge of foods, animals, and objects. Because R.J.'s condition is caused by a developmental disorder, this pattern raises the possibility that there may be mechanisms specialized for acquiring knowledge of one's personality that can remain intact even when the mechanisms for acquiring knowledge of other domains are quite impaired.

K.R. K.R., a patient diagnosed with late-stage Alzheimer's dementia, shows that reliable, accurate knowledge of one's own personality can exist without the ability to update that knowledge (Klein, Cosmides, and Costabile, 2003).

K.R.'s performance on standard tests of cognitive functioning (e.g., the Mini-Mental State Examination) indicated severe dementia. She was disoriented for time and place and experienced difficulties with word finding and object naming. K.R. could not, for example, name simple objects such as batteries and pencils or draw the face of a clock from memory. Her anterograde memory function was severely impaired, leaving her unable to recall events she had in mind moments before. Knowledge of her personal past was sketchy: for example, she sometimes believed her late husband was alive, and her estimates of how long she had lived in her current facility ranged from 2 months to 14 years.

Despite these profound deficits, K.R. had reliable knowledge of her own personality traits. We asked her on two occasions (separated by 2 weeks) to judge a list of personality traits for self-descriptiveness. We also asked K.R.'s daughter and her caregiver at the assisted living facility to rate K.R. on the same traits. The results showed that K.R.'s test-retest ratings were reliable ($r = 0.86$). However, her ratings did not agree with the ratings provided by either her daughter or her caregiver ($r = 0.31$, -0.11 for daughter and caregiver, respectively). This lack of consistency was not because the daughter and caregiver were poor judges of character; when asked to rate other individuals, their judgments correlated strongly with those of others.

How could K.R.'s ratings be so reliable, yet agree so little with those who know her best? According to her family, K.R.'s personality and behavior changed dramatically as the disease progressed, but she seemed unaware of her transformation (a situation fairly common among patients with Alzheimer's dementia; e.g., Siegler, Dawson, and Welsh, 1994; Mills, 1998; Clare, in press). This suggests that the disease may have impaired K.R.'s ability to update the mental records that stored information about her personality. If her self-knowledge was intact but not being updated, then K.R.'s ratings may have reflected her premorbid personality rather than her current one.

To test this hypothesis, we asked K.R.'s daughter to rate her mother on the same list of traits, only this time she was asked to base her ratings on her mother's personality prior to the onset of the disease. These ratings were strongly correlated with those provided by K.R. herself ($r = 0.59$), as were preonset trait ratings of K.R. provided by her son-in-law ($r = 0.79$). Taken together, these findings indicate that K.R.'s ratings were accurate, but reflected her pre-Alzheimer's personality.

K.R. also knew her daughter's personality traits: when asked to rate her daughter on the same list of traits, her ratings correlated strongly with her daughter's self-ratings ($r = 0.65$). This is expected if K.R.'s fund of personality knowledge was created premorbidly and remained intact. But if, as hypothesized, K.R. lost the ability to update her personality files, then her ratings should have been inaccurate for people whom she first met after the onset of her dementia. This was the case. On two occasions (again, 2 weeks apart), K.R. was asked to rate her caregiver, whom she had known for 2.5 years. When the subject was her caregiver, K.R.'s test-retest reliability was low ($r = 0.34$), in striking contrast to the reliablity of her self-ratings ($r = 0.86$). Moreover, K.R.'s ratings of the caregiver did not overlap reliably with the caregiver's ratings of his own personality ($r = 0.18$). This difference was not due to the caregiver having a skewed view of himself: His self-ratings were strongly correlated with those provided by two neurologically healthy women living in the same facility who were similar in age to K.R. and who had known him for about the same length of time ($r = 0.73, 0.68$). This also shows that K.R.'s inability to acquire new personality information was not a simple manifestation of the normal aging process, because the neurologically healthy age-matched controls were quite capable of acquiring accurate knowledge of the personality of someone they had recently met.

Thus, despite profound cognitive deficits, K.R. had intact knowledge of her own premorbid personality and that of her daughter. That her trait knowledge had been preserved and remained retrievable is remarkable, given the difficulties she had retrieving ordinary facts from semantic memory: the names of everyday objects, what a clock looks like, where she was. As in the cases of R.J. and D.B., K.R.'s preserved self-knowledge suggests a dissociation *within* semantic memory, suggesting the presence of a functionally specialized database for the storage and retrieval of information about her personality.

It would appear, however, that the computational machinery responsible for updating personality knowledge was impaired in K.R. by Alzheimer's disease. K.R. did not know her own current, postmorbid personality, nor was she able to learn the personality traits of her primary caregiver. In K.R., trait knowledge of self and other remained intact, but the ability to update that knowledge based on new experiences was no longer functional.

Conclusions

A Semantic Subsystem Specialized for the Storage and Retrieval of Personality Trait Knowledge The results of the neuropsychological case studies support the following inferences:

1. The human mind stores knowledge of its own personality in the form of trait summaries. Retrieving trait summaries from this database does not depend on accessing episodic memories. Accurate trait judgments can be made by amnesic individuals—people who cannot retrieve any episodic memories (K.C., W.J., D.B., R.J.).

2. That K.C. knew his postmorbid personality suggests that trait summaries can be updated without accessing episodic memories. (Perhaps they are updated online, as events unfold.)

3. Intact retrieval of personality trait summaries can occur despite Alzheimer's dementia so severe that it impairs access to knowledge about many semantic domains (K.R.).

4. D.B. and R.J. had intact knowledge of their own personality traits, yet they showed impairments in other domains of semantic knowledge (personal history; general history; facts about animals, foods, objects; etc.). This is a dissociation *between* domains of semantic memory. These dissociations suggest that trait self-knowledge is a functionally isolable subsystem of semantic memory.

5. That D.B. knew his own personality traits but not his daughter's suggests that knowledge about one's own traits is stored separately from knowledge of other people's traits.

6. Taken together, nos. 3–5 suggest that there is a subsystem of semantic memory that is functionally specialized for the storage and retrieval of trait self-knowledge.

The idea of a subsystem within semantic memory specialized for storage and retrieval of personality trait knowledge is consistent with recent findings suggesting that semantic memory can be fractionated into different components, each of which can be damaged independently (e.g., Hodges and Patterson, 1997; Mackenzie Ross, and Hodges, 1997; Cappa et al., 1998; Caramazza and Shelton, 1998). For example, there are cases in which brain damage creates very content-specific patterns of nonretrieval from semantic memory, as seen in patients who (for example) cannot retrieve information about animals but can retrieve information about inanimate objects, whereas others have the opposite pattern of impairment (e.g., Caramazza and Shelton, 1998; Caramazza, 2000), still others have a selective deficit in their ability to retrieve knowledge of types of food (e.g., Hillis and Caramazza, 1991; Hart and Gordon, 1992; Laiacona et al., 1993), and so on. In all cases, the information that is selectively spared or impaired is a type of general world knowledge. It is therefore argued that the inaccessible or missing information is drawn from a semantic memory system, and that category-specific impairments reflect subsystems within a more encompassing semantic system (e.g., Hodges and Patterson, 1997; Caramazza, 2000; but see Martin, Ungerleider, and Haxby, 2000). From this perspective, D.B.'s and R.J.'s normal performance on the trait self-knowledge questionnaire can be seen as reflecting the operation of a specialized subsystem within semantic memory that represents trait knowledge about the self and was not compromised by cortical damage.

A SPECIALIZED ACQUISITION SYSTEM? The neuropsychological case histories also permit drawing some tentative conclusions about how the cognitive architecture learns the personality traits of the individual in which it is situated.

1. Learning personality traits does not require conscious access to episodic memories. K.C. learned about his post-morbid personality despite having no ability to retrieve episodic memories. R.J. also knew his personality traits, yet he could not retrieve behavioral episodes from memory. Indeed, R.J.'s disorder is developmental in origin, suggesting that he had never been able to retrieve episodic memories.

2. Alzheimer's dementia can damage the mechanisms that allow one to learn about personality traits, whether one's own or others. Yet the inability to update personality knowledge need not interfere with the ability to retrieve information from a preexisting store of trait summaries (K.R.).

3. Any dissociation between semantic domains, whether due to brain trauma or to autism, suggests functionally isolable storage and retrieval systems (D.B., R.J., K.R.). But finding a developmental dissociation in R.J. suggests a functionally isolable acquisition system. His semantic dissociation suggests that trait self-knowledge is acquired via learning mechanisms that are functionally distinct from those that cause the acquisition of knowledge about animals, objects, and foods.

Domain-general learning theories, connectionist or otherwise, presume that the same learning mechanisms account for knowledge acquisition across content domains. But a developmental dissociation that impairs the acquisition of knowledge about animals, objects, and foods while having no effect on the acquisition of trait knowledge is difficult to reconcile with such theories. Such results are especially difficult for theories positing equipotential mechanisms that compute correlations between elementary perceptual or conceptual dimensions. Surely the evidence of one's senses is sufficient for R.J. and others to end up concurring that apples are sweet, lemons are not, rocks are hard, and giraffes are tall. Yet R.J. and others did not concur in their judgments of easily observable properties of food, animals, and objects. In stark contrast, R.J.'s judgments about his own personality were consistent with those of others who know him, even though R.J.'s judgments were those of an autistic individual with social deficits.

MIND DESIGN: WHY HAVE A PERSONALITY TRAIT DATABASE ALONGSIDE AN EPISODIC STORE? Trait summaries have a signal virtue: they provide fast answers to trait judgment questions. This is important, because social interaction often requires split-second decisions, and the best course of action may depend on assumptions about how you and others are likely to behave in various situations. Time can be saved if trait summaries—generalizations about how people are

likely to behave—are computed in advance and stored for later use (for discussion, see Klein, Cosmides, Tooby, and Chance, 2002). The alternative—retrieving and then evaluating a series of episodes online each and every time a trait judgment is needed—is more costly in both time and computation (e.g., Klein, Loftus, Trafton, and Fuhrman, 1992; Klein, Babey, and Sherman, 1997).

This view explains three sets of interlocking facts. First, it explains why trait summaries exist. Second, it explains why retrieving a trait summary fails to prime recall of trait-consistent episodes. Because summaries are precomputed answers to trait judgment questions, there is no additional advantage to retrieving trait-consistent episodes in tandem with them; the information that trait-consistent episodes provides is redundant with the summary (Babey, Queller, and Klein, 1998; Klein, Cosmides, Tooby, and Chance, 2001, 2002). Third, and less obviously, it explains why an episodic store is maintained despite trait summaries, and when trait judgments will access the episodic store.

Klein, Cosmides, Tooby, and Chance (2002) argue that an excellent package of speed plus accuracy can be engineered into a decision system by jointly activating a trait summary and episodic memories that are *inconsistent* with it. Trait summaries allow fast access to relevant information. But a trait summary (e.g., "I am usually friendly") gives information about behavior under average circumstances. It does not tell you under what circumstances a behavior deviates from average. In deciding how to behave, one is always facing a particular situation. Accordingly, a generalization is most useful when its scope is delimited, that is, when it is accompanied by information specifying those situations in which it does not apply. Episodic memories that are inconsistent with the generalization can serve this function, because they encode specific situations in which the generalization fails to predict the outcome. Thus, to render judgments that are both fast and accurate, judgment and decision procedures should be designed to search for summary information in semantic memory and, on retrieving it, also search for episodic memories that are inconsistent with that summary, ones that place boundary conditions on the summary's scope. Thus, there is a function to maintaining a store of episodic memories even after a trait summary has been formed: memories of behavioral episodes can provide boundary conditions on the scope of generalizations (Babey, Queller, and Klein, 1998; Cosmides and Tooby, 2000; Klein, Cosmides, Tooby, and Chance, 2001, 2002).

This *scope hypothesis* was tested in a recent series of experiments on trait self-judgments using the priming paradigm described above. Klein, Cosmides, Tooby, and Chance (2001, 2002) showed that when a trait summary is retrieved, trait-inconsistent behavioral episodes are retrieved along with it. More specifically, the time it took subjects to recall a trait-inconsistent episode was faster following a describe task than following a control task. In other words, asking a subject whether he or she is *kind* coactivates memories of episodes in which that person did something *un*kind. Consistent with the scope hypothesis, inconsistent episodes are primed only when a trait summary has been retrieved. When a trait summary is absent, trait-consistent episodes are primed. This makes sense: in the absence of a trait summary, episodes are the only information one has on which to base a judgment.

Many view priming as a functionless by-product of neural activation. The results of these experiments support a quite different view: computational systems will be designed to prime representations when this solves an adaptive problem for the organism. The fact that retrieving trait summaries primes episodic memories that are inconsistent with the summary but not ones that are consistent with it cannot be explained as a by-product of neural activation (for discussion, see Klein, Cosmides, Tooby, and Chance, 2002). It is instead the signature of a functional and adaptive system: one that is designed to deliver just the right mix of information from memory to the right decision rules at the right time.

The human cognitive architecture does seem to contain a database that is functionally specialized for the storage and retrieval of personality trait information. Because social life is so adaptively important for our species, it should not be surprising to find that this database is resilient in the face of trauma and developmental disruptions. Nor should it be surprising to find mechanisms specialized for creating and refreshing this database; people change with time and experience, and the database needs to be constantly updated so that it accurately captures what a person is like at the moment that relevant decisions are made.

By isolating and elucidating the systems and databases that allow us to know ourselves, cognitive neuroscience is making "first-person epistemology" a topic of scientific inquiry rather than just philosophical speculation. As this process continues, the self may gradually reclaim the place William James originally carved out for it: as a central construct in psychology.

ACKNOWLEDGMENTS The work was supported by an Academic Senate Research Grant from the University of California, Santa Barbara (S.B.K.). I thank my primary collaborators, Judith Loftus, John Kihlstrom, and John Tooby, for their invaluable contributions to the work presented here. I also want to thank Leda Cosmides, whose insightful comments, intellectual contributions, and unfailing encouragement played a key role in the development of the ideas in this chapter.

NOTES

1. These conclusions were based on results obtained using the analytic technique known as statistical parametric mapping. However, another technique, partial least-squares analysis, revealed activations of the right and left medial frontal lobes.

2. Although these pioneering studies are provocative and interesting, it is probably too early to conclude that the self is located in the left cerebral hemisphere. Although cognitive science generally has embraced a doctrine of modularity, the neural representation of individual items of declarative knowledge is distributed widely across the cortex. Accordingly, while self-referential processing may be performed by a specialized brain module or system, declarative knowledge of the self, whether episodic or semantic, is likely to be widely distributed over the same neural structures that represent knowledge of other people, as well as objects in the nonsocial domain.

REFERENCES

AHERN, C. A., F. B. WOOD, and C. M. McBRIEN, 1998. Preserved vocabulary and reading acquisition in an amnesic child. In *Brain and Values*, K. Pribram, ed. Mahwah, N.J.: Erlbaum, pp. 277–298.

ALLPORT, G. W., 1961. *Patterns and Growth in Personality.* New York: Holt, Rinehart & Winston.

BABEY, S. H., S. QUELLER, and S. B. KLEIN, 1998. The role of expectancy violating behaviors in the representation of trait-knowledge: A summary-plus-exception model of social memory. *Soc. Cogn.* 16:287–339.

BARON-COHEN, S., 1995. *Mindblindness: An Essay on Autism and Theory of Mind.* Cambridge, Mass.: MIT Press.

BARON-COHEN, S., 2000. The cognitive neuroscience of autism: Evolutionary approaches. In *The New Cognitive Neurosciences*, M. Gazzaniga, ed. Cambridge, Mass.: MIT Press, pp. 1249–1257.

BARON-COHEN, S., A. M. LESLIE, and U. FRITH, 1985. Does the autistic child have a "theory of mind"? *Cognition* 21:37–46.

BERMUDEZ, J. L., 1998. *The Paradox of Self-Consciousness.* Cambridge, Mass.: MIT Press.

BOUCHER, J., 1981. Memory for recent events in autistic children. *J. Autism Dev. Disord.* 11:293–301.

BOUCHER, J., and E. K. WARRINGTON, 1976. Memory deficits in early infantile autism: Some similarities to the amnesic syndrome. *Br. J. Psychol.* 67:73–87.

BOWER, G. H., and S. G. GILLIGAN, 1979. Remembering information related to one's self. *J. Res. Pers.* 13:420–432.

BUSS, D. M., and K. H. CRAIK, 1983. The act frequency approach to personality. *Psychol. Rev.* 90:105–126.

CAPPA, S. F., M. FRUGONI, P. PASQUALI, D. PERANI, and F. ZORAT, 1998. Category-specific naming impairment for artifacts. *Neurocase* 4:391–397.

CARAMAZZA, A., 2000. The organization of conceptual knowledge in the brain. In *The New Cognitive Neurosciences*, M. S. Gazzaniga, ed. Cambridge, Mass.: MIT Press.

CARAMAZZA, A., and J. SHELTON, 1998. Domain-specific knowledge systems in the brain: The animate-inanimate distinction. *J. Cogn. Neurosci.* 10:1–34.

CASSAM, Q., 1994. *Self-Knowledge.* Oxford, England: Oxford University Press.

CERMAK, L. S., 1984. The episodic-semantic memory distinction in amnesia. In *Neuropsychology of Memory*, L. R. Squire and N. Butters, eds. New York: Guilford Press, pp. 45–54.

CERMAK, L. S., and M. O'CONNOR, 1983. The anterograde and retrograde retrieval ability of a patient with amnesia due to encephalitis. *Neuropsychologia* 21:213–234.

Clare, L., in press. Managing threats to self: Awareness in early stage Alzheimer's disease. *Soc. Sci. Med.*

Cohen, N. J., and H. B. Eichenbaum, 1993. *Memory, Amnesia, and Hippocampal Function*, Cambridge, Mass.: MIT Press.

COSMIDES, L., and J. TOOBY, 2000. Consider the source: The evolution of adaptations for decoupling and metarepresentation. In *Metarepresentations: A Multidisciplinary Perspective. Vancouver Studies in Cognitive Science*, D. Sperber, ed. New York: Oxford University Press, pp. 53–115.

CRAIK, F. I. M., T. M. MOROZ, M. MOSCOVITCH, D. T. STUSS, G. WINOCUR, E. TULVING, and S. KAPUR, 1999. In search of the self: A PET investigation of self-referential information. *Psychol. Sci.* 10:26–34.

CRISPIN, W., B. C. SMITH, and C. MACDONALD, eds., 1998. *Knowing Our Own Minds*. Oxford, England: Oxford University Press.

CROVITZ, H. F., and H. SCHIFFMAN, 1974. Frequency of episodic memories as a function of their age. *Bull. Psychon. Soc.* 4(5B): 517–518.

EVAN, J., B. WILSON, E. P. WRAIGHT, and J. R. HODGES, 1993. Neuropsychological and SPECT scan findings during and after transient global amnesia: Evidence for the differential impairment of remote episodic memory. *J. Neurol. Neurosurg. Psychiatry* 56: 1227–1230.

FOSTER, J. K., and M. JELICIC, 1999. *Memory: Systems, Process, or Function?* New York: Oxford University Press.

FRITH, C. D., 1992. *The Cognitive Neuropsychology of Schizophrenia*. East Sussex, England: Erlbaum/Taylor and Francis.

FRITH, C. D., and U. FRITH, 1992. Elective affinities in schizophrenia and childhood autism. In *Social Psychiatry: Theory, Methodology, and Practice*, P. E. Bebbington, ed. New Brunswick, N.J.: Transactions Press.

GALLAGHER, S., 2000. Philosophical conceptions of the self: Implications for cognitive science. *Trends Cogn. Sci.* 4:14–21.

GALLAGHER, S., and J. SHEAR, 1999. *Models of the Self*. Thorverton, England: Academic.

GALTON, F., 1879. Psychometric experiments. *Brain* 2:149–162.

GENNARO, R. J., 1996. *Consciousness and Self-Consciousness*. Philadelphia: John Benjamins.

GREENWALD, A. G., 1981. Self and memory. In *The Psychology of Learning and Motivation*, vol. 15, G. H. Bower, ed. New York: Academic Press, pp. 201–236.

GREENWALD, A. G., and A. R. PRATKANIS, 1984. The self. In *Handbook of Social Cognition*, vol. 3, R. S. Wyer and T. K. Srull, eds. Hillsdale, N.J.: Erlbaum, pp. 129–178.

HART, J., and B. GORDON, 1992. Neural subsystems for object knowledge. *Nature* 6390:60–64.

HIGGINS, E. T., and J. A. BARGH, 1987. Social cognition and social perception. *Ann. Rev. Psychol.* 38:369–425.

HILLIS, A. E., and A. CARAMAZZA, 1991. Category-specific naming and comprehension impairment: A double dissociation. *Brain* 114:2081–2094.

HODGES, J. R., and K. PATTERSON, 1997. Semantic memory disorders. *Trends Cogn. Sci.* 1:68–72.

HUMPHREY, N., 1984. *Consciousness Regained: Chapters in the Development of Mind*. New York: Oxford University Press.

JAMES, W., 1890. *The Principles of Psychology*, vol. 1. New York: Holt.

Keenan, J. M., 1993. An exemplar model can explain Klein and Loftus' results. In *Advances in Social Cognition*, vol. 5, T. K. Srull and R. S. Wyer, eds. Hillsdale, N.J.: Erlbaum, pp. 69–77.

KEENAN, J. P., A. NELSON, M. O'CONNOR, and A. PASCUAL-LEONE, 2001. Self-recognition and the right hemisphere. *Nature* 409:305.

KELLEY, W. M., C. N. MACRAE, C. L. WYLAND, S. CAGLAR, S. INATI, and T. F. HEATHERTON, 2002. Finding the self? An event-related fMRI study. *J. Cogn. Neurosci.* 15:785–794.

KILHSTROM, J. F., 1997. Consciousness and me-ness. In *Scientific Approaches to Consciousness*, J. D. Cohen and J. W. Schooler, eds. Mahwah, N.J.: Erlbaum, pp. 451–468.

KIHLSTROM, J. F., J. S. BEER, and S. B. KLEIN, 2002. Self and identity as memory. In *Handbook of Self and Identity*, M. R. Leary and J. Tangney, eds. New York: Guilford Press, pp. 68–90.

KIHLSTROM, J. F., and S. B. KLEIN, 1994. The self as a knowledge system. In *Handbook of Social Cognition*, vol. 1, *Basic Processes*, R. S. Wyer and T. K. Srull, eds. Hillsdale, N.J.: Erlbaum, pp. 153–208.

KIRCHER, T. T. J., C. SENIOR, M. L. PHILLIPS, P. J. BENSON, E. T. BULLMORE, M. BRAMMER, A. SIMMONS, S. C. R. WILLIAMS, M. BARTELS, and A. S. DAVID, 2000. Towards a functional neuroanatomy of self processing: Effects of faces and words. *Cogn. Brain Res.* 10:133–144.

KLEIN, S. B., 2001. A self to remember: A cognitive neuropsychological perspective on how self creates memory and memory creates self. In *Individual Self, Relational Self, and Collective Self*, C. Sedikides and M. B. Brewer, eds. Philadelphia: Psychology Press, pp. 25–46.

KLEIN, S. B., S. H. BABEY, and J. W. SHERMAN, 1997. The functional independence of trait and behavioral self-knowledge: Methodological considerations and new empirical findings. *Soc. Cognit.* 15:183–203.

KLEIN, S. B., R. L. CHAN, and J. LOFTUS, 1999. Independence of episodic and semantic self-knowledge: The case from autism. *Soc. Cognit.* 17:413–436.

KLEIN, S. B., L. COSMIDES, and K. A. COSTABILE, 2003. Preserved knowledge of self in a case of Alzheimer's dementia. *Soc. Cognit.* 21:157–165.

KLEIN, S. B., L. COSMIDES, K. A. COSTABILE, and L. MEI, 2002. Is there something special about the self? A neuropsychological case study. *J. Res. Pers.* 36:490–506.

KLEIN, S. B., L. COSMIDES, J. TOOBY, and S. CHANCE, 2001. Priming exceptions: A test of the scope hypothesis in naturalistic trait judgments. *Soc. Cognit.* 19:443–468.

KLEIN, S. B., L. COSMIDES, J. TOOBY, and S. CHANCE, 2002. Decisions and the evolution of memory: Multiple systems, multiple functions. *Psychol. Rev.* 109:306–329.

KLEIN, S. B., and J. F. KIHLSTROM, 1986. Elaboration, organization, and the self-reference effect in memory. *J. Exp. Psychol. Gen.* 115: 26–38.

KLEIN, S. B., and J. F. KIHLSTROM, 1998. On bridging the gap between social-personality psychology and neuropsychology. *Pers. Soc. Psychol. Rev.* 2:228–242.

KLEIN, S. B., and J. LOFTUS, 1988. The nature of self-referent encoding: The contributions of elaborative and organizational processes. *J. Pers. Soc. Psychol.* 55:5–11.

KLEIN, S. B., and J. LOFTUS, 1990. The role of abstract and exemplar-based knowledge in self-judgments: Implications for a cognitive model of the self. In *Advances in Social Cognition*, vol. 3, T. K. Srull and R. S. Wyer, eds. Hillsdale, N.J.: Erlbaum, pp. 131–139.

KLEIN, S. B., and J. LOFTUS, 1993a. The mental representation of trait and autobiographical knowledge about the self. In *Advances in Social Cognition*, vol. 5, T. K. Srull and R. S. Wyer, eds. Hillsdale, N.J.: Erlbaum.

KLEIN, S. B., and J. LOFTUS, 1993b. Behavioral experience and trait judgments about the self. *Pers. Soc. Psychol. Bull.* 19:740–745.

KLEIN, S. B., J. LOFTUS, and H. A. BURTON, 1989. Two self-reference effects: The importance of distinguishing between self-descriptiveness judgments and autobiographical retrieval in self-referent encoding. *J. Pers. Soc. Psychol.* 56:853–865.

KLEIN, S. B., J. LOFTUS, and J. F. KIHLSTROM, 1996. Self-knowledge of an amnesic patient: Toward a neuropsychology of personality and social psychology. *J. Exp. Psychol. Gen.* 125:250–260.

KLEIN, S. B., J. LOFTUS, and A. E. PLOG, 1992. Trait judgments about the self: Evidence from the encoding specificity paradigm. *Pers. Soc. Psychol. Bull.* 18:730–735.

KLEIN, S. B., J. LOFTUS, and J. W. SHERMAN, 1993. The role of summary and specific behavioral memories in trait judgments about the self. *Pers. Soc. Psychol. Bull.* 19:305–311.

KLEIN, S. B., J. LOFTUS, R. G. TRAFTON, and R. W. FUHRMAN, 1992. The use of exemplars and abstractions in trait judgments: A model of trait knowledge about the self and others. *J. Pers. Soc. Psychol.* 63:739–753.

KLEIN, S. B., K. ROZENDAL, and L. COSMIDES, 2002. A social-cognitive neuroscience analysis of the self. *Soc. Cognit.* 20:105–135.

KLEIN, S. B., R. W. SHERMAN, and J. LOFTUS, 1996. The role of episodic and semantic memory in the development of trait self-knowledge. *Soc. Cognit.* 14:277–291.

LAIACONA, M., R. BARBAROTTO, K. TRIVELLI, and E. CAPITANI, 1993. Perceptual and associative knowledge in category specific impairment of semantic memory. *Cortex* 4:727–740.

LESLIE, A. M., 1987. Pretense and representation: The origins of "theory of mind." *Psychol. Rev.* 94:412–426.

LESLIE, A. M., 2000. "Theory of mind" as a mechanism of selective attention. In *The New Cognitive Neurosciences*, M. S. Gazzaniga, ed. Cambridge, Mass.: MIT Press, pp. 1235–1247.

LESLIE, A. M., and L. THAISS, 1992. Domain specificity in conceptual development: Neuropsychological evidence from autism. *Cognition* 43:225–251.

LINVILLE, P., and D. E. CARLSTON, 1994. Social cognition of the self. In *Social Cognition: Impact on Social Psychology*, P. G. Devine, D. L. Hamilton, and T. M. Ostrom, eds. San Diego, Calif.: Academic Press, pp. 143–193.

LOCKSLEY, A., and M. LENAUER, 1981. Considerations for a theory of self-inference processes. In *Personality, Cognition, and Social Interaction*, N. Cantor and J. F. Kihlstrom, eds. Hillsdale, N.J.: Erlbaum, pp. 263–277.

LORD, C. G., 1993. The "social self" component of trait knowledge about the self. In *Advances in Social Cognition*, vol. 5, T. K. Srull and R. S Wyer, eds. Hillsdale, N.J.: Erlbaum, pp. 91–100.

MACKENZIE ROSS, S. J., and J. R. HODGES, 1997. Preservation of famous person knowledge in a patient with severe postanoxic amnesia. *Cortex* 33:733–742.

MARTIN, A., L. UNGERLEIDER, and J. HAXBY, 2000. Category specificity and the brain: The sensory/motor model of semantic representations of objects. In *The New Cognitive Neurosciences*, M. S. Gazzaniga, ed. Cambridge, Mass.: MIT Press, pp. 1023–1036.

MAYES, A. R., 2000. Selective memory disorders. In *The Oxford Handbook of Memory*, E. Tulving and F. I. M. Craik, eds. New York: Oxford University Press, pp. 427–440.

McGINN, C., 1991. *The Problem of Consciousness: Essays Toward a Resolution*. Oxford, England: Blackwell.

MILLS, M. A., 1998. *Narrative Identity and Dementia*. Aldershot, England: Ashgate Publishing.

MILLWARD, C., S. POWELL, D. MESSER, and R. JORDAN, 2000. Recall for self and other in autism: Children's memory for events experienced by themselves and their peers. *J. Autism Dev. Disord.* 30: 15–28.

MINSHEW, N. J., and G. GOLDSTEIN, 1993. Is autism an amnesic disorder? Evidence from the California Verbal Learning Test. *Neuropsychology* 7:209–216.

MORIN, A., 2002. Right hemisphere self-awareness: A critical assessment. *Consciousness Cognit.* 11:396–401.

MOSCOVITCH, M., T. YASCHYSHYN, M. ZIEGLER, and L. NADEL, 2000. Remote episodic memory and retrograde amnesia: Was

Tulving right all along? In *Memory, Consciousness, and the Brain: The Tallinn Conference*, E. Tulving, ed. Philadelphia: Psychology Press, pp. 331–345.

OLSON, E. T., 1999. There is no problem of the self. In *Models of the Self*, S. Gallagher and J. Shear, eds. Thorverton, England: Academic, pp. 49–61.

PARKIN, A. J., 1987. *Memory and Amnesia*. New York: Basil Blackwell.

PARKIN, A. J., 1993. *Memory: Phenomena, Experiment and Theory*. Cambridge, England: Blackwell.

PARKIN, A. J., 1996. *Explorations in Cognitive Neuropsychology*. Malden, Mass.: Blackwell.

PARKIN, A. J., and N. R. C. LENG, 1993. *Neuropsychology of the Amnesic Syndrome*. Hillsdale, N.J.: Erlbaum.

PERNER, J., 1991. *Understanding the Representational Mind*. Cambridge, Mass.: MIT Press.

PERNER, J., and T. RUFFMAN, 1994. Episodic memory and autonoetic consciousness: Developmental evidence and a theory of childhood amnesia. *J. Exp. Child Psychol.* 59:516–548.

ROBINSON, J. A., 1976. Sampling autobiographical memory. *Cogn. Psychol.* 8:578–595.

ROGERS, T. B., 1981. A model of the self as an aspect of the human information processing system. In *Personality, Cognition, and Social Interaction*, N. Cantor and J. F. Kihlstrom, eds. Hillsdale, N.J.: Erlbaum, pp. 193–214.

ROGERS, T. B., N. A. KUIPER, and W. S. KIRKER, 1977. Self-reference and the encoding of personal information. *J. Pers. Soc. Psychol.* 35:677–688.

RYLE, G., 1949. *The Concept of Mind*. New York: Barnes and Noble.

SCHACTER, D. L., and E. TULVING, eds., 1994. *Memory Systems 1994*. Cambridge, Mass.: MIT Press.

SCHELL, T. L., S. B. KLEIN, and S. H. BABEY, 1996. Testing a hierarchical model of self-knowledge. *Psychol. Sci.* 7:170–173.

SIEGLER, I. C., D. V. DAWSON, and K. A. WELSH, 1994. Caregiver ratings of personality change in Alzheimer's disease patients: A replication. *Psychol. Aging* 9:464–466.

SHALLICE, T., 1988. *From Neuropsychology to Mental Structure*. New York: Cambridge University Press.

SHERMAN, J. W., 1996. Development and mental representation of stereotypes. *J. Pers. Soc. Psychol.* 70:1126–1141.

SHERMAN, J. W., and S. B. KLEIN, 1994. Development and representation of personality impressions. *J. Pers. Soc. Psychol.* 67: 972–983.

SHERMAN, J. W., S. B. KLEIN, A. LASKEY, and N. A. WYER, 1998. Intergroup bias in group judgment processes: The role of behavioral memories. *J. Exp. Soc. Psychol.* 34:51–65.

SMITH, E. R., and M. A. ZARATE, 1992. Exemplar-based models of social judgment. *Psychol. Rev.* 99:3–21.

STARKSTEIN, S. E., L. SABE, and M. F. DORREGO, 1997. Severe retrograde amnesia after a mild closed head injury. *Neurocase* 3: 105–109.

SUDDENDORF, T., and M. C. CORBALLIS, 1997. Mental time travel and the evolution of the human mind. *Genet. Soc. Gen. Psychol. Monogr.* 123:133–167.

SYMONS, C. S., and B. T. JOHNSON, 1997. The self-reference effect in memory: A meta-analysis. *Psychol. Bull.* 121:371–394.

TULVING, E., 1983. *Elements of Episodic Memory*. New York: Oxford University Press.

TULVING, E., 1985. Memory and consciousness. *Can. Psychol.* 26:1–12.

TULVING, E., 1993a. What is episodic memory? *Curr. Direct. Psychol. Sci.* 2:67–70.

TULVING, E., 1993b. Self-knowledge of an amnesic individual is represented abstractly. In *Advances in Social Cognition*, vol. 5,

T. K. Srull and R. S. Wyer, eds. Hillsdale, N.J.: Erlbaum, pp. 147–156.

TULVING, E., 1995. Organization of memory: Quo vadis? In *The Cognitive Neurosciences*, M. S. Gazzaniga, ed. Cambridge, Mass.: MIT Press, pp. 839–847.

TULVING, E., and D. L. SCHACTER, 1990. Priming and human memory systems. *Science* 247:301–306.

UTTAL, W. R., 2000. *The War Between Mentalism and Behaviorism: On the Accessibility of Mental Processes*. Mahwah, N.J.: Erlbaum.

VARGHA-KHADEM, F., D. G. GADIAN, K. E. WATKINS, A. CONNELLY, W. VAN PAESSCHEN, and M. MISHKIN, 1997. Differential effects of early hippocampal pathology on episodic and semantic memory. *Science* 277:376–380.

WEISKRANTZ, L., 1997. *Consciousness Lost and Found*. New York: Oxford University Press.

WHEELER, M. A., D. T. STUSS, and E. TULVING, 1997. Toward a theory of episodic memory: The frontal lobes and autonoetic consciousness. *Psychol. Bull.* 121:331–354.

WIGGINS, J. S., 1973. *Personality and Prediction: Principles of Personality Assessment*. Reading, Mass.: Addison-Wesley.

WILLIAMS, B., 1973. *Problems of the Self*. Cambridge, England: Cambridge University Press.

WOOD, F. B., I. S. BROWN, and R. H. FELTON, 1989. Long-term follow-up of a childhood amnesic syndrome. *Brain Cogn.* 10: 76–86.

ZHANG, L., J. ZHANG, Z. LIU, T. ZHOU, J. FAN, and Y. ZHU, 2002. *In search of the Chinese self: An fMRI study*. Unpublished manuscript.

ZYSSET, S., O. HUBER, E. FERSTL, and D. Y. VON CRAMON, 2002. The anterior frontomedian cortex and evaluative judgment: An fMRI study. *NeuroImage* 15:983–991.

78   Frontal Lobe Contributions to Executive Control of Cognitive and Social Behavior

JENNIFER S. BEER, ARTHUR P. SHIMAMURA, AND ROBERT T. KNIGHT

ABSTRACT This chapter examines the lateral and medial/orbitofrontal portions of the prefrontal lobes and their distinctive roles in controlling cognitive and social behavior. Evidence from neuropsychological, electrophysiological, and functional neuroimaging research suggests that lateral areas of the frontal lobes are involved in processes that permit the adaptive control of cognition, whereas orbitofrontal and medial prefrontal areas are involved in processes underlying the regulation of social behavior. Future research employing a host of cognitive neuroscience techniques will be critical for understanding how the lateral and orbitofrontal cortices interact to produce adaptive social behavior.

The frontal lobes in humans are critical for executive control of cognition and social behavior. The complex demands of human social interaction raise the issue of how individuals are able to act appropriately to achieve desired outcomes across myriad social situations. Self-regulation, or the ability to modify and control behavior in order to conform to social norms, has been extensively researched and shown to be fundamental to social success (e.g., Carver and Scheier, 1990; Baumeister and Heatherton, 1996). Appropriate social behavior requires individuals to control cognitive processes such as directing attention to relevant information or coping with novel information. After attention has been directed, self-regulation requires individuals to engage in a host of integrative processes such as synthesizing emotional and cognitive information, monitoring behavior in relation to the relevant context, and assessing feedback from others by making inferences about their mental and emotional states. The prefrontal cortex is in a unique position to control both cognitive and social processes through its extensive reciprocal connections with cortical, limbic, and subcortical sites. Evidence from neuropsychological, electrophysiological, and functional neuroimaging research suggests that lateral areas

of the frontal lobes are involved in processes that permit the adaptive control of cognition, whereas orbitofrontal and medial prefrontal areas are involved in processes underlying the regulation of social behavior. This chapter examines the lateral and medial/orbitofrontal portions of the prefrontal lobes and their distinctive roles in controlling cognitive and social behavior.

Lateral prefrontal cortex and control over attention

Cognition must be controlled in various ways; individuals need to filter out what is irrelevant, attend to what is relevant, and monitor novel information for relevance. From an anatomical perspective, the prefrontal cortex is involved in both inhibitory and excitatory control of widespread neural systems, in addition to having a response bias toward novelty. The role of lateral prefrontal areas in controlling online cognition takes two specific forms: the ability to filter out irrelevant information and the ability to orient to, sustain, and manipulate relevant information in working memory. The manipulation of relevant information includes both expected and novel information.

INHIBITION AND LATERAL PREFRONTAL CORTEX Some of the earliest evidence for the role of lateral prefrontal areas in inhibiting irrelevant information comes from the report of a multimodal prefrontal-thalamic sensory gating system in cats (Skinner and Yingling, 1977; Yingling and Skinner, 1977). This prefrontal-thalamic inhibitory system provides a powerful neural substrate for early suppression of extraneous inputs, permitting more effective focusing of attention. In addition to obvious behavioral relevance, this gating system conserves energy expenditure by blocking irrelevant inputs at an early level of processing (Guillery, Feig, and Lozsadi, 1998; Sherman and Guillery, 2003).

Event-related potential (ERP) studies provide similar physiological evidence of an inhibitory mechanism controlled by lateral prefrontal cortex. Recordings of ERPs to irrelevant auditory and somatosensory stimuli in patients with dorsolateral prefrontal damage provide physiological

JENNIFER S. BEER   Department of Psychology and Center for Mind and Brain, University of California at Davis, Davis, Calif.

ARTHUR P. SHIMAMURA and ROBERT T. KNIGHT   Department of Psychology and Helen Wills Neuroscience Institute, University of California at Berkeley, Berkeley, Calif.

evidence of a deficit in inhibitory control. Evoked responses from primary auditory (Kraus, Ozdamar, and Stein, 1982) and somatosensory (Sutherling et al., 1988) cortices were recorded from these patients and both age-matched and brain-lesioned controls (i.e., individuals with lesions of the posterior association cortex, sparing the primary sensory regions). Stimuli elicited a small thumb twitch via monaural clicks or brief electric shocks to the median nerve. Prefrontal damage produced disinhibition of both the primary auditory- and somatosensory-evoked responses (Knight, Scabini, and Woods, 1989; Yamaguchi and Knight, 1990). Spinal cord and brainstem potentials were not affected by prefrontal damage, suggesting that the amplitude enhancement reflected abnormalities in either a prefrontal-thalamic or a prefrontal-sensory cortex mechanism. Damage to primary auditory or somatosensory cortex reduced the early latency (20–40 ms) evoked responses generated in these regions. The attention deficits observed in patients with prefrontal damage have been linked to problems with inhibitory control of posterior sensory and perceptual mechanisms (Lhermitte, 1986; Lhermitte, Pillon, and Serdaru, 1986).

The inability of patients with prefrontal damage to suppress irrelevant information is reflected in their poor performance on target detection and match-to-sample paradigms. Patients who have undergone frontal resections are impaired at detecting multiple visual targets embedded among distracters (Richer et al., 1993). Similarly, patients with focal dorsolateral prefrontal lesions are impaired in simple delay tasks requiring matching of two environmental sounds when distracters intervene between cue and target. For example, patients with prefrontal lesions were tested on an auditory delayed match-to-sample task. Subjects reported whether a cue (S_1) and a subsequent target sound (S_2) were identical. S_1 and S_2 were separated either by a silent period or by distracting, irrelevant tone pips. Distracters impaired the behavioral performance of patients with prefrontal lesions and generated enhanced primary auditory cortex-evoked responses to these irrelevant tones (Chao and Knight, 1995, 1998).

EXCITATION AND LATERAL PREFRONTAL CORTEX   In addition to suppressing response to irrelevant stimuli, subjects must excite and sustain neural activity in distributed brain regions to direct attention to relevant information. Damage to prefrontal areas is associated with deficits in attention. For example, normal subjects generate robust attention effects for left or right ear stimulation. Patients with left prefrontal damage have slightly reduced attention effects in both ears. A different pattern is observed after right prefrontal damage. Patients with right prefrontal damage show electrophysiological and behavioral evidence of a dense hemi-inattention to left ear stimuli (Knight et al., 1981). This observation is consistent with the human hemineglect syndrome, which is

more common after right prefrontal or temporoparietal lesions (Kertesz and Dobrolowski, 1981; Mesulam, 1981; Hier et al., 1983). One theory holds that the contralateral neglect observed after temporoparietal or prefrontal right hemisphere lesions is due to innate hemispheric attention asymmetries. The left frontal lobe is proposed to allocate attention only to the contralateral right hemispace, whereas the right frontal lobe is proposed to allocate attention to both contralateral and ipsilateral hemispaces. Thus, neglect is mild or not apparent after left hemisphere lesions, because the intact right hemisphere is capable of allocating attention to both hemispaces. Dense contralateral neglect is seen after right hemisphere damage, because the left hemisphere is incapable of allocating attention to the left hemispace (Mesulam, 1981).

The increased size of the right frontal lobe in humans may provide the anatomical substrate for the hemi-inattention syndrome in humans (Wada, Clarke, and Hamm, 1975; Weinberger et al., 1982). Posterior association cortex lesions in the temporoparietal junction have comparable attention deficits for left- and right-sided lesions, indicating that these areas are not asymmetrically organized for auditory selective attention (Woods, Knight, and Scabini, 1993). This suggests that the left hemineglect syndrome consequent on right temporoparietal damage may be due to remote effects of disconnection from asymmetrically organized prefrontal regions.

Selective attention to an ear, a region of the visual field, or a digit increases the amplitude of sensory-evoked potentials to all stimuli delivered to that sensory channel (Hillyard et al., 1973). There is evidence that attention reliably modulates neural activity at early sensory cortices, including secondary and perhaps primary sensory cortex (Woldorff et al., 1993; Grady et al., 1997; Somers et al., 1999; Steinmetz et al., 2000). Visual attention involves modulation in the excitability of extrastriate neurons through descending projections from hierarchically ordered brain structures (Hillyard and Anllo-Vento, 1998). The role of prefrontal cortex in the control of extrastriate cortex during visual attention has been shown in single-cell recordings in monkeys (Fuster, Brodner, and Kroger, 2000; Funahashi, Bruce, and Goldman-Rakic, 1993; Rainer et al., 1998a,b), lesion studies in humans (Knight, 1997; Nielsen-Bohlman and Knight, 1999; Barcelo, Suwazono, and Knight, 2000) and monkeys (Rossi et al., 1999), and blood flow studies (McIntosh et al., 1994; Büchel and Friston, 1997; Chawla, Gees, and Friston, 1999; Rees, Frackowiak, and Frith, 1997; Kastner et al., 1999; Corbetta, 1998; Hopfinger, Buonocore, and Mangun, 2000).

The dorsolateral prefrontal cortex controls visual attention by regulating posterior association cortex through predominantly excitatory connections. ERP studies in patients with lateral prefrontal damage have shown that the human lateral prefrontal cortex regulates attention-dependent extrastriate neural activity through three distinct mechanisms. These mechanisms are (1) a tonic excitatory influence on ipsilateral posterior areas for all sensory information, including attended and nonattended sensory inputs, (2) an attention-dependent enhancement of extrastriate cortex, and (3) a phasic excitatory influence of ipsilateral posterior areas to correctly perceived task-relevant stimuli. In these ERP studies, patients with unilateral prefrontal cortex lesions (centered in Brodmann's areas 9 and 46) performed a series of visual attention experiments. In the task, nontarget stimuli consisted of upright triangles, which were presented rapidly to both visual fields. Targets were rarely presented (10% of all stimuli) and consisted of inverted triangles presented randomly in each visual field. In one experiment, patients and age-matched controls were asked to press a button whenever a target appeared in either visual field (Barcelo, Suwazono, and Knight, 2000). In another experiment, subjects were required to allocate attention to only one visual field (Yago and Knight, 2000) (figures 78.1 and 78.2).

An interesting pattern of results emerged from these two experiments. First, both experiments revealed that the lateral prefrontal cortex provides a tonic excitatory influence to ipsilateral extrastriate cortex. Specifically, the P1 component of the visual ERP is markedly reduced in amplitude for all stimuli presented to the contralesional field. Importantly, this tonic influence is attention independent, since a reduced P1 potential in extrastriate cortex was found ipsilateral to prefrontal cortex damage for all visual stimuli (attended and nonattended targets and nontargets) presented to the contralesional field. This tonic component may be viewed as an excitatory modulatory influence on extrastriate activity.

The second experiment (allocating attention to only one visual field) provided evidence of the temporal kinetics of prefrontal-extrastriate interactions. In essence, attention effects on extrastriate cortex were normal in the first 200 ms of processing in patients with lesions of the prefrontal cortex and severely disrupted after 200 ms (Yago and Knight, 2000). This finding suggests that other cortical areas are

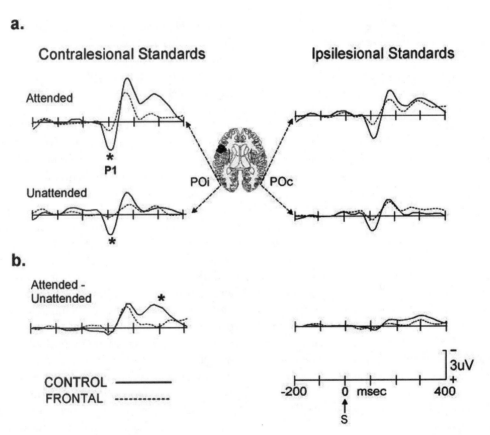

FIGURE 78.1 Visual event-related potentials in patients with lateral frontal lobe damage and healthy control subjects. Patients with dorsolateral prefrontal cortex lesions had to detect upright triangles in a series of inverted triangles (standards, 70%), upright triangles (targets, 20%), and novel stimuli (10%) presented one at time to either side of fixation. Patients ($n = 8$) and controls ($n = 11$) were instructed to attend and respond to targets on the left or the right of fixation. (a) The ERPs elicited by the contralesional standard

stimuli elicited significantly reduced P1 responses in the patients, whether the standards were in the attended or the unattended side. (b) The attention effect, extracted by subtracting the response to unattended standards from the response to the attended ones, revealed a significantly smaller effect for contralesional standards in patients than in controls, starting around 200 ms postonset. (Modified from Yago and Knight, 2000.)

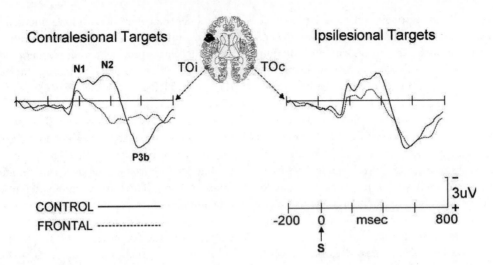

Contralesional Targets   **Ipsilesional Targets**

CONTROL ————
FRONTAL ··············

3uV

-200   0   msec   800

S

FIGURE 78.2   Same paradigm as figure 78.1, except that patients (*n* = 10) and controls (*n* = 10) were attending to both right and left sides in this case. The N1, N2, and P3b peaks, seen in the controls' waveform, were significantly reduced in the patients in response to conralesional targets but not in response to ipsilesional targets (see Yago and Knight, 2000, for more details). TOi = T5 or T6, the one ipsilateral to the lesion in patients; T5 in controls. TOc = T5 or T6, the one contralateral to the lesion in patients, T6 in controls. POi/POc relate in the same manner to P7/8.

responsible for attention-dependent regulation of extrastriate cortex in the first 200 ms. The neuroimaging and clinical literature suggest that the inferior parietal cortex may be responsible for the early reflexive component of attention, whereas the prefrontal cortex is responsible for more controlled and sustained aspects of visual attention onsetting after the parietal signal to extrastriate cortices.

The third observation from these experiments is that lateral prefrontal cortex sends a top-down signal to extrastriate cortex when a task-relevant event is detected during an attention task. Two types of stimuli are typically presented in an attended channel: one task irrelevant and one requiring detection and a behavioral response. The amplitude of both the irrelevant and relevant stimuli is enhanced in an attended channel. Prefrontal cortex is responsible for regulating this channel-specific attention enhancement. When a relevant target event is detected in an attended channel, both a distinct electrophysiological event and a channel-specific enhancement are generated. This top-down signal onsets at about 200 ms after a correct detection, persists for 500 ms and is superimposed on the channel-specific ERP attention enhancement (Suwazono, Machado, and Knight, 2000). Damage to lateral prefrontal cortex reduces the top-down signal and impairs detection ability (Barcelo, Suwazono, and Knight, 2000).

The temporal parameters of this human prefrontal cortex-extrastriate attention modulation are consistent with single-unit recordings in monkeys that reveal enhanced prefrontal stimulus detection-related activity 140 ms poststimulus onset (Rainer, Assad, and Miller, 1998a,b) and with other studies revealing top-down activation of inferior temporal neurons 180–300 ms posttarget detection (Tomita

et al., 1999). Finally, there is a vigorous debate in the single-unit and fMRI research domains over whether lateral prefrontal cortex is organized by modality (Wilson, Scalaidhe, and Goldman-Rakic, 1993; Courtney et al., 1998; Romanski et al., 1999) or whether lateral prefrontal cortex functions in a modality-independent executive manner during working memory and object and spatial integration (Rao, Rainer, and Miller, 1997; Assad, Rainer, and Miller, 1998; D'Esposito et al., 1999; Miller, 1999; Fuster, Brodner, and Kroger, 2000). Evidence from patients with prefrontal cortex lesions (Mueller, Machado, and Knight, 2002) supports the notion that the lateral portion of prefrontal cortex may function in a task-independent manner to control and integrate distributed neural activity in some cognitive tasks.

One manner in which prefrontal cortex may control attention is by modulating the relative excitation and inhibition of neural activity. For example, Desimone (1998) has proposed a competition model of visual attention: visual neurons that process different aspects of the visual world are mutually inhibitory. In this view, an excitatory signal to selective visual neurons inhibits nearby non-task-relevant visual neurons and thereby sharpens attentional focus. A possible glutamatergic pathway by which lateral prefrontal cortex could facilitate visual processing is suggested by projections from prefrontal areas 45 and 8 to inferior temporal (IT) areas TE and TEO in monkeys (Webster, Bachevalier, and Ungerleider, 1994). Patients with focal prefrontal damage fail to maintain excitatory control of these areas, resulting in failure in attention/working memory.

A similar failure of prefrontal excitatory modulation is observed in the auditory modality. Prefrontal lesions markedly reduce the attention-sensitive N100 component throughout the hemisphere ipsilateral to damage (Chao and Knight, 1998). Prefrontal projections to the superior temporal plane may subserve this excitatory prefrontal cortex-auditory cortex input (Alexander, Newman, and Symmes, 1976). The auditory and visual data provide clear evidence that the lateral prefrontal cortex is crucial for maintaining distributed intrahemispheric neural activity during auditory and visual attention/working memory tasks.

VOLUNTARY AND INVOLUNTARY ATTENTION Another manner in which cognition must be controlled is to voluntarily direct attention to relevant information as well as novel stimuli, that is, new and unexpected stimuli.

ERPs, fMRI, and attention to context-relevant stimuli In everyday life, humans continually detect and respond to discrete environmental events. When voluntarily directing attention to a target, people must maintain a template of the target in order to allocate attention to template-matching information. Research suggests that voluntary attention as indexed by the P3b response engages a distributed circuit that includes prefrontal cortex as well as multimodal posterior association cortex, hippocampus, and cingulate cortex (for reviews, see Swick, Kutas, and Neville, 1994; Picton, 1995). In this network, prefrontal activity increases with task difficulty (D'Esposito et al., 1994; Owen, Evans, and Petrides, 1996; Petrides et al., 1993; Swick and Knight, 1994).

Voluntary attention has most often been operationalized using the "oddball" task. In the oddball task, participants detect an infrequent and low-probability event, in other words, an oddball stimulus, in a series of background stimuli. Detection of the oddball generates a prominent parietal maximal P3b. The P3b is the P300 response generated when attention is voluntarily allocated to a task-relevant event (Desmedt, Debecker, and Manil, 1965; Sutton et al., 1965). The P3b is widely believed to reflect an update of activity in corticolimbic circuits or template matching during voluntary attention and working memory (Ruchkin et al., 1992; Chao, Nielsen-Bohlman, and Knight, 1995), but no clear theoretical consensus on the P3b has been reached (Donchin and Coles, 1988; Verleger, 1988).

ERPS and attention to novel stimuli Involuntary orientation to an unexpected and novel stimulus generates a P300 response similar in some regards to the P3b generated by a voluntarily detected stimulus. However, the novel response differs in three important aspects from the P3b. The novelty P300, referred to as P3a, has a more frontocentral scalp distribution than P3b, peaks 60–80 ms earlier in all sensory modalities, and undergoes rapid habituation over the first 5–10 stimulus presentations (Knight, 1984, 1997; Knight, Scabini, Woods, and Clayworth, 1989; Yamaguchi and Knight,

1991a). Just as patients with prefrontal lesions show impairments in both sustained and phasic attention (Knight, 1994), they also show deficits in orienting to unexpected novel stimuli (i.e., P3a response). Prefrontal lesions are associated with reduced P3a responses to unexpected novel stimuli in the auditory (Knight, 1984; Knight and Scabini, 1998), visual (Knight, 1997), and somatosensory modalities (Yamaguchi and Knight, 1991b, 1992; see Soltani and Knight, 2000, for a review) (figure 78.3).

Orbital and medial prefrontal cortex: Integrative processes underlying behavioral regulation

The cognitive control function of the dorsolateral prefrontal regions lays the groundwork for self-regulation; however, many integrative processes must be engaged before behavior can be adaptively controlled. In contrast to the low-level cognitive control function of the dorsolateral prefrontal regions, the orbitofrontal area and medial prefrontal areas are critically involved in the processes that underlie the control of social behavior. From an anatomical perspective, the orbitofrontal cortex is richly connected to areas associated with emotional and social processing, including the amygdala, anterior cingulate, and somatosensory areas I and II (e.g., Brothers, 1996; Adolphs, 1999). Phineas Gage and others like him with orbitofrontal damage are characterized by impaired self-regulation (e.g., Harlow, 1848; Hornak, Rolls, and Wade, 1996; Shimamura, 2002). The regulation of behavior requires various kinds of emotional and social processing, such as the ability to synthesize emotional information (i.e., environmental feedback) with subsequent decisions, the ability to meaningfully monitor one's own behavior, and the ability to make inferences about the mental states and behavior of others. Theory and research suggest that orbitofrontal function is not associated with one specific mechanism underlying behavioral regulation. Rather, orbitofrontal cortex is involved in the synthesis of emotional and cognitive information, the ability to accurately monitor one's own behavior, and possibly the ability to make inferences about others' mental states. In addition, the medial prefrontal cortex is involved in making inferences about others' mental states.

SYNTHESIS OF EMOTION AND COGNITION Three major theories have been proposed to explain the role of the orbitofrontal cortex in the self-regulation of behavior. All three agree that the orbitofrontal cortex is involved in the synthesis of emotional and cognitive information. However, the exact mechanism through which the synthesis is accomplished is somewhat different across theories.

The somatic marker hypothesis The somatic marker hypothesis suggests that poor decision making occurs when somatic

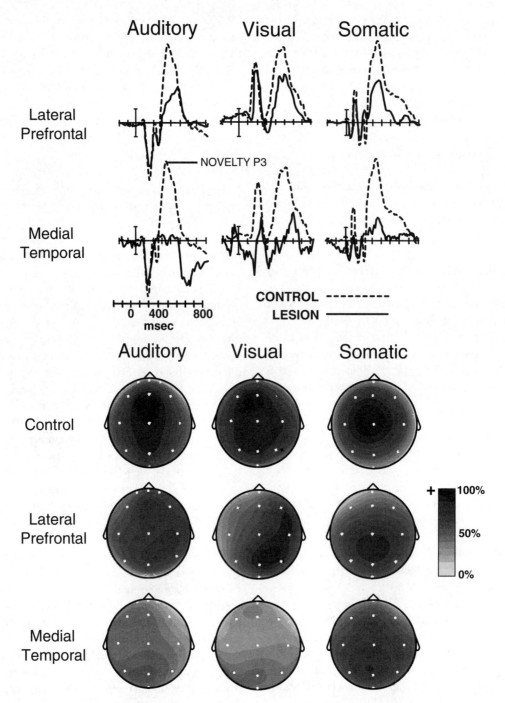

FIGURE 78.3   Results from several studies indicate that lateral pre-frontal and posterior medial temporal regions are crucial for the generation of the scalp-recorded novelty P3. Upper part of figure presents plots of the novelty P3 elicited in the auditory, visual, and somatosensory modalities in patients with lateral prefrontal or posterior medial temporal lesions and in matched control groups. Positive is plotted upward. Scale bar for the auditory and somatosensory plots = 2 μV. Scale bar for the visual plots = 1 μV. Lower part of figure presents topographic maps illustrating the scalp topography of the novelty P3 in the two patient groups and the control group. For illustration purposes, a subset of the electrode locations used to calculate each map is shown as black circles. The novelty P3 had a frontal topography in control subjects across all modalities, whereas the novelty P3 topography was more posterior in patients with prefrontal lesions and was virtually eliminated in patients with medial temporal lesions. (From Ranganath and Rainer, 2003.)

information is not available to guide decision making (e.g., Bechara et al., 1997; Bechara, Damasio, and Damasio, 2000). From this perspective, orbitofrontal structures provide the substrate for learning associations between complex situations and the type of emotional state usually associated with a particular situation. Orbitofrontal cortex modulates a distributed network of activity thought to reflect the brain's attempt to recreate previously experienced associations between internal physiology and external situations. Specifically, orbitofrontal structures are activated in response to complex social situations and then activate somatic effectors in the amygdala, hypothalamus, and brainstem nuclei. Somatic markers are generated for the purpose of rapidly processing option-outcome associations and marking them as good or bad. Decision making can then selectively focus on option-outcome pairings that are potentially rewarding. This process should be particularly helpful when there is ambiguity in the environment and past experience is the primary source for making an informed decision (Bechara, Damasio, and Damasio, 2000; Elliot, Dolan, and Frith, 2000).

Empirical support for the somatic marker hypothesis comes from a series of studies that used a gambling task to examine the relation between somatic markers and decision making (e.g., Bechara et al., 1997). Over time, healthy adults, patients with damage to the dorsolateral prefrontal cortex, and patients with damage outside the prefrontal cortex gradually start to gamble in a manner that maximizes winnings. In contrast, many of the patients with orbitofrontal lesions fail to implement an optimal gambling strategy on a behavioral level, even though some can verbally state the optimal strategy. Furthermore, whereas normal control subjects show an increased SCR in anticipation of making a risky gamble, the group with orbitofrontal damage shows no anticipatory change in SCR. However, both groups do show SCR in response to winning or losing a particular gamble. These results are interpreted as indicating that orbitofrontal damage, particularly to the right side (Tranel, Bechara, and Denburg, 2002), impairs decision making, because somatic markers are not triggered and therefore cannot guide the gambling decisions.

Reinforcement and reversal Another perspective on the role of orbitofrontal cortex in self-regulation focuses on the role of orbitofrontal cortex in reinforcement and reversal processes (Rolls, 2000). From this perspective, the poor decision making and disinhibition of patients with orbitofrontal lesions reflects their inability to change their behavior in response to changing stimulus-reinforcement contingencies. The orbitofrontal cortex computes the reward and punishment value of stimuli as a function of the environmental context. Furthermore, information about the stimulus-reinforcement contingencies is updated continually and

allows for rapid reversal or extinction of stimulus-reinforcement associations. However, with damage to the orbitofrontal cortex, individuals are unable to alter their behavior as a function of these changing stimulus-reinforcement contingencies and presumably cannot inhibit inappropriate responses.

The empirical evidence for this position comes from research with nonhuman primates and humans. Thorpe, Rolls, and Maddison (1983) used single-unit recording in orbitofrontal neurons of three rhesus monkeys during a go/no-go visual discrimination task to examine learning and reversal of stimulus-reinforcement contingencies. The contingencies in the experiment were often reversed during the 4-hour recording session so that the previously rewarded stimuli became aversive. Some neuronal activity in the orbitofrontal cortex was associated with learning a stimulus-reinforcement contingency (e.g., responding to the presence of a reward or responding to the presence of punishment). Furthermore, activity was found (1) in response to behavior that was no longer rewarded and (2) again on the first delivery of a reward in the new paradigm. This activity was interpreted to reflect the detection of a paradigmatic shift. The involvement of the orbitofrontal cortex in reversal learning is also supported by studies in humans. Rolls and colleagues (1994) tested patients with orbitofrontal damage and patients with damage outside the orbitofrontal cortex on a visual discrimination task that examined reversal and extinction. Participants were presented with a go/no-go task involving images of patterns on a computer screen. Throughout the experiment, the reinforcement contingency changed, so that previously rewarded patterns resulted in either loss of points (reversal) or no gain (extinction). The findings suggested that the orbitofrontal group could learn the first pattern-reinforcement contingency much as the other patients and normal controls did. However, on reversal or extinction of the previously learned contingency, patients with orbitofrontal lesions were unable to stop themselves from responding to the previously rewarded patterns. As in the gambling studies, these patients could verbally report that they should no longer touch the screen for those patterns. In contrast, patients with damage outside the orbitofrontal area and normal control subjects did not show this type of perseveration. Staff member ratings of orbitofrontal patients' social disinhibition correlated with their error percentages from the reversal task and the extinction task. The authors interpreted these findings as indicating that patients with orbitofrontal lesions experience social problems because they are unable to alter their behavior in response to changing stimulus-reinforcement contingencies that naturally occur in daily life.

Dynamic filtering theory A third perspective on the role of orbitofrontal cortex in synthesizing emotional and cognitive

Auditory

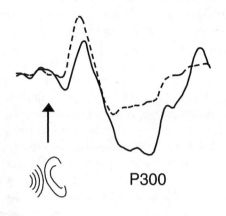

Somatosensory

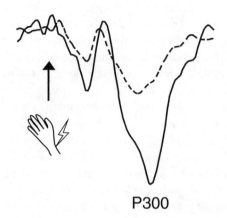

P300

P300

Control - - - - - -
Orbitofrontal ———

-5 uV

100 ms

FIGURE 78.4   ERP recordings at Pz site for abrupt auditory (left panel) and somatosensory (right panel) stimuli. Patients with orbitofrontal damage exhibited heightened P3 amplitudes compared to control participants.

information is dynamic filtering theory (Shimamura, 2000a). According to Shimamura and his colleagues, the prefrontal cortex is responsible for implementing a variety of gating or filtering devices in its role in the monitoring and control of information processing. In other words, the frontal lobes serve an executive function wherein neural activity from other brain regions is filtered or gated based on its relevance to the task at hand. The orbitofrontal cortex is heavily connected to sensory and limbic areas and therefore may be responsible for filtering neural activity associated with emotional response to the environments (Rule, Shimamura, and Knight, 2002). Patients with orbitofrontal damage cannot benefit from this filtering mechanism and cannot inhibit the neural activity associated with emotional processing. Therefore, the disinhibition seen in these patients may be accounted for by their inability to inhibit their response to emotional stimuli in the environment.

Empirical evidence for the dynamic filtering role of the orbitofrontal cortex for emotional stimuli comes from a study that examined ERPs generated in response to unpredictable, aversive stimuli (Rule, Shimamura, and Knight, 2002). Participants with orbitofrontal damage, dorsolateral prefrontal damage, and normal control subjects were presented with mild shocks or distracting noises while watching a silent movie. For both the shock and the noise condition, patients with orbitofrontal damage showed greater P300 amplitudes than the other patient group and the normal control subjects (figure 78.4). Additionally, patients with orbitofrontal damage did not show habituation for the somatosensory stimuli, whereas control subjects did. No significant difference for habituation for the auditory stimuli was found between the orbitofrontal and the control groups. These findings suggest that the orbitofrontal cortex plays a role in regulating neural activity associated with emotional stimuli. Patients with orbitofrontal damage were not able to gate or filter posterior cortical activity in response to aversive stimuli and therefore did not show the habituation characteristic of normal controls.

In summary, close examination of the extant research suggests that these theories are not mutually exclusive. Rather, it may be that the ventromedial portion of the orbitofrontal cortex is involved in decision making (i.e., the somatic marker hypothesis) and the lateral portion is involved in making association reversals (i.e., reinforcement/reversal theory). In this case, both portions could regulate activity from other brain regions involved in socioemotional processing (i.e., dynamic filtering theory).

SELF-MONITORING   Another fundamental process underlying appropriate self-regulation is individuals' ability to accurately perceive their social behavior. Clinical characterizations of damage to various areas of the frontal lobes suggest that the frontal lobes are intricately involved in self-monitoring (e.g., Stuss and Benson, 1986). The impaired self-monitoring associated with frontal damage may be accounted for by faulty monitoring processes such as reality checking (i.e., determining which behaviors are appropriate for a given context), self-insight (i.e., accurate perceptions of one's own behaviors), and encoding self-relevant information.

Reality checking Reality checking has been proposed as a major mechanism underlying different disturbances of self-awareness (Stuss, 1991; Shimamura, 1996, 2000b; Stuss, Gallup, and Alexander, 2001). Reality checking involves a continual assessment of the relationship between behavior and the environment. As an individual acts on the environment, the consequences of the action must be incorporated into existing plans. If the environment deviates from expectations, this change must be detected and plans must be reassessed. Reality checking is necessary for maintaining a flexible repertoire of behavior. Without these monitoring processes, behavior is not under the control of an individual but rather becomes stimulus bound (Luria, 1966/1980; Lhermitte, 1986; Lhermitte, Pillon, and Serdaru, 1986). Stimulus-bound behavior is typical in patients with prefrontal cortex damage (Luria, 1966/1980; Lhermitte, 1986). The patients studied by Lhermitte and colleagues included those with large lateral prefrontal lesions that extended into the orbital and basal ganglia regions in some subjects. Thus, precise behavioral-anatomical conclusions must be tempered. Objects placed in front of patients with damage to the prefrontal cortex in Lhermitte's studies were picked up and used (utilization behavior) without the patient being asked to do so (Lhermitte, 1986). Additionally, patients with prefrontal damage may imitate the behavior of the experimenter even when this behavior is bizarre and socially inappropriate. These observations suggest that prefrontal damage impairs the ability to execute contextually appropriate behavior.

Self-insight Orbitofrontal damage may also impair self-insight, that is, the ability to accurately monitor one's own behavior (figure 78.5). A series of behavioral studies have shown that patients with damage to the orbitofrontal cortex tend to be unaware that their social behavior is inappropriate in comparison to patients with dorsolateral prefrontal damage and healthy control participants (Beer, 2002). In one study, patients with orbitofrontal lesions, patients with dorsolateral prefrontal lesions, and normal subjects participated in a self-disclosure task with an experimenter they did not know. The task (Aron et al., 1997) required participants to regulate how much personal information they disclosed,

because some of the questions were inappropriate for a conversation between two strangers. Trained judges blind to the neurological condition of the participants coded transcripts of the conversations for breadth, appropriateness, and intimacy of self-disclosure. A measure of accurate self-perception was computed by comparing self-reports of self-disclosure with the trained judges' codes. Patients with orbitofrontal damage tended to overestimate the appropriateness of the intimacy of their self-disclosure. No differences were found for patients with dorsolateral prefrontal lesions or normal subjects. A lack of self-insight may also be reflected in orbitofrontal patients' failure to emotionally appraise their behavior in an appropriate way unless their ability to accurately monitor their behavior is facilitated. For example, patients with orbitofrontal damage became embarrassed by their inappropriate social behavior only when experimental methods (e.g., feedback from others, video playback) specifically drew their attention to their behavior. No such failure in emotional appraisal was found in normal subjects (Beer et al., 2001, in press) or patients with dorsolateral lesions (Beer, 2002).

Self-relevant information Imaging research suggests that the medial prefrontal cortex (e.g., BA 9 and 10) is involved in encoding information that is relevant to the self. Decades of behavioral research have shown that information encoded in relation to the self is remembered better than information encoded in relation to other references, including other people (see Symons and Johnson, 1997). Recently, a series of brain imaging studies have suggested that the medial prefrontal cortex is specifically involved in encoding information in relation to one's self. Studies using PET (Craik et al., 1999) and fMRI (Kelley et al., 2002) have found increased activity in the medial prefrontal cortex (BA 9 and 10) when encoding information in relation to the self, compared with encoding information in relation to a famous political figure or syllabic structure. Similarly, a series of fMRI studies has consistently shown that right BA 9 and 10 has increased activity when observing one's own face versus that of a close other or another person (e.g., Keenan et al., 2000).

MAKING INFERENCES ABOUT OTHERS The ability to make inferences about how other people may be reacting to a person or the environment is critical for knowing when to modify one's behavior. Both lesion and imaging research suggest that the medial prefrontal cortex is involved in making inferences about others, such as understanding other people's mental and emotional states.

Theory of mind Both medial prefrontal and orbitofrontal cortex have been implicated in making inferences about others' mental states. Two imaging studies found that left medial prefrontal areas, BA 8 and 9, showed increased

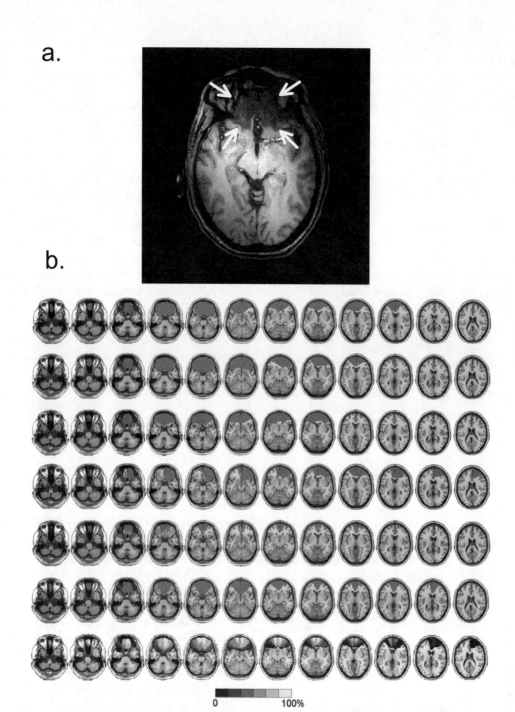

FIGURE 78.5 (*a*) Axial section through orbital prefrontal cortex obtained using a 4T scanner. The lesion has completely destroyed the lateral and medial orbital prefrontal cortex (arrowheads) but has spared the anterior temporal lobes. (*b*) Lesion extent in four patients with bilateral orbital prefrontal cortex damage recon- structed from CT or MRI scans. Each row shows the extent of damage in an individual patient as transcribed onto axial templates using 5-mm sections. Bottom row represents the extent of lesion overlap across subjects.

activation when participants were asked to make a mental inference versus a physical inference. In one study, participants had to decide whether a person living in the fifteenth century would know the function of an object or decide what function an object had. When these two conditions were compared, increased activity in left BA 9 was found (Goel et al., 1997). Another study examined activation in relation to story comprehension that required the participants to make either a mental inference or a physical inference about a character's actions. When these two conditions were compared, increased activity in left BA 8 was found (Fletcher et al., 1995). In contrast, another imaging study showed increased activation in right orbitofrontal regions in comparison with left polar frontal regions during a mental state recognition task that required participants to decide whether a word described a mind state or a body state (Baron-Cohen et al., 1994).

There is also evidence from human lesion research that prefrontal areas are involved in making mental inferences. Price and colleagues (1990) found that patients with damage to the dorsolateral prefrontal cortex were impaired at giving directions to another person, compared with normal subjects. Although some studies suggest that orbitofrontal cortex, particularly the right side, is critically involved in theory of mind on a visual perspective task (Stuss, Gallup, and Alexander, 2001), another study found that patients with orbitofrontal and dorsolateral prefrontal damage did not have trouble with basic-level theory of mind tasks (Stone, Baron-Cohen, and Knight, 1998). However, patients with orbitofrontal lesions were impaired in making inferences about the intentions of characters in vignettes about social faux pas, compared with normal subjects and patients with dorsolateral prefrontal lesions.

Conversational style The lack of insight into others' minds is also reflected in the conversational style of patients with orbitofrontal lesions. Kaczmarek (1984) analyzed lesion patients' utterances as they repeated a story, described pictures, and told a story about both familiar and unfamiliar topics. The study found that damage to the left orbitofrontal cortex was associated with confabulation, misnamings, and digressions from the topic. These findings were interpreted as reflecting a decreased appreciation for the necessity of a coherent description to ensure that the audience understood the speaker.

Empathy It is also possible that prefrontal areas are important for making inferences about the emotional states of others. Empirical support for the role of orbitofrontal cortex in making inferences about the emotional states of others is mixed. Some studies have found that patients with orbitofrontal damage are impaired on paper-and-pencil measures of empathy (Grattan et al., 1994; Shamay-Tsoory

et al., 2003). Two studies found that patients with orbitofrontal lesions were impaired at inferring emotional states from pictures of various emotional facial expressions (Hornak, Rolls, and Wade, 1996), although in one study, this impairment only held for expressions of embarrassment and shame (Beer et al., in press). However, Stone, Baron-Cohen, and Knight (1998) did not find that patients with orbitofrontal lesions had trouble inferring the feelings of story characters who had been on the receiving end of a social faux pas.

Conclusions

The role of the prefrontal cortex in executive control has become a central issue in cognitive neuroscience. The dorsolateral prefrontal cortex is critical in controlling cognition in a manner that permits efficient processing of information. Extensive behavioral and physiological data have confirmed that this area is important not only for filtering out irrelevant information, but also for directing attention and sustaining representations of information that is relevant, including orienting to unexpected stimuli. Additionally, a growing body of research suggests that the orbitofrontal and medial prefrontal regions of the frontal lobes are critical for permitting individuals to control their social behavior appropriately. The bulk of the extant literature consists of lesion studies that suggest that orbitofrontal cortex is fundamentally involved in synthesizing emotional and cognitive information, monitoring one's behavior, and monitoring others' mental states. In addition, neuroimaging studies suggest that prefrontal medial cortex is involved in encoding self-relevant information and making inferences about others' mental states.

The role of the frontal lobes in controlling social behavior is less well developed than its role in cognitive control and is receiving increasing attention. This area will benefit most from future research combining theory and methods from neuroscience and social psychology. For example, psychologists can contribute to neuroscience by providing overarching theories of social and personality constructs that can be used to parsimoniously explain sets of functions associated with a particular network. Neuropsychological and neuroimaging research has shown that orbitofrontal cortex and medial prefrontal areas are involved in such diverse functions as synthesizing emotional information with cognitive information as well as self and other perception. The construct of self-regulation suggests that all of these functions are important for exerting control over social behavior, and therefore suggest a framework for understanding the association between these functions.

Future research employing a host of cognitive neuroscience techniques will be critical for understanding how the lateral and orbital frontal cortices interact online to produce adaptive social behavior. This line of inquiry is expected to yield important insights into the nature of human thought and social interaction.

ACKNOWLEDGMENTS This work was supported by NINDS and NIMH grants NS21135, DA14110, and PO NS40813 and the McDonnell Foundation (R.T.K.). Work was also supported by NSF grant BCS 0121970 and NIMH MH66574 (J.S.B.). Special thanks to Clay C. Clayworth for technical assistance in all phases of the work.

REFERENCES

ADOLPHS, R., 1999. Social cognition and the human brain. *Trends Cogn. Sci.* 3:469–479.

ALEXANDER, G. E., J. D. NEWMAN, and D. SYMMES, 1976. Convergence of prefrontal and acoustic inputs upon neurons in the superior temporal gyrus of the awake squirrel monkey. *Brain Res.* 116:334–338.

AMARAL, D. G., R. INAUSTI, and W. M. COWAN, 1983. Evidence for a direct projection from the superior temporal gyrus to the entorhinal cortex in the monkey. *Brain Res.* 275:263–277.

ARON, A., E. MELINAT, E. N. ARON, R. D. VALLONE, and R. J. BATOR, 1997. The experimental generation of interpersonal closeness: A procedure and some preliminary findings. *Pers. Soc. Psychol. Bull.* 4:363–377.

ASAAD, W. F., G. RAINER, and E. K. MILLER, 1998. Neural activity in the primate prefrontal cortex during associative learning. *Neuron* 21:1399–1407.

BARCELO, P., S. SUWAZONO, and R. T. KNIGHT, 2000. Prefrontal modulation of visual processing in humans. *Nat. Neurosci.* 3: 399–403.

BARON-COHEN, S., H. RING, J. MORIARTY, B. SCHMITZ, D. COSTA, and P. ELL, 1994. Recognition of mental state terms. *B. J. Psychiatry* 165:640–649.

BAUMEISTER, R. F., and T. A. HEATHERTON, 1996. Self-regulation failure: An overview. *Psychol. Inquiry* 7:1–15.

BECHARA, A., H. DAMASIO, and A. R. DAMASIO, 2000. Emotion, decision making, and the orbitofrontal cortex. *Cereb. Cortex* 10:295–307.

BECHARA, A., H. DAMASIO, D. TRANEL, and A. R. DAMASIO, 1997. Deciding advantageously before knowing the advantageous strategy. *Science* 275:1293–1295.

BEER, J. S., 2002. *Self-regulation of social behavior.* Doctoral diss., University of California, Berkeley.

BEER, J. S., E. A. HEEREY, D. KELTNER, D. SCABINI, and R. T. KNIGHT (in press). The regulatory function of self-conscious emotion: Insights from patients with orbitofrontal damage. *J. Pers. Soc. Psychol.*

BEER, J. S., N. A. ROBERTS, K. H. WERNER, R. W. LEVENSON, D. SCABINI, and R. T. KNIGHT, 2001. Orbitofrontal cortex and self-conscious emotion. *Soc. Neurosci. Abstr.* 27:1705.

BROTHERS, L., 1996. Brain mechanisms of social cognition. *J. Psychopharmacol.* 10:2–8.

BÜCHEL, C., and K. J. FRISTON, 1997. Modulation of connectivity in visual pathways by attention: Cortical interactions evaluated with structural equation modeling and fMRI. *Cereb. Cortex* 7:768–778.

CARVER, C. S., and M. SCHEIER, 1990. Principles of self-regulation: Action and emotion. In *Handbook of Motivation and Cognition: Foundations of Social Behavior*, Higgins E. T. and R. M. Sorrentino, eds. New York: Guildford Press, pp. 3–52.

CHAO, L. L., and R. T. KNIGHT, 1995. Human prefrontal lesions increase distractibility to irrelevant sensory inputs. *Neuroreport* 6:1605–1610.

CHAO, L. L., and R. T. KNIGHT, 1998. Contribution of human prefrontal cortex to delay performance. *J. Cogn. Neurosci.* 10:167–177.

CHAO, L. L., L. NIELSEN-BOHLMAN, and R. T. KNIGHT, 1995. Auditory event-related potentials dissociate early and late memory processes. *Electroencephalogr. Clin. Neurophysiol.* 96:157–168.

CHAWLA, D., R. GEES, and K. J. FRISTON, 1999. The physiological basis of attentional modulation in extrastriate visual areas. *Nat. Neurosci.* 2:671–676.

CORBETTA, M., 1998. Frontoparietal cortical networks for directing attention and the eye to visual locations: Identical, independent, or overlapping neural systems? *Proc. Natl. Acad. Sci. U.S.A.* 95: 831–838.

COURTNEY, S. M., L. PETIT, J. M. MAISOG, L. G. UNGERLEIDER, and J. V. HAXBY, 1998. An area specialized for spatial working memory in human frontal cortex. *Science* 279:1347–1351.

CRAIK, F. I. M., T. M. MOROZ, M. MOSCOVITCH, D. T. STUSS, G. WINCOUR, E. TULVING, and S. KAPUR, 1999. In search of the self: A positron emission tomography study. *Psychol. Sci.* 10:26–34.

DESIMONE, R., 1998. Visual attention mediatd by biased competition in extrastriate cortex. *Philos. Trans. R. Soci. Lond. Seri. B Biol. Sci.* 353:1245–1255.

DESMEDT, J. E., J. DEBECKER, and J. MANIL, 1965. Mise en evidence d'un signe electrique cerebral associe a la detection par le sujet d'un stimulus sensoriel tactile. *Bull. Acad. R. Med. Belg.* 5:887–936.

D'ESPOSITO, M., J. DETRE, D. ALSOP, R. SHIN, S. ATLAS, and M. GROSSMAN, 1994. The neural basis of the central executive system of working memory. *Nature* 378:279–281.

D'ESPOSITO, M., B. R. POSTLE, D. BALLARD, and J. LEASE, 1999. Maintenance versus manipulation of information held in working memory: An event-related fMRI study. *Brain Cogn.* 41: 66–86.

DONCHIN, E. and M. G. H. COLES, 1988. Is the P300 component a manifestation of context updating? *Behav. Brain Sci.* 11:357–427.

ELLIOTT, R., R. J. DOLAN, and C. D. FRITH, 2000. Dissociable functions in the medial and lateral orbitofrontal cortex: Evidence from human neuroimaging studies. *Cereb. Cortex* 10:308–317.

FLETCHER, P. C., F. HAPPE, U. FRITH, S. C. BAKER, R. J. DOLAN, R. S. J. FRACKOWIAK, and C. D. FRITH, 1995. Other minds in the brain: A functional imaging study of "theory of mind" in story comprehension. *Cognition* 57:109–128.

FUNIHASHI, S., C. J. BRUCE, and P. S. GOLDMAN-RAKIC, 1993. Dorsolateral prefrontal lesions and oculomotor delayed-response performance: Evidence for mnemonic "scotomas." *J. Neurosci.* 13:1479–1497.

FUSTER, J. M., M. BRODNER, and J. K. KROGER, 2000. Cross-modal and cross-temporal associations in neurons of frontal cortex. *Nature* 405:347–351.

GOEL, V., J. GRAFMAN, J. TAJIK, S. GANA, and D. DANTO, 1997. A study of the performance of patients with frontal lobe lesions in a financial planning task. *Brain* 120:1805–1822.

GRADY, C. L., J. W. VAN METER, J. M. MAISOG, P. PIETRINI, J. KRASUSKI, and J. P. RAUSCHECKER, 1997. Attention-related modulation of activity in primary and secondary auditory cortex. *Neuroreport* 8:2511–2516.

GRATTAN, L. M., R. H. BLOOMER, F. X. ARCHAMBAULT, and P. J. ESLINGER, 1994. Cognitive flexibility and empathy after frontal lobe lesion. *Neuropsychiatry Neuropsychol. Behav. Neurol.* 7:251–259.

GUILLERY, R. W., S. L. FEIG, and D. A. LOZSADI, 1998. Paying attention to the thalamic reticular nucleus. *Trends Neurosci.* 21:28–32.

Harlow, J. M., 1848. Passage of an iron rod through the head. *Boston Med. Surg. J.* 39:389–393.

Hier, D. B., J. Mondlock, and L. R. Caplan, 1983. Behavioral abnormalities after right hemisphere stroke. *Neurology* 33:337–344.

Hillyard, S. A., and L. Anllo-Vento, 1998. Event-related brain potentials in the study of visual selective attention. *Proc. Natl. Acad. Sci. U.S.A.* 95:781–787.

Hillyard, S. A., R. F. Hink, U. L. Schwent, and T. W. Picton, 1973. Electrical signs of selective attention in the human brain. *Science* 182:177–180.

Hopfinger, J. P., M. H. Buonocore, and G. R. Mangun, 2000. The neural mechanisms of top-down attentional control. *Nat. Neurosci.* 3:284–291.

Hornak, J., E. T. Rolls, and D. Wade, 1996. Face and voice expression identification in patients the emotional and behavioural changes following ventral frontal lobe damage. *Neuropsychologia* 34:247–261.

Kaczmarek, B. L. J., 1984. Neurolinguistic analysis of verbal utterances in patients with focal lesions of frontal lobes. *Brain Lang.* 21:52–58.

Kastner, S., M. A. Pinsk, P. de Weerd, R. Desimone, and L. G. Ungerleider, 1999. Increased activity in human visual cortex during directed attention in the absence of visual stimulation. *Neuron* 22:751–761.

Keenan, J. P., M. A. Wheeler, G. G. Gallup, and A. Pasucal-Leone, 2000. Self-recognition and the right prefrontal cortex. *Trends Cogn. Sci.* 4:338–344.

Kelley, W. M., C. N. Macrae, C. L. Wyland, S. Caglar, S. Inati, and T. F. Heatherton, 2002. Finding the self? An event-related fMRI study. *J. Cogn. Neurosci.* 14:785–794.

Kertesz A., and S. Dobrolowski, 1981. Right-hemisphere deficits, lesion size and location. *J. Clin. Neurophysiol.* 3:283–299.

Knight, R. T., 1984. Decreased response to novel stimuli after prefrontal lesions in man. *Electroencephalogr. Clin. Neurophysiol.* 59:9–20.

Knight, R. T., 1994. Attention regulation and human prefrontal cortex. In *Motor and Cognitive Functions of the Prefrontal Cortex. Research and Perspectives in Neurosciences*, A. M. Thierry, J. Glowinski, P. S. Goldman-Rakic, and Y. Christen, eds. Paris: Springer-Verlag, pp. 160–173.

Knight, R. T., 1997. Distributed cortical network for visual stimulus detection. *J. Cogn. Neurosci.* 9:75–91.

Knight, R. T., S. A. Hillyard, D. L. Woods, and H. J. Neville, 1981. The effects of frontal cortex lesions on event-related potentials during auditory selective attention. *Electroencephalogr. Clin. Neurophysiol.* 52:571–582.

Knight, R. T., and D. Scabini, 1998. Anatomic bases of event-related potentials and their relationship to novelty detection in humans. *J. Clin. Neurophysiol.* 15:3–13.

Knight, R. T., D. Scabini, and D. L. Woods, 1989. Prefrontal cortex gating of auditory transmission in humans. *Brain Res.* 504:338–342.

Knight, R. T., D. Scabini, D. L. Woods, and C. C. Clayworth, 1989. Contribution of the temporal-parietal junction to the auditory P3. *Brain Res.* 502:109–116.

Kraus, N., O. Ozdamar, and L. Stein, 1982. Auditory middle latency responses (MLRs) in patients with cortical lesions. *Electroencephalogr. Clin. Neurophysiol.* 54:275–287.

Lhermitte, F., 1986. Human autonomy and the frontal lobes. Part II. Patient behavior in complex and social situations: the "environmental dependency syndrome." *Ann. Neurol.* 19:335–343.

Lhermitte, F., B. Pillon, and M. Serdaru, 1986. Human anatomy and the frontal lobes. Part I. Imitation and utilization behavior: A neuropsychological study of 75 patients. *Ann. Neurol.* 19:326–334.

Luria, A. R., 1966/1980. *Higher Cortical Functions in Man.* New York: Basic Books.

McIntosh, A. R., C. L. Grady, L. G. Ungerleider, J. W. Haxby, S. I. Rapoport, and B. Horwitz, 1994. Network analysis of cortical visual pathways mapped with PET. *J. Neurosci.* 14:655–666.

Mesulam, M. M., 1981. A cortical network for directed attention and unilateral neglect. *Ann. Neurol.* 10:309–325.

Miller, E. K., 1999. The prefrontal cortex: complex neural properties for complex behavior. *Neuron* 22:15–17.

Miller, E. K., L. Li, and R. Desimone, 1991. A neural mechanism for working and recognition memory in inferior temporal cortex. *Science* 254:1377–1379.

Mueller, N. G., L. Machado, and R. T. Knight, 2002. Contribution of subregions of the prefrontal cortex to working memory: Evidence from brain lesions in humans. *J. Cogn. Neurosci.* 14:673–686.

Nielsen-Bohlman, L., and R. T. Knight, 1999. Prefrontal cortical involvement in visual working memory. *Cogn. Brain Res.* 8:299–310.

Owen, A. M., A. C. Evans, and M. Petrides, 1996. Evidence for a two-staged model of spatial working memory processing within the lateral frontal cortex. *Cereb. Cortex* 6:31–38.

Petrides, M., B. Alivisatos, E. Meyer, and A. C. Evans, 1993. Functional activation of the human prefrontal cortex during the performance of verbal working memory tasks. *Proc. Natl. Acad. Sci. U.S.A.* 90:878–882.

Picton, T. W., 1995. The P300 wave of the human event-related potential. *J. Clin. Neurophysiol.* 9:456–479.

Price, B. H., K. R. Daffner, R. M. Stowe, and M. Marsel-Mesulam, 1990. The comportmental learning disabilities of early frontal lobe damage. *Brain* 113:1383–1393.

Rainer, G., W. F. Asaad, and E. K. Miller, 1998a. Memory fields of neurons in the primate prefrontal cortex. *Proc. Natl. Acad. Sci. U.S.A.* 95:15008–15013.

Rainer, G., W. F. Asaad, and E. K. Miller, 1998b. Selective representation of relevant information by neurons in the primate prefrontal cortex. *Nature* 393:577–579.

Ranganath, C., and G. Rainer, 2003. Neural mechanisms for detecting and remember novel events. *Nat. Rev. Neurosci.* 4:193–202.

Rao, S. C., G. Rainer, and E. Miller, 1997. Integration of what and where in the primate prefrontal cortex. *Science* 276:821–824.

Rees, G., R. Frackowiak, and C. Frith, 1997. Two modulatory effects of attention that mediate object categorization in human cortex. *Science* 275:835–838.

Richer, F., A. Decary, M. F. Lapierre, I. Rouleau, G. Bouvier, and J. M. Saint-Hilaire, 1993. Target detection deficits in frontal lobectomy. *Brain Cogn.* 21:203–211.

Rolls, E. T., 2000. The orbitofrontal cortex and reward. *Cereb. Cortex* 10:284–294.

Rolls, E. T., J. Hornak, D. Wade, and J. McGrath, 1994. Emotion-related learning in patients with social and emotional changes associated with frontal lobe damage. *J. Neurol. Neurosurg. Psychiatry* 57:1518–1524.

Romanski, L. M., B. Tian, J. Fritz, M. Mishkin, P. S. Goldman-Rakic, and J. P. Rauschecker, 1999. Dual streams of auditory afferents target multiple domains in the primate prefrontal cortex. *Nat. Neurosci.* 2:1131–1136.

Rossi, A. F., P. S. Rotter, R. Desimone, and L. G. Ungerleider, 1999. Prefrontal lesions produce impairments in feature-cued attention, *Soc. Neurosci.* 29:2.

RUCHKIN, D. S., R. JOHNSON, Jr., J. GRAFMAN, H. CANOUNE, and W. RITTER, 1992. Distinctions and similarities among working memory processes: An event-related potential study. *Cogn. Brain Res.* 1:53–66.

RULE, R., A. SHIMAMURA, and R. T. KNIGHT, 2002. Orbitofrontal damage and dynamic filtering of emotion. *Cogn. Affect. Behav. Neurosci.* 2:264–270.

SHAMAY-TSOORY, S. G., R. TOMER, B. D. BERGER, and J. AHARON-PERETZ, 2003. Characterization of empathy deficits following prefrontal brain damage: The role of the right ventromedial prefrontal cortex. *J. Cogn. Neurosci.* 15:324–337.

SHERMAN, S. M., and R. W. GUILLERY, 2003. The role of thalamus in the flow of information to cortex. *Philosophical Trans. Roy. Soc. Lond. B: Biological Sciences.* 357:1695–1708.

SHIMAMURA, A. P., 1996. The control of monitoring of memory functions. In *Metacognition and Implicit Memory*, L. Reder, ed. Mahwah, N.J.: Erlbaum, pp. 259–274.

SHIMAMURA, A. P., 2000a. The role of the prefrontal cortex in dynamic filtering. *Psychobiology* 28:207–218.

SHIMAMURA, A. P., 2000b. Toward a cognitive neuroscience of metacognition. *Conscious. Cogn.* 9:313–323.

SHIMAMURA, A. P., 2002. Muybridge in motion: Travels in art, psychology, and neurology. *History of Photography* 26:342–350.

SKINNER, J. E., and C. D. YINGLING, 1977. Central gating mechanisms that regulate event-related potentials and behavior. In *Progress in Clinical Neurophysiology*, vol. 1, J. E. Desmedt, ed. Basel: S. Karger, pp. 30–69.

SOLTANI, M., and R. T. KNIGHT, 2000. Neural origins of the P300. *Crit. Rev. Neurobiol.* 14:199–224.

SOMERS, D. C., A. M. DALE, A. E. SEIFFERT, and R. B. TOOTELL, 1999. Functional MRI reveals spatially specific attentional modulation in human primary visual cortex. *Proc. Natl. Acad. Sci. U.S.A.* 96:1663–1668.

STEINMETZ, P. N., A. ROY, P. J. FITZGERALD, S. S. HSIAO, K. O. JOHNSON, and E. NIEBUR, 2000. Attention modulates synchronized neuronal firing in primate somatosensory cortex. *Nature* 404:187–189.

STONE, V. E., S. BARON-COHEN, and R. T. KNIGHT, 1998. Frontal lobe contributions to theory of mind. *J. Cogn. Neurosci.* 10: 640–656.

STUSS, D. T., 1991. Self, awareness, and the frontal lobes: A neuropsychological perspective. In *The Self: Interdisciplinary Approaches*, J. Strauss and G. R. Goethals, eds. New York: Springer-Verlag, pp. 255–278.

STUSS, D. T., and D. F. BENSON, 1986. *The Frontal Lobes*. New York: Raven Press.

STUSS, D. T., G. G. GALLUP, and M. P. ALEXANDER, 2001. The frontal lobes are necessary for "theory of mind." *Brain* 124:279–286.

SUTHERLING, W. W., P. H. CRANDALL, T. M. DARCEY, D. P. BECKER, M. F. LEVESQUE, and D. S. BARTH, 1988. The magnetic and electric fields agree with intracranial localizations of somatosensory cortex. *Neurology* 38:1705–1714.

SUTTON, S., M. BAREN, J. ZUBIN, and E. R. JOHN, 1965. Evoked potentials correlates of stimulus uncertainty. *Science* 150:1187–1188.

SUWAZONO, S., L. MACHADO, and R. T. KNIGHT, 2000. Predictive value of novel stimuli modifies visual event-related potentials and behavior. *Clin. Neurophysiol.* 111:29–39.

SWICK, D., M. KUTAS, and H. J. NEVILLE, 1994. Localizing the neural generators of event-related brain potentials. In *Localization in Neuroimaging in Neuropsychology*, A. Kertesz, ed. New York: Academic Press, pp. 73–121.

SWICK, D., and R. T. KNIGHT, 1994. Recognition memory and cued recall in patients with frontal cortex lesions. *Soc. Neurosci. Abstr.* 20:1003.

THATCHER, R. W., 1992. Cyclic cortical reorganization during early childhood. *Brain Cogn.* 20:24–50.

SYMONS, C. S., and B. T. JOHNSON, 1997. The self-reference effect in memory: A meta-analysis. *Psychol. Bull.* 121:371–394.

THINUS-BLANC, C., E. SAVE, C. ROSSI-ARNAUD, M. TOZZI, and M. AMMASSARI-TEULE, 1996. The differences shown by C57BL/6 and DBA/2 inbred mice in detecting spatial novelty are subserved by a different hippocampal and parietal cortex interplay. *Behav. Brain Res.* 80:33–40.

THORPE, S. J., E. T. ROLLS, and S. MADDISON, 1983. The orbitofrontal cortex: Neuronal activity in the behaving monkey. *Exp. Brain Res.* 49:93–115.

TOMITA, H., M. OHBAYASHI, K. NAKAHARA, I. HASEGAWA, and Y. MIYASHITA, 1999. Top-down signal from prefrontal cortex in executive control of memory retrieval. *Nature* 401:699–703.

TRANEL, D., A. BECHARA, and N. L. DENBURG, 2002. Asymmetric functional roles of right and left ventromedial prefrontal cortices in social conduct, decision-making, and emotional processing. *Cortex* 38:589–612.

VERLEGER, R., 1988. Event-related potentials and cognition: A critique of the context updating hypothesis and an alternative interpretation of P3. *Behav. Brain Sci.* 11:343–356.

WADA, J. A., R. CLARKE, and A. HAMM, 1975. Cerebral hemispheric asymmetry in humans. *Arch. Neurol.* 32:239–246.

WEBSTER, M. J., J. BACHEVALIER, and L. G. UNGERLEIDER, 1994. Connections of inferior temporal areas TEO and TE with parietal and frontal cortex in macaque monkeys. *Cereb. Cortex* 5: 470–483.

WEINBERGER, D. R., D. J. LUCHINS, J. MORISHA, and R. J. WYATT, 1982. Asymmetric volumes of the right and the left frontal and occipital regions of the human brain. *Ann. Neurol.* 11:97–100.

WILSON, F. A. W., S. P. O. SCALAIDHE, and P. S. GOLDMAN-RAKIC, 1993. Dissociation of object and spatial processing in primate prefrontal cortex. *Science* 260:1955–1958.

WOLDORFF, M. G., C. C. GALLEN, S. A. HAMPSON, S. A. HILLYARD, C. PANTEV, D. SOBEL, and F. E. BLOOM, 1993. Modulation of early sensory processing in human auditory cortex during auditory selective attention. *Proc. Natl. Acad. Sci. U.S.A.* 90:8722–8726.

WOODS, D. L, R. T. KNIGHT, and D. SCABINI, 1993. Anatomical substrates of auditory selective attention: Behavioral and electrophysiological effects of temporal and parietal lesions. *Cogn. Brain Res.* 1:227–240.

YAGO, E., and R. T. KNIGHT, 2000. Tonic and phasic prefrontal modulation of extrastriate processing during visual attention. *Soc. Neurosci.* 26:2232.

YAMAGUCHI, S., and R. T. KNIGHT, 1990. Gating of somatosensory inputs by human prefrontal cortex. *Brain Res.* 521:281–288.

YAMAGUCHI, S., and R. T. KNIGHT, 1991a. P300 generation by novel somatosensory stimuli. *Electroencephalogr. Clin. Neurophysiol.* 78:50–55.

YAMAGUCHI, S., and R. T. KNIGHT, 1991b. Anterior and posterior association cortex contributions to the somatosensory P300. *J. Neurosci.* 11:2039–2054.

YAMAGUCHI, S., and R. T. KNIGHT, 1992. Effects of temporal-parietal lesions on the somatosensory P3 to lower limb stimulation. *Electroencephalogr. Clin. Neurophysiol.* 84:139–148.

YINGLING, C. D., and J. E. SKINNER, 1977. Gating of thalamic input to cerebral cortex by nucleus reticularis thalami. In *Progress in Clinical Neurophysiology*, J. E. Desmedt, ed. Basel: S. Karger, pp. 70–96.

X CONSCIOUSNESS

Introduction

CHRISTOF KOCH

CONSCIOUSNESS AND the problem of free will reside at the nexus of the mind–body problem. Consciousness appears as mysterious to twenty-first-century scholars as when humans first started to wonder about their minds several millennia ago. Nevertheless, scientists today are better positioned than ever to investigate the physical basis of consciousness and volition.

The researchers represented in this section take the problem of consciousness, the first-person perspective, as given and assume that brain activity is both necessary and sufficient for biological creatures to experience something. A primary goal is to identify the specific nature of the activity of brains cells that gives rise to any one specific conscious percept, the neuronal correlates of consciousness (Crick and Koch, 1990; Chalmers, 2000; Metzinger, 2000). An auxiliary goal is to determine to what extent these correlates differ from activity that influences behavior without engaging consciousness.

Almost everyone has a general idea of what it means to be conscious. According to the philosopher John Searle, "Consciousness consists of those states of sentience, or feeling, or awareness, which begin in the morning when we awake from a dreamless sleep and continue throughout the day until we fall into a coma or die or fall asleep again or otherwise become unconscious" (Searle, 1997). Some form of attention is probably necessary, but is not sufficient. Operationally, consciousness is needed for nonroutine tasks that require retention of information over seconds. Although provisional and vague, such a definition is good enough to get the process started. As the science of consciousness advances, such definitions will need to be refined and expressed in more fundamental neuronal terms. Until the problem is understood much better, though, a more formal definition of consciousness is likely to be either misleading or overly restrictive, or both. If this seems evasive, try defining a gene (Keller, 2000; Churchland, 2002).

The working hypothesis of brain scientists is that consciousness emerges from neuronal features of the brain. *Emergence* is used here in the sense that the initiation and propagation of the action potential in axonal fibers, a highly nonlinear phenomenon, is the result of, and can be predicted from, the attributes of voltage-dependent ionic channels inserted into the neuronal membrane. Although consciousness is fully compatible with the laws of physics, it is not easy to predict its properties from these interactions.

Understanding the material basis of consciousness is unlikely to require any exotic new physics but rather a much deeper appreciation of how highly interconnected networks of a large number of heterogeneous neurons work. The abilities of groups of neurons to learn from interactions with the environment and from their own internal activities are routinely underestimated. The individual neurons themselves are complex entities with unique morphologies and thousands of inputs and outputs. Humans have no real experience with such vast organization. Hence, even biologists struggle to appreciate the properties and power of the nervous system.

It would be contrary to evolutionary continuity to believe that consciousness is unique to humans. Most brain scientists assume that some species of animals—mammals, in particular—possess some, but not necessarily all, of the features of consciousness; that they see, hear, smell, and otherwise experience the world (Griffin, 2001). This is particularly true for monkeys and apes, whose behavior, development, and brain structure are remarkably similar to those of humans. Of course, each species has its own unique sensorium, matched to its ecological niche, but that is not to deny that animals can have feelings, subjective states. To believe otherwise seems presumptuous and flies in the face of all experimental evidence from split-brain patients, autistic children, evolutionary studies, and animal behavior for the continuity of behaviors between animals and humans.

The focus of much of the empirical work is on sensory forms of consciousness—vision, in particular. More than other aspect of sensation, visual awareness is amenable to empirical investigation. This is so for a variety of reasons. First, humans are visual creatures. This is reflected in the large amount of brain tissue that is dedicated to the analysis of images and in the importance of seeing in daily life. Second, visual percepts are vivid and rich in information. Pictures and movies are highly structured yet easy to manipulate using computer-generated graphics. Third, many visual illusions, such as binocular rivalry, flash suppression, or motion-induced blindness, directly manipulate visual experience while leaving the physical retinal input unchanged. Last, and most important, the neuronal basis of many visual phenomena and illusions has been investigated

throughout the animal kingdom. Perceptual neuroscience has advanced to the point that reasonably sophisticated computational models have been constructed and have proved their worth in guiding experimental agendas and summarizing the data. It is not unlikely that all the different aspects of consciousness—smell, pain, vision, self-consciousness, the feeling of willing an action, and so on—employ one or perhaps a few common mechanisms. Figuring out the neuronal basis for one modality, therefore, will simplify understanding them all.

Similar to the quest to understand life, discovering and characterizing the molecular, biophysical, and neurophysiological operations that constitute the neuronal correlates of consciousness will likely help solve the central enigma, how events in certain privileged systems can be the physical basis of, or even be, feelings.

With this as background, let me briefly introduce the eight chapters. Chalmers summarizes, from the philosopher's point of view, the challenges inherent in coming to grips with the problem of consciousness. He argues for a science that catalogues and quantifies both first-person and third-person data and perspectives and shows how one relates to the other. Schiff reviews the enabling factors needed for any sensation to occur at all. Persistent vegetative states and minimal conscious states are clinical conditions in which affected patients are situated at the borderline between unconscious and consciousness and in which midline structures in the brainstem and thalamus are affected. The next two chapters, by Crick and Koch and by Dehaene and Changeux, provide conceptual frameworks and empirical data for thinking about the neural basis of consciousness. Coming from different directions and traditions (primate electrophysiology versus global workspace theory), the two sets of authors arrive at broadly similar conclusions, emphasizing unconscious processing, the all-or-none aspects of consciousness, interactions among coalitions of neurons that vie for dominance, and the bias exerted on this competition by attention. Goodale defends the two visual streams hypothesis: the idea that "vision for action" is carried out by the dorsal pathway and is quite distinct from the "vision for perception" implemented by the ventral pathway. Whereas the latter is associated with consciousness, the former can proceed without any sensation. This hypothesis explains a great deal of clinical data in neurological patients with their otherwise difficult to interpret patterns of deficits and retained abilities. Among students of the human brain, the most popular tool is functional magnetic resonance imaging (fMRI). The chapter by Rees summarizes what has been learned about the neurology of consciousness from fMRI in normal subjects and in patients, with some intriguing discrepancies that need to be resolved between the interpretation of human imaging data and the results of single-cell studies in monkeys. Split-brain patients have, historically, been of immense importance in demonstrating the brain basis of phenomenal experience, with two conscious minds living in two separate cerebral hemispheres within a single skull. Wolford, Miller, and Gazzaniga investigate the distinct nature of the sensory and more abstract processing in the left and right hemispheres. Finally, Wegner and Sparrow study the conscious perception of willing an action. The feeling of being responsible for some behavior, which forms the cognitive background to everything we do throughout the day, can, under laboratory conditions, be dissociated from its actual execution. This demonstrates that, at least under some conditions, free will is illusory.

Collectively, these studies signal the emergence of a science of consciousness, of the ability to investigate how phenomenal feelings emerge out of excitable brain matter in a rigorous, reliable, and reproducible manner. Needed now are invasive experiments that can close the gap between correlation and causation. Molecular biology is developing methods for deliberately, delicately, transiently, and reversibly dissecting individual components of forebrain circuits in mice and monkeys. The applications of such techniques, in combination with simultaneous recordings from hundreds and more neurons and functional imaging techniques, will do much to advance toward this goal.

REFERENCES

CHALMERS, D. J., 2000. What is a neural correlate of consciousness? In *Neural Correlates of Consciousness: Empirical and Conceptual Questions*, T. Metzinger, ed. Cambridge, Mass.: MIT Press, pp. 17–40.

CHURCHLAND, P. S., 2002. *Brain-Wise: Studies in Neurophilosophy*. Cambridge, Mass.: MIT Press.

CRICK, F. C., and C. KOCH, 1990. Towards a neurobiological theory of consciousness, *Semi. Neurosci.* 2:263–275.

GRIFFIN, D. R., 2001. *Animal Minds: Beyond Cognition to Consciousness*. Chicago: University of Chicago Press.

KELLER, E. F., 2002. *The Century of the Gene*. Cambridge, Mass.: Harvard University Press.

METZINGER, T., ed., 2000. *Neural Correlates of Consciousness: Empirical and Conceptual Questions*. Cambridge, Mass.: MIT Press.

SEARLE, J. R., 1997. *The Mystery of Consciousness. New York Review of Books*, New York.

79 How Can We Construct a Science of Consciousness?

DAVID J. CHALMERS

ABSTRACT   This chapter gives an overview of the projects facing a science of consciousness. Such a science must integrate third-person data about behavior and brain processes with first-person data about conscious experience. Empirical projects for integrating these data include those of contrasting conscious and unconscious processes, investigating the contents of consciousness, finding neural correlates of consciousness, and eventually inferring underlying principles connecting consciousness with physical processes. These projects are discussed with reference to current experimental research on consciousness. Some obstacles that a science of consciousness faces are also discussed.

In recent years there has been an explosion of scientific work on consciousness in cognitive neuroscience, psychology, and other fields. It has become possible to think that we are moving toward a genuine scientific understanding of conscious experience. But what is the science of consciousness all about, and what form should such a science take? This chapter gives an overview of the agenda.

First-person data and third-person data

The task of a science of consciousness, as I see it, is to systematically integrate two key classes of data into a scientific framework: *third-person data*, or data about behavior and brain processes, and *first-person data*, or data about subjective experience. When a conscious system is observed from the third-person point of view, a range of specific behavioral and neural phenomena present themselves. When a conscious system is observed from the first-person point of view, a range of specific subjective phenomena present themselves. Both sorts of phenomena have the status of data for a science of consciousness.

Third-person data concern the behavior and the brain processes of conscious systems. These behavioral and neurophysiological data provide the traditional material of interest for cognitive psychology and of cognitive neuroscience. Where the science of consciousness is concerned, some particularly relevant third-person data are those having to do with the following:

- Perceptual discrimination of external stimuli
- The integration of information across sensory modalities
- Automatic and voluntary actions
- Levels of access to internally represented information
- Verbal reportability of internal states
- The differences between sleep and wakefulness

First-person data concern the subjective experiences of conscious systems. It is a datum for each of us that such experiences exist: we can gather information about them both by attending to our own experiences and by monitoring subjective verbal reports about the experiences of others. These phenomenological data provide the distinctive subject for the science of consciousness. Some central sorts of first-person data include those having to do with the following:

- Visual experience (e.g., the experience of color and depth)
- Other perceptual experiences (e.g., auditory and tactile experiences)
- Bodily experiences (e.g., pain and hunger)
- Mental imagery (e.g., recalled visual images)
- Emotional experience (e.g., happiness and anger)
- Occurrent thought (e.g., the experience of reflecting and deciding)

Both third-person data and first-person data need explanation. An example is provided by the case of musical processing. If we observe someone listening to music, relevant third-person data include those concerning the nature of the auditory stimulus, its effects on the ear and the auditory cortex of the subject, various behavioral responses by the subject, and any verbal reports the subject might produce. All of these third-person data need explanation, but they are not all that needs explanation. As anyone who has listened to music knows, there is also a distinctive quality of subjective experience associated with listening to music. A science of music that explained the various third-person data just listed but that did not explain the first-person data of musical experience would be a seriously incomplete science of music. A complete science of musical experience must explain both sorts of phenomena, preferably within an integrated framework.

DAVID J. CHALMERS   Department of Philosophy, University of Arizona, Tucson, Ariz.

Explaining the data

The problems of explaining third-person data associated with consciousness are sometimes called the "easy problems" of consciousness. The problem of explaining first-person data associated with consciousness is sometimes called the "hard problem" of consciousness. This is not because the problems associated with third-person data are in any sense trivial, but rather because we have a clear model for how we might go about explaining them.

To explain third-person data, we need to explain the objective functioning of a system. For example, to explain perceptual discrimination, we would need to explain how a cognitive process can perform the objective function of distinguishing various different stimuli and produce appropriate responses. To explain an objective function of this sort, we specify a *mechanism* that performs the function. In the sciences of the mind, this is usually a neural or a computational mechanism. For example, in the case of perceptual discrimination, we would specify the neural or computational mechanism responsible for distinguishing the relevant stimuli. In many cases we do not yet know exactly what these mechanisms are, but there seems to be no principled obstacle to finding them, and so to explaining the relevant third-person data.

This sort of explanation is common in many different areas of science. For example, in the explanation of genetic phenomena, what needed explaining was the objective function of transmitting hereditary characteristics through reproduction. Watson and Crick isolated a mechanism that could potentially perform this function: the DNA molecule, through replication of strands of the double helix. As we have come to understand how the DNA molecule performs this function, genetic phenomena have gradually come to be explained. The result is a sort of reductive explanation: we have explained higher-level phenomena (genetic phenomena) in terms of lower-level processes (molecular biology). One can reasonably hope that the same sort of model will apply in the sciences of the mind, at least for the explanation of the objective functioning of the cognitive system in terms of neurophysiology.

When it comes to first-person data, however, this model breaks down. The reason is that first-person data—the data of subjective experience—are not data about objective functioning. One way to see this is to note that even if one has a complete account of all the objective functions in the vicinity of consciousness—perceptual discrimination, integration, report, and so on—there may still remain a further question: Why is all this functioning associated with subjective experience? And further, why is this functioning associated with the particular sort of subjective experience that it is in fact associated with? Merely explaining the objective functions does not answer this question.

Perhaps the lesson is that *as data*, first-person data are irreducible to third-person data, and vice versa. That is, third-person data alone provide an incomplete catalogue of the data that need explaining: if we explain only third-person data, we have not explained everything. Likewise, first-person data alone are incomplete. A satisfactory science of consciousness must admit both sorts of data, and must build an explanatory connection between them.

What form might this connection take? An intermediate position holds that although there are two sorts of data, we can explain first-person data wholly in terms of material provided by third-person data. For example, many think that we might wholly explain the phenomena of subjective experience in terms of processes in the brain. This intermediate position is very attractive, but there are reasons to be skeptical about it. I have discussed this subject at length elsewhere (Chalmers, 1996). Here I will present a simple argument that encapsulates some reasons for doubt, using the following premises:

1. Third-person data are data about the objective structure and dynamics of physical systems.
2. (Low-level) structure and dynamics explain only facts about (high-level) structure and dynamics.
3. Explaining structure and dynamics does not suffice to explain the first-person data.

Therefore,

4. First-person data cannot be wholly explained in terms of third-person data.

Here, premise 1 captures something about the character of third-person data: it always concerns the dynamics of certain physical structures. Premise 2 says that explanations in terms of processes of this sort only explain further processes of that sort. There can be big differences between the processes, as when simple low-level structure and dynamics give rise to highly complex high-level structure and dynamics (in complex systems theory, for example), but there is no escaping the structural/dynamical circle. Premise 3 encapsulates the point, discussed earlier, that explaining structure and dynamics is only to explain objective functions, and that to explain objective functions does not suffice to explain first-person data about subjective experience. From these three premises, the conclusion (4) follows.

Of course, it does not follow that first-person data and third-person data have nothing to do with one another; there is obviously a systematic association between them. There is good reason to believe that subjective experiences are systematically correlated with brain processes and with behavior. It remains plausible that whenever a subject has an appropriate sort of brain process, he or she will have an associated sort of subjective experience. We simply need to distinguish correlation from explanation. Even if first-person data cannot be wholly explained in terms of third-person data, the two sorts of data are still strongly correlated.

It follows that a science of consciousness remains entirely possible. It is just that we should expect this science to take a nonreductive form. A science of consciousness will not reduce first-person data to third-person data, but it will articulate the systematic connections between them. Where there is systematic covariation between two classes of data, we can expect systematic principles to underlie and explain the covariation. In the case of consciousness, we can expect systematic *bridging principles* to underlie and explain the covariation between third-person data and first-person data. A theory of consciousness will ultimately be a theory of these principles.

It should be noted that these foundational issues are controversial, and there are various alternative views. One class of views (e.g., Dennett, 1991) holds that the only phenomena that need explaining are those that concern objective functioning. The most extreme version of this view says that there are no first-person data about consciousness at all. A less extreme version of this view says that all first-person data are equivalent to third-person data (e.g., about verbal reports), so that explaining these third-person data explains everything. Another class of views (e.g., Churchland, 1997) accepts that that first-person data need further explanation, but holds that they might be reductively explained by future neuroscience. One version of this view holds that future neuroscience could go beyond structure and dynamics in ways we cannot currently imagine. Another version holds that if we can find sufficient correlations between brain states and consciousness, that will qualify as a reductive explanation.

I have argued against these views elsewhere (e.g., Chalmers, 2002). In what follows, however, I will focus on constructive projects for a science of consciousness. In this discussion I will sometimes presuppose the reasoning sketched above, but much of what I say will have application even to alternative views.

Projects for a science of consciousness

If what I have said in the previous sections is correct, then a science of consciousness should take first-person data seriously and should proceed by studying the association between first-person data and third-person data, without attempting a reduction. In fact, this is exactly what one finds in practice. The central work in the science of consciousness has always taken first-person data seriously. For example, much central work in psychophysics and perceptual psychology has been concerned with the first-person data of subjective perceptual experience. In research on unconscious perception, the first-person distinction between the presence and absence of subjective experience is crucial. And in recent years, a growing body of research has focused on the correlations between first-person data about subjective experience and third-person data about brain processes and behavior.

In what follows I will articulate what I see as some of the core projects for a science of consciousness, with illustrations drawn from existing research.

PROJECT 1: EXPLAIN THE THIRD-PERSON DATA   One important project for a science of consciousness is that of explaining the third-person data in the vicinity: explaining the difference between functioning in sleep and wakefulness, for example, and explaining the voluntary control of behavior. This sort of project need not engage the difficult issues relating to first-person data, but it may still provide an important component of a final theory.

One example of this sort of project is that of explaining binding in terms of neural synchrony (e.g., Crick and Koch, 1990). Binding is the phenomenon whereby distinct pieces of information (about the color and shape of an object, for example), represented in different areas of the brain, are brought together for the integrated control of behavior. Some researchers theorize that a key role in this process is played by synchronized neural firing: it might be that information about a single object is represented by neurons in different areas that fire in synchrony with each other, enabling later integration. It is not yet clear whether this hypothesis is correct, but if it is correct, it will provide an important component in explaining the integration of perceptual information, which in turn is closely tied to questions about consciousness. Of course, explaining binding will not on its own explain the first-person data of consciousness, but it may help us to understand the associated processes in the brain.

Research on the hypothesis of a "global workspace" also falls into this class. Baars (1988) postulated such a workspace as a mechanism by which shared information can be made available to many different cognitive processes. More recently, other researchers (e.g., Dehaene and Changeux, this volume) have investigated the potential neural basis for this mechanism, postulating a neuronal global workspace. If this hypothesis is correct, it will help to explain third-person data concerning access to information within the cognitive system, as well as data about the information made available to verbal report. Again, explaining these processes will not in itself explain the first-person data of consciousness, but it may well contribute to the project (project 4 below) of finding neural correlates of consciousness.

PROJECT 2: CONTRAST CONSCIOUS AND UNCONSCIOUS PROCESSES   Many cognitive capacities can be exercised both consciously and unconsciously, that is, in the presence or absence of associated subjective experience. For example, the most familiar sort of perceptual processing is conscious, but there is also strong evidence of unconscious perceptual processing (Merikle and Daneman, 2000). One finds a similar contrast in the case of memory, where the now common distinction between explicit and implicit memory (Schacter and Curran, 2000) can equally be seen as a distinction between conscious and unconscious memory. Explicit memory is essentially memory associated with a subjective experience of the remembered information; implicit memory is essentially memory in the absence of such a subjective experience. The same goes for the distinction between explicit and implicit learning (Reber, 1996), which is in effect a distinction between learning in the presence or in the absence of relevant subjective experience.

Conscious and unconscious processes provide pairs of processes that are similar in some respects from the third-person point of view (e.g., both involve registration of perceptual stimuli) but differ from the first-person point of view (e.g., one involves subjective experience of the stimulus, one does not). Of course, there are also differences from the third-person point of view. For a start, a researcher's evidence for conscious processes usually involves a verbal report of a relevant experience, and evidence for unconscious processes usually involves a verbal report of the absence of a relevant experience. At the same time, there are less obvious differences between the behavioral capacities that go along with conscious and unconscious processes, and between the associated neural processes. These differences make for the beginning of a link between the first-person and third-person domains.

For example, evidence suggests that while unconscious perception of visually presented linguistic stimuli is possible, semantic processing of these stimuli seems limited to the level of the single word rather than complex expressions (see Greenwald, 1992). By contrast, conscious perception allows for semantic processing of very complex expressions. Here, experimental results suggest a strong association between the presence or absence of subjective experience and the presence or absence of an associated functional capacity—a systematic link between first-person and third-person data. Many other links of the same sort can be found in the literature on unconscious perception, implicit memory, and implicit learning.

Likewise, there is evidence suggesting distinct neural bases for conscious and unconscious processes in perception. Appealing to an extensive body of research on visuomotor processing, Milner and Goodale (1995; see also Goodale, this volume) have hypothesized that the ventral stream of visual processing subserves conscious perception of visual stimuli for the purpose of cognitive identification of stimuli, while the dorsal stream subserves unconscious processes involved in fine-grained motor capacities. If this hypothesis is correct, one can again draw a systematic link between a distinction in first-person data (presence or absence of conscious perception) and a distinction in third-person data (visual processing in the ventral or dorsal stream). A number of

related proposals have been made in research on memory and learning.

PROJECT 3: INVESTIGATE THE CONTENTS OF CONSCIOUSNESS
Consciousness is not simply an on-off switch. Conscious experiences have a complex structure, with complex representational contents. A conscious subject usually has a manifold of perceptual experiences, bodily sensations, emotional experience, and a stream of conscious thought, among other things. Each of these elements may itself be complex. For example, a typical visual experience has an internal structure representing objects with many different colors and shapes, in varying degrees of detail. We can think of all this complexity as comprising the contents of consciousness.

The contents of consciousness have been studied throughout the history of psychology. Weber's and Fechner's pioneering work in psychophysics concentrated on specific aspects of these contents, such as the subjective brightness associated with a visual experience, and correlated it with properties of the associated stimulus. This provided a basic link between first-person data about sensory experience and third-person data about a stimulus. Later work in psychophysics and Gestalt psychology took an approach of the same general sort, investigating specific features of perceptual experience and analyzing how these covary with properties of a stimulus.

This tradition continues in a significant body of contemporary research. For example, research on visual illusions often uses subjects' first-person reports (and even scientists' first-person experiences) to characterize the structure of perceptual experiences. Research on attention (Mack and Rock, 1998; Treisman, 2003) aims to characterize the structure of perceptual experience inside and outside the focus of attention. Other researchers investigate the contents of consciousness in the domains of mental imagery (Baars, 1996), emotional experience (Kaszniak, 1998), and the stream of conscious thought (Pope, 1978; Hurlburt, 1990).

An important line of research investigates the contents of consciousness in abnormal subjects. For example, subjects with synesthesia have unusually rich sensory experiences. In a common version, letters and numbers trigger reports of extra color experiences, in addition to the standard perceived color of the stimulus. Recent research strongly suggests that these reports reflect the perceptual experiences of the subjects, and not just cognitive associations. For example, Ramachandran and Hubbard (2001) find that certain visual patterns produce a perceptual "pop-out" effect in synesthetic subjects that is not present in normal subjects. When first-person data about the experiences of abnormal subjects are combined with third-person data about brain abnormalities in those subjects, this yields a new source of information about the association between brain and conscious experience.

PROJECT 4: FIND THE NEURAL CORRELATES OF CONSCIOUSNESS
This leads us to what is perhaps the core project of current scientific research on consciousness: the search for neural correlates of consciousness (Metzinger, 2000; Crick and Koch, this volume). A neural correlate of consciousness (NCC) can be characterized as a minimal neural system that is directly associated with states of consciousness. Presumably the brain as a whole is a neural system associated with states of consciousness, but not every part of the brain is associated equally with consciousness. The NCC project aims to isolate relatively limited parts of the brain (or relatively specific features of neural processing) that correlate directly with subjective experience.

It may be that there will be many different NCCs, for different aspects of conscious experience. For example, it might be that there is one neural system that is associated with being conscious as opposed to being unconscious (perhaps in the thalamus or brainstem; see, e.g., Schiff, this volume), another neural system associated with the specific contents of visual consciousness (perhaps in some part of the visual cortex), and other systems associated with the contents of consciousness in different modalities. But any such proposal can be seen as articulating a link between third-person data about brain processes and first-person data about subjective experience.

In recent years, by far the greatest progress has been made on the study of NCCs for visual consciousness. Milner and Goodale's work on the ventral stream provides an example of this sort of research. Another example is the research of Logothetis and colleagues on binocular rivalry in monkeys (e.g., Logothetis, 1998; Leopold, Maier, and Logothetis, 2003). When difference stimuli are presented to the left and right eyes, subjects usually undergo alternating subjective experiences. Logothetis trained monkeys to signal such changes in their visual experience, and correlated these changes with changes in underlying neural processes. The results indicated that changes in visual experience are only weakly correlated with changes in patterns of neural firing in primary visual cortex: in this area, neural firing was more strongly correlated with the stimulus than with the experience. But changes in visual experience were strongly correlated with changes in patterns of neural firing in later visual areas, such as inferior temporal cortex. These results tend to suggest that inferior temporal cortex is a better candidate than primary visual cortex as an NCC for visual consciousness.

Of course, no single experimental result can provide conclusive evidence concerning the location of an NCC, but a large amount of evidence concerning the location of NCCs for vision has accumulated in the last few years (Koch, 2004), and one can expect much more to come. If successful, this project will provide some highly specific connections between brain processes and conscious experiences.

PROJECT 5: SYSTEMATIZE THE CONNECTION   To date, links between first-person data and third-person data have been studied in a somewhat piecemeal fashion. Researchers isolate correlations between specific aspects of subjective experience and certain specific brain processes or behavioral capacities, in a relatively unsystematic way. This is to be expected at the current stage of development. But we can hope that as the science develops, more systematic links will be forthcoming. In particular, we can hope to develop principles of increasing generality that link a wide range of first-person data with a correspondingly wide range of third-person data. For example, there might eventually be an account of the neural correlates of visual consciousness will not only tell us which neural systems are associated with visual consciousness but will also yield systematic principles telling us how the specific content of a visual experience covaries with the character of neural processes in these systems.

A few principles of this sort have been suggested to date in limited domains. For example, Hobson (1997) has suggested a general principle linking certain levels of neurochemical activity with different states of consciousness in wakefulness, sleep, and dreaming. It is likely that any such proposals will be heavily revised as new evidence comes in, but one can expect that in coming decades there will be increasingly well-supported principles of this sort. The possibility of such principles holds out the tantalizing prospect that eventually, we might use them to predict features of an organism's subjective experience based on knowledge of its neurophysiology.

PROJECT 6: INFER FUNDAMENTAL PRINCIPLES   If the previous project succeeds, then we will have general principles connecting third-person data and first-person data. But these general principles will not yet be fundamental principles. The principles might still be quite complex, limited to specific aspects of consciousness, and limited to specific species. A science of consciousness consisting of wholly different principles for different aspects of consciousness and different species would not be entirely satisfactory. It is reasonable to hope that eventually, some unity could be discovered behind this diversity. We should at least aim to maximize the generality and the simplicity of the relevant principles wherever possible. In the ideal situation, we might hope for principles that are maximally general in their scope, applying to any conscious system whatsoever, and applying to all aspects of conscious experience. And we might hope for principles that are relatively simple in their form, in the way that the basic laws of physics appear to be simple.

It is unreasonable to expect that we will discover principles of this sort anytime soon, and it is an open question whether we will be able to discover them at all. Currently, we have little idea what form such principles might take

(Chalmers, 1996, speculates that they might involve the notion of information). But if we can discover them, principles of this sort would be candidates to be fundamental principles: the building blocks of a fundamental theory of consciousness. If what I said earlier is correct, then something about the connection between first-person data and third-person data must be taken as primitive, just as we take fundamental principles in physical theories as primitive. But we can at least hope that the primitive element in our theories will be as simple and as general as possible. If, eventually, we can formulate simple and general principles of this sort, based on an inference from accumulated first-person and third-person data, I think we could be said to have an adequate scientific theory of consciousness.

What would this entail about the relationship between physical processes and consciousness? The existence of such principles is compatible with different philosophical views. One might regard the principles as laws connecting two fundamentally different domains (Descartes, 1641/1996; Popper and Eccles, 1977). One might regard them as laws connecting two aspects of the same thing (Lockwood, 1989; Chalmers, 1996). Or one might regard them as grounding an identification between properties of consciousness and physical properties (Smart, 1959; Papineau, 2002). Such principles could also be combined with different views of the causal relation between physical processes and consciousness (see Chalmers, 2002). But for many purposes, the science of consciousness can remain neutral on these philosophical questions. One can simply regard the principles as principles of correlation, while staying neutral on their underlying causal and ontological status. This makes it possible to have a robust science of consciousness even without a widely accepted solution to the philosophical mind–body problem.

Obstacles to a science of consciousness

The development of a science of consciousness as I have presented it thus far may sound remarkably straightforward. We simultaneously gather first-person data about subjective experience and third-person data about behavior and brain processes, isolate specific correlations between these data, formulate general principles governing these correlations, and infer the underlying fundamental laws. But of course, it is not as simple as this in practice. There are a number of serious obstacles to this research agenda. The most serious obstacles concern the availability of the relevant data, in both the third-person and first-person domains. In what follows I will discuss a few of these obstacles.

OBSTACLES INVOLVING THIRD-PERSON DATA The third-person data relevant to the science of consciousness include both behavioral and neural data. The availability of behavioral data is reasonably straightforward: here, one is constrained only by the ingenuity of the experimenter and by the limitations of experimental contexts. And in practice, researchers have accumulated a rich body of behavioral data relevant to consciousness. But the availability of neural data is much more constrained by technological limitations, and the body of neural data that has been accumulated to date is correspondingly much more limited.

In practice, the most relevant neurophysiological data come from two or three sources: brain imaging via functional magnetic resonance imaging (fMRI) and positron emission tomography (PET) technology, single-cell recording through insertion of electrodes, and surface recording through electroencephalographs (EEG) and magnetoencephalography (MEG). Each of these technologies is useful, but each has serious limitations for the science of consciousness. EEG and MEG have well-known limitations in spatial localization. Brain imaging through fMRI and PET is better in this regard, but these modalities are still spatially quite coarse-grained. Single-cell recording is spatially fine-grained but is largely limited to experimentation on nonhuman animals.

These limitations apply to all areas of cognitive neuroscience, but they are particularly pressing for the science of consciousness, because the science of consciousness relies on gathering third-person data and first-person data simultaneously. By far the most straightforward method for gathering first-person data is verbal report; but verbal report is limited to human subjects. By far the most useful third-person data are data at the level of single neurons, where one can monitor representational content that correlates with the content of consciousness (as when one monitors a neuron with a specific receptive field), but these experiments are largely limited to nonhuman subjects. As a result, it is extremely difficult to discover strong associations between first-person data and corresponding neural data with current techniques.

There have been numerous ingenious attempts to circumvent these limitations. The most well-known include Logothetis's experiments on monkeys, in which they are trained extensively to provide a substitute for a verbal report of visual consciousness by pressing a bar. Research on blindsight in monkeys by Cowey and Stoerig (1995) has done something similar. But the very fact that researchers have to go to such great lengths in order to gather relevant neural data illustrates the problem. Others have performed neuron-level measurements on surgical patients (e.g., Kreiman, Fried, and Koch, 2002), but there are obvious practical limitations here. Many others (e.g., Rees, this volume) have tried to get as much relevant information as they can from the limited resources of brain imaging and surface recording; nevertheless, fewer deep correlations have emerged from this sort of work than from neuron-level studies.

One can hope that this is a temporary limitation imposed by current technology. If a technology is eventually developed that allows for noninvasive monitoring of neuron-level processes in human subjects, we might expect a golden age for the science of consciousness to follow.

OBSTACLES INVOLVING FIRST-PERSON DATA Where the availability of first-person data is concerned, there are a number of related obstacles that run quite deep. I will discuss three of these obstacles here.

1. *Privacy* The most obvious obstacle to the gathering of first-person data concerns the privacy of such data. In most areas of science, data are intersubjectively available: they are equally accessible to a wide range of observers. But in the case of consciousness, first-person data concerning subjective experiences are directly available only to the subject having those experiences. To others, these first-person data are only indirectly available, mediated by observation of the subject's behavior or brain processes. Things would be straightforward if there were a "consciousness meter" that could be pointed at a subject, revealing his or her subjective experiences to all. But in the absence of a theory of consciousness, no such consciousness meter is available. This imposes a deep limitation on the science of consciousness, but it is not a paralyzing limitation. For a start, any subject has direct access to first-person data concerning his or her own conscious experiences. We can imagine that Robinson Crusoe on a desert island (equipped with the latest brain imaging technology) could make considerable progress toward a science of consciousness by first-person observation. More practically, each of us has indirect access to first-person data concerning others' experiences, by relying on behavioral indicators of these data.

In practice, by far the most common way of gathering data about the conscious experiences of other subjects is to rely on their verbal reports. Here, one does not treat the verbal reports just as third-person data (as a behaviorist might, limiting the datum to the fact that a subject made a certain noise). Rather, one treats the report as a report of first-person data that are available to the subject. Just as a scientist can accumulate third-person data by accepting reports of third-person data gathered by others (rather than simply treating those reports as noises), a scientist can also gather first-person data by accepting reports of first-person data gathered by others. This is the typical attitude that researchers adopt toward experimental subjects. If there is positive reason to believe that a subject's report might be unreliable, then a researcher will suspend judgment about it. But in the absence of any such reason, researchers will take a subject's report of a conscious experience as good reason to believe that the subject is having a conscious experience of the sort that the subject is reporting.

In this way, researchers have access to a rich trove of first-person data that is made intersubjectively available. Of course, our access to this data depends on our making certain assumptions: in particular, the assumption that other subjects really are having conscious experiences, and that by and large their verbal reports reflect these conscious experiences. We cannot directly test this assumption; instead, it serves as a sort of background assumption for research in the field. But this situation is present throughout other areas of science. When physicists use perception to gather information about the external world, for example, they rely on the assumption that the external world exists, and that perception reflects the state of the external world. They cannot directly test this assumption; instead, it serves as a sort of background assumption for the whole field. Still, it seems a reasonable assumption to make, and it makes the science of physics possible. The same goes for our assumptions about the conscious experiences and verbal reports of others. These seem to be reasonable assumptions to make, and they make the science of consciousness possible.

Of course, verbal reports have some limits. Some aspects of conscious experience (e.g., the experience of music or of emotion) are very difficult to describe; in these cases we may need to develop a more refined language. And verbal reports cannot be used at all in subjects without language, such as infants and nonhuman animals. In these cases, one needs to rely on other behavioral indicators, as when Logothetis relies on a monkey's bar-pressing. These indicators require further assumptions. For example, Logothetis's work requires the assumption that monkeys are conscious, and the assumption that visual stimuli that the monkey can exploit in the voluntary control of behavior are consciously perceived.

These assumptions appear reasonable to most people, but they go beyond those required in the case of verbal report. The farther we move away from the human case, the more questionable the necessary assumptions become. For example, it would be very difficult to draw conclusions about consciousness from experiments on insects. But in any case, verbal reports in humans, combined with behavioral indicators in primates, give researchers enough access to first-person data to enable a serious body of ongoing research.

2. *Methods* A second obstacle is posed by the fact that our methods for gathering first-person data are quite primitive compared with our methods for gathering third-person data. The latter have been refined by years of scientific practice, but the former have not received nearly as much attention. Where simple first-person data are concerned, this problem is not too pressing: there is usually no great difficulty in determining whether one is having an experience of a certain color in the center of one's visual field, for example. But where more subtle aspects of subjective experience are concerned, the issue arises quickly.

Even with a phenomenon as tangible as visual experience, the issue arises in a number of ways. Visual experiences as a whole usually have a rich and detailed structure, for example, but how can subjects investigate and characterize that detail? Most subjects have great difficulty in introspecting and reporting this detail more than superficially. Particular difficulties arise in investigating the character of consciousness outside attention. To introspect and report this structure would seem to require attending to the relevant sort of experience, which may well change the character of the experience.

Here we can expect that at least some progress can be made by developing better methods for the gathering of first-person data. It may be reasonable to pay attention to traditions where the detailed study of experience has been explored in detail. These traditions include those of Western phenomenology, introspectionist psychology, and even Eastern meditative traditions. Even if one is skeptical of the theories put forward by proponents of these traditions, one might still benefit from attending to their data-gathering methods. This research strategy has been pursued most notably in the "neurophenomenology" of Francisco Varela and colleagues (Varela, 1997; Lutz et al., 2002), in which neurophysiological investigation is combined with phenomenological investigation in the tradition of Husserl. A number of other attempts at refining first-person methods are discussed in the papers collected in Varela and Shear (2001).

Of course, any method has limitations. Subjects' judgments about their subjective experiences are not infallible, and although training may help with this, it also introduces the danger that observations may be corrupted by theory. The introspectionist program of experimental psychology in the nineteenth century famously fell apart when different schools could not agree on the introspective data (Boring, 1929). Still, our ambitions need not be as grand as those of the introspectionists. For now, we are not aiming for a perfect characterization of the structure of consciousness, but simply for a better characterization. Furthermore, we are now in a position where we can use third-person data as a check on first-person investigation. Experimental investigation has helped us to distinguish circumstances in which first-person reports are unreliable from those in which they are more reliable (Schooler and Fiore, 1997), and there is room for much more investigation of this sort in the future. So it is reasonable to hope that there can be at least a modest refinement of our methods for the reliable investigation of first-person data.

3. *Formalisms* A final obstacle is posed by the absence of general formalisms with which first-person data can be expressed. Formalisms are important for two purposes. First, they are needed for data gathering: it is not enough to simply know what one is experiencing, one has to write it down. Second, they are needed for theory construction: to formu-

late principles that connect first-person data with third-person data, we need to represent the data in a way that such principles can exploit.

The main existing formalisms for representing first-person data are quite primitive. Researchers typically rely either on simple qualitative characterizations of data (as in "an experience of red in the center of the visual field") or on simple parameterization of data (as when color experiences are parametrized by hue, saturation, and brightness). These simple formalisms suffice for some purposes, but they are unlikely to suffice for the formulation of systematic theories.

It is not at all clear what form a proper formalism for the expression of first-person data about consciousness should take. The candidates include (1) parametric formalisms, in which various specific features of conscious experience are isolated and parametrized (as in the case of color experience above); (2) geometric and topological formalisms, in which the overall structure of an experience (such as a visual experience) is formalized in geometric or topological terms; (3) informational formalisms, in which one characterizes the informational structure of an experience, specifying it as a sort of bit-by-bit state that falls into a larger space of informational states; and (4) representational formalisms, in which one characterizes an experience by using language for the states of the world that the experience represents (one might characterize an experience as an experience of a yellow cup, for example). All of these formalisms may have limitations, but a detailed study of various alternative formalisms is likely to have significant benefits.

Conclusion

Overall, the prospects for a science of consciousness are reasonably bright. There are numerous clear projects for a science of consciousness that take first-person data seriously. One can recognize the distinctive problems that consciousness poses and still do science. Of course, there are many obstacles, and it is an open question how far we can progress. But the last 10 years have seen many advances, and the next 50 years will see many more. For now, it is reasonable to hope that we may eventually have a theory of the fundamental principles connecting physical processes to conscious experience.

REFERENCES

BAARS, B. J., 1988. *A Cognitive Theory of Consciousness*. New York: Cambridge University Press.

BAARS, B. J., ed., 1996. *Mental Imagery* [Special issue]. *Conscious. Cogn.* 5(3).

BORING, E. G., 1929. *A History of Experimental Psychology*. New York: Century.

CHALMERS, D. J., 1996. *The Conscious Mind: In Search of a Fundamental Theory*. Oxford, England: Oxford University Press.

CHALMERS, D. J., 2002. Consciousness and its place in nature. In *Philosophy of Mind: Classical and Contemporary Readings*. Oxford, England: Oxford University Press.

CHURCHLAND, P. S., 1997. The hornswoggle problem. In *Explaining Consciousness: The Hard Problem*, J. Shear, ed. Cambridge, Mass.: MIT Press.

COWEY, A., and P. STOERIG, 1995. Blindsight in monkeys. *Nature* 373:247–249.

CRICK, F., and C. KOCH, 1990. Towards a neurobiological theory of consciousness. *Semin. Neurosci.* 2:263–275.

DENNETT, D. C., 1991. *Consciousness Explained*. Boston: Little, Brown.

DESCARTES, R., 1641/1996. *Meditations on First Philosophy*, J. Cottingham, trans.-ed. Cambridge, England: Cambridge University Press.

GREENWALD, A. G., 1992. New Look 3: Reclaiming unconscious cognition. *Am. Psychol.* 47:766–779.

HOBSON, J. A., 1997. Consciousness as a state-dependent phenomenon. In *Scientific Approaches to Consciousness*, J. Cohen and J. Schooler, eds. Mahwah, N.J.: Erlbaum.

HURLBURT, R. T., 1990. *Sampling Normal and Schizophrenic Inner Experience*. New York: Plenum Press.

KASZNIAK, A., ed. 1998. *Emotions, Qualia, and Consciousness*. Singapore: World Scientific.

KOCH, C., 2004. *The Quest for Consciousness: A Neuroscientific Approach*. Englewood, Colo.: Roberts.

KREIMAN, G., I. FRIED, and C. KOCH, 2002. Single neuron correlates of subjective vision in the human medial temporal lobe. *Proc. Natl. Acad. Sci. U.S.A.* 99:8378–8383.

LEOPOLD, D. A., A. MAIER, and N. K. LOGOTHETIS, 2003. Measuring subjective visual perception in the nonhuman primate. *J. Conscious. Stud.* 10:115–130.

LOCKWOOD, M., 1989. *Mind, Brain, and the Quantum*. London: Blackwell.

LOGOTHETIS, N. K., 1998. Single units and conscious vision. *Philos. Trans. R. Soc. Lond. Ser. B Biol. Sci.* 353:1801–1818.

LUTZ, A., J. LACHAUX, J. MATRINERIE, and F. VARELA, 2002. Guiding the study of brain dynamics by using first-person data: Synchrony patterns correlate with ongoing conscious states during a simple visual task. *Proc. Natl. Acad. Sci. U.S.A.* 99: 1586–1591.

MACK, A., and I. ROCK, 1998. *Inattentional Blindness*. Cambridge, Mass.: MIT Press.

MERIKLE, P. M., and M. DANEMAN, 2000. Conscious vs. unconscious perception. In *The New Cognitive Neurosciences*, M. S. Gazzaniga, ed. Cambridge, Mass.: MIT Press.

METZINGER, T., 2000. *Neural Correlates of Consciousness: Empirical and Conceptual Questions*. Cambridge, Mass.: MIT Press.

MILNER, D., and M. GOODALE, 1995. *The Visual Brain in Action*. Oxford, England: Oxford University Press.

PAPINEAU, D., 2002. *Thinking about Consciousness*. Oxford, England: Oxford University Press.

POPE, K. S., 1978. *The Stream of Consciousness: Scientific Explorations into the Flow of Human Experience*. New York: Plenum Press.

POPPER, K., and J. ECCLES, 1977. *The Self and Its Brain: An Argument for Interactionism*. New York: Springer-Verlag.

RAMACHANDRAN, V. S., and E. M. HUBBARD, 2001. Psychophysical investigations into the neural basis of synaesthesia. *Proc. R. Soc. Lond.* 268:979–983.

REBER, A., 1996. *Implicit Learning and Tacit Knowledge: An Essay on the Cognitive Unconscious*. Oxford, England: Oxford University Press.

SCHACTER, D. L., and T. CURRAN, 2000. Memory without remembering and remembering without memory: Implicit and false memories. In *The New Cognitive Neurosciences*, M. S. Gazzaniga, ed. Cambridge, Mass.: MIT Press.

SCHOOLER, J. W., and S. M. FIORE, 1997. Consciousness and the limits of language. In *Scientific Approaches to Consciousness*, J. Cohen and J. Schooler, eds. Hillsdale, N.J.: Erlbaum.

SMART, J. J. C., 1959. Sensations and brain processes. *Philos. Rev.* 68:141–156.

TREISMAN, A., 2003. Consciousness and perceptual binding. In *The Unity of Consciousness: Binding, Integration, Dissociation*, A. Cleeremans, ed. Oxford, England: Oxford University Press.

VARELA, F., 1997. Neurophenomenology: A methodological remedy for the "hard problem." In *Explaining Consciousness: The Hard Problem*, J. Shear, ed. Cambridge, Mass.: MIT Press.

VARELA, F., and J. SHEAR, 2001. *The View from Within: First-Person Methodologies*. Exeter, England: Imprint Academic.

80 The Neurology of Impaired Consciousness: Challenges for Cognitive Neuroscience

NICHOLAS D. SCHIFF

ABSTRACT   This chapter examines the contribution of cognitive neuroscience to the study of impaired consciousness. The neurological bases of global disorders of consciousness are considered from the point of view of clinical-pathological correlations and functional neuroimaging studies. The discussion emphasizes the importance of direct measurement of cerebral function in severely brain-injured individuals and highlights several conceptual challenges presented by observational data obtained from such patients. Future directions for research and the wider social and philosophical implications of this field of study are briefly outlined.

Understanding consciousness is a shared goal of neurology and cognitive neuroscience. A scientific account of human consciousness will provide neurologists with accurate information about underlying mechanisms of functional impairments. It will identify distinctions between patients with apparently similar functional disturbances, thus defining the likelihood of improvement and possible therapeutic avenues. At present, such a thorough account of brain mechanisms underlying consciousness is not available. The patient with a persistent disorder of consciousness often brings neurologists to the limits of their professional expertise. In this chapter we explore some of the most diagnostically challenging areas of disorders of consciousness and demonstrate how the methods of the cognitive neurosciences are improving our understanding of this important and difficult topic.

We review functional brain imaging and observational data from neurological cases with a focus on global disorders of consciousness arising from severe brain injuries. These disorders present challenging clinical questions: Do isolated behavioral fragments suggest awareness even if the patient does not respond to environmental stimuli? How aware are patients who show unequivocal responses to their environment, but only intermittently? Do they suffer? What limits the recovery of functional communication in patients who recover the inconsistent ability to follow commands and verbalize? These questions reside at the present boundaries of

NICHOLAS D. SCHIFF   Laboratory for Cognitive Neuromodulation, Department of Neurology and Neuroscience, Weill Medical College of Cornell University, New York, N.Y.

scientific models of consciousness. Complex structural brain injuries produce global disorders of consciousness. Modern neuroimaging methods can extend the traditional method of neuropsychological lesion studies to novel observations of remaining functional brain activity and patterns of recovery. These neurological disorders present a particularly rich and unique framework to address brain structure-function relationships as they relate to the underlying mechanisms of human consciousness and cognition. In addition, this emerging area of cognitive neuroscience will necessarily invite wider social policy and ethical debate.

A brief taxonomy of global disorders of consciousness

The initial brain state produced by a severe brain injury is typically coma. Coma is characterized by lack of arousal or purposeful motor response and reflects overwhelming functional impairment of brainstem arousal mechanisms (Plum and Posner, 1982). A perturbation of the arousal systems sufficient to produce coma can arise from several causes, including anesthesia and the use of other pharmacological agents, and multiple metabolic derangements or physical injuries to the brain that produce large bilateral cortical injuries, either alone or in combination with injury to the higher brainstem (Plum and Posner, 1982). Discrete bilateral structural injuries of either the upper tegmental brainstem (upper pons and midbrain) or the paramedian thalamus may alone produce coma (Plum, 1991; figure 80.1).

If uncomplicated by other factors, the comatose state typically resolves within 7–10 days and is followed by a period of indeterminate duration during which an eyes-open "wakeful" appearance alternates with an eyes-closed, "sleep" state. This limited recovery of a cyclical arousal pattern defines the vegetative state. In other respects the vegetative state is similar to coma in that patients demonstrate no evidence of awareness of self or their environment (Jennett and Plum, 1972). Patients who remain in a vegetative state beyond 30 days are considered to be in a persistent vegetative state (PVS). Vegetative states that are permanent usually result from widespread anoxic injuries or diffuse

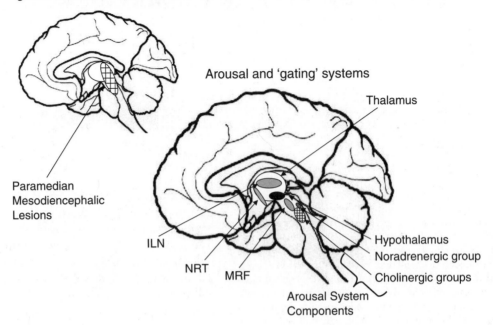

Location of focal injuries producing coma and other global disorders of consciousness

Arousal and 'gating' systems

Thalamus

Paramedian
Mesodiencephalic
Lesions

Hypothalamus
Noradrenergic group
Cholinergic groups

ILN

NRT   MRF

Arousal System
Components

FIGURE 80.1 Overview of paramedian brainstem and thalamus arousal and gating systems. Abbreviations: ILN, intralaminar nuclei; NRT, nucleus reticularis; MRF, mesencephalic reticular formation.

head trauma (Jennett et al., 2001). Quite rarely, despite overwhelming structural brain injury, PVS patients may exhibit fragmentary behaviors that appear to arise from isolated cerebral networks (Schiff, Ribary, et al., 2002). These behavioral fragments are not appropriate or specific to a given behavioral context, nor can they be reliably influenced to establish any evidence of interaction.

The minimally conscious state (MCS) represents the next functional level of improvement. MCS patients exhibit fragments of behavior that may appear similar to those observed in PVS patients. In contrast to PVS patients, however, they demonstrate unequivocal, but typically fluctuating, evidence of awareness of self or the environment (Giacino et al., 2002). Behavioral fragments exhibited by MCS patients include basic verbalization or gestures that demonstrate awareness of self and the environment. Patients emerge from MCS if they can establish consistent functional communication. However, crossing this threshold requires more than the ability to simply follow commands. For example, patients may be able to correctly look toward a card with a printed "yes" or "no" presented by an examiner but not be able to reliably answer any questions using such signaling. In this situation, the patient remains near the borderline of emergence from MCS. This clinical categorization scheme includes patients with a wide range of behavioral patterns and suggests the utility of further refinement, particularly if quantitative indices are developed. Although sometimes confused with MCS patients because of minimal respon-

siveness on examination, patients who have sustained structural injuries limited to the ventral pontine brainstem (see figure 80.1) may enter into a locked-in state (LIS) in which only eye movements may remain under volitional control. These patients are fully conscious but limited by severe motor disabilities (figure 80.2). LIS is not a disorder of consciousness.

Functional origins of global disorders of consciousness: Differing roles of brainstem arousal systems and forebrain "gating" systems

The upper brainstem and midline thalamic regions diagramed in figure 80.1 contain two closely related groups of neuronal populations. The arousal systems include cholinergic, noradrenergic, serotonergic, and histaminergic nuclei located predominantly in the brainstem, basal forebrain, and posterior hypothalamus (Steriade, Jones, and McCormick, 1997; Parvizi and Damasio, 2001). The balanced interactions of these populations control arousal states as judged both by changes in behavior and by brain activity measured by electroencephalography (EEG). These interactions are interdependent on the recently identified hypocretin/orexin system in the hypothalamus, which acts as a "toggle switch" for the large-scale state changes associated with sleep and wakefulness (Sutcliffe and de Lecea, 2002). Earlier models of the arousal systems, however, focused primarily on the role of the mesencephalic reticular formation (MRF) and the

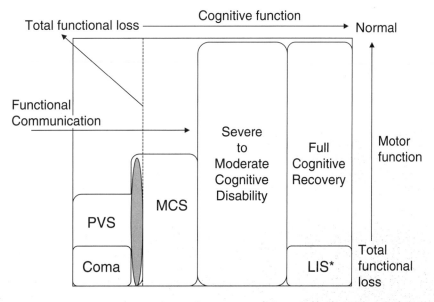

Conceptualizing global disorders of consciousness

FIGURE 80.2   Global disorder of consciousness. Abbreviations: PVS, persistent vegetative state; MCS, minimally conscious state; LIS, locked-in state (see text).

thalamic intralaminar nuclei (ILN) in mediating changes in the sleep-wake cycle and modulating sensory processing and higher integrative brain functions (Morruzi and Magoun, 1949). Electrical stimulation of these paramedian mesodiencephalic (PMD) structures demonstrated their role in both changing EEG patterns and producing arousal as measured by observable changes in behaviors such as eye opening, vigilance, autonomic activity (heart rate, breathing), and even elicited behaviors.

The overall frequency content of the EEG (i.e., the shape of the spectrum of the EEG) is a robust indicator of arousal state in normal subjects. Arousal patterns identified in the ongoing EEG reflect varying degrees of corticothalamic synchronization that are regulated by brainstem and hypothalamic modulation of thalamic reticular neurons, thalamocortical relay neurons, thalamic inhibitory interneurons, and cortical pyramidal cells (Steriade, 2000; Bayer et al., 2002). The background activity changes during arousal states can be precisely identified with shifts in spectral content of the activity of distributed forebrain networks (Contreras and Steriade, 1995). Natural awake attentive states correlate with a shift in spectral power away from a dominance of low frequencies to a mixed state that includes increased synchronized high-frequency activity (Steriade et al., 1996). Such longlasting changes of ongoing background activity, however, are episodically shaped at a finer temporal scale within each frequency range. In wakeful states, such shaping of the dominant EEG frequencies is correlated with several different cognitive functions. For example, low fre-

quencies in the theta range arising over the frontal midline are excited by demands of focused attention and cognitive load (Gevins et al., 1997), and posterior shifts of alpha frequencies correlate with shifts of spatial attention (Worden et al., 2000). Regionally specific modulation of high-frequency oscillatory activity in the 30–80 Hz range is correlated with perceptual awareness (Joliot, Ribary, and Llinás, 1994), visual attention (Fries et al., 2001), motor preparation and exploration (Murthy and Fetz, 1996), and working memory (Pesaran et al., 2002).

Although originally identified as primary arousal systems, the key PMD structures (the ILN, MRF, and nucleus reticularis) appear to link arousal states to the control of moment-to-moment intention or attentional gating (Kinomura et al., 1996; Steriade et al., 1996; Paus et al., 1997; Purpura and Schiff, 1997; Weese, Phillips, and Brown, 1999; Schiff and Purpura, 2002). ILN neurons are powerfully modulated by the hypothalamic orexin system (Bayer et al., 2002) and represent the critical point of interaction of brainstem arousal systems with ongoing cerebral cortical dynamics. In cats, a unidirectional pathway between the MRF and the ILN provides a substrate for generating behavioral arousal and shifting the EEG to higher frequencies during electrical stimulation of these structures (Steriade and Glenn, 1982). Interconnections within the ILN may also be strongly influenced by inhibition through disynaptic connections with the nucleus reticularis (Crabtree and Issac, 2002) and via the connections with the MRF (Steriade and Glenn, 1982). Both the interdependence of these nuclei on brainstem arousal system inputs and their role in the selective integration of large networks with moment-to-moment intentions within the wakeful state suggest that these structures be considered "gating" systems, as diagramed in figure 80.1 (Schiff and Plum, 2000). During wakefulness, the gating systems likely maintain, and facilitate redistribution of, sustained cerebral activity representing behavioral sets (cf. Evarts, Shinoda, and Wise, 1984). Consistent with this view, strong correlations of neuronal firing patterns in the ILN are found in recordings obtained during shifts of attention (Matsumoto et al., 2001), eye movements (Schlag-Rey and Schlag, 1984), and linked to multimodal sensory stimuli (Minamimoto and Kimura, 2002) during goal-directed behaviors.

The ILN include several different nuclei. The rostral group tends to project to prefrontal, posterior parietal, and primary sensory areas and provides a diffuse innervation of the basal ganglia (Macchi and Bentivoglio, 1985); the caudal group forms several strong, in most cases topographically organized, connections with the basal ganglia and premotor and anterior parietal cortices (Sadikot et al., 1992; Groenewegen and Berendse, 1994). Jones (1998) has recently redefined the ILN and other thalamic subdivisions into two classes of neurons on the basis of differential calcium-binding protein expression. One class of thalamic neurons are the "matrix" neurons, which project to superficial cortical layers across relatively wide cortical territories. The other class of thalamic neurons consists of "core" neurons, which project to the middle, or granular, layers of the cortical microcircuit in a more area-specific manner. A large number of matrix neurons populate most ILN subdivisions and are distributed throughout the thalamus, even within primary sensory relay nuclei. Jones proposes that the matrix neurons act collectively as a functional system to organize global patterns of corticothalamic synchronization associated with arousal states (Jones, 2001).

Functional brain imaging of disorders of consciousness

The clinical inference that PVS patients are unconscious first received laboratory support from fluorodeoxyglucose positron emission tomography (FDG-PET) imaging studies that measured overall cerebral metabolism to be reduced by 50% or more below normal levels in PVS patients (Levy et al., 1987). LIS patients also studied, however, maintained near normal metabolic rates in most brain structures. More recently, Laureys and colleagues (2000, 2002) utilized ^{15}O-PET subtraction paradigms to compare responses to elementary auditory and somatosensory stimuli with baseline resting conditions. For both types of stimuli, groups of PVS patients demonstrated a loss of brain activations outside of primary sensory cortices (figure 80.3). "Hierarchically higher-order" cortical regions active in normal control subjects did not show activation in PVS patients. These investigators interpreted their findings as demonstrating multiple functional disconnections along the auditory or somatosensory cortical pathways and concluded that the residual cortical activity seen in PVS patients does not reflect awareness. The findings are consistent with evidence of early sensory processing in PVS patients as measured by evoked potentials and add important additional information about the integrity of cortical sensory processing in PVS.

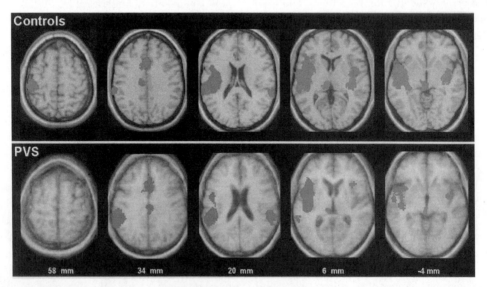

FIGURE 80.3 Brain regions that activated during somatosensory stimulation in normal subjects (top panel) and 15 PVS subjects (bottom panel) are shown in lighter color on mean MRI templates for each group. Darker-colored regions in PVS images correspond to regions that activated significantly less in the patients than in the controls. (Reprinted with permission from S. Laureys et al., Cortical processing of noxious somatosensory stimuli in the persistent vegetative state. *NeuroImage* 17:732–741. © 2002 by Elsevier.) (See color plate 67.)

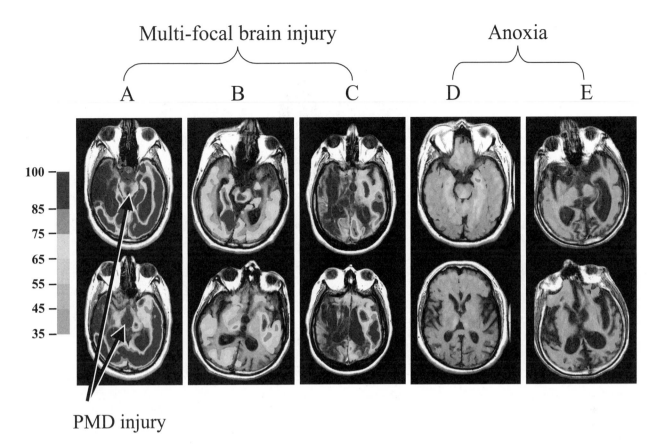

Multi-focal brain injury

A   B   C

Anoxia

D   E

100 —
85 —
75 —
65 —
55 —
45 —
35 —

PMD injury

FIGURE 80.4 Resting brain metabolism in five PVS patients (see text for details). (Reprinted with permission from N. Schiff et al., Residual cerebral activity and behavioral fragments in the persis-tent vegetative state. *Brain* 125:1210–1234. © 2002 by *Brain*.) (See color plate 68.)

The definition of PVS allows for a variety of complex stereotyped responses to be encountered, including rare examples of fragments of behavior that may appear semi-purposeful or inconsistently related to environmental stimuli. Such observations have been left unexplained by previous neurobiological models. We studied a series of PVS patients and identified novel evidence of residual cerebral function in a small number of patients employing FDG-PET, magnetic resonance imaging (MRI), and magnetoen-cephalography (MEG). Figure 80.4 provides an overview of coregistered MRI and FDG-PET images in five chronic PVS patients. The PET data are normalized by region and expressed on a color scale ranging from 35% to 100% of normal regional cerebral metabolic rates. The brackets seg-regate imaging results in three patients who suffered focal brain injuries resulting from trauma (A, B) or deep brain hemorrhage (C) and two patients in PVS following anoxic injuries (D, E). As seen in the marked difference in overall brain metabolism, patients in PVS following anoxic injuries had global reductions of cerebral metabolism in all brain regions. One patient, a 49-year-old woman who suffered suc-cessive hemorrhages from a vascular malformation of the brain, infrequently expressed isolated words (typically epi-thets) in isolation of environmental stimulation despite a 20-year period of PVS (Schiff, Ribary, et al., 1999). Structural brain imaging using MRI (1.5T) showed destruction of the right basal ganglia and thalamus. Resting FDG-PET mea-surements of the patient's brain demonstrated a marked reduction in global cerebral metabolism to less than 50% of normal across most brain regions. Several isolated and relatively small regions in the left hemisphere, however, expressed higher levels of metabolism (patient C). For this patient, only values greater than 55% of normal are displayed.

MEG responses to bilateral auditory stimulation in this patient, shown in figure 80.5, demonstrated an abnormal time-locked response in the gamma range (20–50 Hz) that was restricted to the left hemisphere (Schiff, Ribary, et al., 1999). Compared to normal controls, the pattern has decreased amplitude, coherence, and duration (Joliot, Ribary, and Llinás, 1994). Single-dipole analysis localized the dominant evoked cortical component of the gamma-band activity to primary auditory areas within the left hemi-sphere (Sarvas, 1987). These locations corresponded to the islands of higher resting brain metabolism observed by PET imaging. The incompletely preserved MEG patterns of evoked gamma-band responses indicate that thalamocorti-cal relay connectivity is at least partially spared. Taken

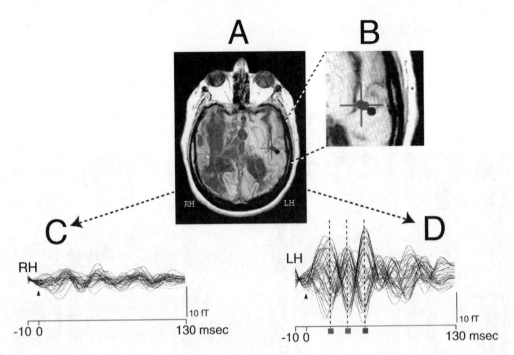

FIGURE 80.5   Combined MRI, FDG-PET, and MEG studies of a single vegetative patient with isolated word production. (*A*) PET activations representing greater than 75% of normal cerebral metabolic rates coregistered with MRI. (*B*) Location of signal generator for average cortical MEG response to bilaterally presented auditory stimuli in left hemisphere. (*C*) MEG recorded cortical response to auditory stimuli over right hemisphere. (*D*) MEG recorded cortical response to auditory stimuli over left hemisphere. (Reprinted with permission from N. D. Schiff et al., words without mind. *J. Cogn. Neurosci.* 11:650–656. © 1999 by the Society for Neuroscience.)

together, the imaging and neurophysiological data suggest isolated sparing of the left-sided thalamocortical-basal ganglia loops that normally support language function, including restricted regions of Heschl's gyrus, the frontal operculum (Broca's area), and corticocortical connections to the left temporoparietal cortex (Wernicke's area) and the left caudate nucleus.

These data provide novel evidence of the modular organization of brain systems (cf. Baynes et al., 1998). Two other patients in this group (D and E) revealed isolated metabolic activity that could be correlated with unusual behavioral patterns. Taken together, these clinical-pathological correlations suggest that remaining residual cerebral activity following severe brain injuries is not random, but rather correlates with regional preservation of cerebral networks. The metabolically active regions may reflect network connectivity and ongoing patterns of neuronal firing.

Evidence from autopsy studies indicates that PVS can result not only from widespread cerebral injuries of varying severity but also from isolated damage to PMD structures (Ingvar and Sourander, 1970; Castaigne et al., 1981; Plum, 1991). Another patient studied had remained in a behaviorally unremarkable vegetative state during a 6-year period following a traumatic injury. Notably, this patient's cerebral cortical metabolism as measured by quantitative FDG-PET was near normal, but there were marked reductions of metabolism in the PMD region that had suffered severe damage (indicated by arrows in figure 80.4, patient A). EEG studies in this patient revealed diffuse low-voltage, low-frequency activity that did not change with behavioral arousal patterns. The unique observation of significantly preserved cortical metabolism in this PVS patient raises the possibility that the metabolic activity indicates multiple preserved but isolated networks. Overwhelming injury to the PMD region in this patient is hypothesized to have resulted in loss of integration of these remaining brain regions. This observation supports the view that subcortical gating systems (intralaminar thalamus and related structures) play a critical role in the precise functional integration of many segregated parallel networks and their interaction with state changes mediated by brainstem and allied arousal systems (Llinás et al., 1994; Steriade, 1997; Schiff and Plum, 2000). Consistent with this interpretation, Laureys, Faymonville, Luxon, and colleagues (2000) identified a normalization of covariation of PET signals between the intralaminar nuclei and prefrontal cortices in a single patient following recovery from a vegetative state. Collectively, the evidence of residual cerebral activity in chronic PVS patients indicates that at least some partially functional cerebral regions can remain in catastrophically injured brains. In addition, the unexpectedly wide variations in resting cerebral metabolism accompanying the vegetative state in these five patients demonstrate that very different mechanisms and underlying substrates may lead to similar phenomenology in brain-injured patients.

A widely discussed case from Menon and colleagues (1998) can be reexamined in the context of these findings (Menon, Owen, and Pickard, 1999; Schiff and Plum, 1999a). A 26-year-old woman near the transition from PVS to MCS 4 months following acute encephalomyelitis was studied using an ^{15}O-PET subtraction paradigm. MRI revealed structural injuries of both cortical and subcortical (brainstem and thalamic) structures. Comparison of brain activation in response to presentation of familiar faces and scrambled images identified selective activation of the right fusiform gyrus and extrastriate visual association areas. No other evidence of cortical processing was reported. The patient became increasingly responsive at 6 months and minimally expressive at 8 months; she eventually made a full cognitive recovery (Wilson, Gracey, and Bainbridge, 2001). Menon and colleagues interpreted the activity measured at 4 months as indicating a recovery of minimal awareness. However, selective identification of relatively complex information processing alone may not demonstrate recovery of cognitive function, or even the potential for recovery (Schiff and Plum, 1999a; Schiff et al., 1999). For example, selective responses of the extrastriate visual areas can be obtained in anesthetized animals (reviewed in Zeki, 1993). Functional imaging studies in severely brain-injured patients are accordingly best interpreted in the context of detailed clinical histories along with baseline structural and functional brain assessment using several clinical tools (MRI, EEG, and evoked potentials). Nonetheless, the findings of Menon and colleagues contrast with those of Laureys and colleagues and suggest that neuroimaging studies may elucidate underlying differences between patients remaining in PVS or transitioning into MCS.

MCS patients who remain near the borderline of emergence raise different questions concerning underlying mechanisms limiting the recovery of functional communication. We studied two male patients, ages 21 and 33, using an fMRI language activation paradigm (N. D. Schiff et al., unpublished observations). Both patients had unremarkable medical histories prior to sustaining sudden brain injuries, which left both in MCS for longer than 18 months at the time of the study. Neither patient demonstrated consistent command following or functional communication (either gestural or verbal) on repeated examinations. Both patients, however, demonstrated significant fluctuations in their responses across examinations. Figure 80.6 shows cortical activity for one patient associated with receptive language comprehension during presentation of 40-s narratives prerecorded by a familiar relative and presented as normal speech and also played time-reversed (backward). Brain activations in response to normal speech are shown in yellow. Selective responses to backward presentations are shown in

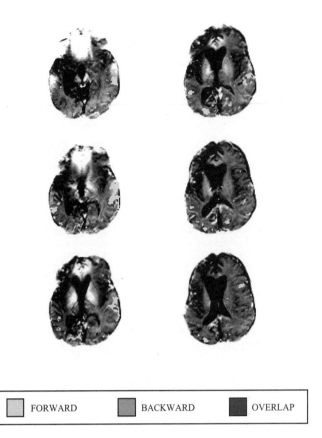

FORWARD   BACKWARD   OVERLAP

FIGURE 80.6 fMRI responses to passive language stimuli (see text for details). (See color plate 69.)

blue, with red regions indicating an overlap. In both patients, normal speech generated robust activity in language-related areas of the superior and middle temporal gyri. In addition, brain activations in the inferior and medial frontal gyri, primary and secondary visual areas (including the calcarine sulcus), and the precuneus in one patient are seen in figure 80.6.

Do the fMRI activations in the MCS patients indicate awareness? Several neuroimaging studies of visual awareness in patients and normal subjects implicate coactivation of prefrontal and parietal cortices along with occipital-temporal cortical areas as a correlate of perceptual awareness (reviewed in Rees, Kreiman, and Koch, 2002). Differences of fMRI activation pattern in aware versus unaware conditions show either elevations of regional activation or changes in the strength of the measured covariance of regional activation in these areas. The activation patterns identified in the MCS patient shown in figure 80.6 preserve the specific regions correlated with awareness in the above imaging studies; however, unlike the patients or the normal subjects evaluated in those studies, MCS patients are unable to communicate their awareness if present. Although the presence of coactivation of prefrontal, parietal, and occipital regions may be suggestive of awareness, it is also consistent with other interpretations.

The results contrast with the ^{15}O-PET studies of Laureys et al. (2000, 2002) of PVS patients who failed to produce activation of polymodal association cortices in response to natural stimuli. Although activation of primary or higher-level cortical areas may occur without evidence of conscious perception (Rees, Kreiman, and Koch, 2002), these findings challenge the cognitive neurosciences to account for the additional details of necessary and sufficient dynamic cerebral interactions that underpin the normal conscious state. It appears that these MCS patients retain connected cerebral networks that underlie language comprehension and expression despite their inability to execute motor commands or communicate reliably. These surprising findings indicate that forebrain networks may remain functional yet fail to establish activity patterns necessary to allow consistent communication in some MCS patients. The preservation of forebrain networks associated with higher cognitive functions such as language provides a clinical foundation for the wide fluctuations sometimes observed in MCS patients.

The fMRI activations observed in these patients must also be placed in the context of their resting cerebral metabolic rates. For both patients, FDG-PET studies showed very low baseline metabolic activity across all cerebral structures (40%–50% of normal values). These regional metabolic rates are comparable to levels measured in patients remaining in a vegetative state following traumatic brain injury (Tomassino et al., 1995; Schiff, Ribary, et al., 2002). The low metabolic rates most likely reflect a marked reduction in baseline neuronal activity and are consistent with a severe deficit in "default" or online self-monitoring processes (Gusnard and Raichle, 2001). Significantly, both MCS patients studied suffered compression injuries of the PMD region due to brain swelling, but neither patient suffered a large complete injury as seen in patient A in figure 80.4. The potential impact of this injury pattern is considered later.

Possible underlying mechanisms of global disorders of consciousness

As further neuroimaging and neurophysiological efforts are applied to study patients with impaired consciousness, it is expected that fundamental questions will arise surrounding different underlying mechanisms of similar functional disabilities. It is likely that some patients will harbor significantly greater residual capacities, and that these may be partially remediable. The findings reviewed in the previous section from several investigative groups indicate that functional integration of modular processing systems is widely disabled across the cerebrum in PVS patients. Although rare examples of identifiable behavioral fragments in PVS can be related to isolated networks, in no case are these fragments organized into purposeful action. At the transition point to MCS, however, it is not clear whether isolated behaviors that

can be inconsistently patterned in response to the environment indicate significantly greater functional capacities. The large variation in structural injury patterns and functional brain activity seen in PVS suggests that a similar if not wider dissociation may exist in MCS. In fact, autopsy studies suggest that at least half of all patients with such severe disability following a traumatic brain injury have suffered diffuse gray and white matter damage comparable to that typically observed in PVS patients (Jennett et al., 2001). In this group of MCS patients, it is likely that evidence of isolated, minimal sensorimotor integration in response to stimuli may indicate only relatively isolated networks as rarely encountered in PVS patients (see gray zone between PVS and MCS in figure 80.2).

The preservation of widely distributed cortical networks in some MCS patients as seen in figure 80.6, however, deserves further consideration. Although it is generally recognized that some aspects of acquired cognitive disabilities may result from functional disturbances disproportionate to the extent of structural injuries, systematic approaches to identifying the mechanisms underlying this dissociation in brain-injured patients have not been developed. An important clue to potential mechanisms underlying the coexistence of functional distributed cerebral networks and MCS is the clinical history of brain swelling and subsequent compression of PMD structures, but not overwhelming direct injury due to brain hemorrhage or loss of blood flow. Direct injuries to the PMD region are associated with PVS, MCS, and other poor outcomes following stroke (Castaigne et al., 1981) or traumatic brain injury (Wedekind et al., 2000). Although it is not well known, some patients do recover from these global disorders of consciousness if they are produced solely as a result of bilateral paramedian thalamic injuries. This observation is a frequently confusing revelation to both neuroscientists and neurologists; it supports the critical, but to a point replaceable, function of the PMD gating systems (Schiff and Plum, 1999b).

A wide range of functional outcomes may be observed following isolated injuries of PMD structures, including sustained PVS or MCS. Although immediate coma following small bilateral lesions of the PMD region is often observed, the coma is typically followed by a rapid recovery of arousal in the form of either a vegetative state or a minimally conscious state characterized by immobility and mutism (akinetic mutism) (Castaigne et al., 1981; Guberman and Stuss, 1983; Katz, Alexander, and Mandel, 1987; van Domburg, ten Donkelaar, and Notermans, 1996). Excessive sleepiness (hypersomnolence) may occur instead of coma (Bassetti et al., 1996) and can be enduring (Steriade, 1997). The clinical course of recovery for patients with bilateral PMD injuries, although infrequently documented, reveals a protracted and dynamically evolving reconstitution of cognitive capacities. An agitated delirious or "manic" phase has been described (Bogousslavsky et al., 1988; van Domburg, ten Donkelaar, and Notermans, 1996), with a variety of unusual hallucinatory or confabulatory behaviors followed by a later stage of recovery characterized by a profound and enduring dementia (Katz, Alexander, and Mandell, 1987; Meissner et al., 1987). One well-documented case of a patient with bilateral paramedian thalamic strokes noted a 2-year time course of recovery (van Domburg, ten Donkelaar, and Notermans, 1996). Beginning with a near comatose state of minimal arousability (stupor) lasting 3 days, the patient progressed to a MCS characterized by akinetic mutism. At 4 weeks, initial interactive behavior was noted and characterized as a delirium with manic features that subsequently evolved into a protracted period of at least 15 months of dementia. Remarkably, the patient regained near normal cognitive function as measured by standard intelligence testing at 24 months after the initial insult. As in this patient, recoveries to a functional level of cognitive "slowing" or baseline neuropsychological function are typically associated with injuries restricted to the thalamus (Katz, Alexander, and Mandell, 1987; Krolak-Salmon et al., 2000).

The early recovery of wakefulness seen following bilateral PMD injuries emphasizes the robust nature of the arousal systems that also directly innervate cortical regions. The slow reconstruction of cognitive functions, however, brings us to the present limits of understanding of brain mechanisms of consciousness and plasticity. This observation raises the important question of what constitutes a necessary and sufficient substrate for consciousness. It has been suggested that outcomes associated with permanent PVS (cf. Castaigne et al., 1981) depend on the rostrocaudal extent of the PMD lesion (Plum, 1991). Jones's matrix neuron concept provides a possible substrate for the rare full recovery of cognitive function and suggests that such a recovery may primarily depend on the reconstitution of dynamic interactions supported by sufficient distribution of remaining matrix neurons to provide a structure to facilitate global patterns of corticothalamic synchronization (Jones, 2001). If the PMD region is overwhelmingly damaged, it may become impossible to generate such patterns of neuronal interaction across the forebrain (Ingvar and Sourander, 1970; Castaigne, 1981; Schiff, Ribary et al., 2002). Van der Werf, Witter, and Groenewegen (2002) have proposed that the ILN provides an anatomical substrate for interactions among all of the segregated corticostriatopallidal-thalamocortical "loop" pathways (Alexander, DeLong, and Strick, 1986) under the control of the prefrontal cortex of the rat (such as the isolated loop proposed for the PVS patient shown in figure 80.4). A related observation is obtained from a multidimensional scaling model of the connections of the entire cat thalamocortical system (Scannell et al., 1999). This model places the matrix neuron-rich regions of the thalamic ILNs in a unique central cluster among all the otherwise segregated thalamocortical loop systems (frontal, limbic, temporal, and parietal); these ILN connections provide a potential shortest path of connection among all cat corticothalamic subsystems. This finding may provide a partial explanation for the importance of the PMD regions in the context of recent studies of abstract, densely connected networks that gain "small world" properties if a limited number of long-range connections arise (Watts, 2000; Braitenberg, 2001). It is possible that a necessary and sufficient number of such long-range connections from the PMD are required to establish the dynamic patterns of activity needed for gating the moment-to-moment intentions of wakeful conscious states.

Patients who do recover from bilateral PMD injuries, however, often demonstrate persistent instability of arousal level and within-state fluctuations of the selective gating of different cognitive functions (Meissner et al., 1987; Mennemeier et al., 1997; van der Werf et al., 1999). Such unstable interactions among the arousal and gating systems may underlie the fluctuations observed in MCS patients, particularly the rare patients who spontaneously emerge for brief periods of time (Burruss and Chacko, 1999). Combinations of PMD damage with other cerebral injuries may lead to several different partially reversible mechanisms of dysfunction in MCS patients (Schiff and Purpura, 2002). For example, strokes involving the intralaminar thalamus are unique in producing widespread hemispheric alterations of blood flow and metabolism following focal lesions (Caselli, Graff-Radford, and Rezai, 1991; Szelies et al., 1991). Both reduction in baseline neuronal activity and alteration of functional interactions across cerebral networks involving wide areas of the cortex, basal ganglia, and thalamus likely play a role. In addition, perhaps the most intriguing hint to the selective contribution of PMD regions to forebrain integrative mechanisms is the generation of absence seizures following direct injuries to these structures (Ingvar, 1955; van Domburg, ten Donkelaar, and Notermans, 1996). Absence seizures represent a unique form of wakeful unconsciousness. A classic absence seizure interrupts ongoing mental or physical activity with a brief period of motionless staring, often accompanied by changes in heart rate, sweating, and twitching facial movements (Penfield and Jasper, 1954). During this behavioral event, a stereotyped large-amplitude spike and wave process overtakes the normal EEG, creating a virtual "brain beat" (running at approximately 3 cps). The seizures are notably differentiated from periods of drowsiness or fainting in that postural stability is maintained, as well as the appearance of wakefulness. Arguably, the episodes may be characterized as momentary vegetative states. After a few seconds, this remarkable disengagement of awareness of self and the environment resolves as quickly as it arises, leaving the trace of prior cognitive and sensorimotor activity sufficiently intact as to not disturb an internal sense of continuity (or continuation of actions). The seizures produce brief periods of amnesia, sensory-motor dissociation, and loss of volition.

As Penfield and Jasper (1954) earlier observed, absence seizures provide a unique window onto brain mechanisms underlying consciousness because of their selective interruption of higher integrative brain functions. The selective disturbance of goal-directed activity, attention, and memory during the absence seizure suggests that normal forebrain gating mechanisms are overwhelmed by the hypersynchronous activity observed in the EEG. Interruption of the brief formation of persistent activity across the corticothalamic interconnections of the PMD regions and the frontal lobe around transient events, such as eye movements or attentional shifts, has been proposed as the gating mechanism disturbed by the seizure (Purpura and Schiff, 1997). An intriguing possibility is that ongoing long-range spatiotemporal interactions across several EEG frequency bands are shaped by these regions. Following incomplete injuries, reconstitution of episodic interactions with the arousal systems may be possible given sufficient matrix cell preservation (and other unknown factors).

We speculate that the frontal midline theta rhythm associated with effortful cognitive tasks demanding attentional control and working memory is the normal functional correlate of the hypersynchronous absence seizure. These lower-frequency rhythms interact with higher-frequency gamma rhythms and posterior alpha rhythms in organizing intentional motor behaviors (Slobounov et al., 2000). Ontogenetically, this rhythm accompanies the first goal-directed activity in early infancy, and a functional role in the regulation of action persists in adults (Luu and Tucker, 2001). Further exploration of the spatiotemporal organization of the EEG during the evolution of complex brain injuries in light of these normal mechanisms may provide a point of entry for developing an understanding of mechanisms of recovery.

Although unstable interactions of arousal and gating systems may limit further recovery from MCS, additional mechanisms are needed to explain why patients who may appear alert and able to respond quickly to commands still fail to emerge from MCS. Here it will be necessary to develop novel measures to quantify cognitive capacities (cf. Friston, 2000; Repucci, Schiff, and Victor, 2001; Sporns, Tononi, and Edelman, 2002) and conceive of neurobiological mechanisms that might limit resources to respond to cognitive loads created by multiple tasks or demands on sustained attention and working memory. Several lines of evidence suggest that these functions are intimately related to the interactions of the arousal and gating systems with specialized distributed networks (Paus et al., 1997; Kinomura et al., 1996), but this area needs significant further development.

Future directions

It is expected that insights from cognitive neuroscience will significantly improve diagnostic precision and suggest new therapeutic avenues for patients with impaired consciousness. Cognitive neuroscience has already significantly informed the development of novel cognitive rehabilitation methods aimed either at improving specific functional deficits (Schindler et al., 2002) or more generally at enhancing cognitive functions, either by utilizing external sensory stimulation techniques (Manly et al., 2002) or by retraining of internally generated behaviors such as eye movement search strategies (Cicerone et al., 2000). For the treatment of the complex brain injuries underlying the disorders reviewed in this chapter, more direct neuromodulation methods such as deep brain stimulation may eventually be extended from their use in the treatment of movement disorders to play a role in treating acquired cognitive disabilities (Schiff, Plum, and Rezai, 2002; Schiff and Purpura, 2002).

Developments in this area of cognitive neuroscience are also likely to have broad implications beyond neurological practice (Fins, 2003). Patients with severe brain injury present the scientific and philosophical problems of consciousness in a unique, operational context. As we advance our understanding of the underlying mechanisms of consciousness in the human brain, it is likely that many assumptions about the possibilities for awareness or functional recovery following injuries, whether optimistic or nihilistic, will be recast. It is the further development of cognitive neuroscience that will ultimately provide a rational basis for the diagnosis and treatment of impaired consciousness.

REFERENCES

ALEXANDER, G. E., M. R. DeLong, and P. L. Strick, 1986. Parallel organization of functionally segregated circuits linking basal ganglia and cortex. *Annu. Rev. Neurosci.* 9:357–381.

Bassetti, C., J. Mathis, M. Gugger, K. O. Lovblad, and C. W. Hess, 1996. Hypersomnia following paramedian thalamic stroke: A report of 12 patients. *Ann. Neurol.* 39: 471–480.

Bayer, L., E. Eggermann, B. Saint-Mleux, D. Machard, B. E. Jones, M. Muhlethaler, and M. Serafin, 2002. Selective action of orexin (hypocretin) on nonspecific thalamocortical projection neurons. *J. Neurosci.* 22:7835–7839.

Baynes, K., J. Eliassen, H. L. Lutsep, and M. S. Gazzaniga, 1998. Modular organization of cognitive systems masked by interhemispheric integration. *Science* 280:902–905.

Bogousslavsky, J., M. Ferrazzini, F. Regli, G. Assal, H. Tanabe, and A. Delaloye-Bischof, 1988. Manic delirium and frontal-like syndrome with paramedian infarction of the right thalamus. *J. Neurol. Neurosurg. Psychiatry* 51:116–119.

Braitenberg, V., 2001. Brain size and number of neurons. *J. Comput. Neurosci.* 10:71–77.

Burruss, J. W., and R. C. Chacko, 1999. Episodically remitting akinetic mutism following subarachnoid hemorrhage. *J. Neuropsychiatry Clin. Neurosci.* 11:100–1002.

CASELLI, R. J., N. R. GRAFF-RADFORD, and K. REZAI, 1991. Thalamocortical diaschisis. *Neuropsych. Neuropsych. Behav. Neurol.* 4: 193–214.

CASTAIGNE, P., F. LHERMITTE, A. BUGE, R. ESCOUROLLE, J. J. HAUW, and O. LYON-CAEN, 1981. Paramedian thalamic and midbrain infarcts: Clinical and neuropathological study. *Ann. Neurol.* 10: 127–148.

CICERONE, K. D., C. DAHLBERG, K. KALMAR, D. M. LANGENBAHN, J. F. MALEC, T. F. BERGQUIST, T. FELICETTI, J. T. GIACINO, J. P. HARLEY, D. E. HARRINGTON, J. HERZOG, S. KNEIPP, L. LAATSCH, and P. A. MORSE, 2000. Evidence-based cognitive rehabilitation. *Arch. Phys. Med. Rehabil.* 81:1596–1615.

CONTRERAS, D., and M. STERIADE, 1995. Cellular basis of EEG slow rhythms. *J. Neurosci.* 15:604–622.

CRABTREE, J. W., and J. T. ISAAC, 2002. New intrathalamic pathways allowing modality-related and cross-modality switching in the dorsal thalamus. *J. Neurosci.* 22:8754–8761.

EVARTS, E. V., Y. SHINODA, and S. P. WISE, 1984. Neurophysiological approaches to higher brain functions. New York: Wiley Interscience.

FINS, J. J., 2003. Constructing an ethical stereotaxy for severe brain injury: Balancing risks, benefits, and access. *Nat. Rev. Neurosci.* 4:323–327.

FRIES, P., J. H. REYNOLDS, A. E. RORIE, and R. DESIMONE, 2001. Modulation of oscillatory neuronal synchronization by selective visual attention. *Science* 291:1560–1563.

FRISTON, K. J., 2000. The labile brain. II. Transients, complexity and selection. *Philos. Trans. R. Soc. Lond. B Biol. Sci.* 355:237–252.

GEVINS, A., M. E. SMITH, L. MCENVOY, and D. YU, 1997. High-resolution EEG mapping of cortical activation related to working memory: Effects of task difficulty, type of processing and practice. *Cereb. Cortex* 7:374–385.

GIACINO, J. T., S. ASHWAL, N. CHILDS, R. CRANFORD, B. JENNETT, D. I. KATZ, J. P. KELLY, J. H. ROSENBERG, J. WHYTE, R. D. ZAFONTE, and N. D. ZASLER, 2002. The minimally conscious state: Definition and diagnostic criteria. *Neurology* 58:349–353.

GRONEWEGEN, H., and H. BERENDSE, 1994. The specificity of the "nonspecific" midline and intralaminar thalamic nuclei. *Trends Neurosci.* 17:52–66.

GUBERMAN, A., and D. STUSS, 1983. The syndrome of bilateral paramedian thalamic infarction. *Neurology* 33:540–546.

GUSNARD, D. A., and M. E. RAICHLE, 2001. Searching for baseline. *Nat. Neurosci.* 685–694.

INGVAR, D. H., 1955. Reproduction of 3 per second spike and wave EEG pattern by subcortical electrical stimulation in cats. *Acta Physiol. Scand.* 33:137–150.

INGVAR, D. H., and P. SOURANDER, 1970. Destruction of the reticular core of the brainstem. *Arch. Neurol.* 23:1–8.

JENNETT, B., J. H. ADAMS, L. S. MURRAY, et al., 2001. Neuropathology in vegetative and severely disabled patients after head injury. *Neurology* 56:486–490.

JENNETT, B., and F. PLUM, 1972. Persistent vegetative state after brain damage: A syndrome in search of a name. *Lancet* 1:734–737.

JOLIOT, M., U. RIBARY, and R. LLINÁS, 1994. Human oscillatory brain activity near 40 Hz coexists with cognitive temporal binding. *Proc. Natl. Acad. Sci. U.S.A.* 91:11748–11751.

JONES, E. G., 1998. A new view of specific and nonspecific thalamocortical connections. *Adv. Neurol.* 77:33–48.

JONES, E. G., 2001. The thalamic matrix and thalamocortical synchrony. *Trends Neurosci.* 24:595–601.

KATZ, D. I., M. P. ALEXANDER, and A. M. MANDELL, 1987. Dementia following strokes in the mesencephalon and diencephalon. *Arch. Neurol.* 44:1127–1133.

KINOMURA, S., J. LARSSEN, B. GULYAS, and P. E. ROLAND, 1996. Activation by attention of the human reticular formation and thalamic intralaminar nuclei. *Science* 271:512–515.

KROLAK-SALMON, P., B. CROISILE, C. HOUZARD, A. SETIEY, P. GIRARD-MADOUX, and A. VIGHETTO, 2000. Total recovery after bilateral paramedian thalamic infarct. *Eur. Neurol.* 44:216.

LAUREYS, S., M. E. FAYMONVILLE, C. DEGUELDRE, G. D. FIORE, P. DAMAS, B. LAMBERMONT, N. JANSSENS, J. AERTS, G. FRANCK, A. LUXEN, G. MOONEN, M. LAMY, and P. MAQUET, 2000. Auditory processing in the vegetative state. *Brain* 123:1589–1601.

LAUREYS, S., M. E. FAYMONVILLE, A. LUXEN, M. LAMY, G. FRANCK, and P. MAQUET, 2000. Restoration of thalamocortical connectivity after recovery from persistent vegetative state. *Lancet* 355: 1790–1791.

LAUREYS, S., M. E. FAYMONVILLE, P. PEIGNEUX, P. DAMAS, B. LAMBERMONT, G. DEL FIORE, C. DEGUELDRE, J. AERTS, A. LUXEN, G. FRANCK, M. LAMY, G. MOONEN, and P. MAQUET, 2002. Cortical processing of noxious somatosensory stimuli in the persistent vegetative state. *NeuroImage* 17:732–741.

LEVY, D. E., J. J. SIDTIS, D. A. ROTTENBERG, D. A. ROTTENBERG, J. O. JARDEN, S. C. STROTHER, V. DHAWAN, J. Z. GINOS, M. J. TRAMO, A. C. EVANS, and F. PLUM, 1987. Differences in cerebral blood flow and glucose utilization in vegetative versus locked-in patients. *Ann. Neurol.* 22:673–682.

LLINÁS, R., U. RIBARY, M. JOLIOT, and X. J. WANG, 1994. Content and context in temporal thalamocortical binding. In *Temporal Coding in the Brain*, G. Buzsaki et al., eds. Heidelberg: Springer-Verlag, pp. 252–272.

LUU, P., and D. M. TUCKER, 2001. Regulating action: Alternating activation of midline frontal and motor cortical networks. *Clin. Neurophysiol.* 112:1295–1306.

MACCHI, G., and M. BENTIVOGLIO, 1985. The thalamic intralaminar nuclei and the cerebral cortex. *Cereb. Cortex* 5:355–389.

MANLY, T., K. HAWKINS, J. EVANS, K. WODLT, and I. H. ROBERTSON, 2002. Rehabilitation of executive function: Facilitation of effective goal management on complex tasks using periodic auditory alerts. *Neuropsychologia* 40:271–281.

MATSUMOTO, N., T. MINAMIMOTO, A. M. GRAYBIEL, and M. KIMURA, 2001. Neurons in the thalamic CM-Pf complex supply striatal neurons with information about behaviorally significant sensory events. *J. Neurophysiol.* 85:960–976.

MEISSNER, I., S. SAPIR, E. KOKMEN, and S. D. STEIN, 1987. The paramedian diencephalic syndrome: A dynamic phenomenon. *Stroke* 18:380–385.

MENNEMEIER, M., B. CROSSON, D. J. WILLIAMSON, S. E. NADEAU, E. FENNELL, E. VALENSTEIN, and K. M. HEILMAN, 1997. Tapping, talking and the thalamus: Possible influence of the intralaminar nuclei on basal ganglia function. *Neuropsychologia* 35(2):183–193.

MENON, D. K., A. M. OWEN, and J. D. PICKARD, 1999. Response from Menon, Owen and Pickard. *Trends Cogn. Sci.* 3:44–46.

MENON, D. K., A. M. OWEN, E. J. WILLIAMS, et al., 1998. Cortical processing in persistent vegetative state. *Lancet* 352:1148–1149.

MINAMIMOTO, T., and M. KIMURA, 2002. Participation of the thalamic CM-Pf complex in attentional orienting. *J. Neurophysiol.* 87:3090–3101.

MORUZZI, G., and H. W. MAGOUN, 1949. Brainstem reticular formation and activation of the EEG. *Electroencephalogr. Clin. Neurophysiol.* 1:455–473.

MURTHY, V. N., and E. E. FETZ, 1996. Synchronization of neurons during local field potential oscillations in sensorimotor cortex of awake monkeys. *J. Neurophysiol.* 76:3968–3982.

PARVIZI, J., and A. DAMASIO, 2001. Consciousness and the brainstem. *Cognition* 79:135–160.

PAUS, T., R. ZATORRE, N. HOFLE, Z. CARAMANOS, J. GOTMAN, M. PETRIDES, and A. EVANS, 1997. Time-related changes in neural systems underlying attention and arousal during the performance of an auditory vigilance task. *J. Cogn. Neurosci.* 9:392–408.

PENFIELD, W. G., and H. H. JASPER, 1954. *Epilepsy and the Functional Anatomy of the Human Brain.* Boston: Little, Brown.

PESARAN, B., J. S. PEZARIS, M. SAHANI, P. P. MITRA, and R. A. ANDERSEN, 2002. Temporal structure in neuronal activity during working memory in macaque parietal cortex. *Nat. Neurosci.* 5: 805–811.

PLUM, F., 1991. Coma and related global disturbances of the human conscious state. *Cereb. Cortex* 9:359–425.

PLUM, F., and J. POSNER, 1982. *Diagnosis of Stupor and Coma.* New York: F.A. Davis.

PURPURA, K. P., and N. D. SCHIFF, 1997. The thalamic intralaminar nuclei: Role in visual awareness. *Neuroscientist* 3:8–14.

REES, G., G. KREIMAN, and C. KOCH, 2002. Neural correlates of consciousness in humans. *Nat. Rev. Neurosci.* 3:261–270.

REPUCCI, M. A., N. D. SCHIFF, and J. D. VICTOR, 2001. General strategy for hierarchical decomposition of multivariate time series: Implications for temporal lobe seizures. *Ann. Biomed. Eng.* 29:1135–1149.

SADIKOT, A. F., A. PARENT, Y. SMITH, and J. P. BOLAM, 1992. Efferent connections of the centromedian and parafascicular thalamic nuclei in the squirrel monkey. *J. Comp. Neurol.* 320:228–242.

SARVAS, J., 1987. Basic mathematical and electromagnetic concepts of the biomagnetic inverse problem. *Phys. Med. Biol.* 32:11–22.

SCANNELL, J. W., G. A. BURNS, C. C. HILGETAG, M. A. O'NEIL, and M. P. YOUNG, 1999. The connectional organization of the cortico-thalamic system of the cat. *Cereb. Cortex* 9:277–299.

SCHIFF, N. D. (MODERATOR), J. J. FINS, J. T. GIACINO, B. LEVINE, D. MENON, and A. M. OWEN, 1999. Persistent vegetative state: A debate. In *HMS Beagle: The BioMedNet Magazine*, no. 72 (Feb. 18) (*http://ny.hmsbeagle.com/hmsbeagle/72/viewpts/overview.htm*).

SCHIFF, N. D., and F. PLUM, 1999a. Cortical processing in the vegetative state. *Trends Cogn. Sci.* 3:43–44.

SCHIFF, N. D., and F. PLUM, 1999b. The neurology of impaired consciousness: Global disorders and implied models (target article). Association for Scientific Study of Consciousness Electronic Seminar Series (*http://athena.english.vt.edu/cgi-bin/netforum/nic/a/1*).

SCHIFF, N. D., and F. PLUM, 2000. The role of arousal and "gating" systems in the neurology of impaired consciousness. *J. Clin. Neurophysiol.* 17:438–452.

SCHIFF, N. D., F. PLUM, and A. R. REZAI, 2002. Developing prosthetics to treat cognitive disabilities resulting from acquired brain injuries. *Neurol. Res.* 24:116–124.

SCHIFF, N. D., and K. P. PURPURA, 2002. Towards a neurophysiological basis for cognitive neuromodulation through deep brain stimulation. *Thalamus Rel. Sys.* 2:55–69.

SCHIFF, N., U. RIBARY, D. MORENO, B. BEATTIE, E. KRONBERG, R. BLASBERG, J. GIACINO, C. MCCAGG, J. J. FINS, R. LLINAS, and F. PLUM, 2002. Residual cerebral activity and behavioral fragments in the persistent vegetative state. *Brain* 125:1210–1234.

SCHIFF, N. D., U. RIBARY, F. PLUM, and R. LLINÁS, 1999. Words without mind. *J. Cogn. Neurosci.* 11:650–656.

SCHINDLER, I., G. KERKHOFF, H. O. KARNATH, I. KELLER, and G. GOLDENBERG, 2002. Neck muscle vibration induces lasting recovery in spatial neglect. *J. Neurol. Neurosurg. Psychiatry* 73:412–419.

SCHLAG-REY, M., and J. SCHLAG, 1984. Visuomotor functions of central thalamus in monkey. I. Unit activity related to spontaneous eye movements. *J. Neurophysiol.* 40:1149–1174.

SLOBOUNOV, S. M., K. FUKADA, R. SIMON, M. REARICK, and W. RAY, 2000. Neurophysiological and behavioral indices of time pressure effects on visuomotor task performance. *Cogn. Brain Res.* 9:287–298.

SPORNS, O., G. TONONI, and G. M. EDELMAN, 2002. Theoretical neuroanatomy and the connectivity of the cerebral cortex. *Behav. Brain Res.* 135:69–74.

STERIADE, M., 1997. Thalamic substrates of disturbances in states of vigilance and consciousness in humans. In *Thalamus*, M. Steriade, E. Jones, and D. McCormick, eds. New York: Elsevier.

STERIADE, M., 2000. Corticothalamic resonance, states of vigilance and mentation. *Neuroscience* 101:243–276.

STERIADE, M., D. CONTRERAS, F. AMZICA, and I. TIMOFEEV, 1996. Synchronization of fast (30–40 Hz) spontaneous oscillations in intrathalamic and thalamocortical networks. *J. Neurosci.* 16:2788–2808.

STERIADE, M., and L. L. GLENN, 1982. Neocortical and caudate projections of intralaminar thalamic neurons and their synaptic excitation from midbrain reticular core. *J. Neurophysiol.* 48:352–371.

STERIADE, M., E. JONES, and D. MCCORMICK, 1997. *Thalamus.* Amsterdam: Elsevier.

SUTCLIFFE, J. G., and L. DE LECEA, 2002. The hypocretins: Setting the arousal threshold. *Nat. Rev. Neurosci.* 3:339–349.

SZELIES, B., et al., 1991. Widespread functional effects of discrete thalamic infarction. *Arch. Neurol.* 48:178–182.

TOMASSINO, C., C. GRANA, G. LUCIGNANI, G. TORRI, and F. FERRUCIO, 1995. Regional metabolism of comatose and vegetative state patients. *J. Neurosurg. Anesthesiol.* 7:109–116.

VAN DOMBURG, P. H., H. J. TEN DONKELAAR, and S. L. NOTERMANS, 1996. Akinetic mutism with bithalamic infarction: Neurophysiological correlates. *J. Neurol. Sci.* 139:58–65.

VAN DER WERF, Y. D., J. G. WEERTS, J. JOLLES, M. P. WITTER, J. LINDEBOOM, and P. SCHELTENS, 1999. Neuropsychological correlates of a right unilateral lacunar thalamic infarction. *J. Neurol. Neurosurg. Psychiatry* 66(1):36–42.

VAN DER WERF, Y. D., M. P. WITTER, and H. J. GROENEWEGEN, 2002. The intralaminar and midline nuclei of the thalamus: Anatomical and functional evidence for participation in processes of arousal and awareness. *Brain Res. Brain Res. Rev.* 39:107–140.

WATTS, D., 2000. *Small Worlds.* Princeton, N.J.: Princeton University Press.

WEDEKIND, C., V. HESSELMANN, M. LIPPERT-GRUNER, and M. EBEL, 2000. Trauma to the pontomesencephalic brainstem: A major clue to the prognosis of severe traumatic brain injury. *Br. J. Neurosurg.* 16:256–260.

WEESE, G. D., J. M. PHILLIPS, and V. J. BROWN, 1999. Attentional orienting is impaired by unilateral lesions of the thalamic reticular nucleus in the rat. *J. Neurosci.* 19:10135–10139.

WILSON, B. A., F. GRACEY, and K. BAINBRIDGE, 2001. Cognitive recovery from "persistent vegetative state." *Brain. Inj.* 15: 1083–1092.

WORDEN, M. S., J. J. FOXE, N. WANG, and G. V. SIMPSON, 2000. Anticipatory biasing of visuospatial attention indexed by retinotopically specific alpha-band electroencephalography increases over occipital cortex. *J. Neurosci.* 20:RC63.

ZEKI, S., 1993. *A Vision of the Brain.* London: Basil Blackwell.

81 A Framework for Consciousness

FRANCIS C. CRICK AND CHRISTOF KOCH

ABSTRACT This chapter summarizes our current thinking on the problem of consciousness. At the moment, the most promising empirical approach is to discover the neuronal correlate of consciousness (NCC) in the mammalian forebrain by electrophysiological means, in combination with interventionist molecular or pharmacological strategies. In this chapter, we set out this general strategy under 10 headings or working hypotheses. This framework offers a coherent scheme for explaining the NCC for sensory consciousness in terms of competing cellular assemblies. Most of the ideas we favor have been suggested before, but their combination is original.

The most difficult aspect of consciousness is the so-called hard problem of qualia (Chalmers, 1995; Shear, 1997; Churchland, 2002; see Chalmers, this volume): what is the relation between subjective sensations—the redness of red, the painfulness of pain, and so on—and their physical basis in electrochemical interactions in the brain? No one has produced any plausible explanation as to how the redness of red could arise from the actions of the brain. It appears fruitless to approach this problem head-on. Instead, we believe that discovering the neural correlates of consciousness (NCCs) is a more fruitful strategy: if we can explain NCCs in causal terms, this may make the problem of qualia clearer (Crick and Koch, 1998a).

In general terms, the NCC is the minimal set of neuronal events that is jointly sufficient for a specific aspect of a conscious percept. We have previously discussed why we think consciousness has to be largely private (Crick and Koch, 1995a). By private we mean that it is impossible for me to convey to you the exact nature of my conscious percepts, such as seeing red, although I can convey whether two shades of red appear to me to be the same or different.

Our main interest is not the enabling factors needed for all forms of consciousness, such as the activity of the ascending reticular system in the upper brainstem and midline thalamic regions, as discussed elsewhere in this volume by Schiff, but the general nature of the neural activities that produce each particular aspect of consciousness, such as an object with a specific color, shape, or movement.

FRANCIS C. CRICK The Salk Institute for Biological Studies, La Jolla, Calif.
CHRISTOF KOCH Division of Biology, California Institute of Technology, Pasadena, Calif.

As a matter of tactics, we have concentrated on the visual system of primates, putting to one side some of the more difficult aspects of consciousness, such as emotion and self-consciousness. However, our framework may well apply to other sensory modalities. We have been especially interested in the alert macaque monkey, because to find the NCC, it is necessary to investigate not only widespread neural activities but also the detailed behavior of single neurons (or small groups of neurons) on very fast time scales. It is difficult to conduct this kind of investigation systematically in human subjects. On the other hand, experiments in visual psychology are much easier to do with humans than with monkeys, and functional magnetic resonance imaging (fMRI) of brain activity in human subjects has proved to be helpful in identifying regions of relevance to conscious perception (see Rees, this volume). Moreover, humans can report what they are conscious of. For these reasons, experiments with monkey and human subjects should be pursued in parallel. For now, we have no convincing explanation of why any phenomenal, conscious state should feel like anything at all, let alone the way it does (see Chalmers, this volume).

What is a framework?

A framework is not a detailed hypothesis or set of hypotheses; rather, it is a point of view for approaching a scientific problem, and one that suggests testable hypotheses. Biological frameworks differ from frameworks in physics and chemistry because of the nature of evolution through natural selection. Biological systems, unlike physical systems, do not have rigid laws. Evolution produces mechanisms and often submechanisms, so that there are few "rules" in biology that do not have occasional exceptions.

A good framework is one that is reasonably plausible relative to available scientific data and that turns out to be largely correct. It is unlikely to be correct in all the details. A framework often incorporates unstated (often unrecognized) assumptions, but this situation is unavoidable.

An example from molecular biology might be helpful. The double-helical structure of DNA immediately suggested, in a novel way, the general nature of gene composition, gene replication, and gene action. This framework turned out to be broadly correct, but it did not foresee, for example, either introns or RNA editing. And who would have guessed that DNA replication usually starts with the synthesis of a short stretch of RNA, which is then removed and replaced by DNA? The broad framework acted as a guide, but only careful experimentation allowed the true details to be discovered. This is a lesson broadly applicable throughout biology.

A preamble on the cerebral cortex

By the cortical system we mean the cerebral cortex plus other regions closely associated with it, such as the thalamus and the claustrum, and probably the basal ganglia, the cerebellum, and the many widespread brainstem projection systems.

We shall refer to the front of the cortex and the back of the cortex, since the terms *frontal* and *prefrontal* can be ambiguous. For example, is the anterior cingulate prefrontal? The dividing line between front and back is somewhat arbitrary. It roughly coincides with the central sulcus. It may turn out that a good operational definition is that the front is all those parts that receive a significant input, via the thalamus, from the basal ganglia. (This simple division is probably not useful for olfaction.)

One general characteristic of the operations of the cortex is the astonishing variety and specificity of the actions performed by the cortical system. The visual system of the higher mammals handles an almost infinite variety of visual inputs and reacts to them in detail with remarkable accuracy. Clearly, the system is highly evolved, is likely to be specified epigenetically in considerable detail, and can learn a large amount from experience.

The main function of the sensory cortex is to construct and use highly specific feature detectors, such as those for orientation, motion, or faces. The features that any cortical neuron responds to are usually highly specific but multidimensional. That is, a single neuron does not respond to a single feature but to a family of related features. Such features are sometimes called the receptive field of that neuron. The visual fields of neurons higher in the visual hierarchy are larger and respond to more complex features than those lower down. The nonclassical receptive field expresses the relevant context of the classical receptive field (Allman, Miezin, and McGuinness, 1985).

An important but neglected aspect of the firing of a neuron (or a small group of associated neurons) is its projective field (Lehky and Sejnowski, 1988). This term describes the perceptual and behavioral consequences of stimulating such a neuron in an appropriate manner (see the work on motor and premotor cortex by Graziano, Taylor, and Moore, 2002). Both the receptive field and the projective field are dynamic, not merely static, and both can be modified by experience.

How are feature detectors formed? A broad answer is that neurons do this by detecting common and significant correlations in their inputs and altering their synapses (and perhaps other properties) so that they can more easily respond to such inputs. In other words, the brain is very good at detecting apparent causation. Exactly how it does this is more controversial. The main mechanism is probably Hebbian, but Hebb's seminal suggestion needs to be expanded.

Everything we have discussed so far might suggest that cortical action is highly local. Nothing could be farther from the truth. In the cortex, there is continual and extensive interaction, both in the near neighborhood and also very widely, thanks to the many long corticocortical and corticothalamocortical routes. This is much less true of the thalamus itself.

The sensory cortex is arranged in a semihierarchical manner. (This is certainly true of the visual cortex [Felleman and Van Essen, 1991]. It is less clear of the front of the brain.) That is, most cortical areas do not detect simple correlations in the sensory input but detect correlations between correlations being expressed by other cortical areas. This remarkable feature of the cortex is seldom emphasized.

There is a great selective advantage, for both predators and prey, in the ability to react very rapidly, and for this reason, the best is the enemy of the good. As a general rule, it is better to achieve a rapid but occasionally imperfect performance than a more prolonged one that produces a perfect result. Another general principle may be that it is better to use several rough-and-ready methods in parallel to reach a conclusion, rather than following just one method very accurately. This appears to be how, for example, people see in depth.

If two brief stimuli are similar, the brain blends them together. If they are different but in contradiction, such as a face and a house, the brain does not blend them but instead selects one of them, as in binocular rivalry.

The incoming visual information is usually not enough to lead to an unambiguous interpretation (Poggio, Torre, and Koch, 1985). In such cases the cortical networks "fill in," that is, they make their best guess, given the incomplete information. Such filling in is likely to happen in many places in the brain. This general principle is an important guide to much of human behavior and appears in many colloquial sayings, such as "jumping to conclusions."

Our present framework

Having outlined a few general points about the cortical system, we will now consider specifically the NCCs and their attendant properties. We are mainly interested in time periods on the order of a few hundred milliseconds, or at most several seconds, so that we can now put to one side processes that take more time, such as the permanent establishment of a new memory. We have listed the main constituents of our framework under 10 headings. These 10 ideas have been published in a recent article (Crick and Koch, 2003), from which most of the material in this chapter is taken.

Our framework leaves out a more detailed consideration of the role of the thalamus (and especially of the intralaminar nuclei), the claustrum, the actions of the basal ganglia and of the diffuse inputs from the brainstem, and the lack of any more detailed scheme for the overall organization of the front of the cortex, and for motor outputs.[1]

On the other hand, concentrating on the NCC while postponing the so-called hard problem of qualia is part of our strategic approach to the overall problem of consciousness (Koch, 2004).

1. The (Nonconscious?) Homunculus A good way to begin to look at the overall behavior of the cerebral cortex is that the front of the brain is "looking at" the sensory systems, most of which are at the back of the brain. This division of labor does not lead to an infinite regress (Attneave, 1961). This idea at this stage is necessarily rather vague (see later discussion under point 3, Coalitions of Neurons).

We have discussed elsewhere (Crick and Koch, 2000) whether the neural activity in the front of the brain is largely inaccessible to consciousness. Jackendoff (1987, 1996), for example, has proposed that humans are not directly conscious of their thoughts, only of sensory representations of them in their imagination. At the moment, there is no consensus about this (see the contributions in Crick and Koch, 2000).

The hypothesis of the homunculus is currently very much out of fashion, but, in broad terms, this is how everyone thinks of him- or herself. It would be surprising if this overwhelming illusion did not in some way reflect the general organization of the brain.

2. Zombie Modes and Consciousness Many actions in response to sensory inputs are rapid, transient, stereotyped, and nonconscious (Milner and Goodale, 1995; Rossetti, 1998; see also Goodale, this volume). They could be thought of as cortical reflexes. We call these actions zombie agents (Koch and Crick, 2001). Consciousness deals more deliberate, more slowly with broader, less stereotyped aspects of the sensory inputs (or a reflection of these in imagery) and takes time to decide on appropriate thoughts and responses. This dual division of labor is needed because otherwise a vast number of different zombie modes would be required. The conscious system may interfere somewhat with the concur-

rent zombie system. It would be a great evolutionary advantage to have both zombie modes that respond rapidly, in a stereotyped manner, and a slightly slower system that allows time for thinking and planning more complex behavior. The slower system would be one of the functions of consciousness.

It seems likely that visual zombie modes in the cortex mainly use the dorsal stream in the parietal region (Milner and Goodale, 1995). However, some parietal activity also affects consciousness by producing attentional effects on the ventral stream, at least under some circumstances, or by generating activity associated with certain attributes of motion perception (Battelli et al., 2001). The conscious mode for vision depends largely on the early visual areas (beyond V1), and especially on the ventral stream. There are no recorded cases of purely parietal damage that led to a complete loss of conscious vision.

In a zombie mode, the main flow of information is probably feedforward. It could be considered a forward traveling net-wave. A net-wave is a propagating wave of neural activity, but it is not the same as a wave in a continuous medium. Neural networks in a cortex have both short and long connections, so a net-wave may, in some cases, jump over intervening regions. In the conscious mode it seems likely that the flow is in both directions (see discussion under point 5, The Higher Levels First), so that it resembles more a standing net-wave.

3. Coalitions of Neurons The cortex is a very highly and specifically interconnected neural network. It has many types of both excitatory and inhibitory interneurons and acts by forming transient coalitions of neurons, the members of which support each other. *Coalitions* implies assemblies—an idea that goes back at least to Hebb (1949)—and competition between them (see also Edelman and Tononi, 2000). Desimone and Duncan (1995) suggested, as a result of experiments on the macaque, that selective attention biases the competition between rivalrous cell assemblies, but they did not explicitly relate this idea to consciousness.

The various neurons in a coalition in some sense support each other, either directly or indirectly, by increasing the activity of their fellow members. The dynamics of coalitions are not simple. In general, at any moment the winning coalition is somewhat sustained, and embodies what we are conscious of.

It may help to make a crude political analogy. The early events in an election and the primaries would correspond roughly to the preliminary nonconscious processing. The winning coalition associated with an object or event would correspond to the winning party, which would remain in power for some time and would attempt to influence and control future events. Attention would correspond to the efforts of journalists, pollsters, and others to focus on certain issues rather than others, and thus attempt to bias the electorate in their favor. The large pyramidal cells in cortical layer V that project to the superior colliculus and the thalamus (both involved in attention) might correspond to electoral polls. These progress from early, tentative polls to later, more accurate ones as the election approaches.

It is unlikely that all this happens in the brain in a fixed time sequence. The brain may resemble more the British system, in which the time between one election and the next can be irregular. Such an analogy should not be pressed too far. Like all analogies, it should be regarded as a possible source of ideas, to be confirmed by experiment.

Coalitions can vary both in size and in character. For example, a coalition produced by visual imagination (with one's eyes closed) may be less widespread than a coalition produced by a vivid and sustained visual input. In particular, it may fail to reach down to the lower echelons of the visual hierarchy. Coalitions in dreams may be somewhat different from waking ones.

If there are coalitions in the front of the cortex, they may have a somewhat different character from those formed at the back of the cortex. There may be more than one coalition that achieves winning status and hence produces conscious experience. The coalitions there may reflect feelings such as happiness and, perhaps, the feeling of "authorship" related to the perception of "freely" initiating motor action (see Wegner and Sparsow, this volume). Such feelings may be more diffuse and may persist for a longer time than coalitions in the back of cortex. Jackendoff (1987) uses the terms affect or valuations for what we have called feelings. Our first working assumption (The homunculus) implies that it is better not to regard the back plus the front as one single coalition, but rather as two or more rather separate coalitions that interact massively, but not in an exactly reciprocal manner.

4. EXPLICIT REPRESENTATIONS AND ESSENTIAL NODES An explicit representation of a particular aspect of the visual scene implies that a small set of neurons exists that responds as a detector for that feature, without further complex neural processing. One possible probe, an operational test, for an explicit representation might be whether a single layer of linear, threshold "units" could deliver the correct answer. For example, if such a layer was fed the activity of retinal neurons, it would not be able to recognize a face. Fed from the relevant parts of inferior temporal cortex, it could reliably signal "face" or "no face." There is much evidence from both humans and monkeys that if such neurons are all lost from brain damage, then the subject is unable to consciously perceive that aspect directly. Well-known clinical examples are achromatopsia (loss of color perception), prosopagnosia (loss of face recognition), and akinetopsia (loss of motion

perception). In all cases, one or a few attributes of conscious experience have been lost, while most other aspects remain intact. In the macaque, a small, irreversible lesion of the motion area MT/V5 leads to a temporal deficit in motion perception that recovers within days. Larger lesions cause a more permanent loss (Newsome and Paré, 1988). We believe that an explicit representation is a necessary but not sufficient condition for the NCC to occur.

One can describe the cortical system in terms of essential nodes (Zeki, 1998; Zeki and Bartels, 1999). The cortical neural networks (at least for perception) can be thought of as having nodes. Each node is needed to express one aspect of one percept or another. An aspect cannot become conscious unless there is an essential node for it. This is a necessary but not a sufficient condition. For consciousness, there may be other necessary conditions, such as projecting to the front of the brain (Crick and Koch, 1995b).

A node by itself cannot produce consciousness. Even if the neurons in that node were firing appropriately, such firing would produce little effect if their output synapses were inactivated. A node is a node, not a network. Thus, a particular coalition is an active network, consisting of the relevant set of interacting nodes that temporarily sustains itself.

Much useful information can be obtained from lesions. In humans, the damaged area is usually fairly large. It is not clear what effects a very small, possibly bilateral, reversible lesion would have in the macaque, because it is difficult to discover exactly what a monkey is conscious of. The smallest useful node may be a cortical column (Mountcastle, 1998), or perhaps a portion of one. The feature which that node represents is (broadly) its columnar property. This is because although a single type of pyramidal cell usually sends its information to only one or two cortical areas, the pyramidal cells in a column project the columnar property collectively to many cortical areas, and thus can lend greater support to any coalition that is forming.

5. THE HIGHER LEVELS FIRST For a new visual input, the neural activity first travels rapidly and *non*consciously up the visual hierarchy to a high level, possibly in the front of the brain (this might instantiate a zombie mode). Signals then start to move backward down the hierarchy, so that the first stages to reach consciousness are at the higher levels (showing the gist of the scene; Biederman, 1972; Wolfe and Bennett, 1997), which send these "conscious" signals again to prefrontal cortex, followed by corresponding activity at successively lower levels (to provide the visual details). This is an oversimplified description. There are also many side connections in the hierarchy (for a similar idea, see Hochstein and Ahissar, 2002). How far up the hierarchy the initial net-wave travels may depend on whether attention is diffused or focused at some particular level.

6. DRIVING AND MODULATING CONNECTIONS   In considering the physiology of coalitions, it is especially important to understand the nature of neural connections (the net is not an undirected one). The classification of neuronal inputs is still somewhat primitive. It is a mistake to think of all excitatory neural connections as being of the same type. Connections to a cortical neuron fall roughly into several different broad classes. An initial classification would divide them into driving and modulating inputs (Crick and Koch, 1998b). For cortical pyramidal cells, driving inputs may largely contact the basal dendrites, whereas modulatory inputs include back-projections (largely to the apical dendrites) or diffuse projections, especially those from the intralaminar nuclei of the thalamus.

This classification may be too simple. In some cases, a single type of input to a neuron may be driving, as in the input from the lateral geniculate nucleus (LGN) to V1. In other cases several types of driving inputs may be needed to make that neuron fire at a significant rate. It is possible that the connections from the back of the brain to the front are largely driving, while the reverse pathways are largely modulatory, but this is not experimentally established. This general pattern would not hold for cross-modal connections.

The tentative classification just proposed is largely for excitatory cells. Strong loops of driving connections probably do not occur under normal conditions (Crick and Koch, 1998b).

It seems likely that cortical layer V cells that project to the thalamus are driving while those from layer VI are modulating (Crick and Koch, 1998b; Sherman and Guillery, 2001).

7. SNAPSHOTS   Has a successful coalition any special characteristics? We propose that conscious awareness (for vision) involves a series of static snapshots, with motion "painted" on them (Zihl, von Cramon, and Mai, 1983; Hess, Baker, and Zihl, 1989; figure 81.1). By this we mean that perception occurs in discrete epochs. It is well established that the mechanisms for position estimation and for motion are largely separate (recall the motion aftereffect.) Thus, a particular motion can be represented by a constant rate of firing of the relevant neurons that represent that motion.

The neurologist Oliver Sacks has reported a rare but dramatic neurological disturbance that he calls cinematographic vision (Sacks, 2004; see also Ffytche and Howard, 1999). It manifests itself during visual migraine, when the subject experiences the world as consisting of a succession of "stills," without any movement between the images, like the flickering of a movie run too slowly. In an earlier work, Sacks (1970) concludes, "The term cinematographic vision denotes the nature of visual experience when the illusion of motion has been lost." It would be important to

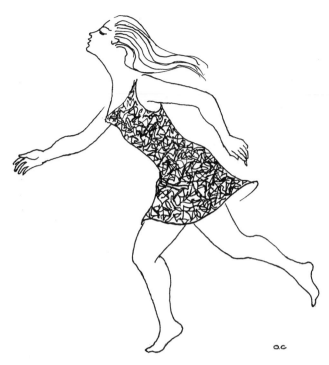

FIGURE 81.1   The snapshot hypothesis proposes that the conscious perception of motion is not represented by the change in firing rate of the relevant neurons, but by the (nearly) constant firing of certain neurons that represent the motion. The figure is an analogy. It shows how a static picture can suggest motion.

replicate such a remarkable phenomenon under controlled conditions.

Purves, Paydarfar, and Andrews (1996) have described several psychological effects, such as an illusion under constant illumination, similar to but distinct from the wagon-wheel effect, that hint that there are some irregular batchlike effects in vision.

The durations of successive snapshots are unlikely to be constant (they are difficult to measure directly). Moreover, the time of a snapshot for shape, say, may not exactly coincide with that for color. It is possible that these durations may be related to the alpha rhythm (Varela et al., 1981) or even the theta rhythm. The theory of the perceptual moment was suggested by Stroud as early as 1955, but in recent years it has been largely forgotten. VanRullen and Koch (2003) review the evidence in favor of discrete perceptual moments

To reach consciousness, some (unspecified) neural activity for that feature has to reach above a threshold. It is unlikely to do so unless it is, or is becoming, the member of a successful coalition. It is held above threshold, possibly as a constant value of the activity, for a certain time (the time of that snapshot). Since specific attributes of conscious perception are all-or-none, so should be the underlying NCC (for instance, either firing at a low or at a high level). This activity may also show hysteresis; that is, it may stay there longer than its support warrants.

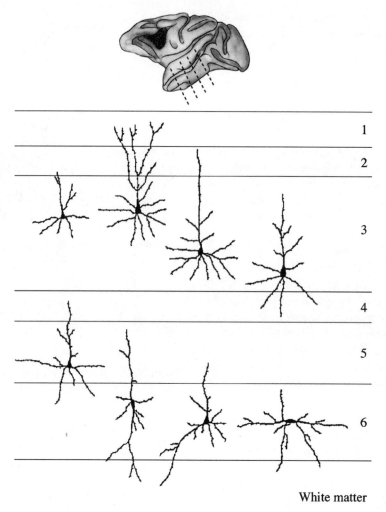

White matter

FIGURE 81.2 Schematic illustrations showing the dendritic arborization of the different types of neurons in the inferior temporal gyrus of the macaque monkey that project to the prefrontal cortex near the principal sulcus (brain diagram at top shows where the injections were made). There will be other types of neurons in this area that project to other places. Only one type of cell has apical dendrites that reach to layer I. (From Koch, 2004, as modified from de Lima, Voigt, and Morrison, 1990.)

What could be special about this form of activity? It might be some particular way of firing, such as a sustained high rate, some sort of synchronized firing, or firing in bursts. Or it might be the firing of special types of neurons, such as those pyramidal cells that project to the front of the brain (de Lima, Voigt, and Morrison, 1990; figure 81.2). This may seem unlikely, but if true, it would greatly simplify the problem, both experimentally and theoretically.

What is required to maintain this special activity above threshold? It might be something special about the internal dynamics of the neuron, perhaps due to the accumulation of chemicals such as Ca^{2+}, either in the neuron itself or in one of its associated inhibitory neurons. It might also be due to reentrant circuits in the cortical system (Edelman, 1989). Positive feedback loops could, by iteratively exciting the neuron, push its activity increasingly upward so that the

activity not only reached above some critical threshold but was maintained there for some time.

There are some complications. The threshold level may depend on the rate of approach to the threshold, or on how long the input is sustained, or both of these. At the beginning of each new snapshot there may be some holdover from the previous one.

Put another way, these are partial descriptions of conscious coalitions forming, growing, or disappearing.

There is no evidence for a regular clock in the brain on the second or fraction of a second time scale. The duration of any snapshot (or fragments of a snapshot) is likely to vary somewhat, depending on factors such as sudden on-signals, off-signals, competition, habituation, and so on.

8. ATTENTION AND BINDING Attention can usefully be divided into rapid, saliency-driven, bottom-up forms and

slower, volitionally controlled, top-down forms. Either form of attention can also be diffused or more focused. Attention probably acts by biasing the competition between rival coalitions, especially in their formation (Desimone and Duncan, 1995). Bottom-up attention may often start from certain layer V neurons that project to parts of the thalamus and the superior colliculus. Top-down attention from the front of the brain may go by somewhat diffuse back-projections to apical dendrites in layers I, II, and III, and perhaps also via the intralaminar nuclei of the thalamus (since these have inputs from the front of the brain). Even though such projections are widespread, it does not follow that they are not specific. To attend to *red* involves specific connections to many places in cortex. An attractive hypothesis is that the thalamus is largely the organ of attention. The reticular nucleus of the thalamus may help select among attentional signals on a broad scale. Whereas attention can produce consciousness of a particular object or event by biasing competition among coalitions, activities associated with nonattended objects are quite transient, giving rise to fleeting consciousness (such as the proto-objects suggested by Rensink, 2000).

Thus, attention and consciousness are separate processes. Some sort of attentional bias is probably necessary to give rise to a single dominant coalition, whose associated representational content the subject is aware of. That is, attention is probably necessary but not sufficient for consciousness (see also Dehaene and Changeux, this volume).

What is binding? (See the special issue of *Neuron*, 1999, on this topic.) This is the term used for the process that brings together rather different aspects of an object/event, such as its shape, color, movement, and so on. Binding can be of several types (Crick and Koch, 1990). If it has been laid down epigenetically or learned by experience, it is already embodied in one or more essential nodes, so no special binding mechanism is needed. If the binding required is (relatively) novel, then in some way the activities of separate essential nodes must be made to act together.

Recent work in psychophysics suggests that "parallel versus serial" search and "preattentive versus attentive" visual processing describe two independent dimensions rather than variations along a single dimension (VanRullen, Reddy, and Koch, 2004). The results can all be expressed in terms of the relevant neural networks. Several objects/events can be handled simultaneously, that is, more than one object/event can be attended to at the same time, if there is no significant overlap in any cortical neural network. In other words, if two or more objects/events have no very active essential nodes in common, they can be consciously perceived. Under such conditions, several largely separate (sensory) coalitions may exist. If there is necessarily such an overlap, then attention is needed to select one of them by biasing the competition between them.

This approach largely solves the classical binding problem, which was mainly concerned with how two different object/events could be bound simultaneously. On this view, the binding of the features of single object/event is simply the membership of a particular coalition. There is no single cortical area where it all comes together. The effects of that coalition are widely distributed over both the back and the front of the brain. Thus, effectively, they bind by interacting in a diffuse manner.

9. STYLES OF FIRING Synchronized firing (including various oscillations) may be used for several purposes to increase the effectiveness of a group of neurons while not necessarily altering their average firing rate (Singer and Gray, 1995). The extent and significance of synchronized firing in cortex remains controversial (Shadlen and Movshon, 1999). Computations show (Salinas and Sejnowski, 2001) that this effectiveness is likely to depend on how the correlated input influences the excitatory and inhibitory neurons in the recipient region to which the synchronized neurons project.

We no longer think (Crick and Koch, 1990) that synchronized firing, such as the so-called 40-Hz oscillations, is a sufficient condition for the NCC.

One likely purpose of synchronized firing is to assist a nascent coalition in its competition with other (nascent) coalitions. If the visual input is simple, such as a single bar in an otherwise empty field, there might be no significant competition, and synchronized firing may not occur. Also, such a bias may not be needed once a successful coalition has reached consciousness, at which point it may be able to maintain itself without the assistance of synchrony, at least for a time (Revonsuo et al., 1997). An analogy: after obtaining tenure, you can relax a little.

At any essential node, the earliest spike to arrive may sometimes have the advantage over spikes arriving shortly thereafter (VanRullen and Thorpe, 2001). In other words, the exact timing of a spike may influence the competition.

10. PENUMBRA AND MEANING Let us consider a set of neurons that fires to, say, some aspect of a face. The experimenter can discover what visual features interest such a set of neurons, but how does the brain know what that firing represents? This is the problem of "meaning" in its broadest sense.

The NCC at any one time will directly involve only a fraction of the total pyramidal cells, but this firing will influence many neurons that are not part of the NCC. These we call the *penumbra*. The penumbra consists of both synaptic effects and firing rates. The penumbra is not the result of just the sum of the effects of each essential node separately, but the effects of that NCC as a whole. This penumbra includes past associations of NCC neurons, the expected consequences of the NCC, movements (or at least possible plans for movement) associated with NCC neurons, and so on. For example, a hammer represented in the NCC is likely to influence plans for hammering.

The penumbra, by definition, is not itself conscious, though part of it may become part of the NCC as the NCC shift. Some of the penumbra neurons may project back to parts of the NCC or their support, and thus help to support the NCC. The penumbra neurons may be the site of non-conscious priming (Schacter, 1992).

Related ideas

In the last 15–20 years there has been an immense flood of publications on consciousness.[2] Many people have said that consciousness is "global" or has a "unity," but have provided few details about such unity. For many years Baars (1997) has argued that consciousness must be widely distributed.

Dennett (1991, 2001) has written at length about his ideas of "multiple drafts," often using elaborate analogies, but he seems not to believe in the existence of aspects of consciousness in the same way as we do. Dennett does consider a limited number of psychological experiments, but neurons, he has told us in a personal communication, "are not my department."

There are two fairly recent books expressing ideas that overlap considerably with ours. The first of these is *Universe of Consciousness*, by Edelman and Tononi (2000). Their "dynamic core" is very similar to our coalitions. They also divide consciousness into "primary consciousness" (which is what we are mainly concerned with) and "higher-order consciousness" (which we have for the moment put to one side). However, in their book, Edelman and Tononi state strongly that they do not think there is a special subset of neurons that alone expresses the NCC.

The other book is Bachmann's *Microgenetic Approach to the Conscious Mind* (2000). For many years, Bachmann has used the term *microgenesis* to mean what is happening in the 100–200 ms leading up to consciousness, which is also our main concern. He considers carefully the relevant psychological phenomena, such as the different types of masking, but has fewer ideas about the detailed behavior of neurons. We agree with much of what he has to say.

A framework somewhat similar to ours has been described by Dehaene and Naccache (2001), by Changeux (2004), and in this volume by Dehaene and Changeux, although they do not elaborate on the snapshot hypothesis or the neural basis of essential nodes. A few key differences are our emphasis on the particular molecular, synaptic, neuronal, or network properties of the mechanisms underlying the NCC, its exclusion from V1, and our hypothesis that many aspects of high-level cognitive processing are not accessible to consciousness

(the homunculus hypothesis). This appears to be at odds with global workspace models.

General remarks

Almost all of the ideas discussed in this chapter have already been suggested, either by us or by others. The framework we have proposed, however, knits all these ideas together, so that for the first time, we have a coherent scheme accounting for the NCC in philosophical, psychological, and neural terms.

What ties these various suggestions together is the idea of competing coalitions. The illusion of a homunculus inside the head looking at the sensory activities of the brain suggests that the coalitions at the back are in some way distinct from the coalitions at the front. The two types of coalitions interact extensively but not exactly reciprocally.

Zombie modes show that not all motor outputs from the cortex are carried out consciously. Consciousness depends on certain coalitions that rest on the properties of very elaborate neural networks. We consider attention to consist of mechanisms that bias the competition between these nascent coalitions.

We suggest that each node in these networks has a characteristic behavior. We speculate that the smallest group of neurons worth considering a node is a cortical column, each with its own characteristic behavior (its receptive and projective fields).

The idea of snapshots is a guess at the dynamic properties of the parts of a successful coalition, since coalitions are not static but are constantly changing. The penumbra, on the other hand, consists of all the neural and synaptic activity produced by the current NCC, but is not strictly part of the NCC.

We also speculate that the actual NCC may be expressed by only a small set of neurons, in particular those that project from the back of cortex to those parts of the front of cortex that are not purely motor and those that project back. However, there is much neural activity leading up to and supporting the NCC, so it is important to study this activity as well as the NCC proper. Moreover, discovering the temporal sequence of such activities (e.g., A precedes B) will help us to move from correlation to causation. This is why it is important to further develop interventionist molecular and genetic strategies applicable to the mammalian forebrain.

The explanation we have provided of this interlocking set of ideas is necessarily abbreviated. A more extended account, together with descriptions of the key experimental data, have been published in book form by one of us (Koch, 2004). The framework we propose is a guide to constructing more detailed hypotheses, so that they can be tested against already existing experimental evidence, and, above all, to suggest new experiments. The aim is to couch all such explanations in terms of the behavior of identified neurons and of the dynamics of very large neural assemblies.

Future experiments

Future experiments fall under several headings. Much further experimental work on small groups of neurons is required in cases in which the percept differs significantly from the sensory input, such as in binocular rivalry (Leopold and Logothetis, 1999; Blake and Logothetis, 2001), flash suppression (Sheinberg and Logothetis, 1997; Kreiman, Fried, and Koch, 2002), and related visual illusions.

Knowledge of the detailed neuroanatomy of the cerebral cortex needs to be greatly expanded, in particular to characterize the many different types of pyramidal cells in any particular cortical area. What do they look like, where do they project, and, eventually, does each have a set of characteristic genetic markers? Are there types of pyramidal cells that do not occur in all cortical areas? When recording spiking activity from a neuron, it would be very desirable to know what type it is, and where this particular cell projects.

Anatomical methods of characterizing types of neurons in the macaque monkey have been available for some years (de Lima, Voigt, and Morrison, 1990; see figure 81.2; for a very promising novel method, see Dacey et al., 2003). In the last two decades, very little additional work has been carried out on cell types and their connectivity, mainly for lack of funds, because such work is not hypothesis-driven. However, because structure is often a clue to function, detailed neuroanatomy is essential background knowledge (of the type the Human Genome Project provided for molecular biology).

On occasion, multiunit electrodes are chronically implanted into alert patients (e.g., to localize seizure onset focus in epileptic patients). With the patients' consent, electrode recording can provide sparse but critical data about the behavior of neurons during conscious perception or imagery (Kreiman, Fried, and Koch, 2002). It would be very valuable if cortical tissue in humans could be microstimulated appropriately with electrodes to generate specific percepts, thoughts, or actions (Fried et al., 1998).

Studying the dynamics of coalitions requires simultaneous recordings on a fast time scale from small groups of neurons in many places in the brain. This might be achieved in a primate with a relatively smooth cortex, such as the owl monkey. It would require recording simultaneously from a thousand or more electrodes, spaced about 1 mm apart, each capable of picking up single cells and the local field potential.

The immense amount of data this stratety would produce could be displayed visually on a two-dimensional map of the cortical surface, either speeded up or slowed down, so that the eye could grasp the nature of the traveling net-waves, as a preliminary to a more detailed study of them. The technical difficulties in recording from so many neurons at once in an alert animal are formidable but not insuperable. To develop the method, one could start with a smaller number of electrodes, more widely spaced, and work on one side of the brain of an animal with the corpus callosum cut. Thus, a judicious combination of molecular, electrophysiological, and imaging methods should ultimately help unravel the last main challenge to the scientific world view, how subjective mind arises out of objective matter.

ACKNOWLEDGMENTS We thank Patricia Churchland, David Eagleman, Gerald Edelman, Nikos Logothetis, Graeme Mitchison, Tomaso Poggio, Vilayanur Ramachandran, Antti Revonsuo, and John Reynolds for thoughtful comments, and Odile Crick for the drawing. This work was supported by the J. W. Kieckhefer Foundation, the W. M. Keck Foundation Fund for Discovery in Basic Medical Research at Caltech, the National Institute of Mental Health, National Institutes of Health, and the National Science Foundation.

NOTES

1. For example, is there some sort of hierarchy in the front? Are there somewhat separate streams of information, as there are in the visual system? Do the neurons in the front of cortex show columnar behavior; and if so, what for?

2. For an extensive bibliography, see Thomas Metzinger's home page at www.philosophie.uni-mainz.de/metzinger.

REFERENCES

ALLMAN, J., F. MIEZIN, and E. McGUINNESS, 1985. Stimulus specific responses from beyond the classical receptive field: Neurophysiological mechanisms for local-global comparisons in visual neurons. *Ann. Rev. Neurosci.* 8:407–430.

ATTNEAVE, F., 1961. In defense of homunculi. In *Sensory Communication*, W. A. Rosenblith, ed. New York: MIT Press and John Wiley, pp. 777–782.

BAARS, B. J., 1997. *In the Theater of Consciousness.* New York: Oxford University Press.

BACHMANN, T., 2000. *Microgenetic Approach to the Conscious Mind.* Amsterdam and Philadelphia: John Benjamins.

BATTELLI, L., P. CAVANAGH, J. INTRILIGATOR, M. J. TRAMO, M. A. HENAFF, F. MICHEL, and J. J. BARTON, 2001. Unilateral right parietal damage leads to bilateral deficit for high-level motion. *Neuron* 32:985–995.

BIEDERMAN, I., 1972. Perceiving real-world scenes. *Science* 177: 77–80.

BLAKE, R., and N. K. LOGOTHETIS, 2001. Visual competition. *Nat. Rev. Neurosci.* 3:13–21.

CHALMERS, D. J., 1995. *The Conscious Mind: In Search of a Fundamental Theory.* New York: Oxford University Press.

CHURCHLAND, P., 2002. *Brain-wise: Studies in Neurophilosophy.* Cambridge, Mass.: MIT Press.

CHANGEUX J.-P., 2004. *The Physiology of Truth: Neuroscience and Human Knowledge.* Cambridge, Mass.: Harvard University Press.

CRICK, F. C., and C. KOCH, 1990. Towards a neurobiological theory of consciousness. *Semin. Neurosci.* 2:263–275.

CRICK, F. C., and C. KOCH, 1995a. Why neuroscience may be able to explain consciousness. *Sci. Am.* 273:84–85.

CRICK, F. C., and C. KOCH, 1995b. Are we aware of neural activity in primary visual cortex? *Nature* 375:121–123.

CRICK, F. C., and C. KOCH, 1998a. Consciousness and neuroscience. *Cereb. Cortex* 8:97–107.

CRICK, F. C., and C. KOCH, 1998b. Constraints on cortical and thalamic projections: The no-strong-loops hypothesis. *Nature* 391:245–250.

CRICK, F. C., and C. KOCH, 2000. The unconscious homunculus. *NeuroPsychoanalysis* 2:3–11.

CRICK, F. C., and C. KOCH, 2003. A framework for consciousness. *Nat. Neurosci.* 6:119–127.

DACEY, D. M., B. B. PETERSON, F. R. RIBISON, and P. D. GAMLIN, 2003. Fireworks in the primate retina: *In vitro* photodynamics reveals diverse LGN-projecting ganglion cell types. *Neuron* 37: 15–27.

DE LIMA, A. D., T. VOIGT, and J. H. MORRISON, 1990. Morphology of the cells within the inferior temporal gyrus that project to the prefrontal cortex in the macaque monkey. *J. Comp. Neurol.* 296:159–172.

DEHAENE, S., and L. NACCACHE, 2001. Towards a cognitive neuroscience of consciousness: Basic evidence and a workspace framework. *Cognition* 79:1–37.

DENNETT, D. C., 1991. *Consciousness Explained.* Boston: Little, Brown.

DENNETT, D. C., 2001. Are we explaining consciousness yet? *Cognition* 79:221–237.

DESIMONE, R., and J. DUNCAN, 1995. Neural mechanisms of selective visual attention. *Annu. Rev. Neurosci.* 18:193–222.

EAGLEMAN, D. M., 2001. Visual illusions and neurobiology. *Nat. Rev. Neurosci.* 2:920–926.

EDELMAN, G. M., 1989. *The Remembered Present: A Biological Theory of Consciousness.* New York: Basic Books.

EDELMAN, G. M., and G. A. TONONI, 2000. *Universe of Consciousness.* New York: Basic Books.

FELLEMAN, D. J., and D. C. VAN ESSEN, 1991. Distributed hierarchical processing in the primate cerebral cortex. *Cereb. Cortex* 1: 1–47.

FFYTCHE, D. H., and R. J. HOWARD, 1999. The perceptual consequences of visual loss: "Positive" pathologies of vision. *Brain* 122:1247–1260.

FRIED, I., C. L. WILSON, K. A. MacDONALD, and E. J. BEHNKE, 1998. Electric current stimulates laughter. *Nature* 391: 650.

GRAZIANO, M. S., C. S. TAYLOR, and T. MOORE, 2002. Complex movements evoked by microstimulation of precentral cortex. *Neuron* 34:841–852.

HEBB, D., 1949. *The Organization of Behavior: A Neuropsychological Theory.* New York: John Wiley.

HESS, R. H., C. L. BAKER, Jr., and J. ZIHL, 1989. The "motion-blind" patient: Low-level spatial and temporal filters. *J. Neurosci.* 9:1628–1640.

HOCHSTEIN, S., and M. AHISSAR, 2002. View from the top: Hierarchies and reverse hierarchies in the visual system. *Neuron* 36:791–804.

JACKENDOFF, R., 1987. *Consciousness and the Computational Mind.* Cambridge, Mass.: MIT Press.

JACKENDOFF, R., 1996. How language helps us think. *Pragm. Cogn.* 4:1–34.

KOCH, C., 2004. *The Quest for Consciousness: A Neurobiological Approach.* Boulder, Colo.: Roberts.

KOCH, C., and F. C. CRICK, 2001. On the zombie within. *Nature* 411:893.

KREIMAN, G., I. FRIED, and C. KOCH, 2002. Single-neuron correlates of subjective vision in the human medial temporal lobe. *Proc. Natl. Acad. Sci. U.S.A.* 99:8378–8383.

LEHKY, S. R., and T. J. SEJNOWSKI, 1988. Network model of shape-from-shading: Neural function arises from both receptive and projective fields. *Nature* 333:452–454.

LEOPOLD, D. A., and N. K. LOGOTHETIS, 1999. Multistable phenomena: Changing views in perception. *Trends Cogn. Sci.* 3:254–264.

MILNER, D. A., and M. A. GOODALE, 1995. *The Visual Brain in Action.* Oxford, England: Oxford University Press.

MOUNTCASTLE, V. B., 1998. *Perceptual Neuroscience.* Cambridge, Mass.: Harvard University Press.

NEWSOME, W. T., and E. B. PARÉ, 1988. A selective impairment of motion perception following lesions of the middle temporal visual area (MT). *J. Neurosci.* 8:2201–2211.

POGGIO, T., V. TORRE, and C. KOCH, 1985. Computational vision and regularization theory. *Nature* 317:314–319.

PURVES, D., J. A. PAYDARFAR, and T. J. ANDREWS, 1996. The wagon wheel illusion in movies and reality. *Proc. Natl. Acad. Sci. U.S.A.* 93:3693–3697.

RENSINK, R. A., 2000. Seeing, sensing, and scrutinizing. *Vision Res.* 40:1469–1487.

REVONSUO, A., M. WILENIUS-EMET, J. KUUSELA, and M. LEHTO, 1997. The neural generation of a unified illusion in human vision. *Neuroreport* 8:3867–3870.

ROSSETTI, Y., 1998. Implicit short-lived motor representations of space in brain damaged and healthy subjects. *Conscious. Cogn.* 7:520–558.

SACKS, O., 1970. *Migraine.* Berkeley, Calif.: University of California Press.

SACKS, O., 2004. In the river of consciousness. *New York Review of Books* 51: January 15.

SALINAS, E., and T. J. SEJNOWSKI, 2001. Correlated neuronal activity and the flow of neural information. *Nat. Rev. Neurosci.* 2:539–550.

SCHACTER, D. L., 1992. Priming and multiple memory systems: Perceptual mechanisms of implicit memory. *J. Cogn. Neurosci.* 4:255–256.

SHADLEN, M. N., and J. A. MOVSHON, 1999. Synchrony unbound: A critical evaluation of the temporal binding hypothesis. *Neuron* 24:67–77, 111–125.

SHEAR, J., 1997. *Explaining Consciousness: The Hard problem.* Cambridge, Mass.: MIT Press.

SHEINBERG, D. L., and N. K. LOGOTHETIS, 1997. The role of temporal cortical areas in perceptual organization. *Proc. Natl. Acad. Sci. U.S.A.* 94:3408–3413.

SHERMAN, S. M., and R. GUILLERY, 2001. *Exploring the Thalamus.* San Diego, Calif.: Academic Press.

SINGER, W., and C. M. GRAY, 1995. Visual feature integration and the temporal correlation hypothesis. *Ann. Rev. Neurosci.* 18:555–586.

STROUD, J. M., 1955. The fine structure of psychological time. In *Information Theory in Psychology*, H. Quastler, ed. Glencoe, Ill.: Free Press, pp. 174–207.

VANRULLEN, R., and C. KOCH, 2003. Is perception discrete or continuous? *Trends Cogn. Sci.* 7:207–213.

VANRULLEN, R., L. REDDY, and C. KOCH, 2004. Visual search and dual tasks reveal two distinct attentional resources. *J. Cogn. Neurosci.* 16:1–11.

VANRULLEN, R., and S. J. THORPE, 2001. The time course of visual processing: From early perception to decision-making. *J. Cogn. Neurosci.* 13:454–461.

VARELA, F. J., A. TORO, E. R. JOHN, and E. L. SCHWARTZ, 1981. Perceptual framing and cortical alpha rhythm. *Neuropsychologia* 19:675–686.

WOLFE, J. M., and S. C. BENNETT, 1997. Preattentive object files: Shapeless bundles of basic features. *Vision Res.* 37:25–43.

ZEKI, S. M., 1998. Parallel processing, asynchronous perception, and a distributed system of consciousness in vision. *Neuroscientist* 4:365–372.

ZEKI, S., and A. BARTELS, 1999. Toward a theory of visual consciousness. *Conscious. Cogn.* 8:225–259.

ZIHL, J., D. VON CRAMON, and N. MAI, 1983. Selective disturbance of movement vision after bilateral brain damage. *Brain* 106: 313–340.

82 Neural Mechanisms for Access to Consciousness

STANISLAS DEHAENE AND JEAN-PIERRE CHANGEUX

ABSTRACT What cerebral events occur when a piece of information, such as an image or a word, crosses the threshold of consciousness and becomes available for conscious report? We postulate that a sensory stimulus becomes reportable when its neural representation in posterior areas is amplified and made available, via long-distance neural connections, to multiple distant sites. Neuronal simulations of this conscious neuronal workspace model suggest that a dynamical phase transition, corresponding to the sudden, all-or-none "ignition" of a large-scale reverberating and self-sustained assembly, underlies the threshold of consciousness. Below this threshold, fast propagation of sensory information remains possible, but without global ignition. This view thus predicts that subliminal processing can be extensive, but remains confined to specialized processors. We confront the model to a variety of behavioral, neurophysiological, and neuroimaging data, particularly from masked priming and attentional blink paradigms, and emphasize the important role of spontaneous, prestimulus fluctuations in top-down activity as a modulator of conscious access.

The challenge of a science of consciousness

Understanding consciousness has become the ultimate intellectual challenge of the new millennium. Even if philosophers now accept the notion that it is a "real, natural, biological phenomenon literally located in the brain" (Revonsuo, 2001), a view in harmony with the neuroscientists' conception that "consciousness is entirely caused by neurobiological processes and realized in brain structures" (Changeux, 1983; Edelman, 1989; Crick, 1994), the real issue becomes how to elaborate a science of consciousness.

This challenging problem raises two questions. The first is how to empirically define experimental paradigms in order to delineate a relevant and ultimately causal relationship between subjective phenomena and objective measurements of neural activity. Cognitive psychologists have now defined a variety of minimal experimental protocols that allow a fair comparison between conscious and nonconscious processing

of information (see Baars, 1989). Moreover, brain imaging and electroencephalographic (EEG) methods in humans and monkeys, as well as electrophysiological recordings at the single-cell level in awake monkeys, provide access to reliable neural correlates of conscious versus nonconscious perceptual processes (see Lamme, 2003). In this chapter, we will restrict the discussion to experimental research on the subliminal processing of visual stimuli under masking and attentional blink paradigms.

The second question is more conceptual. Given the broad diversity of methods required to evaluate neural activity and the extreme, often unresolved complexity of the neuronal architectures involved, it seems risky to draw conclusions simply on the basis of intuitive reasoning. In our opinion, in the present state of affairs, a theoretical framework appears necessary for an in-depth understanding of conscious phenomena. Such a framework will, for instance, consist in formal models, expressed in terms of neuronal networks, that link together the molecular, neuronal, behavioral, and subjective data in a coherent and noncontradictory though minimal form (Changeux and Dehaene, 1989). Such "bridging laws" implemented as formal automata should simultaneously account for the available data and produce experimentally testable predictions at all of those levels. Being minimal, they are not anticipated to give an exhaustive description of reality, but, even if they are wrong, they may give rise to novel theories and as such contribute to the progress of knowledge.

The context of consciousness is so broad and diverse and the issues are often so muddled (see Chalmers, this volume) that we deliberately limit ourselves here to only one aspect of consciousness, the notion of conscious access. This is the observation that a piece of information, once conscious, becomes broadly available for multiple processes, including action planning, voluntary redirection of attention, memory, evaluation, and verbal or nonverbal report. Like others (Weiskrantz, 1997), we emphasize reportability as a key property of conscious representations. This discussion will aim at characterizing the crucial differences between those aspects of neural activity that can be reported by a subject and those that cannot. According to some philosophers, this constitutes an "easy problem" and is irrelevant to the more

STANISLAS DEHAENE Department of Cognitive Neuroimaging, INSERM U562, CEA, Orsay, France.

JEAN-PIERRE CHANGEUX CNRS URA 2182, Récepteurs et Cognition, Institut Pasteur, Paris, France.

1145

central issues of phenomenality and self-awareness (e.g., Block, 1995). Our view, however, is that conscious access is one of the few empirically tractable problems presently accessible to an authentic scientific investigation. We further hope that an understanding of the neural processes that lead to overt report will eventually result in a theory of covert acts of self-report, and thus may ultimately contribute to an explanation of the nature of our private phenomenal world.

In this chapter, we will examine conscious access in the framework of an integrative theory based on the hypothesis of a conscious neuronal workspace (Dehaene, Kerszberg, and Changeux, 1998; Dehaene and Changeux, 2000; Dehaene and Naccache, 2001; Dehaene, Sergent, and Changeux, 2003). The model emphasizes the role of distributed neurons with long-distance connections, particularly dense in prefrontal, cingulate, and parietal regions, that are capable of interconnecting multiple specialized processors and can broadcast signals at the brain scale in a spontaneous and sudden manner. Those neurons form what is referred to here as a conscious *global neuronal workspace* (see Baars, 1989) that breaks the modularity of the nervous system and allows the broadcasting of information to multiple neural targets. This broadcasting creates a global availability that, according to our hypothesis, is experienced as consciousness and results in reportability. The discussion will include a direct comparison of presently available experimental data with the theory, and will stress novel predictions concerning the neural correlates of access consciousness.

At this stage, it may be worth noting a few basic distinctions. First, it is necessary to separate the notions of *state* of consciousness from *content* of consciousness. The English language distinguishes an intransitive meaning of consciousness (e.g., "The patient was still conscious") and a transitive meaning (e.g., "I was conscious *of* motion). The former refers to the state of consciousness, usually considered as a continuous variable (coma, sleep, drowsiness, awake state . . .). The latter refers to the temporary selection of a well-delimited content as the focus of conscious attention. The global neuronal workspace is essentially a theory of conscious content. It specifies the neural conditions under which a given representation is made potentially available to a broad variety of neural processes, thus giving rise to a subjective feeling of conscious access. A prerequisite, however, is that the neuronal workspace within which this global broadcasting occurs be available in an appropriate state of awakeness or readiness. We speculate that the graded states of consciousness correspond to different levels of spontaneous thalamocortical homeostatic regulation contributing to a "conscious milieu" that includes long-distance cortical neurons under the influence of ascending neuromodulatory inputs from, for instance, cholinergic, noradrenergic, or dopaminergic neurons from the basal forebrain and brain-

stem. In the last few years, considerable progress has been made in identifying the electrophysiological correlates of such global state changes, which are consistent with a graded modulation of thalamic and frontocingulate networks (Llinas et al., 1998; Paus, 2000). A detailed review of those findings is beyond the scope of our discussion, which will be limited to how specific content gains access to consciousness (see, however, Schiff, this volume).

The neuronal workspace hypothesis

The concept of a global neuronal workspace (Dehaene, Kerszberg, and Changeux, 1998; Dehaene and Naccache, 2001) is historically rooted in a long neuropsychological tradition, dating back to Hughlings Jackson and perpetuated by, among others, Baddeley, Shallice, Mesulam, and Posner, that emphasizes the hierarchical organization of the brain and separates lower automatized systems from increasingly higher and more autonomous supervisory executive systems. It also builds on Fodor's distinction between the vertical "modular faculties" and a distinct "isotropic central and horizontal system" capable of sharing information across modules. Finally, it relates to Baars's cognitive theory of consciousness, which distinguishes a vast array of unconscious specialized processors running in parallel and a single, limited-capacity, serial workspace that allows them to exchange information (Baars, 1989).

Baars, however, did not specify how the psychological construct of a conscious workspace could be implemented in terms of neuronal networks. By contrast, our views arose progressively from the design of computational neural network models that aimed at specifying the contribution of prefrontal cortex to increasingly higher cognitive tasks (Dehaene and Changeux, 1989, 1991, 1997; Dehaene, Kerszberg, and Changeux, 1998). We successively considered how a network could retain an active memory across a long delay (Dehaene and Changeux, 1989), how it could encode abstract rules that could be selected from external or internal rewards (Dehaene and Changeux, 1991), and finally, how networks based on those principles could pass complex planning tasks such as the Tower of London test or the Stroop test (Dehaene and Changeux, 1997; Dehaene, Kerszberg, and Changeux, 1998). The neuronal workspace model is the last development of the neuronal architectures that we proposed to address those specific problems.

Two Computational Spaces in the Brain   The neuronal workspace hypothesis distinguishes two computational spaces in the brain, each characterized by a distinct pattern of connectivity (figure 82.1).

1. *The network of processors*   Subcortical networks and most of the cortex can be viewed as a collection of specialized

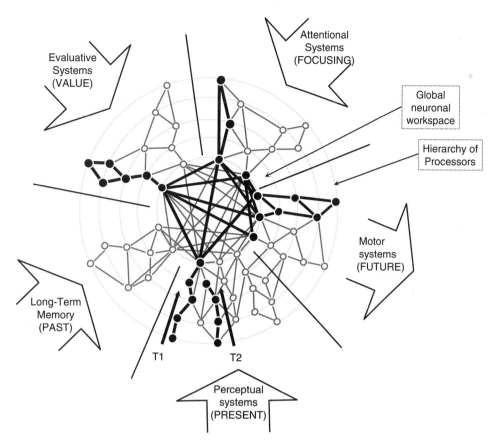

FIGURE 82.1 Schematic depiction of the workspace model. Cortical processors are shown in a state of activity in which a stimulus, T1, has gained access to the conscious workspace, while another stimulus, T2, is only processed nonconsciously up to a limited level. (Redrawn from Dehaene, Kerszberg, and Changeux, 1998.)

processors, each attuned to the processing of a particular type of information. Processors vary widely in complexity, from the elementary line segment detectors in area V1 or the motion processors in area MT to the visual word form processor in the human fusiform gyrus or the mirror neuron system in area F5. Despite this diversity, processors share characteristics of specialization, automaticity, and fast feedforward processing. Their function is made possible by a limited number of local or medium-range connections that bring to each processor the "encapsulated" inputs necessary to its function.

2. *The global neuronal workspace* We postulate the existence of a distinct set of cortical workspace neurons characterized by their ability to send and receive projections to many distant areas through long-range excitatory axons. These neurons therefore no longer obey a principle of local, encapsulated connectivity but rather break the modularity of the cortex by allowing many different processors to exchange information in a global and flexible manner. Information that is encoded in workspace neurons can quickly be made available to many brain systems, in particular the motor and speech-production processors for overt behavioral report.

We hypothesize that the entry of inputs into this global workspace constitutes the neural basis of access to consciousness.

TOP-DOWN AMPLIFICATION AND DYNAMIC MOBILIZATION Among the long-distance connections established by workspace neurons, top-down connections play an essential role in the temporary mobilization of a given content consciousness. Top-down attentional amplification is the mechanism by which modular processors can be temporarily mobilized and made available to the global workspace, and therefore enter consciousness. According to this view, the same brain processes may at different times contribute to the content of consciousness or not. To enter consciousness, it is not sufficient for a processor to be activated; this activity must also be amplified and maintained over a sufficient duration for it to become accessible to multiple other processes. Without such "dynamic mobilization," a process may still contribute to cognitive performance, but only nonconsciously.

A consequence of this hypothesis is the absence of a sharp anatomical delineation of the workspace representations. In time, the contours of the workspace fluctuate as different brain circuits are temporarily mobilized, then abandoned by a given global representation. Workspace neurons are present in many areas, but at any given time only a particular set of these neurons contributes to the mobilized workspace content. They are part of what may be referred to, in a selectionist framework, as a "generator of diversity" (Changeux and Dehaene, 1989). As time elapses, the activity of workspace neurons is characterized by a series of discrete episodes of spontaneous metastable coherent activation separated by sharp transitions. This would fit with the introspective feeling of a stream of consciousness, compared by William James to a sequence of flights and perchings of a bird.

CRITERIA FOR CONSCIOUS ACCESS   To be able to be mobilized in the conscious workspace, a mental object must meet three criteria:

1. *Active firing*   The object must be represented as a firing pattern of neurons. Of course, considerable information is stored in the nervous system in other latent forms, for instance in synaptic connections and weights, neurotransmitter release efficiencies, receptor densities, and so on. The model predicts that such information does not become conscious. It can only be read out very indirectly through its contribution to neural firing.

2. *Long-distance connectivity*   The active neurons must possess a sufficient number of reciprocal anatomical connections to distributed workspace neurons, particularly in prefrontal, parietal, and cingulate cortices. This criterion implies that the activity of many neurons, for instance in subcortical and brainstem nuclei, is excluded from conscious mobilization (e.g., circuits for respiration or emotion). In many cases we become aware of those circuits only through their indirect effects on other representations, such as in somatic cortical areas.

3. *Dynamic mobilization*   At any given moment, workspace neurons can only sustain a single global representation, the rest of workspace neurons being inhibited. This implies that, out of the multiple active cortical representations that could become conscious, only one will receive the appropriate top-down amplification and be mobilized into consciousness. The other representations are temporarily nonconscious. They might be called "preconscious" because it would take only a small reorientation of top-down signals to access them, but, according to our views, until this is achieved, they do not participate in consciousness.

CONSCIOUSNESS AND ATTENTION   Within the framework of the workspace model, the relations between attention and consciousness can be clarified as follows. Top-down attentional selection and amplification are necessary for a representation to become available to consciousness. Thus, subjects cannot become aware of any sensory stimulus unless either (1) they are already attending to the relevant cortical processors or (2) the stimulus itself attracts top-down atten-

tion. The latter is possible because some specialized cortical systems, such as the frontal eye fields, can operate quickly and subliminally (Thompson and Schall, 1999), with the result of reorienting attention and thus forcing a change in the contents of the workspace.

Thus, two modes of conscious access to sensory information should be distinguished: a top-down mode, in which workspace neurons become spontaneously activated and selectively amplify a possibly very small sensory signal, and a bottom-up mode in which initially unattended sensory signals carry sufficient strength to cause a reorienting of top-down amplification toward them.

According to this view, attention and consciousness cannot be equated, for two reasons. First, the orientation of visuospatial attention results from the operation of cortical processors that may operate under voluntary conscious control but also nonconsciously, as when attention is attracted by peripheral stimuli. Second, when attention is present, it may not always be sufficient for a stimulus to gain access to consciousness. In this situation, we expect attention to modulate the depth of subliminal processing, while still failing to make the stimuli conscious (Naccache, Blandin, and Dehaene, 2002, see below). These distinctions are outlined in figure 82.2.

WORKSPACE MODULATION AND SELECTION BY REWARD   Workspace neurons are assumed to be the targets of two different types of neuromodulatory inputs. First, workspace neurons display a constantly fluctuating spontaneous activity whose *intensity* is modulated by ascending activating systems, for instance from cholinergic, noradrenergic, and serotonergic nuclei in the brainstem, basal forebrain, and hypothalamus. Those systems therefore modify the *state* of consciousness through different levels of arousal. Second, the *stability* of workspace activity is modulated by ascending reward inputs arising from the limbic system (via connections to the anterior cingulate, orbitofrontal cortex, and the direct influence of ascending dopaminergic inputs). External or internal goals and rewards may thus stabilize or destabilize particular *contents* of the conscious workspace. Active representations that fit with the current goal of the organism are selected and maintained over a longer period. Conversely, active representations that lead to error are rejected. This "mental selection" process has been simulated in previous models that account for classical cognitive tasks such as the Wisconsin Card Sorting Test (Dehaene and Changeux, 1991), the Tower of London task (Dehaene and Changeux, 1997), and the Stroop task (Dehaene, Kerszberg, and Changeux, 1998).

BRAIN ANATOMY OF THE NEURONAL WORKSPACE   The neuronal workspace hypothesis posits that, as a whole, workspace neurons are reciprocally connected via long-distance axons to many if not all of the cortical processors, thus per-

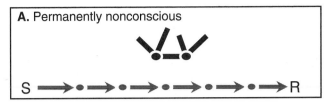

A. Permanently nonconscious

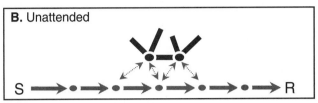

B. Unattended

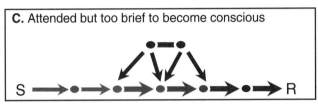

C. Attended but too brief to become conscious

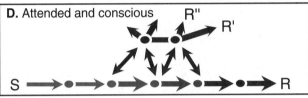

D. Attended and conscious

E. Top-down attention preceeding conscious access

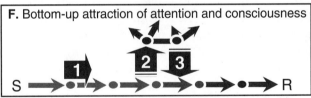

F. Bottom-up attraction of attention and consciousness

FIGURE 82.2 Types of interactions between an automatized stream of processors linking stimulus S and response R, and the workspace system. (*A–C*) Three types of nonconscious processing. In *A*, a processing chain is not connected to workspace neurons and therefore remains permanently inaccessible to consciousness. In *B*, a processing chain is connected reciprocally to workspace neurons but is temporarily not mobilized by top-down amplification. In *C*, the processing chain is attended and subliminal processing is amplified, yet activation is too brief to establish a bidirectional reverberating loop. (*D–F*) Conscious processing. In *D*, the loop is closed, allowing stimulus information to be held online and broadcasted to multiple systems R′, R″, and so on. *E* and *F* illustrate the two orders in which this conscious state can be achieved: a top-down mode (*E*), in which workspace neurons become spontaneously activated first, and selectively amplify a possibly very small sensory signal, and a bottom-up mode (*F*), in which initially unattended sensory signals carry sufficient strength to cause a reorienting of top-down amplification toward them.

mitting locally available information to be brought into consciousness. Nevertheless, these neurons may be more densely accumulated in some areas than in others. Anatomically, long-range corticocortical tangential connections, including callosal connections, originate mostly from the pyramidal cells of layers II and III, which give or receive the so-called "association" efferents and afferents. Those layers are thicker in von Economo's type 2 (dorsolateral prefrontal) and type 3 (inferior parietal) cortical structures. In the monkey, those areas are tightly interconnected together, as well as with the anterior and posterior cingulate, the association cortex of the superior temporal sulcus, and the parahippocampal region, thalamus, and striatum (Goldman-Rakic, 1988). The high concentration of neurons with long-distance axons in those areas may explain why they frequently appear coactivated in neuroimaging studies of conscious effortful processing.

Although we emphasize corticocortical connectivity, it should be noted that corticothalamic columns are the processing units in the brain and in our recent simulation (Dehaene, Sergent, and Changeux, 2003). Thus, connections between thalamic nuclei may also contribute to the establishment of a coherent brain-scale state (Llinas et al., 1998). Studies of split-brain patients should be particularly helpful in delineating the relative contribution of cortical and subcortical connections to workspace coherence.

Our model leads to the prediction that long-distance connections have been the target of a recent evolutionary pressure in the course of hominization and are particularly developed in our species. In that respect, it should be noted that the relative anatomical expansion of cortical areas rich in long-axon neurons, such as the prefrontal cortex, may have contributed to important changes in the functional properties of the workspace (see Changeux, 1983). It is also noteworthy that a particular type of spindle cell, one that establishes long-distance projections, is found in the anterior cingulate cortex of humans and great apes, but not in other primates (Allman et al., 2001). Detailed anatomical studies of transcortical connectivity in the human brain have also revealed the presence of distant transcortical projections that, for instance, link directly the right fusiform gyrus to multiple areas of the left hemisphere, including Broca's and Wernicke's areas (Di Virgilio and Clarke, 1997). It is anticipated that those key components of the verbal reportability system are connected to many cortical areas, given the variety of percepts and concepts that we can name or understand through language.

Comparison with data on subliminal processing of masked words

How can one experimentally test the model's distinction between the substrates of conscious access and the considerable amount of neural activity that can occur spontaneously and nonconsciously within the specialized processors? Our approach has consisted in exploring paradigms in which sensory information is deliberately presented under subliminal conditions. By studying to what extent such information is processed, and what brain areas it contacts, one can progressively draw a negative picture, as it were, of which aspects of brain activity do not suffice to give rise to consciousness. Conversely, one may then ask which particular processes are associated with the crossing of the threshold for consciousness. Here we briefly review those empirical findings and subsequently examine how they fit with the global neuronal workspace theory.

NEUROIMAGING OF SUBLIMINAL WORD PROCESSING In a classic psychological paradigm, the pattern masking of visual words, a word is flashed on a computer screen for a duration of less than 50 ms. If the word is presented alone, it typically remains readable with some effort. However, when the same word is preceded and followed by random geometric shapes or letters at the same retinal location, it may become totally inaccessible to consciousness. In spite of this invisibility, behavioral priming experiments have repeatedly indicated that masked words are processed nonconsciously at orthographic, phonological, and possibly semantic levels (see, e.g., Forster and Davis, 1984; Greenwald, Draine, and Abrams, 1996; Neely and Kahan, 2001).

To identify the brain systems activated by masked words, functional imaging has been combined with masked priming (Dehaene, Naccache, et al., 1998; Dehaene et al., 2001, 2004; Naccache and Dehaene, 2001a). On each trial, a fast sequence comprising a mask, a prime word, another mask, and a target was flashed on screen. Functional magnetic resonance imaging (fMRI) is currently too slow to separate the cerebral activity induced by the prime and by the target. Thus, one necessarily measures the total activity induced by the prime-target pair (relative, say, to a control situation in which only the masks are presented). In spite of this limitation, we can still acquire knowledge of the processing of the prime by varying the type of relation between the prime and target. When the prime and the target are the same word, there is a measurable benefit in both response times and brain activation levels compared to a situation in which the prime and the target are different words. Measuring where this subliminal repetition effect occurs provides an indirect image of the brain areas that have been traversed by the hidden prime word. This can be supplemented by recordings of event-related potentials (ERPs) which have an appropriate temporal resolution to follow the dynamics of prime- and target-induced activations.

Using this method, several cortical stages of word processing have been shown to be activated by subliminal words (figure 82.3):

Early visual activity Extrastriate visual areas reduce their activation in the subliminal repetition priming paradigm, but only if the prime and target words are repeated in the same case and font (Dehaene et al., 2001). Those areas are therefore thought to extract small features of the letter shapes.

Visual word recognition Subliminal repetition priming has a major effect on the activation of a subarea of the left fusiform gyrus, termed the *visual word form area* (Cohen et al., 2000). Contrary to occipital extrastriate cortex, the fusiform visual word form area reduces its activation even when a word is repeated twice in a different case (e.g., prime = RADIO, target = radio). This suggests that a case-independent representation of letter strings can be accessed nonconsciously (Dehaene et al., 2001). By using words made of letters whose upper- and lowercase shapes are arbitrarily related (e.g., A/a, G/g), we have demonstrated that this representation comprises culturally specific information laid down in the course of learning to read (Dehaene et al., 2004).

Subliminal binding The binding of letters in a coherent word is required for reading, because different words can be made up of the same letters. Can such binding occur nonconsciously? We addressed this question by preceding a target word by either a repetition of itself or by an anagram made of the same letters in a different order (Dehaene et al., 2004). In response times, repetition priming occurred for words but not for anagrams, indicating that precise information about the configuration of letters was extracted unconsciously. Furthermore, fMRI separated a posterior fusiform region, sensitive only to the component letters, from a more anterior region that began to be sensitive to letter combinations. Thus, the evidence suggests that the binding of letters into larger units is independent of consciousness, and that an organized structural representation of a word can be constructed in the absence of consciousness.

Semantic access The issue of semantic access from subliminal masked words remains controversial in psychology. Nevertheless, positive evidence for subliminal semantic access was obtained using a small set of high-frequency words with simple semantics: number words. When subjects were engaged in a number comparison task, their responses were accelerated when the prime and the target represented the same quantity, possibly in different notations (e.g., prime = NINE, target = 9) (Dehaene, Naccache, et al., 1998; Koechlin et al., 1999). In this paradigm, fMRI showed "quantity priming" in a bilateral intraparietal region thought to be involved in the semantic representation and manipulation of numerical quantities (Naccache and Dehaene, 2001a).

Motor activation Masked words and digits have a measurable influence down to the motor preparation level. In the number comparison task, where subjects classified targets as

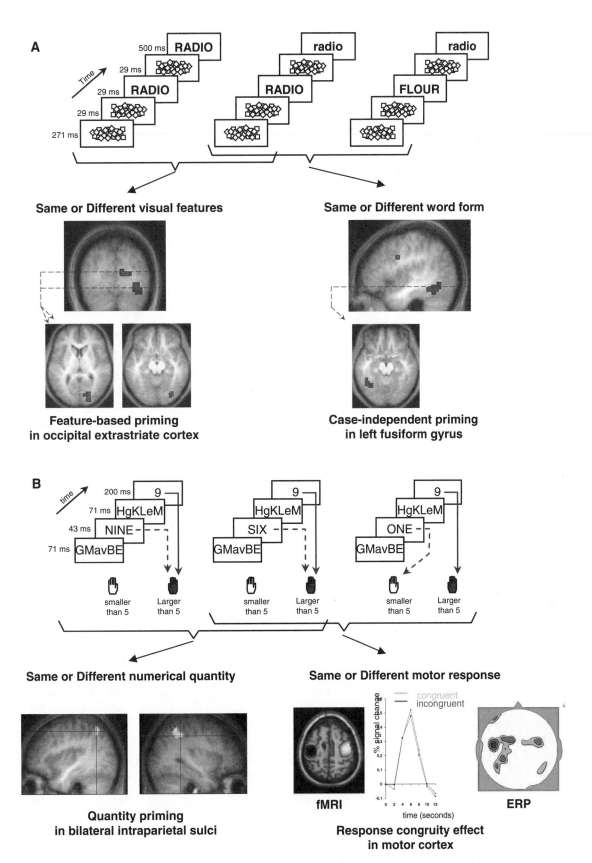

FIGURE 82.3 Main paradigms used in neuroimaging studies of subliminal priming. (*A*) Word repetition paradigm, in which a word prime is flashed for 29 ms, hidden by forward and backward masking shapes (Dehaene et al., 2001, 2004). Repetition of the same physical stimulus as prime and target leads to feature-based priming in occipital cortex, while cross-case word repetition leads to case-independent priming in the left fusiform visual word form area. (*B*) Number comparison paradigm, in which a numerical prime is flashed for 43 ms, hidden by forward and backward letter strings (Dehaene, Naccache et al., 1998; Naccache and Dehaene, 2001a, 2001b; Naccache, Blandin, and Dehaene, 2002). Repeating the same quantity as prime and target leads to quantity-based priming in the left and right intraparietal sulci; repeating the same motor response leads to response priming in the left and right motor cortex. Together, these results indicate that a subliminal prime can proceed through an entire series of visual, semantic, and motor stages without entering consciousness. (See color plate 70.)

larger or smaller than 5 using their left or right hand, the numerical primes could also be larger or small than 5, and thus they could induce a motor response congruent or incongruent with the subsequent target. This response congruity factor interfered with subjects' response times and yielded a response conflict in motor cortex that was measurable in both ERPs and fMRI (Dehaene, Naccache, et al., 1998).

In brief, an entire series of processing stages, highly attuned to the processing of words at the perceptual, semantic, and even the motor level, can be successively activated in a feedforward manner by a subliminal prime. These findings agree with a major tenet of the neuronal workspace theory, the existence of a broad set of distributed specialized processors that, most of the time, process information nonconsciously. Furthermore, examination of the effects of attention on subliminal processing reveals a remarkable dissociation between attention and conscious access. All of the above priming experiments allowed subjects to deploy attention to the target. We recently showed that when the prime-target pair occurs at an unpredictable moment, thus preventing the deployment of temporal attention, then subliminal priming effects disappear (Naccache, Blandin, and Dehaene, 2002). Thus, the idea that subliminal priming reflects a purely passive process of spreading activation can be rejected. Rather, subliminal primes benefit from an attentional amplification, although this is not sufficient from them to enter awareness. Those data imply that subliminal primes are actively processed along consciously prepared routes.

Nevertheless, subliminal processing is not as flexible as conscious processing. As assumed by the neuronal workspace model, functions that depend on central executive control, such as inhibition or conflict detection, appear to require consciousness. When asked to inhibit the dominant strategy of naming the prime words, subjects are unable to comply with this instruction unless the words are consciously accessed (Debner and Jacoby, 1994). Similarly, we contrasted the motor conflict effects generated by subliminal and supraliminal numerical primes (Dehaene et al., 2004). The anterior cingulate showed a conflict effect only with supraliminal primes, not with subliminal primes. Furthermore, schizophrenic subjects with known anterior cingulate pathology showed normal subliminal priming but abnormal supraliminal motor interference. These results indirectly suggest that executive control processes associated with prefrontal and cingulate cortices can operate only on consciously perceived stimuli.

PHYSIOLOGICAL CORRELATES OF NONCONSCIOUS AND CONSCIOUS PROCESSING   The masking paradigm also provides a more direct way of identifying the changes in brain activity that distinguish subliminal and conscious situations. A simple experiment consists in measuring the fMRI or ERP correlates of brain activity evoked by masked or unmasked words,

relative to word-absent trials, under conditions that are as comparable as possible in every other respect (Dehaene et al., 2001). This method looks at the brain activation caused by masked words directly, rather than indirectly, through their priming effects on subsequent words. Using this design, we found that the masked words caused a small, transient, bottom-up activation that was increasingly smaller as one moved from extrastriate cortex to fusiform gyrus and precentral cortex. When the words were unmasked, activation greatly increased in the same areas, but also extended to a distributed network that included distant parietal, inferior prefrontal, and midline precentral/cingulate cortices. Unmasking also enhanced the long-distance correlation between those sites and, in ERP recordings, was associated with an enhanced late positive complex (P300) that was absent or greatly reduced in the masked situation.

Electrophysiologial studies of masking in awake monkeys converge adequately with the research in humans. Lamme, Zipser, and Spekreijse (2002) recorded from V1 neurons while monkeys reported the presence or absence of a visual stimulus with variable degrees of masking. They observed a first peak of neural firing shortly after visual stimulation (~60 ms after stimulus onset). This peak remained unchanged and equally selective for stimulus orientation whether the stimulus was reportable or not, indicating subliminal processing of orientation in V1. However, a second peak of moderate amplification of firing rate (~90–150 ms after stimulus onset) was seen only when the stimulus was reportable. According to Lamme and colleagues (2002), the first period may reflect bottom-up propagation of activation, while the second would reflect top-down signals arising from higher cortical areas. Analogous results were obtained from recordings in monkey inferotemporal cortex (Kovacs, Vogels, and Orban, 1995; Rolls, Tovee, and Panzeri, 1999) and frontal eye field (Thompson and Schall, 1999): a first firing peak (~80 ms after stimulus onset) was left unchanged or only slightly reduced by masking, and the cells maintained their stimulus selectivity, but masking drastically interrupted a later phase of firing starting about 100 ms after the stimulus.

In summary, the following findings fit with the postulates of the neuronal workspace model. First, the same cortical area, such as the left fusiform gyrus, can participate in both subliminal and conscious streams of processing. Second, conscious processing is associated with an amplification of late perceptual activity and its functional correlation with distant parietal, prefrontal, and cingulate sites. Third, consciousness allows the deployment of executive control processes; those seem to be among the few processes that cannot be deployed subliminally.

ALL-OR-NONE DYNAMICS OF WORKSPACE ACTIVITY: COMPARISON OF SUBJECTIVE REPORT AND OBJECTIVE MEASUREMENTS   The neuronal workspace model states that the distinct

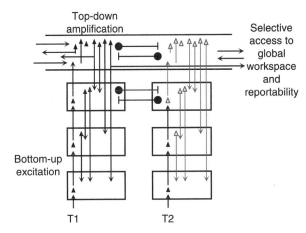

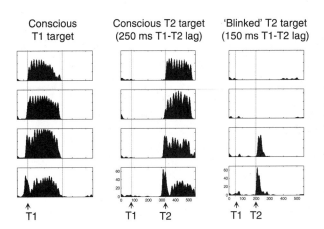

FIGURE 82.4 Anatomical connectivity (left) and functional states of activity (right) in a recent simulation of a subset of the proposed workspace system (for details, see Dehaene, Sergent, and Changeux, 2003). Two hierarchies of pyramidal neurons code for two input stimuli, T1 and T2, at successively higher levels. Higher-level workspace neurons send long-distance axons in a top-down manner all the way down to the earliest cortical area, as well as to many other workspace areas (reportability). At the higher level, cortical representations of T1 and T2 also inhibit each other via inhibitory interneurons. Simulated peristimulus time histograms (right) illustrate that a very brief presentation (40 ms) of either T1 or T2 leads to an initial bottom-up activation through the hierarchy, then a top-down amplification in the reverse direction, finally resulting in a longlasting self-sustained state of coherent activity. When T2 is presented within a short period after T1, however, such "ignition" fails to occur, and only the first stages of bottom-up propagation are seen. This is proposed to constitute the neural basis of the attentional blink.

anatomical connectivity of workspace neurons leads to qualitatively distinct patterns of activity. Because of their global recurrent connectivity, workspace neurons have the capacity of "igniting" suddenly in a self-amplifying manner as soon as a minimum subset of them is activated. At any given moment, the state of activity of workspace is therefore characterized by the intense activation of a subset of workspace neurons, the rest of workspace neurons being actively inhibited. This particular set of active workspace neurons may be viewed as a neuronal correlate of the content of consciousness. For instance, the conscious report of a word might be constituted by the simultaneous, coordinated activation of workspace neurons in a specific processor (the fusiform visual word form area) and in distributed temporal, parietal, prefrontal, and cingulate sites associated with speech production.

Because the entire workspace is globally interconnected, only one such workspace representation can be active at any given time. This property distinguishes it from peripheral processors in which, due to local patterns of connections, several representations with different formats may coexist. Furthermore, the reciprocal excitatory connectivity between workspace neurons imposes a self-amplification of activity that creates a dynamic threshold. Neural activity either is sufficient to trigger a reverberating loop of bottom-up and top-down activity, which quickly amplifies it to a high and self-sustained level, or it remains below this threshold (i.e., "subliminal"), and only a briefly decaying bottom-up activity is seen. Thus, access to the workspace is *all-or-none* and *exclusive* of other representations.

Recently, those nonlinear properties were explicitly demonstrated in a detailed simulation of realistic thalamocortical networks (Dehaene, Sergent, and Changeux, 2003; figure 82.4). The simulations show that a brief thalamic stimulation, T1, could lead to the ignition of a large set of distant cortical areas, which remain active by self-sustaining reverberatory loops for tens of milliseconds beyond the initial stimulus duration. This observation establishes a clear link between the content of working memory and of consciousness and may explain why the maintenance of active information over a short delay is feasible only when the information is conscious.

Crucially, during this period of workspace occupancy by stimulus T1, another stimulus, T2, could still be processed by peripheral thalamocortical processors, but often could not activate workspace neurons until the representation of T1 had vanished. This temporary inability showed many parallels with the "attentional blink," a well-known psychological paradigm in which subjects are temporarily unable to report stimuli while they are attending to another task (Chun and Potter, 1995; Vogel, Luck, and Shapiro, 1998).

An original property of the model is the prediction of a dynamic all-or-none bifurcation in neuronal activity. Across simulated trials, depending on random fluctuations in spontaneous activity prior to stimulus arrival, ascending activity could be sufficient to trigger self-amplifying recurrent activity, or it remained below threshold and only transient bottom-up activity was seen. Thus, for a fixed T1–T2 lag, simulated firing rates in higher areas and other indices of global activity (gamma-band power, long-distance cross-correlation) were found to be distributed bimodally across trials—either global and longlasting, or local and very short-lived.

The neuronal workspace model therefore predicts that the apparent gradual drop in reportability observed during the attentional blink may be an artificial consequence of averaging across trials with full access awareness and others with no awareness. We tested this prediction experimentally using a modified attentional blink paradigm in which subjects reported to what extent they had seen a word (T2) within a rapid letter stream that contained another target letter string (T1) (Dehaene, Sergent, and Changeux, 2003; Sergent and Dehaene, in press). To obtain a continuous measure of subjective perception, we asked subjects to move a cursor on a continuous scale, from "not seen" on the left to "maximal visibility" on the right. The results indicated that subjective perception during the blink is indeed all-or-none. At the peak of the blink, which occurred approximately 260 ms after T1, the very same stimulus T2 was either fully perceived (cursor placed on "maximal visibility"; ~50% of trials), or totally unseen (cursor placed on "not seen"). Participants almost never used intermediate cursor positions, although controls showed that they were able to in other psychophysical situations. This experiment substantiates the hypothesis that conscious states are associated with a fast all-or-none dynamic phase transition in a large-scale neuronal network. More generally, the concept of a sudden "ignition," self-amplified by recurrent top-down/bottom-up interaction, may begin to explain the very notion of a threshold or "limen" of consciousness.

SPONTANEOUS FLUCTUATIONS AND PRECURSORS OF CONSCIOUS ACCESS   What causes the same target T2 to be occasionally perceived or not perceived? In our simulation, thalamic and cortical neurons are permanently subject to spontaneous oscillations, even prior to stimulus presentation. When intrinsic fluctuations are in phase with stimulus presentation, bottom-up activation is enhanced. This coincidence has a cascading effect on subsequent areas and eventually affects the probability of the entire network falling into a global active state. Thus, the resonance of incoming stimuli with spontaneous brain activity is essential for perception. Simulations show that access to consciousness can be partially predicted by random fluctuations in the size of the initial T2-induced bottom-up peak in early areas, or even by the amount of depolarization of T2 neurons 100–200 ms prior to stimulus presentation.

Those observations may shed some light on a recent controversy concerning the earliest correlates of consciousness during visual perception. Many experiments indicate that conscious perception, when contrasted to a nonconscious control, is associated with a sudden increase in parietofrontocingulate activity, in agreement with the predictions of the neuronal workspace model (e.g., Lumer and Rees, 1999;

Beck et al., 2001; Dehaene et al., 2001). However, some studies have also found early differences within occipital cortex. For instance, Pins and ffytche (2003) sorted out trials as a function of whether the same near-threshold grating was or was not reported by human subjects. Using ERPs, they observed an early difference difference, about 100 ms after stimulus onset, that was traced back by fMRI-seeded dipole analysis to area V1 or to the surrounding occipital pole. They also found a later (~260 ms) difference in parietal and frontal regions. Pins and ffytche claimed that the early effect was a "primary correlate of conscious perception," and that the later differences were secondary and reflected contingent processes of attention and report made possible by the first step.

Our model leads to the exactly opposite claim. In our simulation, although conscious access is *defined* by coherent longlasting activity in higher cortical areas, an early difference between seen and unseen trials is present even before this state is attained. This clearly illustrates that this early difference is an indirect consequence of selective averaging over a fluctuating baseline. Likewise, we suggest that the early difference in V1 activation seen by Pins and ffytche (2003) is only a (modest) predictor of subsequent target reportability and does not, in and of itself, constitute the neuronal basis of a conscious state.

According to our view, some neural changes may show statistically significant correlations with the subsequent presence or absence of consciousness, without, however, participating in a *state* of consciousness. This distinction becomes clearer when such correlations are found even before the stimulus is presented. For instance, Super and colleagues (2003) found that changes in the firing rate of V1 neurons 100 ms prior to stimulus presentation partially predicted whether a stimulus would or would not be reported by a macaque monkey. How could the monkey possibly have a conscious state of a target prior to its presentation? The only reasonable interpretation, and one adopted by Super and colleagues (2003), is that the prestimulus differences do not directly indicate access to consciousness but merely a state of attentive readiness that makes it more likely for a subsequent stimulus to become conscious. We suggest that a similar interpretation explains the finding of Pins and ffytche (2003).

In summary, it is not sufficient to merely observe neural *correlates* of consciousness. Ultimately, what is needed is a direct, causal, and contemporaneous link between neuronal activity and conscious perception. Early ventral visual activity, by itself, fails to elicit consciousness because it still occurs in an unchanged form during extinction of visual stimuli in patients with parietal neglect (Vuilleumier et al., 2002). Like us, Vuilleumier and colleagues emphasize that sensory activity alone is not sufficient, and that functional interactions between parietal, frontal, and sensory areas appear necessary for access to consciousness.

Conclusion

It is encouraging that there is increasing empirical and theoretical agreement about the essential ingredients for a theory of consciousness. The proposed neuronal workspace theory can be seen as a physiological implementation of concepts of a central executive, supervisory attentional, or self-regulation system (e.g., Norman and Shallice, 1980; Posner and Rothbart, 1998) that accesses and modulates lower-level processors. At the neuronal network level, a key role is given to connections with the prefrontal cortex, in agreement with the early insights of Bianchi (1922) and with Crick and Koch (1995). Finally, the concept of reverberatory, recurrent or reentrant projections in perceptual awareness has been abundantly mentioned in the past (Changeux, 1983; Edelman, 1993; Di Lollo, Enns, and Rensink, 2000; Lamme and Roelfsema, 2000).

Given this broad convergence, it appears even more critical to keep the theoretical differences among various models clear, to the benefit of decisive experimental tests. First, the present theory departs from other approaches that view the "dynamic core" of consciousness as eminently variable and not directly related to a special subset of neurons (Edelman, 1989; Tononi and Edelman, 1998). On the opposite side, Herbert Jasper has insisted for years that "an anatomically and electrophysiologically separate neuronal system is involved in brain mechanisms of consciousness" (Jasper, 1998). Consistent with Jasper's views, we emphasize that most cerebral processes are nonconscious, and that the neural mechanisms of access to consciousness involve a specific subset of neurons that can be delineated by minimal contrasts between subliminal and supraliminal stimuli.

Second, our theory is not compatible with the statements that prefrontal regions function as an "unconscious homunculus" (Crick and Koch, 2003), that area V1 would not be mobilized by conscious processing (Crick and Koch, 1995), and that strong recurrent loops are avoided in the cortex (Crick and Koch, 1998). On the contrary, we think that prefrontal regions densely contribute to workspace neurons and that their activity usually betrays conscious processing. Moreover, we emphasize that almost all cortical processors (including area V1) can be mobilized into the workspace through joint bottom-up and top-down excitatory links. During fine-grained visual imagery, for instance, our theory predicts that there should be top-down mobilization of V1 neurons and long-distance correlations with prefrontal cortex neurons, and that interference with V1 activity, for instance with transcranial magnetic stimulation, should disrupt the conscious mental image.

Finally, our theory contrasts with the view that consciousness precedes attention (Lamme, 2003). We do not think that a form of "phenomenal consciousness" can be attributed to preattentive contents that cannot be reported (Block, 2001), and that inattentional blindness phenomena such as the attentional blink reflect "brief consciousness followed by amnesia" (Lamme, 2003). Rather, we propose that masked or blinked stimuli never lead to a strong activation of workspace neurons in the first place and thus are simply nonconscious.

The neuronal workspace model proposes that the neural basis of conscious access is a sudden self-amplifying bifurcation leading to a global, brain-scale pattern of activity. We now underline several critical predictions of this view. First, when a stimulus is presented above threshold, we predict that following an initial period of subliminal perceptual processing lasting approximately 100–200 ms, there is a sudden nonlinear transition toward a temporarily metastable state of globally increased brain activity lasting approximately 200–300 ms. This sudden increase should be particularly evident in prefrontal, cingulate, and parietal cortices. It should be accompanied by a synchronous amplification of posterior perceptual activation and by thalamocortical brain-scale synchrony in the gamma range (20–100 Hz). Finer-scale electrophysiological or optical recordings should demonstrate that this state is selective to a subset of neurons coding for the stimulus and is accompanied in higher areas by broad inhibition of neurons cording for other stimuli. Even higher resolution experiments may reveal a layer-specific distribution of active workspace neurons, with intense top-down activity originating from a subpopulation of cells with long axons in supra- and infragranular layers of prefrontal, cingulate, and parietal cortices. The model also predicts that, when presented with a stimulus at threshold, workspace neurons respond in an all-or-none manner, either highly activated or totally inactivated. This all-or-none character should be detectable macroscopically as a bimodal distribution of parameters such as the P300 component of ERPs. Finally, pharmacological interventions or lesions that affect top-down connections or inhibitory interactions in higher cortical areas should alter the dynamics of workspace ignition, and therefore should modify subjective perception in a predictable manner, while possibly leaving subliminal bottom-up processing unaffected (e.g., Granon, Faure, and Changeux, 2003). Through predictions such as these, the road is now paved for a neuroscientific approach to consciousness.

REFERENCES

ALLMAN, J. M., A. HAKEEM, J. M. ERWIN, E. NIMCHINSKY, and P. HOF, 2001. The anterior cingulate cortex: The evolution of an interface between emotion and cognition. *Ann. N.Y. Acad. Sci.* 935:107–117.

BAARS, B. J., 1989. *A Cognitive Theory of Consciousness.* Cambridge, England: Cambridge University Press.

BECK, D. M., G. REES, C. D. FRITH, and N. LAVIE, 2001. Neural correlates of change detection and change blindness. *Nat. Neurosci.* 4:645–650.

BIANCHI, L., 1922. *The mechanism of the Brain and the Functions of the Frontal Lobes*. New York: W. Wood.

BLOCK, N., 1995. On a confusion about a function of consciousness. *Behav. Brain Sci.* 18(2):227–287.

BLOCK, N., 2001. Paradox and cross purposes in recent work on consciousness. *Cognition* 79:197–219.

CHANGEUX, J. P., 1983. *L'homme neuronal*. Paris: Fayard.

CHANGEUX, J. P., and S. DEHAENE, 1989. Neuronal models of cognitive functions. *Cognition* 33:63–109.

CHUN, M. M., and M. C. POTTER, 1995. A two-stage model for multiple target detection in rapid serial visual presentation. *J. Exp. Psychol. Hum. Percept. Perform.* 21:109–127.

COHEN, L., S. DEHAENE, L. NACCACHE, S. LEHÉRICY, G. DEHAENE-LAMBERTZ, M. A. HÉNAFF, et al., 2000. The visual word form area: Spatial and temporal characterization of an initial stage of reading in normal subjects and posterior split-brain patients. *Brain* 123:291–307.

CRICK, F., 1994. *The Astonishing Hypothesis: The Scientific Search for the Soul*. New York: Charles Scribner's Sons.

CRICK, F., and C. KOCH, 1995. Are we aware of neural activity in primary visual cortex? *Nature* 375:121–123.

CRICK, F., and C. KOCH, 1998. Constraints on cortical and thalamic projections: The no-strong-loops hypothesis. *Nature* 391: 245–250.

CRICK, F., and C. KOCH, 2003. A framework for consciousness. *Nat. Neurosci.* 6:119–126.

DEBNER, J. A., and L. L. JACOBY, 1994. Unconscious perception: Attention, awareness, and control. *J. Exp. Psychol. Learn. Mem. Cogn.* 20:304–317.

DEHAENE, S., E. ARTIGES, L. NACCACHE, A. VIARD, and J. L. MARTINOT, 2004. *Conscious and subliminal conflicts in normal and schizophrenic subjects: The role of the anterior cingulate*. Unpublished manuscript.

DEHAENE, S., and J. P. CHANGEUX, 1989. A simple model of prefrontal cortex function in delayed-response tasks. *J. Cogn. Neurosci.* 1:244–261.

DEHAENE, S., and J. P. CHANGEUX, 1991. The Wisconsin Card Sorting Test: Theoretical analysis and modelling in a neuronal network. *Cereb. Cortex* 1:62–79.

DEHAENE, S., and J. P. CHANGEUX, 1997. A hierarchical neuronal network for planning behavior. *Proc. Natl. Acad. Sci. U.S.A.* 94: 13293–13298.

DEHAENE, S., and J. P. CHANGEUX, 2000. Reward-dependent learning in neuronal networks for planning and decision making. *Prog. Brain Res.* 126:217–229.

DEHAENE, S., A. JOBERT, L. NACCACHE, P. CIUCIU, J. B. POLINE, D. LE BIHAN, et al., 2004. Letter binding and invariant recognition of masked words: Behavioral and neuroimaging evidence. *Psychol. Sci.* 15:307–313.

DEHAENE, S., M. KERSZBERG, and J. P. CHANGEUX, 1998. A neuronal model of a global workspace in effortful cognitive tasks. *Proc. Natl. Acad. Sci. U.S.A.* 95:14529–14534.

DEHAENE, S., and L. NACCACHE, 2001. Towards a cognitive neuroscience of consciousness: Basic evidence and a workspace framework. *Cognition* 79:1–37.

DEHAENE, S., L. NACCACHE, L. COHEN, D. LE BIHAN, J. F. MANGIN, J. B. POLINE, et al., 2001. Cerebral mechanisms of word masking and unconscious repetition priming. *Nat. Neurosci.* 4:752–758.

DEHAENE, S., L. NACCACHE, G. LE CLEC H, E. KOECHLIN, M. MUELLER, G. DEHAENE-LAMBERTZ, et al., 1998. Imaging unconscious semantic priming. *Nature* 395:597–600.

DEHAENE, S., C. SERGENT, and J. P. CHANGEUX, 2003. A neuronal model linking subjective reports and objective neurophysiological data during conscious perception. *Proc. Natl. Acad. Sci. U.S.A.* 100:8520–8525.

DI LOLLO, V., J. T. ENNS, and R. A. RENSINK, 2000. Competition for consciousness among visual events: The psychophysics of reentrant visual processes. *J. Exp. Psychol. Gen.* 129:481–507.

DI VIRGILIO, G., and S. CLARKE, 1997. Direct interhemispheric visual input to human speech areas. *Hum. Brain Mapp.* 5:347–354.

EDELMAN, G. M., 1989. *The Remembered Present*. New York: Basic Books.

EDELMAN, G. M., 1993. Neural Darwinism: Selection and reentrant signaling in higher brain function. *Neuron* 10:115–125.

FORSTER, K. I., and C. DAVIS, 1984. Repetition priming and frequency attenuation in lexical access. *J. Exp. Psychol. Learn. Mem. Cogn.* 10:680–698.

GOLDMAN-RAKIC, P. S., 1988. Topography of cognition: Parallel distributed networks in primate association cortex. *Annu. Rev. Neurosci.* 11:137–156.

GRANON, S., P. FAURE, and J. P. CHANGEUX, 2003. Executive and social behaviors under nicotinic receptor regulation. *Proc. Natl. Acad. Sci. U.S.A.* 100:9596–9601.

GREENWALD, A. G., S. C. DRAINE, and R. L. ABRAMS, 1996. Three cognitive markers of unconscious semantic activation. *Science* 273:1699–1702.

JASPER, H. H., 1998. Sensory information and conscious experience. *Adv. Neurol.* 77:33–48.

KOECHLIN, E., L. NACCACHE, E. BLOCK, and S. DEHAENE, 1999. Primed numbers: Exploring the modularity of numerical representations with masked and unmasked semantic priming. *J. Exp. Psychol. Hum. Percept. Perform.* 25:1882–1905.

KOVACS, G., R. VOGELS, and G. A. ORBAN, 1995. Cortical correlate of pattern backward masking. *Proc. Natl. Acad. Sci. U.S.A.* 92: 5587–5591.

LAMME, V. A., 2003. Why visual attention and awareness are different. *Trends Cogn. Sci.* 7:12–18.

LAMME, V. A., and P. R. ROELFSEMA, 2000. The distinct modes of vision offered by feedforward and recurrent processing. *Trends Neurosci.* 23:571–579.

LAMME, V. A., K. ZIPSER, and H. SPEKREIJSE, 2002. Masking interrupts figure-ground signals in V1. *J. Cogn. Neurosci.* 14:1044–1053.

LLINAS, R., U. RIBARY, D. CONTRERAS, and C. PEDROARENA, 1998. The neuronal basis for consciousness. *Philos. Trans. R. Soc. Lond. B Biol. Sci.* 353:1841–1849.

LUMER, E. D., and G. REES, 1999. Covariation of activity in visual and prefrontal cortex associated with subjective visual perception. *Proc. Natl. Acad. Sci. U.S.A.* 96:1669–1673.

NACCACHE, L., E. BLANDIN, and S. DEHAENE, 2002. Unconscious masked priming depends on temporal attention. *Psychol. Sci.* 13: 416–424.

NACCACHE, L., and S. DEHAENE, 2001a. The priming method: Imaging unconscious repetition priming reveals an abstract representation of number in the parietal lobes. *Cereb. Cortex* 11:966–974.

NACCACHE, L., and S. DEHAENE, 2001b. Unconscious semantic priming extends to novel unseen stimuli. *Cognition* 80:215–229.

NEELY, J. H., and T. A. KAHAN, 2001. Is semantic activation automatic? A critical re-evaluation. In *The Nature of Remembering: Essays in Honor of Robert G. Crowder*, H. L. Roediger, J. S. Nairne, I. Neath, and A. M. Surprenant, eds. Washington, D.C.: American Psychological Association, pp. 69–93.

NORMAN, D. A., and T. SHALLICE, 1980. Attention to action: Willed and automatic control of behavior. In *Consciousness and Self-*

Regulation, vol. 4, R. J. Davidson, G. E. Schwartz, and D. Shapiro, eds. New York: Plenum Press.

PAUS, T., 2000. Functional anatomy of arousal and attention systems in the human brain. *Prog. Brain Res.* 126:65–77.

PINS, D., and D. FFYTCHE, 2003. The neural correlates of conscious vision. *Cereb. Cortex* 13:461–474.

POSNER, M. I., and M. K. ROTHBART, 1998. Attention, self-regulation and consciousness. *Philos. Trans. R. Soc. Lond. B Biol. Sci.* 353:1915–1927.

REVONSUO, A., 2001. Can functional brain imaging discover consciousness in the brain? *J. Conscious. Stud.* 8:3–50.

ROLLS, E. T., M. J. TOVEE, and S. PANZERI, 1999. The neurophysiology of backward visual masking: information analysis. *J. Cogn. Neurosci.* 11:300–311.

SERGENT, C., and S. DEHAENE, in press. Is consciousness a gradual phenomenon? Evidence for an all-or-none bifurcation during the attentional blink. *Psychol. Sci.*

SUPER, H., C. VAN DER TOGT, H. SPEKREIJSE, and V. A. LAMME, 2003. Internal state of monkey primary visual cortex (V1) predicts figure-ground perception. *J. Neurosci.* 23:3407–3414.

THOMPSON, K. G., and J. D. SCHALL, 1999. The detection of visual signals by macaque frontal eye field during masking. *Nat. Neurosci.* 2:283–288.

TONONI, G., and G. M. EDELMAN, 1998. Consciousness and complexity. *Science* 282:1846–1851.

VOGEL, E. K., S. J. LUCK, and K. L. SHAPIRO, 1998. Electrophysiological evidence for a postperceptual locus of suppression during the attentional blink. *J. Exp. Psychol. Hum. Percept. Perform.* 24:1656–1674.

VUILLEUMIER, P., J. ARMONY, K. CLARKE, M. HUSAIN, J. DRIVER, and R. DOLAN, 2002. Neural response to emotional faces with and without awareness: Event-related fMRI in a parietal patient with visual extinction and spatial neglect. *Neuropsychologia* 40: 2156.

WEISKRANTZ, L., 1997. *Consciousness Lost and Found: A Neuropsychological Exploration*. New York: Oxford University Press.

83 Perceiving the World and Grasping It: Dissociations Between Conscious and Unconscious Visual Processing

MELVYN A. GOODALE

ABSTRACT Visual systems first evolved not to enable organisms to see, but to provide sensory control of their movements. Vision as "sight" is a relative newcomer on the evolutionary landscape, but its emergence has enabled animals to carry out complex cognitive operations on internal representations of the world in which they live. In the more ancient visuomotor systems, there is a basic iso-morphism between visual input and motor output. In representational vision, there are many cognitive "buffers" between input and output. Thus, the relationship between what is on the retina and the behavior of the organism cannot be understood without reference to other mental states, including those typically described as "conscious." The duplex nature of vision is reflected in the organization of the visual pathways in the primate cerebral cortex. The dorsal "action" stream projecting from primary visual cortex to the posterior parietal cortex provides flexible control of more ancient subcortical visuomotor modules for the control of motor acts. The ventral "perceptual" stream projecting from the primary visual cortex to the temporal lobe provides the rich and detailed representation of the world required for cognitive operations. Both streams work together in the production of goal-directed behavior. The ventral stream identifies goals and together with prefrontal cortical areas plans an appropriate action; the dorsal stream (in conjunction with related circuitry in premotor cortex, basal ganglia, and brainstem) programs and controls those actions.

Most of what we know about the world beyond our immediate body surface comes from vision. But vision does not simply provide information about the objects and events that are out there; it delivers a world so palpable, so real, that it is sometimes difficult to realize that this experience is nothing more than a creation of the central nervous system. Moreover, our visual percepts are so rich and detailed that they appear to contain all the information required for any visually directed thought and action we are capable of making. But, as I will argue in this chapter, this is nothing more than an illusion. The idea that vision delivers a single "general-purpose" representation of the external world is simply not correct. Instead, I will argue, vision consists of a number of separate systems in which the input processing of each system has been shaped by the output mechanisms it serves. The construction of a conscious percept is certainly an important function of vision, but, as will become clear in this chapter, the visual control of actions, from saccadic eye movements to skilled grasping movements of the hand and limb, depends on visual mechanisms that are functionally and neurally separate from those mediating our perception of the world.

One of the themes that I will explore is how consciousness maps onto this distinction between vision for perception and vision for action, and the separate neural pathways that mediate them. Conscious percepts, I will argue, depend on visual processing within the ventral stream, a set of cortical pathways that arise in primary visual cortex and project to the temporal lobe. The percepts constructed by the ventral stream need not be conscious, but we cannot have conscious percepts without a ventral stream. The visual control of skilled actions, such as object-directed grasping with the prehensile hand, depends on a quite separate set of pathways, the dorsal stream of visual projections, which also arises in primary visual cortex but terminates in the posterior parietal cortex. I will argue that we are never conscious of the visual information that is processed by this pathway, even though we are often conscious of the particular actions that the visual information is controlling. But let us first consider how vision came to be.

The evolution of visuomotor control

Vision did not evolve to enable organisms to perceive. It evolved to provide distal control of their movements. Take the case of *Euglena*, a single-cell organism that uses light as a source of energy. *Euglena* alters its pattern of swimming as a function of the ambient light levels in different parts of the

MELVYN A. GOODALE Department of Psychology, University of Western Ontario, London, Ontario, Canada.

pond or puddle in which it lives. Such phototactic behavior ensures that *Euglena* stays longer in regions of its environment where sunlight is available for the manufacture of food (Gould, 1982). To explain this behavior, it is not necessary to argue that *Euglena* "perceives" the light, or even that it has some sort of internal model of the outside world. One simply has to talk about a simple input-output device linking the amount of ambient light to the pattern of locomotion. Of course, a mechanism of this sort, although driven by light, is far less complicated than the visual systems of multicellular organisms. But even in more complex organisms, such as vertebrates, much of vision can be understood entirely in terms of the distal control of movement without reference to experiential perception or any general-purpose representation of the outside world.

As vision evolved in simple vertebrates, visual control systems for different kinds of behavior developed relatively independent neural substrates. Thus, in present-day amphibians such as the frog, there is evidence that visually guided prey catching and visually guided obstacle avoidance are separately mediated by different pathways from the retina right through to the effector systems producing the movements (Ingle, 1973, 1982, 1991). The visual control of prey catching depends on circuitry involving retinal projections to the optic tectum, while the visual control of locomotion around barriers depends on circuitry involving retinal projections to particular regions of the pretectal nuclei. Each of these retinal targets projects in turn to different premotor nuclei in the brainstem and spinal cord. In fact, accumulating evidence from studies in both frog and toad suggests that there are at least five separate visuomotor modules, each responsible for a different kind of visually guided behavior and each having distinct processing routes from input to output (Ewert, 1987; Ingle, 1991). The outputs of these different modules certainly have to be coordinated, but in no sense are they guided by a single, general-purpose visual representation in the frog's brain. (For a discussion of this issue, see Goodale, 1996, and Milner and Goodale, 1995.)

Although there is evidence that the same kind of visuomotor modularity found in the frog also exists in the mammalian brain (for review, see Goodale, 1996), the very complexity of the day-to-day living in many mammals, particularly in higher primates, demands much more flexible organization of the circuitry. In monkeys (and thus presumably in humans as well), many of the visuomotor circuits that are shared with simpler vertebrates appear to be modulated by more recently evolved control systems in the cerebral cortex (for review, see Milner and Goodale, 1995). This Jacksonian circuitry (Jackson, 1875), in which a layer of cortical control is superimposed on more ancient subcortical networks, makes possible much more adaptive visuomotor behavior. Of course, the basic subcortical circuitry has also

changed to some extent, and new visuomotor control systems involving both cortical and subcortical structures have emerged. But even though these complex visuomotor control systems in the primate brain are capable of generating an almost limitless range of visually guided behavior, as we shall see later, there is evidence that these visuomotor modules are functionally and neurally separate from those mediating our perception of the world.

The emergence of visual perception

As interactions with world became more complicated and subtle, direct sensory control of action was not enough. With the emergence of cognitive systems and complex social behavior, a good deal of motor output has become quite arbitrary with respect to sensory input. Many animals, particularly humans and other primates, behave as though their actions are driven by some sort of internal model of the world in which they live. The representational systems that use vision to generate such models or percepts of the world must carry out very different transformations on visual input from the transformations carried out by the visuomotor modules described earlier. For one thing, they are not linked directly to specific motor outputs but access these outputs via cognitive systems involving memory, semantics, spatial reasoning, planning, and communication. Such higher-order representational systems allow us to perceive a world beyond our bodies, to share that experience with other members of our species, and to plan a vast range of different actions. This constellation of abilities is often identified with consciousness, particularly those aspects of consciousness that have to do with higher-order planning and metacognition (e.g., Crick and Koch, 2003). But even though perception allows us to plan an action and choose a particular goal, the actual execution of that action may nevertheless be mediated by dedicated visuomotor modules that are not dissimilar in principle from those found in frogs and toads. In other words, vision in humans and other primates (and perhaps other animals as well) has two distinct but interacting functions: (1) the perception of objects and their relations, which provides a foundation for the organism's cognitive life and its conscious experience of the world, and (2) the control of actions directed at (or with respect to) those objects, in which separate motor outputs are programmed and controlled online.

Dorsal and ventral streams

Beyond area V1, visual information is conveyed to a bewildering number of extrastriate areas. Despite the complexity of the interconnections between these different areas, two broad "streams" of projections from area V1 have been identified in the macaque monkey brain: a ventral stream,

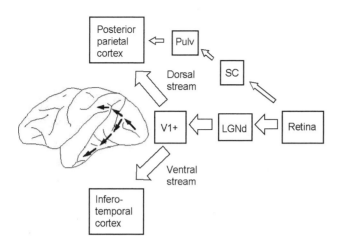

FIGURE 83.1 Major routes whereby retinal input reaches the dorsal and ventral streams. The diagram of the macaque brain (right hemisphere) on the right of the figure shows the approximate routes of the corticocortical projections from primary visual cortex to the posterior parietal and the inferotemporal cortex, respectively. Abbreviations: LGNd, lateral geniculate nucleus, pars dorsalis; Pulv, pulvinar; SC, superior colliculus. (Adapted with permission from Milner and Goodale, 1995.)

projecting eventually to the inferotemporal cortex, and a dorsal stream, projecting to the posterior parietal cortex (Ungerleider and Mishkin, 1982). These regions also receive inputs from a number of other subcortical visual structures, such as the superior colliculus, which sends prominent projections to the dorsal stream (via the thalamus). A schematic diagram of these pathways can be found in figure 83.1. Although some caution must be exercised in generalizing from monkey to human (Crick and Jones, 1993), recent neuroimaging evidence suggests that the visual projections from primary visual cortex to the temporal and parietal lobes in the human brain involve a separation into ventral and dorsal streams similar to that seen in the monkey (Culham and Kanwisher, 2001; Van Essen et al., 2001; Tootell, Tsao, and Vanduffel, 2003; Culham, 2004; Culham et al., 2003; James et al., 2003).

In 1982, Ungerleider and Mishkin argued that the two streams of visual processing play different but complementary roles in the processing of incoming visual information. According to their original account, the ventral stream plays a critical role in the identification and recognition of objects, while the dorsal stream mediates the localization of those same objects. Some have referred to this distinction in visual processing as one between object vision and spatial vision— "what" versus "where." Support for this idea came from work in monkeys. Lesions of the inferotemporal cortex in monkeys produced deficits in their ability to discriminate between objects on the basis of their visual features but did not affect their performance on a spatially demanding "landmark" task (Pohl, 1973; Ungerleider and Brody, 1977). Conversely, lesions of the posterior parietal cortex produced

deficits in performance on the landmark task but did not affect object discrimination learning (for a critique of these studies, see Goodale, 1995; Milner and Goodale, 1995). Although the evidence for the original Ungerleider and Mishkin proposal initially seemed quite compelling, recent findings from a broad range of studies in both humans and monkeys has forced a reinterpretation of the division of labor between the two streams. As will be detailed in subsequent sections, David Milner and I have offered an account of the two streams that emphasizes the differences in the requirements of the output systems that each stream serves.

Vision for perception and vision for action

David Milner and I have suggested, in contrast to Ungerleider and Mishkin (1982), that both streams process information about object features and about their spatial relations. Each stream, however, uses this visual information in different ways (Goodale and Milner, 1992). In the ventral stream, the processing delivers the enduring characteristics of objects and their relations, permitting the formation of long-term perceptual representations. These representations correspond to what we identify as our conscious visual experience of the world (although not all the high-level processing need be conscious). The representations constructed by the ventral stream play an essential role in the identification of objects and enable us to classify objects and events, attach meaning and significance to them, and establish their causal relations. As we saw earlier, such operations are essential for accumulating a knowledge base about the world. Moreover, these representations are necessary (but not sufficient) for delivering our conscious percepts of the world beyond our bodies. In contrast, the transformations carried out by the dorsal stream deal with the moment-to-moment information about the location and disposition of objects with respect to the effector being used and thereby mediate the visual control of skilled actions, such as manual prehension, directed at those objects. As such, the dorsal stream can be regarded as a cortical extension of the dedicated visuomotor modules that mediate visually guided movements in all vertebrates. The visual information that is processed by the dorsal stream for the control of these movements is never accessible to conscious scrutiny. The perceptual representations constructed by the ventral stream interact with various high-level cognitive mechanisms and enable an organism to select a particular course of action with respect to objects in the world, while the visuomotor networks in the dorsal stream (and their associated cortical and subcortical pathways) are responsible for the programming and online control of the particular movements that action entails.

This division of labor between the two cortical visual pathways reflects the fact that different transformations have to be carried out on incoming visual information to meet the requirements for perception and the requirements for the efficient control of action. To be able to grasp an object successfully, for example, it is essential that the brain (i.e., the dorsal stream) compute the actual (absolute) size of the object and its orientation and position with respect to the observer. This explains why an action like object-directed grasping is so refractory to pictorial illusions that by definition affect perception. (For a review of this extensive literature, see Dyde and Milner, 2002; Goodale and Haffenden, 1998; and Haffenden, Schiff, and Goodale, 2001.)

Moreover, the information about the orientation and position of the goal object must be computed in egocentric frames of reference—in other words, in frames of reference that take into account the orientation and position of the object with respect to the effector that is to be used to perform the action. But the time at which these computations are performed is also critical. Observers and goal objects rarely stay in a static relationship with one another, and as a consequence, the egocentric coordinates of a target object can often change dramatically from moment to moment. For this reason, it makes sense that the required coordinates for action be computed immediately before the movements are initiated. Moreover, it would be of little value for these coordinates (or the resulting motor programs) to be stored in memory. In short, the vision-for-action systems in the dorsal stream work best in an online mode.

The situation is quite different for perception, both in terms of the frames of reference used to construct the percept and the time period over which that percept (or some version of it) can be accessed. Vision for perception appears not to rely on computations about the absolute size of objects or their egocentric locations, a fact that explains why we have no difficulty watching television, a medium in which there are no absolute metrics at all. Instead, the perceptual system computes the size, location, shape, and orientation of an object primarily in relation to other objects and surfaces in the scene. Encoding an object in a scene-based frame of reference (sometimes called an allocentric frame of reference) permits a perceptual representation of the object that preserves the relations between the object parts and its surroundings without requiring precise information about the absolute size of the object or its exact position with respect to the observer. Indeed, if our perceptual machinery attempted to deliver the real size and distance of all the objects in the visual array, the computational load on the system would be astronomical. (For a more detailed discussion of these issues, see Goodale and Humphrey, 1998, and Goodale, Jakobson, and Keillor, 1994.)

But perception also operates over a much longer time scale than that used in the visual control of action. We can recognize objects we have seen minutes, hours, days, or even years before. When objects or scenes are coded in allocentric frames of reference, it is much easier to preserve their identity over relatively long periods of time. By making the perceptual representations of objects object- or scene-based, the constancies of size, shape, color, lightness, and relative location can be maintained over time and across different viewing conditions. There is much debate in the object recognition literature about how this is accomplished. Some of the mechanisms driving object perception might use a network of viewer-centered representations of the same object (e.g., Bülthoff and Edelman, 1992); others might use an array of canonical representations (e.g., Palmer, Rosch, and Chase, 1981); still others might be truly "object-centered" (Marr, 1982). But whatever the particular coding might be, it is the identity of the object and its location within the scene, not its disposition with respect to the observer, that is of primary concern to the perceptual system. In other words, we can recognize objects that we have seen before, even though the position of those objects with respect to our body might have changed considerably since the last time we saw them. But of course, not only is this stored information available for mediating recognition of previously encountered objects, it can also contribute to the control of our movements, particularly when we are working in off-line mode, where we have no direct visual information about the size, shape, location, and disposition of the object.

To summarize, then, while similar (but not identical) visual information about object shape, size, local orientation, and location is available to both systems, the transformational algorithms that are applied to these inputs are uniquely tailored to the function of each system. According to our proposal, it is the nature of the functional requirements of perception and action that lies at the root of the division of labor in the ventral and dorsal visual projection systems of the primate cerebral cortex.

Neuropsychological evidence for perception and action streams

In the intact brain, the two streams of processing work together in a seamless and integrated fashion. Nevertheless, by studying individuals who have sustained brain damage that spares one of these systems but not the other, it is possible to get a glimpse of how each stream transforms incoming visual information.

PERCEPTION WITHOUT ACTION   It has been known for a long time that patients with lesions in the superior regions of the posterior parietal cortex, particularly lesions that invade the territory of the intraparietal sulcus (or IPS), can have problems using vision to direct a grasp or aiming movement toward the correct location of a visual target placed in different positions in the visual field, particularly the peripheral visual field. This particular deficit is often described as optic ataxia (Bálint, 1909). But failure to locate an object with the hand should not be construed as a problem in spatial vision; many of these patients can, for example, describe the relative position of the object in space quite accurately, even though they cannot direct their hand toward it (Jeannerod, 1988; Perenin and Vighetto, 1988). Moreover, sometimes the deficit will be seen in one hand but not the other (Bálint, 1909). Problems in the visual control of locomotion and the production of voluntary saccades have also been observed following damage to the posterior parietal region (for review, see Milner and Goodale, 1995). It should be pointed out, of course, that these patients typically have no difficulty using input from other sensory systems, such as proprioception or audition, to guide their movements. In short, their deficit is neither purely visual nor purely motor. It is instead a true visuomotor deficit.

Some of these patients are unable to use visual information to rotate their hand or scale the opening of their fingers when reaching out to pick up an object, even though they have no difficulty describing the size or orientation of objects in that part of the visual field (Jeannerod, 1988; Perenin and Vighetto, 1988; Jakobson et al., 1991; Goodale et al., 1993; Jeannerod, Decety, and Michel, 1994). Similarly, as figure 83.2 illustrates, patients with damage to this region can also show deficits in the selection of stable grasp points on the surface of objects of varying shape (Goodale et al., 1994). These results show that the visuomotor disturbances accompanying damage to the posterior parietal cortex need not be limited to deficits in the spatial control of movements but can extend to object features such as size, shape, and orientation. Nevertheless, it is worth emphasizing once more that the deficits are visuomotor in nature not perceptual; the patients have no trouble discriminating between objects of different size or shape or between objects placed in different orientations. In other words, as far as can be determined, they have conscious percepts of the visual world that they fail to interact with appropriately.

The various visuomotor deficits that have been described in patients with damage to the posterior parietal region are quite dissociable from one another. Some patients are unable to use visual information to control their hand postures but have no difficulty controlling the direction of their grasp; others show the reverse pattern. Some patients are unable to foveate a target object but have no difficulty directing a well-formed grasp in its direction; others may show no evidence of an oculomotor deficit but be unable to guide their hand toward an object under visual control. Indeed, depending on the size and locus of the lesion, a patient can demonstrate any combination of these visuomotor deficits (for review, see Milner and Goodale, 1995). Different subregions of the posterior parietal cortex, it appears, are critical for the visual control of different motor outputs. In fact, as we shall see later, there is clear evidence of specialized visuomotor

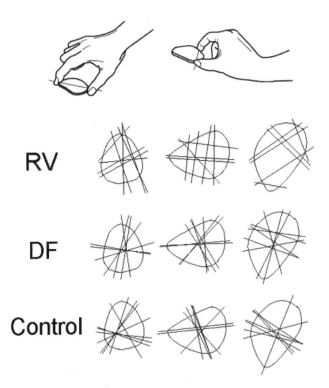

FIGURE 83.2 This figure shows the "grasp lines" (joining points where the thumb and index finger first made contact with the shape) selected by patient with optic ataxia (R.V.), a patient with visual agnosia (D.F.), and a control subject when picking up three of the 12 shapes used in the study. The four different orientations in which each shape was presented have been rotated so that they are aligned. D.F.'s grasp lines are similar to those of the control subject, and both differ from the grasp lines of R.V., who often chose very unstable grasp points. Whereas D.F.'s and the control subject's grasp lines tended to pass through or close to the center of mass of the shape, this was not the case for R.V. (Adapted with permission from Goodale et al., 1994.)

areas for the control of eye movements, head movements, reaching, and grasping in the monkey posterior parietal cortex, with most of these areas located in or around the IPS. Recent neuroimaging evidence suggests that humans, like the monkey, also have areas within IPS and neighboring regions that are specialized for different kinds of visuomotor transformations (Culham and Kanwisher, 2001; Culham, 2004; Culham et al., 2003). A particular motor act, such as reaching out and grasping an object, presumably would engage visuomotor mechanisms in a number of these different areas, including those involved in the control of saccades, visual pursuit, reaching with the limb, and grasping movements of the hands and fingers (for a discussion of the different components of manual prehension, see Jeannerod, 1988). Just how such mechanisms are coordinated is not well understood, although some models have been proposed (e.g., Hoff and Arbib, 1992). In any case, it is clear that the visual control of each of the constituent actions requires different sensorimotor coordinate transformations, and there have been some attempts to specify how the posterior parietal cortex might mediate such transformations (e.g., Cohen and Andersen, 2002; Flanders, Tillery, and Soechting, 1992; Stein, 1992). But again, even though patients with damage to the posterior parietal region may show a variety of different visuomotor deficits, they can often describe (and thus presumably perceive) the intrinsic visual features and the location of the very object they are unable to grasp, foveate, or walk toward.

ACTION WITHOUT PERCEPTION The fact that patients with damage to posterior parietal cortex can perceive objects but cannot grasp them provides one piece of evidence that there are separate neural substrates for perception and action in the human brain. It also suggests that the cortical region in and around the IPS, the human homologue of the monkey dorsal stream, is critical for the visual control of action. But even more compelling evidence for separate visual systems for perception and action comes from patients who show the opposite pattern of deficits and spared visual abilities. Take the case of D.F., now in her late 40s, who at age 34 suffered irreversible brain damage as a result of near asphyxiation by carbon monoxide. When she regained consciousness, it was apparent that D.F.'s visual system had been badly damaged from the hypoxia she had experienced. She was unable to recognize the faces of her relatives and friends or to identify the visual form of common objects. In fact, she could not even tell the difference between simple geometric shapes such as a square and a triangle. At the same time, she had no difficulty recognizing people from their voices or identifying objects placed in her hands; her perceptual problems appeared to be exclusively visual. Even today, nearly 15 years after the accident, she remains quite unable to identify objects or drawings on the basis of their visual form.

The damage in D.F.'s brain is quite diffuse, a common pattern in cases of anoxia. Nevertheless, certain areas of her brain, especially those in the posterior region of her cerebral cortex, appear to be more severely damaged than others. Magnetic resonance imaging (MRI) carried out just over a year after her accident showed that the ventrolateral regions of her occipital lobe are particularly compromised. Primary visual cortex, however, appears to be largely spared in D.F. (for details of the initial structural MRI, see Milner et al., 1991).

D.F.'s perceptual problems are not simply a case of being unable to associate a visual stimulus with meaningful semantic information. For example, while it is true that she cannot find the correct name of or semantic association for the objects depicted in the line drawings shown in the left portion of figure 83.3, she is also completely unable to draw what she sees when she looks at the line drawing. Moreover, her inability to copy drawings is not due to a problem in controlling the movements of the pen or pencil. When she is

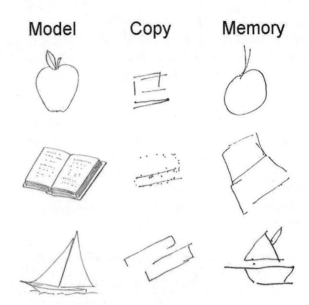

FIGURE 83.3 Patient D.F.'s attempts to draw from models and from memory. D.F. was unable to identify the line drawings of an apple, an open book, and a boat shown on the left. In addition, her copies were very poor. She did incorporate some elements of the line drawing (e.g., the dots indicating the text in the book) into her copy. When she was asked on another occasion to draw an apple, an open book, and a boat from memory, she produced a respectable representation of all three items (drawings on right). When she was later shown her own drawings, she had no idea what they were. (Adapted with permission from Milner and Goodale, 1995.)

asked to draw a particular object from memory, she is able to do so reasonably well, as the drawings on the right side of figure 83.3 illustrate.

Nor is D.F.'s inability to perceive the shape and form of objects in the world due to deficits in basic sensory processing (Milner et al., 1991). She remains quite capable of identifying colors, for example. In addition, perimetric testing carried out quite early after her accident showed that she could detect luminance-defined targets at least as far out as 30° into the visual periphery. Her spatial contrast sensitivity was also normal above 5 Hz and was only moderately impaired at lower spatial frequencies. Of course, even though she could detect the presence of the spatial frequency gratings in these tests, she could not report their orientation. In fact, D.F. has great problems describing or discriminating the orientation and form of any visual contour, no matter how that contour is defined. Thus, she cannot identify shapes whose contours are defined by differences in luminance or color, or by differences in the direction of motion or the plane of depth. Nor can she recognize shapes that are defined by the similarity or proximity of individual elements of the visual array. Nevertheless, information about the spatial distribution of the visual array appeared to reach her primary visual cortex. Thus, when she was shown a high-contrast reversing checkerboard pattern in an electrophysiological assessment carried out just after the accident, the initial components of the evoked response, such as the P100, appeared to be quite normal, suggesting that her primary visual cortex was working normally. In short, D.F.'s deficit seems to be "perceptual" rather than "sensory" in nature. She simply cannot perceive shapes and forms, even though the early stages of her visual system appear to have access to the requisite low-level sensory information.

What is most remarkable about D.F., however, is that despite her profound deficits in form vision, she is able to use visual information about the size, shape, and orientation of objects to control a broad range of visually guided movements. D.F. will reach out and grasp your hand if you offer it when you first meet her. She is equally adept at reaching out for a door handle, even in an unfamiliar environment. She can walk unassisted across a room or patio, stepping easily over low obstacles and walking around higher ones. Even more amazing is the fact that she can reach out and grasp an object placed in front of her with considerable accuracy and confidence, despite the fact that moments before she was quite unable to identify or describe that same object.

These dissociations between D.F.'s perceptual abilities and her ability to use visual information to control skilled movements are also evident in formal testing (Goodale et al., 1991). For example, when she is presented with a series of rectangular blocks that vary in their dimensions but not in their overall surface area, she is unable to say whether or not any two of these blocks are the same or different. Even when a single block is placed in front of her, she is unable to indicate how wide the block is by opening her index finger and thumb a matching amount. Nevertheless, when she reaches out to pick up the block using a precision grip, the opening between her index finger and thumb is scaled in flight to the width of the object, just as it is in subjects with normal vision.

A similar dissociation can be seen in D.F.'s processing of the orientation of objects (Goodale et al., 1991). Thus, even though she cannot discriminate between objects placed in different orientations on a table in front of her, she can rotate her hand in the correct orientation when she reaches out to grasp one of the objects. When presented with a large slot in a vertical surface, she is unable to rotate a hand-held card to match the orientation of that slot (figure 83.4). But again, when she attempts to insert the hand-held card into the slot, she rotates the card in the appropriate way as she moves it toward the slot (see figure 83.4). She can also use information about the shape of an object to locate stable grasp points on its surface when she picks it up (Goodale et al., 1994). Thus, when grasping an object like those shown in figure 83.2, D.F. will place her finger and thumb so that a line joining the opposing points of contact passes through the object's center of mass. And, in contrast to the patient

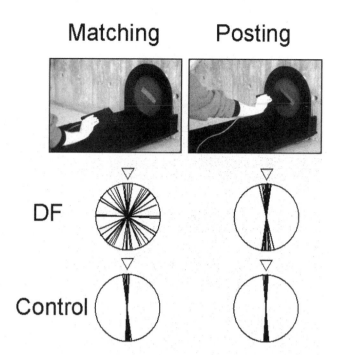

FIGURE 83.4   Photographs at top show the apparatus that was used to test sensitivity to orientation in patient D.F. The slot could be placed in any one of a number of orientations around the clock. Subjects were required either to rotate a hand-held card to match the orientation of the slot (left-hand side) or to "post" the card into the slot (right-hand side). Below are the polar plots of the orientation of the hand-held card on the perceptual matching task (left-hand side) and the visuomotor posting task (right-hand side) for D.F. and an age-matched control subject. The correct orientation on each trial has been rotated to vertical. Although D.F. was unable to match the orientation of the card to that of the slot in the perceptual matching card, she did rotate the card to the correct orientation as she attempted to insert it into the slot on the posting task.

with posterior parietal damage whose performance is also illustrated in figure 83.2, D.F. chooses points on the object's boundary where her fingers are the least likely to slip, such as points of high convexity or concavity, just as the control subject with normal vision does. Needless to say, D.F. is quite unable to tell these objects apart in a same-different discrimination. In short, D.F. can use visual information about the size, orientation, and shape of objects to program and control her goal-directed movements even though she has no conscious perception of those same object features.

As I mentioned earlier, D.F.'s spared visuomotor skills are not limited to reaching and grasping movements; D.F. can also walk around quite well under visual control. When she was tested more formally, we found that she is able to negotiate obstacles during locomotion as well as control subjects (Patla and Goodale, 1997). Thus, when obstacles of different heights were randomly placed in her path on different trials, she stepped over these obstacles quite efficiently, and the elevation of her toe increased linearly as a function of obstacle height, just as it does in neurologically intact individuals. Yet when she was asked to give verbal estimates of the height of the obstacles, the slope of the line relating estimated and actual obstacle height was much shallower in her case than in normal subjects. Similar dissociations between perceptual judgments about the pitch of the visual field and its effect on eye position have also been observed in D.F. (Servos, Matin, and Goodale, 1995).

To summarize, even though D.F.'s brain damage has left her unable to perceive the size, shape, and orientation of objects, her visuomotor outputs remain quite sensitive to these same object features. There appears to have been an interruption in the normal flow of shape and contour information into her perceptual system without affecting the processing of shape and contour information by her visuomotor control systems. But where is the damage in D.F.'s brain? If, as was suggested earlier, the perception of objects and events is mediated by the ventral stream of visual projections to inferotemporal cortex, then D.F. should show evidence for damage relatively early in this pathway.

As described earlier, an MRI taken shortly after her accident showed evidence of damage in the ventrolateral region of her occipital lobe on both sides of D.F.'s brain. More recent high-resolution anatomical MRIs of D.F.'s brain have confirmed that this is indeed the case (James et al., 2003). In fact, the damage is remarkably localized to the lateral

occipital area (LO) part of the lateral occipital complex (LOC), a heterogeneous collection of visual areas that have been implicated in object recognition in a number of functional imaging studies (Malach et al., 2002; Kanwisher et al., 2001; James et al., 2000; Grill-Spector, 2003; James, 2002). As figure 83.5 shows, the LO lesions are bilateral and do not include that part of LOC extending into the fusiform gyrus on the ventral surface of the brain. As we shall see later, it is these lesions in area LO that are undoubtedly responsible for her deficit in form and shape perception.

The recent anatomical MRI also shows that, with the exception of a unilateral lesion in the parieto-occipital area, D.F.'s dorsal stream is relatively intact. In other words, visual information from primary visual cortex presumably still projects to visuomotor areas in D.F.'s posterior parietal cortex. But in addition, the dorsal stream, unlike the ventral stream, also receives visual input from the superior colliculus via the pulvinar, a nucleus in the thalamus (see figure 83.1). Indeed, experiments by Perenin and Rossetti (1996) suggests that this collicular-pulvinar route to the dorsal stream may be able to support object-directed grasping movements even without input from area V1. They tested a patient who was completely blind (by conventional testing) in one-half of his visual field following a medial occipital lesion that included

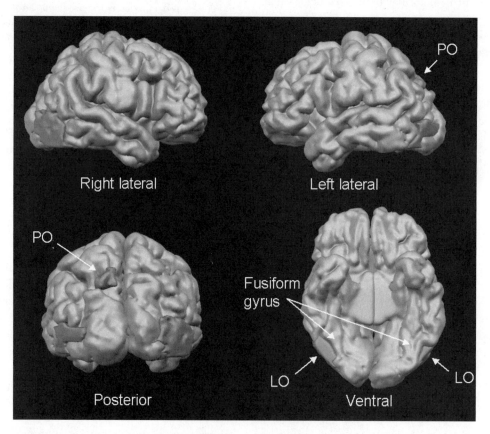

FIGURE 83.5   Four views of D.F.'s brain, mathematically rendered to show pial surface. The lesions were reconstructed from high-resolution MRI sections and were then rendered on the pial surface in pale blue. Abbreviations: LO, lateral occipital area; PO, parieto-occipital area. (Adapted with permission from James et al., 2003.) (See color plate 71.)

all of area V1. The patient could not see any objects in his blind field. Nevertheless, when he was persuaded to reach out and grasp objects placed in his blind field, he showed some evidence of sensitivity to the size and orientation of objects. Thus, there are at least two routes whereby information about object form could reach the dorsal stream in D.F.: from the superior colliculus (via the pulvinar) and from the lateral geniculate nucleus (via the primary visual cortex). Either or both of these pathways could be continuing to mediate the well-formed visuomotor responses that D.F. exhibits.

In summary, the neuropsychological findings can be accommodated quite well by the proposal that the division of labor between the ventral and dorsal streams of visual processing is based on the distinction between visuomotor control and the more visuocognitive functions of vision. Moreover, as we shall see in the next two sections, this new way of looking at the organization of the visual system is also consistent with the story that is emerging from anatomical, neurophysiological, and behavioral work in the monkey, as well as with findings from recent functional neuroimaging experiments with D.F.

Evidence from monkey studies

A broad range of different studies on the dorsal and ventral streams in the monkey lend considerable support to the distinction outlined in the previous section. [For a detailed account of this work, see Milner and Goodale, 1995). For example, monkeys with lesions of inferotemporal cortex, who show profound deficits in object recognition, are nevertheless as capable as normal animals are at picking up small objects (Klüver and Bucy, 1939) and at catching flying insects (Pribram, 1967). More recent formal testing has revealed that these monkeys can orient their fingers in a precision grip to grasp morsels of food embedded in small slots placed at different orientations, even though their orientation discrimination abilities are profoundly impaired (Glickstein, Buchbinder, and May, 1998). In short, these animals behave much the same way as D.F.: they are unable to discriminate between objects on the basis of visual features that they can clearly use to direct their grasping movements.

In addition to the lesion studies, there is a long history of electrophysiological work showing that cells in inferotemporal cortex and neighboring regions of the superior temporal sulcus are tuned to specific objects and object features (see, e.g., Tanaka, 2003; Logothetis, 1998), and some of them maintain their selectivity irrespective of viewpoint, retinal image size, and even color (for review, see Milner and Goodale, 1995). Moreover, the responses of these cells are not affected by the animal's motor behavior but are instead sensitive to the reinforcement history and significance of the visual stimuli that drive them. It has been suggested that cells in this region might play a role in comparing current visual inputs with internal representations of recalled images (e.g., Eskandar, Richmond, and Optican, 1992), which are themselves presumably stored in other regions, such as neighboring regions of the medial temporal lobe and related limbic areas (Fahy, Riches, and Brown, 1993; Nishijo et al., 1993). In fact, sensitivity to particular objects can be created in ensembles of cells in inferotemporal cortex simply by training the animals to discriminate between different objects (Logothetis, Pauls, and Poggio, 1995). There is also evidence for a specialization within separate regions of the ventral stream for the coding of certain categories of objects, such as faces and hands, which are of particular social significance to the monkey. Finally, recent studies using a binocular rivalry paradigm, in which competing images are presented at the same time to the two eyes, have shown that cells in the monkey's inferotemporal cortex are tuned to what the monkey reports seeing on a particular trial, not simply to what is present on the two eyes (Logothetis, 1998). But neurons earlier in the visual system, such as area V1, do not show these correlations. They respond in the same way no matter what the monkey indicates that it sees. Even in intermediate areas, such as V4, early in the ventral stream, the correlations are relatively weak. These results again provide indirect support for the claim that the ventral stream plays a critical role in delivering the contents of our visual consciousness (insofar as activity in the monkey's inferotemporal cortex reflects what the monkey indicates that it sees). These and other studies lend considerable support to the suggestion that the object-based descriptions provided by the ventral stream form the basic raw material for visual perception, recognition memory, and other long-term representations of the visual world, and that activity in higher regions of this pathway may be correlated with visual consciousness. Interested readers are directed to Milner and Goodale (1995), Perrett and colleagues (1995), Logothetis and Sheinberg (1996), Logothetis, (1998), and Tanaka (2003).

In sharp contrast to the activity of cells in the ventral stream, the responses of cells in the dorsal stream are greatly dependent on the concurrent motor behavior of the animal. Thus, separate subsets of visual cells in the posterior parietal cortex, the major terminal zone for the dorsal stream, have been shown to be implicated in visual fixation, pursuit, and saccadic eye movements, visually guided reaching, and the manipulation of objects (Hyvärinen and Poranen, 1974; Mountcastle et al., 1975). In reviewing these studies, Andersen (1987) has pointed out that most neurons in these areas exhibit both sensory-related and movement-related activity. Moreover, the motor modulation is quite specific. Recent work in Andersen's laboratory, for example, has shown that visual cells in the posterior parietal cortex that code the location of a target for a saccadic eye movement are quite separate from cells in this region that code the location for a manual aiming movement to the same target (Snyder, Batista, and Andersen, 1997). In other experiments (Taira et al., 1990), cells in the anterior intraparietal region of parietal cortex (area AIP), which fire when the monkey manipulates an object, have also been shown to be sensitive to the intrinsic object features, such as size and orientation, that determine the posture of the hand and fingers during a grasping movement. Lesions in this region of the posterior parietal cortex produce deficits in the visual control of reaching and grasping similar in many respects to those seen in humans following damage to the homologous region (e.g., Ettlinger, 1977). In a recent study, small reversible pharmacological lesions were made directly in area AIP. When the circuitry in this region was inactivated, there was a selective interference with preshaping of the hand as the monkey reached out to grasp an object (Gallese et al., 1994). The posterior parietal cortex is also intimately linked with the premotor cortex, the superior colliculus, and the pontine nuclei—brain areas that have also been implicated in various aspects of the visual control of eye, limb, and body movements (for review, see Goodale, 1996). In short, the networks in the dorsal stream have the functional properties and interconnections that one might expect to see in the system concerned with the moment-to-moment control of visually guided actions. (Of necessity, this review of the monkey literature on the dorsal stream is far from complete. Interested readers are directed to Milner and Goodale, 1995, and Cohen and Andersen, 2002.)

Functional Neuroimaging Studies in D.F. As we saw earlier, D.F. has relatively circumscribed lesions in area LO on both sides of her brain. Because area LO has been implicated in object recognition, we suspected that these lesions were responsible for D.F.'s difficulty in recognizing the shape and form of objects. To test this more directly, we carried out a functional MRI (fMRI) study in which we presented D.F. with line drawings of objects versus scrambled versions of the same line drawings. With these stimuli, D.F. was expected to do very poorly, because the only information about the object was conveyed by form and contour information. There were no color or surface cues. When D.F. was shown the line drawings, she was unable to recognize any of them. Not surprisingly, as can be seen in figure 83.6, her brain also showed no differential activation with the line drawings. Neurologically intact observers, of course, showed robust activation with the line drawings. In fact, when a normal observer's brain was stereotactically aligned onto D.F.'s brain, the differential activation with line drawings fell neatly into D.F.'s area LO lesions (see figure 83.6).

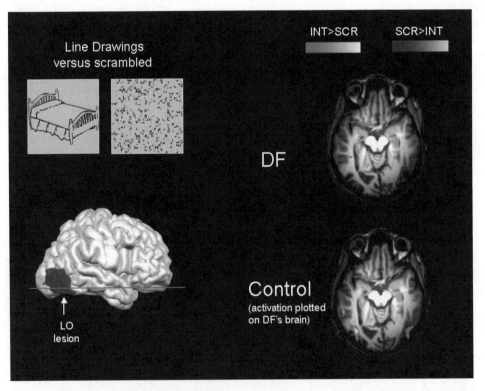

FIGURE 83.6   An fMRI study of activation in D.F. on presentation of line drawings versus scrambled line drawings. D.F. shows essentially no differential activation with line drawings, whereas a control subject shows robust activation. The activation in the control subject has been stereotactically morphed to fit onto D.F.'s brain. Activation to the line drawings falls neatly into the LO lesions. (Adapted with permission from James et al., 2003.) (See color plate 72.)

Although D.F. did not show any activation to line drawings of objects, we suspected that she might show activation to images of objects in which color and texture cues were available, since she was often able to identify the material or "stuff" from which objects were made. Indeed, as figure 83.7 illustrates, when we tested her with such stimuli she showed robust (but somewhat atypical) activation in the fusiform gyrus and other ventral stream areas. Normal subjects, of course, showed robust activation in area LO, and much less in the neighboring fusiform region. Interestingly, though, the activation that D.F. showed in the fusiform region was higher for objects that she could identify than for objects she could not.

So D.F., who has bilateral lesions of area LO, shows no differential activation for line drawings of objects but continues to show robust activation for colored and textured images of objects. These results not only conform extremely well with her behavioral performance with such objects, but also indicate that area LO may play a special role in processing the geometric structure of objects, whereas regions in the fusiform might be more involved in processing information about the material properties of objects, the stuff from which they are made. (For an extended discussion of these issues, see James et al., 2003.) In any case, fMRI results and the structural MRI evidence discussed earlier provide a strong confirmation of our original conjecture (Goodale and Milner, 1992), namely, that D.F.'s problem is related to damage to the ventral stream of visual processing.

But what about the visual control of actions such as grasping, in which D.F. shows relatively normal behavior? To answer this question we carried out an event-related fMRI study of grasping in D.F. Recent neuroimaging experiments have shown that there appears to be a human homologue of monkey area AIP that is activated during visually guided grasping (Binkofski et al., 1998; Culham and Kanwisher, 2001; Culham, 2004; Culham et al., 2003). In our laboratory, Culham and colleagues (2003) have devised an apparatus (the "grasparatus") that permits the presentation of target objects in the scanner in a pseudo-random schedule. As illustrated in figure 83.8, the two most critical tasks in these experiments has been a grasping condition in which the subject reaches out and grasps a small rectangular object that varies in size and orientation and a reaching condition in which the subject simply reaches out and touches the object with the back of the knuckles without forming a grasp at all. When these two conditions are compared, and a number of somatosensory and motor control tasks are carried out, an area in the posterior parietal cortex in the more anterior part of the IPS has been identified that appears to be homologous with area AIP. Interestingly, normal subjects show no differential activation in area LO when they grasp an object, indicating that the analysis of object structure for grasping may be mediated by the dorsal stream, quite independently from any ventral stream processing (see figure 83.8).

When D.F. was tested with the grasparatus, she showed robust activation, when she grasped the target objects, in a

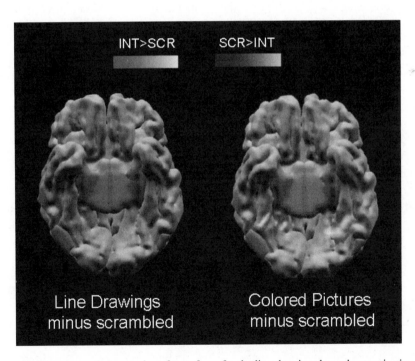

FIGURE 83.7   Activation maps drawn on the ventral surface of D.F.'s brain that represent the comparison of intact line drawing with scrambled line drawing (left) and intact colored pictures with scrambled colored pictures (right). D.F. shows no fMRI activation for the line drawings but robust activation in the fusiform gyrus for the colored pictures. (Adapted with permission from James et al., 2003.) (See color plate 73.)

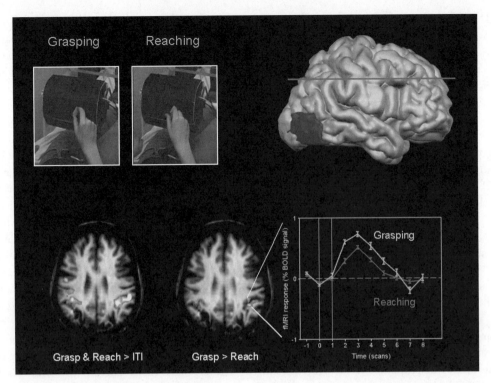

FIGURE 83.8 The "grasparatus" devised by Culham and colleagues (2003) is shown in the upper left. The subject lies in the dark inside the MRI magnet. The solid shapes appear in front of the subject as the cylinder is made to rotate stepwise by a pneumatic motor. The target shape is presented by turning on a superbright LED behind the shape. The task is either to grasp the target shape or, in a control condition, to simply touch it with the knuckles. A section imaged through D.F.'s parietal lobe reveals selective activation in an anterior part of the IPS (area AIP) when she grasps the target object. This activation is similar to that seen in control subjects. (Adapted with permission from James et al., 2003.) (See color plate 74.)

region that appears to correspond to area AIP, despite the fact that moderate degeneration was evident in the IPS (see figure 83.8). This result, coupled with the observation that area LO is damaged bilaterally in D.F., provides strong support for the argument that the visual control of object-directed grasping does not depend on object recognition mechanisms in the ventral stream but instead is mediated by object-driven visuomotor systems in the dorsal stream.

In short, the new MRI and fMRI findings with D.F. provide a striking confirmation of our earlier proposal that visual perception and the visual control of action depend on separate visual pathways in the cerebral cortex, and confirm the respective roles of the ventral and dorsal visual streams in these functions.

The integration of perception and action

Although the dorsal action stream and the ventral perception stream are anatomically and functionally distinct, the two streams must work together in everyday life. Indeed, an argument can be made that the two streams play complementary roles in the production of adaptive behavior.

A useful metaphor for understanding the different contributions of the dorsal and ventral stream to visually guided behavior can be found in robotic engineering. That metaphor is *teleassistance* (Pook and Ballard, 1996). In teleassistance, a human operator identifies the goal and then uses a symbolic language to communicate with a semiautonomous robot that actually performs the required motor act on the identified goal object. Teleassistance is much more flexible than completely autonomous robotic control, which is limited to the working environment for which it has been programmed and cannot cope easily with novel events. Teleassistance is also more efficient than teleoperation, in which a human operator simply controls the movement of a manipulandum at a distance. As Pook and Ballard (1996) have demonstrated, teleoperation (i.e., with a human operator) cannot cope with sudden changes in scale or a delay between action and feedback from that action. In short, teleassistance combines the flexibility of teleoperation with the precision of autonomous routines.

The interaction between the ventral and dorsal streams is an excellent example of the principle of teleassistance, but in this case instantiated in biology. The perceptual-cognitive systems in the ventral stream, like the human operator in teleassistance, identify different objects in the scene, using a representational system that is rich and detailed but not metrically precise. When a particular goal object has been flagged, dedicated visuomotor networks in the dorsal stream (in conjunction with related circuits in premotor cortex, basal ganglia, and brainstem) are activated to perform the desired motor act. Thus, the networks in the dorsal stream, with their precise egocentric coding of the location, size, orientation, and shape of the goal object, are like the robotic component of teleassistance. Thus, both systems are required for purposive behavior—one system to select the goal object from the visual array, the other to carry out the required metrical computations for the goal-directed action. One of the most important questions yet to be addressed is how the two streams communicate with one another (Goodale and Milner, 2004).

REFERENCES

ANDERSEN, R. A., 1987. Inferior parietal lobule function in spatial perception and visuomotor integration. In *Handbook of Physiology*, Sect. 1, *The Nervous System*, Vol. V, *Higher Functions of the Brain, Pt. 2*, V. B. Mountcastle, F. Plum, and S. R. Geiger, eds. Bethesda, Md.: American Physiological Association, pp. 483–518.

BÁLINT, R., 1909. Seelenlämung des "Schauens," optische Ataxie, räumliche Störung der Aufmerksamkeit. *Monatsch. Psychiatr. Neurolog.* 25:51–81.

BINKOFSKI, F., C. DOHLE, S. POSSE, K. M. STEPHAN, H. HEFTER, R. J. SEITZ, et al., 1998. Human anterior intraparietal area subserves prehension: A combined lesion and functional MRI activation study. *Neurology* 50:1253–1259.

BÜLTHOFF, H. H., and S. EDELMAN, 1992. Psychophysical support for a two-dimensional view interpolation theory of object recognition. *Proc. Natl. Acad Sci. U.S.A.* 89:60–64.

COHEN, Y. E., and R. A. ANDERSEN, 2002. A common reference frame for movement plans in the posterior parietal cortex. *Nat. Rev. Neurosci.* 3:553–562.

CRICK, F., and E. JONES, 1993. Backwardness of human neuroanatomy. *Nature* 361:109–110.

CRICK, F., and C. KOCH, 2003. A framework for consciousness. *Nat. Neurosci.* 6:119–126.

CULHAM, J. C., 2004. Human brain imaging reveals a parietal area specialized for grasping. In *Attention and Performance XX. Functional Brain Imaging of Visual Cognition*, N. Kanwisher and J. Duncan, eds. Oxford, England: Oxford University Press.

CULHAM, J. C., S. L. DANCKERT, J. F. X. DESOUZA, J. S. GATI, R. S. MENON, and M. A. GOODALE, 2003. Visually-guided grasping produces activation in dorsal but not ventral brain areas. *Exp. Brain Res.* 153:180–189.

CULHAM, J. C., and N. G. KANWISHER, 2001. Neuroimaging of cognitive functions in human parietal cortex. *Curr. Opin. Neurobiol.* 11:157–163.

DYDE, R. T., and A. D. MILNER, 2002. Two illusions of perceived orientation: One fools all of the people some of the time; the other fools all of the people all of the time. *Exp. Brain Res.* 144:518–527.

ESKANDAR, E. M., B. J. RICHMOND, and L. M. OPTICAN, 1992. Role of inferior temporal neurons in visual memory. I. Temporal encoding of information about visual images, recalled images, and behavioral context. *J. Neurophysiol.* 68:1277–1295.

ETTLINGER, G., 1977. Parietal cortex in visual orientation. In *Physiological Aspects of Clinical Neurology*, F. C. Rose, ed. Oxford, England: Blackwell.

EWERT, J.-P., 1987. Neuroethology of releasing mechanisms: Prey-catching in toads. *Behav. Brain Sci.* 10:337–405.

FAHY, F. L., I. P. RICHES, and M. W. BROWN, 1993. Neuronal signals of importance to the performance of visual recognition memory tasks: Evidence from recordings of single neurones in the medial thalamus of primates. *Prog. Brain Res.* 95:401–416.

FLANDERS, M., S. I. H. TILLERY, and J. F. SOECHTING, 1992. Early stages in a sensorimotor transformation. *Behav. Brain Sci.* 15: 309–362.

GALLESE, V., A. MURATA, M. KASEDA, N. NIKI, and H. SAKATA, 1994. Deficit of hand preshaping after muscimol injection in monkey parietal cortex. *Neuroreport* 5:1525–1529.

GLICKSTEIN M., S. BUCHBINDER, and J. L. MAY 3rd, 1998. Visual control of the arm, the wrist and the fingers: Pathways through the brain. *Neuropsychologia* 36:981–1001.

GOODALE, M. A., 1995. The cortical organization of visual perception and visuomotor contol. In *An Invitation to Cognitive Science*, vol. 2, *Visual Cognition and Action*, 2nd ed., S. Kosslyn, ed. Cambridge, Mass: MIT Press.

GOODALE, M. A., 1996. Visuomotor modules in the vertebrate brain. *Can. J. Physiol. Pharm.* 74:390–400.

GOODALE, M. A., and A. M. HAFFENDEN, 1998. Frames of reference for perception and action in the human visual system. *Neurosci. Biobehav. Rev.* 22:161–172.

GOODALE, M.A., and G. K. HUMPHREY, 1998. The objects of action and perception. *Cognition* 67:181–207.

GOODALE, M. A., L. S. JAKOBSON, and J. M. KEILLOR, 1994. Differences in the visual control of pantomimed and natural grasping movements. *Neuropsychologia* 32:1159–1178.

GOODALE, M. A., J. P. MEENAN, H. H. BÜLTHOFF, D. A. NICOLLE, K. S. MURPHY, and C. I. RACICOT, 1994. Separate neural pathways for the visual analysis of object shape in perception and prehension. *Curr. Biol.* 4:604–610.

GOODALE, M. A., and A. D. MILNER, 1992. Separate visual pathways for perception and action. *Trends Neurosci.* 15:20–25.

GOODALE, M. A, and A. D. MILNER (2004). *Sight Unseen: An Exploration of Conscious and Unconscious Vision*. Oxford, England: Oxford University Press.

GOODALE, M. A., A. D. MILNER, L. S. JAKOBSON, and D. P. CAREY, 1991. A neurological dissociation between perceiving objects and grasping them. *Nature* 349:154–156.

GOODALE, M. A., K. MURPHY, J. P. MEENAN, C. I. RACICOT, and D. A. NICOLLE, 1993. Spared object perception but poor object-calibrated grasping in a patient with optic ataxia. *Soc. Neurosci. Abstr.* 19:775.

GOULD, J. L., 1982. *Ethology: The Mechanisms and Evolution of Behavior*. New York: Norton.

GRILL-SPECTOR, K., 2003. The neural basis of object perception. *Curr. Opin. Neurobiol.* 13:159–166.

HAFFENDEN, A. M., K. C. SCHIFF, and M. A. GOODALE, 2001. The dissociation between perception and action in the Ebbinghaus illusion: Nonillusory effects of pictorial cues on grasp. *Curr. Biol.* 11:177–181.

HOFF, B., and M. A. ARBIB, 1992. A model of the effects of speed, accuracy and perturbation on visually guided reaching. In *Control of Arm movement in Space: Neurophysiological and Computational Approaches*, R. Caminiti, P. B. Johnson, and Y. Burnod, eds. New York: Springer-Verlag, pp. 285–306.

HYVÄRINEN, J., and A. PORANEN, 1974. Function of the parietal associative area 7 as revealed from cellular discharges in alert monkeys. *Brain* 97:673–692.

INGLE, D. J., 1973. Two visual systems in the frog. *Science* 181: 1053–1055.

INGLE, D. J., 1982. Organization of visuomotor behaviors in vertebrates. In *Analysis of Visual Behavior*, D. J. Ingle, M. A. Goodale, and R. J. W. Mansfield, eds. Cambridge, Mass.: MIT Press, pp. 67–109.

INGLE, D. J., 1991. Functions of subcortical visual systems in vertebrates and the evolution of higher visual mechanisms. In *Vision and Visual Dysfunction*, Vol. 2: *Evolution of the Eye and Visual System*, R. L. Gregory and J. Cronly-Dillon, eds. London: Macmillan, pp. 152–164.

JACKSON, J. H., 1875. *Clinical and Physiological Researches on the Nervous System*. London: Churchill.

JAKOBSON, L. S., Y. M. ARCHIBALD, D. P. CAREY, and M. A. GOODALE, 1991. A kinematic analysis of reaching and grasping movements in a patient recovering from optic ataxia. *Neuropsychologia* 29:803–809.

JAMES, T. W., G. K. HUMPHREY, J. S. GATI, R. S. MENON, and M. A. GOODALE, 2000. The effects of visual object priming on brain activation before and after recognition. *Curr. Biol.* 10:1017–1024.

JAMES, T. W., G. K. HUMPHREY, J. S. GATI, R. S. MENON, and M. A. GOODALE, 2002. Differential effects of viewpoint on object-driven activation in dorsal and ventral streams. *Neuron* 35:793–801.

JAMES, T. W., J. CULHAM, G. K. HUMPHREY, D. A. MILNER, and M. A. GOODALE, 2003. Ventral occipital lesions impair object recognition but not object-directed grasping: An fMRI study. *Brain* 126:2463–2475.

JEANNEROD, M., 1988. *The Neural and Behavioural Organization of Goal-directed Movements*. Oxford, England: Oxford University Press.

JEANNEROD, M., J. DECETY, and F. MICHEL, 1994. Impairment of grasping movements following bilateral posterior parietal lesion. *Neuropsychologia* 32:369–380.

KANWISHER, N., P. DOWNING, R. EPSTEIN, and Z. KOURTZI, 2001. Functional neuroimaging of visual recognition. In *Handbook of Functional Neuroimaging of Cognition*, R. Cabeza and A. Kingstone, eds. Cambridge, Mass.: MIT Press, pp. 109–152.

KLÜVER, H., and P. C. BUCY, 1939. Preliminary analysis of functions of the temporal lobes of monkeys. *Arch. Neurol. Psychiatry* 42:979–1000.

LOGOTHETIS, N., 1998. Object vision and visual awareness. *Curr. Opin. Neurobiol.* 8:536–544.

LOGOTHETIS, N. K., J. PAULS, and T. POGGIO, 1995. Shape representation in the inferior temporal cortex of monkeys. *Curr. Biol.* 5:552–563.

LOGOTHETIS, N. K., and D. L. SHEINBERG, 1996. Visual object recognition. *Ann. Rev. Neurosci.* 19:577–621.

MALACH, R., I. LEVY, and U. HASSON, 2002. The topography of high-order human object areas. *Trends Cogn. Sci.* 6:176–184.

MARR, D., 1982. *Vision.* San Francisco: Freeman.

MILNER, A. D., and M. A. GOODALE, 1995. *The Visual Brain in Action.* Oxford, England: Oxford University Press.

MILNER, A. D., D. I. PERRETT, R. S. JOHNSTON, P. J. BENSON, T. R. JORDAN, D. W. HEELEY, D. BETTUCCI, F. MORTARA, R. MUTANI, E. TERAZZI, and D. L. W. DAVIDSON, 1991. Perception and action in visual form agnosia. *Brain* 114:405–428.

MOUNTCASTLE, V. B., J. C. LYNCH, A. GEORGOPOULOS, H. SAKATA, and C. ACUNA, 1975. Posterior parietal association cortex of the monkey: Command functions for operations within extrapersonal space. *J. Neurophysiol.* 38:871–908.

NISHIJO, H., T. ONO, R. TAMURA, and K. NAKAMURA, 1993. Amygdalar and hippocampal neuron responses related to recognition and memory in monkey. *Prog. Brain Res.* 95:339–358.

PALMER, S., E. ROSCH, and P. CHASE, 1981. Canonical perspective and the perception of objects. In *Attention and Performance IX*, J. Long and A. Baddeley A, eds. Hillsdale, N.J.: Earlbaum, pp. 135–151.

PATLA, A., and M. A. GOODALE, 1997. Visuomotor transformation required for obstacle avoidance during locomotion is unaffected in a patient with visual form agnosia. *Neuroreport* 8:165–168.

PERENIN, M.-T., and Y. ROSSETTI, 1996. Grasping without form discrimination in a hemianopic field. *Neuroreport* 7:793–797.

PERENIN, M.-T., and A. VIGHETTO, 1988. Optic ataxia: A specific disruption in visuomotor mechanisms. I. Different aspects of the deficit in reaching for objects. *Brain* 111:643–674.

PERRETT, D., P. J. BENSON, J. K. HIETANEN, M. W. ORAM, and W. H. DITTRICH, 1995. When is a face not a face? In *The Artful Eye*, R. Gregory, J. Harris, P. Heard, and D. Rose, eds. Oxford, England: Oxford University Press, pp. 95–124

POHL, W., 1973. Dissociation of spatial discrimination deficits following frontal and parietal lesions in monkeys. *J. Comp. Physiol. Psychol.* 82:227–239.

POOK, P. K., and D. H. BALLARD, 1996. Deictic human/robot interaction. *Robot. Auton. Syst.* 18:259–269.

PRIBRAM, K. H., 1967. Memory and the organization of attention. In *Brain Function and Learning*, Vol. IV, *UCLA Forum in Medical Sciences 6*, D. B. Lindsley and A. A. Lumsdaine, eds. Berkeley: University of California Press, pp. 79–122.

SERVOS, P., M. A. GOODALE, and G. K. HUMPHREY, 1993. The drawing of objects by a visual form agnosic: Contribution of surface properties and memorial representations. *Neuropsychologia* 31:251–259.

SERVOS, P., L. MATIN, and M. A. GOODALE, 1995. Dissociations between two forms of spatial processing by a visual form agnosic. *Neuroreport* 6:1893–1896.

SNYDER, L. H., A. P. BATISTA, and R. A. ANDERSEN, 1997. Coding of intention in the posterior parietal cortex. *Nature* 386:167–170.

STEIN, J. F., 1992. The representation of egocentric space in the posterior parietal cortex. *Behav. Brain Sci.* 15:691–700.

TAIRA, M., S. MINE, A. P. GEORGOPOULOS, A. MURATA, and H. SAKATA, 1990. Parietal cortex neurons of the monkey related to the visual guidance of hand movement. *Exp. Brain Res.* 83:29–36.

TANAKA, K. 2003. Columns for complex visual object features in the inferotemporal cortex: clustering of cells with similar but slightly different stimulus selectivities. *Cereb. Cortex* 13:90–99.

TOOTELL, R., D. TSAO, and W. VANDUFFEL, 2003. Neuroimaging weighs in: Humans meet macaques in "primate" visual cortex. *J. Neurosci.* 23:3981–3989.

UNGERLEIDER, L. G., and B. A. BRODY, 1977. Extrapersonal spatial orientation: The role of posterior parietal, anterior frontal, and inferotemporal cortex. *Exp. Neurol.* 56:265–280.

UNGERLEIDER, L. G., and M. MISHKIN, 1982. Two cortical visual systems. In *Analysis of Visual Behavior*, D. J. Ingle, M. A. Goodale, and R. J. W. Mansfield, eds. Cambridge, Mass.: MIT Press, pp. 549–586.

VAN ESSEN, D. C., J. W. LEWIS, H. A. DRURY, N. HADJIKHANI, R. B. TOOTELL, M. BAKIRCIOGLU, and M. I. MILLER, 2001. Mapping visual cortex in monkeys and humans using surface-based atlases. *Vision Res.* 41:1359–1378.

84 Neural Correlates of Visual Consciousness in Humans

GERAINT REES

ABSTRACT The immediacy and directness of conscious experience belies the complexity of the underlying neural mechanisms, which remain incompletely understood. This chapter focuses on the neural correlates of visual consciousness in humans. Activity in functionally specialized areas of ventral visual cortex is necessary for visual awareness, but recent evidence suggests that such activity may not be sufficient to support conscious vision without a contribution from parietal and prefrontal areas, reflecting processes such as selective attention and working memory. Reciprocal interactions between parietal and ventral visual cortex can serve to selectively integrate internal representations of visual events in the broader behavioral context in which they occur. Such network interactions may account for the richness of our conscious experience and may provide a fundamental neural substrate for visual consciousness.

We all have first-hand knowledge of what it is to be conscious, as opposed to not being conscious (for example, in deep dreamless sleep). When we are conscious, our experiences have specific phenomenal content, and when consciousness is absent, phenomenal content is also absent. During waking, the phenomenal content of our experience is constantly changing. Yet at the same time, our sense of self, of the person having the experience, remains constant. These phenomenal differences highlight a useful distinction between factors that influence the overall *level* of consciousness, those that determine its *content*, and those associated with *self-awareness*. The contents of consciousness can vary independently of the level of consciousness. Specific brain lesions can alter the contents of consciousness without having any effect on the level of consciousness. For example, lesions of the fusiform and lingual gyri can result in loss of awareness of color (achromatopsia) while the awareness of other aspects of the world remains normal (Verrey, 1888; Pearlman, Birch, and Meadows, 1979; Damasio, 1980). This chapter describes what is known about the neural correlates of the contents of consciousness in humans.

Questions about the neural correlates of the contents of consciousness are invariably questions about the relationship between mental representations and neural representations (Frith, Perry, and Lumer, 1999). It is generally accepted (though see O'Regan and Noe, 2001, for a contrasting view) that a neural representation of a particular feature or object is necessary for that feature or object to be present in consciousness. Some property of a neural population (for example, instantaneous spike rate or coherence) may encode a specific dimension of conscious visual experience. The search for neural correlates of consciousness is therefore a search for those neural populations and neural properties that encode a corresponding dimension of the contents of consciousness. It is assumed that a change in a mental representation of some phenomenal property entails a corresponding change in its neural representation, but the converse is not true: changes in neural representations may occur in the absence of changes in mental representations (Frith, Perry, and Lumer, 1999). Such an account necessarily eschews many philosophical debates (see Noe and Thompson, 2002) in favor of a pragmatic, empirical approach (Crick and Koch, 2003).

The neural correlates of the contents of consciousness have been studied most extensively in the visual system (Rees, Wojciulik, et al., 2002) and will be focused on here. The primate visual system is organized in a distributed and hierarchical fashion; in the monkey, different aspects of the visual scene are analyzed in different cortical areas (Zeki, 1978; Felleman and Van Essen, 1991). An organization into dorsal and ventral streams leading away from primary visual cortex is apparent (Ungerleider and Mishkin, 1982). In humans, the organization of visual cortex appears broadly similar to that in monkeys, including retinotopically mapped striate and extrastriate visual areas (Engel et al., 1994; Sereno et al., 1995; Brewer et al., 2002) with specific functional specializations (e.g., Zeki et al., 1991). However, there also appear to be differences in both overall organization and specific functional roles between human and macaque monkey visual cortex (Culham and Kanwisher, 2001), including substantial differences in the organization and relative size of parietal and prefrontal cortex. These differences should be borne in mind when comparing both the study of visual perception (Povinelli and Vonk, 2003) and physiological data (Tootell, Tsao, and Vanduffel, 2003) in human and nonhuman primates. This chapter will focus almost entirely on data from humans.

GERAINT REES   Institute of Cognitive Neuroscience and Wellcome Department of Imaging Neuroscience, University College London, London, U.K.

Human primary visual cortex

Human primary visual cortex (V1) is located in the calcarine sulcus in occipital cortex (Henschen, 1893). Damage to this area leads to a circumscribed retinotopic visual field defect (scotoma) in which conscious perception of all visual attributes, including form, brightness, and contrast, is typically absent. There is a topographic mapping between field defects and the physical location of cortical damage (Inouye, 1909; Holmes and Lister, 1916), consistent with the retinotopic representation observed in monkeys (Hubel and Wiesel, 1968, 1974) that was subsequently revealed in humans by functional imaging (Engel et al., 1994; Sereno et al., 1995) and the distribution of phosphenes (perceived flashes of light) produced by direct electrical stimulation (Brindley and Lewin, 1968; Dobelle et al., 1979).

Within a scotoma, conscious perception of all visual properties, including brightness, contrast, and form, is lost, and cannot be induced in patients with striate lesions by transcranial magnetic stimulation (TMS) over ipsilesional extrastriate cortex (Cowey and Walsh, 2000). By comparison, phenomenal experience in the remainder of the visual field appears to be well preserved, although there may be subtle abnormalities detectable psychophysically (Rizzo and Robin, 1996). Some patients with primary visual cortex damage can show a surprising range of preserved abilities to detect and discriminate stimuli within a phenomenally blind scotoma. This ability, in the absence of awareness, has become known as blindsight (Weiskrantz, 1986). An apparently similar phenomenon, dissociating awareness and discrimination performance, can be seen with dichoptic displays in normal observers (Kolb and Braun, 1995), though this has not always been replicated (Morgan, Mason, and Solomon, 1997; Robichaud and Stelmach, 2003). These data suggest that intact primary visual cortex may be necessary for conscious awareness of brightness, contrast, and at least some aspects of form. However, whether altered awareness following damage to primary visual cortex reflects disruption of neural representations just in V1 itself, impaired onward passage of signals to extrastriate cortex, or altered feedback from extrastriate areas is unclear.

The relationship between neural representations in intact primary visual cortex and the contents of consciousness has been studied directly using functional imaging techniques (Rees, Kreiman, and Koch, 2002; Tong, 2003). Binocular rivalry provides a powerful experimental paradigm with which to study the neural correlates of visual awareness (e.g., Levelt, 1965; Leopold and Logothetis, 1999). When dissimilar images are presented to the two eyes, they compete for perceptual dominance. Each image may be visible in turn for a few seconds while the other is suppressed. Because perceptual transitions between each monocular view occur spontaneously without any change in the physical stimulus,

neural correlates of consciousness may be distinguished from neural correlates attributable to stimulus characteristics. In nonhuman primates, most visually responsive neurons early in visual cortex show patterns of firing that mirror the stimulus, rather than the contents of consciousness. In contrast, human functional magnetic resonance imaging (fMRI) studies have shown quantitatively much stronger modulations of primary visual cortex. Over the whole of V1, fluctuations in activity during rivalry have been measured for monocular stimuli differing in contrast, and can be about half as large as those evoked by real stimulus alternation (Polonsky et al., 2000; Lee and Blake, 2002). In a region of primary visual cortex corresponding to the blind spot (a monocular representation corresponding to just the other eye), fluctuations during rivalry and physical stimulus alternations are approximately equal (Tong and Engel, 2001) (figure 84.1). Such an association between V1 activity (as measured with fMRI in humans) and visual experience is not restricted to bistable perception. In a contrast detection task, false alarms (i.e., incorrect reports of seeing a stimulus in its absence) evoke more activity in primary visual cortex than misses, despite the stimuli being physically identical (Ress and Heeger, 2003). Neuromagnetic responses localized to V1 correspond more closely to the perceived than the physical contrast of a briefly flashed stimulus (Haynes et al., 2003). Taken together, these data suggest that hemodynamic activity in human primary visual cortex (as measured with fMRI) can more closely reflect the contents of consciousness than the physical properties of the stimulus, at least for certain stimulus features (e.g., perceived brightness or contrast). However, the discrepancy between some monkey electrophysiological results, which show minimal perceptual modulation among V1 or V2 cells during binocular rivalry (Leopold and Logothetis, 1996), and the corresponding human fMRI results, with strong perceptual modulation in V1, remains to be resolved. Such an understanding will depend on the exact relationship between spiking activity in cortical neurons and the corresponding fMRI blood-oxygen-level-dependent (BOLD) activity (see Logothetis, this volume).

Necessity and sufficiency of striate cortex activity

The data discussed in the previous section could be taken to suggest that when certain visual features are represented in consciousness, activity is present in primary visual cortex. However, awareness of other stimulus features appears possible even when V1 is damaged. Some patients with blindsight seem to have residual impressions of salient moving stimuli (Riddoch, 1917; Barbur et al., 1993; Stoerig and Barth, 2001), and one such patient has awareness of visual afterimages despite his inability to perceive the original adapting stimulus (Weiskrantz, Cowey, and Hodinott-Hill,

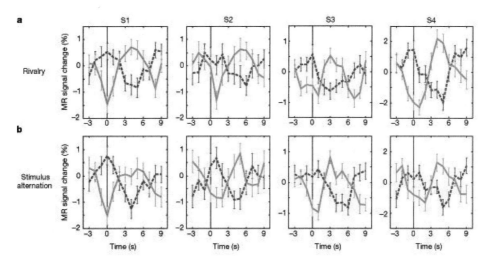

FIGURE 84.1   Rivalry in the V1 blind-spot representation. Average fMRI activity in the V1 blind-spot representation is shown for four subjects during perceptual switches to a grating presented ipsilaterally (solid line) or blind-spot grating (dotted line) for both rivalry (*a*) and physical stimulus alternation (*b*). Vertical lines at time zero indicate the time of the subject's response. Activity during binocular rivalry and physical stimulus alternation is very similar. (*a*) During rivalry, fMRI activity increases sharply soon after the ipsi-lateral grating becomes dominant in awareness and decreases when the blind-spot grating becomes dominant. (*b*) Very similar fMRI responses occur during stimulus alternations between the two monocular gratings. (fMRI responses typically peak 2–6 s after stimulus onset because of haemodynamic lag.) (Reprinted with permission from F. Tong and S. A. Engel, Interocular rivalry revealed in the human cortical blind-spot representation. *Nature* 411:195–199. © 2001 by the Nature Publishing Group.)

2002). Thus, phenomenal vision within scotomas in blindsight is severely degraded but not always completely absent. Consequently, V1 damage may impair only the contents of consciousness whose neural representation is contingent on V1 activity, specifically brightness, contrast, and some aspects of form.

It is also apparent that not all features that are neurally represented in V1 are also represented in consciousness. For example, signals from the two eyes remain segregated as they arrive at the input layers of V1 (Hubel and Weisel, 1968, 1974). However, although this information is available unconsciously (for example, in the computation of perceived depth; von Helmholtz, 1867), psychophysical studies suggest that reliable eye-of-origin discriminations are not possible (Ono and Barbeito, 1985). Thus, eye-of-origin information is strongly represented in some layers of V1 but not ordinarily in the contents of consciousness. Similar conclusions have been reached from the study of orientation-specific adaptation. Such adaptation is presumed to reflect changes in the activity in V1, the first location in the visual pathway where neurons respond to oriented stimuli (Hubel and Wiesel, 1974). The orientation of a grating can be rendered invisible and impossible to discriminate when it is presented in the periphery, with four similar gratings positioned above and below it, due to crowding. However, adaptation to such a grating can result in an orientation-dependent aftereffect (where the earlier adaptation influences the perceived orientation of a subsequently presented stimulus) that is indistinguishable from that produced when it is presented alone with its orientation clearly (and consciously) perceived (He, Cavanagh, and Intriligator, 1996). Similarly, very high-frequency gratings that are perceptually indistinguishable from a uniform field can nevertheless produce robust orientation-dependent aftereffects (He and MacLeod, 2001). The presence of aftereffects from stimuli that are not consciously perceived (Blake and Fox, 1974) indicates that stimulus properties must be represented outside awareness. Thus, the mere presence of a feature representation in V1 is not a useful guide to whether V1 activity correlates well with the contents of consciousness for that feature.

Moreover, physiological observations of human V1 indicate that activity in V1 is not always well correlated with the contents of consciousness. A lesion of the extrastriate visual cortex that isolates primary visual cortex can result in blindness, yet evoked potentials from V1 can still be recorded (Bodis-Wollner et al., 1977). In normal observers, some V1 activity can be evoked even when a stimulus is judged to be phenomenally absent (Ress, Backus, and Heeger, 2000), and activity in primary visual cortex may also be evoked during a period of expectation when visual stimulation (and phenomenal experience) is absent (Kastner et al., 1999). Following damage to parietal cortex causing visual extinction (deficient awareness for contralesional visual stimuli, particularly when a competing stimulus is also present ipsilesionally), visual stimulation can evoke activity in primary visual cortex in the absence of awareness (Rees, Wojciulik, et al., 2000; Vuilleumier et al., 2002). Finally, high-frequency flickering stimuli evoke responses from human V1 despite being above the flicker fusion frequency and hence consciously perceived as of constant brightness (Maier et al., 1987; Krolak-Salmon et al., 2003). Thus, some changes in activity in primary visual cortex can be seen in the absence of changes in the contents of consciousness.

Taken together, these data suggest that activity in V1 may be necessary but not sufficient for awareness of some stimulus features such as brightness, contrast, and some aspects of form (Crick and Koch, 1995). For awareness of other stimulus features, such as some aspects of motion, V1 activity may not be necessary at all (Riddoch, 1917; Zeki and ffytche, 1998).

Human extrastriate and ventral visual cortex

Extrastriate visual cortex in humans consists of multiple functionally specialized areas, many of which are retinotopically organized (Wandell, 1999), as in monkey (Felleman and Van Essen, 1991). A prominent clinical finding is that damage to cortical areas containing neurons that represent particular features of the visual environment leads to remarkably specific deficits in the corresponding contents of visual consciousness. For example, damage to V5/MT leads to akinetopsia (the inability to see fast movement; Zihl, von Cramon, and Mai, 1983), but has no effect on color perception (Vaina, 1994). Indeed, the clinical syndrome of akinetopsia following V5/MT damage may be specific for particular types of motion perception. Patients with bilateral V5/MT lesions may have some preservation of conscious perception of motion at low velocities (Hess, Baker, and Zihl, 1989; McLeod et al., 1989; Zihl, von Cramon, and Mai, 1983; Zihl et al., 1991; Rizzo, Nawrot, and Zihl, 1995) and spared perception of biological motion (McLeod et al., 1989; Vaina et al., 1990). Nevertheless, the general principle appears to be that damage to an area specific for the analysis of visual motion leads to a specific deficit in the conscious representation of visual motion. Similarly, damage to different areas of the fusiform or lingual gyri may cause prosopagnosia (the inability to recognize faces) or achromatopsia (the inability to see color; Verrey, 1888; Pearlman, Birch, and Meadows, 1979; Damasio, Tranel, and Rizzo, 2000), which may be restricted to particular quadrants of the visual field (Gallant, Shoup, and Mazer, 2000). In each case, although a specific aspect of phenomenal awareness is impaired, contents of consciousness reflecting undamaged feature representations remain intact. This suggests that appropriate activity in a functionally specialized cortical visual area is required to evoke consciousness of the attribute analyzed in that area (Zeki, 2003).

Neuroimaging data appear consistent with this general notion. Phenomenal contingent aftereffects based on color or motion activate either V4 (Sakai et al., 1995; Hadjikhani et al., 1998; Barnes et al., 1999) or V5/MT (Tootell et al.,

1995; He, Cohen, and Hu, 1998; Culham et al., 1999; though see Huk, Ress, and Heeger, 2001), respectively, and the time course of such activation reflects phenomenal experience (Tootell et al., 1995; He, Cohen, and Hu, 1998; but see Huk, Ress, and Heeger, 2001). Perception of illusory or implied motion in a static visual stimulus results in activation of V5/MT (Zeki, Watson, and Frackowiak, 1993; Kourtzi and Kanwisher, 2000). Disruption of activity in V5/MT using TMS disrupts motion perception (Beckers and Zeki, 1995) and perception and storage of the motion aftereffect (Theoret et al., 2002). Both transcranial and direct electrical stimulation of V5/MT in the absence of visual stimulation can induce motion hallucinations (Penfield and Rasmussen, 1950; Lee et al., 2000; Pascual-Leone and Walsh, 2001). Perception of subjective figures activates extrastriate cortex (Hirsch et al., 1995; ffytche and Zeki, 1996; Stanley and Rubin, 2003). Finally, differential activity in word-processing areas is present when subjects are consciously aware of visually presented words versus consonant letter strings, and absent when they are not due to inattention (Rees et al., 1999) (figure 84.2). Common to all these experimental paradigms are changes in subjects' phenomenal experience without corresponding physical stimulus changes. Altered brain activity is observed in areas of the brain known (or suspected) to contain neurons whose stimulus specificities encompass the attribute represented in consciousness.

Activity corresponding to phenomenal experience can also be seen in the absence of visual stimulation. Patients with schizophrenia who experience visual and auditory hallucinations show activity in modality-specific cortex during hallucinatory episodes (Silbersweig et al., 1995; Dierks et al., 1999). Similarly, patients with damage to the peripheral visual system who experience hallucinations with specific phenomenal content show activity in functionally specialized areas of visual cortex corresponding to the content of their hallucinations (ffytche et al., 1998). In normal subjects, visual imagery activates category-specific areas of visual cortex (D'Esposito et al., 1997; Goebel et al., 2001; Howard et al., 1998; O'Craven and Kanwisher, 2000; Ishai, Ungerleider, and Haxby, 2000).

Investigations of bistable perception are consistent with the general picture outlined above. Responses in fusiform face area (FFA) or parahippocampal place area (PPA) as a function of awareness for faces or houses during binocular rivalry are larger than those in VI, and equal in magnitude to responses evoked by real alternation of stimuli (Tong et al., 1998). This suggests that neural competition during rivalry has been resolved by these later stages of visual processing, and that activity in FFA (or PPA) therefore reflects the contents of consciousness rather than the retinal stimulus. In addition, fluctuations in activity in human V5/MT are seen during reversals in the motion of a bistable stimu-

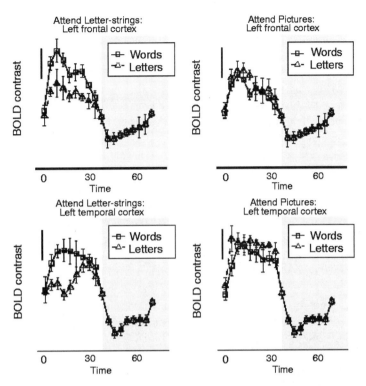

FIGURE 84.2 Attention is necessary for conscious word perception. Time course of activity in left frontal (upper) and left posterior basal temporal cortex (the visual word form area; lower). All four panels use the same plotting conventions. Average BOLD contrast evoked at each locus is plotted as a function of time, collapsing across epochs and participants. The areas whose time courses are shown were identified as those areas showing a maximal simple main effect of words under attention to letters. Unshaded areas represent scans acquired in the experimental conditions and shaded areas represent those acquired during the passive fixation baseline. Error bars indicate interparticipant standard error and dark scale bar represents 0.5% BOLD signal change. Activity evoked when the letter stream contained meaningful words is plotted with black squares and a solid line, and activity when the same stream included only meaningless letter strings is plotted with triangles and a dotted line. (Reprinted with permission from G. Rees et al., Inattentional blindness versus inattentional amnesia for fixated but ignored words. *Science* 286:2504–2507. © 1999 by the American Association for the Advancement of Science.)

lus (Muckli et al., 2002; Sterzer et al., 2002). Qualitatively, these observations are compatible with findings in monkeys demonstrating that the majority of neurons in inferior temporal cortex show responses that reflect the monkey's percept rather than the retinal stimulus (Logothetis and Schall, 1989; Leopold and Logothetis, 1996).

The activity of single neurons can be recorded in even more anterior regions of the medial temporal lobe in epileptic patients in whom electrodes have been implanted for presurgical mapping. Category-specific neural responses are seen both during visual stimulation (Kreiman, Koch, and Fried, 2000a) and during visual imagery (Kreiman, Koch, and Fried, 2000b), and such neurons fire selectively when their preferred stimulus is perceived, but not when it is perceptually suppressed (and so invisible), during binocular rivalry or flash suppression (Kreiman, Fried, and Koch, 2002). These single-cell findings complement neuroimaging studies that show activation of common brain areas during both visual processing and recall during imagery of specific types of stimulus (O'Craven and Kanwisher, 2000; Kosslyn, Ganis, and Thompson, 2001).

Necessity and sufficiency of extrastriate neural activity

The data discussed in the previous section suggest that for visual features such as color, motion, or facial category to be represented in consciousness, appropriate activity must be present in the relevant functionally specialized area of extrastriate ventral visual cortex. However, activation of extrastriate ventral visual cortex may be necessary but not sufficient for awareness of a corresponding specific property. When volunteers incorrectly report the absence of a visual stimulus, some stimulus-specific activity can nevertheless still be seen in extrastriate visual cortex (Ress, Backus, and Heeger, 2000). In FFA, changes in the identity of a face stimulus can evoke some activity even when the subject is blind to the change (Beck et al., 2001). Masked words of which a subject is unaware can nevertheless still evoke some activity in the ventral visual pathway (Dehaene et al., 2001). Objects presented dichoptically in complementary colors, so that they are not consciously perceived during binocular vision, nevertheless evoke activity in appropriate specialized areas of ventral extrastriate cortex (Moutoussis and Zeki, 2002).

Event-related potential (ERP) components that are thought to have generators in ventral visual cortex can also be seen in some form for stimuli that are not consciously perceived. For example, the P300 response to "oddball" stimuli that are not consciously perceived is reduced, but not totally absent (Bernat, Shevrin, and Snodgrass, 2001). Semantically anomalous words that are not perceived when presented during the attentional blink nevertheless evoke an N400 response (Luck, Vogel, and Shapiro, 1996), as do masked words that are not consciously perceived (Kiefer and Spitzer, 2000; Stenberg et al., 2000). Consistent with this observation, words that are masked or unseen due to the attentional blink can produce semantic priming effects (Maki, Frigen, and Paulson, 1997; Dehaene et al., 1998). Finally, prior to conscious detection of change, ERPs indicate a cortical signature of unconscious change detection (Niedeggen, Wichmann, and Stoerig, 2001).

These findings complement recent work addressing the neural correlates of visual extinction, a common component of the neglect syndrome following right parietal damage (see Driver and Mattingley, 1998; Driver et al., this volume). Patients with visual extinction show deficient awareness for contralesional visual stimuli, particularly when a competing stimulus is also present ipsilesionally. Extinction illustrates that visual awareness can be lost even when V1 and extrastriate cortex are structurally intact. Two neuroimaging studies show that areas of both primary and extrastriate visual cortex that are activated by a seen left visual field stim-

ulus can also be activated to some extent by an unseen and extinguished left visual field stimulus (Rees, Wojciulik, et al., 2000; Vuilleumier et al., 2001, 2002) (figure 84.3). Indeed, the unconscious processing of an extinguished face stimulus extends even to the FFA (Rees, Wojciulik, et al., 2002) (figure 84.4), and, for emotional faces, to the amygdala and orbitofrontal cortex (Vuilleumier et al., 2002). Thus, the presence of some activity in these areas is not sufficient to evoke awareness following right parietal damage.

Conscious and unconscious representations in visual cortex

The data just reviewed give strong support to a direct link between neural representations in both primary and extrastriate ventral visual cortex and the contents of visual consciousness. The link is stronger for some features, such as motion, than for others. However, it is also apparent that the mere presence of feature-specific activity in primary or extrastriate cortex is not always sufficient for awareness. Conscious and unconscious representations may differ in several respects, including the overall level of activity that is evoked (as measured with fMRI) in a given visual area. For example, conscious recognition of objects shows a strong correlation with fMRI signal strength in object-responsive regions of visual cortex (Grill-Spector et al., 2000). Dichoptically presented objects that are not perceived evoke lower levels of activity than objects that are consciously identified (Moutossis and Zeki, 2002). The P300 potential evoked by

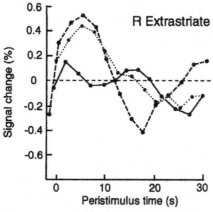
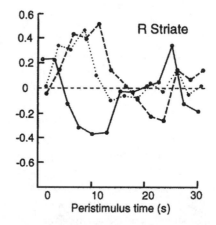
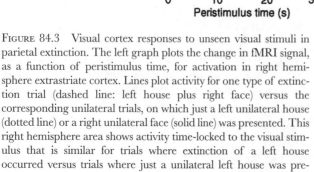

FIGURE 84.3 Visual cortex responses to unseen visual stimuli in parietal extinction. The left graph plots the change in fMRI signal, as a function of peristimulus time, for activation in right hemisphere extrastriate cortex. Lines plot activity for one type of extinction trial (dashed line: left house plus right face) versus the corresponding unilateral trials, on which just a left unilateral house (dotted line) or a right unilateral face (solid line) was presented. This right hemisphere area shows activity time-locked to the visual stimulus that is similar for trials where extinction of a left house occurred versus trials where just a unilateral left house was presented. There is little differential activity when a right-sided face is presented. The right graph shows a similar peristimulus time plot

of mean cortical activity for right striate cortex. Lines plot activity for one type of extinction trial (dashed line: now a left face plus a right house) versus the corresponding unilateral trials, on which just a left unilateral face (dotted line) or a right unilateral house (solid line) was presented. Note again that this area also increases its activity following a left visual field stimulus, whether unilateral or extinguished, with no such increase for a right visual stimulus (if anything, some tendency for a decrease is apparent). (Reprinted with permission from G. Rees et al., Unconscious activation of visual cortex in the damaged right hemisphere of a parietal patient with extinction. *Brain* 123:1624–1633. © 2000 by Oxford University Press.)

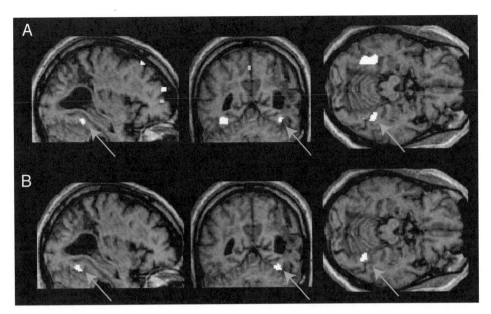

FIGURE 84.4 Category-specific unconscious activation in ventral visual cortex. (*A*) Loci activated by foveally presented and consciously perceived faces (versus houses) are superimposed in white on three sections (sagittal, coronal, and axial) of an anatomical image of the brain of a patient with parietal extinction. Bilateral activation of areas in the fusiform gyrus consistent with the locus of the fusiform face area (FFA) is seen, with the gray arrows indicating the right FFA. (*B*) Three equivalent anatomical sections on which are superimposed loci that showed greater activity for an extinguished left visual field face stimulus compared to an extinguished left visual field house stimulus. The gray arrows indicate activation in a location consistent with the right FFA shown in *A*. These data demonstrate unconscious category-specific activation of the FFA in parietal extinction. (Reprinted with permission from G. Rees et al., Neural correlates of conscious and unconscious vision in parietal extinction. *Neurocare* 8:387–393. © 2002 by Swets and Zeitlinger.)

oddball stimuli that are not consciously perceived is smaller than the P300 for consciously perceived oddball stimuli (Bernat, Shevrin, and Snodgrass, 2001). Activity evoked by masked and unseen words in ventral visual cortex is significantly lower than activity evoked by unmasked and consciously perceived words (Dehaene et al., 2001). These data suggest that one difference between conscious and unconscious representations in visual cortex may be quantitative, differing in the amount of activity (or its time course, or the specific neurons involved) that is evoked, rather than qualitatively in the topographic distribution of activity. In this sense, cortical areas that process visual stimuli appear also to be involved in their conscious perception (Zeki and Bartels, 1998).

Although it is clear that brain activity can differ in a quantitative fashion in human visual cortex when comparing conscious and unconscious representations, the interpretation of this activity in neural terms is not yet clear. Methodological caution in interpretation is appropriate for many of the techniques used in humans. For example, direct electrical stimulation and TMS may have remote effects distant from the site of stimulation (Paus et al., 1997). The mapping between electrical measurements on the scalp and their underlying neural generators in cortex and subcortical structures is indeterminate (Phillips, Rugg, and Friston, 2002). And the physiological link between functional MRI signals and underlying neuronal activity is only just starting to be elucidated (Rees, Kreiman, and Koch, 2002; Smith et al., 2002; Logothetis, 2003; see also Logothetis, this volume). In addition, the spatial resolution of fMRI (on the order of millimeters) may be insufficient to distinguish activity in interdigitating populations of neurons. Thus a quantitative difference in fMRI activity may reflect activation of a separate population of neurons, rather than more activity in the same population of neurons.

It is therefore not clear exactly what aspect of underlying neural activity differs when comparing conscious and unconscious representations that reveal a quantitative difference in fMRI signal (or, for that matter, ERP signals). In addition to overall differences in level of spiking, there are several other possibilities. For example, a minimum duration of neural activity might be required for conscious experience (Libet et al., 1964). In potential agreement with this possibility, patients experiencing visual hallucinations show a rise in fMRI signal in visual cortex some time before they report the presence of the hallucination (ffytche et al., 1998). The precise timing of neural activity might also be important. For example, in humans, the perception of moving phosphenes caused by stimulation of area V5/MT with TMS can be reduced by stimulation of V1, but only if stimulation of V1 is applied after the TMS pulse to V5/MT (Pascual-Leone and Walsh, 2001). Finally, a specific form of neural activity such as recurrent processing or synchrony might be required (von der Malsburg, 1981; Engel et al., 1991; Lamme and Roelfsema, 2000). For example, it has been suggested that synchronized electroencephalographic (EEG) oscillations in the high-frequency range (40–150 Hz) might underlie feature integration (thus representing a candidate solution to the binding problem; Singer and Gray, 1995) and form one potential substrate for visual awareness (Crick and Koch, 1990; Engel and Singer, 2001), although this idea remains controversial (Shadlen and Movshon, 1999). In support of this theory, cognitive processes that are thought to be closely associated with awareness, such as attention (Rock et al., 1992; Rees and Lavie, 2001), can modulate neural synchrony in monkey (Steinmetz et al., 2000; Fries et al., 2001). In humans, neuromagnetic responses show a correlation between perception of a visual stimulus during binocular rivalry and both interhemispheric and intrahemispheric coherence (Tononi et al., 1998). Viewing ambiguous visual stimuli that can be perceived as either faces or meaningless shapes leads to a long-distance pattern of synchronization in the scalp EEG that is specific for face perception and corresponds to the moment of conscious perception itself (Rodriguez et al., 1999). These findings suggest a possible role for synchronous processes in human conscious vision, but a clear synthesis has not yet emerged.

Parietal and prefrontal correlates of visual awareness

Conscious vision does not depend solely on the integrity of posterior and ventral visual cortex (Driver and Mattingley, 1998; Le et al., 2002). The longstanding clinical observation that disturbances of visual awareness may follow parietal damage provides strong evidence for a contribution of cortical areas distant from striate and extrastriate cortex to conscious vision (Driver and Mattingley, 1998). Although it has been argued that dorsal frontoparietal cortex activity might be related only to unconscious processing associated with visually guided action (Milner and Goodale, 1995), there is now compelling evidence to support a direct role for frontal and parietal cortex in visual awareness. In monkeys, chronic blindness follows a massive cortical ablation of parietal and frontal areas that spares most of the modality-specific visual cortex (Nakamura and Mishkin, 1986). Similarly, removal of frontoparietal cortex in cats produces as much or more decrement in visual discrimination than does removal of temporal cortex (Sperry, Myers, and Schrier, 1960). Furthermore, anatomical and electrophysiological studies show that parietal and prefrontal cortex are reciprocally connected and act together with visual cortex (Friedman and Goldman-Rakic, 1994). Direct evidence in normal humans for parietal and prefrontal correlates of visual awareness has come from recent studies of bistable perception. Brain activity during spontaneous fluctuations in awareness has been examined both for binocular rivalry and for a variety of bistable figures (Kleinschmidt et al., 1998; Lumer, Friston, and Rees, 1998; Lumer and Rees, 1999) (figure 84.5). Unlike the rivalry studies discussed previously (Tong et al., 1998; Polonsky et al., 2000), these studies focused on activity that was time-locked to the transitions between different perceptual states rather than to the contents of one or other perceptual state. Cortical regions whose activity reflects perceptual transitions include not only ventral extrastriate cortex, but also parietal and frontal regions previously implicated in the control of attention (Lumer, Friston, and Rees, 1998). However, whereas extrastriate areas are also engaged by nonrivalrous perceptual changes, activity in frontal and parietal cortex is specifically associated with the perceptual alternations during rivalry. Similar parietal and frontal regions are active during perceptual transitions that occur while subjects view a range of bistable figures such as the Necker cube and Rubins face/vase (Kleinschmidt et al., 1998), and during fluctuations in the direction of motion of a bistable motion stimulus (Sterzer et al., 2002). Clinically, it has been observed that patients with prefrontal cortex lesions typically exhibit abnormal bistable perception (Wilkins, Shallice, and McCarthy, 1987; Ricci and Blundo, 1990; Meenan and Miller, 1994) and that patients with parietal neglect exhibit abnormal patterns of transitions in binocular rivalry (Bonneh, Pavlovskaya, and Soroker, 2002). These data suggest that activity in frontal and parietal cortex might be causally associated with the generation of transitions between different percepts.

A number of other paradigms reveal a similar association between frontoparietal activity and awareness. The pop-out in depth of stereographic images activates areas of superior parietal and prefrontal cortex, compared with regions active during continued stable viewing of the same figures (Portas et al., 2000). In addition, similar areas of frontal and parietal cortex are activated when subjects become consciously aware of the presence of a change in a visual scene, compared with when they are blind to that change (Beck et al., 2001) (figure 84.6). During visual imagery, fMRI reveals content-independent activity in frontal and parietal cortex (Ishai, Ungerleider, and Haxby, 2000). Unmasked and consciously perceived visual words, compared with masked and unseen words, also evoke activity in frontal and parietal cortex (Dehaene et al., 2001) (figure 84.7). Finally, the attentional blink may be associated with right intraparietal sulcus and prefrontal cortical activations (Marois, Chun, and Gore, 2000).

These data are complemented by experiments on patients with visual extinction resulting from right parietal damage. As mentioned earlier, fMRI evidence suggests that extinguished stimuli are processed and activate contralesional ventral visual cortex in the absence of awareness (Rees,

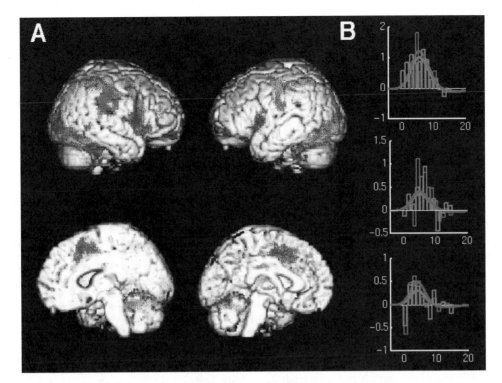

FIGURE 84.5 Event-related activity associated with binocular rivalry perceptual switches. (*A*) Four views of the medial and lateral surfaces of a rendering of an anatomical template image in Talairach space, on which are superimposed areas where evoked activity was specifically related to perceptual transitions in either binocular rivalry (red) or physical stimulus alternation (green). Areas modulated by perception during both rivalrous and physical stimulus alternation, and the bilateral symmetry of the evoked activity are apparent. (*B*) Illustrative postevent histograms of the modulation of activity produced by transition events in rivalry (red) and physical stimulus alternation (green) conditions from three different subjects. The evoked activity (percent change in BOLD contrast) is shown as a function of postevent time (in seconds) for each subject, with the fitted models of hemodynamic response function superimposed in solid lines. The modulation of activity shown here is taken from a voxel in right anterior fusiform gyrus. (Reprinted with permission from E. D. Lumer et al., Neural correlates of perceptual rivalry in the human brain. *Science* 280:1930–1934. © 1998 by the American Association for the Advancement of Science.) (See color plate 75.)

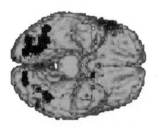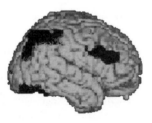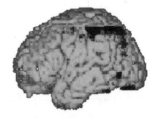

FIGURE 84.6 Conscious awareness of change. Three views of an anatomical template brain on which are superimposed loci (in black) where evoked activity was greater when subjects consciously detected a change in two sequentially presented visual images, compared to when the same physical change remained undetected. Conscious change detection activates not only the ventral visual cortex but also areas of right dorsolateral prefrontal and bilateral parietal cortex. (Reprinted with permission from D. M. Beck et al., Neural correlates of change detection and change blindness. *Nat. Neurosci.* 4:645–650. © 2001 by the Nature Publishing Group.)

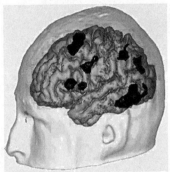
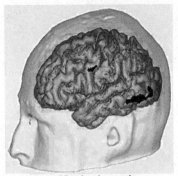

Visible words   **Masked words**

FIGURE 84.7 fMRI activations to visible and masked words. Activations produced by single words that are either masked and not consciously perceived (right) or visible and consciously perceived (left). Only the left hemisphere is shown, as seen through a translucent three-dimensional reconstruction of the skull and brain of one of the participants. In these transparent views, the deep activations in fusiform, parietal, and mesial frontal cortex appear through the overlying lateral cortices. Masked words that are not consciously perceived activate a large area of the left fusiform gyrus, while visible words produce greater activation in this area combined with widespread activity in left parietal and prefrontal cortex. (Reprinted with permission from S. Dehaene et al., Cerebral mechanisms of word masking and unconscious repetition priming. *Nat. Neurosci.* 4:752–758. © 2001 by the Nature Publishing Group.)

Wojciulik, et al., 2000, 2002; Vuilleumier et al., 2001). However, because extinction does not arise on all bilateral trials, this also affords an opportunity to compare trials in which the patient reports awareness with physically identical trials when awareness of one of the stimuli is absent. In trials in which one patient (correctly) reports seeing bilateral stimulation, awareness is specifically associated with covariation of activity in a distributed network involving primary visual cortex, inferior temporal cortex, and areas of prefrontal and left parietal cortex (Driver et al., 2001; Vuilleumier et al., 2001; Rees, Wojciulik, et al., 2002). Conscious perception of emotional faces leads to enhanced activity in fusiform, parietal, and prefrontal areas of the left hemisphere, independent of emotional expression (Vuilleumier et al., 2002).

Loss of awareness for objects in the contralesional visual field in parietal extinction is typically complete, affecting all stimulus features (even those such as color and motion thought to be represented in extrastriate visual cortex). In this respect, the effects of parietal damage on phenomenal experience are distinct from the effects of extrastriate damage, where awareness of only an isolated visual feature may be lost. This profound loss of the ability to consciously represent different objects in different egocentric spatial locations may depend on the putative function of parietal cortex in remapping retinotopic space represented in ventral visual cortex into more complex head-and-body-centered representations (Cohen and Andersen, 2002). Bilateral parietal lesions can give rise to even more pronounced visual deficits, with unpredictable perception and recognition of only parts of the visual field (simultanagnosia), together with impairments of visually guided reaching and visual scanning (Balint, 1909; Husain and Stein, 1988). Patients with simultanagnosia may show nonspatial extinction, failing to per-

ceive the second of two objects presented simultaneously in overlapping locations (Humphreys et al., 1994). Of course, patients with parietal extinction (and even patients with bilateral parietal damage) remain conscious of *some* kinds of phenomenal experience, such as in the ipsilesional visual field. But the lesions encountered in patients are typically too small to stand comparison with the large ablations of the dorsal stream that render monkeys blind (Nakamura and Mishkin, 1986). The effect on phenomenal awareness in humans of bilateral damage to the entire frontal and parietal cortex therefore remains an open question.

Despite varied paradigms and types of visual stimulation, the anatomical location of the areas in parietal and prefrontal cortex activated by changes in the contents of visual consciousness is relatively consistent. Meta-analysis suggests two prominent foci in the superior parietal lobule and dorsolateral prefrontal cortex (Rees, 2001; Rees, Kreiman, and Koch, 2002) (figure 84.8). These observations suggest the existence of a general mechanism in these areas that is specifically related to visual consciousness, active during transitions between different types of perceptual experience, and associated with content-independent spatial representation rather than content-specific visual features (e.g., Driver and Mattingley, 1998; Driver and Vuilleumieur, 2001; Kanwisher, 2001). Although frontal and parietal areas play a prominent role in the organization of behavior, their involvement in rivalry is independent of motor report (Lumer and Rees, 1999). During transitions in binocular rivalry, activity is coordinated between ventral visual areas, parietal areas, and prefrontal areas in a way that is not linked to external motor or sensory events but instead varies in strength with the frequency of perceptual events. In parietal extinction, awareness of bilateral visual stimulation is specifically associated with covariation of activity in a distributed

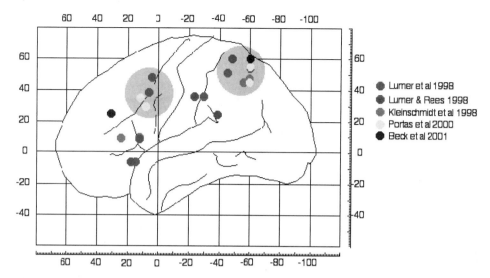

FIGURE 84.8   Neural correlates of conscious vision in parietal and prefrontal cortex. Areas of parietal and prefrontal cortex that show activation correlated with changes in visual awareness in a number of selected studies (Lumer et al., 1998; Lumer and Rees, 1999; Kleinschmidt et al., 1998; Portas et al., 2000; Beck et al., 2001) are plotted on a standardized brain in Talairach space (Talairach and Tournoux, 1988). Each circle is placed at the center of a cluster of activation, with different shades representing different studies; overlapping loci from the same study are omitted for clarity. There is prominent clustering of activations in superior parietal and dorsolateral prefrontal cortex, highlighted by large, light circles. (See color plate 76.)

network involving primary visual cortex, inferior temporal cortex, and areas of prefrontal and left parietal cortex (Driver et al., 2001; Vuilleumier et al., 2001). These observations represent direct evidence that awareness may be specifically associated with covariation between visual cortex and nonvisual areas of cortex, complementing earlier studies showing similar distributed interactions associated with consciousness in normal subjects (Dolan et al., 1997; Lumer and Rees, 1999; McIntosh, Rajah, and Lobaugh, 1999). This suggests that functional interactions between visual and frontoparietal cortex may make an important contribution to the contents of consciousness. Such an interaction has been proposed on theoretical (Crick and Koch, 1995) and empirical (Driver and Mattingley, 1998) grounds; one possibility is that this represents activity in a global neuronal workspace (Baars, 1988; Dehaene and Naccache, 2001; Baars and Franklin, 2003; Dehaene, Sergent, and Changeux, 2003).

Synthesis

The evidence reviewed in this chapter suggests that although activity in visual cortex may be necessary, it does not appear sufficient for conscious vision without some contribution from parietal and/or prefrontal cortex. What is the nature of that contribution? It is striking that the studies reviewed here all focused on transitions between experiences with different types of phenomenal content. James (1890) made a phenomenal distinction between the experience of rapid changes in perceptual awareness (transitive states) and stable contemplation (substantive states). Both are part of our everyday experience of the visual environment. Perhaps the

neural correlates of conscious experience in parietal cortex are thus more specifically correlates of transitive states? The anatomical loci associated with these correlates substantially overlap areas previously associated with covert spatial attention (Corbetta et al., 1995). Indeed, the deployment of spatial attention and the phenomenal experience of binocular rivalry both entail the suppression of visual information from conscious perception. Monocular stimuli become periodically invisible during rivalry; sensory events associated with unattended (or neglected) stimuli have a diminished impact on awareness. Both phenomena may call on common neural machinery in frontoparietal cortex that is involved in the selection of neuronal activity leading to visual awareness (Rees, 2001; Rees and Lavie, 2001).

This phenomenological distinction raises the possibility that the maintenance of a conscious perceptual state may involve different cortical mechanisms from those involved in generating transitions (Portas et al., 2000). Sustained perceptual experience is an obvious feature of consciousness but is inconsistent with the observation that the brain is designed to represent only the unexpected (Friston, 2002). For a percept to be sustained requires either the filling in of missing information or prevention of adaptation when stimulation remains constant. Such mechanisms might depend on top-down signals from higher-level brain regions. Future work in this area may prove rewarding, as there are tantalizing indications that such mechanisms do exist. For example, when a stereo image becomes visible, transient activity is seen in frontal and parietal cortex (Portas et al., 2000). However, in a subsequent period where perception of the same image is sustained, activity is seen in different regions of prefrontal cortex and in the hippocampus. Thus, sustaining a visual percept recruits different anatomical loci from those associated with immediate conscious recognition. Similarly, regions of brain activation in frontal and parietal cortex associated with transient selection of an item from spatial working memory differ from those associated with sustained maintenance of items in working memory (Rowe et al., 2000). Finally, as previously reviewed, brain areas activated during epochs of sustained face perception in binocular rivalry include the FFA (Lumer, Friston, and Rees, 1998; Tong et al., 1998; Lumer, 2000). However, several prefrontal areas also show greater activity during sustained face perception (Lumer, 2000). These areas show strong overlap with those previously implicated in maintaining working memory for faces in a delayed match-to-sample task (Courtney et al., 1997). The phenomenological distinction between transitive and substantive states of mind may perhaps reflect the involvement of distinct regions of dorsal and ventral frontoparietal cortex associated with attention and working memory.

Concluding remarks

The evidence reviewed here suggests that ventral visual cortex is undeniably (and unremarkably) crucial for conscious vision in humans; both primary visual cortex and ventral extrastriate cortex contain neuronal populations whose activity closely correlates with the contents of consciousness. Different areas emphasize different features in consciousness; primary visual cortex appears to be more important for brightness and contrast, while V5/MT and areas of the fusiform gyrus are more important for motion and color, respectively. Within these areas, level of activation is one factor that may distinguish conscious and unconscious representations. However, even strong activation in visual cortex can be insufficient for awareness without a contribution from parietal and/or prefrontal cortex. The minimal sufficient conditions (in humans) for a visual scene to be represented in consciousness may therefore be the combination of an activated representation of its constituent features in striate and extrastriate visual cortex, coupled with activity in specific regions of parietal and prefrontal cortex.

ACKNOWLEDGMENTS   This work was supported by the Wellcome Trust. I thank Jon Driver for helpful comments.

REFERENCES

BAARS, B. J., 1988. *A Cognitive Theory of Consciousness*. Cambridge, England: Cambridge University Press.

BAARS, B. J., and S. FRANKLIN, 2003. How conscious experience and working memory interact. *Trends. Cogn. Sci.* 7:166–172.

BALINT, R., 1909. Seelenlähmung des "Schauens," optische Ataxie, raumlich Störung der Augmerksamkeit. *Monatsschr. Psychiatr. Neurol.* 25:51–81.

BARBUR J. L., J. D. WATSON, R. S. FRACKOWIAK, and S. ZEKI, 1993. Conscious visual perception without V1. *Brain* 116:1293–1302.

BARNES, J., R. J. HOWARD, C. SENIOR, M. BRAMMER, E. T. BULLMORE, A. SIMMONS, and A. S. DAVID, 1999. The functional anatomy of the McCollough contingent colour after-effect. *Neuroreport* 10:195–199.

BECK, D. M., G. REES, C. D. FRITH, and N. LAVIE, 2001. Neural correlates of change detection and change blindness. *Nat. Neurosci.* 4:645–650.

BECKERS, G., and S. ZEKI, 1995. The consequences of inactivating areas V1 and V5 on visual motion perception. *Brain* 118:49–60.

BERNAT, E., H. SHEVRIN, and M. SNODGRASS, 2001. Subliminal visual oddball stimuli evoke a P300 component. *Clin. Neurophysiol.* 112:159–171.

BLAKE, R., and R. FOX, 1974. Adaptation to invisible gratings and the site of binocular rivalry suppression. *Nature* 249:488–490.

BODIS-WOLLNER, I., A. ATKIN, E. RAAB, and M. WOLKSTEIN, 1977. Visual association cortex and vision in man: Pattern-evoked occipital potentials in a blind boy. *Science* 198:629–631.

BONNEH, Y., M. PAVLOVSKAYA, and N. SOROKER, 2002. Slow binocular rivalry in hemispatial neglect (abstr.). *J. Vision* 2:278a (*http://journalofvision.org/2/7/278/, DOI 10.1167/2.7.278*).

BREWER, A. A., W. A. PRESS, N. K. LOGOTHETIS, and B. A. WANDELL, 2002. Visual areas in macaque cortex measured using functional magnetic resonance imaging. *J. Neurosci.* 22:10416–10426.

BRINDLEY, G. S., and W. S. LEWIN, 1968. The sensations produced by electrical stimulation of the visual cortex. *J. Physiol.* 196:479–493.

COHEN, Y. E., and R. A. ANDERSEN, 2002. A common reference frame for movement plans in the posterior parietal cortex. *Nat. Rev. Neurosci.* 3:553–562.

CORBETTA, M., G. L. SHULMAN, F. M. MIEZIN, and S. E. PETERSEN, 1995. Superior parietal cortex activation during spatial attention shifts and visual feature conjunction. *Science* 270:802–805.

COURTNEY, S. M., L. G. UNGERLEIDER, K. KEIL, and J. V. HAXBY, 1997. Transient and sustained activity in a distributed neural system for human working memory. *Nature* 10:608–611.

COWEY, A., and V. WALSH, 2000. Magnetically induced phosphenes in sighted, blind and blindsighted observers. *Neuroreport* 11: 3269–3273.

CRICK, F., and C. KOCH, 1990. Some reflections on visual awareness. *Cold Spring Harb. Symp. Quant. Biol.* 55:953–962.

CRICK, F., and C. KOCH, 1995. Are we aware of neural activity in primary visual cortex? *Nature* 375:121–123.

CRICK, F., and C. KOCH, 2003. A framework for consciousness. *Nat. Neurosci.* 6:119–126.

CULHAM, J. C., S. P. DUKELOW, T. VILIS, F. A. HASSARD, J. S. GATI, R. S. MENON, and M. A. GOODALE, 1999. Recovery of fMRI activation in motion area MT following storage of the motion aftereffect. *J. Neurophysiol.* 81:388–393.

CULHAM, J. C., and N. G. KANWISHER, 2001. Neuroimaging of cognitive functions in human parietal cortex. *Curr. Opin. Neurobiol.* 11:157–163.

DAMASIO, A. R., T. YAMADA, H. DAMASIO, J. CORBETT, and J. McKEE, 1980. Central achromatopsia: Behavioral, anatomic, and physiologic aspects. *Neurology* 30:1064–1071.

DAMASIO, A. R., D. TRANEL, and M. RIZZO, 2000. Disorders of complex visual processing. In *Principles of Cognitive and Behavioral Neurology*, 2nd ed. M.-M. MESULAM, ed. Oxford, England: Oxford University Press, pp. 332–372.

DEHAENE, S., and L. NACCACHE, 2001. Towards a cognitive neuroscience of consciousness: Basic evidence and a workspace framework. *Cognition* 79:1–3.

DEHAENE, S., L. NACCACHE, L. COHEN, D. L. BIHAN, J. F. MANGIN, J. B. POLINE, and D. RIVIERE, 2001. Cerebral mechanisms of word masking and unconscious repetition priming. *Nat. Neurosci.* 4:752–758.

DEHAENE, S., L. NACCACHE, H. G. LE CLEC, E. KOECHLIN, M. MUELLER, G. DEHAENE-LAMBERTZ, P. F. VAN DE MOORTELE, and D. LE BIHAN, 1998. Imaging unconscious semantic priming. *Nature* 395:597–600.

DEHAENE, S., C. SERGENT, and J. P. CHANGEUX, 2003, June 26. A neuronal network model linking subjective reports and objective physiological data during conscious perception. *Proc. Natl. Acad. Sci. U.S.A.* (Epub ahead of print).

D'ESPOSITO, M., J. A. DETRE, G. K. AGUIRRE, M. STALLCUP, D. C. ALSOP, L. J. TIPPET, and M. J. FARAH, 1997. A functional MRI study of mental image generation. *Neuropsychologia* 35:725–730.

DIERKS, T., D. E. LINDEN, M. JANDL, E. FORMISANO, R. GOEBEL, H. LANFERMANN, and W. SINGER, 1999. Activation of Heschl's gyrus during auditory hallucinations. *Neuron* 22:615–621.

DOBELLE, W. H., J. TURKEL, D. C. HENDERSON, and J. R. EVANS, 1979. Mapping the representation of the visual field by electrical stimulation of human visual cortex. *Am. J. Ophthalmol.* 88:727–735.

DOLAN, R. J., G. R. FINK, E. ROLLS, M. BOOTH, A. HOLMES, R. S. FRACKOWIAK, and K. J. FRISTON, 1997. How the brain learns to see objects and faces in an impoverished context. *Nature* 389:596–599.

DRIVER, J., and P. VUILLEUMIER, 2001. Perceptual awareness and its loss in unilateral neglect and extinction. *Cognition* 79:39–88.

DRIVER, J., and J. B. MATTINGLEY, 1998. Parietal neglect and visual awareness. *Nat. Neurosci.* 1:17–22.

DRIVER, J., P. VUILLEUMIER, M. EIMER, and G. REES, 2001. Functional magnetic resonance imaging and evoked potential correlates of conscious and unconscious vision in parietal extinction patients. *NeuroImage* 14:S68–75.

EIMER, M., A. MARAVITA, J. VAN VELZEN, M. HUSAIN, and J. DRIVER, 2002. The electrophysiology of tactile extinction: ERP correlates of unconscious somatosensory processing. *Neuropsychologia* 40:2438–2447.

ENGEL, A. K., P. KONIG, A. K. KREITER, and W. SINGER, 1991. Interhemispheric synchronization of oscillatory neuronal responses in cat visual cortex. *Science* 24:1177–1179.

ENGEL, A. K., and W. SINGER, 2001. Temporal binding and the neural correlates of sensory awareness. *Trends Cogn. Sci.* 5:16–25.

ENGEL, S. A., D. E. RUMELHART, B. A. WANDELL, A. T. LEE, G. H. GLOVER, E. J. CHICHILNISKY, and M. N. SHADLEN, 1994. fMRI of human visual cortex. *Nature* 369:525.

FELLEMAN, D. J., and D. C. VAN ESSEN, 1991. Distributed hierarchical processing in the primate cerebral cortex. *Cereb. Cortex* 1:1–47.

FFYTCHE, D. H., R. J. HOWARD, M. J. BRAMMER, A. DAVID, P. WOODRUFF, and S. WILLIAMS, 1998. The anatomy of conscious vision: An fMRI study of visual hallucinations. *Nat. Neurosci.* 1:738–742.

FFYTCHE, D. H., and S. ZEKI, 1996. Brain activity related to the perception of illusory contours. *NeuroImage* 3:104–108.

FRIEDMAN, H. R., and P. S. GOLDMAN-RAKIC, 1994. Coactivation of prefrontal cortex and inferior parietal cortex in working memory tasks revealed by 2DG functional mapping in the rhesus monkey. *J. Neurosci.* 14:2775–2788.

FRIES, P., J. H. REYNOLDS, A. E. RORIE, and R. DESIMONE, 2001. Modulation of oscillatory neuronal synchronization by selective visual attention. *Science* 291:1560–1563.

FRISTON, K. J., 2002. Beyond phrenology: What can neuroimaging tell us about distributed circuitry? *Ann. Rev. Neurosci.* 25:221–250.

FRITH, C. D., R. PERRY, and E. LUMER, 1999. The neural correlates of conscious experience: An experimental framework. *Trends Cogn. Sci.* 3:105–114.

GALLANT, J. L., R. E. SHOUP, and J. A. MAZER, 2000. A human extrastriate area functionally homologous to macaque V4. *Neuron* 27:227–235.

GOEBEL, R., L. MUCKLI, F. E. ZANELLA, W. SINGER, and P. STOERIG, 2001. Sustained extrastriate cortical activation without visual awareness revealed by fMRI studies of hemianopic patients. *Vision Res.* 41:1459–1474.

GRILL-SPECTOR, K., T. KUSHNIR, T. HENDLER, and R. MALACH, 2000. The dynamics of object-selective activation correlate with recognition performance in humans. *Nat. Neurosci.* 3:837–843.

HADJIKHANI, N., A. K. LIU, A. M. DALE, P. CAVANAGH, and R. B. TOOTELL, 1998. Retinotopy and color sensitivity in human visual cortical area V8. *Nat. Neurosci.* 1:235–241.

HAYNES, J. D., G. ROTH, M. STADLER, and H. J. HEINZE, 2003. Neuromagnetic correlates of perceived contrast in primary visual cortex. *J. Neurophysiol.* 89:2655–2666.

HE, S., P. CAVANAGH, and J. INTRILIGATOR, 1996. Attentional resolution and the locus of visual awareness. *Nature* 383:334–337.

HE, S., E. R. COHEN, and X. HU, 1998. Close correlation between activity in brain area MT/V5 and the perception of a visual motion aftereffect. *Curr. Biol.* 8:1215–1218.

HE, S., and D. I. MACLEOD, 2001. Orientation-selective adaptation and tilt after-effect from invisible patterns. *Nature* 411:473–476.

HOWARD, R. J., D. H. FFYTCHE, J. BARNES, D. MCKEEFRY, Y. HA, P. W. WOODRUFF, E. T. BULLMORE, A. SIMMONS, S. C. WILLIAMS, A. S. DAVID, and M. BRAMMER, 1998. The functional anatomy of imagining and perceiving colour. *Neuroreport* 9:1019–1923.

HENSCHEN, S. E., 1893. On the visual path and centre. *Brain* 16:170–180.

HESS, R. H., C. L. BAKER, JR., and J. ZIHL, 1989. The "motion-blind" patient: Low-level spatial and temporal filters. *J. Neurosci.* 9:1628–1640.

HIRSCH, J., R. L. DELAPAZ, N. R. RELKIN, J. VICTOR, K. KIM, T. LI, P. BORDEN, N. RUBIN, and R. SHAPLEY, 1995. Illusory contours activate specific regions in human visual cortex: Evidence from functional magnetic resonance imaging. *Proc. Natl. Acad. Sci. U.S.A.* 92:6469–6473.

HOLMES, G., and W. T. LISTER, 1916. Disturbances of vision from cerebral lesions with special reference to the cortical representation of the macula. *Brain* 39:34–73.

HOWARD, R. J., D. H. FFYTCHE, J. BARNES, D. MCKEEFRY, Y. HA, P. W. WOODRUFF, E. T. BULLMORE, A. SIMMONS, S. C. WILLIAMS, A. S. DAVID, and M. BRAMMER, 1998. The functional anatomy of imagining and perceiving colour. *Neuroreport* 9:1019–1023.

HUBEL, D. H., and T. N. WIESEL, 1968. Receptive fields and functional architevture of monkey striate cortex. *J. Physiol. (Lond.)* 195:215–243.

HUBEL, D. H., and T. N. WIESEL, 1974. Sequence regularity and geometry of orientation columns in the monkey striate cortex. *J. Comp. Neurol.* 158:267–293.

HUK, A. C., D. RESS, and D. J. HEEGER, 2001. Neuronal basis of the motion aftereffect reconsidered. *Neuron* 32:161–172.

HUMPHREYS, G. W., C. ROMANI, A. OLSON, M. J. RIDDOCH, and J. DUNCAN, 1994. Non-spatial extinction following lesions of the parietal lobe in humans. *Nature* 372:357–359.

HUSAIN, M., and J. STEIN, 1988. Rezso Balint and his most celebrated case. *Arch. Neurol.* 45:89–93.

INOUYE, T., 1909. *Die Sehstörungen bei Schussverletzungen der kortikalen Sehsphare nach Beobachtungen an Verwundeten der letzten japanischen Kriege.* Leipzig: W. Engelmann.

ISHAI, A., L. G. UNGERLEIDER, and J. V. HAXBY, 2000. Distributed neural systems for the generation of visual images *Neuron* 28:979–990.

JAMES, W., 1890. *The Principles of Psychology.* Cambridge, Mass.: Harvard University Press.

KANWISHER, N., 2001. Neural events and perceptual awareness. *Cognition* 79:89–113.

KASTNER, S., M. A. PINSK, P. DE WEERD, R. DESIMONE, and L. G. UNGERLEIDER, 1999. Increased activity in human visual cortex during directed attention in the absence of visual stimulation. *Neuron* 22:751–761.

KIEFER, M., and M. SPITZER, 2000. Time course of conscious and unconscious semantic brain activation. *Neuroreport* 11:2401–2407.

KLEINSCHMIDT, A., C. BUCHEL, S. ZEKI, and R. S. J. FRACKOWIAK, 1998. Human brain activity during spontaneously reversing perception of ambiguous figures. *Proc. R. Soc. Lond. B* 265:2427–2433.

KOLB, F. C., and J. BRAUN, 1995. Blindsight in normal observers. *Nature* 377:336–338.

KOSSLYN, S. M., G. GANIS, and W. L. THOMPSON, 2001. Neural foundations of imagery. *Nat. Rev. Neurosci.* 2:635–642.

KOURTZI, Z., and N. KANWISHER, 2000. Activation in human MT/MST by static images with implied motion. *J. Cogn. Neurosci.* 12:48–55.

KREIMAN, G., C. KOCH, and I. FRIED, 2000a. Category-specific visual responses of single neurons in the human medial temporal lobe. *Nat. Neurosci.* 3:946–953.

KREIMAN, G., C. KOCH, and I. FRIED, 2000b. Imagery neurons in the human brain. *Nature* 408:357–361.

KREIMAN, G., I. FRIED, and C. KOCH, 2002. Single-neuron correlates of subjective vision in the human medial temporal lobe. *Proc. Natl. Acad. Sci. U.S.A.* 99:8378–8383.

KROLAK-SALMON, P., M.-A. HÈNAFF, C. TALLON-BAUDRY, B. YVERT, M. GUÈNOT, A. VIGHETTO, F. MAUGUIÈRE, and O. BERTRAND, 2003. Human lateral geniculate nucleus and visual cortex respond to screen flicker. *Ann. Neurol.* 53:73–80.

LAMME, V. A., and P. R. ROELFSEMA, 2000. The distinct modes of vision offered by feedforward and recurrent processing. *Trends Neurosci.* 23:571–579.

LE, S., D. CARDEBAT, K. BOULANOUAR, M. A. HENAFF, F. MICHEL, D. MILNER, C. DIJKERMAN, M. PUEL, and J. F. DEMONET, 2002. Seeing, since childhood, without ventral stream: A behavioural study. *Brain* 125:58–74.

LEE, H. W., S. B. HONG, D. W. SEO, W. S. TAE, and S. C. HONG, 2000. Mapping of functional organization in human visual cortex: Electrical cortical stimulation. *Neurology* 54:849–854.

LEE, S. H., and R. BLAKE, 2002. V1 activity is reduced during binocular rivalry. *J. Vision* 2:618–626.

LEOPOLD, D. A., and N. K. LOGOTHETIS, 1996. Activity changes in early visual cortex reflect monkeys' percepts during binocular rivalry. *Nature* 379:549–553.

LEOPOLD, D. A., and N. K. LOGOTHETIS, 1999. Multistable phenomena: Changing views in perception. *Trends Cogn. Sci.* 3: 254–264.

LEVELT, W. J. M., 1965. *On Binocular Rivalry.* Assen, The Netherlands: Royal VanGorcum.

LIBET, B., W. W. ALBERTS, E. W. WRIGHT, Jr., L. D. DELATTRE, G. LEVIN, and B. FEINSTEIN, 1964. Production of threshold levels of conscious sensation by electrical stimulation of human somatosensory cortex. *J. Neurophysiol.* 27:546–578.

LOGOTHETIS, N. K. 2003. The underpinnings of the BOLD functional magnetic resonance imaging signal. *J. Neurosci.* 23: 3963–3971.

LOGOTHETIS, N. K., and J. D. SCHALL, 1989. Neuronal correlates of subjective visual perception. *Science* 245:761–763.

LUCK, S. J., E. K. VOGEL, and K. L. SHAPIRO, 1996. Word meanings can be accessed but not reported during the attentional blink. *Nature* 383:616–618.

LUMER, E., 2000. Binocular rivalry and human visual awareness. In *Neural Correlates of Consciousness: Conceptual and Empirical Questions,* T. Metzinger, ed. Cambridge, Mass.: MIT Press.

LUMER, E. D., K. J. FRISTON, and G. REES, 1998. Neural correlates of perceptual rivalry in the human brain. *Science* 280:1930–1934.

LUMER, E. D., and G. REES, 1999. Covariation of activity in visual and prefrontal cortex associated with subjective visual perception. *Proc. Natl. Acad. Sci. U.S.A.* 96:1669–1673.

MAIER, J., G. DAGNELIE, H. SPEKREIJSE, and B. W. VAN DIJK, 1987. Principal components analysis for source localization of VEPs in man. *Vision Res.* 27:165–177.

MAKI, W. S., K. FRIGEN, and K. PAULSON, 1997. Associative priming by targets and distractors during rapid serial visual presentation: Does word meaning survive the attentional blink? *J. Exp. Psychol. Hum. Percept. Perform.* 23:1014–1034.

MAROIS, R., M. M. CHUN, and J. C. GORE, 2000. Neural correlates of the attentional blink. *Neuron* 28:299–308.

McINTOSH, A. R., M. N. RAJAH, and N. J. LOBAUGH, 1999. Interactions of prefrontal cortex in relation to awareness in sensory learning. *Science* 284:1531–1533.

McLEOD, P., C. HEYWOOD, J. DRIVER, and J. ZIHL, 1989. Selective deficit of visual search in moving displays after extrastriate damage. *Nature* 339:466–467.

MEADOWS, J. C., 1974. Disturbed perception of colours associated with localized cerebral lesions. *Brain* 97:615–632.

MEENAN, J. P., and L. A. MILLER, 1994. Perceptual flexibility after frontal or temporal lobectomy. *Neuropsychologia* 32:1145–1149.

MENDOLA, J. D., A. M. DALE, B. FISCHL, A. K. LIU, and R. B. TOOTELL, 1999. The representation of illusory and real contours in human cortical visual areas revealed by functional magnetic resonance imaging. *J. Neurosci.* 19:8560–8572.

MILNER, A. D., and M. A. GOODALE, 1995. *The Visual Brain in Action.* Oxford, England: Oxford University Press.

MORGAN, M. J., A. J. MASON, and J. A. SOLOMON, 1997. Blindsight in normal subjects? *Nature* 385:401–402.

MOUTOUSSIS, K., and S. ZEKI, 2002. The relationship between cortical activation and perception investigated with invisible stimuli. *Proc. Natl. Acad. Sci. U.S.A.* 99(14):9527–9532.

MUCKLI, L., N. KRIEGESKORTE, H. LANFERMANN, F. E. ZANELLA, W. SINGER, and R. GOEBEL, 2002. Apparent motion: Event-related functional magnetic resonance imaging of perceptual switches and States. *J. Neurosci.* 22:RC219.

NAKAMURA, R. K., and M. MISHKIN, 1980. Blindness in monkeys following non-visual cortical lesions. *Brain Res.* 188:572–577.

NAKAMURA, R. K., and M. MISHKIN, 1986. Chronic "blindness" following lesions of nonvisual cortex in the monkey. *Exp. Brain Res.* 63:173–184.

NIEDEGGEN, M., P. WICHMANN, and P. STOERIG, 2001. Change blindness and time to consciousness. *Eur. J. Neurosci.* 14: 1719–1726.

NOE, A., and E. T. THOMPSON, 2002. *Vision and Mind: Selected Readings in the Philosophy of Perception.* Cambridge, Mass.: MIT Press.

O'CRAVEN, K. M., and N. KANWISHER, 2000. Mental imagery of faces and places activates corresponding stimulus-specific brain regions. *J. Cogn. Neurosci.* 12:1013–1023.

Ono, H., and R. Barbeito, 1985. Utrocular discrimination is not sufficient for utrocular identification. *Vision Res.* 25:289–299.

O'Regan, J. K., and A. Noe, 2001. A sensorimotor account of vision and visual consciousness. *Behav. Brain Sci.* 24:939–973 [discussion 973–1031].

Pascual-Leone, A., and V. Walsh, 2001. Fast backprojections from the motion to the primary visual area necessary for visual awareness. *Science* 292:510–512.

Paus, T., R. Jech, C. J. Thompson, R. Comeau, T. Peters, and A. C. Evans, 1997. Transcranial magnetic stimulation during positron emission tomography: A new method for studying connectivity of the human cerebral cortex. *J. Neurosci.* 17:3178–3184.

Pearlman, A. L., J. Birch, and J. C. Meadows, 1979. Cerebral color blindness: An acquired defect in hue discrimination. *Ann. Neurol.* 5:253–261.

Penfield, W., and T. Rasmussen, 1950. *The Cerebral Cortex of Man.* New York: Macmillan.

Perry, R. J., and S. Zeki, 2001. Functional specialization for perceptual binding between different visual submodalities. *Soc. Neurosci. Abstr.* 250.1.

Phillips, C., M. D. Rugg, and K. J. Friston, 2002. Anatomically informed basis functions for EEG source localization: Combining functional and anatomical constraints. *NeuroImage* 16:678–695.

Polonsky, A., R. Blake, J. Braun, and D. J. Heeger, 2000. Neuronal activity in human primary visual cortex correlates with perception during binocular rivalry. *Nat. Neurosci.* 3:1153–1159.

Portas, C. M., B. A. Strange, K. J. Friston, R. J. Dolan, and C. D. Frith, 2000. How does the brain sustain a visual percept? *Proc. R. Soc. Lond. B Biol. Sci.* 267:845–850.

Povinelli, D. J., and J. Vonk, 2003. Chimpanzee minds: Suspiciously human? *Trends Cogn. Sci.* 7:157–160.

Rees, G., 2001. Neuroimaging of visual awareness in patients and normal subjects. *Curr. Opin. Neurobiol.* 11:150–156.

Rees, G., K. Friston, and C. Koch, 2000. A direct quantitative relationship between the functional properties of human and macaque V5. *Nat. Neurosci.* 3:716–723.

Rees, G., G. Kreiman, and C. Koch, 2002. Neural correlates of consciousness in humans. *Nat. Rev. Neurosci.* 3:261–270.

Rees, G., and N. Lavie, 2001. What can functional imaging reveal about the role of attention in visual awareness? *Neuropsychologia* 39:1343–1353.

Rees, G., C. Russell, C. D. Frith, and J. Driver, 1999. Inattentional blindness versus inattentional amnesia for fixated but ignored words. *Science* 286:2504–2507.

Rees, G., E. Wojciulik, K. Clarke, M. Husain, C. Frith, and J. Driver, 2000. Unconscious activation of visual cortex in the damaged right hemisphere of a parietal patient with extinction. *Brain* 123:1624–1633.

Rees, G., E. Wojciulik, K. Clarke, M. Husain, C. Frith, and J. Driver, 2002. Neural correlates of conscious and unconscious vision in parietal extinction. *Neurocase* 8:387–393.

Ress, D., B. T. Backus, and D. J. Heeger, 2000. Activity in primary visual cortex predicts performance in a visual detection task. *Nat. Neurosci.* 3:940–945.

Ress, D., and D. J. Heeger, 2003. Neuronal correlates of perception in early visual cortex. *Nat. Neurosci.* 6:414–420.

Ricci, C., and C. Blundo, 1990. Perception of ambiguous figures after focal brain lesions. *Neuropsychologia* 28:1163–1173.

Riddoch, G., 1917. Dissociation of visual perceptions due to occipital injuries, with especial reference to appreciation of movement. *Brain* 40:15–57.

Rizzo, M., M. Nawrot, and J. Zihl, 1995. Motion and shape perception in cerebral akinetopsia. *Brain* 118:1105–1127.

Rizzo, M., and D. A. Robin, 1996. Bilateral effects of unilateral visual cortex lesions in human. *Brain* 119:951–963.

Robichaud, L., and L. B. Stelmach, 2003. Inducing blindsight in normal observers. *Psychon. Bull. Rev.* 10:206–209.

Rock, I., C. M. Linnett, P. Grant, and A. Mack, 1992. Perception without attention: Results of a new method. *Cognit. Psychol.* 24:502–534.

Rodriguez, E., N. George, J. P. Lachaux, J. Martinerie, B. Renault, and F. J. Varela, 1999. Perception's shadow: Long-distance synchronization of human brain activity. *Nature* 397:430–433.

Rowe, J. B., I. Toni, O. Josephs, R. S. Frackowiak, and R. E. Passingham, 2000. The prefrontal cortex: Response selection or maintenance within working memory? *Science* 288:1656–1660.

Sahraie, A., L. Weiskrantz, J. L. Barbur, A. Simmons, S. C. Williams, and M. J. Brammer, 1997. Pattern of neuronal activity associated with conscious and unconscious processing of visual signals. *Proc. Natl. Acad. Sci. U.S.A.* 94:9406–9411.

Sakai, K., E. Watanabe, Y. Onodera, I. Uchida, H. Kato, E. Yamamoto, H. Koizumi, and Y. Miyashita, 1995. Functional mapping of the human colour centre with echo-planar magnetic resonance imaging. *Proc. R. Soc. Lond. B Biol. Sci.* 261:89–98.

Sereno, M. I., A. M. Dale, J. B. Reppas, K. K. Kwong, J. W. Belliveau, T. J. Brady, B. R. Rosen, and R. B. Tootell, 1995. Borders of multiple visual areas in humans revealed by functional magnetic resonance imaging. *Science* 268:889–893.

Shadlen, M. N., and J. A. Movshon, 1999. Synchrony unbound: A critical evaluation of the temporal binding hypothesis. *Neuron* 24:67–77, 111–125.

Silbersweig, D. A., E. Stern, C. Frith, C. Cahill, A. Holmes, S. Grootoonk, J. Seaward, P. McKenna, S. E. Chua, L. Schnorr, et al., 1995. A functional neuroanatomy of hallucinations in schizophrenia. *Nature* 378:176–179.

Smith, A. J., H. Blumenfeld, K. L. Behar, D. L. Rothman, R. G. Shulman, and F. Hyder, 2002. Cerebral energetics and spiking frequency: The neurophysiological basis of fMRI. *Proc. Natl. Acad. Sci. U.S.A.* 99:10765–10770.

Sperry, R. W., R. E. Myers, and A. M. Schrier, 1960. Perceptual capacity of the isolated visual cortex in the cat. *Q. J. Exp. Psychol.* 12:65–71.

Stanley, D. A., and N. Rubin, 2003. fMRI activation in response to illusory contours and salient regions in the human lateral occipital complex. *Neuron* 37:323–331.

Steinmetz, P. N., A. Roy, P. J. Fitzgerald, S. S. Hsiao, K. O. Johnson, and E. Niebur, 2000. Attention modulates synchronized neuronal firing in primate somatosensory cortex. *Nature* 404:187–190.

Stenberg, G., M. Lindgren, M. Johansson, A. Olsson, and I. Rosen, 2000. Semantic processing without conscious identification: Evidence from event-related potentials. *J. Exp. Psychol. Learn. Mem. Cogn.* 26:973–1004.

Sterzer, P., M. O. Russ, C. Preibisch, and A. Kleinschmidt, 2002. Neural correlates of spontaneous direction reversals in ambiguous apparent visual motion. *Neuroimage* 15:908–916.

Stoerig, P., and E. Barth, 2001. Low-level phenomenal vision despite unilateral destruction of primary visual cortex. *Conscious. Cogn.* 10:574–587.

Talairach, J., and P. Tournoux, 1988. *Co-planar Stereotaxic Atlas of the Human Brain,* New York: Thieme Medical.

Theoret, H., M. Kobayashi, G. Ganis, P. Di Capua, and A. Pascual-Leone, 2002. Repetitive transcranial magnetic stimulation of human area MT/V5 disrupts perception and storage of the motion aftereffect. *Neuropsychologia* 40:2280–2287.

TONG, F., 2003. Primary visual cortex and visual awareness. *Nat. Rev. Neurosci.* 4:219–229.

TONG, F., and S. A. ENGEL, 2001. Interocular rivalry revealed in the human cortical blind-spot representation. *Nature* 411: 195–199.

TONG, F., K. NAKAYAMA, J. T. VAUGHAN, and N. KANWISHER, 1998. Binocular rivalry and visual awareness in human extrastriate cortex. *Neuron* 21:753–759.

TONONI, G., R. SRINIVASAN, D. P. RUSSELL, and G. M. EDELMAN, 1998. Investigating neural correlates of conscious perception by frequency-tagged neuromagnetic responses. *Proc. Natl. Acad. Sci. U.S.A.* 95:3198–3203.

TOOTELL, R. B., J. B. REPPAS, A. M. DALE, R. B. LOOK, M. I. SERENO, R. MALACH, T. J. BRADY, and B. R. ROSEN, 1995. Visual motion aftereffect in human cortical area MT revealed by functional magnetic resonance imaging. *Nature* 375:139–141.

TOOTELL, R. B., D. TSAO, and W. VANDUFFEL, 2003. Neuroimaging weighs in: Humans meet macaques in "primate" visual cortex. *J. Neurosci.* 15:3981–3989.

UNGERLEIDER, L. G., and M. MISHKIN, 1982. Two cortical visual systems. In *Analysis of Visual Behavior*, D. J. Ingle, M. A. Goodale, and R. J. W. Mansfield, eds. Cambridge, Mass.: MIT Press, pp. 549–586.

VAINA, L. M., 1994. Functional segregation of color and motion processing in the human visual cortex: Clinical evidence. *Cereb. Cortex.* 4:555–572.

VAINA, L. M., M. LEMAY, D. C. BIENFANG, A. Y. CHOI, and K. NAKAYAMA, 1990. Intact "biological motion" and "structure from motion" perception in a patient with impaired motion mechanisms: A case study. *Vis. Neurosci.* 5:353–369.

VERREY, D., 1888. Hemiachromatopsie droite absolue. *Arch Ophthalmol (Paris)* 8:289–300.

VON DER MALSBURG, C., 1981, 1994. The correlation theory of brain function. MPI Biophysical Chemistry, Internal Report 81–2. Reprinted in *Analysis of Visual Behavior* II, E. Domany, J. L. van Hemmen, and K. Schulten, eds. Berlin: Springer.

VON HELMHOLTZ, H., 1867. *Handbuch der physiologischen Optik*. In *Allgemeine Encyklopädie der Physik*, vol. 9, G. Karsten, ed. Leipzig: Voss.

VUILLEUMIER, P., J. L. ARMONY, K. CLARKE, M. HUSAIN, J. DRIVER, and R. J. DOLAN, 2002. Neural response to emotional faces with and without awareness: Event-related fMRI in a parietal patient with visual extinction and spatial neglect. *Neuropsychologia* 40:2156–2166.

VUILLEUMIER, P., N. SAGIV, E. HAZELTINE, R. A. POLDRACK, D. SWICK, R. D. RAFAL, and J. D. GABRIELI, 2001. Neural fate of seen and unseen faces in visuospatial neglect: A combined event-related functional MRI and event-related potential study. *Proc. Natl. Acad. Sci. U.S.A.* 98:3495–3500.

WANDELL, B. A., 1999. Computational neuroimaging of human visual cortex. *Annu Rev. Neurosci.* 22:145–173.

WEISKRANTZ, L., 1986. Blindsight: *A case study and Its Implications.* Oxford, England: Oxford University Press.

WEISKRANTZ, L., A. COWEY, and I. HODINOTT-HILL, 2002. Primesight in a blindsight subject. *Nat. Neurosci.* 5:101–102.

WILKINS, A. J., T. SHALLICE, and R. MCCARTHY, 1987. Frontal lesions and sustained attention. *Neuropsychologia* 25:359–365.

ZEKI, S. M., 1978. Functional specialisation in the visual cortex of the rhesus monkey. *Nature* 274:423–428.

ZEKI, S., 2003. The disunity of consciousness. *Trends Cogn. Sci.* 7:214–218.

ZEKI, S., and A. BARTELS, 1998. The autonomy of the visual systems and the modularity of conscious vision. *Philos. Trans. R. Soc. Lond. B Biol. Sci.* 353:1911–1914.

ZEKI, S., and D. H. FFYTCHE, 1998. The Riddoch syndrome: Insights into the neurobiology of conscious vision. *Brain* 121:25–45.

ZEKI, S., J. D. WATSON, C. J. LUECK, K. J. FRISTON, C. KENNARD, and R. S. FRACKOWIAK, 1991. A direct demonstration of functional specialization in human visual cortex. *J. Neurosci.* 11: 641–649.

ZEKI, S., J. D. WATSON, and R. S. FRACKOWIAK, 1993. Going beyond the information given: the relation of illusory visual motion to brain activity. *Proc. R. Soc. Lond. B Biol. Sci.* 252:215–222.

ZIHL, J., D. VON CRAMON, and N. MAI, 1983. Selective disturbance of movement vision after bilateral brain damage. *Brain* 106(Pt. 2):313–340.

ZIHL, J., D. VON CRAMON, N. MAI, and C. SCHMID, 1991. Disturbance of movement vision after bilateral posterior brain damage. Further evidence and follow up observations. *Brain* 114(Pt. 5):2235–2252.

85 Split Decisions

GEORGE WOLFORD, MICHAEL B. MILLER, AND
MICHAEL S. GAZZANIGA

ABSTRACT Split-brain patients provide a fascinating look at some of the issues surrounding consciousness. We briefly review past findings and insights gained from studying these patients. We discuss in more detail some of the more interesting (to us) findings since the last edition of this volume. We conclude by suggesting a modified version of signal detection theory that may shed some light on aspects of consciousness in these patients.

Consciousness in the split brain

Split-brain patients offer a unique perspective on some aspects of conscious experience, and perhaps on the nature of consciousness itself. Roger Sperry once referred to the brain as "two separate realms of conscious awareness; two sensing, perceiving, thinking and remembering systems." There were early fears that severing the callosum was a bad idea and would lead to dire consequences. The operation might create a person with the ultimate split personality, just like having two persons inside the same body. One of the big early surprises was the seemingly complete absence of any splitness in the consciousness or personality of these patients (Akelaitis, 1941; Gazzaniga, Bogen, and Sperry, 1962). Most of the patients seemed blithely unaware that anything had changed in their mental processes, with the pleasant exception that their seizures had lessened or even stopped. Why don't split-brain patients experience dual consciousness? Possibly consciousness is housed in neural tissue that is completely lateralized to one hemisphere or the other. Perhaps consciousness is completely tied to language, and since language is generally lateralized, consciousness is as well. Perhaps the two hemispheres have worked out a division of labor such that consciousness follows the task or materials and that different hemispheres are consciously aware at different times. We will explore that final possibility later in this chapter.

GEORGE WOLFORD and MICHAEL S. GAZZANIGA Department of Psychological and Brain Sciences, Dartmouth College, Hanover, N.H.

MICHAEL B. MILLER Department of Psychological and Brain Sciences, Dartmouth College, Hanover, N.H., and Department of Psychology, University of California at Santa Barbara, Santa Barbara, Calif.

The split-brain operation

Split-brain surgery is a treatment for certain types of intractable epilepsy. Seizures in epilepsy are caused by an abnormal electrical discharge that leads to a reverberating or rhythmic discharge. In some individuals, the rhythmic discharges recruit tissue in both hemispheres. The split surgery involves severing all or part of the corpus callosum, the major fiber tract connecting the two cerebral hemispheres, and on occasion other forebrain commisures as well. The corpus callosum is the largest fiber tract in the brain. The human corpus callosum contains about 200 million axons, originating from layer 2/3 pyramidal neurons (Aboitiz et al., 1992). The first reported use of splitting the corpus callosum to control epilepsy was by Van Wagenen and Herren (1940). Van Wagenen got the idea for the surgery by observing that one of his patients with severe seizures experienced considerable relief after developing a tumor in his corpus callosum. Based on that observation, he and his colleague severed part or all of the callosi in 10 patients and reported considerable relief from seizures. They performed the surgery on a second set of 14 patients as well. After a hiatus of a couple of decades, the procedure was tried in a new set of patients in California (Bogen and Vogel, 1962). The behavior of these patients was studied extensively by Gazzaniga and his colleagues (Gazzaniga, Bogen, and Sperry, 1962, 1963, 1965). The treatment was effective in reducing seizures in these patients. Overall there was about a 60%–70% seizure reduction in 80% of the patients. However, there were serious complications in many of these earlier cases. More than 50% of the early patients experienced aseptic meningitis or hydrocephalus, often resulting in death. Among other difficulties, the wall separating the bottom of the corpus callosum from the ventricles is only four cells thick in places and is easily punctured. D. H. Wilson at Dartmouth perfected the use of microsurgery in splitting the corpus callosum and revived the use of the procedure in controlling seizures (Wilson et al., 1977). Split-brain surgery was never performed at a high rate and was considered a treatment of last resort. The procedure is less common today, with the availability of newer and better pharmacological treatments coupled with advances in neurolocation and more focused neurosurgery. Further, a higher percentage of recent split-brain operations have involved only a portion of the corpus callosum. In theory, patients who have undergone a complete callosotomy form an ideal population for studying the independent functioning of the two hemispheres. In practice, only a relatively small percentage of these patients are appropriate for behavioral studies. All of the patients have had a long history of severe epileptic seizures, and many suffer from other cognitive deficits. Although relatively rare, there are more split-brain patients than there are patients for many of the other interesting brain anomalies.

Hemispheric asymmetries

Since at least the time of Broca, we have believed that some behavioral functions such as language are lateralized in the brain. Broca studied a patient who was paralyzed on the right side and had lost the ability to speak. The man died shortly thereafter, and his brain was preserved. Most of our knowledge about hemispheric asymmetries over the next century came from studying people with various types of brain injuries. Researchers also examined hemispheric differences in people without brain damage, using tachistoscopic presentation to one visual field or the other. The research on neurologically intact subjects confirmed much of the patient work, but interpretation of the results obtained in such subjects is always clouded by the fact that any information presented to a specific hemisphere can cross to the other hemisphere at will, and that crossing takes only a few milliseconds (Berlucchi et al., 1971).

Split-brain patients provided an ideal environment for studying these hemispheric asymmetries, because information presented to a specific hemisphere more or less had to stay there. Early studies with split-brain patients confirmed that language was usually lateralized to the left hemisphere and confirmed advantages in the right hemisphere for spatial processing. There has been interesting evidence that processing in the right hemisphere is relatively more literal, while processing in the left is more constructive (Metcalfe, Funnell, and Gazzaniga, 1995). Several studies over the last few years have helped clarify those asymmetries. In this chapter, we will focus on several new developments concerning the role of the two hemispheres in attention and memory, and we will present some intriguing studies aimed at clarifying the precise advantages of the right hemisphere in spatial processing.

PERCEPTUAL PROCESSING It has been known at least since the time of John Hughlings Jackson (1874/1915), a contemporary of Broca, that many perceptual processes are lateralized to the right hemisphere. Current research has shown that not all perceptual processing is superior in the right hemisphere. The presence of asymmetries is quite specific to both the particular stimuli and the particular task. For example, Corballis, Funnell, and Gazzaniga (2000a) found

that both hemispheres of two split-brain patients (one with a complete split, the other a partial split) could discriminate two objects with different identities equally well, but that the right hemisphere performed better than the left hemisphere in discriminating two identical objects with different spatial locations. In subsequent studies they found that the right hemisphere was better at line orientation and vernier acuity, but that both hemispheres performed equally well in size comparisons and luminance discrimination (Corballis, Funnell, and Gazzaniga, 1999, 2000a).

Furthermore, Corballis and colleagues have suggested that these hemispheric asymmetries in visuospatial processing are not entirely due to hemispheric specializations for particular types of sensory input but involve lateralization of specific types of processing, such as visual grouping. One piece of evidence for this idea involves the line motion effect. This occurs when a line is presented briefly between two squares. Just prior to the appearance of the line, one of the squares flashes. To observers, it appears that the line is propagating from the flashing square. Hikosaka, Miyauchi, and Shimojo (1993) proposed a low-level visual process to explain the effect in which the flashing square draws attention to the location prior to the onset of the line. However, subsequent researchers have demonstrated that changing the properties of the stimuli can create quite different illusions (von Grünau and Faubert, 1994; Tse, Cavanagh, and Nakayama, 1998). For example, using a red line between a red and green square will create the illusion that the red line is propagating from the red square. In this case, the effect of apparent motion must rely on visual grouping after the onset of the line. Corballis and colleagues found that the left hemisphere in a split-brain patient was indifferent to the color manipulation but that the right hemisphere almost always perceived the line as moving away from the square with the matching color (Corballis, Funnell, and Gazzaniga, 2000b; Corballis, Barnett, and Corballis, 2004).

Corballis and colleagues reached similar conclusions using paradigms involving the perception of subjective figures by modal and amodal boundary completion (Corballis et al., 1999). Modal completion can be solved by relying solely on low-level visual processing. Two split-brain patients were found to perform modal completion equally well in both hemispheres. Amodal completion relies on visual grouping to resolve the spatial ambiguity, since there are no subjective contours, and, in this case, the right hemisphere was superior to the left. Corballis refers to this lateralization of visual grouping in the right hemisphere as the "right hemisphere interpreter" (Corballis, in press).

A recent study that is consistent with the idea of a right hemisphere interpreter involves the perception of causality using the Michotte task. Short movies were shown to patient J.W., who had a complete split. Each movie showed one disk moving toward a second disk and coming to a standstill when it touched the second disk. The second disk then moved away from the first disk. To most observers, it would appear that the movement of the second disk is caused by the first disk. However, if a large enough gap, either spatial or temporal, is inserted between the two circles, the motion of the disks does not appear causally related. The left hemisphere of a split-brain patient, J.W., was indifferent to the manipulation of the magnitude of the gap, but the right hemisphere responses were affected by the magnitude of the gaps in an appropriate fashion (Roser et al., in press).

Despite the right hemisphere advantage for some forms of visuospatial processing and evidence for a right hemisphere interpreter, there are some visual processes in which the left hemisphere has an advantage. For example, recent neuroimaging studies have shown that mentally rotating an object activates parietal and frontal regions in both hemispheres, but that imagining yourself in a different spatial perspective relative to an object may involve different parietal and frontal regions located primarily in the left hemisphere (Wraga, Church, and Badre, 2002; Zacks et al., 2002). Funnell and colleagues have tested this distinction in a split-brain patient using a paradigm in which an identical stimulus can be mentally rotated or imagined from a different perspective. They found that while the right hemisphere appeared to be better at mental rotation, the left hemisphere appeared to be better at perspective taking (Funnell, Johnson, and Gazzaniga, 2001).

For these relatively low-level perceptual paradigms, the hemispheric asymmetries appear to be driven by top-down processes. In contrast, many hemispheric differences with higher-order cognitive processes, such as attention and memory, appear to be driven by specialization for stimulus properties. Kingstone, Friesen, and Gazzaniga (2000) performed several fascinating studies on reflexive attention using eye gaze direction in split-brain patients. As in the Posner cuing paradigm, a schematic face was presented as the cue. The direction of the eyes may point to a target, or it may not. In the case of primary interest, the direction of eye gaze was not predictive of the target location. Yet in the right hemisphere, but not the left, the patient was faster to respond to a target in the path of the eye gaze. This effect was obtained with schematic faces and with eyes alone, but not when the schematic faces were presented upside down (figure 85.1). When the face was actually predictive of target location or when the stimulus was a nonpredictive arrow, both hemispheres showed a similar effect. These finding suggest that reflexive joint attention is mediated by cortical processes that are lateralized to the hemisphere responsible for face processing, which in these two patients is the right hemisphere. Parenthetically, this work with split-brain patients led to the surprising finding that nonpredictive arrows did orient attention in normal subjects, a finding that runs counter to a basic assumption (and never explicitly tested) in the field of attention since the start of the Posner cuing paradigm in the 1970s (Kingstone et al., in press).

MEMORY Hemispheric specialization in particular low-level cognitive processes can affect episodic memory formation, the memory for real-world events, as well. Retrieving episodic memories often involves decision processes that are affected by a variety of influences, just like any other decision process, and the underlying brain regions engaged during retrieval can vary greatly from subject to subject, depending on individual strategies (Miller et al., 2001; Miller, Kingstone, and Gazzaniga, 2002; Windmann, Urbach, and Kutas, 2002). The encoding of episodic memories, as opposed to retrieval, appears to be elicit more consistent neural activations across subjects (for review, see Cabeza and Nyberg, 2000). Hemispheric asymmetries play a role in memory formation, as evidenced by neuropsychological studies (Milner, Corkin, and Tueber, 1968; Milner, 1972) and more recently by neuroimaging studies (Tulving et al., 1994; Kelley et al., 1998; Nyberg, Cabeza, and Tulving, 1998; Wagner et al., 1998; Nyberg et al., 2000). However, many memory researchers debate the nature of those asymmetries. Some investigators have argued that episodic encoding is predominantly a left prefrontal function and that episodic retrieval is predominantly a right prefrontal function (Tulving et al., 1994). Typically these neuroimaging studies rely on the encoding and retrieval of familiar verbal material (Cabeza and Nyberg, 2000). Other researchers have suggested that hemispheric asymmetries, particularly episodic encoding, are material-specific rather than process-specific. For example, recent neuroimaging research has found predominantly right hemisphere activations in the prefrontal cortex during the encoding of unfamiliar faces (Kelley et al., 1998) and textures (Wagner et al., 1998). Nevertheless, proponents of a lateralized episodic encoding region argue that the bulk of neuroimaging research, including some studies using nonverbal material, is consistent with episodic encoding being predominantly a left hemisphere process (Nyberg, Cabeza, and Tulving, 1998; Nyberg et al., 2000).

The testing of split-brain patients can play a role in resolving this debate. If encoding and retrieval are predominantly lateralized processes in opposite hemispheres, then split-brain patients should have major memory impairment, because the information is encoded in one hemisphere and retrieved by the other and the two hemispheres are disconnected. Yet these patients demonstrate only minor deficits in episodic memory (Zaidel and Sperry, 1974; LeDoux et al., 1977; Phelps, Hirst, and Gazzaniga, 1991; Metcalfe, Funnell, and Gazzaniga, 1995; see Viskontas, Zaidel, Knowlton, 2003, for a recent case of a patient with more severe impairments in autobiographical memory). Split-brain patients perform normally on most recognition tests yet often have slight impairments on free recall tasks that

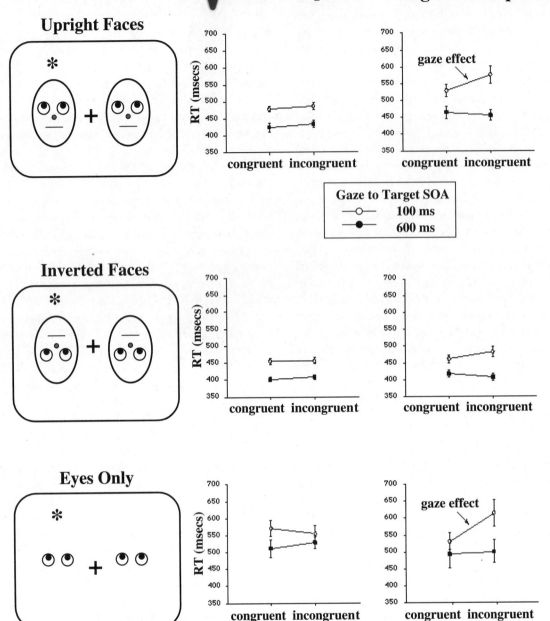

FIGURE 85.1   The graphs represent split-brain patient J.W.'s performance. Two faces (upright or inverted) or two pairs of eyes were presented concurrently to the left of a central fixation cross and to the right of the cross. The task was to maintain central fixation and to press a left-hand key when the target asterisk was presented to the left visual field (right hemisphere) and a right-hand key when the target was in the right visual field (left hemisphere). Gaze direction did not predict target location. The gaze effect (responding significantly faster to a congruency between target location and gaze direction than to an incongruency) was evident only in the right hemisphere, and only for upright faces and eyes. Patient V.P. had similar results (Kingstone, Friesen, and Gazzaniga, 2000).

require additional recruitment of strategic resources (Phelps, Hirst, and Gazzaniga, 1991). These findings in split-brain patients suggest that activations seen on neuroimaging studies may indeed be material-specific rather than process-specific, as suggested by Kelley and colleagues (1998) and Wagner and colleagues (1998).

We directly tested this hypothesis by manipulating the encoding of words and faces in each hemisphere of two split-brain patients, one with a complete split and the other with a partial split (Miller, Kingstone, and Gazzaniga, 2002). If episodic encoding is predominantly a left hemisphere function independent of material type, then only the left hemisphere in these patients should benefit from more elaborate encoding of words and faces. However, because language is preferentially lateralized to the left hemisphere and face processing is lateralized to the right hemisphere in these patients (Gazzaniga, 2000), we hypothesized that the left hemisphere, but not the right, would benefit from the deeper encoding of familiar words, and that the right hemisphere, but not the left, would benefit from the deeper encoding of unfamiliar faces. Our hypothesis would work only if encoding processes were available in both hemispheres.

As shown in figure 85.2, we found in both patients a significant difference in recognition performance after deep processing during encoding of words versus shallow processing during encoding of words in the left hemisphere, but no difference as a function of depth of encoding in the right hemisphere. Unfamiliar faces yielded the opposite result. There was a significant difference in recognition performance after deep encoding of faces versus shallow encoding of faces in the right hemisphere, but no difference in the left hemisphere. Our results clearly indicated that manipulations of episodic encoding differentially affect the performance of the hemispheres, depending on the type of material being processed. Each hemisphere seems to be fully capable of supporting episodic memory, and some asymmetries seem to be based on the type of material being processed. A more recent fMRI study of normal subjects regarding hemispheric asymmetries during encoding of faces (Wig et al., in press), along with previous patient studies (Milner, 1972) and sodium amytal studies (Kelley et al., 2002), demonstrate functionally separable routes to memory within prefrontal cortex that depend on both the intrinsic properties of the to-be-remembered materials and on the specific cognitive operations required by the task.

Wig and colleagues (in press) also suggest that memorization of namable objects (materials with fluent access to both verbal and pictorial codes) engages both hemispheres, and that these materials are remembered better than materials that have access to single codes—the "picture superiority" effect (Paivio and Csapo, 1973).

We conducted a study (Cooney et al., 2002) with a split-brain patient using a simple full-field, nonlateralized

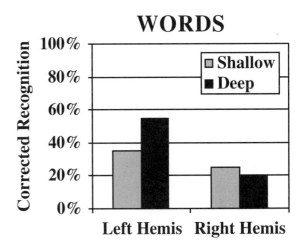

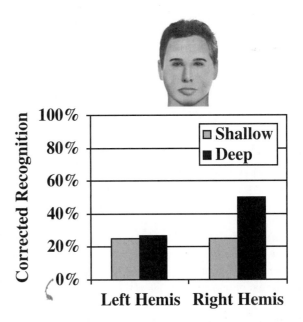

FIGURE 85.2 The top graph represents recognition performance using words for the left and right hemispheres of split-brain patient J.W., while the bottom graph represents recognition performance using unfamiliar faces. Gray bars represent a shallow level of processing during encoding (for words: does the word contain the letter *a*? for faces: is the face female?), and black bars represent a deep level of processing (for words: does the word represent a living object? for faces: is the face the face of a healthy person?). Both the study and the test sessions were lateralized to one hemisphere. The left hemisphere's recognition performance improved significantly after deep processing of words compared to shallow processing, while the right hemisphere showed no improvement. In contrast to word processing, the right hemisphere's recognition performance improved significantly after deep processing compared to shallow processing, but the left hemisphere's recognition performance did not. Patient V.P. had similar results (Miller, Kingstone, and Gazzaniga, 2002).

presentation with responses collected separately for the right and left hands. In three separate conditions, the patient memorized words, namable objects, and unfamiliar faces. Following the presentation of each stimulus set, the patient was given a recognition memory test with responses for each hand. Consistent with dual-coding predictions, when the subject used the right hand, memory for namable objects was no better than for words, and when the subject used the left hand, memory for namable objects was no better than for faces. These findings suggest that the picture superiority effect results from the collective contribution of left and right hemisphere brain regions during memorization.

Looking for patterns

Gazzaniga and his colleagues have long argued for the existence of a structure in the left hemisphere referred to as the interpreter. The interpreter was the process that tried to make sense out of incomplete or ambiguous information. The existence of such an interpreter has been demonstrated in several experiments in which the left hemisphere apparently "felt" the need to explain responses made by the left hand under control of the right hemisphere (Gazzaniga, 2000). We recently developed a new technique for examining the existence and characteristics of the interpreter in the left hemisphere (Wolford, Miller, and Gazzaniga, 2000). The technique is quite simple and involves having the participant guess which of two events will happen on the next trial. This paradigm, referred to as probability guessing, was examined extensively in the middle of the twentieth century. One curious and easily replicable finding is that humans tend to frequency match in this paradigm. Frequency matching means that humans tend to guess the alternatives in the proportion at which they have been presented in the past. So, if the two alternatives are "left" and "right," and left occurs on 70% of the trials, participants will tend to guess "left" about 70% of the time. Frequency matching is curious because it is nonoptimal and because animals from almost every other species maximize the optimal strategy (Hinson and Staddon, 1983). Maximizing is always guessing the most frequent alternative.

The likely reason that humans frequency match is that they believe there is a deterministic pattern, and they are determined to find that pattern even when told there isn't one. Yellott (1969) provided a striking demonstration that people were looking for patterns in these experiments. In his experiment, a stimulus appeared either on the left or on the right, on each trial, and subjects had to predict which light would appear. The probability of the lights was varied across blocks. Subjects matched the frequency of the actual presentations (frequency matching), changing when the frequency changed. In the last block of 50 trials, the light appeared wherever the subject predicted it would, regardless

of the subjects' guesses. Subjects continued to frequency match during these last 50 trials. When Yellott stopped the experiment and asked subjects for their impressions, they overwhelmingly responded that there was a fixed pattern to the light sequences and that they had finally figured it out. They proceeded to describe elaborate and complex sequences of right and left choices that resulted in their responses always being correct. These verbal reports support the contention that subjects had been searching for fixed sequences all along and were fooled into thinking they had succeeded.

We reasoned that if frequency matching results from searching for patterns even when there are none, and if the left hemisphere interpreter postulated by Gazzaniga is a neural structure that tries to make sense of the world around it, then there might be an intimate relationship between frequency matching and the left hemisphere. To test this hypothesis, we lateralized the probability guessing paradigm, presenting the stimuli to either the right or left visual field of two split-brain patients and collecting the predictions from the appropriate contralateral hand. We reasoned that if the interpreter were responsible for frequency matching, then we should see frequency matching with left hemisphere presentation and maximizing with right hemisphere presentation.

That is what we found. We replicated the paradigm using patients with unilateral frontal brain damage, reasoning that a patient with unilateral but widespread damage to the right frontal cortex would perform similar to the left hemisphere of a split-brain patient, and vice versa for a patient with unilateral damage to the left hemisphere. As predicted, the patient with unilateral left frontal damage maximized, but the patients with unilateral right frontal damage frequency matched. Figure 85.3 shows the data averaged across the two split-brain patients and the patients with frontal lesions (see original article for individual graphs).

Recognition of self

Various researchers have argued that the concept of self is intimately related to consciousness (Kihlstrom and Klein 1997; Turk et al., in press). Leaving aside the notion of consciousness during visual perception as portrayed by Crick and Koch (see Crick and Koch, this volume), the self as agent seems to be a major part of much conscious experience. Is processing or awareness of self really different from other forms of semantic processing? Are there neural circuits specifically related to self processing? Could there be a connection between the left hemisphere interpreter and the self? There have been interesting findings related to all three of these questions over the last few years.

Many investigators, following the level-of-processing tradition, have shown that self-relevant processing leads to

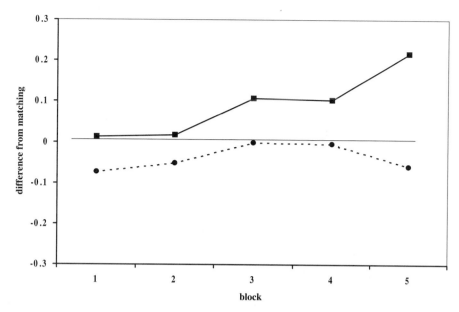

FIGURE 85.3   The graph represents the probability of guessing the most frequent stimulus as a function of hemisphere for each block of 100 trials. The data are averaged over two split-brain patients and five patients with unilateral frontal damage. The most frequent stimulus appeared 70% of the time in all cases, and the horizontal line in the middle of the graph represents frequency matching or guessing the most frequent stimulus 70% of the time. Left hemisphere presentations yielded frequency matching, but right hemisphere presentations yielded maximizing or guessing the most frequent stimulus most of the time. (The data, broken down by individuals, are presented in Wolford, Miller, and Gazzaniga, 2000.)

better subsequent memory than even deep semantic processing (see review by Lockhart and Craik, 1990). Some investigators have argued that self-relevant processing is not qualitatively different from other forms of semantic processing (Kihlstrom and Klein, 1997). They argue that its advantage comes from increased familiarity with self and the broader array of associations that are available. Kelley and colleagues (2002) compared self-relevant processing to other-relevant processing and to upper- and lowercase judgments. They found that both self-relevant and other-relevant processing produced greater activation in the left inferior frontal cortex and in the anterior cingulate when compared to case judgments, but there was no difference between self and other in these regions. They did find one area, the medial prefrontal cortex, in which self processing was substantially higher in activation level than either other or case processing. Taken together, these findings suggest that self processing is similar in some ways but qualitatively different in other ways from deep semantic processing.

What about the possible relationship between the left hemisphere interpreter and the processing of self? The findings from Kelley and colleagues (2002) were ambiguous as to laterality, and the medial prefrontal activation straddled the midline. Given the smoothing algorithms used, the activation might have been bilateral or might have been lateralized to one of the two sides. The previous literature has been mixed with respect to the laterality of self processing. Using WADA tests, Keenan argued that the right hemi-

sphere was more apt to remember having seen one's self following presentation of morphed photographs in which the self was part of the morph (Keenan et al., 2001). Of necessity, perception and memory are confounded in a WADA paradigm. Generally, face processing is better in the right hemisphere (Kanwisher, McDermott, and Chun, 1997), but not necessarily processing of one's own face. Other studies have shown a left hemisphere advantage for autobiographical memory and for pictures of one's face (Conway and Pleydell-Pearce, 2000).

In a recent study, Turk and colleagues (2002) examined the perceptual recognition of self in a split-brain patient. They presented morphs of the patient and one of three familiar others to the patient, varying the percentage of self in the morph. They went through each sequence of morphs from 0% self to 100% self twice. On some sequences the patient was asked to respond "yes" if he saw himself. On other sequences, he was asked if he saw a particular familiar other. They found a strong dissociation in that the patient was more likely to identify the other familiar person in right hemisphere presentations but substantially more likely to identify himself in left hemisphere presentations. These data do not necessarily resolve the ambiguity in the previous literature, but they do suggest that the left hemisphere may be biased to perceive one's self. Such was not the case in the right hemisphere.

The foregoing data do not necessarily speak to the involvement of the interpreter, but the link between a structure that tries to make sense of the world and the perception of self is compelling. Both appear to reside in the left hemisphere, and a large part of making sense of the world seems to involve thoughts about one's self. Continuing in the speculative vein, it is possible that consciousness, the self, and the left hemisphere interpreter are intimately connected. As compelling as these relationships seem to us, we are going to do our best in the next couple of sections to complicate the picture.

A two-stage signal detection model

We noticed an interesting aspect to the data on self perception presented by Turk and colleagues (2002) that was not discussed by the authors. A reanalysis of the data confirmed our impression and meshed with previous observations of working with split-brain patients. The split-brain patient went through each of the morphed sequences several times using one of two response options. On one-half of the trials the patient was instructed to respond "yes" if he saw himself in the picture. On the other half of the trials he responded "yes" if he saw the familiar other in the photograph. We reanalyzed the data by adding together the number of yes responses for a given morph stimulus across the two different response formats. For example, on one morph sequence for the stimulus that contained 90% of the patient's face, the patient responded "yes" a sum of 110% of the time (100% of the time when asked about self and 10% when

asked about the familiar other) when the morph was presented to the left hemisphere, but only 75% of the time (60% and 15%) when the morph was presented to the right hemisphere. The average rate of yes responses across the different morph fractions is presented in figure 85.4.

As the figure shows, presentations to the left hemisphere were more likely to yield a yes response, regardless of morph fraction or response required. We concluded that presentations to the left hemisphere are biased to yield a perception of "self," but they are also more likely to yield a yes response in general (92% yes responses in left hemisphere vs. 72% in the right). Treating different morphs as replications, this difference was significant ($t(10) = 2.82$, $P = 0.018$).

We are suggesting that willingness to respond and bias for a particular response given that a response is made are separable parameters. This separability is not observable in most paradigms, as the subject is forced to respond in most paradigms. The separation between willingness to respond and bias for a particular response seems well captured by a two-stage signal detection model. Subjects first decide to respond, and once they have decided to respond, the traditional signal detection model would apply. In order to avoid this possible confound, one would have to use a paradigm that allowed a nonresponse on each trial. However, even in paradigms that do not permit a nonresponse, we believe that in some conditions, the subjects may essentially decide not to respond, even though they hit a button. In those cases, the subjects would choose responses with little or no thought.

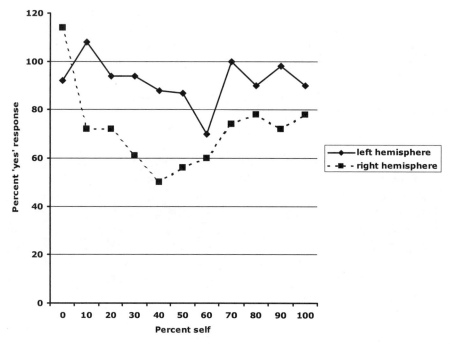

FIGURE 85.4 The graph represents the percentage of yes responses summed over trials on which patient was asked to say "yes" if he saw himself and on trials in which he was asked to say "yes" if he saw a familiar other as a function of percentage of self in the morphed image. If the patient always said yes in both response categories, the measure would sum to 200%. The graph shows that yes responses are significantly more common in the left hemisphere.

We present a rough idea of this model in the context of a recognition memory experiment requiring an old/new response in which the test is presented to different hemispheres on some schedule. The first stage would be a decision about whether to bother trying. The subject might decide that the task was too difficult in the right hemisphere and would not even to try to decide whether the item was old or new. The subject would make that decision with probability g. If the subject chose not to try, then he or she would make some response that required little thought or effort. Such a response might be pure guessing (50/50), perseveration on a single response, and so on. If the subject chose to try (say on tests in the left hemisphere), then he would assess the position of the item on some dimension of strength and respond "old" if that strength exceeded a criterion value and "no" otherwise. The decision to bother trying would be based on several factors such as the strength and quality of the available information, the context, the subject's a priori confidence in being able to perform the task, and so on.

In most standard tasks, it is difficult or impossible to disentangle the two processes with the usual data as collected. A decision not to try in some conditions of a standard recognition or judgment paradigm would show up as a reduced d' and an altered criterion, depending on the exact type of low-effort response that the subject chose to use. The paradigm of Turk and colleagues was unusual as it consisted of what could be described as two separate go/no-go tasks, one for each response option. By combining them, one obtains an estimate of the willingness to respond, the first stage, and in addition an estimate of the bias for or against the "self" response in the two hemispheres once a decision to try is made. To test the model systematically, one would need to run a standard recognition or signal detection paradigm and add the response option "don't know" on each trial. The "don't know" responses would be excluded from the estimation of the traditional signal detection parameters.

Our sense from testing split-brain patients in a number of diverse paradigms is that it seems that in many cases one hemisphere defers to the other hemisphere. The responses from the unfavored hemisphere look random and yield low estimates of d', but we have the sense that the low sensitivity often reflects an unwillingness to try. For example, the patient may believe that face recognition is the responsibility of the right hemisphere and may not try very hard on faces presented to the left.

We replicated our probability guessing paradigm with numerous variations on one of the split-brain patients. The typical result was frequency matching in the left hemisphere, but the behavior of the right hemisphere was quite inconsistent. We observed maximizing, minimizing (both forms of single-response perseveration), 50/50 responding, and simple alternation. As a group, we would characterize these responses as not trying with that hemisphere.

One of those probability guessing paradigms was particularly revealing. In addition to exploring new variables, one reason we kept varying the paradigm was to keep our subject from the depths of boredom. On one occasion we used facial hair as the event to predict. So the split-brain patient, J.W., was asked to predict on each trial whether the face that would appear had facial hair or not. For the only time in our lengthy series, the patient frequency matched with the right hemisphere and responded randomly with the left hemisphere. Our interpretation was as above. Faces were seen as the purview of the right hemisphere, so only that hemisphere took the task seriously.

The asymmetries discussed in this and in the preceding sections have implications for the nature and location of consciousness. There are undoubtedly specific modules in the brain both for different types of processing and for different types of stimuli. At least to some extent, these individual modules seem to be related to conscious experience (Cooney and Gazzaniga, 2003). The modular specificity of consciousness is further indicated by awareness of one's deficits or the lack thereof. With certain types of brain damage, the patient is fully aware of problems and bothered by them. With other types of brain damage, there is little or no awareness. A passage from Stuss and Alexander (2000) illustrates this specificity: "This domain specificity is the reason why impaired disorders of awareness within a specific module can exist. For example, a lesion in the left posterior temporal lobe typically results in Wernicke's aphasia (Benson, 1979) . . . the patient is unaware of the comprehension failure or the abnormal speech. If damage occurs to the right parietal lobe, the patient may neglect the left side with total unawareness of this neglect (Heilman et al., 1985)." We suggested earlier that for some tasks, a part of the brain assumes that it is its job to handle that task. We now suggest that when that occurs, that part of the brain is also responsible for any awareness that accompanies the task.

ACKNOWLEDGMENTS This work was supported in part by NIH grant No. P50 NS17778-19, Section 5 (G.W. and M.M.). We thank Paul Corballis, Margaret Funnell, Alan Kingstone, and Gagan Wig for their contributions.

REFERENCES

ABOITIZ, F., A. B. SCHEIBEL, R. S. FISHER, and E. ZAIDEL, 1992. Fiber composition of the human corpus callosum. *Brain Res.* 598: 143–153.

AKELAITIS, A. J., 1941. Studies on the corpus callosum: Higher visual functions in each homonymous field following complete section of the corpus callosum. *Arch. Neurol. Psychiatry* 45:788.

BENSON, D., 1979. Aphasia rehabilitation. *Arch. Neurol.* 36:187–189.

BERLUCCHI, G., W. HERON, R. HYMAN, G. RIZZOLATTI, C. UMILTÀ, 1971. Simple reaction times of ipsilateral and contralateral hand to lateralized visual stimuli. *Brain* 94:419–449.

BOGEN, J. E., and P. J. VOGEL, 1962. Cerebral commissurotomy in man: Preliminary case report. *Bull. L.A. Neurol. Soc.* 27:169–172.

CABEZA, R., and L. NYBERG, 2000. Imaging cognition. II. An empirical review of 275 PET and fMRI studies. *J. Cogn. Neurosci.* 12:1–47.

CONWAY, M. A., and C. W. PLEYDELL-PEARCE, 2000. The construction of autobiographical memories in the self memory system. *Psychol. Rev.* 107:325–339.

COONEY, J., M. B. MILLER, M. S. GAZZANIGA, and W. M. KELLEY, 2002. Picture superiority and the role of the left and right hemisphere during memory formation. Paper presented at the annual meeting of the Cognitive Neuroscience Society, San Francisco.

COONEY, J. W., and M. GAZZANIGA, 2003. Neurological disorders and the structure of human consciousness. *Trends Cogn. Sci.* 7: 161–165.

CORBALLIS, P. M., K. BARNETT, and M. C. CORBALLIS, 2004. *Line-motion illusions in the normal and divided brain.* Unpublished manuscript.

CORBALLIS, P. M., R. FENDRICH, R. SHAPLEY, and M. S. GAZZANIGA, 1999. Illusory contours and amodal completion: Evidence for a functional dissociation in callosotomy patients. *J. Cogn. Neurosci.* 11:459–466.

CORBALLIS, P. M., M. G. FUNNELL, and M. S. GAZZANIGA, 1999. A dissociation between spatial and identity matching in callosotomy patients. *Neuroreport* 10:2183–2187.

CORBALLIS, P. M., M. G. FUNNELL, and M. S. GAZZANIGA, 2000a. Hemispheric asymmetries for simple visual judgments in the split brain. *Neuropsychologia* 40:401–410.

CORBALLIS, P. M., M. G. FUNNELL, and M. S. GAZZANIGA, 2000b. An investigation of the line motion effect in a callosotomy patient. *Brain Cogn.* 48:327–332.

CORBALLIS, P. M. (in press). Visuospatial processing and the right-hemisphere interpreter. *Brain Cogn.*

FUNNELL, M. G., S. H. JOHNSON, and M. S. GAZZANIGA, 2001. Hemispheric differences in egocentric and allocentric mental rotation: evidence from fMRI and a split-brain patient. Paper presented at the annual meeting of the Cognitive Neuroscience Society, New York.

GAZZANIGA, M. S., 2000. Cerebral specialization and interhemispheric communication: Does the corpus callosum enable the human condition? *Brain* 7:1293–1326.

GAZZANIGA, M. S., J. E. BOGEN, and R. W. SPERRY, 1962. Some functional effects of sectioning the cerebral commissures in man. *Proc. Natl. Acad. Sci. U.S.A.* 48:1765–1769.

GAZZANIGA, M. S., J. E. BOGEN, and R. W. SPERRY, 1963. Laterality effects in somesthesis following cerebral commissurotomy in man. *Neuropsychologia* 1:209–215.

GAZZANIGA, M. S., J. E. BOGEN, and R. W. SPERRY, 1965. Observations on visual perception after disconnexion of the cerebral hemispheres in man. *Brain* 88:221–236.

HEILMAN, K. M., R. T. WATSON, and E. VALENSTEIN, 1985. Neglect and related disorders. In *Cinical Neuropsychology*, K. M. Heilman and E. Valenstein, eds. 2nd ed, New York: Oxford University Press, pp. 243–294.

HIKOSAKA, O., S. MIYAUCHI, and S. SHIMOJO, 1993. Focal visual attention produces illusory temporal order and motion sensation. *Vision Res.* 33:1219–1240.

HINSON, J. M., and J. E. R. STADDON, 1983. Matching, maximizing and hill-climbing. *J. Exp. Anal. Behav.* 40:321–331.

JACKSON, J. H., 1874/1915. On the nature of the duality of the brain. *Brain* 38:80–103.

KANWISHER, N., J. MCDERMOTT, and M. M. CHUN, 1997. The fusiform face area: A module in human extrastriate cortex specialized for face perception. *J. Neurosci.* 17:4302–4311.

KEENAN, J. P., A. NELSON, M. O'CONNOR, and A. PASCAULE-LEONE, 2001. Self-recognition and the right hemisphere. *Nature* 409:305.

KELLEY, W. M., F. M. MIEZIN, K. B. MCDERMOTT, R. L. BUCKNER, M. E. RAICHLE, N. J. COHEN, J. M. OLLINGER, E. AKBUDAK, T. E. CONTURO, A. Z. SNYDER, and S. E. PETERSEN, 1998. Hemispheric specialization in human dorsal frontal cortex and medial temporal lobe for verbal and nonverbal memory encoding. *Neuron* 20:927–936.

KELLEY, W. M., J. G. OJEMANN, R. D. WETZEL, C. P. DERDEYN, C. J. MORAN, D. T. CROSS, J. L. DOWLING, J. W. MILLER, and S. E. PETERSEN, 2002. Wada testing reveals frontal lateralization for the memorization of words and faces. *J. Cogn. Neurosci.* 14:116–125.

KIHLSTROM, J. F., and S. B. KLEIN, 1997. Self-knowledge and self-awareness, *Ann. N.Y. Acad. Sci.* 818:4–17.

KINGSTONE, A., C. K. FRIESEN, and M. S. GAZZANIGA, 2000. Reflexive joint attention depends on lateralized cortical connections. *Psychol. Sci.* 11:159–166.

KINGSTONE, A., D. SMILEK, J. RISTIC, C. K. FRIESEN, and J. D. EASTWOOD (in press). Attention researchers! It's time to pay attention to the real world. *Curr. Direct. Psychol. Sci.*

LEDOUX, J. E., G. RISSE, S. SPRINGER, D. H. WILSON, and M. S. GAZZANIGA, 1977. Cognition and commissurotomy. *Brain* 110:87–104.

LOCKHART, R. S., and F. I. M. CRAIK, 1990. Levels of processing: A retrospective commentary of a framework for memory research. *Cana. J. Psychol.* 44:87–112.

METCALFE, J., M. FUNNELL, and M. S. GAZZANIGA, 1995. Right-hemisphere superiority: Studies of a split-brain patient. *Psychol. Sci.* 6:157–163.

MILLER, M. B., T. C. HANDY, J. CUTLER, S. INATI, and G. L. WOLFORD, 2001. Brain activations associated with shifts in response criterion on a recognition test. In *Cognitive Neuroscience* [special issue]. *Can. J. Exp. Psychol.* 55:164–175.

MILLER, M. B., A. KINGSTONE, and M. S. GAZZANIGA, 2002. Hemispheric encoding asymmetries are more apparent than real. *J. Cogn. Neurosci.* 14:702–708.

MILNER, B., 1972. Disorders of learning and memory after temporal lobe lesions in man. *Clin. Neurosurg.* 19:421–446.

MILNER, B., S. CORKIN, and H. L. TEUBER, 1968. Further analysis of the hippocampal amnesic syndrome: 14-year follow-up study of H. M. *Neuropsychologia* 6:215–234.

NYBERG, L., R. CABEZA, and E. TULVING, 1998. Asymmetric frontal activation during episodic memory: What kind of specificity? *Trends Cogn. Sci.* 2:419–420.

NYBERG, L., R. HABIB, E. TULVING, R. CABEZA, S. HOULE, J. PERSSON, and A. R. MCINTOSH, 2000. Large scale neurocognitive networks underlying episodic memory. *J. Cogn. Neurosci.* 12:163–173.

PAIVIO, A., and K. CSAPO, 1973. Picture superiority in free recall: Imagery or dual coding? *Cogn. Psychol.* 5:176–206.

PHELPS, E. A., W. HIRST, and M. S. GAZZANIGA, 1991. Deficits in recall following partial and complete commissurotomy. *Cereb. Cortex* 1:492–498.

ROSER, M., J. FUGELSANG, K. DUNBAR, P. M. CORBALLIS, and M. S. GAZZANIGA (in press). Understanding causality. Perception and inference in a split-brain patient. *Nat. Neurosci.*

STUSS, D. T., and M. P. ALEXANDER, 2000. Executive functions and the frontal lobes: A conceptual view. *Psychol. Res.* 63:289–298.

TSE, P., P. CAVANAGH, and K. NAKAYAMA, 1998. The role of parsing in high-level motion processing. In *High Level Motion Processing: Computational, Neurobiological, and Psychophysical Perspectives*, T. Watanabe, ed. Cambridge, Mass: MIT Press, pp. 249–266.

TULVING, E., S. KAPUR, F. I. M. CRAIK, M. MOSCOVITCH, and S. HOULE, 1994. Hemispheric encoding/retrieval asymmetry in episodic memory: Positron emission tomography findings. *Proc. Natl. Acad. Sci. U.S.A.* 91:2016–2020.

TURK, D. J., T. F. HEATHERTON, W. M. KELLEY, M. G. FUNNELL, M. S. GAZZANIGA, and C. N. MACRAE, 2002. Mike or me? Self-recognition in a split-brain patient. *Nat. Neurosci.* 5:841–842.

TURK, D. J., T. F. HEATHERTON, C. N. MACRAE, W. M. KELLEY, and M. S. GAZZANIGA (in press). Out of contact, Out of mind: The distributed nature of self. *Ann. N.Y. Acad. Sci.*

VISKONTAS, I. V., E. ZAIDEL, and B. J. KNOWLTON, 2003. Severe episodic memory impairments in a commissurotomy patient. Paper presented at the annual meeting of the Cognitive Neuroscience Society, New York.

VAN WAGENEN, W. P., and R. Y. HERREN, 1940. Surgical division of commissural pathways in the corpus callosum: Relation to spread of an epileptic seizure. *Arch. Neurol. Psychiatry* 44:740–759.

VON GRÜNAU, M., and J. FAUBERT, 1994. Intraattribute and inter-attribute motion induction. *Perception* 23:913–928.

WAGNER, A. D., R. A. POLDRACK, L. L. ELDRIDGE, J. E. DESMOND, G. H. GLOVER, and J. D. E. GABRIELI, 1998. Material-specific lateralization of prefrontal activation during episodic encoding and retrieval. *Neuroreport* 9:3711–3717.

WIG, G. S., M. B. MILLER, A. KINGSTONE, and W. M. KELLEY (in press). Separable routes to human memory formation: Dissociating task and material contributions in prefrontal cortex. *J. Cogn. Neurosci.*

WILSON, D. H., A. G. REEVES, M. GAZZANIGA, and C. CULVER, 1977. Cerebral commissurotomy for control of intractable seizures. *Neurology* 27:708–715.

WINDMANN, S., T. P. URBACH, and M. KUTAS, 2002. Cognitive and neural mechanisms of decision biases in recognition memory. *Cereb. Cortex* 12:808–817.

WOLFORD, G. L., M. B. MILLER, and M. GAZZANIGA, 2000. The left hemisphere's role in hypothesis formation. *J. Neurosci.* 20:1–4.

WRAGA, M., J. CHURCH, and D. BADRE, 2002. Event-related FMRI study of imaginal self and object rotations. Paper presented at the annual meeting of the Cognitive Neuroscience Society, San Francisco.

YELLOTT, J. I., Jr., 1969. Probability learning with noncontingent success. *J. Math. Psychol.* 6:541–575.

ZACKS, J. M., J. M. OLLINGER, M. A. SHERIDAN, and B. TVERSKY, 2002. A parametric study of mental spatial transformations of bodies. *NeuroImage* 16:857–872.

ZAIDEL, D., and R. W. SPERRY, 1974. Memory impairment after commissurotomy in man. *Brain* 97:263–272.

86 Authorship Processing

DANIEL M. WEGNER AND BETSY SPARROW

ABSTRACT Authorship processing supports the perception of events, actions, and thoughts as issuing from the self as a causal agent. To discern whether a given item is authored by self or has arisen from some other source, this processing mechanism consults authorship indicators—sources of information about the likely origin of the item. The elemental indicators include body and environment orientation, direct bodily feedback, direct bodily feedforward, visual and other indirect sensory feedback, social cues, action consequences, and action-relevant thought.

How can you tell that you're reading this sentence? Why is it so clear to you that it is not someone else who is doing this? For that matter, how do you know it is not just an event happening without anyone doing it at all?

Each of us can typically offer reliable answers to many questions of our own authorship, sometimes with remarkable rapidity ("Of course I was reading the sentence!"). This suggests that there is an efficient system of mind that deploys ready answers to questions of one's own agency. The topic of this chapter is this system for *authorship processing*, the set of mental processes that monitors indications of authorship to judge whether an event, action, or thought should be ascribed to self as a causal agent.

To explore how authorship is assessed, we begin by examining what authorship is and why authorship could be unclear. We then examine a series of authorship indicators—sources of information that influence the judgment of authorship—examining how these indicators inform the experience of authorship of action and thought. As we shall see, one of the main authorship indicators is intention. The person uses the previews of action that occur in mind as signs that the action emanated from the self (if I had the thought of doing it and then it occurred, I must have done it).

Why is authorship ever unclear?

Many people assume that authorship is a given, a kind of knowledge that arises in the very process whereby actions are produced. If I do something, how could I not know that I did it? The process through which mind causes an action seems to require knowledge of the action for the causation even to happen, so knowledge of authorship appears simply inherent in the way the action is produced. The usual experience of action as following directly from our conscious will suggests that we should always be intrinsically informed of our authorship. Indeed, an auxiliary system for discerning our authorship would be redundant, perhaps even likely to create confusion. Yes, we might occasionally forget about having caused an action and thus report its authorship incorrectly, but by and large, we should be able to report our authorship of actions we consciously will. If the self causes actions, it must know them.

The idea that authorship needs processing, then, only makes sense if we suspect that conscious will does not cause action. In this sense, the study of authorship processing is built on the assumption that our intuition about how actions occur is deeply flawed, an illusion created by a lack of insight into mental causation. It is only if we do not consciously cause our actions but only come to feel that we do that we might need a mental system for authorship processing—the ascription of the movements of our bodies and workings of our minds to our selves (Wegner and Wheatley, 1999; Wegner, 2002, 2003). Authorship processing, in this light, may be the mechanism that produces our experience of a self as a cause of our actions (Spence and Frith, 1999; Wegner and Wheatley, 1999; Metzinger, 2003; Wegner, in press). In contrast to the Cartesian dictum, *cogito ergo sum* (I think, therefore I am), the struggle to find an author for our actions may yield a quite different path to self, *ago ergo sum* (I act, therefore I am).

As a first step in the analysis of authorship processing, then, it is useful to ask whether and when people make mistakes in appreciating the authorship of their actions or thoughts. Does conscious will always illuminate actions to us as we do them, intrinsically informing us of our authorship, or do we make enough mistakes in authorship that this is something that indeed requires special processing? The following examples are illuminating:

- Normal people often report losing consciousness of acting, particularly when the action is repetitive or well-learned (Schooler, 2002).
- Patients with schizophrenia may say that their actions feel as though they were under the control of someone else. As one patient said, "When I reach for the comb, it is my hand and arm which move. . . . But I don't control them. I sit watching them move and they are quite independent, what they do is nothing to do with me. I am just a puppet

DANIEL M. WEGNER and BETSY SPARROW Department of Psychology, Harvard University, Cambridge, Mass.

manipulated by cosmic strings" (Graham and Stephens, 1994, p. 99).

• Patients with brain damage leading to alien hand syndrome experience one hand acting without their conscious will, with a "mind of its own" (Geschwind et al., 1995).

• Normal individuals helping someone communicate at a keyboard can create messages on the other's behalf, fully believing that the other is the author, when they themselves are actually originating the communications (Wegner, Fuller, and Sparrow, 2003).

• Survivors of life-threatening danger often report that the event led to an experience of depersonalization, a sense of strangeness and unreality that included the perception that their actions were involuntary or automatic (Noyes and Kletti, 1977).

• People who are susceptible to hypnosis describe the actions they perform in the state as involuntary, even though the actions appear complex, multifaceted, and temporally extended. Even behaviors performed in waking that result from posthypnotic suggestion are described as occurring without conscious will (Lynn, Rhue, and Weekes, 1990).

• When people are asked to try not to think about their intention before performing a simple task (such as winding thread on a spool), they report an increased sense that the action just seems to "happen," rather than that they did it on purpose (Wegner and Erksine, 2003).

There are a variety of anomalies of authorship, errors produced not only by brain damage or psychopathology but also occurring in normal individuals responding in special situations. These examples suggest that authorship knowledge is not a "given" when people produce apparently voluntary actions, and instead that resolving the question of authorship for any action may require considerable information and inference. What exactly is it that people are trying to judge when they describe their sense of authorship?

The nature of authorship

Authorship processing is a form of causal inference in which events are attributed to entities that are perceived to cause them. The idea that people are entities that cause things to happen is an old one, of course, but the idea that this is a unique form of causal judgment is somewhat more contemporary (Michotte, 1963). Fritz Heider (1958; Heider and Simmel, 1944) emphasized that the perception of agency or authorship in animate objects is quite unlike the perception of causation that occurs for physical events or inanimate objects (as when one marble rolls into another). Agents are seen as first causes or uncaused causes, origins of action to which authorship can be ascribed. Authorship is not of concern in determining the causal underpinnings of events caused by prior events, then, and only arises when events are traced to agents.

Agents are entities that cause events through self-movement. Agents of all kinds (humans, animals, plants, and even artificially intelligent software devices) can be described in terms of the operation of sensors, processors, and actuators. Agents input information through sensors, process the information, and output behavior through actuators (Russell and Norvig, 2003). An agent may sense a flying object, recognize it as a housefly, and dart out a tongue to snatch it (ideally, this particular agent is not a human). Quite simply, agents appear to cause events "on purpose," and this facility is the basis for authorship ascriptions (Johnson, 2003). An observer asked about this event, for example, would likely mention that "the frog ate the fly," rather than describing the mechanism of causes and effects underlying the event.

Processing one's own authorship is a subset of the general problem of processing the authorship of any agent. However, there is an important difference. When we ascribe an act to another person, we often do so dispassionately, noting merely that this is something they have done ("he hit the ball"). Part of authorship processing involves just such judgments pertaining to our selves. However, when we sense our own authorship of an action, there is an additional quality present, a feeling of doing, that marks the event uniquely. The feeling of doing adds a psychological exclamation point to the action ("I hit the ball!"). This experience of consciously willing the action is the feeling that anchors our pesky intuition that we might not even need to analyze authorship at all—that we are intrinsically informed of authorship in causing our actions.

The experience of consciously willing an action is an *authorship emotion* (Wegner, 2002), a feeling that ties the basic fact of the causal event to a bodily response and lends it a sense of "embodiment" (Barsalou et al., 2003). Knocking in a nice pool shot, opening up a box of candy, or typing the letter T can each be remembered and identified as "my own" more readily because of the experience of conscious will. This experience need not be a veridical expression of how the action came about (although we tend to interpret it this way), but it does serve to authenticate the action as something done by the self. Authorship seems to be a self-recognition of agency, then, that has both a rational component (knowledge that one was the agent causing the action) and an experiential component (the feeling of consciously willing the action).

Authorship should be distinguished from ownership. Several of the thought anomalies that occur in schizophrenia, for example, give rise to experiences of thoughts occurring in one's own mind but which are seemingly authored by someone else (Frith and Fletcher, 1995). When this happens, the thought may still seem owned by the self, in that it occurs to the self and can be self-reported, but it can seem not caused by the self, in that another mind was the agent that made it occur (Stephens and Graham, 2000;

Gerrans, 2001). The simple fact of having a thought occur in mind may not be sufficient to guarantee that the thought is something one authored. An experience of authorship involves an ascription of a thought or action to an agent as cause.

Authorship indicators

Authorship processing normally seems unproblematic and transparent, yielding rapid-fire judgments of what one has done. Yet these judgments must take into account bits of information from multiple sources that often arrive in varied order (Georgieff and Jeannerod, 1998; Frith, Blakemore, and Wolpert, 2000). Authorship cues arrive from the environment, direct bodily feedback, indirect bodily feedback, direct bodily feedforward, social situations, knowledge of action consequences, and knowledge of action-relevant thoughts. Often these authorship indicators converge and complement each other, and sometimes they conflict, but each may be sufficient to support inferred authorship in the absence of others.

THE BODY IN THE ENVIRONMENT   The relationship between body and environment provides cues to authorship. Actions often require props or tools, for example, or they can only be done by someone who is in a particular place or has a certain vantage point. Cooking happens in kitchens, yelling happens at sports stadiums, painting happens when a brush is at hand, and so on. Any environment affords some actions and not others, so knowing one's relation to the environment is a clue to authorship. This realization is part of the ecological approach to perception and action (Gibson, 1977), and has also been described in accounts of action identification (Goldman, 1970; Vallacher and Wegner, 1985). An action alone in a room may be "pursing lips," for instance, whereas the same action in the presence of a lover may be "puckering up for a kiss." Knowing what the action is, in turn, may contribute to understanding who did it.

Environments can be sufficient to stimulate relevant actions. In patients with certain forms of frontal lobe damage, for example, environmental stimuli can cause action in what has been called "utilization behavior" (Lhermitte, 1983). One patient was induced by the mere presence of a glass of water to drink repeatedly, eventually downing a whole liter even though he said he was not thirsty. In normal individuals, in turn, contextual primes suggesting thoughts of aging can prompt people to walk slowly (Bargh, Chen, and Burrows, 1996) and primes suggesting intelligence can lead people to perform well in a game of Trivial Pursuit (Dijksterhuis and van Knippenberg, 1998). However, the stimuli that prompt behavior do not simultaneously and automatically induce knowledge of authorship. A stimulus to behave may yield the behavior and also prompt a secondary processing of the stimulus to yield an authorship

judgment, but these pathways are separable. Beyond their influence on behavior per se, environments serve as cues to authorship inference.

Ambiguities in authorship occur when environmental cues do not distinguish one author from another. One case of such confusion can be observed when two people are in a position to perform the coaction of moving a Ouija board pointer. Both place their fingers on the pointer and attempt together to "receive messages" from some spirit agent. This circumstance obscures whether any particular movement is one's own or belongs to the other (or is that of the imagined spirit), and the sense of authorship may be lost while the pointer spells out messages. A study modeled on the Ouija board setting found that the authorship confusion is sufficient in this context to make people lose the capacity to track their causal influence (Wegner and Wheatley, 1999). In general, however, the perception of one's body in its environment can be a helpful authorship clue. The person standing near the elevator buttons, after all, is likely to be the culprit who pushed them all.

BODILY ACTION FEEDBACK   The most widely studied authorship indicators are the forms of sensory feedback about action that the brain receives directly from the body. Such proprioceptive or kinesthetic feedback includes sensations derived from muscles, skin, joints, and tendons, as well as from the vestibular system (Gandevia and Burke, 1992). These indicators not only point to what was done, but may subtly contribute to judgments of authorship. Obviously, we lack such feedback for the movements of others, so this authorship indicator is only helpful for discerning authorship other than our own by a process of elimination. If I didn't feel I did it, perhaps you did it.

Much of the study of proprioception has been carried out under the assumption that bodily processes are the sole basis of the processing of authorship. Historical arguments about topics such as muscle sense, innervation sensations, efference copy, and the like have raged in part because it seemed that the pathway from mind to action and back for simple voluntary actions could yield a full understanding of how authorship is determined (Scheerer, 1987). However, two key observations suggest that such direct perception of the body is only a part of authorship processing.

First, there is no proprioception for thought, but thoughts certainly vary in the degree to which they seem authored by the self. Creative insights, for example, often strike as "bolts from the blue," and are experienced as much less willed than are other thoughts (Schooler and Melcher, 1995). And as mentioned earlier, thoughts experienced as authored by other agents are common in schizophrenia (Hoffman, 1986; Frith, 1992). Unless a muscle connection is suggested for all mental events, authorship processing for thoughts cannot involve any of the standard pathways assumed for proprioception. A second reason for doubting the primary influence of proprioception in authorship processing is that proprioceptive influences are often weak in comparison with other sources of feedback (Fourneret and Jeannerod, 1998). Indirect sources of feedback can eclipse proprioception in producing authorship ascriptions.

DIRECT BODILY FEEDFORWARD   A great deal of research in the history of psychology and physiology has been devoted to establishing the origins of proprioception. The focus has been on whether we sense our movements by virtue of outgoing or efferent signals from brain to body, through incoming or afferent signals from body to brain, or through some combination of these. The question has been whether knowledge of what will be done is ever necessary for authorship processing, or whether authorship is determined solely by information about what has been done. Current answers suggest that the combination of outgoing and incoming signals is often required (Jones, 1988; Gandevia and Burke, 1992; Jeannerod, 1997).

The role of outgoing or efferent signals is demonstrated, for example, in research on the central cancellation of the tickle sensation (Blakemore, Wolpert, and Frith, 1998). The feeling of being tickled is more pronounced when the tickle stimulus is not self-produced. Signals originating in the process of producing the tickling movement must somehow operate to cancel the tickle sensation. Blakemore and colleagues (1998) provide evidence that this form of authorship processing occurs on the way to the sensation of being tickled through deactivation of cerebellar function by the tickling action. The conclusion suggested is that authorship of action is influenced by motor plans, not only by sensations returning to the brain from peripheral sensation.

VISUAL ACTION FEEDBACK   People can be fooled by indirect visual feedback about the authorship of their own actions. To begin with, visual feedback can be sufficiently compelling that it influences the perceived locus of sensations. Botvinick and Cohen (1998) found that people who watched a rubber hand being stimulated while their own hand was similarly stimulated out of view came over time to sense that they were feeling the stimulus being applied to the rubber hand (see also Pavani, Spence, and Driver, 2000).

False visual feedback can also influence the experience of authorship. In an early study, Nielson (1963) had participants view what appeared to be their own gloved hand, but which was actually the hand of an experimenter projected in its place. When the experimenter's hand went astray in drawing a line, participants regularly attempted to compensate. Subsequent research finds that such misperception is increased when the other's hand is oriented in the same way as one's own hand (fingers pointing away from the body), and is particularly increased when the other's hand is performing the same action as one's own hand (van den Bos and Jeannerod,

2002). Similar brain activations have been found in a positron emission tomography study when one's own and other's hands have similar orientations (Farrer et al., 2003). The readiness to accept visual feedback in place of proprioception makes sense in view of the finding that in monkeys, visual cues and proprioceptive cues for limb position act on the same neurons (Graziano, 1999).

Normal individuals have been found to be moderately susceptible to misleading visual feedback, whereas people with schizophrenia are far more susceptible, often showing exaggerated tendencies to mistake others' visually presented hand movements for their own (Daprati et al., 1997). Both normal and schizophrenic individuals make more errors when their own and the other's hand movements are presented with temporal delays (Franck et al., 2001). Individuals whose parietal cortex lesions have led to certain forms of apraxia are also susceptible to visual overshadowing of proprioception. Apraxic and control participants in one study were asked to produce simple and complex hand movements to be viewed on video, and were to judge whether it was their own or the experimenter's hand. Apraxics were worse than control subjects when experimenter movement was consistent with their own planned movement, for complex movements. These errors occurred when subjects performed the movement inaccurately and the experimenter performed the movement correctly (Sirigu et al., 1999). It is as though subjects preferred to claim authorship for the experimenter's correct movement when their own movement was faulty. Overall, the susceptibility of both normal and special-population participants to misperceptions of own hand movement in these paradigms suggests that visual feedback can have a profound influence on authorship.

SOCIAL CUES   When the prom queen and king get tangled up and fall to the floor during the spotlight dance, people want to know who did it. Questions of authorship are often social questions. Authorship processing in social situations involves the presence of other agents, of course, and so introduces layers of complexity beyond "whose hand was that?" Other people have not only other hands but also other minds, and the many processes involved in mind perception can affect how authorship is understood (Wellman, 1992; Baron-Cohen, 1994; Gilbert, 1997; Flavell, 1999; Blakemore and Decety, 2001).

The issue of authorship in social settings is most acute in cases of *obedience* and *imitation*. In the case of obedience, when one person instructs another to act, the first person may be understood as deserving a share of authorship ascription for the second person's action. This sharing of authorship influences individuals' perceptions of their own authorship and seems to affect even the most basic aspects of authorship processing. If you pick up a pen to write, for example, your experience of authorship may be strongly undermined by the mere fact that another person picked up a pen just before you did, or that another person asked you to pick it up. When people obey or follow others, they experience an "agentic shift" such that their sense of authorship is reduced (Milgram, 1974). Chaminade and Decety (2002) have observed differential brain activity underlying the experience of leading versus following the actions of another. The dramatic reductions in experienced voluntariness of action accompanying hypnosis (Lynn, Rhue, and Weekes, 1990) provide another example of this phenomenon.

Imitation is a second social situation in which authorship processing becomes complicated. A variety of recent studies suggest that there are important interrelations among the cognitive processes and brain structures that support the perception of others' actions and the production and perception of own actions (e.g., Jeannerod, 1999; Dijksterhuis and Bargh, 2001; Ruby and Decety, 2001; Decety et al., 2002; Prinz and Hommel, 2002). The discovery of mirror neurons in monkeys, which are activated both by performing an action and by watching another perform an action, also points to the possibility that imitation may be supported by a common neural substrate (Gallese et al., 1996; Rizzolatti et al., 1996). The question of whether action and perception of action are entirely enmeshed in the brain, however, remains a matter of discussion (Gallese and Goldman, 1998; Gallagher, Cole, and McNeill, 2002).

One conclusion suggested by this work is that authorship processing may occur at early stages of action perception and production, rather than requiring high-level cognitive processing or rational inference. The potential common coding of action and perceived action may promote distinctions between self and nonself early in the production of action, as in the case of the aforementioned cancellation of self-produced tickle sensations (Blakemore, Wolpert, and Frith, 1998). However, the common coding of one's own and other's action might also provide occasions for the confusion of own and other authorship. In imitating another person or empathizing with the other, the individual may lose track of one's own authorship because the neural bases of self's action and the perception of other's action are enmeshed.

ACTION CONSEQUENCES Sometimes the consequences of actions help to establish authorship. When individuals are known to have preferences for action (e.g., Reeder et al., 2002), consequences consistent with preferences are telling. If you want a cup of soup and your friend wants a big steak, for example, you will likely perceive your friend as the author of your travels if you end up making a joint trip to a steakhouse. Information indicating what self and other agents want can figure prominently in authorship processing because the assumption that agents are self-interested guides inferences of authorship (Miller, 1999). People are likely to locate causality in the self when they have succeeded

in performing an action, and less likely to do so when they have failed (Jenkins and Ward, 1965; Langer and Roth, 1975). Success is normally defined in terms of the self-interest of an individual, so the person for whom things turn out well is likely to be seen as having been "behind" the course of events. When things go particularly well, however, people may be tempted to ascribe authorship to an external agent such as God who could have caused the good fortune (Gilbert et al., 2000).

The consequence of an action may increase the person's experience of willing the action when the consequence lends purpose to the action. Wheatley (2001) asked participants to perform each of a variety of different simple actions (e.g., put hands out, facing each other). They were subsequently asked to perform an action enabled by this prior act (e.g., clap) or an action unrelated to the prior act (e.g., reach arms over head), and then to report their experience of intentionality for the initial action. Those who performed the enabled action reported greater feelings of intentionality for the initial action. When the initial action had an apparently reasonable consequence, it was experienced as more likely to be authored by the self.

Action consequences can become bound to action even more concretely, as discovered by Haggard, Clark, and Kalogeras (2002). Participants performed either a voluntary finger movement or an involuntary finger movement (instigated by transcranial magnetic stimulation), which was followed by a tone 250 ms later. Participants shifted their perceptions of both the timing of the finger movement and the corresponding tone, depending on the voluntariness of the action. In the voluntary movement-tone pair, participants perceived that the finger movement occurred later and the tone occurred earlier. The opposite pattern was found for the involuntary movement-tone pair. This pair repelled each other, with participants perceiving an earlier movement and a later tone. A perceptual binding of action and consequence might conceivably influence authorship judgments as well.

ACTION-RELEVANT THOUGHTS A person's own thoughts about action are a key source for understanding action authorship. The person who thinks of suicide in advance and writes a note before plummeting from a cliff, for example, is likely to be understood as the author of his or her own death, whereas the person who has no prior mental output may be viewed as merely clumsy.

In nonscientific intuitions about the mind, of course, some thoughts about action—intentions—are presumed to have the special status of causing action. Other thoughts may not be seen as causal but can bear on whether an action was intended or not, such as when legal or moral interpretations hinge on issues of *mens rea*, or guilty mind, or when religious opprobrium is attached to "unclean thoughts." In understanding how people use thoughts to arrive at judgments of authorship, however, these special mental states may be no different from garden variety thoughts about an action such as self-predictions, hopes, desires, beliefs, expectations, action identifications, or conscious perceptions of the environment. All the various things a person might think about that are relevant to a particular action could conceivably influence the perception of action authorship. By the same token, the processing of authorship for a thought may take into account the constellation of other thoughts relevant to the target thought.

The idea that thought could influence the experience of authorship was recognized by Hume (1888). He held that the "constant union" and "inference of the mind" that underlies the perception of causality between physical events must also give rise to perceived causality in "actions of the mind." Drawing on this idea, the theory of *apparent mental causation* (Wegner and Wheatley, 1999; Wegner, 2002) suggests that the experience we have of causing our own actions arises when we draw a causal inference linking our thought to our action. When thought seems to cause action, we experience will. Principles guiding such inferences follow principles of attribution and inference that govern cause perception more generally (Heider, 1958; Michotte, 1963; Kelley, 1972; Gilbert, 1997).

According to this theory, when a thought appears in consciousness just prior to an action, is consistent with the action, and is not accompanied by salient alternative causes of the action, we experience conscious will and ascribe authorship to ourselves for the action. In contrast, when thoughts do not arise with such priority, consistency, and exclusivity, we experience the ensuing actions as less willed or voluntary. The theory suggests that authorship is experienced primarily when thought about action is the primary candidate for having caused the action that is observed.

For many actions, we often do have thoughts of action that are consistent, prior, and exclusive. We may think of driving to work before we do so, for example, so when we indeed go, we quickly conclude that we did it. If we were not thinking of driving to work but nonetheless found ourselves suddenly on the way to the office, the lack of consistency between our thought and action would undermine our feeling of conscious will for the action. If we thought of going to work only after the action, in turn, we would have the requisite consistent thought, but its lack of appropriate priority would yield little sense of will for the action. And, of course, if we were led to drive to work by other forces—say, a series of oddly placed detour signs—even if we had thought of going and had been contented with the idea, we might find our experience of will undermined because the thought was not an exclusive cause.

Evidence from several experiments has accumulated relevant to this theory. Tests of the consistency principle, for example, examined whether people accept authorship of actions merely because they have had thoughts consistent with those actions (Gibson and Wegner, 2003). Participants were asked to type letters randomly at a computer keyboard without seeing the screen. They were told that the experiment examined "automatic typing" and that their random responses would be analyzed. Just before this, participants were exposed to the word *deer* in an ostensibly unrelated task. Then the "automatic typing" began and participants typed for 5 minutes. The experimenter ostensibly ran a program on the typed text to extract the words that had been typed, and then asked participants to rate words to indicate the degree to which they felt they had authored that word. None of the words rated were actually produced, yet participants reported higher authorship ratings for the word they had seen in the prior computer task (*deer*) relative to other words, and also reported relatively higher ratings that they had authored an associated word, *doe*. These findings suggest that people can experience will for an action that was never performed, merely when they have prior thoughts consistent with the action (see also Aarts, Custers, and Wegner, 2004).

In a study of the priority principle, Wegner and Wheatley (1999) presented people with thoughts (e.g., a tape-recorded mention of the word *swan*) relevant to their action (moving an on-screen cursor to select a picture of a swan). The movement participants performed was not their own, as they shared the computer mouse with an experimental confederate who gently forced the action without the participants' knowledge. Nevertheless, when the relevant thought was provided either 1 s or 5 s before the action, participants reported feeling that they acted intentionally in making the movement. The operation of the priority principle in this case was clear because on other trials, thoughts of the swan prompted 30 s before the forced action or 1 s afterward did not yield an inflated experience of will. So, even when the action is forced and thought of the action is baldly prompted by an outside stimulus—in this case, over headphones—the timely occurrence of thought before action leads to an erroneous experience of apparent mental causation.

In view of such studies, it appears that knowledge of one's own thoughts can have a pivotal influence on the experience of authorship. Beyond concrete perceptions of environment, the proprioceptive and visual experience of the body, and the perception of the social context and the consequences of action, the world of the mind offers a range of further authorship indicators. Each of us is in the unusual position of knowing the previews our mind offers us for what our bodies do, and we are thus able to make causal inferences about actions that can take those previews into account.

Counterfeit authorship

The authorship of action and thought is something people find out about, not something they know immediately and intrinsically. The evidence surveyed in this chapter makes this point in various ways, and suggests that there may be many instances in which action authorship is experienced incorrectly. People can feel they have done things that they did not do, and can feel they were not authors of things they did. Authorship must be indicated because it is not given in the process of acting or thinking.

HELPING HANDS STUDIES   The interplay of authorship indicators is illustrated in studies we have recently conducted on the counterfeit experience of authorship—the sense that one has authored actions actually performed by another (Wegner, Sparrow, and Winerman, 2004). In these studies, participants were led to experience the arm movements of another as if the movements were their own. The participant was attired in a robe and positioned in front of a mirror such that the arms of a second person standing behind the participant could be extended through the robe to look as though they were the arms of the participant (figure 86.1). The second person wore gloves to aid in this illusion. (You might recognize this circumstance as the "helping hands" pantomime sometimes used as a party game.) Participants kept their own arms at their sides and were instructed not to move. Both participant and "hand helper" wore headphones.

For the experiment, the helper's arms performed a series of 32 movements (e.g., snap the fingers of your right hand,

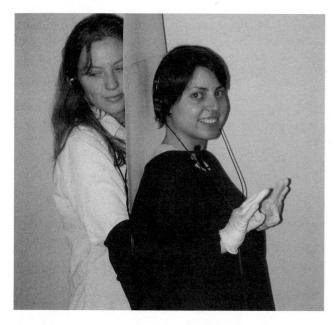

FIGURE 86.1.   Hand helper (left) and participant (right) in the helping hands experiments.

wave hello with both hands) in response to a series of instructions the helper was given via the headphones. In the first experiment, participants also heard the instructions for each of the arm movements through their own headphones, or they heard nothing. Those who heard the instructions thus were provided with consistent previews (prior thoughts) for actions they perceived visually to be occurring in the position their own actions might occur. Participants in the second experiment also participated in these preview and no-preview conditions, or heard inconsistent previews (i.e., the instructions would say "wave your left hand" but what would be seen was hands clapping).

In both experiments, the consistent previews led participants to report an enhanced feeling of control over the arm movements as compared with other participants. Participants did not feel that they had full control of the arms, of course, as they had no control at all, but they reported a significantly enhanced *impression* of such control.

This impression was found to have psychophysiological consequences. Participants in the second experiment had skin conductance measurements taken while the hand helper twice snapped a rubber band on the wrist of one arm. These snaps occurred before and after the hand movement portion of the experiment. All participants showed significant skin conductance responses (SCRs) to the first snap of the rubber band, perhaps revealing a startle response to the snap. The preview conditions had an interesting effect on the reaction to the second snap. Participants who had heard consistent previews maintained the strong SCR they had shown for the first snap, whereas participants who heard no preview or inconsistent previews apparently had habituated, as they showed reduced SCR to the second snap. Hearing a consistent preview seemed to cause an empathic entrainment and enhanced sensitivity to the other's arm that coincided with the enhanced feeling of control over the arm's movement.

In these studies, authorship indicators were arranged so as to counterfeit the experience of authorship for participants. Environmental cues were deemphasized by having the participant see the helper's arms in place of the participant's own arms. Proprioceptive cues were not manipulated specifically, but visual cues to arm movement were provided by having participants see the helper's arms perform the actions. Social cues to imitation or obedience were not manipulated, and the consequences of the actions were also kept constant across conditions. The key variation, then, was the presence of thoughts consistent with the action—thoughts provided merely by hearing instructions for arm movements—and this variation was found to yield both subtle changes in the experience of authorship and enhanced psychophysiological sensitivity to insult to the observed limbs. In the context of a host of authorship indicators, the occurrence of thoughts relevant to action can be sufficient to induce an experience of authorship that is reflected both in self-reports and in bodily responses.

New directions

There remain many challenges for research in authorship processing. The measurement of brain activations associated with experiences of authorship is one important avenue for progress (Farrer and Frith, 2002). The rapid development of technologies for creating virtual realities in turn suggests that it will be useful to examine how authorship processing occurs when actions occur in simulated environments with simulated consequences, and perhaps even simulated social contexts (Blascovich et al., 2002). And eventually the invention of techniques for prosthetic actions—the control of mechanical devices by neural activation (e.g., Chapin et al., 1999)—will yield a brave new world for authorship processing as well. Eventually it may be possible to specify at the neuronal level the processes underlying the processing of authorship. As people can do more and more in ways that transcend all the usual authorship indicators, the challenges for authorship processing will grow apace.

ACKNOWLEDGMENT   This work was supported in part by NIMH grant No. MH 49127.

REFERENCES

AARTS, H., R. CUSTERS, and D. WEGNER, 2004. *Attributing the cause of one's own actions: Priming effects in agency judgments.* Unpublished manuscript.

BARGH, J. A., M. CHEN, and L. BURROWS, 1996. Automaticity of social behavior: Direct effects of trait construct and stereotype activation on action. *J. Pers. Soc. Psychol.* 71:230–244.

BARON-COHEN, S., 1994. How to build a baby that can read minds: Cognitive mechanisms in mindreading. *Cahiers Psychol. Cogn.* 13:513–552.

BARSALOU, L. W., P. M. NIEDENTHAL, A. K. BARBEY, and J. A. RUPPERT, 2003. Social embodiment. In *The Psychology of Learning and Motivation*, vol. 43, B. H. Ross, ed. San Diego, Calif.: Academic Press. pp. 43–92.

BLAKEMORE, S. J., and J. DECETY, 2001. From the perception of action to the understanding of intention. *Nat. Rev. Neurosci.* 2: 561–567.

BLAKEMORE, S. J., D. M. WOLPERT, and C. FRITH, 1998. Central cancellation of self-produced tickle sensation. *Nat. Neurosci.* 1: 635–640.

BLASCOVICH, J., J. LOOMIS, A. C. BEALL, K. R. SWINTH, C. L. HOYT, and J. N. BAILENSON, 2002. Immersive virtual environment technology as a methodological tool for social psychology. *Psychol. Inquiry* 13:103–124.

BOTVINICK, M., and J. COHEN, 1998. Rubber hands "feel" touch that eyes see. *Nature* 391:756.

CHAMINADE, T., and J. DECETY, 2002. Leader or follower? Involvement of the inferior parietal lobule in agency. *Neuroreport* 13: 1975–1978.

CHAPIN, J. K., K. A. MOXON, R. S. MARKOWITZ, and M. A. L. NICOLELIS, 1999. Real-time control of a robot arm using simul-

taneously recorded neurons in the motor cortex. *Nat. Neurosci.* 2:664–670.

DAPRATI, E., N. FRANCK, N. GEORGIEFF, J. PROUST, E. PACHERIE, J. DALERY, et al., 1997. Looking for the agent: An investigation into consciousness of action and self-consciousness in schizophrenic patients. *Cognition* 65:71–86.

DECETY, J., T. CHAMINADE, J. GREZES, and A. MELTZOFF, 2002. A PET exploration of neural mechanisms involved in reciprocal imitation. *NeuroImage* 15:265–272.

DIJKSTERHUIS, A., and J. A. BARGH, 2001. The perception-behavior expressway: Automatic effects of social perception on social behavior. *Adv. Exp. Soc. Psychol.* 33:1–40.

DIJKSTERHUIS, A., and A. VAN KNIPPENBERG, 1998. The relation between perception and behavior or how to win a game of Trivial Pursuit. *J. Pers. Soc. Psychol.* 74:865–877.

FARRER, C., N. FRANCK, N. GEORGIEFF, C. FRITH, J. DECETY, and M. JEANNEROD, 2003. Modulating the experience of agency: A positron emission tomography study. *NeuroImage* 18:324–333.

FARRER, C., and C. FRITH, 2002. Experiencing oneself vs another person as being the cause of an action: The neural correlates of the experience of agency. *NeuroImage* 15:596–603.

FLAVELL, J. H., 1999. Cognitive development: Children's knowledge of the mind. *Annu. Rev. Psychol.* 50:21–45.

FOURNERET, P., and M. JEANNEROD, 1998. Limited consciousness monitoring of motor performance in normal subjects. *Neuropsychologia* 36:1133–1140.

FRANCK, N., C. FARRER, N. GEORGIEFF, M. MARIE-CARDINE, J. DALÉRY, T. D'AMATO, et al., 2001. Defective recognition of one's own actions in patients with schizophrenia. *Am. J. Psychiatry* 158: 454–459.

FRITH, C. D., 1992. *The Cognitive Neuropsychology of Schizophrenia.* Hove, England: Erlbaum.

FRITH, C., S. J. BLAKEMORE, and D. M. WOLPERT, 2000. Abnormalities in the awareness and control of action. *Philos. Trans. R. Soc. Lond. Ser. B* 355:1771–1788.

FRITH, C. D., and P. FLETCHER, 1995. Voices from nowhere. *Critical Quarterly* 37:71–83.

GALLAGHER, S., J. COLE, and D. MCNEILL, 2002. Social cognition and primacy of movement revisited. *Trends Cogn. Sci.* 6:155–156.

GALLESE, V., L. FADIGA, L. FOGASSI, and G. RIZZOLATTI, 1996. Action recognition in the premotor cortex. *Brain* 119:593–609.

GALLESE, V., and A. GOLDMAN, 1998. Mirror neurons and the simulation theory of mindreading. *Trends Cogn. Sci.* 2:493–501.

GANDEVIA, S., and D. BURKE, 1992. Does the nervous system depend on kinesthetic information to control natural limb movements? *Behav. Brain Sci.* 15:614–632.

GEORGIEFF, N., and M. JEANNEROD, 1998. Beyond consciousness of external reality: A "who" system for consciousness of action and self-consciousness. *Conscious. Cogn.* 7:465–477.

GERRANS, P., 2001. Authorship and ownership of thoughts. *Psychiatry Philos. Psychol.* 8:231–237.

GESCHWIND, D., M. IACOBONI, M. MEGA, D. ZAIDEL, T. CLOUGHESY, and E. ZAIDEL, 1995. Alien hand syndrome: Interhemispheric motor disconnection due to a lesion in the midbody of the corpus callosum. *Neurology* 45:802–808.

GIBSON, J. J., 1977. The theory of affordances. In *Perceiving, Acting, and Knowing*, R. E. Shaw and J. Bransford, eds. Hillsdale, N.J.: Erlbaum.

GIBSON, L., and D. M. WEGNER, 2003. *Believing we've done what we were thinking: An illusion of authorship.* Paper presented at the Society for Personality and Social Psychology, Los Angeles.

GILBERT, D., R. BROWN, E. PINEL, and T. WILSON, 2000. The illusion of external agency. *J. Pers. Soc. Psycho.* 79:690–700.

GILBERT, D. T., 1997. Ordinary personology. In *Handbook of Social Psychology*, 4th ed., D. T. Gilbert, S. T. Fiske, and G. Lindzey, eds. New York: McGraw-Hill.

GOLDMAN, A. I., 1970. *A Theory of Human Action*. Princeton, N.J.: Princeton University Press.

GRAHAM, G., and G. L. STEPHENS, 1994. Mind and mine. In *Philosophical Psychology*, G. Graham and G. L. Stephens, eds. Cambridge, Mass.: MIT Press, pp. 91–109.

GRAZIANO, M. S. A., 1999. Where is my arm? The relative role of vision and proprioception in the neuronal representation of limb position. *Proc. Natl. Acad. Sci. U.S.A.* 96:10418–10421.

HAGGARD, P., S. CLARK, and J. KALOGERAS, 2002. Voluntary action and conscious awareness. *Nat. Neurosci.* 5:382–385.

HEIDER, F., 1958. *The Psychology of Interpersonal Relations*. New York: Wiley.

HEIDER, F., and M. SIMMEL, 1944. An experimental study of apparent behavior. *Am. J. Psychol.* 57:243–259.

HOFFMAN, R. E., 1986. Verbal hallucinations and language production processes in schizophrenia. *Behav. Brain Sci.* 9:503–548.

HUME, D., 1888. *A Treatise of Human Nature*. London: Oxford University Press.

JEANNEROD, M., 1997. *The Cognitive Neuroscience of Action*. Oxford, England: Blackwell.

JEANNEROD, M., 1999. The 25th Bartlett Lecture: To act or not to act: Perspectives on the representation of actions. *Q. J. Exp. Psychol. A* 52A:1–29.

JENKINS, H. M., and W. C. WARD, 1965. Judgments of contingency between responses and outcomes. *Psychol. Monogr.* 79(1).

JOHNSON, S. C., 2003. Detecting agents. *Philos. Trans. R. Soc. Lond. Ser. B* 358:549–559.

JONES, L. A., 1988. Motor illusions: What do they reveal about proprioception? *Psychol. Bull.* 103:72–86.

KELLEY, H. H., 1972. Causal schemata and the attribution process. In *Attribution: Perceiving the Causes of Behavior*, E. E. Jones, D. E. Kanouse, H. H. Kelley, R. E. Nisbett, S. Valins, and B. Weiner, eds. Morristown, N.J.: General Learning Press, pp. 151–174.

LANGER, E., and J. ROTH, 1975. Heads I win, tails it's chance: The illusion of control as a function of the sequence of outcomes in a pure chance task. *J. Pers. Soc. Psychol.* 32:951–955.

LHERMITTE, F., 1983. "Utilization behaviour" and its relation to lesions of the frontal lobes. *Brain* 106(Pt. 2):237–255.

LYNN, S. J., J. W. RHUE, and J. R. WEEKES, 1990. Hypnotic involuntariness: A social cognitive analysis. *Psychol. Rev.* 97:169–184.

METZINGER, T., 2003. *Being No One*. Cambridge, Mass.: MIT Press.

MICHOTTE, A., 1963. *The Perception of Causality* T. R. Miles and E. Miles, trans. New York: Basic Books.

MILGRAM, S., 1974. *Obedience to Authority*. New York: Harper and Row.

MILLER, D. T., 1999. The norm of self-interest. *Am. Psychol.* 54:1053–1060.

NIELSON, T. I., 1963. Volition: A new experimental approach. *Scand. J. Psychol.* 4:215–230.

NOYES, R., JR., and R. KLETTI, 1977. Depersonalization in response to life-threatening danger. *Compr. Psychiatry* 18:375–384.

PAVANI, F., C. SPENCE, and J. DRIVER, 2000. Visual capture of touch: Out of body experiences with rubber gloves. *Psychol. Sci.* 11:353–359.

PRINZ, W., and B. HOMMEL, eds., 2002. *Common Mechanisms in Perception and Action*. Oxford, England: Oxford University Press.

REEDER, G. D., S. KUMAR, M. HESSON-McINNIS, and D. TRAFIMOW, 2002. Inferences about the morality of an aggressor: The role of perceived motive. *J. Pers. Soc. Psychol.* 83:789–803.

RIZZOLATTI, G., L. FADIGA, V. GALLESE, and L. FOGASSI, 1996. Premotor cortex and the recogntion of motor actions. *Cogn. Brain Res.* 3:131–141.

RUBY, P., and J. DECETY, 2001. Effect of subjective perspective taking during simulation of action: A PET investigation of agency. *Nat. Neurosci.* 4:546–550.

RUSSELL, S. J., and P. NORVIG, 2003. *Artificial Intelligence: A Modern Approach*, 2nd ed. Englewood Cliffs, N.J.: Prentice-Hall.

SCHEERER, E., 1987. Muscle sense and innervation feelings: A chapter in the history of perception and action. In *Perspectives on Perception and Action*, H. Heuer and A. F. Sanders, eds. Hillsdale, N.J.: Erlbaum. pp. 171–194.

SCHOOLER, J. W., 2002. Re-representing consciousness: Dissociations between experience and meta-consciousness. *Trends Cogn. Sci.* 6:339–344.

SCHOOLER, J. W., and J. MELCHER, 1995. The ineffability of insight. In *The Creative Cognition Approach*, S. M. Smith and T. B. Ward, eds. Cambridge, Mass.: MIT Press, pp. 97–133.

SIRIGU, A., E. DAPRATI, P. PRADAT-DIEHL, N. FRANCK, and M. JEANNEROD, 1999. Perception of self-generated movement following left-parietal lesion. *Brain* 122:1867–1874.

SPENCE, S. A., and C. FRITH, 1999. Toward a functional anatomy of volition. *J. Conscious. Stud.* 6(8–9):11–29.

STEPHENS, G. L., and G. GRAHAM, 2000. *When Self-Consciousness Breaks: Alien Voices and Inserted Thoughts*. Cambrdge, Mass.: MIT Press.

VALLACHER, R. R., and D. M. WEGNER, 1985. *A Theory of Action Identification*. Hillsdale, N.J.: Erlbaum.

VAN DEN BOS, E., and M. JEANNEROD, 2002. Sense of body and sense of action both contribute to self-recognition. *Cognition* 85:177–187.

WEGNER, D. M., 2002. *The Illusion of Conscious Will*. Cambridge, Mass.: MIT Press.

WEGNER, D. M., 2003. The mind's best trick: How we experience conscious will. *Trends Cogn. Sci.* 7:65–69.

WEGNER, D. M. in press. Who is the controller of controlled processes? In *The New Unconscious*, 2nd ed., R. Hassin, J. Uleman, and A. Bargh, eds. New York: Oxford University Press.

WEGNER, D. M., and J. ERKSINE, 2003. Voluntary involuntariness: Thought suppression and the regulation of the experience of will. *Conscious. Cogn.* 12:684–694.

WEGNER, D. M., V. A. FULLER, and B. SPARROW, 2003. Clever hands: Uncontrolled intelligence in facilitated communication. *J. Pers. Soc. Psychol.* 85:5–19.

WEGNER, D. M., B. SPARROW, and L. WINERMAN, 2004. Vicarious agency: Experiencing control over the movements of others. *J. Pers. Soc. Psychol.* 86:838–848.

WEGNER, D. M., and T. P. WHEATLEY, 1999. Apparent mental causation: Sources of the experience of will. *Am. Psychol.* 54:480–492.

WELLMAN, H. M., 1992. *The Child's Theory of Mind*. Cambridge, Mass.: MIT Press.

WHEATLEY, T. P., 2001. *When unintentional acts feel intentional: The power of an illusory purpose*. Doctoral diss., University of Virginia, Charlottesville.

XI PERSPECTIVES AND NEW DIRECTIONS

Introduction

MICHAEL S. GAZZANIGA

OVER THE COURSE of publishing three editions of this book, we have centered each section on a recognized topic in cognitive neuroscience. The whole idea behind the book was to assess the state of the field every 5 years. Regular publication provided a time to reflect on what we have learned and what we still need to know.

In this edition, for the first time, we wanted to capture more explicitly a variety of issues that lend themselves to a larger perspective. This section, therefore, is not thematic in the traditional sense in that it does not reflect the systematic exploration of a single topic. Rather, the authors offer a wider view of selected topics. We are attempting to look ahead to possible future paths for the discipline.

We begin with two chapters on the rich discoveries that are being made in primate neurophysiology. First, Glimcher and Dorris probe how the brain makes decisions and how it values the outcomes of the choices to be made. This groundbreaking work drives to the core function of the brain, namely, its decision-making faculty. In a similar vein, Shadlen and Gold investigate the neurons working to transform sensory signals into motor commands; their goal is to gain an understanding of cognitive processes.

Steven and Blakemore then review the work on adult cortical plasticity and make a compelling case for its presence and for its underlying mechanism. The implications of this work for rehabilitative medicine are enormous.

Cognitive neuroscience attempts to understand the biological underpinnings of complex cognition. It is rare when one can offer mechanistic analysis of cognition from gene expression up to cognition. In the chapter by Fosella and Posner, this goal is met.

Gusnard and Raichle tackle the complex problem of the physiological baseline in metabolic studies and how it must be understood in relationship to a task challenge. They urge that all functional imaging studies take a resting baseline into account.

All of biological science is undergoing a quiet revolution. With the advent of the capacity for aggregating large sets of data in databases, neuroinformatics is beginning to play a central role in cognitive neuroscience research. Van Horn, director of the fMRI Data Center at Dartmouth College, begins to show us the way.

Cosmides and Tooby then remind us of the complex social nature of our species. Building on their early work, they continue to show how an evolutionary perspective helps us understand complex human cognition.

Finally, Farah ponders the ethical implications of research in cognitive neuroscience. As cognitive neuroscience moves forward, the ethical issues that arise from a wide variety of new capacities are dense and worrying. Everything from cognitive privacy to enhancing our biological capacity is up for grabs.

With each passing decade, more and more is known about the mechanistic action of the nervous system and how it produces perceptual, attentional, and mnemonic function and decisions. While this assertion serves as the motivating aspiration of modern neuroscience, it should also be observed that the actual goal is nowhere in sight.

As a final word, I would like to observe the following: at the conclusion of a conference attended by more than 80 leading scientists who presented their research on how brain enables mind, it became obvious that the central question of cognitive neuroscience remains not only unanswered, but worse: it remains unexamined. The brain scientists who are addressing issues of human cognition are producing work that illuminates which brain systems correlate with particular measurable human behaviors. Thus, a series of studies might investigate which areas of the visual system become activated when the subject attends to a particular visual stimulus. While these correlations are of interest, and some have been found, the question of how the brain knows whether, when, and how to increase the gain of a particular neuronal system remains unknown. Overall, modern studies always seem to leave room for the homunculus, the ghost in the machine, that does all the directing of brain traffic. In the field of cognitive neuroscience, it is commonplace to hear discussions of "top-down processes" versus "bottom-up processes"—that is, processes driven by feedback from "higher" areas of the brain rather than by direct input from the sensory stimuli—but the fact of the matter is, no one knows anything about the "top" in "top-down." This is a major problem of cognitive neuroscience today, and we hope that it will become the subject of research in the near future. There is a universe of knowledge yet untapped.

87 Neuronal Studies of Decision Making in the Visual-Saccadic System

PAUL W. GLIMCHER AND MICHAEL DORRIS

ABSTRACT Making a behaviorally relevant decision of any kind involves selecting and ultimately executing a course of action. To accomplish this, organisms must combine available sensory data with stored information about the structure of the environment in a manner appropriate to the type of decision that they face. Over the past few decades neuroscientists have examined decision making by focusing on conditions in which sensory signals identify a single response as rewarded, or in which learned information about the probabilities and magnitudes of rewards associated with each possible action specifies the best single response. These studies have yielded insights into the sensorimotor pathways and computational processes that underlie these forms of decision making, and the basic outlines of the circuits responsible for simple decision making are now beginning to emerge. We have, however, only just begun to study the kinds of decisions that are made when environmental conditions do not uniquely identify a best single response from among a set of alternatives. It is at present unclear how the neural architecture produces decisions under such free choice conditions. Some of the most promising research aimed at this problem has begun to employ analytic techniques developed in the social sciences, and these studies have begun to define a rigorous approach that can be used to study even the most complicated forms of decision making. Although real theoretical and experimental challenges remain, these approaches are laying the biological foundations for studying one of the most elusive properties of mind, the neural basis of voluntary choice.

Introduction

SIMPLE DECISION MAKING: IDENTIFYING AND EXECUTING THE BEST RESPONSE   Over the past decade, studies on the primate visual-saccadic system, the brain network that uses visual data to guide the selection and execution of orienting eye movements, have made significant progress toward explaining the neurobiological basis of simple decision making (see Glimcher, 2001, 2003a). Several sets of studies have, for example, succeeded in identifying the neuronal processes underlying the selection of a rewarded saccadic target from a number of unrewarded alternatives (Newsome et al., 1995; Hikosaka et al., 2000; Schall, 2001). One line of this research has demonstrated that the extrastriate visual cortices play a critical role in stimulus analysis and that the outputs of these areas can be used to identify saccades that will yield rewards (Newsome et al., 1989, 1995). In the frontal cortices, another line of research has identified mechanisms that appear to initiate or withhold saccades in response to reward contingencies signaled by visual stimuli (Schall, 2001). These experiments, together with others that have shown how the neural circuitry transforms sensory signals into coordinate frameworks appropriate for movement generation (Sparks and Mays, 1990; Colby et al., 1995; Colby and Goldberg, 1999; Andersen and Buneo, 2002), have provided us with a preliminary understanding of how the nervous system selects courses of action based on sensory cues.

In a similar way, neurobiological studies have also begun to describe the processes by which neuronal activity encodes variables that play an important role in guiding choice behavior but are not present in the immediate sensory environment (Hikosaka et al., 2000; Glimcher, 2001; Gold and Shadlen, 2001). Several lines of evidence have identified neuronal circuits that lie between sensory and motor brain regions that appear to encode the value of the behavioral responses available to an animal. Signals have been identified in parietal cortex and basal ganglia, for example, that encode either the amount of reward that a movement will produce or the likelihood that a movement will produce a reward (Kawagoe et al., 1998; Platt and Glimcher, 1999; Handel and Glimcher, 2000).

There are, however, classes of behavior that these studies have failed to engage, behaviors in which a single most valuable response is not fully specified by the information available in the stimulus or environment. It is not yet clear how the neural architecture accomplishes movement selection under these free choice conditions. One problem faced by these inquiries is that traditional physiological conceptualizations of the sensory-to-motor process offer very few tools for describing such free choice behavior. This situation has

PAUL W. GLIMCHER   Center for Neural Science, New York University, New York, N.Y.
MICHAEL DORRIS   Department of Physiology, Queens University, Kingston, Ontario.

recently led a group of physiologists to turn to social scientific theories of decision making, which provide a powerful corpus of mathematical techniques specifically designed for the study of these classes of behavior.

ECONOMIC MODELS OF DECISION MAKING A central goal of the social sciences has been to define the decision-making process in general. Economic models in particular have been quite successful in formally describing simple decision making for more than a century (e.g., Kreps, 1990). Only recently, however, have these social scientists developed tools for characterizing decision making under conditions in which subjects are free to make any of several responses that have incompletely specified values. Of particular interest to economists in this regard are situations in which humans interact with other decision makers whose behavior is unpredictable (e.g., Fudenberg and Tirole, 1991). Consider two opponents repeatedly playing the childhood game of rock-paper-scissors. In each round, both players must simultaneously choose either rock, paper, or scissors; paper beats rock, scissors beats paper, and rock beats scissors. The responses of the players are not constrained because no response is uniquely correct. Without knowing in advance exactly how one's opponent will behave, a subject cannot produce a fixed single strategy that will always yield a maximal reward under a given set of conditions.

The economic theory of games approaches the formal study of this type of behavior by assuming that all players desire strategies that will maximize their gains, given the assumption that other players seek to do the same. Thus, when faced with the opportunity to make a decision, players are assumed to consider the sensory and environmental cues that might influence the values of the options available to them, and then to adopt a behavioral strategy that combines this information with a strategic consideration of their opponent's likely behavior. Economists refer to strategies of this type as rational. If two humans playing rock-paper-scissors behave rationally, they each settle on the strategy of choosing each possible action roughly one-third of the time.

QUANTIFYING THE VALUE OF A STRATEGY In games like rock-paper-scissors, a stable behavioral strategy arises when the average subjective value of each available option, rock or paper or scissors, is rendered equivalent by the behavior of one's opponent. As long as one's opponent is equally likely to choose rock or paper or scissors, then choosing any response has an equal probability of winning, and hence an equal subjective value. Economists employ two related but distinct measures to estimate the value of any course of action. The first is an objective measure, known as *expected value*, which is determined by multiplying the gain that could be realized from an action by the probability that the gain would be realized. The second is a subjective measure,

expected utility, which is computed by adjusting the expected value to reflect subjective considerations, typically an aversion to risky courses of action. In practice, economists presume that this second measure guides choice.

The rationale for the first of these measures derives from the work of Blaise Pascal (Arnauld and Nicole, 1662/1994; Pascal, 1670/1966). If one chooses rock, there is a 50% chance of winning one dollar and a 50% chance of losing one dollar (assuming that if the other player also picks rock, the game is repeated). Therefore, over many repeated plays the average value, or expected value, of rock is 0 cents. Behavioral studies (Bernoulli, 1738/1954; Stephens and Krebs, 1986; Kreps, 1990) have demonstrated, however, that in many situations, humans and animals reliably select courses of action that do not yield the maximal expected value, particularly when the option yielding maximal expected value involves significant risk. Under these conditions, subjective and objective measures of value can be shown to differ empirically. Consider choosing between two actions, one that offers a 100% chance of earning $250,000 and a second one that offers a 50% chance of earning $500,000 and a 50% chance of earning nothing. Both actions have equal expected values ($250,000), but most humans do not view them as equally desirable, preferring the certain gain of $250,000. Most humans, however, do find a 50% chance of winning $8 million preferable to a guaranteed $250,000. The subjective value, or *utility*, of $500,000 is thus less than twice the subjective value of $250,000 for most decision makers, whereas the subjective value of $8 million is significantly more than twice the subjective value of $250,000. The subjective estimate of average value, or *expected utility*, is presumed to reflect, among other things, a natural aversion to risk by human and animal decision makers. Thus a decision maker's utility function, which can vary with his internal state, provides a means for combining sensory data and a representation of environmental uncertainty in a manner that encapsulates subjective preference.

Importantly, in tasks of the kind used most extensively by neuroscientists to study decision making, both the probability and the values of all possible rewards are fully specified by the experimental paradigm. Under these conditions the probability and value of any reward can be viewed as fixed, if imperfectly known, quantities from which expected utility can be computed. During strategic interactions with an intelligent opponent, however, a new type of uncertainty enters the decision-making process. The opponent may at any time alter the probability that he will produce a particular response, making expected utility more fundamentally uncertain and much more difficult to calculate on a trial-by-trial basis. While acknowledging this difficulty, the mathematician John Nash developed a powerful approach to the problem of computing expected utility during strategic interactions. Nash (1950) proved that whenever all the players engaged in a strategic interaction behave *rationally*, average behavior must converge to an equilibrium state at which the relative expected utilities of available courses of action can often be specified. Nash's approach abandoned any attempt to describe the trial-by-trial dynamics of strategic decision making and worked instead to at least describe the average, or molar, behavior of rational players.

Although not all strategic behavior is perfectly predicted by the mathematical formalisms that Nash and later theorists developed, under many conditions these theories do define rational decision making when that process involves an assessment of the unpredictable actions of one's opponents. Both empirical and theoretical studies have built on this foundation to show that game theory can be used both to describe the variables that must guide strategic behavior and to rigorously analyze the properties of empirically observed human voluntary actions. These observations suggest that approaches to the study of free choice behavior rooted in economic theory may ultimately provide the theoretical leverage necessary for a rigorous neurobiological study of unconstrained decision making.

Behavioral and physiological studies of unconstrained choice

Together, these observations led us to ask whether game theory could be used to develop an animal model for examining how the economic variables that should guide free choice toward behavioral equilibrium in strategic interactions might be represented in the primate nervous system. The larger goal of this approach was to examine the neurobiological substrate for decision making under conditions that begin to approximate human voluntary choice behavior.

Our goal was to develop a behavioral task that (1) engaged humans in what could be considered voluntary decision making, (2) could be well described by game theory, and (3) could also be employed in a neurophysiological setting with nonhuman primates. To this end, we had both human and monkey subjects play the *inspection game*. In this game, two players must each select one of two possible actions, and the payoffs they receive on each trial depend on both their own choice and that of their opponent (figure 87.1A). The experimental subject played the role of the *employee* and decided either to *work*, which resulted in a guaranteed payoff of one unit of reward, or to *shirk*, which resulted either in a reward twice that size or in no reward at all, depending on the action of the *employer*. The role of the employer was played either by another human or by a dynamic computer algorithm that tracked the employee's behavior and tried to maximize its own virtual reward. The employer decided whether to *inspect* or *not inspect* on each trial, and the utility of this action depended on the behavior of employee.

Like rock-paper-scissors, when this game is played repeatedly, rational players should converge on an equilibrium solution in which each response is produced a certain proportion of the time. However, unlike rock-paper-scissors, the proportion of choosing each response at equilibrium need not be always fixed at a single value but can be manipulated experimentally. Somewhat counterintuitively, the proportion of choices that the employee should devote to each response at equilibrium is controlled not by changing the employee's payoffs, but by changing those of the employer (Fudenberg and Tirole, 1991; Glimcher, 2003b). This reflects the fact that altering the employer payoff changes the utility of the options available to the employer and thus changes employer behavior, a change for which the employee ultimately compensates. The employee uses his own behavior as a lever, driving the employer back toward the equilibrium state. By holding the payoff structure for the employee constant, we can therefore ensure the employer's rational strategy will always be to inspect 50% of the time (see figure 87.1A) while systematically varying the rational strategy for the employee. In the inspection game, the employee faces a task in which the payoffs associated with each action remain constant while the proportion of responses that should be devoted to each action varies whenever we manipulate the cost of inspection to the employer.

In games like this one, trial-by-trial uncertainty derives for both players from incomplete knowledge of the future actions of one's opponent. The economic analysis presumes that rational decision makers will choose the option with the highest expected utility, but on a *trial-by-trial basis* there seems no obvious way for the choosers to compute this parameter. The equilibrium approach addresses this problem more globally by presuming that if both subjects act rationally, a stable average rate of working and shirking will be reached when on average the expected utilities for working and shirking are driven toward equality over many trials by the dynamic behavior of one's opponent.[1]

STUDIES OF HUMAN AND MONKEY BEHAVIOR   Across blocks of trials we varied the employer's cost of inspection from 0.1 to 0.9 in steps of 0.2, and according to the Nash formulation this should have had the effect of varying the probability that the employee would shirk from roughly 10% to 90% in 20% steps. Humans competed in the inspection game for real monetary rewards, which were delivered at the end of the experiment, and in a typical session a subject would compete 300 times over about 30 minutes. Figure 87.1B shows a 20-trial running average of the typical behavior of a human employee playing a computer employer during two sequentially presented blocks of trials. The Nash equilibrium predicts a 70% shirk rate in the first block of trials (payoff matrix in figure 87.1A, middle panel) and a 30% shirk rate in the second block of trials (figure 87.1A, right

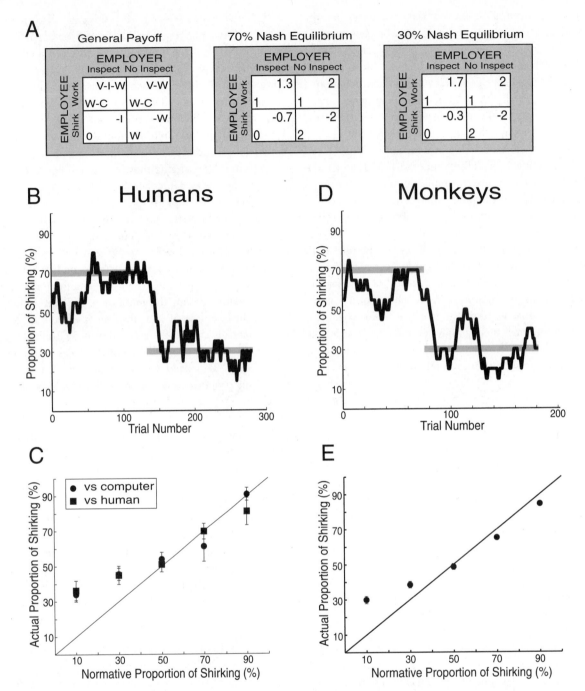

FIGURE 87.1 Behavior during the inspection game. (*A*) In left panel is the general form of the payoff matrix for the inspection game for both the experimental subject (employee) and the opponent (employer). The variables in the bottom left of each cell determine the employee's payoffs and the variables in the top right of each cell determine the employer's payoffs for each combination of player's responses. V = value of hypothetical product to the employer, fixed at 4; W = wage paid by employer to employee, fixed at 2; C = cost of working to employee, fixed at 1; I = cost of inspection to the employer, varied from 0.1 to 0.9 in steps of 0.2. Middle and right panels show payoff matrices for 70% and 30% employee shirk rates. The predicted equilibrium strategy for the employer remains constant at a 50% inspect for all blocks of trials. 1 unit of

payoff = 0.25 mL of water for monkey = $0.05 for human. (*B*) The behavior of an individual human subject playing the role of employee during two Nash equilibrium blocks of the inspection game. The jagged black line represents a running average of the shirk choices over the last 20 trials. The gray bars represent the predicted Nash equilibrium strategy. (*C*) The average shirk rate (± SEM) for human subjects calculated for the last half of each Nash equilibrium block. The proportion of shirking predicted at Nash equilibrium is denoted by the line of unity (black). Filled squares, human vs. human (N = 6 subjects); filled circles, human vs. computer (N = 5 subjects). (*D*) Same plot as *B* for an individual monkey subject. (*E*) Same plot as *C* for monkey subjects. 29 blocks/point: 13 blocks from monkey 1, 16 blocks from monkey 2.

panel). Although both players freely chose either of two actions on every trial, we found that the overall behavior of our human subjects was well predicted by these Nash equilibriums (gray lines).[2]

During the last half of each block, once subjects had reached a stable strategy, we determined the average shirk rate produced in response to changes in employer inspection costs and plotted this against the shirk rate predicted at equilibrium (figure 87.1C). We found that the responses of humans generally tracked the theoretical shirk rate but tended to overshirk at the lowest predicted rates, a phenomenon that may reflect a sampling strategy intended to maximize the accuracy with which employees estimate the rate at which their employer inspects.

We then trained monkeys to play a version of the inspection game against our computer employer and assessed whether their behavior was comparable to that of humans. In these experiments, thirsty monkeys competed for a water reward and indicated their choices on each trial with a saccadic eye movement directed to one of two eccentric visual targets. On all trials, a red shirk target appeared in the center of the neuronal response field (Gnadt and Andersen, 1988; Platt and Glimcher, 1998) and a green work target appeared opposite the neuronal response field. Despite the difference in species and response modality, monkeys tracked the Nash equilibrium solutions (figure 87.1D, E) and deviated from those solutions when shirking rates of 30% or less were efficient strategies, just as humans do when playing the inspection game.

STUDIES OF NEURONAL ACTIVITY We studied lateral intraparietal (area LIP) neurons with a mixture of inspection game trials and instructed trials. In instructed trials, after an initial delay, the color of the fixation stimulus changed from yellow to either red or green with equal probability. The monkey was rewarded for making a saccade to the eccentric target (work target or shirk target) that matched the color of the fixation stimulus. By examining the same neurons with blocks of both instructed trials and inspection game trials, we were able to examine LIP neurons both inside and outside the context of a strategic game.

Figure 87.2A examines the relationship among expected utility, behavior, and firing rate of a single LIP neuron. A great deal of work has suggested that the responses of these neurons reflect the intention to make an eye movement (Andersen and Buneo, 2002) or the saliency of stimuli (Colby and Goldberg, 1999; Kusonoki et al., 2000; Gottlieb, 2002). Here we tested whether these neurons are in fact sensitive to the expected utility of movements or movement targets. For the remainder of this analysis, we restrict our discussion to trials that ended with a movement toward the target in the response field, trials on which all sensory stimuli and movements were essentially identical. This control

ensures that any changes in neuronal activity were unlikely to result from differences in aspects of sensory or motor processing but instead reflected differences in the decision-making process itself. The lower axis of figure 87.2A plots the trial numbers during which six sequential blocks of trials were presented. In the first block, only instructed trials were presented, in which a visual cue specified what movement would be reinforced. For this block, a movement to the shirk target was reinforced with twice as much water as a movement to the work target (0.5 mL vs. 0.25 mL). The second block also presented instructed trials, but this time the rewards were reversed, such that a movement to the shirk target yielded half as much juice as a movement to the other target. Blocks 3–6 presented game theoretic inspection trials in which the monkey was free to select any response and in which dynamic interactions of the two players should have maintained an expected utility for the two movements near equivalence. (During these trials, working yielded 0.25 mL of water while shirking yielded either 0.5 or 0 mL of fluid.) The solid gray lines plot the trial-to-trial probability of the shirk target being the rewarded target during the first two instructed blocks, followed by the Nash equilibrium response strategies during the four free choice inspection trial blocks. At a purely behavioral level, the animal seemed to closely approximate the rational response strategies predicted by theory. Initially the probability of looking at the shirk target was fixed at 50% during the instructed blocks, and then shifted dynamically to each of the Nash equilibrium strategies in the subsequent four inspection trial blocks. The dots plot the running average of neuronal firing rate during the visual epoch, a period shortly after target onset on each of these shirk trials. Note that when the expected utility of the shirk target is high in the first block, firing rate is high. When the expected utility is low in the second block, firing rate is low. Finally, when the expected utility is assumed to be at equivalence, according to the Nash formulation, the firing rate is at a fairly constant and intermediate level. This is the specific result that would be expected if LIP neurons encode the expected utility of movements into their response fields.

These results suggest that the activity of this LIP neuron is modulated by the expected utilities of the available courses of action. To assess whether this was consistently true across our neuronal sample, we performed a similar analysis on the activity of our sample of neurons. Once again we analyzed only those trials in which the monkeys were either instructed (figure 87.2B—instructed task) or freely chose (figure 87.2C—inspection game) to look at the shirk target that was placed inside the response field. Twenty neurons were tested in two blocks of the instructed task with a high and low level of expected utility associated with the shirk response, as in the first two blocks of figure 87.2A. Average neuronal activity was high when the expected utility associated with the

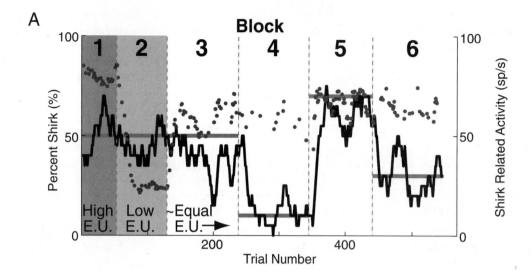

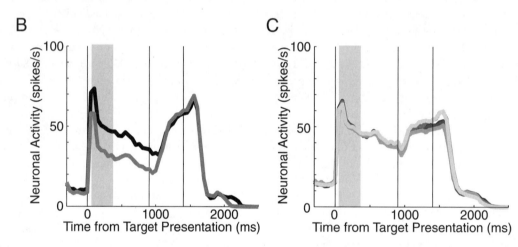

FIGURE 87.2 Activity of LIP neurons during instructed and free choice tasks. (*A*) Proportion of monkey's choices devoted to shirking and corresponding activity of a single LIP neuron. The monkey performed six successive blocks of trials; the first two were during the instructed task and the final four were during the free choice task with four different payoff matrices. During both blocks of the instructed task, the rate of shirking was fixed at 50% (gray bars). In the first block, the reward associated with the shirk target was twice as large as that associated with the work target (high expected utility [E.U.]) and in the second block, the rewards were switched such that the reward associated with the shirk target was half as much as that associated with the work target (low E.U.). During the four free choice blocks, the monkey's shirk rate was near that predicted by the Nash equilibrium (gray bars), and the expected utility is assumed to be approximately equal (~equal E.U.) between movements for these blocks. The black line represents the running average of shirking over the last 20 trials. The black dots represent the running average of neuronal activity on shirk trials produced during the last 20 trials. This neuronal activity was sampled 50–350 ms after the visual stimuli were presented (see gray bars in *B* and *C*). (*B*) The average post-stimulus time histograms (bin width 50 ms) for 20 neurons that were tested in the two blocks of the instructed task with different expected utilities in the response field as shown in *A*. The dark gray line represents the average activity during the high E.U. block and the light gray line represents the average activity during the low E.U. block. (*C*) The average post-stimulus time histograms for 41 neurons that were tested in five blocks of the free choice task in which the Nash equilibrium strategy ranged from responding with a shirk rate of 10% (lightest line) to 90% (darkest line) in steps of 20%. A direct comparison of the figures in *C* and *D* is not possible because they describe separate populations of neurons. However, similar results were obtained for 13 neurons that were tested in both the free and forced choice tasks (not shown).

shirk target was larger than the expected utility of the work target (figure 87.2B, black line). This average neuronal activity was low when the expected utility associated with the shirk target was smaller than the expected utility of the work target (figure 87.2B, gray line). Forty-one neurons were tested in five blocks of trials of the inspection game (figure 87.2C) in which the strategy at Nash equilibrium ranged from responding 10% (lightest gray line) to 90% (darkest line) of the time in the neuronal response field. Of these 41 neurons, 13 were also tested in the instructed task described above. As discussed previously, at equilibrium the expected utilities are roughly equal between the two targets, regardless of the actual proportion of responses devoted to the target in the neuronal response field. Correspondingly, we found that the average neuronal activity remained unchanged, as indicated by the superimposed post-stimulus time histograms that plot the average population firing rate across different Nash equilibrium blocks.

DISSOCIATING DECISION VARIABLES In a subset of 20 neurons we also examined the effects of reversing the locations of the work and shirk targets during 50% Nash equilibrium blocks of the inspection game each of which was about 100 trials long (figure 87.3A). This changed both the probability and magnitude of reward associated with the target in the neuronal response field, while the relative expected utility remained constant. Firing rates should differ across blocks if they reflect either probability of reward or magnitude of reward alone, but they should remain constant if they reflect expected utility. In fact, the firing rates did not change, which bolsters the hypothesis that LIP firing rates encode the expected utility of choices.

ENCODING RELATIVE VERSUS ABSOLUTE EXPECTED UTILITY The preceding results suggest that neurons in LIP encode expected utility, the product of probability and the subjective value of reward. It is not clear from these observations, however, whether the firing rates of LIP neurons encode expected utility for the movement in the response field or the relative expected utilities of all available options. A number of authors have suggested that when humans and animals make decisions, they consider the relative expected utility of each available action rather than the absolute expected utility of each action (Flaherty, 1996; Herrnstein, 1997). In order to test the hypothesis that LIP neurons encode the relative expected utility of movements rather than the absolute expected utility of movements, we examined 18 neurons while monkeys completed a block of about 100 trials in which the magnitude of both working and shirking rewards was doubled. If LIP activity is sensitive to absolute expected utility, it should increase when the rewards are doubled. If, however, LIP activity is sensitive only to relative expected utility, then the firing rate should be the same for both blocks

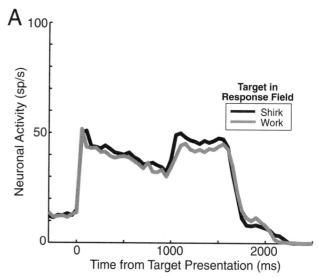

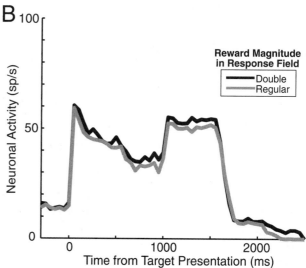

FIGURE 87.3 Two additional experiments support the notion that LIP activity is correlated with relative expected utility. (A) Switching work and shirk targets. Average neuronal activity in the standard inspection game when the shirk target was placed in the neuronal response field (black line) was compared with average neuronal activity on a block of trials in which the work target was placed in the neuronal response field (gray line). In both blocks the Nash equilibrium strategy was to choose each response 50% of the time. Across blocks, the expected utility remained constant despite differences in the probability and magnitude of reward. (B) Relative versus absolute expected utility. The monkeys performed two blocks of trials with the shirk target in the neuronal response field. In one block, the magnitude of reward for the work trials was 1 unit and for the shirk trials 2 units (gray). In the other block, the absolute magnitudes of reward were doubled for both movements (black). Although the absolute expected utility in the neuronal response fields changed across blocks, the relative expected utility between the two choices was approximately equal ($N = 18$).

of trials. As figure 87.3B shows, there was no change in the firing rate of LIP neurons when absolute reward magnitude was doubled. This result suggests that LIP neurons encode the relative expected utility of movements.

Relative Expected Utility versus Relative Expected Value   Throughout this discussion we have assumed that the expected utilities of the monkeys' actions are reasonably approximated by the expected values of those actions. Although this may be reasonable, we did not test this assumption. It is critical to remember that this lack of information renders a direct quantitative comparison between the instructed task data and the inspection game data impossible. In the inspection game, according to the Nash equilibrium prediction, the expected utilities of the two available movements are roughly equal. However, in the instructed task we have no direct measure that would allow us to determine the expected utility of each response. Instead, we can only compute the expected value of each response from the actual juice volumes and probabilities we employed and then presume that the subjective values of these responses approximate that objective measure. Although it is probably reasonable to assume that the utility of juice is close to the value of juice in the range of volumes and at the range of animal satiety selected for these experiments, the inability to directly compare these two experiments highlights an outstanding issue in most neurobiological studies of decision making. The underlying utility functions on which choices in decision-making experiments are based are rarely measured. Instead, experimentalists report expected values, or closely related quantities. One exception is work by Gallistel and colleagues, who have used elegant techniques based on Herrnstein's (1997) matching law to directly measure the utility of electrical stimulation of the medial forebrain bundle in rats (reviewed in Gallistel, 1994). It seems clear that similar techniques could also be used to quantify expected utility during decision making in other species. Future studies of decision making will have to begin to include direct measurements of utility.

Summary   One of the problems that some neurobiological studies of decision making have faced is the absence of a theoretical framework for describing the computational process involved in generating free choice behavior. This has been evident in studies of voluntary behavior, where the relationship between events in the outside world and internally generated decisions often appears unpredictable. Social scientists working in economics and psychology have, however, developed a theoretical corpus for describing choice behavior both when it is predictable on a trial-by-trial basis and when it is predictable only on an average, or molar, level.

The data discussed above suggest that we can begin to use game theoretic approaches to examine the control of free choice behavior at the level of single neurons. Recently, a number of other closely related techniques have also been used to achieve this same goal in other electrophysiological studies. For example, Coe and colleagues (2002) used a dynamic, free choice task to show that the activity of neurons in the frontal and supplementary eye fields and area LIP predicted the choice a monkey would make well before the movement was executed. Researchers using functional magnetic resonance imaging are also beginning to adopt closely related approaches. In one experiment, Montague and Berns (2002) used a free choice task to divide human subjects into two groups, risky and conservative, depending on their willingness to accept negative payoffs. They were able to show that the nucleus accumbens was differentially active in the risky and conservative subjects.

These examples present a small sample of the growing number of studies that are beginning to use economic-style models and techniques for studying voluntary choice behavior (Breiter et al., 2001; McCabe et al., 2001; Sugrue et al., 2001; Montague and Berns, 2002; Montague et al., 2002). Together, these parallel lines of inquiry suggest a growing synthesis of social scientific and neuroscientific approaches that are beginning to define the outlines of the neural system for unconstrained decision making.

Implications for the neural basis of unconstrained choice

These experiments suggest that we can begin to use theoretical approaches from the social sciences to examine the macroscopic pattern of individual free choice behavior at a neurobiological level, but they tell us very little about the trial-by-trial process from which this aggregate behavior emerges. The inability of equilibrium formulations like these to describe the dynamics of choice behavior is, however, hardly unique to neurophysiology. Almost since the inception of equilibrium models, psychologists and economists have been developing alternative frameworks that seek to complement the equilibrium approach with explainations of how free choice behaviors are generated at a trial-by-trial level. Unfortunately, even for the social scientists who have devoted significant resources to achieving this goal, it is not yet possible to accurately predict whether a subject will select rock, paper, or scissors on the next round of play (see, e.g., Bush and Mosteller, 1955; Luce, 1959; Herrnstein, 1997; Erev and Roth, 1998; Fudenberg and Levine, 1998; McKelvey and Palfrey, 1998; Dragoi and Staddon, 1999; Camerer, 2003). Does behavior produced under these conditions defy trial-by-trial prediction because we still lack adequate models for describing these processes, or are some classes of behavior truly and irreducibly unpredictable, defying trial-by-trial prediction in principle? Traditionally that has been a difficult question to answer, but neurobiologists may now be able to engage this issue in a novel way. It may now be possible to ask whether behavior can be driven by irreducibly stochastic processes that operate at the neuronal or subneuronal level. We may now be able to determine whether the apparent unpredictability with which a subject chooses to play rock reflects the action of a fundamentally stochastic underlying process.

RANDOMNESS AT THE NEURONAL AND SUBNEURONAL LEVEL
One known source of stochasticity at the neuronal level is the mechanism by which synaptic inputs give rise to action potentials in cortical neurons. Abundant evidence indicates that when cortical neurons are repeatedly activated by precisely the same stimulus, the neurons do not deterministically generate action potentials in precisely the same pattern. Instead, the pattern of stimulation delivered to cortical neurons appears to determine only the average firing rates of those neurons; the instant-by-instant dynamics of action potential generation are highly variable and appear to defy precise prediction (Tolhurst, Movshon, and Dean, 1981; Dean, 1981). The available data suggest that this moment-by-moment variation, the overall variance in cortical firing rate, is related to mean firing rate by a roughly fixed constant of proportionality that has a value near 1.07 over a very broad range of mean rates (Tolhurst et al., 1981; Dean, 1981; Zohary, Shadlen, and Newsome, 1994; Lee et al., 1998), and this seems to be true of essentially all cortical areas that have been examined, including parietal cortex (Lee et al., 1998). This has led to the suggestion that action potential production can be described as something like a stochastic Poisson process,[3] a truly probabilistic operation for which the stimulus specifies an average rate but which generates action potentials in a fundamentally stochastic manner.

More recently, there have even been several efforts to identify the biophysical source of this Poisson-like stochasticity. Mainen and Sejnowski (1995), for example, sought to determine whether the process of action potential generation in the cell body was the source of this stochasticity. Their work led to the conculsion that action potential generation is quite deterministically tied to membrane voltage, and thus that this process was not a source of intrinsic action potential variability. Subsequent studies have begun to suggest that it may instead be the process of synaptic transmission which imposes a stochastic pattern on cortical action potential production (for review, see Stevens, 1994). We now know, for example, that presynaptic action potentials lead to postsynaptic depolarizations with surprisingly low probabilities in many cortical synapses, and that the sizes of the postsynaptic depolarizations that do occur can be quite variable. The actual pattern of instant-by-instant membrane voltage seems thus to be influenced by irreducible stochasticity at the level of the synapse, a stochasticity imposed by fluctuations in the amount of transmitter encapsulated by the kinetic processes that fill synaptic vesicles and by the dynamics of calcium diffusion, among other things. All of these data suggest that the precise pattern of activity in cortical neurons is stochastic. Exactly when an action potential is generated seems to depend on apparently random molecular and atomic-level processes. So the nervous system does seem to include stochastic elements at a very low level. The times at which action potentials occur seem to be fundamentally stochastic. What implications, if any, might this have for the generation of behavior?

RANDOMNESS IN COMPUTATIONAL SYSTEMS   One of the most influential studies of how this randomness in the activity of individual neurons might affect behavior is Shadlen and colleagues' (1996) landmark model of visual-saccadic decision making. Their model sought to explain, at a computational level, a series of experiments (reviewed in Newsome et al., 1995) in which trained monkeys viewed a display of chaotically moving spots of light. On any given trial, a subset of the spots moved coherently in a single direction while the remaining spots moved randomly. The direction of the coherent motion indicated which of two possible saccadic eye movements would yield a reward, and at the end of each trial animals were free to make a saccade. If they made the correct movement, they then received that reward. Physiological data from those experiments indicated that the firing rates of single neurons in the middle temporal visual area (area MT) were correlated with the fraction of spots that moved coherently in a particular direction and thus with the movement produced by the subject at the end of the trial.

Shadlen and colleagues (1996) found, however, that the combination of signals from as few as 50–100 of these area MT neurons could be used to identify the reinforced direction of motion with greater accuracy than was actually evidenced by the choice behavior of the monkeys. The trial-by-trial choices of the monkeys seemed to be slightly less accurate, or more unpredictable, than might be expected from an analysis of the area MT firing rates. To account for this finding, Shadlen and colleagues proposed that the MT signal was, at a later stage in the neuronal architecture, corrupted by a noise source that effectively placed an upper limit on the efficiency with which the cortical signals could be combined during the moving spot task. Their model proposed that the cortical targets of MT neurons further randomized the behavior of the animals under the circumstances they had examined. From this, one might speculate that the physiological cost of more deterministically generating behavior from MT activity in later cortical areas may simply have been greater than the benefits that could have been accrued by the animal had the stochasticity of those later elements in the cortical architecture been reduced.

To further explore this notion that computational elements may impose quite specific levels of unpredictability on

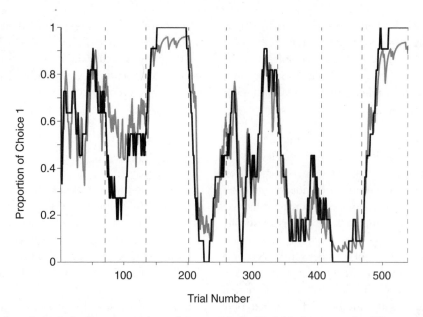

FIGURE 87.4 Monkey free choice behavior on a variant of the Platt and Glimcher (1999) task. Monkey chose between two possible movements, each of which provided a different magnitude and probability of fluid reward. Black line plots an 11-trial running average of the monkey's choice behavior over eight sequential blocks. Each block presented a different expected utility for each of the two movements. Block transitions were unsignaled. Gray line plots the trial-by-trial prediction of a reinforcement learning model that estimates the utilities of the two movements and employs a simple stochastic decision rule. See text for details.

behavior, we can consider a variant of Platt and Glimcher's (1999) free choice experiments that we recently performed. In this behavioral experiment, monkeys once again chose to make one of two possible saccades, and the expected utility of each movement was manipulated by varying both the magnitude and probability of fluid reward (associated with each movement) across blocks of trials. Figure 87.4 (black line) plots the behavior of a monkey performing this task. In an effort to examine the unpredictability of this relatively simple nonstrategic behavior, we modeled the monkey's decisions on a trial-by-trial basis as an estimation process followed by a decision rule. In the estimation process, an exponentially weighted average of the recently obtained rewards was used to determine the expected utilities of each of the two possible movements. The time constant of this exponential weighted average, which determined how many previous trials influenced the current estimate of movement value, was left as a free parameter. The decision rule used a sigmoidal function to convert the difference in value of the two movements to a probability of choosing each movement. The slope of the sigmoid, which we refer to as the stochastic transfer function, was left as the second free parameter in this model. The steepness of the slope thus described the model's sensitivity to the differences in the utility of the two possible movements. Put another way, the slope of the stochastic transfer function employed by the model quantified the level of trial-by-trial unpredictability evidenced by the monkey's decisions as a function of the relative utility of the two possible responses. (This is a variant of models that have been used extensively to describe choice behavior in animals

and humans.[4] For examples, see Luce, 1959; Killeen, 1981; Dow and Lea, 1987; Shadlen et al., 1996; Egelman et al., 1998; Sugrue et al., 2001; Montague and Berns, 2002; Sugrue and Newsome, 2002.)

The gray line in figure 87.4 plots the predictions of the model when both the time constant of the exponential weighted average and the stochastic transfer function were fitted to the accompanying data. The model does a reasonable job of predicting the monkey's choice behavior under these nonstrategic conditions by employing these two free parameters. This suggests that under these circumstances, decisions may be based on a dynamic estimate of relative expected utility computed as a weighted average of recent reward history. But much more interesting is the observation that the slope of the sigmoid, which stochastically relates expected utility to behavior, is quite shallow. The model achieves the best possible prediction by incorporating a significant degree of randomness that would, in principle, defy trial-by-trial prediction.

Even given a biophysical basis for neural stochasticity, and that successful models employ this stochasticity to generate behavior, should we actually believe that real animals are unpredictable because stochastic neural elements make them so, or is it more realistic to assume that behavior is predictable and that with the appropriate model, this predictability will become obvious? At one level this is a philosophical question, but at another it can certainly be viewed as an evolutionary issue: could natural selection have preserved stochastic neural mechanisms that produce unpredictable behaviors if unpredictable behaviors yield greater evolutionary fitness? To begin to answer that question we need to be able to more quantitatively determine the costs and benefits of behavioral stochasticity to real animals.

ASSESSING THE COSTS AND BENEFITS OF RANDOMNESS Let us consider once more the game of rock-paper-scissors. If one player uses a determinate strategy of playing rock, then scissors, then paper, repeatedly in that order, the opponent could win every time by detecting this pattern and playing paper, then rock, then scissors. For this reason, the production of any trial-by-trial pattern, no matter how subtle, puts a player at a potential disadvantage. This highlights the fact that an efficient mixed strategy equilibrium of the type Nash described does not simply require specific proportions of each choice, but also requires that the dynamic process by which choices are allocated must be unpredictable. Unlike the experiments of Newsome and colleagues (1995), Shadlen and colleagues (1996), and Platt and Glimcher (1999), under these specific conditions, *increasing* the unpredictability of behavior would increase the gains achieved by a player. This seems a critical point, because if under some conditions unpredictability is efficient, and we know of stochastic subneuronal mechanisms that could generate unpredictable behavior, then we might usefully begin to search for environmental conditions that call for specific levels of unpredictability. Under these conditions, we might measure the difference between observed levels of unpredictability and efficient levels of unpredictability in order to begin to test the hypothesis that unpredictability is an evolved feature of behavior.

Daeyeol Lee and his colleagues (Barraclough et al., 2002) have recently begun to examine this issue by studying the decisions of monkeys playing a game called *matching pennies* against a variable computer opponent. They found that the behavior of these monkeys did indeed depend on the properties of the computer opponent they faced. If the computer opponent was constructed with an ability to identify and exploit nonrandom patterns in the behavior of the monkeys, the animals produced behaviors that were more random. In contrast, if the computer opponent was only weakly able to detect patterns in the trial-by-trial dynamics of the monkeys' behavior, then the animals adopted a less random strategy. These observations indicate that the level of trial-by-trial randomness produced by an animal can reflect the task that it faces; the level of randomness expressed by behavior may represent an adjustable process governed by an internal set of costs at each level of the neural architecture that we have not yet measured.

Stochastic events occur at the subneuronal level. Models of behavior often must employ stochastic components if they are to simulate behavior accurately. In order to be efficient, some behaviors must be unpredictable. In sum, it seems that a number of elements point toward true randomness as an important feature of vertebrate behavior.

What remains unclear, however, is how all of these processes are connected. How might largely fixed stochastic subneuronal processes give rise to variably random behavior? The answer to that critical last question is far from certain but there are some hints that we may be beginning to uncover at least one basic mechanism that could accomplish this linkage. Whether this mechanism actually serves to link neuronal stochasticity and behavioral unpredictability is still very unclear, but the existence of a mechanism of this general type within the primate neural architecture suggests that these linkages are at least possible.

LINKING THE STOCHASTICITY OF NEURONS AND BEHAVIOR Shadlen and colleagues' 1996 model demonstrated that relating neuronal firing rates to behavior required a knowledge of two critical parameters, the intrinsic variance in instantaneous firing rate evidenced by each cortical neuron (the Poisson-like variability of the action potential generation process) and the correlation in action potential patterns between the many neurons that participate in any neural computation (the interneuronal cross-correlation). Shadlen and colleagues demonstrated that both of these properties contribute to the unpredictability evidenced by behavior. The variability in the firing rate of each neuron contributes to the unpredictability of behavior by producing an initial stochasticity in the neuronal architecture, and the degree to which that stochasticity influences behavior depends on how tightly correlated are the firing patterns of the many neurons in a population.

To make this insight clear, consider a population of 1000 neurons, all of which fire with the same mean rate and have the same level of intrinsic variability but are generating action potentials independently of each other. The members of such a population generate moment-by-moment patterns of action potentials that are completely uncorrelated; the only thing that they share is a common underlying mean firing rate. Because of this independence, globally averaging the activity of all of these independent neurons would allow one to recover the underlying mean rate at any instant. A cortical target receiving diffuse inputs from these 1000 source neurons would therefore accurately and instantaneously have access to the underlying mean rate at which the population was firing; there would be nothing necessarily stochastic about the behavior of such a neuron. However, a circuit in which a population of 1000 neurons all fire with the same mean rate and still have the same level of intrinsic variability, but in which each of the 1000 source neurons is tightly correlated in their activity patterns, would behave differently. Under these conditions, it is the stochastic and synchronous pattern of activity shared by all of the neurons in the population that is available to the target neuron at any moment, rather than the underlying mean rate. In a highly correlated system of this type, the output at any moment is irreducibly stochastic. Of course, these are just two extreme conditions along a continuum. Many levels of correlation between neurons are possible, and each would provide the target with a slightly different level of access to the underlying mean rate, and a different level of instrinsic randomness.

To address these issues of stochasticity in their original model, Shadlen and his colleagues (1996) were able to use available data to estimate both the intrinsic stochasticity of cortical neurons and the actual level of interneuronal correlation in area MT during the moving-dot task they studied. A number of studies had shown that the intrinsic variance in the firing rates of cortical neurons, the cortical coefficient of variation, is largely fixed at 1.07 (Tolhurst, Movshon, and Dean, 1981; Dean, 1981; Zohary et al., 1994; Lee et al., 1998) and Zohary, Shadlen, and Newsome (1994) had demonstrated that under the behavioral conditions being modeled, pairs of MT neurons that were close enough to be studied with the same electrode showed an interneuronal correlation of about 0.19. It was by using this number and knowledge of the unpredictability of the animal's actual behavior that Shadlen and his colleagues were able to estimate the magnitude of the later randomizing element that they believed intervened between MT activity and the generation of behavior.

More recently, Parker, Krug, and Cumming (2002; Dodd et al., 2001) examined the activity of this same population of MT neurons but in a different behavioral task that imposed different environmental contingencies. Like Zohary and colleagues, they were also able to record the activity of pairs of MT neurons and to determine both the coefficient of variation and the interneuronal correlation between these pairs under their behavioral conditions. They found that the coefficient of variation was essentially the same in their task but that the interneuronal correlation was quite different, a correlation coefficient of 0.44. At a behavioral level they also found that the stochastic firing rates of individual neurons were more tightly correlated with the stochastic behavior of their subjects than in the Zohary study (a choice probability of 0.67 rather than the 0.56 measured by Britten and colleagues [1996]). In other words, MT neurons in the Parker task showed a higher level of interneuronal correlation and the behavior of the animals was more tightly coupled to the stochastic behavior of individual neurons. Just as one might have predicted, the level of observed interneuronal correlation in a single cortical area and the level of randomness in behavior appear to be related. Futhermore, the level of interneuronal correlation appears to be variable, dependent on the task the animal is asked to perform.

These results may be very important, not because they definitively explain how neurons and behavior are linked but because they demonstrate that such linkages are at least conceptually possible. We now know that in order to be efficient, some behaviors must be unpredictable, and that the level of

this unpredictability is, and should be, adjustable. We also know that there are intrinsic sources of stochasticity in the vertebrate nervous system. Evolution could, at least in principle, have yielded mechanisms that link these processes.

SUMMARY   Over the last century, social scientists have made significant progress toward describing the underlying computational processes that guide decision making. While their early successes focused on predictable forms of decision making, more recent studies have examined the kinds of unpredictable decision making that occur under conditions such as strategic interaction. The equilibrium approaches used in the social sciences to describe unpredictable decision making have, however, been unable to determine the ultimate source of the randomness evidenced in strategic behavior.

Over the past decade, neuroscientists have begun to employ many of the mathematical formulations developed by social scientists. Their rich set of computational mechanisms has provided powerful tools for understanding the neural architecture. The most recent studies of this architecture seem, however, to go beyond the insights available from the social sciences. These newest studies suggest that some irreducible level of randomness may be an essential feature of the vertebrate nervous system and may play a critical role in the generation of behavior. If the mechanism by which neuronal firing rates yield behavior can preserve a variable fraction of the neuronal stochasticity that we and others have observed, then the level of unpredictability expressed by behavior could be a reflection of this variable underlying physical process. Limitations imposed by that process could reflect an implicit cost function against which behavior is optimized. These observations may therefore hint that the randomness captured in our neuroscientific models by elements like the stochastic transfer function may be the instantiation of an intrinsic stochasticity in the neurobiological architecture. Indeed, these observations may even suggest that the precise slope of the stochastic transfer function under a given set of environmental conditions represents some kind of adjustable neurophysiological process by which stochastic neuronal firing rates lead to the efficient generation of unpredictable behavior. Neuroscience may thus soon be able to provide a final answer to the social scientific question of whether some classes of behavior are truly and irreducibly unpredictable. Under some conditions, behavior may well be irreducibly unpredictable, and this unpredictability may extend down to the molecular level at which synapses operate.

Conclusions

The ultimate goal of neurobiological studies of decision making is to explain human voluntary choice, a process often attributed to the agency of free will. When a real human employee faces a real human employer, she must make a voluntary decision about whether to go to work or to stay at home and shirk. Many clear factors influence her decision: how recently and how often she has been inspected, how much she stands to gain by successfully shirking, and her own predispositions or biases. Were she, however, always to work and then shirk and then work and then shirk, alternating deterministically between these two actions, her behavior would seem less than voluntary. In large measure, what makes the decision seem voluntary to an outside observer is that her response defies prediction on a decision-by-decision basis. Explaining the neurobiological source of that unpredictability will probably pose the greatest challenge for students of this process and will yield fundamental insights into the causal processes that underlie human action.

ACKNOWLEDGMENTS The authors wish to thank Brian Lau for helpful discussions, for thoughtful comments on earlier drafts of the manuscript, and for providing the model fit illustrated in figure 87.4. We would also like to thank David Heeger, Hannah Bayer, Michael Platt, Daeyeol Lee, and Maggie Grantner for helpful discussions. This work was supported by the Klingenstein Foundation and the National Eye Institute.

NOTES

1. Thus at Nash equilibrium for the employee:

$$EU(\text{Shirk}) = EU(\text{Work}) \qquad (1)$$

which given the payoff matrix (Fig. 1A, left panel) expands to

$$p(\text{Inspect}) * 0 + (1 - p(\text{Inspect})) * W =$$
$$p(\text{Inspect}) * (W - C) + (1 - p(\text{Inspect})) * (W - C) \qquad (2)$$

solving for p(Inspect)

$$p(\text{Inspect}) = C/W \qquad (3)$$

where EU(Shirk) is the expected utility for choosing to shirk, EU(Work) is the expected utility for choosing to work, p(Inspect) is the probability of the employer inspecting and $1 - p(\text{Inspect})$ is the probability of the employer not inspecting when at equilibrium, W is the wage paid by the employer to the employee, and C is the cost of work to the employee.

Similarly, at Nash equilibrium, the expected utility for inspecting is equal to the expected utility for not inspecting for the employer. Solving for p(Shirk)

$$p(\text{Shirk}) = I/W \qquad (4)$$

where p(Shirk) is the probability of the employee shirking when at equilibrium and I is the cost of inspection.

Unfortunately, using these equations to predict the behavior of rational players with precision requires knowledge of the subjective functions that relate value to utility. The equilibrium points occur when expected utilities are precisely equivalent, even though it is objective value that is most easily measured by an experimenter. For the purposes of the computations presented here we assume a linear utility function in the subsequent analysis. Although this would be expected to produce small metrical

errors in our computations, it should not have any effect on the ordinal representations we compute, which form the core of this presentation.

2. Given the assumptions about the relationship of value and utility stated in the preceding footnote.

3. To be more precise, the process of action potential generation appears to be a skewed Poisson process.

4. In Shadlen and colleagues' model, for example, the magnitude of the secondary noise source is essentially equivalent to the slope term for our stochastic transfer function.

REFERENCES

ANDERSEN, R. A., and C. A. BUNEO, 2002. Intentional maps in posterior parietal cortex. *Annu. Rev. Neurosci.* 25:189–220.

ARNAULD, A., and P. NICOLE, 1662/1994. *Logic or the Art of Thinking*. Cambridge, England: Cambridge University Press.

BARRACLOUGH, D. J., M. L. CONROY, et al., 2002. Stochastic decision-making in a two-player competitive game. *Soc. Neurosci. Abstr.* 285.16.

BERNOULLI, D., 1738/1954. Exposition on a new theory on the measurement of risk. *Econometrica* 22:23–36.

BREITER, H. C., I. AHARON, et al., 2001. Functional imaging of neural responses to expectancy and experience of monetary gains and losses. *Neuron* 30(2):619–639.

BRITTEN, K. H., W. T. NEWSOME, M. N. SHADLEN, S. CELEBRINI, and J. A. MOVSHON, 1996. A relationship between behavioral choice and the visual responses of neurons in macaque area MT. *Vis. Neurosci.* 13:87–100.

BUSH, R. R., and F. MOSTELLER, 1955. *Stochastic Models for Learning*. New York: Wiley.

CAMERER, C. F., 2003. *Behavioral Game Theory: Experiments in Strategic Interaction*. Princeton, N.J.: Princeton University Press.

COE, B., K. TOMIHARA, et al., 2002. Visual and anticipatory bias in three cortical eye fields of the monkey during an adaptive decision-making task. *J. Neurosci.* 22:5081–5090.

COLBY, C. L., J. R. DUHAMEL, et al., 1995. Oculocentric spatial representation in parietal cortex. *Cereb. Cortex* 5:470–481.

COLBY, C. L., and M. E. GOLDBERG, 1999. Space and attention in parietal cortex. *Annu. Rev. Neurosci.* 22:319–349.

DEAN, A. F., 1981. The variability of discharge of simple cells in the cat striate cortex. *Exp. Brain Res.* 44:437–440.

DODD, J. V., K. KRUG, B. G. CUMMING, and A. J. PARKER, 2001. Perceptually bistable figures lead to high choice probabilities in cortical area MT. *J. Neurophysiol.* 21:4809–4821.

DORRIS, M. C., and P. W. GLIMCHER, 2002. A neural correlate for the relative expected value of choices in the lateral intraparietal area. *Soc. Neurosci. Abstr.* 28:280.6.

DOW, S. M., and S. E. G. LEA, 1987. Foraging in a changing environment: Simulations in the operant laboratory. In *Quantitative Analyses of Behavior*, M. L. Commons, A. Kacelnik, and S. J. Shettleworth, eds. Hillsdale, N.J.: Erlbaum.

DRAGOI, V., and J. E. STADDON, 1999. The dynamics of operant conditioning. *Psychol. Rev.* 106:20–61.

EGELMAN, D. M., C. PERSON, et al., 1998. A computational role for dopamine delivery in human decision-making. *J. Cogn. Neurosci.* 10:623–630.

EREV, I., and A. ROTH, 1998. Prediction how people play games: Reinforcement learning in games with unique strategy equilibrium. *Am. Econ. Rev.* 88:848–881.

FLAHERTY, C. F., 1996. *Incentive Relativity*. New York: Cambridge University Press.

FUDENBERG, D., and D. K. LEVINE, 1998. *The Theory of Learning in Games*. Cambridge, Mass.: MIT Press.

FUDENBERG, D., and J. TIROLE, 1991. *Game Theory*. Cambridge, Mass.: MIT Press.

GALLISTEL, C. R., 1994. Foraging for brain stimulation: Toward a neurobiology of computation. *Cognition* 50:151–170.

GLIMCHER, P. W., 2001. Making choices: The neurophysiology of visual-saccadic decision making. *Trends Neurosci.* 24:654–659.

GLIMCHER, P. W., 2003a. Neural correlates of primate decision-making. *Annu. Rev. Neurosci.* 26:133–179.

GLIMCHER, P. W., 2003b. *Decisions, Uncertainty, and the Brain: The Science of Neuroeconomics*. Cambridge, Mass.: MIT Press.

GNADT, J. W., and R. A. ANDERSEN, 1988. Memory related motor planning activity in posterior parietal cortex of macaque. *Exp. Brain. Res.* 70:216–220.

GOLD, J. I., and M. N. SHADLEN, 2001. Neural computations that underlie decisions about sensory stimuli. *Trends. Cogn. Sci.* 5:10–16.

GOTTLIEB, J., 2002. Parietal mechanisms of target representation. *Curr. Opin. Neurobiol.* 12:134–140.

HANDEL, A., and P. W. GLIMCHER, 2000. Contextual modulation of substantia nigra pars reticulata neurons. *J. Neurophysiol.* 83:3042–3048.

HERRNSTEIN, R. J., 1997. *The Matching Law: Papers in Psychology and Economics*, Harvard University Press.

HIKOSAKA, O., Y. TAKIKAWA, et al., 2000. Role of the basal ganglia in the control of purposive saccadic eye movements. *Physiol. Rev.* 80:953–978.

KAWAGOE, R., Y. TAKIKAWA, et al., 1998. Expectation of reward modulates cognitive signals in the basal ganglia. *Nat. Neurosci.* 1:411–416.

KILLEEN, P. R., 1981. Averaging theory. In *Recent Developments in the Quantification of Steady-State Operant Behavior*, C. M. Bradshaw, E. Szabadi, and C. F. Lowe, eds. New York: Elsevier.

KREPS, D. M., 1990. *A Course in Microeconomic Theory*. Princeton, N.J.: Princeton University Press.

KUSUNOKI, M., J. GOTTLIEB, et al., 2000. The lateral intraparietal area as a salience map: The representation of abrupt onset, stimulus motion, and task relevance. *Vision Res.* 40:1459–1468.

LEE, D., N. L. PORT, W. KRUSE, and A. P. GEORGOPOULOS, 1998. Variability and correlated noise in the discharge of neurons in motor and parietal areas of the primate cortex. *J. Neurosci.* 18:1161–1170.

LUCE, R. D., 1959. *Individual Choice Behavior: A Theoretical Analysis*. New York: Wiley.

LUCE, R. D., and H. RAIFFA, 1957. *Games and Decisions*. New York: Wiley.

MAINEN, Z. F., and T. J. SEJNOWSKI, 1995. Reliability of spike timing in neocortical neurons. *Science* 268:1503–1506.

McCABE, K., D. HOUSER, et al., 2001. A functional imaging study of cooperation in two-person reciprocal exchange. *Proc. Natl. Acad. Sci. U.S.A.* 98:11832–11835.

McKELVEY, R. D., and T. R. PALFREY, 1998. Quantal response equilibria in extensive form games. *Exp. Econ.* 1:9–41.

MILLER, G. F., 1997. Protean primates: The evolution of adaptive unpredictability in competition and courtship. In *Machiavellian Intelligence II: Extensions and Evaluations*, A. Whiten and R. W.

Byrne, eds. Cambridge, England: Cambridge University Press, pp. 312–340.

MONTAGUE, P. R., and G. S. BERNS, 2002. Neural economics and the biological substrates of valuation. *Neuron* 36:265–284.

MONTAGUE, P. R., G. S. BERNS, et al., 2002. Hyperscanning: Simultaneous fMRI during linked social interactions. *NeuroImage* 16:1159–1164.

MYERS, J. L., 1976. Probability learning and sequence learning. In *Handbook of Learning and Cognitive Processes: Approaches to Human Learning and Motivation*, W. K. Estes. Hillsdale, N.J.: Erlbaum, pp. 171–205.

NASH, J. F., 1950. Equilibrium points in N-person games. *Proc. Natl. Acad. Sci. U.S.A.* 36:48–49.

NEURINGER, A., 2002. Operant variability: Evidence, functions, and theory. *Psychon. Bull. Rev.* 9:672–705.

NEWSOME, W. T., K. H. BRITTEN, et al., 1989. Neuronal correlates of a perceptual decision. *Nature* 341:52–54.

NEWSOME, W. T., M. N. SHADLEN, et al., 1995. Visual motion: Linking neuronal activity to psychophysical performance. *The Cognitive Neurosciences*, M. S. Gazzaniga, ed. Cambridge, Mass.: MIT Press.

PARKER, A. J., K. KRUG, and B. G. CUMMING, 2002. Neuronal activity and its links with the perception of multi-stable figures. *Philos. Trans. R. Soc. Lond. B* 357:1053–1062.

PASCAL, B., 1670/1966. *Pensées*. New York: Penguin Books.

PLATT, M. L., and P. W. GLIMCHER, 1998. Response fields of intraparietal neurons quantified with multiple saccadic targets. *Exp. Brain Res.* 121:65–75.

PLATT, M. L., and P. W. GLIMCHER, 1999. Neural correlates of decision variables in parietal cortex. *Nature* 400:233–238.

RAPOPORT, A., and D. V. BUDESCU, 1992. Generation of random binary series in strictly competitive games. *J. Exp. Psychol. Gen.* 121:352–364.

SCHALL, J. D., 2001. Neural basis of deciding, choosing and acting. *Nat. Rev. Neurosci.* 2:33–42.

SHADLEN, M. N., K. H. BRITTEN, et al., 1996. A computational analysis of the relationship between neuronal and behavioral responses to visual motion. *J. Neurosci.* 16:1486–1510.

SPARKS, D. L., and L. E. MAYS, 1990. Signal transformations required for the generation of saccadic eye movements. *Annu. Rev. Neurosci.* 13:309–336.

STEPHENS, D. W., and J. R. KREBS, 1986. *Foraging Theory*. Princeton, N.J.: Princeton University Press.

STEVENS, C. F., 1994. Neuronal communication: Cooperativity of unreliable neurons. *Curr Biol.* 4:268–269.

SUGRUE, L. P., W. T. NEWSOME, et al., 2001. Matching behavior in rhesus monkeys. *Soc. Neurosci. Abstr.* 59.3.

SUGRUE, L. P., and W. T. NEWSOME, 2002. Neural correlates of experienced value in area LIP of the rhesus monkey. *Soc. Neurosci. Abstr.* 121.5.

TOLHURST, D. J., J. A. MOVSHON, and A. F. DEAN, 1981. The statistical reliability of signals in single neurons in cat and monkey visual cortex. *Vision Res.* 23:775–785.

ZOHARY, E., M. N. SHADLEN, and W. T. NEWSOME, 1994. Correlated neuronal discharge and its implications for psychophysical performance. *Nature* 370:140–143.

88 The Neurophysiology of Decision Making as a Window on Cognition

MICHAEL N. SHADLEN AND JOSHUA I. GOLD

ABSTRACT Neurobiology has begun to uncover the brain mechanisms responsible for such higher cognitive functions as planning, remembering, and deciding. Progress has come, in part, from measurements of neural activity in brain regions that link sensory input to motor output. In this chapter we summarize a body of experimental work that has examined the neural basis of a simple sensory decision that uses visual input to instruct an oculomotor response. The decision is formed by transforming the visual input into a weight of evidence that supports or opposes the alternative outcomes. This evidence accumulates until a criterion level is reached. The neural processing architecture for forming the decision is closely tied to the motor intention. These principles seem likely to provide insight into a wide variety of higher brain functions.

Would any one trust in the convictions of a monkey's mind, if there are any convictions in such a mind?

—Charles Darwin, letter to W. Graham, 1881

Nervous systems extract sensory information from the environment to guide behavior. The underlying neural mechanisms have been studied extensively, in part by identifying neurons with responses linked deterministically to sensory and motor events. Higher nervous systems are also capable of widespread cognitive abilities, including interpretation, decision making, valuation, intention, language, and learning. The mechanisms underlying these abilities are less clear, in part because they seem beyond the scope of the machine-like behavior of sensory and motor neurons. This chapter examines this conundrum: How do properties of neurons and neural circuits give rise not just to reflexive sensory and motor abilities, but to cognition as well? We suggest that an answer can be found in circuits that link sensory input to motor output. Here, transformations of sensory and motor

signals reflect the kinds of nuance and flexibility that are hallmarks of cognition.

Several lines of evidence show that sensorimotor and cognitive mechanisms interact in the brain. Psychophysical measurements illustrate the many ways in which mechanisms that link sensation and action are not reflexive: they take a variable amount of time that can depend on the subject's strategy and other factors (Luce, 1986), they can involve flexible associations between different sensory stimuli and different actions (Murray, Bussey, and Wise, 2000; Wise and Murray, 2000), and they can be influenced by psychological factors such as bias, attention, and expected costs and benefits (Carpenter and Williams, 1995; Reddi and Carpenter, 2000). Clinical observations of patients with damage to association areas of cortex, particularly in the parietal and frontal lobes, have shown deficits in both sensory-guided behavior and cognitive functions (Mesulam, 1985; Feinberg and Farah, 1997). Neuroimaging studies have also shown colocalization of function, with similar patterns of activation in these association areas during certain sensorimotor and cognitive tasks (Corbetta et al., 1998; Acuna et al., 2002; Simon et al., 2002; Astafiev et al., 2003).

Combined electrophysiological and psychophysical studies in monkeys provide an opportunity to investigate the neural basis of these sensorimotor and cognitive abilities. In this chapter, we describe advances in understanding the neural mechanisms responsible for making a decision about visual motion (figure 88.1). In the first part of the chapter, we quantify decision formation in terms of a tradeoff between speed and accuracy. In the second part, we show that the underlying mechanisms involve neural activity that (1) persists beyond sensory and motor events, (2) accumulates over time a "weight of evidence" that supports or opposes the alternative decisions, and (3) is related to motor intention. In the third part, we discuss the broader implications of these findings. The mechanisms of decision formation appear well-suited for a variety of roles, from sensorimotor processing to more complex aspects of cognition.

MICHAEL N. SHADLEN Howard Hughes Medical Institute, Department of Physiology and Biophysics and National Primate Research Center, University of Washington Medical School, Seattle, Wash.
JOSHUA I. GOLD Department of Neuroscience, University of Pennsylvania, Philadelphia, Penn.

A
Variable Viewing Duration

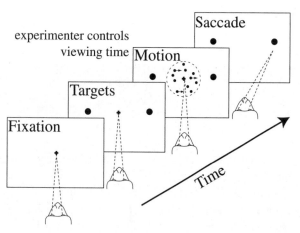

B
Response Time

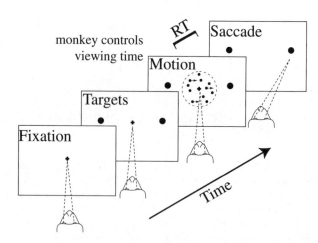

FIGURE 88.1 Two versions of the motion task used to study decision making in monkeys. This task was formerly used to study the relationship between the properties of neurons in the visual cortex and the limits of perception (see Parker and Newsome, 1998). The monkey decides whether the net direction of random-dot motion is in one of two directions—here, right or left. The ease and difficulty of the task can be controlled by varying the percentage of dots that are moving coherently in one of the two directions. The remaining dots merely appear and disappear at random locations. The monkey does not know beforehand what percentage of dots will be moving coherently or in which direction they will be moving. Even the moving dots are not shown for more than about 40 ms before being replotted elsewhere. Thus, the decision depends on assessing the net motion across all the dots and across time. The monkey is trained to look at a target to the right for rightward

motion, to the left for leftward motion, and so on. The monkey is also trained to handle stimuli with different directions, speeds, and locations in the visual field. To study sensory processing, the random-dot stimulus is placed in the receptive field of a direction-selective neuron. To study decision making, one of the targets that signals the monkey's commitment to a particular choice is placed in a neuron's response field. (*A*) In the variable-duration version of the task, the viewing time is a random value drawn from an exponential distribution. The experimenter controls the duration of motion viewing. The monkey indicates its choice when the fixation point is extinguished. (*B*) In the response-time (RT) version of the task, the monkey controls the viewing duration. Whenever ready, the monkey makes an eye movement to one of the choice targets. The RT is the time from the onset of random-dot motion to the beginning of the eye movement.

Psychophysics of decision making

Decisions about noisy sensory signals involve an inherent tradeoff between speed and accuracy. Deciding quickly can mean missing important signals. Taking more time can provide more or better signals, but that time might be wasted. We use the motion task to study the mechanisms responsible for this tradeoff. The random-dot stimulus supplies a continuous source of noisy signals that can take hundreds of milliseconds for the brain to accumulate and interpret. Thus, we can study the underlying mechanisms on a time scale that is relatively long for neurons. Here we analyze performance and show that information from the motion stimulus appears to accumulate over time until sufficient evidence has been gathered to render a decision.

Direct evidence for a temporal accumulation of motion information comes from experiments in which the time given to view the stimulus was varied randomly from trial to trial (figure 88.1*A*). The percentage of coherently moving

dots was also varied. Performance accuracy was affected by both variables (figure 88.2). At high motion coherence (top curve in figure 88.2), accuracy was perfect (no errors) with greater than approximately 200 ms of motion viewing. At lower motion coherences, performance improved with increased viewing time, measured out to 700 ms, but never reached perfect accuracy. The smooth curves fit to the data allow us to infer properties of the signals in the brain that are used to make the decision (Gold and Shadlen, 2000, 2003). Information from the stimulus appears to be accumulated throughout motion viewing without loss, as long as it is needed to improve performance. Information gained in the first 100 ms is simply added to information gained in the next 100 ms, and so forth. This accumulation persists over a time scale that is at least an order of magnitude greater than the time scale of neural computations in the sensory cortex, which must keep up with changes in the environment.

In a second set of experiments, the monkey rather than the experimenter controlled the period of motion viewing

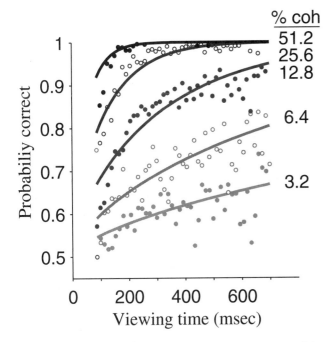

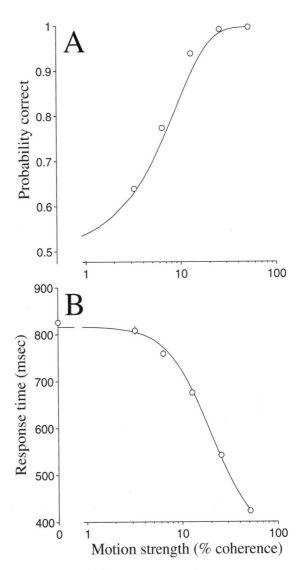

FIGURE 88.2 Performance on the variable-duration version of the discrimination task depends on motion coherence and viewing time. Solid lines are best-fitting functions based on a model for the decision using signal detection theory. The best fits suggest that the internal signals are proportional to motion strength and viewing time. N = 45,511 trials from 32 experiments in two monkeys. (Reprinted with permission from J. I. Gold and M. N. Shadlen, The influence of behavioral context on the representation of a perceptual decision in developing oculomotor commands. *J. Neurosci.* 23:632–651. © 2003 by the Society for Neuroscience.)

FIGURE 88.3 Accuracy and speed of decisions in the response-time (RT) version of the motion task. Data points are from two monkeys. (*A*) Psychometric function depicting accuracy as a function of motion strength. (*B*) Chronometric function depicting RT as a function of motion strength. The solid curve in *B* is the fit of Equation 1 to the data. It describes the amount of time it would take accumulating evidence to reach a criterion level were it to diffuse like a particle in Brownian motion with average drift proportional to motion coherence (see figure 88.4). The sigmoid curve in *A* is the predicted psychometric function based on the model fit to the RT data.

(figure 88.1*B*). The results from this type of experiment are shown in figure 88.3. In addition to a psychometric function describing accuracy (figure 88.3*A*), we also obtain a chronometric function of behavioral response time (RT) versus motion strength (figure 88.3*B*). The RT was measured from the time the random dots first appeared to the time that the monkey initiated an eye movement to indicate its choice of direction. For high coherences, the task was easy and the monkey took a short time to reach a decision. For progressively lower coherences, the task was more difficult and the monkey took progressively longer to reach a decision.

Performance on the RT task is also consistent with a decision process that accumulates noisy motion evidence over time. In this case, the accumulation terminates and the monkey issues a response when the amount of evidence in favor of one of the alternatives reaches a criterion level. The analysis of this kind of process has roots in sequential analysis (a branch of statistical hypothesis testing) and psychology (Wald, 1947; Stone, 1960; Laming, 1968; Link, 1992; Ratcliff and Rouder, 1998; Gold and Shadlen, 2002; Usher, Olami, and McClelland, 2002). Here we emphasize an analogy to the diffusion of a particle toward absorbing barriers that lie on either side of its starting point (figure 88.4).

Random-dot motion causes the brain to generate signals that depend on the direction and strength of the motion stimulus but are highly variable from moment to moment (Shadlen and Newsome, 1994, 1998). We assume that the accumulation of these signals will tend to drift in one direction or the other, depending on the stimulus, but because of the variability will meander like a particle in Brownian motion. The process stops when the accumulation reaches one of two barriers at ±B (see figure 88.4; here the barriers

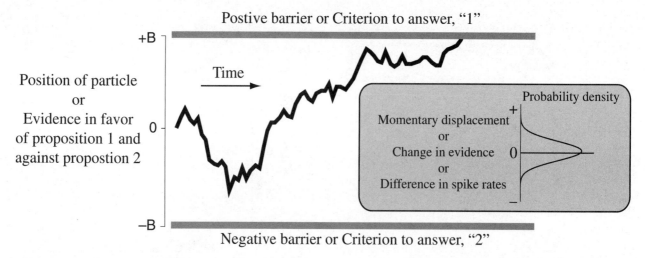

Positive barrier or Criterion to answer, "1"

Position of particle or Evidence in favor of proposition 1 and against propostion 2

Time

Momentary displacement or Change in evidence or Difference in spike rates

Probability density

Negative barrier or Criterion to answer, "2"

FIGURE 88.4   Diffusion-to-barrier as a model for decision making. In one-dimensional Brownian motion of a particle, random displacements are accumulated in a trajectory that stops at ±B. The displacements at each moment are drawn from a normal distribu- tion (insert). Decisions about direction are based on an accumula- tion of evidence, which is the difference in spike rates from ensem- bles of direction-selective neurons in the visual cortex.

are stationary as a function of time, but in principle, that does not need to be the case). If the accumulation reaches +B, the brain renders a decision in favor of one direction; if the accumulation reaches −B, the brain renders the opposite decision. The value of B controls the tradeoff between speed and accuracy: larger values imply more time to reach the barrier and thus more time to accumulate signals, resulting in fewer errors (i.e., crossing the wrong barrier). The vari- ability in the signals being accumulated ensures that one of the barriers will be reached, even when the evidence favors neither alternative on average (i.e., 0% coherence). This variability accounts for both errors and trial-by-trial differences in RT.

The smooth curves in figure 88.3 illustrate how well the diffusion-to-barrier model can account for performance on the RT task. The sigmoid curve fit to the RT data (figure 88.3B) describes the hitting time of a particle in one- dimensional Brownian motion:

$$t(c) = \frac{B}{kc} \tanh(Bkc) + t_{nd} \qquad (1)$$

where c is motion strength (percent coherence) and k, B, and t_{nd} are fitted parameters (for derivations of Equations 1 and 2, see Link, 1992; Ross, 1996). t_{nd} is the nondecision compo- nent of the RT; it includes, for example, the time needed to propagate information from the stimulus to the circuits that form the decision and to execute the eye movement once the decision has been made. The term involving tanh describes the amount of time for an accumulation at one sample per millisecond of a normally distributed random number with mean kc and variance 1 to reach a criterion level, ±B.

The same diffusion-to-barrier model also predicts the monkey's choices. It specifies how often the accumulation will reach +B first. This is quantified as a logistic function for the probability of correct choices:

$$p(c) = \frac{1}{1 + e^{-2k|c|B}} \qquad (2)$$

Equation 2 describes the sigmoid curve in figure 88.3A, but it is not a fit to the data. It is a prediction from the chrono- metric function. The scaling factor, k, and barrier distance, B, were determined by fitting the RTs. This leaves no free parameters to fit the psychometric function, which nonethe- less lies close to the data points. This close match is emblem- atic of the success this kind of model has had in explaining psychophysical data, including percent correct, mean RT, and distributions of RT, on a wide range of perceptual tasks (Link, 1992; Ratcliff and Rouder, 1998).

Both the variable-duration and the RT experiments suggest that there is a gradual evolution of a quantity, termed a decision variable, that determines the monkey's decision. The decision variable grows, on average, in pro- portion to the motion strength and viewing time. It repre- sents the accumulated evidence in favor of one proposition and against another. As described in the next section, such a decision variable has been identified in the brain of the monkey.

Neurophysiology of decision making

Early brain mapping studies using electrical microstimula- tion in awake patients undergoing brain surgery exposed extensive "silent" regions of neocortex that did not seem tied to particular sensations or motor outputs (Penfield and Roberts, 1959). These regions, found in the parietal, tem- poral, and frontal lobes, were eventually assumed to subserve higher associative functions. Electrophysiological measurements in alert monkeys have shown that neurons in these areas have complicated response properties that are not simply locked to sensory or motor events. Instead, the neural activity tends to persist throughout delay periods. Such persistent activity is likely to be a hallmark of the capacity for temporal integration—holding a level of response until perturbed to a new value—that underlies the computation of decision variables. Here we describe neural signals that appear to integrate over time a "weight of evidence" that supports or opposes the alternative direction interpretations on the motion task, thereby linking the interpretation of sensory input to a motor output (in this case, the eye movement response).

In one set of experiments, we recorded from neurons in the lateral intraparietal area (LIP; figure 88.5A) (for reviews, see Colby and Goldberg, 1999; Andersen and Buneo, 2002). Using a saccade-to-target task, we selected neurons with activity that persisted in a delay period between flashing the target in the periphery and instructing the monkey to initiate an eye movement to the target (figure 88.5B). These neurons are not purely sensory because they respond when there is nothing present in the visual scene (after the target has been turned off). They are also not purely motor, because their discharge does not obligate an immediate action. In our experiments, the persistent activity corresponded to particular target locations, termed the neuron's response field (RF). This term is a descriptive hybrid of "receptive field," which implies visual processing of the target, and "motor field," which implies processing the metrics of the impending eye movement.

We used the motion task to test whether this persistent activity represented a decision variable. Instead of a flashed target, the direction of random-dot motion indicated which eye movement to make. Not surprisingly, the LIP neuron predicted whether or not the monkey made an eye movement into the RF; that is, it reflected the outcome of the process that formed the direction decision. What is perhaps more surprising is that the LIP responses also reflected the computations underlying the decision process itself.

This result is best appreciated in the RT version of the motion task (Roitman and Shadlen, 2002). The advantage of this task is that the monkey indicates the end of the decision process on every trial. Thus, we can study LIP activity in the time epoch in which the monkey is forming a decision but has not yet committed to an answer. The results are summarized in figure 88.5C. Following onset of the targets (not shown), activity is robust (~35 spikes/s on average) until approximately 100 ms following onset of the motion stimulus. The activity then undergoes a stereotyped dip and recovery that does not reflect the motion stimulus or the eye movement response. We think this activity might represent a reset of an integration process that appears to begin

approximately 200 ms after motion onset and continues until the decision is formed.

The integration process is evident as ramplike changes in LIP activity. The ramps represent accumulations of motion evidence that support the monkey's decisions. For the decision associated with the target in the neuron's RF, the activity ramps upward (solid curves in figure 88.5C). For the alternative decision, the activity ramps downward (dashed curves). Higher coherence provides more evidence, corresponding to steeper ramps. Lower coherence provides less evidence, corresponding to shallower ramps. Even zero coherence, which provides no net motion information but still must be interpreted by the monkey to reach a decision, is treated as noisy evidence that ramps gradually toward the monkey's choice. Note that the responses in figure 88.5C are averages from many individual trials. For any one trial, LIP activity is probably more like the meandering path of a particle in Brownian motion.

The upward and downward ramps, apparent for individual neurons, suggest that the motion evidence being accumulated is a difference in activity favoring the two directions. For example, an LIP neuron with a rightward RF would accumulate the difference between rightward and leftward direction signals. Rightward motion would tend to cause a positive (upward) accumulation, whereas leftward motion would tend to cause a negative (downward) accumulation. A recent study provided direct experimental support for this difference operation (Ditterich, Mazurek, and Shadlen, 2003). Importantly, such a difference approximates the logarithm of the likelihood ratio—or "weight of evidence"—in favor of one or the other alternative (Gold and Shadlen, 2001). Thus, accumulating this difference to a criterion value approximates a statistical process known as the sequential probability ratio test (Wald, 1947; Stone, 1960; Laming, 1968; Link, 1992).

Consistent with the sequential probability ratio test and the diffusion-to-barrier model (see figure 88.4), the LIP activity appears to reach a criterion value that indicates the end of the decision process. On the right side of figure 88.5C, the same responses are shown aligned to the beginning of the eye movement response. In contrast to the ramps on the left, the rising responses are stereotyped. They seem to reach a common value approximately 100 ms before the eye movement response, regardless of their trajectory to this point. This is more apparent when the data are sorted by RT instead of motion strength (figure 88.5D): the responses reach an apparent decision threshold rapidly for fast decisions but take a more meandering approach to the same threshold when the decision takes longer. In contrast, there is no common end point for the declining responses associated with the opposite decision (figure 88.5C, dashed curves). Presumably, a second set of neurons accumulates evidence in the opposite direction. When their activity reaches the

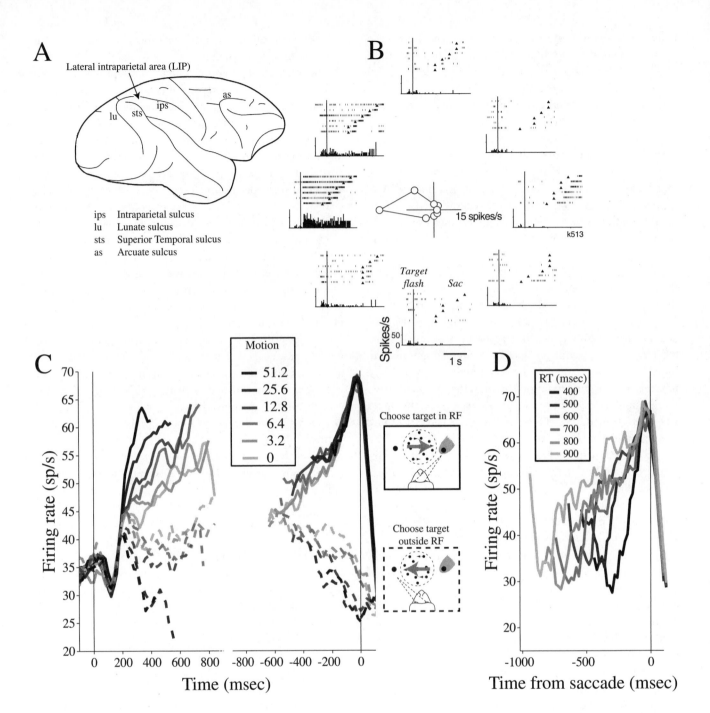

FIGURE 88.5 A neural correlate of a decision process in the parietal cortex. (A) The right hemisphere of the macaque brain. Experiments focus on neurons in the LIP, which lies on the lateral bank of the intraparietal sulcus. It receives input from direction-selective neurons in area MT, along the superior temporal sulcus, and projects to structures involved in eye movement control. (B) Persistent activity from an LIP neuron recorded during memory-guided saccadic eye movements. Targets appeared in one of eight locations arranged around a circle. The responses are aligned to the onset of the target that was flashed on and immediately off. The monkey made an eye movement to the remembered location of the target when the fixation point was extinguished (triangles). Rasters and peristimulus time histograms are arranged to illustrate the position of the target. The response histograms do not include activity after the initiation of the saccadic eye movement. The polar graph at the center of the figure shows the memory period response as a function of target location. This neuron exhibited activity in the delay period before saccadic eye movements to the left. (Adapted with permission from M. N. Shadlen and W. T. Newsome, Neural basis of a perceptual decision in the parietal cortex (area LIP) of the rhesus monkey. *J. Neurophysiol.* 86:1916–1936. © 2001 by the American Physiological Society.) (C) Time course of LIP activity in the RT version of the motion task. Traces are averaged responses from 54 LIP neurons. Responses are grouped by motion strength and choice as indicated by color and line type, respectively. The task is arranged so that one of the choice targets is in the neuron's RF. The other target and the random dots are outside the RF, as indicated by the icons. On the left, responses are aligned to the onset of stimulus motion. Response averages in this portion of the graph show only activity accompanying motion viewing. They stop at the median RT for each motion strength and exclude any activity within 100 ms of eye movement initiation. On the right, responses are aligned to initiation of the eye movement response. Response averages in this portion of the graph show the build-up and decline in activity at the end of the decision process. They exclude any activity within 200 ms of motion onset. The average firing rate was smoothed using a 60-ms running mean. (D) Time course of activity on trials with similar RT. Curves are population average responses for trials that end with an eye movement to the choice target in the RF. The responses are aligned to saccade initiation. Color designates the RT of the trials included in the average that fall within 25 ms of the time indicated (e.g., 400–425 ms). All spikes are included in these averages ($N = 54$ neurons). Average firing rate was smoothed using a 60-ms running mean. (Panels C and D adapted with permission from J. D. Roitman and M. N. Shadlen, Response of neurons in the lateral intraparietal area during a combined visual discrimination reaction time task. *J. Neurosci.* 22:9475–9489. © 2002 by the Society for Neuroscience.) (See color plate 77.)

criterion value, a movement into their RF is triggered and all decision processes are terminated.

LIP is just one of several brain structures with neurons that show this kind of activity on the motion task. Similar activity has been found in other cortical association areas, including the frontal eye field (FEF) and dorsolateral prefrontal cortex, and in subcortical structures, including the superior colliculus (Kim and Shadlen, 1999; Horwitz and Newsome, 2001). The relative contributions these different structures make to the decision process are not known. For example, it is not clear whether they all help to compute the decision variable or some simply reflect computations performed elsewhere. Nevertheless, one common feature of these structures is evident: they are all involved in preparing the eye movement response (Funahashi, Bruce, and Goldman-Rakic, 1991; Schall, 1997; Sparks, 2002).

Thus, a decision that links sensation to action appears to be formed by structures involved in motor preparation. From one perspective, this seems odd. The direction decision clearly depends on the sensory input but seems like it ought to be unrelated to how the answer will be communicated. Indeed, one might predict that the motor systems that control the behavioral response should be engaged only after the decision is reached. These motor systems should not be concerned with the evolving sensory evidence. This prediction turns out to be incorrect.

We examined how much of the decision process is communicated to the oculomotor system while the monkey performs the motion task (figure 88.6A). In effect, we perturbed the oculomotor system to find evidence of the decision variable. As in some of the behavioral experiments, the monkey

was given a variable amount of time to view the motion stimulus. At the exact time that the motion was turned off, a brief train of microstimulation pulses was applied to the FEF. These pulses evoked a short-latency saccadic eye movement. After another approximately 100 ms, the monkey, having recognized the offset of random-dot motion and thus the end of the trial, made a second, voluntary eye movement to one of the choice targets to indicate its direction decision.

The trajectory of the evoked saccade was influenced by an evolving decision variable. The trajectory was similar to those measured on control trials when the monkey simply fixated a central spot (figure 88.6B, *fix*). However, on discrimination trials, the trajectory tended to deviate in the direction of the subsequent voluntary eye movement (figure 88.6B, *up* and *down*). This deviation appeared to reflect an ongoing plan to make this movement while viewing the motion stimulus. Importantly, this deviation was not an all or none phenomenon but instead, like the decision variable, depended on the strength and duration of motion (figure 88.6C). Thus, the accumulated weight of evidence in favor of one direction versus the other is represented in the commands related to the behavioral response.

A window on cognition: Perspectives and future directions

Several principles appear to govern the formation of decisions about motion. Sensory input is converted into a weight of evidence to support or oppose the alternative direction decisions. The weight of evidence is accumulated over time. The accumulation stops when a criterion value is reached.

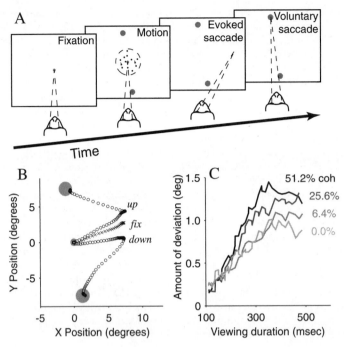

FIGURE 88.6 An evolving decision variable is represented in brain structures that prepare the motor response. Microstimulation of the FEF (located in the anterior bank of the arcuate sulcus; see figure 88.5A) evokes a stereotyped saccadic eye movement. When evoked at a random time during motion viewing, this eye movement reflects the evolving direction decision. (A) The monkey performs the motion task as in figure 88.1A. The axis of the direction discrimination is aligned perpendicular to the direction of stimulation-evoked eye movements. On some trials, a brief train of stimulating current (50 ms of biphasic stimulation, 20–70 µA) evokes an eye movement. After ~100 ms, the monkey makes a second, voluntary eye movement to indicate its direction decision. (B) Examples of eye movement trajectories. Fixation point is at the origin. The two larger circles are the choice targets. The random-

dot stimulus (not shown) was centered on the fixation point. The symbols mark eye position in 2-ms steps. Stimulation during fixation, in the absence of motion and choice targets, elicited a rightward saccade (trace marked *fix*). Stimulation while viewing upward and downward motion induced saccades that deviated in the direction of the subsequent, voluntary eye movements. (C) The average amount of deviation depends on motion strength and viewing time. The amount of deviation toward the chosen target was estimated using the evoked saccades from 32 stimulation sites (14,972 trials). This result shows that the oculomotor system is privy to information about the evolving decision, not just the final outcome of the decision process. (Adapted with permission from J. I. Gold and M. N. Shadlen, Neural computations that underlie decisions about sensory stimuli. *Trends Cogn. Sci.* 5:10–16. © 2001 by Elsevier.)

This process is represented in structures that prepare the behavioral response. Here we discuss the broader implications of these principles for sensorimotor processing and cognition.

SENSORY INFORMATION AS WEIGHT OF EVIDENCE The monkey's direction decisions appear to be based on the difference in activity between pools of motion-sensitive neurons with preferences for the two alternative directions. This difference provides a weight of evidence that quantifies the relative likelihoods of the alternatives given the sensory activity. Thus, the decision is not simply a reflex that associates a pattern of sensory activity with an appropriate behavioral response (an eye movement). Instead, the decision is a process of interpretation that uses the weight of evidence to make sense of noisy, distributed sensory information to reach a categorical judgment.

The usefulness of the weight of evidence is not limited to decisions about motion. In general, it can be used to maxi-

mize the probability of deciding correctly between two alternatives (Good, 1979; Gold and Shadlen, 2001, 2002). The basic principles can even be extended to decisions with many alternatives (Laming, 1968; Usher, Olami, and McClelland, 2002), although it is unknown whether the brain uses this method for such complicated problems.

The weight of evidence is also easy to compute. Motion direction is represented systematically in the middle temporal area (MT or V5) of extrastriate visual cortex (Zeki, 1974; Albright, Desimone, and Gross, 1984). Other sensory parameters, including location, orientation, and disparity, are similarly mapped in sensory cortex. A simple difference in activity within any of these maps represents a weight of evidence that can distinguish between different values of the mapped parameter. In principle, differences computed from other representations can also be used as a weight of evidence (Link, 1992); for example, the difference between sensory activity and memory activity could help to distinguish between sequentially presented stimuli.

Finally, the weight of evidence constitutes a currency that allows signals with dissimilar origins to be compared and combined. By analogy, monetary currency can define the relative values of seemingly unrelated quantities, such as an hour's labor versus a new car. Similarly, the weight of evidence can, in principle, be used to compare the information provided by different sources, sensory or otherwise, to make decisions. For example, the evidence provided by a sensory stimulus can be weighed against other factors, such as bias, reward expectation, and utility (Gold and Shadlen, 2001, 2002; Montague and Berns, 2002; Glimcher, 2003). Indeed, such a confluence of factors is evident in the activity of neurons in association areas of cortex (Leon and Shadlen, 1999; Platt and Glimcher, 1999; Amador, Schlag-Rey, and Schlag, 2000; Hikosaka and Watanabe, 2000; Tremblay and Schultz, 2000).

ACCUMULATION OF EVIDENCE OVER TIME   Time is needed to form the direction decision. At any given moment, the weight of evidence provided by the stochastic motion stimulus is too vague to reach a decision. However, the motion signals are presented continuously over time. Appropriately, the decision appears to be formed by accumulating over time the moment-by-moment weight of evidence. Thus, less time implies less accumulated evidence and lower accuracy. More time implies more evidence and higher accuracy.

Accumulation is undoubtedly just one of many strategies that the brain uses to interpret incoming sensory information. For the motion task, a continuous accumulation is appropriate for a continuously arriving signal. For other tasks, different temporal functions might be more appropriate if, for example, information arrives at separate, predictable intervals. The point is that decisions about stochastic stimuli like the dots are not simply processes that take time. Rather, they are processes that can use strategies like accumulation to interpret information that arrives at different times. This capacity is central to organizing behavior that is not tied to the immediacy of a particular sensory input or motor output (Fuster, 1985).

In general, mechanisms that establish a logical relationship between sensory input and motor output but are not invariably tied to either exemplify the close relationship between sensorimotor and cognitive function in the brain. For example, in the association cortex, activity that persists between sensory and motor events has been implicated in short-term (working) memory (Fuster and Alexander, 1971; Miyashita and Chang, 1988; Goldman-Rakic, Funahashi, and Bruce, 1990; Quintana and Fuster, 1992; Miller, Erickson, and Desimone, 1996; Graziano, Hu, and Gross, 1997; Romo et al., 1999), allocation of attention (Colby and Goldberg, 1999), motor planning (Crammond and Kalaska, 1989; Andersen and Buneo, 2002), motor sequencing (Shima and Tanji, 2000), the representation of motor set or rules (Evarts and Tanji, 1974; di Pellegrino and Wise, 1993; Hoshi, Shima, and Tanji, 2000; Tanji and Hoshi, 2001; Wallis, Anderson, and Miller, 2001), and, as we have discussed, the formation of decisions (Schall, 2001; Glimcher, 2003; Romo and Salinas, 2003). It is intriguing to think that these higher functions have coopted mechanisms that evolved to solve more mundane problems in sensorimotor processing. For example, persistent activity in certain brainstem nuclei holds the gaze in a fixed position. This activity arises through a process resembling integration with respect to time: eye position is the integral of a pulselike motor command signal that controls eye velocity (Robinson, 1989). By analogy, neurons in association areas might integrate over time the "pulses" of evidence that bear on decisions.

Thus, cognition appears to rest, in part, on mechanisms that liberate the brain from time constraints imposed by the environment and the body. However, this freedom poses new problems. How does the brain organize in time computations that are not linked to immediate sensory or motor events? When do the computations begin and end? How can they take into account sensory input from the past? Or affect future behavior? To solve these problems, time itself is likely to be represented explicitly in brain structures with persistent activity. Indeed, recent experiments suggest that elapsed time is represented in the parietal cortex (Leon and Shadlen, 2003). The representation of time will likely emerge as an important future direction in the pursuit of the neural mechanisms of higher brain function.

COMMITMENT TO ONE ALTERNATIVE WHEN A CRITERION LEVEL OF EVIDENCE IS REACHED   To form the direction decision, the weight of evidence appears to be accumulated until a criterion level or "barrier height" is reached. Setting the barrier height controls the tradeoff between speed and accuracy. A low barrier provides fast but uncertain decisions. A high barrier provides slow but certain decisions. This process—accumulating a difference to a barrier—can explain not just decisions about motion, but also a wide variety of laws of sensation and perception. These include Weber's law, which governs the appreciation of increments, and both Fechner's law and Stevens' law, which explain estimates of subjective magnitude of sensory experience (Link, 1992).

The barrier crossing also represents a form of temporal control. For the RT task, it determines the end point of decision processing and the beginning of motor execution. In principle, a barrier crossing could help control how cognitive processing is organized in time, as well. It could determine the end point of decision processing and a commitment to a more abstract proposition than an immediate behavior, such as more computations. In this sense, accumulations to barriers seem intimately related to internal representations of time. This mechanism could help control the brain's ability to process sequences of sensory inputs, plan sequences of behavior, and in general cascade sequences of operations on a flexible time scale.

REPRESENTATION OF THE DECISION VARIABLE IN BRAIN STRUCTURES THAT CONTROL THE MOTOR RESPONSE In monkeys trained to indicate their direction decision with an eye movement to a predictable location in the same direction, formation of the decision and formation of the eye movement response seem to be closely linked in the brain. Neurons in several structures involved in oculomotor preparation, including area LIP, the FEF, the dorsolateral prefrontal cortex, and the superior colliculus, represent both the impending eye movement response and the accumulation of motion evidence used to select that response. Indeed, the decision variable appears to be represented in the very motor commands that ultimately generate the eye movement response.

These results certainly reflect the design of the task. If the monkeys were trained to indicate their decision with an arm movement, not an eye movement, we would expect the decision variable to be represented in neurons that prepare arm movements. It seems to be, in part, a matter of efficiency. When the decision is associated with a particular, predictable, and impending motor response, there is a continuous flow of up-to-date information about the decision, both sensory and psychological, in the circuits that prepare the response (Bichot, Chenchal Rao, and Schall, 2001).

The same principles can be extended to include decisions not linked to specific movements. This is illustrated with a new version of the motion task. This task requires the monkey to indicate its direction decision with an eye movement to a target not at a particular location but of a particular color: red for rightward motion, green for leftward motion. Critically, the locations of the targets are not known until after the decision is formed. FEF microstimulation confirms that, for this task, the decision variable is not represented in commands to generate a specific eye movement (Gold and Shadlen, 2003). Instead, the brain might construe incoming motion information as evidence for implementing a particular behavioral rule. The possible rules are "when two targets appear, look at the red one" or "look at the green one." Thus, the decision can still be formed in an intention-oriented framework (Horwitz, Batista, and Newsome, 2004), but the intention, a behavioral rule, is more abstract than a specific movement.

An obvious question is whether intention-related structures form the decisions or simply reflect computations performed elsewhere. As a practical issue of determining what those computations are, the answer might not matter: studying the computations themselves or their faithful reflections will yield similar insights. To understand the flow of information in the brain, however, the answer certainly does

matter. Is information that arrives in intention-related structures already processed thoroughly, having been sent there by higher-order circuits that do the hard work of cognition? If so, where are those circuits? If not, what are the implications of high-order brain function being processed in an intention-oriented framework?

We do not know the answers to these questions. However, there is reason to speculate that intention-related structures indeed play pivotal roles in forming decisions. In our view, the most compelling reason is that decision making implies a goal. The most obvious goals are behaviors and consequences of behaviors: to get from here to there, to avoid bad things, to get good things. Thus, brain structures involved in achieving these goals—that is, structures that determine what to do and how and when to do it—seem likely to make decisions. With flexible representations of behaviors and behavioral goals, along with a flexible currency like the weight of evidence, it seems unnecessary to posit other structures to do the hard work.

The generalization of this principle shifts the emphasis of brain function from the descriptive analysis of sensory data to the informed control of behavior. Intention-related mechanisms provide goals. These goals establish the utility and meaning of sensory and psychological signals, which are used as evidence to help decide among alternatives and achieve these goals. Thus, intention-related structures provide the framework for both sensorimotor processing and the rudiments of higher cognitive function (Jeannerod, 1994; Rizzolatti, Fogassi, and Gallese, 2002). These ideas on the centrality of intention to perception and higher brain function have a long tradition. For example, Helmholtz suggested that the perception of space, including the interpretation of curvature and straightness, could be understood in terms of the way our motor systems are organized to rotate our eyes along great circles (Helmhotz, 1925). These ideas also emerge under various guises in philosophy, notably in the writings of Merleau-Ponty and other descendants of Heidegger, who recognized that our perception of the properties of things are related in a profound sense to their utility (Heidegger, 1962; Merleau-Ponty, 1962; Clark, 1997; O'Regan and Noë, 2001).

An intention-based framework for information processing might also point the way toward understanding one of the deepest mysteries of neuroscience, consciousness. Our understanding of consciousness seems stymied by the same conundrum posed at the beginning of this article. Consciousness, like cognition, seems unrelated to the operations that neurons perform. There seem to be too few constraints to explain the leap from raw sensory information to the coherence and salience of conscious perception. For example, how can we group the elements of visual scenes into meaningful wholes and background, despite the combinatorial complexity posed by the raw data of light, edges,

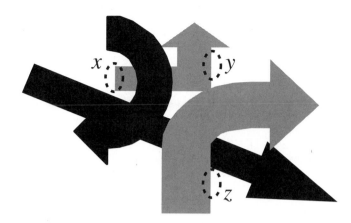

FIGURE 88.7 An example of a binding problem. A famous problem in visual perception concerns the ability to combine the elements of the representation of vision into appropriate groups, that is, to determine which elements are bound to a common object and which are not. To perceive this scene, the brain must combine information from small regions of the visual field (dashed ellipses) corresponding to the receptive fields of neurons in visual cortex. For example, the contours falling in the receptive fields x and y are bound to a common object. The contours falling in y and z are not bound, despite their colinearity and shared color. The brain performs this task with little effort, despite the large number of ways that information about surface order, border ownership, and other properties of the objects could be combined in principle. An intention-based architecture would tame this combinatorial explosion by restating the problem in terms of potential actions that could be performed, interrogating the visual cortex for evidence supporting hypotheses of the form: if the topmost arrowhead is moved, which other contours are likely to be displaced? The answer is presumably based on the way the contours trace paths that support or oppose a hypothesis of continuity. The underlying mechanisms seem likely to resemble those that form the motion decision, because in both cases, sensory evidence is assembled across space and time to support a particular action. (Adapted with permission from M. N. Shadlen and J. A. Movshon, Synchrony unbound: A critical evaluation of the temporal binding hypothesis. *Neuron* 24:67–77. © 1999 by Elsevier.)

and color (figure 88.7)? To solve this kind of problem, many theories of consciousness posit a central interpreter, or homunculus. The intention-based framework provides an alternative view. According to this view, our conscious experience is indeed constrained. Conscious perception derives from, in effect, questions related to behavior (Is that something I can grab? Can I walk there?). Sensory and memory signals are interrogated for evidence that can be used to provide answers. Thus, our conscious experiences, and the underlying neural computations, are constrained to what is being asked and what is answered. Because the questions are determined from the repertoire of possible behaviors, the underlying mechanisms of consciousness are intimately tied to the fact that the brain controls a body.

This intention-based architecture seems to take some of the hard work of consciousness away from the homunculus. However, another, equally mysterious mechanism seems to

be required. If sensory information flows to circuits where it can exert leverage on intentions, plans, and rules, what controls the flow? Which intentions, plans, and rules are under consideration at any moment? The need for a homunculus has apparently been replaced by the need for a traffic cop.

We speculate that, unlike for the homunculus, we already have insights into the brain mechanisms that serve as traffic cop. These are the same mechanisms that allow an animal to explore its environment, that is, to forage. Foraging is about connecting data in the environment to a prediction of reward through complex behavior (Gallistel, 2000). However, in principle, the mechanisms of foraging, like the mechanisms of decision making, do not need to be tied to overt behaviors. The same principles that apply to visits to flowers could direct the parietal lobe to query the visual cortex for evidence needed to answer a question about motion. More generally, foraging might be related to the leaps our brains make to replace one percept with another (e.g., binocular rivalry), to escape one behavioral context for another, or to explore new ideas. For cognitive neuroscientists, these ideas inspire research on how reward expectation influences sensorimotor and higher processing in association areas of the brain. For the philosopher of mind, these ideas provide an inkling of how properties of the brain give rise to agency and, perhaps, free will.

Conclusions

When designing an experiment to study decision making and other cognitive functions, among the critical questions we ask is, where should we put our electrodes? That is, where in the brain will we find neurons that contribute to these higher functions? We and others are finding success by recording from neurons at the nexus of sensorimotor processing. By studying how sensory information is converted into a categorical decision that guides behavior, we gain insight into flexible and efficient mechanisms that could subserve cognitive functions as well. These mechanisms provide a common currency for integrating information from a variety of sources, sensory or otherwise; they disengage information processing from the immediacy of sensory and motor events; and they establish rules for committing to a proposition. The mechanisms we study also hint at a broad principle of brain organization: behavior and behavioral goals are the hubs around which other information is organized. These hubs define, for example, how utility and meaning should be ascribed to sensory signals. This organization lights the path to future research in cognition and perhaps even consciousness.

ACKNOWLEDGMENTS We thank Jochen Ditterich, William Newsome, and Alex Huk for helpful comments on the manuscript. This work was supported by the Howard Hughes Medical

Institute, the National Eye Institute (EY11378), the National Center for Research Resources (RR00166), the McKnight Foundation, and the Burroughs-Wellcome Fund.

REFERENCES

ACUNA, B. D., J. C. ELIASSEN, J. P. DONOGHUE, and J. N. SANES, 2002. Frontal and parietal lobe activation during transitive inference in humans. *Cereb. Cortex* 12:1312–1321.

ALBRIGHT, T. D., R. DESIMONE, and C. G. GROSS, 1984. Columnar organization of directionally selective cells in visual area MT of macaques. *J. Neurophysiol.* 51:16–31.

AMADOR, N., M. SCHLAG-REY, and J. SCHLAG, 2000. Reward-predicting and reward-detecting neuronal activity in the primate supplementary eye field. *J. Neurophysiol.* 84:2166–2170.

ANDERSEN, R. A., and C. A. BUNEO, 2002. Intentional maps in posterior parietal cortex. *Annu. Rev. Neurosci.* 25:189–220.

ASTAFIEV, S. V., G. L. SHULMAN, C. M. STANLEY, A. Z. SNYDER, D. C. VAN ESSEN, and M. CORBETTA, 2003. Functional organization of human intraparietal and frontal cortex for attending, looking, and pointing. *J. Neurosci.* 23:4689–4699.

BICHOT, N. P., S. CHENCHAL RAO, and J. D. SCHALL, 2001. Continuous processing in macaque frontal cortex during visual search. *Neuropsychologia* 39:972–982.

CARPENTER, R. H., and M. L. WILLIAMS, 1995. Neural computation of log likelihood in control of saccadic eye movements. *Nature* 377:59–62.

CLARK, A., 1997. *Being There: Putting Brain, Body, and World Together Again*. Cambridge, Mass.: MIT Press.

COLBY, C. L., and M. E. GOLDBERG, 1999. Space and attention in parietal cortex. *Annu. Rev. Neurosci.* 22:319–349.

CORBETTA, M., E. AKBUDAK, T. E. CONTURO, A. Z. SNYDER, J. M. OLLINGER, H. A. DRURY, M. R. LINENWEBER, S. E. PETERSEN, M. E. RAICHLE, D. C. VAN ESSEN, and G. L. SHULMAN, 1998. A common network of functional areas for attention and eye movements. *Neuron* 21:761–773.

CRAMMOND, D. J., and J. F. KALASKA, 1989. Neuronal activity in primate parietal cortex area 5 varies with intended movement direction during an instructed-delay period. *Exp. Brain Res.* 76:458–462.

DI PELLEGRINO, G., and S. P. WISE, 1993. Visuospatial versus visuomotor activity in the premotor and prefrontal cortex of a primate. *J. Neurosci.* 13:1227–1243.

DITTERICH, J., M. MAZUREK, and M. N. SHADLEN, 2003. Microstimulation of visual cortex affects the speed of perceptual decisions. *Nat. Neurosci.* 6:891–898.

EVARTS, E. V., and J. TANJI, 1974. Gating of motor cortex reflexes by prior instruction. *Brain Res.* 71:479–494.

FEINBERG, T. E., and M. J. FARAH, eds., 1997. *Behavioral Neurology and Neuropsychology*. New York: McGraw-Hill.

FUNAHASHI, S., C. J. BRUCE, and P. S. GOLDMAN-RAKIC, 1991. Neuronal activity related to saccadic eye movements in the monkey's dorsolateral prefrontal cortex. *J. Neurophysiol.* 65:1464–1483.

FUSTER, J., 1985. The prefrontal cortex and temporal integration. In *Cerebral Cortexm*, A. Peters and E. Jones, eds. New York: Plenum Press, pp. 151–177.

FUSTER, J. M., and G. E. ALEXANDER, 1971. Neuron activity related to short-term memory. *Science* 173:652–654.

GALLISTEL, C. R., 2000. Time, rate, and conditioning. *Psychol. Rev.* 107:289–344.

GLIMCHER, P., 2003. The neurobiology of visual-saccadic decision making. *Annu. Rev. Neurosci.* 26:133–179.

GOLD, J. I., and M. N. SHADLEN, 2000. Representation of a perceptual decision in developing oculomotor commands. *Nature* 404:390–394.

GOLD, J. I., and M. N. SHADLEN, 2001. Neural computations that underlie decisions about sensory stimuli. *Trends Cogn. Sci.* 5: 10–16.

GOLD, J. I., and M. N. SHADLEN, 2002. Banburismus and the brain: Decoding the relationship between sensory stimuli, decisions, and reward. *Neuron* 36:299–308.

GOLD, J. I., and M. N. SHADLEN, 2003. The influence of behavioral context on the representation of a perceptual decision in developing oculomotor commands. *J. Neurosci.* 23:632–651.

GOLDMAN-RAKIC, P. S., S. FUNAHASHI, and C. J. BRUCE, 1990. Neocortical memory circuits. *Cold Spring Harb. Symp. Quant. Biol.* 55:1025–1038.

GOOD, I. J., 1979. Studies in the history of probability and statistics. XXXVII. A.M. Turing's statistical work in World War II. *Biometrika* 66:393–396.

GRAZIANO, M. S. A., X. T. HU, and C. G. GROSS, 1997. Visuospatial properties of ventral premotor cortex. *J. Neurophysiol.* 77:2268–2292.

HEIDEGGER, M., 1962. *Being and Time*. New York: Harper and Row.

HELMHOTZ, H. V., 1925. The monocular field of vision. In *Helmholtz's Treatise on Physiological Optics*, J. P. C. Southall, ed. Menasha, Wis.: Optical Society of America and George Banta Publishing.

HIKOSAKA, K., and M. WATANABE, 2000. Delay activity of orbital and lateral prefrontal neurons of the monkey varying with different rewards. *Cereb. Cortex* 10:263–271.

HORWITZ, G. D., and W. T. NEWSOME, 2001. Target selection for saccadic eye movements: Prelude activity in the superior colliculus during a direction-discrimination task. *J. Neurophysiol.* 86:2543–2558.

HORWITZ, G. D., A. P. BATISTA, and W. T. NEWSOME, 2004. Representation of an abstract perceptual decision in macaque superior colliculus. *J. Neurophysiol.* 91:2281—2296.

HOSHI, E., K. SHIMA, and J. TANJI, 2000. Neuronal activity in the primate prefrontal cortex in the process of motor selection based on two behavioral rules. *J. Neurophysiol.* 83:2355–2373.

JEANNEROD, M., 1994. The representing brain: Neural correlates of motor intention and imagery. *Behav. Brain Sci.* 17:187–245.

KIM, J.-N., and M. N. SHADLEN, 1999. Neural correlates of a decision in the dorsolateral prefrontal cortex of the macaque. *Nat. Neurosci.* 2:176–185.

LAMING, D. R. J., 1968. *Information Theory of Choice-Reaction Times*. London: Academic Press.

LEON, M. I., and M. N. SHADLEN, 1999. Effect of expected reward magnitude on the response of neurons in the dorsolateral prefrontal cortex of the macaque. *Neuron* 24:415–425.

LEON, M. I., and M. N. SHADLEN, 2003. Representation of time by neurons in the posterior parietal cortex of the macaque. *Neuron* 38:317–327.

LINK, S. W., 1992. *The Wave Theory of Difference and Similarity*. Hillsdale, N.J.: Erlbaum.

LUCE, R. D., 1986. *Response Times: Their Role in Inferring Elementary Mental Organization*. New York: Oxford University Press.

MERLEAU-PONTY, M., 1962. *Phenomenology of Perception*. London: Routledge and Kegan Paul.

MESULAM, M.-M., 1985. *Principles of Behavioral Neurology*. Philadelphia: F.A. Davis.

MILLER, E. K., C. A. ERICKSON, and R. DESIMONE, 1996. Neural mechanisms of visual working memory in prefrontal cortex of the macaque. *J. Neurosci.* 16:5154–5167.

MIYASHITA, Y., and H. S. CHANG, 1988. Neuronal correlate of pictorial short-term memory in the primate temporal cortex. *Nature* 331:68–70.

MONTAGUE, P. R., and G. S. BERNS, 2002. Neural economics and the biological substrates of valuation. *Neuron* 36:265–284.

MURRAY, E. A., T. J. BUSSEY, and S. P. WISE, 2000. Role of prefrontal cortex in a network for arbitrary visuomotor mapping. *Exp. Brain Res.* 133:114–129.

O'REGAN, J. K., and A. NOË, 2001. A sensorimotor account of vision and visual consciousness. *Behav. Brain Sci.* 24:939–973.

PARKER, A. J., and W. T. NEWSOME, 1998. Sense and the single neuron: probing the physiology of perception. *Annu. Rev. Neurosci.* 21:227–277.

PENFIELD, W., and L. ROBERTS, 1959. *Speech and Brain-Mechanisms.* Princeton, N. J.: Princeton University Press.

PLATT, M. L., and P. W. GLIMCHER, 1999. Neural correlates of decision variables in parietal cortex. *Nature* 400:233–238.

QUINTANA, J., and J. FUSTER, 1992. Mnemonic and predictive functions of cortical neurons in a memory task. *Neuroreport* 3:721–724.

RATCLIFF, R., and J. N. ROUDER, 1998. Modeling response times for two-choice decisions. *Psychol. Sci.* 9:347–356.

REDDI, B. A., and R. H. CARPENTER, 2000. The influence of urgency on decision time. *Nat. Neurosci.* 3:827–830.

RIZZOLATTI, G., L. FOGASSI, and V. GALLESE, 2002. Motor and cognitive functions of the ventral premotor cortex. *Curr. Opin. Neurobiol.* 12:149–154.

ROBINSON, D. A., 1989. Integrating with neurons. *Annu. Rev. Neurosci.* 12:33–45.

ROITMAN, J. D., and M. N. SHADLEN, 2002. Response of neurons in the lateral intraparietal area during a combined visual discrimination reaction time task. *J. Neurosci.* 22:9475–9489.

ROMO, R., C. BRODY, A. HERNANDEZ, and L. LEMUS, 1999. Neuronal correlates of parametric working memory in the prefrontal cortex. *Nature* 399:470–473.

ROMO, R., and E. SALINAS, 2003. Flutter discrimination: Neural codes, perception, memory and decision making. *Nat. Rev. Neurosci.* 4:203–218.

ROSS, S., 1996. *Stochastic Processes*, 2nd ed. New York: Wiley.

SCHALL, J. D., 1997. Visuomotor areas of the frontal lobe. In *Cerebral Cortex*, K. Rockland, A. Peters, J. Kass, eds. New York: Plenum Press, pp. 527–638.

SCHALL, J. D., 2001. Neural basis of deciding, choosing and acting. *Nat. Rev. Neurosci.* 2:33–42.

SHADLEN, M. N., and W. T. NEWSOME, 1994. Noise, neural codes and cortical organization. *Curr. Opin. Neurobiol.* 4:569–579.

SHADLEN, M. N., and W. T. NEWSOME, 1998. The variable discharge of cortical neurons: Implications for connectivity, computation and information coding. *J. Neurosci.* 18:3870–3896.

SHADLEN, M. N., and W. T. NEWSOME, 2001. Neural basis of a perceptual decision in the parietal cortex (area LIP) of the rhesus monkey. *J. Neurophysiol.* 86:1916–1936.

SHADLEN, M. N., and J. A. MOVSHON, 1999. Synchrony unbound: A critical evaluation of the temporal binding hypothesis. *Neuron* 24:67–77.

SHIMA, K., and J. TANJI, 2000. Neuronal activity in the supplementary and presupplementary motor areas for temporal organization of multiple movements. *J. Neurophysiol.* 84:2148–2160.

SIMON, S. R., M. MEUNIER, L. PIETTRE, A. M. BERARDI, C. M. SEGEBARTH, and D. BOUSSAOUD, 2002. Spatial attention and memory versus motor preparation: Premotor cortex involvement as revealed by fMRI. *J. Neurophysiol.* 88:2047–2057.

SPARKS, D. L., 2002. The brainstem control of saccadic eye movements. *Nat. Rev. Neurosci.* 3:952–964.

STONE, M., 1960. Models for choice-reaction time. *Psychometrika* 25:251–260.

TANJI, J., and E. HOSHI, 2001. Behavioral planning in the prefrontal cortex. *Curr. Opin. Neurobiol.* 11:164–170.

TREMBLAY, L., and W. SCHULTZ, 2000. Reward-related neuronal activity during Go-nogo task performance in primate orbitofrontal cortex. *J. Neurophysiol.* 83:1864–1876.

USHER, M., Z. OLAMI, and J. L. MCCLELLAND, 2002. Hick's law in a stochastic race model with speed-accuracy tradeoff. *J. Math. Psychol.* 46:704–715.

WALD, A., 1947. *Sequential Analysis.* New York: Wiley.

WALLIS, J. D., K. C. ANDERSON, and E. K. MILLER, 2001. Single neurons in prefrontal cortex encode abstract rules. *Nature* 411:953–956.

WISE, S. P., and E. A. MURRAY, 2000. Arbitrary associations between antecedents and actions. *Trends Neurosci.* 23:271–276.

ZEKI, S. M., 1974. Functional organization of a visual area in the posterior bank of the superior temporal sulcus of the rhesus monkey. *J. Physiol.* 236:549–573.

89 Cortical Plasticity in the Adult Human Brain

MEGAN S. STEVEN AND COLIN BLAKEMORE

ABSTRACT The idea that the cerebral cortex of the adult brain is capable of massive reorganization, once virtually unthinkable, is now firmly established. The past 20 years have produced myriad demonstrations of such plasticity, first in animals and then in humans. We now understand much about which specific areas of the cortex are capable of plasticity, what sensory or motor activity is necessary to evoke cortical remapping, and whether or not the changes are functionally valuable. In this chapter, we review recent findings on plasticity in the motor, somatosensory, visual, auditory, and olfactory cortices of the adult human brain. We consider possible mechanisms for these changes, address the implications of these findings for the amelioration of stroke, developmental disabilities, and other disorders, and make suggestions for the direction of future research.

Until recently, most neuroscientists believed that the adult brain was rigidly organized and incapable of great change. The demonstration of specific early sensitive periods for language development and visual cortical organization led to the prevailing view that certain areas of the cortex pass through periods of activity-dependent plasticity in the infant or young child, but that once experience has played its part in guiding maturation, cortical circuits become fixed. Indeed, it seemed to make sense that such stability should be achieved, in order for each cortical area to provide reliable signals to other regions of the brain.

However, research in animals, mainly starting some 20 years ago, produced evidence of remarkable plasticity in adult mammals. Some examples were not so surprising, because they involved areas of association cortex thought to be involved in long-term memory. Miyashita and colleagues, for example, showed that individual neurons of the monkey's anterior inferotemporal cortex can change their stimulus preferences while the animal is engaged in a visual discrimination task (Miyashita, 1999). More unexpected was evidence that the spatial representations of sensory input or motor output in primary sensory and motor areas can undergo dramatic and rapid reorganization simply as a result of modified sensory input or motor activity (see Buonomano and Merzenich, 1998).

These observations in animals, as well as the emergence of the new functional imaging techniques, stimulated the search for similar phenomena in humans. Research over the past 10 years has revealed that parts of the adult human cortex can indeed be remapped as a result of experience, as if to meet ever-changing sensory and motor demands. A couple of striking examples can be mentioned here. There is evidence that somatosensory and motor areas of the cortex of an active musician become reorganized to allocate more space to those fingers that are used most to play their musical instrument, and that the otherwise indolent visual cortex of a blind person can apparently be used to help process information about touch, audition, and even language. Indeed, in many other domains, experience-driven cortical plasticity seems to occur throughout life.

An 80-year-old person can learn to play the piano. Some stroke victims recover function remarkably well. Do these forms of learning depend on changes in cortical mapping? Which areas of the cortex can undergo such plasticity? What are the exact circumstances and patterns of stimulation that encourage such plasticity? Are some individual brains more plastic than others? Might it be possible to enhance the plastic process, perhaps to facilitate learning or to promote recovery from stroke? And are there other diseases and disorders that might benefit from artificial encouragement of cortical plasticity?

Plasticity in the motor cortex

Each part of the body has a specific division of motor cortex devoted to it, and the relative volume of cortex concerned with each set of muscles depends on the density of innervation and the fineness of control of the muscles. The nonlinear map of the body across the motor cortex is called the motor homunculus. Interestingly, even short amounts of practice affect body representation in the homunculus. Motor skill acquisition, by repeated practice, has distinct and measurable effects on the map. Extensive training of specific limb movements leads to reorganization of the motor cortex, giving preference to the exercised limbs (Pascual-Leone et al., 1995; see also Karni et al., 1995). Classen and colleagues (1998) used transcranial magnetic stimulation (TMS) of the

MEGAN S. STEVEN and COLIN BLAKEMORE University Laboratory of Physiology, University of Oxford, Oxford, U.K.

motor cortex to evoke a consistent movement of the thumb in one direction. Then subjects practiced a thumb movement in the opposite direction. After 15–30 minutes of this practice (and in two cases after only 5–10 minutes), TMS of the same area of motor cortex that evoked the original thumb movement now produced a thumb movement in the newly learned direction. Motor cortex reorganization can thus be triggered even by short amounts of practice.

Even artificially stimulating a muscle can induce an expansion of its cortical representation. Hamdy and colleagues (1998) stimulated the pharyngeal muscles and found that the area of motor cortex representing the pharynx increased while the representation of the adjacent esophagus decreased. This reorganization lasted for at least 30 minutes after the cessation of the stimulation. Conversely, denervation of muscles can cause shrinkage of their representation in the motor cortex. A positron emission tomography (PET) study of people with facial palsy showed that the hand area of the motor cortex, which is situated adjacent to the face area, expands by taking over part of the cortical area that formerly represented the face (Rijntjes et al., 1997). Giraux and colleagues (2001) asked whether such shrinkage of motor representation caused by disuse can be reversed. They found that transplantation to replace an amputated hand causes the hand representation to be restored and to expand to reoccupy cortical territory previously taken over by other body regions as a result of the loss of the hand.

Muellbacher and colleagues (2002) showed that activity in the primary motor cortex is necessary for early consolidation of motor skills. Low-frequency repetitive TMS (rTMS), which is thought to disrupt neural processing, inhibits retention of a newly acquired motor skill, indicating a functional role for the motor cortex in the neural plasticity that underlies this form of learning.

Changes in cortical organization as a result of motor activity can involve more than just rescaling of the homunculus in the motor cortex. When movement is combined with visual attention (a combination that frequently occurs in sports), cortical activation is more extensive than the sum of activations during either movement alone or visual attention alone. The combination of attention and movement leads to supernumerary regions of cortical activation, including the left superior parietal lobule, right fusiform gyrus, and left insula (Indovina and Sanes, 2001). Athletes, by practicing skilled motor movements and by combining motor movements with visual attention, might then display increased cortical plasticity.

Plasticity in the somatosensory cortex

Reorganization can also occur in the somatosensory cortex (S1; the postcentral gyrus) as a result of somatic stimulation, especially during learning tasks. The somatosensory cortex has its own homunculus: input from the body is laid out in a sequence that parallels the arrangement in the adjacent motor cortex. Each part of the somatosensory cortex processes information about a particular part of the body, and the representation of the fingers is particularly large and distinct. When a person's fingers are deprived of stimulation, there appears to be a decrease in the area of sensory cortex devoted to those unused fingers. Rossini and colleagues (1994) reported that following ischemic anesthesia of the second and fourth fingers of each hand, the somatosensory representations of those fingers shrank and the area of cortex previously representing them was taken over by the adjacent first, third, and fifth fingers.

Conversely, in well-practiced musicians, the area of cortex devoted to the particular fingers that they use to play their instrument is enlarged (Pantev et al., 2001). Magnetic source imaging shows that, in right-handed string players, the representation of the fingers of the left hand, which are used for fingering, is increased compared with that of the other (bowing) hand or the hands of non-string-playing control subjects (Elbert et al., 1995). Similarly, the cortical representation of the reading fingers in blind Braille readers is increased compared with that of nonreading fingers and the fingers of sighted and blind non-Braille readers (Pascual-Leone and Torres, 1993).

Is the expansion of finger representation causative of the improved performance, or is it an epiphenomenon, merely correlated with increased tactile skill? This is a central issue in the field: Does adult cortical plasticity actually support changes in behavior? A recent study by Goldreich and Kanics (2003) confirms long-standing anecdotal evidence that tactile acuity is significantly greater in blind than in sighted subjects, which might be taken to imply that the expansion of cortical plasticity in S1 of blind Braille readers supports their superior functional capacity. In this study, tactile acuity was tested in the index finger (used for Braille reading) but, interestingly, Goldreich and Kanics found that tactile acuity of the reading finger in blind Braille readers was not significantly greater than the tactile acuity of the same finger in blind non-Braille readers. Thus, changes in S1 are likely related to the increased dependence on touch for all blind persons. Intriguing results from work by Cohen and colleagues (1997) suggest that the increased representation in S1 contributes to, but is unlikely to be the sole cause of, the enhanced performance. They showed that low-frequency rTMS of S1 in blind subjects caused a decline in tactile discrimination ability; however, blind Braille readers undergoing this procedure could still perform tactile discrimination tasks better than sighted controls receiving TMS to S1. It therefore seems likely that the changes in S1 are not essential for improved discrimination performance. Perhaps functional changes elsewhere in the brain (possibly the visual cortex) also contribute to the increased ability in blind Braille readers.

Plasticity in S1 is not always related to functional improvement, and in some cases it might even be maladaptive. Lim, Altenmüller, and Bradshaw (2001) reported that overpractice of motor skill can lead to focal hand dystonia, an impairment of fine control of organized movements seen particularly in the fingers of musicians (1% of active musicians develop this disorder). Elbert and colleagues (1998) used neuroimaging to show that the expanded representations of digits overlap each other in S1 of people with focal hand dystonia and that the distance between the cortical regions subserving the little finger and the index finger is decreased, compared with that in healthy musicians. Perhaps the expansion of a digit's representation to involve neurons that originally analyzed input from other digits, and the confusion caused by overlap of representation of neighboring digits, interferes with the encoding of tactile information. Writer's cramp produces similar maladaptive reorganization (Sanger et al., 2002; see also Münte, Altenmüller, and Jäncke, 2002, and Elbert and Heim, 2001, for discussions of maladaptive plasticity).

In the somatosensory homunculus, the area of representation of the forearm is adjacent to the representation of the face, on one side, and to that of the upper arm, on the other. Ramachandran, Rogers-Ramachandran, and Stewart (1992) report that, following forelimb amputation, tactile stimulation of the face or the upper arm produced two sensations, one veridically located and the other on the missing forearm. This finding implies that cortical areas corresponding to the amputated limb become "invaded" by input from the adjacent regions of the homunculus. Tactile stimulation of the face or remaining upper arm activates the hand region and hence elicits the illusory sensation on the hand. Indeed, Yang and colleagues (1994), using magneto-encephalography (MEG), showed that amputation does indeed lead to such a reorganization of the somatosensory map. Interestingly, Borsook and colleagues (1998) discovered that the illusory perceptual experiences can occur very quickly, less than 24 hours after amputation. In the context of the debate over whether changes in cortical maps actually have behavioral consequences, it would be interesting to know whether cortical mapping can be detected with neuroimaging methods so soon after amputation.

It seems, then, that the proportions of representation within the somatosensory homunculus are being continuously updated, based on both sensory experience and the acquisition of skills, throughout our lives (Ramachandran and Rogers-Ramachandran, 2000).

Plasticity in the visual cortex

In animals, there is evidence that local remapping occurs in the primary visual cortex (V1) in response to discrete retinal lesions, similar to the modification of the somatosensory homunculus after amputation (e.g., Gilbert and Wiesel, 1992). Although some comparable studies exist in humans (see Dreher, Burke, and Calford, 2001, for a review), most of our knowledge of plasticity in visual areas of the adult human cortex comes from studies of people deprived of sight either from birth (congenital or early blindness) or after an initial period of relatively normal vision, usually for some years (late blindness). It appears that the visual cortex does not remain completely inactive in blind people. At least some parts of the array of visual areas in the posterior half of the cerebral hemispheres become responsive to tactile and, perhaps to a lesser extent, auditory stimulation. Does this mean that cortical regions constructed to deal with vision can become functionally reorganized, not only to respond to but also to play a part in processing signals from other senses, represented far away in the hemisphere?

Sadato and colleagues (1996) used PET to measure the blood flow in the visual cortex during a tactile discrimination task in both blind and sighted subjects. They found that in the blind subjects, blood flow increased in primary and secondary visual cortices that normally respond only to visual stimulation, whereas blood flow decreased in these areas in sighted subjects during the task. Other studies have confirmed that visual cortex is activated during tactile discrimination in the blind (Büchel et al., 1998; Sadato et al., 1998; Burton, Snyder, Conturo, et al., 2002).

Further studies using functional magnetic resonance imaging (fMRI) have generally confirmed that visual cortical areas are recruited during Braille reading and non-Braille tactile stimulation in blind subjects, although there has been some debate about the extent to which visual cortical areas are activated in early-blind persons and those who became blind later in life. Some studies have reported no significant activation in the primary visual cortex in late-blind subjects during Braille reading (Cohen et al., 1999), while others have found that Braille reading activates primary visual cortex in both early- and late-blind individuals (Sadato et al., 1996; Burton, Snyder, Conturo, et al., 2002). Büchel and colleagues (1998) confirmed that tactile stimulation causes extensive extrastriate activation in the blind, but reported that it extends to V1 only in late-blind subjects. They suggested that this activation might be due to visual imagination of the touched surface. By contrast, Sadato and colleagues (1998) reported that the earlier the onset of blindness, the more strongly V1 is activated by touch, and they suggested that the underlying neural plasticity of V1 might decline with age.

A study on the effects of extended blindfolding of sighted volunteers suggests that such deprivation of vision in sighted adults improves tactile discrimination (Kauffman, Théoret, and Pascual-Leone, 2002). The study included four groups of participants. Two groups were continuously blindfolded for 5 days, during which one group received intensive Braille training and the other group did not. There were also matched controls groups that were not blindfolded. Regardless of whether or not the blindfolded subjects were trained, they could discriminate Braille letters better than nonblindfolded subjects after only 5 days of visual deprivation. This finding implies that, once deprived of normal input, the adult visual system can become engaged in tactile analysis in a very short period of time. Pascual-Leone and Hamilton (2001) reported that fMRI of these subjects revealed activation in the visual cortex during tactile stimulation of the right or left fingertips using a loofah brush (to reduce the likelihood of visual imagery) during the last day of the study (day 5). Interestingly, just 20 hours after the blindfold was removed (on day 6) the activation in visual cortex disappeared. Furthermore, TMS of the occipital cortex disrupted tactile discrimination abilities during the last day of blindfolding, but not after the blindfold was removed on day 6 (A. Pascual-Leone, personal correspondence), suggesting a functional role of the visual cortex activation in tactile discrimination during blindfolding. Similarly, auditory stimulation was shown to activate the visual cortex in blindfolded subjects: left-lateralized activations of the mesial occipital lobe and the posterior extension of the superior temporal lobe were found in the blindfolded population during tone and phoneme matching tasks (Schlaug et al., 1999, 2000).

Kujala and colleagues (1995) reported, with data from MEG, that early-blind subjects also activated the visual cortex during sound frequency discrimination, but unfortunately, the researchers were unable to accurately specify the areas of visual cortex involved. Activation of primary and association areas of the visual cortex in the blind was detected with PET during auditory tasks involving sound localization (Weeks et al., 2000) and during a pattern recognition task using a sensory substitution device that translates the visual world into auditory stimuli and is being developed as a tool for the blind (Arno et al., 2001). Primary and association areas of the visual cortex were also detected with event-related potentials (ERPs) while blind subjects listened to meaningful and meaningless sentences (Roder, Roslwe, and Neville, 2000) and during a sound localization task (Leclerc et al., 2000). Indeed, this activation may be functional, since Lessard and colleagues (1998) demonstrated that the early blind are better at localizing sources of sound than sighted individuals. It would be interesting to know if this superior ability is influenced by TMS of the occipital cortex.

Neville and Lawson (1987) measured ERPs with a dense array of scalp electrodes (to enable source localization) and compared the effects of attention to peripheral and central visual stimuli in normal hearing and congenitally deaf subjects. Whereas each group performs similarly when attending to stimuli in the foveal area, deaf subjects displayed attention effects over the occipital lobe that were several times larger than the hearing controls. Moreover, they displayed attentional modulation of ERPs over the occipital regions several times larger than that of hearing subjects during attention to peripheral stimuli. This attentional difference might reflect the need of the deaf to rely more on the visual system to orient to peripheral stimuli when no auditory cues are available.

Although studies such as those of Weeks and colleagues (2000) and Arno and colleagues (2001) indicate that striate and extrastriate visual areas can be activated by auditory stimulation in the blind, the general impression from the literature is that the takeover of visual cortex in the blind is more extensive and intensive for tactile stimulation (see Sadato et al., 1996; Kauffman, Théoret, and Pascual-Leone, 2002). If this is true, it might reflect the more similar computational tasks of visual and somatosensory systems: both are involved in analyzing form, three-dimensional shape, and movement of objects.

This raises the question of whether the remarkably rapid "invasion" of visual areas by the other senses (as with the more local, activity-dependent plastic remapping within sensory and motor areas described earlier) is functionally valuable. There is indeed some evidence that the neural machinery of the visual cortex can be recruited to assist the analysis of other sensory modalities.

TMS of the occipital (early) visual cortex of the blind has been reported to disrupt Braille reading ability (Cohen et al., 1997) in the blind, and rTMS of the occipital visual cortex at a rate that is known to cause excitation, increased Braille reading speed in early-blind subjects (Hamilton and Pascual-Leone, 1998). In fact, the amount of increased tactile perception accuracy found in Braille readers correlated with the amount of striate activation in the occipital cortex during tactile stimulation (Kiriakopoulos et al., 1999). This result suggests that early visual areas might indeed serve a functional role in the tactile task of Braille reading in the blind.

There is even evidence that V1 plays some part in processing tactile stimuli in normal sighted people without visual deprivation. Zangaladze and colleagues (1999) found that when the occipital visual cortex is disrupted with low-frequency TMS, sighted subjects have difficulty discriminating the orientation of ridged patterns felt with the fingers. Again, it could be that interference with visual imagery of the touched surface is responsible for this effect (Sathian and Zangaladze, 2001). While this result is interesting with respect to the possible collaboration of different sensory areas in the analysis of stimuli, it raises concerns about the reliability or sensitivity of neuroimaging techniques, since Zangaladze and colleagues (1999), like Sadato and colleagues (1996), showed that V1 is not significantly activated during tactile stimulation in sighted subjects.

	Sighted	Late-onset Blind	Congenitally Blind			Sighted	Late-onset Blind	Congenitally Blind

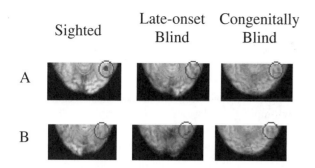

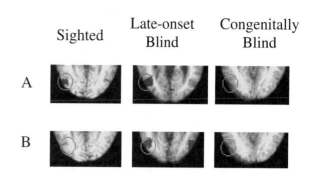

FIGURE 89.1 (*A*) Horizontal MRI images of the posterior part of the hemisphere at the level of the fusiform gyrus (right side on the right). Shown is the effect of visual imagery of a face for 10 s, compared with the effect of imagining a static, nonface pattern. In both sighted individuals and those with late-onset blindness (even though they had been blind for decades), there was clear and specific activation (red voxels) in the right FFA. (*B*) Effect of touching a doll's face on activity in FFA in the sighted (but blindfolded) late and congenitally blind, compared with the effect of touching a "scrambled" doll's face. (See color plate 78.)

FIGURE 89.2 (*A*) The effect of imagining, for 10 s, the visual impression of curtains opening and closing, compared with the effect of imagining the same curtains closed and stationary. The level of this section is through the visual motion area, V5 or MT, and this is clearly activated, at least on the left side, by this motion imagery in both sighted and late-blind individuals. (*B*) The effect of touching the surface of the palm with an unidentifiable moving object, compared with the effect of static placement of the same object on the hand. The visual motion area, MT/V5, is strongly activated only in the late blind. (See color plate 79.)

A recent fMRI study from our own laboratory also supports the view that the tactile activation of visual areas in the late blind is appropriate to the particular tactile discrimination task. Goyal and colleagues (in press) looked at cortical activity evoked by palpation of the face of a doll's head, compared with touching a deformed doll's head that did not feel like a face but had the similar textural features. In late-blind subjects, the tactile face stimulus caused specific activation of a region of the right fusiform gyrus known as the fusiform face area (FFA). This region is thought to be involved in visual face recognition (Kanwisher et al., 1996) and mental imagery of faces (O'Craven and Kanwisher, 2000) in sighted people. Interestingly, the FFA was not activated when early-blind or sighted subjects touched the doll's face, although it was strongly activated in both sighted and late-blind subjects when they tried to imagine the visual impression of a face (figure 89.1).

Goyal and colleagues (in press) also showed that, in late-blind people, movement of an object over the palm of the hand, when compared with static placement of the object on the skin, caused specific bilateral activation of the lateral occipital area V5 or human MT (figure 89.2), which is implicated in the analysis of visual motion in sighted people (Zeki et al., 1991). Again, this activation did not occur in early-blind people or in sighted people, which argues against its being due to visual imagery of the tactile stimulus. On the other hand, Hagen and colleagues (2002) showed activation of V5 in normal sighted subjects when an object was brushed along the whole length of the forearm, but perhaps this particular stimulus was more effective in evoking visual imagination.

Further evidence that activation of visual cortex by touch in the blind is related to function comes from a recent study by Gizewski and colleagues (2003). They confirmed that primary, secondary, and higher visual cortices are activated during both Braille reading and the tactile discrimination of non-Braille dot patterns in the blind, but not during electrical stimulation of the skin of the relevant finger or during meaningless tapping of the finger.

Interestingly, the visual cortex of the blind, even V1, appears to be involved not only in simple tactile and auditory analysis but also in processing language. Amedi and colleagues (2003) reported that congenitally blind subjects activate the visual cortex during verb generation and verbal memory tasks. They then compared these specific sites to activations in the same subjects during Braille reading. They found that anterior regions of visual cortex are preferentially activated during Braille reading, whereas posterior regions (including V1) are more strongly activated during verbal memory and verb generation tasks (see also Burton, Snyder, Diamond, et al., 2002). Moreover, the magnitude of V1 activation correlated with the subject's ability on the tasks, suggesting that this reorganization is functionally important. These data could be taken to indicate that the activation of visual cortex during Braille reading reflects the processing of language-related information. On the other hand, meaningless tactile texture can also cause activation of V1 (Sadato et al., 1996; Büchel et al., 1998; Gizewski et al., 2003), which implies that this ectopic activity is not specifically related to linguistic analysis.

Plasticity in the auditory and olfactory cortices

The auditory cortex, like the somatosensory cortex, is modified as a result of musical practice, but, not surprisingly, the changes reflect practice in discriminating the auditory tones, not in touching the strings. Pantev and colleagues

(2001), recording auditory N1 evoked field potentials, found that the auditory cortex of musicians becomes specialized (responding with larger neuronal excitation) for processing the complex tones produced by musical instruments as opposed to pure sinusoidal tones. The auditory system of musicians also learns to process very slight pitch changes: musicians can detect pitch changes faster and more accurately than nonmusicians (Tervaniemi, 2001). In fact, violinists seem to have the greatest ability to detect small pitch changes, as they are in greatest need of such ability among all musicians. Not only do violinists perform more accurately on pitch discrimination tasks, but they also show earlier onset of N2b and P3b EEG components, indicating that automated neural functions in pitch discrimination are most sensitive in this group of musicians (Tervaniemi, 2001). Indeed, the volume of gray matter in Heschl's gyrus (the site of the primary auditory cortex) is greater in musicians than in nonmusicians (Schneider et al., 2002). However, the direction of causation is unclear. It is possible that practice causes reorganization of connectivity at the boundaries of the auditory cortex, leading to an enlargement of Heschl's gyrus. On the other hand, it could be that people with a relatively large Heschl's gyrus have greater aptitude for music.

Finney, Fine, and Dobkins (2001) reported that the auditory cortex is activated when deaf subjects view visual stimuli (moving-dot patterns). This result implies that auditory deprivation allows for reorganization of the auditory cortex, perhaps to help process other types of sensory information, as seems likely for the reorganization of visual cortex in the blind.

The olfactory cortex also appears to be capable of plasticity. Mainland and colleagues (2002) reported that olfactory learning as a result of repeated smelling through one nostril can be transferred to the other "naive" nostril through cortical mechanisms. In this study, they exposed one nostril to androstenone (a scent that, in some people, cannot be detected when first smelled, but can be detected after learning through repetitive presentation); air was injected into the other nostril to prevent retronasal circulation. After the subject learned to detect the smell through one nostril, androstenone was delivered through the naive nostril and the subject was immediately more sensitive to the smell than when briefly tested at the start of the experiment. It seems likely that experience-dependent functional plasticity in the olfactory cortex is responsible for this transfer of learning.

Mechanisms of plasticity

The responses of cortical neurons are determined by their afferent inputs, from the thalamus and from other cortical cells (both intrinsic, within the same cortical area, and associational, from other areas in the same or the opposite hemisphere). Thalamocortical projections and intrinsic cortico-cortical connections are, at least for primary sensory areas, rather tightly topographically distributed. This exact, localized connectivity is presumed to underpin the discrete receptive fields of cortical neurons and the precise spatial organization that characterizes the retinotopic, somatotopic, and tonotopic maps. How, then, can peripheral deafferentation or hyperstimulation cause shifts or expansions of activation, over distances of several millimeters or more, within individual cortical areas? Some of the changes in mapping seen in the human cortex occur across distances far larger than the typical spread of thalamic axons or intracortical connections.

Even more puzzling is the way in which regions of cortex that appear to be normally unresponsive to a particular stimulus come to respond to it as a result of a loss of their normal input. In some cases (e.g., the takeover of the visual cortex in the blind), cortical areas respond to sensory inputs for which there are no classical afferent connections, either thalamic or associational.

Most of the evidence for the mechanisms of cortical plasticity comes from animal studies. The results suggest a cascade of effects, operating on different time scales. Incidentally, the existence of a variety of mechanisms that all contribute to the same basic outcome is good circumstantial evidence that the phenomenon has evolved through selective pressure and is functionally important. The same argument can be applied to the various mechanisms that are known to contribute to the modification of synaptic strength in the hippocampus, some involving short-term changes in transmitter release or receptor efficacy, others engaging gene expression and protein synthesis to enlarge the region of synaptic apposition (Capogna, 1998). The existence of a mechanistic cascade strengthens the argument that modification of synaptic efficacy is functionally important.

It is important to remember that the responses of sensory areas of the cortex reflect the functional connectivity of the entire sensory pathway from the periphery—through the spinal cord, brainstem, and thalamus, for the somatosensory cortex, for example. Changes at the level of the cortex might depend on reorganization at a more peripheral level. In animals, there is indeed evidence that some components of remapping after deafferentation do occur peripherally, for instance in the spinal cord and somatosensory thalamus (Wall, 1975). However, there is general agreement that at least some elements of reorganization seen in the cortex depend on mechanisms inherent to the cortex itself.

In both humans and other animals, changes in cortical mapping can be detected essentially immediately after the change in sensory input or motor activity (e.g., Rossini et al., 1994; Borsook et al., 1998; Classen et al., 1998; Hamdy et al., 1998; Mainland et al., 2002), but further components of the plasticity take longer to appear (e.g., Pascual-Leone and

Torres, 1993; Elbert et al., 1995; Lim, Altenmüller, and Bradshaw, 2001). There might be at least three distinct mechanisms—two that account for short-term changes, and a separate mechanism for very long-term effects.

Rapid changes probably reflect the unveiling of weak connections that already exist in the cortex, through both release from inhibition and changes in the efficacy of synapses (Borsook et al., 1998; Ramachandran, Rogers-Ramachandran, and Stewart, 1992; although Pons et al., 1991, and Rajan, 1998, are more skeptical). More long-term plasticity may result from the growth of new synapses and/or axons.

Immediate effects (e.g., as a result of amputation) are likely to be due to a sudden reduction in the level of inhibitory synaptic activity in the cortex, which normally suppresses weak inputs on to cortical cells from regions of the receptor surface beyond their classical receptive fields (see Donaghue, Hess, and Sanes, 1996; Huntley, 1997; Levy et al., 2002). Ziemann and colleagues (2001) report that reorganization in the motor cortex is dependent on the level of γ-aminobutyric acid (GABA, the principal inhibitory neurotransmitter). They showed that, as the level of GABAergic inhibition was increased by administering a GABA receptor agonist drug (lorazepam), the capacity for plasticity decreased. The opposite was true when GABA levels were lowered with an ischemic nerve block in the hand (the decrease in GABA is due to deafferentation; see Levy et al., 1999, for details). These data suggest that short-term plasticity, at least in the motor cortex, is controlled by a release of tonic inhibition on synaptic input (thalamic or intracortical) from remote sources.

Changes in cortical mapping over a period of days following increased or decreased sensory or motor activity probably involve modulation of the effectiveness of initially weak excitatory synapses. After loss of normal sensory input (e.g., through amputation or peripheral nerve section), cortical neurons that previously responded to that input might undergo "denervation hypersensitivity," or upregulation of the strength of their responses to any remaining weak excitatory input. But remapping as a result of more subtle changes in activity (e.g., through motor or sensory learning) might well depend on regulated changes in synaptic efficacy similar to the forms of long-term potentiation and depression in the hippocampus that are thought to underlie the formation of spatial and episodic memories (see Rosenbaum, Winocur, and Moscovitch, 2001, for a review).

There is a great deal of evidence that activation of the *N*-methyl-D-aspartate (NMDA) glutamate receptor is involved in modulation of synaptic efficacy in the hippocampus (see Bliss and Collingridge, 1993; Nicoll and Malenka, 1995). A recent study by Dinse and colleagues (2003) implicates the NMDA receptor in cortical plasticity in humans. They found that administration of NMDA antagonists decreases both the effectiveness of perceptual learning and the cortical remapping that accompanies such learning after only brief periods of stimulation. It is thus likely that changes in synaptic efficacy similar to long-term potentiation in the hippocampus are, at least in part, responsible for the relatively short-term plastic changes seen in sensory areas of the adult human cerebral cortex.

In other animals, electrophysiological recording indicates that the body map in the somatosensory cortex continues to change, albeit more slowly, over months or even years after amputation (Pons et al., 1991). The distance over which afferent activation spreads can extend to several millimeters, or even more than 1 cm across the cortical surface—enormously more than the scatter and arborization of individual afferent thalamic axons or intrinsic cortical connections (Pons et al., 1991). There is some evidence in animals that the growth of intracortical axonal connections and even sprouting of new axons might contribute to these very slow changes (Darian-Smith and Gilbert, 1994).

Less is known about the basis of changes in activity beyond individual cortical areas, such as the tactile activation of visual areas in the blind. It is conceivable, but seems very unlikely, that there is wholesale growth of new long-range corticocortical association connections. More plausible is the hypothesis that the plasticity occurs because of changes in the efficacy of existing circuitry, but there is little evidence and no general agreement about which particular form of connections might be involved. There is massive feedback connectivity from "higher" to "lower" sensory areas in the cortex. It is possible that this recurrent network comes under the control of inputs from other sensory areas, enabling them to activate regions of cortex normally used for a different sensory system. Alternatively, the long-range influences might be mediated through facilitation of multiple, serial intrinsic connections, or even of descending and ascending loops via the thalamus.

Bavelier and Neville (2002) pointed out that some of the areas that show unusual responses after sensory loss (e.g., in the blind and deaf) are normally involved in multimodal sensory processing (including higher visual cortical areas in the temporal lobe and the inferior parietal lobe, among others). A recent study on the tactile and visual cross-modal processing of "what" and "where" information found that activity during the what task was greater in the right superior temporal gyrus, and during the where task in the left inferior parietal lobule, suggesting that these areas are both important for multimodal processing (Calvert et al., 2003). In fact, the left inferior parietal lobe is also the site of enhanced activity in people with anomia as they regain the ability to name words after therapy (Cornelissen et al., 2003). Since multimodal areas already have input from several senses, it is not so surprising that loss of input from one sense should lead to the enhancement of response to a remaining sensory input, perhaps through modulation of the strength of synapses from association connections.

New imaging methods, particularly diffusion tensor imaging, that allow for the noninvasive mapping of white matter tracts within the human brain, offer great promise in this area of research.

Implications of these findings and directions for future research

One interesting question that has not been extensively researched has to do with the dilemma of the subjective interpretation of a shift of representation in sensory or motor cortex. Presumably, we perceive the form and position of objects that touch our skin, or appear in our visual or auditory field, because of some kind of perceptual "tag" attached to the activity of each cortical neuron or area of cortex—a sort of subjective "local sign" of the activity that helps us to determine the location of the object on our skin or in our visual or auditory field (Hering, 1865; Mioche and Perenin, 1986). Equally, when we decide to make a movement, the brain selects a set of neurons in the motor cortex with a motor tag corresponding to the desired action. What happens to subjective experience, then, when the input or output connectivity of a region of cortex shifts as a result of plasticity? What happened to the local subjective sign associated with activity of that area? Does it shift to match the new input or output?

If local perceptual tags are fixed, one would predict that the sensations associated with activity in a remapped area would be appropriate to the original function of the given region of cortex. This is the obvious explanation for the illusory phantom sensations on an amputated hand when touching the person's face causes activity in the hand area of the cortex (Ramachandran, Rogers-Ramachandran, and Stewart, 1992). Yet most of the literature on cortical remapping implies that the expansion of an area of representation is useful for the particular receptor area or set of muscles whose representation is expanded. For instance, when a musician's left finger representations get bigger, he or she does not feel as though the strings are touching the wrong fingers or even areas outside the hand. When the visual cortex of the blind is activated by tactile stimulation, they do not "see" it (except in the case of synesthesia). What is the difference between the plasticity that occurs in phantom limbs and synesthesia, which seems functionally irrelevant and appears to reflect rigid local sign, and the plasticity that occurs in musicians or in the blind, which might well be functionally valuable and which implies a change in local sign? Understanding how the local sign is shifted during plasticity in musicians and in the blind might provide the key to understanding why some plasticity is functional while some is maladaptive.

Beyond scientific fascination with the plastic capacity of the human cortex and the possibility that the kinds of reorganization described here are important for aspects of learning, there is hope that cortical plasticity might be harnessed for therapeutic purposes. However, controversy remains as to whether or not plastic changes in the cortex are causatively related to behavioral changes. Determining in which circumstances plasticity is adaptive will greatly influence the field and will help build the foundation on which clinical applications of plasticity research can grow.

A few studies have begun to address how techniques such as direct peripheral sensory stimulation and TMS might encourage functional plastic changes (particularly in primary motor or somatosensory cortex). Stimulating muscles, such as the pharyngeal musculature (Hamdy et al., 1998; see earlier discussion), can cause long-term reorganization of motor cortex, and this might have implications for the treatment of movement disorders. Sensory stimulation might also provide a route to beneficial therapy, not only through its effects on regions of sensory cortex but also through its indirect effects on the motor cortex.

Direct stimulation of the cortex is also currently used for experimental treatment in a variety of clinical populations. rTMS is known to produce longlasting effects in the cortex, the nature of which depends on the frequency of stimulation. Frequencies of 5 Hz and higher are generally thought to be excitatory (Pascual-Leone, Valls-Solé, Wassermann, et al., 1994), but frequencies of 1 Hz can produce inhibition (Chen et al., 1997; Lee et al., 2003). Some results suggest that rTMS of the motor cortex might help patients with Parkinson's disease, either by speeding up reaction time (Pascual-Leone, Valls-Solé, Brasil-Neto, et al., 1994) or by improving pointing abilities (Siebner, Mentschel, et al., 1999), but these results have not been replicated (see Ghabra, Hallett, and Wassermann, 1999). There is also some preliminary evidence that rTMS of the motor cortex can benefit people with writer's cramp (Siebner, Tormos, et al., 1999), and stimulation of the prefrontal cortex has been used to ameliorate depression (George et al., 1995; see also Hallett, 2000, for a discussion of the uses of TMS for research and therapy).

Further investigation into the ability of cortical stimulation to induce functional cortical plasticity, either directly with rTMS or indirectly via sensory and motor activity, is warranted and holds promise for clinical application. It might be useful not only for the treatment of stroke, Parkinson's disease, and depression, but also for the prevention of developmental disabilities associated with poor motor function.

Johansen-Berg, Dawes, and colleagues (2002) imaged the brains of stroke patients before and after they received conventional rehabilitative therapy. They found that therapy-related improvements in hand function correlated with increased activity in certain cortical areas (including premotor and secondary somatosensory cortices). They then applied disruptive low-frequency TMS to these areas to find out which ones mediated the improved performance (Johansen-Berg, Rushworth, et al., 2002). They found that disrupting the ipsilateral primary motor or dorsal premotor cortex significantly reduced function, indicating that the enhanced activity in these areas underpins the recovery of function. This raises the possibility that higher-frequency rTMS applied to cortical regions known to mediate recovery from the effects of stroke might enhance such recovery, or even achieve recovery in patients who are unable to participate in conventional rehabilitation programs. However, Ward and colleagues in 2003 found a negative correlation between outcome after stroke and the degree of task-related activation in regions including those shown to be beneficial to outcome in the studies by Johansen-Berg and colleagues. More work is needed to define the neural correlates of outcome following stroke before rTMS stimulation can be effectively used for therapy.

An intriguing puzzle concerns the enormous variability in outcome after stroke. Patients with apparently similar initial lesions, treated in the same manner, vary greatly in the speed and extent of their recovery. What might account for the individual differences in brain reorganization that are presumed to underlie recovery? It will be interesting to learn what aspects of cortical plasticity serve as predictors of the effectiveness of recovery, and whether encouragement of the more highly correlated changes actually enhance recovery.

An important issue, all too easily masked by enthusiasm for exploiting the potential benefits of cortical plasticity, is the risk of maladaptive cortical organization. Elbert and Heim (2001), in their essay on the light and dark sides of cortical plasticity, discuss Michael Merzenich's conjecture (Buonomano and Merzenich, 1998) that dyslexia and autism might, like dystonia, be the result of aberrant cortical organization. More work is needed to test this hypothesis, but if it is correct, new therapeutic programs might be developed that utilize cortical plasticity to correct maladaptive organization and hence to ameliorate these disorders, which are currently intractable or difficult to treat.

One particular phenomenon that might aid in answering questions about cortical plasticity is synesthesia. This neurological phenomenon, which occurs in at least one in every 2000 individuals (Baron-Cohen et al., 1996) and runs in families, is characterized by idiosyncratic and inappropriate union of sensory modalities (most often the perception of color in association with sounds or the sight of particular graphemes). This curious experience seems to be neither clearly functional nor obviously maladaptive. There is evidence from neuroimaging (Nunn et al., 2002) that the inappropriate sensation is associated with ectopic activity in the corresponding sensory area (the visual color area, V4/V8, in the case of illusory colored percepts). One possibility is that a genetic mutation codes for inappropriate corticocortical association connections, which lead to the aberrant activations. However, synesthetes within a single family can differ in the nature of their synesthetic perceptions, and some stimuli that induce synesthesia (e.g., letters) are themselves learned. It therefore seems that while there is a genetic predisposition for synesthesia, the corticocortical connectivity, leading to the development of the specific and unusual connections (e.g., red with the letter "A") is dependent on a mechanism of plasticity.

We are currently studying a cohort of late-blind visual synesthetes who, although blind, have vivid visual experiences in association with hearing or thinking about words, reading Braille, and so on (Steven and Blakemore, 2003). We have found that visual synesthesia can persist even following long-term sensory deprivation. Although all the subjects had at least 4 years of sight postnatally, some have been blind for more than 40 years, yet their synesthesia persists. This implies that inappropriate cross-sensory responsiveness, once established, does not require natural stimulation through both modalities to support some kind of continuous associative learning. The phenomenon of synesthesia contrasts with the superficially similar takeover of visual cortical areas in the blind. Synesthetes have visual experiences in association with the ectopic activation of visual cortex, while late-blind people who are not synesthetes do not visually experience the aberrant activity in their visual cortex.

There are many questions about synesthesia whose answers might cast light more generally on the nature of cortical plasticity. If a gene or genes can be identified, the function of the proteins could provide insight into the mechanism of cortical plasticity. Synesthetes might have quite normal anatomical connectivity but might differ in the local inhibition or potentiation of weak inputs. If that is the case, then might it be possible to induce synesthesia-like experiences in normal individuals by modulation of inhibition or potentiation? Anecdotal evidence from Cytowic (2002) suggests that the answer might be yes: people who take the hallucinogenic drug LSD often report mixing of the senses and synesthesia-like experiences.

Finally, it will be important to define the similarities and differences between developmental and adult cortical plasticity in humans. Much research has focused on a comparison of the degree of plasticity in the brains of infants and adults, the general conclusion (particularly on the basis of recovery from stroke) being that the young brain is much more plastic (see Payne and Lomber, 2001). It might be, however, that some forms of plasticity are more potent in the adult brain. Just as for hearing, vision, and language, where there is compelling evidence for early sensitive periods in which functional organization is driven by the nature of the sensory input, there could be other aspects of behavioral performance that can benefit best from heightened plasticity later in life.

Conclusions

Plastic changes can occur on a continuous basis in many areas of the adult human cortex. Practicing of motor skills, increased or decreased use of body parts, and artificial stimulation of the cortex, sense organs, or muscles can all yield cortical reorganization. Nevertheless, for reasons that are not yet clear, plasticity occurs more in some people than in others, and aberrations of plastic reorganization might underlie such conditions as synesthesia and autism. Although some forms of plasticity are certainly more pronounced in the child's brain, others persist, with remarkable sensitivity, throughout life. We have yet to define the exact mechanisms of plastic change, and we are not yet certain that these phenomena are of functional importance in matching the organization of the cortex to the behavioral demands of the world. Still, the field holds great promise for the amelioration of various brain disorders, and the next few years of investigation are likely to see striking advances in the clinical application of research on adult plasticity.

ACKNOWLEDGMENTS This work was supported by the Medical Research Council and the Rhodes Trust.

REFERENCES

AMEDI, A., N. RAZ, P. PIANKA, R. MALACH, and E. ZOHARY, 2003. Early "visual" cortex activation correlates with superior verbal memory performance in the blind. *Nat. Neurosci.* 6:758–766.

ARNO, P., A. G. DE VOLDER, A. VANLIERDE, M.-C. WANET-DEFALQUE, E. STREEL, A. ROBERT, S. SANABRIA-BOHORQUEZ, and C. VERAART, 2001. Occipital activation by pattern recognition in the early blind using auditory substitution for vision. *NeuroImage* 13:632–645.

BARON-COHEN, S., L. BURT, F. SMITH-LAITTAN, J. HARRISON, and P. BOLTON, 1996. Synaesthesia: Prevalence and familiality. *Perception* 25:1073–1079.

BAVELIER, D., and H. J. NEVILLE, 2002. Cross-modal plasticity: Where and how? *Nat. Rev. Neurosci.* 3:443–452.

BLISS, T. V., and G. L. COLLINGRIDGE, 1993. A synaptic model of memory: Long-term potentiation in the hippocampus. *Nature* 361:31–39.

BORSOOK, D., L. BECERRA, S. FISHMAN, A. EDWARDS, C. L. JENNINGS, M. STOJANOVIC, L. PAPINICOLAS, V. S. RAMACHANDRAN, R. G. GONZALEZ, and H. BREITER, 1998. Acute plasticity in the human somatosensory cortex following amputation. *Neuroreport* 9:1013–1017.

BÜCHEL, C., C. PRICE, R. S. J. FRACKOWIAK, and K. FRISTON, 1998. Different activation patterns in the visual cortex of late and congenitally blind subjects. *Brain* 121:409–419.

BUONOMANO, D. V., and M. M. MERZENICH, 1998. Cortical plasticity: From synapses to maps. *Annu. Rev. Neurosci.* 21:149–186.

BURTON, H., 2003. Visual cortex activity in early and late blind people. *J. Neurosci.* 23:4005–4001.

BURTON, H., A. Z. SNYDER, T. E. CONTURO, E. AKBUDAK, J. M. OLLINGER, and M. E. RAICHLE, 2002. Adaptive changes in early and late blind: A fMRI study of Braille reading. *J. Neurophysiol.* 87:589–607.

BURTON, H., A. Z. SNYDER, J. B. DIAMOND, and M. E. RAICHLE, 2002. Adaptive changes in early and late blind: A fMRI study of verb generation to heard nouns. *J. Neurophysiol.* 88:3359–3371.

CALVERT, G., P. C. HANSEN, M. S. STEVEN, and F. NEWELL, 2003. An fMRI comparative study of visual, tactile and visuo-tactile "what" and "where" systems. *Soci. Neurosci. Abstr.* 912.11.

CAPOGNA, M., 1998. Presynaptic facilitation of synaptic transmission in the hippocampus. *Pharmacol. Therapeut.* 77:203–223.

CHEN, R., J. CLASSEN, C. GERLOFF, P. CELNIK, E. M. WASSERMANN, M. HALLETT, and L. G. COHEN, 1997. Depression of motor cortex excitability by low-frequency transcranial magnetic stimulation. *Neurology* 48:1398–1403.

CLASSEN, J., J. LIEPERT, S. P. WISE, M. HALLETT, and L. G. COHEN, 1998. Rapid plasticity of human cortical movement representation induced by practice. *J. Neurophysiol.* 79:1117–1123.

COHEN, L. G., P. CELNIK, A. PASCUAL-LEONE, B. CORWELL, L. FAIZ, J. DAMBROSIA, M. HONDA, N. SADATO, C. GERLOFF, M. D. CATALA, and M. HALLETT, 1997. Functional relevance of cross-modal plasticity in blind humans. *Nature* 389:180–183.

COHEN, L. G., R. A. WEEKS, N. SADATO, P. CELNIK, K. ISHII, and M. HALLETT, 1999. Period of susceptibility for cross-modal plasticity in the blind. *Ann. Neurol.* 45:451–460.

CORNELISSEN, K., M. LAINE, A. TARKIAINEN, T. JARVENSIVU, N. MARTIN, and R. SALMELIN, 2003. Adult brain plasticity elicited by anomia treatment. *J. Cogn. Neurosci.* 15:444–461.

CYTOWIC, R. E., 2002. *Synesthesia: A Union of the Senses*, 2nd ed. Cambridge, Mass.: MIT Press.

DARIAN-SMITH, C., and C. D. GILBERT, 1994. Axonal sprouting accompanies functional reorganization in adult cat striate cortex. *Nature* 368:737–740.

DONAGHUE, J. P., G. HESS, and J. N. SANES, 1996. In *The Acquisition of Motor Behavior in Vertebrates*, J. R. Bloedel, T. J. Ebner, and S. P. Wise, eds. Cambridge, Mass.: MIT Press.

DINSE, H. R., P. RAGERT, B. PLEGER, P. SCHWENKREIS, and M. TEGENTHOFF, 2003. Pharmalogical modulation of perceptual learning and associated cortical reorganization. *Science* 301:91–94.

DREHER, B., W. BURKE, and M. B. CALFORD, 2001. Cortical plasticity revealed by circumscribed retinal lesions or artificial scotomas. *Prog. Brain Res.* 134:217–246.

ELBERT, T., and S. HEIM, 2001. A light and a dark side. *Nature* 411:139.

ELBERT, T., C. PANTEV, C. WIENBRUCH, B. ROCKSTROH, and E. TAUB, 1995. Increased cortical representation of the fingers of the left hand in string players. *Science* 270:305–307.

ELBERT, T., V. CANDIA, E. ALTENMÜLLER, H. RAU, A. STERR, B. ROCKSTROH, C. PANTEV, and E. TAUB, 1998. Alteration of digital representations in somatosensory cortex in focal hand dystonia. *Neuroreport* 9:3671–3575.

FINNEY, E. M., I. FINE, and K. R. DOBKINS, 2001. Visual stimuli activate auditory cortex in the deaf. *Nat. Neurosci.* 4:1171–1175.

GEORGE, M. S., E. M. WASSERMANN, W. A. WILLIAMS, A. CALLAHAN, T. A. KETTER, P. BASSER, M. HALLETT, and R. M. POST, 1995. Daily repetitive transcranial magnetic stimulation (rTMS) improves mood in depression. *Neuroreport* 6:1853–1856.

GHABRA, M. B., M. HALLETT, and E. M. WASSERMANN, 1999. Simultaneous repetitive transcranial magnetic stimulation does not speed fine movement in PD. *Neurology* 52:768–770.

GILBERT, C. D., and T. N. WIESEL, 1992. Receptive field dynamics in adult primary visual cortex. *Nature* 356:150–152.

GIRAUX, P., A. SIRIGU, F. SCHNEIDER, and J.-M. DUBERNARD, 2001. Cortical reorganization in motor cortex after graft of both hands. *Nat. Neurosci.* 4:691–692.

GIZEWSKI, E. R., T. GASSER, A. DE GREIFF, A. BOEHM, and M. FORSTING, 2003. Cross-modal plasticity for sensory and motor activation patterns in blind subjects. *NeuroImage* 19:968–975.

GOLDREICH, D., and I. M. KANICS, 2003. Tactile acuity is enhanced in blindness. *J. Neurosci.* 23:3439–3445.

GOYAL, M., M. S. STEVEN, P. C. HANSEN, and C. BLAKEMORE (in press).

HAGEN, M. C., O. FRANZEN, F. MCGLONE, G. ESSICK, C. DANCER, and J. V. PARDO, 2002. Tactile motion activates the human middle temporal/V5 (MT/V5) complex. *Eur. J. Neurosci.* 16: 957–964.

HALLETT, M., 2000. Transcranial magnetic stimulation and the human brain. *Nature* 406:147–150.

HAMDY, S., J. C. ROTHWELL, Q. AZIZ, K. D. SINGH, and D. G. THOMPSON, 1998. Long-term reorganization of human motor cortex driven by short-term sensory stimulation. *Nat. Neorosci.* 1:64–68.

HAMILTON, R. H., and A. PASCUAL-LEONE, 1998. Cortical plasticity associated with Braille learning. *Trends Cogn. Sci.* 2:168–174.

HERING, E., 1865. Vom binocularen Tiefsehen. In *Beiträge zur Physiologie*, Part 5. Leipzig: Engelmann.

HUNTLEY, G. W., 1997. Correlation between patterns of horizontal connectivity and the extent of short-term representational plasticity in rat motor cortex. *Cereb. Cortex* 7:143–156.

INDOVINA, I., and J. N. SANES, 2001. Combined visual attention and finger movement effects on human brain representations. *Exp. Brain Res.* 140:265–279.

JÄNCKE, L., G. SCHLAUG, and H. STEINMETZ, 1997. Hand skill asymmetry in professional musicians. *Brain Cogn.* 34:424–432.

JOHANSEN-BERG, H., H. DAWES, C. GUY, S. M. SMITH, D. T. WADE, and P. M. MATTHEWS, 2002. Correlation between motor improvements and altered fMRI activity after rehabilitative therapy. *Brain* 124:2731–2742.

JOHANSEN-BERG, H., M. F. RUSHWORTH, M. D. BOGDANOVIC, U. KISCHKA, S. WIMALARATNA, and P. M. MATTHEWS, 2002. The role of ipsilateral premotor cortex in hand movement after stroke. *Proc. Natl. Acad. Sci. U.S.A.* 99:14518–14523.

KANWISHER, N., M. M. CHUN, J. MCDERMOTT, and P. LEDDEN, 1996. Functional imaging of human visual recognition. *Cogn. Brain Res.* 5:55–67.

KARNI, A., G. MEYER, P. JEZZARD, M. M. ADAMS, R. TURNER, and L. G. UNGERLEIDER, 1995. Functional MRI evidence for adult motor cortex plasticity during motor skill learning. *Nature* 377: 155–158.

KAUFFMAN, T., H. THÉORET, and A. PASCUAL-LEONE, 2002. Braille character discrimination in blindfolded human subjects. *Neuroreport* 13:571–574.

KIRIAKOPOULOS, E., J. BAKER, R. HAMILTON, and A. PASCUAL-LEONE, 1999. Relationship between tactile spatial acuity and brain activation in brain functional magnetic resonance imaging. *Neurology* 52(Suppl. 2):A307.

KUJALA, T., M. HUOTILAINEN, J. SINKKONEN, A. I. AHONEN, K. ALHO, M. S. HAMALAINEN, R. J. ILMONIEMI, M. KAJOLA, J. E. T. KNUTILA, J. LAVIKAINEN, O. SALONEN, J. SIMOLA, C.-G. STANDERTSKJÖLD-NORDENSTAM, H. TIITINEN, S. O. TISSARI, and R. NAATANEN, 1995. Visual cortex activation in blind humans during sound discrimination. *Neurosci. Lett.* 183:143–146.

LECLERC, C., D. SAINT-AMOUR, M. E. LAVOIE, M. LASSONDE, and F. LEPORE, 2000. Brain functional reorganization in early blind humans revealed by auditory event-related potentials. *Neuroreport* 11:545–550.

LEE, L., H. R. SIEBNER, J. B. ROWE, V. RIZZO, J. C. ROTHWELL, R. S. FRACKOWIAK, and K. J. FRISTON, 2003. Acute remapping within the motor system induced by low-frequency repetitive transcranial magnetic stimulation. *J. Neurosci.* 23:5308–5318.

LESSARD, N., M. PARÉ, F. LEPORE, and M. LASSONDE, 1998. Early-blind human subjects localize sound sources better than sighted subjects. *Nature* 395:278–280.

LEVY, L. M., U. ZIEMANN, R. CHEN, and L. G. COHEN, 1999. Rapid modulation of GABA in human cortical plasticity demonstrated by magnetic resonance spectroscopy (abstract). *Neurology* 52(6 Suppl. 2):A88.

LEVY, L. M., U. ZIEMANN, R. CHEN, and L. G. COHEN, 2002. Rapid modulation of GABA in sensorimotor cortex induced by acute deafferentation. *Ann. Neurol.* 52:755–761.

LIM, V. K., E. ALTENMÜLLER, and J. L. BRADSHAW, 2001. Focal dystonia current theories. *Hum. Move. Sci.* 20:870–914.

MAINLAND, J. D., E. A. BREMNER, N. YOUNG, B. N. JOHNSON, R. M. KHAN, M. BENSAFI, and N. SOBEL, 2002. One nostril knows what the other one learns. *Nature* 418:802.

MIOCHE, L., and M. T. PERENIN, 1986. Central and peripheral residual vision in humans with bilateral deprivation amblyopia. *Exp. Brain Res.* 62:259–272.

MIYASHITA, Y., 1999. Visual associative long-term memory: Encoding and retrieval in inferotemporal cortex of the primate. In *The New Cognitive Neurosciences*, 2nd ed., M. S. Gazzaniga, ed. Cambridge, Mass.: MIT Press.

MOORE, C. E. G., and W. SCHADY, 2000. Investigation of the functional correlates of reorganization within the human somatosensory cortex. *Brain* 123:1883–1895.

MUELLBACHER, W., U. ZIEMANN, J. WISSEL, N. DANG, M. KOFLER, S. FACCHINI, B. BOROOJERDI, W. POEWE, and M. HALLETT, 2002. Early consolidation in human primary motor cortex. *Nature* 415:640–644.

MÜNTE, T. F., E. ALTENMÜLLER, and L. JÄNCKE, 2002. The musician's brain as a model of neuroplasticity. *Nat. Rev. Neurosci.* 3:473–478.

NEVILLE, H. J., and D. LAWSON, 1987. Attention to central and peripheral visual space in a movement detection task. III. Separate effects of auditory deprivation and acquisition of a visual language. *Brain Res.* 405:284–294.

NICOLL, R. A., and R. C. MALENKA, 1995. Contrasting properties of two forms of long-term potentiation in the hippocampus. *Nature* 377:115–118.

NUNN, J. A., L. J. GREGORY, M. BRAMMER, S. C. WILLIAMS, D. M. PARSLOW, M. J. MORGAN, R. G. MORRIS, E. T. BULLMORE, S. BARON-COHEN, and J. A. GRAY, 2002. Functional magnetic resonance imaging of synesthesia: Activation of V4/V8 by spoken words. *Nat. Neurosci.* 5:371–375.

O'CRAVEN, K. M., and N. KANWISHER, 2000. Mental imagery of faces and places activates corresponding stimulus-specific brain regions. *J. Cogn. Neurosci.* 12:1013–1023.

PANTEV, C., A. ENGELIEN, V. CANDIA, and T. ELBERT, 2001. Representational cortex in musicians: Plastic alterations in response to musical practice. *Ann. N.Y. Acad. Sci.* 930:300–314.

PASCUAL-LEONE, A., and R. HAMILTON, 2001. The metamodal organization of the brain. *Prog. Brain Res.* 134:427–445.

PASCUAL-LEONE, A., D. NGUYET, L. G. COHEN, J. P. BRASIL-NETO, A. CAMMAROTA, and M. HALLETT, 1995. Modulation of muscle responses evoked by transcranial magnetic stimulation during the acquisition of new fine motor skills. *J. Neurophysiol.* 74:1037–1045.

PASCUAL-LEONE, A., and F. TORRES, 1993. Sensorimotor cortex representation of the reading finger of Braille readers: An example of activity-induced cerebral plasticity in humans. *Brain* 116:39–52.

PASCUAL-LEONE, A., J. VALLS-SOLÉ, J. P. BRASIL-NETO, A. CAMMAROTA, J. GRAFMAN, and M. HALLETT, 1994. Akinesia in Parkinson's disease. II. Effects of subthreshold repetitive transcranial motor cortex stimulation. *Neurology* 48:1398–1403.

PASCUAL-LEONE, A., J. VALLS-SOLÉ, E. M. WASSERMANN, and M. HALLET, 1994. Responses to rapid-rate transcranial magnetic stimulation of the human motor cortex. *Brain* 117:847–858.

PAYNE, B. R., and S. G. LOMBER, 2001. Reconstructing functional systems after lesions of cerebral cortex. *Nat. Rev. Neurosci.* 2:911–919.

PONS, T. P., P. E. GARRAGHTY, A. K. OMMAYA, J. H. KAAS, E. TAUB, and M. MISHKIN, 1991. Massive reorganization of the primary somatosensory cortex after peripheral sensory deafferation. *Science* 252:1857–1860.

RAJAN, R., 1998. Receptor organ damage causes loss of cortical surround inhibition without topographic map plasticity. *Nat. Neurosci.* 1:138–143.

RAMACHANDRAN, V. S., and D. ROGERS-RAMACHANDRAN, 2000. Phantom limbs and neural plasticity. *Arch. Neurol.* 57:317–320.

RAMACHANDRAN, V. S., D. ROGERS-RAMACHANDRAN, and M. STEWART, 1992. Perceptual correlates of massive cortical reorganization. *Science* 258:1159–1160.

RIJNTJES, M., M. TEGENTHOFF, J. LIEPERT, G. LEONHARDT, S. KOTTERBA, S. MULLER, S. KIEBEL, J. P. MALIN, H. C. DIENER, and C. WEILLER, 1997. Cortical reorganization in patients with facial palsy. *Ann. Neurol.* 41:621–630.

RODER, B., F. ROSLWE, and H. J. NEVILLE, 2000. Event-related potentials during auditory language processing in congenitally blind and sighted people. *Neuropsychologia* 38:1482–1502.

ROSENBAUM, R. S., G. WINOCUR, and M. MOSCOVITCH, 2001. New views on old memories: Re-evaluating the role of the hippocampal complex. *Behav. Brain Rese.* 127:183–197.

ROSSINI, P. M., G. MARTINO, L. NARICI, A. PASQUARELLI, M. PERESSON, V. PIZZELLA, F. TECCHIO, G. TORRIOLI, and G. L. ROMANI, 1994. Short-term brain "plasticity" in humans: Transient finger representation changes in sensory cortex somatotopy following ischemic anesthesia. *Brain Res.* 642:169–177.

SADATO, N., A. PASCUAL-LEONE, J. GRAFMAN, M. P. DEIBER, V. IBANEZ, and M. HALLETT, 1998. Neural networks for Braille reading by the blind. *Brain* 121:1213–1229.

SADATO, N., A. PASCUAL-LEONE, J. GRAFMAN, V. IBANEZ, M. P. DEIBER, G. DOLD, and M. HALLETT, 1996. Activation of primary visual cortex by Braille reading in blind subjects. *Nature* 380:562–568.

SANGER, T. D., A. PASCUAL-LEONE, D. TARSY, and G. SCHLAUG, 2002. Nonlinear sensory cortex response to simultaneous tactile stimuli in writer's cramp. *Move. Disord.* 17:105–111.

SATHIAN, K., and A. ZANGALADZE, 2001. Feeling with the mind's eye: The role of visual imagery in tactile perception. *Optom. Vision Sci.* 78:276–281.

SCHLAUG, G., C. CHEN, D. Z. PRESS, A. WARDE, Q. CHEN, and A. PASCUAL-LEONE, 2000. Hearing with the mind's eye. *Hum. Brain Mapp.* 11:S57.

SCHLAUG, G., A. R. HALPERN. D. Z. PRESS, J. T. BAKER, R. R. EDELMAN, and A. PASCUAL-LEONE, 1999. Changes in cortical auditory processing after blindfolding. *Soci. Neurosci. Abstr.* 25:1628.

SCHNEIDER, P., M. SCHERG, H. G. DOSCH, H. J. SPECHT, A. GUTSCHALK, and R. RUPP, 2002. Morphology of Heschl's gyrus reflects enhanced activation in the auditory cortex of musicians. *Nat. Neurosci.* 5:688–694.

SIEBNER, H. R., C. MENTSCHEL, C. AUER, and B. CONRAD, 1999. Repetitive transcranial magnetic stimulation has a beneficial effect on bradykinesia in Parkinson's disease. *Neuroreport* 10:589–594.

SIEBNER, H. R., J. M. TORMOS, A. O. CEBALLOS-BAUMANN, C. AUER, M. D. CATALA, B. CONRAD, and A. PASCUAL-LEONE, 1999. Low-frequency repetitive transcranial magnetic stimulation of the motor cortex in writer's cramp. *Neurology* 52:529–537.

STEVEN, M. S., and C. BLAKEMORE, 2003. Visual synesthesia in the blind. *Soc. Neurosci. Abstr.* 934.6.

TERVANIEMI, M., 2001. Musical sound processing in the human brain: Evidence from electric and magnetic recordings. *Ann. N.Y. Acad. Sci.* 930:259–272.

WALL, P. D., 1975. Signs of plasticity and reconnection in spinal cord damage. *Ciba Found. Symp.* 34:35–63.

WALSH, V., and A. COWEY, 2000. Transcranial magnetic stimulation and cognitive neuroscience. *Nat. Rev. Neurosci.* 1:73–79.

WARD, N. S., M. M. BROWN, A. J. THOMPSON, and R. S. J. FRACKOWIAK, 2003. Neural correlates of outcome after stroke: A cross-sectional fMRI study. *Brain* 126:1430–1448.

WEEKS, R., B. HORWITZ, A. AZIZ-SULTAN, B. TIAN, C. M. WESSINGER, L. G. COHEN, M. HALLETT, and J. P. RAUSCHECKER, 2000. A positron emission tomographic study of auditory localization in the congenitally blind. *J. Neurosci.* 20:2664–2672.

YANG, T. T., C. C. GALLEN, V. S. RAMACHANDRAN, S. COBB, B. J. SCHWARTZ, and F. E. BLOOM, 1994. Noninvasive detection of cerebral plasticity in adult human somatosensory cortex. *Neuroreport* 5:701–704.

ZANGALADZE, A., C. M. EPSTEIN, S. T. GRAFTON, and K. SATHIAN, 1999. Involvement of visual cortex in tactile discrimination of orientation. *Nature* 401:587–590.

ZEKI S., J. D. WATSON, C. J. LUECK, K. J. FRISTON, C. KENNARD, and R. S. FRACKOWIAK, 1991. A direct demonstration of functional specialization in human visual cortex. *J. Neurosci.* 11:641–649.

ZIEMANN, U., W. MUELBACHER, M. HALLETT, and L. G. COHEN, 2001. Modulation of practice-dependent plasticity in human motor cortex. *Brain* 124:1171–1181.

90 Genes and the Development of Neural Networks Underlying Cognitive Processes

JOHN FOSSELLA AND MICHAEL I. POSNER

ABSTRACT The influence of genetic factors on normal and abnormal mental development has been well established so it is appropriate to begin to explore in more detail the biological bases of these phenomena. The influence of genes on the development of neural networks that are related to cognitive processes can be accomplished using tools developed by the Human Genome Project. One approach to this question examines individual differences in the efficiency and activity of various neural networks related to attention as a function of genetic variation in specific candidate genes. This chapter reviews what has been accomplished using this appoach and presents some of its limitations.

In the last 10 years, separate neural networks active during cognitive tasks such as orienting to sensory stimuli (Corbetta and Shulman, 2002), processing faces (Liu, Harris, and Kanwisher, 2002), reading words (Shaywitz et al., 2002), music (Janata et al., 2002), calculation (Dehaene et al., 1999), and many others have been reported extensively. With the use of appropriate imaging methods it is possible to work out the time course and connectivity of these networks (Posner and McCandliss, 1999; Formisano et al., 2002). As the general outlines of cognitive networks are understood in terms of anatomy and circuitry, it becomes important to ask how they differ among individuals and how these differences arise.

Neuroimaging studies have shown that the general outlines of networks underlying cognitive and emotional processes are sufficiently common among individuals that they can be averaged together to produce a common network. That does not mean that all subjects are identical. Reliable individual differences in the functional anatomy of such networks are being revealed in fMRI studies (Miller et al., 2002). However, the commonalties that exist suggest that many features of these networks are specified genetically. In addition, while genetic variation may play a role in the differences between individuals in these networks, it is also likely that these differences can arise or be modified by life experiences.

Most of the studies of genetic variation conducted so far have involved attempts at understanding the basis of psychopathologies. These include developmental pathologies such as attention deficit/hyperactivity disorder (ADHD, Faraone, 2001) and dyslexia (Fisher and DeFries, 2002) that are likely to be continuous with normal function, as well as pathological conditions such as autism (Cook, 2001), schizophrenia (Bassett et al., 2002), and Williams syndrome (Donnai and Karmiloff-Smith, 2000) that are more clearly due to states not found within the normal range (Pennington, 2002; Rothbart and Posner, in press). In this chapter our major emphasis will be on variations in attentional networks, memory, and reading skill that are clearly in the normal range. Our goal is to describe research that can eventually lead to an understanding of how genes work together in development with specific experience to shape individual variation in the networks of brain areas that underlie cognitive and emotional processes.

A major change in the opportunity to conduct research with normal human subjects arises from the cooperative worldwide efforts of the Human Genome Project and human genome diversity projects. These programs have provided new tools for neurobiologists and cognitive neuroscientists. Genome-wide sequence information, sequence diversity information, and a variety of analytic tools are freely accessible and openly available via the Internet (see Wolfsberg, 2003). Public databases (see list of Web sites at end of chapter), such as Gene Expression Omnibus, the Expressed Gene Anatomy Database, the Gene Expression Database, and other gene expression atlases dedicated to brain anatomy, provide information about the time and spatial location of gene expression in the developing brain and body.

In addition, there have been numerous published reports cataloguing changes in gene expression during brain development (Johnston et al., 2001; Mody et al., 2001), during sustained neural activity (French et al., 2001), in response to

JOHN FOSSELLA and MICHAEL I. POSNER Sackler Institute, Department of Psychiatry, Weill Medical College of Cornell University, New York, N.Y., and University of Oregon, Eugene, Ore.

pharmacological challenge (Kontkanen et al., 2002), in normal versus pathological states (Mirnics et al., 2000; Mandel, Grünblatt, and Youdim, 2000; Shilling and Kelsoe, 2002), and in awake subjects (Blasberg, 2002). These tools allow investigators to focus on candidate genes whose expression is specific to a process or structure of interest or perhaps to a particular pathological state or pharmacological challenge. Further converging evidence can be readily obtained from the animal research literature, in particular the mouse gene-targeting literature, where a wide array of functional and developmental data are catalogued (see TBASE Web site).

Finally, genotyping continues to get cheaper and easier, permitting small- and medium-scale exploratory genetic analyses to be conducted on modest budgets. Commercial, government, and foundation-supported genotyping services now routinely provide genetic analyses on DNA obtained from cheek swabs (see reference list of Web sites). Cheek swabs can be collected in a sterile and noninvasive manner, pretty much like brushing one's teeth. The free and open access to genomic information and the ease and low cost of genetic analyses make it an attractive tool for the study of individual differences. It is important that cognitive neuroscientists use these new tools in developing an understanding of the neural networks underlying important aspects of cognition.

Measurement of individual variation

There are several methods for examining individual variation in cognition. One approach involves the use of a test or a self-report scale that samples the domain widely with many different types of questions or problems pooled into an overall score. Examples are self-report of personality, parent or teacher report of child temperament, and intelligence tests. A somewhat different approach is to study the distribution of performance on a single experimental marker task in which a number of identical trials are pooled. The task is usually thought to represent prototypical performance within the domain of study. For example, a letter-matching test has been used to study individual differences in a component skill of verbal intelligence (Hunt, Lunneborg, and Lewis, 1975), the Stroop test has been used to study differences in one component of attention (Fan et al., 2002), and a cued detection task has been used to study another component of attention (Posner, 1980). The methods are complementary in that the scales tend to sample a wide range of natural behaviors, while the experimental method provides clearer analysis of the particular computations involved in the skill. In some cases the two methods have been used together to provide a broader basis for individual differences (Hunt, Lunneborg, and Lewis, 1975; Posner and Rothbart, 1998).

Moreover, both of these methods have been used as phenotypes for genetic studies. Scale scores based on symptom counts have been a frequent method for probing the genetic basis of ADHD (Swanson et al., 2001). In examining dyslexia, rhyming tests have been used as a phenotype related to the critical dimension of phonological skill. Rather than study all of the symptoms of schizophrenia, some studies have focused on the difficulty shown by patients in filtering input information and have used the ability of a cue to suppress the startle response (prepulse inhibition) as a surrogate for the disorder (Geyer and Braff, 1987).

There have already been several efforts to relate scores of normal differences in personality or performance to brain activity. One example involves the mapping of extroversion by showing that it correlates with activity in frontotemporal networks (Canli et al., 2001). Another study examined a measure of persistence from a temperament and personality test developed by Cloninger (1987). Persistence is related to conscientiousness and effortful control, and is one of the so-called big five personality dimensions. They found very high correlations between scores on the test and a particular brain network that involved midline prefrontal and lateral areas (Gusnard et al., 2003).

In our work, we have been trying to link the brain networks underlying attention to the study of individual differences. To do this, we used neuroimaging data to argue for three anatomically separate networks of attention. We then devised a marker task that allows us to measure individual differences in efficiency in each of the networks (Attention Network Test, Fan et al., 2002). We found that the measures of the three networks were reliable and for the most part independent. Scanning studies showed that the networks activated by the test were similar to those found in previous studies using individual components of the test (Fan et al., 2001).

These initial efforts are a few examples of efforts to show that specific brain activity can be associated with individual differences as measured by psychological scales and experimental tasks. How do these individual differences arise? Many neural networks develop in early life under genetic control, and it is likely that genetic differences account for a portion of developmental variation.

Genetic influences on cognitive networks

HERITABILITY One major method for demonstrating a genetic influence on individual differences in cognitive processes compares the performance of monzygotic twins, who have identical genomes, with dizygotic twins, who share only as much genetic similarity as siblings do. A heritability index can be computed from the differences between these two correlations. In this way, performance on many commonly used cognitive tasks has been shown to be influenced by genetic factors. Studies using the Continuous Performance Task (CPT) have shown that the d' signal detection component of CPT performance has a heritability among normal subjects of 0.49 (Cornblatt et al., 1988). The Span of Apprehension task (SPAN), a visual search task, has been shown to have a heritability among normal subjects of 0.65 (Bartfai et al., 1991) and the P/N ratio of the Spontaneous Selective Attention Task (SSAT) was shown to have a heritability among normal subjects of 0.41 (Myles-Worsley and Coon, 1997). Twin studies using normal control twins show that spatial working memory, divided attention, choice reaction time (RT) and selective attention (Cannon et al., 2000), attentional set shifting (Pardo et al., 2000), sensorimotor gating (Geyer and Braff, 1987), smooth pursuit eye tracking (Katsanis et al., 2000), and executive attention (Fan, Wu, et al., 2001) are underlain by inherited factors. In addition, anatomical studies in rodents, nonhuman primates, and humans have established that genes are major determinants of overall brain size (Cheverud et al., 1990; Thompson et al., 2002) and structural aspects of specific brain regions such as the frontal cortex (Tramo et al., 1998; Thompson et al., 2000) and corpus callosum (Oppenheim et al., 1989).

BEYOND HERITABILITY   How can we go from evidence of the heritability of networks to an understanding of the specific genes involved? With approximately 30,000 genes in the human genome, it remains a challenge to identify the genes of critical importance for any network.

Two general approaches have been used to make these connections. The first involves genetic linkage analysis. Linkage studies are used when there are no good hypotheses about candidate genes. The basic approach is to evaluate the genotypes of a collection of related individuals using a set of neutral genetic markers spread evenly across the human genome. Siblings with extreme values such as symptoms of psychopathology or extreme scores on an individual differences measure are examined to determine if the marker is overrepresented among those family members having the common phenotype. If such a linkage occurs, it suggests that a nearby gene may be related to the common extreme value. For example, families with many dyslexic members have been studied genetically and found to have common linkage to chromosome 6, suggesting a gene nearby related to the disorder (Fisher and DeFries, 2002).

A second method that is increasingly possible is to use existing knowledge about neural networks, pharmacology, gene expression patterns, animal models, and human genetic anomalies to define candidate genes. Once the candidate genes are proposed, individuals with specific alleles of the genes associated with a network can be tested with the appropriate measures to determine if the allele influences performance of that network. In the next section we explore current research using the method of relating differences in brain networks to alleles associated with them.

Candidate molecular pathways

By now there are several examples of the candidate gene strategy applied to networks underlying cognitive processes. One example is the work of Egan and colleagues (2001, 2003) in the study of working and episodic memory. Schizophrenia is a complex disorder that has often been associated with dopamine, partly because of the types of drugs that work to remediate the disorder. This link led Egan and colleagues to examine genes related to schizophrenia that might involve the dopamine pathway. Because schizophrenia is highly heritable, studies of families of patients had led to genetic linkage to several chromosomal areas. One of these areas is on chromosome 22, in the 22q11 region that contains the catechol-*O*-methyl transferase (COMT) gene that produces an enzyme important in the metabolism of dopamine. Egan and colleagues found that a variant of the COMT gene was related to performance on cognitive tasks involving working memory. This gene accounted for about 4% of the variance in perseveration errors during the Wisconsin Card Sorting task. The COMT gene is likely to be important in many aspects of executive function. Not only did we find a trend for its relation to resolving conflict in our ANT, but a major developmental pathology (R22q11 syndrome) involves a deletion of this gene among others. The syndrome displays many physical abnormalities and carries an increased risk for schizophrenia, and experimental studies suggest that performance on the conflict aspect of the ANT is greatly impaired in these children (Sobin et al., 2003).

A different approach to the analysis of candidate genes is found in a study of episodic memory storage (Egan et al., 2003). Animal and human studies have shown that storage of information in episodic memory is affected by lesions of the midtemporal areas, including the hippocampus. Animal models revealed that brain-derived neurotrophic factor (BDNF) was an important protein involved in changes in plasticity that accompany learning and memory in the hippocampus. This led the investigators to study the performance of normal subjects on a task of memory of episodic information from the Wechsler Adult Memory Scale. They showed that alleles of the BDNF gene were related to performance on this task and were unrelated to performance on many similar tasks less clearly dependent on episodic memory. In this case, animal models were critical to understanding the genes involved.

We have pursued a somewhat similar strategy to identify genes involved in attention. Three attentional networks have been identified in human neuroimaging studies (Corbetta and Shulman, 2002) and associated with specific biochemicals that serve to modulate neuronal activity within the network (Marrocco and Davidson, 1998; Davidson and Marrocco, 2000). Studies of alert monkeys have suggested that alerting produced by warning signals is modulated by the norepinepherine system. Orienting appears to involve modulation by the cholinergic system. For the executive network, the focus is on dopamine (DA). This rests in part on the important role of the anterior cingulate within this network. Moreover, the cingulate gyrus is also implicated in a number of psychiatric disorders. Interestingly, all of these disorders show familial patterns of inheritance, increased risk among first-degree relatives of affected patients, and increased concordance in identical versus fraternal twins.

To obtain precise measures of the efficiency of individual performance in each network, we employed the ANT (Fan et al., 2002) as a measure that would be (1) highly heritable (Fan, Wu, et al., 2001), (2) highly sensitive to several core dimensions of various psychiatric disorders (Posner and Rothbart, 2000), and (3) dependent on specific anatomical brain areas (Fan et al., 2003). The ANT is advantageous for genetic studies insofar as it distinguishes between separate functions of attention (alerting, orienting, and executive) that are correlated with the activation of these specific neuroanatomical circuits. As a first step in evaluating the suitability of the ANT, we chose to examine polymorphisms in the dopamine D4 receptor (DRD4), dopamine transporter (DAT1), monoamine oxidase A (MAOA), and COMT genes. These candidates, as discussed earlier, are ideal, because (1) they have been repeatedly associated with disorders where attention is disrupted, (2) they have been pharmacologically related to the executive attention network, and (3) they have been biochemically characterized so that each allelic class is associated with a difference in biochemical activity or expression level.

In Fossella and colleagues (2002), variation in the DRD4 gene at the exon III variable nucelotide tandem repeat (VNTR) and the single nucleotide polymorphism (SNP) at -521 showed a modest influence on executive attention efficiency as measured by the speed of resolving conflict, but no such association with RT or alerting. The finding that the 4-repeat-absent group showed lower executive attention scores is consistent with previous findings on ADHD populations. Swanson and colleagues (2000) showed that ADHD subjects with the 7-repeat allele did not show cognitive deficits on cued-detection, color-word, and go/no-go neuropsychological tasks designed to measure various attentional functions. Although the 7-repeat allele has often been associated with ADHD, it may not contribute to a loss of attentional efficiency, but perhaps to other dimensions that underlie the development of ADHD. Moreover, recent studies on the phylogenetic history of the DRD4 exon III VNTR suggest that the 4-repeat is phylogenetically ancient and that the 7- and 2-repeat alleles appeared in human populations more

recently (see later discussion under Evolution). Based on these data, the differences in executive attention between the 4-present versus 4-absent groups may relate in some way to the disparate geographic dispersal of these alleles (Ding et al., 2002).

Polymorphisms in MAOA were also found to be associated with executive attention. This was expected, mainly because of the important role of MAOA in catecholamine metabolism. The additional finding of an association with alerting efficiency is consistent with a role of MAOA in the clearance of noradrenaline as well as dopamine. This role of MAOA in alerting may be related to the findings of Lim and colleagues (1995) showing a significant association of the MAOA locus to susceptibility for bipolar disorder. Also, the recent findings showing that the low-activity allele of the MAOA-LPR polymorphism is associated with aggression in maltreated children may be consistent with the lower efficiency of executive attention seen in normal subjects with this allele (Caspi et al., 2002).

Nonsignificant trends were observed for DAT and COMT in measures of executive attention, and no trends or significant associations were observed for the other attentional network scores, mean RT, and/or accuracy. The lack of any association with COMT was surprising, given previous reports of association with various disorders, the results of Egan and colleagues (2001), and functional imaging studies showing that the dorsolateral prefrontal cortex (DLPFC) is activated during the flanker task, and that the anatomical structure of DLPFC is highly heritable (Thompson et al., 2001). It should be noted that although we observed a statistical trend for the COMT gene, COMT accounted for 4% of the variance in the study by Egan and colleagues (2001), and thus it may be difficult to reach a significant threshold without relatively large subject populations.

Many such design and implementation issues become apparent when conducting genetic association studies. Genetic modeling studies suggest that when many genes underlie a complex trait such as attention, or a disorder such as ADHD, great difficulty should be expected in detecting significant associations of single candidate genes (Suarez et al., 1995; Lohmueller et al., 2003). Moreover, individual polymorphisms can exert extremely weak main effects. The results of Fossella and colleagues (2002) showed that a population of 200 subjects lacked the needed statistical power, because the modest statistical associations were well below the standards set for the reporting of true associations (Lohmueller et al., 2003). An encouraging aspect of this study, however, was the finding that no associations or statistical trends were observed for global measures of performance such as overall RT. This suggests that there may be specificity in the role of genetic factors in contributing to specific neural functions. In addition, it is possible to replicate any result with new populations, owing to the relatively inexpensive and noninvasive genetic methods that are available.

Despite these difficulties, the current findings illustrate the kinds of strategies that can be used to assess candidate genes. We believe that all cognitive and emotional networks are influenced by genes, and for most if not all of them, reasonable candidates should be found. For attention networks, a clue to candidate genes came from pharmacological studies of alert monkeys. As we have indicated, areas of research such as attention and memory can often rely on animal models to provide appropriate candidates. However, there are many human functions for which animal models are absent or more difficult. An example is the ability to read printed words. Here, statistical association studies have attempted to find regions of various chromosomes associated with orthographic and phonological features of word reading (Olson et al., 1999). As these efforts yield fruit, the human genome databases can provide information on which genes are related to the areas discovered. In the next section we consider the use of neuroimaging to obtain converging evidence on these gene × behavior associations.

Neuroimaging of genetic effects

Functional magnetic resonance imaging (fMRI) can be used to confirm and extend the association between genes and particular underlying networks. Egan and colleagues (2001) showed that a methionine/valine polymorphism in the COMT gene correlated with performance on a cognitive task involving some aspects of working memory. When fMRI measurements were made on subjects performing a working memory task, those subjects with the valine allele showed worse performance and higher levels of brain activation in the prefrontal cortex. Furthermore, the valine allele accounted for a portion of the genetic risk toward schizophrenia.

The use of fMRI data in a genetic study has been further explored using the BDNF gene. Egan and colleagues (2003) studied normal subjects in an fMRI study of working memory. They were able to show that performance and the level of activation in the scanner within the hippocampus were related to alleles of the gene, as would be predicted from their behavioral results. One interesting aspect of these data that could have important implications for the candidate gene approach is that the number of subjects needed to obtain the result in the scanner was far less than predicted from the behavioral study. The authors speculated that the behavior was affected by many additional factors beyond those related to the role of the gene.

In our studies of the attentional networks, we found that polymorphisms in the DRD4 and MAOA genes showed significant associations with efficiency of handling conflict as measured by RT differences on the ANT (Fossella et al.,

2002). To examine whether this genetic variation might contribute to differences in brain activation, subjects who performed the ANT while in the scanner were genotyped for the DRD4 and MAOA genes. We found that the DRD4 and MAOA alleles that were associated with more efficient handling of conflict in the RT experiment also differed in amount of activation in the anterior cingulate while subjects were performing the ANT task (Fan et al., 2003). Because we studied 16 genotypically unselected subjects, we did not have sufficient data to subdivide groups equally based on genotype at the several genes we found to be related to conflict in our behavioral study. However, we did find significant differences in activation in alleles that we believe have considerable influence on dopamine activity within the network being studied. Moreover, our scanning data showed significant differences with about eight subjects per cell, while the same alleles only approached significance in a behavioral study with nearly 100 subjects in each cell. These data support the speculation by Egan and colleagues that a combination of behavioral and fMRI work can provide statistical confirmation, even though the influence of any individual gene is rather small.

A number of other studies have exploited the advantages of the cognitive, genetic, and neuroimaging approach. Positron emission tomography (PET) is a well-established method suitable for measuring specific biochemical processes in the body over time and in three dimensions. Individual differences in radioligand binding are often observed. One of the best examples of this are seen for two genes, DAT and DRD2. Each of these genes contains genetic polymorphisms that have been associated with psychiatric illness. The protein encoded by each gene can be probed using specific radioligands suitable for quantitative measures of ligand binding. The dopamine transporter carries a polymorphic 40-base-pair repeat that varies in length across human populations. The ability of radioligands to bind to the transporter in subjects with different versions of this polymorphic repeat seems to be influenced by the number of repeats. Subjects homozygous for the 10-repeat allele showed significantly lower dopamine transporter binding than carriers of the 9-repeat allele (Jacobsen et al., 2000). Such findings have been applied to alcoholism, where DAT polymorphisms are associated with the severity of withdrawal (Heinz et al., 2000). Similarly, genetic polymorphisms in the DRD2 gene have been associated with differences in DRD2 receptor levels (Pohjalainen et al., 1999; Jonsson et al., 1999). Some evidence shows that these polymorphisms contribute to the risk of schizophrenia and to alcoholism. It would be desirable to extend the PET studies to all genes implicated in mental illness.

Electroencephalographic (EEG) and event-related potential (ERP) measurements have long been used to probe psychological and cognitive processes in normal subjects and in studies of mental illness and genetics. For example, in alcoholism, a reduction in the P300 amplitude in patients and in first-degree relatives has been found (Porjesz et al., 1998). Other family studies and twin studies show that individual differences in the P300 are at least moderately heritable (Boomsma, 1994; Vogel, 2000). Similarly, the P50 has been used to study early sensory processing of paired stimuli in schizophrenia (Geyer and Braff, 1987) and has been shown to be heritable (Myles-Worsley et al., 1996; Young et al., 1996).

Development of neural networks

It is a long way from identifying a gene related to some network and showing how that gene actually influences the development of the ability to perform a high-level cognitive task. It is at this point that the understanding of the development of neural networks is likely to be extremely important.

DEVELOPMENT OF EXECUTIVE ATTENTION   Using the child ANT, we have assayed the developmental course of the attentional networks (Fan et al., unpublished observations). As in the adult data, the child study also revealed independence between the three network scores. Network scores of five groups of children between 6 and 10 years of age and a group of adults were measured by the child ANT. Overall performance measures (RT and accuracy) are fundamental to interpreting the network scores, especially when comparing populations with differences in overall RT and accuracy.

There were large declines in overall RT and accuracy with increasing age. Despite this common decline in RT, each network showed a different developmental course. There was a significant improvement in conflict resolution at age 7 compared with younger children, but a remarkable stability in both RT and accuracy conflict scores from the age 7 to adulthood. The alerting scores show some improvement in late childhood and continued development between age 10 and adulthood. Finally, the orienting score was similar to adult levels at the age of 6.

SYNAPTOGENESIS   The time course of development of attention networks can also be explored using molecular genetic tools in humans and accompanying animal models. For example, the "A not B" task normally shows a postnatal increase in performance. Frequently, this is associated with a change in DA levels, because behavioral performance is paralleled by a postnatal increase in DA levels (Goldman-Rakic, 1981) and an increase in DA receptor gene expression (Lidow et al., 1991). In addition, tyrosine hydroxylase (TH)-positive processes in prefrontal areas 9 and 46 show a gradual maturation of axons and varicosities (Rosenberg and Lewis, 1995). Such changes in cellular arborization

suggest that dopaminergic synapse formation plays a role in the normal development of inhibitory control. Mouse models in which these processes are disrupted, such as the orphan nuclear, nur-related receptor (NURR1)-deficient mice, may yield clues to the molecular players involved in postnatal dopaminergic function (Buervenich et al., 2000).

In addition to the postnatal changes in dopaminergic networks, other cellular processes such as synaptogenesis have been explored. Human postnatal development proceeds with a period of synaptic overgrowth followed by a period of synaptic pruning near adolescence (Huttenlocher et al., 1982). A relatively delayed period of synaptic and dendritic development occurs in the prefrontal cortex (PFC) (Huttenlocher, 1979; Conel, 1939/1963). Whereas a delay in synaptogenesis and dendritic arborization in the PFC correlates with a relative delay in the onset of executive function, it is not yet clear exactly how the regulation of synaptogenesis influences normal cognitive development.

Abnormal pre- and postnatal synaptogenic processes have been implicated in disorders in which executive function is diminished or severely developmentally delayed. The most striking example is seen in fragile X mental retardation (FMR). This genetic disorder (reviewed in Irwin, Galvez, and Greenough, 2000) arises from the loss of function of a single gene that encodes the fragile X mental retardation protein (FMRP). This protein is locally translated in synaptic spines in response to neuronal stimulation (Weiler et al., 1997). Golgi-histochemical studies of postmortem tissue from patients with FMR show no gross anatomical disturbances, but rather abnormalities in the quantity and morphology of dendritic spines in pyramidal cells (Wisniewski et al., 1991). An excess of dendritic spines in fragile X patients indicates a deficit in synaptic pruning. This pathology is also seen in mice that are deficient in FMRP, whose pyramidal neurons show an excess of spines (Kooy et al., 1996). Other forms of mental retardation seem to implicate synaptogenesis as a key step in cognitive development. Mutations in the *rho*-family of small GTPases, which are key regulators of synaptogenesis, are implicated in mental retardation syndromes. *oligophrenin-1*, a *rho* activator, has been associated with X-linked mental retardation, and *synaptojanin*, a *rho*-family effector, is overexpressed in Down syndrome (Billuart et al., 1998; Arai et al., 2002).

Further evidence of disruption of normal synaptogenic processes can be found in longitudinal brain structure studies of patients with early-onset schizophrenia. An accelerated loss of gray matter seems to appear early in parietal areas and spreads through adolescence to temporal and frontal areas (Thompson et al., 2001). A loss of gray matter may be related to decreases in input from the mediodorsal thalamic nucleus, given the evidence for a decreased number of these neurons (Manaye et al., 1995) and reduced thalamic size (Andreasen et al., 1994). Gene expression assays show that the regulator of G-protein-coupled signaling (RGS4) gene was reduced in expression in subjects with schizophrenia (Mirnics et al., 2000). In addition to the loss of expression in schizophrenia, RGS4 was found to reside on chromosome 1q21–22, a well-known schizophrenia susceptibility locus (Brzustowicz et al., 2000). This suggests that the loss of expression might be underlain not by environmental factors but perhaps by genetic variation unique to the affected patients. Alleleic variants of RGS4 were examined in a population-based gene association study, and several polymorphisms were found to be preferentially transmitted to affected probands (Chowdari et al., 2002). Similarly, BDNF shows increases in expression in response to neural stimulation (Rocamora et al., 1996) and influences dendritic morphology (McAllister, Katz, and Lo, 1996). As with RGS4, allelic variants in this gene have been associated with schizophrenia (Krebs et al., 2000), MRI-based brain volume (Wassink et al., 1999), and fMRI measures of hippocampal activity (Egan et al., 2003). Last, the SNAP25 gene, like RGS4, was found to be differentially expressed in schizophrenia (Hemby et al., 2002). Developmentally, it may play a key regulatory role, because selective inhibition via antisense oligonucleotides blocks cortical neurite elongation (Osen-Sand et al., 1993). A mutant mouse, *Coloboma*, carrying a deletion of this gene shows high levels of hyperactivity (Wilson, 2000) and disruptions of dopaminergic signaling (Jones et al., 2001). Gene association studies have related allelic variants of SNAP25 with ADHD (Brophy et al., 2002; Mill et al., 2002; Barr et al., 2000) and decrements in executive attention (Fossella et al., 2003).

CINGULATE FORMATION   The far-reaching connectivity of the cingulate gyrus implicates this brain area in a number of psychiatric disorders with high heritabilities. Tasks that activate the anterior cingulate cortex, such as spatial working memory tasks, divided attention tasks, and attentional set shifting, have been examined in identical and fraternal twin populations and found to have high heritabilities (Cannon et al., 2000; Pardo et al., 2000). Several candidate genes may be of particular interest to studies of cingulate function. The neurotrophin-3 (NT-3) gene, a molecule involved in the growth and survival of developing neurons, shows enriched expression in the anterior cingulate cortex during development (Vigers, Baquet, and Jones, 2000). Variation in the NT-3 gene was associated with schizophrenia (Hattori and Nanko, 1995). Similarly, the neurotensin (NTS) gene shows enriched expression in the cingulate cortex at birth (Sato et al., 1991). Recent gene association studies on the promoter of the neurotensin receptor (NTSR1) have also shown associations with schizophrenia (Austin et al., 2000). Other genes whose expression is enriched in the developing cingulate cortex include *Emx2* and ER-81 (Cecchi and Boncinelli, 2000; Yun, Potter, and Rubenstein, 2001). Mutations in the *Emx2* gene have been shown to cause schizencephaly (Brunelli et al., 1996).

Role of experience

INDIVIDUAL   Gene expression studies have shown that the anterior cingulate cortex is highly sensitive to environmental stress. Anoxia (Mehmet et al., 1994), maternal separation (Avishai-Eliner et al., 1999), amyloid protein expression (Dodart et al., 1999), and drug abuse (Ladenheim et al., 2000) induce hypometabolism, gliosis, and programmed cell death in the anterior cingulate cortex. Exposure to stress induces the expression of glucocorticoid receptor (GR), a transcription factor that mediates the cellular response to stress (McEwen, 2000). Stress-induced excititoxic damage has been noted in the anterior cingulate cortex in schizophrenia (Benes, 2000). Specifically, dopaminergic innervation of interneurons in layers II and V is elevated in postmortem analyses of schizophrenia (Benes, 2000). The hyperinnervation of interneuronal DRD2 contacts is suspected to disable local inhibition of pyramidal cells and lead to excess glutamatergic signaling and excitotoxicity in downstream brain areas. Because this type of excitotoxic damage is mediated by GR, variation in this gene and/or its downstream targets may contribute to the gene × environment interactions seen in many psychiatric disorders. The importance of such environmental factors in the discovery of genetic origins of brain disorders has been recognized (Chakravarti and Little, 2003).

Specific educational experiences in children influence the development of neural networks, and these forms of plasticity might involve changes in gene expression. Evidence of important changes in brain networks with specific training has begun to arise in neuroimaging studies. For example, studies of children with specific difficulties in reading have shown that a brief period of training with a commercial program focused on improving phonemic knowledge can change the areas of the brain activated by real words and pseudowords (Temple et al., 2003). This kind of evidence for the plasticity of neural networks underlying cognition by specific training raises the issue of whether individual differences related to specific genes may be important determinants of the success of such training. If so, understanding these differences could help developing improved methods for treatment optimization. For example, Swanson and colleagues (2000) speculated that there might be two groups of children with ADHD, one characterized by genetic abnormalities and the other characterized by brain structure abnormalities from nongenetic causes, and that these groups might respond differently to behavioral versus medication therapy. Structural MRI studies on persons with ADHD consistently show reduced caudate nucleus volumes

(Castellanos et al., 1996, 2002). Caudate volume can be an accurate predictor of performance (Casey et al., 1997; Mataro et al., 1997). Filipek and colleagues (1997) found that subjects with smaller and more symmetrical caudate nuclei had a more favorable response to treatment with stimulant medication. If specific training can influence neural networks in pathological conditions it seems likely that this can also do so in normal development.

EVOLUTION One of the most interesting uses of genetic data is for phylogenetic analyses of genes and human history (Templeton, 2002). Genetic influences on functions such as language and executive attention are of great interest since genetic variation can be compared with primate species and used to roughly date the emergence of function (Enard et al., 2003). For example, the anterior cingulate cortical microstructure in humans shows a remarkable leap of recent evolution. Betz (1881) first noted the presence of large motor neurons in the cingulate region of humans but not in other great ape species. Similarly, spindle cells, so named for their elongate and gradually tapering morphology, have been found predominantly in layer Vb in the medial wall of the cingulate gyrus. These cells are not seen in Old World primates but are found in bonobos, chimpanzees, and humans (Nimchinsky et al., 1999).

Phylogenetic studies comparing human and primate genomic sequence data attempt to explain such recent evolutionary leaps. For example, Chen and colleagues (1999) evaluated the role of the DRD4 gene in human evolution and migration. They reported a high correlation (0.8) between the frequency of the exon III 7-repeat allele and miles of migration estimated for ethnic groups around the world as the human population expanded out of Africa. Ding and colleagues (2002) and Seaman and colleagues (2000) have shown that the DRD4 gene has undergone strong positive selection during primate evolution. Similarly, the FOXP2 gene has been noted for its role in a severe form of speech impairment that showed monogenic inheritance (Lai et al., 2001). Phylogenetic studies showed a similar pattern of rapid evolution and positive selection in the hominid lineage (Enard et al., 2003). Additional studies of genes that contribute to the development of various neural networks underlying cognition may help in the effort to understand the evolution of mind.

Summary

The study of individuality has a long history within psychology. Advances in neuroimaging have made it possible to examine differences among people using a variety of morphological and functional imaging methods. It seems clear that reliable individual differences must have their origin in genetic variability among people and that genetic expression

is itself subject to change by specific experiences. The Human Genome Project has provided the basis for adding molecular genetic analysis to the everyday laboratory procedures of cognitive neuroscience. In this chapter, we have reviewed approaches designed to link individual differences in the genome to differences in neural networks among individuals. One sign of the acceptance of these new approaches is a new initiative sponsored by the National Institutes of Mental Health that aims to build on the interface of molecular genetics, pharmacology, and cognitive neuroscience to bridge gaps between clinical diagnosis and the molecular processes that influence susceptibility to psychiatric disorders (Hyman and Fenton, 2003).

REFERENCES

ANDREASEN, N. C., S. ARNDT, V. SWAYZE, 2nd, T. CIZADLO, M. FLAUM, D. O'LEARY, J. C. EHRHARDT, and W. T. YUH, 1994. Thalamic abnormalities in schizophrenia visualized through magnetic resonance image averaging. *Science* 266:294–298.

ARAI, Y., T. IJUIN, T. TAKENAWA, L. E. BECKER, and S. TAKASHIMA, 2002. Excessive expression of synaptojanin in brains with Down syndrome. *Brain Dev.* 24:67–72.

AUSTIN, J., P. BUCKLAND, A. G. CARDNO, N. WILLIAMS, G. SPURLOCK, B. HOOGENDOORN, S. ZAMMIT, G. JONES, R. SANDERS, L. JONES, G. MCCARTHY, S. JONES, N. J. BRAY, P. MCGUFFIN, M. J. OWEN, and M. C. O'DONOVAN, 2000. The high affinity neurotensin receptor gene (NTSR1): Comparative sequencing and association studies in schizophrenia. *Mol. Psychiatry* 5:552–557.

AVISHAI-ELINER, S., C. G. HATALSKI, E. TABACHNIK, M. EGHBAL-AHMADI, and T. Z. BARAM, 1999. Differential regulation of glucocorticoid receptor messenger RNA (GR-mRNA) by maternal deprivation in immature rat hypothalamus and limbic regions. *Brain Res. Dev. Brain Res.* 114:265–268.

BARR, C. L., Y. FENG, K. WIGG, S. BLOOM, W. ROBERTS, M. MALONE, R. SCHACHAR, R. TANNOCK, and J. L. KENNEDY, 2000. Identification of DNA variants in the SNAP-25 gene and linkage study of these polymorphisms and attention-deficit hyperactivity disorder. *Mol. Psychiatry* 5:405–409.

BARTFAI, A., N. L. PEDERSEN, R. F. ASARNOW, and D. SCHALLING, 1991. Genetic factors for the span of apprehension test: A study of normal twins. *Psychiatry Res.* 38:115–124.

BASSETT, A. S., E. W. CHOW, R. WEKSBERG, and L. BRZUSTOWICZ, 2002. Schizophrenia and genetics: New insights. *Curr. Psychiatry Rep.* 4:307–314.

BENES, F. M., 2000. Emerging principles of altered neural circuitry in schizophrenia. *Brain Res. Brain Res. Rev.* 31:251–269.

BETZ, W., 1881. *Zentralbl. Med. Wiss.* 19:193–195, 209–213, 231–234.

BILLUART, P., T. BIENVENU, N. RONCE, V. DES PORTES, M. C. VINET, R. ZEMNI, A. CARRIE, C. BELDJORD, A. KAHN, C. MORAINE, and J. CHELLY, 1998. Oligophrenin 1 encodes a rho-GAP protein involved in X-linked mental retardation. *Pathol. Biol. (Paris)* 46:678.

BLASBERG, R., 2002. Pet imaging of gene expression. *Eur. J. Cancer* 38:2137–2146.

BOOMSMA, D. I., J. R. KOOPMANS, L. J. VAN DOORNEN, and J. F. ORLEBEKE, 1994. Genetic and social influences on starting to smoke: A study of Dutch adolescent twins and their parents. *Addiction* 89:219–226.

BROPHY, K., Z. HAWI, A. KIRLEY, M. FITZGERALD, and M. GILL, 2002. Synaptosomal-associated protein 25 (SNAP-25) and attention deficit hyperactivity disorder (ADHD): Evidence of linkage and association in the Irish population. *Mol. Psychiatry* 7:913–917.

BRUNELLI, S., A. FAIELLA, V. CAPRA, V. NIGRO, A. SIMEONE, A. CAMA, and E. BONCINELLI, 1996. Germline mutations in the homeobox gene EMX2 in patients with severe schizencephaly. *Nat. Genet.* 12:94–96.

BRZUSTOWICZ, L. M., K. A. HODGKINSON, E. W. CHOW, W. G. HONER, and A. S. BASSETT, 2000. Location of a major susceptibility locus for familial schizophrenia on chromosome 1q21–q22. *Science* 288:678–682.

BUERVENICH, S., A. CARMINE, M. ARVIDSSON, F. XIANG, Z. ZHANG, O. SYDOW, E. G. JONSSON, G. C. SEDVALL, S. LEONARD, R. G. ROSS, R. FREEDMAN, K. V. CHOWDARI, V. L. NIMGAONKAR, T. PERLMANN, M. ANVRET, and L. OLSON, 2000. Nurrl mutations in cases of schizophrenia and manic-depressive disorder. *Am. J. Med. Genet.* 96:808–813.

CANLI, T., Z. ZHAO, J. E. DESMOND, E. J. KANG, J. GROSS, and J. D. E. GABRIELI, 2001. An fMRI study of personality influences on brain reactivity to emotional stimuli. *Behav. Neurosci.* 115:33–42.

CANNON, T. D., M. O. HUTTUNEN, J. LONNQVIST, A. TUULIO-HENRIKSSON, T. PIRKOLA, D. GLAHN, J. FINKELSTEIN, M. HIETANEN, J. KAPRIO, and M. KOSKENVUO, 2000. The inheritance of neuropsychological dysfunction in twins discordant for schizophrenia. *Am. J. Hum. Genet.* 67:369–382.

CASEY, B. J., F. X. CASTELLANOS, J. N. GIEDD, W. L. MARSH, S. D. HAMBURGER, A. B. SCHUBERT, Y. C. VAUSS, A. C. VAITUZIS, D. P. DICKSTEIN, S. E. SARFATTI, and J. L. RAPOPORT, 1997. Implication of right frontostriatal circuitry in response inhibition and attention-deficit/hyperactivity disorder. *J. Am. Acad. Child Adolesc. Psychiatry* 36:374–383.

CASPI, A., J. MCCLAY, T. E. MOFFITT, J. MILL, J. MARTIN, I. W. CRAIG, A. TAYLOR, and R. POULTON, 2002. Role of genotype in the cycle of violence in maltreated children. *Science* 297(5582): 851–854.

CASTELLANOS, F. X., J. N. GIEDD, W. L. MARSH, S. D. HAMBURGER, A. C. VAITUZIS, D. P. DICKSTEIN, S. E. SARFATTI, Y. C. VAUSS, N. LANGE, D. KAYSEN, A. L. KRAIN, G. F. RITCHIE, J. W. SNELL, J. C. PAJAPAKSE, and J. L. RAPOPORT, 1996. Quantative brain magnetic resonance imaging iin attention-deficit hyperactivity disorder. *Arch. Gen. Psychiatry* 53:607–616.

CASTELLANOS, F. X., P. P. LEE, W. SHARP, N. O. JEFFRIES, D. K. GREENSTEIN, L. S. CLASEN, J. D. BLUMENTHAL, R. S. JAMES, C. L. EBENS, J. M. WALTER, A. ZIJDENBOS, A. C. EVANS, J. N. GIEDD, and J. L. RAPOPORT, 2002. Developmental trajectories of brain volume abnormalities in children and adolescents with attention-deficit/hyperactivity disorder. *JAMA* 288:1740–1748.

CECCHI, C., and E. BONCINELLI, 2000. Emx homeogenes and mouse brain development. *Trends Neurosci.* 23:347–352.

CHAKRAVARTI, A., and P. LITTLE, 2003. Nature, nurture and human disease. *Nature* 421:412–414.

CHEN, C., M. BURTON, E. GREENBERGER, and J. DMITRIEVA, 1999. Population migration and the variation of dopamine D4 receptor (DRD4) allele frequencies around the globe. *Evol. Hum. Behav.* 20:309–324.

CHEVERUD, J. M., D. FALK, M. VANNIER, L. KONIGSBERG, R. C. HELMKAMP, and C. HILDEBOLT, 1990. Heritability of brain size and surface features in rhesus macaques (macaca mulatta). *J. Hered.* 81:51–57.

CHOWDARI, K. V., K. MIRNICS, P. SEMWAL, J. WOOD, E. LAWRENCE, T. BHATIA, S. N. DESHPANDE, B. K. THELMA, R. E. FERRELL, F. A. MIDDLETON, B. DEVLIN, P. LEVITT, D. A. LEWIS, and V. L. NIMGAONKAR, 2002. Association and linkage analyses of RGS4 polymorphisms in schizophrenia. *Hum. Mol. Genet.* 11:1373–1380.

CLONINGER, C. R., 1987. A systematic method for clinical description and classification of personality variants. *Arch. Gen. Psychiatry* 44:573–588.

CONEL, J. L., 1939/1963. *The Postnatal Development of the Human Cerebral Cortex.* Cambridge, Mass: Harvard University Press.

COOK, E. H., Jr., 2001. Genetics of autism. *Child Adolesc. Psychiatr. Clin. North Am.* 10:333–350.

CORBETTA, M., and G. L. SHULMAN, 2002. Control of goal-directed and stimulus-driven attention in the brain. *Nat. Neurosci. Rev.* 3:201–215.

CORNBLATT, B. A., N. J. RISCH, G. FARIS, D. FRIEDMAN, and L. ERLENMEYER-KIMLING, 1988. The Continuous Performance Test, identical pairs version (CPT-IP). I. New findings about sustained attention in normal families. *Psychiatry Res.* 26:223–238.

DAVIDSON, M. C., and R. T. MARROCCO, 2000. Local infusion of scopolamine into intraparietal cortex slows covert orienting in rhesus monkeys. *J. Neurophysiol.* 83:1536–1549.

DEHAENE, S., E. SPELKE, P. PINEL, R. STANESCU, and S. TSIVKIN, 1999. Sources of mathematical thinking: Behavioral and brain-imaging evidence. *Science* 284:970–974.

DING, Y. C., H. C. CHI, D. L. GRADY, A. MORISHIMA, J. R. KIDD, K. K. KIDD, P. FLODMAN, M. A. SPENCE, S. SCHUCK, J. M. SWANSON, Y. P. ZHANG, and R. K. MOYZIS, 2002. Evidence of positive selection acting at the human dopamine receptor D4 gene locus. *Proc. Natl. Acad. Sci. U.S.A.* 99:309–314.

DODART, J. C., C. MATHIS, K. R. BALES, S. M. PAUL, and A. UNGERER, 1999. Early regional cerebral glucose hypometabolism in transgenic mice overexpressing the V717F beta-amyloid precursor protein. *Neurosci. Lett.* 277:49–52.

DONNAI, D., and A. KARMILOFF-SMITH, 2000. Williams syndrome: From genotype through to the cognitive phenotype. *Am. J. Med. Genet.* 97:164–171.

EGAN, M. F., T. E. GOLDBERG, B. S. KOLACHANA, J. H. CALLICOTT, C. M. MAZZANTI, R. E. STRAUB, D. GOLDMAN, and D. R. WEINBERGER, 2001. Effect of COMT Val108/158 Met genotype on frontal lobe function and risk for schizophrenia. *Proc. Natl. Acad. Sci. U.S.A.* 98:6917–6922.

EGAN, M. F., M. KOJIMA, J. H. CALLICOTT, T. E. GOLDBERG, B. S. KOLACHANA, A. BERTOLINO, E. ZAITSEV, B. GOLD, D. GOLDMAN, M. DEAN, B. LU, and D. R. WEINBERGER, 2003. The BDNF val66met polymorphism affects activity-dependent secretion of BDNF and human memory and hippocampal function. *Cell* 112:257–269.

ENARD, W., M. PRZEWORSKI, S. E. FISHER, C. S. LAI, V. WIEBE, T. KITANO, A. P. MONACO, and S. PAABO, 2002. Molecular evolution of FOXP2, a gene involved in speech and language. *Nature* 418:869–872.

FAN, J., J. I. FLOMBAUM, B. D. MCCANDLISS, K. M. THOMAS, and M. I. POSNER, 2003. *NeuroImage* 18:42–57.

FAN, J., J. FOSSELLA, T. SOMMER, Y. WU, and M. I. POSNER, 2003. Mapping the genetic variation of executive attention onto brain activity. *Proc. Natl. Acad. Sci. U.S.A.* 100:7406–7411.

FAN, J., B. D. MCCANDLISS, J. I. FLOMBAUM, and M. I. POSNER, 2001. Paper presented atte Society for Neuroscience 2001 Annual Meeting, San Diego.

FAN, J., B. D. MCCANDLISS, T. SOMMER, A. RAZ, and M. I. POSNER, 2002. Testing the efficiency and independence of attentional networks. *J. Cogn. Neurosci.* 14:340–347.

FAN, J., M. R. RUEDA, J. HALPARIN, D. GRUBER, L. P. LERCARI, B. D. McCANDLISS, and M. I. POSNER (unpublished observations). Asssaying the develoment of attentional networks in six to ten year old children. *Neuropsychologia.*

FAN, J., Y. WU, J. A. FOSSELLA, and M. I. POSNER, 2001. Assessing the heritability of attentional networks. *BMC Neurosci.* 2:14.

FARAONE, S. V., A. E. DOYLE, E. MICK, and J. BIEDERMAN, 2001. Meta-analysis of the association between the 7-repeat allele of the dopamine d(4) receptor gene and attention deficit hyperactivity disorder. *Am. J. Psychiatry* 158:1052–1057.

FILIPEK, P. A., M. SEMRUD-CLIKEMAN, R. J. STEINGARD, P. F. RENSHAW, D. N. KENNEDY, and J. BIEDERMAN, 1997. Volumetric MRI analysis comparing subjects having attention-deficit hyperactivity disorder with normal controls. *Neurology* 48:589–601.

FISHER, S. E., and J. C. DEFRIES, 2002. Developmental dyslexia: Genetic dissection of a complex cognitive trait. *Nat. Rev. Neurosci.* 3:767–780.

FORMISANO, E., D. E. J. LINDEN, F. DI SALLE, L. TROJANO, F. ESPOSITO, A. T. SACK, D. GROSSI, F. E. ZANELLA, and R. GOEBEL, 2002. Tracking the mind's image in the brain. I. Time-resolved fMRI during visuospatila mental imagery. *Neuron* 35:185–194.

FOSSELLA, J. A., T. SOMMER, J. FAN, D. PFAFF, and M. I. POSNER, 2003. Synaptogenesis and heritable aspects of executive attention. *Ment. Retard. Dev. Disabil. Res. Rev.* 9:178–183.

FOSSELLA, J., T. SOMMER, J. FAN, Y. WU, J. M. SWANSON, D. W. PFAFF, and M. I. POSNER, 2002. Assessing the molecular genetics of attention networks. *BMC Neurosci.* 3:14.

FRENCH, P. J., V. O'CONNOR, M. W. JONES, S. DAVIS, M. L. ERRINGTON, K. VOSS, B. TRUCHET, C. WOTJAK, T. STEAN, V. DOYERE, M. MAROUN, S. LAROCHE, and T. V. BLISS, 2001. Subfield-specific immediate early gene expression associated with hippocampal long-term potentiation in vivo. *Eur. J. Neurosci.* 13:968–976.

GUSNARD, D. A., J. M. OLLINGER, G. L. SHULMAN, C. R. CLONINGER, J. L. PRICE, D. C. VAN ESSEN, and M. E. RAICHLE, 2003. Persistance and brain circuitry. *Proc. Natl. Acad. Sci. U.S.A.* 100:3479–3484.

GEYER, M. A., and D. L. BRAFF, 1987. Startle habituation and sensorimotor gating in schizophrenia and related animal models. *Schizophr. Bull.* 13:643–668.

GOLDMAN-RAKIC, P. S., 1981. Prenatal formation of cortical input and development of cytoarchitectonic compartments in the neostriatum of the rhesus monkey. *J. Neurosci.* 1:721–735.

HATTORI, M., and S. NANKO, 1995. Association of neurotrophin-3 gene variant with severe forms of schizophrenia. *Biochem. Biophys. Res. Commun.* 209:513–518.

HEINZ, A., D. GOLDMAN, D. W. JONES, R. PALMOUR, D. HOMMER, J. G. GOREY, K. S. LEE, M. LINNOILA, and D. R. WEINBERGER, 2000. Genotype influences in vivo dopamine transporter availability in human striatum. *Neuropsychopharmacology* 22:133–139.

HEMBY, S. E., S. D. GINSBERG, B. BRUNK, S. E. ARNOLD, J. Q. TROJANOWSKI, and J. H. EBERWINE, 2002. Gene expression profile for schizophrenia: Discrete neuron transcription patterns in the entorhinal cortex. *Arch. Gen. Psychiatry* 59:631–640.

HUNT, E., C. LUNNEBORG, and J. LEWIS, 1975. What does it mean to be high verbal? *Cogn. Psychol.* 7:194–227.

HUTTENLOCHER, P. R., 1979. Synaptic density in human frontal cortex: Developmental changes and effects of aging. *Brain Res.* 163:195–205.

HUTTENLOCHER, P. R., C. DE COURTEN, L. J. GAREY, and H. VAN DER LOOS, 1982. Synaptic development in human cerebral cortex. *Int. J. Neurol.* 16:144–154.

HYMAN, S. E., and W. S. FENTON, 2003. Medicine. What are the right targets for psychopharmacology? *Science* 299:350–351.

IRWIN, S. A., R. GALVEZ, and W. T. GREENOUGH, 2000. Dendritic spine structural anomalies in fragile-X mental retardation syndrome. *Cereb. Cortex* 10:1038–1044.

JACOBSEN, L. K., J. K. STALEY, S. S. ZOGHBI, J. P. SEIBYL, T. R. KOSTEN, R. B. INNIS, and J. GELERNTER, 2000. Prediction of dopamine transporter binding availability by genotype: A preliminary report. *Am. J. Psychiatry* 157:1700–1703.

JANATA, P., J. L. BIRK, J. D. VAN HORN, M. LEMAN, B. TILLMANN, and J. J. BHARUCHA, 2002. The cortical topography of tonal structures underlying Western music. *Science* 298:2167–2170.

JOHNSTON, M. V., O. H. JEON, J. PEVSNER, M. E. BLUE, and S. NAIDU, 2001. Neurobiology of Rett syndrome: A genetic disorder of synapse development. *Brain. Dev.* 23(Suppl. 1):S206–S213.

JONES, M. D., M. E. WILLIAMS, and E. J. HESS, 2001. Expression of atecholaminergic mrnas in the hyperactive mouse mutant coloboma. *Brain Res. Mol. Brain Res.* 96:114–121.

JONSSON, E. G., M. M. NOTHEN, H. NEIDT, K. FORSLUND, G. RYLANDER, M. MATTILA-EVENDEN, M. ASBERG, P. PROPPING, and G. C. SEDVALL, 1999. Association between a promoter polymorphism in the dopamine D2 receptor gene and schizophrenia. *Schizophr. Res.* 40:31–36.

KATSANIS, J., J. TAYLOR, W. G. IACONO, and M. A. HAMMER, 2000. Heritability of different measures of smooth pursuit eye tracking dysfunction: a study of normal twins. *Psychophysiology* 37:724–730.

KONTKANEN, O., P. TORONEN, M. LAKSO, G. WONG, and E. CASTREN, 2002. Antipsychotic drug treatment induces differential gene expression in the rat cortex. *J. Neurochem.* 83:1043–1053.

KOOY, R. F., R. D'HOOGE, E. REYNIERS, C. E. BAKKER, G. NAGELS, K. DE BOULLE, K. STORM, G. CLINCKE, P. P. DE DEYN, B. A. OOSTRA, and P. J. WILLEMS, 1996. Transgenic mouse model for the fragile X syndrome. *Am. J. Med. Genet.* 64:241–245.

KREBS, M. O., O. GUILLIN, M. C. BOURDELL, J. C. SCHWARTZ, J. P. OLIE, M. F. POIRIER, and P. SOKOLOFF, 2000. Brain derived neurotrophic factor (BDNF) gene variants association with age at onset and therapeutic response in schizophrenia. *Mol. Psychiatry* 5:558–562.

LADENHEIM, B., I. N. KRASNOVA, X. DENG, J. M. OYLER, A. POLETTINI, T. H. MORAN, M. A. HUESTIS, and J. L. CADET, 2000. Methamphetamine-induced neurotoxicity is attenuated in transgenic mice with a null mutation for interleukin-6. *Mol. Pharmacol.* 58:1247–1256.

LAI, C. S., S. E. FISHER, J. A. HURST, F. VARGHA-KHADEM, and A. P. MONACO, 2001. A forkhead-domain gene is mutated in a severe speech and language disorder. *Nature* 413:519–523.

LIDOW, M. S., T. S. GOLDMAN-RAKIC, D. W. GALLAGER, and P. RAKIC, 1991. Distribution of dopaminergic receptors in the primate cerebral cortex: Quantitative autoradiographic analysis using [³H] raclopride and [³H] SCH23390. *J. Neurosci.* 40:657–671.

LIM, L. C., J. POWELL, P. SHAM, D. CASTLE, N. HUNT, R. MURRAY, and M. GILL, 1995. Evidence for a genetic association between alleles of monoamine oxidase A gene and bipolar affective disorder. *Am. J. Med. Genet.* 60:325–331.

LIU, J., A. HARRIS, and N. KANWISHER, 2002. Stages of processing in face perception: An MEG study. *Nat. Neurosci.* 5:910–916.

LOHMUELLER, K. E., C. L. PEARCE, M. PIKE, E. S. LANDER, and J. N. HIRSCHHORN, 2003. Meta-analysis of genetic association studies supports a contribution of common variants to susceptibility to common disease. *Nat. Genet.* 33:177–182.

LUO, Z., and D. H. GESCHWIND, 2001. Microarray applications in neuroscience. *Neurobiol. Dis.* 8:183–193.

MANAYE, K. F., D. D. MCINTIRE, D. M. MANN, and D. C. GERMAN, 1995. Locus coeruleus cell loss in the aging human brain: a nonrandom process. *J. Comp. Neurol.* 358:79–87.

MANDEL, S., E. GRÜNBLATT, and M. YOUDIM, 2000. cDNA microarray to study gene expression of dopaminergic neurodegeneration and neuroprotection in MPTP and 6-hydroxydopamine models: Implications for idiopathic Parkinson's disease. *J. Neural. Transm. Suppl.* 60:117–124.

MARROCCO, R. T., and M. C. DAVIDSON, 1998. Neurochemistry of attention. In *The Attention Brain*, R. Parasuraman, ed. Cambridge, Mass.: MIT Press, pp. 35–50.

MATARO, M., C. GARCIA-SANCHEZ, C. JUNQUE, A. ESTEVEZ-GONZALEZ, and J. PUJOL, 1997. Magnetic resonance imaging measurement of the caudate nucleus in adolescents with attention-deficit hyperactivity disorder and its relationship with neuropsychological and behavioral measures. *Arch. Neurol.* 54:963–968.

MCALLISTER, A. K., L. C. KATZ, and D. C. LO, 1996. Neurotrophin regulation of cortical dendritic growth requires activity. *Neuron* 17:1057–1064.

MCEWEN, B. S., 2000. The neurobiology of stress: From serendipity to clinical relevance. *Brain. Res* 886:172–189.

MEHMET, H., X. YUE, M. V. SQUIER, A. LOREK, E. CADY, J. PENRICE, C. SARRAF, M. WYLEZINSKA, V. KIRKBRIDE, C. COOPER, et al., 1994. Increased apoptosis in the cingulate sulcus of newborn piglets following transient hypoxia-ischaemia is related to the degree of high energy phosphate depletion during the insult. *Neurosci. Lett.* 181:121–125.

MILL, J., S. CURRAN, L. KENT, A. GOULD, L. HUCKETT, S. RICHARDS, E. TAYLOR, and P. ASHERSON, 2002. Association study of a SNAP-25 microsatellite and attention deficit hyperactivity disorder. *Am. J. Med. Genet.* 114:269–271.

MILLER, M. B., J. D. VAN HORN, G. L. WOLFORD, T. C. HANDY, M. VALSANGKAR-SMYTH, S. INATI, S. GRAFTON, and M. S. GAZZANIGA, 2002. Extensive individual differences in brain activations associated with episodic retrieval are reliable over time. *J. Cogn. Neurosci.* 14:1200–1214.

MIRNICS, K., F. A. MIDDLETON, A. MARQUEZ, D. A. LEWIS, and P. LEVITT, 2000. Molecular characterization of schizophrenia viewed by microarray analysis of gene expression in prefrontal cortex. *Neuron* 28:53–67.

MODY, M., Y. CAO, Z. CUI, K. Y. TAY, A. SHYONG, E. SHIMIZU, K. PHAM, P. SCHULTZ, D. WELSH, and J. Z. TSIEN, 2001. Genome-wide gene expression profiles of the developing mouse hippocampus. *Proc. Natl. Acad. Sci. U.S.A.* 98:8862–8867.

MYLES-WORSLEY, M., and H. COON, 1997. Genetic and developmental factors in spontaneous selective attention: A study of normal twins. *Psychiatry Res.* 71:163–174.

MYLES-WORSLEY, M., H. COON, W. BYERLEY, M. WALDO, D. YOUNG, and R. FREEDMAN, 1996. Developmental and genetic influences on the P50 sensory gating phenotype. *Biol. Psychiatry* 39:289–295.

NIMCHINSKY, E. A., E. GILISSEN, J. M. ALLMAN, D. P. PERL, J. M. ERWIN, and P. R. HOF, 1999. A neuronal morphologic type unique to humans and great apes. *Proc. Natl. Acad. Sci. U.S.A.* 96:5268–5273.

OLSON, R. K., H. DATTA, J. GAYAN, and J. C. DEFRIES, 1999. A behavioral-genetic analysis of reading disabilities and component processes. In *Converging Methods for Understanding Reading and Dyslexia*, R. Klein and P. McMullen, eds. Cambridge, Mass.: MIT Press, pp. 133–151.

OPPENHEIM, J. S., J. E. SKERRY, M. J. TRAMO, and M. S. GAZZANIGA, 1989. Magnetic resonance imaging morphology of the corpus callosum in monozygotic twins. *Ann. Neurol.* 26:100–104.

OSEN-SAND, A., M. CATSICAS, J. K. STAPLE, K. A. JONES, G. AYALA, J. KNOWLES, G. GRENNINGLOH, and S. CATSICAS, 1993. Inhibition of axonal growth by SNAP-25 antisense oligonucleotides in vitro and in vivo. *Nature* 364:445–448.

PARDO, P. J., M. A. KNESEVICH, G. P. VOGLER, J. V. PARDO, B. TOWNE, C. R. CLONINGER, and M. I. POSNER, 2000. Genetic and state variables of neurocognitive dysfunction in schizophrenia: A twin study (in process citation). *Schizophr. Bull.* 26:459–477.

PENNINGTON, B. F., 2002. *The Development of Psychopathology: Nature and Nurture.* New York: Guilford Press.

POHJALAINEN, T., K. NAGREN, E. K. SYVALAHTI, and J. HIETALA, 1999. The dopamine D2 receptor 5′-flanking variant, −141C Ins/Del, is not associated with reduced dopamine D2 receptor density in vivo. *Pharmacogenetics* 9:505–509.

PORJESZ, B., H. BEGLEITER, T. REICH, P. VAN EERDEWEGH, H. J. EDENBERG, T. FOROUD, A. GOATE, A. LITKE, D. B. CHORLIAN, A. STIMUS, J. RICE, J. BLANGERO, L. ALMASY, J. SORBELL, L. O. BAUER, S. KUPERMAN, S. J. O'CONNOR, and J. ROHRBAUGH, 1998. Amplitude of visual P3 event-related potential as a phenotypic marker for a predisposition to alcoholism: Preliminary results from the COGA Project. Collaborative Study on the Genetics of Alcoholism. *Alcohol Clin. Exp. Res.* 22:1317–1323.

POSNER, M. I., 1980. Orienting of attention. The 7th Sir F. C. Bartlett Lecture. *Q. J. Exp. Psychol.* 32:3–25.

POSNER, M. I., and B. D. MCCANDLISS, 1999. In *Converging Methods for Understanding Reading and Dyslexia*, R. Klein and P. McMullen, eds. Cambridge, Mass.: MIT Press, pp. 305–337.

POSNER, M. I., and M. K. ROTHBART, 1998. Attention, self regulation and consciousness. *Philoso. Trans. R. Soc. Lond. B* 353:1915–1927.

POSNER, M. I., and M. K. ROTHBART, 2000. Developing mechanisms of self regulation. *Dev. Psychopathol.* 12:427–441.

ROCAMORA, N., E. WELKER, M. PASCUAL, and E. SORIANO, 1996. Upregulation of BDNF mRNA expression in the barrel cortex of adult mice after sensory stimulation. *J. Neurosci.* 16:4411–4419.

ROSENBERG, D. R., and D. A. LEWIS, 1995. Postnatal maturation of the dopaminergic innervation of monkey prefrontal and motor cortices: A tyrosine hydroxylase immunohistochemical analysis. *J. Comp. Neurol.* 358:383–400.

ROTHBART, M. K., and ••. ••. BATES, 1998. Temperament. In *Handbook of Child Psychology*, W. Damon, series ed., vol. 3, *Social, Emotional, and Personality Development* N. Eisenberg, vol. ed., 5th ed. New York: Wiley, pp. 105–176.

ROTHBART, M. K., and M. I. POSNER (in press). Temperament, attention, and developmental psychopathology. In *Manual of Developmental Psychopathology*, 2nd ed., D. Cicchetti, ed. New York: Wiley.

RUEDA, M. R., M. I. POSNER, and M. K. ROTHBART (in press). Attentional control and self regulation. In *Handbook of Self Regulation*, R. F. Baumeister and K. D. Vohs, eds. New York: Guilford Press.

SATO, M., H. KIYAMA, S. YOSHIDA, T. SAIKA, and M. TOHYAMA, 1991. Postnatal ontogeny of cells expressing prepro-neurotensin/neuromedin N mRNA in the rat forebrain and midbrain: A hybridization histochemical study involving isotope-labeled and enzyme-labeled probes. *J. Comp. Neurol.* 310:300–315.

SEAMAN, M. I., F. M. CHANG, A. T. QUINONES, and K. K. KIDD, 2000. Evolution of exon 1 of the dopamine D4 receptor (DRD4) gene in primates. *J. Exp. Zool.* 288:32–38.

SHAYWITZ, S. E., B. A. SHAYWITZ, K. R. PUGH, R. K. FULBRIGHT, R. T. CONSTABLE, W. E. MENCL, D. P. SHANKWEILER, A. M. LIBERMAN, P. SKUDLARSKI, J. M. FLETCHER, L. KATZ, K. E. MARCHIONE, C. LACADIE, C. GATENBY, and J. C. GORE, 1998. *Proc. Natl. Acad. Sci. U.S.A.* 95:2636–2641.

SHAYWITZ, B. A., S. E. SHAYWITZ, K. R. PUGH, W. E. MENCL, R. K. FULBRIGHT, P. SKUDLARSKI, R. T. CONSTABLE, K. E. MARCHIONE, J. M. FLETCHER, G. R. LYON, and J. C. GORE, 2002. Disruption of posterior brain systems for reading in children with developmental dyslexia. *Biol. Psychiatry* 52:101–110.

SHILLING, P. D., and J. R. KELSOE, 2002. Functional genomics approaches to understanding brain disorders. *Pharmacogenomics* 3:31–45.

SOBIN, C., K., KILEY-BRABECK, S. DANIELS, M. BLUNDELL, and KARAYIORGOU, 2003. Networks of attention in children with the 22q11 deletion syndrome. Unpublished manuscript.

SUAREZ, B. K., C. L. HAMPE, D. O'ROURKE, P. VAN EERDEWEGH, and T. REICH, 1995. Sib-based detection of qtls. *Genet. Epidemiol.* 12:675–680.

SWANSON, J., C. DEUTSCH, D. CANTWELL, M. POSNER, J. KENNDY, C. BARR, R. MOYZIS, S. SCHUCK, P. FLODMAN, and A. SPENCE, 2001. Genes and attention-deficit hyperactivity disorder. *Clin. Neurosci. Res.* 1:207–216.

SWANSON, J., J. OOSTERLAAN, M., MURIAS, R. MOYZIS, S. SCHUCK, M. MANN, P. FELDMAN, M. A. SPENCE, J. SERGEANT, M. SMITH, J. KENNEDY, and M. I. POSNER, 2000. ADHD children with 7-repeat allele of the DRD4 gene have extreme behavior but normal performance on critical neuropsychological tests of attention *Proc. Natl. Acad. Sci. U.S.A.* 97:4754–4759.

TEMPLE, E., G. K. DEUTSCH, R. A. POLDRACK, S. L. MILLER, P. TALLAL, M. M. MERZENICH, and J. A. GABRELI, 2003. Neural deficits in dyslexic children ameliorated by behavioral remediation: An fMRI study. *Proc. Natl. Acad. Sci. U.S.A.* 100:2860–2865.

TEMPLETON, A., 2002. Out of Africa again and again. *Nature* 416:45–51.

THOMPSON, P. M., T. D. CANNON, K. L. NARR, T. VAN ERP, V. P. POUTANEN, M. HUTTUNEN, J. LONNQVIST, C. G. STANDERTSKJOLD-NORDENSTAM, J. KAPRIO, M. KHALEDY, R. DAIL, C. I. ZOUMALAN, and A. W. TOGA, 2001. Genetic influences on brain structure. *Nat. Neurosci.* 4:1253–1258.

THOMPSON, P., T. D. CANNON, and A. W. TOGA, 2002. Mapping genetic influences on human brain structure. *Ann. Med.* 34:523–536.

THOMPSON, P. M., J. N. GIEDD, R. P. WOODS, D. MACDONALD, A. C. EVANS, and A. W. TOGA, 2000. Growth patterns in the developing brain detected by using continuum mechanical tensor maps. *Nature* 404:190–193.

TRAMO, M. J., W. C. LOFTUS, T. A. STUKEL, R. L. GREEN, J. B. WEAVER, and M. S. GAZZANIGA, 1998. Brain size, head size, and intelligence quotient in monozygotic twins. *Neurology* 50:246–252.

VIGERS, A. J., Z. C. BAQUET, and K. R. JONES, 2000. Expression of neurotrophin-3 in the mouse forebrain: Insights from a targeted LacZ reporter. *J. Comp. Neurol.* 416:398–415.

VOGEL, G. Development: Brain cells reveal surprising versatility. *Science* 288:1559–1560.

WASSINK, T. H., J. J. NELSON, R. R. CROWE, and N. C. ANDREASEN, 1999. Heritability of BDNF alleles and their effect on brain morphology in schizophrenia. *Am. J. Med. Genet.* 88:724–728.

WEILER, I. J., S. A. IRWIN, A. Y. KLINTSOVA, C. M. SPENCER, A. D. BRAZELTON, K. MIYASHIRO, T. A. COMERY, B. PATEL, J. EBERWINE, and W. T. GREENOUGH, 1997. Fragile X mental retardation protein is translated near synapses in response to neurotransmitter activation. *Proc. Natl. Acad. Sci. U.S.A.* 94: 5395–5400.

WILSON, M. C., 2000. Coloboma mouse mutant as an animal model of hyperkinesis and attention deficit hyperactivity disorder. *Neurosci. Biobehav. Rev.* 24:51–57.

WISNIEWSKI, K. E., S. M. SEGAN, C. M. MIEZEJESKI, E. A. SERSEN, and R. D. RUDELLI, 1991. The Fra(X) syndrome: Neurological, electrophysiological, and neuropathological abnormalities. *Am. J. Med. Genet.* 38:476–480.

WOLFSBERG, T. G., K. A. WETTERSTRAND, M. S. GUYER, F. S. COLLINS, and A. D. BAXEVANIS, 2003. A user's guide to the human genome. *Nat. Genet.* 35(Suppl 1):4.

YOUNG, D. A., M. WALDO, J. H. RUTLEDGE, 3rd, and R. FREEDMAN, 1996. Heritability of inhibitory gating of the P50 auditory-evoked potential in monozygotic and dizygotic twins. *Neuropsychobiology* 33:113–117.

YUN, K., S. POTTER, and J. L. RUBENSTEIN, 2001. Gsh2 and Pax6 play complementary roles in dorsoventral patterning of the mammalian telencephalon. *Development* 128:193–205.

Web Sites for gene expression, gene targeting, and genotyping

Gene Expression Omnibus
http://www.ncbi.nlm.nih.gov/geo/

Expressed Gene Anatomy Database
http://www.tigr.org/tdb/egad/egad.shtml

Gene Expression Database
http://www.informatics.jax.org/mgihome/GXD/aboutGXD.shtml

Edinburgh mouse atlas project
http://genex.hgu.mrc.ac.uk/

Princeton Brain Genomics
http://braingenomics.princeton.edu/tsien/index.html

TBASE (database of gene targeted mice)
http://tbase.jax.org/

Bioserve Inc. (genotyping)
http://www.bioserve.com/

Sequenom Inc. (genotyping)
http://www.sequenom.com/

91 Functional Imaging, Neurophysiology, and the Resting State of the Human Brain

DEBRA A. GUSNARD AND MARCUS E. RAICHLE

ABSTRACT In this chapter, the physiological underpinnings of functional imaging signals and their significance for a more complete understanding of functional imaging studies are described. The physiological basis of brain functional imaging studies is related to a remarkable relationship between local brain blood flow, metabolism, and cellular function. When cell function changes, blood flow and metabolism change as well, making it possible for brain imaging to monitor local changes in cellular actively with great fidelity. Recent advances in our understanding of brain energy consumption at "rest" are beginning to inform us about the nature of ongoing brain activity and how such local changes are to be considered in relation to it. In this context, the physiological basis for understanding imaging activations versus so-called deactivations will also be discussed.

Thirty years ago, the introduction of x-ray computed tomography (CT) set in motion a revolution in medical imaging that changed forever the practice of medicine (Hounsfield, 1973). The introduction of CT also proved to be an immediate and powerful catalyst for the development of other imaging techniques, particularly positron emission tomography (PET) and magnetic resonance imaging (MRI) (for historical perspectives, see Kevles, 1997; Webb, 1990). With the development of PET and MRI came the opportunity to noninvasively image not only the anatomy of organs within the living human but also their function (Raichle, 2000).

With these new imaging techniques, researchers interested in the function of the human brain were presented with an unprecedented opportunity to examine the neurobiological correlates of human behaviors. As a result, not only has there been an exponential increase in the number of publications on functional brain imaging, there is also a worldwide movement to establish research imaging centers in which expensive imaging equipment, primarily MRI scanners, and teams of investigators are devoted exclusively to

research. Currently there are more than 60 such centers (for a partial listing, see Raichle, 2003).

Despite this success, some researchers have questioned the ability of functional imaging techniques to truly enlighten us about the relationship between human behavior and brain function (see, e.g., Nichols and Newsome, 1999; Uttal, 2001). One way to address such concerns is to relate and compare work in cognitive neuroscience and imaging with parallel work in other areas of neuroscience.

In this chapter, we address some of the issues that are currently confronting researchers using functional imaging techniques. These include the relationship between imaging signals and brain neurophysiology, and the implications of this relationship for interpreting functional imaging studies. In addition, we will define the concept of a physiological baseline of the brain from the perspective of functional imaging and consider some of its properties on the basis of information derived from neurophysiology and computational neuroscience. Finally, we will discuss the resting state—unconstrained cognition associated with being awake with the eyes closed—and its relationship to the physiological baseline.

Imaging and brain cellular neurophysiology

Cognitive neuroscientists might well question why they need to know anything about the relationship between the cellular neurophysiology of the brain and the imaging signals that they employ in their quest to understand the relationship between brain function and human behaviors at the systems level. After all, we have known for more than a century that local changes in brain blood flow accompany changes in local neuronal activity in a remarkably consistent manner (Raichle, 2000). What more do cognitive neuroscientists need to know? As always, the answer to such a question lies in the details. Until recently, these details were available only in sketchy form and in obscure sources. Recently, they have begun to emerge in clearer form, and have been clarified and elaborated in specific experiments (for recent reviews, see Logothetis, 2003; Lauritzen and Gold, 2003).

DEBRA A. GUSNARD Departments of Radiology and Psychiatry, Washington University, St. Louis, Mo.

MARCUS E. RAICHLE Departments of Radiology, Neurology, and Neurobiology, Washington University, St. Louis, Mo.

1267

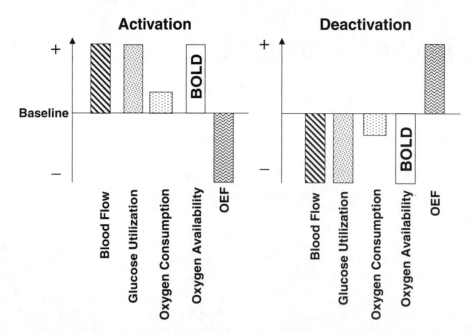

FIGURE 91.1 From a functional brain imaging perspective, activations and deactivations are defined in terms of regional changes in blood flow, oxygen consumption, and glucose utilization. Activation, or an increase in neuronal activity, is associated with increases in blood flow and glucose utilization to about the same degree. Oxygen consumption, while it may increase, does so to a much lesser degree. This results in an increase in the baseline ratio of oxygen consumption to blood flow, referred to as the oxygen extraction fraction (OEF), such that the increased supply of oxygen during activation exceeds the increased demand. As a result, the tissue oxygen availability increases and results in the BOLD signal of fMRI. Deactivation is simply the reverse of these phenomena.

IMAGING SIGNAL INCREASES We begin by reviewing the basic features of the functional imaging signal (figure 91.1). The imaging signal reflects changes in local blood flow within the brain (Raichle, 1998). In addition, there is an increase in the metabolism of glucose that parallels in magnitude and spatial extent the change in blood flow (see, e.g., Hand and Greenberg, cited in Woolsey et al., 1996; Ueki, Linn, and Hossmann, 1988). The change in local consumption of oxygen is much smaller in magnitude than either the increase in blood flow or glucose utilization (Fox and Raichle, 1986; Fox et al., 1988). As a result, there is an increase in the local blood oxygen content (i.e., the supply of oxygen exceeds the demand). This local increase in blood oxygen content forms the basis for the blood-oxygen-level-dependent (BOLD) signal of fMRI (Ogawa et al., 1990; Raichle, 1998; see figure 91.1).

Early in the course of trying to understand how such changes might relate to underlying neurophysiological events, researchers made two rather important observations. First, in early calculations of the amount of energy used by a neuron to fire an action potential (i.e., to spike), Creutzfeldt estimated that the spike activity of neurons accounted for a small fraction of the total energy consumption of the vertebrate brain (i.e., <3%) (Creutzfeldt, 1975). At the time, this was a most puzzling observation to those considering the energy requirements associated with behaviorally induced changes in blood flow. For the most part this observation was ignored because of the general belief that changes in blood flow reflected changes in the spiking activity or output of neurons.

In 1979, Schwartz and colleagues made a second important observation. Using a newly developed method for autoradiographically measuring brain glucose metabolism in animal experiments (Schwartz et al., 1979), they observed that stimulating the activity of neurons in the hypothalamus of rodents resulted not in increased glucose utilization in the area of the cell bodies of the stimulated neurons but, rather, in increased glucose metabolism in the terminal fields of these neurons some distance away, in the anterior pituitary gland.

These two early and important observations suggested that imaging signals would be directly related not to the spiking activity of neurons (i.e., their output) but to changes in their input occurring in axon terminals and dendrites. Despite the importance of these observations, they were little appreciated in the early days of imaging.

Recent experimental results have dramatically refocused our attention on the implications of these earlier data and the interpretation of modern functional imaging signals. Work by Logothetis and colleagues (2001) provided the first truly comprehensive look at the relationship between the fMRI signal and the underlying neural activity. Their results emerge from pioneering work on the development of functional MRI in monkeys instrumented to record, simultaneously with imaging, the cellular electrical activity within the brain (Logothetis et al., 1999; Logothetis, 2003).

Their work has shown that a spatially localized increase in the fMRI signal, in this instance in the visual cortex of the monkey while the latter sat in an MRI scanner viewing checkerboard patterns, directly and monotonically reflects an increase in neural activity. The time course of the fMRI signal, which is based on a vascular response to the neural activity and begins about 2 s after the onset of the electrical activity and reaches a plateau in about 7 s, was shown to be a temporally delayed and dispersed reflection of the underlying neuronal activity (see also Boynton et al., 1996).

Several aspects of the neuronal activity were analyzed by Logothetis and colleagues (Logothetis et al., 2001; Logothetis, 2003). With their electrical recording techniques, they were able to distinguish between the all-or-none instantaneous firing rates of individual neurons and groups of neurons (i.e., action potentials) reflecting their output, and relatively slowly varying electrical potentials (i.e., local field potentials, LFPs) arising from the input to and integrative processes within and among neurons. The electrophysiological measure most highly correlated with the fMRI signal turned out to be the LFP. Thus, activation of an area of the brain as seen by fMRI predominantly reflects the incoming input to and the local information processing within an area of the brain, a finding that had been anticipated by Schwartz and colleagues (1979) more than 20 years earlier.

Complementary work by Lauritzen and colleagues in the rat cerebellar cortex (Mathiesen et al., 1998; Mathiesen, Caesar, and Lauritzen, 2000; Lauritzen and Gold, 2003) has demonstrated unequivocal dissociations between the spiking rates of neurons and changes in local blood flow. That is, stimulating inhibitory inputs to cerebellar Purkinje cells caused spiking to cease yet blood flow to rise in a stimulation-dependent manner. Likewise, stimulating excitatory inputs to the Purkinje cells changed the pattern of firing without changing the total number of spikes per unit time. Again, blood flow increased in a stimulation-dependent manner.

Thus, the degree to which spiking activity is correlated with imaging signals probably depends on the balance of excitatory and inhibitory activity in their input during activations.

IMAGING SIGNAL DECREASES Although most of the work analyzing the relationship between neurophysiology and functional brain imaging signals has focused on the neural correlates of imaging signal increases (activations), researchers have become increasingly aware of the fact that signal decreases (so-called deactivations) also occur. The interpretation of these decreases has been challenging and

has resulted in differing opinions as to their origin and significance (Tootell et al., 1998; Smith, Singh, and Greenlee, 2000; Shmuel et al., 2002). In discussing these signal decreases, we note at the outset that they are very unlikely to be due to local inhibitory processes, because the latter are known to require energy and are as likely to be associated with signal increases as are excitatory processes (Ackerman et al., 1984; Lauritzen, 2001; Lauritzen and Gold, 2003).

In this section, we review evidence concerning the underlying physiology of signal decreases as they occur in a task-specific manner in some imaging paradigms. We refer to these decreases as *task-dependent* decreases (TDDs) because the areas of the brain involved vary with the task. In the next section, we examine other signal decreases. These signal decreases we refer to as *task-independent* decreases (TIDs) because they are relatively independent of the details (e.g., sensory input, motor responses, cognitive operations) of any particular goal-directed behavior. Interestingly, TIDs, in contrast to TDDs, occur outside of primary sensory cortices. This distinction is likely to be of considerable conceptual importance as we consider functional distinctions between TDDs and TIDs.

TDDs in imaging signal intensity have been noted for some time. They appear to occur exclusively within or between perceptual systems (e.g., visual, somatosensory, or auditory). Thus, subjects may exhibit decreases in activity in auditory or somatosensory cortices when engaging in a task involving visual perception (e.g., Haxby et al., 1994; Kawashima, O'Sullivan, and Roland, 1995; Ghatan et al., 1998). Likewise, tasks involving elements of the visual or somatosensory systems, but not others within the same sensory system, will induce increases in some elements and decreases in others (e.g., Drevets et al., 1995; Shmuel et al., 2001, 2002; Tootell, Tsao, and Vanduffel, 2003).

An initial speculation by some investigators was that decreases in imaging signal merely represented the stealing of nutritive resources from areas adjacent to those experiencing an increased need for blood flow. Such a concept appeared to receive some support from work on the brain microvasculature at the capillary level (Woolsey et al., 1996), but other evidence has suggested that these observations cannot be extrapolated to the larger areas of brain normally seen in functional imaging studies. For example, the actual changes in local blood flow associated with increased cognitive activity are very small (a few percent locally in the cortex) relative to the overall blood flow to the brain. In fact, these local changes are so small that changes in total brain blood flow cannot be measured during cognitive activity (Sokoloff et al., 1955; Fox et al., 1985; Fox, Burton, and Raichle, 1987; Fox, Miezin, et al., 1987). A second argument against the stealing of nutritive resources is that the hemodynamic reserve of the brain is very large (Heistad and Kontos, 1983). Thus, the brain can double its blood flow when the need arises (e.g., during an epileptic seizure; Plum, Posner, and Troy, 1968). Finally, the decreases can occur remote from the site of the increases (G. L. Shulman, Corbetta, Buckner, Fiez, et al., 1997; G. L. Shulman, Corbetta, Buckner, Raichle, et al., 1997; G. L. Shulman, Fiez, et al., 1997) or in the absence of increases altogether (Raichle et al., 2001), making a steal within a given vascular territory an unlikely explanation.

Recent neurophysiological observations (Gold and Lauritzen, 2002; Shmuel, Augath, Oeltermann, et al., 2003; Shmuel, Augath, Rounis, et al., 2003) indicate that these signal decreases are the result of decreases in neuronal activity, in particular, decreases in LFPs. Thus, TDDs are reasonably posited to reflect the suppression or "gating" of information processing in areas not engaged in task performance, as has been suggested (see, e.g., Drevets et al., 1995). This gating in turn may facilitate the processing of information expected to carry behavioral significance by filtering out unattended sensory input.

SUMMARY There are clear lessons for cognitive neuroscientists from these many observations on the neurophysiological correlates of functional imaging signals. First, increases and decreases in imaging signals unequivocally reflect changes in neuronal activity. Second, neurophysiology traditionally has emphasized recording the output of neurons in a particular brain area, while imaging informs us about the input to and the local information processing within it. The absence of a correlation between the signals obtained with single-cell recording studies and functional imaging studies (when they occur) does not necessarily invalidate the results of either approach. Third, the imaging signal changes that are observed may consist of both increases and decreases as the information processing architecture is sculpted to address particular task demands.

The physiologic baseline

OVERALL BRAIN METABOLISM It is important to maintain a sense of proportion when it comes to viewing functional imaging signals. In the average adult human, the brain represents about 2% of the total body weight. Remarkably, despite its relatively small size, the brain accounts for about 20% of the oxygen consumed, and hence of the calories consumed, by the body (Clark and Sokoloff, 1999), 10 times that predicted by its weight alone. In relation to this very high rate of baseline metabolism, regional imaging signals are remarkably small, in metabolic terms often less than 5% of the ongoing metabolism of the brain in that particular area (figure 91.2). These are modest modulations in ongoing or baseline activity and do not appreciably effect the overall metabolic rate of the brain (Sokoloff et al., 1955; Fox et al., 1985; Fox, Burton, et al., 1987; Fox, Miezin, et al., 1987).

The modest nature of activations and deactivations compared to the brain's baseline metabolic rate and blood flow is further emphasized when we consider their relative energy consumption. The baseline metabolic activity is largely (~99%) supported (Siesjo, 1978) by the complete oxidation of glucose to carbon dioxide and water, where one molecule of glucose produces energy in the form of 30 ATP molecules. Activations, on the other hand, exhibit a disproportionate increase in glycolysis (Fox et al., 1988) (i.e., the metabolism of glucose to lactate without the consumption of oxygen), which produces a meager 2 ATPs per molecule of glucose consumed. An important advantage to the glycolytic route is that its rate of ATP production is much faster (twice that of oxidative metabolism), which would be in keeping with the speed required for activations that occur on a time scale of milliseconds, far faster than the characteristic vascular response time (Boynton et al., 1996; Buckner et al., 1996).

Presently, the most parsimonious explanation for this increase in glycolysis during brain activation is that it is related to metabolic changes in astrocytes associated with increased clearance of glutamate from the synapse (see, e.g., Magistretti et al., 1999; Shulman, Hyder, and Rothman, 2001; see also Mintun et al., 2001). It has recently been suggested that the astrocyte provides a critical link between neurons and blood vessels in orchestrating the changes in blood flow associated with changes in neuronal activity (Zonta et al., 2003). Thus, currently available information suggests an important role for the astrocyte, along with neurons and blood vessels, in the cell biology of functional brain imaging signals.

DEFINING A PHYSIOLOGICAL BASELINE Before exploring the potential functions of the very large baseline energy consumption of the brain, it is important to define more precisely what we mean by a physiological baseline and how it is to be distinguished from activations and deactivations.

The definition of a baseline that we use here is physiologically based. It has arisen in the context of a functional imaging framework. Although this perspective and the terminology used to define it may be unfamiliar to many in cognitive neuroscience, we believe they have utility for developing a more complete understanding of the true role of functional imaging in probing brain function. We suggest that familiarity with the concept of a physiological baseline expands the possibility of exploring many issues, including aspects of individual differences, changes consequent on disease, and complex functions such as spontaneous thought processes, consciousness, and subjectivity.

To begin, researchers interested in blood flow and metabolic relationships in the brain have appreciated the close match between local blood flow and oxygen utilization aver-

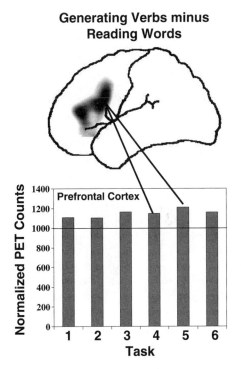

**Generating Verbs minus
Reading Words**

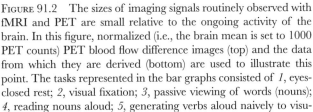

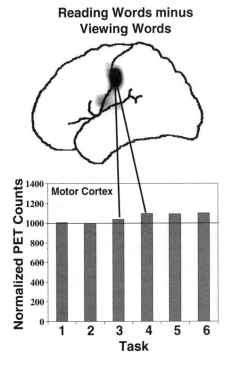

**Reading Words minus
Viewing Words**

FIGURE 91.2   The sizes of imaging signals routinely observed with fMRI and PET are small relative to the ongoing activity of the brain. In this figure, normalized (i.e., the brain mean is set to 1000 PET counts) PET blood flow difference images (top) and the data from which they are derived (bottom) are used to illustrate this point. The tasks represented in the bar graphs consisted of *1*, eyes-closed rest; *2*, visual fixation; *3*, passive viewing of words (nouns); *4*, reading nouns aloud; *5*, generating verbs aloud naively to visu- ally presented nouns; and *6*, generating verbs aloud to the same nouns after practice (data from Petersen et al., 1988). Task-induced changes in blood flow are small relative to the overall regional blood flow. Also, the resting mean blood flow in the two areas (Task 1 in both graphs) is different. The prefrontal cortex mean (left) is sig- nificantly above the brain mean, whereas the motor cortex mean (right) is not. (The horizontal line in both graphs indicates the brain mean.)

aged over time (data obtained with PET usually over ~30 minutes; Mintun et al., 1984) in normal adult humans lying quietly in a PET scanner with eyes closed but awake (Raichle et al., 2001; figure 91.3). This relationship is often expressed in terms of the ratio of oxygen consumption to oxygen deliv- ery. This ratio (~0.40 in the adult human) is known as the oxygen extraction fraction (OEF) and is characterized by its spatial uniformity. This spatial uniformity in the OEF exists despite marked regional differences in both blood flow and oxygen consumption between gray matter and white matter, as well as among gray matter areas (see figure 91.3). It is important to emphasize that this uniformity exists only when data are averaged across time and individuals, a point to which we will return later.

Activation in the context of functional brain imaging may be defined as a fall in the average resting OEF that results from a local increase in blood flow that is not accompanied by a commensurate increase in oxygen consumption (Fox and Raichle, 1986; Fox et al., 1988; see figure 91.1). This leads to increased local blood oxygen content, which is responsible for the fMRI BOLD signal (Ogawa et al., 1990). Activation in these terms represents a regional change in the relationship between oxygen delivery (i.e., blood flow ×

blood oxygen content = oxygen delivery per unit time), which increases because blood flow increases, and oxygen utilization, which does not increase as much (Fox and Raichle, 1986; Fox et al., 1988).

From the above it follows that a physiological baseline can be defined as the *average* OEF obtained across individuals or within an individual across time while they rest quietly with eyes closed, but awake. Activations are deviations from this baseline as reflected in local reductions in the OEF or increases in the fMRI BOLD signal (Raichle et al., 2001). Put simply, we are here defining the physiological baseline as the absence of activation in terms of an average OEF.

Heretofore, the OEF has been used almost exclusively to characterize the relationship between regional blood flow and oxygen consumption in the diseased brain, particularly where various forms of cerebrovascular disease have com- promised blood flow (Grubb et al., 1998; Marchal et al., 1993). Historically, the uniformity of the averaged OEF at rest in the normal brain and its implications were not con- sidered for the defining of a physiologic baseline.

IMPLICATIONS OF A PHYSIOLOGIC BASELINE   The uniformity of the OEF in averaged data obtained at rest in the normal

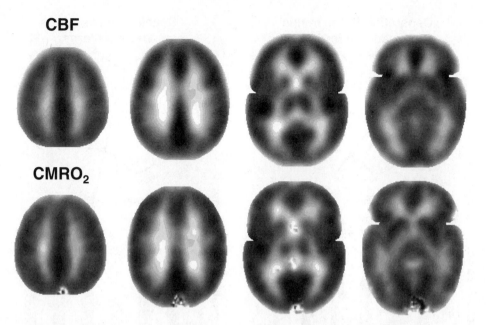

CBF

CMRO₂

FIGURE 91.3   Averaged resting measurements of cerebral blood flow (CBF) and the cerebral metabolic rate for oxygen (CMRO₂) in 19 normal adult subjects resting quietly awake in the scanner with eyes closed. Of note is the remarkably close correspondence between CMRO₂ and CBF. This relationship is reflected in the OEF, which is the ratio of these two images (see text for further discussion). As a result of their similarity, there is remarkable uniformity in OEF throughout the brain despite the large regional differences in both CBF and CMRO₂. (Data are from Group 1 in Raichle et al., 2001.)

brain suggests that equilibrium exists between the local metabolic requirements necessary to sustain an ongoing level of neural activity and the blood flow in that region. We have suggested (Gusnard and Raichle, 2001; Raichle et al., 2001) that this equilibrium state identifies a baseline level of neuronal activity. Consequently, areas with a reduction in this equilibrium OEF (i.e., an increase in the BOLD signal of fMRI; see figure 91.1) are defined as *activated* (i.e., neural activity is increased above baseline level). Those areas not differing from the brain mean OEF are considered to be at *baseline*. In this scheme, increases in the OEF (i.e., decreases in the BOLD signal; see figure 91.1) define areas of *deactivation* (i.e., neural activity is decreased below the baseline level). It is important to note that obvious decreases in the OEF from the brain mean, which would indicate areas of activation (Raichle, 1998), are *not* present in averaged data from subjects resting quietly with eyes closed.

When subjects' eyes are closed, areas of apparent deactivation (increased OEF) primarily in extrastriate visual areas are clearly present, however (see Figure 4 in Raichle et al., 2001). These regional increases in OEF were also noted in some of the earliest PET work on normal humans (Lebrun-Grandie et al., 1983), although their possible significance was not appreciated. Their presence suggests that the physiological baseline for these extrastriate visual areas may well be associated with eyes open. In support of this hypothesis, eye opening appears to increase blood flow in these areas (Raichle et al., 2001).

Thus, we propose that there exists a physiological baseline of the human brain that is closely approximated in data averaged across time and subjects when they are awake and resting with eyes closed. (An exception exists for some extrastriate visual areas, as noted earlier.) Further, this physiological baseline accounts for the majority of the brain's metabolic requirements. Evidence suggests that this physiological baseline may inhere functionally significant signaling processes. We now turn to a consideration of the evidence.

UNACCOUNTED-FOR NEURONAL ACTIVITY   Several lines of evidence strongly suggest that the baseline metabolic activity of the brain may be related, at least in part, to functionally significant signaling processes. From an imaging perspective, measurements of brain energy metabolism using magnetic resonance spectroscopy (MRS) (Sibson et al., 1998; R. G. Shulman, Hyder, and Rothman, 2001; Hyder, Rothman, and Shulman, 2002) in a variety of experimental settings have indicated that up to 80% of the entire energy consumption of the brain is devoted to glutamate cycling, and hence to signaling processes. In a parallel analysis of extant anatomical and physiological data, Attwell and Laughlin (2001) assessed the energy expenditure on different components of excitatory signaling in the gray matter. Their analysis suggests a similar distribution of components of energy consumption as that measured with MRS (Sibson et al., 1998; R. G. Shulman, Hyder, and Rothman, 2001;

Hyder, Rothman, and Shulman, 2002), with approximately 75% of the total consumption being devoted to various aspects of signaling. A considerable portion of the remaining energy consumption is thought to relate to housekeeping functions—protein synthesis, axonal transport, and so on.

Another line of evidence comes from neurophysiological studies. Specifically, neurophysiologists have noted electrical activity that does not bear any obvious relationship to specific sensory or motor tasks, and have usually referred to this as spontaneous activity (Arieli et al., 1996; McCormick, 1999; Tsodyks et al., 1999; Sanchez-Vives and McCormick, 2000; Shu, Hasenstaub, and McCormick, 2003). There has been increasing interest in the possibility that in the adult brain this spontaneous activity is not merely noise (see, e.g., Ferster, 1996; McCormick, 1999).

When recorded in terms of spikes, this spontaneous activity is relatively low in frequency and seemingly random, compared with vigorous bursts of activity seen during task performance. It has been suggested that this difference in activity may bear a relationship to the nature of representation or neural coding of information, which offers differential economies of energy use as well (Attwell and Laughlin, 2001). The representation of information as the simultaneous activity of a large number of neurons has been referred to as distributed coding and is highly energy-efficient. By contrast, sparse coding, which has been related to the firing of fewer neurons, has the advantage of higher temporal resolution and hence may be more appropriate for activations, but is much more costly in terms of energy use (Attwell and Laughlin, 2001).

One might posit that in the physiological baseline, where oxidative metabolism is the primary source of energy, there has developed a very efficient strategy to manage large amounts of information on a sustained or long-term basis. This would complement the situation for activations, in which glycolysis assumes an important role as a source of energy (Fox et al., 1988), which may have the potential for supporting more specific, rapidly varying, and time-limited information processing required for immediate purposes (table 91.1).

The nature of unaccounted-for neuronal activity Thus, in addition to the signaling revealed to cognitive neuroscientists as activations and to neurophysiologists as changes in the spiking activity of neurons, there remains a large reservoir of unaccounted-for neuronal activity that commands a large percentage of the brain's energy resources, and whose functional significance remains to be fully explained.

Are there any clues to the nature of this baseline neuronal activity? In one view, it may serve a preparatory or facilitatory processing role. Thus, from a physiological perspective, it has been suggested that the response of neuronal circuits

TABLE 91.1

Suggested features of brain activity relevant to the distinction between a physiologic baseline and activations*

Feature	Physiological Baseline	Activations
Energy consumption	High	Low
Energy source	Oxidative metabolism	Glycolysis
Temporal features	Sustained	Transient
Neural coding	Distributed	Sparse
Representation of information	More abstract (?)	Less abstract (?)

* These suggestions provide a potential basis for hypothesis generation and future research.

is dramatically affected by a continuous and balanced input of both inhibitory and excitatory activity (for review, see Salinas and Sejnowski, 2001). This balanced activity has been implicated in the generation of spontaneous activity (Steriade, Timofeev, and Grenier, 2001; Shu, Hasenstaub, and McCormick, 2003) and has been demonstrated to facilitate the responsivity of neurons to other incoming signals (Shadlen and Newsome, 1994; van Vreeswijk and Sompolinsky, 1996; Salinas and Sejnowski, 2001; Shu, Hasenstaub, and McCormick, 2003).

From this perspective it might be argued that such a facilitatory process may be a necessary and expensive component of brain function, but not one that directly involves information processing with inherent functionality. However, some have suggested that information processing might in fact be a property of such a state (e.g., Tononi and Edelman, 1998; Shu, Hasenstaub, and McCormick, 2003). Here, functional brain imaging with both PET and fMRI provides a potentially unique perspective. This emanates directly from the observation of the previously mentioned *task-independent decreases* (TIDs) that occur from the physiological baseline during the performance of a wide variety of goal-directed tasks.

TASK-INDEPENDENT DECREASES (TIDs) As already stated, functional brain imaging has demonstrated not only task-dependent increases (activations) and TDDs, but also the presence of a unique set of areas that exhibit decreases in activity in averaged data obtained relative to a passive resting state condition (see figure 91.4 and figure 91.6). These occur across a wide spectrum of goal-directed tasks and so are referred to here as task-independent decreases. They have been seen in medial prefrontal and parietal cortices, as well as in lateral parietal cortex bilaterally and the amygdalae (G. L. Shulman, Fiez, et al., 1997; Mazoyer et al., 2001). The magnitude of some of these decreases in activity has been noted to vary with such factors as task difficulty (McKiernan

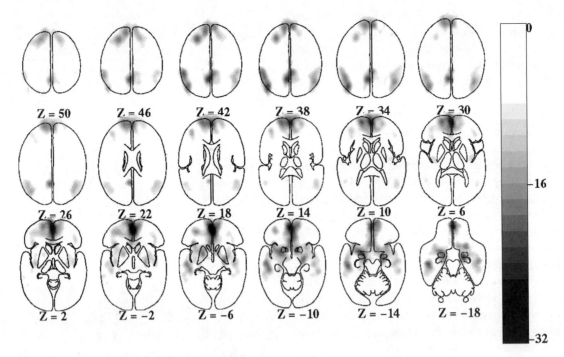

FIGURE 91.4 Areas of the brain observed to have task-independent decreases in activity during a wide variety of goal-directed behaviors. In this instance, data from nine different PET imaging experiments involving a total of 134 subjects were averaged (G. L. Shulman, Fiez, et al., 1997).

et al., 2003) and the emotional state of the subject (Simpson et al., 2001).

Current evidence (Raichle et al., 2001) indicates that the TIDs noted on functional imaging studies do not correspond to activations in the resting state, as has been suggested (Mazoyer et al., 2001), but arise from the physiological baseline (for a more detailed defense of this assertion, see Raichle et al., 2001). This suggests to us that they might more appropriately be referred to as areas that, in the resting state, are active rather than activated. This would be consistent with functions that are spontaneous and virtually continuous, being attenuated only when we engage in goal-directed behaviors; hence our designation of them as "default" functions (Raichle et al., 2001).

Binder and colleagues have suggested that these areas contribute to the "thought" processing that humans experience during resting consciousness (Binder et al., 1999), while Mazoyer and colleagues (Mazoyer et al., 2001) have suggested that they represent "cortical networks for working memory and executive functions that sustain the conscious resting state" in humans. Interestingly, David Ingvar articulated similar notions many years ago (Ingvar, 1985).

Consideration of the TID areas together rather than separately may suggest the need for descriptions that do not simply emerge from their individual functions. Accumulating evidence (for review, see Gusnard and Raichle, 2001) suggests, for example, that these ongoing processes are likely to be involved in activities having strong survival value for the individual in a passive state, such as detection and evaluation of novelty and biological motion in the environment as well as monitoring of his or her own internal states (including bodily states and thought processes). These processes would only be attenuated as the individual reallocated resources, including attentional resources, in the service of engaging in goal-directed behaviors. A possible mechanism by which such reallocation might be accomplished is through modulation of cortical regional activity by subcortical structures (figure 91.5).

Interestingly, evidence suggests that some of the areas involved in TIDs, particularly posteriorly, are also attenuated in their activity during normal REM and non-REM sleep (for review, see Maquet, 2000) and general anesthesia (Fiset et al., 1999). Also, recent reports indicate that many of the areas of TID exhibit reduced activity during absence seizures (Salek-Haddadi et al., 2003) and during generalized spike-and-wave discharges in patients with generalized epilepsy (Khani et al., 2003). Such findings raise the possibility of these areas having some relationship to states of awareness.

The resting state

One of the challenges of determining whether TIDs indicate the presence of default functions within the physiological baseline is to know how they relate to resting state cognition. In this regard, two recent observations using novel

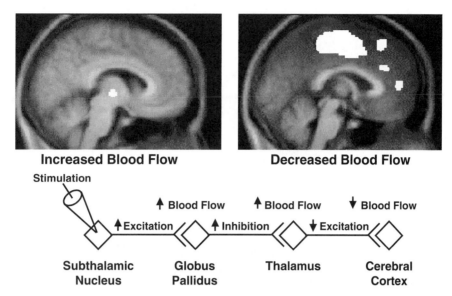

Increased Blood Flow   **Decreased Blood Flow**

FIGURE 91.5   PET images of blood flow differences during the stimulation of the subthalamic nucleus in 13 patients with Parkinson's disease. The voxel clusters that achieved statistical significance are shown on composite MRI structural (sagittal) images. During this procedure, blood flow increased in the subthalamic nucleus (site of stimulation, not shown), globus pallidus (not shown), and thalamus (upper left), and decreased in areas of the cerebral cortex (upper right). A diagram of the circuitry involved in these changes is presented schematically. Two points relating imaging signals and neurophysiology are nicely illustrated by these data. First, blood flow changes (and BOLD in fMRI) reflect the input to neurons.

When input activity increases, whether as excitation or inhibition, blood flow increases (globus pallidus and thalamus) even though output activity may decrease (as in this case from the thalamus). When input activity decreases, blood flow decreases (cerebral cortex). Second, with regard to activity decreases from the physiologic baseline (both TDDs and TIDs), the relationships depicted in this example provide a means of thinking about potential subcortical mechanisms underlying such decreases in the cerebral cortex. (Data were adapted from Hershey et al., 2003, by permission of the authors.)

approaches to the study of the resting state (i.e., awake, eyes closed, unconstrained cognition) provide interesting new information relevant to the relationships among the resting state, TIDs, and a physiological baseline as we have defined it.

Using an imaging strategy that has been used in several laboratories (Coren, 1969; Biswal et al., 1995; Lowe, Mock, and Sorenson, 1998; Xiong et al., 1999), Greicius and colleagues (2002) explored the interregional temporal correlations of spontaneous BOLD signal fluctuations in the resting state using regions of interest (ROIs) in posterior cingulate and precuneus, as well as the ventral anterior cingulate cortex. These ROIs are among those regularly exhibiting TIDs. What emerged was evidence for significant correlations in the spontaneous activity among a group of areas almost identical with those that have been identified with the TIDs (see figure 91.4 and figure 91.6).

Up to this point, the evidence for a network of interrelated areas exhibiting coordinated activity in the resting state has been indirect. This evidence has consisted of demonstrations of TIDs, which represent areas that are attenuated in their activity relative to the resting state condition. This paper by Greicius and colleagues (2002) is the first to provide direct evidence of coordinated activity in the same network of areas in the resting state.

These results make it clear that the resting state is not equivalent to the physiological baseline state of the brain. This is because the correlated regional temporal variations in the BOLD signal, an approximate surrogate for the OEF, indicate changes in brain activity during the resting state that could potentially be in the form of either activations (increases) or deactivations (decreases) from the physiological baseline (the direction of change from the physiological baseline cannot be determined from the fMRI signal). Does this then argue, as Mazoyer and colleagues (2001) have done, that TIDs merely represent activations in the resting state that return to the physiological baseline during goal-directed behaviors? We think not. Our reasoning is as follows.

Averaging such variable resting state activity across time and individuals, as has been done using PET and fMRI, could result in the presence of a mean signal change relative to the baseline. If the changes were, on average, increases above the baseline, activations should be detectable in the averaged resting state image, as predicted by Mazoyer and colleagues (2001). Alternatively, if the changes were, on average, decreases from the baseline, deactivations should be detectable in the averaged resting state image. However, we have actually measured the OEF in averaged resting state PET images in two groups of normal individuals (Raichle et al., 2001). Neither activations nor deactivations were

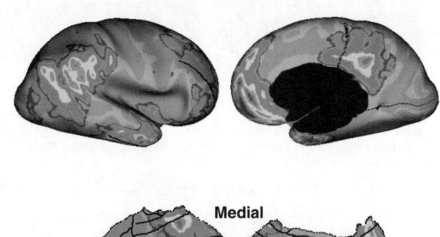

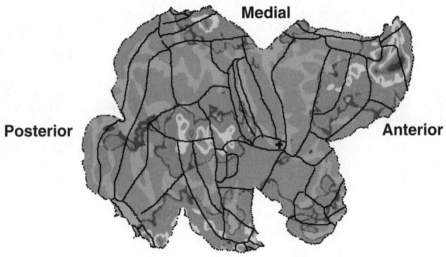

Medial

Posterior

Anterior

FIGURE 91.6 Areas of the brain observed to decrease their activity during a wide variety of goal-directed behaviors and referred to in the text as task-independent decreases (TIDS). Here these data, representing nine different PET imaging experiments and 134 subjects (G. L. Shulman, Fiez, et al., 1997), are mapped to surface reconstructions of the right cerebral hemisphere from the *Human.colin* atlas (Holmes et al., 1998; Van Essen, 2002). The PET data are mapped to fiducial (3D) surface reconstructions registered to Talairach space (Talairach and Tournoux, 1988) and are displayed on inflated surfaces (top) and on a flat map (bottom). The fiducial markers on the flat map reflect Brodmann areas. Those of particular interest here are designated by their appropriate number. (For further details concerning these mapping strategies, see Van Essen, 2002.) (See color plate 80.)

found in the TID areas. From these data we are able to draw two conclusions. First, on average, activations are not present in the resting state in the TID areas. Second, fMRI BOLD signal fluctuations in these areas during the resting state as observed in the study of Greicius and colleagues (2002) must be nearly equally above and below the baseline, since if they were not, one would see mean signal changes representing activations or deactivations. Thus, because activations are not present in averaged resting state images, TIDs must represent activity reductions from the physiological baseline level of brain activity.

The second study, by Laufs and colleagues (2003), followed a novel approach to resting state fMRI data employing an analysis driven by variations in EEG frequency bands (for examples and review of the literature, see Goldman et al., 2002; Moosmann et al., 2003). Their study provides additional new data on changes occurring in the resting state by means of a novel combination of fMRI and EEG. In this study, simultaneous EEG and fMRI measurements were obtained in subjects in the resting state (eyes closed, awake, unconstrained cognition). The EEG was analyzed in terms of activity (power) within the alpha frequency band (8–13 Hz) and subsets of the beta frequency band (13–16 Hz, 17–23 Hz, and 24–30 Hz). (For technical reasons related to recording EEG in the MR scanner, Laufs and colleagues were unable to obtain recordings of gamma band activity.) Changes in the power within these bands over time were correlated with magnitude variations in regional BOLD within the brain. The authors observed that areas in dorsolateral parietal and prefrontal cortices varied inversely with alpha power, whereas a significant number of the areas traditionally associated with TIDs varied directly with beta power in the 17–23 Hz range.

In interpreting these results, the authors equated alpha activity with "inattention" and beta activity with "spontaneous cognition" in the resting state. Based on this hypothesis and their data, the authors concluded that the resting state is characterized by temporal fluctuations in functional activity involving "inattention" and "spontaneous cognition," and that these states are associated with changes in activity in specific brain systems.

In the present context, two aspects of this study deserve comment. First, the higher BOLD activity observed in regions that correspond to TID areas, which was associated with increased EEG power in a segment of the beta frequency band (i.e., 17–23 Hz), could be interpreted as consistent with an overall role for these areas in spontaneous mental processes in the resting state. Such processes may include monitoring of one's own internal states (including bodily states and thought processes; Damasio, 1994; Andreasen et al., 1995; McGuire et al., 1996; Binder et al., 1999; Gusnard and Raichle, 2001), as well as the detection and evaluation of novelty and biological motion in the environment (Allison, Puce, and McCarthy, 2000; Gusnard and Raichle, 2001; Corbetta and Shulman, 2002).

Second, additional brain areas in parietal and prefrontal cortices, which are traditionally associated with visual attention (Corbetta et al., 1998), negatively correlated with alpha power. This suggests that these areas might play some role in the spontaneous mental activity of rest as well. In particular, these areas might play a role in attention directed toward introspective activities, as well as attending to or monitoring the external environment (Gusnard and Raichle, 2001).

From both of the aforementioned studies (Greicius et al., 2002; Laufs et al., 2003), it is apparent that there are fluctuations in brain activity during the resting state that, as suggested by the study of Laufs and colleagues (2003), may be related to changes in the power of EEG frequency bands.

Slow spontaneous fluctuations in brain activity (~0.1 Hz) have also been noted by neurophysiologists while recording the activity of single cells and LFPs with microelectrodes (Tsodyks et al., 1999; Leopold, Murayama, and Logothetis, 2003; Shu, Hasenstaub, and McCormick, 2003) and optical techniques (Arieli et al., 1996; Tsodyks et al., 1999). The exact relationships between these directly recorded electrical phenomenon and the fluctuations of the BOLD signal in the resting state and the EEG remain to be firmly established.

Conclusions

In this chapter, we have discussed our current knowledge of the physiology of functional imaging signals and their relationship to the underlying neurophysiology, the concept of a physiological baseline, and the relationships of activations and deactivations, as well as the resting state, to this physiological baseline.

With regard to the relationship between imaging signals and neurophysiology, one of the important conclusions to be drawn is that imaging is not a simple proxy for the spiking of neurons but, rather, represents a unique and complementary view of physiological events underlying neural information processing. Recent PET blood flow measurements obtained during stimulation of the subthalamic nucleus in humans (Hershey et al., 2003) provide a particularly nice example of the intricacies of this relationship and illustrate the benefits to be derived by cognitive neuroscientists and neurophysiologists understanding them as fully as possible (see figure 91.5).

We have emphasized the importance of considering the possible functionality of the brain's baseline level of neuronal activity. In pursuing this, the existence of an acceptable definition of a baseline becomes essential. We reviewed efforts to establish such a definition and the implications of using it in the analysis of functional imaging data. As a practical matter, we would also urge the inclusion of a simple control condition, such as eyes-closed rest or visual fixation, in functional imaging studies. To do so enriches the yield of functional imaging experiments by allowing investigators to unequivocally establish the direction of changes induced by their complex control and task states relative to the physiological baseline.

We also noted that baseline measurements of brain blood flow and metabolism have a long history in brain imaging, beginning in the late 1970s. Many groups used these measurements to characterize differences between individuals with psychiatric (e.g., Bench et al., 1990; Drevets and Botteron, 1997) and neurological diseases (e.g., Berent et al., 1988; Silverman et al., 2001) and normals, but the implications of these findings beyond denoting particular areas of brain involvement were not pursued. Revisiting the study of individual differences in the physiological baseline in health and disease would, we believe, be an important adjunct to current imaging work in cognitive neuroscience.

Even as combined EEG and functional imaging studies expand our knowledge in important new ways concerning the nature of the resting state and underscore its dynamic nature, they suggest important questions to be answered by future research. It is clear that we will need more detailed information on the possible cognitive operations associated with enhanced power in specific EEG frequency bands. How, for example, do definable spontaneous mental processes relate to EEG and BOLD changes?

Although the long-term goal of both cognitive neuroscientists and neurophysiologists is to understand the nature of information processing in the brain, it is important to appreciate their complementary roles in this endeavor. Cognitive neuroscientists who remain informed on this evolving dialogue will have an enriched understanding of their imaging results and will be able to draw more informed conclusions from the work that they do.

REFERENCES

ACKERMAN, R. F., D. M. FINCH, T. L. BABB, and J. J. ENGEL, 1984. Increased glucose utilization during long-duration recurrent inhibition of hippocampal pyramidal cells. *J. Neurosci.* 4: 251–264.

ALLISON, T., A. PUCE, and G. MCCARTHY, 2000. Social perception from visual cues: Role of the STS region. *Trends Cogn. Sci.* 4: 267–278.

ANDREASEN, N. C., D. S. O'LEARY, T. CIZADLO, S. ARNDT, K. REZAI, G. L. WATKINS, et al., 1995. Remembering the past: Two facets of episodic memory explored with positron emission tomography. *Am. J. Psychiatry* 152:1576–1585.

ARIELI, A., A. STERKIN, A. GRINVALD, and A. AERTSENT, 1996. Dynamics of ongoing activity: Explanation of the large variability in evoked cortical responses. *Science* 273:1868–1871.

ATTWELL, D., and S. B. LAUGHLIN, 2001. An energy budget for signaling in the grey matter of the brain. *J. Cereb. Blood Flow Metabol.* 21:1133–1145.

BENCH, C. J., R. J. DOLAN, K. J. FRISTON, and R. S. J. FRACKOWIAK, 1990. Positron emission tomography in the study of brain metabolism in psychiatric and neurosychiatric disorders. *Br. J. Psychiatry* 157(Suppl. 9):82–95.

BERENT, S., B. GIORDANI, S. LEHTINEN, D. MARKEL, J. B. PENNEY, H. A. BÜCHTEL, et al., 1988. Postron emission tomographic scan investigations of Huntington's disease: Cerebral metabolic correlates of cognitive function. *Ann. Neurol.* 23:541–546.

BINDER, J. R., J. A. FROST, T. A. HAMMEKE, P. S. F. BELLGOWAN, S. M. RAO, and R. W. COX, 1999. Conceptual processing during the conscious resting state: A functional MRI study. *J. Cogn. Neurosci.* 11:80–93.

BISWAL, B., F. YETKIN, V. HAUGHTON, and J. HYDE, 1995. Functional connectivity in the motor cortex of resting human brain using echo-planar MRI. *Magn. Reson. Med.* 34:537–541.

BOYNTON, G. M., S. A. ENGEL, G. H. GLOVER, and D. J. HEEGER, 1996. Linear systems analysis of functional magnetic resonance imaging in human V1. *J. Neurosci.* 16:4207–4221.

BUCKNER, R. L., P. A. BANDETTINI, K. M. O'CRAVEN, R. L. SAVOY, S. E. PETERSEN, M. E. RAICHLE, et al., 1996. Detection of cortical activation during averaged single trials of a cognitive task using functional magnetic resonance imaging. *Proc. Natl. Acad. Sci. U.S.A.* 93:14878–14883.

CLARK, D. D., and L. SOKOLOFF, 1999. Circulation and energy metabolism of the brain. In *Basic Neurochemistry: Molecular, Cellular and Medical Aspects*, 6th ed., G. J. Siegel, B. W. Agranoff, R. W. Albers, S. K. Fisher, and M. D. Uhler, eds. Philadelphia: Lippincott-Raven, pp. 637–670.

CORBETTA, M., E. AKBUDAK, T. E. CONTURO, A. Z. SNYDER, J. M. OLLINGER, H. A. DRURY, M. R. LINENWEBER, S. E. PETERSEN, M. E. RAICHLE, D. C. VAN ESSEN, and G. L. SHULMAN, 1998. A common network of functional areas for attention and eye movements. *Neuron* 21:761–773.

CORBETTA, M., and G. L. SHULMAN, 2002. Control of goal-directed and stimulus-driven attention in the brain. *Nat. Rev. Neurosci.* 3: 201–215.

COREN, S., 1969. Brightness contrast as a function of figure-ground relations. *J. Exp. Psychol.* 80:517–524.

CREUTZFELDT, O. D., 1975. Neurophysiological correlates of different functional states of the brain. In *Brain Work: The Coupling of Function, Metabolism and Blood Flow in the Brain*, D. H. Ingvar and N. A. Lassen, eds. Copenhagen: Munksgaard, pp. 22–47.

DAMASIO, A. R., 1994. *Descartes' Error: Emotion, Reason, and the Human Brain*. New York: Avon Books.

DREVETS, W. C., and K. BOTTERON, 1997. Neuroimaging in psychiatry. In *Adult Psychiatry*, S. B. Guze, ed. St. Louis: Mosby.

DREVETS, W. C., H. BURTON, T. O. VIDEEN, A. Z. SNYDER, J. R. SIMPSON, Jr., and M. E. RAICHLE, 1995. Blood flow changes in human somatosensory cortex during anticipated stimulation. *Nature* 373:249–252.

FERSTER, D., 1996. Is neural noise just a nuisance? *Science* 273:1812.

FISET, P., T. PAUS, T. DALOZE, G. PLOURDE, P. MEURET, V. BONHOMME, et al., 1999. Brain mechanisms of propofol-induced loss of consciousness in humans: A positron emission tomographic study. *J. Neurosci.* 19:5506–5513.

FOX, P. T., H. BURTON, and M. E. RAICHLE, 1987. Mapping human somatosensory cortex with positron emission tomography. *J. Neurosurg.* 67:34–43.

FOX, P. T., J. M. FOX, M. E. RAICHLE, and R. M. BURDE, 1985. The role of cerebral cortex in the generation of voluntary saccades: A positron emission tomographic study. *J. Neurophysiol.* 54: 348–369.

FOX, P. T., F. M. MIEZIN, J. M. ALLMAN, D. C. VAN ESSEN, and M. E. RAICHLE, 1987. Retinotopic organization of human visual cortex mapped with positron emission tomography. *J. Neurosci.* 7:913–922.

FOX, P. T., and M. E. RAICHLE, 1986. Focal physiological uncoupling of cerebral blood flow and oxidative metabolism during somatosensory stimulation in human subjects. *Proc. Natl. Acad. Sci. U.S.A.* 83:1140–1144.

FOX, P. T., M. E. RAICHLE, M. A. MINTUN, and C. DENCE, 1988. Nonoxidative glucose consumption during focal physiologic neural activity. *Science* 241:462–464.

GHATAN, P. H., J.-C. HSIEH, K. M. PETERSSON, S. STONE-ELANDER, and M. INGVAR, 1998. Coexistence of attention-based facilitation and inhibion in human cortex. *NeuroImage* 7:23–29.

GOLD, L., and M. LAURITZEN, 2002. Neuronal deactivation explains decreased cerebellar blood flow in response to focal cerebral ischemia or suppressed neocortical function. *Proc. Natl. Acad. Sci. U.S.A.* 99:7699–7704.

GOLDMAN, R. I., J. M. STERN, J. J. ENGEL, and M. S. COHEN, 2002. Simultaneous EEG and fMRI of the alpha rhythm. *Neuroreport* 13:2487–2492.

GREICIUS, M. D., B. KRASNOW, A. L. REISS, and V. MENON, 2002. *Neural connectivity in the resting brain: Further evidence for a default mode of brain activity*. Paper presented at a meeting of the Organization for Human Brain Mapping, Sendai, Japan.

GRUBB, R. L. J., C. P. DERDEYN, S. M. FRITSCH, D. A. CARPENTAR, K. D. YUNDT, T. O. VIDEEN, et al., 1998. Importance of hemodynamic factors in the prognosis of symptomatic carotid occlusion. *JAMA* 280:1055–1060.

GUSNARD, D. A., and M. E. RAICHLE, 2001. Searching for a baseline: Functional imaging and the resting human brain. *Nat. Rev. Neurosci.* 2:685–694.

HAXBY, J. V., B. HORWITZ, L. G. UNGERLEIDER, J. M. MAISOG, P. PIETRINI, and C. L. GRADY, 1994. The functional organization of human extrastriate cortex: A PET-rCBF study of selective attention to faces and locations. *J. Neurosci.* 14:6336–6353.

HEISTAD, D. D., and H. A. KONTOS, 1983. Cerebral circulation. In J. T. Sheppard and F. M. Abboud, eds. *Handbook of Physiology: The Cardiovascular System*. vol. 3, Bethesda, Md.: American Physiological Society, pp. 137–182.

HERSHEY, T., F. J. REVILLA, A. R. WERNLE, L. MCGEE-MINNICH, J. V. ANTENOR, T. O. VIDEEN, et al., 2003. Cortical and subcortical blood flow effects of subthalamic nucleus stimulation in PD. *Neurology* 61:816–821.

HOLMES, C. J., R. HOGE, L. COLLINS, R. WOODS, A. W. TOGA, and A. C. EVENS, 1998. Enhancement of MR images using registration for signal averaging. *J. Comput. Assist. Tomogr.* 22: 324–333.

HOUNSFIELD, G. N., 1973. Computerized transverse axial scanning (tomography). Part I. Description of system. *Br. J. Radiol.* 46:1016–1022.

HYDER, F., D. L. ROTHMAN, and R. G. SHULMAN, 2002. Total neuroenergetics support localized brain activity: implications for the interpretation of fMRI. *Proc. Natl. Acad. Sci. U.S.A.* 99: 10237–10239.

INGVAR, D. H., 1985. Memory of the future: An essay on the temporal organization of conscious awareness. *Hum. Neurobiol.* 4:127–136.

KAWASHIMA, R., B. T. O'SULLIVAN, and P. E. ROLAND, 1995. Positron-emission tomography studies of cross-modality inhibition in selective attentional tasks: Closing the "mind's eye." *Proc. Natl. Acad. Sci. U.S.A.* 92:5969–5972.

KEVLES, B. H., 1997. *Naked to the Bone: Medical Imaging in the Twentieth Century.* New Brunswick, N.J.: Rutgers University Press.

KHANI, Y. A., F. DUBEAU, C.-G. BENAR, M. VEILLEUX, F. ANDERMANN, and J. GOTMAN, 2003. *EEG-fMRI findings in patients with idiopathic generalized epilepsy.* Paper presented at a meeting of the Organization for Human Brain Mapping, New York.

LAUFS, H., K. KRAKOW, P. STERZER, E. EGGER, A. BEYERLE, A. SALEK-HADDADI, et al., 2003. Electroencephalographic signatures of attentional and cognitive default modes in spontaneous brain activity fluctuations at rest. *Proc. Natl. Acad. Sci. U.S.A.* 100:11053–11058.

LAURITZEN, M., 2001. Relationship of spikes, synaptic activity and local changes of cerebral blood flow. *J. Cereb. Blood Flow Metab.* 21:1367–1383.

LAURITZEN, M., and L. GOLD, 2003. Brain function and neurophysiological correlates of signals used in functional neuroimaging. *J. Neurosci.* 23:3972–3980.

LEBRUN-GRANDIE, P., J.-C. BARON, F. SOUSSALINE, C. LOCH'H, J. SASTRE, and M.-G. BOUSSER, 1983. Coupling between regional blood flow and oxygen utilization in the normal human brain. *Arch. Neurol.* 40:230–236.

LEOPOLD, D. A., Y. MURAYAMA, and N. K. LOGOTHETIS, 2003. Very slow activity fluctuations in monkey visual cortex: Implications for functional brain imaging. *Cereb. Cortex* 13:423–433.

LOGOTHETIS, N. K., 2003. The underpinnings of the BOLD functional magnetic resonance imaging signal. *J. Neurosci.* 23: 3963–3971.

LOGOTHETIS, N. K., H. GUGGENBERGER, S. PELED, and J. PAULS, 1999. Functional imaging of the monkey brain. *Nat. Neurosci.* 2: 555–562.

LOGOTHETIS, N. K., J. PAULS, M. AUGATH, T. TRINATH, and A. OELTERMANN, 2001. Neurophysiological investigation of the basis of the fMRI signal. *Nature* 412:150–157.

LOWE, M. J., B. J. MOCK, and J. A. SORENSON, 1998. Functional connectivity in single and multislice echoplanar imaging using resting-state fluctuations. *NeuroImage* 7:119–132.

MAGISTRETTI, P. J., L. PELLERIN, D. L. ROTHMAN, and R. G. SHULMAN, 1999. Energy on demand. *Science* 283:496–497.

MAQUET, P., 2000. Functional neuroimaging of normal human sleep by positron emission tomography. *J. Sleep Res.* 9:207–231.

MARCHAL, G., C. SERRATI, P. RIOUX, M. C. PETIT-TABOUE, F. VIADER, V. DE LA SAYETTE, et al., 1993. PET imaging of cerebral perfusion and oxygen consumption in acute ischaemic stroke: Relation to outcome. *Lancet* 341:925–927.

MATHIESEN, C., K. CAESAR, N. AKJOREN, and M. LAURITZEN, 1998. Modification of activity-dependent increases of cerebral blood flow by excitatory synaptic activity and spikes in rat cerebellar cortex. *J. Physiol.* 512:555–566.

MATHIESEN, C., K. CAESAR, and M. LAURITZEN, 2000. Temporal coupling between neuronal activity and blood flow in rat cereballar cortex as indicated by field potential analysis. *J. Physiol.* (*Lond.*) 523:235–246.

MAZOYER, B., L. ZAGO, E. MELLET, S. BRICOGNE, O. ETARD, O. HOUDE, et al., 2001. Cortical networks for working memory and executive functions sustain the conscious resting state in man. *Brain Res. Bull.* 543:287–298.

MCCORMICK, D. A., 1999. Spontaneous activity: Signal or noise? *Science* 285:541–543.

MCGUIRE, P. K., E. PAULESU, R. S. J. FRACKOWIAK, and C. D. FRITH, 1996. Brain activity during stimulus independent thought. *Neuroreport* 7:2095–2099.

MCKIERNAN, K. A., J. N. KAUFMAN, J. KUCERA-THOMPSON, and J. R. BINDER, 2003. A parametric manipulation of factors affecting task-induced deactivation in functional neuroimaging. *J. Cogn. Neurosci.* 15:394–408.

MINTUN, M. A., B. N. LUNDSTROM, A. Z. SNYDER, A. G. VLASSENKO, G. L. SHULMAN, and M. E. RAICHLE, 2001. Blood flow and oxygen delivery to human brain during functional activity: Theoretical modeling and experimental data. *Proc. Natl. Acad. Sci. U.S.A.* 98:6859–6864.

MINTUN, M. A., M. E. RAICHLE, W. R. MARTIN, and P. HERSCOVITCH, 1984. Brain oxygen utilization measured with O–15 radiotracers and positron emission tomography. *J. Nucl. Med.* 25:177–187.

MOOSMANN, M., P. RITTER, I. KRASTEL, A. BRINK, S. THEES, F. BLANKENBURG, et al., 2003. Correlates of alpha rhythm in functional magnetic resonance imaging and near infrared spectroscopy. *NeuroImage* 20:145–158.

NICHOLS, M. J., and W. T. NEWSOME, 1999. The neurobiology of cognition. *Nature* 402:C35–C38.

OGAWA, S., T. M. LEE, A. R. KAY, and D. W. TANK, 1990. Brain magnetic resonance imaging with contrast dependent on blood oxygenation. *Proc. Natl. Acad. Sci. U.S.A.* 87:9868–9872.

O'GORMAN, R., V. KUMARI, S. E. J. CONNOR, D. C. ALSOP, T. HARTKENS, J. GRAY, et al., 2003. *Personality scores correlate with resting cerebral perfusion.* Paper presented at a meeting of the Organization for Human Brain Mapping, New York.

PETERSEN, S. E., P. T. FOX, M. I. POSNER, M. MINTUN, and M. E. RAICHLE, 1988. Positron emission tomographic studies of the cortical anatomy of single-word processing. *Nature* 331:585–589.

PLUM, F., J. B. POSNER, and B. TROY, 1968. Cerebral metabolic and circulatory responses to induced convulsions in animals. *Arch. Neurol.* 18:1–13.

RAICHLE, M. E., 1998. Behind the scenes of functional brain imaging: A historical and physiological perspective. *Proc. Natl. Acad. Sci. U.S.A.* 95:765–772.

RAICHLE, M. E., 2000. A brief history of human functional brain mapping. In *Brain Mapping: The Systems*, A. W. Toga and J. C. Mazziotta, eds. San Diego: Academic Press, pp. 33–75.

RAICHLE, M. E., 2003. Functional brain imaging and human brain function. *J. Neurosci.* 23:3959–3962.

RAICHLE, M. E., A. M. MACLEOD, A. Z. SNYDER, W. J. POWERS, D. A. GUSNARD, and G. L. SHULMAN, 2001. A default mode of brain function. *Proc. Natl. Acad. Sci. U.S.A.* 98:676–682.

SALEK-HADDADI, A., L. LEMIEUX, M. MERSCHEMKE, K. J. FRISTON, J. S. DUNCAN, and D. R. FISH, 2003. Functional magnetic resonance imaging of human absence seizures. *Ann. Neurol.* 53:663–667.

SALINAS, E., and T. J. SEJNOWSKI, 2001. Correlated neuronal activity and the flow of neural information. *Nat. Rev. Neurosci.* 2:539–550.

SANCHEZ-VIVES, M. V., and D. A. McCORMICK, 2000. Cellular and network mechanisms of rhythmic recurrent activity in neocortex. *Nat. Neurosci.* 3:1027–1034.

SCHWARTZ, W. J., C. B. SMITH, L. DAVIDSEN, H. SAVAKI, L. SOKOLOFF, M. MATA, et al., 1979. Metabolic mapping of functional activity in the hypothalamo-neurohypophysial system of the rat. *Science Washington DC* 205:723–725.

SHADLEN, M. N., and W. T. NEWSOME, 1994. Noise, neural codes and cortical organization. *Curr. Opin. Neurobiol.* 4:569–579.

SHMUEL, A., M. AUGATH, A. OELTERMANN, J. PAULS, Y. MURAYAMA, and N. K. LOGOTHETIS, 2003. *The negative BOLD response in monkey V1 is associated with decreases in neuronal activity.* Paper presented at a meeting of the Organization for Human Brain Mapping, New York.

SHMUEL, A., M. AUGATH, E. ROUNIS, N. K. LOGOTHETIS, and S. SMIRNAKIS, 2003. *Negative BOLD response ipsilateral to the visual stimulus: Origin is not blood stealing.* Paper presented at a meeting of the Organization for Human Brain Mapping, New York.

SHMUEL, A., E. YACOUB, J. PFEUFFER, P.-F. VAN DE MOORTELE, G. ADRIANY, X. HU, et al., 2002. Sustained negative BOLD, blood flow and oxygen consumption response and its coupling to the positive response in the human brain. *Neuron* 36:1195–1210.

SHMUEL, A., E. YACOUB, J. PFEUFFER, P.-F. VAN DE MOORTELE, G. ADRIANY, K. UGURBIL, et al., 2001. Negative BOLD response and its coupling to the positive response in the human brain. *Neuroimage* 13:S1005.

SHU, Y., A. HASENSTAUB, and D. A. McCORMICK, 2003. Turning on and off recurrent balanced cortical activity. *Nature* 423:288–293.

SHULMAN, G. L., M. CORBETTA, R. L. BUCKNER, J. A. FIEZ, F. M. MIEZIN, M. E. RAICHLE, et al., 1997. Common blood flow changes across visual tasks. I. Increases in subcortical structures and cerebellum, but not in non-visual cortex. *J. Cogn. Neurosci.* 9:624–647.

SHULMAN, G. L., M. CORBETTA, R. L. BUCKNER, M. E. RAICHLE, J. A. FIEZ, F. M. MIEZIN, et al., 1997. Top-down modulation of early sensory cortex. *Cereb. Cortex* 7:193–206.

SHULMAN, G. L., J. A. FIEZ, M. CORBETTA, R. L. BUCKNER, F. M. MIEZIN, M. E. RAICHLE, et al., 1997. Common blood flow changes across visual tasks. II. Decreases in cerebral cortex. *J. Cogn. Neurosci.* 9:648–663.

SHULMAN, R. G., F. HYDER, and D. L. ROTHMAN, 2001. Cerebral energetics and the glycogen shunt: Neurochemical basis of functional imaging. *Proc. Natl. Acad. Sci. U.S.A.* 98:6417–6422.

SIBSON, N. R., A. DHANKHAR, G. F. MASON, D. L. ROTHMAN, K. L. BEHAR, and R. G. SHULMAN, 1998. Stoichiometric coupling of brain glucose metabolism and glutamatergic neuronal activity. *Proc. Natl. Acad. Sci. U.S.A.* 95:316–321.

SIESJO, B. K., 1978. *Brain Energy Metabolism.* New York: Wiley.

SILVERMAN, D. H. S., G. W. SMALL, C. Y. CHANG, C. S. LU, M. A. K. DE ABURTO, W. CHEN, et al., 2001. Positron emission tomography in evaluation of dementia: Regional brain metabolism and long-term outcome. *JAMA* 286:2120–2126.

SIMPSON, J. R. J., A. Z. SNYDER, D. A. GUSNARD, and M. E. RAICHLE, 2001. Emotion-induced changes in human medial prefrontal cortex. I. During cognitive task performance. *Proc. Natl. Acad. Sci. U.S.A.* 98:683–687.

SMITH, A. T., K. D. SINGH, and M. W. GREENLEE, 2000. Attentional suppression of activity in the human visual cortex. *Neuroreport* 11:271–277.

SOKOLOFF, L., R. MANGOLD, R. WECHSLER, C. KENNEDY, and S. S. KETY, 1955. The effect of mental arithmetic on cerebral circulation and metabolism. *J. Clin. Invest.* 34:1101–1108.

SOKOLOFF, L., M. REIVICH, C. KENNEDY, M. H. DES ROSIERS, C. S. PATLAK, K. D. PETTIGREW, et al., 1977. The [^{14}C]deoxyglucose method for the measurement of local glucose utilization: Theory, procedure and normal values in the conscious and anesthetized albino rat. *J. Neurochem.* 28:897–916.

STERIADE, M., I. TIMOFEEV, and F. GRENIER, 2001. Natural waking and sleep states: A view from inside neocortical neurons. *J. Neurophysiol.* 85:1969–1985.

TALAIRACH, J., and P. TOURNOUX, 1988. *Co-Planar Stereotaxic Atlas of the Human Brain,* M. Rayport, trans. New York: Thieme.

TONONI, G., and G. M. EDELMAN, 1998. Consciousness and the integration of information in the brain. In *Consciousness: At the Frontiers of Neuroscience,* vol. 77, H. H. Jasper, J. L. Descarries, V. F. Castellucci, and S. Rossignol, eds. Philadelphia: Lippincott-Raven.

TOOTELL, R. B. H., N. HADJIKHANI, E. K. HALL, S. MARRETT, W. VANDUFFEL, J. T. VAUGHN, et al., 1998. The retinotopy of visual spatial attention. *Neuron* 21:1409–1422.

TOOTELL, R. B. H., D. TSAO, and W. VANDUFFEL, 2003. Neuroimaging weighs in: Humans meet macaques in primate visual cortex. *J. Neurosci.* 23:3981–3989.

TSODYKS, M., T. KENET, A. GRINVALD, and A. ARIELI, 1999. Linking spontaneous activity of single cortical neurons and the underlying functional architecture. *Science* 286:1943–1946.

UEKI, M., F. LINN, and K.-A. HOSSMANN, 1988. Functional activation of cerebral blood flow and metabolism before and after global ischemia of rat brain. *J. Cereb. Blood Flow Metabol.* 8:486–494.

UTTAL, W. R., 2001. *The New Phrenology.* Cambridge, Mass.: Bradford Books/MIT Press.

VAN ESSEN, D. C., 2002. Windows on the brain: The emerging role of atlases and databases in neuroscience. *Curr. Opin. Neurobiol.* 12:574–579.

VAN VREESWIJK, C., and H. SOMPOLINSKY, 1996. Chaos in neuronal networks with balanced excitatory and inhibitory activity. *Science* 274:1724–1726.

WEBB, S., 1990. *From the Watching of Shadows.* New York: Adam Hilger.

WOOLSEY, T. A., C. M. ROVAINEN, S. B. COX, M. H. HENEGAR, G. E. LIANG, D. LIU, et al., 1996. Neuronal units linked to microvascular modules in cerebral cortex: Response elements for imaging the brain. *Cereb. Cortex* 6:647–660.

XIONG, J., L. M. PARSONS, J. H. GAO, and P. T. FOX, 1999. Interregional connectivity to primary motor cortex revealed using MRI resting state images. *Hum. Brain Mapp.* 8:151–156.

ZONTA, M., M. C. ANGULO, S. GOBBO, B. ROSENGARTEN, K.-A. HOSSMANN, T. POZZAN, et al., 2003. Neuron-to-astrocyte signaling is central to the dynamic control of brain microcirculation. *Nat. Neurosci.* 6:43–50.

92 Cognitive Neuroimaging: History, Developments, and Directions

JOHN DARRELL VAN HORN

ABSTRACT Over the past two decades, the field of cognitive neuroscience has flourished as the leading scientific discipline seeking to rigorously understand the relationship between mind and brain. Central to the excitement surrounding the cognitive neuroscientific revolution has been the advent of in vivo imaging of the brain using fMRI during the performance of cognitive tasks. With this technique for mapping the distribution of brain blood flow over time, researchers are making progress in identifying the networks of brain areas responsible for many fundamental cognitive functions (e.g., memory encoding and retrieval, processing visual information, cognitive functions in complex motor processes). However, the union of psychology, brain neurophysiology, and particle physics that led to functional brain imaging did not happen overnight; the seeds of it can be traced back for more than a century. The symbiotic relationship that has developed among these coevolving fields is a unique story in science, unified through the mutual interest in measuring and mapping the neurophysiological signature of human cognitive function. Ever greater sophistication in designing efficient experimental paradigms and an improved data collection ability are being brought to bear in teasing apart subtle differences between task-related and control states. At the same time, brain energetics and combined neurophysiological approaches are being explored for clues to the origins of the BOLD response. Moreover, raw data repositories are enabling others to mine previously published data in new and clever ways that will further aid in understanding these rich sources of information. As cognitive neuroscience grows, so too will functional neuroimaging, but there are still considerable challenges to meet. This chapter provides an overview of the past and present on fMRI research while speculating on the future for studies of mapping human cognitive function.

Since the first edition of this book, interest in understanding the cognitive processes at work in the human brain has grown remarkably. Much attention has been focused on the cognitive revolution (Mandler, 2002; Miller, 2003) and the emergence of cognitive neuroscience as driving forces in attributing mental function to brain structure (Posner and DiGirolamo, 2000; McIntosh, Fitzpatrick, and Friston, 2001; Shulman, Hyder, and Rothman, 2002; Adolphs, 2003). Techniques of functional brain imaging, in particular positron emission tomography (PET) and, more recently, functional magnetic resonance imaging (fMRI), have been at the forefront of cognitive neuroscientific research. Noninvasive means of examining the brain in vivo not only allow the capture of detailed information about cerebral anatomy but also measurements related to the time course of neural activity. Indeed, more than a century after Broca's original observations localizing language function to the left cerebral hemisphere, neuroimaging has itself revolutionized the localization of cognitive function and has contributed much to our knowledge of how fundamental processes are organized in the brain. The increased use of fMRI in particular to examine brain processes is evident in the increasing number of peer-reviewed publications on fMRI that have been published in the past decade (figure 92.1).

The increasing interest in cognitive neuroscience and the growing number of fMRI papers published each year suggest that neuroscientists are rising to the challenge set forth by Michael Gazzaniga in his introduction to the first edition of this book:

> The future of the field, however, is in working toward a science that truly relates brain and cognition in a mechanistic way. That task is not easy, and many areas of research in the mind sciences are not ready for that kind of analysis. Yet that is the objective.

In the years since this challenge was made, researchers have discovered that whole-brain functional neuroimaging methods, more than any other means of measuring brain function, have the potential to finally reveal the manner in which the brain begets complex thought, language, emotion, the retrieval of memories, movement representation, and so forth. Largely because of neuroimaging, cognitive neuroscience has become the nexus of an eclectic mix of scientific disciplines, each contributing its own unique components to the quest for relating function to form in brain science.

Neuroimaging experiments are becoming easier to carry out with the increasing availability of MRI scanners. Preprocessing steps are being streamlined and automated (Toga, Rex, and Ma, 2001; Rex and Toga, 2002), enabling data to be processed faster and more easily. However, functional neuroimaging is by no means a turnkey operation. The tools of brain imaging are highly technical, and cognitive neuroscientists today must be comfortable with the high degree of

JOHN DARRELL VAN HORN Center for Cognitive Neuroscience, Dartmouth College, Hanover, N.H.

1281

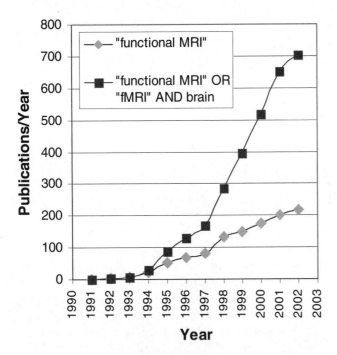

FIGURE 92.1   The growth of fMRI to examine brain function can be gauged by the number of articles published on the topic over time. This figure shows the number of PubMed (http://www.ncbi.nlm.nih.gov/PubMed/) references per year between 1991 and 2002 returned for searches on ["functional MRI"] and ["functional MRI" OR "fMRI" AND brain].

expertise needed to conduct these studies. They must be acquainted with the physics of proton spin (Budinger and Lauterbur, 1984; Pipe, 1999), how MR images are obtained (Xu et al., 1999), the sources of the blood-oxygen-level-dependent (BOLD) signal (Turner, 1997), how to correct data for the effects of subject movement (Woods, Grafton, Holmes, et al., 1998; Woods, Grafton, Watson, et al., 1998), multivariate statistical methods (Aguirre, Zarahn, and D'Esposito, 1997; Friston, Phillips, et al., 2000; Kherif et al., 2002), and Bayesian inference (Friston, Glaser, et al., 2002; Friston, Penny, et al., 2002), in addition to keeping up with the literature on cognitive neuroanatomy. Future computational advances could also require brain researchers to understand the foundations of communications systems and the axioms of complex variable theory! The technical knowhow required in modern cognitive neuroimaging approaches for understanding the working mind is indeed vast.

This chapter provides a brief overview of the origins of modern functional neuroimaging and the coevolution of brain neurophysiology, cognitive research, and the science of particle physics that gave rise to it. Also discussed are some of the cognitive domains in which fMRI has played an important role in recent years. Experimental design considerations are discussed, with a brief mention of statistical parameter estimation efficiency. Several extant and emerging technologies that complement fMRI studies are described. Finally, the chapter considers future directions for cognitive neuroimaging, the limits of these techniques, caveats to be held in mind in interpreting their results, and whether the algorithms driving "structural neural elements into the physiological activity that results in perception, cognition, and perhaps even consciousness" (Gazzaniga, 1997, p. xiii) are, in fact, being identified.

The coevolution of modern functional neuroimaging and cognitive neuroscience

The emergence of neuroimaging to examine in vivo neurological function represents a unique cooperation between researchers in the brain and physical sciences. Although several reviews point to the discovery of BOLD effects using MRI (Ogawa and Lee, 1990; Ogawa, Lee, Kay, et al., 1990; Ogawa, Lee, Nayak, et al., 1990) and how this discovery led to a subsequent explosion of research using fMRI to investigate cognitive function (Di Salle et al., 1999; D'Esposito, 2000; Detre and Floyd, 2001), the origins of magnetic resonance and cerebral blood flow measurement extend back to the beginning of the twentieth century. In fact, the development of fMRI technology for examining brain processes has benefited from contributions from different sciences, beginning with the breakthroughs in the early days of particle physics (Pais, 2002), continuing through physiological investigation of brain blood flow and cerebral energetics (Sokoloff, 1999; Mintun et al., 2001; Raichle and Gusnard, 2002), and incorporating research from brain-injured and neurosurgical subjects (Milner, 1963, 1982; Phelps, Hirst, and Gazzaniga, 1991).

Early pioneers in psychology, such as Wilhelm Wundt in Germany and William James in the United States, who were interested in normal "mental faculties" and the damaged brain, provided the impetus for academe to include psychology as a formal study (Schwehn, 1982; Taylor, 1982, 1984; Ziche, 1999). At about the same time, Roy and Sherrington (1890) made their initial investigations into cerebral blood flow (CBF) measurement. The timeline depicted in figure 92.2, a limited historical record of neuroimaging, arbitrarily begins with Pauli's 1924 prediction that protons possess the property of spin—the effect that forms the basis of MRI. During this period, the science of particle physics was growing quickly (Pais, 2002), and the discovery of the proton in 1911 and of the positron in 1936 resulted in considerable excitement that physics was making critical inroads toward understanding the fundamental properties of matter. These different fields of study could not have seemed farther apart on the continuum of scientific exploration than they did in the early days of the twentieth century.

Advances in the measurement of regional cerebral blood flow (rCBF) were made in the 1950s and 1960s by Seymour Kety and Louis Sokoloff (Kety, 1963, 1966; Sokoloff, 1981,

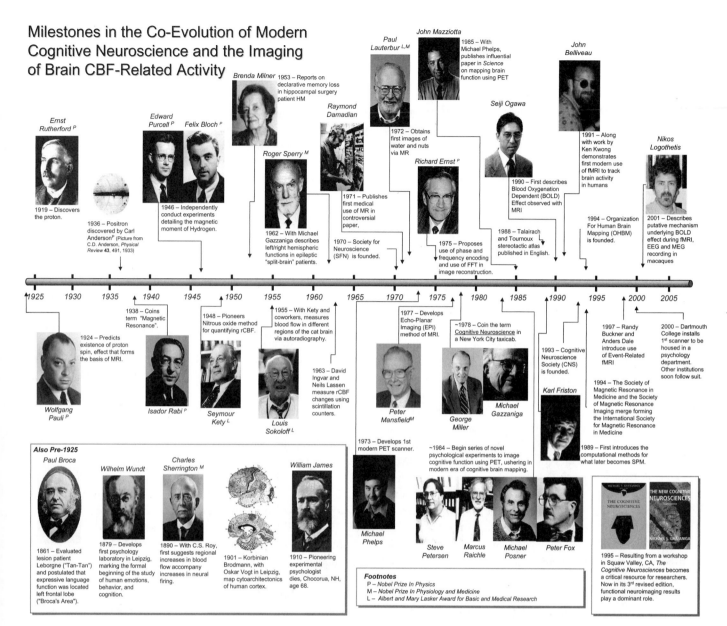

Milestones in the Co-Evolution of Modern Cognitive Neuroscience and the Imaging of Brain CBF-Related Activity

Ernst Rutherford [P]
1919 – Discovers the proton.

1936 – Positron discovered by Carl Anderson [P] (Picture from C.D. Anderson, *Physical Review* **43**, 491, 1933)

Edward Purcell [P] **Felix Bloch** [P]
1946 – Independently conduct experiments detailing the magnetic moment of Hydrogen.

Brenda Milner 1953 – Reports on declarative memory loss in hippocampal surgery patient HM

Roger Sperry [M]
1962 – With Michael Gazzaniga describes left/right hemispheric functions in epileptic "split-brain" patients.

Raymond Damadian
1971 – Publishes first medical use of MR in controversial paper.

1970 – Society for Neuroscience (SFN) is founded.

Paul Lauterbur [L,M]
1972 – Obtains first images of water and nuts via MR

John Mazziotta
1985 – With Michael Phelps, publishes influential paper in *Science* on mapping brain function using PET

Richard Ernst [P]
1975 – Proposes use of phase and frequency encoding and use of FFT in image reconstruction.

Seiji Ogawa
1990 – First describes Blood Oxygenation Dependent (BOLD) Effect observed with MRI

1988 – Talairach and Tournoux stereotactic atlas published in English.

John Belliveau
1991 – Along with work by Ken Kwong demonstrates first modern use of fMRI to track brain activity in humans

1994 – Organization For Human Brain Mapping (OHBM) is founded.

Nikos Logothetis
2001 – Describes putative mechanism underlying BOLD effect during fMRI, EEG and MEG recording in macaques

1925 1930 1935 1940 1945 1950 1955 1960 1965 1970 1975 1980 1985 1990 1995 2000 2005

Wolfgang Pauli [P]
1924 – Predicts existence of proton spin, effect that forms the basis of MRI.

Isador Rabi [P]
1938 – Coins term "Magnetic Resonance".

Seymour Kety [L]
1948 – Pioneers Nitrous oxide method for quantifying rCBF.

Louis Sokoloff [L]
1955 – With Kety and coworkers, measures blood flow in different regions of the cat brain via autoradiography.

1963 – David Ingvar and Neils Lassen measure rCBF changes using scintillation counters.

Peter Mansfield [M]
1977 – Develops Echo-Planar Imaging (EPI) method of MRI.
1973 – Develops 1st modern PET scanner.

~1978 – Coin the term Cognitive Neuroscience in a New York City taxicab.

George Miller   **Michael Gazzaniga**
~1984 – Begin series of novel psychological experiments to image cognitive function using PET, ushering in modern era of cognitive brain mapping.

1993 – Cognitive Neuroscience Society (CNS) is founded.

Karl Friston
1989 – First introduces the computational methods for what later becomes SPM.

1997 – Randy Buckner and Anders Dale introduce use of Event-Related fMRI

1994 – The Society of Magnetic Resonance in Medicine and the Society of Magnetic Resonance Imaging merge forming the International Society for Magnetic Resonance in Medicine

2000 – Dartmouth College installs 1st scanner to be housed in a psychology department. Other institutions soon follow suit.

Michael Phelps

Steve Petersen **Marcus Raichle** **Michael Posner** **Peter Fox**

Also Pre-1925

Paul Broca
1861 – Evaluated lesion patient Leborgne ("Tan-Tan") and postulated that expressive language function was located left frontal lobe ("Broca's Area").

Wilhelm Wundt
1879 – Develops first psychology laboratory in Leipzig, marking the formal beginning of the study of human emotions, behavior, and cognition.

Charles Sherrington [M]
1890 – With C.S. Roy, first suggests regional increases in blood flow accompany increases in neural firing.

1901 – Korbinian Brodmann, with Oskar Vogt in Leipzig, map cytoarchitectonics of human cortex.

William James
1910 – Pioneering experimental psychologist dies, Chocorua, NH, age 68.

1995 – Resulting from a workshop in Squaw Valley, CA, *The Cognitive Neurosciences* becomes a critical resource for researchers. Now in its 3rd revised edition, functional neuroimaging results play a dominant role.

Footnotes
P – Nobel Prize In Physics
M – Nobel Prize In Physiology and Medicine
L – Albert and Mary Lasker Award for Basic and Medical Research

FIGURE 92.2   This figure represents a limited historical time line of the coevolution of particle physics and brain sciences from their individual origins to eventual combination to form modern functional neuroimaging. The contributions of numerous disciplines, researchers, and events contributing to and advancing the study of cognitive function are shown.

1982) and gave rise to the later development of PET by Phelps, Ter-Pogossian, and co-workers in the 1970s (Ter-Pogossian et al., 1975; Phelps et al., 1977; Hoffman and Phelps, 1979). During the 1980s, the first modern cognitive neuroscientific experiments using PET were conducted by Marcus Raichle, Michael Posner, Steve Peterson, and Peter Fox and their co-workers. In a series of papers, they described PET brain mapping experiment tasks such as word reading (Petersen et al., 1988), visual stimulation (Fox and Raichle, 1985), attention (Posner and Petersen, 1990), and mental imagery and memory (Posner et al., 1988). A few years later, early versions of the computational and statistical methods used in what was to become statisti-

cal parametric mapping (SPM), the most widely used set of software tools for analyzing brain imaging data, were first described (Friston et al., 1989; Friston et al., 1990a,b). Without question, the current methods of mapping brain function using fMRI owe much to pioneering work done prior to the wide availability of fMRI in the twenty-first century.

What can neuroimaging tell us about cognitive function?

Using fMRI to visualize brain function in vivo, neuroscientists have demonstrated that the mental operations carried out by the human brain can be empirically measured. New insights into higher cognitive functions, such as episodic and working memory (Carpenter, Just, and Reichle, 2000; Cabeza et al., 2002) and linguistic processes (Binder et al., 1997; Büchel, Price, and Friston, 1998; Crosson et al., 1999), have been described, to name just a few salient domains. Face perception is one particular cognitive operation that has been extensively explored using fMRI (Haxby, Hoffman, and Gobbini, 2000). Face processing appears to be governed principally by the ventral portion of the temporal lobe, the so-called fusiform face area (FFA; Kanwisher, McDermott, and Chun, 1997). Areas bordering this region may be sensitive to the spatial properties of pictures of other objects, such as chairs and houses (Ishai et al., 2000). Recent work suggests that representations of faces and objects in ventral temporal cortex are spatially distributed but with overlapping portions (Haxby et al., 2001). Research has also investigated the social context of face perception, in particular with respect to the perception of threat (Haxby, Hoffman, and Gobbini, 2002; Adolphs, 2003), the familiarity of faces (Leveroni et al., 2000), and the processing of faces in disorders such as autism (Adolphs, Sears, and Piven, 2001). Visuospatial attention has also received considerable examination using fMRI (Kanwisher and Wojciulik, 2000; Culham, Cavanagh, and Kanwisher, 2001; Binkofski et al., 2002; Hamalainen, Hiltunen, and Titievskaja, 2002). Imaging studies have indicated that a cortical network of visuospatial and oculomotor control areas, specifically the precentral sulcus, intraparietal sulcus, and lateral occipital cortex, is active for covert shifts of spatial attention (Beauchamp et al., 2001). In parietal and frontal cortical areas, activation increased with attentional load, suggesting that these areas are directly involved in attentional processes, though this was not evident in the fusiform gyrus (Culham, Cavanagh, and Kanwisher, 2001).

Measuring evoked neurophysiological changes during cognition

The signal measured using PET is based on the fact that changes in the cellular activity of the brain of normal, awake humans and laboratory animals are almost invariably accompanied by changes in local blood flow (Raichle, 1975; Sokoloff, 1981). This robust empirical relationship has intrigued researchers for well over a hundred years (Raichle, 2001b). Early PET studies of the brain's response to cognitive tasks provided a level of precision in the measurement of blood flow that opened up the modern era of functional human brain mapping (Raichle, 2003). fMRI is distinguished from PET in that it capitalizes on the endogenous contrast of hemoglobin to track rCBF (Hoppel et al., 1993; Rosen et al., 1993). Since the early 1990s, fMRI has replaced PET as the most widely used method for brain mapping and studying the neural basis of human cognition. Although the

method is now widely used throughout the world, an incomplete understanding of the physiological basis of the fMRI signal has prevented a confident interpretation of the data with respect to neuronal activity. The biological origin of these signals is an area of much interest to those involved in cognitive neuroscience research and modeling (Raichle, 2001a; Woo and Hathout, 2001). Understanding the origins of the BOLD signal is useful for building models of the hemodynamic response function (Buxton and Frank, 1997; Buxton, Wong, and Frank, 1998) and to guide characterization of the neurophysiological processes that occur in advance of the BOLD signal change (Friston and Price, 2001b; Friston, 2002; Price and Friston, 2002).

Among the factors that have been implicated in the origins of the BOLD response are energetics, oxygen consumption, and parameters such as blood volume and flow (Buxton, Wong, and Frank, 1998). The question of whether the BOLD response is the result of neuronal output or is due to internal communication among localized populations of cells has also been addressed. In an experimental tour de force, Logothetis and co-workers (2001) conducted the first simultaneous intracortical recordings of neural signals and hemodynamic responses. Varying the temporal characteristics of the stimulus, they observed a moderate to strong association between the neural activity measured with microelectrodes and the pooled BOLD signal from around a small area near the microelectrode tips. However, the BOLD signal showed significantly higher variability than the neural activity, indicating that human fMRI, coupled with traditional statistical methods, underestimates the reliability of the neuronal activity. To further characterize the relative contribution of several types of neuronal signals to the hemodynamic response, Logothetis and colleagues compared local field potentials (LFPs), single- and multiunit activity (MUA) with high spatiotemporal fMRI responses recorded simultaneously in primate visual cortex. After selecting recording sites having transient responses, Logothetic and colleagues found that only the LFP signal showed significant correlation with the hemodynamic response, and was superior to MUA in predicting the fMRI response. Thus, BOLD signal is putatively measuring the input and processing of neuronal information within brain foci, not the output signal transmitted to other brain areas.

In many cognitive neuroimaging experiments, a baseline or control state is fundamental to providing the context in which relative activation can be interpreted. Many feel that resting state activity, if left unconstrained, varies unpredictably or, worse, is systematically dependent on previous task-related stimuli (Stark and Squire, 2001). Clearly, however, the brain is actively consuming glucose even when not actively engaged in a demanding cognitive task. Work by Hyder, Rothman, and Shulman (2002) underscored the role of brain energetics in determining brain activity, a topic of long interest in the study of cortical function (see Kety, 1963), and its potential in determining alterations in baseline brain activity. In anesthetized rats, Hyder and colleagues measured changes in the BOLD signal and the relative spiking frequency of a neuronal ensemble in the somatosensory cortex during forepaw stimulation after two different baseline conditions (see also Smith et al., 2002). Changes in cerebral oxygen consumption were measured from the BOLD signal at 7.0 T via independent determinations in CBF and cerebral blood volume, while the spiking frequency was measured using extracellular recordings in cortical layer 4. Changes in all three parameters were found to be higher during the deep anesthesia baseline condition. For both baselines, cerebral oxygen consumption and relative spiking frequency were approximately one order of magnitude larger than BOLD signal change, but the final values of oxygen consumption and neuronal spiking reached during stimulation were approximately the same from both baselines. These results indicate that particular magnitudes of activity may be needed to support neuronal function. This implies that disregarding baseline activity in fMRI experiments through differencing may remove a large and critical component of the total neural activity (for an overview, see Gusnard et al., 2001).

Raichle and co-workers have explored a baseline state of the normal adult human brain in terms of the brain oxygen extraction fraction (OEF), or the ratio of oxygen used by the brain to the oxygen delivered via blood flow. The OEF typically remains uniform in the conscious resting state (e.g., in an eyes-closed, supine position) (Ito et al., 2001). Local variations in OEF form the physiological basis of signal changes in neuronal activity obtained using fMRI during a wide variety of cognitive and behavioral tasks (An et al., 2001). Raichle and colleagues performed quantitative metabolic and circulatory measurements using PET to obtain the regional OEF throughout the brain. They observed that significant departures from the average hemispheric OEF were all positive, suggesting relative rCBF deactivation, which was present predominantly in the visual system. Decreases such as these suggest a default baseline mode of brain physiological processes that may be being overridden during specific goal-directed behaviors and cognitive tasks. In a related study, Greicius and colleagues (2003) investigated whether a resting-state network exists in the human brain, whether it can be modulated by simple sensory processing, and how it is modulated during higher cognitive processing. They examined posterior cingulate cortex (PCC) and ventral anterior cingulate (vACC) regions that showed decreased activity during a cognitive (working memory) task, then examined their functional connectivity during rest. PCC was found to be strongly coupled with vACC and several other brain regions implicated in the default mode network. Three lateral prefrontal regions showed increased activity during a visual task, and the investigators found inverse correlations among all three lateral prefrontal regions and PCC. Taken together, these findings suggest a mechanism for a default-mode network modulation during cognitive processing.

Experimental paradigm design considerations in fMRI

Epoch or block experimental designs have been the workhorse of fMRI experimentation. In these designs, stimuli are presented for a period of seconds (several TRs) and alternated randomly or pseudo-randomly over the course of the data acquisition period. These experiments are easy to conduct and tend to provide robust activation in most tasks, but the number of stimulus types that can be presented may be limited. Conversely, event-related experimental designs are characterized by having a baseline time course that is punctuated by stimulus events. Event-related methods have permitted a broad array of task designs to be explored with brain imaging techniques (Buckner et al., 1996; Buckner, 1998; Rosen, Buckner, and Dale, 1998). Individual trial events can be presented rapidly, in random or intermixed order, and the hemodynamic responses associated with individual trial events can be estimated (Dale and Buckner, 1997). The basis of event-related studies is that the hemodynamic response tracks neuronal activity on a temporal scale of seconds and, in many situations, summates over trials in a manner well predicted by a linear model that is sufficient even for very briefly spaced stimuli (e.g., ~2 s). With the increased interest in event-related paradigms in fMRI, considerable effort has been made to identify the optimal stimulus timing, especially when the interstimulus interval (ISI) is varied during the imaging acquisition run (Birn, Cox, and Bandettini, 2002; Dreher et al., 2002).

Experimental designs for event-related fMRI can be characterized by both their detection power, a measure of the ability to detect activation, and their estimation efficiency, a measure of the ability to estimate the shape of the hemodynamic response. Computer simulation studies have indicated that estimation of the hemodynamic response function is optimized when stimuli are frequently alternated between task and control states, having shorter ISIs and stimulus durations, while the overall detection ability of activated areas is optimized when blocked designs are used (Mohamed et al., 2000; Birn, Cox, and Bandettini, 2002). This implies that event-related designs may provide more accurate estimates of the HRF than epoch-related designs, with the maximal response to events occurring sooner and returning to baseline later than in a stimulus epoch (Mechelli et al., 2003).

Since the dispersion and delay of the hemodynamic response will govern the BOLD signal that is recovered from any series of input stimulus events, several methods have been proposed for measuring the relative efficiency of event-related designs (Dale, 1999; Friston, Josephs, Zarahn, et al., 2000; Liu et al., 2001; Buracas and Boynton, 2002). Most notably, the method of Dale (1999) expresses the event-related parameter estimation efficiency as the reciprocal of the trace of the inverted experimental design covariance matrix. When this ratio is maximized, the ability to unambiguously compute parameter estimates for event sequences is greatest. However, this is always the case when the eigenvalues of the covariance matrix are equivalent, indicating an orthogonal design (Liu et al., 2001). Thus, ensuring that the collection of regressors is not linearly dependent is essential to being able to determine the unique contribution of each regressor to experimentally induced variation in the BOLD signal.

One additional though very little explored means for examining event-related and other discrete stimulus experimental designs is by calculating the state transition entropy of the event sequence. For any collection of **k** stimulus event types in an experimental run, having $n_1, n_2, \ldots, n_k$ instances over time, respectively, there will be $N!/(n_1!n_2!\ldots n_k!)$ mutually exclusive arrangements of the events that can be realized, where $N = \Sigma_{i=1}^{k} n_i$ is the number of time steps. A set of event-related regressors based on such sequences will always have a known cross-correlation matrix dependent only on the probabilities of each stimulus type. Therefore, the computed efficiency will be fixed for all arrangements of stimuli within a run in the absence of temporal filtering. Thus, simply determining a design measured to be maximally efficient does not guarantee that it is the only such sequence of events that could be identified. Of these event sequences, however, there will be only a small number in which the transitions between stimuli are maximally unpredictable relative to any constraints imposed on the sequence. From information theory it can be demonstrated that there are approximately 2^{NH} sequences that will satisfy the transition probabilities, where H is the conditional entropy measured on the transition probability matrix, and that are worthy of further attention (for review, see Cover and Thomas, 1991). Constraints on event sequences can be applied with a computable decrease in the transition entropy and therefore in the number of available event sequences. Moreover, by determining the conditional entropy, it should be possible to identify cases in which there is no sequence that can satisfy a collection of constraints. Maximum entropy event transition sequences have been used in fMRI studies of the BOLD response to nonverbal stimuli (Bischoff-Grethe et al., 2000) and in studies of motor sequence learning (Bischoff-Grethe et al., 2001). A detailed examination of the information theoretic aspects of fMRI experimental design are beyond the scope of this chapter. However, their use may prove fruitful for designing event sequences that minimize subject habituation and expecta-tion, potentially maximizing stimulus-induced BOLD activation.

Beyond modularity: Functional connectivity and causal modeling

The current portrait of cognitive localization is often at odds with the continually changing, plastic nature of the central nervous system. Occurring at multiple levels of neural organization, from the molecular scale to that of large-scale neural networks, neural connectivity is continuously being altered on the basis of development, aging, and experience throughout a person's life span (Johnston et al., 2001). Functional dynamics and neural plasticity refer to the manner in which the role of neurons in the cerebral cortex adapt to meet changing functional demands following learning and memory encoding (Eichenbaum, 2001). Investigators are now beginning to utilize functional neuroimaging to characterize the functional organization, connectivity, and alteration of the nervous system (Kujala, Alho, and Näätanen, 2000; Jancke et al., 2001; Pascual-Leone, 2001).

A recent theoretical model proposed by Friston and Price (2001a; see also Price et al., 2001) posits that the representational capacity and inherent function of any neuron, neuronal ensemble, or cortical region is dynamic and context-sensitive. This adaptive and contextual specialization is mediated by functional integration or the interactions among brain systems, with a special emphasis on backward or top-down connections. Neuronal responses in any given cortical area may represent different things at different times (McIntosh, 2000; McIntosh, Fitzpatrick, and Friston, 2001). Thus, the specialization of any region may be determined through bottom-up driving inputs as well as by top-down predictions. Conflict between the two is resolved by alterations in the higher-level representations, driven by the resulting perceptual or behaviorally mediated errors detected in lower regions, until the mismatch has been nullified (e.g., visual response competition; Desimone, 1998). Therefore, functional specialization may not be an intrinsic property of any region but is dependent on both forward and backward connections with other areas. This important concept has also been suggested as playing an important role in the formation of motor programs (Desmurget et al., 1999; Desmurget and Grafton, 2000; Van Horn, 2002a). Thus, ongoing neural plasticity is the result of adaptive connectivity within and between upper- and lower-level brain regions. This important conjecture deserves greater attention and empirical study and may help to elucidate the developmental and dynamic properties underlying connectivity and functional plasticity.

One manner in which to examine adaptations due to the neural representation for cognitive processes is through the use of advanced multivariate analyses. Functional connectivity modeling is the most important approach for tracking the changes associated with long-term learning and the adaptation of the brain with experience. Structural equation modeling may be used to identify the strength of connectivity between brain regions, thereby describing patterns of brain activity not in terms of how much regions are activated but in terms of their extent of correlation (McIntosh, 1999). Additionally, to take into account subject task performance variables, partial least-squares (PLS) analysis may also be performed. This methodology has been used previously to identify sensorimotor-specific brain systems that jointly embody learning-related responses to stimuli and the subsequent change in behavior (McIntosh et al., 1998). Also, the application of network-theory-based analytic techniques can illustrate minimum-cost paths of connectivity that may result on the basis of neural requirements for minimal metabolic expenditure at maximal transfer of neural information. Figure 92.3 shows an example of the application of a simple network-analytical approach. These methods will all be critical to the modeling, representation, and characterization of

changes due to functional dynamics accompanying behavioral experience.

Because imaging can be used to measure the whole brain, it is possible to examine the operations of large-scale neural systems and their relation to cognition. McIntosh, Horwitz, and others (McIntosh, 1998, 1999, 2000; Horwitz, Tagamets, and McIntosh, 1999) have pointed out that one approach uses the partial least-squares method. This multivariate method decomposes the covariance between brain images and exogenous variables representing either the experiment design or a simultaneously collected behavioral measure. The patterns obtained are believed to represent large-scale neural models of brain activity, specific to the experimental manipulation in question. This approach differs markedly from other statistical methods for neuroimaging data analysis in that rather than trying to predict the individual values of the image pixels, PLS attempts to explain the relation between image pixels and task or behavior. Therefore, PLS serves as an important extension by extracting new information from imaging data that is not

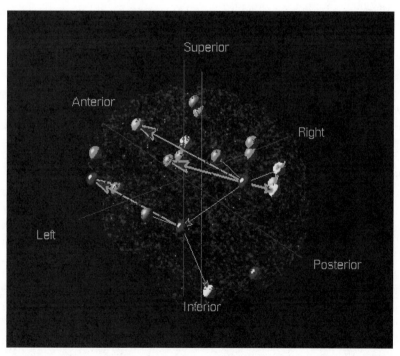

FIGURE 92.3   In a connected network it is often useful to identify the optimal route by which to propagate a message through the system. Analytical techniques permit the assessment of the minimum-cost path (the path in which information loss is minimal or propagation delay is smallest) between a node in a connected network to other surrounding nodes. In this figure, the brain regions identified in a study of face processing by McIntosh (1998) are shown as spheroids in the standardized Talairach space. In the McIntosh study, path weights were determined through decomposition of the covariance matrix between brain regions. To examine the minimum-cost path from the region of the fusiform gyrus to its

neighbors, the reported path weights may be subjected to Djikstra's Minimum-cost path analysis. The resulting paths shown here indicate both direct and indirect paths connecting the fusiform area to other regions distributed throughout the brain. This suggests the existence of both functional and effective connectivity in the processing of faces, in particular connectivity between FFA and regions of the frontal lobe putatively involved in executive functions. The strength of the connection is indicated by line thickness, and no connectivity is evident where two brain regions are not connected by a path. (See color plate 81.)

accessible through other currently used univariate and multivariate image analysis tools.

The archiving and mining of fMRI data

Meta-analyses of neuroimaging study results have helped to synthesize the literature on cognitive function (Koski and Paus, 2000; Joseph, 2001; Chein et al., 2002; Phan et al., 2002; Turkeltaub et al., 2002) but have also highlighted a number of parameters that may influence the results of these studies (Cabeza and Nyberg, 2000). Of particular use for determining study variables to be included in this ontology are analyses of the study parameters that may influence fMRI statistical findings. For example, in a study of the processing parameters that can affect the interpretation of fMRI data, Hopfinger and colleagues (2000) noted that the choice of spatial smoothing filter was an important factor in predicting the extent of reported activation, as was the choice of basis set used in the statistical design matrix. Indeed, the choice of parameters made in the data processing stream can greatly influence the results (for review, see Brett, Johnsrude, and Owen, 2002). Investigations in patient groups versus control subjects in studies of brain structural anomalies have noted that the year of publication of a study can be a strong indicator of the reported statistical effect size (Van Horn and McManus, 1992), presumably related to the increasing experimental control over time.

The increasing application of imaging methods for mapping patterns of brain activation has spurred the development of brain databasing tools (Van Horn et al., 2002) and population-based digital atlases (Toga and Thompson, 2001). Archives of functional imaging data permit others to mine and explore data from published experiments (Van Horn and Gazzaniga, 2002). Digital atlases contain information on how the brain varies across age, sex, and time, in health and disease, and in large human populations. The fMRI Data Center (fMRIDC, *http://www.fmridc.org*) began making data sets publicly available in 2001. At present, the archive contains 70 complete data sets (over 3 terabytes worth of data) which researchers may request online and have sent to them free of charge (Van Horn et al., 2001). Authors of studies from the peer-reviewed literature provide as much detail as possible about their study: a description of the subjects (e.g., age, handedness, clinical diagnosis), the MRI scanner (e.g., manufacturer, model, software revision, field strength), scanner parameters (e.g., number of slices acquired, TR, TE), the specifics of the experimental design (e.g., stimulus time course information, number of experimental runs), and imaging data—raw, preprocessed, and final results. Researchers then request and mine these data to explore human consciousness (Lloyd, 2002), top-down and bottom-up visual processing (Mechelli et al., 2003), and the robustness of patterns of activation (Liou et al., 2003).

Further examination of previously obtained data may reveal effects not observed in the original study, or may help develop novel analysis methods, or may be combined to perform a large-scale meta-analysis across cognitive domains.

Future directions

BOLD RESPONSE LATENCY MAPPING   Recent computational advancements have made it possible to determine the latency and temporal structure of the HRF activation function at a temporal scale of few hundreds of milliseconds. Despite the sluggishness of the hemodynamic response, fMRI can detect a temporal ordering of neural activations over the cortex potentially indicative of corticocortical communication (Calhoun et al., 2000; Formisano and Goebel, 2003). Estimates of hemodynamic amplitude, delay, and width have been combined to investigate the system dynamics involved in lexical decision making (Bellgowan, Saad, and Bandettini, 2003), visual processing (Huettel and McCarthy, 2001), and temporally dependent behavior (Nobre, 2001). These methods aid in the linear-system analyses of fMRI data, contain information about neural processing rate, and can be used to improve parameter estimates of the HRF.

DIFFUSION TENSOR IMAGING   Diffusion tensor MRI (DTI) permits determination of the dominant orientation of structured tissue within an image voxel. This has led to the development of computational and graphical methods for representing fiber orientation and DTI "tractography" (Bammer, Acar, and Moseley, 2003), which aims to reconstruct the three-dimensional (3D) trajectories of white matter fiber bundles. Most contemporary fiber orientation mapping schemes and tractography algorithms employ the directional information contained in the eigenvectors of the diffusion tensor to approximate white matter fiber orientation (Basser and Jones, 2002). There is, however, an uncertainty associated with every estimate of the tensor directionality (Pajevic and Basser, 2003), although recent techniques have become available that allow simultaneous viewing of fiber orientation and its uncertainty, and examination of the relationship between orientation uncertainty and tissue anisotropy (Jones, 2003). Although DTI is largely considered an anatomically based form of imaging, several articles have described its utility in helping to interpret cognitive function (Moseley, Bammer, and Illes, 2002), its role in measuring the effects of aging on white matter connectivity (Moseley, 2002), and its predictive power of reaction time on mental rotation (Baird et al., in press; figure 92.4).

MR SPECTROSCOPY   Although fMRI techniques have traditionally been used to investigate sensory, motor, and cognitive functions, they are also very attractive for investigating

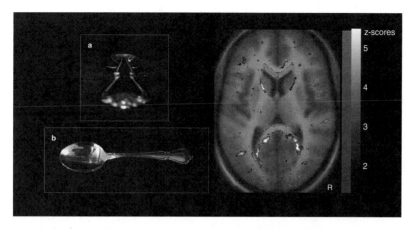

FIGURE 92.4   Example object, a spoon, used in the study of Baird and colleagues. The spoon is shown in both unusual and usual perspectives. At right is a *z*-score statistical parametric map illustrating the results of a multiple regression analysis using DTI anisotropy and BOLD activation, in which the splenium of the corpus callosum is predictive of relatively faster reaction times and

decreased BOLD response. Conversely, the genu of the corpus callosum was significantly predictive of longer reaction times and increased BOLD response in cortical regions of interest on a task that required individuals to name objects presented from unusual perspectives. (Images courtesy of Abigail Baird, Dartmouth College, Hanover, N.H.) (See color plate 82.)

the distribution of neurochemically related signals in the brain, using MRS (Rothman et al., 2003). These methods allow the determination of metabolic processes that support neurotransmission and neurotransmission rates (Ugurbil et al., 2000). Spectroscopic methods have been employed in examinations of schizophrenia and psychiatric patients (Bertolino et al., 2001; Frank and Pavlakis, 2001), HIV infection (Pfefferbaum, Rosenbloom, and Sullivan, 2002), and stroke (Cramer and Bastings, 2000). These methods hold promise for helping to guide understanding of the neurochemical makeup of brain regions found to activate under different cognitive tasks in BOLD imaging studies. Pharmacological investigations of drug activity are also promising. In these studies a drug is administered and its effects on brain chemistry are examined, although special experimental control considerations exist (Salmeron and Stein, 2002). These concerns notwithstanding, careful attention to experimental detail and verification procedures promises to make neurochemically and pharmacologically based MRI valuable tools for understanding the neurochemical basis and the actions of drugs on the brain at many levels.

MR PERFUSION   Emerging fMRI methods based on BOLD contrast and arterial spin labeling (ASL) perfusion contrast have now enabled imaging of changes in blood oxygenation and CBF. Whereas BOLD contrast has been widely used as a surrogate for true neuronal activation, recent evidence suggests that perfusion contrast is also suitable for studying relatively long-term effects on CBF, both at rest or during activation (Detre and Wang, 2002; Liu et al., 2002). Special considerations need to be given to designing cognitive task paradigms for use with perfusion imaging that seek to capitalize on the beneficial properties of the perfusion signal that are quite distinct from BOLD. For instance, whereas the

BOLD signal has a substantial temporal autocorrelation function, the perfusion signal's autocorrelation FWHM is much less, potentially meaning greater single-stimulus response resolvability in BOLD event-related studies (Aguirre et al., 2002). Comparisons of BOLD and perfusion imaging during event-related scanning have indicated that the perfusion response curve may precede the BOLD curve in well under a second (Yang et al., 2000).

Discussion

The identification of links between the observable phenomena of mental processes and the measurable neural activity in the human brain has long been a fundamental goal in cognitive neuroscience (Posner et al., 1988; Posner, 1993). The examination of processes governing functional dynamics of these cognitive processes has been of considerable interest in both normal and patient groups. As cognitive neuroscience continues to grow, so too will techniques for functional neuroimaging, and vice versa. The symbiotic relationship between cognitive science, neurophysiology, and MRI physics is unique in science, wherein technological sophistication enhances neuroimaging data collection and neuroscientific questions help drive technological innovation. This is an inherent and desirable strength.

There is a slight danger, however, that the rapid growth and ease of conducting neuroimaging studies will have unfortunate effects. Rightly or wrongly, the field has already been criticized as representing "neophrenology," interested only in blindly localizing cognitive processes to neurologically defined modules (Uttal, 2001). The critics of cognitive neuroimaging contend that nothing more has been learned about brain function from these methods than was already known from studies of lesion patients. The "pure insertion" model tends to be at the root of such complaints (Friston et al., 1996). Cognitive neuroscience, with its heavy dependence on neuroimaging technology, could view this critique defensively and argue that such missives are coming from researchers who have not kept up with the times. A more healthy approach would be to recognize the onus to produce credible and convincing evidence of brain function that could not have been achieved without brain mapping techniques. Greater demand should be placed on more rigidly defining the goals in examining the functional correlates of certain "higher cognitive functions" lest we later be accused of simply chasing phantoms. Vigilance should be heightened to ensure that cognitive neuroimaging studies that make it into the literature are unique in their merit, rigorously conducted, parsimoniously and cautiously interpreted, and the data from them made open to public scrutiny. Investigators should avoid overly derivative and perhaps banal fMRI studies where they are not needed. The integrity and continued maturity of cognitive neuroscience depends on our own ability to be self-critical if neuroimaging is to move forward toward meeting Gazzaniga's challenge.

Studies using several modalities have reported changes in the organization of cortical representations, both on the basis of developmental processes as well as on the basis of experience in mature animals as well as in humans (Buonomano and Merzenich, 1998). This process of adaptive specialization and plasticity is believed to be mediated through functional integration and interactions among brain systems, with an emphasis on feedback and top-down connections (e.g., visual attention and memory; Desimone, 1998). Evidence from functional neuroimaging investigations further suggests that higher-level systems provide predictive inputs to lower-level regions in goal-oriented tasks such as visuomotor tracking. These findings imply that functional plasticity is a fundamental property of the brain, dependent on both feedforward and feedback connections distributed widely throughout the brain. It is possible for these dynamical effects to be measured using functional imaging, thereby shedding light on the processes underlying these adaptive changes in both normal subjects and in those who have suffered from neurological disease or insult (Poldrack, 2000). Functional imaging examination focused on the motor system is of particular interest, given its interest to clinicians for patients recovering from stroke (see, e.g., Cramer et al., 1997, 2000).

The data from neuroimaging studies of cognitive function are a rich source of spatial, temporal, and empirical information that may be more useful in examining the properties of blood oxygenation changes evoked by cognition than for what is reported in any individual study. Rigorous computational approaches can be employed to move beyond simple pure insertion-based activation models of regional localization to those that might mathematically characterize distributed circuitry and regional communication underlying cognitive function (Friston, 2002). This would involve analysis of not only how activity in a brain area is modulated by task requirements but also how that area is influenced by top-down and bottom-up inputs from other brain areas. Though there are undoubtedly brain regions with specialized function, it is likely the manner in which brain regions exchange information that underlies many cognitive processes (McIntosh, 1998).

Finally, the cognitive neuroscience field has matured to the point of requiring that greater importance be placed on the sharing of neuroimaging study data so that data may be combined with the data from other studies (Van Horn, 2002b). It might be argued that a single fMRI study is like peering at brain function through a drinking straw. However, it would be pedestrian to claim that combining fMRI studies would have the effect of simply increasing the diameter of the straw. Rather, combining studies permits a view of the broader landscape of cognitive activation patterns across the brain specific to individual cognitive domains but that also involve common regions of cortex. This relative increase in our cognitive neuroscientific field of view, to borrow a term from neuroimaging, can permit greater understanding of just which brain areas are unique in cognitive processes, such as attention episodic memory, and in what brain regions do the neural systems underlying these processes overlap.

REFERENCES

ADOLPHS, R., 2003. Cognitive neuroscience of human social behaviour. *Nat. Rev. Neurosci.* 4:165–178.

ADOLPHS, R., L. SEARS, and J. PIVEN, 2001. Abnormal processing of social information from faces in autism. *J. Cogn. Neurosci.* 13:232–240.

AGUIRRE, G. K., J. A. DETRE, E. ZARAHN, and D. C. ALSOP, 2002. Experimental design and the relative sensitivity of BOLD and perfusion fMRI. *Neuroimage* 15:488–500.

AGUIRRE, G. K., E. ZARAHN, and M. D'ESPOSITO, 1997. Empirical analyses of BOLD fMRI statistics. II. Spatially smoothed data collected under null-hypothesis and experimental conditions. *NeuroImage* 5:199–212.

AN, H., W. LIN, A. CELIK, and Y. Z. LEE, 2001. Quantitative measurements of cerebral metabolic rate of oxygen utilization using MRI: A volunteer study. *NMR Biomed.* 14:441–447.

BAIRD, A. A., M. K. COLVIN, H. L. GORDON, S. INATI, and M. S. GAZZANIGA (in press). Predicting interhemispheric communication speed using cortical activation and callosal anisotropy. *Psychol. Sci.*

BAMMER, R., B. ACAR, and M. E. MOSELEY, 2003. In vivo MR tractography using diffusion imaging. *Eur. J. Radiol.* 45:223–234.

BASSER, P. J., and D. K. JONES, 2002. Diffusion-tensor MRI: Theory, experimental design and data analysis. A technical review. *NMR Biomed.* 15:456–467.

BEAUCHAMP, M. S., L. PETIT, T. M. ELLMORE, J. INGEHOLM, and J. V. HAXBY, 2001. A parametric fMRI study of overt and covert shifts of visuospatial attention. *NeuroImage* 14:310–321.

BELLGOWAN, P. S., Z. S. SAAD, and P. A. BANDETTINI, 2003. Understanding neural system dynamics through task modulation and measurement of functional MRI amplitude, latency, and width. *Proc. Natl. Acad. Sci. U.S.A.* 100:1415–1419.

BERTOLINO, A., J. H. CALLICOTT, V. S. MATTAY, K. M. WEIDENHAMMER, R. RAKOW, M. F. EGAN, and D. R. WEINBERGER, 2001. The effect of treatment with antipsychotic drugs on brain *N*-acetylaspartate measures in patients with schizophrenia. *Biol. Psychiatry* 49:39–46.

BINDER, J. R., J. A. FROST, T. A. HAMMEKE, R. W. COX, S. M. RAO, and T. PRIETO, 1997. Human brain language areas identified by functional magnetic resonance imaging. *J. Neurosci.* 17:353–362.

BINKOFSKI, F., G. R. FINK, S. GEYER, G. BUCCINO, O. GRUBER, N. J. SHAH, J. G. TAYLOR, R. J. SEITZ, K. ZILLES, and H. J. FREUND, 2002. Neural activity in human primary motor cortex areas 4a and 4p is modulated differentially by attention to action. *J. Neurophysiol* 88:514–519.

BIRN, R. M., R. W. COX, and P. A. BANDETTINI, 2002. Detection versus estimation in event-related fMRI: Choosing the optimal stimulus timing. *NeuroImage* 15:252–264.

BISCHOFF-GRETHE, A., M. MARTIN, H. MAO, and G. S. BERNS, 2001. The context of uncertainty modulates the subcortical response to predictability. *J. Cogn. Neurosci.* 13:986–993.

BISCHOFF-GRETHE, A., S. M. PROPER, H. MAO, K. A. DANIELS, and G. S. BERNS, 2000. Conscious and unconscious processing of nonverbal predictability in Wernicke's area. *J. Neurosci.* 20:1975–1981.

BRETT, M., I. S. JOHNSRUDE, and A. M. OWEN, 2002. The problem of functional localization in the human brain. *Nat. Rev. Neurosci.* 3:243–249.

BÜCHEL, C., C. PRICE, and K. FRISTON, 1998. A multimodal language region in the ventral visual pathway. *Nature* 394:274–277.

BUCKNER, R. L., 1998. Event-related fMRI and the hemodynamic response. *Hum. Brain Mapp.* 6:373–377.

BUCKNER, R. L., P. A. BANDETTINI, K. M. O'CRAVEN, R. L. SAVOY, S. E. PETERSEN, M. E. RAICHLE, and B. R. ROSEN, 1996. Detection of cortical activation during averaged single trials of a cognitive task using functional magnetic resonance imaging. *Proc. Natl. Acad. Sci. U.S.A.* 93:14878–14883.

BUDINGER, T. F., and P. C. LAUTERBUR, 1984. Nuclear magnetic resonance technology for medical studies. *Science* 226:288–298.

BUONOMANO, D. V., and M. M. MERZENICH, 1998. Cortical plasticity: From synapses to maps. *Annu. Rev. Neurosci.* 21:149–186.

BURACAS, G. T., and G. M. BOYNTON, 2002. Efficient design of event-related fMRI experiments using M-sequences. *NeuroImage* 16(3 Pt. 1):801–813.

BUXTON, R. B., and L. R. FRANK, 1997. A model for the coupling between cerebral blood flow and oxygen metabolism during neural stimulation. *J. Cereb. Blood Flow Metab.* 17:64–72.

BUXTON, R. B., E. C. WONG, and L. R. FRANK, 1998. Dynamics of blood flow and oxygenation changes during brain activation: The balloon model. *Magn. Reson. Med.* 39:855–864.

CABEZA, R., F. DOLCOS, R. GRAHAM, and L. NYBERG, 2002. Similarities and differences in the neural correlates of episodic memory retrieval and working memory. *NeuroImage* 16:317–330.

CABEZA, R., and L. NYBERG, 2000. Imaging cognition. II. An empirical review of 275 PET and fMRI studies. *J. Cogn. Neurosci.* 12:1–47.

CALHOUN, V., T. ADALI, M. KRAUT, and G. PEARLSON, 2000. A weighted least-squares algorithm for estimation and visualization of relative latencies in event-related functional MRI. *Magn. Reson. Med.* 44:947–954.

CARPENTER, P. A., M. A. JUST, and E. D. REICHLE, 2000. Working memory and executive function: Evidence from neuroimaging. *Curr. Opin. Neurobiol.* 10:195–199.

CHEIN, J. M., K. FISSELL, S. JACOBS, and J. A. FIEZ, 2002. Functional heterogeneity within Broca's area during verbal working memory. *Physiol. Behav.* 77:635–639.

COVER, T. M., and J. A. THOMAS, 1991. *Elements of Information Theory.* New York: Wiley.

CRAMER, S. C., and E. P. BASTINGS, 2000. Mapping clinically relevant plasticity after stroke. *Neuropharmacology* 39:842–851.

CRAMER, S. C., C. I. MOORE, S. P. FINKLESTEIN, and B. R. ROSEN, 2000. A pilot study of somatotopic mapping after cortical infarct. *Stroke* 31:668–671.

CRAMER, S. C., G. NELLES, R. R. BENSON, J. D. KAPLAN, R. A. PARKER, K. K. KWONG, D. N. KENNEDY, S. P. FINKLESTEIN, and B. R. ROSEN, 1997. A functional MRI study of subjects recovered from hemiparetic stroke. *Stroke* 28:2518–2527.

CROSSON, B., S. M. RAO, S. J. WOODLEY, A. C. ROSEN, J. A. BOBHOLZ, A. MAYER, J. M. CUNNINGHAM, T. A. HAMMEKE, S. A. FULLER, J. R. BINDER, R. W. COX, and E. A. STEIN, 1999. Mapping of semantic, phonological, and orthographic verbal working memory in normal adults with functional magnetic resonance imaging. *Neuropsychology* 13:171–187.

CULHAM, J. C., P. CAVANAGH, and N. G. KANWISHER, 2001. Attention response functions: Characterizing brain areas using fMRI activation during parametric variations of attentional load. *Neuron* 32:737–745.

DALE, A. M., 1999. Optimal experimental design for event-related fMRI. *Hum. Brain Mapp.* 8:109–114.

DALE, A. M., and R. L. BUCKNER, 1997. Selective averaging of rapidly presented individual trials using fMRI. *Hum. Brain Mapp.* 5:329–340.

DESIMONE, R., 1998. Visual attention mediated by biased competition in extrastriate visual cortex. *Philos. Trans. R. Soc. Lond. B Biol. Sci.* 353:1245–1255.

DESMURGET, M., C. M. EPSTEIN, R. S. TURNER, C. PRABLANC, G. E. ALEXANDER, and S. T. GRAFTON, 1999. Role of the posterior parietal cortex in updating reaching movements to a visual target. *Nat. Neurosci.* 2:563–567.

DESMURGET, M., and S. GRAFTON, 2000. Forward modeling allows feedback control for fast reaching movements. *Trends Cogn. Sci.* 4:423–431.

D'ESPOSITO, M., 2000. Functional neuroimaging of cognition. *Semin. Neurol.* 20:487–498.

DETRE, J. A., and T. F. FLOYD, 2001. Functional MRI and its applications to the clinical neurosciences. *Neuroscientist* 7:64–79.

DETRE, J. A., and J. WANG, 2002. Technical aspects and utility of fMRI using BOLD and ASL. *Clin. Neurophysiol.* 113:621–634.

DI SALLE, F., E. FORMISANO, D. E. LINDEN, R. GOEBEL, S. BONAVITA, A. PEPINO, F. SMALTINO, and G. TEDESCHI, 1999. Exploring brain function with magnetic resonance imaging. *Eur. J. Radiol.* 30:84–94.

DREHER, J. C., E. KOECHLIN, S. O. ALI, and J. GRAFMAN, 2002. The roles of timing and task order during task switching. *NeuroImage* 17:95–109.

EICHENBAUM, H., 2001. The long and winding road to memory consolidation. *Nat. Neurosci.* 4:1057–1058.

FORMISANO, E., and R. GOEBEL, 2003. Tracking cognitive processes with functional MRI mental chronometry. *Curr. Opin. Neurobiol.* 13:174–181.

FOX, P. T., and M. E. RAICHLE, 1985. Stimulus rate determines regional brain blood flow in striate cortex. *Ann. Neurol.* 17:303–305.

FRANK, Y., and S. G. PAVLAKIS, 2001. Brain imaging in neurobehavioral disorders. *Pediatr. Neurol.* 25:278–287.

FRISTON, K., 2002. Beyond phrenology: What can neuroimaging tell us about distributed circuitry? *Annu. Rev. Neurosci.* 25: 221–250.

FRISTON, K. J., C. D. FRITH, P. F. LIDDLE, R. J. DOLAN, A. A. LAMMERTSMA, and R. S. FRACKOWIAK, 1990a. The relationship between global and local changes in PET scans. *J. Cereb. Blood Flow Metab.* 10:458–466.

FRISTON, K. J., C. D. FRITH, P. F. LIDDLE, R. J. DOLAN, A. A. LAMMERTSMA, and R. S. J. FRACKOWIAK, 1990b. The relationship between global and local changes in PET scans. *J. Cereb. Blood Flow Metab.* 10:458–466.

FRISTON, K. J., D. E. GLASER, R. N. HENSON, S. KIEBEL, C. PHILLIPS, and J. ASHBURNER, 2002. Classical and Bayesian inference in neuroimaging: Applications. *NeuroImage* 16:484–512.

FRISTON, K. J., O. JOSEPHS, E. ZARAHN, A. P. HOLMES, S. ROUQUETTE, and J. POLINE, 2000. To smooth or not to smooth? Bias and efficiency in fMRI time-series analysis. *NeuroImage* 12:196–208.

FRISTON, K. J., R. E. PASSINGHAM, J. G. NUTT, J. D. HEATHER, G. V. SAWLE, and R. S. FRACKOWIAK, 1989. Localisation in PET images: Direct fitting of the intercommissural (AC-PC) line. *J. Cereb. Blood Flow Metab.* 9:690–695.

FRISTON, K. J., W. PENNY, C. PHILLIPS, S. KIEBEL, G. HINTON, and J. ASHBURNER, 2002. Classical and Bayesian inference in neuroimaging: Theory. *NeuroImage* 16:465–483.

FRISTON, K., J. PHILLIPS, D. CHAWLA, and C. BUCHEL, 2000. Nonlinear PCA: Characterizing interactions between modes of brain activity. *Philos. Trans. R. Soc. Lond. B Biol. Sci.* 355:135–146.

FRISTON, K. J., and C. J. PRICE, 2001a. Dynamic representations and generative models of brain function. *Brain Res. Bull.* 54:275–285.

FRISTON, K. J., and C. J. PRICE, 2001b. Generative models, brain function and neuroimaging. *Scand. J. Psychol.* 42:167–177.

FRISTON, K. J., C. J. PRICE, P. FLETCHER, C. MOORE, R. S. FRACKOWIAK, and R. J. DOLAN, 1996. The trouble with cognitive subtraction. *NeuroImage* 4:97–104.

GAZZANIGA, M., 1997. Preface. In *The Cognitive Neurosciences*, M. Gazzaniga, ed. Cambridge, Mass.: MIT Press.

GREICIUS, M. D., B. KRASNOW, A. L. REISS, and V. MENON, 2003. Functional connectivity in the resting brain: A network analysis of the default mode hypothesis. *Proc. Natl. Acad. Sci. U.S.A.* 100: 253–258.

GUSNARD, D. A., E. AKBUDAK, G. L. SHULMAN, and M. E. RAICHLE, 2001. Medial prefrontal cortex and self-referential mental activity: Relation to a default mode of brain function. *Proc. Natl. Acad. Sci. U.S.A.* 98:4259–4264.

HAMALAINEN, H., J. HILTUNEN, and I. TITIEVSKAJA, 2002. Activation of somatosensory cortical areas varies with attentional state: An fMRI study. *Behav. Brain Res.* 135:159.

HAXBY, J. V., M. I. GOBBINI, M. L. FUREY, A. ISHAI, J. L. SCHOUTEN, and P. PIETRINI, 2001. Distributed and overlapping representations of faces and objects in ventral temporal cortex. *Science* 293:2425–2430.

HAXBY, J. V., E. A. HOFFMAN, and M. I. GOBBINI, 2000. The distributed human neural system for face perception. *Trends Cogn. Sci.* 4:223–233.

HAXBY, J. V., E. A. HOFFMAN, and M. I. GOBBINI, 2002. Human neural systems for face recognition and social communication. *Biol. Psychiatry* 51:59–67.

HOFFMAN, E. J., and M. E. PHELPS, 1979. Positron emission tomography. *Med. Instrum.* 13:147–151.

HOPFINGER, J. B., C. BÜCHEL, A. P. HOLMES, and K. J. Friston, 2000. A study of analysis parameters that influence the sensitivity of event-related fMRI analyses. *NeuroImage* 11:326–333.

HOPPEL, B. E., R. M. WEISSKOFF, K. R. THULBORN, J. B. MOORE, K. K. KWONG, and B. R. ROSEN, 1993. Measurement of regional blood oxygenation and cerebral hemodynamics. *Magn. Reson. Med.* 30:715–723.

HORWITZ, B., M. A. TAGAMETS, and A. R. MCINTOSH, 1999. Neural modeling, functional brain imaging, and cognition. *Trends. Cogn. Sci.* 3:91–98.

HUETTEL, S. A., and G. MCCARTHY, 2001. Regional differences in the refractory period of the hemodynamic response: An event-related fMRI study. *NeuroImage* 14:967–976.

HYDER, F., D. L. ROTHMAN, and R. G. SHULMAN, 2002. Total neuroenergetics support localized brain activity: Implications for the interpretation of fMRI. *Proc. Natl. Acad. Sci. U.S.A.* 19: 19.

ISHAI, A., L. G. UNGERLEIDER, A. MARTIN, and J. V. HAXBY, 2000. The representation of objects in the human occipital and temporal cortex. *J. Cogn. Neurosci.* 12(Suppl. 2):35–51.

ITO, H., I. KANNO, H. IIDA, J. HATAZAWA, E. SHIMOSEGAWA, H. TAMURA, and T. OKUDERA, 2001. Arterial fraction of cerebral blood volume in humans measured by positron emission tomography. *Ann. Nucl. Med.* 15:111–116.

JANCKE, L., N. GAAB, T. WUSTENBERG, H. SCHEICH, and H. J. HEINZE, 2001. Short-term functional plasticity in the human auditory cortex: An fMRI study. *Brain Res. Cogn. Brain Res.* 12: 479–485.

JOHNSTON, M. V., A. NISHIMURA, K. HARUM, J. PEKAR, and M. E. BLUE, 2001. Sculpting the developing brain. *Adv. Pediatr.* 48: 1–38.

JONES, D. K., 2003. Determining and visualizing uncertainty in estimates of fiber orientation from diffusion tensor MRI. *Magn. Reson. Med.* 49:7–12.

JOSEPH, J. E., 2001. Functional neuroimaging studies of category specificity in object recognition: A critical review and meta-analysis. *Cogn. Affect. Behav. Neurosci.* 1:119–136.

KANWISHER, N., J. MCDERMOTT, and M. M. CHUN, 1997. The fusiform face area: A module in human extrastriate cortex specialized for face perception. *J. Neurosci.* 17:4302–4311.

KANWISHER, N., and E. WOJCIULIK, 2000. Visual attention: Insights from brain imaging. *Nat. Rev. Neurosci.* 1:91–100.

KETY, S. S., 1963. The circulation and energy metabolism of the brain. *Clin. Neurosurg.* 9:56–66.

KETY, S. S., 1966. Recent approaches to the measurement of cerebral blood flow and their underlying principles. *Res. Publ. Assoc. Res. Nerv. Ment. Dis.* 41:226–236.

KHERIF, F., J. B. POLINE, G. FLANDIN, H. BENALI, O. SIMON, S. DEHAENE, and K. J. WORSLEY, 2002. Multivariate model specification for fMRI data. *NeuroImage* 16:1068–1083.

KOSKI, L., and T. PAUS, 2000. Functional connectivity of the anterior cingulate cortex within the human frontal lobe: A brain-mapping meta-analysis. *Exp. Brain Res.* 133:55–65.

KUJALA, T., K. ALHO, and R. NÄÄTANEN, 2000. Cross-modal reorganization of human cortical functions. *Trends Neurosci.* 23: 115–120.

LEVERONI, C. L., M. SEIDENBERG, A. R. MAYER, L. A. MEAD, J. R. BINDER, and S. M. RAO, 2000. Neural systems underlying the recognition of familiar and newly learned faces. *J. Neurosci.* 20:878–886.

LIOU, M., H.-R. SU, J.-D. LEE, and P. E. CHENG, 2003. Bridging functional MR images and scientific inference: Reproducibilty maps. *J. Cogn. Neurosci.* 15:934–945.

LIU, T. T., L. R. FRANK, E. C. WONG, and R. B. BUXTON, 2001. Detection power, estimation efficiency, and predictability in event-related fMRI. *NeuroImage* 13:759–773.

LIU, T. T., E. C. WONG, L. R. FRANK, and R. B. BUXTON, 2002. Analysis and design of perfusion-based event-related fMRI experiments. *NeuroImage* 16:269–282.

LLOYD, D., 2002. Functional MRI and the study of human consciousness. *J. Cogn. Neurosci.* 14:818–831.

LOGOTHETIS, N. K., J. PAULS, M. AUGATH, T. TRINATH, and A. OELTERMANN, 2001. Neurophysiological investigation of the basis of the fMRI signal. *Nature* 412:150–157.

MANDLER, G., 2002. Origins of the cognitive (r)evolution. *J. Hist. Behav. Sci.* 38:339–353.

MCINTOSH, A. R., 1998. Understanding neural interactions in learning and memory using functional neuroimaging. *Ann. N.Y. Acad. Sci.* 855:556–571.

MCINTOSH, A. R., 1999. Mapping cognition to the brain through neural interactions. *Memory* 7:523–548.

MCINTOSH, A. R., 2000. Towards a network theory of cognition. *Neural Netw.* 13:861–870.

MCINTOSH, A. R., S. M. FITZPATRICK, and K. J. FRISTON, 2001. On the marriage of cognition and neuroscience. *NeuroImage* 14: 1231–1237.

MCINTOSH, A. R., N. J. LOBAUGH, R. CABEZA, F. L. BOOKSTEIN, and S. HOULE, 1998. Convergence of neural systems processing stimulus associations and coordinating motor responses. *Cereb. Cortex* 8:648–659.

MECHELLI, A., R. N. HENSON, C. J. PRICE, and K. J. FRISTON, 2003. Comparing event-related and epoch analysis in blocked design fMRI. *NeuroImage* 18:806–810.

MECHELLI, A., C. PRICE, U. NOPPENEY, and K. FRISTON, 2003. A dynamic causal modelling study on category effects: Bottom-up or top-down mediation? *J. Cogn. Neurosci.* 15:925–934.

MILLER, G. A., 2003. The cognitive revolution: A historical perspective. *Trends Cogn. Sci.* 7:141–144.

MILNER, B., 1963. Effects of different brain lesions on card sorting: The role of the frontal lobes. *Arch. Neurol.* 9:100–110.

MILNER, B., 1982. Some cognitive effects of frontal-lobe lesions in man. *Proc. R. Soc. Lond.* 298(1089):211–226.

MINTUN, M. A., B. N. LUNDSTROM, A. Z. SNYDER, A. G. VLASSENKO, G. L. SHULMAN, and M. E. RAICHLE, 2001. Blood flow and oxygen delivery to human brain during functional activity: Theoretical modeling and experimental data. *Proc. Natl. Acad. Sci. U.S.A.* 98:6859–6864.

MOHAMED, F. B., J. I. TRACY, S. H. FARO, J. EMPERADO, R. KOENIGSBERG, A. PINUS, and F. Y. TSAI, 2000. Investigation of alternating and continuous experimental task designs during single finger opposition fMRI: A comparative study. *J. Comput. Assist. Tomogr.* 24:935–941.

MOSELEY, M., 2002. Diffusion tensor imaging and aging—a review. *Nucl. Med. Reson. Biomed.* 15:553–560.

MOSELEY, M., R. BAMMER, and J. ILLES, 2002. Diffusion-tensor imaging of cognitive performance. *Brain Cogn.* 50:396–413.

NOBRE, A. C., 2001. Orienting attention to instants in time. *Neuropsychologia* 39:1317–1328.

OGAWA, S., and T. M. LEE, 1990. Magnetic resonance imaging of blood vessels at high fields: In vivo and in vitro measurements and image simulation. *Magn. Reson. Med.* 16:9–18.

OGAWA, S., T. M. LEE, A. R. KAY, and D. W. TANK, 1990. Brain magnetic resonance imaging with contrast dependent on blood oxygenation. *Proc. Natl. Acad. Sci. U.S.A.* 87:9868–9872.

OGAWA, S., T. M. LEE, A. S. NAYAK, and P. GLYNN, 1990. Oxygenation-sensitive contrast in magnetic resonance image of rodent brain at high magnetic fields. *Magn. Reson. Med.* 14:68–78.

PAIS, A., 2002. *Inward Bound: Of Matter and Forces in the Physical World.* Oxford, England: Oxford University Press.

PAJEVIC, S., and P. J. BASSER, 2003. Parametric and non-parametric statistical analysis of DT-MRI data. *J. Magn. Reson.* 161:1–14.

PASCUAL-LEONE, A., 2001. The brain that plays music and is changed by it. *Ann. N.Y. Acad. Sci.* 930:315–329.

PETERSEN, S. E., P. T. FOX, M. I. POSNER, M. MINTUN, and M. E. RAICHLE, 1988. Positron emission tomographic studies of the cortical anatomy of single-word processing. *Nature* 331:585–589.

PFEFFERBAUM, A., M. ROSENBLOOM, and E. V. SULLIVAN, 2002. Alcoholism and AIDS: Magnetic resonance imaging approaches for detecting interactive neuropathology. *Alcohol Clin. Exp. Res.* 26:1031–1046.

PHAN, K. L., T. WAGER, S. F. TAYLOR, and I. LIBERZON, 2002. Functional neuroanatomy of emotion: A meta-analysis of emotion activation studies in PET and fMRI. *NeuroImage* 16:331–348.

PHELPS, E. A., W. HIRST, and M. S. GAZZANIGA, 1991. Deficits in recall following partial and complete commissurotomy. *Cereb. Cortex* 1:492–498.

PHELPS, M. E., E. J. HOFFMAN, S. C. HUANG, and D. E. KUHL, 1977. Positron tomography: "In vivo" autoradiographic approach to measurement of cerebral hemodynamics and metabolism. *Acta. Neurol. Scand. Suppl.* 64:446–447.

PIPE, J. G., 1999. Basic spin physics. *Magn. Reson. Imaging. Clin. North Am.* 7:607–627.

POLDRACK, R. A., 2000. Imaging brain plasticity: Conceptual and methodological issues: A theoretical review. *NeuroImage* 12:1–13.

POSNER, M. I., 1993. Seeing the mind. *Science* 262:673–674.

POSNER, M. I., and G. J. DIGIROLAMO, 2000. Cognitive neuroscience: Origins and promise. *Psychol. Bull.* 126:873–889.

POSNER, M. I., and S. E. PETERSEN, 1990. The attention system of the human brain. *Annu. Rev. Neurosci.* 13:25–42.

POSNER, M. I., S. E. PETERSEN, P. T. FOX, and M. E. RAICHLE, 1988. Localization of cognitive operations in the human brain. *Science* 240:1627–1631.

PRICE, C. J., and K. J. FRISTON, 2002. Degeneracy and cognitive anatomy. *Trends Cogn. Sci.* 6:416–421.

PRICE, C. J., E. A. WARBURTON, C. J. MOORE, R. S. FRACKOWIAK, and K. J. FRISTON, 2001. Dynamic diaschisis: Anatomically remote and context-sensitive human brain lesions. *J. Cogn. Neurosci.* 13:419–429.

RAICHLE, M. E., 1975. Cerebral blood flow and metabolism. *Ciba Found. Symp.* 34:85–96.

RAICHLE, M. E., 2001a. Cognitive neuroscience: BOLD insights. *Nature* 412:128–130.

RAICHLE, M. E., 2001b. Functional neuroimaging: A historical and physiological perspective. In *Handbook of Functional Neuroimaging of Cognition*, R. Cabeza and A. Kingstone, eds. Cambridge, Mass: MIT Press, pp. 3–26.

RAICHLE, M. E., 2003. Functional brain imaging and human brain function. *J. Neurosci.* 23:3959–3962.

RAICHLE, M. E., and D. A. GUSNARD, 2002. Appraising the brain's energy budget. *Proc. Natl. Acad. Sci. U.S.A.* 99:10237–10239.

REX, D. E., and A. TOGA, 2002. *A fully automated comparison of the Brain Surface Extractor and the Brain Extraction Tool using the LONI pipeline.* Paper presented at a meeting of the Organization for Human Brain Mapping, Sendai, Japan.

ROSEN, B. R., H. J. ARONEN, K. K. KWONG, J. W. BELLIVEAU, L. M. HAMBERG, and J. A. FORDHAM, 1993. Advances in clinical neuroimaging: Functional MR imaging techniques. *Radiographics* 13:889–896.

ROSEN, B. R., R. L. BUCKNER, and A. DALE, 1998. Event-related functional MRI: Past, present, and future. *Proc. Natl. Acad. Sci. U.S.A.* 95:773–780.

ROTHMAN, D. L., K. L. BEHAR, F. HYDER, and R. G. SHULMAN, 2003. In vivo NMR studies of the glutamate neurotransmitter flux and neuroenergetics: Implications for brain function. *Annu. Rev. Physiol.* 65:401–427.

ROY, C. S., and C. S. SHERRINGTON, 1890. On the regulation of blood supply of the brain. *J. Physiol.* 11:85–108.

SALMERON, B. J., and E. A. STEIN, 2002. Pharmacological applications of magnetic resonance imaging. *Psychopharmacol. Bull.* 36:102–129.

SCHWEHN, M. R., 1982. Making the world: William James and the life of the mind. *Harv. Libr. Bull.* 30:426–454.

SHULMAN, R. G., F. HYDER, and D. L. ROTHMAN, 2002. Biophysical basis of brain activity: Implications for neuroimaging. *Q. Rev. Biophys.* 35:287–325.

SMITH, A. J., H. BLUMENFELD, K. L. BEHAR, D. L. ROTHMAN, R. G. SHULMAN, and F. HYDER, 2002. Cerebral energetics and spiking frequency: The neurophysiological basis of fMRI. *Proc. Natl. Acad. Sci. U.S.A.* 99:10765–10770.

SOKOLOFF, L., 1981. Relationships among local functional activity, energy metabolism, and blood flow in the central nervous system. *Fed. Proc.* 40:2311–2316.

SOKOLOFF, L., 1982. New techniques in the study of local brain activity in animal and man. *Prog. Brain Res.* 55:331–347.

SOKOLOFF, L., 1999. Energetics of functional activation in neural tissues. *Neurochem. Res.* 24:321–329.

STARK, C. E., and L. R. SQUIRE, 2001. When zero is not zero: The problem of ambiguous baseline conditions in fMRI. *Proc. Natl. Acad. Sci. U.S.A.* 98:12760–12766.

TAYLOR, E., 1982. William James on psychopathology: The 1896 Lowell lectures on Exceptional Mental States. *Harv. Libr. Bull.* 30:455–479.

TAYLOR, E., 1984. William James on psychopathology: An archival memoir. *Rev. Hist. Psicol.* 5:357–365.

TER-POGOSSIAN, M. M., M. E. PHELPS, E. J. HOFFMAN, and N. A. MULLANI, 1975. A positron-emission transaxial tomograph for nuclear imaging (PETT). *Radiology* 114:89–98.

TOGA, A., D. E. REX, and J. MA, 2001. *A graphical interoperable processing pipeline.* Paper presented at the annual meeting of the Organization for Human Brain Mapping, Brighton, England.

TOGA, A. W., and P. M. THOMPSON, 2001. Maps of the brain. *Anat. Rec.* 265:37–53.

TURKELTAUB, P. E., G. F. EDEN, K. M. JONES, and T. A. ZEFFIRO, 2002. Meta-analysis of the functional neuroanatomy of single-word reading: Method and validation. *NeuroImage* 16(3 Pt. 1):765–780.

TURNER, R., 1997. Signal sources in bold contrast fMRI. *Adv. Exp. Med. Biol.* 413:19–25.

UGURBIL, K., G. ADRIANY, P. ANDERSEN, W. CHEN, R. GRUETTER, X. HU, H. MERKLE, D. S. KIM, S. G. KIM, J. STRUPP, X. H. ZHU, and S. OGAWA, 2000. Magnetic resonance studies of brain function and neurochemistry. *Annu. Rev. Biomed. Eng.* 2:633–660.

UTTAL, W. R., 2001. *The New Phrenology: The Limits of Localizing Cognitive Processes in the Brain.* Cambridge, Mass.: MIT Press.

VAN HORN, J. D., 2002a. Imaging the motor brain. In *The Handbook of Brain Theory and Neural Networks*, M. A. Arbib, ed. Cambridge, Mass.: MIT Press.

VAN HORN, J. D., 2002b. Maturing as a Science: The new perspectives in fMRI research award. *J. Cogn. Neurosci.* 14:817.

VAN HORN, J. D., and M. S. GAZZANIGA, 2002. Databasing fMRI studies: Toward a "discovery science" of brain function. *Nat. Rev. Neurosci.* 3:314–318.

VAN HORN, J. D., J. S. GRETHE, P. KOSTELEC, J. B. WOODWARD, J. A. ASLAM, D. RUS, D. ROCKMORE, and M. S. GAZZANIGA, 2001. The functional magnetic resonance imaging data center (fMRIDC): The challenges and rewards of large-scale databasing of neuroimaging studies. *Philos. Trans. R. Soc. Lond. B Biol. Sci.* 356:1323–1339.

VAN HORN, J. D., and I. C. MCMANUS, 1992. Ventricular enlargement in schizophrenia: A meta-analysis of studies of the ventricle: brain ratio (VBR). *Br. J. Psychiat.* 160:687–697.

VAN HORN, J. D., J. B. WOODWARD, G. SIMONDS, B. VANCE, J. S. GRETHE, M. MONTAGUE, J. A. ASLAM, D. RUS, D. ROCKMORE, and M. S. GAZZANIGA, 2002. The fMRI data center: Software tools for neuroimaging data management, inspection, and sharing. In *A Practical Guide to Neuroscience Databases and Associated Tools*, R. Kotter, ed. Amsterdam: Kluwer.

WOO, J. H., and G. M. HATHOUT, 2001. Systems analysis of functional magnetic resonance imaging data using a physiologic model of venous oxygenation. *J. Cereb. Blood Flow Metab.* 21:517–528.

WOODS, R. P., S. T. GRAFTON, C. J. HOLMES, S. R. CHERRY, and J. C. MAZZIOTTA, 1998. Automated image registration. I. General methods and intrasubject, intramodality validation. *J. Comput. Assist. Tomogr.* 22:139–152.

WOODS, R. P., S. T. GRAFTON, J. D. WATSON, N. L. SICOTTE, and J. C. MAZZIOTTA, 1998. Automated image registration. II. Intersubject validation of linear and nonlinear models. *J. Comput. Assist. Tomogr.* 22:153–165.

XU, C., D. L. PHAM, M. E. RETTMANN, D. N. YU, and J. L. PRINCE, 1999. Reconstruction of the human cerebral cortex from magnetic resonance images. *IEEE Trans. Med. Imag.* 18:467–480.

YANG, Y., W. ENGELIEN, H. PAN, S. XU, D. A. SILBERSWEIG, and E. STERN, 2000. A CBF-based event-related brain activation paradigm: Characterization of impulse-response function and comparison to BOLD. *NeuroImage* 12:287–297.

ZICHE, P., 1999. Neuroscience in its context: Neuroscience and psychology in the work of Wilhelm Wundt. *Physis Riv. Int. Stor. Sci.* 36:407–429.

93 Social Exchange: The Evolutionary Design of a Neurocognitive System

LEDA COSMIDES AND JOHN TOOBY

ABSTRACT How functionally specialized is the evolutionary design of our neural circuitry? Neuropsychological and cognitive research on human reasoning about social exchange indicates that at least some neurocomputational adaptations are quite narrow in scope. Evolutionary game theory shows that social exchange—cooperation for mutual benefit—can evolve and persist only if the cognitive programs that cause it conform to a narrow and complex set of design specifications. These design features were tested for and found, in experiments that simultaneously falsified theories claiming that more domain-general cognitive procedures cause reasoning about social exchange. The complex pattern of functional and neural dissociations found reveal so close a fit between adaptive problem and computational solution that a neurocognitive specialization for reasoning about social exchange is implicated, including a subroutine for cheater detection. This subroutine develops precocially (by ages 3–4) and appears cross-culturally: hunter-horticulturalists in the Amazon detect cheaters as reliably as adults who live in advanced market economies. The computational specialization found in adults appears to have been built by developmental mechanisms that evolved for that function; its design, ontogenetic timetable, and cross-cultural distribution are not consistent with any known domain-general learning process. In sum, the system that causes reasoning about social exchange shows evidence of being a cognitive instinct (Pinker, 1994): it is complexly organized for solving a well-defined adaptive problem our ancestors faced in the past, it reliably develops in all normal human beings, it develops without any conscious effort and in the absence of explicit instruction, it is applied without any conscious awareness of its underlying logic, and it is functionally and neurally distinct from more general abilities to process information or behave intelligently.

Everything should be made as simple as possible, but no simpler.
—Albert Einstein

LEDA COSMIDES Department of Psychology and Center for Evolutionary Psychology, University of California, Santa Barbara, Santa Barbara, Calif.
JOHN TOOBY Department of Anthropology and Center for Evolutionary Psychology, University of California, Santa Barbara, Santa Barbara, Calif.

Designed for social exchange?

By exchanging benefits—goods, services, acts of help and kindness—people can make themselves better off than they were before. This very basic fact of human social life is easy to take for granted. But when placed in zoological perspective, social exchange stands out as a strange phenomenon whose existence requires explanation.

ZOOLOGICAL DISTRIBUTION Despite widespread investigation, social exchange (reciprocity, reciprocal altruism) has been reported in only a tiny handful of species, such as chimpanzees, baboons, lions, and vampire bats (see Dugatkin, 1997, and Hauser, in press, for contrasting views on the animal findings). Most species do not engage in this very useful form of mutual help.

In contrast, social exchange is a characteristic of our species as language or tool use. Not only is social exchange found in every documented culture, but it is a feature of virtually every human life within each culture, taking on a multiplicity of forms, such as returning favors, sharing food, reciprocal gift giving, market exchange, and extending acts of help with the (implicit) expectation that they will be reciprocated (Cashdan, 1989; Fiske, 1991; Gurven, 2002). Paleoanthropological evidence suggests that certain forms of social exchange were present in hominids at least two million years ago (Isaac, 1978), and its presence in other primates suggests it may be even more ancient than that.

The fact that social exchange is an ancient and pervasive feature of human social life, yet rare in other species, is informative. It means that the neurocognitive machinery necessary for social exchange exists in humans, but not in most animals. But what, exactly, is the nature of the neurocognitive machinery that enables exchange, and how specialized is it for this function?

Is social exchange a by-product of neural circuitry that causes one to reason logically? To think intelligently? To reason about all conditional rules? To reason about deontic rules—moral rules involving obligation and entitlement? Or does the ability to engage in social exchange require evolved mechanisms that were tailored by natural selection specifically for social exchange?

The research discussed in this chapter explores a simple hypothesis: that the evolved, species-typical design of the human mind includes computational adaptations specialized for reasoning about social exchange.

EVOLUTIONARY FUNCTION AND DESIGN EVIDENCE Social exchange clearly produces beneficial effects for those who successfully engage in it. I offer to provide a benefit to you, contingent on your satisfying a requirement that I specify. I impose that requirement in the hope that your satisfying it will create a situation that benefits me in some way. These conditional agreements—social contracts—are offered and accepted in the expectation that they will be rewarding for each party.

This means that the neurocognitive system that enables social exchange is beneficial. But this is not sufficient for showing that it was designed by natural selection to produce social exchange. Social exchange may simply be a side effect of a system that was designed for some entirely different function. How can one tell?

To demonstrate that the neurocognitive system that enables social exchange is an adaptation for that function, design evidence is needed. Computational systems, whether in brains or in computers, are composed of design features: properties that exist because they solve computational problems well. Natural selection is a causal feedback process that retains and discards properties from a species' design on the basis of how well they solve adaptive problems (evolutionarily recurrent problems whose solution promotes reproduction). To show that a system is an adaptation that evolved for a particular function, one must demonstrate that its properties solve a well-specified adaptive problem in a well-engineered way (Williams, 1966; Dawkins, 1986; Tooby and Cosmides, 1992).

The expectation of a fit between problem and solution can also be used to discover facts previously unknown. From a good specification of a computational problem one can predict and then look for representations and procedures that solve that problem well. In the reseach described here, we applied that approach to social exchange by (1) examining the selection pressures that arise in social exchange, (2) developing a task analysis of the computational problems that must be solved by a brain that was sculpted by these selection pressures, (3) using neuropsychological and cognitive methods to test for the presence of computational units that appear well designed for solving these problems, and (4) empirically testing to see whether performance is better explained as the by-product of mechanisms designed to solve some different, larger, or more general class of problems.

Selection pressures and design features

Selection pressures favoring social exchange exist whenever one organism (the provisioner) can change the behavior of a target organism to the provisioner's advantage by making the target's receipt of a provisioned benefit *conditional* on the target acting in a required manner. This mutual provisioning of benefits, each conditional on the other's compliance, is what is meant by social exchange or reciprocation (Cosmides, 1985; Cosmides and Tooby, 1989; Tooby and Cosmides, 1996). In social exchange, individuals agree, either explicitly or implicitly, to abide by a particular *social contract*. For ease of explication, let us define a social contract as a conditional rule that fits the following template: "If you accept a benefit from X, then you must satisfy X's requirement" (where X is an individual or set of individuals).

An evolutionarily stable strategy, or ESS, is a strategy (a decision rule) that can arise and persist in a population because it produces fitness outcomes greater than or equal to alternative strategies (Maynard Smith, 1982). Whatever the decision rules are that guide social exchange in humans, it is likely that they embody an ESS (because they would not exist unless they had outcompeted alternatives). By using game theory and conducting computer simulations of the evolutionary process, one can determine which strategies for engaging in social exchange are ESSs.

In such simulations, social exchange is usually modeled as a repeated Prisoners' Dilemma (Trivers, 1971; Axelrod and Hamilton, 1981; Boyd, 1988; but see Tooby and Cosmides, 1996). The results show that the behavior of cooperators must be generated by programs that perform certain specific tasks very well if they are to be evolutionarily stable (Cosmides, 1985; Cosmides and Tooby, 1989). Here, we will focus on one of these requirements—cheater detection. A *cheater* is an individual who fails to reciprocate: who accepts the benefit specified by a social contract without satisfying the requirement that provision of that benefit was made contingent upon.

The ability to reliably and systematically detect cheaters is a necessary condition for cooperation in the repeated Prisoners' Dilemma to be an ESS (e.g., Williams, 1966; Trivers, 1971; Axelrod and Hamilton, 1981; Axelrod, 1984; Boyd, 1988). To see this, consider the fate of a program that, because it cannot detect cheaters, bestows benefits on others unconditionally. These unconditional helpers will increase the fitness of any nonreciprocating design they meet in the population. But when a nonreciprocating design is helped, the unconditional helper never recoups the expense of helping: the helper design incurs a net fitness cost while conferring a net fitness advantage on a design that does not help. As a result, a population of unconditional helpers is easily invaded and eventually outcompeted by designs that accept the benefits helpers bestow without reciprocating them.

In contrast, program designs that cause *conditional* helping—that help those who reciprocate the favor, but not those who fail to reciprocate—can invade a population of nonreciprocators and outcompete them. Moreover, a population of such designs can resist invasion by designs that do not nonreciprocate (cheater designs). Therefore, conditional helping, which requires the ability to detect cheaters, is an ESS.

Based on ESS analyses and the behavioral ecology of hunter-gatherers, one can define some of the computational requirements of an evolutionarily stable program for engaging in social exchange (Cosmides, 1985; Cosmides and Tooby, 1989). This task analysis of the required computations is what we mean by social contract theory. Social contract theory provides a standard of good design for this domain. That is, well-designed programs for engaging in social exchange should include features that execute the computational requirements specified in social contract theory.

Among the design features predicted by social contract theory are D1–D6:

D1. Social exchange is cooperation for mutual *benefit*. If there is nothing in a conditional rule that can be interpreted as a rationed benefit, then interperative procedures should not classify that rule as a social contract.

D2. Cheating is a specific way of violating a social contract: it is taking the benefit when you are not entitled to do so. Consequently, the cognitive architecture must define the concept of *cheating* using contentful representational primitives, referring to illicitly taken *benefits*. This implies that a system designed for cheater detection will not know what to look for if the rule specifies no benefit to the potential violator.

D3. The definition of cheating is also perspective dependent, because the item or action that one party views as a benefit is viewed as a requirement by the other party. The system needs to be able to compute a cost-benefit representation from the perspective of each participant, and define cheating with respect to that perspective-relative representation.

D4. To be an ESS, a design for conditional helping must not be outcompeted by alternative designs. Accidents and innocent mistakes that result in an individual being cheated are not markers of a design difference. A cheater detection system should look for cheaters: designs that cheat by intention rather than by accident. (Mistakes that result in one being cheated are relevant only insofar as they may not be true mistakes.)

D5. However unfamiliar the situation may be, rules that fit the template of a social contract should elicit cheater detection.

D6. Inferences made about social contracts should not follow the rules of a content-free formal logic. They should follow a content-specific adaptive logic, evolutionarily tailored for the domain of social exchange (described in Cosmides and Tooby, 1989).

Not only does cheating involve the violation of a conditional rule, but it involves a particular *kind* of violation of a particular *kind* of conditional rule. The rule must fit the template for a social contract; the violation must be one in which an individual intentionally took what that individual considered to be a benefit, and did so without satisfying the requirement.

Formal logics (e.g., the propositional calculus) are content-free; the definition of violation in standard logics applies to all conditional rules, whether they are social contracts, threats, or descriptions of how the world works. But, as we will see later, the definition of cheating implied by design features D1–D4 does not map onto this content-free definition of violation. What counts as cheating in social exchange is so content dependent that a detection mechanism equipped only with a domain-general definition of violation would not be able to solve the problem of cheater detection. This suggests that there should be a program specialized for cheater detection. To operate, this would have to function as a subcomponent of a system that, because of its domain-specialized structure, is well designed for detecting social conditionals involving exchange, interpreting their meaning, and successfully solving the inferential problems they pose: social contract algorithms.

Conditional reasoning and social exchange

Reciprocation is, by definition, social behavior that is conditional: you agree to deliver a benefit conditionally (conditional on the other person doing what you required in return). Understanding it therefore requires conditional reasoning.

Because engaging in social exchange requires conditional reasoning, investigations of conditional reasoning can be used to test for the presence of social contract algorithms. The hypothesis that the brain contains social contract algorithms predicts a dissociation in reasoning performance by content: a sharply enhanced ability to reason adaptively about conditional rules when those rules specify a social exchange. The null hypothesis is that there is nothing specialized in the brain for social exchange. This null hypothesis follows from the traditional assumption that reasoning is caused by content-independent processes. It predicts no enhanced conditional reasoning performance specifically triggered by social exchanges as compared to other contents.

A standard tool for investigating conditional reasoning is the Wason selection task, which asks one to look for potential violations of a conditional rule of the form *If P then Q*

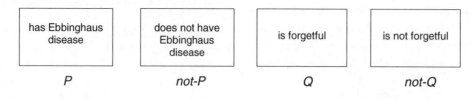

Ebbinghaus disease was recently identified and is not yet well understood. So an international committee of physicians who have experience with this disease were assembled. Their goal was to characterize the symptoms, and develop surefire ways of diagnosing it.

Patients afflicted with Ebbinghaus disease have many different symptoms: nose bleeds, headaches, ringing in the ears, and others. Diagnosing it is difficult because a patient may have the disease, yet not manifest all of the symptoms. Dr. Buchner, an expert on the disease, said that the following rule holds:

"If a person has Ebbinghaus disease, then that person will be forgetful."
If   P   then   Q

Dr. Buchner may be wrong, however. You are interested in seeing whether there are any patients whose symptoms violate this rule.

The cards below represent four patients in your hospital. Each card represents one patient. One side of the card tells whether or not the patient has Ebbinghaus disease, and the other side tells whether or not that patient is forgetful.

Which of the following card(s) would you definitely need to turn over to see if any of these cases violate Dr. Buchner's rule: "If a person has Ebbinghaus disease, then that person will be forgetful." Don't turn over any more cards than are absolutely necessary.

has Ebbinghaus disease	does not have Ebbinghaus disease	is forgetful	is not forgetful
P	*not-P*	*Q*	*not-Q*

FIGURE 93.1 The Wason selection task (descriptive rule, familiar content). In a Wason task, there is always a rule of the form *If P then Q*, and four cards showing the values *P*, *not-P*, *Q*, and *not-Q* (respectively) on the side that the subject can see. From a logical point of view, only the combination of *P* and *not-Q* can violate this rule, so the correct answer is to check the *P* card (to see if it has a *not-Q* on the back), the *not-Q* card (to see if it has a *P* on the back), and no others. Few subjects answer correctly, however, when the conditional rule is descriptive (indicative), even when its content is familiar. For example, only 26% of subjects answered the above problem correctly (by choosing "has Ebbinghaus disease" and "is not forgetful"). Most choose either *P* alone, or *P&Q*. (The italicized *P*s and *Q*s are not in problems given to subjects.)

(Wason, 1966, 1983; Wason and Johnson-Laird, 1972). Using this task, an extensive series of experiments has been conducted that address the following questions:

1. Do our minds include cognitive machinery that is specialized for reasoning about social exchange? (alongside some other domain-specific mechanisms, each specialized for reasoning about a different adaptive domain involving conditional behavior?) Or,

2. Is the cognitive machinery that causes good conditional reasoning general—does it operate well regardless of content?

If the human brain had cognitive machinery that causes good conditional reasoning regardless of content, then people should be good at tasks requiring conditional reasoning. For example, they should be good at detecting violations of conditional rules. Yet studies with the Wason selection task show that they are not. The Wason task in figure 93.1 is illustrative. The correct answer (choose *P*, choose *not-Q*) would be intuitively obvious if our minds were equipped with reasoning procedures specialized for detecting *logical* violations of conditional rules. But this is not obvious. Studies in many nations have shown that reasoning performance on descriptive (indicative) rules like this is low: only 5%–30% of people give the logically correct answer, even when the rule involves familiar terms drawn from everyday life (Wason, 1966, 1983; Manktelow and Evans, 1979; Cosmides, 1989; Sugiyama, Tooby, and Cosmides, 2002).

A DISSOCIATION BY CONTENT People are poor at detecting violations of conditional rules when their content is descriptive. Does this result generalize to conditional rules that express social contracts? No. People who ordinarily cannot detect violations of if-then rules can do so easily and accurately when that violation represents cheating in a situation of social exchange. This pattern—good violation detection for social contracts but not for descriptive rules—is a dissociation in reasoning elicited by differences in the conditional rule's content. It provides (initial) evidence that the mind has reasoning procedures specialized for detecting cheaters.

More specifically, when asked to look for violations of a conditional rule that fits the social contract template—"If you take benefit B, then you must satisfy requirement R" (e.g., "If you borrow my car, then you have to fill up the tank

A.

Teenagers who don't have their own cars usually end up borrowing their parents' cars. In return for the privilege of borrowing the car, the Carter's have given their kids the rule,

"If you borrow my car, then you have to fill up the tank with gas."

Of course, teenagers are sometimes irresponsible. You are interested in seeing whether any of the Carter teenagers broke this rule.

The cards below represent four of the Carter teenagers. Each card represents one teenager. One side of the card tells whether or not a teenager has borrowed the parents' car on a particular day, and the other side tells whether or not that teenager filled up the tank with gas on that day.

Which of the following card(s) would you definitely need to turn over to see if any of these teenagers are breaking their parents' rule: "If you borrow my car, then you have to fill up the tank with gas." Don't turn over any more cards than are absolutely necessary.

borrowed car	did not borrow car	filled up tank with gas	did not fill up tank with gas

B.

The mind translates social contracts into representations of benefits and requirements, and it inserts concepts such as "entitled to" and "obligated to", whether they are specified or not.

How the mind "sees" the social contract above is shown in **bold italics**.

"If you borrow my car, then you have to fill up the tank with gas."

If you take the benefit, then you are obligated to satisfy the requirement.

borrowed car	did not borrow car	filled up tank with gas	did not fill up tank with gas
= accepted the benefit	**= did not accept the benefit**	**= satisfied the requirement**	**= did not satisfy the requirement**

FIGURE 93.2 Wason task with a social contract rule. (*A*) In response to this social contract problem, 76% of subjects chose *P & not-Q* ("borrowed the car" and "did not fill the tank with gas"), the cards that represent potential cheaters. Yet only 26% chose this (logically correct) answer in response to the descriptive rule in figure 93.1. Although this social contract rule involves familiar items, unfamiliar social contracts elicit the same high performance. (*B*)

How the mind represents the social contract shown in *A*. According to inferential rules specialized for social exchange (but not according to formal logic), "If you take the benefit, then you are obligated to satisfy the requirement" implies "If you satisfy the requirement, then you are entitled to take the benefit." Consequently, the rule in *A* implies: "If you fill the tank with gas, then you may borrow the car" (see figure 93.4, switched social contracts).

with gas")—people check the individual who accepted the benefit (borrowed the car; *P*) and the individual who did not satisfy the requirement (did not fill the tank; *not-Q*), that is, the cases that represent potential cheaters (figure 93.2*A*). The adaptively correct answer is immediately obvious to most subjects, who commonly experience a pop-out effect. No formal training is needed. Whenever the content of a problem asks one to look for cheaters in a social exchange, subjects experience the problem as simple to solve, and their performance jumps dramatically. In general, 65%–80% of subjects get it right, the highest performance found for a task of this kind (for reviews, see Cosmides, 1985, 1989; Cosmides and Tooby, 1992, 1997; Gigerenzer and Hug, 1992; Platt and Griggs, 1993; Fiddick, Cosmides, and Tooby, 2000).

Given the content-free syntax of formal logic, investigating the person who borrowed the car (*P*) and the person who did not fill the gas tank (*not-Q*) is logically equivalent to investigating the person in figure 93.1 with Ebbinghaus disease (*P*) and the person who is not forgetful (*not-Q*). But everywhere it has been tested (adults in the United States, United Kingdom, Germany, Italy, France, Hong Kong, Japan; schoolchildren in Quito, Ecuador; Shiwiar hunter-horticulturalists in the Ecuadorian Amazon), people do not treat social exchange problems as equivalent to other kinds of reasoning problems (Cheng and Holyoak, 1985; Cosmides, 1989; Platt and Griggs, 1993; Hasegawa and Hiraishi, 2000; Sugiyama, Tooby, and Cosmides, 2002; supports D5, D6). Their minds distinguish social exchange contents, and reason as if they were translating these situations into representational primitives such as *benefit, cost, obligation, entitlement, intentional,* and *agent* (figure 93.2*B*; Cosmides and Tooby, 1992; Fiddick, Cosmides, and Tooby, 2000). Reasoning problems and their elements could be sorted into indefinitely many categories based on their content or structure (including the propositional calculus's two content-free categories, antecedent and consequent). Yet even in remarkably different cultures, the same mental categorization occurs. This cross-culturally recurrent dissociation by content was predicted by social contract theory's adaptationist analysis.

In the next section we review experiments conducted to test for design features that should be present in a system specialized for social exchange. Each experiment testing for a design feature was also constructed to pit the adaptive specialization hypothesis against at least one alternative by-product hypothesis, so design feature and by-product implications will be discussed in tandem. As we will show, reasoning performance on social contracts is not explained by familiarity effects, by a content-free formal logic, by a permission schema, or by a general deontic logic (table 93.1).

Do unfamiliar social contracts elicit cheater detection (D5)?

One needs to understand each new opportunity to exchange as it arises, so it was predicted that social exchange reasoning should operate even for unfamiliar social contract rules (D5). (This distinguishes social contract theory strongly from theories that explain reasoning performance as the product of general learning strategies plus experience: The most natural prediction for such skill acquisition theories is that performance should be a function of familiarity.) Surprisingly, social contract theory is supported: cheater detection

Table 93.1

Alternative (by-product) hypotheses eliminated

B1	That familiarity can explain the social contract effect
B2	That social contract content merely activates the rules of inference of the propositional calculus (logic)
B3	That any problem involving payoffs will elicit the detection of logical violations
B4	That permission schema theory can explain the social contract effect
B5	That social contract content merely promotes "clear thinking"
B6	That a content-independent deontic logic can explain social contract reasoning
B7	That a single mechanism operates on all deontic rules involving subjective utilities
B8	That relevance theory can explain social contract effects (see also Fiddick et al., 2000)

occurs even when the social contract is wildly unfamiliar (figure 93.3*A*). For example, the rule "If a man eats cassava root, then he must have a tattoo on his face" can be made to fit the social contract template by explaining that the people involved consider eating cassava root to be a benefit (the rule then implies that having a tattoo is the requirement one must satisfy to be eligible for that benefit). When this is done, this outlandish, culturally alien rule elicits the same high level of cheater detection as highly familiar social exchange rules (Cosmides, 1985, 1989; Gigerenzer and Hug, 1992; Platt and Griggs, 1993).

ELIMINATING FAMILIARITY (B1) The dissociation by content—good performance for social contract rules but not for descriptive ones—has nothing to do with the familiarity of the rules tested. Surprisingly, familiarity is neither necessary nor sufficient for eliciting high performance (B1 of table 93.1).

First, familiarity does not produce high levels of performance for descriptive rules (Manktelow and Evans, 1979; Cosmides, 1989). For example, the Ebbinghaus problem in figure 93.1 involves a familiar causal relationship, a disease causing a symptom, embedded in a real-world context. Yet only 26% of 111 college students that we tested produced the logically correct answer, *P & not-Q*, for this problem. If familiarity fails to elicit high performance on descriptive rules, then it also fails as an explanation for high performance on social contracts.

Second, the fact that unfamiliar social contracts elicit high performance shows that familiarity is not necessary for eliciting violation detection. Third, and most surprising, people are just as good at detecting cheaters on culturally unfamiliar or imaginary social contracts as they are at detecting cheaters on completely familiar social contracts (Cosmides, 1985). This provides a challenge for any counterhypothesis resting on a general-learning skill acquisition account (most of which rely on familiarity and repetition).

Adaptive logic, not formal logic (D3, D6)

Social contract problems can be constructed so as to elicit a logically correct answer (*P & not-Q*; see figure 93.2*A*). This has led some to conclude that social exchange content simply activates a dormant content-free logical faculty. But this is not the case.

Good cheater detection is not the same as good detection of logical violations (and vice versa). Hence, problems can be created in which the search for cheaters will result in a logically incorrect response (and the search for logical violations will fail to detect cheaters; figure 93.4). When given such problems, people look for cheaters, thereby giving a logically incorrect answer (*Q & not-P*). Experiments with perspective change and switched social contracts provide examples.

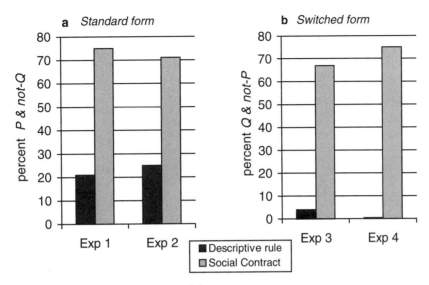

a *Standard form*

b *Switched form*

■ Descriptive rule
□ Social Contract

Exp 1 & 3: Social contract = social rule
Exp 2 & 4: Social contract = personal exchange

FIGURE 93.3   Detecting violations of unfamiliar conditional rules: social contracts versus descriptive rules. In these experiments, the same unfamiliar rule was embedded either in a story that caused it to be interpreted as a social contract or in a story that caused it to be interpreted as a rule describing some state of the world. For social contracts, the correct answer is always to pick the *benefit accepted* card and the *requirement not satisfied* card. (*A*) For standard social contracts, these correspond to the logical categories *P* and *not-Q. P & not-Q* also happens to be the logically correct answer. More than 70% of subjects chose these cards for the social contracts, but fewer than 25% chose them for the matching descriptive rules. (*B*) For switched social contracts, the *benefit accepted* and *requirement not satisfied* cards correspond to the logical categories *Q* and *not-P*. This is not a logically correct response. Nevertheless, about 70% of subjects chose it for the social contracts; virtually no one chose it for the matching descriptive rule (see figure 93.4).

PERSPECTIVE CHANGE   As predicted (D3), the mind's automatically deployed definition of cheating is tied to the perspective one is taking (Gigerenzer and Hug, 1992). For example, consider the following social contract:

(1) *If an employee is to get a pension, then that employee must have worked for the firm for over 10 years.*

This rule elicits different answers depending on whether subjects are cued into the role of employer or employee. Those in the employer role look for cheating by employees, investigating cases of *P* and *not-Q* (employees with pensions; employees who have worked for fewer than 10 years). Those in the employee role look for cheating by employers, investigating cases of *not-P* and *Q* (employees with no pension; employees who have worked more than 10 years). *Not-P & Q* is correct if the goal is to find out whether the employer is a cheater. But it is not *logically* correct. Content-free logical rules would always look for the co-occurrence of *P* and *not-Q*; perspective, a content-rich concept, is irrelevant to logic.

SWITCHED SOCIAL CONTRACTS   Assume you are the employer looking for cheating by employees. You are looking for violations of this social contract:

(2) *If an employee has worked for the firm for over 10 years, then that employee gets a pension.*

The mind recognizes (1) and (2) as expressing the same social contract (figures 93.2*B*, 93.4). For (2), as for (1), finding employees who cheat involves checking the employee who took the benefit (the pension) without meeting the requirement (worked < 10 years). But now these fall into the logical categories *not-P* and *Q*. When given social contracts with the benefit in the consequent clause (a "switched" format), subjects overwhelmingly choose *Q & not-P*—an answer that is adaptively correct but logically incorrect (Cosmides, 1989; Gigerenzer and Hug, 1992; supports D2, D6) (fig. 93.3*B*).

ELIMINATING LOGIC (B2, B3)   In these experiments, people did not follow the inferential rules of a content-free logic; by doing so they would have failed to detect cheaters (see figure 93.4). They applied inferential rules specific to social exchange, and therefore detected cheaters. The results show that performance on social contract problems is not caused by the activation of a dormant logic faculty (also see Fiddick et al., 2000).

In fact, social contract reasoning can be maintained in the face of impairments in general logical reasoning. Individuals with schizophrenia manifest deficits on virtually any test of general intellectual functioning they are given (McKenna, Clare, and Baddeley, 1995), yet their ability to detect cheaters can remain intact. Maljkovic (1987) tested the rea-

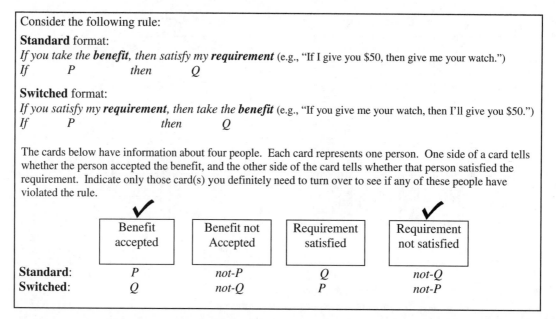

Consider the following rule:

Standard format:
*If you take the **benefit**, then satisfy my **requirement*** (e.g., "If I give you $50, then give me your watch.")
If   *P*   *then*   *Q*

Switched format:
*If you satisfy my **requirement**, then take the **benefit*** (e.g., "If you give me your watch, then I'll give you $50.")
If   *P*   *then*   *Q*

The cards below have information about four people. Each card represents one person. One side of a card tells whether the person accepted the benefit, and the other side of the card tells whether that person satisfied the requirement. Indicate only those card(s) you definitely need to turn over to see if any of these people have violated the rule.

	Benefit accepted ✔	Benefit not Accepted	Requirement satisfied	Requirement not satisfied ✔
Standard:	*P*	*not-P*	*Q*	*not-Q*
Switched:	*Q*	*not-Q*	*P*	*not-P*

FIGURE 93.4   Generic structure of a Wason task when the conditional rule is a social contract. A social contract can be translated into either social contract terms (benefits and requirements) or logical terms (*P*s and *Q*s). Checkmarks indicate the correct card choices if one is looking for cheaters; these cards should be chosen by a cheater detection subroutine, whether the exchange was expressed in a standard or switched format. This results in a logically incorrect answer (*Q & not-P*) when the rule is expressed in the switched format and a logically correct answer (*P & not-Q*) when the rule is expressed in the standard format. By testing switched social contracts, one can see that the reasoning procedures activated cause one to detect cheaters, not logical violations (see figure 93.3*B*). A logically correct response to a switched social contract, where *P = requirement satisfied* and *not-Q = benefit not accepted*, would fail to detect cheaters.

soning of patients exhibiting positive symptoms of schizophrenia and compared their performance with that of hospitalized control patients. Compared to the control patients, the schizophrenic patients were impaired on more general (non-Wason) tests of logical reasoning, in a way typical of individuals with frontal lobe dysfunction. But their ability to detect cheaters on Wason tasks was unimpaired: it was indistinguishable from that of the controls, and showed the typical dissociation by content. This selective preservation of social exchange reasoning is consistent with the notion that reasoning about social exchange is handled by a dedicated system that can operate even when the systems responsible for more general reasoning are damaged.

Benefits are necessary for cheater detection (D1, D2)

The function of a social exchange for each participant is to gain access to a benefit that would otherwise be unavailable to them. Therefore, an important cue that a conditional rule is a social contract is the presence in it of a desired benefit under the control of an agent.

In social exchange, this agent *permits* you to take a benefit from him or her, conditonal upon your having met the agent's requirement. There are, however, many situations other than social exchange in which an action is permitted conditionally. A *permission rule* is any deontic conditional that fits the template "If one is to take action A, then one must

TABLE 93.2

The four production rules of the permission schema*

Rule 1:	If the action is to be taken, then the precondition must be satisfied.
Rule 2:	If the action is not to be taken, then the precondition need not be satisfied.
Rule 3:	If the precondition is satisfied, then the action may be taken.
Rule 4:	If the precondition is not satisfied, then the action must not be taken.

Social contracts and precautions fit the template of Rule 1:

If the benefit is to be taken, then the requirement must be satisfied.

If the hazardous action is to be taken, then the precaution must be taken.

* Permission schema of Cheng and Holyoak (1985).

satisify precondition R"[1] (table 93.2; Cheng and Holyoak, 1985, 1989). All social contracts are permission rules, but there are many permission rules that are not social contracts (see table 93.2, figure 93.5). *Permission schema theory* proposes that the reasoning system that causes cheater detection is not specialized for that purpose. According to this theory, good violation detection is elicited by the entire class of permission rules—a far more inclusive and general set (Cheng and Holyoak, 1985, 1989).

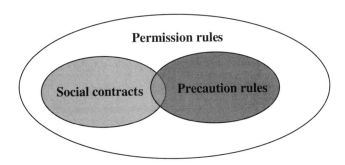

FIGURE 93.5 The class of permission rules is larger than, and includes, social contracts and precautionary rules. Many of the permission rules we encounter in everyday life are neither social contracts nor precautions (white area). Rules of civil society (etiquette, customs, traditions), bureaucratic rules, corporate rules—many of these are conditional rules that do not regulate access to a benefit or involve a danger. Permission schema theory (see table 93.2) predicts high performance for all permission rules; however, permission rules that fall into the white area do not elicit the high levels of performance that social contracts and precaution rules do. Neuropsychological and cognitive tests show that performance on social contracts dissociates from other permission rules (white area), from precautionary rules, and from the general class of deontic rules involving subjective utilities. These dissociations would be impossible if reasoning about social contracts and precautions were caused by a single schema that is general to the domain of permission rules.

Just how precise and functionally specialized is the reasoning system that causes cheater detection? Permission schema theory predicts uniformly high performance for all permission rules, whether they are social contracts or not. In contrast, social contract theory predicts dissociations *within* the class of permission rules: being a permission rule will not be sufficient, and large subsets of permission rules will fail to elicit the effect. For example, according to social contract theory, removing benefits (D1, D2) and/or intentionality (D4) from a social contract will result in a permission rule that does not elicit violation detection.

The benefit prediction was tested by Cosmides and Tooby (1992), who constructed Wason tasks involving a fictitious culture in which the elders made laws governing the conditions under which adolescents were permitted to take certain actions. For all tasks, the law fit the template for a permission rule. What varied was whether the action to be taken was a benefit or an unpleasant chore.

A cheater detection subroutine looks for benefits illicitly taken; without a benefit, it doesn't know what kind of violation to look for (D1, D2). When the permitted action was a benefit, 80% of subjects answered correctly; when it was a chore, only 44% did so. This dramatic decrease in violation detection was predicted in advance by social contract theory; in contrast, it violates the central prediction of permission schema theory, that being a permission rule is sufficient to facilitate violation detection. For similar results, see

Manktelow and Over (1991), Platt and Griggs (1993), and Barrett (1999).

This dissociation within the domain of permission rules supports the psychological reality of social contract categories; it shows that the representations necessary to trigger differential reasoning are more content-specific than those of the permission schema.

Social contract violations must be intentional (D4)

Evolutionarily, the function of a cheater detection subroutine is to correctly connect an attributed disposition (to cheat) with a person (a cheater), not simply to recognize instances wherein an individual did not get what she was entitled to. This is because the fitness benefit of cheater detection is the ability to avoid squandering costly future cooperative efforts on those who will not reciprocate. Violations of social contracts are relevant only insofar as they reveal individuals disposed to cheat—individuals who cheat by design, not by accident. Noncompliance caused by factors other than disposition, such as accidental violations and other innocent mistakes, do not reveal the disposition or design of the exchange partner; they may result in someone being cheated, but without indicating the presence of a cheater. Therefore, social contract theory predicts another additional level of cognitive specialization beyond detecting compliance or noncompliance with a social contract. The subroutine should look for *intentional* violations (D4).

Given the same social contract rule, one can manipulate contextual factors to change the nature of the violation from intentional cheating to an innocent mistake. One experiment, for example, compared a condition in which the potential rule violator was well-meaning but inattentive to one in which she had an incentive to intentionally cheat. Varying intentionality caused a radical change in performance, from 68% correct in the intentional cheating condition to 27% correct in the innocent mistake condition (Cosmides, Barrett, and Tooby, 2004; supports D4; disconfirms B1–B8). Fiddick (1998, 2004) found the same effect (as did Gigerenzer and Hug, 1992, using a different context manipulation).

Barrett (1999) conducted a series of parametric studies to find out whether the drop in performance in the innocent mistake condition was caused by the violator's lack of intentionality or by her inability to benefit from her mistake (see D2). He found that both factors contributed, independently and additively, to the drop.

ELIMINATING PERMISSION SCHEMA THEORY (B4) Cheng and Holyoak (1985, 1989) speculate that repeated encounters with permission rules cause domain-general learning mechanisms to induce a *permission schema*, consisting of four production rules (see table 93.2). This schema generates inferences about any conditional rule that fits the permission rule template, resulting in good violation detection for permission rules. However, permission schema theory cannot explain the above results.

According to permission schema theory, (1) all permission rules should elicit high levels of violation detection, whether the action term is a benefit or a chore; and (2) all permission rules should elicit high levels of violation detection, whether the violation was committed intentionally or accidentally. Both predictions fail. Permission rules fail to elicit high levels of violation detection when the action term is neutral or unpleasant (yet not hazardous; see later discussion). Moreover, people are poor at detecting accidental violations of social contract rules (which are a species of permission rule; see figure 93.5). Taken together, these results cast doubt on the hypothesis that the mind contains or develops a permission schema of the kind postulated by Cheng and Holyoak (1985, 1989).

The same results also falsify B6, that cheater detection on social contracts is caused by a content-free deontic logic (for discussion, see Manktelow and Over, 1987), as well as a proposal by Fodor (2000). All the rules tested above were deontic rules, but not all elicited violation detection. B5—that social contract rules elicit good performance because we understand their implications (e.g., Almor and Sloman, 1996)—is eliminated by the intention versus accident dissociation (the same social contract failed to elicit violation detection in the accident condition).

In short, it is not enough to admit that moral reasoning or social reasoning is special; the specificity implicated is far narrower in scope.

A neuropsychological dissociation between social contracts and precautions

The notion of multiple adaptive specializations is commonplace in physiology: the body is composed of many organs, each designed for a different function. Nevertheless, many cognitive neuroscientists are skeptical of multiple evolved specializations when these involve high-level cognitive operations such as reasoning. From an evolutionary perspective, however, social contracts are not the only conditional rules for which we should have specialized mechanisms (e.g., Tooby and Cosmides, 1989, on threats). Alongside specializations for reasoning about social exchange and threats, the human cognitive architecture should contain computational machinery specialized for managing hazards that causes good violation detection on precautionary rules. A system well designed for reasoning about hazards and precautions should have properties different from one for detecting cheaters (some of which have been tested for and found; Fiddick, 1998, 2004; Fiddick, Cosmides, and Tooby, 2000; Stone et al., 2002).

Precautionary rules are conditional rules that fit the template, *If one is to engage in hazardous activity H, then one must take precaution R* (e.g., "If you are working with toxic gases, then you must wear a gas mask"; Fiddick, Cosmides, and Tooby, 2000; Stone et al., 2002). Being able to detect when someone is in danger from having violated a precautionary rule is of obvious adaptive value. Tests with the Wason task show that precautionary rules strongly elicit the search for potential violators: subjects look for people who have engaged in the hazardous activity without taking the appropriate precaution (e.g., the "worked with toxic gases" card (*P*) and the "did not wear gas mask" card (*not-Q*)).

Like social contracts, precautionary rules are conditional, deontic, involve subjective utilities, and have the same pragmatic implications for Wason tasks (see table 93.2). Moreover, people are as good at detecting violators of precautionary rules as they are at detecting cheaters on social contracts. This has led some to conclude that reasoning about social contracts and precautions is caused by a single more general mechanism (e.g., general to permissions or to deontic rules involving subjective utilities; Manktelow and Over, 1988, 1990, 1991; Cheng and Holyoak, 1989; Sperber, Cara, and Girotto, 1995).

One Mechanism or Two? If reasoning about social contracts and precautions is caused by a single mechanism, then neurological damage to this mechanism should lower performance on both rules. But if reasoning about these two domains is caused by two functionally distinct mechanisms, then it is possible for social contract algorithms to be damaged while leaving precautionary mechanisms unimpaired, and vice versa.

Stone and colleagues (2002) developed a battery of Wason tasks that tested social contracts, precautionary rules, and descriptive rules. The social contracts and precautionary rules elicited equally high levels of violation detection from normal subjects (who got 70% and 71% correct, respectively). For each subject, a difference score was calculated: percent correct for precautions minus percent correct for social contracts. For normal subjects, these difference scores were close to zero (mean = 1.2 percentage points, SD = 11.5).

Stone and colleagues (2002) administered this battery of Wason tasks to R.M., a patient with bilateral damage to his medial orbitofrontal cortex and anterior temporal cortex (which had disconnected both amygdalae). R.M.'s performance on the precaution problems was 70% correct: equivalent to that of the normal controls. In contrast, his performance on the social contract problems was only 39% correct. Whereas the average difference score for control subjects was 1.2, R.M.'s difference score (precaution minus social contract) was 31 percentage points. This is 2.7 SD larger than the control mean (*P* < 0.005).

Double dissociations are helpful in ruling out differences in task difficulty as a counterexplanation for a given dissociation (Shallice, 1988), but here the tasks were perfectly matched for difficulty. The social contracts and precautionary rules given to R.M. were logically identical, posed identical task demands, and were equally difficult for normal subjects. Moreover, because the performance of the normal controls was not at ceiling, ceiling effects could not be masking real differences in the difficulty of the two sets of problems. In this case, a single dissociation is telling.

R.M.'s dissociation supports the hypothesis that reasoning about social exchange is caused by a different computational system than reasoning about precautionary rules—a two-mechanism account.

Although tests of this kind cannot conclusively establish the anatomical location of a mechanism, tests with other patients suggest that amygdalar disconnection was important in creating this selective deficit.[2]

ELIMINATING ONE MECHANISM HYPOTHESES (B6–B8; B1–B4) Every alternative explanation of cheater detection proposed so far claims that reasoning about social contracts and precautions is caused by the same computational system. R.M.'s dissociation is inconsistent with these one-mechanism accounts. These include mental logic (Rips, 1994), mental models (Johnson-Laird and Byrne, 1991), decision theory/optimal data selection (Kirby, 1994; Oaksford and Chater, 1994), permission schema theory (Cheng and Holyoak, 1989), relevance theory (Sperber, Cara, and Girotto, 1995[3]), and Manktelow and Over's (1991) view implicating a system that is general to any deontic rule that involves subjective utilities.

Indeed, no other reasoning theory even distinguishes between precautions and social contract rules; the distinction is derived from evolutionary-functional analyses, and is purely in terms of content. These results indicate the presence of a very narrow, content-based cognitive specialization within human reasoning.

The development of social contract reasoning

The evidence strongly supports the claim that reasoning about social exchange is caused by computational machinery that is specialized for this function in adults: in other words, social contract algorithms. But how was this computational specialization produced? Do humans have domain-specific mechanisms that are designed to cause the development of social contract algorithms? Or are they the outcome of a domain-general learning process?

PRECOCIOUS DEVELOPMENT OF CHEATER DETECTION Children understand what counts as cheating on a social contract by age 3 (Harris and Núñez, 1996; Núñez and Harris, 1998b; Harris, Núñez, and Brett, 2001). This has been shown repeatedly in experiments by Harris and Núñez using an evaluation task, in which the child must identify the picture in which a character is violating the rule. For social contracts, British 3-year-olds chose the correct picture 72%–83% of the time and 4-year-olds chose correctly 77%–100% of the time (Harris and Núñez, 1996; Núñez and Harris, 1998a; Harris, Núñez, and Brett, 2001). The same effects were found for preschoolers from the United Kingdom, Colombia, and (with minor qualifications) from rural Nepal.

The performance of the preschoolers was adult-like in other ways. Like adults, the preschoolers did well whether the social contract was familiar or unfamiliar, and understood that taking the benefit was conditional on meeting the requirement. Also like adults, intentionality mattered to the children: intentional violations were viewed as "naughty" far more often than accidental ones (80% vs. 10% by age 4; 65% vs. 17% at age 3; Núñez and Harris, 1998a). Moreover, the children tested by Harris and Núñez (1996) showed the same dissociation between social contract and descriptive rules as adults: 3–4-year-olds chose the correct violation condition only 40% of the time for descriptive rules but 72%–83% of the time for social contracts. By age 5, children could solve the full array, four-card Wason task when the conditional rule expressed a social contract (Núñez and Harris, 1998b).

CROSS-CULTURAL INVARIANCES AND DISSOCIATIONS The ESS concept carries predictions about development. Because detecting cheaters is necessary for social exchange to maintain itself in an evolving species—to be an ESS (D4)—its development should be buffered against cultural variation. The hypothesis that social exchange reasoning is caused by an evolved specialization therefore predicts that cheater detection will be found in all human cultures. In contrast, the development of ESS-irrelevant aspects of Wason performance are under no selection to be uniform across cultures.

Sugiyama, Tooby, and Cosmides (2002) tested this prediction among the Shiwiar, a hunter-horticultural population in a remote part of the Ecuadorian Amazon. Good cheater detection had already been established in the United States, Europe, Hong Kong, and Japan. But adults in advanced market economies engage in more trade, especially with strangers, than people who hunt and garden in remote parts of the Amazon. Anonymity facilitates cheating; markets increase the volume of transactions experienced by each individual. If no evolved specialization is involved—that is, if the mechanism is induced through repeated experience with cheating—then it may not be found outside the industrialized world.

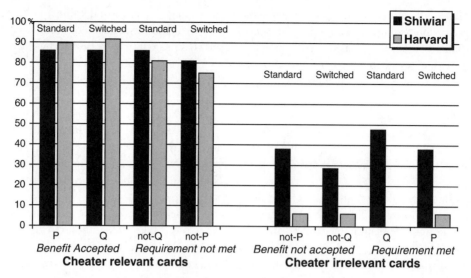

FIGURE 93.6   Performance of Shiwiar hunter-horticulturalists and Harvard undergraduates on standard and switched social contracts. Graphed is the percentage of subjects choosing each card. There was no difference between the two populations in their choice of cheater-relevant cards (*benefit accepted, requirement not satisfied*). They differed only in their choice of cheater-irrelevant cards (Shiwiar showing some interest in cards that could reveal acts of generosity or fair play). Shiwiar high performance on cheater-relevant cards is not caused by indiscriminate interest in all cards. Holding logical category constant, Shiwiar always chose a card more frequently when it was relevant to cheater detection than when it was not. This can be shown by comparing performance on standard versus switched social contracts. (For example, the *P* card is cheater relevant for a standard social contract but not for a switched one; see figure 93.4.)

The Shiwiar live in a culture as different from that of Western subjects as any remaining on the planet. Yet the Shiwiar were just as good at detecting cheaters on Wason tasks (figure 93.6). For cheater-relevant cards, the performance of Shiwiar hunter-horticulturalists was identical to that of Harvard undergraduates. Shiwiar differed only in that they were slightly more likely to show interest in cheater-irrelevant cards, the ones that could reveal acts of generosity.

The Shiwiar results suggest that the brain mechanism responsible for cheater detection reliably develops even in disparate cultural contexts—just what one would expect of a universal feature of human nature. There was no dissociation between cultures in the parts of the mechanism necessary to its performing its evolved function. The only "cultural dissociation" was in ESS-irrelevant aspects of performance.

Conclusion: Does domain-general learning build this computational specialization?

Reasoning about social exchange narrowly dissociates from other forms of reasoning, both cognitively and neurally. It displays design features specially tailored to fit the computational requirements necessary to produce an evolutionarily stable form of conditional helping (as opposed to the many kinds of helping that are culturally encouraged).

However, many psychologists believe that high-level cognitive competences like this emerge from general-purpose cognitive abilities trained by culturally specific activities. Such domain-general accounts rely on experience, familiarity, and repetition as explanatory variables. But the counterhypothesis that social exchange reasoning developed through some form of domain-general learning runs into a series of difficulties:

1. There is no evidence that familiarity, experience, or repetition improves conditional reasoning in any domain.

2. Neither experience with type of rule nor familiarity with specific rules accounts for which reasoning skills develop and which do not. For example, humans do not appear to develop the ability to reason well about large classes of rules with which they have far more experience than they do with social exchanges. We know this because social exchanges are a small subset of (for example) conditional rules, deontic rules, and permission rules; so, by class inclusion, humans necessarily have far more experience with these more general domains of rules (caption, figure 93.5). It was on this basis that Cheng and Holyoak (1985, 1989) argued that domain-general inductive processes *should* produce the more abstract and inclusive permission schema rather than social contract algorithms. Yet careful tests show that the permission schema does not exist, nor any of the other more inclusive competences that this view predicts.

3. Preschoolers have a limited base of experience, yet in reasoning about social exchange, they show virtually all the features of special design that adults do. It is difficult to understand why a domain-general learning process would cause the early and uniform acquisition of reasoning in

this domain yet fail to do so for others (Cosmides and Tooby, 1997).

4. Culture is often invoked as a schema-building factor. Yet, despite a massive difference in experience with trade and cheating, there was no difference between Shiwiar and American adults in cheater detection.

5. That people are good at detecting intentional cheating but not accidental mistakes is a prediction of the evolutionary task analysis of exchange. It is specifically the detection of intentional cheaters that makes contingent exchange evolutionarily stable against exploitation by cheaters (i.e., an ESS). In contrast, nonevolutionary theories of the origin of social exchange reasoning should predict good violation detection regardless of cause. A single inference procedure that scrutinizes cases in which the benefit was accepted and the requirement was not met indiscriminately reveals both accidental and intentional violations. Both represent damage to personal utility, both are useful to know, and both require detection if the participant is to get what she wants and is entitled to. From a pragmatic, utility-based perspective, it represents a strange addition to the competence to have the ordinarily deployed procedure inactive when there is evidence that the mistake would not have been intentional.

6. Similarly, it is not clear how or why domain-general learning would cause a cultural dissociation in the ESS irrelevant aspects of Wason-based social exchange reasoning, but not in the ESS-relevant aspects of cheater detection.

In contrast, the hypothesis that social contract algorithms were built by a developmental process designed for that function neatly accounts for all the developmental facts: that cheater detection develops invariantly across widely divergent cultures (whereas other aspects dissociate); that social exchange reasoning and cheater detection develop precocially; that they operate smoothly regardless of experience and familiarity; that they detect cheating and not other kinds of violations; that the developmental process results in a social contract specialization rather than one for more inclusive classes such as permissions.

The simplest, most parsimonious explanation that can account for all the results—developmental, neuropsychological, and cognitive—is that social contract algorithms are a reliably developing component of a universal human nature, designed by natural selection to produce an evolutionarily stable strategy for conditional helping.

NOTES

1. Cheng and Holyoak (1985) also propose an obligation schema, but for most rules tested (especially social contracts), this leads to the same predictions as the permission schema (see Cosmides, 1989).

2. Stone and colleagues tested two other patients with overlapping but different patterns of brain damage. R.B. had more extensive bilateral orbitofrontal damage than R.M., but his right temporal pole was largely spared (thus he did not have bilateral disconnection of the amygdalae): his scores were 85% correct for precautions and 83% correct for social contracts. B.G. had extensive bilateral temporal pole damage compromising (though not severing) input into both amygdalae, but his orbitofrontal cortex was completely spared: he scored 100% on both sets of problems.

3. For a full account of the problems relevance theory has explaining social contract reasoning, see Fiddick and colleagues (2000).

REFERENCES

ALMOR, A., and S. SLOMAN, 1996. Is deontic reasoning special? *Psychol. Rev.* 103:374–380.

AXELROD, R., 1984. *The Evolution of Cooperation.* New York: Basic Books.

AXELROD, R., and W. D. HAMILTON, 1981. The evolution of cooperation. *Science* 211:1390–1396.

BARRETT, H. C., 1999. *Guilty minds: How perceived intent, incentive, and ability to cheat influence social contract reasoning.* Paper presented at the 11th Annual Meeting of the Human Behavior and Evolution Society, Salt Lake City, Utah.

BOYD, R., 1988. Is the repeated prisoner's dilemma a good model of reciprocal altruism? *Ethol. Sociobiol.* 9:211–222.

CASHDAN, E., 1989. Hunters and gatherers: Economic behavior in bands. In *Economic Anthropology*, S. Plattner, ed. Stanford, Calif.: Stanford University Press, pp. 21–48.

CHENG, P., and K. HOLYOAK, 1985. Pragmatic reasoning schemas. *Cogn. Psychol.* 17:391–416.

CHENG, P., and K. HOLYOAK, 1989. On the natural selection of reasoning theories. *Cognition* 33:285–313.

COSMIDES, L., 1985. *Deduction or Darwinian algorithms? An explanation of the "elusive" content effect on the Wason selection task.* Doctoral diss., Department of Psychology, Harvard University; University Microfilms, 86-02206.

COSMIDES, L., 1989. The logic of social exchange: Has natural selection shaped how humans reason? Studies with the Wason selection task. *Cognition* 31:187–276.

COSMIDES, L., H. C. BARRETT, and J. TOOBY, 2004. Social contracts elicit the detection of intentional cheaters, not innocent mistakes. Unpublished manuscript.

COSMIDES, L., and J. TOOBY, 1989. Evolutionary psychology and the generation of culture. Part II. Case study: A computational theory of social exchange. *Ethol. Sociobiol.* 10:51–97.

COSMIDES, L., and J. TOOBY, 1992. Cognitive adaptations for social exchange. In *The Adapted Mind*, J. Barkow, L. Cosmides, and J. Tooby, eds. New York: Oxford University Press, pp. 163–228.

COSMIDES, L., and J. TOOBY, 1997. Dissecting the computational architecture of social inference mechanisms. In *Characterizing Human Psychological Adaptations Ciba Found. Symp.* 208:132–156.

DAWKINS, R., 1986. *The Blind Watchmaker.* New York: Norton.

DUGATKIN, L. A., 1997. *Cooperation Among Animals: A Modern Perspective.* New York, Oxford University Press.

FIDDICK, L., 1998. *The Deal and the Danger: An Evolutionary Analysis of Deontic Reasoning.* Doctoral diss., Department of Psychology, University of California, Santa Barbara.

FIDDICK, L., 2004. Domains of deontic reasoning: Resolving the discrepancy between the cognitive and moral reasoning literatures. *Q. J. Exp. Psychol.* 57(3):447–474.

FIDDICK, L., L. COSMIDES, and J. TOOBY, 2000. No interpretation without representation: The role of domain-specific representations and inferences in the Wason selection task. *Cognition* 77:1–79.

FISKE, A., 1991. *Structures of Social Life: The Four Elementary Forms of Human Relations*. New York: Free Press.

FODOR, J., 2000. Why we are so good at catching cheaters. *Cognition* 75:29–32.

GIGERENZER, G., and K. HUG, 1992. Domain specific reasoning: Social contracts, cheating, and perspective change. *Cognition* 43:127–171.

GURVEN, M., 2002. To give and to give not: The behavioral ecology of human food transfers. *Behav. Brain Sci.*

HARRIS, P., and M. NÚÑEZ, 1996. Understanding of permission rules by preschool children. *Child Dev.* 67:1572–1591.

HARRIS, P., M. NÚÑEZ, and C. BRETT, 2001. Let's swap: Early understanding of social exchange by British and Nepali children. *Mem. Cogn.* 29:757–764.

HAUSER, M. D., in press. *Ought! The Inevitability of a Universal Moral Grammar*. New York: Holt.

HASEGAWA, T., and K. HIRAISHI, 2000. Ontogeny of the mind from an evolutionary psychological viewpoint. In *Comparative Cognitive Science of Mind*, S. Watanabe, ed. (in Japanese). Kyoto: Minerva Publications, pp. 413–427.

ISAAC, G., 1978. The food-sharing behavior of protohuman hominids. *Sci. Am.* 238:90–108.

JOHNSON-LAIRD, P., and R. BYRNE, 1991. *Deduction*. Hillsdale, N.J.: Erlsbaum.

KIRBY, K., 1994. Probabilities and utilities of fictional outcomes in Wason's four-card selection task. *Cognition* 51:1–28.

MALJKOVIC, V., 1987. *Reasoning in evolutionarily important domains and schizophrenia: Dissociation between content-dependent and content independent reasoning*. Thesis, Department of Psychology, Harvard University.

MANKTELOW, K. I., and J. St. B. T. EVANS, 1979. Facilation of reasoning by realism: Effect or non-effect? *Br. J. Psychol.* 70:477–488.

MANKTELOW, K., and D. OVER, 1987. Reasoning and rationality. *Mind Lang.* 2:199–219.

MANKTELOW, K., and D. OVER, 1988. *Sentences, stories, scenarios, and the selection task*. Paper presented at the First International Conference on Thinking, Plymouth, U.K.

MANKTELOW, K., and D. OVER, 1990. Deontic thought and the selection task. In *Lines of Thinking*, vol. 1, K. J. Gilhooly, M. T. G. Keane, R. H. Logie, and G. Erdos, eds. London: Wiley.

MANKTELOW, K., and D. OVER, 1991. Social roles and utilities in reasoning with deontic conditionals. *Cognition* 39:85–105.

MAYNARD SMITH, J., 1982. *Evolution and the Theory of Games*. Cambridge, England: Cambridge University Press.

MCKENNA, P., L. CLARE, and A. BADDELEY, 1995. Schizophrenia. In *Handbook of Memory Disorders*, A. D. Baddeley, B. A. Wilson, and F. N. Watts, eds. New York: Wiley.

NÚÑEZ, M., and P. HARRIS, 1998a. Psychological and deontic concepts: Separate domains or intimate connections? *Mind Lang.* 13:153–170.

NÚÑEZ, M., and P. HARRIS, 1998b. *Young children's reasoning about prescriptive rules: Spotting transgressions through the selection task*. Paper presented at the XVth Biennial Meeting of the International Society for the Study of Behavioral Development, Berne, Switzerland.

OAKSFORD, M., and N. CHATER, 1994. A rational analysis of the selection task as optimal data selection. *Psychol. Rev.* 101:608–631.

PINKER, S., 1994. *The Language Instinct*. New York: Morrow.

PLATT, R., and R. GRIGGS, 1993. Darwinian algorithms and the Wason selection task: A factorial analysis of social contract selection task problems. *Cognition* 48:163–192.

RIPS, L., 1994. *The Psychology of Proof*. Cambridge, Mass.: MIT Press.

SHALLICE, T., 1988. *From Neuropsychology to Mental Structure*. Cambridge, England: Cambridge University Press.

SPERBER, D., F. CARA, and V. GIROTTO, 1995. Relevance theory explains the selection task. *Cognition* 57:31–95.

STONE, V., L. COSMIDES, J. TOOBY, N. KROLL, and R. KNIGHT, 2002. Selective impairment of reasoning about social exchange in a patient with bilateral limbic system damage. *Proc. Natl. Acad. Sci. U.S.A.* 99:11531–11536.

SUGIYAMA, L., J. TOOBY, and L. COSMIDES, 2002. Cross-cultural evidence of cognitive adaptations for social exchange among the Shiwiar of Ecuadorian Amazonia. *Proc. Natl. Acad. Sci. U.S.A.* 99:11537–11542.

TOOBY, J., and L. COSMIDES, 1989. The logic of threat. Paper presented at a meeting of the Human Behavior and Evolution Society, Evanston, Ill., August.

TOOBY, J., and L. COSMIDES, 1992. The psychological foundations of culture. In *The Adapted Mind*, J. Barkow, L. Cosmides, and J. Tooby, eds. New York: Oxford University Press, pp. 19–136.

TOOBY, J., and L. COSMIDES, 1996. Friendship and the Banker's Paradox: Other pathways to the evolution of adaptations for altruism. In *Evolution of Social Behaviour Patterns in Primates and Man*, W. G. Runciman, J. Maynard Smith, and R. I. M. Dunbar, eds. *Proceedings of the British Academy*, vol. 88, pp. 119–143.

TRIVERS, R., 1971. The evolution of reciprocal altruism. *Q. Rev. Biol.* 46:35–57.

WASON, P., 1966. Reasoning. In *New Horizons in Psychology*, B. M. Foss, ed. Harmondsworth: Penguin.

WASON, P., 1983. Realism and rationality in the selection task. In *Thinking and Reasoning: Psychological Approaches*, J. St. B. T. Evans, ed. London: Routledge, pp. 44–75.

WASON, P., and P. JOHNSON-LAIRD, 1972. *The Psychology of Reasoning: Structure and content*. Cambridge, Mass.: Harvard University Press.

WILLIAMS, G., 1966. *Adaptation and Natural Selection*. Princeton, N.J.: Princeton University Press.

94 Bioethical Issues in the Cognitive Neurosciences

MARTHA J. FARAH

ABSTRACT From the visualization of mental processes with functional neuroimaging to their manipulation with ever more selective drugs, the new capabilities of cognitive neuroscience have the potential to transform our individual lives and our society. This chapter reviews the state of the art in monitoring and enhancing brain function and analyzes some of the ethical issues that accompany these developments. In addition, neuroethical issues concerning the treatment of criminal offenders, the determination of guilt, and the definition of death are briefly mentioned.

Most cognitive neuroscientists view their field as in its infancy. Despite the remarkable progress detailed in the chapters of this book, understanding the physical basis of the human mind remains a daunting goal. We are all too aware of the limits of our understanding, and as a result we often assume that our research has few implications beyond academic science. This assumption is looking increasingly questionable, however. From the visualization of mental processes with functional neuroimaging to their manipulation with ever more selective drugs, the new capabilities of cognitive neuroscience have the potential to transform our individual lives and our society.

Like the field of genetics, cognitive neuroscience concerns the biological foundations of who we are, of our essence. Indeed, the relation of self to brain is, if anything, more direct than that of self to genome. More important, neural interventions are more easily accomplished than genetic interventions. Yet compared to the field of molecular genetics, in which ethical issues have been at the forefront since the days of the Asilomar meeting in 1975, little attention has been paid to the bioethics of neuroscience.

Our field's neglect of its own ethical implications is now being replaced by awareness and concern. In the Society for Neuroscience's recently formulated mission statement, bioethical issues figure prominently. Numerous articles, meetings, and symposia have appeared on the subject (Farah, 2002; Marcus, 2002; Roskies, 2002; Illes, Kirschen, and Gabrieli, 2003; Moreno, 2003; Farah et al., 2004). The term *neuroethics*, which was used earlier in discussions of

bioethical issues in clinical neurology, has now been adopted to refer to ethical issues in neuroscience more generally.

Many of the new social and ethical issues in neuroscience result from one of two broad classes of development. The first is the ability to monitor brain function in living humans with a spatial and temporal resolution sufficient to capture psychologically meaningful fluctuations of activity. The second is the ability to alter human brain function with a chemical or anatomical selectivity sufficient to induce specific psychological changes. These developments are the focus of the next two sections of this chapter. The final section provides a brief review of other current neuroethical issues.

Neuroimaging as mind reading

The history of modern brain imaging began in the 1970s, with computed tomography (CT), and proceeded at a rapidly accelerating rate for the remaining decades of the twentieth century. The idea of passing x-rays through the head from multiple directions and reconstructing a three-dimensional structural image, revolutionary at the time, was quickly adapted to radiological signals other than x-rays. These included radiation from exogenous tracers to enable imaging of brain function, as in positron emission tomography (PET) and single-photon emission computed tomography (SPECT), and the use of endogenously generated magnetic fields to image either structure or function, as in magnetic resonance imaging (MRI). Pioneering research on cognition and emotion was undertaken with PET and SPECT in the 1980s (reviewed by Posner and Raichle, 1994), and by the 1990s, MRI had become commonplace as the noninvasive alternative to PET in research.

In MRI, atoms are first aligned by a strong static magnetic field, then knocked out of alignment by a radiofrequency pulse, and then allowed to realign. The fluctuating field created as the atoms relax to the aligned state is the signal that is measured. Although early functional MRI used an injected contrast agent, current methods use the magnetic properties of the blood itself as a tracer, and therefore are entirely noninvasive. In blood-oxygen-level-dependent (BOLD) MRI, the different magnetic susceptibility of

MARTHA J. FARAH Center for Cognitive Neuroscience, University of Pennsylvania, Philadelphia, Penna.

oxygenated and deoxygenated hemoglobin provides a measure of regional brain activity. In arterial spin labeling (ASL) MRI, the atoms are aligned by a magnetic field at the neck and relax as they circulate through the brain, indicating regional perfusion. The spatial and temporal resolution of fMRI are limited by hemodynamics rather than by the physics of the method; blood flow changes over seconds in response to neural activity, and these changes extend into nearby tissue. In practice, fMRI has a spatial resolution of 1 mm and a temporal resolution of about 1 s, which is adequate to distinguish among psychologically meaningful differences in brain activity (Aguirre, 2003).

A few additional methods figure in the cognitive neuroimaging revolution. One is structural MRI, from which precise measurements of brain size and shape can be made. Combined with reliable methods for delineating and measuring particular brain structures, this capability has opened up the field of brain morphometry, in which slight anatomical variations are correlated with psychological traits. The venerable techniques of electroencephalography (EEG) and event-related potential (ERP) recording have acquired new capabilities with the application of signal processing techniques in the same family as for CT, PET, and MRI, allowing better localization of brain activity and analysis of temporal patterns of activity. Optical methods, such as near infrared spectroscopy (NIRS), provide another noninvasive measure of regional brain activity, based on the absorption of different wavelengths of light as it passes through the head.

By and large, these methods have been developed for long-standing clinical and scientific goals, from localizing seizure foci to studying the neurochemical abnormalities in psychiatric illness. These uses are associated with ethical issues of a familiar nature: for example, the risks of radiation exposure, the nature of informed consent (especially from the mentally ill), and the possibility of discovering incidental brain anomalies. However, neuroimaging also yields information that can be used for different purposes, raising new ethical issues. In principle, and increasingly in practice, imaging can be used to infer people's psychological traits and states, in many cases without the person's cooperation or consent. It is, in effect, a crude form of mind reading.

Imaging of Personal Information

Imaging psychiatric history Our society's attitude toward mental illness has come a long way since 1972, when Senator Thomas Eagleton was forced to withdraw his vice presidential candidacy after his history of depression became known. Nevertheless, psychiatric illness continues to carry a stigma, and a currently healthy individual might well wish to avoid disclosing a psychiatric history. The finding that depression, schizophrenia, and other illnesses leave their marks on the

brain raises the possibility that psychiatric history and risk could be inferred from a brain scan without an individual's knowledge or consent. For the most part, the relevant markers are morphometric, relying on structural rather than functional imaging (e.g., Botteron et al., 2002; Ho et al., 2003). Although the abnormalities that characterize particular illnesses can be demonstrated when small groups of patients are compared with control subjects, they are not currently diagnostic at the individual patient level. Nevertheless, diagnostic imaging is currently the goal of many research groups, with encouraging results for some disorders, for example ADHD (Dougherty et al., 1999).

Imaging personality A number of recent studies have sought neuroimaging correlates of the dimensions of personality found in classic theories of normal personality, including extraversion/introversion, neuroticism, novelty seeking, harm avoidance, and reward dependence (Fischer, Wik, and Fredrikson, 1997; Johnson et al., 1999; Sugiura et al., 2000; Youn et al., 2002; see Canli and Amin, 2002, for a review). Most of the studies employed resting scans of groups of 15–30 healthy subjects, not selected for being especially extreme on any dimension, and performed correlations between personality scale scores and brain activation throughout the brain, with no a priori regions of interest. Despite the seemingly low power of such designs, a number of positive results have been reported, with both converging and diverging results among the studies. The areas that distinguish normal people with differing personality at rest include a large number of cortical and subcortical areas, particularly paralimbic cortical areas such as the insula, orbital frontal cortex, and the anterior cingulate, as well as subcortical structures such as the amygdala and putamen.

Canli and colleagues have sought correlates of personality in the brain's response to emotionally evocative stimuli. Given that many aspects of personality are most apparent in the context of frightening, happy, sad, or temping stimuli, such an approach has the potential to demonstrate important differences not apparent in resting scans. In one study (Canli et al., 2001), they focused on two personality traits: extraversion, the tendency to seek out and enjoy social contact and maintain an upbeat outlook, and neuroticism, the tendency to worry and focus on negative information. They found that extraversion was correlated with brain response in several areas to pictures with positive emotional valence, such as puppies, ice cream, and sunsets. Figure 94.1 shows this relation for several brain areas. The effect was specific to positive and not negative stimuli, and this was confirmed in a later study with pictures of happy and fearful faces (Canli et al., 2002). Neuroticism, in contrast, is associated with differences in response to negative but not positive stimuli. Photographs of spiders, cemeteries, crying people, and other negatively valenced images evoked more response

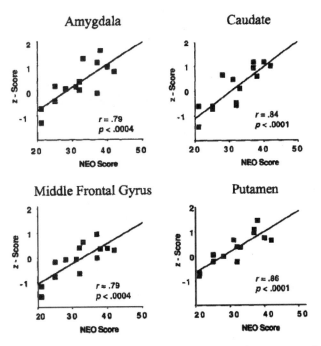

FIGURE 94.1   Relation of extroversion to BOLD signal change in various brain areas in response to happy faces relative to neutral faces. (From Canli et al., 2001.)

in certain brain areas the more neurotic the subject; positive pictures did not induce such an effect.

Imaging social and moral attitudes   In a well-known study of white subjects' attitudes toward unfamiliar black people, Phelps and colleagues (2000) recruited white subjects for a study that used both behavioral measures of evaluation and fMRI. Using previously developed behavioral measures, they were able to estimate the degree of unconscious negative evaluation of unfamiliar black as opposed to white faces. They then measured brain response to unfamiliar black and white faces and found a moderately strong correlation between amygdala activation and negative evaluation of black faces, as shown by figure 94.2.

Racial group identity also has neural correlates that are roughly measurable with current brain imaging methods. In a study of black and white subjects viewing photographs of black and white faces, significant differences in response to ingroup and outgroup faces were found.

Differences in the way people view particular actions as right or wrong, across specific moral dilemmas and across individuals, have measurable neural correlates. In particular, Greene and colleagues (2001) used fMRI to demonstrate different patterns of brain activation associated with the logical weighing of rights and wrongs, on the one hand, and the more visceral reaction against certain kinds of wrong, on the other.

Imaging preferences   The objects of a person's desires are also discernible in some cases with function neuroimaging.

The first experiments to demonstrate this concerned drug craving. Drug-free cocaine addicts experience a craving state when shown pictures of drug paraphernalia, which results in reliable group differences in PET activation of the amygdala, anterior cingulate, and orbitofrontal cortex (Childress et al., 1999). Although some of the individual scans in the patient group will be indistinguishable from normal, others will clearly differ from normal.

Drug use is not unique in this respect; other stimuli to which individuals are strongly attracted have been found to evoke activity in similar circuits. Subjects aroused by sexually explicit videos activate many of the same limbic system areas (Garavan et al., 2000). Furthermore, the conscious

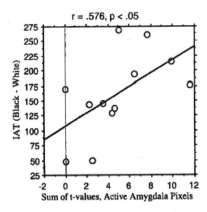

FIGURE 94.2   Relation of behavioral measure of unconscious racial attitudes to BOLD signal change in amygdala. (From Phelps et al., 2000.)

attempt to suppress arousal may also engender a distinct pattern of brain activation (Beauregard et al., 2001), suggesting an advantage of such scans over more peripheral measures capable of revealing sexual preferences.

Forensic imaging The ability to know a person's attitudes and thoughts and to predict his or her actions would be particularly useful in the criminal justice, intelligence, and immigration communities, where interviewees are often motivated to lie or to withhold needed information. For this reason, several different applications of functional neuroimaging are being explored with support from these communities. Lie detection is one of the most sought-after applications. The work of Langleben and colleagues (2002) attracted tremendous media attention when it showed differences in subjects' brain activation when bluffing versus telling the truth about symbols on playing cards. Lee and colleagues (2002) mapped the differences in brain activation in a memory task between honest test performance and simulated malingering. Such research has a long way to go before it can be used to detect spontaneous, genuine deception. The forms of deception being detected in these studies involve highly constrained questions and may reflect nothing more than the additional cognitive effort required to deceive.

The "guilty knowledge test," used for decades with peripheral measures of autonomic response, has been adapted for use with scalp-recorded ERPs and marketed by Lawrence Farwell. This method is based on the difference in P300 evoked by familiar and unfamiliar stimuli such as people, objects, or scenes that would associate an individual with a crime. It was admitted as evidence in a murder trial (GAO Report, 2001) and is being promoted as a means of screening for terrorists (e.g., *www.skirsh.com*), despite the reservations of some leading ERP researchers such as Emmanual Donchin (GAO Report, 2001).

A related research program uses brain activity to discriminate false from veridical memories. A false memory is a kind of memory error that occurs when a person mistakenly believes that he or she remembers an event that did not happen. When false memories are induced in the laboratory, they evoke patterns of activity in memory-related areas of the brain that are distinct from both veridical memories and correct judgments that an event did not happen. In one study, for example, it was found that whereas both veridical and false memories activate the hippocampus, the parahippocampal region is more activated by veridical memories (Cabeza et al., 2001).

Finally, the effort to predict future violent crime may eventually be aided by functional neuroimaging. Some offenders commit one violent crime and live the rest of their lives without harming anyone, whereas others continue to be violent. Personality factors correlate with these tendencies,

but more recently PET and fMRI have been used on an experimental basis to distinguish these two populations (Raine et al., 1998).

Imaging specific thoughts Perhaps the most science-fictionesque example of brain imaging as mind reading comes from studies of high-level vision. Although visual object recognition does not have the obvious personal and social relevance that we associate with social attitudes, emotions, or tendencies to violence, the striking thing about work in this area is the specificity of the mental content that can be recovered by analyzing a brain image. Haxby and colleagues (2001) scanned subjects while the subjects viewed numerous pictures each of faces, cats, houses, chairs, scissors, shoes, and bottles. They found that the overall pattern of activation in ventral extrastriate cortex enabled them to classify the stimulus category viewed by the subject with 96% accuracy.

Working with a reduced set of stimulus categories, O'Craven and Kanwisher (2000) accomplished a similar feat with subjects' mental images, formed in response to verbal command in the absence of a visual stimulus. The researchers were able to classify a majority of the scans as thoughts of faces or houses on the basis of the locations of activation maxima relative to localizer scans of visually presented faces and houses.

ETHICAL ISSUES IN NEUROIMAGING

Privacy The main ethical problem posed by the scientific trends just reviewed concerns privacy. As with any testing method that reveals new kinds of information about an individual (e.g., genetic testing for breast cancer risk), it may not always be in the individual's best interest to have that information available to others. However, there is an added dimension of ethical significance when the information concerns the kinds of personal psychological traits and states that neuroimaging may reveal. In the near future it is possible that employers, juries, parole boards, and law enforcement agents will attempt to use brain imaging to answer such questions as: How conscientious are you? To whom are you attracted? How do you feel about other races? What scares you? Are you prone to depression?

What obstacles lie between the present state of imaging technology and the ability to reliably read personality, psychiatric history, truthfulness, and so on from an individual's brain scan? One important limitation of the current technology is the need to aggregate data over multiple observations. When the individual subject is the unit of analysis, the need for multiple trials of data collection may render the approach impractical. Although fears or cravings can be evoked repeatedly if necessary, the recall of a specific memory cannot be repeated without changing the nature of the memory itself. For most of the examples cited here, groups of subjects must be compared in order to obtain reliable differences between groups (e.g., formerly depressed and never depressed individuals) or to detect a relation to a trait (e.g., extraversion).

Nevertheless, even when a scanning protocol is incapable of reliably classifying all individuals, it may allow certain individuals with relatively extreme patterns of brain activity to be classified. In one laboratory, at least half of recently detoxified cocaine users can be identified by differential amygdala response to drug-related versus non-drug-related pictures (A. R. Childress, personal communication). In another, simple visual examination of whole-brain activity patterns allows at least a fraction of the subjects to be sorted by personality trait (T. Canli, personal communication). Even when patterns of brain activation are not extreme, they provide information sufficient to narrow down the range of an individual's likely values on psychological traits of interest. Using only the published data in reports of imaging correlates of personality traits, a new individual's trait level could be bracketed within a range of 2.0–3.5 standard deviations (depending on the study), compared to the 4 standard deviation range of the population (Farah, Foster, and Gawuga, 2004).

Illusory accuracy In addition to privacy concerns, neuroimaging raises another issue of social concern, namely, overreliance on information from brain scans. Physiological measures, especially brain-based measures, possess an illusory accuracy and objectivity as perceived by the general public. One commentator, in proposing the use of brain fingerprinting as a screening tool at airports, wrote, "Although people lie . . . brainwaves do not" (www.skirsh.com). Although brainwaves do not lie, neither do they tell the truth; they are simply measures of brain activity. Whether based on regional cerebral bloodflow or electrical activity, brain images must be interpreted like any other correlate of mental activity, behavioral or physiological. Brain images and waveforms give an impression of concreteness and directness compared to behavioral measures of psychological traits and states, and high-tech instrumentation lends an aura of accuracy and objectivity. Nevertheless, the inference from these measures to their psychological interpretations is far from direct or intrinsically objective. As the foregoing review suggests, progress has been made in the use of such measures, and some inferences to socially relevant traits and states can now be made with a degree of certainty under specific and highly controlled conditions. However, the current state of the art does not allow reliable screening, profiling, or lie detection.

Brain-based measures do, in principle, have an advantage as indices of psychological traits and states over more familiar behavioral or autonomic measures. They are one causal

step closer to these traits and states than responses on personality questionnaires or polygraph tracings. Imaging may therefore one day provide the most sensitive and specific measures available of psychological processes. For now, however, this is not the case, and there is a risk that juries, judges, parole boards, the immigration service, and so on will weight such measures too heavily in their decision making.

From therapy to enhancement

TECHNICAL ADVANCES The psychopharmacology of the mid-twentieth century depended entirely on serendipity. The antihistamine chlorpromazine was accidentally found to calm agitated schizophrenic patients and even reduce their psychosis. Another early drug investigated for its antipsychotic properties, imipramine, turned out to be ineffective for that purpose but was observed to lift the mood of some of the patients taking it. When a small number of patients with major depression tried it, the therapeutic effect was dramatic, and imipramine continues to be used as an antidepressant today. The second antidepressant to be discovered, iproniazid, was being used as an antibiotic to treat tuberculosis when its mood-elevating properties were observed. Similar accidental discoveries led to the identification of amphetamine as a stimulant in the course of refining a treatment for asthma, and meprobamate as an antianxiety treatment in the course of testing an antibiotic (see Barondes, 2003, for a review of psychiatric drug discovery).

Such lucky accidents were then augmented by trial-and-error tests with other molecules of similar structure. In parallel, researchers began to understand the effects of these drugs on brain function, identifying the specific neurotransmitter systems affected by the drugs and the mechanisms by which the drugs interacted with these systems. The advent of direct binding assays in the 1960s provided the first direct approach to testing and comparing the affinity of a drug for different neurotransmitter receptors, and the tools of the molecular biology revolution, including the cloning of rare subtypes of receptors, allowed the design of highly selective agonists, antagonists, and other molecules to selectively influence the process of neurotransmission.

The continual improvement in side effect profile of modern psychotropic medications is due to the increasing selectivity of drug action, made possible by the methods of molecular neuroscience. "Selective" is the first S in SSRI (selective serotonin reuptake inhibitor), the class of drugs to which fluoxetine (Prozac) belongs. New drugs with ever more selective actions on the neurochemistry of mood, anxiety, attention, and memory are in development.

The enhancement potential of some medications is, in itself, nothing new. Until recently, however, psychotropic drugs had significant risks and side effects that limited their attractiveness. This situation is changing as side effects become more tolerable. In addition, adjuvant therapy with other drugs is increasingly used to counteract the remaining side effects. For example, the most troublesome side effect for users of SSRIs is sexual dysfunction, which responds well to the drug sildenafil (Viagra). Other drugs specifically developed to counteract the sexual side effects of SSRIs are in development and clinical trials. The result of both new designer drugs and adjuvant drugs is the same: increasingly selective alteration of our mental states and abilities through neurochemical intervention, with correspondingly less downside to their use by anyone, sick or well.

Technical advances in nonpharmaceutical methods for altering brain function are also potential enhancement tools. Transcranial magnetic stimulation (TMS), and more rarely vagus nerve stimulation and deep brain stimulation, have already been used to improve mental function or mood in patients with medically intractable neuropsychiatric illnesses (Mahli and Sachdev, 2002). Research on the effects of non-pharmacuetical methods on brain function in normal individuals has been limited to the relatively less invasive TMS. Mood effects in normal healthy subjects have been investigated in the context of basic research on mood and brain function (e.g., George, Wasserman, and Post, 1996; Mosimann et al., 2000), and at least one laboratory is working to develop TMS methods for enhancing normal cognition (Snyder et al., 2003).

Finally, there is growing research interest in the cyborg-like computer augmentation of brains. Most research on brain–machine interfaces currently focuses on capturing and using movement command signals from the brain and carrying sensory inputs to the brain (Donoghue, 2002). The motivation for this research is partly scientific, to better understand neural coding of sensory and motor, information, and partly clinical, to help patients with paralysis and peripheral sensory impairments. Nevertheless, the presence of substantial research support in this area from the military suggests that, in some minds at least, normal healthy individuals might some day incorporate neural prostheses (Hoag, 2003).

Enhancement of Normal Brain Function

Enhancement of mood   Amphetamines, barbituates, benzodiazepenes, and other "mother's little helpers" have long been used to improve the moods of healthy, normal people. However, the high potential for addiction and tolerance with these drugs dissuade most people from using them. Pre-SSRI antidepressants, while presenting no such risks, have unpleasant side effects that limit their appeal to all but those faced with clinical depression as the alternative. The SSRIs, in contrast, have relatively narrower neurochemical effects and consequently fewer side effects. The result, as Peter

Kramer described in *Listening to Prozac*, is that many people who would never have taken a tricyclic antidepressant are taking SSRIs.

Of course, most people using SSRIs meet *DSM-IV* criteria for some psychiatric disorder, although not necessarily major depression: dysthymia (a mild depression), social phobia (an extreme form of shyness and self-consciousness), premenstrual dysphoric disorder (a recurrent negative mood associated with PMS), and various eating disorders respond well to SSRIs. Nevertheless, it remains controversial whether some of these diagnostic categories are medicalized labels for normal variants of human personality that do not necessarily require treatment. Other people using SSRIs have no recognized illness. Some have suffered from depression in the past and choose to continue medication prophylactically. Others have simply decided that, in Peter Kramer's words, they feel "better than well" when taking an antidepressant.

What is the nature of the enhancement experienced by normal, healthy individuals taking SSRIs? No systematic studies have assessed the effects on individuals who choose to take these medications. However, a handful of studies have assessed the effects of SSRIs on mood and personality in randomly selected healthy subjects over short periods of a few months or less (Knutson et al., 1998; Tse and Bond, 2002). Effects on mood are relatively selective, reducing self-reported negative affect (e.g., fear, hostility) while leaving positive affect (e.g., happiness, excitement) neither increased nor decreased. The drugs also increased affiliative behavior in laboratory social interactions and cooperative/competitive games played with confederates. For example, subjects on drugs spoke fewer commands and instead made more suggestions. In one double-blind crossover design, subjects were not only more cooperative in a game but showed real-world changes in behavior as well: flatmates found them less submissive on citalopam, though no more dominant or hostile (Tse and Bond, 2002). Much more research is needed to clarify the effects of SSRIs and other antidepressant agents on the mood and behavior of normal healthy subjects, but the evidence so far suggests subtle but salutary effects.

Enhancement of cognition   Our current ability to enhance cognition by the direct alteration of brain function involves two types of cognitive function: attention and memory (Farah et al., 2004). *Attention* is used here in its broadest sense, including the active use of working memory, executive function, and other forms of cognitive self-control. These are the cognitive abilities most obviously deficient in the syndrome of ADHD. These same abilities vary in their strength within the normal population. Indeed, it seems likely that ADHD represents the lower tail of the whole population distribution rather than a qualitatively different state of functioning, discontinuous with the normal population (NIH Consensus Statement, 1998).

Drugs targeting the neurotransmitter systems dopamine and norephinephrine are effective in treating ADHD and have been shown to improve normal attentional function as well. Methylphenidate (Ritalin) and amphetamine (Adderall) have been shown to enhance attention across a variety of different tests in healthy young volunteers (e.g., Elliot et al., 1997; Mehta et al., 2000). Figure 94.3 shows the anatomical specificity with which methylphenidate modulates the spatial working memory of normal healthy subjects.

Do these laboratory-measured improvements translate into a noticeable improvement of real world cognitive performance? No experimental evidence is available, but the growing illicit use of ADHD medications on college campuses (Babcock and Bryne, 2000) suggests that many young adults believe their cognition to be enhanced by the drugs. Parents also appear to find real-world benefits for their normal children with ADHD medication: in certain school districts, the proportion of boys taking methylphenidate exceeds the most generous estimates of ADHD prevalence (Diller, 1996).

Memory is the other cognitive ability that can, at present, be manipulated to some degree by drugs. Interest in memory enhancement has so far been confined to the middle-aged and elderly, whose memory ability undergoes a gradual decline even in the absence of dementia. The most com-

monly used method involves manipulation not of memory circuits per se but of cerebrovascular function. Herbal supplements such as *Gingko biloba* affect memory mainly by increasing blood flow within the brain. However, the effectiveness of this treatment is questionable (Gold, Cahill, and Wenk, 2002). How close are we to more specific and effective memory enhancement for healthy older adults?

As the molecular biology of memory progresses, it presents drug designers with a variety of entry points through which to influence the specific processes of memory formation. A huge research effort is now being directed to the development of memory-boosting drugs (Lynch, 2002). The candidate drugs target various stages in the molecular cascade that underlies memory formation, including the initial induction of long-term potentiation and the later stages of memory consolidation. These drugs are currently envisioned as treatments for dementia and so-called "mild cognitive impairment," which is more severe than normal age-related cognitive decline. However, there is reason to believe that some of the products under development would work for that purpose as well. For example, treatment of healthy older human subjects with an ampakine, which enhances long-term potentiation, improved performance in a dose-dependent manner (figure 94.4).

Few consider memory enhancement for the young to be a goal. Although certain specialized pursuits such as competitive card games could conceivably benefit from super-memory, evidence suggests that the forgetting rates of normal young humans are optimal for most purposes (Anderson, 1990). Empirically, prodigious memory has been linked to difficulties with thinking and problem solving (Luria, 1968), and computationally, the effect of boosting the durability of individual memories is to decrease the ability to generalize (McClelland, McNaughton, and O'Reilly,

sagittal

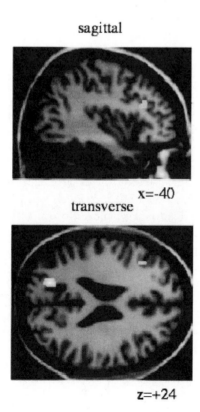

x=-40

transverse

z=+24

FIGURE 94.3 Effects of methylphenidate on brain activity underlying working memory in normal subjects. (From Mehta et al., 2000.)

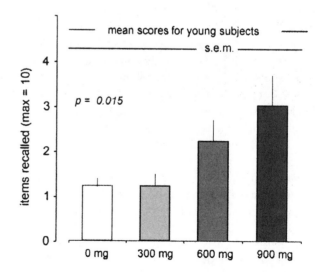

FIGURE 94.4 Effect of ampakine on memory performance of normal subjects. (From Lynch, 2002.)

1995). Indeed, in some circumstances, reduced learning would confer benefit.

Memories of traumatic events can cause lifelong suffering in the form of posttraumatic stress disorder (PTSD), and methods are being sought to prevent the consolidation of such memories by intervening pharmacologically immediately following the trauma (Pittman et al., 2002). Drugs that interfere with the consolidation of memories in general, such as benzodiazepines, are well known (Buffett-Jerrott and Stewart, 2002). Extending these methods beyond the victims of trauma to anyone wishing to avoid remembering an unpleasant event is yet another way in which the neural bases of memory could be altered to enhance normal function.

ETHICAL ISSUES IN ENHANCEMENT Although the upside of enhancement is easy to identify—smarter, more cheerful, and more capable people—the downside is harder to articulate. Most people feel at least some ambivalence about neuropsychological enhancement, but it takes some discussion and analysis to identify the underlying ethical issues.

Many of the ethical issues raised by neuropsychological enhancement also arise with other types of enhancement (Elliot, 2003; Parens, 2000). Examples of medically based enhancements that do not affect brain function include cosmetic surgery and the use of human growth hormone for healthy children who are naturally short. Examples of enhancements that affect psychological function, and hence brain function, through more familiar and non-neuroscience-based interventions include tutoring and psychotherapy. When thinking through the ethical pros and cons of these practices, we encounter in a familiar context many of the issues that arise in the less familiar realm of neuropsychological enhancement. In addition, some genuinely new issues may be raised by direct enhancement of brain function.

Problems with enhancement per se Neuropsychological enhancement, like any medically based form of enhancement, raises safety issues in the minds of many. Perhaps a youth spent scaling the heights of academic and job success thanks to enhancement by Ritalin will be followed by a middle age of premature memory loss and cognitive decline. Risks weigh especially heavily with enhancement compared to therapy. We naturally require lower levels of risk for interventions that have lower levels of benefit, and we assume that the benefit of enhancing is smaller than the benefit of treating an impairment. How safe an enhancement is, as opposed to whether enhancement should be practiced given a certain level of safety, is an empirical question. So far, medications such as SSRIs and stimulants have good safety records, and their long-term effects may even be positive. For example, SSRIs have been shown to be neuroprotective over the long term (Sanchez et al., 2001). A recent study of the effects of Ritalin on rat brain development showed both desirable and undesirable effects on later adult behavior (Carlezon, Mague, and Andersen, 2003). Nevertheless, drug safety testing does not routinely address long-term use, and relatively little evidence is available on long-term use by healthy subjects.

Another objection common to all forms of enhancement centers on the problem of gain without pain. Our culture places value on earning one's happiness, success, and so on. Improving attention or mood with a pill seems wrong to some people because it requires so little effort.

However, while we all recognize the value of earning life's rewards, our lives are full of shortcuts to looking and feeling better. We don't disapprove of people who dislike vegetables improving their health by taking vitamin pills. Nor do we begrudge college applicants their SAT prep books or Stanley Kaplan classes. The idea of just deserts is certainly alive and well in our culture, but it coexists with other values: we feel good about embracing opportunities and admire the ingenuity that helps us do things more quickly and easily.

Other objections to enhancement stem from potential harm to society. One such worry is that enhancement will not be fairly distributed. It is likely that the wealthy and privileged will have access to enhancement and the less privileged will not. Is this what lies at the root of our unease with enhancement? Probably not, given that our society is already full of such inequities. No one would seek to prohibit private tutoring or cosmetic surgery on the grounds that these benefits are inequitably distributed. Besides, consider a scenario in which the entire populace is given full and equal access to Ritalin, Prozac, and other enhancers. If our qualms about enhancement were linked to equal opportunity, then this should set our minds at ease, but more than likely it does not.

Another potential problem with enhancement is that widespread enhancement might raise our standards of normalcy. This would put individuals who choose not to enhance at a disadvantage, in effect a form of indirect coercion. Even the enhancement of mood, which at first glance lacks a competitive function, appears to be associated with increased social ability, which does confer an advantage in many walks of life. Such indirect coercion may already be felt by parents whose children attend schools with high rates of Ritalin use. Direct coercion is also possible: employers could pressure their employees to enhance attention or mood on the job. Clearly coercion is not a good thing. However, to prevent people from practicing a safe form of enhancement, for the sake of people who might not want it, is also coercive.

Problems with neuropsychological enhancement The objections to enhancement just reviewed apply to neuropsychological enhancement, but they are not unique to it. Other objections pertain to neuropsychological enhancement exclusively. These objections include a variant of the safety concerns with which the previous section began. The brain is a far more complex system than the face or even the endocrine system (targets of cosmetic surgery and growth hormone treatments). One could argue that we are therefore at greater risk of unanticipated problems when we tinker. In addition, we understand little about the evolutionary constraints that were satisfied in the process of creating a modern human brain. We therefore do not know which "limitations" are there for a good reason. As already mentioned, normal forgetting rates appear to be optimal for information retrieval.

There is a variant of the "no pain, no gain" objection that is specific to enhancement of mood and most trenchant in the case of pharmacologic interventions. Some people believe that one cannot experience the beauty and joy of life unless one is also acquainted with life's pain. This is an empirical claim, of course, and evidence for it has yet to be presented. Anecdotal reports of generalized emotional blunting caused by SSRIs have not been replicated in systematic research (Furlan et al., 2004) and the small literature on short-term SSRI effects in normal subjects suggests no decrease or increase in positive affect, only a selective decrease in negative affect. In any case, even if emotional blunting were a side effect of current mood enhancers, it is not a basis for rejecting mood enhancement in general. There is no a priori reason that newer medications would have the same effect.

Finally, neuropsychological enhancement challenges some of our intuitions about personhood and selfhood. We are not the same when on Ritalin or Prozac as when off. Of course, we are also not the same on vacation as before an exam, but our intuitions about personal identity seem accommodate such situational variation more easily than pharmacologic variation. Peter Kramer's classic book, *Listening to Prozac* (1993), is a meditation on antidepressant-initiated transformation of the self, and he quotes patients who feel that they are their "true" selves only on medication. As alteration and enhancement of mood and other psychological states become more common, Kramer predicts that our notions of selfhood will evolve and reach "a point at which such concepts as mood, personality and self become . . . unstable" (p. xi). In other words, neuropsychological enhancement may eventually dissolve the notion of an essential, fixed self.

Other neuroethical issues

It would take a book to explore all of the ethical issues raised by recent progress in cognitive neuroscience. Of the many remaining issues, some relate to other biomedical sciences as well, and others are particular to cognitive neuroscience.

Neuroethical issues with clear parallels in other fields include the following: How safe are the new methods of cognitive neuroscience, such as TMS or high-field MRI, and who should decide? What is the appropriate course of action when an incidental neurological abnormality is found in the course of research scanning? How should promising new therapies be rationed? When and why should predictive testing be offered for future neurological or neuropsychiatric illness when no cure is available, as is the case with Alzheimer's and Huntington's diseases?

Other ethical issues arise exclusively in cognitive neuroscience because of the particular subject matter of our field. The brain is the organ of the mind, consciousness, and selfhood. A few more of these issues, beyond brain imaging as mind reading and enhancement of brain function, will be mentioned briefly here.

An issue related to enhancement concerns the use of brain-based methods for behavior change in the criminal justice system. State-imposed rehabilitation, along with punishment, has long been an option for sentencing within the criminal justice system. Furthermore, court-ordered therapy or rehabilitation is not confined to medically diagnosed illnesses. Judges may require healthy individuals to undergo interventions such as parenting classes or anger management therapy. As pharmacologic interventions prove their effectiveness in modulating tendencies to criminal acts such as violent aggression or sexual predation, it seems logical to incorporate them into sentencing as well. Impulsive violence has been linked to serotonergic abnormalities, and SSRIs have accordingly been tried as a treatment for aggressive behavior, and are generally found to be helpful (Walsh and Dinan, 2001).

How close do our current practices come to directly altering brain function under the rubric of court-ordered rehabilitation? Criminals who are deemed a threat to self or others are routinely medicated by court order, and this strikes most people as reasonable. Several states in the United States have enacted laws that either allow or require sex offenders to take testosterone-lowering drugs to reduce their sex drive, and the use of serotonergic drugs for this purpose is being explored in research studies (Grossman, Martis, and Fichtner, 1999). As more such methods become available, society will have to weigh the value of individual freedom of thought, personality, and sexual interest against the value of protecting the populace.

The criminal justice system must also come to grips with the deterministic view of human behavior that emerges from neuroscience and reconcile it with the notions of responsibility and blame that undergird our legal system, as well as our personal ethics. Although the perceived conflict between free will and determinism does not hinge on the particulars of any specific deterministic account, progress in cognitive neuroscience certainly increases the salience of the deterministic view. The abstraction that all human behavior is explainable in terms of the laws of physics does not encroach much on our intuitions about a defendant's responsibility for his actions. In contrast, a detailed account of the mechanisms linking childhood abuse to diminished impulse control seems much more likely to temper our intuitions about responsibility and blame.

Death criteria have focused on brain function since the 1960s, and have been critiqued and revised in the interim. With our growing understanding of mind–brain relations and our ability to assess them with functional neuroimaging, a narrower focus on the status of higher brain functions seems indicated. However, any such move will raise profound questions about personhood and the brain. Similarly, the theories and methods of cognitive neuroscience hold potential for refining our conceptions of competence. The ability to provide informed consent for research participation or for treatment can be especially crucial in our field because in many cases, the subjects or patients in question will have brain disorders that affect their decision-making ability.

As cognitive neuroscience reaches out of the ivory tower and into society, it is vital that cognitive neuroscientists take a share of responsibility for the results. One important task that falls to us alone is to communicate our ideas and methods accurately to policy makers and the public. The abruptly formulated and, to many, ill-considered U.S. policy on stem cell research emerged in the context of virtually nonexistent public understanding of the method. A rush to embrace "brain reading" as an objective tool for screening terrorists, or to lump safe mood- and cognition-enhancing drugs with drugs of abuse, are examples of social policy that a well-informed public can avoid.

REFERENCES

AGUIRRE, G. K., 2003. Functional imaging in behavioral neurology and neuropsychology. In *Behavioral Neurology and Neuropsychology*, 2nd ed., T. E. Feinberg and M. J. Farah, eds. New York, McGraw-Hill, pp. 85–96.

ANDERSON, J., 1990. *The Adaptive Characteristics of Thought* Hillsdale, N.J.: Erlbaum.

BABCOCK, Q., and T. BYRNE, 2000. Student perceptions of methylphenidate abuse at a public liberal arts college. *J. Am. Coll. Health* 49:143–145.

BARONDES, S. H. 2003. *Better than Prozac: Creating the Next Generation of Psychiatric Drugs*. London: Oxford University Press.

BEAUREGARD, M., J. LEVESQUE, and P. BOURGOUIN, 2001. Neural correlates of conscious self-regulation of emotion. *J. Neurosci.* 21:RC165.

BOTTERON, K. N., M. E. RAICHLE, W. C. DREVETS, A. C. HEATH, and R. O. TODD, 2002. Volumetric reduction in left subgenual prefrontal cortex in early onset depression. *Biol. Psychiatry* 15:342–344.

BUFFETT-JERROTT, S. E., and S. H. STEWART, 2002. Cognitive and sedative effects of benzodiazepine use. *Curr. Pharmaceutical Design* 8:45–58.

CABEZA, R., S. M. RAO, A. D. WAGNER, A. R. MAYER, and D. L. SCHACTER, 2001. Can medial temporal regions distinguish true from false? *Proc. Natl. Acad. Sci. U.S.A.* 98:4805–4810.

CANLI, T., and Z. AMIN, 2002. Neuroimaging of emotion and personality: Scientific evidence and ethical considerations. *Brain Cogn.* 50:414–431.

CANLI, T., H. SIVERS, S. L. WHITFIELD, I. H. GOTLIEB, and J. D. GABRIELI, 2002. Amygdala response to happy faces as a function of extraversion. *Science* 296:2191.

CANLI, T., Z. ZHAO, J. E. DESMOND, E. KANG, J. GROSS, and J. D. GABRIELI, 2001. An fMRI study of personality influences on brain reactivity to emotional stimuli. *Behav. Neurosci.* 115:33–42.

CARLEZON, W. A., JR., M. D. MAGUE, and S. L. ANDERSEN, 2003. Enduring behavioral effects of early exposure to methylphenidate in rats. *Biol. Psychiatry* 54:1330–1337.

CHILDRESS, A. R., P. D. MOZLEY, W. MCELGIN, J. FITZGERALD, M. REIVICH, and C. P. O'BRIEN, 1999. Limbic activation during cue-induced cocaine craving. *Am. J. Psychiatry* 156:11–18.

DILLER, L. H., 1996. The run on Ritalin: Attention deficit disorder and stimulant treatment in the 1990s. *Hastings Center Rep.* 26:12–14.

DONOGHUE, J. P., 2002. Connecting cortex to machines: recent advances in brain interfaces. *Nat. Neurosci.* 5(Suppl.):1085–1088.

DOUGHERTY, D. D., A. A. BONAB, T. J. SPENCER, S. L. RAUCH, B. K. MADRAS, and A. J. FISCHMAN, 1999. Dopamine transporter density in patients with attention deficit hyperacivity disorder. *Lancet* 354: 2132–2133.

ELLIOT, C., 2003. *Better Than Well: American Medicine Meets the American Dream*. New York: Norton.

ELLIOTT, R., B. J. SAHAKIAN, et al., 1997. Effects of methylphenidate on spatial working memory and planning in healthy young adults. *Psychopharmacology* 131:196–206.

FARAH, M. J., 2002. Emerging ethical issues in neuroscience. *Nat. Neurosci.* 5:1123–1129.

FARAH, M. J., J. ILLES, R. COOK-DEEGAN, H. GARDNER, E. KANDEL, P. KING, E. PARENS, B. SAHAKIAN, and P. R. WOLPE, 2004. Neurocognitive enhancement: What can we do? What should we do? *Nat. Rev. Neurosci.* 5:421–425.

FISCHER, H., G. WIK, and M. FREDRIKSON, 1997. Extraversion, neuroticism, and brain & function: A pet study of personality. *Personality and Individual Differences* 23:345–352.

FURLAN, P. M., M. J. KALLAN, T. TEN HAVE, I. LUCKI, and I. KATZ, 2004. SSRIs do not cause affective blunting in healthy elderly volunteers. *Am J. Ger. Psychiat.* 12:323–330.

GAO Report, 2001. *Investigative Contacts: Federal Agency Views on the Potential Application of "Brain Fingerprinting."* Washington, D.C., U.S. General Accounting Office, pp. 1–24.

GARAVAN, H., et al., 2000. Cue-induced cocaine craving: Neuroanatomical specificity for drug users and drug stimuli. *Am. J. Psychiatry* 157:1789–1798.

GEORGE, M., E. WASSERMAN, and R. POST, 1996. Transcranial magnetic stimulation: A neuropsychiatric tool for the 21st century. *J. Neuropsychiatry Clin. Neurosci.* 8:373–382.

GOLD, P. E., L. CAHILL, and G. L. WENK, 2002. *Ginkgo biloba*: A cognitive enhancer? *Psychol. Sci. Public Interest* 3:2–11.

GREENE, J., et al., 2001. An fMRI investigation of emotional engagement in moral judgement. *Science* 293:2105–2108.

GROSSMAN, L. S., B. MARTIS, and C. G. FICHTNER, 1999. Are sex offenders treatable? A research overview. *Psychiatr. Serv.* 50: 349–361.

HART, A. J., P. J. WHALEN, L. M. SHIN, S. MCINERNEY, H. FISCHER, and S. RAUCH, 2000. Differential response in the human amygdala to racial outgroup vs. ingroup face stimuli. *Neuroreport* 11:2351–2355.

HAXBY, J. V., M. I. GOBBINI, M. L. FUREY, A. ISHAI, J. L. SCHOUTEN, and P. PIETRINI, 2001. Distributed and overlapping representations of faces and objects in ventral temporal cortex. *Science* 293:2425–2430.

HO, B. C., N. C. ANDREASEN, P. NOPOULOS, S. ARNDT, V. MAGNOTTA, and M. FLAUM, 2003. Progressive structural brain abnormalities and their relationship to clinical outcome: A longitudinal magnetic resonance imaging study early in schizophrenia. *Arch. Gen. Psychiatry* 60:585–594.

HOAG, H., 2003. Remote control. *Nature* 423:796–798.

ILLES, J., M. P. KIRSCHEN, and J. O. GABRIELI, 2003. From neuroimaging to neuroethics. *Nat. Neurosci.* 6:205.

JOHNSON, D. L., J. S. WIEBE, S. M. GOLD, N. C. ANDREASEN, R. D. HICHWA, G. L. WATKINS, and L. L. BOLES PONTO, 2001. Cerebral blood flow and personality: A positron emission tomography study. *Am. J. Psychiatry* 156:252–257.

KNUTSON, B., et al., 1998. Selective alteration of personality and social behavior by serotonergic intervention. *Am. J. Psychiatry* 155:373–379.

KRAMER, P. D., 1993. *Listening to Prozac*. New York: Penguin.

LANGLEBEN, D. D., L. SCHROEDER, J. A. MALDJIAN, R. C. GUR, S. MCDONALD, J. D. RAGLAND, C. P. O'BRIEN, and A. R. CHILDRESS, 2002. Brain activity during simulated deception: An event-related functional magnetic resonance study. *NeuroImage* 15:727–732.

LEE, T. M., H. L. LIU, L. H. TAN, C. C. CHAN, S. MAHANKALI, C. M. FENG, J. HOU, P. T. FOX, and J. H. GAO, 2002. Lie detection by functional magnetic resonance imaging. *Hum. Brain Mapp.* 15:157–164.

LURIA, A. R., 1968. *The Mind of a Mnemomist*. Cambridge, Mass.: Harvard University Press.

LYNCH, G., 2002. Memory enhancement: The search for mechanism-based drugs. *Nat. Neurosci.* 5:1035–1038.

MAHLI, G. S., and P. SACHDEV, 2002. Novel physical treatments for the management of neuropsychiatric disorders. *J. Psychosom. Res.* 53:709–719.

MARCUS, D., ed., 2002. *Neuroethics Mapping the Field Conference. Proceedings of the Dana Foundation*. Washington, D.C.: Dana Press.

MCCLELLAND, J. L., B. L. MCNAUGHTON, and R. C. O'REILLY, 1995. Why there are complementary learning systems in the hippocampus and neocortex: Insights from the successes and failures of connectionist models of learning and memory. *Psychol. Rev.* 102:419–457.

MEHTA, M. A., A. M. OWEN, et al., 2000. Methylphenidate enhances working memory by modulating discrete frontal and parietal lobe regions in the human brain. *J. Neurosci.* 20:RC65.

MEHTA, M. A., A. M. OWEN, B. J. SAHAKIAN, N. MAVADDAT, J. D. PICKARD, and T. W. ROBBINS, 2000. Methylphenidate enhances working memory by modulating discrete frontal and parietal lobe regions in the human brain. *J. Neurosci.* 20:RC65.

MORENO, J. 2003. Neuroethics: An agenda for neuroscience and society. *Nat. Rev. Neurosci.* 4:149–153.

MOSIMANN, U. P., T. A. RIHS, J. ENGELER, H. FISCH, and T. E. SCHLAEPFER, 2000. Mood effects of repetitive transcranial magnetic stimulation of left prefrontal cortex in healthy volunteers. *Psychiatry Res.* 94:251–256.

NIH Consensus Statement, 1998. Diagnosis and Treatment of Attention Deficit Hyperactivity Disorder. Nov. 16–18; 16(2):1–37.

O'CRAVEN, K. M., and N. KANWISHER, 2000. Mental imagery of faces and places activates corresponding stimulus-specific brain regions. *J. Cogn. Neurosci.* 12:1013–1023.

PARENS, E., ed. 2000. *Enhancing Human Traits: Social and Ethical Implications*. Washington: Georgetown University Press.

PHELPS, E., et al., 2000. Performance on indirect measures of race evaluation predicts amygdala activation. *J. Cogn. Neurosci.* 12:729–738.

PITTMAN, R. K., K. M. SANDERS, R. M. ZUSMAN, A. R. HEALY, F. CHEEMA, and N. B. LASKO, 2002. Pilot study of secondary prevention of posttraumatic stress disorder with propranolol. *Biol. Psychiatry* 15:189–192.

POSNER, M. I., and M. E. RAICHLE, 1994. *Images of the Mind*. New York: Scientific American Books.

RAINE, A., J. R. MELOY, S. BIHRLE, J. SODDARD, L. LACASSE, and M. S. BUCHSBAUM, 1998. Reduced prefrontal and increased subcortical brain functioning assessed using positron emission tomography in predatory and affective murderers. *Behav. Sci. Law* 16:319–332.

ROSKIES, A., 2002. Neuroethics for the new millenium. *Neuron* 35:21–23.

SANCHEZ, V., J. CAMARERO, B. ESTEBAN, M. J. PETER, A. R. GREEN, and M. I. COLADO, 2001. The mechanisms involved in the long-lasting neuroprotective effect of fluoxetine against MDMA ("ecstasy")-induced degeneration of 5-HT nerve endings in rat brain." *Br. J. Pharmacol.* 134:46–57.

SNYDER, A. W., E. MULCAHEY, J. L. TAYLOR, D. J. MITCHELL, P. SACHDEV, and S. GANDEVIA, 2003. Savant-like skills exposed in normal people by suppressing the left fronto-temporal lobe. *J. Integr. Neurosci.* 2:149–158.

SUGIURA, M., R. KAWASHIMA, M. NAKAGAWA, K. OKADA, T. SATO, R. GOTO, K. SATO, S. ONO, T. SCHORMANN, K. ZILLES, and H. FUKUDA, 2001. Correlation between human personality and neural activity in cerebral cortex. *NeuroImage* 11:541–546.

TSE, W. S., and A. J. BOND, 2002. Serotonergic intervention affects both social dominance and affiliative behaviour. *Psychopharmacology* 161:324–330.

WALSH, M. T., and T. G. DINAN, 2001. Selective serotonin reuptake inhibitors and violence: A review of the available evidence. *Acta Psychiatry Scand* 104:84–91.

YOUN, T., I. K. LYOO, J. K. KIM, H. J. PARK, K. S. HA, D. S. LEE, K. Y. ABRAMS, M. C. LEE, and J. S. KWON, 2002. Relationship between personality trait and regional cerebral glucose metabolism assessed with positron emission tomography. *Biol. Psychol.* 60:109–120.

CONTRIBUTORS

ADELSON, EDWARD H.   Department of Brain and Cognitive Science, Massachusetts Institute of Technology, Cambridge, Massachusetts

ADOLPHS, RALPH   Division of Humanities and Social Sciences, California Institute of Technology, Pasadena, California

ANDERSEN, RICHARD   Division of Biology, California Institute of Technology, Pasadena, California

ANG, EUGENIUS S. B. C.   Department of Neurobiology, Yale University School of Medicine, New Haven, Connecticut

BADRE, DAVID   Department of Brain and Cognitive Sciences, Massachusetts Institute of Technology, Cambridge, Massachusetts

BAILEY, CRAIG H.   Center for Neurobiology and Behavior, College of Physicians and Surgeons of Columbia University, New York, New York

BAIRD, ABIGAIL   Department of Psychology, Dartmouth College, Hanover, New Hampshire

BAYLEY, PETER J.   Veterans Affairs Healthcare System, Department of Psychiatry, University of California, San Diego, California

BEAR, MARK F.   The Picower Center for Learning and Memory, Massachusetts Institute of Technology, Cambridge, Massachusetts

BEER, JENNIFER S.   Department of Psychology and Center for Mind and Brain, University of California, Davis, California

BENSAFI, MOUSTAFA   Department of Neuroscience, University of California, Berkeley, California

BERNTSON, GARY G.   Departments of Psychology and Psychiatry, Ohio State University, Columbus, Ohio

BIZZI, EMILIO   McGovern Institute for Brain Research, Department of Brain and Cognitive Science, Massachusetts Institute of Technology, Cambridge, Massachusetts

BLACK, IRA B.   Stem Cell Research Center, Department of Neuroscience and Cell Biology, University of Medicine and Dentistry of New Jersey, Robert Wood Johnson Medical School, Piscataway, New Jersey

BLAKEMORE, COLIN   University Laboratory of Physiology, University of Oxford, Oxford, U.K.

BOETTIGER, CHARLOTTE A.   Keck Center for Integrative Neuroscience, and Departments of Physiology and Psychiatry, University of California, San Francisco, California; Helen Wills Neuroscience Institute, University of California, Berkeley, California

BOUDREAU, C. ELIZABETH   Department of Neurobiology and Physiology, Northwestern University, Evanston, Illinois

BREITER, HANS C.   Departments of Psychiatry and Radiology, Harvard Medical School, and Athinoula Martinos Center for Biomedical Imaging, Massachusetts General Hospital, Boston, Massachusetts

BREUNIG, JOSHUA   Department of Neurobiology, Yale University School of Medicine, New Haven, Connecticut

BREZNEN, BORIS   Division of Biology, California Institute of Technology, Pasadena, California

BUCKNER, RANDY L.   Department of Psychology, Howard Hughes Medical Institute at Washington University, St. Louis, Missouri

BUNEO, CHRISTOPHER   Division of Biology, California Institute of Technology, Pasadena, California

BUNGE, SILVIA A.   Department of Psychology and Center for Mind and Brain, University of California, Davis, California

CACIOPPO, JOHN T.   Department of Psychology, University of Chicago, Chicago, Illinois

CARAMAZZA, ALFONSO   Cognitive Neuropsychology Laboratory, and Department of Psychology, Harvard University, Cambridge, Massachusetts

CARANDINI, MATTEO   Smith-Kettlewell Eye Research Institute, San Francisco, California

CHAFEE, MATTHEW V.   Department of Neuroscience, Minnesota Medical School, Minneapolis, Minnesota

CHALMERS, DAVID J.   Department of Philosophy, University of Arizona, Tucson, Arizona

CHALUPA, LEO M.   Department of Ophthalmology, School of Medicine; Section of Neurobiology, Physiology and Behavior; Division of Biological Sciences; and Center for Neuroscience; University of California, Davis, California

CHANGEUX, JEAN-PIERRE   CNRS URA 2182, Récepteurs et Cognition, Institut Pasteur, Paris, France

CLARK, ROBERT E.   Veterans Affairs Healthcare System, and Department of Psychiatry, University of California, San Diego, California

COSMIDES, LEDA   Department of Psychology and Center for Evolutionary Psychology, University of California, Santa Barbara, California

CRICK, FRANCIS C.   The Salk Institute for Biological Studies, La Jolla, California

CROZIER, ROBERT A.   The Picower Center for Learning and Memory, Massachusetts Institute of Technology, Cambridge, Massachusetts

CUTLER, ANNE   Max Planck Institute for Psycholinguistics, Nijmegen, The Netherlands

DACEY, DENNIS   Department of Biological Structure and the National Primate Research Center, University of Washington, Seattle, Washington

DAVACHI, LILA   Department of Psychology, New York University, New York, N.Y.

DEHAENE, STANISLAS   Department of Cognitive Neuroimaging, INSERM U562, CEA, Orsay, France

DE LAFUENTE, VICTOR   Instituto de Fisiología Celular, Universidad Nacional Autónoma de México, Mexico City, Mexico

DORRIS, MICHAEL   Department of Physiology, Queens University, Kingston, Ontario, Canada

DOUPE, ALLISON J.   Keck Center for Integrative Neuroscience, and Departments of Physiology and Psychiatry, University of California, San Francisco, California

DRIVER, JON   Institute of Cognitive Neuroscience, University College London, London, U.K.

EICHENBAUM, HOWARD   Center for Memory and Brain, Boston University, Boston, Massachusetts

FARAH, MARTHA J.   Center for Cognitive Neuroscience, University of Pennsylvania, Philadelphia, Pennsylvania

FERSTER, DAVID   Department of Neurobiology and Physiology, Northwestern University, Evanston, Illinois

FITCH, W. TECUMSEH   School of Psychology, University of St. Andrews, Fife, Scotland

FOGASSI, LEONARDO   Dipartimento di Neuroscienze, Sezione di Fisiologia,University of Parma, Parma, Italy

FOSSELLA, JOHN   Sackler Institute, Department of Psychiatry, Weill Medical College of Cornell University, New York, New York

FREIWALD, WINRICH A.   Department of Neurobiology, Harvard Medical School, Boston, Massachusetts

FRIEDERICI, ANGELA D.   Max Planck Institute for Human Cognitive and Brain Sciences, Leipzig, Germany

FUJIMICHI, RYOKO   The University of Tokyo School of Medicine, Hongo, Tokyo, Japan

GAGE, FRED H.   The Salk Institute for Biological Studies, La Jolla, California

GALLESE, VITTORIO   Dipartimento di Neuroscienze, Sezione di Fisiologia, University of Parma, Parma, Italy

GANIS, GIORGIO   Department of Psychology, Harvard University, Cambridge, Massachusetts, and Department of Radiology, Massachusetts General Hospital, Boston, Massachusetts

GARAVAN, HUGH   Department of Psychology and Institute of Neuroscience, Trinity College, Dublin, Ireland

GAREL, SONIA   INSERUM U368, Département de Biologie, Ecole Normale Supérieure, Paris, France

GASIC, GREGORY P.   Departments of Psychiatry and Radiology, Harvard Medical School, and Athinoula Martinos Center for Biomedical Imaging, Massachusetts General Hospital, Boston, Massachusetts

GAZZANIGA, MICHAEL S.   Department of Psychological and Brain Sciences, Dartmouth College, Hanover, New Hampshire

GEORGOPOULOS, APOSTOLOS P.   Brain Sciences Center, Veterans Affairs Medical Center, and Departments of Neuroscience, Neurology, and Psychiatry, University of Minnesota Medical School, Minneapolis, Minnesota

GHAHRAMANI, ZOUBIN   Gatsby Computational Neuroscience Unit, University College London, London, U.K.

GHOSE, GEOFFREY M.   Division of Neuroscience, Baylor College of Medicine, Houston, Texas

GLIMCHER, PAUL W.   Center for Neural Science, New York University, New York, New York

GOBBINI, M. IDA   Department of Psychology, Princeton University, Princeton, New Jersey

GOLD, JOSHUA I.   Department of Neuroscience, University of Pennsylvania, Philadelphia, Pennsylvania

GOLDMAN-RAKIC, PATRICIA S.   Section of Neurobiology, Yale University, New Haven, Connecticut

GOODALE, MELVYN A.   Department of Psychology, University of Western Ontario, London, Ontario, Canada

GOULD, ELIZABETH   Department of Psychology, Princeton University, Princeton, New Jersey

GRAFTON, SCOTT T.   Department of Psychological and Brain Sciences, Dartmouth College, Hanover, New Hampshire

GRAYBIEL, ANN M.   Department of Brain and Cognitive Sciences, and McGovern Institute for Brain Research, Massachusetts Institute of Technology, Cambridge, Massachusetts

GUSNARD, DEBRA A.   Departments of Radiology and Psychiatry, Washington University, St. Louis, Missouri

HACKETT, TROY A.   Department of Hearing and Speech Sciences, Vanderbilt University School of Medicine, Nashville, Tennessee

HAUSER, MARC D.   Department of Psychology, Harvard University, Cambridge, Massachusetts

HAXBY, JAMES V.   Department of Psychology, Princeton University, Princeton, New Jersey

HAYES, NANCY L.   Department of Neuroscience and Cell Biology, UMDNJ-Robert Wood Johnson Medical School, Piscataway, New Jersey

HEATHERTON, TODD F.   Department of Psychological and Brain Sciences, Dartmouth College, Hanover, New Hampshire

HEEGER, DAVID J.   Department of Psychology and Center for Neural Science, New York University, New York, New York

HERNÁNDEZ, ADRIÁN   Instituto de Fisiología Celular, Universidad Nacional Autónoma de México, Mexico City, Mexico

HESSLER, NEAL A.   RIKEN Brain Science Institute, Lab for Vocal Behavior Mechanisms, Wako-Shi, Japan

HILLIS, ARGYE E.   Department of Neurology, Johns Hopkins University School of Medicine, and Department of Cognitive Science, Johns Hopkins University, Baltimore, Maryland

HILLYARD, STEVEN A.   Department of Neuroscience, University of California, San Diego, California

HOPFINGER, JOSEPH B.   Department of Psychology, University of North Carolina, Chapel Hill, North Carolina

HORTON, JONATHAN C.   Beckman Vision Center, University of California, San Francisco, California

HUBERMAN, ANDREW D.   Department of Ophthalmology, School of Medicine; Section of Neurobiology, Physiology and Behavior; Division of Biological Sciences; and Center for Neuroscience; University of California, Davis, California

HUMPHREYS, GLYN W.   Behavioural Brain Sciences Centre, School of Psychology, University of Birmingham, Birmingham, U.K.

HUSAIN, MASUD   Institute of Cognitive Neuroscience, University College London, London, U.K., and Division of

Neuroscience and Psychological Medicine, Imperial College London, London, U.K.

INDEFREY, PETER   Max Planck Institute for Psycholinguistics, Nijmegen, The Netherlands

IVRY, RICHARD B.   Department of Psychology, University of California, Berkeley, California

JOHNSON, BRAD   Department of Bioengineering, University of California, Berkeley, California

KAAS, JON H.   Department of Psychology, Vanderbilt University School of Medicine, Nashville, Tennessee

KAGAN, JEROME   Department of Psychology, Harvard University, Cambridge, Massachusetts

KANDEL, ERIC R.   Howard Hughes Medical Institute and Center for Neurobiology and Behavior, College of Physicians and Surgeons of Columbia University, New York, New York

KANWISHER, NANCY G.   Department of Cognitive and Brain Sciences, Massachusetts Institute of Technology, Cambridge, Massachusetts

KELLEY, WILLIAM M.   Department of Psychological and Brain Sciences, Dartmouth College, Hanover, New Hampshire

KHAN, REHAN   Department of Neuroscience, University of California, Berkeley, California

KLEIN, RAYMOND   Department of Psychology, Dalhousie University, Halifax, Nova Scotia, Canada

KLEIN, STANLEY B.   Department of Psychology, University of California, Santa Barbara, California

KNIGHT, ROBERT T.   Department of Psychology and Helen Wills Neuroscience Institute, University of California, Berkeley, California

KOCH, CHRISTOF   Division of Biology, Caltech, Pasadena, California

KORNACK, DAVID R.   Center for Aging and Developmental Biology, Department of Neurobiology and Anatomy, University of Rochester School of Medicine and Dentistry, Rochester, New York

KOSSLYN, STEPHEN M.   Department of Psychology, Harvard University, Cambridge, Massachusetts, and Department of Neurology, Massachusetts General Hospital, Boston, Massachusetts

KRISTJANSSON, ARNI   Institute of Cognitive Neuroscience, London, U.K.

LAUGHLIN, SIMON B.   Department of Zoology, University of Cambridge, Cambridge, England

LEDOUX, JOSEPH E.   W.M. Keck Foundation Laboratory of Neurobiology, Center for Natural Science, New York University, New York, New York

LIU, GUOFA   Department of Anatomy and Neurobiology, Washington University School of Medicine, St. Louis, Missouri

LOGOTHETIS, NIKOS K.   Max Planck Institute for Biological Cybernetics, Tübingen, Germany

LUCK, STEVEN J.   Department of Psychology, University of Iowa, Iowa City, Iowa

MACRAE, C. NEIL   Dartmouth College; Massachusetts General Hospital, Hanover, New Hampshire

MAINLAND, JOEL   Department of Neuroscience, University of California, Berkeley, California

MALJKOVIC, VERA   Department of Psychology, University of Chicago, Chicago, Illinois

MAST, FRED   Department of Psychology, University of Zurich, Zurich, Switzerland

MAUNSELL, JOHN H. R.   Howard Hughes Medical Institute and Division of Neuroscience, Baylor College of Medicine, Houston, Texas

MCDERMOTT, JOSH   Department of Brain and Cognitive Science, Massachusetts Institute of Technology, Cambridge, Massachusetts

MCEWEN, BRUCE S.   Harold and Margaret Milliken Hatch Laboratory of Neuroendocrinology, Rockefeller University, New York, New York

MEEKER, DANIELLA   Division of Biology, California Institute of Technology, Pasadena, California

MEHLER, JACQUES   Cognitive Neuroscience Sector, International School for Advanced Studies, Trieste, Italy, and CNRS, Paris, France

MILLER, MICHAEL B.   Department of Psychological and Brain Sciences, Dartmouth College, Hanover, New Hampshire, and Department of Psychology, University of California, Santa Barbara, California

MIYASHITA, YASUSHI   The University of Tokyo School of Medicine, Hongo, Tokyo, Japan

MONTGOMERY, K.   Department of Psychology, Princeton University, Princeton, New Jersey

MOVSHON, J. ANTHONY,   Center for Neural Science, New York University, New York, N.Y.

MUSSA-IVALDI, FERDINANDO A.   Department of Physiology and Sensory Motor Performance Program, Northwestern University Medical School, Chicago, Illinois

NAKAYAMA, KEN   Department of Psychology, Harvard University, Cambridge, Massachusetts

NAYA, YUJI   The University of Tokyo School of Medicine, Hongo, Tokyo, Japan

NESPOR, MARINA   Department of Linguistics, Ferrara University, Ferrara, Italy

NOWAKOWSKI, RICHARD S.   Department of Neuroscience and Cell Biology, UMDNJ-Robert Wood Johnson Medical School, Piscataway, New Jersey

PANINSKI, LIAM   Center for Neural Science and Courant Institute of Mathematical Sciences, New York University, New York, New York

PESARAN, BIJAN   Division of Biology, California Institute of Technology, Pasadena, California

PESSOA, LUIZ   Department of Psychology, Brown University, Providence, Rhode Island

PHELPS, ELIZABETH A.   Department of Psychology, New York University, New York, New York

PHILPOT, BENJAMIN D.   Department of Cell and Molecular Psychology, University of North Carolina, Chapel Hill, North Carolina

PIAZZA, MANUELA   Service Hopitalier Frédéric Joliot and Department of Cognitive Neuroimaging, INSERIM U562, Orsay, France

PILLOW, JONATHAN   Center for Neural Science and Courant Institute of Mathematical Sciences, New York University, New York, New York

POSNER, MICHAEL I.   Department of Psychology, University of Oregon, Eugene, Oregon

PREUSS, TODD M.   Center for Behavioral Neuroscience and Division of Neuroscience, Yerkes Primate Research Center, Emory University, Atlanta, Georgia

RAICHLE, MARCUS E.   Division of Radiological Sciences, Washington University, St. Louis, Missouri

RAKIC, PASKO   Department of Neurobiology, Yale University School of Medicine, New Haven, Connecticut

RAMUS, FRANCK   Laboratoire de Sciences Cognitives et Psycholinguistique (EHESS/ENS/CNRS), Paris, France

RAO, YI   Department of Anatomy and Neurobiology, Washington University School of Medicine, St. Louis, Missouri

RAPP, BRENDA C.   Department of Cognitive Science, Johns Hopkins University, Baltimore, Maryland

RECANZONE, GREGG H.   Center for Neuroscience and Section of Neurobiology, Physiology and Behavior, University of California, Davis, California

REES, GERAINT   Institute of Cognitive Neuroscience and Wellcome Department of Imaging Neurosience, University College London, London, U.K.

RESS, DAVID   Department of Psychology, Stanford University, Stanford, California

RIZZOLATTI, GIACOMO   Dipartimento di Neuroscienze, Sezione di Fisiologia, University of Parma, Parma, Italy

ROBERTSON, IAN H.   Department of Psychology and Institute of Neuroscience, Trinity College, Dublin, Ireland

ROMANSKI, LIZABETH M.   Department of Neurobiology and Anatomy and the Center for Navigation and Communication Sciences, University of Rochester, Rochester, New York

ROMO, RANULFO   Instituto de Fisiología Celular, Universidad Nacional Autónoma de México, Mexico City, Mexico

RUBENSTEIN, JOHN L. R.   Nina Ireland Laboratory of Developmental Neurobiology, University of California, San Francisco, California

RUGG, MICHAEL D.   Center for the Neurobiology of Learning and Memory and Department of Neurobiology, University of California, Irvine, California

SAKA, ESEN   Department of Brain and Cognitive Sciences, and the McGovern Institute for Brain Research, Massachusetts Institute of Technology, Cambridge, Massachusetts

SAMSON, DANA   Behavioural Brain Sciences Centre, School of Psychology, University of Birmingham, Birmingham, U.K.

SAPOLSKY, ROBERT M.   Department of Biological Sciences, Stanford University, and Department of Neurology and Neurological Sciences, Stanford University School of Medicine, Stanford, California

SAWTELL, NATHANIEL B.   Neurological Sciences Institute, Oregon Health and Science University, Beaverton, Oregon

SCHACTER, DANIEL L.   Department of Psychology, Harvard University, Cambridge, Massachusetts

SCHAFE, GLENN E.   Department of Psychology, Yale University, New Haven, Connecticut

SCHERBERGER, HANS   Division of Biology, California Institute of Technology, Pasadena, California

SCHIFF, NICHOLAS D.   Laboratory of Cognitive Neuromodulation, Department of Neurology and Neuroscience, Weill Medical College of Cornell University, New York, New York

SCHWARTZ, ODELIA   The Salk Institute for Biological Studies, La Jolla, California

SEBASTIÁN-GALLÉS, NÚRIA   Department of Psychology, Universitat de Barcelona, Barcelona, Spain

SHADLEN, MICHAEL N.   Howard Hughes Medical Institute, Department of Physiology and Biophysics, and National Primate Research Center, University of Washington Medical School, Seattle, Washington

SHADMEHR, REZA   Department of Biomedical Engineering, Johns Hopkins School of Medicine, Baltimore, Maryland

SHALLICE, TIM   Institute of Cognitive Neuroscience, University College London, London, U.K.

SHAPIRO, KEVIN   Cognitive Neuropsychology Laboratory and Department of Psychology, Harvard University, Cambridge, Massachusetts

SHIMAMURA, ARTHUR P.   Department of Psychology and Helen Wills Neuroscience Institute, University of California, Berkeley, California

SIMONCELLI, EERO P.   Center for Neural Science and Courant Institute of Mathematical Sciences, New York University, New York, New York

SINCICH, LAWRENCE C.   Beckman Vision Center, University of California, San Francisco, California

SOBEL, NOAM   Departments of Neuroscience, Biophysics, Bioengineering and Psychology, University of California, Berkeley, California

SOLIS, MICHELE M.   Keck Center for Integrative Neuroscience, and Departments of Physiology and Psychiatry, University of California, San Francisco, California; Department of Otolaryngology, University of Washington, Seattle, Washington

SPARROW, BETSY   Department of Psychology, Harvard Cambridge, Massachusetts

SPELKE, ELIZABETH   Department of Psychology, Harvard University, Cambridge, Massachusetts

SQUIRE, LARRY R.   Veterans Affairs Healthcare System, and Departments of Psychiatry, Neurosciences, and Psychology, University of California, San Diego, California

STEVEN, MEGAN S.   University Laboratory of Physiology, University of Oxford, Oxford, U.K.

STRICK, PETER L.   Department of Veterans Affairs Medical Center and Center for the Neural Basis of Cognition, Department of Neurobiology, University of Pittsburgh School of Medicine, Pittsburgh, Pennsylvania

TANAKA, JAMES W.   Department of Psychology, University of Victoria, Victoria, British Columbia, Canada

TIPPER, STEVEN P.   Centre for Cognitive Neuroscience, School of Psychology, University of Wales, Bangor, Gwynedd, U.K.

THOMPSON, WILLIAM L.   Department of Psychology, Harvard University, Cambridge, Massachusetts

TOOBY, JOHN   Department of Anthropology and Center for Evolutionary Psychology, University of California, Santa Barbara, California

TREISMAN, ANNE   Psychology Department, Princeton University, Princeton, New Jersey

UNGERLEIDER, LESLIE G.   Laboratory of Brain and Cognition, National Institute of Mental Health, National Institutes of Health, Bethesda, Maryland

VAN HORN, JOHN DARRELL   Center for Cognitive Neuroscience, Dartmouth College, Hanover, New Hampshire

VAN PRAAG, HENRIETTE   The Salk Institute for Biological Studies, La Jolla, California

VUILLEUMIER, PATRIK   Institute of Cognitive Neuroscience, University College London, London, U.K., and Department of Neuroscience, Medical Center, University of Geneva, Geneva, Switzerland

WAGNER, ANTHONY D.   Department of Psychology and Neurosciences Program, Stanford University, Stanford, California

WANDELL, BRIAN   Department of Psychology, Stanford University, Stanford, California

WEGNER, DANIEL M.   Department of Psychology, Harvard University, Cambridge, Massachusetts

WISE, STEVEN P.   Laboratory of Systems Neuroscience, National Institute of Mental Health, Bethesda, Maryland

WOLFORD, GEORGE   Department of Psychological and Brain Sciences, Dartmouth College, Hanover, New Hampshire

WOLPERT, DANIEL M.   Sobell Department of Motor Neuroscience, Institute of Neurology, University College London, London, U.K.

WOODBURY, DALE   Stem Cell Research Center, Department of Neuroscience and Cell Biology, University of Medicine and Dentistry of New Jersey, Robert Wood Johnson Medical School, Piscataway, New Jersey

YOST, WILLIAM A.   Parmly Hearing Institute, Loyola University, Chicago, Illinois

ZELANO, CHRISTINA   Department of Biophysics, University of California, Berkeley, California

ZHAO, XINYU   University of New Mexico School of Medicine, Albuquerque, New Mexico

INDEX

CXCR4, in neuronal migration, 55
Cyborg-like augmentation, 1313
Cyclic adenosine monophosphate (cAMP)
    in adult neurogenesis, 130
    in long-term facilitation, in *Aplysia*, 653–655
    in long-term memory, 647, 660
    in long-term sensitization, in *Aplysia*, 653
    in neural differentiation of peripheral stem cells, 164
    in olfaction, 262
Cyclin-dependent kinase 5 (cdk5), in cortical lamination, 57–58
Cystatin, and adult neurogenesis, 133
Cytochrome oxidase studies
    in auditory cortex, 217–218
    in visual system, 234–235, 240
Cytoplasmic polyadenylation element binding protein (CPEB),
        homologue in *Aplysia*, 658

D

Darwin, Charles, 837
Database, for neuroimaging, 1288
d-dimensional stimulus space, in linear-nonlinear-Poisson model, 329
Deafness
    cortical plasticity in, 1248
    and reading acquisition, 818, 820
Death criteria, neuroimaging and ethical issues in, 1318
Decision making, 1215–1227, 1229–1239
    amygdala in, 1020
    commitment to alternative in, 1237–1238
    criterion level or barrier height in, 1237–1238
    criterion value in, 1233–1235
    diffusion-to-barrier model of, 1231–1232
    dissociating decision variables in, 1221
    economic models of, 1216–1222
    expected utility in, 1216
        encoding relative versus absolute, 1221–1222
        versus expected value, 1222
        and neuronal activity, 1219–1221
    expected value in, 1216
    free choice, 1215–1217
        behavioral and physiological studies of, 1217–1222
        neural basis of, implications of social science approaches for,
            1222–1226
    games theory in, 1216–1222
    goals in, 1238–1239
    identifying and executing best response in, 1215–1216
    and insight into cognition, 1229–1239
    intention-related mechanisms in, 1238–1239
    in monkeys and humans, 1217–1219
    motion, 1229–1239
        principles in, 1235–1236
    Nash equilibrium model of, 1216–1219
    neuronal activity in, 1219–1221
    neurophysiology of, 1229, 1232–1235
    orbitofrontal cortex in, 1095–1097
    perspectives on and future directions in, 1235–1239
    psychophysics of, 1230–1232
    quantifying value of strategy in, 1216–1218
    randomness in
        in computational systems, 1223–1225
        cost versus benefits of, 1225
        evolutionary advantage of, 1224–1225
        at neuronal and subneuronal levels, 1223
        of neurons, and behavior, 1225–1226
    rational, 1216–1217
    rewarded versus unrewarded, 1215

simple, 1215–1226
    in somatosensory discrimination, 204–208
    speed versus accuracy in, 1230–1232, 1237
    temporal accumulation for, 1230, 1237
    trial-by-trial basis in, 1217
    variable representation in motor response structures, 1238–1239
    in visual-saccadic system, 1215–1227, 1233–1235, 1238
    weight of evidence for, 1233, 1235–1237
        as comparative currency, 1237
        computation of, 1236
        sensory information as, 1236–1237
Declarative memory, 647, 679–680, 905, 1078, 1113–1114
    assessment in animals, 682
    cognitive control and, 714–718
    conscious recollection of, 679–680
    hippocampal processing of, 647, 679–689
    medial temporal lobe in, 691–705
    neural localization of, 647
    stress and, 1031–1034
    sex differences in, 1037–1038
Deep brain stimulation, for enhancement, 1313
Deep cerebellar nuclei, 453
Default mode network, in neuroimaging, 1274, 1285
Deficit states, and reward/aversion, 1046
Degrees-of-freedom problem, in motor control, 491
Delay conditioning, 701–705
Dementia
    drug therapy for, 1315–1316
    false recognition in, 745–746
    in Huntington's disease, 498
    in Parkinson's disease, 498
    semantic, 770
        number sense in, 869, 871
        temporal variant of, 715
    temporal, noun deficits in, 806
Dendrite atrophy/retraction, stress and, 1034–1035
Dendrite remodeling, in hippocampus, adrenal steroids and, 175–176
Dentate gyrus, 171–172
    adrenal steroids and, 141–142, 174–175
    adult, neurogenesis in, 23–26, 127–134, 139–147, 151, 154–157,
            172, 175
        and anxiety, 146
        brain damage and, 141
        cell cycle in, 155–157
        cell turnover in, 141
        and endocrine control, 146
        enrichment versus deprivation in, 144
        environment and, 143–144
        experience and, 142–144
        functional significance of, 145–147, 157–158
        hormonal regulation of, 141–143
        learning effects of, 145–146
        learning effects on, 143–144
        proliferative capacity in, 155–157
        and psychiatric disorders, 26
        sex differences in, 176
        stress and, 142–143, 175–177
    connections/circuits of, 453–454
        to amygdala, 172
        and CA3 pyramidal neurons, 174–175
        to premotor areas, 455–456
    development of, during infancy, 94
    long-term depression in, 117
    long-term potentiation in, 172
    maturation of, 172
    plasticity of, 23, 25, 151

Pavlovian, 997–999
  as model system, 987
  stress hormones in, 174
  synaptic plasticity and, 989, 995–996
Fear extinction, 996–997
Fear learning
  instructed, amygdala in, 1006–1007
  instrumental, 997–999
Feature(s)
  in attention selection, 403–405, 538, 564, 578–579
  evaluation, in motivation, 1046
  in motion perception, 370–371
  neuronal detection of, 1134
  in object categorization, 880–882, 886
Feature integration
  attention in, 538–539, 621
  EEG findings in, 1180
  in neglect, 599
Fechner's law, 1237
Feedback error learning, in motor control, 491
Feedback learning, basal ganglia in, 503–504
Feeling-of-knowing paradigm, 914
Ferrets, eye-specific projections in, 87–90
Fetal brain
  cell proliferation in, 152–154
  neurogenesis in, quantitative analysis of, 149–157
Fgf8
  and cortical arealization, 77–78
  and cortical patterning, 72–73
Fibroblast growth factor (FGF)
  in adult neurogenesis, 129, 131, 132, 133
  in cortical patterning, 72–73
Fight-or-flight response, 1031
Fingers, cortical representation of, plasticity in, 1244–1245
Finnish language, acquisition of, 827–828
Firing rates/patterns
  in attention, 344, 347, 579–581, 584
  characterization with stochastic stimuli, 327–336
  in consciousness, 1113, 1139, 1148
  curse of dimensionality in computation of, 329
  in decision making, 1219–1221, 1225–1226
  energy-efficient, in neural signaling, 194
  intracortical recording of, 960
  as neural code for frequency of vibrotactile stimuli, 199–201, 210–211
  in perceptual priming, 719–720
First-person data
  in consciousness, 1111
    connections with third-person data, 1113, 1115
    explanation of, 1112–1113
    formalisms for, 1118
    as "hard" problems, 1112
    methods for collecting, 1117–1118
    obstacles involving, 1117–1118
    privacy of, 1117
    as subjective experience, 1112–1113
  in memory, sources of, 1079
First-person epistemology, 1077, 1080, 1086
FIT task, constructional praxis in, 480–483
Fixation-centered frame, for reaching, 516
Fluoxetine (Prozac), 129–130, 1313–1314, 1317
Flutter discrimination, 199
FMRFamide, in long-term facilitation, in *Aplysia,* 655–657
fMRI. *See* Functional magnetic resonance imaging
fMRI Data Center, 1288
Focal hand dystonia, 1245

Foraging, 398, 407, 1239
Foraging facilitator hypothesis, of inhibition of return, 549–551
Force field(s), in motor control, 416–418, 488–489
Force field approximation, motor control as, 419–422
Forebrain
  basal
    in evaluative processes, 983
    in social cognition, 979
  in fear conditioning, 989
  gating systems of, and consciousness, 1122–1124
  primate, adult neurogenesis in, 23–28
Foreground-background distinctions, stress/stress hormones and, 1033–1034
Forensic neuroimaging, 1312
Form, visual processing of
  cytochrome oxidase studies of, 234–235
  and motion perception, 369–382
  prevailing view of, 233–234
  V1 interpatches in, 234–235
  V2 stripe type and, 240–241
  V1-to-V2 projections in, 234–241
Formalisms, for first-person data, in consciousness, 1118
Forward kinematics, in reaching, 511
Forward models, for reaching, 518
Fovea, retinal, 282
FOXP2 gene
  and language evolution, 843, 1261
  sequence evolution of, 18
Fragile X mental retardation, 1260
Frames of reference
  in action representation, 442
  allocentric, 1162
  egocentric, 1162
  for inhibition of return (IOR), 549
  for reaching, 516, 1162
    shared with saccades, 471–472
Framework. *See also specific concepts and processes*
  definition of, 1133–1141
Free-choice decisions, 1215
  behavioral and physiological studies of, 1217–1222
  economic models of, 1216–1222
  neural basis of, implications of social science approaches for, 1222–1226
  studies in monkeys and humans, 1217–1219
Freezing response, 987, 989
French language, acquisition of, 827–828
  in Korean adoptees, 833–834
Frequency discrimination, 199–211, 385–388
  periodicity and firing rate as neural codes for, 199–201
  S1 microstimulation studies of, 201–203
Frequency domains, in olfaction, 266–267
Frequency matching, 1194, 1197
Frequency modulation, 393
Frontal cortex
  in attentional control, 569–570, 923–925, 928, 1284
  auditory-visual interactions in, 365–368
  basal ganglia connections to, 455–456, 496–497
  in categorization, 811–812
  cerebellar connections to, 455–456
  in cognitive neuroscience, 811–812
  in consciousness, 1154, 1180–1183
  in decision making, 1215
  development of
    during adolescence, 98–99
    during infancy, 94–95
  evolution of, 8–9, 978

Observer, in motor control, 487
Obsessive-compulsive disorder, 444
    basal ganglia in, 459, 498, 500–502, 504
    learning in, 504
    reward/aversion circuitry in, 1056
Occipital cortex
    in blind persons, auditory and tactile processing in, 1246
    in consciousness, 1154
    in imitation, 437
    lateral, in attention, 1284
    in memory retrieval, 744
    in mental imagery, 935
    in object/face representation, 890, 896–898
    in visual mental imagery, 932
    in visual perception, 1164–1167
Occipitotemporal cortex
    in face processing, 1020
    object/face representations in, 892–896
    in reading acquisition, 821–822
    in working memory, spatial and object, 711
Occlusion, in motion perception, 369–382
Ocular dominance columns
    activity and, 85–86
    deprivation studies of, 85–86
    development of, 85–86
Oculomotor delayed-response (ODR), spatial working memory in, 666–668
Oddball task, 1178–1179
    voluntary attention in, 1095
Odor(s)
    definition of, 259
    discrimination of
        neuronal migration and, 59
        in rodents, adult neurogenesis and, 27
        spatial encoding for, 264–266
    encoding of, 263–264
    metric of, 265–266
    from molecule to percept, 259–260
    transduction of, 260–262
Odorant-binding protein (OBP), 260
Odotopes, 264
Olfaction, 259–275
    explosion in research, 275
    hierarchy in, 260
    in humans, 259
    mammalian, 259–275
    metric of smell in, 265–266
    from molecule to percept in, 259–260
    odor encoding in, 263–264
    primacy, in animals, 259
    retronasal, 260
    in rodents, adult neurogenesis and, 27
    sniff in, 260, 267–275
        airflow rate and, 272–275
        odorant concentration and, 269
        sorption rates and, 269–275
    spatial encoding (odor maps) in, 264–266
    temporal coding in, 266–267
    transduction of odors in, 260–262
Olfactory bulb, 260, 262–263
    adult, neurogenesis in, 23, 26–28, 140, 141, 146
    cellular layers of, 262–263
    neuronal migration to, 26–27, 52–54, 59
    odor encoding in, 263–264
    spatial encoding (odor maps) in, 264–266
    temporal coding in, 266–267

Olfactory constancy, 269
Olfactory cortex, 260, 263
    habituation in, 267–269
    odor encoding in, 263–264
    plasticity of, 1247–1248
    primary versus secondary, 260
    sniff and, 267–275
    spatial encoding (odor maps) in, 264–266
    temporal coding in, 266–267
Olfactory epithelium, 260–262
    cell types in, 260
    mucous layer of, 260
    odor encoding in, 263–264
    spatial encoding (odor maps) in, 264–266
    transduction of odors to, 260
Olfactory memory, relational hypothesis of, 682–685
Olfactory nerve, 260, 262–263
    odorant response in, 272
Olfactory receptors, 260–262, 275
    in odor encoding, 263–264
    in spatial encoding, 264–266
Olfactory tubercle, 263
    adult, neurogenesis in, 139
Oligonucleotide microarrays, brain studies with, 18
Oligophrenin-1, 1260
Onsets and offsets, in auditory scene analysis, 392–393
Open field geometric arrangement, of cells, 961
Opiates, and adult neurogenesis, 130
Oppositional behavior, reward/aversion circuitry in, 1056
Optical imaging, 959
Optical topography, in language acquisition, 828
Optic aphasia, 806
Optic ataxia, 1162–1163
Optimality, in motor control, 485–487
Orbitofrontal cortex
    and conversational style, 1101
    in decision making, 1095–1097
    dynamic filtering theory of, 1097–1098
    emotion-cognition synthesis in, 1095–1098
    and empathy, 1101
    in reality checking, 1099
    in reinforcement and reversal, 1097
    in reward/aversion system, 1043, 1049–1053
    in selective attention, 539
    in self-insight, 1099
    in self-monitoring, 1098–1099
    in self-regulation, 1095–1101
    in social cognition, 979
    somatic marker hypothesis of, 1095–1097
    and theory of mind, 1101
Orexin, in arousal states, 1122–1123
"Organ pipe" formation, of auditory cortex, 218
Orientation, and attention, 632
Orientation selectivity, 303–311, 1175
    action potential threshold and, 305
    contrast invariance of, 305–307
    cortical input to, 307–309
        estimating contribution of, 308–309
    distribution of, 311
    dynamics of, 310
    feedback models of, 307–309
    feedback versus feedforward models of, 308–310
    feedforward models of, 304–305
        refinement of, 305
    iceberg effect in, 305, 307
    implementation of, species variations in, 303

and positional information in cortical primordium, 74–75
   regulation by signaling centers, 73
Transdifferentiation, of stem cells, 162–167
Transfer-appropriate processing, in memory retrieval, 728
Transformation, of mental images, 938–939
   egocentric, 938
   object-based, 938
Transgermal differentiation, of stem cells, 162–167
   apparent, in humans, 165
   debate over, 166–167
Transient attention, 398–407
   as elemental memory event, 403–405
   flexible deployment of, 398–400
   learning in, 400–401
      as associative, modulatory process, 406
      contingent relations lacking in, 401–402
      neural substrates for, 405–407
      versus other forms of learning, 405–407
      piecemeal nature of, 406
   versus sustained attention, 398–399
"Transit-amplifying cell," as neuronal progenitor, 35
Transitive states, in visual consciousness, 1183–1184
Translocation
   neuronal migration via, 37–39, 51–52
   nuclear, 51–52
   somal, 51–52
Traumatic brain injury
   and adult neurogenesis, 131
   and consciousness, 1121–1130
   and self-knowledge, 1081–1082, 1084–1085
   and social cognition, 977–978
   and vigilant attention, 631–632
Trial-and-error learning, basal ganglia in, 503–504
Trial-by-trial basis, in decision making, 1217
Trigeminal system, in olfaction, 260
TrkB receptor, in cortical lamination, 58
Tuberin, in tuberous sclerosis, 59
Tuberous sclerosis, 59
Tubulin
   in adult neurogenesis, 24, 140
   in long-term facilitation, in *Aplysia*, 659
Tufted cell axons, of olfactory bulb, 263
Turkish language, acquisition of, 827–828
Turner's syndrome, 1057
   number sense in, 870
Twin studies, 1256–1257

U

Uncertainty, in motor control, 422–423, 486, 492
Universal Grammar, 843–844
Universe of Consciousness (Edelman and Tononi), 1140
Upper rhombic lip (URL), neuronal migration from, 51, 55
Urbach-Wiethe syndrome, 980, 1021–1022
Utilization behavior, 443–444, 610–612, 1203

V

Vagus nerve, in stress response, 1036–1037
Vagus nerve stimulation, for enhancement, 1313
Vakayala (good sense), development of, 96
Variance buffer, in motor control, 423
Vector summation, of spinal force fields, 416–417
Vegetative state, 1121
   persistent, 1121–1122
      functional brain imaging of, 1124–1128

Ventral anterior cingulate cortex, in default mode network, 1285
Ventral intraparietal (VIP) area
   auditory processing in, 224
   homologue in nonhuman primates, 12
Ventral pallidum, 453
Ventral taenia tecta, 263
Ventral tegmentum, in reward/aversion system, 1043, 1049–1053
Ventral telencephalon, neuronal migration from, 52
Ventral visual stream, 233, 1160–1161, 1173
   in action representation, 445, 448–449
   in attention, 582
   and bimanual actions, 448–449
   in consciousness, 1154
   interaction with dorsal stream, 1170–1171
   in object categorization, 889–892, 894
   as perception stream, 1159, 1161–1171
      neuropsychological evidence for, 1162–1167
      studies in monkeys, 1167–1168
   in reach and grasp, 445, 620
   in visual mental imagery, 935–937
   as "what" system, 233, 1161
Ventricular zone (VZ), cell proliferation in, 152–154
Ventriloquism effect, 363–364
Ventrobasal nucleus (VBN)
   cortical connections of, 70
   evolution of, 9, 10
Ventrolateral prefrontal cortex (VLPFC), 953
   in auditory processing, 670–671
   connections of, 670
   versus dorsolateral, 713–714, 947
   in memory retrieval, 716–717
   in working memory, 669–671
      spatial and object, 711
      verbal, 710–711
Verb(s)
   argument processing, 795–796
   in blind persons, visual cortex and, 1247
   cerebral representation of, 803–809
   deficits in, 804–809
      electrophysiology of, 807–808
      lexical-grammatical hypothesis of, 804
      modality-specific, 805
      morphologic hypothesis of, 804
      morphosyntactic, 805–807
      neurophysiology of, 804–807
      semantic hypothesis of, 804
Verbal communication, for fear learning, 1006–1007
Verbal reports, in consciousness research, 1117–1118
Verbal span task, prefrontal cortex in, 943
Verbal working memory, 709–711
Vernier acuity, in split brain, 1190
Vibrotactile discrimination, 197–211
   chain of operations for, 197, 199
   comparison and decision-making processes in, 204–208
   complementary, dual representation for, 197, 210–211
   decision motor responses in, 208–209
   S1 microstimulation studies of, 201–203
Vibrotactile stimuli
   coding of
      in frontal cortex, 203
      peripheral and central, 199
      in S2, 203
      during working memory, 203–204
   frequency of, periodicity and firing rate as neural codes for, 199–201

Vocal learning (cont.)
  adult neurogenesis and, 127–128, 129, 161
  anterior forebrain pathway (AFP) in, 246–256
  bird's own song (BOS) in, 246
  combination sensitivity in, 247
  efference copy and, 252
  in juveniles, 246–251
  long-term potentiation in, 253–255
  as model system, 245–246, 255
  sensorimotor phase of, 246
  sensory phase of, 246
  singing-related AFP activity in, 251–258
  song selectivity in, 246–251
  synaptic plasticity underlying, 252–255
  template for, 246, 248
  tutor's song in, 246
Voltage-gated ion channels
  in long-term potentiation, 991
  in neuronal migration, 39, 40
Voltage-to-action potential transformation, in orientation selectivity, 307
Vomeronasal system, 260
Vowel space, in bilingual acquisition, 830–831
Voxel-based morphometry, in number tasks, 869–870

W

Walker's area 12 and 45, 670
Walker-Warburg syndrome (WWS), 58–59
Wason selection task
  precautionary rules in, 1304
  social exchange in, 1297–1298
Wavelength coding, midget cell hypothesis of, 286
Weber's fraction, 866
Weber's law, 855–858, 866–867, 873, 1237
Weighted-sum model, of receptive fields, 313, 317
Wernicke's aphasia, 770
Wernicke's area
  asymmetry of, 13
  auditory processing in, 226
  homologue in nonhuman primates, 12
  in listening, 769
  and speech development, 95
  in syntactic processing, 791, 793
Wheat germ-conjugated horseradish peroxidase (WGA-HRP), for tracing V1-to-V2 projections, 235
White ensemble, in linear-nonlinear-Poisson model, 329
White noise analysis
  experimental caveats with, 331–335
  future directions for, 336
  of neuronal response, 327–336
  realistic spike dynamics modifying, 335–336
Whole language instruction, 818
Whole object assumption, in language, 841
Wiener-Volterra series, 328, 329, 330
Williams syndrome, 19, 1255
Win-shift behavior, 503
Win-stay learning, 503, 505
Wisconsin Card Sort Test (WCST), 609, 714, 1148, 1257
Withdrawal reflex, 981–982
Wnt3a, and cortical patterning, 72–73
Word(s)
  auditory processing of, 759, 764, 770
  function, in grammar, 809–811
  grammatical properties of, cerebral representation of, 803–812

subliminal processing of
  versus conscious access, 1149–1154
  early visual activity in, 1150
  motor activity in, 1150–1152
  neuroimaging of, 1149–1152
  physiological correlates of, 1152
  semantic access in, 1150
  subliminal binding in, 1150
  visual word recognition in, 1150
Word blindness, congenital, 819
Word list, syntax versus, 792
Working memory, 709–714
  and attention, 343–344, 347, 568–569, 607–610, 616
    overlap in neural control of, 923–924, 928
  and attentional control of behavior, 607–610, 616
  central executive in, 709–710, 711
  cognitive control and, 709–714
  components of, 709–710
  and consciousness, 1153
  control of, 919–925
  delay interval in, 919–922
  development of, during infancy, 94–95
  as distinctive human property, 100
  faces in, 669–671
  frontal lobes and, 607–610
  genetics of, 1257–1259
  maintaining information in, 608, 919
  manipulating information in, 608–610, 712
  monitoring of, 712
  network specificity in, 668–669
  neural signature of, 919
  neurotransmitters in, 668
  objects in, 669–674, 709–711
  prefrontal cortex in, 203–204, 209–210, 607–609, 665, 709–711, 919, 921–922, 943–944
    areal specificity of, 669–671
    cellular specificity of, 665–668
    domain specificity of, 665–675
    interaction with parietal cortex, 668–669
    necessity of, 674
  and response selection, 612
  spatial, 665–668
    versus faces, 671–674
    in neglect, 599
    neural activity patterns in, 668–669
    versus nonspatial, 669–671
    versus object, 671–674
  spatial and object, 709, 711
  stress/stress hormones and, 1033
  successful performance in, determinants of, 920–922
  sustained neuronal response in, 919
  in task switching, 609–610
  top-down processes for, 919–928
  verbal, 709–711
  vibrotactile discrimination during, 203–204, 209–210
  and visual attention/perception, 343–344, 347
Workplace neurons, in consciousness, 1113, 1146–1149, 1155
  all-or-none dynamics of, 1152–1154, 1155
  critical predictions of, 1155
  dynamic mobilization of, 1147
  ignition of, 1153–1154
  intensity of, 1148
  modulation of and selection by reward, 1148
  network of processors for, 1146–1147
  stability of, 1148
  top-down amplification of, 1147–1155

Writer's cramp, 1245, 1250
Written language
  acquisition of, 815–822
  cognitive and neural substrates in, 775–784
  noun-verb deficits in, 805
Wundt, Wilhelm, 1282

X

X-linked mental retardation, 1260

Y

Yerkes-Dodson law, of arousal, 634–635
Yotari mice, cortical lamination in, 57

Z

Zajonc, Robert, on cognition and emotion, 1005
Zellweger syndrome, 58–59
*zif*268, in associative memory, 910
Zombie modes, and consciousness, 1135, 1140